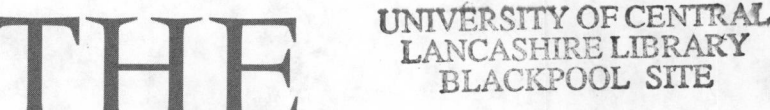
KT-231-020

UNIVERSITY OF CENTRAL
LANCASHIRE LIBRARY
BLACKPOOL SITE

THE
LIPPINCOTT
MANUAL OF
NURSING PRACTICE

This book is due for return on or before the last date shown below.

-7. MAY 1997
15. AUG. 1997
18. SEP. 1997
11. NOV. 1997
10. MAR. 1998
16. OCT 1998
16. JUN 2000
-5. JAN. 2001
-6. AUG. 2001
10. SEP. 2001
0. OCT 2002

23. APR 2002
19. JUN. 2003
-3. MAR. 2004
-9. JAN. 2006
11. NOV. 06
27 NOV 2008
28 FEB 2012
29 MAY 2014

Don Gresswell Ltd., London, N.21   Cat. No. 1208   DG 02242/71

Blackpool, Fylde and Wyre NHS
Library

TV09056

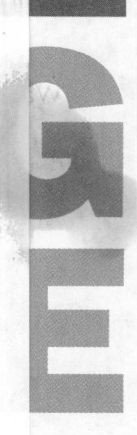

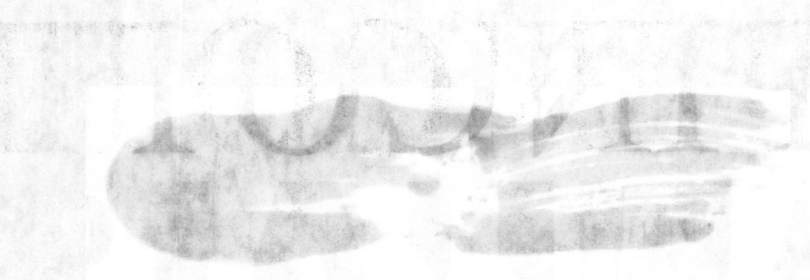

Sandra M. Nettina, RN,C, MSN, ANP

Adjunct Faculty
George Washington University
Washington, D.C., and George Mason University, Fairfax, Virginia
Primary Care Nurse Practitioner
Greenbelt, Maryland

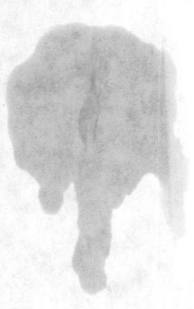

THE
LIPPINCOTT
MANUAL OF
NURSING
PRACTICE

Sixth Edition

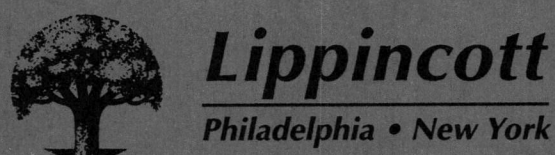

Lippincott
Philadelphia • New York

UNIVERSITY OF CENTRAL
LANCASHIRE LIBRARY
BLACKPOOL SITE

Acquisitions Editor: Lisa Stead
Editorial Assistant: Brian MacDonald
Project Editor: Amy P. Jirsa
Production Manager: Helen Ewan
Production Coordinator: Kathryn Rule
Design Coordinator: Doug Smock
Indexer: Ellen Murray

6th Edition

Copyright © 1996 by Lippincott-Raven Publishers.
© 1991, 1986, 1982, 1978, 1974 by J. B. Lippincott Company. All
rights reserved. This book is protected by copyright. No part of it
may be reproduced, stored in a retrieval system, or transmitted,
in any form or by any means—electronic, mechanical,
photocopy, recording, or otherwise—without the prior written
permission of the publisher, except for brief quotations embodied
in critical articles and reviews. Printed in the United States of
America. For information write Lippincott-Raven Publishers, 227
East Washington Square, Philadelphia, PA 19106.

Library of Congress Cataloging-in-Publication Data

The Lippincott manual of nursing practice.—6th ed./[edited by]
    Sandra M. Nettina
        p.   cm.
    Includes bibliographical references and index.
    ISBN 0-397-55163-0
    1. Nusing—Handbooks, manuals, etc.   I. Nettina, Sandra M.
    [DNLM: 1. Nursing Care—handbooks.   WY 491 L765   1996]
RT51.B78 1996
610.73—dc20
DNLM/DLC
for Library of Congress   95-20484
                                                          CIP

The material contained in this volume was submitted as
previously unpublished material, except in the instances in
which credit has been given to the source from which some of
the illustrative material was derived.

Any procedure or practice described in this book should be
applied by the health-care practitioner under appropriate
supervision in accordance with professional standards of care
used with regard to the unique circumstances that apply in each
practice situation. Care has been taken to confirm the accuracy
of information presented and to describe generally accepted
practices. However, the authors, editors, and publisher cannot
accept any responsibility for errors or omissions or for any
consequences from application of the information in this book
and make no warranty, express or implied, with respect to the
contents of the book.

The authors and publisher have exerted every effort to ensure
that drug selection and dosage set forth in this text are in
accordance with current recommendations and practice at the
time of publication. However, in view of ongoing research,
changes in government regulations, and the constant flow of
information relating to drug therapy and drug reactions, the
reader is urged to check the package insert for each drug for any
change in indications and dosage and for added warnings and
precautions. This is particularly important when the
recommended agent is a new or infrequently employed drug.

Materials appearing in this book prepared by individuals as part
of their official duties as U.S. Government employees are not
covered by the above-mentioned copyright.

9 8 7 6 5 4 3 2 1

007567

610.73 NETSL

Dedicated to my husband, Dan Nettina,
and my children, Adam and Carolyn, whose love and support
have made this edition a reality

CONTRIBUTORS

Susan E. Appling, RN, MS, CRNP
Assistant Professor
The Johns Hopkins University School of Nursing
Baltimore, Maryland

Marie Brown, RN, PNP, PhD
Professor of Family Nursing
Oregon Health Science Center
Portland, Oregon

Susan E. Brown, RN, MS
Faculty
Harbor Hospital Center School of Nursing
Baltimore, Maryland

Cynthia A. Bumgarner, RN, MSN
Clinical Nurse Specialist—Critical Care
Formerly of Holy Cross Hospital
Silver Spring, MD

Jeanette Campbell, RN, MS, PNP
Developmental Nurse Practitioner
Quaker Medical Associates
Buffalo, New York

Barbara W. Case, RN, CNN
Pediatric Renal Nurse
The Johns Hopkins University
Baltimore, Maryland

JoAnn Coleman, MS, RN, CS, OCN
Clinical Nurse Specialist, Gastrointestinal Surgery
The Johns Hopkins Hospital
Baltimore, Maryland

Dale Ellen Drucker, MSN, CRNP
Nurse Practitioner—Adolescent Medicine
St. Christopher's Hospital for Children
Philadelphia, Pennsylvania

Susan Katharine Fallen, RN, MS
Instructor
Villa Julie College/Union Memorial Hospital
Stevenson, Maryland

Carolyn D. Farrell, MS, CNP
Adjunct Instructor, School of Nursing
State University of New York at Buffalo
Clinical Instructor, School of Medicine
    and Biomedical Sciences
Roswell Park Cancer Institute
Buffalo, New York

Joel C. Farwell, RN, BSN, ONC, MBA
Orthopedic Nurse Clinician
The Children's Hospital of Buffalo
Buffalo, New York

Susan Dill Fischera, RN, MSN
Family Nurse Practitioner
Southeastern Surgical Group
Tallahassee, Florida

Charles Gilkison, RN, MSN, FNP
Clinical Faculty
University of Texas School of Nursing at Galveston
Galveston, Texas

Gina Limardi Hass, RN, BSN
Registered Nurse, Department of Obstetrics
    and Childbirth Education
The George Washington University Medical Center
Washington, D.C.

Joan Hebden, RN, MS, CIC
Infection Control Manager
University of Maryland Medical System
Baltimore, Maryland

Sharon Ann Hyland, RN, MS, NP
Nurse Practitioner, Solid Tumor Division
Roswell Park Cancer Institute
Buffalo, New York

Kathleen Gault Kellinger, PhD, CRNP
Adjunct Professor, School of Nursing
University of Pittsburgh
Pittsburgh, Pennsylvania

Carol A. Kilmon, PhD, RN, CPNP
Associate Professor
University of Texas School of Nursing at Galveston
Galveston, Texas

Debra Kosko, MN, FNP-C
Director of Ambulatory Services, Adult HIV Program
Associate Faculty, School of Nursing
Division of Infectious Diseases, Department of Medicine
University of Maryland
Baltimore, Maryland

Susan Krupnik, RN, MSN, CARN, CS
Psychiatric Consultation Liaison Nurse
Bay State Medical Center
Springfield, Massachusetts
Program Consultant

Comprehensive Behavioral Health Care Home
    Care Program
Skilled Nursing, Inc.
Flourtown, Pennsylvania

Ruth M. Lebet, MSN, RN, CCRN
Clinical Nurse Specialist, Pediatric Emergency Department
The Johns Hopkins Children's Center
Baltimore, Maryland

Mary E. Maciejewski, RN, MS, CNS
Clinical Nurse Specialist, Pediatrics
Children's Hospital of Buffalo
Buffalo, New York

Ruth G. Manchester, RN, MA, OCN, CRNI
IV Therapist
Holy Cross Hospital
Silver Spring, Maryland

Sally Matson, RN, MS, CETN
Enterostomal Nurse Consultant—Education
Formerly of St. Luke's Hospital
Jacksonville, Florida

Cheryl W. McGinnis, MA, MSN, ARNP
Nurse Educator/Nurse Practitioner, Pediatric Liver
    Transplant Program
University of Florida
Gainesville, Florida

Lynn Menza, RN, MS, PNP
Nurse Coordinator, Hemophilia Center
Division of Hematology and Oncology
Children's Hospital
Buffalo, New York

Nancy E. Mooney, MA, RN, ONC
Director of Nursing
Beth Israel Medical Center, North Division
New York, New York

Patricia A. Mosko, MSN, CRNP
Instructor, Adult Nurse Practitioner Program
Temple University
Adult Nurse Practitioner, Primary Care Clinic
Philadelphia Veterans Affairs Medical Center
Philadelphia, Pennsylvania

Zoe Stough O'Brien, MS, CRNP-Ped
Certified Pediatric Nurse Practitioner
The Walkersville Family Medical Center
Walkersville, Maryland

Margaret M. O'Connor, RN
Staff Nurse, P.I.C.U.
Children's Hospital of Buffalo
Buffalo, New York

Lana Parsons, MS, ANP-C
Burn Trauma Coordinator
Baltimore Regional Burn Center, Johns Hopkins Bayview
    Medical Center
Baltimore, Maryland

Nancy J. Reilly, RN, MSN, CURN
GI/GU Clinical Nurse Specialist
University of Pennsylvania Medical Center
Philadelphia, Pennsylvania

Barbara Resnick, MSN, CRNP
Doctoral Candidate, School of Nursing; Nurse Practitioner,
    Department of Family Practice; Faculty Nurse
    Practitioner Program
University of Maryland School of Nursing
Baltimore, Maryland

Beth H. Rodgers, RN, BSN, CNOR
Full Partner: Neurosurgical Operating Room
University of Maryland Hospital
Baltimore, Maryland

Laurie E. Scudder, MS, CPNP
Curriculum Coordinator
Nurse Practitioner Education Associates, Ltd.
Columbia, Maryland

Jane C. Shivnan, RN, MSCN
Nurse Manager, Bone Marrow Transplant
The Johns Hopkins Hospital
Baltimore, Maryland

Sylvia Siegel, RN, CPNP
Pediatric Nurse Practitioner
East Aurora, New York

Joan Bauman Skawski, RN, MA, CCRN
Staff Nurse, Intensive Care Unit
Cayuga Medical Center at Ithaca
Ithaca, New York

Gayla P. Smith, RN, MS, CCRN
Critical Care Clinical Nurse Specialist
Holy Cross Hospital
Silver Spring, Maryland

Geralyn R. Spollett, MSN, C-ANP, CDE
Assistant Professor
Yale University School of Nursing
New Haven, Connecticut

Thom Stuart, RN, BSN
Clinical Coordinator, Pediatric Endocrinology
Children's Health Center of St. Joseph's Hospital
Phoenix, Arizona

Julie N. Tackenberg, RN, MA, MAOM
Clinical Nurse Specialist
University Medical Center
Tucson, Arizona

Dianne M. Whyne, RN, MS
Clinical Specialist
The Johns Hopkins Hospital
Baltimore, Maryland

REVIEWERS

Marie Dobyns, MD
Private Practice
Internal Medicine and Gerontology
Baltimore, Maryland

D. Kim Drake, RN,C, MSN, ANP
Nurse Practitioner
Baltimore, Maryland

Susan Katharine Fallen, RN, MS
Instructor
Villa Julie College/Union Memorial Hospital
Stevenson, Maryland

Ruth M. Lebet, MSN, RN,C, CRN
Clinical Nurse Specialist,
Pediatric Emergency Department
The Johns Hopkins Children's Center
Baltimore, Maryland

Linda L. Rath, RN, MSN, CNNP
Assistant Professor of Nursing
University of Texas Medical Branch—Galveston
Galveston, Texas

David Spott, MD
Private Practice
Dermatology
Clinton, Maryland

Harriet Tootle, RN, BSN, CRNP
Nurse Practitioner, Gynecology
Kaiser Permanente
Baltimore, Maryland

PREFACE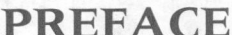

As the *Lippincott Manual of Nursing Practice* begins its 20th year and sixth edition, profound changes are occurring in nursing and in health care delivery. The downsizing of acute care facilities, the growth of managed care, and the increased emphasis on outpatient care all reflect the latest attempts to control the mammoth cost of health care. Because nursing represents a large portion of the health care dollar, the nurse's role is in the spotlight more than ever before.

As I began my nursing career, the first edition of the *Lippincott Manual of Nursing Practice* was published. Just as my nursing career grew and expanded from diploma RN to critical care nurse, to advanced practice nurse and educator, the Manual grew and changed as well. Each edition grew in breadth and depth of information: the maturing nursing process was more carefully outlined in each edition as it developed; guidelines were continually added and updated, reflecting the nurse's increased involvement in technical procedures performed at the bedside; and with each edition nurses replaced physicians as contributors and writers. Throughout its six editions, the *Lippincott Manual of Nursing Practice* has been a comprehensive and reliable reference to nurses at every stage in their careers. The contributors and I have prepared this edition with the needs of contemporary nurses in mind.

◆ ORGANIZATION

The basic organization and easy-to-read outline format of the *Lippincott Manual of Nursing Practice* remain unchanged. However, the focus of the sixth edition is expanded to include information that will enable the nurse to provide care wherever the patient is—in the hospital, the extended care facility, outpatient facility, at home, or on the streets (as with the homeless). Some chapters have been rearranged to promote understanding and ease of use. For example, chapters on Hematologic Disorders and Transfusion Therapy and Bone Marrow Transplantations have been grouped under a separate new section on Blood Disorders. Similarly, conditions of the nose and throat have been merged with material on conditions of the ear, because these disorders often present concurrently.

The heading "discharge planning" has been purposely omitted because many of the problems discussed no longer involve a hospital stay. Instead, care is outlined as it would be provided by the nurse in a variety of settings or as it would be taught by the nurse to the patient or care giver. Because the patient's role on the health care team is greater than ever before, and because the nurse is responsible for fostering that role, Patient Education and Health Maintenance appears as a distinct heading throughout the Manual. Discussion of most disorders begins with the necessary background information, followed by the complete nursing process for care of patients with that disorder.

The Manual is a comprehensive reference for nurses in all areas of care. It is divided into five sections: Nursing Process and Practice, Medical/Surgical Nursing, Maternal and Neonatal Nursing, Pediatric Nursing, and Psychiatric Nursing.

Part 1 discusses the role of the nurse in the health care delivery system. It is comprised of chapters on Nursing Practice and the Nursing Process and on Health Promotion and Preventative Care. An introduction to managed care and an example of a Critical Pathway appear in this unit.

Part 2 comprises the bulk of the book, beginning with chapters on Physical Assessment, IV Therapy, Perioperative Nursing, Cancer, and Care of the Older Adult. The remaining chapters in Unit 2 of this section deal with diseases and disorders of adults, grouped by body system. Most disorders contain the completely developed nursing process, including a discussion of Nursing Assessment, Nursing Diagnosis, Nursing Intervention, and Evaluation. Procedure Guidelines are interspersed throughout the Manual, outlining clinical techniques for procedures performed in all aspects of care and detailing collaborative problems that may occur when performing them.

Part 3 covers Maternal and Neonatal Nursing, and includes chapters on Maternal and Fetal Health, Nursing Management During Labor and Delivery, Care of the Mother and Newborn During the Postpartum Period, and Complications of the Childbearing Experience.

Part 4 is devoted to Pediatric Nursing. It begins with a discussion of General Pediatric Considerations, including chapters on Pediatric Growth and Development, Pediatric Physical Assessment, Pediatric Primary Care, and Care of the Sick or Hospitalized Child. This is followed by a unit on Pediatric Disorders, organized by body system. Where appropriate, the reader is referred to chapters in the medical/surgical section for related information or procedures.

Part 5 is new to this edition and contains information on Psychiatric Nursing, including the most up-to-date information from DSM-IV. Charts on Diagnostic Studies and Their Meaning, Conversion Tables, and Pediatric Laboratory Values appear in the appendices.

◆ NEW AND EXPANDED MATERIAL

A new chapter, Health Promotion and Preventative Care, has been developed for Unit 1. This chapter addresses the nurse's role in the "Healthy People 2000" initiative, as outlined by the U.S. government, and contains practical patient teaching tools that the nurse can use when educating about nutrition, smoking cessation, exercise, and stress management.

Also new to this edition is a separate chapter on Psychiatric Disorders, including DSM-IV classifications and nursing interventions.

In addition, the chapter on HIV Disease and AIDS has been greatly expanded and revised to reflect current research and knowledge of this disease. And for the first time, the Manual includes selected examples of Nursing Care Plans.

◆ PROCEDURE GUIDELINES

The sixth edition of the Manual includes over 100 Procedure Guidelines, making it suitable for use as a procedure manual. New Guidelines on Giving an Allergy Injection, Administering an Enema, Measurement of Cardiac Output by Thermodilution Method, Intracranial Pressure Monitoring, and Diabetic Foot Care are presented for the first time. All Guidelines contain Rationales and many also include a discussion of Collaborative Problems.

◆ NURSING ALERTS

Nursing Alerts appear throughout the Manual, drawing the reader's attention to vital information or pointing out possible life-threatening conditions.

◆ COMMUNITY-BASED NURSING TIPS

For the first time, Community-Based Nursing Tips are included throughout the Lippincott Manual to provide the reader with specific information related to caring for the patient in the non-hospital setting.

◆ GERONTOLOGIC ALERTS

Gerontologic Alerts also appear throughout the Manual to illustrate differences in older adults in both wellness and illness, and to alert the reader to special situations faced by older people.

It is my hope that the sixth edition of the *Lippincott Manual of Nursing Practice* continues to serve as a reassuring reference for today's nurse, as it did for me, and that it promotes the knowledge, skills, and love of nursing that we all possess.

Sandra M. Nettina, RN, MSN, ANP

ACKNOWLEDGMENTS ◆

I would like to thank Janet Peterka, RN, MBA, consultant and editor, for her hours of work, support, and friendship during this project; Diana Rhoads and Linda Shine who spent many hours typing; the faculty members from Sisters of Charity Hospital, Buffalo, NY, Marymount University, Arlington, VA, and the University of Pennsylvania, Philadelphia, PA, from whom I have learned along the way; Lillian S. Brunner and Doris S. Suddarth for their unmeasurable contribution to nursing science; and the past contributors to the *Lippincott Manual of Nursing Practice*. At Lippincott, I would like to thank Lisa Stead, acquisitions editor; Amy P. Jirsa, project editor; Donna Hilton, vice president and publisher; Diana Intenzo, former vice president; Sarah Andrus, developmental editor; and Brian Mac-Donald, editorial assistant.

CONTENTS ◆

PART III ◆ Maternity and Neonatal Nursing   973

PART IV ◆ Pediatric Nursing   1053

UNIT 14   General Practice Considerations   1055

UNIT 15   Pediatric Disorders   1165

PART V ◆ Psychiatric Nursing   1421

LIST OF
PROCEDURE
GUIDELINES ◆

COMMUNITY-BASED
CARE TIPS ◆

THE LIPPINCOTT MANUAL OF NURSING PRACTICE

PART I

Nursing Process and Practice

CHAPTER 1

Nursing Practice and the Nursing Process

Nursing Practice

◆ BASIC CONCEPTS IN NURSING PRACTICE

Understanding basic concepts in nursing practice such as roles of nursing, theories of nursing, licensing, and legal issues help enhance performance.

Definition of Nursing

1. Nursing is an art and a science.
2. Earlier emphasis was on care of sick; now promotion of health is being stressed.
3. American Nurses Association definition, 1980: Nursing is the diagnosis and treatment of human responses to actual and potential health problems.

Roles of Nursing

Whether in hospital-based or community health care setting, nurses assume three basic roles:

1. Practitioner—involves actions that directly meet the health care and nursing needs of patients, families, and significant others; includes staff nurses at all levels of the clinical ladder, advanced practice nurses, and community-based nurses.
2. Leadership—involves actions such as deciding, relating, influencing, and facilitating that affect the actions of others and are directed toward goal determination and achievement; may be a formal nursing leadership role or an informal role periodically assumed by the nurse.
3. Researcher—involves actions taken to implement studies to determine the actual effects of nursing care to further the scientific base of nursing; can include all nurses, not just academicians, nurse scientists, and graduate nursing students.

History of Nursing

1. First nurses were trained by religious institutions to care for patients; no standards or educational basis.
2. In 1873, Florence Nightingale developed a model for independent nursing schools to teach critical thinking, attention to patient's individual needs, and respect for patient's rights.
3. During the early 1900s, hospitals used nursing students as cheap labor and most graduate nurses worked in private duty in homes.
4. After World War II, technological advancements brought more skilled and specialized care to hospitals, requiring more experienced nurses.
5. Development of intensive and coronary care units during the 1950s brought forth specialty nursing and advanced practice nurses.
6. Greater interest in health promotion and disease prevention since the 1960s along with a shortage of physicians serving rural areas helped create the role of nurse practitioner.

Theories of Nursing

1. Nursing theories help define nursing as a scientific discipline of its own.
2. The elements of nursing theories are uniform—nursing, person, environment, and health; also known as the paradigm or model of nursing.
3. Nightingale was the first nursing theorist; she believed the purpose of nursing is to put the person in the best condition for nature to restore or preserve health.
4. More recent nursing theorists include:
   a. Levine—nursing supports person's adaptation to change due to internal and external environmental stimuli.
   b. Orem—nurses assist the person to meet universal, developmental, and health deviation self-care requisites.
   c. Roy—nurses manipulate stimuli to promote adaptation in four modes—physiologic, self-concept, role function, and interdependence relations.
   d. Neuman—nurses affect a person's response to stressors in the areas of physiologic, psychological, sociocultural, and developmental variables.
   e. King—nurses exchange information with clients who are open systems, to attain mutually set goals.
   f. Rogers—nurses promote harmonious interaction between the person and environment to maximize health; both are four-dimensional energy fields.

Nursing in the Health Care Delivery System

1. Technology, education, society values, demographics, and health care financing all have an impact on where and how nursing is practiced.

a. It is predicted that the elderly population of the United States will almost double by the year 2010.
b. Almost 50% of the U.S. population has one or more chronic conditions.
c. The annual cost of medical care in the United States is greater than $900 billion and growing at a rate twice that of inflation.

2. Current trends to use health care dollars for primary care of many, rather than specialized care for a few, has shifted nursing care out of the acute care hospital and into the home and outpatient setting.

3. Inpatient staff nurses are now responsible for a greater number of patients who may be older, more acutely ill, and hospitalized for shorter stays.
a. Diagnosis-related groups (DRGs), implemented in 1983, set rates for Medicare payment for inpatient services, fixing reimbursement based on diagnosis, not on actual charges. This set the standard for shorter hospital stays and other cost-cutting measures.

4. The concept of managed care has expanded for health maintenance organizations (HMOs) and preferred provider organizations (PPOs) to case management and reimbursement control for most insurance plans. Hence, more nurses are working in utilization management or for hospitals or insurance companies, to determine the need for specialist consultations, costly procedures, surgeries, and hospitalizations.

5. More nurses are working for large outpatient centers run by hospitals or HMOs; responsibilities include less "hands on" care, but more assessment and health education for patients and their families.

6. The nursing role has expanded to meet health care challenges more efficiently with certification in a variety of specialties to provide direct care or support and educate other nurses in their roles (Table 1-1).

Advanced Practice Nursing

1. Registered professional nurses with advanced training, education, and certification are allowed to practice in expanded scope.

2. This includes nurse practitioners, nurse midwives, nurse anesthetists, and clinical nurse specialists.

3. Scope of practice and legislation vary by state.
a. Clinical nurse specialists are included in advanced practice nurse (APN) legislation in at least 25 states (some of these just include psychiatric/mental health clinical nurse specialists).
b. APNs in at least 45 states have some form of prescriptive authority.
c. APNs in most states are eligible for Medicare reimbursement and in 34 states can receive some form of third-party reimbursement.
d. Most states give authority to APNs through the Board of Nursing with some degree of physician collaboration/supervision required.

4. Master's degree preparation is becoming the requirement for most APN roles; however, many certificate programs have trained APNs in the past 30 years.

5. Regulation of Canadian APNs has been slower than in the United States, except for midwives, so practice of ANPs has been restricted.

TABLE 1-1 American Nurses Association Credentialing Center Certification Programs

Generalist Programs
Psychiatric and Mental Health Nurse
Medical Surgical Nurse
Gerontologic Nurse
College Health Nurse
Community Health Nurse
School Nurse
General Nursing Practice
Pediatric Nurse
Perinatal Nurse
High-Risk Perinatal Nurse
Maternal-Child Nurse

Clinical Specialist Programs
Clinical Specialist in Adult Psychiatric and Mental Health Nursing
Clinical Specialist in Child and Adolescent Psychiatric Mental Health
Clinical Specialist in Medical–Surgical Nursing
Clinical Specialist in Gerontologic Nursing
Clinical Specialist in Community Health Nursing

Nursing Practitioner Programs
Adult Nurse Practitioner
Family Nurse Practitioner
Gerontologic Nurse Practitioner
School Nurse Practitioner
Pediatric Nurse Practitioner

Nursing Administration Programs
Nursing Administration
Nursing Administration, Advanced

Licensing/Continuing Education

1. Every professional registered nurse must be licensed through the state Board of Nursing in the United States to practice in that state or the College of Nursing to practice in a Canadian province.

2. Continuing education requirements vary depending on state laws, institutional policies, and area of specialty practice. Continuing education units (CEUs) can be obtained through a variety of professional nursing organizations and commercial educational services.

3. Many professional nursing organizations exist to provide education, certification, support, and communication among nurses; for more information contact your state nurses' association, state Board of Nursing, or the American Nurses Association, 600 Maryland Avenue S.W., Suite 100, Washington, DC 20024-2571, 202-554-4444.

Legal/Ethical Issues in Nursing Practice

A. *Malpractice*
1. Nurses have the responsibility to follow a reasonable, professional standard of care; if they fail to do this and injury to the patient results, malpractice may be claimed.

2. To obtain the American Nurses Association Standards for Clinical Nursing, call 1-800-637-0323 and order publication #NP 79.
3. All nurses should be covered by malpractice insurance, either through the institution or employer or through a malpractice policy of their own offered by many commercial and professional groups, including the American Nurses Association, 202-554-4444.
4. Most lawsuits, whether justified or not, are initiated because the patient or family is dissatisfied with *how* they were treated, rather than with *what* care they did or did not receive. To avoid lawsuits, make your bedside manner compassionate, caring, and sensitive to the patient.
5. Documentation is the key to protecting yourself if a lawsuit is filed; include all pertinent data with times and dosages and sites of your actions, patient assessment data, your response to change in condition, specific actions you took, if and when you notified the physician or other health care team members, and what their responses were.
6. Patient rights
   a. Nursing is accountable to provide health care within the framework of society's beliefs and values.
   b. The National League for Nursing has issued a statement on patients' rights that is incorporated into nursing education programs and should be upheld by practicing nurses (Table 1-2).

The Nursing Process

The *nursing process* is a deliberate, problem-solving approach to meeting the health care and nursing needs of patients. It involves assessment (data collection), nursing diagnosis, planning, implementation, and evaluation, with subsequent modifications used as feedback mechanisms that promote the resolution of the nursing diagnoses. The process as a whole is cyclical, the steps being interrelated, interdependent, and recurrent.

◆ Steps in the Nursing Process

Assessment—systematic collection of data to determine the patient's health status and to identify any actual or potential health problems. (Analysis of data is included as part of the assessment. For those who wish to emphasize its importance, analysis may be identified as a separate step of the nursing process.)
Nursing Diagnosis—identification of actual or potential health problems that are amenable to resolution by means of nursing actions
Planning—development of goals and a plan of care designed to assist the patient in resolving the nursing diagnoses
Implementation—actualization of the plan of care through nursing interventions or supervision of others to do the same
Evaluation—determination of the patient's responses to the nursing interventions and of the extent to which the goals have been achieved

TABLE 1-2 National League of Nursing Statement on Patients' Rights

Nurses have a responsibility to uphold the following rights of patients:
To health care that is accessible and that meets professional standards, regardless of the setting.
To courteous and individualized health care that is equitable, humane, and given without discrimination as to race, color, creed, sex, national origin, source of payment, or ethical or political beliefs.
To information about their diagnosis, prognosis, and treatment—including alternatives to care and risks involved—in terms they and their families can readily understand, so that they can give their informed consent.
To informed participation in all decisions concerning their health care.
To information about the qualifications, names, and titles of personnel responsible for providing their health care.
To refuse observation by those not directly involved in their care.
To privacy during interview, examination, and treatment.
To privacy in communicating and visiting with persons of their choice.
To refuse treatment, medications, or participation in research and experimentation, without punitive action being taken against them.
To coordination and continuity of health care.
To appropriate instruction or education from health care personnel so that they can achieve an optimal level of wellness and an understanding of their basic health needs.
To confidentiality of all records (except as otherwise provided for by law or third party payer contracts) and all communications, written or oral, between patients and health care providers.
To access to all health records pertaining to them, and the right to challenge and correct their records for accuracy, and the right to transfer all such records in the case of continuing care.
To information on the charges for services, including the right to challenge these.
To be fully informed as to all their rights in all health care settings.

Assessment

A. *The Nursing History* (see details p. 19)

1. Obtains subjective data through interviewing the patient, family members, or significant other and reviewing old records.
2. Also provides the opportunity to convey interest, support, and understanding to the patient and to establish a rapport based on trust.

B. *The Physical Examination* (see details p. 23)

1. Objective data obtained to determine the patient's physical alterations, limitations, and assets.
2. Should be done in a private, comfortable environment with efficiency and respect.

Nursing Diagnosis

1. Organize, analyze, synthesize, and summarize the collected data.

TABLE 1-3 North American Nursing Diagnosis Association-Accepted Nursing Diagnoses

Activity Intolerance	Knowledge Deficit (Specify)
Activity Intolerance, Risk for	Loneliness, Risk for
Adaptive Capacity: Intracranial, Decreased	Memory, Impaired
Adjustment, Impaired	Noncompliance (Specify)
Airway Clearance, Ineffective	Nutrition, Altered: Less than Body Requirements
Anxiety	Nutrition, Altered: More than Body Requirements
Aspiration, Risk for	Nutrition, Altered: Potential for More than Body Requirements
Body Image Disturbance	Oral Mucous Membrane, Altered
Body Temperature, Risk for Altered	Organized Infant Behavior, Potential for Enhanced
Breastfeeding, Effective	Pain
Breastfeeding, Ineffective	Pain, Chronic
Breastfeeding, Interrupted	Parent/Infant/Child Attachment, Risk for Altered
Breathing Pattern, Ineffective	Parental Role Conflict
Cardiac Output, Decreased	Parenting, Altered
Caregiver Role Strain	Parenting, Risk for Altered
Caregiver Role Strain, Risk for	Perioperative Positioning Injury, Risk for
Communication, Impaired Verbal	Peripheral Neurovascular Dysfunction, Risk for
Community Coping, Ineffective	Personal Identity Disturbance
Community Coping, Potential for Advanced	Physical Mobility, Impaired
Confusion, Acute	Poisoning, Risk for
Confusion, Chronic	Post-Trauma Response
Constipation	Powerlessness
Constipation, Colonic	Protection, Altered
Constipation, Perceived	Rape Trauma Syndrome
Coping, Defensive	Rape Trauma Syndrome: Compound Reaction
Coping, Ineffective Individual	Rape Trauma Syndrome: Silent Reaction
Decisional Conflict (Specify)	Relocation Stress Syndrome
Denial, Ineffective	Role Performance, Altered
Diarrhea	Self-Care Deficit
Disorganized Infant Behavior	Bathing/Hygiene
Disorganized Infant Behavior, Risk for	Feeding
Disuse Syndrome, Risk for	Dressing/Grooming
Diversional Activity Deficit	Toileting
Dysreflexia	Self-Esteem, Chronic Low
Energy Field Disturbance	Self-Esteem, Situational Low
Family Coping: Compromised, Ineffective	Self-Esteem, Disturbance
Family Coping: Disabling, Ineffective	Self-Mutilation, Risk for
Family Coping: Potential for Growth	Sensory/Perceptual Alterations (Specify) (visual, auditory, kinesthetic, gustatory, tactile, olfactory)
Family Process: Alcoholism, Altered	Sexual Dysfunction
Family Processes, Altered	Sexuality Patterns, Altered
Fatigue	Skin Integrity, Risk for Impaired
Fear	Skin Integrity, Impaired
Fluid Volume Deficit	Sleep Pattern Disturbance
Fluid Volume Deficit, Risk for	Social Interaction, Impaired
Fluid Volume Excess	Social Isolation
Gas Exchange, Impaired	Spiritual Distress
Grieving, Anticipatory	Spiritual Well-being, Potential for Enhanced
Grieving, Dysfunctional	Suffocation, Risk for
Growth and Development, Altered	Swallowing, Impaired
Health Maintenance, Altered	Therapeutic Regimen, Ineffective Management of
Health-Seeking Behaviors (Specify)	Therapeutic Regimen: Community, Ineffective Management of
Home Maintenance Management, Impaired	Therapeutic Regimen: Families, Ineffective Management of
Hopelessness	Therapeutic Regimen: Individual, Ineffective Management of
Hyperthermia	Thermoregulation, Ineffective
Hypothermia	Thought Processes, Altered
Impaired Environmental Interpretation Syndrome	Tissue Integrity, Impaired
Incontinence, Bowel	Tissue Perfusion, Altered (Specify type) (renal, cerebral, cardiopulmonary, gastrointestinal, peripheral)
Incontinence, Functional	Trauma, Risk for
Incontinence, Reflex	Unilateral Neglect
Incontinence, Stress	Urinary Elimination, Altered
Incontinence, Total	Urinary Retention
Incontinence, Urge	Ventilation, Inability to Sustain Spontaneous
Infant Feeding Pattern, Ineffective	Ventilatory Weaning Response, Dysfunctional
Infection, Risk for	Violence, Risk for: Self-Directed or Directed at Others
Injury, Risk for	

TABLE 1-4 **Example of a Nursing Care Plan**

Mr. John Preston, a 52-year-old businessman, was admitted to the hospital with a diagnosis of angina pectoris. He stated that he had experienced substernal chest pain and weakness in his arms and hands after having lunch with a business associate. The pain had lessened by the time he arrived at the hospital. The nursing history revealed that he had been hospitalized 5 months previously with the same complaints and had been told by his physician to go to the emergency department if the pain ever recurred. He had been placed on a low-fat diet and had stopped smoking. Physical examination revealed that Mr. Preston's vital signs were within normal ranges and that his chest pain had been relieved with nitroglycerin. He stated that he had feared he was having a "heart attack" until his pain subsided and until he was told that his ECG was normal. He verbalized that he wanted to find out how he could prevent the attacks of pain in the future. The physician's requests on admission included activity as tolerated, low-cholesterol diet, and nitroglycerin 0.4 mg. ($^{1}/_{150}$ gr) sublingually PRN.

**NURSING
DIAGNOSIS:** Pain related to myocardial ischemia

GOALS:
   Short-term: Relief of pain
   Long-term: Altered lifestyle to include measures that decrease myocardial oxygen demands
                        Compliance with therapeutic regimen

NURSING INTERVENTIONS	EXPECTED OUTCOMES (GOALS)	CRITICAL TIME*	OUTCOMES (EVALUATION)
Continue assessment of cardiac function: Monitor blood pressure (BP), pulse (P), respirations (R) q4h.	BP, P, R will remain within normal limits.	24 h	BP: stable at 116–122/72–84 P: stable at 68–82 R: stable at 16–20
Assess frequency of chest pain and precipitating events.	Patient will remain free of chest pain.	24 h	Denies chest pain; able to walk length of hall, eat meals, and visit with family and friends without chest discomfort.
Encourage food and fluid intake that promotes normal nutrition, digestion, and elimination and that does not precipitate chest pain: light, regular meals; foods low in cholesterol; 1500–2000 mL fluid/d.	Will tolerate dietary regimen. Will not experience chest pain after meals. Will maintain normal bowel elimination. Will have intake of 1500–2000 mL fluid/d.	48 h	Denies chest pain after meals; no constipation or diarrhea; fluid intake 1700–2100 mL/d.
Request consultation with dietitian—for diet teaching.	Will identify foods low in cholesterol and those foods that are to be avoided. Will select well balanced diet within prescribed restrictions.	48 h	Selects and eats a balanced diet consisting of foods low in cholesterol; dietitian reviewed diet restrictions with patient and wife; wife counseled in meal planning.
Encourage alterations in activities and exercise that are necessary to prevent episodes of anginal pain.	Will identify activities and exercises that could precipitate chest pain: those that require sudden bursts of activity and heavy effort. Will identify emotionally stressful situations; will explain the necessity for alternating periods of activity with periods of rest.	3 d	Patient and wife have identified activities and situations that should be avoided; patient and wife have studied their usual daily routine and have made plans to alter the routine to allow for rest periods; teenage son has volunteered to assist with strenuous home-maintenance chores.
Teach nitroglycerin regimen.	Will describe action, use, and correct administration of nitroglycerin.		Accurately stated action, use, and dosage of nitroglycerin; demonstrated correct administration.

* These times have not been standardized, but are individualized according to the patient's needs.

TABLE 1-5 Clinical Pathway

Mastectomy	Day 1 (LOS 3.6)	O*	C*	Day 2 (DRG 258)	O*	C*	Day 3	O*	C*	Day 4	O*	C*
Special Orders Tests (Consults)	PAT: CBC, SMA6, urinalysis, CXR, EDG (>40 y or H/O cardiac disease).						Liver scan, CBC if increase blood loss during OR. Post for bone scan as outpatient.					
Nutrition	Clear liquids/advance as tolerated.			Increase diet as tolerated.									
Treatment	VS q4h. IM pain med q4h PRN. Assess dressing and reinforce arm. No Rx or needlesticks affected arm (post-sign). Empty & measure J.P. drain q8h. I&O. Respiratory care—q2h while awake q4h at night (turn, cough, and deep breathe, use incentive spirometry).			VS q shift. PO pain meds if tolerating food and fluids. Change dressing, assess incision. Measure J.P. outputs. Respiratory care q4h while awake q8h at night. Liver scan if indicated. Schedule for outpatient bone scan before discharge (if indicated). Demonstrate or begin postmastectomy exercises (per surgeon request).			Change dressing, assess incision measure J.P. output. Matectomy exercises (per surgeon).					
Activity	OOB with assistance.			OOB ambulating with assistance. Encourage "normal" use of arm.			OOB ambulating in hall. Increase use of arm affected side as tolerated, ie, abduction. Reinforce walking fully erect and not guarding on affected side.					
Teaching	Instruct incentive spirometry and pulmonary toilet. Verbalizes understanding of rationale for pulmonary toilet.			Verbalizes how to care for affected arm, prevent infection, manage lymphadema. Verbalizes rationale for exercises. Demonstrates postmastectomy exercises (per surgeon request). Views incision and verbalizes feelings.			Demonstrate how to empty & care for J.P. drain. Demonstrate mastectomy exercises correctly. Verbalize S&S infection, when to contact MD. Acknowledge change in body image.			Importance of mammography.		
Discharge Planning	Explain Reach for Recovery Organization contact per patient's request. Explain Arm in Arm support group at HHC—give pamphlet.						Give pamphlet or literature for Reach for Recovery, Arm in Arm and mastectomy exercises and arm care.					
Variance												

Expected Outcomes
1. The patient will _____ date
2. The patient will _____ date
3. The patient will _____ date

* O, ordered; C, completed
Courtesy of Harbor Hospital Center, Baltimore, MD.

2. Identify the patient's health problem(s), its (their) particular characteristic(s) and etiology(ies).
3. State nursing diagnoses based on the North American Nursing Diagnosis Association (NANDA) list (Table 1-3).

Planning (Tables 1-4 and 1-5)

1. Assign priorities to the nursing diagnoses. Highest priority is given to problems that are the most urgent and critical.
2. Establish goals or expected outcomes derived from the nursing diagnoses.
   a. Specify short-term, intermediate, and long-term goals as established by nurse and patient together.
   b. Goals should be specific, measurable, and patient focused and should include a time frame.
3. Identify nursing interventions as appropriate for goal attainment.
   a. Include independent nursing actions as well as medical orders.
   b. Should be detailed to provide continuity of care.
4. Formulate the nursing care plan.
   a. Include nursing diagnoses, expected outcomes, interventions, and a space for evaluation.
   b. May use a standardized care plan—check off appropriate data and fill in target dates for expected outcomes and frequency and other specifics of interventions.
   c. May use a protocol that gives specific sequential instructions for treating patients with a particular problem, including who is responsible and what specific actions should be taken in terms of assessment, planning, interventions, teaching, recognition of complications, evaluation, and documentation.
   d. May use a clinical pathway (also called critical pathway) in which the nurse as case manager is responsible for outcomes, length of stay, and use of equipment during the patient's illness; includes the patient's medical diagnosis, length of stay allowed by DRG, expected outcomes, and key events that must occur for the patient to be discharged by that date. Key events are not as specific as nursing interventions but are categorized by day of stay and who is responsible—the nurse, physician, other health care team member, or patient or family.

Implementation

1. Coordinate the activities of the patient, the family, significant others, nursing team members, and other health team members.
2. Delegate specific nursing interventions to other members of the nursing team, as appropriate.
   a. Consider the capabilities and limitations of the members of the nursing team.
   b. Supervise the performance of the nursing interventions.
3. Record the patient's responses to the nursing interventions precisely and concisely.

Evaluation

Determines the success of nursing care and need to alter care plan.

1. Collect assessment data.
2. Compare the patient's behavioral outcomes to the expected outcomes to determine to what extent goals have been achieved.
3. Include the patient, family or significant others, nursing team members, and other health team members in the evaluation.
4. Identify alterations that need to be made in the goals and the nursing care plan.

Continuation of the Nursing Process

1. Continue all steps of the nursing process: assessment, nursing diagnosis, planning, implementation, and evaluation.
2. Continuous evaluation provides the means for maintaining the viability of the entire nursing process and for demonstrating accountability for the quality of nursing care rendered.

Selected References

Alfaro, R. (1989). *Applying nursing diagnoses and nursing process: A step-by-step guide.* Philadelphia: J. B. Lippincott.

Birkholz, G., & Walker, D. (1994). Strategies for state statutory language changes granting fully independent nurse practitioner practice. *The Nurse Practitioner, 19*(1), 54-58.

Carpenito, L. J. (1993). *Handbook of nursing diagnosis* (5th ed.). Philadelphia: J. B. Lippincott.

Carpenito, L. J. (1993). *Nursing diagnosis: Application to clinical practice* (5th ed.). Philadelphia: J. B. Lippincott.

Clark, M. D. (1991). Toward safer nursing practice. *Nursing Management, 2*(3), 88-90.

Doenges, M. E., & Moorhouse, M. F. (1993). *Nurse's pocket guide: Nursing diagnoses with interventions* (4th ed.). Philadelphia: F. A. Davis.

Fawcett, J. (1989). *Analysis and evaluation of conceptual models of nursing.* Philadelphia: F. A. Davis.

Fitzpatrick, J. J., & Whall, A. L. (1989). *Conceptual models of nursing: Analysis and application.* East Norwalk, CT: Appleton & Lange.

Mundinger, M. O. (1994). Advanced-practice nursing—good medicine for physicians? *New England Journal of Medicine, 330*(3), 211-214.

Nursing Process in Clinical Practice. (1993). Springhouse, PA: Springhouse.

Pearson, L. (1994). Annual update of how each state stands on legislative issues affecting advanced nursing practice. *The Nurse Practitioner, 19*(1), 11.

Safriet, B. J. (1992). Health care dollars and regulatory sense: The role of advanced practice nursing. *Yale Journal of Regulation, 9*(2), 417-487.

CHAPTER 2 ◆

Health Promotion/Preventive Care

Concepts in Promotion and Prevention

◆ PRINCIPLES OF HEALTH PROMOTION

Health promotion is defined as the actions taken to develop a high level of wellness and is accomplished by influencing individual behavior and the environment in which people live.

Levels of Prevention

1. Disease prevention is aimed at avoidance of problems or minimizing problems once they occur.
    a. Primary prevention is the total prevention of a condition.
    b. Secondary prevention is the early recognition of a condition and measures taken to speed recovery.
    c. Tertiary prevention is the care given to minimize the effects of the condition and prevent long-term complications.
2. Preventive care should involve risk assessment to focus interventions at persons at risk for specific disorders.

Healthy People 2000

1. Health promotion goes beyond prevention to help people manage their health and live longer and feel better.
2. Health promotion has become a priority since the U.S. Department of Health and Human Services launched the Healthy People 2000 campaign in 1990 to focus public and health care worker attention on 21 health objectives, such as reducing tobacco use, reducing alcohol abuse, improving nutrition, improving environmental public health, preventing and controlling human immunodeficiency virus (HIV) infection and acquired immunodeficiency syndrome (AIDS), and improving maternal and infant health (Table 2-1).

Nursing Role in Health Promotion

1. Nurses have played key roles in prevention in areas such as prenatal care, immunization programs, occupational health and safety, cardiac rehabilitation and education, and public health case finding and early intervention.
2. Nurses in all settings can meet health promotion needs of patients, whether practice is in the hospital, clinic, patient's home, health maintenance organization, private office, or community setting.
3. Health promotion is primarily accomplished through patient education, an independent function of nursing.
4. Health promotion should occur through the life cycle, with topics focused for infancy, childhood, adolescence, adulthood, and older age.
    a. For infancy, teach parents about the importance of prenatal care, basic care of infants, breast-feeding, nutrition, and infant safety.
    b. For childhood, stress the topics of immunizations; proper nutrition to enhance growth and development; and safety practices such as use of carseats and seat belts, fire prevention, and poison proofing the home.
    c. For adolescence, focus topics on motor vehicle safety; avoidance of drug, alcohol, and tobacco use; sexual decision-making and contraception; and prevention of suicide.
    d. For adulthood, teach patients about nutrition, exercise, and stress management to help them feel better; also teach cancer screening techniques such as breast and testicular self-examination, and risk factor reduction for the leading causes of death—heart disease, stroke, and cancer.
    e. For older age, stress the topics of nutrition and exercise to help them live longer and stay fit, safety measures to help them compensate for decreasing mobility and sensory function, and ways to stay active and independent.

◆ PATIENT TEACHING/HEALTH EDUCATION

Health education is included in the American Nurses Association Standards of Care and is defined as an essential component of nursing care. It is directed toward promotion, maintenance, and restoration of health and toward adaptation to the residual effects of illness.

Learning Readiness

1. Assist the patient in physical readiness to learn by trying to alleviate any physical distress that may distract the patient's attention and prevent effective learning.

TABLE 2-1 Health Objectives
of *Healthy People 2000*

1. Reduce tobacco use
2. Reduce alcohol and other abuse
3. Improve nutrition
4. Increase physical activity and fitness
5. Improve mental health and prevent mental illness
6. Reduce violent and abusive behavior
7. Increase access to family planning services
8. Promote health education and community-based health programs
9. Improve environmental public safety
10. Improve occupational health and safety
11. Prevent and control unintentional injuries
12. Improve oral health
13. Improve food and drug safety
14. Increase clinical preventive health services
15. Prevent and control HIV infection and AIDS
16. Prevent and control sexually transmitted diseases
17. Immunize against and control infectious diseases
18. Improve maternal and infant health
19. Prevent, detect, and control hypertension, heart disease, and stroke
20. Prevent, detect, and control cancer
21. Prevent, detect, and control diabetes and other disabling conditons

U.S. Department of Health and Human Services (1991). *Healthy people 2000: National health promotion and disease prevention objectives.* Washington, DC: Author. (DHHS Publication PHS 91-50212).

2. Assess and promote the patient's emotional readiness to learn.
   a. Motivation to learn depends on acceptance of the illness or that illness is a threat, recognition of the need to learn, values related to social and cultural background, and a therapeutic regimen comparable with the patient's lifestyle.
   b. Promote motivation to learn by creating a warm, accepting, positive atmosphere; encouraging the patient to participate in the establishment of acceptable, realistic, and attainable learning goals; and providing constructive feedback about progress.
3. Assess and promote the patient's experiential readiness to learn.
   a. Determine what past experiences the patient has had with health and illness, what success or failure the patient has had with learning, and what basic knowledge the patient has on related topics.
   b. Provide the patient with any prerequisite knowledge necessary to begin the learning process.

Teaching Strategies

1. Patient education can occur at any time and in any setting; however, you must consider how conducive the environment is to learning, how much time you are able to schedule, and what other family members or significant others can attend the teaching session.
2. Use a variety of techniques that are appropriate to meet the needs of each individual.
   a. Lecture or explanation should include discussion or a question and answer period.
   b. Group discussion is effective for individuals with

similar needs; participants often gain support, assistance, and encouragement from other members.
   c. Demonstration and practice should be used when skills need to be learned; ample time should be allowed for practice and return demonstration.
   d. Teaching aids include books, pamphlets, pictures, slides, videos, tapes, and models and should be supplemental to verbal teaching. These can be obtained from government agencies such as the Department of Health and Human Services, the Centers for Disease Control and Prevention, and the National Institutes of Health; not-for-profit groups such as the American Heart Association or the March of Dimes; or pharmaceutical and insurance companies.
   e. Reinforcement and follow-up sessions offer time for evaluation and additional teaching if necessary and can greatly increase effectiveness of teaching.
3. Document patient teaching including what was taught and how the patient responded; use standardized patient teaching checklists if available.

◆ SELECTED AREAS OF HEALTH PROMOTION

Counsel patients on the topics of proper nutrition, smoking cessation, exercise, relaxation, and sexual health to promote health.

Nutrition/Diet

1. It is projected that 35% of all cancer could be prevented with an improved diet recommended by the National Cancer Institute.
2. A low-fat, high-fiber diet is recommended.
   a. Fat should account for no more than 30% of calories.
   b. Fiber content should be 20 to 30 g daily.
   c. Five servings of fruits and vegetables should be included daily.
   d. Six servings of breads, cereals, and legumes should be included daily.
3. Dietary modifications are also necessary to treat and prevent disease such as hypertension, type II diabetes mellitus, coronary artery disease, and hyperlipidemia, as well as to promote optimal weight, energy, and well-being.
4. Educate patients about the five basic food groups and their placement on the food pyramid, optimum weight, calorie requirements, and ways to increase fiber and decrease fat in the diet.
   a. Total fat content can be reduced by cutting down on red and fatty cuts of meat; bacon and sausage; cooking oils; whole dairy products; eggs; baked goods; cookies and candy; and sauces, soups, and dressings made with cream, eggs, or oil. Also teach patients to save high-fat foods for a special treat, reduce portion size, use fat substitutes, and prepare dishes at home using low-fat recipes.
   b. Teach patients to add fiber to the diet by choosing whole grain breads and cereals; raw or minimally cooked fruits and vegetables (especially citrus fruits, squash, cabbage, lettuce and other greens, beans); and any nuts, skins, and seeds. Fiber can also be increased by adding several teaspoons of whole bran to meals each day or taking an over-the-

counter fiber supplement such as psyllium (Metamucil), as directed.

5. Encourage patients to keep diaries of their food intake and review them periodically to determine if other adjustments should be made.

6. If weight loss is desired, have the patient weigh in monthly, and review the diet and give praise or constructive criticism at this visit.

7. Use and refer patients to resources such as:
TOPS (Take Off Pounds Sensibly)
P.O. Box 07360
4575 South Fifth Street
Milwaukee, Wisconsin 53207
414-482-4620
United States Department of Agriculture
Room 344
6505 Belcrest Road
Hyattsville, MD 20782
301-436-8617

Smoking Prevention/Cessation

1. It has been estimated that 30% of all cancer is linked to smoking and is preventable.

2. Studies show that 60% of all current smokers began by age 14 and that more than 3,000 children each day begin to use tobacco in the United States.

3. Smoking is a risk factor for hypertension, heart disease, peripheral vascular disease, chronic obstructive pulmonary disease (COPD), and cancer of the lung, colon, larynx, oral cavity, esophagus, bladder, pancreas, and kidney. It also worsens such conditions as respiratory infections, peptic ulcers, hiatal hernia, and gastroesophageal reflux.

4. Not smoking promotes health by increasing exercise tolerance; enhancing taste bud function; and avoiding facial wrinkles, bad breath, and odor on clothes.

5. Smoking prevention education should begin during childhood and stressed during adolescence, a time when peer modeling and confusion over self-image may lead to smoking.

6. Smoking cessation can be accomplished through an individualized, multidimensional program including:
   a. Information on the short- and long-term health effects of smoking.
   b. Practical behavior modification techniques to help break the habit—gum chewing, munching on carrot and celery sticks, sucking on mints and hard candy to provide oral stimulation; working modeling clay, knitting, or other ways to keep provide tactile stimulation; avoiding coffee shops, bars, or other situations that smokers frequent; incentive plans such as saving money for each cigarette not smoked and rewarding oneself when a goal is reached.
   c. Use of medications designed to reduce physical dependence and minimize withdrawal symptoms such as nicotine chewing gum or nicotine transdermal patches.
   d. Use of support groups, frequent reinforcement, and follow-up.

7. Use and refer patients to agencies such as:
American Cancer Society
19 West 56th Street
New York, NY 10019
212-586-8700

American Lung Association
1740 Broadway
New York, NY 10019
212-315-8700

Exercise/Fitness

1. Regular exercise as part of a fitness program helps achieve optimal weight, control blood pressure, increase high-density lipoprotein (HDL), lower risk of coronary artery disease, increase endurance, and improve the sense of well-being.

2. Long-term goals of regular exercise include decreased absenteeism from work, less disability, and reduced health care costs.

3. Studies have shown that both high-intensity exercise and low- to moderate-intensity exercise performed at least three times a week have positive effects.
   a. High-intensity exercise achieving 70% to 90% of maximum heart rate produces lactic acid in the muscles, which inhibits fat burning; however, calories will be burned at a high rate because carbohydrate is used for energy.
   b. Low- to moderate-intensity exercise achieving 50% to 70% of maximum heart rate begins to access fat stores for fuel after 30 minutes of exercise; with longer duration of exercise fewer calories but more fat will be burned.

4. Individual tolerance, time allotment, interests, and physical impairment must be figured into exercise planning.

5. Suggest walking, jogging, bicycling, swimming, water aerobics, and low-impact aerobic dancing as good low- to moderate- intensity exercise, performed three to five times a week for 45 minutes. Walking can be done safely and comfortably by most patients if the pace is adjusted to the individual's physical condition.
   a. Exercise programs should include 5- to 10-minute warm-up and cool-down periods with stretching activities to prevent injuries.
   b. Full intensity and duration of exercise should be worked up to gradually over a period of several weeks to months.

GERONTOLOGIC ALERT
Due to physiologic limitations of old age, maximum effective exercise for the elderly is 20 to 40 minutes at 50% to 60% of maximum heart rate.

6. Advise patients to stop if pain, shortness of breath, dizziness, palpitations, or excessive sweating is experienced.

7. Advise patients with cardiovascular, respiratory, and musculoskeletal disorders to check with their health care provider about specific guidelines or limitations for exercise.

COMMUNITY-BASED CARE TIP
Severe cases of COPD, osteoarthritis, and coronary artery disease are contraindications for unsupervised exercise; check with the patient's health care provider to see if a physical therapy or occupational therapy referral would be helpful.

8. Use and refer patients to resources such as:
American Heart Association
772 Greenville Avenue
Dallas, TX 75231
214-373-6300

UNIVERSITY OF CENTRAL
LANCASHIRE LIBRARY
BLACKPOOL SITE

Relaxation/Stress Management

1. *Stress* is a change in the environment that is perceived as a threat, challenge, or harm to the person's dynamic equilibrium. In times of stress, the sympathetic nervous system is activated to produce immediate changes of increased heart rate, peripheral vasoconstriction, and increased blood pressure. This response is prolonged by adrenal stimulation and secretion of epinephrine and norepinephrine, and is known as "the fight or flight" reaction.
2. A limited amount of stress can be a positive motivator to take action; however, excessive or prolonged stress can cause emotional discomfort, anxiety, possible panic, and illness.
3. Prolonged sympathetic-adrenal stimulation may lead to high blood pressure, arteriosclerotic changes, and cardiovascular disease; stress has also been implicated in acute asthma attack, peptic ulcer disease, irritable bowel syndrome, migraine headaches, and other illnesses.
4. Stress management can help control these illnesses as well as help individuals improve self-esteem, gain control over their lives, and enjoy life more fully.
5. Stress management involves identification of physiologic and psychosocial stressors through assessment of the patient's education, finances, job, family, habits, activities, personal and family health history, and responsibilities. Positive and negative coping methods should also be identified.
6. Relaxation therapy is one of the first steps in stress management; it can be used to reduce anxiety brought on by stress. Relaxation techniques include:
   a. *Relaxation breathing*—the simplest technique that can be performed at any time. The patient breathes slowly and deeply until relaxation is achieved; however, it can lead to hypoventilation if done incorrectly.
   b. *Progressive muscle relaxation*—relieves muscle tension related to stress. The patient alternately tenses, then relaxes muscle groups until the entire body feels relaxed.
   c. *Autogenic training*—can help relieve pain and induce sleep. The patient replaces painful or unpleasant sensations with pleasant ones through self-suggestions; may require extensive coaching at first.
   d. *Imagery*—uses imagination and concentration to take a "mental vacation." The patient imagines a peaceful, pleasant scene involving multiple senses. It can last as long as patient decides.
   e. *Distraction*—uses patient's own interests and activities to divert attention from pain or anxiety and includes listening to music, watching television, reading a book, singing, knitting, doing crafts or projects, or physical activities.
7. To assist patients with relaxation therapy, follow these steps:
   a. Review the techniques and encourage a trial with several techniques of the patient's choice.
   b. Teach the chosen technique(s) and coach the patient until effective use of the technique is demonstrated.
   c. Suggest that the patient practice relaxation techniques for 20 minutes a day to feel more relaxed and to be prepared to use them confidently when stress increases.
   d. Encourage the patient to combine techniques such as relaxation breathing before and after imagery or progressive muscle relaxation along with autogenic training to achieve better results.
8. Additional steps in stress management include dealing with the stressors or problem areas and increasing coping behaviors.
   a. Assist the patient to recognize specific stressors and determine if they can be altered. Then develop a plan for managing that stressor such as changing jobs, postponing taking an extra class, hiring a babysitter once a week, talking to the neighbor about his dog, or getting up an hour earlier to exercise.
   b. Teach the patient to avoid negative coping behaviors such as smoking, drinking, using drugs, overeating, cursing, and using abusive behavior toward others. Teach positive coping mechanisms such as continued use of relaxation techniques, fostering of support systems—family, friends, church groups, social groups, or professional support groups.

Sexual Health

1. Because sexuality is inherent to every person and sexual functioning is a basic physiologic need of human beings, nurses must provide care in a way that is promotional to sexual health.
2. As a health educator and counselor in the area of sexual health, the nurse helps the patient gain knowledge, validate normalcy, prepare for changes in sexuality throughout the life cycle, and prevent harm gained through sexual activity.
3. Education about sexual activity should begin during school age, heighten during adolescence, and continue through adulthood.
4. Topics to cover include:
   a. Normal reproduction—the menstrual cycle, ovulation, fertilization (see p. 644)
   b. Unwanted pregnancy—approximately one million teen pregnancies occur in the United States each year.
   c. Contraception—ideally should begin before sexual activity is started, various methods, side effects, effectiveness, convenience (see p. 650)
   d. Sexually transmitted diseases (STDs)—mode of transmission, prevalence, signs and symptoms, methods of prevention (see p. 667)
      (1) Over 20 million people have genital herpes in the United States.
      (2) Chlamydia is now the most common sexually transmitted pathogen and is often asymptomatic.
      (3) Genital warts are highly recurrent and may lead to cervical dysplasia.
      (4) Approximately 400,000 cases of AIDS were reported in the United States in 1993.
   e. Safer sex/abstinence—primarily adopted to prevent HIV transmission, but can also prevent other STDs and pregnancy
      (1) Abstinence is the only 100% effective method

007567

for HIV prevention related to sexual transmission.

(2) Mutual monogamy can also be 100% effective if both partners enter the relationship HIV negative.

(3) Use of female or male latex condoms correctly and consistently is also highly effective.

(4) Use of spermicide containing nonoxynal-9 in addition to condoms provides additional protection.

(5) For individuals infected with HIV, avoid vaginal, anal, and oral intercourse, deep kissing, and any practices that may injure tissues, if possible.

5. Other areas in which nurses can help promote healthy sexual functioning:

a. Discuss with teenagers the value of delaying sexual activity—prevention of pregnancy and STDs, saving money on contraception, greater enjoyment of first sexual encounter when older, greater control of relationship and decision-making if not sexually involved.

b. Assist men to have greater respect for women, to allow women partnership in relationship, and to not equate sex with violence as often depicted in movies and television.

c. Assist women to understand their sexuality needs, become comfortable with their bodies, communicate with sexual partners about their satisfaction, and seek medical help for gynecologic problems.

6. Use and refer patients to resources such as:
American Foundation for the Prevention of Venereal Disease
Suite 638
799 Broadway
New York, NY 10003
212-759-2069

Ortho Pharmaceutical Corporation
Patient Education Coordinator
Route 202
P.O. Box 300
Raritan, NJ 08869
1-800-722-7786

National AIDS Clearinghouse
1-800-458-5231

Patient Teaching Aids

Copy and distribute the following patient teaching aids to enhance your counseling and promote health.

PATIENT TEACHING AID ◇ Stress Management

Stress is a common phenomenon among most individuals today, and can be related to job, relationship, financial, and other pressures. Known as the "fight or flight" reaction, the physiologic and emotional response to stress can lead to tension, anxiety, and a variety of health threats. Stress can be minimized by better coping with it and adapting to its causes. Follow this guide to better manage stress.

RECOGNIZE STRESS

1. First, identify signs that you may be under stress, for example, irritability, tension, fatigue, insomnia, loss of interest in activities, feeling overwhelmed, or fighting with spouse and others.

2. Next, try to identify the true cause of stress. For example, you may snap at your children for playing the stereo too loudly, but what is the underlying cause of your irritability?

3. Examine areas of your job, family life, financial stability, and other roles and responsibilities that may be demanding or problematic.

DO SOMETHING ABOUT IT

1. Try to manage stressful areas better—be assertive, negotiate, and say no if necessary. For example, confront the person with whom you are at odds and work out a mutual agreement, put the plan in writing, and try to stick to it.

2. Make more time for yourself and important relationships. Say no to responsibilities that you don't have time for and get help from a familymember or friend, or hire a babysitter when necessary.

RELAX

When you enter a stressful situation or you feel tension rising, practice the following relaxation techniques; you will be able to think more clearly and function more effectively.

Relaxation Breathing

Concentrate on breathing slowly and deeply with eyes closed (if possible) for several minutes when you need a quick tension reducer or before beginning one of the other methods.

1. Breathe in through your nose and mouth with face relaxed for a count of 1 and 2 and 3 and 4.

2. Hold your breath for 4 seconds, without straining.

3. Breathe out through your nose and pursed lips for a count of 6.

4. Repeat two or three times, breathe naturally for about 30 seconds, then repeat one or more sequences.

5. If you feel dizzy or tingling in your fingertips, you may be hyperventilating; slow down your breathing and don't take such deep breaths.

Progressive Muscle Relaxation

Because stress may cause you to subconsciously contract your muscles, in this exercise you will alternately tense and relax your muscle groups one by one, until your entire body is in a state of relaxation.

1. Assume a comfortable position, either sitting or reclining, and close your eyes.

2. Start with your forehead and tense the muscles so that you feel tightness or strain; hold this position for 5 to 10 seconds.

PATIENT TEACHING AID ◇ Stress Management (continued)

3. Next, relax your forehead, noting the relief; concentrate on this for 10 to 15 seconds.
4. Progress from head to toe with each muscle group, including your jaw next, then shoulders, arms, hands, abdomen, buttocks, legs, and feet (you can do both sides simultaneously).
5. Note the feeling of total relaxation in your body once you have relieved tension from all your muscles.
6. Complete the exercise by opening your eyes, taking a few deep breaths, stretching, and arising slowly.

Imagery
Imagery allows you to take a mental vacation by using your imagination and diverting your attention from stressful thoughts.

1. Assume a comfortable position, breathe deeply, and close your eyes.
2. Count backward from 5 and begin to imagine a pleasant place such as a beach or garden.
3. Put yourself in that place by imagining it with all your senses, for example, hear the sound of waves washing up on the beach, feel the warm sun saturating your skin, or taste a tangy drink of lemonade.

4. Stay in that place for about 5 minutes, imagining different images.
5. Slowly let the images fade, breathe deeply, and count to 5 before opening your eyes.

Distraction
You can use many methods of distraction to block your concentration from anxiety and stressful matters. Using your senses to listen to music, petting your dog, or reading can be relaxing.

1. Choose activities that you enjoy—reading, watching television, listening to music, taking a walk, playing an instrument, knitting, doing a craft, or drawing or painting.
2. Adjust the distraction method to your mood—if you are extremely tense do not attempt a complex project or listen to loud, lively music. Rather, listen to quiet, soothing music or sketch a free-form design.
3. Use a variety of methods, some reserved for longer periods of time, and others that can be used on the spot when needed (eg, a portable tape player with headphones and your favorite music or a book of poetry).

PATIENT TEACHING AID ◇ Smoking Cessation

Cigarette smoking is the single most preventable cause of death and disability today. Smoking is related to about 30% of all cancer deaths, is the leading risk factor for coronary artery disease and emphysema, and has many other effects on health and hygiene. People who smoke tend to have more dental problems, premature aging of the skin, increased acid in the stomach, decreased exercise tolerance, loss of taste bud function, problems with pregnancy and fetal growth, more frequent respiratory infections, and bad breath.

Smoking cessation, however, will reverse most of these risks and allow you to breathe more easily and feel better.

PLAN TO QUIT
1. Make a list of all the positive things and all the negative things about smoking; consider the short- and long-term health risks on your list.
2. Talk to your health care provider about the use of nicotine chewing gum or skin patch to aid your stop smoking program by reducing withdrawal symptoms and cravings for a cigarette.
3. Talk to family and friends and form a support network of people who have quit smoking.
4. Set the date to quit and don't make any excuses.
5. Stock up on low-calorie treats such as raw vegetables, sugarless gum, popcorn, and sugar-free soft drinks to enjoy when the urge to smoke hits.
6. Remove all ashtrays, cigarettes, matches, and lighters from your home, car, and office.

STICK WITH IT
1. Avoid smoky environments such as bars and coffee shops and the smoking section of restaurants.
2. Restructure your routine to eliminate times you previously enjoyed a cigarette.
3. Anticipate feeling irritable for several days to several weeks while quitting, so avoid stressful situations.
4. Increase exercise, such as walking, biking, or sporting activities to relieve tension, fill free time, and concentrate on healthy activity.
5. Occupy your hands with modeling clay, knitting, doodling, or a craft project.
6. Brush your teeth often and enjoy fresher breath.
7. Reward yourself for not smoking.

TRY, TRY AGAIN
1. If you start smoking again, don't be discouraged; many people are successful the second time around.
2. Review and revise your plan and pick a new quit date.
3. For more information on smoking cessation programs, contact:
   American Cancer Society 800-ACS-2345
   American Heart Association 214-373-6300
   American Lung Association 212-315-8700

PATIENT TEACHING AID ◇ *Exercise Guidelines*

Aerobic exercise provides a wide range of benefits including weight loss, muscle toning, endurance building, improved circulation, increased HDL (the "good" cholesterol), lowered risk of a heart attack, better controlled blood pressure, and a sense of reduced tension and feeling better. Aerobic exercise refers to any type of activity that uses oxygen to produce energy. The cardiovascular system is stimulated and fat is burned. Most people can do aerobic exercise of some kind, adjusting the intensity as necessary. Follow these guidelines to develop your own exercise program.

1. Choose an activity that you enjoy, is convenient, and you are capable of; consider walking, bicycle riding, jogging, swimming, aerobics or step aerobics, sporting activities, or use of fitness equipment such as the rowing machine, stair stepper, or cross country ski machine.
2. Start out exercising 15 to 20 minutes at a time for the first week or two, then gradually increase the intensity and length of exercise time over several weeks to months.
3. Include 5- to 10-minute warm-up and cool-down periods with each exercise session, doing stretching of major muscles, deep breathing, and light calisthenics.
4. Exercise at least three times a week and be consistent.
5. Exercise at 50% to 70% of your maximum heart rate for moderate intensity or 70% to 90% for high intensity, as tolerated.

CALCULATING TARGET HEART RATE

To get the most out of exercise, calculate your heart rate. First subtract your age from 220. This is your maximum heart rate; do not exceed this rate while exercising to avoid strain on your heart.

If you are 40 years old, your maximum heart rate 220 minus 40, or 180. Your target heart rate is 40% to 50% of maximum for low-intensity exercise, 50% to 70% of maximum for moderate-intensity exercise, or 70% to 90% of maximum for high-intensity exercise. So if you want to exercise at moderate intensity, 60% of 180 is 108 (180 × 0.6). Your target heart rate is 108. By taking your pulse several times during exercise, you can adjust your pace to stay close to your target heart rate and exercise optimally but safely.

TAKING YOUR PULSE

First take your resting pulse before you begin exercise, counting for 30 seconds and multiplying by 2.

To take your pulse during exercise, slow down and find the carotid pulse point in your neck. Place two or three fingers on your trachea (windpipe) near the base of your neck and then move them over to the left or right about 2 to 3 inches until you feel the beating of your pulse. Press lightly so you do not cause an irregular heartbeat or interrupt circulation to your brain. Use a watch with a second hand to count the number of beats in 6 seconds. Now multiply by 10 to get an estimate of your true 60-second pulse.

If you counted 10 beats in 6 seconds, your working heart rate is 100 (10 × 10). As you continue to exercise, you can work a little harder to reach your target rate. If your working heart rate is 10 beats or more greater than your target rate, slow down your pace and check your pulse again in 5 to 10 minutes.

When you complete your exercise, your pulse should be no more than 15 beats above your resting pulse; if it is, continue your cool-down activity.

WHEN TO STOP

You should usually never stop exercising abruptly; you must allow the heart to slow down and the blood to redistribute appropriately. You should slow down if you experience muscle cramps, shortness of breath, or fatigue. You should stop, however, if you experience chest pain, a cold sweat, dizziness, nausea or vomiting, heart palpitations, or fainting. Seek help and notify your health care provider immediately.

PATIENT TEACHING AID ◇ *Eating a Healthier Diet*

To help maintain optimal weight, feel better, and reduce the risk of heart disease, cancer, and a variety of health problems, the following dietary changes are recommended:

1. Increase fiber in diet to 20 to 30 g daily.
2. Reduce fat content to no more than 30% of total calories each day.
3. Eat five servings of fruits and vegetables each day. A serving consists of:
   a. One medium piece of fruit, ½ cup of cut up fruit, or 6 oz of juice
   b. One-half cup of cooked or raw vegetable, or 1 cup of leafy greens
4. Include six or more servings of cereal or bread per day.
5. Maintain moderate protein intake of fish, beans, nuts, or no more than 5 to 7 oz of lean meat per day.
6. Limit salt and alcohol consumption.

REDUCING FAT

To determine how many grams of fat you should eat in your diet, first identify how many calories you should eat each day. This will vary depending on your body build and activity level, but approximately 2,100 calories is an average amount for an active medium-sized man or woman who is not trying to lose weight. Next, figure that 30% of 2,100 is 630 calories of fat. There are 9 calories per gram of fat, so 630 divided by 9 equals 70 g of fat. Now you are ready to read food labels to see how many grams of fat are in each serving of food you eat. Margarine, for example, contains 11 g of fat per tablespoon, and cheddar cheese contains about 8 g of fat per ounce. You will find that 70 g will add up quickly unless you include a variety of low-fat foods in your diet. Note: If you are trying to lose weight and are on a lower calorie diet with a lower percentage of fat, this figure will be much lower.

Follow this guide to reduce fat:

Breads, Cereals, and Grains

1. Eat whole grain (oat, bran, multigrain), light, wheat, or rye bread rather than pure white bread or other breads that list eggs as a major ingredient.
2. Eat pasta or rice rather than egg noodles, serve with light tomato sauce or vegetables as main dish, rather than meat.
3. Substitute angel food cake, low-fat cookies, crackers, and home-baked goods made with low-fat ingredients for higher fat pies, cakes, cookies, doughnuts, biscuits, and muffins.

Eggs and Dairy Products

1. Use only skim or 1% milk, no cream or half and half.
2. Use part skim and reduced fat cheeses sparingly, substitue low-fat cottage cheese.
3. Use low-fat yogurt and frozen yogurt, pudding made from skim milk, and fat-free dessert items.

Fats and Oils

1. Never use butter, lard, or coconut, palm, or palm kernel oil.
2. Use unsaturated vegetable oils sparingly (especially, canola, safflower, sesame, soybean, sunflower, and olive).
3. Substitue margarine, especially diet or light margarine, for butter, but use sparingly.
4. Avoid egg yolks, chocolate, and bacon or beef fat for cooking; substitue two egg whites for one whole egg in recipes.
5. Use only low-fat mayonnaise and salad dressings.

Meats, Fish, and Poultry

1. Use lean cuts of beef, lamb, and pork sparingly.
2. Eat white meat (chicken and turkey) with skin and fat removed before cooking, if possible.
3. Avoid organ meat, ribs, chicken wings, sausage, hot dogs, and bacon.
4. Use fillets of sole, salmon, mackerel, tuna, haddock, or canned tuna packed in water; avoid sardines, roe, and shrimp (high in cholesterol).
5. Eat small portions; bake or broil; blot with paper towel after cooking; and discard drained fat.

INCREASING FIBER

Fiber is a plant cell wall component that is not broken down by the digestive system. It absorbs fluid and moves through the intestines in a bulky mass with the ability to absorb cholesterol and carcinogens. It decreases intestinal transit time, therefore decreasing constipation and related problems. Increase fiber in your diet gradually to prevent gas. Here are good sources of fiber:

1. Cereal containing 4 g or more of fiber per serving (read package label)
2. Whole grain breads and muffins
3. Fresh or frozen fruits and vegetables, not overcooked, with skin on
4. Nuts, seeds, and popcorn
5. Bran; add 1 teaspoon to food three times a day.
6. Legumes (pods) such as peas or beans

Selected References

Anderson, J., & Yuhos, R. (1993). Health promotion in rural settings. *Nursing Clinics of North America, 28*(1), 145-155.

Bal, D. G., & Forester, S. B. (1993). Dietary strategies for cancer prevention. *Cancer, 72*(3, supplement), 1005-1010.

Blair, J. E. (1993). Social learning theory: Strategies for health promotion. *AAOHN Journal, 41*(5), 245-249.

Blair, S. N., Cohl, H. W., Paffenbarger, R. S., et al. (1989). Physical fitness and all-cause mortality: A prospective study of healthy men and women. *Journal of the American Medical Association, 262*, 2395-2401.

Cohen, R. Y., Sattler, J., Felix, M. R. J., & Brownell, K. D. (1987). Experimentation with smokeless tobacco and cigarettes by children and adolescents: Relationships to beliefs, peer use, and prenatal use. *American Journal of Public Health, 77*, 1454-1456.

Cordell, B., & Smith-Blair, N. (1994). Streamlined charting for patient education. *Nursing 94*, January, 57-59.

Dwyer, J. T. (1993). Diet and nutritional strategies for cancer risk reduction: Focus on the 21st century. *Cancer, 72*(3, supplement), 1024-1031.

Epps, R. P., & Manley, M. W. (1993). Prevention of tobacco use during childhood and adolescence. *Cancer, 72*(3, supplement), 1002-1004.

Goeppinger, J. (1993). Health promotion for rural populations: Partnership interventions. *Family and Community Health, 16*(1), 1-10.

Grubbs, L. (1993). The critical role of exercise in weight control. *Nurse Practitioner, 18*(4), 20-29.

Healthy people 2000. National health promotion and disease prevention objectives. (1990). Washington, DC: U.S. Department of Health and Human Services. Public Health Service, 5, 416-417.

Heimendinger, J. (1993). Community nutrition intervention strategies for cancer risk reduction. *Cancer, 72*(3, supplement, 1019-1023.

Karle, H., Shenassa, E., Edwards, C., et al. (1994). Tobacco control for high-risk youth: Tracking and evaluation issues. *Family and Community Health, 16*(4), 10-17.

Kritchevsky, D. (1993). Dietary guidelines. *Cancer, 72*(3, supplement, 1011-1014.

Manson, J. E., Nathan, D. M., Krolewski, A. S., et al. (1992). A prospective study of exercise and incidence of diabetes among US male physicians. *Journal of the American Medical Association, 268*, 63-67.

Redland, A. R., & Stuifbergen, A. K. (1993). Strategies for maintenance of health-promoting behaviors. *Nursing Clinics of North America, 28*(2), 427-442.

PART II ◆

Medical-Surgical Nursing

UNIT 1

◆

General Considerations

The Patient History

General Principles

1. The first step in caring for a patient and in soliciting his active cooperation is to gather a careful and complete history.
    a. In *all* patient concerns and problems, an accurate history is the foundation on which data collection and the process of assessment are based.
    b. The comprehensiveness of the history elicited will depend on the information available in the patient's record.
2. Time spent early in the nurse–patient relationship gathering detailed information about what the patient knows, thinks, and feels about the problems will prevent time-consuming errors and misunderstandings later.
3. Skill in interviewing will affect both the accuracy of information elicited and the quality of the relationship established with the patient.
        This point cannot be overemphasized; the reader is encouraged to consult other sources for detailed discussion of techniques of health interviewing.
4. The purpose of the interview is to encourage an interchange of information between the patient and the nurse. The patient must feel that his words are understood and that his concerns are being heard and dealt with sensitively.

Interviewing Techniques

1. Provide privacy in as quiet a place as possible and see that the patient is comfortable.
2. Begin the interview with a courteous greeting and an introduction. Explain who you are and why you are there.
3. Be sure that facial expressions, body movements, and tone of voice are pleasant, unhurried, and nonevaluative, and that they convey the attitude of a sensitive listener, so that the patient will feel free to express thoughts and feelings.
4. Avoid reassuring the patient prematurely (before you have adequate information about the problem). This only cuts off discussion; the patient may then be unwilling to bring up a problem causing concern.
5. At times a patient gives cues or suggests information, but does not tell enough. It may be necessary to probe for more information to obtain a thorough history; the patient must realize that this is done for his or her benefit.
6. Guide the interview so that the necessary information is obtained, without cutting off discussion. Controlling the rambling patient is often difficult, but with practice, it can be done skillfully, without jeopardizing the quality of the information gained.

Identifying Information

A. **Purposes**
1. To eliminate confusion about the patient's identity; to obtain the information required for contacting patient if the need arises
2. To provide an introduction to the patient and some indication of habits, lifestyle, and beliefs, which may be explored in greater depth in the personal and social history
3. To initiate a relationship based on recognition of the importance of the informant's role in sharing in the care of the patient (when this is the case)

B. **Types of Information Needed**
1. Date and time
2. Patient's name, address, telephone number, race, religion, birth date, and age
3. Name of referring practitioner
4. Insurance data
5. Name of informant—the patient may be the person giving this history; if not, record the name, address, telephone number, and relationship to the patient of the person giving the history.
6. Accuracy and reliability of informant—this is a judgment based on the consistency of responses to questions and on a comparison of information in the history with your own observations in the physical examination.

C. **Method of Collecting Data**
1. Careful interviewing of the patient or caregiver will provide most of the information.

2. The patient's hospital or clinic record may also be a valuable source.
3. Repeat information when necessary to verify accuracy (eg, to ensure that there has been no change in address or telephone number).
4. Assume a direct and courteous manner.
5. Explain the reasons why the information is needed—to help put the patient at ease.

Chief Complaint

A. Purposes
1. To allow the patient to describe his or her own problems and expectations with little or no direction from the interviewer
2. To identify the overriding problem for which the person is seeking help
   a. Adults with chronic conditions often have numerous complaints.
   b. If possible, focus on a single problem or concern—the one most important to the patient.
3. To identify the patient's feelings about symptoms. The patient may show fear, guilt, or defensiveness in this first statement.

B. Types of Information Needed
The patient's primary problem(s) or concern in the patient's own words. A statement describing the duration of the complaint.

C. Method of Collecting Data
1. Ask the patient a direct question, for example, "How may I help you?" or "For what reason have you come to the hospital (clinic, etc.)?"
2. Avoid confusing questions, for example, "What brings you here?" ("The bus.") or "Why are you here?" ("That's what I came to find out.")
3. Ask how long the concern or problem has been present. If necessary, establish the time of onset precisely by offering such clues as "Did you feel this way a month (6 months or 2 years) ago?"
4. Let the patient speak freely without offering your opinion until he has had an opportunity to identify the problem as clearly as possible.
5. Write down what the patient says, using quotation marks to identify patient's words.

History of Present Illness

A. Purposes
1. To amplify the description of the chief complaint and to clarify its relationship to other symptoms and events
2. To carefully describe a symptom or problem that may be a clue to future diagnosis

B. Types of Information Needed
1. A *detailed chronological* picture beginning with the time the patient was last well (or, in the case of a problem with an acute onset, the patient's condition just before the onset of the problem) and ending with a description of the patient's current condition.
2. If there is more than one important problem, each is described in a separate, chronologically organized paragraph in the written history of present illness.
3. The outline for reporting the present illness will vary with each case.

C. Method of Collecting Data
1. For each problem investigate the following:
   a. Quality (eg, sharp, dull, knife-like—referring to pain)
   b. Quantity (eg, $\frac{1}{2}$ cup sputum)
   c. Location of symptoms, intensity, periodicity (eg, epigastric area; daily; after meals)
   d. Aggravating and alleviating factors (eg, medications, prescribed and over-the-counter; rest; diet)
   e. Associated phenomena (eg, shortness of breath)
2. Date the onset of the problem as accurately as possible because chronology is of the utmost importance (see Chief Complaint).
3. Describe the character of the symptoms and state whether they have changed over time.
4. In the case of acute infections, inquire about possible exposure or an incubation period.
5. When the present illness has been characterized by attacks separated by free intervals, obtain the history of a typical attack: onset, duration, and associated symptoms—pain; fever; chills; relation to any activity, either physical or emotional, or to such factors as diet, medication, etc.
6. In both acute and chronic illnesses, note whether and when the patient stopped working or went to bed.
7. Get the patient's subjective appraisal of whether the symptom or problem is getting better or worse.
8. When a particular organ or system is disturbed, ask for a review of that system and related systems so that important negative and positive information may be included in the written history. For instance, if a patient complains of chest pain, ask about both the respiratory and cardiac systems, as well as the musculoskeletal history of the chest.
9. Questioning may reveal that other systems must also be reviewed.
10. Ask about previous treatment, including medications, prescribing physician or practitioner, and place where treatment was obtained (name of hospital, clinic, etc.).
11. At the end, review the chronology and specifics and ask patient to affirm or correct the information.
12. Organize the information for recording or presentation.

Past Medical History

A. Purposes
1. To determine any change in the patient's normal patterns of living that may or may not be caused by illness
2. To identify clues that may aid in diagnosing the present illness
3. To participate in gathering and recording information that may be helpful in making a diagnosis, even though the nurse may not have the final responsibility for diagnosing the patient's particular problem

B. Types of Information Needed
1. *General health and strength*—sleeping patterns, appetite, stability of weight, usual activities
2. *Acute infectious diseases*—measles, mumps, whooping cough, chickenpox, pneumonia, pleurisy, tuberculosis, scarlet fever, acute rheumatic fever, rheumatic heart disease, tonsillitis, hepatitis, polio, sexually transmitted disease, tropical or parasitic diseases, any other acute infectious problem the patient describes
3. *Immunization*—polio, diphtheria, pertussis, tetanus, measles, mumps, rubella, hepatitis B, pnemococcal in-

fluenza, last PPD or other skin test, any abnormal or unusual reactions. Give date when possible
4. *Operation*—indications, diagnosis, dates, hospital, surgeon, complications
5. *Previous hospitalizations*—physician, hospital data (year), diagnosis, treatment
6. *Injuries*—type; resulting disabilities
7. *Major illnesses* (any prolonged illnesses not requiring hospitalization)—dates, symptoms, course, treatment
8. *Allergies* (may appear in review of systems)—asthma, hay fever, hives, food allergies, drug reactions, previous treatment with penicillin and any reactions
9. *Obstetric history* (may appear in review of systems)
   a. Pregnancies, miscarriages, abortions
   b. Describe course of pregnancy, labor, and delivery; date, place of delivery.
10. *Psychiatric history* (may appear in review of systems)—treatment by a psychiatrist or psychologist, indications, date, place, medications for "nerves"

C. Method of Collecting Data
1. Begin by explaining the purpose and type of questions you will be asking; for example, "I am now going to ask you some questions about your past health."
2. Explain that these questions are important to obtain an accurate picture of all the events that affected or that *did not* affect the patient's health in the past.
3. Use direct questions; for example, "How would you describe your general health?" and then proceed with more specific queries, such as "Has your weight been stable over the past 5 years?"

Family History

A. Purposes
1. To present a picture of the patient's family health, including specifically that of grandparents, parents, brothers, sisters, aunts, and uncles. It also involves the health of close relatives because some diseases show a familial tendency or are hereditary.
2. To describe the health of the patient's spouse and children because this may give clues about possible communicable disease problems. It also will be important in determining what sort of condition a family is in and how this affects the patient.

B. Types of Information Needed
1. Age and health status of (or age at and cause of death of) parent, sibling
2. History, in immediate and close relatives, of heart disease, hypertension, stroke, diabetes, gout, kidney disease or stones, thyroid disease, asthma or other allergies, blood problems, cancer (types), epilepsy, mental illness, arthritis, alcoholism, obesity
3. Hereditary diseases such as hemophilia or sickle cell disease
4. Age and health status of spouse and children

C. Method of Collecting Data
1. Begin with an explanation of what you are asking and why because the patient may not understand the purpose of your questions. For example:

"I am going to ask now about the health of your immediate family and relatives. It is important to know if there are any conditions which tend to or could occur in your family, or in you as a member of the family."

2. Ask direct questions.
   a. Begin with the patient's siblings.

   "Do you have any brothers and sisters?"
   "How old are they and what is the state of their health?"

   b. List each sibling separately, giving age and state of health.

Review of Systems

A. Purpose
To obtain detailed information about the current state of the patient and any past symptoms, or lack of symptoms, patient may have experienced related to a particular body system.

B. Types of Information Needed
Subjective information about what the patient feels or sees with regard to the major systems of the body.
1. *Skin*—rash, itching, change in pigmentation or texture, sweating, hair growth and distribution, condition of nails
2. *Skeletal*—stiffness of joints, pain, deformity, restriction of motion, swelling, redness, heat. If there are problems, ask the patient to specify any activities of daily life that are difficult or impossible to perform.
3. *Head*—headaches, dizziness, syncope, head injuries
4. *Eyes*—vision, pain, diplopia, photophobia, blind spots, itching, burning, discharge, recent change in appearance or vision, glaucoma, cataracts, glasses/contact lenses worn, date of last refraction, infection
5. *Ears*—hearing acuity, earache, discharge, tinnitus, vertigo
6. *Nose*—sense of smell, frequency of colds, obstruction, epistaxis, postnasal discharge, sinus pain or therapy, use of nose drops or sprays (type and frequency)
7. *Teeth*—pain; bleeding, swollen or receding gums; recent abscesses, extractions; dentures; dental hygiene practices
8. *Mouth and tongue*—soreness of tongue or buccal mucosa, ulcers, swelling
9. *Throat*—sore throat, tonsillitis, hoarseness, dysphagia
10. *Neck*—pain, stiffness, swelling, enlarged glands or lymph nodes
11. *Endocrine*—goiter, thyroid tenderness, tremors, weakness, tolerance to heat and cold, changes in hat or glove size, changes in skin pigmentation, libido, bruisability, muscle cramps, polyuria, polydipsia, polyphagia, hormone therapy
12. *Respiratory*
    a. Pain in the chest and relationship to respirations
    b. Dyspnea, wheezing, cough, sputum (character, quantity), hemoptysis
    c. Night sweats (Does the patient have to change his bedding?)
    d. Last chest x-ray and result (indicate where obtained)
    e. Exposure to tuberculosis
13. *Cardiac*
    a. Presence of pain or distress and location (have patient point to location); radiation of pain; precipitating/aggravating causes; alleviating measures; timing and duration
    b. Palpitations, dyspnea, orthopnea (note number of pillows required for sleeping), edema, cyanosis
    c. Exercise tolerance (determine in relation to pa-

tient's regular activities—how much can he do before stopping to rest?)

d. Blood pressure (if known): last electrocardiogram (ECG) and results (indicate where obtained)

14. *Hematologic*—anemia (if so, treatment received), tendency to bruise or bleed, thromboses, thrombophlebitis, any known abnormalities of blood cells

15. *Lymph nodes*—enlargement, tenderness, suppuration, duration and progress of abnormality

16. *Gastrointestinal*
   a. Appetite and digestion, intolerance to certain classes of foods
   b. Pain associated with hunger or eating, eructation, regurgitation, heartburn, nausea, vomiting, hematemesis
   c. Regularity of bowel movement (describe normal bowel habits and whether they have changed recently or not); diarrhea, flatulence, stools (color—brown, black, clay; tarry, fresh blood, mucus, etc.)
   d. Hemorrhoids, jaundice, dark urine, use of laxatives—type; frequency. (This should be included under past medical history with medications, but may be repeated here.)
   e. History of ulcer, gallstones, polyps, tumors
   f. Previous x-rays—where, when, results

17. *Genitourinary*—dysuria, pain, urgency, frequency, hematuria, nocturia, polydipsia, polyuria, oliguria, edema of the face, hesitancy, dribbling, loss in size or force of stream, passage of stones, stress incontinence, hernias, human immunodeficiency virus (HIV) status, history of sexually transmitted disease
   a. Males
      (1) Puberty—onset, voice change, erections, emissions
      (2) Libido—satisfaction with sexual relations
   b. Females
      (1) Menses—onset, regularity, duration of flow, dysmenorrhea, last period, intermenstrual bleeding or discharge, dyspareunia
      (2) Libido—satisfaction with sexual relations
      (3) Pregnancies (see past medical history)
      (4) Methods of contraception
      (5) Breasts—pain, tenderness, discharge, lumps, mammograms, breast self-examination—techniques and timing with regard to menstrual cycle

18. *Neuromuscular*
   a. Mental status—orientation to time, place, person, and distance. "How far is your home from the hospital?" (Interviewer must be able to verify the answer.)
   b. Memory
      (1) Distant memory shown by recalling past medical history
      (2) Recent memory shown by recalling what was eaten for breakfast
   c. Cognition, or ability of patient to conceptualize (very useful information in determining a health education plan for the patient)
   d. Patient's description of personality—how patient views self.
   e. Presence of tics, twitching, weakness, paralysis, tremor, wasting of muscles, incoordination, fatigue, sensory loss with respect to pain, temperature, touch, muscle pain, cramps
   f. Psychiatric history may be entered here.

19. *General constitutional symptoms*—fever, chills, malaise, fatigability, recent loss or gain of weight

C. *Method of Collecting Data*
1. Begin by explaining to the patient—"I am going to ask you many questions about your body that will help in understanding your present problem."
2. Ask direct questions about each system, using terms that the patient understands.
3. Whenever the patient complains or suggests a symptom, ask the questions outlined under method of collecting data about the present illness (onset, duration, etc.).
4. Never assume that things are "OK" if the patient fails to mention something.
   a. Ask about every aspect of the function of a particular system and be sure to record the patient's responses.
   b. Often the fact that a body system has been free of any symptoms is as important as any symptoms that have been experienced.
5. If necessary, memorize a list of questions for each system or use a list when interviewing the patient. Knowing what to ask about each system is based on knowledge of the function of each body system and of the way that normal function manifests itself.

Personal and Social History

A. *Purposes*
1. To describe the patient's life situation—may have bearing on the present condition or the patient's ability to cope with this problem
2. To develop a plan of care that "fits" the patient. Here the interviewer finds out the many personal and family resources an individual has to aid in coping with the situation—both long term and short term.
3. To have some idea of how the patient patterns his life
   a. Certain habits and patterns are more easily assimilated and changed, when necessary, than others.
   b. Knowing the patient's patterns is useful in helping to organize hospital routine in ways that will be least disruptive to the patient.
4. To help the patient develop a workable plan of care at home, based on knowledge of home conditions
5. To determine if the patient's occupation is directly or indirectly related to his condition
6. To determine if the patient's religious affiliation may affect therapy

B. *Types of Information Needed*
1. *Personal status*—birth place, education, armed service affiliation, position in the family, satisfaction with life situations (home and job), personal concerns
2. *Habits/patterns*
   a. Sleeping, activities/hobbies, nutrition/eating habits (diet for a typical day)
   b. Consumption of alcohol, coffee, tea, drugs (marijuana, over-the-counter medications)
   c. Tobacco (what form; how long)
   d. Sexual habits (can be part of genitourinary history)—relationships, frequency, satisfaction, HIV prevention
3. *Home conditions*
   a. Marital status, nature of family relationships
   b. Economic conditions—source of income; health insurance, Medicare, Medicaid
   c. Living arrangements and housing (owning/renting, heating, sewage, pets, etc.)

d. Involvement with agencies (name, case worker, etc.)
4. *Occupation*
    a. Past and present employment and working conditions, including exposure to stress/tension, noise, pollution
    b. Working hours
    c. Job satisfaction
5. *Religion*—name, whether practicing or not, any stipulations with regard to health practices
C. *Method of Collecting Data*
1. Begin by explaining that you are now going to ask questions about the patient's life situation to gain a clearer perspective of the patient's condition and of how you might help.
2. Your manner should be matter-of-fact, yet concerned. If you are uncomfortable asking the questions, most likely the patient will sense that and be uneasy answering them.
3. A sensitive interviewer can ask most of the questions listed above in an initial interview without alienating the patient. For instance, ask "What has been your education?" instead of "How far have you gone in school?"

Ending the History

When you have completed the history, it is often helpful to say: "Is there anything else you would like to tell me?" or "What do you think is the matter with you?" This allows the patient to end the history by saying what is on his or her mind and what concerns the patient most.

Physical Examination

General Principles

1. A complete or partial physical examination is conducted following a careful comprehensive or problem-related history.
2. It is conducted in a quiet, well-lit room with consideration for patient privacy and comfort.

Approach to the Patient

1. When possible, begin with the patient in a sitting position, so that both front and back can be examined.
2. Completely expose the part to be examined but drape the rest of the body appropriately.
3. Conduct the examination systematically from head to foot so as not to miss observing any system or body part.
4. While examining each region, consider the underlying anatomic structures, their function, and possible abnormalities.
5. Because the body is bilaterally symmetrical, for the most part, compare findings on one side with those on the other.
6. Explain all procedures to the patient while the examination is being conducted—to avoid alarming or worrying the patient and to encourage cooperation.

Techniques of Examination and Assessment

Use the following techniques of examination as appropriate for eliciting findings.
INSPECTION
1. Begins with first encounter with the patient and is the most important of all the techniques.
2. Is an organized scrutiny of the patient's behavior and body.
3. With knowledge and experience, the examiner can become highly sensitive to visual clues.
4. The examiner begins each phase of the examination by inspecting the particular part with the eyes.
PALPATION
1. Involves touching the region or body part just observed and noting what the various structures feel like.
2. With experience comes the ability to distinguish variations of normal from abnormal.
3. Is performed in an organized manner from region to region.
PERCUSSION
1. By setting underlying tissues in motion, percussion helps in determining whether the underlying tissue is air filled, fluid filled, or solid.
2. Audible sounds and palpable vibrations are produced, which can be distinguished by the examiner.

There are five basic notes produced by percussion, which can be distinguished by differences in the qualities of sound, pitch, duration, and intensity.

	Relative Intensity	Relative Pitch	Relative Duration	Example Location
Flatness	Soft	High	Short	Thigh
Dullness	Medium	Medium	Medium	Liver
Resonance	Loud	Low	Long	Normal lung

| Hyperresonance | Very loud | Lower | Longer | Emphysematous lung |
| Tympany | Loud | * | * | Gastric air bubble or puffed out cheek |

* Distinguished mainly by its musical timbre.
(From Bates, B. L. (1995). *A guide to physical examination* (6th ed.). Philadelphia: J.B. Lippincott.)

3. The technique for percussion may be described as follows:
   a. Hyperextend the middle finger of your left hand, pressing the distal portion and joint firmly against the surface to be percussed.
      (1) Other fingers touching the surface will damp the sound.
      (2) Be consistent in the degree of firmness exerted by the hyperextended finger as you move it from area to area or the sound will vary.
   b. Cock the right hand at the wrist, flex the middle finger upward, and place the forearm close to the surface to be percussed. The right hand and forearm should be as relaxed as possible.
   c. With a quick, sharp, relaxed wrist motion, strike the extended left middle finger with the flexed right middle finger, using the tip of the finger, not the pad. (A very short fingernail is a must!)
      Aim at the end of the extended left middle finger (just behind the nail bed) where the greatest pressure is exerted on the surface to be percussed.
   d. Lift the right middle finger rapidly to avoid damping the vibrations.
   e. The movement is at the wrist, not at the finger, elbow, or shoulder; the examiner should use the lightest touch capable of producing a clear sound.

AUSCULTATION
1. This method uses the stethoscope to augment the sense of hearing.
2. The stethoscope must be constructed well and must fit the user. Earpieces should be comfortable, the length of the tubing should be 25 to 38 cm (10–15 inches), and the head should have a diaphragm and a bell.
   a. The bell is used for low-pitched sounds such as certain heart murmurs.
   b. The diaphragm screens out low-pitched sounds and is good for hearing high-frequency sounds such as breath sounds.
   c. Extraneous sounds can be produced by clothing, hair, and movement of the head of the stethoscope.

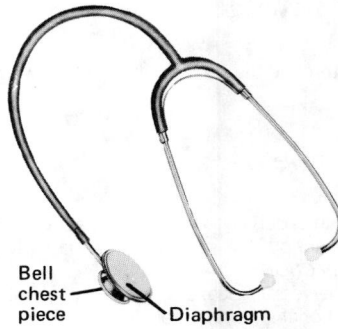

Bell chest piece — Diaphragm

Equipment

Thermometer
Sphygmomanometer
Oto-ophthalmoscope
Flashlight
Tongue depressor

Cotton applicator stick
Stethoscope
Reflex hammer
Tuning fork
Safety pin

Additional items include disposable gloves and lubricant for rectal examination and a speculum for examination of female pelvis.

| TECHNIQUE | FINDINGS |

Vital Signs

Importance—Many major therapeutic decisions are based on the vital signs; therefore, accuracy is essential.

TEMPERATURE

Routinely, where accuracy is not crucial, an oral temperature will suffice.
A rectal temperature is the most accurate.
Unless contraindicated (as in a patient with a severe cardiac arrhythmia), a rectal temperature is often preferred.

Temperature—may vary with the time of day.
  Oral: 37°C (98.6°F) is considered normal.
May vary from 35.8°C to 37.3°C (96.4°–99.1°F).
  Rectal: Higher than oral by 0.4°C to 0.5°C (0.7°–0.9°F).

TECHNIQUE	*FINDINGS*

PULSE

Palpate the radial pulse and count for at least 30 seconds.

If the pulse is irregular, count for a full minute and note the number of irregular beats/min.

Note whether the beat of the pulse against your finger is strong or weak, bounding or thready.

Pulse—Normal adult pulse is 60 to 80 beats/min; regular in rhythm. Elasticity of the arterial walls, blood volume, and mechanical action of the heart muscle are some of the factors that affect strength of the pulse wave, which normally is full and strong.

RESPIRATION

Count the number of respirations taken in 15 seconds and multiply by 4.

Note rhythm and depth of breathing.

Respiration—Normally 16 to 20 respirations/min.

BLOOD PRESSURE

Measure the blood pressure in both arms.

Palpate the systolic pressure before using the stethoscope in order to detect an auscultatory gap.*

Apply cuff firmly; if too loose, it will give a falsely high reading.

Use cuff in appropriate size: a pediatric cuff for children; a leg cuff for obese people.

The cuff should be approximately 2.5 cm (1 inch) above the antecubital fossa.

Normal range
  Systolic—95–140 mm Hg
  Diastolic—60–90 mm Hg
A difference of 5 to 10 mm Hg between arms is common.
Systolic pressure in lower extremities is usually 10 mm Hg higher than reading in upper extremities.
Going from a recumbent to a standing position can cause the systolic pressure to fall 10 to 15 mm Hg and the diastolic pressure to rise slightly (by 5 mm Hg).

Height and Weight

Determine the patient's height and weight.

General Appearance

Begin observation on first contact with the patient (in the waiting room or while the patient is in bed); continue throughout the interview systematically—as the first step in the examination of each body part.

INSPECTION

Observe for: race, sex, general physical development, nutritional state, mental alertness, evidence of pain, restlessness, body position, clothes, apparent age, hygiene, grooming.

Careful observation of the general state of the individual provides many clues about a person's body image and how he behaves and also some idea of how well or ill he is.

Skin

1. Examination of the skin is correlated with the information obtained in the history and other parts of the physical examination.
2. Examine the skin as you proceed through each body system.

INSPECTION

Observe for: skin color, pigmentation, lesions (distribution, type, configuration, size), jaundice, cyanosis, scars, superficial vascularity, moisture, edema, color of mucous membranes, hair distribution, nails.

1. "Normal" varies considerably depending on racial or ethnic background, exposure to sun, complexion, pigmentation tendencies (eg, freckles).

---

* Auscultatory gap:
  1. The first sound of blood in the artery is usually followed by continuous sound until nothing is audible with the stethoscope.
  2. Occasionally the sound is not continuous and there is a gap after the first sound, after which the sound of blood in the vessel is heard again.
  3. If one uses only the auscultatory method and pumps the cuff up until the sound is no longer heard, it is possible, when there is a gap in the sound or when the sound is not continuous, to get a falsely low systolic reading.

TECHNIQUE	FINDINGS

PALPATION
Examine skin for temperature, texture, elasticity, turgor.

2. The skin is normally warm, slightly moist, and smooth and returns quickly to its original shape when picked up between two fingers and released. There is a characteristic hair distribution over the body associated with gender and normal physiologic function. Nails are present and smooth and cared for in some way.

Head

INSPECTION
Observe for: symmetry of face, configuration of skull, hair color and distribution, scalp.

1. Normally, the skull and face are symmetrical, with distribution of hair varying from person to person. (However, determine by history if there has been any change.)

PALPATION
Examine: hair texture, masses, swelling or tenderness of scalp, configuration of skull.

2. The scalp should be free of flaking, with no signs of nits (small, white louse eggs), lesions, deformities, or tenderness.

Eyes and Vision

Equipment
Ophthalmoscope
Anatomic Landmarks
Globes
Palpebral fissures
Lid margins
Conjunctivae
Sclerae
Pupils
Iris

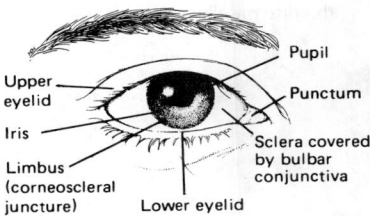

INSPECTION
1. *Globes*—for protrusion.
2. *Palperbral fissures* (longitudinal openings between the eyelids)—for width and symmetry.

2. *Palpebral fissures*—appear equal in size when the eyes are open.
    Upper lid—covers a small portion of the iris and cornea.
    Lower lid—margin is just below the junction of the cornea and sclera (limbus).
    Ptosis—drooping of eyelids.

3. *Lid margins*—for scaling, secretions, erythema, position of lashes.

3. *Lid margins*—are clear; the lacrimal duct openings (puncta) are evident at the nasal ends of the upper and lower lids.
    Eye lashes—normally are evenly distributed and turn outward.

4. *Bulbar and palpebral conjunctivae*—for congestion and color.
    Bulbar conjunctiva—membranous covering of the sclera (contains blood vessels).
    Palpebral conjunctiva—membranous covering of the inside of the upper and lower lids (contains blood vessels).

4. *Bulbar conjunctiva* (cover of sclera)—consists of transparent red blood vessels, which may become dilated and produce the characteristic "bloodshot" eye.
    Palpebral conjunctivae—are pink and clear.
    Conjunctivitis—inflammation of the conjunctival surfaces.

5. *Sclerae*—for color; *iris*—for color
6. *Pupils*—for size, shape, symmetry, reaction to light and accommodation (ability of the lens to adjust to objects at varying distances).

5. *Sclerae*—should be white and clear.
6. *Pupils*—normally constrict with increasing light and accommodation. Pupils are normally round and can range in size from very small ("pinpoint") to large (occupying the entire space of the iris).

7. *Eye movement*—extraocular movements, nystagmus, convergence.
    (Nystagmus: rapid, lateral, horizontal, or rotary movement of the eye.)
    (Convergence: ability of the eye to turn in and focus on a very close object.)
    (See neurologic examination, p. 49.)

7. *Extraocular movement*—movement of the eyes in conjugate fashion. (Six muscles control the movement of the eye.) Eyes normally move in conjugate fashion, except when converging on an object that is moving closer.
    Nystagmus—may be seen normally as a result of eye fatigue.
    Convergence—fails when double vision occurs, usually 10 to 15 cm (4–6 inches) from nose.

TECHNIQUE	*FINDINGS*

8. *Gross visual fields*—by confrontation. (See neurologic examination, p. 49.)
9. *Visual acuity*
   Check with a Snellen chart (with and without glasses).

8. *Peripheral vision*—is full (medially and laterally, superiorly and inferiorly) in both eyes.
9. *Normal vision*—20/20.
   Myopia—nearsightedness
   Hyperopia—farsightedness

PALPATION

1. Determine strength of upper lids by attempting to open closed lids against resistance.
2. Palpate globes through closed lids for tenderness and tension.

1. The examiner should not be able to open the lids when the patient is squeezing them shut.
2. Globes normally are not tender when palpated.

FUNDOSCOPIC EXAMINATION

1. *Red retinal reflex*—check the transparency of the anterior and posterior chambers.
2. *Cornea*—check for transparency.
3. *Lens*—check for transparency.
4. *Retina*—check for color, pigmentation, hemorrhages, and exudates.
5. *Optic disc*—check for color, distinction of margins, pigmentation, degree of elevation, cupping.
6. *Macula*—check for color. (Lies at a distance of 2 optic disc diameters laterally from the optic disc.)
7. *Blood vessels*—check for diameter; arteriovenous (A/V) ratio; origin and course; venous-arterial crossings. (Both arteries and veins are present and move outward from the disc nasally and temporally.)

1. *Red retinal reflex*—can be spotted by the examiner while standing 30 cm (12 inches) from the eye.
2. *Cornea*—should be transparent.
3. *Lens*—should be transparent (ie, retina can be seen).
4. *Retina*—color varies according to the amount of pigment present. There should be no hemorrhages or exudates.
5. *Optic disc*—is circular and has a yellowish pink color. Although disc appearance may vary, the margins are normally distinct and regular, with varying amounts of pigment.
6. *Macula*—because it is free of blood vessels, it is lighter in color than the rest of the retina.
7. *Retinal arteries and veins*—arteries are approximately $\frac{4}{5}$ the size of the veins and lighter in color. Where arteries and veins cross, there is usually no disturbance in the course of either. Pulsations may occur in the vein near the optic disc.

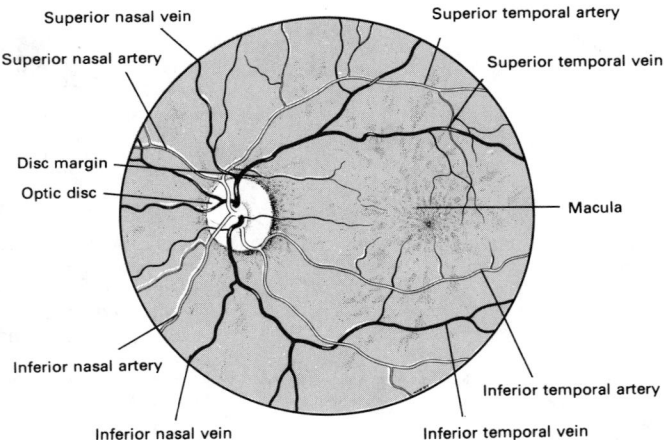

Superior nasal vein
Superior nasal artery
Disc margin
Optic disc
Inferior nasal artery
Inferior nasal vein
Superior temporal artery
Superior temporal vein
Macula
Inferior temporal artery
Inferior temporal vein

USE OF THE OPHTHALMOSCOPE

1. Hold the instrument in your right hand and use your right eye to examine the patient's right eye.
   a. Reverse the procedure to examine the patient's left eye.
   b. This approach allows you to get close to the patient without bumping noses.
2. Hold the instrument so that your last two fingers are straight, rather than curved around the handle.
   You can place these fingers against the patient's cheek to steady the instrument and to avoid hitting the patient with it.
3. Begin the fundoscopic examination standing about 30 cm (a foot) from the patient. The room should be darkened.
4. Turn the dial on the head of the ophthalmoscope to +8 or +10 (black numbers).

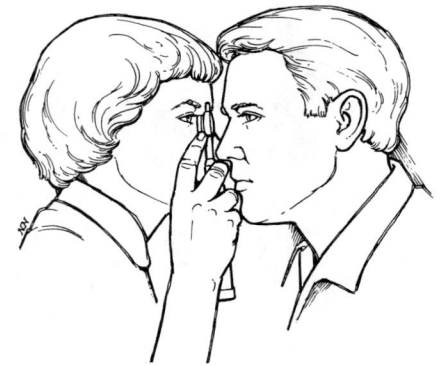

TECHNIQUE	FINDINGS

5. Turn on the ophthalmoscope light and place the eyepiece up to your eye.
   If you wear glasses or contact lenses, it is best to wear them during the examination so that you do not have to accommodate for your vision by turning the dial on the ophthalmoscope.
6. Aim the light at the pupil of the eye. You should see the red reflex immediately.
7. Slowly move in toward the patient, continuing to look through the eyepiece and keeping the light directed at the pupil, beyond which is the fundus.
8. With the index finger of the hand holding the ophthalmoscope, turn the dial toward zero as you move in.
   a. This allows you to focus on the various chambers of the eye.
   b. A way to find the eye and pupil is to put your hand on top of the patient's head and your thumb at the outer corner of the eye. If you lose the fundus, you can return to your thumb and get your bearings by moving medially from the thumb nail.
9. Once your hand is resting on the patient's cheek, continue to turn the dial until you can focus on the retina, and the blood vessels and the optic disc appear sharp.
10. Once you are focused on the optic disc, it is possible to follow the blood vessels out from the disc inferiorly and superiorly, medially and laterally. (See Chapter 30 [Eye Disorders] for visual fields, color vision tests, refraction, tonometry.)

Ears and Hearing

Equipment
Tuning fork, otoscope

TO *EXAMINE WITH OTOSCOPE*

1. Hold the helix of the ear and gently pull the pinna upward and back toward the occiput to straighten the external canal.
2. Gently insert the lighted otoscope, using an earpiece that is a comfortable size for the patient.
3. Once the otoscope is in place, put your eye up to the eyepiece and examine the external canal.

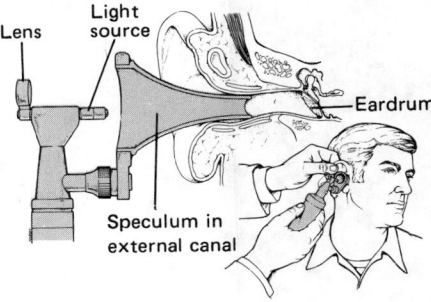

Techniques of Examination

INSPECTION

1. *Pinna*—examine for size, shape, color, lesions, masses.
2. *External canal*—examine with the otoscope for discharge, impacted cerumen, inflammation, masses, or foreign bodies.
3. *Tympanic membrane*—examine for color, luster, shape, position, transparency, integrity, and scarring.
4. *Landmarks*—note cone of light, umbo, handle and short process of the malleus, pars flaccida, and pars tensa.
   Gently move the otoscope to observe the entire drum. (Cerumen may obscure visualization of the drum.)

2. *External canal*—is normally clear with perhaps minimal cerumen.

3. *Tympanic membrane and landmarks.*

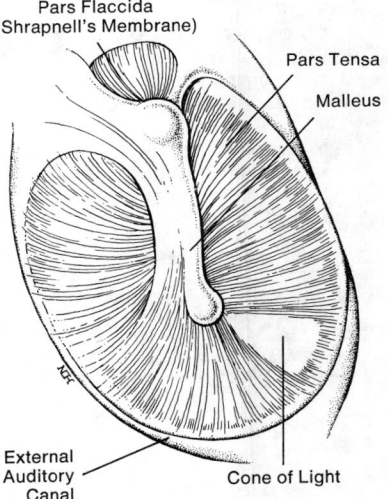

TECHNIQUE	*FINDINGS*

PALPATION

Pinna—examine for tenderness, consistency of cartilage, swelling.

MECHANICAL TESTS

1. Test each ear for gross hearing acuity using whispered word or watch. Cover the ear not being tested.

2. *Weber test*—test for lateralization of vibration. Place tuning fork in the center of the scalp near the forehead (*A*). (Also see Chapter 31 [Ear Disorders]).

3. *Rinne Test*—compares air and bone conduction.
   a. Place vibrating tuning fork on the mastoid process behind the ear and have the patient tell you when the vibration stops (*B*).
   b. Then quickly hold the buzzing end of the tuning fork *near* the ear canal and ask if patient can hear it (*C*).

1. A person with normal hearing can hear a whispered word from approximately 4.5 meters (15 feet) and a watch from 30 cm (12 inches). The patient should hear the sound equally well in both ears, that is, there is no lateralization.

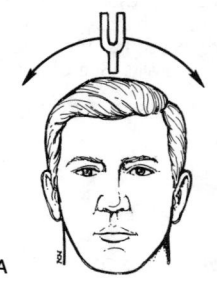

A

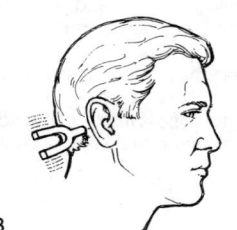
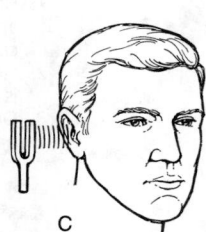

B   C

Normally, sound should be heard after vibration can no longer be felt, that is, air conduction is greater than bone conduction. Lateralization and conduction findings are altered by damage to the 8th cranial nerve and damage to the ossicles in the middle ear.

Nose and Sinuses

Equipment
Otoscope, nasal speculum
Techniques of Examination

INSPECTION

1. Observe for general deformity.
2. With nasal speculum (otoscope, if speculum is unavailable) examine for:
   a. Nasal septum (position and performation)

   b. Discharge (anteriorly and posteriorly)
   c. Nasal obstruction and airway patency
   d. Mucous membranes for color
   e. Turbinates for color and swelling

Nasal septum—is normally straight and not perforated.
Discharge—none should be present.
Airways—are patent.
Mucous membranes—are normally pink.
Turbinates—3 bony projections on each lateral wall of the nasal cavity covered with well vascularized, mucous-secreting membranes. They warm the air going into the lungs and may become swollen and pale with colds and allergies.

— Inferior turbinate

TECHNIQUE	*FINDINGS*

PALPATION

Sinuses (frontal and maxillary)—for tenderness

Frontal—direct manual pressure upward toward wall of sinus. Avoid pressure on eyes.

Maxillary—with thumbs, direct pressure upward over lower edge of maxillary bones.

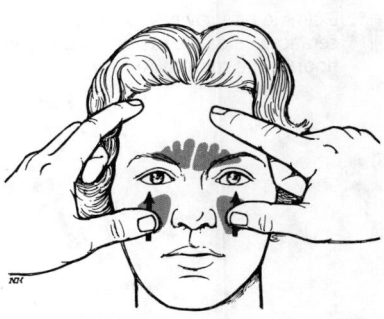

Mouth

Equipment

Flashlight, tongue depressor, gloves, gauze sponges

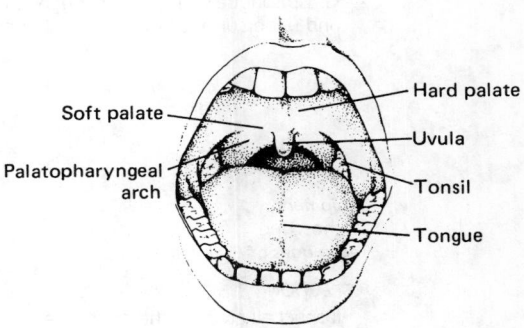

Techniques of Examination

INSPECTION

1. Observe lips for color, moisture, pigment, masses, ulcerations, fissures.
2. Use tongue depressor and penlight to examine:
   a. *Teeth*—number, arrangement, general condition
   b. *Gums*—for color, texture, discharge, swelling, or retraction

Teeth—the adult normally has 32 teeth.
Gums—commonly recede in adults.
Gums—bleeding is fairly common and may result from trauma, gingival disease, or systemic problems (less common).

   c. *Buccal mucosa*—for discoloration, vesicles, ulcers, masses
   d. *Pharynx*—for inflammation, exudate, and masses
   e. *Tongue* (protruded)—for size, color, thickness, lesions, moisture, symmetry, deviations from midline, fasciculations

Tongue—is normally midline and covered with papillae, which vary in size from the tip of the tongue to the back. (The circumvallate papillae are large and posterior.)

   f. *Salivary glands*—for patency
      Parotid glands

      Sublingual and submaxillary glands

Parotid glands—open in the buccal pouch at the level of the upper teeth halfway back
Sublingual and submaxillary glands—open underneath the tongue.

   g. *Uvula*—for symmetry when patient says ''ah''
   h. *Tonsils*—for size, ulceration, exudates, inflammation

Lingual tonsils—can often be seen on the posterior portion of the tongue.
Odor of breath—may indicate dental caries.

   i. *Odor of breath*
   j. *Voice*—for hoarseness

TECHNIQUE	FINDINGS

PALPATION

1. Examine oral cavity with gloved hand for masses and ulceration. Palpate beneath tongue and explore laterally the floor of the mouth (A).

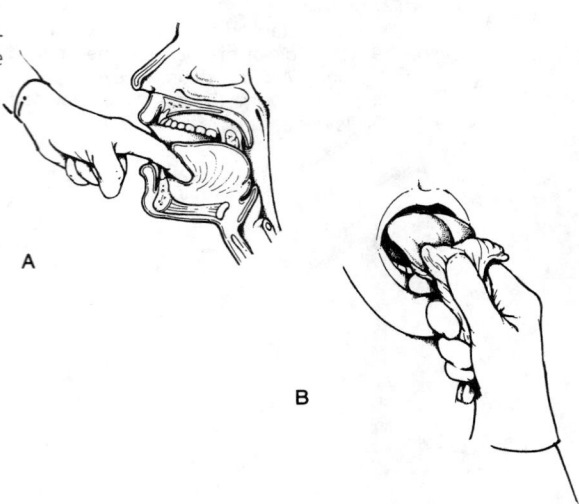

2. Grasp tongue with gauze sponge to retract; inspect sides and undersurface of tongue and floor of mouth (B).

Neck

Equipment
Stethoscope
Techniques of Examination

INSPECTION

1. Inspect all areas of the neck anteriorly and posteriorly for muscular symmetry, masses, unusual swelling or pulsations, and range of motion.

2. *Thyroid*—ask the patient to swallow and observe for movement of an enlarged thyroid gland at the suprasternal notch.

3. *Muscular strength*
   a. *Cervical muscles*—have patient turn his chin forcefully against your hand.
   b. *Trapezius muscles*—exert pressure on the patient's shoulders while he shrugs his shoulders.

4. *External jugular veins*—observe with patient sitting and then lying at 30° to 40° angle; patient's neck should not be flexed.

1. *Range of motion*—normally, the chin can touch the anterior chest, the head can be extended at least 45° from the vertical position and can be rotated 90° from midline to side.

2. *Thyroid*—is not usually visible, except in extremely thin persons.

3. *Strength*—see Findings, 11th cranial nerve.

Jugular veins—when the patient is lying with head elevated 30° to 40°, the jugular veins are approximately at the level of the right atrium, and pulsations that are transmitted from the right atrium can normally be seen with tangential lighting. Veins are not distended when the patient is sitting.

This serves as a fairly constant and therefore reliable landmark, when patient is supine or sitting, for estimating venous pressure, that is, the height in cm measured from level of distended internal jugular veins to level of sternal angle.

Note the sternal angle, the point on the surface anatomy that is approximately 5 to 7 cm (2–2.75 inches) above the right atrium.

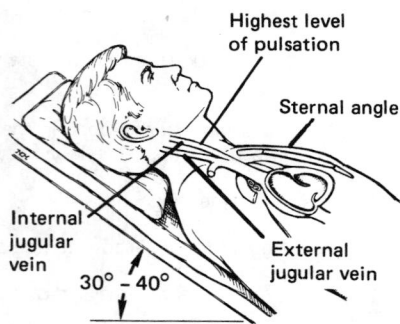

TECHNIQUE	*FINDINGS*

PALPATION

1. *Cervical nodes and salivary glands.*

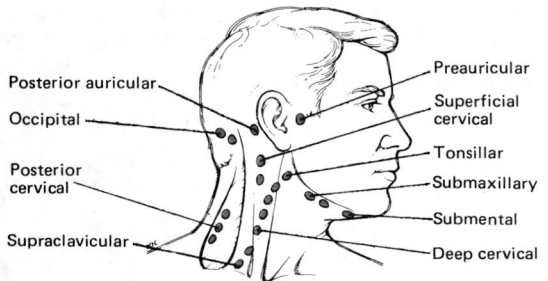

1. *Cervical nodes*—in the adult, the cervical lymph nodes are not normally palpable unless the patient is very thin, in which case the nodes are felt as small, freely movable masses.

2. *Trachea*—palpate at the sternal notch. Stand behind (or in front of) patient and allow the middle finger of each hand to glide off the head of the clavicle into the sternal notch.
Palpate for deviation and tracheal tug.

3. *Thyroid*
   a. Stand behind the patient and have him flex his neck to relax the cervical muscles.
   b. Place the fingertips of your left hand behind the left sternocleidomastoid muscle adjacent to the trachea just below larynx.

2. *Trachea*—should be midline.
Landmarks are easy to identify using this procedure.

This is the downward pull synchronous with cardiac pulsation, usually the result of aneurysm of aorta.

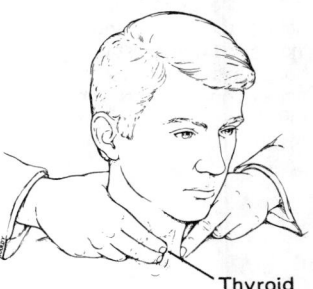

To discern the outline of the isthmus of the left lobe of the thyroid gland.

   c. Palpate the area over the trachea and to the left of the trachea.
   d. Note any enlargement, nodules, masses, consistency.
   e. Reverse the procedure and examine the right lobe of the thyroid.
   f. Because the thyroid gland moves upward on swallowing, have the patient swallow to facilitate examination.

If the thyroid is palpable, it is normally smooth, without nodules, masses, or irregularities, or bruits (gushing sound produced by blood moving through a narrow vessel).

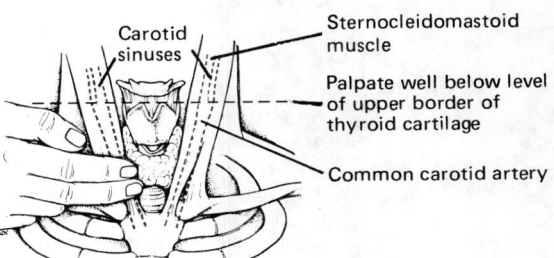

4. *Carotid arteries*
   a. Palpate the carotids one side at a time.
   b. The carotids lie anterolaterally in the neck—avoid palpating the carotid sinuses at the level of the thyroid cartilage just below the angle of the jaw because this may cause slowing of heart rate.
   c. Note symmetry of pulsations, strength, and amplitude.

Lymph Nodes

1. It is important at some point in the examination to palpate all areas where lymphadenopathy might appear.
2. Often this is done as each region of the body is examined, for example, the cervical nodes are examined when the neck is examined.
3. However, in the record, the condition of the lymph nodes is described under a separate heading.

Techniques of Examination

INSPECTION
Note size, shape, mobility, consistency, tenderness, and inflammation.

PALPATION
1. *Cervical, supra- and infraclavicular nodes.*

   Cervical nodes and supra- and infraclavicular nodes—are not normally palpable.
   Axillary nodes—are not normally palpable.

2. *Axillary nodes*
   a. Examine while the patient is sitting.
   b. Place the patient's arm at his side and insert the examining fingers to the apex of the patient's axilla. (Use the fingers of your right hand to examine the left axilla and vice versa.)
   c. Rotate the examining hand, so that the fingers can palpate the anterior and posterior axillary fossae pressing against the chest wall. Press against the humerus bone in the axilla to examine the lateral fossa for nodes. Conclude the axillary examination by moving the fingers from the apex of the axilla downward in the midline along the chest wall.

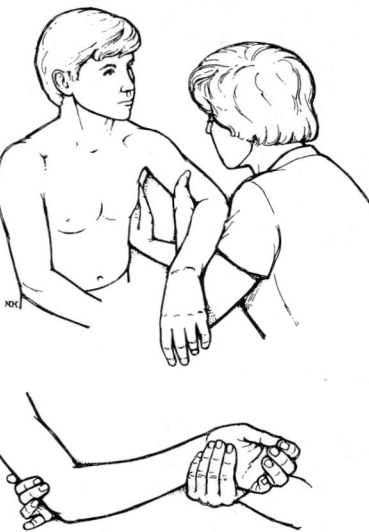

3. *Inguinal nodes*—are located in inguanal and are usually examined when the abdomen is examined.
4. *Epitrochlear nodes*—are palpated just above the olecranon process.

Inguinal nodes—a few may be felt, but are small, movable, and nontender.
Epitrochlear nodes—not usually palpable.

Breasts *(Male and Female)*

FEMALE BREAST

INSPECTION
(With the patient sitting, arms relaxed at sides.)
1. Inspect the areolae and nipples for position, pigmentation, inversion, discharge, crusting, and masses.
   Extra, or supernumerary, nipples may occur normally, most commonly in the anterior axillary region or just below the normal breasts.
2. Examine the breast tissue for size, shape, color, symmetry, surface, contour, skin characteristics, and level of breasts. Note any retraction or dimpling of the skin.

3. Ask the patient to elevate her hands over her head; repeat the observation.

4. Have patient press her hands to her hips; repeat the observation.

1. The *nipples* should be at the same level and protrude slightly. An *inverted nipple* (one that turns inward), if present since puberty, may be normal.
   A *supernumerary nipple* usually consists of a nipple and a small areola and may be mistaken for a mole.
2. *Breast size*—in the female it is not uncommon to find a difference in the size of the two breasts. Normal asymmetry has usually been present since puberty and is not a recent phenomenon.
3. If there is a mass attached to the pectoral muscles, contracting the muscles will cause retraction of the breast tissue.

TECHNIQUE	*FINDINGS*

PALPATION

(This is best done with the patient recumbent.)

1. The patient with pendulous breasts should be given a pillow to place under the ipsilateral scapula of the breast being palpated so that the tissue is distributed more evenly over the chest wall.

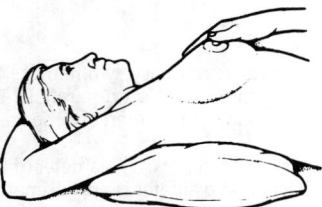

2. The arm on the side of the breast being palpated should be raised above the patient's head.
3. Palpate one breast at a time, beginning with the "asymptomatic" breast if the patient complains of symptoms.
4. To palpate, use the palmar aspects of the fingers in a rotating motion, compressing the breast tissue against the chest wall. (This is done quadrant by quadrant until the entire breast has been palpated—including the "tail" of the breast tissue which extends into the axillary region in the upper outer quadrant of the breast.)

5. Note skin texture, moisture, temperature, or masses.

6. Gently squeeze the nipple and note any expressible discharge.
7. Repeat examination on the opposite breast and compare findings.

3. This allows the examiner to palpate the "normal" breast first and then compare the "symptomatic" breast to it.
4. *Breast texture*—varies according to the amount of subcutaneous tissue present.
   a. In young females, tissue is fairly soft and homogeneous; in postmenopausal women, tissue may feel nodular or stringy.
   b. Consistency also varies with menstrual cycle, being more nodular and edematous just prior to menstruation.*
5. *Masses*—If a mass is palpated, its location, size, shape, consistency, mobility, and associated tenderness are reported.
6. *Discharge*—In the normal nonpregnant or nonlactating female, there is no nipple discharge.

MALE BREAST

Examination of the male breast can be brief and should never be omitted.

1. Observe the nipple and areola for ulceration, nodules, swelling, or discharge.
2. Palpate the areola for nodules and tenderness.

1. There should be no discharge.

Thorax and Lungs

General Information

1. Methodical inspection of the thorax requires reference to established "landmarks" to locate specific structures and to report significant findings.
2. The same structural landmarks are used in examining both the lung and the heart.
3. It is important to visualize the underlying structures and organs when examining the thorax.

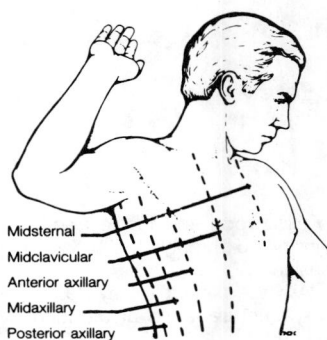

Midsternal
Midclavicular
Anterior axillary
Midaxillary
Posterior axillary

---

* In teaching women about breast self-examination, explain that the best time for performing the examination is a week after the menstrual period, when the breasts are least engorged and tender.

TECHNIQUE	*FINDINGS*

Techniques of Examination

POSTERIOR THORAX AND LUNGS

Begin the examination with the patient seated; examine posterior chest and lungs.

INSPECTION

1. Inspect the spine for mobility and any structural deformity.
2. Observe the symmetry of the posterior chest and the posture and mobility of the thorax on respiration. (Note any bulges or retractions of the costal interspaces on respiration or any impairment of respiratory movement.)
3. Note the anteroposterior diameter in relation to the lateral diameter of the chest.

PALPATION

1. Palpate the posterior chest with the patient sitting; identify areas of tenderness, masses, inflammation.
2. Palpate the ribs and costal margins for symmetry, mobility, and tenderness and the spine for tenderness and vertebral position.
3. To assess respiratory excursion—place the thumbs at the level of the 10th vertebra; with hands held parallel to the 10th ribs as they grasp the lateral rib cage, ask the patient to inhale deeply. Observe the movement of the thumbs while feeling the range, and observe the symmetry of the hands.

2. The thorax is normally symmetrical; it moves easily and without impairment on respiration. There are no bulges or retractions of the intercostal spaces.

3. The anteroposterior (AP) diameter of the thorax in relation to the lateral diameter is approximately 1:2.

2. On palpation there should be no tenderness; chest movement should be symmetrical and without lag or impairment.

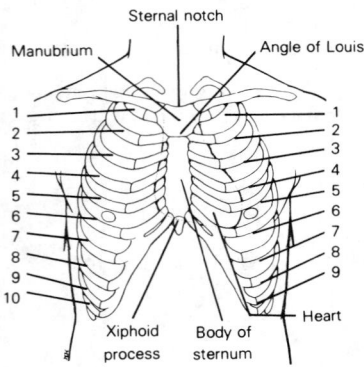

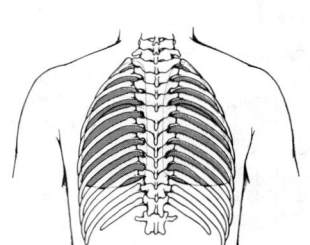

4. To elicit vocal and tactile *fremitus* (palpable vibrations transmitted through the bronchopulmonary system on speaking).
   a. Ask the patient to say ''99''; palpate and compare symmetrical areas of the lungs with the ball of one hand.
   b. Note any areas of increased or decreased fremitus.
   c. If fremitus is faint, ask the patient to speak louder and in a deeper voice.

4. Posteriorly, fremitus is generally equal throughout the lung fields.
   It may be increased near the large bronchi.
      It may be decreased or absent anteriorly and posteriorly when vocal loudness is decreased, when posture is not erect, or when excessive tissue or underlying structures are present.

   One must distinguish the various normal causes of increased or decreased fremitus from the pathologic causes.

TECHNIQUE	*FINDINGS*

PERCUSSION

As with palpation, the posterior chest is percussed with the patient sitting.

1. Percuss symmetrical areas, comparing sides.
2. Begin across the top of each shoulder and proceed down between the scapulae and then under the scapulae, both medially and laterally in the axillary lines.
3. Note and localize any abnormal percussion sound.
4. For diaphragmatic excursion, percuss by placing the pleximeter (stationary) finger parallel to the approximate level of the diaphragm below the right scapula.
   a. Ask the patient to inhale deeply and hold his breath; percuss downward to the point of dullness. Mark this point.
   b. Let the patient breathe normally and then ask him to exhale deeply; percuss upward from the mark to the point of resonance.
   c. Mark this point and measure between the 2 marks—normally 5 to 6 cm (2–2.3 inches).
   d. Repeat this procedure medially and laterally on the right and left sides of the chest.

The lower border of the lungs on normal respiration is approximately at the level of the 10th thoracic spinous process.

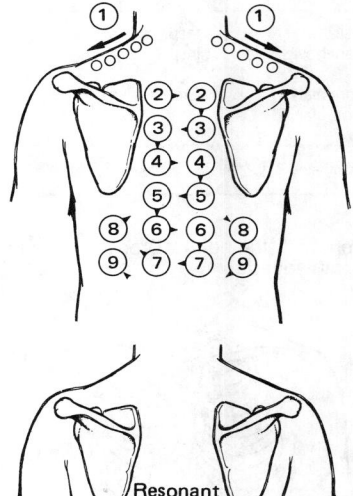

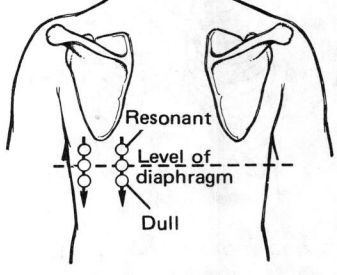

Percussion normally reveals resonance over symmetrical areas of the lung.

Percussion sound may be altered by poor posture and/or presence of excessive tissue.

BREATH SOUNDS

On auscultation, breath sounds vary according to proximity of the large bronchi.

   a. They are louder and coarser near the large bronchi and over the anterior.
   b. They are softer and much finer (vesicular) at the periphery over the alveolae.

Breath sounds also vary in duration with inspiration and expiration.

Sounds may normally decrease in obese individuals.

Pathology will alter the normal bronchial, bronchovesicular, and vesicular breath sounds. (Abnormal breath sounds or adventitious sounds are to be noted and localized.)

AUSCULTATION

Aids in assessing air flow through the lungs, the presence of fluid or mucus, and the condition of the surrounding pleural space and lungs.

1. Have patient sit erect.*
2. With a stethoscope, listen to the lungs as the patient breathes somewhat more deeply than normally with mouth open. (Let the patient pause, as needed, to avoid hyperventilation.)
3. Place the stethoscope in the same areas on the chest wall as those percussed, and listen to a complete inspiration and expiration in each area.
4. Compare symmetrical areas methodically from the apex to the lung bases.
5. It should be possible to distinguish three types of normal breath sounds as indicated in the following table.

* Note: if patient is unable to sit with or without assistance for examination of the posterior chest and lungs, position the patient first on one side and then on the other as you examine the lung fields.

	TECHNIQUE			FINDINGS
Breath Sounds	**Duration of Inspiration and Expiration**	**Pitch of Expiration**	**Intensity of Expiration**	**Normal Location**
Vesicular	Insp. > Exp.	Low	Soft	Most of lungs
Bronchovesicular	Insp. = Exp.	Medium	Medium	Near the main stem bronchi, ie, below the clavicles and between the scapulae, especially on the right
Bronchial or tubular	Exp. > Insp.	High	Usually loud	Over the trachea

(From Bates, B. L. (1995). *A guide to physical examination* (6th ed.) Philadelphia; J. B. Lippincott.)

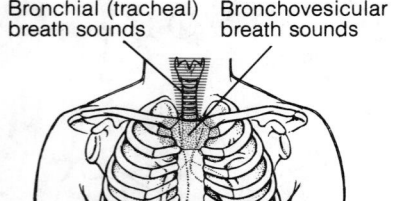

Bronchial (tracheal) breath sounds   Bronchovesicular breath sounds

ANTERIOR THORAX AND LUNGS

(The patient should be recumbent with arms at sides and slightly abducted.)

INSPECTION

1. Inspect the chest for any structural deformity.
2. Note the width of the costal angle.

3. Observe rate and rhythm of breathing, any bulging or retraction of intercostal spaces on respiration, use of accessory muscles of respiration (sternocleidomastoid and trapezius on inspiration and abdominal muscles on expiration).
4. Note any asymmetry of chest wall movement on respiration.

PALPATION

(Serves the same purposes in examining the anterior chest as in the posterior chest.)

1. To assess diaphragmatic excursion, place hands along the costal margins and note symmetry and degree of expansion as the patient inhales deeply.
2. Palpate for fremitus with the ball of the hand anteriorly and laterally.
   (Underlying structures, eg, heart, liver, etc., may damp, or decrease, fremitus.)
3. Compare symmetrical areas.
4. If necessary, displace the female breast gently.

2. The angle at the tip of the sternum is determined by the right and left rib margins at the xiphoid process. Normally, the angle is less than 90°.
3. The thorax is normally symmetrical and moves easily without impairment on respiration. There are no bulges or retractions of the intercostal spaces.

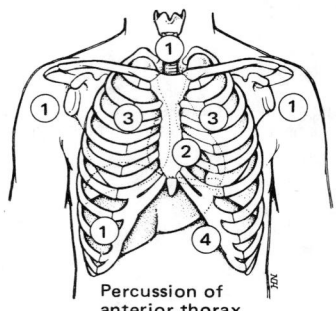

Percussion of anterior thorax

① Flat   ③ Resonant

② Dull   ④ Tympanic

TECHNIQUE	*FINDINGS*

PERCUSSION

1. With patient's arms resting comfortably at his sides, examiner percusses the anterior and lateral chest.
   Begin just below the clavicles and percuss downward from one interspace to the next, comparing the sound from the interspace on one side with that of the contralateral interspace.

2. Displace the female breast, so that breast tissue does not damp the vibration. Continue downward, noting the intercostal space where hepatic dullness is percussed on the right and cardiac dullness on the left.

3. Note effect of underlying structures.

2. A tympanic sound is produced over the gastric air bubble on the left somewhat lower than the point of liver dullness on the right.

3. Percussion over heart will produce a dull sound. The upper border of the liver will be percussed on the right side, producing a dull note.

AUSCULTATION

Listen to the chest anteriorly and laterally for the distribution of resonance and any abnormal or adventitious sounds.

Heart

General Approach

1. The examiner must visualize the position of the heart under the sternum and the ribs and know certain landmarks for identification of specific structures and significant findings.

2. It is also important to identify those "areas" on the chest wall that will yield the most information initially about the function of the heart and its valves.
   a. In locating the intercostal spaces, begin by identifying the angle of Louis, which is felt as a slight ridge approximately 2.5 cm (1 inch) below the sternal notch, where the manubrium and the body of the sternum are joined.
   b. The 2nd ribs extend to the right and left of this angle.
   c. Once the 2nd rib is located, palpate downward and obliquely away from the sternum to identify the remaining ribs and intercostal spaces.

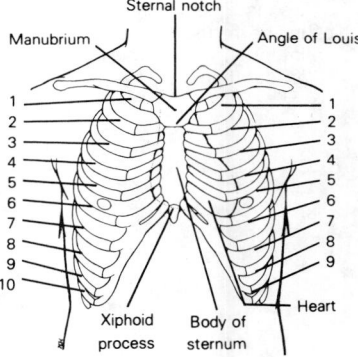

INSPECTION

1. Inspect the precordium for any bulging, heaving, or thrusting.

2. Look for the apical impulse approximately in the 5th or 6th intercostal space at or just medial to the midclavicular line.

3. Note any other pulsations. Tangential lighting is most helpful in detecting pulsations.

PALPATION

1. Use the ball of the hand to detect vibrations, or "thrills," which may be caused by murmurs. (Use the fingertips or palmar surface to detect pulsations.)

2. Proceed methodically through the examination so that no area is omitted. Palpate for thrills and pulsations in each area (aortic, pulmonic, tricuspid, mitral).
   a. Begin in the aortic area (2nd right intercostal space, close to the sternum) and proceed downward to the apex of the heart. (The mitral area is considered the apex of the heart.)
   b. In the tricuspid area, use the palm of the hand to detect any heaving or thrusting of the precordium (tricuspid area—5th intercostal space next to the sternum).
   c. In the mitral area (5th intercostal space, at or just medial to the midclavicular line) palpate for the apical beat; identify the point of maximal impulse (PMI) and note its size and force.

1. Normally there are no bulges.

2. An apical impulse may or may not be observable.

3. There should be no other pulsations.

1. There should be no thrills or other pulsations. (Thrills are vibrations [caused by turbulence of blood moving through valves] that are transmitted through the skin—feels similar to a purring cat.)

Ordinarily, no heaving of the ventricle is felt, except, possibly, in the pregnant female.

The apical pulse should be felt approximately in the 5th intercostal space, at or just medial to the midclavicular line. In the young, thin person, it is a sharp, quick impulse no larger than the intercostal space. In the older person, the impulse may be less sharp and quick.

TECHNIQUE	*FINDINGS*

PERCUSSION

1. Outline the border of the heart or area of cardiac dullness.
    a. The left border generally does not extend beyond 4, 7, and 10 cm left of the midsternal line in the 4th, 5th, and 6th intercostal spaces, respectively.
    b. The right border usually lies under the sternum.
2. Percuss outward from the sternum with the stationary finger parallel to the intercostal space until dullness is no longer heard. Measure the distance from the midsternal line in centimeters.

AUSCULTATION

1. Place the stethoscope in the pulmonic or aortic area.
2. Begin by identifying the 1st (S_1) and 2nd (S_2) heart sounds.
    a. S_1 is caused by the closing of the tricuspid and mitral valves.
    b. S_2 results from the closing of the aortic and pulmonary valves.

    The two sounds are separated by a short systolic interval; each pair of sounds is separated from the next pair by a longer diastolic interval. Normally, two sounds are heard—"lub," "dub."
    a. In the aortic and pulmonic areas, S_2 is usually louder than S_1. In this way, each of the paired sounds can be distinguished from the other.
    b. In the tricuspid area, S_1 and S_2 are of almost equal intensity, and in the mitral area, S_1 is often slightly louder than S_2.

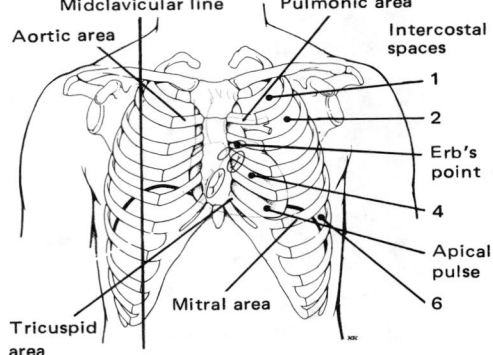

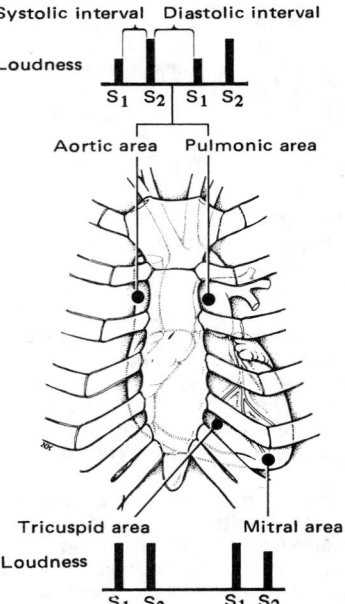

3. Once the heart sounds are identified, count the rate and note the rhythm as discussed under vital signs.
    If there is an irregularity, try to determine if there is any pattern to the irregularity in relation to the intervals, heart sounds, or respirations.
4. Once rate and rhythm are determined, listen in each of the four areas and at Erb's point (3rd left interspace, close to the sternum) systematically, first with the diaphragm (detects higher pitched sounds) and then with the bell (detects lower pitched sounds).

Normally, the heart sounds are regular, with a rate of 60 to 80 beats/min (in the adult). In the athlete or jogger, the resting pulse may be between 40 and 60 beats/min.

TECHNIQUE	*FINDINGS*
a. In each area, listen to S_1 and then to S_2 for intensity and splitting.	a. Occasionally, there may be a splitting of S_2 in the pulmonary area. This is normal. Splitting of S_2 (two contiguous sounds are heard instead of one) is best heard at the end of inspiration, when right ventricular stroke volume is sufficiently increased to delay closure of the pulmonic valve *slightly* behind closure of the aortic valve.
b. Listen to the intervals one at a time and note any extra sounds or murmurs.	b. There are usually no extra sounds.

Peripheral Circulation

JUGULAR VEINS

Evaluation of jugular venous distention is most useful in patients with suspected compromise of cardiac function.

INSPECTION

1. Inspect neck for internal jugular venous pulsations.

1. Jugular venous pulsations can be distinguished from carotid pulsations by the following chart:

Internal Jugular Pulsations	Carotid Pulsations
Rarely palpable	Palpable
Soft, undulating quality, usually with 2 or 3 outward components (a, c, and v waves)	A more vigorous thrust with a single outward component
Pulsation eliminated by light pressure on the vein just above the sternal end of the clavicle	Pulsation not eliminated
Level of pulsation usually descends with inspiration	Pulsation not affected by inspiration
Pulsations vary with position	Pulsations are unchanged by position

(From Bates, B. L. (1995). *A guide to physical examination* 6th ed. Philadelphia: J. B. Lippincott.)

2. Identify the highest point at which the pulsations can be seen and measure the vertical line between the point and the sternal angle.

    With the head raised to 45° the internal jugular venous pulsations should not be visible above 3 cm (1.18 inch).

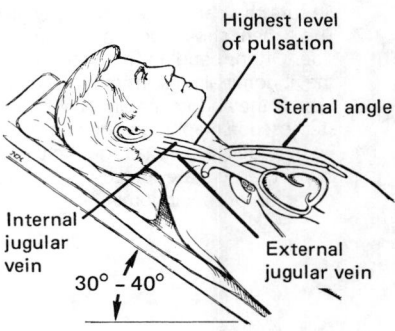

Highest level of pulsation

Sternal angle

Internal jugular vein

External jugular vein

30° – 40°

EXTREMITIES

INSPECTION

1. Observe skin over extremities for color, pallor, rubor, hair distribution.
2. Inspect for any superficial vessels.

1. Extremities should be symmetrically even in color, warmth, and moisture, without swelling.

    Swelling of feet may occur after prolonged standing or sitting, but will disappear readily when extremity is elevated.

TECHNIQUE	FINDINGS

PALPATION

1. Note temperature of skin over extremities, comparing one side to the other.
2. Palpate pulses (radial, femoral, posterior tibial, dorsalis pedis), comparing symmetry from side to side.

2. There should be no arterial bruits.

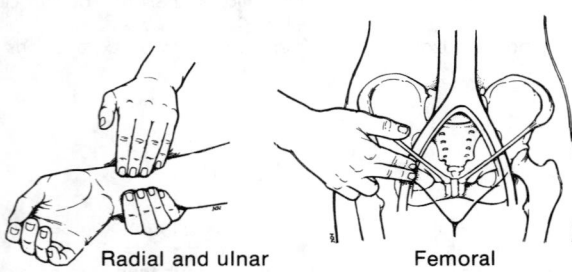

Radial and ulnar   Femoral

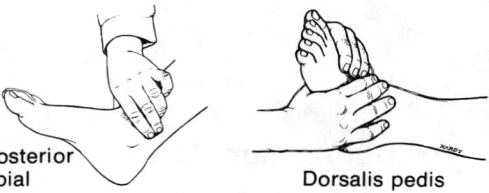

Posterior tibial   Dorsalis pedis

3. Palpate skin over the tibia for edema by pressing skin between thumb and index finger for 30 seconds to 1 minute.
   Then run pads of fingers over the area pressed and note indentation.
   If indentation is noted, repeat procedure, moving up the extremity, and note the point at which no more swelling is present.

3. Edema is usually graded from trace to 3+ or 4+ pitting (note scale used when recording data). Trace is a slight indentation that disappears in a short time. Grade 3+ or 4+, depending on the scale, is *deep* pitting that does not disappear readily. At best, these are subjective measurements, which are tried and confirmed through practice and comparison of findings with associates.

Abdomen

General Approach

1. Be sure the patient has an empty bladder.
2. The patient should be lying comfortably with arms at the side. Often, bending the knees slightly will help to relax the abdominal muscles and make palpation easier.
3. Expose the abdomen fully. Make sure your hands and the stethoscope diaphragm are warm.
4. Be methodical in visualizing the underlying organs as you inspect, auscultate, percuss, and palpate each quadrant or region of the abdomen.

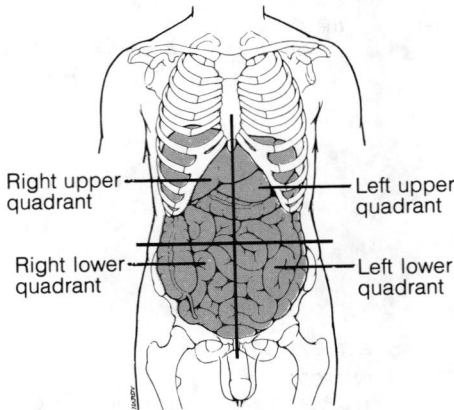

Right upper quadrant   Left upper quadrant

Right lower quadrant   Left lower quadrant

INSPECTION

1. Observe the general contour of the abdomen (flat, protuberant, scaphoid, or concave; local bulges). Also note symmetry, visible peristalsis, aortic pulsations.
2. Check the umbilicus for contour or hernia and the skin for rashes, striae, and scars.

AUSCULTATION

1. This is done before percussion and palpation because palpation may alter the character of bowel sounds.
2. Note the frequency and character of bowel sounds (pitch, duration).
3. Listen over the aorta and renal arteries (either side of the umbilicus) for bruits.

1. The abdomen may or may not have any scars and should be flat or slightly rounded in the nonobese person.

2. Anywhere from 5 to 35 bowel sounds/minute. May have familiar sound of "growling."
3. There should be no bruits or rubs.

TECHNIQUE	FINDINGS

PERCUSSION

1. Percussion provides a general orientation to the abdomen.
2. Proceed methodically from quadrant to quadrant, noting tympany and dullness.
3. In right upper quadrant (RUQ) in the midclavicular line, percuss the borders of the liver.

   a. Begin at a point of tympany in the midclavicular line of the right lower quadrant (RLQ) and percuss upward to the point of dullness (the lower liver border); mark the point.
   b. Percuss downward from the point of lung resonance above the RUQ to the point of dullness (the upper border of the liver); mark the point.
   c. Measure in centimeters the distance between the two marks in the midclavicular line (the liver span).
   d. Tympany of the gastric air bubble can be percussed in the left upper quadrant (LUQ) over the anterior lower border of the rib cage.

2. Tympany should predominate.

3. Percussion of the liver should help guide subsequent palpation. The liver border in the midclavicular line should normally range from 6 to 12 cm (2.3–4.6 inches).

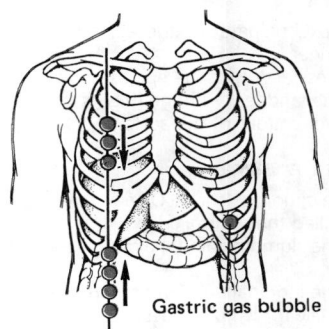

Gastric gas bubble

Midclavicular line

PALPATION

1. Perform light palpation in an organized manner to detect any muscular resistance (guarding), tenderness, or superficial organs or masses.
2. Perform deep palpation to determine location, size, shape, consistency, tenderness, pulsations, and mobility of underlying organs and masses.
3. Move slowly and gently from one quadrant to the next to relax and reassure the patient.
4. Use two hands if the abdomen is obese or muscular, with one hand on top of the other. The upper hand exerts pressure downward while the lower hand feels the abdomen.

1. Tenderness and involuntary guarding indicate peritoneal inflammation

2. Rebound tenderness (pain on quick withdrawal of the fingers following palpation) suggests peritoneal irritation, as in acute appendicitis.

LIVER

1. Palpate the liver by placing the left hand under the patient's lower right rib cage and the right hand on the abdomen below the level of liver dullness. Press gently inward and upward with your fingertips while the patient takes a deep breath.

1. A normal liver edge may be palpable as a smooth, sharp, regular surface. An enlarged liver will be palpable and may be tender, hard or irregular.

SPLEEN

1. Place your left hand around and under the patient's left lower rib cage and press your right hand below the left costal margin inward toward the spleen while the patient takes a deep breath.
2. Double check for an enlarged spleen by percussing in the lowest interspace in the left anterior axillary line as the patient takes a deep breath. An enlarged spleen will cause a change in percussion note from tympany to dullness.

1. A normal spleen is usually not palpable.

2. Be sure to start low enough so as not to miss the border of an enlarged spleen.

KIDNEY

1. Next palpate for the left and right kidneys.
2. Place the left hand under the patient's back between the rib cage and the iliac crest.
3. Support the patient while you palpate the abdomen with the right palmar surface of the fingers facing the left side of the body.
4. Palpate by bringing the left and right hands together as much as possible slightly below the level of the umbilicus on right and left.

4. The kidney is usually felt only in persons with very relaxed abdominal muscles (the very young, the aged, multiparous women). The right kidney is slightly lower than the left. The kidney is felt as a solid, firm, smooth elastic mass.

TECHNIQUE	*FINDINGS*

5. If the kidney is felt, describe its size and shape, and any tenderness.

6. Costal vertebral angle (CVA) tenderness is palpated with the patient sitting—usually during the examination of the posterior chest. Locate the CVA in the flank region and strike firmly with the ulnar surface of your hand. Note any tenderness over the area.

    6. There should be no CVA tenderness.

AORTA

1. Next, palpate for the aorta with the thumb and index finger.

2. Press deeply in the epigastric region (roughly in the midline) and feel with the fingers for pulsations, as well as for the contour of the aorta.

    1. The aorta is soft and pulsatile.

OTHER FINDINGS

1. Palpation of the RLQ may reveal the part of the bowel called the cecum.

2. The sigmoid colon may be palpated in the LLQ.

3. The inguinal and femoral areas should be palpated bilaterally for lymph nodes.

    1. The cecum will be soft.

    2. The sigmoid colon is ropelike and vertical and, if filled with feces, may be quite firm.

    3. Often small inguinal nodes are present; they are nontender freely movable, and firm.

Male Genitalia and Hernias

This part of the examination, especially for hernias, is best done with the patient standing. (A *hernia* is the protrusion of a portion of the intestine through an abnormal opening.)

1. Drape the patient's chest and abdomen.
2. Expose the groin and genitalia.

INSPECTION

1. Inspect the pubic hair distribution and the skin of the penis.
2. Retract or have the patient retract the foreskin, if present.

3. Observe the glans penis and the urethral meatus. Note any ulcers, masses, or scars.
4. Note the location of the urethral meatus and any discharge.

5. Observe the skin of the scrotum for ulcers, masses, redness, or swelling. Note size, contour, and symmetry. Lift the scrotum to inspect the posterior surface.
6. Inspect the inguinal areas and groin for bulges (without and with the patient bearing down—as though having a bowel movement).

    2. The foreskin of the penis, if present, should be easily retractable.
    3. The skin of the glans penis is smooth, without ulceration.
    4. The urethral meatus normally is located ventrally on the end of the penis. Normally, there is no discharge from the urethra.
    5. The scrotum descends approximately 4 cm (1.5 inches) in the adult; the left side is often larger than the right side.

PALPATION

Wear gloves.

1. Palpate any lesions, nodules, or masses, noting tenderness, contour, size, and induration. Palpate the shaft of the penis for any induration (firmness in relation to surrounding tissues).

2. Palpate each testis and epididymis separately between the thumb and first two fingers, noting size, shape, consistency, and undue tenderness (pressure on the testis normally produces pain).

3. Also palpate the spermatic cord, including the vas deferens within the cord, from the testis to the inguinal ring. Note any nodules or tenderness.

4. Palpate for inguinal hernias, using the left hand to examine the patient's left side and the right hand to examine the patient's right side.

    2. The testes are usually rubbery and of equal size. The epididymis is located posterolaterally on each testis and is most easily palpable on the superior portion of the testis.

    4. Normally, there is no palpable herniating mass in the inguinal area.

TECHNIQUE	FINDINGS

a. Insert the right index finger laterally, invaginating the scrotal sac to the external inguinal ring.

b. If the external ring is large enough, insert the finger along the inguinal canal toward the internal ring and ask the patient to strain down, noting any mass that touches the finger.

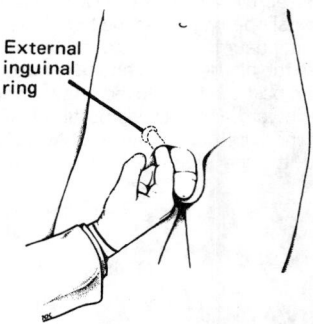

External inguinal ring

5. Also palpate the anterior thigh for a herniating mass in the femoral canal. Ask patient to strain down. (Femoral canal—not palpable, but is a potential opening in the anterior thigh, medial to the femoral artery below the inguinal ligament.)

5. Ordinarily, there is no palpable mass in the femoral area.

Female Genitalia

Equipment

Disposable gloves, lubricant, speculum of appropriate size, excellent direct lighting, cervical scraper, glass slide, fluid for fixing Papanicolaou smear, cotton-tip applicator

General Approach

1. The patient's bladder should be empty.
2. The patient should lie in the lithotomy position with her buttocks extending slightly over the end of the examining table.
3. Her thighs are flexed and abducted; her feet are in the stirrups.
4. Her arms are at her side or crossed over her chest.
5. If a man is performing the examination, a female attendant must be present.
6. The examination will be most successful if the patient is relaxed. This can best be accomplished by draping the patient well so that the drape extends over the knees.
7. Explain each step of the procedure and avoid any quick, unexpected movements.
8. Be sure that your hands and the speculum are warm.

INSPECTION AND PALPATION

(These are performed almost simultaneously through the course of the examination.)

1. Begin with inspection of the pubic hair distribution.

2. Inspect the labia majora, the mons pubis, and the perineum (tissue between the anus and the vaginal opening).
3. With gloved hand, separate the labia majora and inspect the clitoris, urethral meatus, and vaginal opening. Note skin color, ulcerations, nodules, discharge, or swelling.
4. Note the area of the Skene's and Bartholin's glands. If there is any history of swelling of the latter, palpate the glands by placing the index finger in the vagina at the posterior end of the opening and the thumb outside the posterior portion of the vagina. Palpate between the finger and thumb for nodules, tenderness, or swelling. Repeat on each side of the posterior vaginal opening.

1. Normally, the pubic hair is distributed in an inverted triangle over the symphysis pubis.
2. In the virgin, the labia majora are full and rounded. They become thinner in older and multiparous women.
3. The labia minora and the prepuce around the clitoris are pinkish.

4. The hymen, or membranous fold that may partially occlude the vaginal opening, may or may not be present.

SPECULUM EXAMINATION

1. Have the appropriate size speculum available and lubricated with warm water. (Other lubricants may interfere with cytologic studies.)
2. Begin by inserting the first two fingers of the gloved hand into the vagina; locate the cervix, noting the angle of the fingers and the distance from the vaginal opening to the cervix.

2. Normally, the uterus is positioned forward with the cervix at almost a right angle to the vagina.

TECHNIQUE	*FINDINGS*

3. Proceed by removing the two fingers to the edge of the vaginal opening. Press the two fingers downward against the perineum. Take the speculum in your other hand and, with the blades closed and help obliquely, guide the speculum past the two gloved fingers while exerting pressure downward. (This avoids putting painful pressure on the anterior urethral structures.) Avoid pinching the vagina with the speculum.

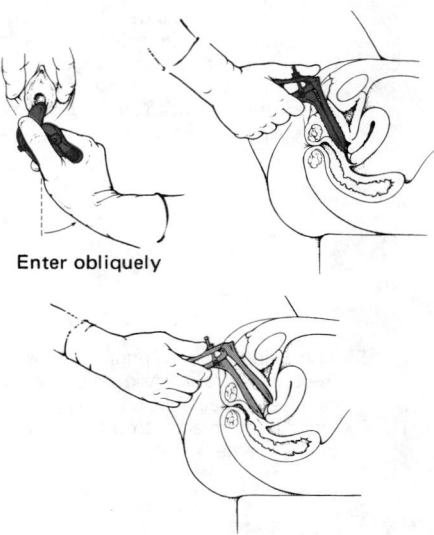

Enter obliquely

4. Once the speculum is inserted, remove the gloved fingers from the introitus (vaginal opening) and return the speculum blades to a horizontal position, maintaining pressure posteriorly.
5. Next, open the speculum blades and, with direct light, visualize the cervix. Maneuver the speculum, so that the cervix comes into full view.
   (The cervix lies within the *fornix,* or posterior portion of the vagina, dividing the fornix into the anterior, posterior, right, and left fornices.)
6. Inspect the cervix and its opening (os), noting position, color, and shape of the os, ulceration, nodules, bleeding, and discharge. (For Papanicolaou smear, see p. 646).
7. As you slowly pull the speculum out of the vagina, inspect the vaginal mucosa for color, inflammation, ulcers, masses, or discharge.
8. Close the blades before reaching the introitus, and remove the speculum without pinching the vaginal wall. (Also see Guidelines in Chapter 20, p. 645).

6. The cervix of the nonpregnant woman is pink and smooth.

7. A small amount of clear lubricating mucus is normal in the vagina. Normally, there is no bleeding from the nonmenstruating female.

PALPATION (BIMANUAL EXAMINATION)
1. Lubricate the index and middle fingers of the gloved hand and insert them into the vagina, noting nodules, masses, or irregularities anteriorly and posteriorly.
2. Locate the cervix and fornices and note tenderness, shape, size, consistency, regularity, and mobility of the cervix.
3. Place the gloved finger in the posterior fornix and the ungloved hand on the abdomen approximately midway between the umbilicus and the symphysis pubis.

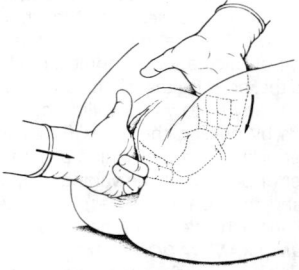

4. Press the two hands toward one another and palpate the uterus, noting its size, shape, regularity, consistency, mobility and tenderness, and any masses.
5. Next, place the gloved fingers in the right lateral fornix and the ungloved hand in the right lower quadrant. Palpate the ovaries, if possible, noting shapes, sizes, consistency, regularity, mobility, pain (the ovary is usually tender), or masses. Repeat the procedure on the left side.
6. Next, withdraw the gloved hand, leaving the index finger in the vagina and placing the middle finger in the rectum. Repeat the procedure of the bimanual examination.

The cervix of the nonpregnant women is smooth, firm, and slightly movable. It is nontender. The uterus is firm, smooth, and nontender.
5. The ovaries vary in size considerably, but average about 3.5 × 2 × 1.5 cm (1.4 × 0.8 × 0.6 inches). The uterine (fallopian) tubes are generally not palpable.

6. Explain what you are doing because this is uncomfortable for the patient and may produce the sensation of wanting to defecate.

TECHNIQUE	FINDINGS

7. If possible, press the uterus downward toward the rectal finger, so that as much of the posterior surface of the uterus as possible can be examined.
8. Proceed with the rectal examination (see below).
9. On completing the examination, wipe genitalia and perineum with a tissue or offer the patient one so that she may do it herself.

Rectum

Equipment
Glove, lubricant
Techniques of Examination

MALE

General Approach
1. If the patient is ambulatory, have him stand and bend over the edge of the table.
2. It is also possible to examine the anus and rectum with the patient lying on his left side, knees drawn up and buttocks close to the edge of the table. (This is generally an uncomfortable position, and the patient should be told that he may feel as though he wants to move his bowels.)
3. The patient should be draped so that only his buttocks are exposed.

INSPECTION
Spread the buttocks and inspect the anus, perianal region, and sacral region for inflammation, nodules, scars, lesions, ulcerations, or rashes. Ask the patient to bear down; note any bulges.

In males and females, the perianal and sacrococcygeal areas are dry, with varying amounts of hair covering them. In the sacrococcygeal region, it is not uncommon to find a small opening or sinus surrounded by a tuft of hair. This is a *pilonidal cyst;* it should be nontender and noninflamed.

PALPATION
1. Palpate any abnormal area noted on inspection.
2. Lubricate the index finger of the gloved hand. Rest the finger over the anus as the patient bears down and, as the sphincter relaxes, insert finger slowly into the rectum.

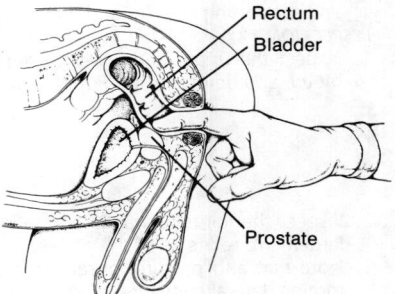

3. Note sphincter tone, any nodules or masses, or tenderness.

4. Insert the finger further and palpate the walls of the rectum laterally and posteriorly while rotating your index finger. Note irregularities, masses, nodules, tenderness.
5. Anteriorly, palpate the two lateral lobes of the prostate gland and its median sulcus for irregularities, nodules, swelling, or tenderness.
6. If possible, palpate the superior portion of the lateral lobe, where the seminal vesicles are located. Note induration, swelling, or tenderness.
7. Just above the prostate anteriorly, the rectum lies adjacent to the peritoneal cavity. If possible, palpate this region for peritoneal masses and tenderness.
8. Continue to insert the finger as far as possible and have the patient bear down so that more of the bowel can be palpated.
9. Gently withdraw your finger. Any fecal material on the glove should be tested for occult blood.

3. The anal canal is approximately 2.5 cm (1 inch) long; it is bordered by the external and internal anal sphincters, which are normally firm and smooth.
4. The wall of the rectum in males and females is smooth and moist.
5. The male prostate gland is approximately 2.5 cm (1 inch) long, smooth, regular, nonmovable, nontender, and rubbery.
6. The seminal vesicles are generally not palpable unless swollen.

9. There is normally no occult blood in the stools.

TECHNIQUE	*FINDINGS*

FEMALE

General Approach

1. The examination is usually performed following the pelvic examination with the patient still in the lithotomy position.
2. If only the rectal examination is done, the patient may be positioned laterally, as for examination of the male.
   The lateral position permits better visualization of the sacral region.
3. The technique is basically the same for the female as for the male.
4. Anteriorly, the cervix, and perhaps a retroverted uterus, may be felt.

4. Anteriorly, the cervix is round and smooth.

Musculoskeletal System

General Approach

1. Examine the muscles and joints, keeping in mind the structure and functions of each.
2. This discussion will center on the technique for examining the patient who is asymptomatic and, therefore, will not present in detail the techniques for inspecting and palpating joints that are symptomatic or deformed.
3. It is important to ask in the history and to note in the examination whether the patient has difficulty performing activities of daily living:
   a. Bathing
   b. Dressing (buttoning, using zippers, tying shoelaces)
   c. Combing hair
   d. Brushing teeth
   e. Walking up and down stairs
   f. Bending
   g. Sitting
   h. Grasping and holding items without dropping them
   i. Standing from a sitting position, unaided
4. Once the above facts have been ascertained, the examination proceeds. Observe and palpate joints and muscles for symmetry and then examine each joint individually as indicated.
5. The examination is performed with the joints both at rest and in motion—moving through a full range of motion; joints and supporting muscles and tissues are noted.

INSPECTION

1. Inspect the upper and lower extremities for size, symmetry, and deformity, and muscle mass.

For the purpose of this text, it is sufficient to say that in the course of the history and examination, the examiner should not find any compromise or restriction of the patient's activities of daily living or any other normal activities. If any activity is restricted because of muscular or skeletal problems, the reader is referred to a more detailed text on physical examination.

2. Inspect the joints for range of motion (in degrees), enlargement, redness.
3. Note gait and posture; observe the spine for range of motion, lateral curvature, or any abnormal curvature.
4. Observe the patient for signs of pain during the examination.

PALPATION

1. Palpate the joints of the upper and lower extremities and the neck for tenderness, swelling, temperature, and range of motion.
2. Hold the palm of the hand over the joint as it moves, or move the joint through the fullest range of motion and note any crepitation (crackling feeling within the joint).
3. Palpate the muscles for size, tone, strength, and tenderness.
4. Palpate the spine for bony deformities and crepitation. Gently tap the spine with the ulnar surface of your fist from the cervical to the lumbar region and note any pain or tenderness.

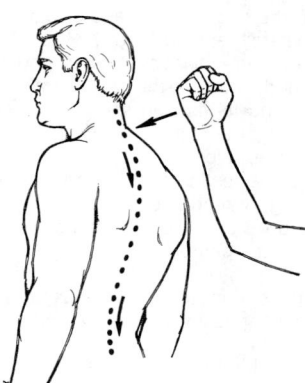

Neurologic System

Equipment

Safety pin, cotton, tuning fork, reflex hammer, flashlight, tongue blade, ophthalmoscope, vision screener, cloves, coffee, or other scented items

General Information

1. The examination described in this section is a screening neurologic examination.
   a. It is performed on individuals without specific neurologic complaints.
   b. A more detailed examination is used for patients with specific signs and symptoms.
   c. The student is referred to another text for the content and technique of a detailed neurologic examination.
2. The examination is performed with the patient in either the sitting or supine position.
3. Much of the neurologic examination can be performed as different regions of the body are being examined. This facilitates the flow of the entire examination.
   Example: The cranial nerves can be examined at the same time as the head and neck.
   A mental status evaluation can be done while the history is elicited and while the entire physical examination is performed.

Components of the Neurologic Examination

There are six components of the neurologic examination:

1. Mental status (cerebral function)
2. Cranial nerve function
3. Cerebellar function
4. Motor function
5. Sensory function
6. Deep tendon reflexes (DTRs)

The screening neurologic examination involves testing all of these components at least superficially. Learning these components in order will help in organizing the examination and in avoiding the omission of any part.

Basic Principles

1. Symmetry of function and findings on both sides of the body is important to note.
   Always compare one side of the body with the other side (eg, compare degree of motor strength of the right biceps with that of the left biceps).
2. Integrating the neurologic examination into the examination of the various body regions is advisable, although the results of the neurologic findings should be recorded together as an entity.

Carrying Out the Examination

MENTAL STATUS

Components of the mental status examination include the following:

—State of consciousness (alert, somnolent, stuporous, comatose)

—Memory (short-term, long-term, intermediate)

—Cognition (calculations, current events)

—Affect (mood)

—Ideational content (hallucinations)

In a screening examination, mental status is evaluated by observing the patient's affect during the history and the content of what he or she says.

1. While recording the history ask the patient for identifying information (how to spell his name, where he lives), and ask what the date is. This tests orientation.

2. The patient's ability to remember is also evaluated as the history is taken—by asking for his past medical history (long-term memory) and dietary habits: "What did you eat for breakfast?" (intermediate memory).

3. Cognition and ideational content are evaluated throughout the history by what the patient says and by his articulateness, consistency, and reliability in reporting events.

4. Affect or mood is evaluated by observing the patient's verbal and nonverbal behavior in response to questions asked, to sudden noises, to interruptions—for example, does the patient laugh or smile when talking about normally sad events; is he easily startled by unexpected noises?

1. Normally the individual is alert, knows who he is and where he lives, and can tell you the date.

2. The patient remembers recent and past events consistently, and willingly admits forgetting something.
   Elderly people often have much better long-term memory than recent memory.

4. Mood should be appropriate to the content of the conversation.

CRANIAL NERVE FUNCTION

FIRST (OLFACTORY) NERVE

(Is not usually tested unless the patient complains of a disturbance in sense of smell.)

TECHNIQUE	*FINDINGS*

1. The airway must be patent.
2. Occlude one nostril; ask the patient to close his eyes and then present various substances to smell (eg, coffee, tobacco). Occlude the other nostril and repeat.
3. Use substances that do not have a lingering effect.

SECOND (OPTIC) NERVE
(Includes tests of visual acuity and of gross visual fields and examination of the optic disc with a fundoscope.)
Visual acuity
    Is tested with the use of a Snellen chart (patient uses glasses if required).
1. Have the patient cover one eye at a time and read the smallest print possible on the chart from a distance of 6 meters (20 feet).

1. Normal vision and corrected vision should be 20/20.

Visual fields
1. Measure by having patient cover his right eye with his right hand. (You cover your left eye with your left hand.)
2. Stand approximately 60 cm (2 feet) from the patient and have him fix his gaze on your nose.
3. Bring two wagging fingers in from the periphery (in a plane equidistant from the patient and you) in all quadrants of the visual field and ask the patient to tell you when he sees your wagging fingers.

3. Assuming your visual fields are grossly normal, the patient and you should see the wagging fingers approximately simultaneously. (The patient's peripheral vision should approximate the examiner's, assuming that it is normal.)

Optic disc
Is visualized as part of the fundoscopic examination (see p. 27).

THIRD (OCULOMOTOR), FOURTH (TROCHLEAR), AND SIXTH (ABDUCENS) NERVES
(Are tested together.) These nerves control the movements of the extraocular muscles of the eye—the superior and inferior oblique and the medial and lateral rectus muscles.
    The oculomotor nerve also controls pupillary constriction.
1. Hold your index finger approximately 30 cm (1 foot) from the patient's nose. Ask the patient to hold his head steady.
2. Ask the patient to follow your finger with his eyes.
3. Move your finger to the right as far as the patient's eye moves. Before bringing your finger back to the center, move it up and then down, so that the patient glances up and peripherally and then down and peripherally.
4. Repeat the test, moving your finger to the left.

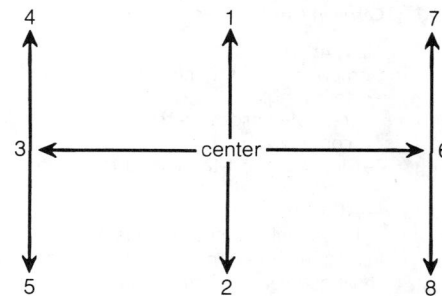

FIFTH (TRIGEMINAL) NERVE
(Has motor component that controls muscles of mastication and a sensory component that controls sensations of the face.)
Motor
1. Have the patient bite down on a tongue depressor with one side of his mouth while you try to pull the blade out.
2. Repeat the test on the other side of the mouth and compare muscle strength of the two sides.

Muscle strength in the face should be present and should be symmetrical.

Sensory
(Sensation to light touch.)
1. Have the patient close his eyes.
2. Touch first one side of the patient's face and then the other (forehead, cheek, and chin), asking the patient if the sensation is present and feels the same on both sides.

Sensation should be present and symmetrical. Always demonstrate to the patient how and with what you are testing sensation—to avoid startling the patient and to encourage cooperation.

3. Sensation to pain (pinprick) is tested similarly.

SEVENTH (FACIAL) NERVE
(Motor function is tested by observing facial expression and symmetry of facial movement.)
    Ask the patient to frown, close his eyes, and smile.

The facial muscles should look symmetrical when the patient frowns, closes his eyes, and smiles. Notice particularly the symmetry of the nasolabial folds.

TECHNIQUE	FINDINGS

EIGHTH (ACOUSTIC) NERVE

(Has 2 branches.)

  Cochlear (mediates hearing). See ear examination, page 28.

  Vestibular (helps control equilibrium).

Romberg test: Have the patient stand erect with his eyes closed and feet close together.

Slight swaying may occur, but the patient should not fall. (Stand close to the patient, so that you can assist if he begins to fall.)

NINTH (GLOSSOPHARYNGEAL) AND TENTH (VAGUS) NERVES

(Are tested together because both have a motor portion innervating the pharynx.)

1. *Ninth:* Test the presence of the gag reflex.

The gag reflex should be present, and there should be no difficulty in swallowing.

2. *Tenth:* Ask the patient to say ''ah'' and observe the movement of the uvula and palate for deviation and asymmetry.

The palate and uvula should move symmetrically without deviation.

ELEVENTH (SPINAL ACCESSORY) NERVE

(Mediates the sternocleidomastoid and upper portion of the trapezius muscles.)

1. Ask the patient to turn his head to the side against resistance while your fingers apply pressure to the jaw.
2. Palpate the sternocleidomastoid muscle on the opposite side.

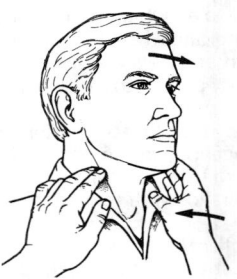

3. Then have the patient shrug his shoulders while you place your hands on his shoulders and apply slight pressure.

Neck and shoulder muscle strength should be symmetrical.

TWELFTH (HYPOGLOSSAL) NERVE

(Innervates muscles of the tongue.)

Test by noting articulation and by having the patient stick out his tongue, noting any deviation or asymmetry.

The tongue should be symmetrical and should not deviate.

CEREBELLAR FUNCTION

(Purpose: to screen for coordination.)

1. Observe posture and gait.
2. Ask the patient to walk forward (and then backward) in a straight line.

The patient should be able to perform all the tests described with smooth, even movement and without losing balance.

3. To test for muscle coordination in the lower extremities, have the patient run his right heel down his left shin and vice versa.
4. To test coordination in upper extremities, have the patient close his eyes and touch his nose with his index finger (starting position: arms outstretched) first left, then right, in rapid succession.

The normal person can do this with rapid, smooth movements without undershooting or overshooting the target.

MOTOR FUNCTION

(Tested in conjunction with the skeletal system because any bony deformity will affect motor function.)

  Evaluate muscle mass, tone, strength, and any abnormal movements (tics, fasciculations, twitching).

Muscle mass: Note symmetry between sides of the body and distribution distally and proximally.

Tone: Test by noting the resistance the muscle offers to movement on passive motion.

Muscle mass: Is usually considered in relation to sex and body build and to use of various muscle groups.

Tone: Generally there is slight resistance to passive movement of muscles as opposed to flaccidity (no resistance) or rigidity (increased muscle tone).

TECHNIQUE	FINDINGS

Strength
 	
    Lower extremity—have the patient do deep knee bends; walk on his toes and then his heels; hop on one foot and then the other.
    Upper extremity—have the patient squeeze your fingers with both hands; compare sides of the body.
    Also, apply resistance to the patient's outstretched arms and when the patient flexes the wrist and elbow; compare sides.
	Strength: Will vary from person to person.

Unusual muscle movements: If present, are noted both when muscle is at rest and when it is moving.	Normally, tremors, tics, or fasciculations are not present either at rest or with movement.

SENSORY FUNCTION

(Should test sensitivity to light touch [cotton], pain [pinprick], vibration [tuning fork], and position.) Compare both sides of body.

Light touch: Ask the patient to close his eyes. Brush his skin with a piece of cotton (on back of hands, forearms, upper arms, dorsal portion of foot laterally and medially; and along the tibia and thigh laterally and medially). Ask the patient to indicate when he feels the cotton and to compare the sensation bilaterally.

Pain: Use a safety pin; touch the skin as lightly as possible to elicit a sharp sensation.

| *Vibration sense:* Test by placing a vibrating tuning fork on a bony prominence (wrist, medial and lateral malleoli). Ask the patient to tell you when he no longer feels vibration. Stop the vibration with your hand. | The patient should normally feel no vibration within a very short time. |

Position sense

1. Have the patient close his eyes.

| 2. Move the patient's digit (finger, great toe) up or down and ask the patient to say in what direction his finger or toe is pointing. | Normally the patient can tell you without hesitation in what direction his digit is pointing. |

3. Place your thumb and index finger on either side of the digit being moved, so that the patient will not sense any pressure from your finger in the direction in which you are moving the digit.

DEEP TENDON REFLEXES

1. Have the patient relax; provide support for the extremity being tested.

| 2. Compare reflex amplitude of the same tendons on either side of the body. | Amplitude of the reflex may vary for different tendons. |

UPPER EXTREMITIES

Biceps

1. Place your right thumb on the patient's right biceps tendon (located in the antecubital fossa).
2. Rest the patient's forearm on your left hand and strike your thumb with the pointed end of the hammer head. (Hold the hammer loosely, so that it pivots in your hand when it is moved with a wrist action.)

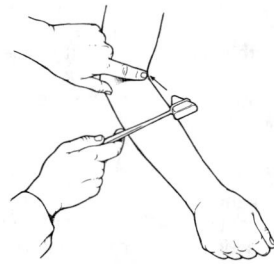

| 3. Strike your thumb with the least amount of pressure needed to elicit the reflex. | The forearm may move, and your thumb should feel the tendon jerk. |

TECHNIQUE	*FINDINGS*

Triceps tendon
1. Hold the patient's arm abducted and bent at the elbow.
2. Posteriorly, about 2.5 cm (1 inch) above the olecranon process, strike the tendon directly, using the pointed end of the hammer.

The forearm should move slightly.

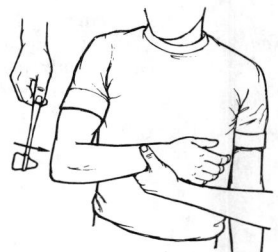

Brachioradialis tendon
1. Strike the forearm with the hammer about 2.5 cm (1 inch) above the wrist over the radius.
2. Be sure the forearm is supported and relaxed.

The thumb may be observed moving downward.

LOWER EXTREMITIES

Quadriceps reflex
1. Have the patient sitting with his legs hanging over the edge of the table or lying down while you support the legs at the knee (slightly bent).
2. Strike the tendon just below the patella.
3. If reflexes are difficult to elicit, have the patient interlace the fingers of both hands and then have patient try to pull his hands apart. While he is thus distracted, inhibition of the quadriceps reflex is diminished, and the reflex can be elicited more easily. If such a distraction is used to elicit the reflex, record this fact with the physical findings.

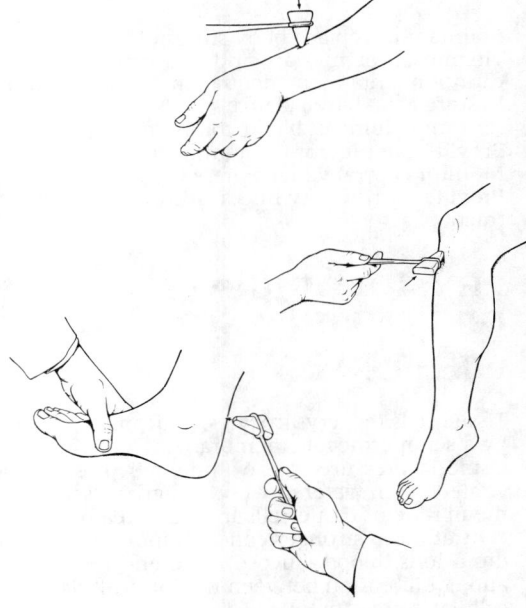

Achilles reflex
1. Support the foot in dorsiflexed position.
2. Tap the Achilles tendon with the hammer head.

The foot should move downward into your hand.

Selected References

Bates, B. L. (1995). *A guide to physical examination and history taking* (6th ed.). Philadelphia: J. B. Lippincott.

DeGowin, R. L. (1994). *DeGowin & DeGowin's bedside diagnostic examination.* New York: Macmillan.

Fuller, J. & Schaller-Ayers, J. (1994). *Health assessment: A nursing approach* (2nd ed.). Philadelphia: J. B. Lippincott.

Owen, K. Listen to what patients don't say. (1994). *RN, 57*(1), 96.

Williams, J., Schneiderman, H., & Algranati, P. (1994). *Physical diagnosis: Bedside evaluation of diagnosis and function.* Baltimore: Williams & Wilkins.

CHAPTER 4 ◆

IV Therapy

General Considerations

◆ GOALS

The goals of intravenous (IV) therapy include:

1. Maintain or replace body stores of water, electrolytes, vitamins, proteins, fats, and calories in the patient who cannot maintain an adequate intake by mouth.
2. Restore acid–base balance.
3. Restore volume of blood components.
4. Provide avenues for the administration of medications.
5. Monitor central venous pressure (CVP).
6. Provide nutrition while resting the gastrointestinal tract.

◆ PHYSIOLOGIC ASSIMILATION OF INFUSION SOLUTIONS

Principles

1. Tissue cells (eg, erythrocytes, neurons) are surrounded by a semipermeable membrane.
2. Osmotic pressure is the ''pulling'' pressure demonstrated when water moves through the semipermeable membrane of tissue cells from an area of weaker concentration to stronger concentration of solute (eg, sodium ions, blood glucose). The end result is dilution and equilibration between the intracellular and extracellular compartments.
3. Extracellular compartment fluids primarily include plasma and interstitial fluid.

Types of Fluids

1. Isotonic—a solution that exerts the same osmotic pressure as that found in plasma.
   a. Normal saline 0.9%
   b. Lactated Ringer's
   c. Blood components
      (1) Albumin 5%
      (2) Plasma
   d. 5% dextrose in water (D5W)
2. Hypotonic—a solution that exerts less osmotic pressure than that of blood plasma. Administration of this fluid generally causes dilution of plasma solute concentration and forces water movement into cells to reestablish intracellular and extracellular equilibrium; cells will then expand or swell.
   a. Dextrose 2.5% in half-strength normal saline, 0.45%
   b. Half-strength normal saline, 0.45%
   c. Quarter-strength normal saline, 0.2%
3. Hypertonic—a solution that exerts a higher osmotic pressure than that of blood plasma. Administration of this fluid increases the solute concentration of plasma, drawing water out of the cells and into the extracellular compartment to restore osmotic equilibrium; cells will then shrink.
   a. Dextrose 5% in normal saline 0.9%
   b. Dextrose 5% in half-strength normal saline (only slightly hypertonic because dextrose is rapidly metabolized and renders only temporary osmotic pressure)
   c. Dextrose 10% in water
   d. Dextrose 20% in water
   e. Saline, 3% and 5%
   f. Hyperalimentation solutions
   g. Dextrose 5% in lactated Ringer's
   h. Albumin 25%

Composition of Fluids (Table 4-1)

1. Saline solutions—water and electrolytes (Na^+, Cl^-)
2. Dextrose solutions—water or saline and calories
3. Lactated Ringer's—water and electrolytes (Na^+, K^+, Cl^-, Ca^{++}, lactate)
4. Balanced isotonic—varies; water, electrolytes, some calories (Na^+, K^+, Mg^{++}, Cl^-, HCO_3^-, gluconate)
5. Whole blood and blood components
6. Plasma expanders—albumin, dextran, plasma protein fraction 5% (Plasmanate), hetastarch (Hespan) (exert increased oncotic pressure, pulling fluid from interstitium into the circulation and temporarily increasing blood volume)
7. Parenteral hyperalimentation—fluid, electrolytes, amino acids, and calories

Uses and Precautions With Common Types of Infusions

1. D5W
   a. Used to replace water (hypotonic fluid) losses, sup-

TABLE 4-1 Composition of Selected IV Solutions

Solution	Tonicity	Na⁺	K⁺	Cl⁻ (mEq/L)	Ca⁺⁺	pH	mOsm/L	Calories
5% DW	Isotonic	—	—	—	—	5.0	253	170
10% DW	Hypertonic	—	—	—	—	4.6	561	340
0.9% NS	Isotonic	154	—	154	—	5.7	308	—
0.45% NS	Hypotonic	77	—	77	—	5.3	154	—
5% D and 0.9% NS*	Slightly hypertonic	154	—	154	—	4.2	561	170
5% and 0.45% NS	Slightly hypertonic	77	—	77	—	4.2	407	170
5% and 0.2% NS	Hypotonic	34	—	34	—	4.2	290	170
Lactated Ringer's†	Isotonic	148	4	156	4.5	6.7	309	9
5% D and lactated Ringer's	Slightly hypertonic	130	4	109	3.0	5.1	527	170
Normosol-R	Isotonic	140	5	96	—	6.4	295	—
Sodium lactate 1/6 molar	Slightly hypertonic	167	—	—	—	6.9	333	55
6% Dextran 75 and 0.9% NS	Isotonic	154	—	154	—	4.3	309	—

DW, dextrose in water, NS, normal saline
* 5% Dextrose metabolizes rapidly in the blood and, in reality, produces minimal osmotic effects.
† Lactate converts to bicarbonate in the liver.

ply some caloric intake, administer as carrying solution for numerous medications, or function as a slow "keep-vein-open" infusion.
b. Cautious use in patients with water intoxication (hyponatremia, syndrome of inappropriate antidiuretic hormone release). Should not be used as concurrent solution infusion with blood or blood components. Table 4-2 lists signs and symptoms of water excess or deficit.
2. Normal saline
a. Used to replace saline (isotonic fluid) losses, administer with blood components, or treat patients in hemodynamic shock.
b. Cautious use in patients with isotonic volume excess (eg, heart failure, renal failure). See Table 4-3 for signs and symptoms of isotonic fluid excess or deficit.
3. Lactated Ringer's
a. Used to replace isotonic fluid losses, replenish specific electrolyte losses, and moderate metabolic acidosis

Types of IV Administration

◆ IV "PUSH"

Intravenous "push" (or "IV bolus") refers to the administration of a medication from a syringe and needle directly into an ongoing IV infusion. It may also be given directly into a vein or heparin lock.

Indications

1. For emergency administration of cardiopulmonary resuscitative procedures, allowing rapid concentration of a medication in the patient's bloodstream
2. When quicker response to the medication is required (eg, furosemide [Lasix], digoxin [Lanoxin])
3. To administer "loading" doses of a drug that will be continued via infusion (eg, lidocaine [Xylocaine])

TABLE 4-2 Signs and Symptoms of Water Excess or Deficit

Site	Hyponatremia (Water Intoxication)	Hypernatremia (Water Deficit)
CNS	Muscle twitching	Restlessness
	Hyperactive tendon reflexes	Weakness
	Convulsions	Delirium
	Increased intracranial pressure, coma	Coma
CV	Increased BP and pulse, if severe	Tachycardia
		Hypotension (if severe)
Tissues	Increased salivation, tears	Decreased saliva and tears
	Watery diarrhea	Dry, sticky mucous membranes
	Fingerprinting of skin	Red, swollen tongue
		Flushed skin
Renal	Oliguria	Oliguria
Other	None	Fever

TABLE 4-3 Signs and Symptoms of Isotonic Fluid Excess or Deficit

Site	Deficit	Excess
CNS	Fatigue, apathy Anorexia Stupor, coma	Confusion (if severe)
CV	Orthostatic hypotension Flat neck veins Fast, thready pulse Hypotension Cool, clammy skin	Elevated venous pressure Distended neck veins Increased cardiac output Heart gallops Pulmonary edema
GI	Anorexia Thirst Silent ileus	Anorexia, nausea and vomiting Edema of stomach, colon, and mesentery
Tissues	Soft, small tongue with longitudinal wrinkling Sunken eyes Decreased skin turgor	Pitting edema Moist pulmonary crackles
Metabolism	Mild decrease in temperature	None

4. To reduce patient discomfort by limiting need for intramuscular injections
5. To avoid incompatibility problems that may occur when several medications are mixed in one bottle
6. To deliver drugs to patients unable to take them orally (eg, coma) or intramuscularly (eg, coagulation disorder)

Precautions and Recommendations

1. Before administration of the medication:
   a. Determine that the medication matches the order.
   b. Dilute the drug as indicated by pharmacy references. Many medications are irritating to veins and require sufficient dilution.
   c. Determine the correct (safest) rate of administration. Consult pharmacy or pharmaceutical text. Most medications are given slowly (rarely over less than 1 minute); sometimes as long as 30 minutes is required. Too rapid administration may result in serious side effects.
   d. If IV push is to be given with an ongoing IV infusion or to follow another IV push medication, check pharmacy for possible incompatibility. It is always wise to flush the IV tubing or cannula with saline before and after administration of a drug.
   e. Assess patient's condition and ability to tolerate the drug.
   f. Assess patency of IV line by presence of blood return.
      (1) Lower running IV bottle.
      (2) Withdraw with syringe before injecting medication.
      (3) Pinch IV tubing gently.
   g. Ascertain dwell time of catheter. For infusion of vesicants (some chemotherapy agents), a catheter placement of 24 hours or less is advisable.
2. Watch patient's reaction to the drug.
   a. Are there major side effects, such as anaphylaxis, respiratory distress, tachycardia, bradycardia, or seizures?
   b. What about minor side effects such as nausea, flushing, skin rash, or confusion?
   c. Stop medication and consult health care provider if any such reactions occur.
3. Vesicants are always given through the side port of a running IV infusion.
4. Be familiar with hospital policies and guidelines regarding how, where, and by whom IV push medications can be given.

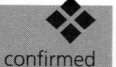

NURSING ALERT:
Unusual dosages or unfamiliar drugs should always be confirmed with the health care provider or pharmacist before administration. The nurse is ultimately accountable for the drug that he or she administers.

◆ CONTINUOUS INFUSION USING INFUSION CONTROL DEVICES

Continuous IV infusions may be given through traditionally hung bags of solution and tubing, with or without flow rate regulators. IV, intra-arterial, and intrathecal (spinal) infusion may be accomplished through the use of special external or implantable pumps. See Procedure Guidelines 4-1, p. 66.

General Considerations

A. Advantages
1. Ability to infuse large and small volumes of fluid with accuracy.
2. An alarm warns of problem, such as air in line or occlusion.
3. Reduces nursing time in constantly readjusting flow rates.

B. Disadvantages
1. Requires special tubing.
2. There may be added cost to therapy.

3. Infusion pumps will continue to infuse despite presence of infiltration.

C. *Nursing Responsibilities*
1. Remember that a mechanical infusion regulator is only as effective as the nurse operating it.
2. Continue to check the patient regularly for complications, such as infiltration or infection.
3. Follow the manufacturer's instruction carefully when inserting the tubing.
4. Double-check the flow rate.
5. Be sure to flush all air out of the tubing before connecting it to the patient.
6. Explain purpose of the device and the alarm system. Added machines in the room can evoke greater anxiety in the patient and family.

Types

A. *Electronic Flow-Rate Regulators*
1. Controller—an electronic flow-rate regulator infusion by monitoring drop rate (drops/min) or monitoring volume passage (mL/min); the latter is currently more commonly used because it is not affected by drop size, temperature, or fluid viscosity. The delivery of fluid will stop if the line is occluded or if infiltration is detected.
2. Infusion pump—an electronic flow-rate regulator that exerts pressure on the tubing or on fluid. It continually pumps against a pressure gradient, providing a constant, accurate delivery of a preselected rate of fluid volume. The high-pressure pumping capability is particularly useful for arterial infusions.
3. Use of electronic flow-rate regulators is indicated for:
   a. Continuous infusions of medications of hyperalimentation
   b. Chemotherapy
      (1) Use only a controller for peripheral IV infusions.
      (2) Use a pump for central line and intra-arterial infusions.
   c. Small volume infusions such as pediatric infusion
   d. Critical care fluid and medication management

B. *Battery-Powered Ambulatory Infusion Pumps*
1. Example: CADD 1™ pump (Pharmacia Deltec, Inc.)
2. These external pumps deliver continuous or intermittent medications via IV, subcutaneous, or spinal routes.
3. If used for pain control, patient may deliver a "bolus" injection if relief is not obtained from continuous, prescribed dose.

C. *Freon-Controlled Spring Pump (Implanted)*
1. Example: Infusaid™ (Pfizer)
2. This pump is placed subcutaneously, usually in the left lower quadrant of the abdomen.
3. It will deliver continuous pain medication or chemotherapy via an artery, vein, or the spinal canal.

◆ Intermittent Infusions

Intermittent IV infusions may be given through a heparin lock, "piggyback" to a continuous IV infusion, or for long-term therapy through a venous access device. See Procedure Guidelines 4-2, 4-3, and 4-4, pp. 68-71.

Heparin Lock

1. This intermittent infusion reservoir permits administration of periodic IV medications and solution without continuous fluid administration.
2. Many institutions do not use heparin solutions to keep short peripheral catheters open. A saline flush (2 mL) is administered and a clamp is tightened or the needle is withdrawn while injecting to create negative pressure and keep vein open.

"Piggyback" IV Administration

1. Means of administering medication via the fluid pathway of an established primary infusion line.
2. Drugs may be given on an intermittent basis through a primary infusion.
3. When a check-valve is present on the primary tubing, it performs the following functions:
   a. Permits the primary infusion to flow after the medication has been administered.
   b. Prevents air from entering the system.
   c. Prevents secondary fluid from " running dry."
   d. Permits less mixing of primary fluid with secondary solution.
4. Use of an infusion pump or controller will permit rate changes between primary and secondary infusates.

Venous Access Devices

A. *Indications*
1. Long-term therapy—weeks, months, even years
2. Chemotherapy, medication, or blood product infusion; blood specimen collection
3. IV fluids in the home
4. Limited peripheral venous access due to extensive previous IV therapy, surgery, or previous tissue damage

B. *Types* (Figure 4-1)
1. Central catheter—nontunneled; often called percutaneous
   a. Has one to four lumens
   b. Dwell time usually less than a month
   c. May be inserted in femoral, jugular, or subclavian veins

NURSING ALERT:
An x-ray to determine placement of central catheter is necessary for all devices that deliver fluid into the subclavian vein or superior vena cava.

2. Central catheter—tunneled
   a. A tunneled catheter is inserted into a central vein (usually the subclavian, then the superior vena cava) and subcutaneously tunneled to an exit site approximately 10 cm from the insertion site.
   b. A Dacron cuff is located approximately 2 to 3 cm from the exit site, providing a barrier against microorganisms.
   c. Examples of the tunneled catheters in current use are Hickman, Broviac, and Groshong.
3. Central implanted device
   a. A subcutaneous pocket is formed and a reservoir is placed; a catheter is attached to the reservoir and

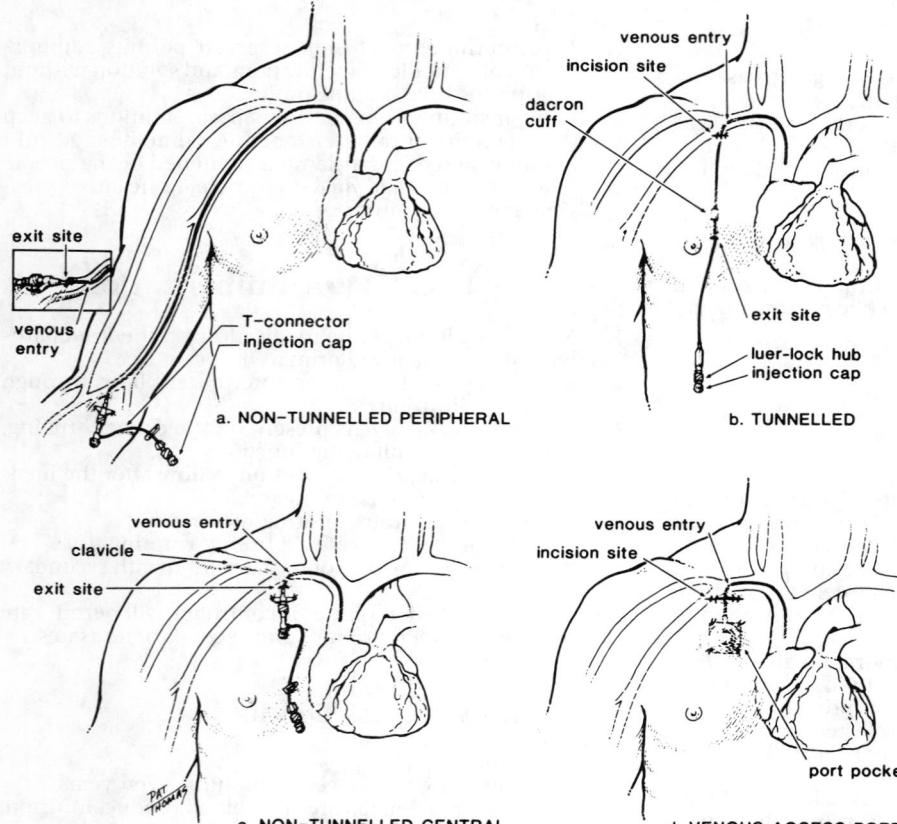

a. NON-TUNNELLED PERIPHERAL

exit site
venous entry
T-connector
injection cap

b. TUNNELLED

venous entry
incision site
dacron cuff
exit site
luer-lock hub
injection cap

c. NON-TUNNELLED CENTRAL

venous entry
clavicle
exit site

d. VENOUS ACCESS PORT

venous entry
incision site
port pocket

FIGURE 4-1 *Common sites for long-term venous access devices. (Courtesy American Cancer Society.)*

tunneled subcutaneously and inserted into a central vein (usually the catheter tip is in the superior vena cava). This device cannot be visualized exteriorly.
  b. Examples of implanted devices in current use include the Port-A-Cath, Medi-Port, Infuse-A-Port, and Hickman Port.
4. Peripheral central—nontunneled
  a. Peripherally inserted central catheter (PICC line)
    (1) Inserted in basilic or cephalic vein
    (2) May be inserted by nurses with special education
    (3) Delivers fluid centrally into superior vena cava
  b. PAS Port™
    (1) Inserted in basilic vein
    (2) Connected to a subcutaneously implanted port in the forearm
    (3) Delivers fluid centrally into superior vena cava

NURSING ALERT: ❖

If central catheters are placed too deeply and extend into the right atrium, an irregular heartbeat may result. Notify health care provider immediately.

5. Midline catheters
  a. These catheters are inserted into the basilic or cephalic vein and extend 6 to 7 inches up the arm.

  b. They are inserted by specially educated nurses.
  c. Dwell time—for intermediate therapy of 2 to 6 weeks
  d. They are not appropriate for hyperosmolar solutions such as hyperalimentation and some antibiotics such as erythromycin (Ilotycin) and nafcillin (Unipen).
  e. An example of a midline catheter is the Landmark™ catheter.

Nursing Role in IV Therapy

◆ INITIATING AN IV

Nurses must be familiar with the procedure as well as the equipment involved in initiating an IV to provide effective therapy and prevent complications.

Selecting a Vein

1. First verify the order for IV therapy unless it is an emergency situation.
2. Explain the procedure to the patient.

3. Select a vein suitable for venipuncture.
   a. Back of hand—metacarpal vein (Fig. 4-2A). Avoid digital veins, if possible.
      (1) The advantage of this site is that it permits arm movement.
      (2) If later a vein problem develops at this site, another vein higher up the arm may be used.
   b. Forearm—basilic or cephalic vein (see Figure 4-2B)
   c. Inner aspect of elbow, antecubital fossa—median basilic and median cephalic for relatively short-term infusion

---

NURSING ALERT: ◆◆
The median basilic and cephalic veins are not recommended for chemotherapy administration due to potential for extravasation and poor healing resulting in impaired joint movement. In addition, these veins may be needed for intermediate or long-term indwelling catheters.

---

   d. Lower extremities
      (1) Foot—venous plexus of dorsum, dorsal venous arch, medial marginal vein
      (2) Ankle—great saphenous vein

NURSING ALERT: ◆◆
Use lower extremities as a last resort. A patient with diabetes is not a suitable candidate. Monitor lower extremity closely for signs of phlebitis and thrombosis.

---

4. Central veins are used:
   a. When medications and infusions are hypertonic or highly irritating, requiring rapid, high-volume dilution to prevent systemic reactions and local venous damage (eg, chemotherapy, hyperalimentation).
   b. When peripheral blood flow is diminished (eg, shock) or when peripheral vessels are not accessible (eg, obese patients).
   c. When CVP monitoring is desired.
   d. When moderate or long-term fluid therapy is expected.

Methods of Distending a Vein

1. Apply manual compression above site where cannula is to be inserted.
2. Have the patient periodically clench the fist (if arm is used).
3. Massage area in direction of venous flow.
4. Apply tourniquet (made of soft rubber tubing) at least 5 to 15 cm (2–6 inches) above planned insertion site, fastening it with a slip knot or hemostat.
5. An alternative is to apply blood pressure cuff (keep pressure just below systolic pressure).
6. Lightly tap vein site; this is to be done gently so that the vein is not injured.
7. Allow extremity to be dependent (below heart level) for a few minutes.
8. Apply heat to a possible needle site by using a moist, warm towel.

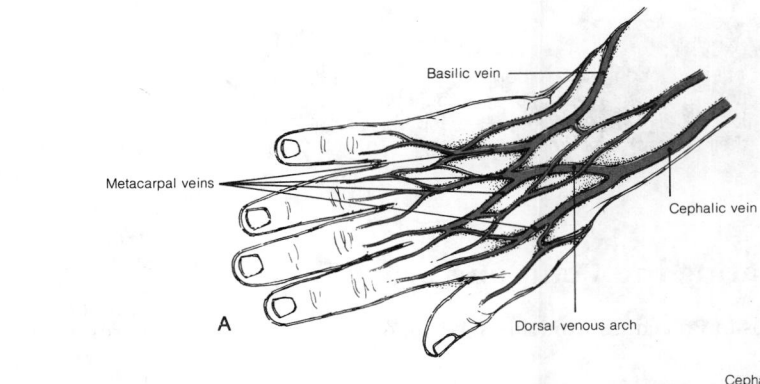

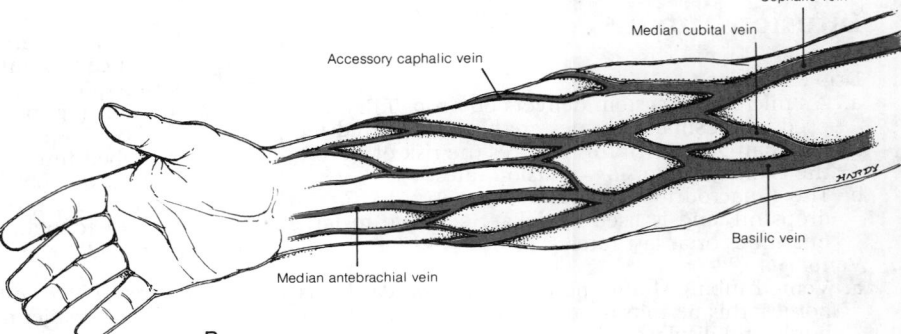

FIGURE 4-2 (**A**) *Superficial veins, dorsal aspect of hand.* (**B**) *Superficial veins, forearm.*

Selecting Needle or Catheter

1. Use the smallest gauge catheter suitable for type and location of infusion.
2. If blood transfusion is to be given, use a larger bore catheter, preferably a 20 gauge.
3. For very small veins and an infusion rate below 50 mL/h, a 24-gauge catheter may be appropriate.
4. Consider local anesthesia.
   a. If large-bore needle (greater than 18 gauge) is being inserted in an unusually sensitive patient, 0.1 mL 1% lidocaine (without epinephrine) may be ordered and infiltrated intradermally around the site to provide local anesthesia.
   b. Local anesthesia is best avoided because it may cause collapse of desired veins, allergic reactions, and increased cost of the procedure.
5. For a short-term infusion of 1 hour or less, a steel needle may be used.
6. For longer-term therapy, chose a flexible catheter. These may be made of Teflon™, Vialyon™, Aquavene™, etc.

Cleansing the Infusion Site

1. If skin is unusually soiled, cleanse infusion site thoroughly with a good surgical soap and rinse.
2. Cleanse IV site with effective topical antiseptic (according to hospital protocol).
   a. Three alcohol swabs, used one at a time, in a circular movement from site outward and for 1 minute is an appropriate cleansing.
   b. Povidone-iodine, used for 1 minute and allowed to dry, is also appropriate, especially for the neutropenic patient.

NURSING ALERT: ❖
Iodine solutions and iodophors (an iodine compound) may cause allergic reactions in some patients. Patient should be assessed for iodine allergies before IV insertion. Iodine and iodophor should dry to facilitate their antimicrobial properties.

Initiating the Venipuncture

Follow steps in Procedure Guidelines 4-1, p. 66.

Infusion Tubing

1. Drip chambers
   a. A "microdrip" system delivers 60 drops/mL and is used when small volumes are being delivered (eg, less than 50 mL/h); this reduces the risk of clotting the IV line due to slow infusion rates.
   b. The "macrodrip" system delivers 10, 15, or 20 drops/mL and is used to deliver solution in large quantities or at fast rates.
2. Vents
   a. Vented tubing should be used with standard glass bottles; this permits air to enter the vacuum in the bottle and displace solution as it flows out.
   b. Nonvented tubing should be used for IV bags and glass bottles that have a built-in air vent.
3. Filters
   a. Filters help minimize the risk of contamination from certain microorganisms and particulate matter.
   b. Filters should be changed every 24 to 48 hours because bacteria may become trapped in the filter and release endotoxin, a small pyrogen capable of passing through the filter.
   c. Filters are found "in line" on conventional IV and hyperalimentation tubing. Check your institution's equipment and protocols to see if an additional filter is warranted. (An additional filter is needed for mannitol infusions.)
4. Special tubing
   a. Most mechanical infusion pumps and controllers require specialized tubing to fit their particular pumping chamber. Need for such a device should be determined before initiating infusion therapy.
   b. If added tubing length is required (especially for children and restless patients), extension tubing is available; this should be added at the time of IV setup.
   c. Secondary tubing is used for administration of intermittent "piggyback" medications that are connected to the port closest to the drip chamber.
   d. Special coated tubing, designed to prevent leaching of polyvinyl chloride, is used for delivering medications such as nitroglycerin (Tridil), tamoxifen (Taxol), and cyclosporine (Sandimmune).
5. Tubing change
   a. Check your institutional protocol for time of tubing change. Standard is 48 to 72 hours.
   b. Label new tubing with date, time hung, and your initials.
6. Dressing changes and flushing of IV—varies depending on type of IV (Table 4-4).

Adjusting Rate of Flow

The health care provider prescribes the flow rate. However, the nurse is responsible for regulating and maintaining the proper rate.

A. *Patient-Determining Factors*
1. Surface area of the patient—the larger the patient, the more fluid may be required and tolerated.
2. Patient condition—a patient in hypovolemic shock requires greater amounts of fluids, whereas the patient with heart or renal failure should receive fluids judiciously.
3. Age of patient—fluids should be administered more slowly in the very young and elderly.
4. Tolerance to solutions—fluids containing medications causing potential allergic reactions or intense vascular irritation (eg, potassium chloride) should be well diluted or given slowly.
5. Prescribed fluid composition—efficacy of some drugs is based on speed of infusion (eg, antibiotics); other solutions are given at a rate titrated to the patient's response to them (eg, dopamine [Intropin], sodium nitroprusside [Nipride], heparin [Heparin].)

B. *Factors Affecting Rate of Flow*
1. Pressure gradient—the difference between two levels in a fluid system

TABLE 4-4 IV Catheter Maintenance Guidelines

Catheter	Dressing Change	Flush (Maintenance)	Flush (After Blood Draw)
Short peripheral	3d when site changed	If used as a lock, 2 mL saline every shift or heparin 1:10 units/mL	N/A
Midline (ie, Landmark)	q 3–5d	3 mL 1:10 units/mL heparin qd	5 mL normal saline 3 mL 1:100 units/mL heparin
PICC	3 times/wk postinsertion, weekly after that	2–3 mL 1:100 units/mL heparin qd	10 mL normal saline 3 mL 1:10 units/mL heparin
Groshong	q 1–2d postinsertion for a week postop, then q 3d until site fully healed, then every week. When site healed, no dressing. Secure catheter to chest with tape.	10 mL normal saline weekly	10 mL normal saline
Hickman/Broviac	Same as Groshong	3 mL 1:100 units qd * if accessed q 8h or more frequently, no need for heparin between infusions.	10 mL normal saline 3 mL 1:100 units/mL heparin
Implanted ports (including PAS Port)	Needle and dressing change every week when accessed	If accessed and locked: 5 mL normal saline and 5 mL 1:100 units/mL heparin after each infusion. Terminal flush: 5–7 mL 1:100 units/mL heparin and q 4wk thereafter	5 mL normal saline 5 mL 1:100 units/mL heparin
Percutaneous catheters (triple/double lumen)	q 2–3d	3 mL normal saline 2 mL 1:10 units heparin twice per day or after each infusion	3 mL normal saline 3 mL 1:10 units heparin
Quinton/Perm-A catheter (blue lumen, use only with order)	q 2–3d	2 mL 1000 units/mL heparin q 2–3d (always withdraw heparin first when using catheter)	10 mL normal saline 2 mL 1000 units/mL heparin

2. Friction—the interaction between fluid molecules and surfaces of inner wall of tubing
3. Diameter and length of tubing; gauge of cannula
4. Height of column of fluid
5. Size of opening through which fluid leaves receptacle
6. Characteristics of fluid
   a. Viscosity
   b. Temperature—refrigerated fluids may cause diminished flow and vessel spasm; bring fluid to room temperature.
7. Vein trauma, clots, plugging of vents, venous spasm, vasoconstriction, etc.
8. Flow-control clamp derangement
   a. Some clamps may slip and loosen, resulting in a rapid, or "runaway," infusion.
   b. Plastic tubing may distort, causing "creep" or "cold flow"—the inside diameter of tubing will continue to change long after clamp is tightened or relaxed.
   c. Marked stretching of tubing may cause distortions of tubing and render clamp ineffective (may occur when patient turns over and pulls on a short tubing).
9. If there is any question regarding rate of fluid administration, check with the health care provider.

C. *Calculation of Flow Rate*
1. Most infusion rates are prescribed to be given at a certain volume per hour.

2. The delivery of the prescribed volume is determined by calculating the necessary drops per minute to deliver the volume.
3. Drops per mL will vary with commercial parenteral sets (eg, 10, 15, 20, or 60 drops/mL) Check directions on set.
4. Calculate infusion rate using the following formula:

$$\text{Drops/minute} = \frac{\text{total volume infused} \times \text{drops/mL}}{\text{total time for infusion in minutes}}$$

Example: Infuse 150 mL of D5W in 1 hour (set indicates 10 drops/mL)

$$\frac{150 \times 10 = 25 \text{ drops/minute}}{60 \text{ minutes}}$$

5. The nurse hanging a new IV solution should record date, time, and his or her initials on the container label.

NURSING ALERT:
Never write directly on the IV bag to avoid leaks. Write on label or tape using a regular pen. Do not use magic markers because they are absorbed into the plastic bag and perhaps into the solution.

◆ COMPLICATIONS OF IV THERAPY

Infiltration

A. Cause
1. Dislodgment of the IV cannula from the vein results in infusion of fluid into the surrounding tissues.

B. Clinical Manifestations
1. Swelling, blanching, and coolness of surrounding skin and tissues
2. Discomfort, depending on nature of solution
3. Fluid flowing more slowly or ceasing
4. Absence of blood backflow in IV catheter and tubing

C. Preventive Measures
1. Ensure that IV and distal tubing are secured sufficiently with tape to prevent movement.
2. Splint arm or hand as necessary.
3. Check IV site frequently for complications.

D. Nursing Interventions
1. Stop infusion immediately and remove IV needle or catheter.
2. Restart IV in the other arm.
3. If infiltration is moderate to severe, apply warm, moist compresses and elevate limb.
4. If a vasoconstrictor agent (eg, norepinephrine bitartrate [Levophed], dopamine [Intropin], or a vesicant [eg, various chemotherapy agents]) has infiltrated, initiate emergency local treatment as directed; serious tissue injury, necrosis, and sloughing may result if actions are not taken.
5. Document interventions and assessments.

Thrombophlebitis

A. Causes
1. Injury to vein during venipuncture, large-bore needle/catheter use, or prolonged needle/catheter use
2. Irritation to vein due to rapid infusions or irritating solutions (eg, hypertonic glucose solutions, cytotoxic agents, strong acids or alkalis, potassium, and others). Smaller veins are more susceptible.
3. Clot formation at the end of the needle or catheter due to slow infusion rates
4. More often seen with synthetic catheters than steel needles

B. Clinical Manifestations
1. Tenderness at first, then pain along course of the vein
2. Swelling, warmth, and redness at infusion site; the vein may appear as a red streak above insertion site.

C. Preventive Measures
1. Anchor needle or catheter securely at insertion site.
2. Change insertion site at least every 72 hours.
3. Use large veins for irritating fluid because of higher blood flow, which rapidly dilutes irritant.
4. Sufficiently dilute irritating agents before infusion.

D. Nursing Interventions
1. Apply cold compresses immediately to relieve pain and inflammation.

2. Later follow with moist, warm compresses to stimulate circulation and promote absorption.
3. Document interventions and assessments.

Bacteremia

A. Causes
1. Underlying phlebitis increases risk 18-fold.
2. Contaminated equipment or infused solutions (Fig. 4-3)
3. Prolonged placement of an IV device (catheter/needle, tubing, solution container)
4. Nonaseptic IV insertion or dressing change
5. Cross-contamination by patient with other infected areas of body
6. The critically ill or immunosuppressed patient is at greatest risk of bacteremia.

B. Clinical Manifestations
1. Elevated temperature, chills
2. Nausea, vomiting
3. Malaise, increased pulse

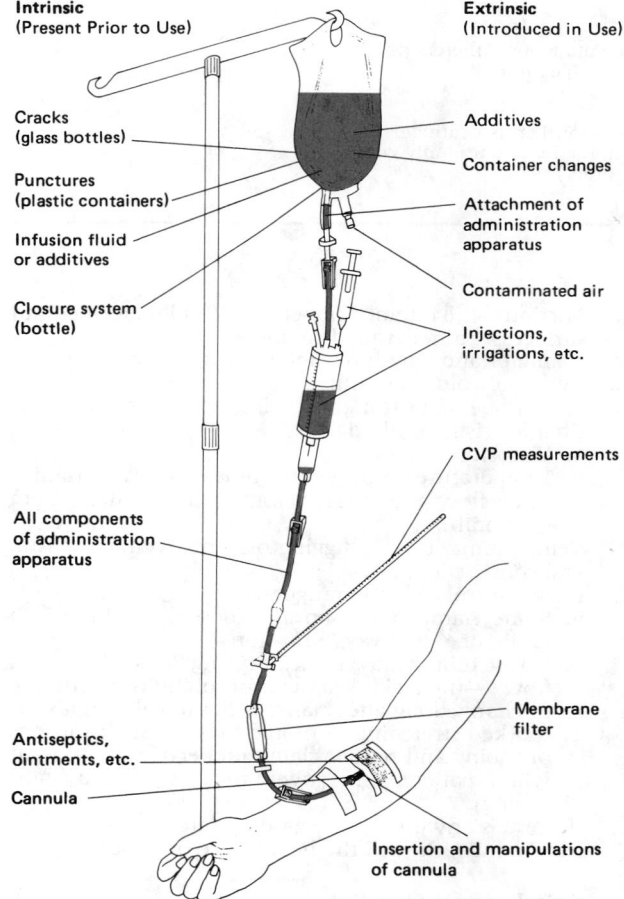

FIGURE 4-3 Potential mechanisms for contamination of IV infusion systems.

4. Backache, headache
5. May progress to septic shock with profound hypotension
6. Possible signs of local infection at IV insertion site (eg, redness, pain, foul drainage)

C. *Preventive Measures*
1. Follow same measures as outlined for thrombophlebitis.
2. Use strict asepsis when inserting IV or changing IV dressing.
3. Solutions should never hang longer than 24 hours.
4. Change insertion site at least every 48 to 72 hours.
5. Change IV administration set every 48 to 72 hours.
6. Change IV dressing every 48 to 72 hours.
7. Maintain integrity of infusion system.

D. *Nursing Interventions*
1. Discontinue infusion and IV cannula.
2. IV device should be aseptically removed and the tip cut off with sterile scissors, placed in a dry sterile container, and immediately sent to the laboratory for analysis.
3. Check vital signs; reassure patient.
4. Obtain white blood cell count, as directed, and assess for other sites of infection (urine, sputum, wound).
5. Start appropriate antibiotic therapy immediately after receiving orders.
6. Document interventions and assessments.

Circulatory Overload

A. *Cause*
1. Delivery of excessive amounts of IV fluid (especially a risk for elderly patients, infants, or patients with cardiac or renal insufficiency).

B. *Clinical Manifestations*
1. Increased blood pressure and pulse
2. Increased CVP, venous distention (engorged neck veins)
3. Headache, anxiety
4. Shortness of breath, tachypnea, coughing
5. Pulmonary crackles
6. Chest pain (if history of coronary artery disease)

C. *Preventive Measures*
1. Know whether patient has existing heart or kidney condition. Be particularly vigilant in the high-risk patient.
2. Closely monitor infusion flow rate.
3. Splint arm or hand if IV flow rate fluctuates too widely with movement.

D. *Nursing Interventions*
1. Slow infusion to a ''keep-open'' rate and notify health care provider.
2. Monitor closely for worsening condition.
3. Raise patient's head to facilitate breathing.
4. Document interventions and assessments.

Air Embolism

A. *Causes*
1. A greater risk exists in central venous lines, when air enters catheter during tubing changes (air sucked in during inspiration due to negative intrathoracic pressure).

2. Air in tubing delivered by IV push or infused by infusion pump

B. *Clinical Manifestations*
1. Drop in blood pressure, elevated heart rate
2. Cyanosis, tachypnea
3. Rise in CVP
4. Changes in mentation, loss of consciousness

C. *Preventive Measures*
1. Clear all air from tubing before infusion to patient.
2. Change solution containers before they run dry.
3. Ensure that all connections are secure.
4. Use filter unless contraindicated.
5. Change IV tubing during expiration.

D. *Nursing Interventions*
1. Immediately turn patient on left side and lower head of bed; in this position, air will rise to right atrium.
2. Notify health care provider immediately.
3. Administer oxygen as needed.
4. Reassure patient.
5. Document interventions and assessments.

Mechanical Failure (Sluggish IV Flow)

A. *Causes*
1. Needle lying against the side of the vein, cutting off fluid flow
2. Clot at the end of the catheter or needle
3. Infiltration of IV cannula
4. Kinking of tubing or catheter

B. *Clinical Manifestations*
1. Sluggish IV flow
2. Alarm of flow regulator sounding
3. May be signs of local irritation—swelling, coolness of skin

C. *Preventive Measures*
1. Check IV often for patency, kinking, excessive movement by patient.
2. Secure IV well with tape and armboard, if necessary.

D. *Nursing Assessment and Interventions*
1. Remove tape and check for kinking of tubing or catheter.
2. Pull back cannula because it may be lying against wall of vein, vein valve, or vein bifurcation.
3. Elevate or lower needle to prevent occlusion of bevel.
4. Move patient's arm to new position.
5. Lower solution container below level of patient's heart and observe for blood backflow.
6. If electronic flow-rate regulator is in use, check its integrity.
7. If none of the preceding steps produces the desired flow, remove needle or catheter and restart infusion.

Hemorrhage

A. *Causes*
1. Loose connection of tubing or injection port
2. Inadvertent or accidental removal of peripheral or central catheter
3. Anticoagulant therapy

B. Clinical Manifestations
1. Oozing or trickling of blood from IV site or catheter
2. Hematoma

C. Preventive Measures
1. Cap all central lines with PRN adapters and connect tubing to the cap—not directly to the line.
2. Tape all catheters securely—use transparent dressing when possible for peripheral and central catheters. Then tape the remaining catheter lumens and tubing in a loop so tension is not directly on the catheter.
3. Keep pressure on sites where catheters have been removed—10 minutes for an anticoagulated patient.

Venous Thrombosis

The vein in which the peripheral or central catheter lies becomes partially or fully occluded by a thrombus.

A. Causes
1. Infusion of irritating solutions
2. Infection along catheter may preclude this syndrome.

B. Clinical Manifestations
1. Slowing of IV infusion or inability to draw blood from the central line
2. Swelling and pain in the area of catheter or in the extremity proximal to the IV line

C. Preventive Measures
1. Ensure proper dilution of irritating substances.

D. Nursing Interventions
1. Stop fluids immediately and notify health care provider.
2. Reassure patient and institute appropriate therapy:
   a. Anticoagulants
   b. Heat
   c. Elevation of affected extremity
   d. Antibiotics

PROCEDURE GUIDELINES 4-1 ◆ Venipuncture Using Needle or Catheter

EQUIPMENT

Rubber tourniquet
Disposable gloves
Antiseptic swab (alcohol, iodine, povidone-iodine)
If continuous infusion:
    IV solution
    Tubing
If heparin lock:
    Heparin lock cap
    Heparin or normal saline solution (1–2 mL) in sterile syringe

Tape
Transparent IV dressing or other dressing supplies
Covered armboard (if necessary)
Desired cannula:
    Catheter (Teflon, Silastic polyurethane, or polyvinylchloride) in chosen bore size (gauges 14–25)
    Winged ("butterfly") needle

Note: Thorough handwashing is required before handling sterile supplies and initiating venipuncture.

PROCEDURE

NURSING ACTION	RATIONALE
PREPARATORY PHASE	
1. Explain procedure to patient. Have patient lie in bed. Ascertain whether patient is left- or right-handed.	1. Helps alleviate anxiety about the procedure. Determining "handedness" of patient suggests the infusion be started in opposite arm if possible.
2. Clear all IV tubing of air; winged needle tubing as well (may clear air with fluid from infusion tubing by attaching needle to it, or by irrigating needle with saline in sterile syringe).	2. To prevent infusion of air and potential air embolus.
3. Don gloves.	3. Complies with CDC requirements to minimize passing of blood-borne pathogens between the patient and nurse.
4. Select site for insertion (see discussion on Site Selection, p. 60).	
5. Apply tourniquet 5–10 cm (2–6 inches) above desired insertion site and ascertain satisfactory distention of the vein. Distal pulses should remain palpable.	5. The vein must be visible or palpable before venipuncture is attempted. The tourniquet should not be applied too tightly as to interfere with arterial blood flow.
6. Have patient open and close fist several times.	6. To increase blood supply in the area. Further techniques to aid in vein distention are discussed on p. 61. A tourniquet may not be necessary on greatly distended veins.
7. Cleanse the site: a. Cleanse the skin with an alcohol swab. b. Prepare skin with povidone-iodine (an iodophor) swab for 1 min, working from the center of proposed site to the periphery until a circle of 5–10 cm (2–4 inches) has been disinfected. c. Allow area to air dry. d. Clip hair if site is too obscured.	7. To reduce number of skin microorganisms and minimize risk of infection. If a 1–2% iodine solution is used, it should be used to prep the skin first (30–60 s), allowed to dry.

PROCEDURE (cont'd)	NURSING ACTION	RATIONALE

PERFORMANCE PHASE: CATHETER INSERTION

1. Remove needle guard.
2. Grasp patient's arm so that the nurse's thumb is positioned approximately 5 cm (2 inches) from the site. Exert traction on skin in direction of hand.
3. Insert the needle, bevel up, through the skin at a 45° angle. Use a slow, continuous motion.
4. If the vessel rolls, it may be necessary to penetrate the skin first at a 20° angle and then apply a second thrust parallel to the skin.
5. When the vein is entered, lower the catheter to skin level.
6. When inserting, always hold the catheter by the clear plastic flashback chamber and not by the colored hub.
7. Advance the catheter approximately 0.6–1.3 cm. (¼–½ inch) into the vein.
8. Pull back on needle to separate needle from catheter 0.6 cm. (about ¼ inch) and advance catheter into vein.
9. If resistance is met while attempting to thread catheter, stop, release tourniquet, and carefully remove both needle and catheter. Attempt another venipuncture with a *new* catheter.

2. To stabilize the vein and facilitate successful cannulation.

3. Bevel up position allows for the smallest and sharpest point of the needle to enter the vein first.
4. Satisfactory penetration is evidenced by a sudden decrease in resistance and by appearance of blood coming back into syringe.
5. This will prevent puncturing through the vessel wall.

7. To ensure entry into the vein.

8. Pulling back on needle prevents inadvertent puncture of vein and provides stability of catheter for insertion.
9. The catheter may have become dislodged or encountered a turn or valve in the vein. It is better to start again than to cause further damage to vessel.

NURSING ALERT: ◆◆◆
Never reinsert stylet back into catheter once it has been removed. You may puncture or sever catheter.

a. Alternately, if catheter does not freely advance, attach IV tubing or heparin lock and flush, attempting to float catheter into vein.
10. Apply pressure on vein beyond catheter tip with the small or ring finger (see accompanying figure); release tourniquet and slowly remove needle while holding catheter hub in place.

a. Flow of flush solution may advance catheter.

10. This will reduce blood leakage while removing needle and connecting tubing to infusion set.

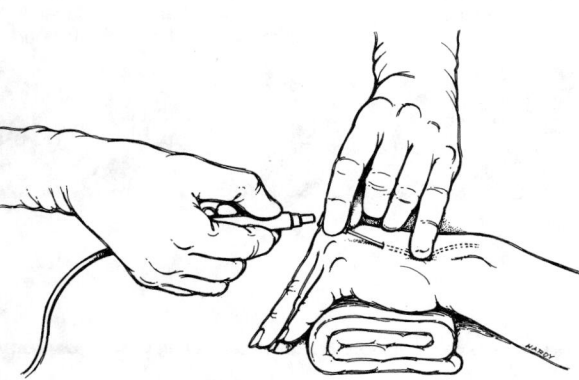

Finger palpation of dorsal venous arch.

11. *If an IV,* attach the cleared administration set to the hub of the catheter and adjust the infusion flow at the prescribed rate.
12. *If a heparin lock,* attach heparin lock cap, taking care to maintain sterility of the cap. Flush with 0.5 mL heparin or normal saline solution.

(continued)

PROCEDURE GUIDELINES 4-1 ◆ Venipuncture Using Needle or Catheter
(continued)

PROCEDURE (cont'd)	NURSING ACTION	RATIONALE
	13. Apply transparent dressing to site or use dressing according to institutional protocol (see accompanying figure).	13. Transparent dressing secures IV catheter in place and prevents infection.
	14. Loop tubing and tape to dressing or arm.	14. Prevents tension on IV catheter itself.

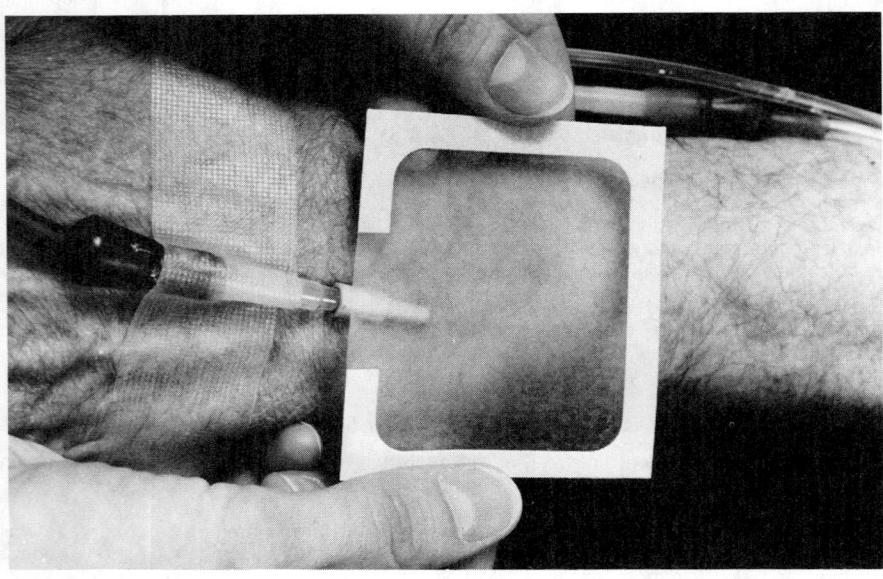

Transparent IV dressing.

	15. Label strip of tape with an arrow indicating the path of the catheter, size of catheter, date, time of insertion and inserter's initials. Affix to dressing. Prepare similar label with each dressing change.	15. Labeling of dressing is dictated by hospital policy. Such a practice provides information useful in determining next dressing change and capability of needle to accommodate various types of infusion.

NURSING ALERT:
Standard dwell time for short peripheral catheter is 3 days. However, exceptions may be made due to patient's venous access, type of solution, and catheter material. If the catheter is not rotated according to institution policy, document reason.

PROCEDURE GUIDELINES 4-2 ◆ Heparin Lock

Heparin lock is an intermittent infusion reservoir that permits administration of periodic IV medications and solution without continuous fluid administration and aspiration of blood samples for laboratory analysis.

EQUIPMENT

Antiseptic swabs (usually alcohol)
2 syringes containing 2 mL sterile normal saline solution
Tape (if "piggyback" medication is to be infused)
Unsterile gloves

Optional:
Syringe containing 1–2 mL heparin solution 1:10 units/ mL

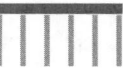

PROCEDURE TO ADMINISTER MEDICATION

NURSING ACTION	RATIONALE
1. Wash hands.	
2. Explain procedure to patient.	2. To minimize patient anxiety.
3. Don gloves.	
4. Cleanse port of the heparin lock with alcohol. Insert normal saline syringe needle into port and aspirate slightly.	4. Use either a protected needle or a blunt-end syringe to access port. This equipment avoids accidental needle sticks. If small gauge catheter does not show a positive blood return, monitor site carefully.
5. Inject normal saline solution slowly to flush reservoir of saline or heparin solution and blood.	5. Not all institutions use heparin to maintain peripheral locks.
6. Check with patient to ensure no pain on flushing.	6. May indicate a clot or infiltration.
7. Check for swelling at needle site when flushing.	7. May indicate a clot or infiltration.
8. Insert medication tubing, administer drug, infuse at prescribed rate.	
9. Following drug or solution administration, insert saline syringe and flush reservoir slowly. Remove needle while still pushing plunger of syringe to ensure positive pressure.	9. To prevent blood clotting in the IV cannula. Central venous catheters require greater than 2.5 mL of solution to be effective.
10. Optional: Insert heparin solution into reservoir.	

FOLLOW-UP PHASE

1. Maintain patency of heparin lock by flushing it q8–12 h, regardless of use.	1. If resistance is met, device should not be flushed. Attempt to remove occlusion via aspiration. If unable to restore patency, remove IV device.
2. IV administration set for intermittent therapy should be changed according to institutional policy. A new sterile needle should be used for each entry into the heparin lock. The tubing should only be used for the same medication.	2. It is recommended that the tubing be changed q24 h because the tubing is not maintained as a closed system and therefore poses a risk for infection.

PROCEDURE GUIDELINES 4-3 ◆ Setting Up an Automatic Intravenous "Piggyback"

EQUIPMENT
Sterile infusion set (primary)
Sterile infusion set (secondary)
Alcohol prep pad
Admixture

PROCEDURE
Follow procedure of particular manufacturer of "piggyback" infusion set.
In general, most procedures are similar to the following:

NURSING ACTION	RATIONALE
1. Wash hands thoroughly.	1. Minimizes possibility of infection.
2. Set up primary infusion set; this may have a check-valve (see A in accompanying figure).	2. The primary set should be functioning effectively before the secondary (piggyback) set can be attached.
3. Lower the primary flask on the IV pole; usually, an extension hook accompanies the set.	3. This will permit the check-valve to function.

(continued)

PROCEDURE GUIDELINES 4-3 ◆ Setting Up an Automatic Intravenous "Piggyback" (continued)

PROCEDURE (cont'd)	NURSING ACTION	RATIONALE

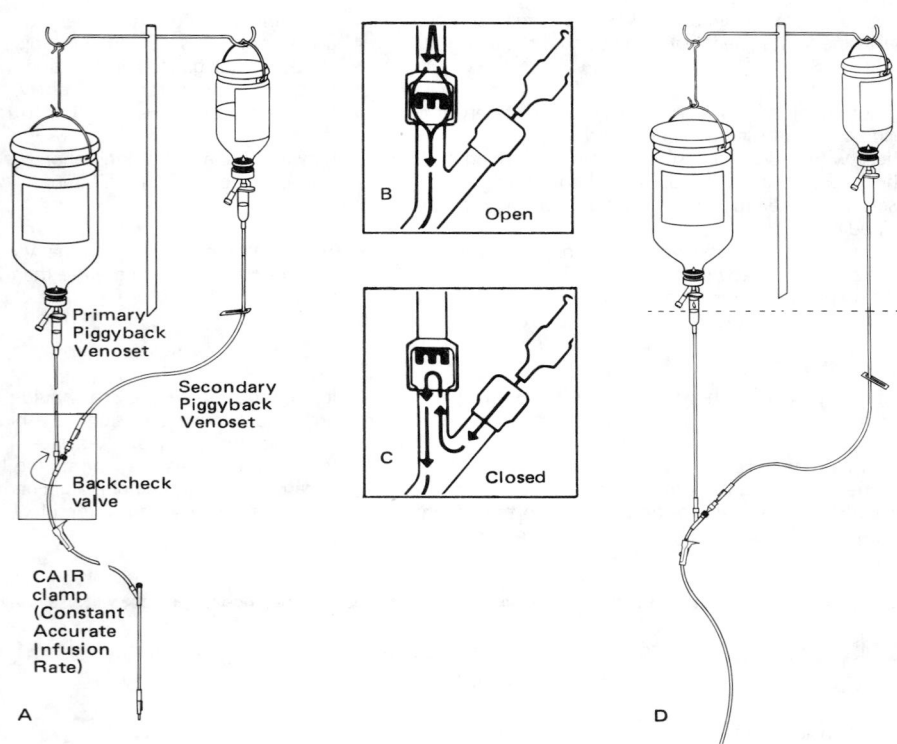

(**A**) "Piggyback" IV. On left is the primary infusion flask. Note use of extension hook (hanging from IV pole) to suspend primary flask. Backcheck valve is seen more clearly in B and C. Secondary "piggyback" source is seen on the right. (**B**) Open check-valve. Fluid from primary source flows down on either side of movable disc. Fluid from secondary source is closed off with clamp (not visible). (**C**) Closed check-valve. Note that fluid source from secondary flask (where pressure is greater because flask source is higher) is forcing movable disc upward, thereby closing off fluid from primary source. (**D**) When last of fluid from secondary source reaches the level of the fluid in the primary set drip chamber (as indicated by broken line), hydrostatic pressure between both sets will equalize. This releases check-valve; flow will shift from secondary to primary source. (Adapted from Abbott Laboratories)

4. Use alcohol swab to carefully cleanse injection site.
5. Attach secondary tubing to primary tubing—preferably with a protected needle—at entry port.
6. Lower secondary bottle, open clamp, and allow infusate from primary bottle to prime secondary tubing. Close clamp.
7. Then hang secondary bottle higher than primary solution. Open roller clamp (see D in accompanying figure).
8. Program pump or controller for rate of infusion for secondary medication.

FOLLOW-UP PHASE

1. Change IV administration tubing according to your institutional guidelines.
2. If possible, do not disattach secondary tubing from primary after infusion regimen started.

4. Usually this is a Y-connection on the primary site.

6. This clears secondary tubing of air and prevents any loss of medication from secondary line.

8. To ensure medication administration over appropriate time period.

2. If using more than one secondary medication, the same tubing may be used. Back-flush tubing into old secondary bag or bottle. Dispose of bag or bottle. Hang new secondary medication to same tubing.

PROCEDURE GUIDELINES 4-4 ◆ Accessing an Implanted Port

Implanted ports are becoming increasingly popular for patients with diseases such as cancer, sickle cell anemia, or cystic fibrosis to administer medications and continuous or intermittent IV fluids.

EQUIPMENT
5–10-mL syringes filled with normal saline
Noncoring Huber needle
Heparin flush solution 1:100 units/mL

Alcohol prep pads
3 povidone-iodine swab sticks
Sterile gloves

PROCEDURE

NURSING ACTION	RATIONALE
1. Wash hands thoroughly.	
2. Explain procedure to patient.	2. To minimize anxiety and facilitate learning.
3. Palpate port—feel septum.	3. To ensure placement and patency.
4. Select appropriate Huber needle—gauge and length.	
5. Flush Huber needle and extension with normal saline, leaving 5-mL syringe attached, being careful not to touch needle with unsterile gloves or fingers.	5. Priming of needle is essential to prevent infusion of air and ensure patency.
6. Don sterile gloves and cleanse site with alcohol and 3 povidone-iodine swabs. Allow to dry.	6. To prevent introduction of organisms into central line.
7. Grasp Huber needle with one hand and stabilize port with other hand—again locating septum.	
8. With a firm, steady motion, insert needle into port.	
9. Aspirate. If unable to aspirate, flush port with saline and try to aspirate blood again.	9. By aspirating first, you withdraw heparin solution that has been in port.
10. After aspirating blood, flush with 10 mL normal saline.	10. Presence of blood confirms correct needle placement in port.
11. If still no blood return, repeat port access or report findings to health care provider.	11. May order a radiologic study or urokinase declotting procedure.
12. When placement of needle confirmed, attach IV or "heparin lock" the port.	

FOLLOW-UP PHASE
1. Maintain patency by flushing according to your institutional guidelines. Change needle every 7 days.
2. Instruct patient to have port flushed monthly and notify health care provider of any problems.

Selected References

Fontaine, P. J. (1991, March/April). Performance of a new softening expanding midline catheter in home intravenous therapy. *Journal of Intravenous Therapy, 14,* 91-99.

Green, L., & Gerlach, C. J. (1994, May). Central lines have moved out. *RN, 57,* 26-31.

Hastings-Tolsma, M. & Yucha, C. (1994). IV infiltration: no clear signs, no treatment? *RN, 57* (12), 34-37.

Holcombe, B. J., Forloines-Lynn, S., & Garmhausen, L. W. (1992, January/February). Restoring patency of long-term central venous access devices. *Journal of Intravenous Therapy, 15,* 36-41.

Metheny, N. M. (1992). *Fluid and electrolyte balance* (2nd ed.). Philadelphia: J. B. Lippincott.

Messner, R. L. (1992, June). Preventing a peripheral I.V. infection. *Nursing 92, 22,* 34-41.

Orr, M. E., & Ryder, M. A. (1993, August). Vascular access devices: Perspectives on designs, complications, and management. *Nutrition in Clinical Practice, 8,* 145-152.

Richardson, D., & Brusso, P. (1993, January/February). Vascular access devices: Management of common complications. *Journal of Intravenous Therapy, 16,* 44-49.

Weinstein, S. M. (1993). *Plumer's Principles and Practice of Intravenous Therapy* (5th ed.). Philadelphia: J. B. Lippincott.

Winters, V., Peters, B., Coila, S., & Jones, L. (1990). A trial with a new peripheral implanted vascular device. *Oncology Nursing Forum, 17,* 891-896.

CHAPTER 5

Perioperative Nursing

Perioperative Overview

◆ INTRODUCTORY INFORMATION

Perioperative nursing is a term used to describe the nursing functions in the total surgical experience of the patient: preoperative, intraoperative, and postoperative.

Preoperative phase—from the time the decision is made for surgical intervention to the transfer of the patient to the operating room.

Intraoperative phase—from the time the patient is received in the operating room until admitted to the recovery room.

Postoperative phase—from the time of admission to the recovery room to the follow-up home/clinic evaluation.

Types of Surgery

1. *Optional*—Surgery is scheduled completely at the preference of the patient (eg, cosmetic surgery).
2. *Elective*—The approximate time for surgery is at the convenience of the patient; failure to have surgery is not catastrophic (eg, superficial cyst).
3. *Required*—The condition requires surgery within a few weeks (eg, eye cataract).
4. *Urgent*—The surgical problem requires attention within 24 to 48 hours (eg, cancer).
5. *Emergency*—Situation requires immediate surgical attention without delay (eg, intestinal obstruction).

Common surgical incisions are pictured in Figure 5-1.

◆ AMBULATORY (DAY) SURGERY

Ambulatory surgery (day surgery, in-and-out surgery, outpatient surgery) is becoming a common occurrence for certain types of procedures. The office nurse is in a key position to assess patient status; plan perioperative experience; and monitor, instruct, and evaluate the patient.

Advantages

1. Reduced cost to patient, hospital, and insuring and governmental agencies
2. Reduced psychological stress to the patient
3. Less evidence of hospital-acquired infection
4. Less time lost from work by patient; minimal disruption of patient's activities and family life

Disadvantages

1. Less time to assess patient and perform preoperative teaching
2. Less time to establish rapport between patient and health personnel
3. Less opportunity to assess for late postoperative complications. This responsibility is primarily with the patient although telephone and home care follow-up is possible.

Patient Selection

Criteria for selection include:

1. Surgery of short duration (15–90 minutes)
2. Noninfected conditions
3. Type of operation in which postoperative complications are predictably low
4. Age is usually not a factor although too risky in a premature infant
5. Types of frequently performed procedures:
   a. Ear-nose-throat (ENT; tonsillectomy, adenoidectomy)
   b. Gynecology (diagnostic laparoscopy, tubal ligation, dilatation and curettage)
   c. Orthopedics (arthroscopy, fracture or tendon repair)
   d. Oral surgery (wisdom teeth extraction, dental restorations)
   e. Urology (circumcision, cystoscopy, vasectomy)
   f. Ophthalmology (cataract)
   g. Plastic surgery (rhinoplasty, blepharoplasty, face lift)
   h. General surgery (laparoscopic hernia repair, lap-assisted cholecystectomy, biopsy, cyst removal)

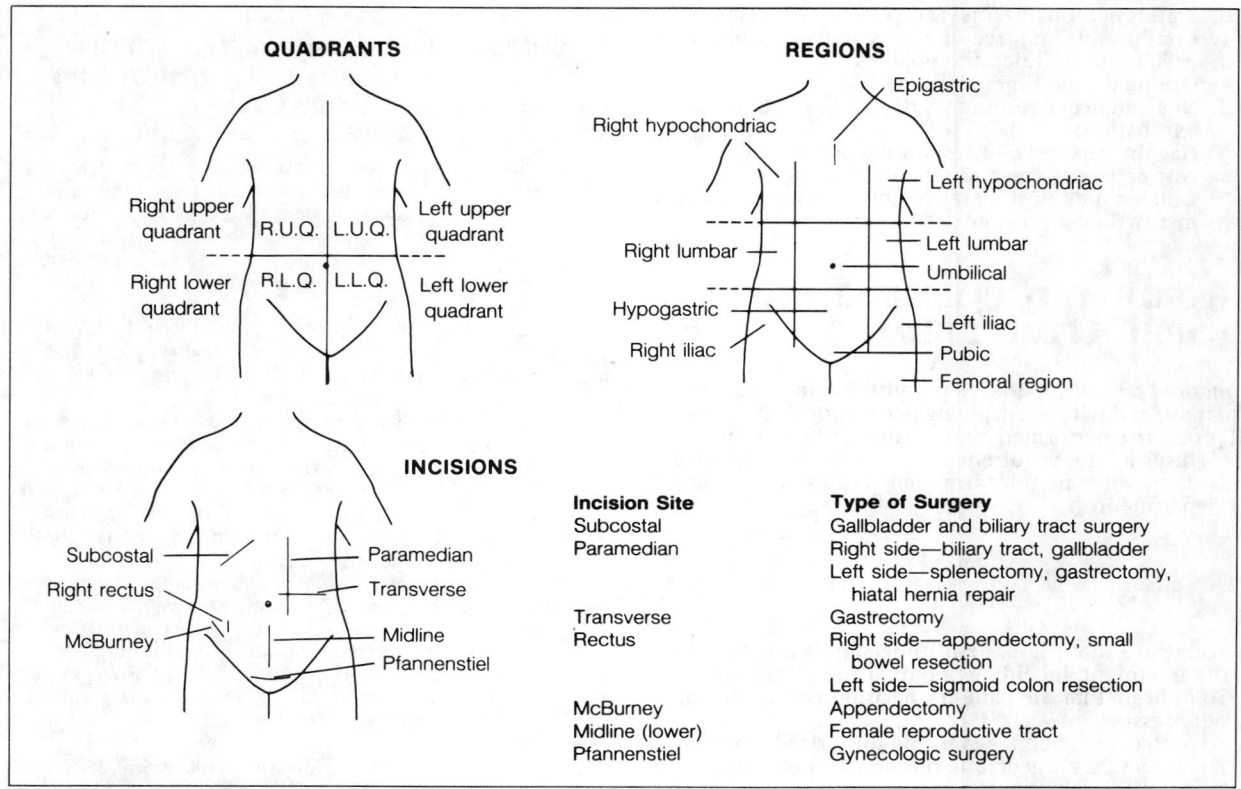

FIGURE 5-1 *Regions and incisions of the abdomen.*

Ambulatory Surgery Settings

Ambulatory surgery is performed in a variety of settings. A high percentage of outpatient surgery occurs in traditional hospital operating rooms in hospital-integrated facilities. Other ambulatory surgery settings may be hospital affiliated or independently owned and operated. Some types of outpatient surgeries can be performed safely in the health care provider's office.

Nursing Management

A. Initial Assessment
1. Develop a nursing history for the day surgical patient; this may be initiated in the health care provider's office.
2. Obtain a signed informed consent form.
3. Explain what laboratory studies are needed and why.
4. Determine the following during initial assessment of the patient's physical and psychological status: Calm or agitated? Overweight? Disabilities or limitations? Clean or dirty? Allergies? Medications being taken? Condition of teeth (dentures, caps, crowns)? Blood pressure problems? Major illnesses? Other surgeries? Seizures? Severe headaches? Smoker?
5. Begin health education regimen. Instructions to patient:

   a. Notify health care provider and surgical unit immediately if you get a cold, have a fever, or have any illness before date of surgery.
   b. Arrive at specified time.
   c. Do not ingest food or fluid from midnight previous to day of surgery.
   d. Do not wear make-up or nail polish.
   e. Wear comfortable, loose clothing and low-heeled shoes.
   f. Leave valuables or jewelry at home.
   g. Brush teeth in morning, rinse, but do not swallow liquid.
   h. Shower the night before or day of surgery.
   i. Have a responsible adult accompany you and drive you home—have person stay with you for 24 hours after surgery.

B. Preoperative Preparation
1. Administer preanesthetic medication; check vital signs.
2. Escort the patient to surgery after patient has urinated.

C. Postoperative Care
1. Check vital signs frequently until stable.
2. Administer oxygen if necessary; check temperature.
3. Change patient's position and progress activity—head of bed elevated, dangling, ambulating. Watch for dizziness or nausea.
4. Ascertain, using the following criteria, that the patient has recovered adequately to be discharged:
   a. Vital signs stable for at least 1 hour

b. Stands without dizziness and nausea; begins to walk
c. Comfortable and free of excessive pain or bleeding
d. Able to drink fluids and void
e. Oriented as to time, place, person
f. No evidence of respiratory depression (2 hours after extubation)
g. Has the services of a responsible adult who can escort patient home and remain at home
h. Understands postoperative instructions and takes instruction sheet home (Box 5-1)

◆ INFORMED CONSENT (OPERATIVE PERMIT)

An *informed consent* (operative permit) is a form signed by the patient, and witnessed, giving permission to have a surgical procedure performed by the patient's health care provider. This is a legal requirement. Hospitals usually have a standard operative permit form approved by the hospital's legal department.

Purposes

1. To ensure that the patient understands the nature of the treatment, including potential complications
2. To indicate that the patient's decision was made without pressure
3. To protect the patient against unauthorized procedures
4. To protect the surgeon and hospital against legal action by a patient who claims that an unauthorized procedure was performed

Adolescent Patient and Informed Consent

1. An emancipated minor is usually recognized as one who is not subject to parental control:
   a. Married minor
   b. Those in military service
   c. College student under 18 but living away from home
   d. Minor who has a child
2. Most states have statutes regarding treatment of minors.
3. Standards for informed consent are the same as for adults.

Procedures Requiring a Permit

1. Surgical procedures where scalpel, scissors, suture, hemostats, or electrocoagulation may be used
2. Entrance into a body cavity, such as paracentesis, bronchoscopy, cystoscopy
3. Radiologic procedure, particularly if contrast material is required (eg, myelogram, magnetic resonance imaging with contrast, angiography)
4. General anesthesia, local infiltration, and regional block

---

> **BOX 5-1** *Outpatient Postanesthesia and Postsurgery Instructions and Information*
>
> 1. Although you will be awake and alert in the Recovery Room, small amounts of anesthetic will remain in your body for at least 24 hours and you may feel tired and sleepy for the remainder of the day. Once you are home, take it easy and rest as much as possible. It is advisable to have someone with you at home for the remainder of the day.
> 2. Eat lightly for the first 12 to 24 hours, then resume a well-balanced, normal diet. Drink plenty of fluids. Alcoholic beverages are to be avoided for 24 hours after your anesthesia or intravenous sedation.
> 3. Nausea or vomiting may occur in the first 24 hours. Lie down on your side and breathe deeply. Prolonged nausea, vomiting, or pain should be reported to your surgeon.
> 4. Medications, unless prescribed by your physician, should be avoided for 24 hours. Check with your surgeon or anesthesiologist for specific instructions if you have been taking a daily medication.
> 5. Your surgeon will discuss your postsurgery instructions with you and prescribe medication for you as indicated. You will also receive additional instructions specific to your surgical procedure prior to leaving the hospital.
> 6. Your family will be waiting for you in the hospital's waiting room area near the Outpatient Surgery Department. Your surgeon will speak to them in this area prior to your discharge.
> 7. DO NOT OPERATE A MOTOR VEHICLE OR ANY MECHANICAL OR ELECTRICAL EQUIPMENT FOR *24 HOURS* AFTER YOUR ANESTHESIA.
> 8. DO NOT MAKE ANY IMPORTANT DECISIONS OR SIGN LEGAL DOCUMENTS FOR 24 HOURS FOLLOWING YOUR ANESTHESIA.
>
> (Courtesy of Doctor's Hospital of Prince George's County, Lanham, Maryland)

Obtaining Informed Consent

1. Before signing an informed consent, the patient should:
   a. Be told in clear and simple terms by the surgeon or other appropriate personnel (eg, anesthesiologist) what is to be done.
   b. Be aware of the risks, possible complications, disfigurement, and removal of parts.
   c. Have a general idea of what to expect in the early and late postoperative periods.
   d. Have a general idea of the time frame involved from surgery to recovery.
   e. Have an opportunity to ask any questions.
   f. Sign a separate form for each procedure or operation.
2. Written permission is best and is legally acceptable.
3. Signature is obtained with the patient's complete understanding of what is to occur; it is obtained before the patient receives sedation and is secured without pressure or duress.

4. A witness is desirable—nurse, health care provider, or other authorized person.
5. In an emergency, permission via telephone or telegram is acceptable.
6. For a minor (or a patient who is unconscious or irresponsible), permission is required from a responsible member of the family—parent or legal guardian.
7. For married minor, permission from the husband or wife is acceptable.
8. If the patient is unable to write, an "X" to indicate his sign is acceptable if there are two signed witnesses to his mark.

◆ SURGICAL RISK FACTORS AND PREVENTIVE STRATEGIES

Obesity

A. *Danger*
1. Increases difficulty involved in technical aspects of performing surgery (eg, sutures are difficult to tie because of fatty secretions); wound dehiscence is greater.
2. Increases likelihood of infection because of lessened resistance.
3. Increases postoperative pneumonia and other pulmonary complications because greatly obese patients chronically hypoventilate.
4. Increases demands on the heart, leading to cardiovascular compromise.
5. Increases possibility of renal, biliary, hepatic, and endocrine disorders.
6. Decreases ability to conserve heat due to radiant heat loss.
7. Has altered response to many drugs and anesthetics.

B. *Therapeutic Approach*
1. Encourage weight reduction if time permits.
2. Consult with health care provider about obtaining preoperative pulmonary function test and arterial blood gases (to assess baseline pulmonary status).
3. Anticipate postoperative obesity-related complications.
4. Be extremely vigilant for respiratory complications.
5. Carefully splint abdominal incisions when moving or coughing; for large patients, sling a drawsheet around the patient's back and pull ends firmly together in front.
6. Be aware that some drugs should be dosed according to ideal body weight versus actual weight, or an overdose may occur (eg, digoxin [Lanoxin], lidocaine [Xylocaine], aminoglycosides, and theophylline [Theo-Dur]).
7. Avoid intramuscular injections in morbidly obese individuals (intravenous [IV] or subcutaneous routes preferred).
8. Never attempt to move an impaired patient without assistance or without using proper body mechanics.
9. Obtain dietary consultation early in patient's postoperative course.

Poor Nutrition

A. *Danger*
1. Preoperative malnutrition (especially protein and calorie deficits) greatly impairs wound healing.
2. Increases the risk of infection and shock.

B. *Therapeutic Approach*
1. Any recent (within 4–6 weeks) weight loss of 10% of patient's normal body weight should alert health care staff to poor nutritional status.
2. Attempt to improve nutritional status before and after surgery. Unless contraindicated, provide diet high in proteins, calories, and vitamins (especially vitamins C and A); this may require enteral and parenteral feeding.
3. Recommend repair of dental caries and proper mouth hygiene to prevent respiratory tract infection.

Fluid and Electrolyte Imbalance

A. *Danger*
Dehydration and electrolyte imbalances can have adverse effects in terms of general anesthesia and the anticipated volume losses associated with surgery; this can cause shock and cardiac dysrhythmias.

NURSING ALERT:
Patients undergoing major abdominal operations (eg, colectomies, aortic repairs) often experience a massive fluid shift into tissues around the operative site in the form of edema (as much as a liter may be lost from circulation). Watch for the fluid shift to reverse (from tissue to circulation) around the third postoperative day. Patients with heart disease may develop failure due to the excess fluid "load."

B. *Therapeutic Approach*
1. Scrupulously assess patient's fluid and electrolyte status.
2. Rehydrate patient parenterally and orally as prescribed.
3. Monitor for evidence of electrolyte imbalance, especially Na^+, K^+, Mg^{++}, Ca^{++}.
4. Be aware of expected drainage amounts and composition; report excess and abnormalities.
5. Monitor the patient's intake and output; be sure to include all body fluid losses.

Aging

A. *Danger*
1. Recognize that reactions to injury are not as obvious and are slower in appearing.
2. Be aware that the cumulative effect of medications is greater in the older person than it is in younger people.
3. Note that medications such as morphine and barbiturates in the usual dosages may cause confusion and disorientation; morphine may cause more noticeable respiratory depression than with the younger patient.

B. *Therapeutic Approach*
1. Consider using lesser doses for desired effect.
2. Anticipate problems from chronic disorders such as anemia, obesity, diabetes, hypoproteinemia.
3. Adjust nutritional intake to conform to higher protein and vitamin needs.
4. When possible, cater to set patterns in older patients, such as sleeping and eating.

Presence of Cardiovascular Disease

A. Danger
Many surgical problems may be complicated in the presence of cardiovascular compromise.

B. Therapeutic Approach
1. Maintain increased diligence in nursing assessment.
2. Avoid fluid overload (oral, parenteral, blood products) because of possible myocardial infarction, angina, congestive failure, and pulmonary edema.
3. Prevent prolonged immobilization, which results in venous stasis. Monitor for potential deep vein thrombosis or pulmonary embolus.
4. Encourage change of position but avoid sudden exertion.
5. Use antiembolic hose and pneumatic stockings intraoperatively and postoperatively.
6. Note evidence of hypoxia and initiate therapy.

Presence of Diabetes Mellitus

A. Danger
Hyperglycemia is potentiated by increased catecholamines and glucocorticoids due to surgical stress.

B. Therapeutic Approach
1. Recognize the signs and symptoms of ketoacidosis and glucosuria, which can threaten an otherwise smooth surgical experience.
2. Reassure the diabetic patient that when the disease is controlled, the surgical risk may be no greater than it is for the nondiabetic person.

Presence of Alcoholism

A. Danger
Additional problem of malnutrition may be present in the presurgical patient with alcoholism. The patient may also have an increased tolerance to anesthetics.

B. Therapeutic Approach
1. Be prepared to perform gastric lavage on the intoxicated patient if surgery cannot be postponed; this may lessen the chance of vomiting and aspiration during anesthesia induction.
2. Note that risk due to surgery is greater for the individual who has chronic alcoholism.
3. Anticipate the acute withdrawal syndrome (delirium tremens) within 72 hours of the last alcoholic drink.

Presence of Pulmonary and Upper Respiratory Disease

A. Danger
Surgery may be contraindicated in the patient who has an upper respiratory infection because it might potentiate a more serious illness, such as pneumonia.

B. Therapeutic Approach
1. Patients with chronic pulmonary problems such as emphysema or bronchiectasis should be treated for several days preoperatively with bronchodilators, aerosol medications, and conscientious mouth care, along with a reduction in weight and smoking, and methods to control secretions.
2. Chronic pulmonary disease increases the risk of atelectasis and pneumonia and potentiates respiratory depression from narcotics.

Concurrent or Prior Pharmacotherapy

A. Danger
Hazards exist when certain medications are given concomitantly with others (eg, interaction of some drugs with anesthetics can lead to arterial hypotension and circulatory collapse).

B. Therapeutic Approach
1. An awareness of drug therapy is essential.
2. Notify health care provider and anesthesiologist if the patient is taking any of the following drugs:
    a. Certain antibiotics may interrupt nerve transmission when combined with a curariform muscle relaxant. This may cause respiratory paralysis and apnea.
    b. Antidepressants, particularly monoamine oxidase inhibitors (MAOs), increase hypotensive effects of anesthesia.
    c. Phenothiazines increase hypotensive action of anesthesia.
    d. Diuretics, particularly thiazides, cause electrolyte imbalance and respiratory depression during anesthesia.
    e. Steroids inhibit wound healing.

Preoperative Care

◆ PATIENT EDUCATION

Patient education is a vital component of the surgical experience. *Preoperative patient education* may be offered through conversation, discussion, the use of audiovisual aids, demonstrations, and return demonstrations. It is designed to help the patient understand the surgical experience to minimize anxiety and promote full recovery from surgery and anesthesia. The educational program may be initiated before hospitalization by the physician, nurse practitioner or office nurse, or other designated personnel. This is particularly important for patients who are admitted the day of surgery or undergo outpatient surgical procedures. The perioperative nurse can assess the patient's knowledge base and use this information in developing a plan for an uneventful perioperative course.

Teaching Strategies

A. Obtain a Data Base
1. Determine what the patient already knows or wants to know. This can be accomplished by reading the patient's chart, by interviewing the patient, and by com-

municating with the health care provider, family, and other members of the health team.

2. Ascertain patient's psychosocial adjustment to impending surgery.
3. Determine cultural or religious health beliefs and practices that may have an impact on the patient's surgical experience, such as refusal of blood transfusions, burial of amputated limbs within 24 hours, or special healing rituals.

B. *Plan and Implement Teaching Program*
1. Begin at the patient's level of understanding and proceed from there.
2. Plan a presentation, or series of presentations, for this individual patient or a group of patients.
3. Include family members and significant others in the teaching process.
4. Encourage active participation of patients in their care and recovery.
5. Demonstrate essential techniques; provide opportunity for patient practice and return demonstration.
6. Provide time for and encourage patient to ask questions and express concerns; make every effort to answer all questions truthfully and in basic agreement with the overall therapeutic plan.
7. Provide general information and assess the patient's level of interest in or reaction to it.
   a. Explain details of preoperative preparation and provide tour of area and view of equipment when possible.
   b. Offer general information on the surgery. Explain that the health care provider is the primary resource person.
   c. Tell when surgery is scheduled (if known) and approximately how long it will take; explain that afterward the patient will go to the recovery room. Emphasize that delays may be attributed to many factors other than a problem developing with this patient (eg, previous case in the operating room may have taken longer than expected or an emergency case has been given priority).
   d. Let patient know that family will be kept informed and that they will be told where to wait and when they can see patient; note visiting hours.
   e. Explain how a procedure or test may feel during or after.
   f. Describe the recovery room; what personnel and equipment the patient may expect to see and hear (specially trained personnel, monitoring equipment, tubing for various functions, and a moderate amount of activity by nurses and health care providers).
   g. Stress the importance of active participation in postoperative recovery.
8. Use other resource persons: health care providers, therapists, chaplain, interpreters, and so forth.
9. Document what has been taught or discussed, as well as the patient's reaction and level of understanding.

C. *Use Audiovisual Aids if Available*
1. Videotapes with sound or film strips with narration are effective in giving basic information to a single patient or group of patients. Many hospitals provide a television channel dedicated to patient instruction.
2. Booklets, brochures, and models, if available, are helpful.
3. Demonstrate any equipment that will be specific for the particular patient. Examples:
   Drainage equipment

Monitoring equipment
Side rails
Incentive spirometer
Ostomy bag

General Instructions

Preoperatively, the patient will be instructed in the following postoperative activities. This will allow a chance for practice and familiarity.

A. *Diaphragmatic Breathing*
This is a mode of breathing in which the dome of the diaphragm is flattened during inspiration, resulting in enlargement of the upper abdomen as air rushes into the chest. During expiration, abdominal muscles and the diaphragm relax. It is an effective relaxation technique.
   Instruct the patient to:

1. Assume bed position similar to that most likely to be used postoperatively (semi-Fowler's).
2. Place both hands over lower rib cage; make a loose fist and rest the flat surface of the fingernails against the chest (to feel chest movement).
3. Exhale gently and fully; ribs will sink downward and inward toward midline.
4. Inhale deeply through mouth and nose; permit abdomen to rise as lungs fill with air.
5. Hold this breath through a count of 5.
6. Exhale and let all air out through mouth and nose.
7. Repeat 15 times with a brief rest following each group of five.
8. Practice this twice each day preoperatively.

B. *Incentive Spirometry*
Preoperatively, the patient uses a spirometer to measure deep breaths (inspired air) while exerting maximum effort. The preoperative measurement becomes the goal to be achieved as soon as possible after the operation.

1. Postoperatively, the patient is encouraged to use the incentive spirometer about 10 to 12 times an hour.
2. Deep inhalations expand alveoli, which, in turn, prevents atelectasis and other pulmonary complications.
3. There is less pain with inspiratory concentration than with expiratory concentration, such as with coughing and using blow bottles.

C. *Coughing*
Coughing promotes the removal of chest secretions. Instruct the patient to:

1. Interlace the fingers and place the hands over the proposed incision site; this will act as a splint during coughing and not harm the incision.
2. Lean forward slightly while sitting in bed.
3. Breathe, using the diaphragm as described under diaphragmatic breathing (see above, item A).
4. Inhale fully with the mouth slightly open.
5. Let out three or four sharp "hacks."
6. Then, with mouth open, take in a deep breath and quickly give one or two strong coughs.
7. Secretions should be readily cleared form the chest to prevent respiratory complications (pneumonia, obstruction). Note: Certain position changes may be contraindicated following some surgeries (eg, craniotomy and eye or ear surgery).

D. Turning
Changing positions from back to side-lying (and vice versa) stimulates circulation, encourages deeper breathing, and relieves pressure areas.

1. Assist the patient to move onto side if assistance is needed.
2. Place the uppermost leg in a more flexed position than that of the lower leg and place a pillow comfortably between the legs.
3. Ensure that the patient is turned from one side to back and onto the other side every 2 hours.

E. Foot and Leg Exercises
Moving the legs improves circulation and muscle tone.

1. Have the patient lie on back, instruct patient to bend the knee and raise the foot—hold it a few seconds, extend the leg, and lower it to the bed.
2. Repeat above for about five times with one leg and then with the other. Repeat the set five times every 3 to 5 hours.
3. Then have the patient lie on side; exercise the legs by pretending to pedal a bicycle.
4. Suggest the following foot exercise. Trace a complete circle with the great toe.

F. Evaluation of Teaching Program
1. Observe patient for correct demonstration of expected postoperative behaviors, such as foot and leg exercises and special breathing techniques.
2. Ask pertinent questions to determine patient's level of understanding.
3. Reinforce information when necessary.

◆ PREPARATION OF THE OPERATIVE AREA

Skin

1. Human skin normally harbors transient and resident bacterial flora, some of which are pathogenic.
2. Skin cannot be sterilized without destroying skin cells.
3. Friction enhances the action of detergent antiseptics; however, friction should not be applied over a superficial malignancy (causes seeding of malignant cells) or areas of carotid plaque (causes plaque dislodgment and emboli).
4. It is ideal for the patient to bathe or shower, using a bacteriostatic soap (eg, povidone-iodine), on the day of surgery. The surgical schedule may require that the shower be taken the night before.
5. The Centers for Disease Control and Prevention recommend that hair not be removed near the operative site unless it will interfere with surgery. Skin is easily injured during shaving and often results in a higher rate of postoperative wound infection.
6. If requested, shaving should be performed as close to the operative time as possible. The longer the interval between the shave and operation, the higher the incidence of postoperative wound infection.
   a. Use of electrical clippers is preferable. Hair should be removed within 1 to 2 mm of the skin to avoid skin abrasion. Thorough cleaning of the clippers, after use, is essential.
   b. A sharp disposable razor, with a recessed blade, may be used as long as a "wet shave" is done. It is im-

portant that the shave be done in the direction of hair growth.
   c. Depilatory creams (hair-removing chemicals) offer the advantage of eliminating possible abrasions and cuts and producing clean, smooth, intact skin. Many patients even find this form of skin preparation relaxing. The depilatory creams may cause transient skin reactions in some patients, especially when used near the rectal and scrotal areas.
   d. Scissors may be used to remove hair greater than 3 mm in length.
7. For head surgery, obtain specific instructions from the surgeon concerning the extent of shaving.

Gastrointestinal Tract

1. Preparation of the bowel is imperative for intestinal surgery because escaping bacteria can invade adjacent tissues and cause sepsis.
   a. Cathartics and enemas remove gross collections of stool.
   b. Oral antimicrobial agents (eg, neomycin, erythromycin) suppress the colon's potent microflora.
   c. Enemas "until clear" are prescribed the evening of elective surgery. Not more than three enemas should be given because of negative effects on fluid and electrolyte balance. (It is also exhausting to the patient.) Notify the health care provider if the enemas never return clear.
2. Solid food is withheld from the patient for 8 to 10 hours before surgery. Patients having morning surgery are kept NPO overnight. Clear fluids (water) may be given up to 4 hours of surgery if ordered.

Genitourinary Tract

A medicated douche may be prescribed preoperatively if the patient is to have a gynecologic (eg, hysterectomy) or urologic operation.

◆ PREOPERATIVE MEDICATION

Medication will be prescribed postoperatively to facilitate the following goals:
1. To facilitate the administration of any anesthetic
2. To minimize respiratory tract secretions and changes in heart rate
3. To relax the patient and reduce anxiety

Types

1. Opiates—such as morphine (Roxanol) and meperidine (Demerol) are given to relax the patient and potentiate anesthesia.
2. Anticholinergics—such as atropine, scopolamine, and glycopyrrolate (Robinul) are given primarily to reduce respiratory tract secretions and to prevent severe reflex slowing of the heart during anesthesia. Typically given in conjunction with an opiate less than an hour before the patient's trip to the operating room.
3. Barbiturates/tranquilizers—such as pentobarbital (Nembutal) and other hypnotic agents are given the

night before surgery to help ensure a restful night's sleep. It is important to note that reassurance from the nurse, anesthesiologist, and health care provider can do much to alleviate the patient's anxiety and insomnia.

4. Prophylactic antibiotics—are administered just before or during surgery when bacterial contamination is expected.

Administering "On Call" Medications

> **NURSING ALERT:**
> Administer preanesthetic medication precisely at the time it is prescribed. If given too early, the maximum potency will have passed before it is needed; if given too late, the action will not have begun before anesthesia is started.

1. Have medication ready and administer as soon as call is received from the operating room.
2. Proceed with remaining preparation activities.
3. Indicate on the chart or preoperative checklist the time when medication was administered and by whom.

◆ ADMITTING THE PATIENT TO SURGERY

Final Checklist

The preoperative checklist is the last procedure before taking the patient to the operating room. Most facilities have a standard form for this check.

A. Identification and Verification
This includes verbal and written documentation (eg, name band) of the patient's identity, the procedure to be performed, the surgeon, and the type of anesthesia.

B. Review of Patient Record
Check for inclusion of the face sheet, allergies, history and physical, completed preoperative checklist, laboratory values, including most recent ones, electrocardiogram (ECG) if necessary, chest x-rays, preoperative medications, and other preoperative orders by either the surgeon or anesthesiologist.

C. Consent Form
All nurses involved with patient care in the preoperative setting should be aware of the individual state laws regarding informed consent and the specific hospital policy. Obtaining informed consent is the responsibility of the surgeon performing the specific procedure. Consent forms should contain the stated procedure, the various risks, and alternatives to surgery, if any. It is a nursing responsibility to make sure the consent form has been obtained and is in the chart.

D. Patient Preparedness
1. NPO status
2. Proper attire (hospital gown)
3. Skin preparation
4. IV started with correct gauge needle
5. Dentures or plates removed
6. Jewelry, contact lenses, glasses removed and secured in locked area or given to family member
7. Allow patient to void.

Transporting Patient to the Operating Room

1. Adhere to the principle of maintaining the comfort and safety of the patient.
2. Accompany operating room attendants to the patient's bedside for introduction and proper identification.
3. Assist in transferring the patient from bed to stretcher (unless bed goes to operating room floor).
4. Complete chart and preoperative checklist; include laboratory reports and x-rays as required by hospital policy or health care provider's directive.
5. Recognize importance of coordinating team effort to ensure arrival of the patient in the operating room at the proper time.

The Patient's Family

1. Direct the patient's family to the proper waiting room where magazines, television, and coffee may be available.
2. Inform the family that the surgeon will probably contact them there immediately after surgery to inform them of the operation.
3. Acquaint the family with the fact that a long interval of waiting does not mean the patient is in the operating room all the while; anesthesia preparation and induction take time, and after surgery the patient is taken to the recovery room.
4. Tell the family what to expect postoperatively when they see the patient—tubes; monitoring equipment; and blood transfusion, suctioning, and oxygen equipment.

Intraoperative Care

◆ ANESTHESIA AND RELATED COMPLICATIONS

The goals of anesthesia are to provide analgesia, sedation, and muscle relaxation appropriate for the type of operative procedure, as well as to control the autonomic nervous system.

Common Anesthetic Techniques

A. Conscious Sedation
1. Patient remains conscious with some alteration of mood, drowsiness, and sometimes analgesia.
2. Protective reflexes remain intact.

B. Deep Sedation
1. Patient is asleep but easily arousable.
2. Protective reflexes are minimally depressed.

C. General Anesthesia
1. Complete loss of consciousness, unarousable
2. A reversible state that provides analgesia, muscle relaxation, and sedation
3. Protective reflexes partially or (more commonly) completely lost
4. Produced by IV or inhaled anesthetics

D. Regional Anesthesia
1. Production of analgesia in a specific body part
2. Achieved by placing local anesthetics in close proximity (usually by injection) to appropriate nerves

E. Spinal Anesthesia
1. Local anesthetic is injected into lumbar intrathecal space.
2. Anesthetic blocks conduction in spinal nerve roots and dorsal ganglia; paralysis and analgesia occur below level of injection.

F. Epidural Anesthesia
1. Achieved by injecting local anesthetic into extradural space via a lumbar puncture
2. Results similar to spinal analgesia

G. Peripheral Nerve Blocks
1. Achieved by injecting local anesthetic at a specific site to render a defined area of anesthesia

Intraoperative Complications

1. **Hypoventilation** (hypoxemia, hypercarbia)—inadequate ventilatory support following paralysis of respiratory muscles and ensuing coma
2. **Oral trauma** (broken teeth, oropharyngeal, or laryngeal trauma)—due to difficult endotracheal intubation
3. **Hypotension**—due to preoperative hypovolemia or untoward reactions to anesthetic agents
4. **Cardiac dysrhythmia**—due to preexisting cardiovascular compromise, electrolyte imbalance, or untoward reactions to anesthetic agents
5. **Hypothermia**—due to exposure to cool ambient operating room environment and loss of normal thermoregulation capability from anesthetic agents
6. **Peripheral nerve damage**—due to improper positioning of patient (eg, full weight on an arm) or restraints
7. **Malignant hyperthermia**
   a. This is a rare reaction to anesthetic inhalants (notably cyclopropane, enflurane, ether, fluroxene, halothane, isoflurane) and muscle relaxants (eg, succinylcholine [Anectine]).
   b. Such drugs as theophylline (Theo-Dur), aminophylline (Aminophyllin), epinephrine (Adrenalin), and digoxin (Lanoxin) may also induce or intensify this reaction.
   c. This deadly complication is most apt to occur in younger individuals with an inherited muscle disorder (eg, forms of muscular dystrophy) or a history of subluxating joints, scoliosis.
   d. Malignant hyperthermia is due to abnormal and excessive intracellular accumulations of calcium with resulting hypermetabolism and increased muscle contraction.
   e. Clinical manifestations—tachycardia, pseudotetany, muscle rigidity, high fever, cyanosis, heart failure, and central nervous system damage.
   f. Treatment—dantrolene sodium (Dantrium), oxygen, dextrose 50% (with extra insulin to enhance its utilization), diuretics, antiarrhythmics, sodium bicarbonate (for severe acidosis), and hypothermic measures (eg, cooling blanket, iced IV saline solutions, or iced saline lavages of stomach, bladder, or rectum).

Postoperative Care

◆ RECOVERY ROOM OR POSTANESTHESIA CARE UNIT (PACU)

To ensure continuity of care from the intraoperative phase to the immediate postoperative phase, the circulating nurse, anesthesiologist, or nurse anesthetist will give a thorough report to the PACU nurse. This should include the following:

1. Type of surgery performed and any intraoperative complications
2. Type of anesthesia (eg, general, local, sedation)
3. Drains and type of dressings
4. Presence of endotracheal (ET) tube or type of oxygen to be administered (eg, nasal cannula, T-piece)
5. Types of lines and locations (eg, peripheral IV, arterial line)
6. Catheters or tubes such as Foley, T-tube
7. Administration of blood, colloids, and fluid and electrolyte balance
8. Drug allergies
9. Preexisting medical conditions

Initial Nursing Assessment

Before receiving the patient, note proper functioning of monitoring and suctioning devices, oxygen therapy equipment, and all other equipment. The following initial assessment is made by the nurse in the PACU:

1. Verify the patient's identity, the operative procedure, and the surgeon who performed the procedure.
2. Evaluate the following signs and verify their level of stability with the anesthesiologist:
   a. Respiratory status
   b. Circulatory status
   c. Pulses
   d. Temperature
   e. Oxygen saturation level
   f. Hemodynamic values
3. Determine swallowing, gag reflexes, and level of consciousness, including patient's response to stimuli.
4. Evaluate any lines, tubes, or drains, estimated blood loss, condition of the wound (open, closed, packed), medications used, infusions, including transfusions, and output.
5. Evaluate the patient's level of comfort and safety by indicators such as pain and protective reflexes.
6. Perform safety checks to verify that padded side rails are in place, and restraints properly applied, as needed, for infusions, transfusions, etc.

7. Evaluate activity status; movement of extremities
8. Review health care provider's orders
Note: It is important for the nurse to know the patient's native language to provide an accurate assessment. Interpreters are available at many facilities.

Initial Nursing Diagnoses

A. Ineffective Airway Clearance related to effects of anesthesia
B. Impaired Gas Exchange related to ventilation perfusion imbalance
C. Altered Tissue Perfusion (Coronary) related to hypotension postoperatively
D. Risk for Altered Body Temperature related to medications, sedation, and cool environment
E. Risk for Fluid Volume Deficit related to blood loss, food and fluid deprivation, vomiting, and indwelling tubes
F. Pain related to surgical incision and tissue trauma
G. Impaired Skin Integrity related to invasive procedure, immobilization, and altered metabolic and circulatory state
H. Risk for Injury related to sensory dysfunction and physical environment
I. Sensory Alterations related to effects of medications and anesthesia

Initial Nursing Interventions

A. *Maintaining a Patent Airway*
1. Allow metal, rubber, or plastic airway to remain in place until the patient begins to waken and is trying to eject the airway.
  a. The airway keeps the passage open and prevents the tongue from falling backward and obstructing the air passages.
  b. Leaving the airway in after the pharyngeal reflex has returned may cause the patient to gag and vomit.
  Note: Many seriously ill patients return from the operating room with an endotracheal tube in place; this may be left in place for hours or days and requires special management.
2. Aspirate excessive secretions when they are heard in the nasopharynx and oropharynx.

B. *Maintaining Adequate Respiratory Function*
1. Place patient in the lateral position with neck extended (if not contraindicated), and the upper arm supported on a pillow.
  a. This will promote chest expansion.
  b. Turn the patient every hour or two to facilitate breathing and ventilation.
2. Encourage patient to take deep breaths to aerate lungs fully and prevent hypostatic pneumonia; use incentive spirometer to aid in this function.
3. Assess lung fields frequently by auscultation.
4. Evaluate periodically the patient's orientation—response to name or command.
  Note: Alterations in cerebral function may suggest impaired oxygen delivery to tissues.
5. Administer humidified oxygen if required.
  a. Heat and moisture are normally lost during exhalation.

  b. Dehydrated patients may require oxygen and humidity because of higher incidence of irritated respiratory passages in these patients.
  c. Secretions can be kept moist to facilitate removal.
6. Use mechanical ventilation to maintain adequate pulmonary ventilation if required.

C. *Assessing Status of Circulatory System*
1. Take vital signs (blood pressure, pulse, and respiration) frequently, as clinical condition indicates, until the patient is well stabilized. Then check every 4 hours thereafter or as ordered.
  a. Know the patient's preoperative blood pressure to make significant comparisons.
  b. Report immediately a falling systolic pressure and an increasing heart rate.
  c. Report variations in blood pressure, cardiac arrhythmias, and respirations over 30.
  d. Evaluate pulse pressure to determine status of perfusion. (A narrowing pulse pressure indicates impending shock.)
2. Monitor intake and output closely.
3. Recognize the variety of factors that may alter circulating blood volume.
  a. Reactions to anesthesia and medications
  b. Blood loss and organ manipulation during surgery
  c. Moving the patient from one position on the operating table to another on the stretcher
4. Recognize early symptoms of shock or hemorrhage.
  a. Cool extremities, decreased urine output (less than 30 mL/h), slow capillary refill (greater than 3 seconds), lowered blood pressure, narrowing of pulse pressure, and increased heart rate are often indicative of decreased cardiac output.
  b. Initiate oxygen therapy to increase oxygen availability from the circulating blood.
  c. Increase parenteral fluid infusion as prescribed.
  d. Place the patient in shock position with feet elevated (unless contraindicated).
  e. See Chapter 33 for more detailed consideration of shock.

D. *Assessing Thermoregulatory Status*
1. Monitor temperature hourly to be alert for malignant hyperthermia or to detect hypothermia.
2. A temperature over 37.7°C (100°F) or under 36.1°C (97°F) is reportable.
3. Monitor for postanesthesia shivering (PAS). It is most significant in hypothermic patients 30 to 45 minutes after admission to the PACU. It represents a heat-gain mechanism and relates to regaining thermal balance.
4. Provide a therapeutic environment with proper temperature and humidity; when cold, provide the patient with warm blankets.

E. *Maintaining Adequate Fluid Volume*
1. Administer IV solutions as ordered.
2. Monitor electrolytes and recognize evidence of imbalance, such as nausea and vomiting, weakness.
3. Evaluate mental status, skin color and turgor, and body temperature.
4. Recognize signs of fluid imbalance.
  a. Hypovolemia—decreased blood pressure and urine output, decreased central venous pressure (CVP), increased pulse
  b. Hypervolemia—increased blood pressure, changes in lung sounds such as crackles in the bases, and changes in heart sounds (eg, S_3 gallop), increased CVP

5. Monitor intake and output, including all drains. Observe for bladder distention.
6. Inspect skin and tissue surrounding maintenance lines to detect early infiltration. Restart lines immediately to maintain fluid volume.

F. *Promoting Comfort*
1. Assess pain by observing behavioral and physiologic manifestations.
2. Administer analgesics (change in vital signs may be a result of pain) and document efficacy.
3. Position the patient to maximize comfort.

G. *Minimizing Complications of Skin Impairment*
1. Perform handwashing before and after contact with patient.
2. Inspect dressings routinely and reinforce if necessary.
3. Record amount and type of wound drainage (refer to wound care, p. 90).
4. Turn the patient frequently and maintain good body alignment.

H. *Maintaining Safety*
1. Place side rails in protecting position until the patient is fully awake.
2. Protect the extremity into which IV fluids are running so that the needle will not become accidentally dislodged.
3. Avoid nerve damage and muscle strain by properly supporting and padding pressure areas.
4. Recognize that the patient may not be able to complain of injury such as the pricking of an open safety pin or a clamp that is exerting pressure.
5. Check dressing for constriction.
6. Determine return of motor control following anesthesia—indicated by how the patient responds to a pinprick or a request to move a part.

I. *Minimizing the Stress Factors of Sensory Deficits*
1. Know that the ability to hear returns more quickly than other senses as the patient emerges from anesthesia.
2. Avoid saying anything in the patient's presence that may be disturbing; patient may appear to be sleeping but still consciously hears what is being said.
3. Explain procedures and activities at the patient's level of understanding.
4. Minimize the patient's exposure to emergency treatment of nearby patients by drawing curtains and lowering voice and noise levels.
5. Treat the patient as a person who needs as much attention as the equipment and monitoring devices.
6. Respect the patient's feeling of sensory deprivation and overstimulation; make adjustments to minimize this fluctuation of stimuli.
7. Demonstrate concern for and understanding of the patient and anticipate needs and feelings.
8. Tell the patient repeatedly that the surgery is over and that he or she is in the recovery room.

Evaluation

A. Breathes easily
B. Lung sounds clear to auscultation
C. Vital signs stable
D. Body temperature remains stable; minimal chills or shivering
E. Intake and output are equal; no signs of volume imbalance
F. Reports adequate pain control
G. Wound edges intact without drainage
H. Side rails up; positioned carefully
I. Quiet, reassuring environment maintained

NURSING ALERT:
This phase of nursing care is geared to recognizing the significance of signs and anticipating and preventing postoperative difficulties. Carefully monitor the patient coming out of general anesthesia until:
1. Vital signs are stable for at least 30 minutes and are within normal range.
2. Patient is breathing easily.
3. Reflexes have returned to normal.
4. Patient is out of anesthesia, responsive, and oriented to time and place.
For the patient who had regional anesthesia, observe carefully until:
1. Sensation has been recovered.
2. Reflexes have returned.
3. Vital signs have stabilized for at least 30 minutes.

Transferring the Patient From the PACU

A. *Transfer Criteria*
Each facility may have an individual checklist or scoring guide used to determine a patient's readiness for transfer from the PACU based on the following:

1. Uncompromised cardiopulmonary status
2. Stable vital signs
3. Adequate urine output (at least 30 mL/h)
4. Orientation to person, place, events, and time
5. Satisfactory response to commands when asked to cough, breathe deeply, or move
6. Movement of extremities following regional anesthesia
7. Control of pain
8. Control or absence of vomiting

B. *Transfer Responsibilities*
1. Relay appropriate information to the unit nurse regarding condition; point out significant needs (eg, drainage, fluid therapy, incision and dressing requirements, intake needs, urinary output).
2. Physically assist in the transfer of the patient.
3. Orient patient to room, attending nurse, call light, and therapeutic devices.

◆ POSTOPERATIVE DISCOMFORTS

Most patients experience some discomforts postoperatively. These are usually related to the general anesthetic and the surgical procedure. The most common discomforts are nausea, vomiting, restlessness, sleeplessness, thirst, constipation, flatulence, and pain.

Nausea and Vomiting

A. Causes
1. Occurs in many postoperative patients.
2. Most often related to inhalation (volatile) anesthetics, which may irritate the stomach lining and stimulate the vomiting center in the brain.
3. Results from an accumulation of fluid or food in the stomach before peristalsis returns.
4. May occur as a result of abdominal distention, which follows manipulation of abdominal organs.
5. Likely to occur if the patient believes preoperatively that vomiting will occur (psychological induction).
6. May be a side effect of narcotics.

B. Preventive Measures
1. Insert nasogastric tube preoperatively for operations on gastrointestinal tract to prevent abdominal distention, which triggers vomiting.
2. Determine whether patient is sensitive to morphine, meperidine (Demerol), or other narcotic because they may induce vomiting in some patients.
3. Be alert for any significant comment such as, "I just know I will vomit under anesthesia." Report such a comment to the anesthesiologist, who may prescribe an antiemetic drug and also talk to the patient before the operation.

C. Nursing Interventions
1. Encourage patient to breathe deeply to facilitate elimination of anesthetic.
2. Support the wound during retching and vomiting; turn head to side to avoid aspiration.
3. Discard vomitus and refresh patient—mouthwash for mouth, clean linens for bed, etc.
4. Offer hot tea with lemon or small sips of a carbonated beverage such as ginger ale, if tolerated or permitted.
5. Report excessive or prolonged vomiting so that the cause may be investigated.
6. Maintain accurate intake and output record and replace fluids as ordered.
7. Detect presence of abdominal distention or hiccups, suggesting gastric retention.
8. Administer medications as ordered. Antiemetic medication such as prochlorperazine (Compazine) or promethazine (Phenergan) may be given; be aware that these drugs may potentiate the hypotensive effects of narcotics.

Note: Suspect idiosyncratic response to a drug if vomiting is worse when a medication is given (but diminishes thereafter).

Thirst

A. Causes
1. Inhibition of secretions by preoperative medication with atropine.
2. Fluid lost via perspiration, blood loss, and dehydration due to preoperative fluid restriction.

B. Preventive Measures
Unfortunately, postoperative thirst is a common and troublesome symptom that is often unavoidable due to anesthesia. The immediate implementation of nursing interventions is most helpful.

C. Nursing Interventions
1. Administer fluids by vein or by mouth if tolerated and permitted.
2. Offer sips of hot tea with lemon juice to dissolve mucus if diet orders allow.
3. Apply a moistened gauze square over lips occasionally to humidify inspired air.
4. Allow the patient to rinse mouth with mouthwash.
5. Obtain hard candies or chewing gum, if allowed, to help in stimulating saliva flow and in keeping the mouth moist.

Constipation and Gas Cramps

A. Causes
1. Trauma and manipulation of the bowel during surgery, as well as narcotic use, will retard peristalsis.
2. Local inflammation, peritonitis, or abscess.
3. Long-standing bowel problem; this may lead to fecal impaction.

B. Preventive Measures
1. Encourage early ambulation to aid in promoting peristalsis.
2. Provide adequate fluid intake to promote soft stools and hydration.
3. Advocate proper diet to promote peristalsis.
4. Encourage early use of nonnarcotic analgesia because many opiates increase chance of constipation.
5. Assess lower sounds frequently.

C. Nursing Interventions
1. Ask patient about usual remedy for constipation and try it, if appropriate.
2. Insert gloved finger and break up the fecal impaction manually, if necessary.
3. Administer an oil retention enema (180–200 mL), if prescribed, to help soften the fecal mass and facilitate evacuation.
4. Administer a return-flow enema (if prescribed) or a rectal tube to decrease painful flatulence.
5. Administer gastrointestinal stimulants, laxatives, suppositories, and stool softeners may be prescribed.

◆ POSTOPERATIVE PAIN

Pain is a subjective symptom in which the patient exhibits a feeling of distress. Stimulation of, or trauma to, certain nerve endings as a result of surgery causes pain.

General Principles

1. Pain is one of the earliest symptoms that the patient expresses on return to consciousness.
2. Maximal postoperative pain occurs between 12 and 36 hours after surgery and usually diminishes significantly by 48 hours.
3. Soluble anesthetic agents are slow to leave the body and therefore control pain for a longer time than insoluble agents; the latter produce rapid recovery, but the patient is more restless and complains more of pain.

4. Older persons seem to have a higher tolerance for pain than younger or middle-aged persons.
5. There is no documented proof that one sex tolerates pain better than the other.

Clinical Manifestations

1. Autonomic
   a. Outpouring of epinephrine
   b. Elevation of blood pressure
   c. Increase in heart and pulse rate
   d. Rapid and irregular respiration
   e. Increase in perspiration
2. Skeletal muscle
   a. Increase in muscle tension or activity
3. Psychological
   a. Increase in irritability
   b. Increase in apprehension
   c. Increase in anxiety
   d. Attention focused on pain
   e. Complaints of pain
4. Patient's reaction depends on:
   a. Previous experience
   b. Anxiety or tension
   c. State of health
   d. Ability to concentrate away from the problem or be distracted
   e. Meaning that pain has for the patient

Preventive Measures

1. Reduce anxiety of pain anticipation.
2. Teach patient about pain and expectations.
3. Review analgesics with patient and reassure that the pain relief will be available quickly.
4. Establish a trusting relationship and spend time with patient.

Nursing Interventions

A. *Use Basic Comfort Measures*
1. Provide therapeutic environment—proper temperature and humidity, ventilation, visitors.
2. Massage the patient's back and pressure points with soothing strokes—move patient easily and gently and with prewarning.
3. Offer diversional activities, soft radio music, or favorite quiet television program.
4. Provide for fluid needs by giving a cool drink, offering a bedpan.
5. Investigate possible causes of pain such as bandage or adhesive that is too tight, full bladder, cast that is too snug, or elevated temperature suggestive of inflammation or infection.
6. Instruct patient to splint wound when moving.
7. Keep bedding clean, dry, and free of wrinkles and debris.

B. *Recognize the Power of Suggestion*
1. Provide reassurance that the discomfort is temporary and that the medication will aid in pain reduction.
2. Clarify patient's fears regarding the perceived significance of pain.

3. Assist patient in maintaining a positive, hopeful attitude.

C. *Assist in Relaxation Techniques*
Imagery, meditation, controlled breathing, self-hypnosis/suggestion (autogenic training), and progressive relaxation.

D. *Apply Cutaneous Counterstimulation (Unless Contraindicated)*
1. Vibration—a vigorous form of massage that is applied to a nonoperative site. It lessens patient's perception of pain. (Avoid applying this to calf, which may dislodge an unheralded thrombus.)
2. Heat or cold—apply to operative or nonoperative site as prescribed. This works best for well localized pain. Cold has more advantages than heat and fewer unwanted side effects (ie, burns). Heat works well with muscle spasm.

E. *Give Analgesics as Prescribed in a Timely Manner*
1. Instruct patient to request analgesic before the pain becomes severe.
2. If pain occurs consistently and predictably throughout a 24-hour period, analgesics should be given around the clock—avoiding the usual "demand cycle" of dosing that sets up eventual dependency and provides less adequate pain relief.
3. Administer prescribed medication to patient before anticipated activities and painful procedures (eg, dressing changes).
4. Monitor for possible side effects of analgesic therapy (eg, respiratory depression, hypotension, nausea, skin rash). Administer naloxone hydrochloride (Narcan) to relieve significant narcotic-induced respiratory depression.

> **NURSING ALERT:**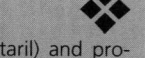
> Narcotic "potentiators," such as hydroxyzine (Vistaril) and promethazine (Phenergan), may further sedate the patient.

5. Assess and document efficacy of analgesic therapy.

Pharmacologic Management

A. *Oral and Parenteral Analgesia*
1. Surgical patients are often prescribed a parenteral analgesic for 2 to 4 days or until incisional pain abates. At that time an oral analgesic, narcotic or nonnarcotic, will be prescribed.
2. Although the health care provider is responsible for prescribing the appropriate medication, it is the nurse's responsibility to ensure the drug is given safely and assessed for efficacy.

B. *Patient-Controlled Analgesia (PCA)*
1. Benefits
   a. Bypasses the delays inherent in traditional analgesic administration (the "demand cycle").
   b. Medication is administered by IV, producing more rapid pain relief and greater consistency in patient response.
   c. The patient retains control over pain relief (added placebo and relaxation effects).
   d. Decreased nursing time in frequent delivery of analgesics.
2. Contraindications
   a. Patients under 10 to 11 years of age

b. Patients with cognitive impairment (delirium, dementia, mental illness, hemodynamic or respiratory impairment)
3. A portable PCA device delivers a preset dosage of narcotic (usually morphine). An adjustable "lockout interval" controls the frequency of dose administration, preventing another dose from being delivered prematurely. An example of PCA settings might be a dose of 1 mg morphine with a lockout interval of 6 minutes (total possible dose is 10 mg/h).
4. Patient pushes a button to activate the device.
5. Instruction about PCA should occur preoperatively; some patients fear being overdosed by the machine and require reassurance.

C. Epidural Analgesia
1. Requires injections of narcotics into the epidural space via a catheter inserted by an anesthesiologist under aseptic conditions (Fig. 5-2).
2. Benefits
   a. Produces effective analgesia without sensory, motor, or sympathetic changes.
   b. Provides for longer periods of analgesia.
3. Disadvantages
   a. The epidural catheter's proximity to the spinal nerves and spinal canal, along with its potential for catheter migration, make correct injection technique and close patient assessment imperative.
   b. Requires specific hospital protocol for injection and verification of nursing staff's injection technique.
   c. Side effects include generalized pruritus (common), nausea, urinary retention, respiratory depression, hypotension, motor block, and sensory/sympathetic block. These side effects are related to the narcotic used (usually a morphine derivative [Duramorph] or fentanyl [Sublimaze]) and catheter position.
4. Strict asepsis is necessary when injecting the epidural catheter.

5. The catheter is initially aspirated gently; if blood or greater than 1 mL clear fluid is aspirated, hold injection and notify health care provider of possible catheter migration into spinal column.
6. Narcotic-related side effects are reversed with naloxone hydrochloride (Narcan).
7. The nurse ensures proper integrity of both the catheter and the dressing.
8. Occasionally, concurrent use of low-dose anesthetics such as bupivacaine (Marcaine) may be added to potentiate efficacy of epidural analgesia; this is most common following thoracic trauma.

◆ POSTOPERATIVE COMPLICATIONS

Postoperative complications are a risk inherent in surgical procedures. They may interfere with the expected outcome of the surgery and may extend the patient's hospitalization and convalescence. The nurse plays a critical role in attempting to prevent complications and in recognizing their signs and symptoms immediately. Implementing nursing interventions at an early stage of a complication is also of utmost importance.

Shock

Shock is a response of the body to a decrease in the circulating volume of blood; tissue perfusion is impaired culminating, eventually, in cellular hypoxia and death. See page 952 for classification and emergency management of shock.

A. Preventive Measures
1. Have blood available if there is any indication that it may be needed.

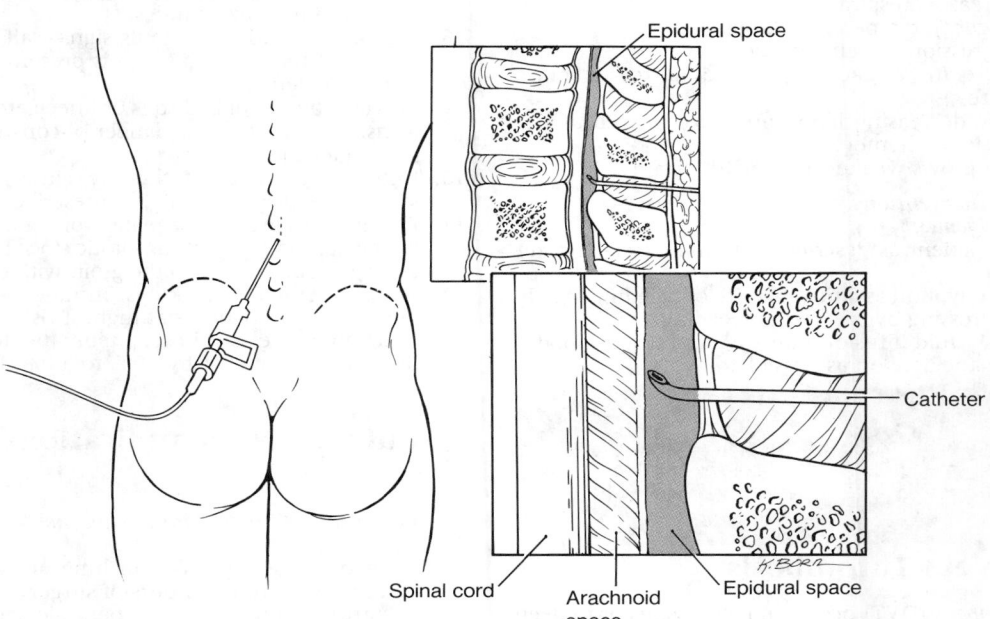

Epidural space

Catheter

Spinal cord

Arachnoid space

Epidural space

FIGURE 5-2 Epidural catheter placement.

2. Measure accurately any blood loss.
3. Anticipate progression of symptoms on earliest manifestation.
4. Monitor vital signs frequently until they are stable.
5. Assess vital sign deviations; evaluate blood pressure in relation to other physiologic parameters of shock and patient's premorbid values. Orthostatic hypotension is an important indicator of hypovolemic shock.
6. Prevent infection (eg, indwelling catheter care, wound care, pulmonary care) because this will minimize septic shock.

Hemorrhage

Hemorrhage is copious escape of blood from a blood vessel.

A. **Classification**
1. General
   a. *Primary*—occurs at the time of operation.
   b. *Intermediary*—occurs within the first few hours after surgery. Blood pressure returns to normal and causes loosening of some ligated sutures and flushing out of weak clots from unligated vessels.
   c. *Secondary*—occurs some time after surgery due to ligature slip from blood vessel and erosion of blood vessel.
2. According to Blood Vessels
   a. *Capillary*—slow general oozing from capillaries
   b. *Venous*—bleeding that is dark in color and bubbles out
   c. *Arterial*—bleeding that spurts and is bright red in color
3. According to Location
   a. *Evident or external*—visible bleeding on the surface
   b. *Internal (concealed)*—bleeding that cannot be seen

B. **Clinical Manifestations**
1. Apprehension; restlessness; thirst; cold, moist, pale skin; and circumoral pallor
2. Pulse increases, respirations become rapid and deep ("air hunger"), temperature drops.
3. With progression of hemorrhage:
   a. Decrease in cardiac output and narrowed pulse pressure
   b. Rapidly decreasing blood pressure, as well as hematocrit and hemoglobin
   c. Patient grows weaker until death occurs.

C. **Nursing Interventions and Management**
1. Treat the patient as described for shock (see Chapter 33).
2. Inspect the wound as a possible site of bleeding. Apply pressure dressing over external bleeding site.
3. Increase IV fluid infusion rate and administer blood if necessary and as soon as possible.

> **NURSING ALERT:** ❖
> Numerous, rapid blood transfusions may induce coagulopathy and prolonged bleeding time. The patient should be monitored closely for signs of increased bleeding tendencies following such transfusions.

Deep Vein Thrombosis

Deep vein thrombosis (DVT) occurs in pelvic veins or in deep veins of the lower extremities in postoperative patients. The incidence of DVT varies between 10% and 40% depending on the complexity of the surgery or the severity of the underlying illness. DVT is most common after hip surgery, followed by retropubic prostatectomy, and general thoracic or abdominal surgery. Venous thrombi located above the knee are considered the major source of pulmonary emboli.

A. **Causes**
1. Injury to intimal layer of the vein wall
2. Venous stasis
3. Hypercoagulopathy, polycythemia
4. High risks include obesity, prolonged immobility, cancer, smoking, advancing age, varicose veins, dehydration, splenectomy, and orthopedic procedures.

B. **Clinical Manifestations**
1. Majority of DVT are asymptomatic.
2. Pain or cramp in the calf or thigh, progressing to painful swelling of entire leg
3. Slight fever, chills, perspiration
4. Marked tenderness over anteromedial surface of thigh
5. Intravascular clotting without marked inflammation may develop, leading to phlebothrombosis.
6. Circulation distal to the DVT may be compromised if sufficient swelling is present.

C. **Nursing Interventions and Management**
1. Hydrate the patient adequately postoperatively to prevent hemoconcentration.
2. Encourage leg exercises and ambulate the patient as soon as permitted by the surgeon.
3. Avoid any restricting devices such as tight straps that can constrict and impair circulation.
4. Avoid rubbing or massaging calves and thighs.
5. Instruct patient to avoid standing or sitting in one place for prolonged periods or crossing legs when seated.
6. Refrain from inserting IV catheters into legs or feet of adults.
7. Assess distal peripheral pulses, capillary refill, and sensation of lower extremities.
8. Check for positive Homan's sign—calf pain on dorsiflexion of the foot. This sign is present in nearly 30% of DVT patients.
9. Prevent the use of bed rolls or knee gatches in patients at risk because there is danger of constricting the vessels under the knee.
10. Initiate anticoagulant therapy either intravenously, subcutaneously, or orally, as prescribed.
11. Prevent swelling and stagnation of venous blood by applying appropriately fitting elastic stockings or wrapping the legs from the toes to the groin with elastic bandage.
12. Apply pneumatic stockings, intraoperatively or postoperatively, to patients at highest risk of DVT. In conjunction with elastic hose, pneumatic stockings can reduce the risk of DVT by 30% to 50% (Fig. 5-3).

Pulmonary Complications

A. **Causes and Clinical Manifestations**
1. Atelectasis
   a. Incomplete expansion of lung or portion of it occurring within 48 hours of surgery
   b. Attributed to absence of periodic deep breaths
   c. A mucous plug closes a bronchiole, causing alveoli distal to plug to collapse.

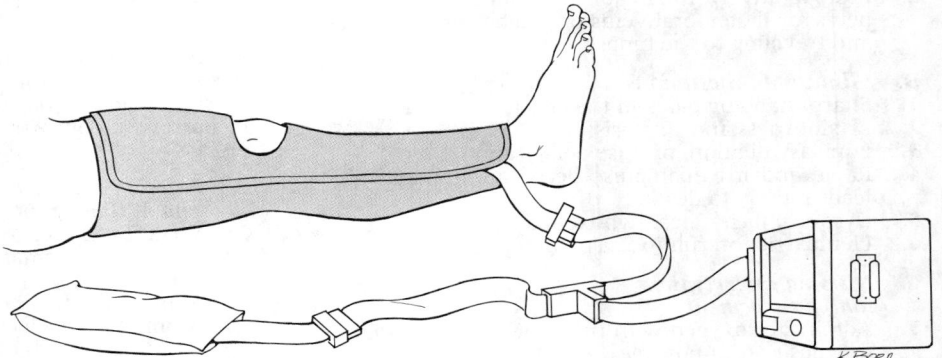

FIGURE 5-3 *Pneumatic hose. Pressures of 35 mm Hg to 20 mm Hg are sequentially applied from ankle to thigh, producing an increase in blood flow velocity and improved venous clearing.*

    d. Symptoms are often absent—may comprise mild to severe tachypnea, tachycardia, cough, fever, hypotension, and decreased breath sounds and chest expansion of affected side.

2. Aspiration

    a. Caused by inhalation of food, gastric contents, water, or blood into the tracheobronchial system.

    b. Anesthetic agents and narcotics depress the central nervous system, causing inhibition of gag or cough reflexes.

    c. Nasogastric tube insertion renders both upper and lower esophageal sphincters partially incompetent.

    d. Gross aspiration has a 50% mortality.

    e. Symptoms depend on severity of aspiration; it may be silent. Usually evidence of atelectasis occurs within 2 minutes of aspiration. Other symptoms include tachypnea, dyspnea, cough, bronchospasm, wheezing, rhonchi, crackles, hypoxia, and frothy sputum.

3. Pneumonia

    a. This is an inflammatory response in which cellular material replaces alveolar gas.

    b. In postoperative patient, most often caused by gram-negative bacilli due to impaired oropharyngeal defense mechanisms.

    c. Predisposing factors include atelectasis, upper respiratory infection, copious secretions, aspiration, dehydration, prolonged intubation or tracheostomy, history of smoking, impaired normal host defenses (cough reflex, mucociliary system, alveolar macrophage activity).

    d. Symptoms include dyspnea, tachypnea, pleuritic chest pain, fever, chills, hemoptysis, cough (rusty or purulent sputum), and decreased breath sounds over involved area.

B. *Preventive Measures*

1. Report any evidence of upper respiratory infection to the surgeon.

2. Suction nasopharyngeal or bronchial secretions if patient is unable to clear own airway.

3. Prevent regurgitation and aspiration through proper patient positioning.

4. Recognize the predisposing causes of pulmonary complications:

    a. Infections—mouth, nose, sinuses, throat

    b. Aspiration of vomitus

    c. History of heavy smoking, chronic pulmonary disease

    d. Obesity

C. *Nursing Interventions and Management*

1. Monitor the patient's progress carefully on a daily basis for the first postoperative week to detect early signs and symptoms of respiratory difficulties.

    a. Slight temperature, pulse, and respiration elevations

    b. Apprehension and restlessness or a decreased level of consciousness

    c. Complaints of chest pain, signs of dyspnea or cough

2. Promote full aeration of the lungs.

    a. Turn the patient frequently.

    b. Encourage the patient to take 10 deep breaths hourly, holding each breath to a count of 5 and exhaling.

    c. Use a spirometer or any device that encourages the patient to ventilate more effectively.

    d. Assist the patient in coughing in an effort to bring up mucous secretions. Have patient splint chest or abdominal wound to minimize discomfort associated with deep breathing and coughing.

    e. Encourage and assist the patient to ambulate as early as the health care provider will allow.

3. Initiate specific measures for particular pulmonary problems.

    a. Provide cool mist or heated nebulizer for the patient exhibiting signs of bronchitis or thick secretions.

    b. Encourage patient to take fluids to help ''liquefy'' secretions and facilitate expectoration (in pneumonia).

    c. Elevate the head of bed and ensure proper administration of prescribed oxygen.

    d. Prevent adbominal distention—nasogastric tube insertion may be necessary.

    e. Administer prescribed antibiotics for pulmonary infections.

Pulmonary Embolism (PE)

A. *Causes*

1. *Pulmonary embolism* is caused by the obstruction of one or more pulmonary arterioles by an embolus originating somewhere in the venous system or in the right side of the heart.

2. Postoperatively, the majority of emboli develop in the pelvic or iliofemoral veins before becoming dislodged and traveling to the lungs.

B. *Clinical Manifestations*
1. Sharp, stabbing pains in the chest
2. Anxiousness and cyanosis
3. Pupillary dilation, profuse perspiration
4. Rapid and irregular pulse becoming imperceptible—leads rapidly to death
5. Dyspnea, tachypnea, hypoxemia
6. Pleural friction rub (occasionally)

C. *Nursing Interventions and Management*
1. Administer oxygen with the patient in an upright sitting position (if possible).
2. Reassure and quiet the patient.
3. Monitor vital signs, ECG, and arterial blood gases.
4. Treat for shock or heart failure as needed.
5. Give analgesics or sedatives to control pain or apprehension.
6. Prepare for anticoagulation or thrombolytic therapy or surgical intervention. Management depends on the severity of the PE.

> **NURSING ALERT:**
> Massive PE is life threatening and requires immediate interventions to maintain the patient's cardiorespiratory status. Refer to page 220.

Urinary Retention

A. *Causes*
1. Occurs most frequently after operations of the rectum, anus, vagina, or lower abdomen.
2. Caused by spasm of bladder sphincter.
3. More common in male patients due to inherent increases in urethral resistance to urine flow.

B. *Clinical Manifestations*
1. Inability to void
2. Voiding small amounts at frequent intervals
3. Palpable bladder
4. Lower abdominal discomfort

C. *Nursing Interventions and Management*
1. Assist patient to sit or stand (if permissible) because many patients are unable to void while lying in bed.
2. Provide the patient with privacy.
3. Run the tap water—frequently the sound or sight of running water relaxes spasm of the bladder sphincter.
4. Use warmth to relax sphincters (ie, sitz bath, warm compresses).
5. Administer bethanechol chloride (Urecholine) intramuscularly, if prescribed.
6. Catheterize only when all other measures are unsuccessful.

> **NURSING ALERT:**
> Recognize that when a patient voids small amounts (30–60 mL every 15–30 minutes), this may be a sign of an overdistended bladder with "overflow" of urine.

Intestinal Obstruction

Bowel obstructions result in a partial or complete impairment to the forward flow of intestinal contents. Most obstructions occur in the small bowel, especially at its narrowest point—the ileum. See page 529 for full discussion of intestinal obstruction.

A. *Nursing Intervention and Management*
1. Treat the cause.
2. Relieve abdominal distention by passing a nasoenteric suction tube.
3. Replace fluid and electrolytes.
4. Monitor fluid, electrolyte (especially potassium and sodium), and acid–base status.
5. Administer narcotics judiciously because these medications may further suppress peristalsis.
6. Prepare the patient for surgical intervention if obstruction continues unresolved.
7. Closely monitor patient for signs of shock.
8. Provide frequent reassurance to patient; use nontraditional methods to promote comfort (touch, relaxation, imagery).
9. Assess bowel tones and degree of abdominal distention (may need to measure abdominal girth); document these findings every shift.
10. Monitor and document characteristics of emesis and nasogastric drainage.

Hiccups (Singultus)

Hiccups are intermittent spasms of the diaphragm causing the sound ("hic") that results from the vibration of closed vocal cords as air rushes suddenly into the lungs.

A. *Causes*
Irritation of the phrenic nerve between the spinal cord and terminal ramifications on undersurface of diaphragm.

1. *Direct*—distended stomach, peritonitis, abdominal distention, chest pleurisy, tumors, pressing on nerves
2. *Indirect*—toxemia, uremia
3. *Reflex*—exposure to cold, drinking very hot or very cold liquids, intestinal obstruction

B. *Clinical Manifestations*
1. Audible "hic"
2. Distress and fatigue
3. Vomiting
4. Wound dehiscence in severe cases

C. *Nursing Interventions and Management*
1. Remove the cause, if possible.
2. When removal of cause if not possible, favorite remedies may be tried, if appropriate.
   a. Swallow a large glass of water.
   b. Place tablespoon of coarse, granulated sugar on back of tongue and swallow it.
   c. Medicate with a phenothiazine drug such as prochlorperazine (Compazine) or chlorpromazine (Thorazine).
   d. Introduce a small catheter into the patient's pharynx (about 8–10 cm [3–4 inches]); rotate gently and jiggle back and forth.
   e. For rare, intractable hiccups, an extreme procedure is surgical crush of the phrenic nerve.

Wound Infection

Wound infections are the second most common nosocomial infection. The infection may be limited to the surgical site (60–80%) or may affect the patient systemically.

A. Causes
1. Drying tissues by long exposure, operations on contaminated structures, gross obesity, old age, chronic hypoxemia, and malnutrition are directly related to an increased infection rate.
2. The patient's own flora is most often implicated in wound infections (*Staphylococcus aureus*).
3. Other common culprits in wound infection include *Escherichia coli*, *Klebsiella*, *Enterobacter*, and *Proteus*.
4. Wound infections typically present 5 to 7 days postoperatively.
5. Factors affecting the extent of infection include:
   a. Kind, virulence, and quantity of contaminating microorganisms
   b. Presence of foreign bodies or devitalized tissue
   c. Location and nature of the wound
   d. Amount of dead space or presence of hematoma
   e. Immune response of the patient
   f. Presence of adequate blood supply to wound
   g. Presurgical condition of the patient (eg, elderly, alcoholism, diabetes, malnutrition)

B. Clinical Manifestations
1. Redness, excessive swelling, tenderness, warmth
2. Red streaks in the skin near the wound
3. Pus or other discharge from the wound
4. Tender, enlarged lymph nodes in axillary region or groin closest to wound
5. Foul smell from wound
6. Generalized body chills or fever
7. Elevated temperature and pulse

NURSING ALERT:
Mild, transient fevers appear postoperatively due to tissue necrosis, hematoma, or cauterization. Higher sustained fevers arise with the following four most common postoperative complications: atelectasis (within the first 48 hours); wound infections (in 5–7 days); urinary infections (in 5–8 days); and thrombophlebitis (in 7–14 days).

C. Nursing Interventions and Management
1. Preoperative
   a. Encourage the patient to achieve an optimal nutritional level. Provide for enteral or parenteral alimentation if patient has hypoproteinemia with weight loss.
   b. Reduce preoperative hospitalization to a minimum to avoid acquiring nosocomial infections.
2. Operative
   a. Follow strict asepsis throughout the operative procedure.
   b. When a wound has exudate, fibrin, desiccated fat, or nonviable skin, it is not approximated by primary closure but approximation is delayed (secondary closure).
3. Postoperative
   a. Keep dressings intact, reinforcing if necessary, until prescribed otherwise.
   b. Use strict asepsis when dressings are changed.
   c. Monitor and document amount, type, and location of drainage. Ensure that all drains are working properly. (See Table 5-1 for expected drainage amounts from common types of drains and tubes.)
4. Postoperative Care of an Infected Wound
   a. The surgeon removes one or more stitches, separates wound edges, and examines for infection using a hemostat as a probe.
   b. A culture is taken and sent to the laboratory for bacterial analysis.
   c. Wound irrigation may be done; have asepto syringe and saline available.
   d. A drain may be inserted, or the wound may be packed with sterile gauze.
   e. Antibiotics are prescribed.
   f. Wet-to-dry dressings may be applied (see p. 92).

Wound Dehiscence (Evisceration)

A. Causes
1. Commonly occurs between fifth and eighth day postoperatively when incision has weakest tensile strength; greatest strength is found between the first and third postoperative day.
2. Chiefly associated with abdominal surgery.

TABLE 5-1 Expected Drainage From Tubes and Catheters

Device	Substance	Daily Drainage
Foley catheter Ileal conduit Suprapubic catheter	Urine	500–700 mL/24 h first 48 h; then 1500–2500 mL/24 h
Gastrostomy tube	Gastric contents	Up to 1500 mL/24 h
Chest tube	Blood, pleural fluid, air	Varies: 500–1000 mL first 24 h
Ileostomy	Small bowel contents	Up to 4000 mL in first 24 h; then <500 mL/24 h
Miller-Abbott tube	Intestinal contents	Up to 3000 mL/24 h
Nasogastric tube	Gastric contents	Up to 1500 mL/24 h
T-tube	Bile	500 mL/24 h

3. This catastrophe is often related to the following:
  a. Inadequate sutures or excessively tight closures (the latter compromises blood supply)
  b. Hematomas; seromas
  c. Infections
  d. Excessive coughing, hiccups, retching, distention
  e. Poor nutrition; immunosuppression
  f. Uremia; diabetes mellitus
  g. Steroid use

B. *Preventive Measures*
1. Apply abdominal binder for heavy or elderly patients or those with weak or pendulous abdominal walls.
2. Encourage patient to splint incision while coughing.
3. Monitor for and relieve abdominal distention.
4. Encourage proper nutrition with emphasis on adequate amounts of protein and vitamin C.

C. *Clinical Manifestations*
1. Dehiscence is heralded by sudden discharge of serosanguineous fluid from wound.
2. Patient complains that something suddenly "gave way" in the wound.
3. In an intestinal wound, the edges of the wound may part and the intestines may gradually push out—observe for drainage of peritoneal fluid on dressing (clear or serosanguineous fluid).

D. *Nursing Interventions and Management*
1. Stay with the patient and have someone notify the surgeon immediately.
2. If intestines are exposed, cover with sterile moist saline dressings.
3. Monitor vital signs and watch for shock.
4. Keep the patient on absolute bed rest.
5. Instruct patient to bend knees, with head of bed elevated in semi-Fowler's position to relieve tension on abdomen.
6. Assure the patient that the wound will be properly cared for; attempt to keep patient quiet and relaxed.
7. Prepare the patient for surgery and repair of the wound.

Psychological Disturbances

A. *Depression*
1. Cause—perceived loss of health or stamina, pain, altered body image, various drugs, and anxiety about an uncertain future.
2. Clinical manifestations—withdrawal, restlessness, insomnia, nonadherence to therapeutic regimens, tearfulness, and expressions of hopelessness.
3. Nursing interventions and management
  a. Clarify misconceptions about surgery and its future implications.
  b. Listen to, reassure, and support patient.
  c. If appropriate, introduce patient to representatives of ostomy, mastectomy, or amputee clubs.
  d. Involve patient's partner and support persons in care; psychiatric consultation is obtained for severe depression.

B. *Delirium*
1. Cause—prolonged anesthesia, cardiopulmonary bypass, drug reactions, sepsis, alcoholism (delirium tremens), electrolyte imbalances, and other metabolic disorders.

2. Clinical manifestations—disorientation, hallucinations, perceptual distortions, paranoid delusions, reversed day-night pattern, agitation, insomnia; delirium tremens often appears within 72 hours of last alcoholic drink and may include autonomic overactivity—tachycardia, dilated pupils, diaphoresis, and fever.
3. Nursing interventions and management
  a. Treat the underlying cause (restore fluid and electrolyte balance).
  b. Reorient to environment and time.
  c. Keep surroundings calm.
  d. Explain in detail every procedure done to patient.
  e. Sedate patient to reduce agitation, prevent exhaustion, and promote sleep.
  f. Allow for extended periods of uninterrupted sleep.
  g. Reassure family members with clear explanations of patient's aberrant behavior.
  h. Apply restraints to patient if safety is in question.

Wound Care

◆ WOUNDS AND WOUND HEALING

A *wound* is a disruption in the continuity and regulatory processes of tissue cells; *wound healing* is the restoration of that continuity. Wound healing, however, may or may not restore normal cellular function.

Wound Classification

A. *Mechanism of Injury*
1. *Incised wounds*—made by a clean cut of a sharp instrument, such as a surgical incision with a scalpel.
2. *Contused wounds*—made by blunt force that typically does not break the skin but causes considerable tissue damage with bruising and swelling.
3. *Lacerated wounds*—made by an object that tears tissues producing jagged, irregular edges; examples include glass, jagged wire, and blunt knife.
4. *Puncture wounds*—made by a pointed instrument, such as an ice pick, bullet, and nail.

B. *Degree of Contamination*
1. *Clean*—an aseptically made wound, as in surgery, that does not enter the alimentary, respiratory, or genitourinary tracts.
2. *Clean–contaminated*—an aseptically made wound that enters the respiratory, alimentary, or genitourinary tracts. These wounds have slightly higher probability of wound infection than do clean wounds.
3. *Contaminated*—wounds exposed to excessive amounts of bacteria. These wounds may be open (avulsive) or accidentally made, or the result of surgical operations in which there are major breaks in aseptic techniques or gross spillage from the gastrointestinal tract.
4. *Infected*—a wound that retains devitalized tissue or involves preoperatively existing infection or perforated viscera. Such wounds are often left open to drain.

Physiology of Wound Healing

The phases of wound healing—inflammation, reconstruction (proliferation), and maturation—involve continuous and overlapping processes.

A. **Inflammatory Phase**
(lasts 1–5 days)

1. Vascular and cellular responses are immediately initiated when tissue is cut or injured.
2. Transient vasoconstriction occurs immediately at the site of injury, lasting 5 to 10 minutes, along with deposition of a fibrinoplatelet clot to help control bleeding.
3. Subsequent dilation of small venules occurs; antibodies, plasma proteins, plasma fluids, leukocytes, and red blood cells leave the microcirculation to permeate the general area of injury, causing edema, redness, warmth, and pain.
4. Localized vasodilation is the result of direct action by histamine, serotonin, and prostaglandins.
5. Polymorphic leukocytes (neutrophils) and monocytes enter the wound to engage in destruction and ingestion of wound debris. Monocytes predominate during this phase.
6. Basal cells at the wound edges undergo mitosis; resultant daughter cells enlarge, flatten, and creep across the wound surface to eventually approximate the wound edges.

B. **Proliferative Phase**
(lasts 2–20 days)

1. Fibroblasts (connective tissue cells) multiply and migrate along fibrin strands that are thought to serve as a matrix.
2. Endothelial budding occurs on nearby blood vessels, forming new capillaries that penetrate and nourish the injured tissue.
3. The combination of budding capillaries and proliferating fibroblasts is called granulation tissue.
4. Active collagen synthesis by fibroblasts begins by the fifth to seventh day and the wound gains tensile strength.
5. By 3 weeks, skin obtains 30% of its preinjury tensile strength, the intestinal tissue about 65%, and fascia 20%.

C. **Maturation Phase**
(21 days to months and even years)

1. Scar tissue is composed primarily of collagen and ground substance (mucopolysaccharide, glycoproteins, electrolytes, and water).
2. From the start of collagen synthesis, collagen fibers undergo a process of lysis and regeneration. The collagen fibers become more organized, aligning more closely to each other and increasing in tensile strength.
3. The overall bulk and form of the scar continues to change once maturation has started.
4. Typically, collagen production drops off; however, if collagen production greatly exceeds collagen lysis, keloid (greatly hypertrophied, deforming scar tissue) will form.
5. Normal maturation of the wound is clinically observed as an initial red, raised, hard immature scar that molds into a flat, soft, and pale mature scar.
6. The scar tissue will never achieve greater than 80% of its preinjury tensile strength.

Types of Wound Healing (Fig. 5-4)

A. **First Intention Healing (Primary Union)**
1. Wounds are made aseptic by with a minimum of tissue damage and tissue reaction; wound edges are properly approximated with sutures.
2. Granulation tissue is not visible and scar formation is typically minimal (keloid may still form in susceptible individuals).

B. **Second Intention Healing (Granulation)**
1. Wounds are left open to heal spontaneously or surgically closed at a later date; they need not be infected.
2. Examples in which wounds may heal by second intention include burns, traumatic injuries, ulcers, and suppurative infected wounds.
3. The cavity of the wound fills with a red, soft, sensitive tissue (granulation tissue), which bleeds easily. A scar (cicatrix) eventually forms.
4. In infected wounds, drainage may be accomplished by use of special dressings and drains. Healing is thus improved.
5. In wounds that are later resutured, two opposing granulation surfaces are brought together.
6. Second intention healing produces a deeper, wider scar.

◆ WOUND MANAGEMENT

Many factors promote wound healing, such as adequate nutrition, cleanliness, rest, and position, along with the patient's underlying psychological and physiologic state. Of added importance is the application of appropriate dressings and drains. See Procedure Guidelines 5-1 and 5-2.

Dressings

A. **Purpose of Dressings**
1. To protect the wound from mechanical injury
2. To splint or immobilize the wound
3. To absorb drainage
4. To prevent contamination from bodily discharges (feces, urine)
5. To promote hemostasis, as in pressure dressings
6. To debride the wound by combining capillary action and the entwining of necrotic tissue within its mesh
7. To inhibit or kill microorganisms by using dressings with antiseptic or antimicrobial properties
8. To provide a physiologic environment conducive to healing
9. To provide mental and physical comfort for the patient

B. **Advantages for Not Using Dressings**
When the initial dressing on a clean, dry, and intact incision is removed, it is often not replaced. This may occur within 24 hours after surgery.

1. Permits better visualization of wound.
2. Eliminates conditions necessary for growth of organisms (warmth, moisture, and darkness).
3. Minimizes adhesive tape reaction.
4. It is economical.

C. **Types of Dressings**
1. Dry-to-dry dressings

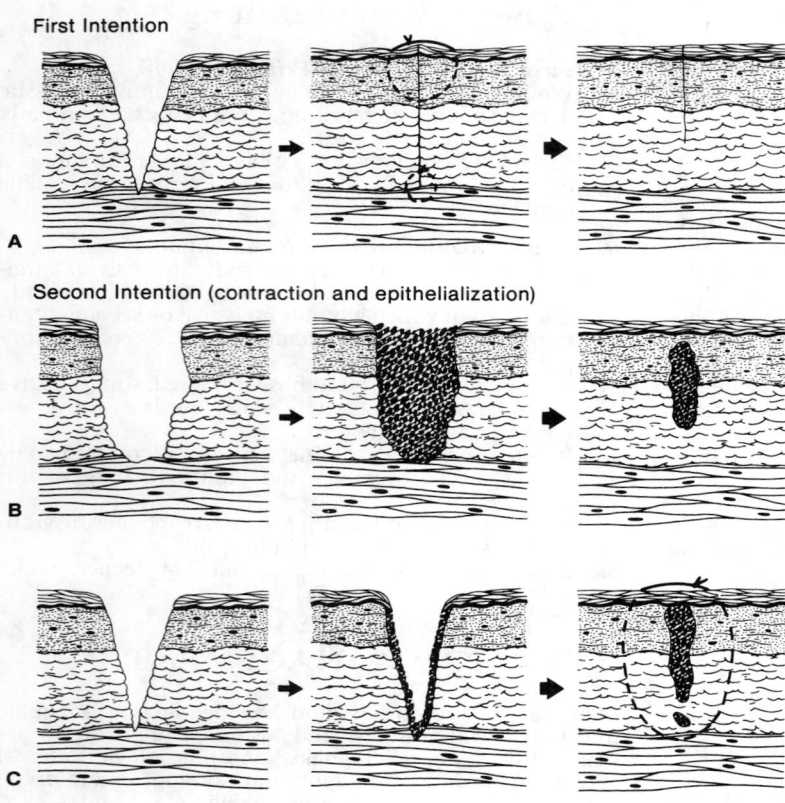

First Intention

A

Second Intention (contraction and epithelialization)

B

C

*FIGURE 5-4 Classification of wound healing. (**A**) First intention: A clean incision is made with primary closure; there is minimal scarring. (**B** and **C**) Second intention: The wound is left open so that granulation can occur; a large scar results, (**B**) or the wound is initially left open and later closed when there is no further evidence of infection (**C**).*

a. Used primarily for wounds closing by primary intention.
b. Offers good wound protection, absorption of drainage, and esthetics for the patient and provides pressure (if needed) for hemostasis.
c. Disadvantage—they adhere to the wound surface when drainage dries. Removal can cause pain and disruption of granulation tissue.
2. Wet-to-dry dressings
a. These are particularly useful for untidy or infected wounds that must be debrided and closed by secondary intention.
b. Gauze saturated with sterile saline (preferred) or an antimicrobial solution is packed into the wound, eliminating dead space.
c. The wet dressings are then covered by dry dressings (gauze sponges or absorbent pads).
d. As drying occurs, wound debris and necrotic tissue are absorbed into the gauze dressing by capillary action.
e. The dressing is changed when it becomes dry (or just before). If there is excessive necrotic debris on the dressing, more frequent dressing changes are required.
3. Wet-to-wet dressings
a. Used on clean open wounds or on granulating surfaces. Sterile saline or an antimicrobial agent may be used to saturate the dressings.
b. Provide a more physiologic environment (warmth, moisture), which can enhance the local healing processes as well as ensure greater patient comfort. Thick exudate is more easily removed.

c. Disadvantage—surrounding tissues can become macerated, the risk of infection may rise, and bed linens become damp.

Types of Surgical Dressing Supplies

1. Hydrophobic occlusive (petrolatum gauze)
a. This is an impermeable, nonadhering dressing that protects wounds from air- and moisture-borne contamination.
b. It is used around chest tubes and any fistula or stoma that drains digestive juices.
c. It is relatively nonabsorptive.
2. Hydrophilic permeable (oil-based gauze, Telfa pads)
a. Allows drainage to penetrate dressing but remains somewhat nonadhering.
b. For wounds with light to moderate exudate.
c. Oil-based gauze used on abraded and open ulcerated or granulating wounds.
d. May also be used to pack "caverns and sinuses" of large open wounds.
e. Telfa pads are generally reserved for simple, closed, stable wounds.
3. Dressing sponges (Topper sponges or general-use gauze sponges)
a. General-use gauze sponges come in various sizes (most commonly 2 × 2, 4 × 4 inches) and may be used for simple dry dressings, wet-to-dry dressings,

or wet-to-wet dressings. Large-pore mesh allows for better absorption of drainage and necrotic wound debris.

   b. Topper sponges are primarily used over stable surgical incisions. Their smaller pore size and cotton filling make them less suitable for debriding activities.

4. All-absorbent combined dressing (Surgipad, ABD)
   a. Large (5 × 9 to 8 × 10 inches) cotton-filled dressing that is typically used as an "over-dressing," covering gauze or hydrophilic dressings for added wound protection, stabilization of dressings, and drainage absorption.
   b. May also be used unaccompanied over intact surgical wounds.

5. High-bulk gauze bandage ("fluffs")—primarily used for packing of large wounds undergoing healing by secondary intention

6. Drain sponge—similar to the Topper sponge except for the premade slit, which makes the dressing highly suitable for drain sites and tracheostomy sites.

7. Transparent film dressing (Tegaderm, Op-Site)
   a. Highly elastic dressing, adjusts exceptionally well to body contours. It is permeable to oxygen and water vapor but generally impermeable to liquids and bacteria.
   b. Controversies surrounding its use (related to incidence of infection) have reduced its usage.
   c. Most common indications include covering arterial and venous catheter sites as well as protecting vulnerable skin exposed to shearing forces.
   d. It is not commonly used for surgical wounds.

Drains

A. Purpose of Drains
1. Drains are placed in wounds only when abnormal fluid collections are present or expected.
2. Drains are placed near the incision site:
   a. Usually in compartments (such as joints and pleural space) that are intolerant to fluid accumulation
   b. In areas with a large blood supply (such as the neck and kidney)
   c. In infected draining wounds
   d. In areas that have sustained large superficial tissue dissection (such as the breast)
3. Collection of body fluids in wounds can be harmful in the following ways:
   a. Provides culture media for bacterial growth.
   b. Causes increased pressure at surgical site, interfering with blood flow to area.
   c. Causes pressure on adjacent areas.
   d. Causes local tissue irritation and necrosis (due to fluids such as bile, pus, pancreatic juice, and urine).

B. Wound Drainage
1. Drains are commonly made of soft rubber or plastic and placed either within wounds or body cavities.
2. Drains placed within wounds are typically attached to portable (or, rarely, wall) suction with a collection container.
   a. Examples include the Hemovac, Jackson-Pratt, and Surgivac drainage system.
3. Drains may also be used postoperatively to form hollow connections from internal organs to the outside to drain a body fluid, such as the T-tube (bile drainage), nephrostomy, gastrostomy, jejunostomy, and cecostomy tubes.

4. Drains act as foreign bodies; granulation tissue forms around them, walling them off rapidly.
5. Drains within wounds are removed when the amount of drainage decreases over a period of days or rarely weeks.
6. Fistula-forming tubes are often left in for longer periods of time.
   a. Careful handling of these drains and collection bags is essential.
   b. Accidental early removal may result in caustic drainage leaking within the tissues.
   c. The risk is reduced within 7 to 10 days when a wall of fibrous tissue has been formed.
7. The amount of drainage will vary with the procedure. Most common surgical procedures (eg, appendectomy, cholecystectomy, abdominal hysterectomy) have minimal wound drainage by the third to fourth postoperative day. Drains are not commonly used following these operations.

NURSING ALERT:
The greatest amount of drainage is expected during the first 24 hours; closely monitor dressing and drains.

◆ NURSING PROCESS OVERVIEW

Assessment

The wound should be assessed every 15 minutes while the patient is in the recovery room. Thereafter, the frequency of wound assessment is determined by the nature of the wound, the degree of drainage, and the hospital protocol. Assessment and documentation of the wound's status should occur at least every shift until patient discharge.

Determine the following which will impact on wound healing:
1. What type of surgery did the patient have?
2. Was hemostasis in the operating room effective?
3. Has the patient received blood to sustain an adequate hematocrit (and promote perfusion to wound)?
4. What is the patient's age?
5. What is the nutritional status? What was it preoperatively?
   a. Is current intake of protein and vitamin C adequate?
   b. Is patient obese or cachectic?
6. What underlying medical conditions does patient have, and what medications is patient taking that could affect wound healing (eg, diabetes mellitus; steroids)?
7. How long has the patient been hospitalized preoperatively? (Longer preoperative hospital stays can increase complications.)
8. How is the wound held together?
   a. Staples, nylon sutures, adhesive strips, tension sutures?
   b. If the wound is left open, how is it being treated? Is granulation tissue present?
9. Are drains in place? What kind? How many?
   a. Is portable suction being used?
   b. Is the amount of drainage consistent with the nature of surgery?
10. What kind of dressings are being used?
    a. Are they saturated with exudate?
    b. Is the amount and type of drainage consistent with nature of the surgery?
11. How does the wound appear?
    a. Is there evidence of edema, irritation, inflammation?

b. Are the wound edges well approximated?

c. Is the wound clean and dry?

12. How does the patient appear?

a. Are there signs of wound pain or discomfort?

b. Is fever or elevated white blood cell count present?

c. Does patient express concern about the wound and potential disfigurement?

13. Does patient understand purpose of wound therapies, and can patient or significant other effectively carry out discharge instructions about wound care?

Nursing Interventions

1. Ensure asepsis during dressing changes.

2. Reinforce or change dressings promptly when saturated with drainage.

3. Give patient prescribed medication before painful dressing changes.

4. Minimize strain on incision site:

a. Use appropriate tape, bandages, and binders.

b. Have patient splint abdominal and chest incision when coughing.

c. Instruct patient in proper way to get out of bed while minimizing incision strain (eg, for abdominal incision, turn on side and push self up with dependent elbow and opposite hand).

5. Keep drainage tubing away from actual incision site.

6. Instruct patient to avoid touching incision to minimize wound contamination and injury.

7. Assess patient's nutritional intake; consult with patient's health care provider if supplemental nutritional intake is required.

8. Assess and accurately document condition of incision site each shift.

9. Clarify patient's misconceptions of surgery and surgical incision.

10. Discuss the patient's feelings regarding the wound appearance and perceived disfigurement.

Patient Education

Before discharge, instruct patient and significant other on techniques and rationale for wound care.

1. Report immediately to health care provider if the following signs of infection occur:

a. Redness, marked swelling (beyond $\frac{1}{2}$ inch from incision site), tenderness, and increased warmth around wound

b. Pus or unusual discharge, foul odor from wound

c. Red streaks in skin near wound

d. Chills or fever (over 37.7°C or 100°F)

2. Follow directives of the nurse or health care provider regarding activity allowances.

3. Keep suture line clean (may shower unless contraindicated by health care provider; avoid tub bathing until wound heals); never vigorously rub near suture line, pat dry.

4. Report to health care provider if after 2 months the incision site continues to be red, thick, and painful to pressure (probable beginning of keloid formation).

PROCEDURE GUIDELINES 5-1 ♦ Changing Surgical Dressings

GENERAL CONSIDERATIONS

1. The procedure of changing dressings, then examining and cleansing the wound, uses principles of asepsis.

2. The initial dressing change is frequently done by the physician, especially for craniotomy, orthopedic, or thoracotomy procedures; subsequent dressing changes are the nurse's responsibility.

EQUIPMENT

STERILE

Gloves—disposable

Scissors, forceps (disposable packs available)

Appropriate dressing materials

Sterile saline

Cotton-tipped swabs

Culture tubes (if infection suspected)

For draining wound: add extra gauze and packing material, absorbent pads, and irrigation set

UNSTERILE

Gloves

Plastic bag for discarded dressings

Tape, proper size and type

Pads to protect patient's bed

Gown for nurse if wound is purulent/infected

PROCEDURE

PREPARATORY PHASE

1. Inform patient of dressing change. Explain procedure and have patient lie in bed.

2. Avoid changing dressings at mealtime.

3. Ensure privacy by drawing the curtains or closing the door; expose the dressing site.

4. Respect patient's modesty and prevent patient from being chilled.

5. Wash hands thoroughly.

6. Place dressing supplies on a clean, flat surface (overbed table).

7. If linen protection is needed, place clean towel or plastic bag under part of the body where wound is located.

8. Cut (or tear) off pieces of tape to be used in dressing change.

9. Place disposable bag nearby to collect soiled dressings.

10. Determine how many and what types of dressings are necessary. Open each dressing by peeling apart the edges of package (MAINTAIN STERILITY OF DRESSING). Leave each dressing within the open package.

PROCEDURE (cont'd)	NURSING ACTION	RATIONALE

REMOVING OLD DRESSING

1. Don disposable gloves.

2. Loosen all tape and gently pull tape ends toward the wound. It helps to hold skin taut with one hand while carefully peeling up an edge of the tape with the other hand. Wiping the back of tape with alcohol will hasten removal of "stuck" tape.
3. Remove old dressings, one layer at a time, and place in disposable bag.
4. Removal of adherent dressings may be facilitated by moistening dressing with sterile saline.

1. Unsterile gloves are sufficient if care is used not to touch wound.
2. This process is less painful and less disturbing to the healing process (avoids pulling the wound edges apart and traumatizing sensitive skin).

3. Hasty removal of dressings can cause trauma to wound and dislodge existing drains.
4. This process is less painful and less traumatic to the delicate healing tissues.

OBTAINING A WOUND CULTURE

1. Use aseptic technique.

2. Open sterile package of gloves; open package containing sterile syringe and needle; open package containing cotton-tipped culture swab. Keep all products within their sterile open packages until use.
3. Don sterile gloves.
4. Aspirate generous amount of drainage liquid into syringe; inject into anaerobic tube. If liquid material is unobtainable, swab desired area with cotton-tipped culture swab, attempting to get maximum saturation.
5. See that specimen is properly labeled and sent to laboratory for study.

1. To prevent contamination of a clean wound or culture media, or to prevent further contamination of a "dirty" wound.
2. Preparation for septic procedure.

4. It is important to collect culture specimen before wound is cleansed. The swab is the more common approach to wound cultures.

CLEANSING THE SIMPLE SURGICAL WOUND

1. Use aseptic technique.
2. Open package of sterile gloves; open sterile cleaning supplies (cotton-tipped applicators, sterile gauze sponges, sterile solution cup, sterile saline).
3. Don sterile gloves.
4. Clean along wound edges using a small circular motion from one end of the incision to the other; be sure to clean each side of the wound separately. Repeat the process using another moistened gauze or swab until the entire incision is cleansed. DO NOT SCRUB BACK AND FORTH ACROSS THE INCISION LINE.
5. Sterile saline is the cleansing agent of choice. Topical antiseptics (eg, povidone-iodine, hexachlorophene, alcohol, and boric acid) may be used on intact skin surrounding the wound but SHOULD NEVER BE USED WITHIN THE WOUND.
6. Repeat the same process with the drain site. Always clean the drain site separately from the primary incision site.
7. Discard used cleaning supplies in the disposable bag.
8. Pat the incision site and drain site dry with a sterile dressing sponge.

2. Preparation for aseptic procedure. Pour sterile cleansing solution (preferably saline) into the solution cup before donning sterile gloves.

4. To prevent contamination and mechanical trauma of wound.

5. Most of the antiseptic agents are caustic to tissues and impair healing. The old saying, "Never put anything in a wound that you couldn't put in your eye," is a truthful one.

6. Reduces chance of cross-contamination.

7. This will be incinerated later.
8. To prepare wound for final dressing.

DRESSING THE WOUND

1. Maintain asepsis with use of sterile gloves.
2. After wound is dry, apply appropriate dressing, taking into consideration the nature of wound.
3. Tape dressing, using only the amount of tape required for secure attachment of dressing. Applying a "skin prep" on site to be taped can facilitate fixation and reduce irritation.

3. Excessive use of tape can cause irritation and trauma to intact skin.

(continued)

PROCEDURE GUIDELINES 5-1 ◆ Changing Surgical Dressings *(continued)*

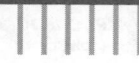

PROCEDURE (cont'd)	NURSING ACTION	RATIONALE

4. When *dressing the drain site:*
   a. Use premade drain sponge (can be prepared by making 5 cm (2-inch) slit, with sterile scissors, in 4 × 4 inch gauze sponge).
   b. Gently slip sponge around drain; repeat process with second drain sponge, placing it at a right angle to the other sponge (see accompanying figure).

   a. The slit allows gauze to fit around the drainage tube.

   b. Placement of the drain sponges in this manner allows for circumferential coverage of the drain site.

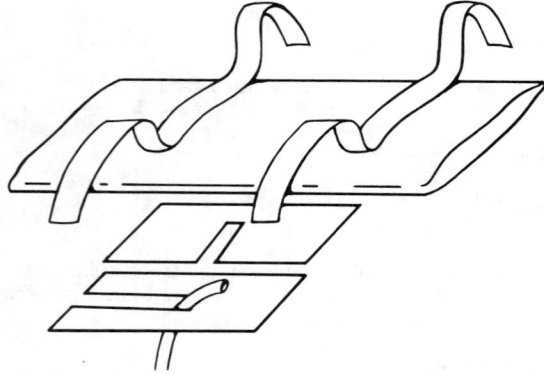

Dressing the drainage tube insertion site. Be sure that one sponge is placed at a right angle to the second sponge so that the slits are going in different directions. If drainage is heavy, a sterile absorbent pad or extra gauze may be placed overall.

5. When *dressing an excessively draining wound:*
   a. Consider need for extra dressings and packing material.
   b. Use Montgomery straps if frequent dressing changes are required (see accompanying figure).

   a. More dressing materials are needed to absorb excess fluid.
   b. Frequent dressing changes can damage surrounding, intact skin due to the frequent application and removal of tape. Montgomery straps alleviate the problem.

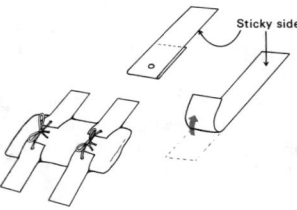 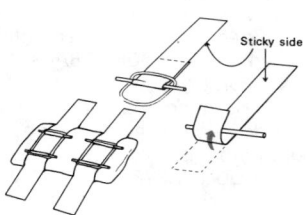

Montgomery straps; two styles are shown.

   c. Excessively draining wounds may be "pouched," much like an ostomy bag.
   d. Protect skin surrounding wound from copious or irritating drainage (eg, gastrointestinal drainage), by applying some type of skin barrier.

   c. To protect surrounding skin, save nursing time, and facilitate accurate assessment of drainage.
   d. Maintaining the cleanliness and integrity of surrounding tissue is essential for successful overall wound healing.

FOLLOW-UP CARE

1. Assess patient's tolerance to the procedure and help make patient more comfortable.
2. Discard disposable items according to hospital protocol and clean equipment that is to be reused.
3. Wash hands.
4. Record nature of procedure and condition of wound, as well as patient reaction.

2. To prevent transmission of pathogenic organisms.

NURSING ACTION	RATIONALE

SKIN CARE TIPS

1. Apply protective "screens" to skin surrounding wounds with copious or irritating secretions (eg, gastrointestinal secretions):
   a. Hydrophobic gauze (eg, vaseline gauze)
   b. Stomahesive (by Squibb)
   c. Skin Barrier (by Bard)
   d. Transparent film dressing

1. Some drainage can be quite damaging to normal or sensitive skin surrounding draining wound sites—adding another risk of infection. Acids and proteolytic enzymes from gastrointestinal drainage are especially caustic.

PROCEDURE GUIDELINES 5-2 ◆ Using Portable Wound Suction

EQUIPMENT A calibrated collection container
Nonsterile gloves

NURSING ACTION	RATIONALE

1. When evacuator is full (200–800 mL—depending on size of evacuator), it is time to empty. A good rule is to empty every 8 hours, or more frequently if necessary.
2. Carefully remove plug, maintaining its sterility.
3. Empty contents of evacuator into calibrated container.
4. Place evacuator on flat surface.
5. Cleanse opening, as well as plug, with an alcohol sponge.
6. Compress evacuator completely (see accompanying figure).

1. Negative pressure is dissipated as the evacuator fills.

2. Minimizes risk of wound infection.
3. Measure drainage.
4. To permit adequate compression.
5. To maintain cleanliness of outlet.
6. To remove air.

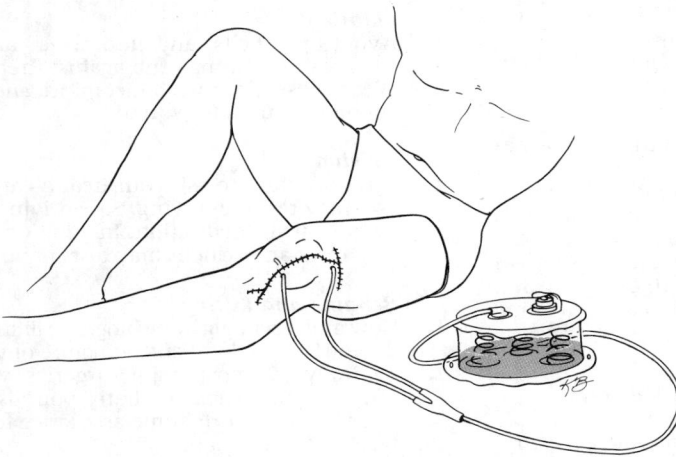

Portable wound suction. Two perforated catheters are draining the incisional area following knee surgery. Drainage is drawn into the portable wound suction unit.

7. Replace plug while evacuator is compressed.
8. As spring expands, a negative pressure of approximately 45 mm Hg is produced.

9. Check system for proper operation.

10. Secure evacuator to patient's dressing; if patient is ambulatory, may fasten evacuator to clothing.
11. Ensure that the drainage catheters are positioned off of incisional site.
12. Wash hands thoroughly.
13. Record character and amount of drainage.

7. To reestablish negative pressure (suction).
8. Any fluid and blood in tissues is sucked into evacuator. Negative pressure is not great enough to suck the soft tissues into the holes of the drainage catheter.
9. Look for fluid entering system; if none, look for disconnections.
10. This permits patient to move without disturbing closed suction.
11. Minimizes trauma and contamination of wound.

12. To prevent cross-contamination with other patients and staff.

Postoperative Discharge Instructions

It is of primary importance that the nurse ensure that the patient has been given specific and individualized discharge instructions. These should be written by a provider and reinforced verbally by the nurse. A provider telephone contact should be included, as well as information regarding follow-up care and appointments. The instructions should be signed by the patient, provider, and nurse and a copy becomes part of the patient's chart. Forms and procedures for discharge instructions may vary per facility.

General Nursing Responsibilities

The nurse should reinforce the following items with the patient as a discharge summary.

A. Rest and Activity
1. It is common to feel tired and frustrated about not feeling able to do all the things you want; this is normal.
2. Plan regular naps and quiet activities, gradually increasing your exercise over the following weeks.
3. When you begin to exercise more, start by taking a short walk two or three times a day. Consult your health care provider if more specific exercises are required.
4. Climbing stairs in your home may be surprisingly tiring at first. If you have difficulty with this activity, try going upstairs backward ("scooching") on your "bottom" until your strength has returned.
5. Consult your health care provider to determine the appropriate time to return to work.

B. Eating
1. Follow dietary instructions provided at the hospital before your discharge.
2. It is not surprising to find that your appetite is limited at first or that you may feel bloated after meals; this should become less a problem as you become more active. (Some prescribed medications can cause this.) If symptoms persist, consult your health care provider.
3. Eat small, regular meals and make them as nourishing as possible to promote wound healing.

C. Sleeping
1. If sleeping is difficult because of wound discomfort, try taking your pain medication at bedtime.
2. Attempt to get sufficient sleep to aid in your recovery.

D. Wound Healing
1. Your wound will go through several stages of healing. After initial pain at the site, the wound may feel tingling, itchy, numb, or tight (a slight pulling sensation) as healing occurs.
2. Do not pull off any scabs because they protect the delicate new tissues underneath. They will fall off without any help when ready.
3. Consult your health care provider if the amount of pain in your wound increases or if you notice increased redness, swelling, or discharge from wound.

E. Bowels
1. Irregular bowel habits can result from changes in activity and diet or the use of some drugs.
2. Avoid straining because it can intensify discomfort in some wounds; instead, use a rocking motion while trying to pass stool.
3. It may be helpful to take a mild laxative. Consult your health care provider if you have any questions.

F. Bathing, Showering
1. You may get your wound wet within 3 days of your operation (unless otherwise advised).
2. Showering is preferable because it allows for thorough rinsing of the wound.
3. If you are feeling too weak, place a plastic or metal chair in the shower so that you may be seated during showering.
4. Be sure to dry your wound thoroughly with a clean towel and dress it as instructed before discharge.

G. Clothing
1. Avoid tight belts, and underwear and other clothes with seams that may rub against the wound.
2. Wear loose clothing for comfort and to reduce mechanical trauma to wound.

H. Driving
1. It is important to ask your health care provider when you may resume driving. Safe driving may be affected by your pain medication. In addition, any violent jarring from an accident may disrupt your wound.

I. Bending and Lifting
1. How much bending, stretching, and lifting you are allowed depends on the location and nature of your surgery.
2. Typically, for most major surgeries, you should avoid lifting anything heavier than 5 pounds for 4 to 8 weeks.
3. It is ideal to secure home assistance for the first 2 to 3 weeks after discharge.

Selected References

American Society of Post Anesthesia Nurses. (1991). *Standards of Post Anesthesia Nursing Practice.* Richmond, VA: Author.

Association of Operating Room Nurses. (1993). *AORN Standards and Recommended Practices for Perioperative Nursing.* Denver: the Association.

Drain, C. B. (1994). *The post anesthesia care unit* (3rd ed.). Philadelphia: W. B. Saunders.

Erwin-Toth, P. & Hocevar, J. (1995). Wound care: Selecting the right dressing. *AJN, 95* (2), 46–51.

Fairchild, S. S. (1993). *Perioperative nursing, principles and practice.* Boston: Jones and Bartlett Publishers.

Kaiser, K. S. (1992). Assessment and management of pain in the critically ill trauma patient. *Critical Care Nursing Quarterly, 15* (2), 14-34.

Litwick, K. (1994). *Core curriculum for post anesthesia nursing practice* (3rd ed.). Philadelphia: W. B. Saunders.

Meeker, M. H. (1995). *Alexander's care of the patient in surgery* (10th ed.). St. Louis: C. V. Mosby.

Pica-Furey, W. (1993). Ambulatory surgery—hospital based versus freestanding. *AORN Journal, 57* (5), 1119–1127.

Cancer Nursing

General Considerations

Cancer is a disease of the cell in which the normal mechanisms of control of growth and proliferation are disturbed. This results in distinctive morphologic alterations of the cell and aberrations in tissue patterns.

The malignant cell is able to invade the surrounding tissue and regional lymph nodes. Primary cancer usually has a predictable natural history and pattern of spread.

Metastasis is the secondary growth of the primary cancer in another organ. The cancer cell migrates through a series of steps to another area of the body. This is the reason that cancer cannot always be cured by surgical removal alone. Most patients die as a result of metastases rather than progression of the primary cancer. Metastasis begins with local invasion followed by detachment of cancer cells that disseminate via the lymphatics and blood vessels and eventually establish a secondary tumor in another area of the body. Lymph nodes are often the first site of distant spread (Table 6-1).

◆ ETIOLOGY, DETECTION, AND PREVENTION

Epidemiology

1. Age is the most outstanding risk factor for cancer.
    a. Cancer incidence increases progressively with age.
    b. Approximately 55% of persons diagnosed with cancer are over 65 years of age.
2. The elderly often have inadequate knowledge about cancer.
    a. Their attitudes and perceptions toward cancer and screening tests pose significant barriers to early detection.
    b. The largest barrier may be lack of symptoms.
3. Five-year survival rates are increasing with improved therapy and earlier detection.
4. Smoking is related to 85% of all cancers.
5. Ongoing genetic research is searching for the ability to correct and modify hereditary susceptibility.
6. Patterns of incidence and death rates vary with sex, age, race, and geographic location (Table 6-2).

Nutrition and Cancer

> **GERONTOLOGIC ALERT:**
> Elderly patients, especially those who live alone, may be malnourished before the initiation of therapy. Dietary consultation may be crucial before therapy.

1. Diet does influence the risk of cancer.
2. The National Research Council (NRC) recommends a diet moderate in total saturated fat, high in complex carbohydrates and fiber, low in sugars, and moderate in protein, especially animal proteins.
    a. High intake of fats is associated with breast, colon, and prostate cancer.
    b. Low intake of fruit, vegetables, complex carbohydrates, and fiber is linked with cancer of the colon, larynx, esophagus, prostate, bladder, stomach, and lung.
    c. Salt-cured foods may influence cancers of the esophagus and stomach.
    d. Alcohol use can increase the risk of cancer of the mouth, larynx, throat, esophagus, and liver.
    e. Obesity is linked to cancers of the breast, colon, uterus, and gallbladder.
    f. The role of heredity also is acknowledged.
3. Table 6-3 compares the dietary guidelines for cancer prevention from the National Cancer Institute (NCI), the American Cancer Society (ACS), and the NRC.

Detection and Prevention

1. Early detection and prevention are effective in decreasing mortality and morbidity of many cancers. The ACS recommends specific screening measures to reduce an individual's risk of cancer (Table 6-4).
2. Prevention
    a. Elimination of smoking is key to reduction of risk for many cancers.
    b. Consideration should be given to reducing overall fat intake in the diet.
    c. Avoidance of sun exposure helps to prevent actinic skin damage.
3. Early detection and screening—most cancers are diagnosed after a reported symptom(s).

TABLE 6-1 Differences Between Malignant and Benign Tumors

Characteristic	Benign	Malignant
Type of cell	Mature, differentiated	Immature; poorly differentiated
Growth	Slowly expansile	Invasive
Metastasis	Absent	Present

a. Performing routine screening blood tests or radiologic work-up should be based on whether these tests are adequate to detect a potentially curable cancer in an otherwise asymptomatic person and are also cost effective.

b. One must consider the family history of cancer, age, sex, ethnic group or race, genetic predisposition, psychological factors, previous iatrogenic factors (prior radiation therapy or drugs such as estrogen replacement therapy) and physical environment (place of employment, exposure to industrial agents such as nickel, chromate, asbestos, vinyl chloride).

c. Women with first or second degree relatives with breast cancer are at increased risk. Women with family histories develop breast cancer at younger ages. Other risk factors include early age of menarche, late age at first pregnancy, and nulliparity.

d. Testicular cancer is the most common cancer of men between the ages of 15 and 34. Men with undescended testicles are at greatest risk.

Diagnostic Evaluation

1. Complete past medical history, social history, and physical examination

2. Biopsy of tumor site to determine pathologic diagnosis
   a. The malignancy is classified according to anatomic extent and histopathologic analysis.
   b. Biopsy is obtained from the most accessible site (eg, lymph node versus lung biopsy).
   c. All original slides should be reviewed with the pathologist. Clinical information should correlate with pathologic diagnosis. Be aware of possible errors and differences in interpretation.
   d. Classification of tumor type is based on tissue and cellular staining. Differences in cytoplasmic and nuclear staining distinguish one cell type from another and identify their stage of differentiation. The grade of the tumor (rating of 1–4) is based on how well differentiated the tissue or cells appear. For most tumors, the higher grade the less differentiated, which is associated with poorer prognosis.
   e. Flow cytometry testing of tumor tissue determines DNA content and indicates potential risk of recurrence.
   f. Estrogen/progesterone levels are obtained from breast tissue.

3. Laboratory tests including complete blood count (CBC) with differential, platelet count, blood chemistries including liver function tests, blood urea nitrogen (BUN), and creatinine are done to determine baseline values.
   a. Further tests depend on cancer diagnosis.
   b. Blood markers (α-fetoprotein, β-human chorionic gonadotropin, CA15-3, CA125) may be appropriate to follow response to therapy.

4. Imaging procedures: chest x-ray, nuclear medicine scan, computed tomography (CT) scans, magnetic resonance imaging (MRI) all to determine evidence or extent of metastasis

Staging

Staging is done to determine the extent of disease (local versus metastatic) to be able to best proceed in proper management.

TABLE 6-2 Leading Sites of Cancer Incidence and Death— 1995 Estimates

Cancer Incidence by Site and Sex*		Cancer Deaths by Site and Sex	
Male	Female	Male	Female
Prostate 244,000	Breast 182,000	Lung 95,400	Lung 62,000
Lung 96,000	Colon & rectum 73,900	Prostate 40,400	Breast 46,000
Colon & rectum 70,700	Lung 73,900	Colon & rectum 27,200	Colon & rectum 28,100
Bladder 37,300	Uterus 48,600	Pancreas 13,200	Ovary 14,500
Lymphoma 34,000	Ovary 26,600	Lymphoma 12,820	Pancreas 13,800
Oral 18,800	Lymphoma 24,700	Leukemia 11,100	Lymphoma 11,330
Melanoma of the skin 18,700	Melanoma of the skin 15,400	Stomach 8,800	Uterus 10,700
Kidney 17,100	Pancreas 13,200	Esophagus 8,200	Leukemia 9,300
Leukemia 14,700	Bladder 13,000	Liver 7,700	Liver 6,500
Stomach 14,000	Leukemia 11,000	Bladder 7,500	Brain 6,000
Pancreas 11,000	Kidney 11,700	Brain 7,300	Stomach 5,900
Larynx 9,000	Oral 9,350	Kidney 7,100	Multiple myeloma 5,000
All sites 677,000	All sites 575,000	All sites 289,000	All sites 258,000

* Excluding basal and squamous cell skin cancer and carcinoma in situ.
(American Cancer Society, 1995.)

TABLE 6-3 Dietary Guidelines for Cancer Prevention*

	NCI	ACS	NRC
Fats	30% or less of total calories	Decrease total fat	30% or less of total calories
Carbohydrates Breads, cereals, and legumes	20–30 g fiber daily 3–5† servings	Increase foods high in fiber, and foods high in vitamins A and C, such as whole grain cereals, fruits, and vegetables. Include cruciferous vegetables.	6+ servings
Fruits	2–3 servings		5+ servings (especially citrus, and green and yellow vegetables)
Vegetables	3–5 servings		

* A comparison of the fat and carbohydrate recommendations from the dietary guidlines of the National Cancer Institute (NCI), American Cancer Society (ACS), and the National Research Council (NRC).
† Serving = 1 cup or 2 slices. **Note:** All other servings = ¹/₂ cup or 1 slice.
(From 1989. *Journal of the National Cancer Institute, 81*(7), 4.)

1. No standard evaluation exists for all cancers. Work-up depends on the patient, tumor type, symptoms, and medical knowledge of the natural history of that cancer.
2. Includes extent of primary cancer (size, invasion of surrounding tissues, involvement of nerves, blood vessels, or lymphatic system), sites of metastases, and overall performance status of the patient.
3. There is no standard long-term follow-up. Routine laboratory and radiologic testing should be cost effective and based on known patterns of spread or recurrence. Usual timing is every 3 months for the first year.

TABLE 6-4 Recommendations for the Early Detection of Cancer in Asymptomatic Persons

Cancer Site	Test	Sex	Age	Frequency
Skin	Self-exam	M/F	Any age	Regularly; by health care provider when changes in size, shape, or color of moles, or a new growth
Colon/Rectum	Fecal occult blood test	M/F	50 and over	Yearly
	Digital rectal exam	M/F	50 and over	Yearly
	Sigmoidoscopy	M/F	50 and over	Every 3–5 y
Cervix	Pelvic exam, PAP smear	F	18 or sexually active	Yearly
Mouth	Oral exam	M/F	Over 50 or any age if use of alcohol or smoker	Regularly; when change in color, sore, swelling, or bleeding
Prostate	Digital rectal exam	M	Over 40	Yearly
Testicle	Self-exam	M	15–34	Regularly; by health care provider when lump felt
Breast	Self-exam	M/F	Any age	Regularly; by health care provider when lump felt and yearly. (Monthly self-exam for female)
	Mammogram	F	35–39	Baseline
			40–49	Every 1–2 y
			50 and over	Yearly

Management

The method of treatment depends on the type of malignancy, the specific histologic cell type, stage, presence of metastasis, and condition of the patient. Cancer is treated by surgery, chemotherapy, radiation, immunotherapy, or a combination of these modalities.

◆ SURGICAL MANAGEMENT

The principles of surgical management are based on a cooperative, multidisciplinary approach to various surgical resources. This is key to the management of the cancer patient. A surgical intervention usually provides the initial diagnosis and subsequent procedures may be needed for treatment.

Types of Surgical Procedures

1. *Biopsy*—surgical removal of a piece of tissue from the questionable area; the tissue sample is sent to the pathology laboratory for diagnostic verification.
2. *Reconstructive/rehabilitative surgery*—repair of defects from previous radical surgical resection. Can be performed early (breast reconstruction) or delayed (head and neck surgery).
3. *Palliative surgery*—surgery that attempts to relieve the complications of cancer (eg, obstruction of the gastrointestinal tract, pain produced by tumor extension into surrounding nerves).
4. *Adjuvant surgery*—use of various surgical techniques to facilitate the overall management. These procedures include vascular access devices, radiotherapy implants, peritoneal access, ventricular access, drainage of peritoneal or pleural effusions.
5. *Treatment of primary tumor*—the removal of the primary site of malignancy. The goal of therapy is cure. This depends on the biology of that particular cancer (eg, basal cell carcinoma of the skin, early tumors of the rectum or colon).
6. *Resection of metastases*—used only in selected cases when a cure can be obtained or a reasonable prolongation of survival is possible. The primary cancer must be under control. The decision to proceed is influenced by the type of histology, number of lesions, their location, and whether they are bilateral.
7. *Preventive/prophylactic surgery*—removal of lesions that if left in the body are apt to develop into cancer. An example is polyps in the rectum.
8. *Curative surgery*—the removal of the primary site of malignancy and any lymph nodes to which the neoplasm has extended. Such surgery may be all that is required.
9. *Debulking surgery*—removal of bulk of the tumor; should be performed before the start of chemotherapy whenever possible.

◆ CHEMOTHERAPY FOR CANCER

Chemotherapy is the use of antineoplastic drugs to promote tumor cell destruction by interfering with cellular function and reproduction. It includes the use of various chemotherapeutic agents and hormones.

Indications and Precautions

1. The goal of chemotherapy is to destroy as many tumor cells as possible with minimal effect on healthy cells.
2. Chemotherapy can be used for cure, control, or palliation.
   a. It may be curative for certain malignancies (testicular cancer, acute lymphocytic leukemia, Hodgkin's disease).
   b. It is a palliative measure with the goal of maintaining optimum functioning.
   c. *Adjuvant therapy*—administered when no detectable disease is present. The goal is to decrease the rate of relapse and improve disease-free survival as well as maximizing potential for cure.
   d. *Neoadjuvant*—administration of several courses of chemotherapy before definitive surgical intervention (eg, large breast masses). The goal of therapy is to decrease the amount of tissue that needs to be removed as well as attempt to maximize cure potential.
   e. *High dose/intensive*—administration of high doses of chemotherapy usually in association with growth factor support or before bone marrow transplant.
3. Should not be administered if there is no reasonable benefit or the patient's condition is moribund.
4. Asymptomatic patients with slow-growing tumors should have treatment postponed until symptoms are worse than potential side effects of chemotherapy.
5. Many chemotherapeutic agents have associated toxicities that can be dose limiting and require nursing interventions (Table 6-5).
6. Dosage can be accurately calculated in adults and children using body surface area (mg/m^2).
7. Many types of cancers respond to chemotherapy, including specific types of leukemia and lymphomas, breast cancer, small cell lung cancer, Ewing's sarcoma, retinoblastoma, and Wilms' tumor.
8. Can be given as single agents or in combination. Combinations of chemotherapeutic agents are often more effective.
9. Toxicity is the limiting factor when using chemotherapy; therefore, it is imperative that the toxicities be recognized by the nurse. Chemotherapy predictably affects normal, rapidly growing cells (eg, bone marrow, gastrointestinal tract lining, hair follicles).
10. Certain chemotherapeutic agents can be effective on one of the four phases of the cell cycle or during any phase of the cell cycle. The cell cycle is divided into four stages:
    a. G1 (Gap one) phase (Postmitotic): Enzymes for DNA synthesis are manufactured.
    b. S (Synthesis) phase: During a long time period the DNA component doubles for the chromosomes in preparation for cell division.
    c. G2 (Gap two) phase: This is a short time period; protein and RNA synthesis occurs, and the mitotic spindle apparatus is formed.
    d. M (Mitosis) phase: In an extremely short time period, the cell actually divides into two identical daughter cells.
    e. Cells not active in the cell cycle are designated as "resting" (G0).
11. Malignant cells may exhibit resistance to some antineoplastic agents, thus limiting their usefulness. The tumor can be resistant to certain drugs from the start of therapy (natural resistance) or become resistant after therapy has begun (acquired resistance).

12. Drugs may be given by the following routes:
   a. Oral—capsule, tablet or liquid
   b. Intravenous (IV)—push (bolus) or infusion over a specified time period
   c. Intramuscular
   d. Subcutaneous
   e. Intrathecal/intraventricular—given by injection through an Ommaya reservoir or by spinal tap
   f. Intra-arterial
   g. Intracavitary—such as peritoneal cavity
   h. Intravesicle—into uterus or bladder
   i. Topical

Safety Measures in Handling Chemotherapy

Cytotoxic drugs may be irritating to the skin, eyes, and mucous membranes. See Procedure Guidelines 6-1, p. 109.

A. Personal Safety to Minimize Exposure via Inhalation
1. Chemotherapeutic agents should be prepared in a class II biologic safety cabinet (vertical laminar flow hood).
2. If no class II safety cabinet is available, prepare chemotherapy in a well ventilated area. Wear gloves, goggles, and a gown of low-permeability fabric with cuffed long sleeves and closed front.
3. Vent vials with filter needle to equalize the internal pressure or use negative-pressure techniques.
4. Wrap gauze or alcohol pads around the neck of ampules when opening to decrease droplet contamination.
5. Wrap gauze or alcohol pads around injection sites when removing syringes or needles from IV injection ports.
6. Do not dispose of materials by clipping needles or removing needles from syringes.
7. Use puncture- and leak-proof containers for noncapped, nonclipped needles.

B. Personal Safety to Minimize Exposure via Skin Contact
1. Wear latex gloves at all times when preparing or working with chemotherapeutic agents.
2. Wash hands before putting on gloves and after removing gloves.
3. Change latex gloves frequently (as often as every 30 minutes) because no conclusive data exist for permeability of chemotherapeutic agents via gloves.
4. Wear a gown of low-permeability fabric with a closed front and cuffed long sleeves.
5. Use syringes and IV tubing with Luer locks (which have a locking device to hold needle firmly in place).
6. Label all syringes and IV tubing containing chemotherapeutic agents as hazardous material.
7. Place an absorbent pad directly under the injection site to absorb any accidental spillage.
8. If any contact with the skin occurs, immediately wash the area thoroughly with soap and water.
9. If eye contact is made, immediately flush the eye with water and seek medical attention.

C. Personal Safety to Minimize Exposure via Ingestion
1. Do not eat, drink, chew gum, or smoke while preparing or handling chemotherapy.
2. Keep all food and drink away from preparation area.
3. Wash hands before and after handling chemotherapy.
4. Avoid hand-to-mouth or hand-to-eye contact while handling chemotherapeutic agents or body fluids of the person receiving chemotherapy.

D. Safe Disposal of Antineoplastic Agents, Body Fluids, and Excreta
1. Discard gloves and gown into a leak-proof container, which should be marked as contaminated or hazardous waste.
2. Use puncture- and leak-proof containers for noncapped, nonclipped needles and other sharp or breakable objects.
3. Wear latex gloves for disposing of body excreta and handling soiled linens.
4. The literature pertaining to this topic has not been conclusive.

Complications of Chemotherapy

1. Complications include the side effects or toxicity to chemotherapy (see Table 6-5).
   a. Side effects are usually not life threatening; vary in degree, but can be annoying; they follow a predictable course.
      (1) Nausea and vomiting—usually delayed, vary in intensity depending on drug and dose.
      (2) Alopecia—partial or complete, resolves after drug stopped.
      (3) Change in taste sensation
      (4) Mucositis—usually delayed
   b. Toxic effects usually refer to a life-threatening reaction. Medication dosage may have to be reduced or therapy may be postponed or discontinued.
      (1) Hematologic toxicity—severe bone marrow depression or anemia; delayed and may be prolonged.
      (2) Nephrotoxicity, hepatotoxicity, etc.
2. Grading—scale ranges from 0 to 4 with 0 being normal and 4 indicating life threatening. Score of side effects can determine delay in therapy until the patient returns to normal, dose modification of drug(s), or cessation of therapy.
3. Grade 4 usually requires completion of adverse drug reaction (ADR) notification if drug is investigational.
4. Expected toxicities—known to occur with specific drug(s).
5. Unexpected or ADR should be reported to drug company or study chairperson.

Nursing Assessment

A. Integumentary System
1. Inspect for pain, swelling, with inflammation or phlebitis, necrosis or ulceration.
2. Inspect for skin rash, characteristics, whether pruritus, general or local.
3. Assess areas of erythema and associated tenderness or pruritus. Instruct patient to avoid irritation to skin and to avoid sun exposure or irritating soaps.
4. Assess changes in skin pigmentation.
5. Note reports of photosensitivity, tearing of the eyes.
6. Assess condition of gums, teeth, buccal mucosa, and tongue.
   a. Determine if any taste changes have occurred.
   b. Check for evidence of stomatitis, erythematous areas, ulceration, infection, or pain on swallowing.
   c. Determine if the patient has any complaints of pain or burning of the oral mucosa or on swallowing.

B. Gastrointestinal System
1. Assess for frequency, timing of onset, duration, and severity of nausea and vomiting episodes before and after chemotherapy.
   a. Usually occurs from 1 to 24 hours after chemotherapy but may be delayed. Anticipatory vomiting occurs after at least one course of therapy. Can be initiated by various cues including thoughts, smell, or even sight of the medical personnel.
2. Observe for alterations in hydration, electrolyte balance.
3. Assess for diarrhea or constipation.
   a. Ascertain any changes in bowel patterns.
   b. Discuss the consistency of stools.
   c. Consider the frequency and duration of diarrhea (the number of stools each day for the number of days).
   d. Evaluate any dietary changes or use of medications such as narcotics that have had an impact on the diarrhea or constipation.
4. Assess for anorexia.
   a. Discuss taste changes and changes in food preferences.
   b. Ask about daily food intake and normal eating patterns.
5. Assess for jaundice, right upper quadrant abdominal pain, changes in the stool or urine, and elevated liver function tests that indicate hepatotoxicity.

C. Hematopoietic System
1. Assess for neutropenia—absolute granulocyte count less than 500/mm³.
   a. Assess for any signs of infection (pulmonary, integumentary, central nervous system [CNS], and urinary).
   b. Auscultate lungs for any changes including crackles, wheezes, or rhonchi.
   c. Determine if patient has productive cough or shortness of breath.
   d. Ask if patient has experienced urinary frequency, pain, or odor.
   e. Monitor for an elevation of a temperature above 38.3°C (101°F), chills.
2. Assess for thrombocytopenia—platelet count less than 50,000/mm³ (mild risk of bleeding); less than 20,000/mm³ (severe risk of bleeding).
   a. Assess skin and oral mucous membranes for petechiae, bruises on extremities.
   b. Determine if patient has episodes of bleeding (including nose, urinary, rectal, or hemoptysis).
   c. Assess if any blood in stools or urine, or if emesis has been detected.
   d. Assess for signs and symptoms of intracranial bleeding if platelet count is less than 20,00/mm³; monitor for changes in level of responsiveness, vital signs, and pupillary reaction.
3. Assess for anemia.
   a. Assess skin color, turgor, and capillary refill.
   b. Ascertain if patient has experienced dyspnea on exertion, fatigue, weakness, palpitations, or vertigo. Advise rest periods as needed.

D. Respiratory and Cardiovascular Systems
1. Assess for pulmonary fibrosis evidenced by a dry, nonproductive cough with increasing dyspnea. Patients at risk include: those over 60 years old, smokers, those receiving or having had pulmonary radiation, those receiving cumulative dose of bleomycin (Blenoxane), or any preexisting lung disease.
2. Assess for signs and symptoms of congestive heart failure or irregular apical or radial pulses.
3. Verify baseline cardiac studies (eg, electrocardiogram, multiple gated acquisition scan/ejection fraction) before administering doxorubicin (Adriamycin) or high-dose cyclophosphamide (Cytoxan).

E. Neuromuscular System
1. Ascertain if patient is having difficulty with fine motor activities, such as zipping pants, tying shoes, or buttoning a shirt.
2. Determine the presence of paresthesia (tingling, numbness) of fingers or toes.
3. Evaluate deep tendon reflexes.
4. Evaluate patient for weakness, ataxia, or slapping gait.
5. Determine impact on activities of daily living and discuss changes.
6. Discuss symptoms of urinary retention or constipation.
7. Assess for ringing in ears or decreased hearing acuity.

> **NURSING ALERT:**
> Anorexia, nausea, vomiting along with lethargy, weakness, personality changes, and tetany signal hypomagnesemia caused by cisplatin (Platin) therapy. Administer magnesium promptly.

F. Genitourinary System
1. Assess if patient has increased urinary frequency.
2. Evaluate any changes in odor, color, or clarity of urine sample.
3. Assess for hematuria, oliguria, or anuria.
4. Monitor BUN, creatinine.

Nursing Diagnoses

A. Risk for Infection related to neutropenia
B. Risk for Injury related to thrombocytopenia
C. Fatigue related to anemia
D. Altered Nutrition (Less than Body Requirements) related to side effects of therapy
E. Altered Oral Mucous Membranes related to stomatitis
F. Altered Body Image related to alopecia and weight loss

Nursing Interventions

A. Preventing Infection
1. Monitor vital signs every 4 hours; report any occurrence of fever greater than 38.3°C (101.0°F) and chills.
2. Instruct patient about signs and symptoms of infection including:
   a. Mouth lesions, swelling, or redness
   b. Redness, pain, or tenderness at rectum
   c. Any change in bowel habits
   d. Any areas of redness, swelling, induration, or pain on skin surface
   e. Any pain or burning when urinating or odor from urine
   f. Any cough or shortness of breath
   g. Monitor white blood cell count (WBC) and differential
3. Avoid performing invasive procedures—rectal temperatures, enemas, or insertion of indwelling urinary catheters.
4. Reinforce good personal hygiene habits (routine bathing, preferably a shower, clean hair, nails, and mouth care).

5. Stress importance of strict handwashing.
6. Be aware that nadirs (lowest level) generally occur within 7 to 14 days after drug administration. Length of myelosuppression depends on specific drug. Institution of further therapy usually depends on an adequate WBC and absolute neutrophil count (ANC).
7. Calculate ANC to determine the number of leukocytes capable of fighting an infection by:

$$\text{Total WBC} \times (\% \text{ polys} + \% \text{ bands}) = \text{ANC}$$

$$\text{Example: } 700 \times (10\% + 5\%) = 105$$

Interpretation: 105 of the 700 white blood cells are mature and capable of fighting an infection (indicates severe neutropenia).
8. Administer prophylactic antibiotics as prescribed (if WBC is less than 500) and growth colony-stimulating factor with subsequent courses of chemotherapy to hasten neutrophil maturity.

B. Preventing Bleeding
1. Avoid invasive procedures when platelet count is less than 100,000 mm^3, including intramuscular injections, suppositories, enemas, and insertion of indwelling urinary catheters.
2. Apply pressure on injection sites for 5 minutes.
3. Avoid aspirin-containing products.
4. Monitor platelet count; administer platelets as prescribed.
5. Monitor and test all urine, stools, and emesis for blood.
6. Advise patient to avoid dental work or other invasive procedures while thrombocytopenic.

C. Minimizing Fatigue
1. Monitor blood counts (hemoglobin and hematocrit).
2. Explain why fatigue and shortness of breath may occur.
3. Plan frequent rest periods between daily activities.
4. Administer blood products as prescribed.
5. Caution the patient about physical overexertion; encourage rest frequently and warn patient to expect a tired feeling.
6. Explain that blood transfusions, if given, are a part of therapy and not necessarily an indication of a setback.
7. Observe skin color.

D. Promoting Nutrition
1. Start antiemetics before chemotherapy. Administer on a schedule (not PRN) for highly and moderately emetogenic chemotherapy regimens.
2. For highly emetogenic regimens consider premedication with ondansetron (Zofran), a single dose, or in combination with droperidol (Inapsine) or dexamethasone (Decadron). Failures to this regimen may require metoclopramide (Reglan) with droperidol, dexamethasone, or lorazepam (Ativan).
3. For moderately emetogenic regimens start with droperidol or dexamethasone with metoclopramide plus diphenhydramine (Benadryl). Failures may receive ondansetron.
4. For low emetogenic regimens, consider oral prochlorperazine (Compazine).
5. Extrapyramidal reactions occur frequently in patients under age 30. Treat dystonic reactions with diphenhydramine; restlessness with lorazepam.
6. If delayed nausea and vomiting begin 8 hours after acute prophylactic antiemetic therapy and continue for 24 to 36 hours, administer agents such as metoclopramide with dexamethasone plus diphenhydramine or haloperidol (Haldol) or prochlorperazine or lorezapam.
7. Consider alternative measures for relief of anticipatory nausea such as relaxation therapy, imagery, and distraction.
8. Encourage small, frequent meals, appealing to patient preferences.
9. Encourage patient to eat a diet high in calories and proteins. Provide high-protein supplement as needed.
10. Discourage smoking and alcoholic beverages, which may irritate mucous membranes.
11. Encourage fluid intake to prevent constipation.
12. Monitor intake and output including emesis.
13. Consult dietitian concerning patient's food preferences, intolerances, and individual dietary interventions.
14. Provide emesis basin and tissues; empty and clean basin after each use.
15. Recognize that the patient may have alterations in taste perception, such as a keener taste of bitterness and loss of ability to detect sweet tastes.

E. Minimizing Stomatitis
1. Report signs of infection—erythematous areas, white patches, ulcers.
2. Perform frequent mouth care with soft toothbrush and dilute mouthwash.
3. Assess need for antifungal, antibacterial, or antiviral therapy (each has a different appearance).
4. Administer local oral therapy (combinations with viscous lidocaine [Xylocaine]) for symptomatic control and maintenance of calorie intake.

F. Strengthening Coping With Altered Body Image
1. Reassure patient that hair will usually grow back. It may grow back a different texture or different color.
2. Suggest wearing a turban, wig, or head scarf, preferably purchased before hair loss occurs.
3. Encourage patient to stay on therapeutic program.
4. Be honest with the patient.

Patient Education/Health Maintenance

1. Ensure that patient uses good hygiene, knows symptoms of infection to report, and avoids crowds and persons with infection while neutropenic.
2. Advise patient to avoid use of razor blade to shave, contact sports, manipulation of sharp articles, use of hard bristle toothbrush, and passage of hard stool to prevent bleeding while thrombocytopenic.
3. Advise women to report symptoms of vaginal infection such as pain, discharge, ulceration, or inflammation due to opportunistic fungal or viral infection.
4. Encourage patient participation in treatment plan for chemotherapy and to set realistic goals for work and activities.
5. Assure patient that changes in menses, libido, and sexual function are usually temporary during therapy.

Evaluation

A. Afebrile, no signs of infection
B. No bruising or bleeding noted; stool and urine heme-test negative
C. Denies shortness of breath or severe fatigue
D. Tolerating small, frequent meals following antiemetic
E. No oral lesions or pain on swallowing
F. Dressed, wearing wig and make-up

TABLE 6-5 Frequently Used Chemotherapeutic Agents

Drug	Dose, Route, and Frequency	How Supplied	Major Side Effects			Other Side Effects or Comments
			Myelosuppression	Thrombocytopenia	Risk for Nausea and Vomiting	
Alkylators						
Cyclophosphamide (Cytoxan)	500–1500 mg/m² IV q3–4wk 100 mg/m² PO daily for 14 d	25 mg, 50 mg tablets 100 mg, 200 mg, 500 mg, 1 g, 2 g vials	Marked	Mild	Moderate	Hemorrhagic cystitis, alopecia Monitor liver function Drink 3 L fluids daily
Busulfan (Myleran)	2–8 mg PO, daily	2 mg tablets	Marked	Marked	Mild	Pulmonary fibrosis, skin pigmentation
BCNU (Carmustine)	75–100 mg/m² IV for 1–3 d q6wk	100 mg vial with 3 mL alcohol diluent	Marked delayed	Marked	Marked	Local pain during infusion, pulmonary fibrosis, crosses blood–brain barrier/irritant Requires reconstitution with supplied diluent
CBCDA (Carboplatin)	200–400 mg/m² IV q4wk	50 mg, 150 mg, 450 mg vials	Marked	Marked	Mild	Possible anaphylaxis, thrombocytopenia can be severe and prolonged
CCNU (Lomustine CeeNu)	130 mg/m² PO q6wk	10 mg, 40 mg, 100 mg capsules	Marked delayed	Marked	Moderate	Myelosuppression can be cumulative. Crosses blood–brain barrier. Take at bedtime on empty stomach
Chlorambucil (Leukeran)	0.1–0.2 mg/kg PO daily Usually 2 mg maintenance	2 mg tablet	Moderate	Moderate	Mild	Infertility. Leukopenia delayed up to 3 wk
Cisplatin (Platinol)	50–120 mg/m² IV q3–4wk 20 mg/m² IV daily for 5 d q3–4wk	10 mg, 50 mg vial	Moderate	Moderate	Severe	Nephrotoxicity/neurotoxicity, magnesium wasting, ototoxicity, anemia. Requires antiemetics before and after
Dacarbazine (DTIC)	150 mg/m² daily IV for 5 d q4wk 375 mg/m² on day 1 q15d	100 mg, 200 mg vial	Mild	Mild	Marked	Flulike syndrome, alopecia, facial flushing, parethesia, vesicant
Ifosfamide (Ifex)	1200 mg/m² IV for 5 d q3w	1 g, 2 g, 3 g	Moderate	Moderate	Mild	Neurotoxicity, hemorrhagic cystitis, alopecia, concomitant uroprotection with MESNA
Mesna	20 mg/kg 15 min before Ifex, repeated q3h for 4 doses	200 mg vial	None	None	None	Not an antineoplastice agent. Binds to reactive metabolite of Ifex or Cytoxan without affecting antitumor activity
MeCCNU (Semustine, Methyl CCNU)	130 mg/m² q6wk	10 mg, 40 mg, 100 mg capsules	Marked	Marked	Moderate	Delayed and cumulative myelosuppression, stomatitis, anorexia
Mechlorethamine hydrochloride (nitrogen mustard)	0.4 mg/kg intracavitary or 10 mg/m² q3–6wk	10 mg vials	Marked	Marked	Severe	Vesicant, stomatitis, alopecia, chemical thrombophlebitis
Melphalan (L-Pam, Alkeran)	6 mg orally, daily for 2–4 wk	2 mg tablet	Moderate	Moderate	Mild	Leukemia, second malignancies. Given on empty stomach.

Drug	Dose	Supplied				Toxicity
Streptozocin (Zanosan)	500 mg/m² IV daily for 5 d q6wk	1 g vial	Mild	Mild	Moderate-marked	Irritant, renal failure, reactive hypoglycemia due to insulin release, diarrhea
Antibiotics						
Bleomycin (Blenoxane)	10–20 units/m² IV, IM, SQ weekly Total dose not to exceed 400 units 60–120 units in 100 mL normal saline for intracavitary therapy	15 unit vial	Rare	Rare	Mild	Skin reaction, pulmonary fibrosis, fever, allergic reaction, alopecia, stomatitis
Dactinomycin (Actinomycin D, Cosmegen)	0.010–0.015 µg/kg IV for 5 d q3–4wk	0.5 mg vial	Marked	Marked	Moderate-severe	Alopecia, stomatitis, skin rash, hepatic dysfunction, vesicant, radiation recall
Daunorubicin (Cerubidine)	60 mg/m² IV for 3 d q3–4wk 550 mg/m² total IV dose	20 mg vial	Marked	Marked	Moderate-severe	Cardiomyopathy, alopecia, red urine, radiation recall, vesicant 450–550 mg/m² total dose with mediastinal radiation
Doxorubicin (Adriamycin)	60–75 mg/m² IV q3wk 30 mg/m² for 3 d q3–4 wk Total cumulative dose 550 mg/m²	10 mg, 20 mg, 50 mg vial	Marked	Marked	Moderate	Alopecia, cardiomyopathy, radiation recall, red urine, hepatic dysfunction, vesicant
Mitomycin (Mutamycin)	10–20 mg/m² IV q6–8wk	5 mg, 20 mg vial	Marked	Marked	Moderate	Renal and pulmonary dysfunction, alopecia, stomatitis, delayed myelosuppression, vesicant
Plant Alkaloids						
Vinblastine (Velban)	5 mg/m² IV q1–2wk	10 mg vial	Marked	Marked	Mild	Elevated uric acid, neurotoxicity, mucositis, alopecia, vesicant
Vincristine (Oncovin)	1–2 mg/m² IV maximum single dose 2 mg IV	1 mg/mL vial, 2 mg/mL vial	Mild	Mild	Mild	Distal neuropathy, constipation, vesicant
Vindesine (Eldisine)	2–4 mg/m² IV q1–2wk	10 mg ampule	Moderate	Mild	Mild	Neurotoxicity—can be cumulative if administered with other plant alkaloids, vesicant
Teniposide (VM 26)	50–100 mg/m² IV weekly for 4–6 wk	10 mg/mL ampule	Moderate	Mild	Mild	Distal neuropathy, can have cumulative neurotoxicity if administered with other plant alkaloids, alopecia, vesicant
Etoposide (VePesid) (VP-16)	45–75 mg/m²/d 3–5 d q3–5wk 125–140 mg/m² PO 3 times/wk q5wk	50 mg capsule, 100 mg/5 mL vial	Moderate	Mild	Mild-moderate	Distal neuropathy, alopecia, hypotension can occur following rapid infusion, headache, give over 30 minutes, irritant
Antimetabolites						
Azacytidine (5-azacytidine)	150 mg/m² IV for 5 d by continuous infusion	100 mg vial	Marked	Marked	Severe	Diarrhea, neurotoxicity, mucositis

(continued)

TABLE 6-5 Frequently Used Chemotherapeutic Agents (continued)

Drug	Dose, Route, and Frequency	How Supplied	Major Side Effects			Other Side Effects or Comments
			Myelosuppression	Thrombocytopenia	Risk for Nausea and Vomiting	
Cytarabine (Cytosar, ARA-C)	100 mg/m² continuous IV infusion q12h for 7 d	100 mg vial	Marked	Marked	Moderate	Stomatitis, headaches; anorexia, arachnoiditis with intrathecal. Cerebellar complications with high dose
5-Fluorouracil (5FU, Efudex)	50–100 mg in 100 mL saline for intrathecal; 300–500 mg/m² IV weekly or daily ×5	500 mg ampule cream, 1%, 5%	Moderate-marked	Mild	Mild	Stomatitis, diarrhea, alopecia, vein discoloration, photosensitivity, nail color changes
Hydroxyurea (Hydrea)	80 mg/kg PO daily	500 mg tablet	Marked	Marked	Mild	Alopecia, diarrhea, stomatitis. Crosses blood–brain barrier
6-Mercaptopurine (6 MP, Purinethol)	1.5–2.5 mg/kg PO	50 mg tablet	Moderate-marked	Moderate-marked	Mild	Stomatitis, hepatoxicity. Reduce dose if giving alopurinol concurrently
Methotrexate (Mexate)	2.5–5.0 mg PO daily; IV or IM dose varies 25–50 mg/m² intrathecal 5–10 mg/m² q3–7d	2.5 mg tablets 25 mg, 50 mg injection	Moderated-marked	Moderate-marked	Mild	Stomatitis, nephrotoxicity, diarrhea, crosses blood–brain barrier. Creatinine clearance must be >60 mL/min
Thioguanine (6 TG, Tabloid)	2 mg/kg daily PO	40 mg tablet	Moderate	Moderate	Mild	Cholestasis, stomatitis, diarrhea, hepatotoxicity
Miscellaneous Drugs						
Procarbazine (Matulane)	2–4 mg/kg daily PO	50 mg capsule	Moderate	Moderate	Mild	Sensitive to amines, neurotoxicity, crosses blood–brain barrier
Mitoxantrone (Novantrone)	12 mg/m² IV day 1–3	2 mg/mL in 10 mL, 12.5 mL, 15 mL vial	Moderate	Mild	Mild	Tachycardia, mucositis. Use extreme caution in preparation of drug
Paclitaxel (Taxol)	175 mg/m² IV over 3 h q3wk	30 mg vial, 6 mg/mL with 5 mL	Marked	Mild	Mild	Peripheral neuropathy, alopecia, fatigue. Observe closely for allergic response; premedicate with Benadryl and steroids; heart block, arrhythmia. Requires non-PVC IV tubing

PROCEDURE GUIDELINES 6-1 ◆ Administering IV Chemotherapy

EQUIPMENT
Supplies to start IV infusion or a running IV line
Specific antidote for extravasation (if indicated)
10 mL syringe with needle
Alcohol swabs
Cold or warm compresses

PROCEDURE

NURSING ACTION	RATIONALE
PREPARATORY PHASE	
1. If the patient is receiving chemotherapy for the first time, review understanding of treatment plan and the drug side effects.	
2. If the drug is investigational, verify informed consent.	
3. Check for appropriate dose and route of administration. Verify the patient's identification. Assess if blood counts are adequate (CBC, differential and platelet count).	3. Drug may be withheld in severe neutropenia or thrombocytopenia.
4. Review previous side effects as to their type and severity.	
5. Consider antiemetic therapy before chemotherapy administration.	5. Antiemetics are more effective if given before administration and on a regular dosing schedule thereafter.
6. Be aware of agents that cause anaphylactic reaction such as asparginase (Elspar). Have emergency resuscitation equipment and drugs available.	
7. Review patient's medication history including over-the-counter medications for possible interactions.	
PERFORMANCE PHASE	
1. Select venipuncture site free of sclerosis, thrombosis, or scar formation if at all possible.	1. Prevention is the best treatment approach to avoid extravasation or possible edema of the arm.

NURSING ALERT:
Avoid venipuncture in an arm where dissection of the axillary lymph nodes has been performed or where radiation therapy has caused marked fibrosis in the axillary area.

NURSING ACTION	RATIONALE
2. Use a running IV (flush solution) while administering a vesicant (blistering or necrotic) chemotherapeutic agent IV push.	2. A vesicant is a chemotherapeutic agent capable of causing blistering of tissues and possible tissue necrosis if it extravasates. Some agents are irritants, which cause pain along the vein wall, with or without inflammation.

NURSING ALERT:
If a small focal hematoma develops during insertion of the needle into the vein, DO NOT use this site for chemotherapeutic administration because of the increased risk for extravasation and infiltration.

NURSING ACTION	RATIONALE
3. Maintain constant supervision during administration of IV push vesicant chemotherapy.	3. To identify and treat extravasation immediately.
4. If any doubt exists regarding vein patency or safety of chemotherapy administration, discontinue the administration and treat as an extravasation if a vesicant chemotherapeutic agent has been used.	4. Tissue necrosis and sloughing may lead to permanent disability of an extremity.
a. Monitor for pain, which the patient may describe as localized to severe burning and radiating along the vein.	
b. Examine the site for erythema or swelling. Over a period of days to weeks, the site can become mottled and lead to necrosis.	
c. Stop the infusion of the chemotherapeutic agent.	

(continued)

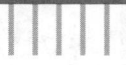

PROCEDURE GUIDELINES 6-1 ◆ Administering IV Chemotherapy
(continued)

PROCEDURE *(cont'd)*	**NURSING ACTION**	**RATIONALE**
	d. Aspirate all residual chemotherapeutic agent in the IV needle/catheter.	
	e. Administer antidote (see accompanying table). Inject intradermally in circular motion around the extravasation site to prevent leakage of drug to surrounding tissues (if appropriate or inject via the IV catheter).	e. Antidote may prevent tissue necrosis. If unable to aspirate from IV catheter, catheter may be blocked and antidote will not reach extravasation.

Management of an Extravasation

CHEMOTHERAPEUTIC AGENT	LOCAL ANTIDOTE	METHOD OF ADMINISTRATION
Dacarbazine (DTIC) Dactinomycin (Actinomycin D) Mitomycin C (Mutamycin) Mechlorethamine (nitrogen mustard)	Isotonic sodium thiosulfate 10% Mixing 4.0 mL of sodium thiosulfate 10% with 6.0 mL sterile water for injection	1. Inject 5–6 mL of mixture through the existing line and SQ in divided doses into the extravasated site with multiple injections. Repeat SQ dosing over several hours. 2. Apply cold compresses 6–12 h after the extravasation.
Vinblastine (Velban) Vincristine (Oncovin) Teniposide (Vm26) Etoposide (VePesid) Streptozocin (Zanosar) Mithramycin (Mithracin)	Hyaluronidase (Wydase) 150 units/mL Add 1 mL USP NaCl	1. Inject 1–6 mL (150–900 units) SQ into extravasated site with multiple injections. 2. Apply warm compresses.
Daunorubicin (Cerubidine) Doxorubicin (Adriamycin) Mitoxantrone (Navantrone) AMSA	Hydrocortisone 50–100 mg/mL	1. Inject ½ mL (50–100 mg) IV through the existing line and SQ into the extravasated site with multiple injections. Total dose not to exceed 100 mg. 2. Apply cold compresses for 15 min 4 times in a 24-h period.
BCNU (Carmustine)	Sodium bicarbonate (0.5 mEq/1 mL) prefilled syringe	1. Inject 2–6 mL of mixture (1.0–3.0 mEq) IV through the existing IV line and into the extravasated site with multiple injections. 2. Total dose not to exceed 10 mL of 0.5 mEq/mL solution (5.0 mEq). 3. Apply cold compresses. Do not apply pressure.
Paclitaxel (Taxol)	None	1. Apply warm compresses to the extravasation site for 24 h.

NURSING ALERT:
Do not inject an antidote via the IV catheter if unable to aspirate the chemotherapeutic agent.

   f. Remove the needle.
   g. Apply ice or heat to the site, depending on the chemotherapeutic agent that has extravasated.

FOLLOW-UP PHASE

1. Document drug dosage, site, and any occurrence of extravasation including estimated amount of drug extravasated, management. Photograph if possible.
2. Observe regularly after administration for pain, erythema, induration, and necrosis.

3. Monitor for other side effects of infusion.
   a. Patient may describe sensations of pain, stretching, or pressure within the vessel, originating near the venipuncture site or extending 7.5–12.5 cm (3–5 inches) along the vein.
   b. Discoloration—red streak following the line of the vein (called a flare reaction) or darkening of the vein
   c. Itching, urticaria, muscle cramps, or pressure in the arm

2. If only a small amount of drug extravasated and frank necrosis does not occur, phlebitis may still result, causing pain for several days or induration at the site that may last for weeks or months.
3.
   a. Caused by irritation to the vein

   b. Flare reaction common with doxorubicin (Adriamycin). Darkening of vein may occur with 5-fluorouracil (5-FU).
   c. Caused by irritation of surrounding subcutaneous tissue

◆ RADIATION THERAPY

Radiation therapy is the use of high-energy, ionizing beams to treat cancer and certain benign disorders. It causes molecular damage and biochemical changes and eventual cell death from disruption of the reproductive cycle.

General Considerations

A. Principles of Therapy
To deliver a precise dose of ionizing radiation without affecting healthy tissue.

1. *Radiosensitivity*—degree and speed of response. This measure of susceptibility of cells to injury or death by radiation depends on cancer diagnosis and its inherent biologic activity. It is directly related to reproductive capability of the cell. Radiosensitive tumors include seminoma, Hodgkin's disease, and lymphomas. Sensitive normal tissues are bone marrow, skin, gonads, mucous membrane, and lymph nodes.
2. *Role of oxygen*—required to be present for maximal killing effect. Poor circulation with resultant hypoxia can reduce cellular radiosensitivity. Giving multiple, daily doses allows reoxygenation and enhances radiosensitivity. The dose should allow for repair of normal tissues.
3. *Cellular response*—can be modified by changes in dose rate, manipulating the process of cell repair, recruiting cells into replication cycle and use of hyperthermia (above 104°F).
4. *Radioresistance*—lack of tumor response to radiation because of tumor characteristics (slow-growing tumor, less responsive), tumor cell proliferation, and circulation. Radiation is most effective during mitotic stage of cell cycle.
5. *Radioresistant tumors*—squamous cell, ovarian, soft tissue sarcoma, gliomas. Normal radioresistant tissues—mature bone, cartilage, liver, thyroid, muscle, brain, and spinal cord.
6. *Beam energy and penetration*—majority of therapeutic radiation is administered using the cobalt 60 source or high-energy photons from linear accelerators. The radiation beam decreases its intensity with increasing depth. The penetration of the radiation into the body is directly proportional to the generating energy. Linear energy transfer (LET) is the rate at which energy is deposited per unit distance. High-energy electrons are used for tumors on or near the skin surface.

B. Types of Radiation Therapy
1. *Teletherapy*—external beam irradiation. Administered by machines a distance from the body (80–100 cm).
   a. Types of machines—cobalt 60 teletherapy units and high energy x-ray sources (linear accelerator, photons)
   b. Most common use of radiation—local therapy.
2. *Brachytherapy*—high dose to a small tissue volume with less dose to adjacent normal tissue. The use of radioactive sources close to or within the tumor. Need direct access to the tumor.
   a. *Interstitial*—implants with solid material such as seeds. May be temporary implants that are removed after several days or permanent. The permanent ones remain in place with gradual decay. Implant procedure is performed under local or general anesthesia. Used in breast and prostate disease.
   b. *Intracavitary*—used in cancers of uterine cervix.
   c. *Surface radiation* is used in choroid cancer.
   d. *Systemic irradiation*—parenteral or IV, oral ^{131}I for thyroid cancer, intraperitoneal.
3. Future trends
   a. *Intraoperative radiation therapy*—surgically removing tumor followed by single high dose to tumor bed. Usually prophylactic.
   b. *Hyperthermia*—combined with radiation. Use a variety of sources (ultrasound, microwaves).
   c. *Radiation sensitizers and radioprotectors*—use of medications to modify the radiation effect.

C. Units for Measuring Radiation Exposure or Absorption
1. *Gray* (Gy)—a unit to measure absorbed dose. One Gy equals 100 rads. (Rad—term used in the past to measure absorbed dose). Joules/kg is also used to measure absorbed dose. 1 joule/kg = Gy.
2. *Roentgen* (R)—standard unit of exposure (usually applied to x-ray or gamma rays)
3. *Radiation dose equivalent* (Rem)—unit of measure that relates to biologic effectiveness (roentgen equivalent in human beings). Standards were established by the International Committee on Radiation Protection (ICRP). The recommendation for maximum permissible dose (MPD) for radiation workers is 5 rems for persons over age 18 and maximum dose for women of reproductive capacity is 1.25 rems per quarter at an even rate.

Clinical Considerations

A. Nature and Indications for Use
Used alone or in combination with surgery or chemotherapy depending on the stage of disease and goal of therapy.

1. *Adjuvant radiation therapy*—used when a high risk of local recurrence or large primary tumor exists.
2. *Curative radiation therapy*—used in anatomically limited tumors (retina, optic nerve, certain brain tumors, skin, oral cavity).
   a. Course is usually longer and the dose higher.
3. *Palliative*—for treatment of symptoms.
   a. Provides excellent pain control for bone metastases.
   b. Used to relieve obstruction.
   c. Relief of neurologic dysfunction for brain metastases.
   d. Given in short, intensive courses.

B. Treatment Planning
1. Accurate diagnosis is established by biopsy and extent of disease is determined.
2. Goal of therapy is decided. Cure versus palliation versus adjuvant.
3. All patients undergo simulation and treatment planning.
   a. Target volume is identified by x-ray, scans, or physical examination.
   b. Treatment unit is selected.
   c. The design and pattern of delivery, total dose to be administered, time, and dose per day are determined.
   d. Usual schedule is Monday through Friday.
   e. Actual therapy lasts minutes. Most time is spent on positioning.
4. Computerized treatment plans are devised.
   a. Lead blocks are made to shape the beam and protect normal tissues.

b. Immobilization devices (casts, head holders) are designed to ensure accurate positioning.
c. Skin markings are applied to define the target and portal. These are replaced later by permanent tattoos.

Complications

Complications depend on site of radiation therapy, type of radiation therapy (brachytherapy or teletherapy), total radiation dose, daily fractionated doses, and overall health of the patient. Side effects are predictable, depending on the normal organs and tissues involved in the field.

GERONTOLOGIC ALERT:
Side effects may be prolonged due to decreased ability of the body to repair cellular damage.

A. Acute Side Effects
During treatment to 6 months after treatment:

1. Erythema at the site, possible dry-to-wet desquamation
2. Fatigue and malaise
3. Gastrointestinal effects: nausea and vomiting, diarrhea, and esophagitis
4. Oral effects: changes in taste, mucositis, dryness and xerostomia (dryness of mouth from lack of normal secretions)
5. Pulmonary effects: dyspnea, productive cough, pneumonitis
6. Renal and bladder effects: cystitis
7. Recall reactions—acute skin and mucosal reactions when concurrent or past chemotherapy (doxorubicin [Adriamycin], dactinomycin [Actinomycin D])

B. Chronic Side Effects
After 6 months with a variability in time of expression:

1. Skin effects: fibrosis, telangiectasia, permanent darkening of the skin, and atrophy
2. Gastrointestinal effects: fibrosis, adhesions, obstruction, ulceration, and strictures
3. Oral effects: permanent xerostomia, permanent taste alterations, and dental caries
4. Pulmonary effects: fibrosis
5. Renal and bladder effects: radiation nephritis, fibrosis
6. Second primary cancer—patients who have received combined radiation and chemotherapy with alkylating agents have a 5% to 7% risk of acute leukemia.

Nursing Assessment

1. Assess skin and mucous membranes for side effects of radiation.
2. Assess gastrointestinal, respiratory, and renal function for signs of side effects.
3. Assess patient's understanding of treatment and emotional status.

Nursing Diagnoses

A. Risk for Impaired Skin Integrity related to radiation effects
B. Altered Protection (for nurse and others) related to brachytherapy

Nursing Interventions

A. Maintaining Optimal Skin Care
1. Inform the patient that some skin reaction can be expected but that it varies from patient to patient. Examples include dry erythema, dry desquamation, wet desquamation, epilation, and tanning.
2. Do not apply lotions, ointments, or cosmetics to the site of radiation unless prescribed. Cornstarch may be used when the skin is dry and itchy.
3. Discourage vigorous rubbing, friction, or scratching because this can destroy skin cells. Apply ointments as instructed by health professionals.
4. Avoid wearing tight-fitting clothing over the treatment field; prevent irritation by not using rough fabric such as wool and corduroy.
5. Take precautions against exposure of radiation field to sunlight and extremes in temperature.
6. Do not apply adhesive or other tape to the skin.
7. Avoid shaving the skin in the treatment field.
8. Do not wash the area of radiation if possible.
9. If the area must be washed, use lukewarm water only.

B. Ensuring Protection from Radiation
1. Post a radioactive symbol on patient's chart and door; use radiation instruction sheet as provided.
2. Consider the following:
   a. Your distance from the patient. Note: The inverse square law applies—doubling the distance from a radiation source cuts intensity received to one-fourth.
   b. Amount of time spent in actual contact with the patient
   c. Degree of shielding used (chosen according to type of radiation—alpha, beta, gamma)

NURSING ALERT:
During the period of greatest radioactivity (24–72 hours), limit amount of time spent with the patient to that required for essential care. Require the patient to remain in the bed or room during course of treatment.

3. If exposed to penetrating radiation (x-ray or gamma rays), wear film badges on front of the body.
4. Take appropriate measures associated with sealed sources of radiation implanted within a patient (sealed internal radiation).
   a. Follow directives on precaution sheet that is placed on chart of all patients receiving radiotherapy.
   b. Do not remain within 1 meter (3 feet) of the patient any longer than required to give essential care.
5. Know that the casing material absorbs all alpha radiation and most beta radiation, but that a hazard concerning gamma radiation may exist.
6. Do not linger longer than necessary in giving patient care, even though all precautions are followed.

7. Be alert for implants that may have become loosened (those inserted in cavities that have access to the exterior); for example, check the emesis basin following mouth care for a patient with an oral implant.
8. Notify the radiation therapist of any implant that has moved out of position.
9. Use long-handled forceps or tongs and hold at arm's length when picking up any accidentally dislodged radium needle, seeds, or tubes that may appear on dressings, bed, or floor. *Never* pick up a radioactive source with your hands.
10. Do not discard any dressings or linens unless you are sure that no radioactive source is present.
11. Wash hands with soap and water after caring for a patient who is being treated with a radioisotope.
12. After the patient is discharged from the hospital, it is a good policy for the radiologist to check the room with a radiograph or survey meter to be certain that all radioactive materials have been removed.
13. Continue radiation precautions when a patient has a permanent implant, until the radiologist declares precautions unnecessary.

Evaluation

A. Skin without breakdown or signs of infection
B. Radiation precautions maintained

◆ CANCER IMMUNOTHERAPY

Cancer immunotherapy, or the use of biologic response modifiers (BMRs), involves the transfer to the patient of previously sensitized immunologic substances that can directly or indirectly mediate an antitumor response (eg, interleukin-2 or α-interferon). Cancer immunotherapy is rapidly becoming a fourth modality for cancer treatment.

Underlying Principles

A. Function
The primary function of the immune system is to detect and eliminate substances that are recognized as "non-self."

B. The Immune System
Has two major components: nonspecific (innate) and specific (acquired).

1. *Nonspecific* or *innate immunity* is inherent in all individuals. The largest component of the nonspecific system is the skin. Other nonspecific defense mechanisms include mucous membranes, cilia, tears, sebaceous glands, and acidic urine.
2. *Specific immunity* or *acquired immunity* has two primary features—specificity and memory. It is composed of three groups: cell-mediated immunity, humoral immunity, and null cells.
   a. *Cell-mediated immunity* is the T cells: T4 (helper/inducer cells) and T8 (cytotoxic and suppressor).
   b. *Humoral immunity* is the B cells, which ultimately secrete antibodies.
   c. *Null cells* are cells that are neither T nor B cells. The principal function is still unknown. Natural killer (NK) cells and lymphokine activated killer (LAK) cells are included in this group.

C. Cytokines
Cytokines are proteins produced by mononuclear cells of the immune system (usually the lymphocytes and monocytes) that have regulatory actions on other cells in the immune system or target cells involved in the immune reaction.

1. Cytokines include lymphokines (produced by lymphocytes) and monokines (produced by monocytes or macrophages).
2. Examples of cytokines include interleukins, interferons, and colony-stimulating factors (CSFs). Six different interleukins (1–6) have been identified, three types of interferon (α, β, and γ), and three different types of CSFs (granulocyte-macrophage CSF, granulocyte CSF, and macrophage CSF).

Nursing Assessment

1. Review patient's chart to determine site of cancer, previous cancer therapies, current medications, and other medical conditions.
2. Assess patient's current cardiovascular and respiratory status.
3. Assess patient's understanding of immunotherapy and the associated toxicities.

Nursing Diagnoses

A. Hyperthermia as a side effect of immunotherapy
B. Altered Tissue Perfusion (Cardiopulmonary) related to capillary permeability leak syndrome (third spacing of fluid) caused by immunotherapy

Nursing Interventions

A. Controlling Hyperthermia
1. Discuss the overall goal of immunotherapy, expected side effects, and the method of administration.
2. Instruct the patient to report any discomfort including fever, chills, diarrhea, nausea and vomiting, itching, or weight gain.
3. Administer or advise self-administration of antipyretics such as acetaminophen (Tylenol) for fever.
4. Emphasize that the side effects are temporary and will usually cease within 1 week after treatment ends.

B. Maintaining Tissue Perfusion
1. Monitor vital signs at least every 4 hours for hypotension, tachycardia, tachypnea, and fever.
   a. Instruct patient to remain in bed if blood pressure is low.
   b. Monitor apical heart rate.
2. Assess respirations for rate and depth, and auscultate breath sounds for evidence of pulmonary edema.
3. Assess for signs of restlessness, apprehension, discomfort, or cyanosis, which may indicate respiratory distress.
4. Administer oxygen as prescribed.
5. Maintain patent IV line and administer serum albumin as prescribed.
6. Check extremities for warmth, color, and capillary refill.

Evaluation

A. Relief of fever following medication
B. Blood pressure stable; lungs clear

Special Considerations in Cancer Care

◆ PAIN MANAGEMENT

Pain related to cancer may be caused by direct tumor infiltration of bones, nerves, viscera, or soft tissue or prior therapeutic measures (surgery, peripheral neuropathy).

Types of Pain

A. *Acute Pain—Self-limited, Mild to Moderate*
1. Has a beginning and an end, duration less than 6 months.
2. Can be readily described by the patient.
3. Can be managed with nonopioid analgesia administered "around the clock" using: acetaminophen or aspirin or nonsteroidal anti-inflammatory drug (NSAID) such as ibuprofen [Motrin] or naproxen [Naprosyn].
4. Radiation may be helpful.
5. Narcotics are used for short courses.

B. *Chronic Pain*
1. This is persistent or episodic pain.
2. Underlying cause is not always resolvable.
3. It does not have a beginning or an end.
4. Duration is greater than 6 months.
5. Treatment requires frequent reevaluation. Goal of therapy is to improve or stabilize patient's performance status.
6. Several different measures may be needed.

Clinical Manifestations

1. Pain of varying degrees and severity including:
   a. *Visceral*—poorly localized, frequently referred (eg, right shoulder pain from liver metastases).
      (1) May be described as deep, squeezing, or pressure.
      (2) Acute onset associated with nausea and vomiting can signal bowel obstruction.
      (3) Usually requires opioid drugs.
   b. *Somatic*—caused by direct tumor involvement of sensory receptors in cutaneous and deep tissues.
      (1) May be described as dull, gnawing, aching.
      (2) Most common form of pain.
      (3) Associated with bone and liver metastases.
      (4) Pain decreases if a response to chemotherapy or radiation.
      (5) Use combination therapy with NSAIDs and opioids. Medications can be tapered and stopped if response to antineoplastic therapy.
   c. *Neuropathic*—results from nerve injury or compression (eg, metastatic or radiation-induced brachial plexopathies, postherpetic neuralgia, spinal cord compression).

      (1) May be described as burning, stabbing, sharp.
      (2) Symptoms can be diverse and range from pain to paresthesia to sensory loss.
      (3) Responds to combinations of opioid plus tricyclic antidepressant or anticonvulsant.
2. Fatigue from sleep disturbances; most patients may not have slept for extended periods of time.
3. Loss of appetite or weight loss; anxiety or depression.
4. Change in self-concept, change in quality of life.

Management

A. *Pharmacologic Management*
1. NSAIDs such as indomethacin (Indocin) and ibuprofen (Motrin) act on the peripheral neurotransmitters. For mild pain.
2. Aspirin has antipyretic and anti-inflammatory activity.
3. Acetaminophen (Tylenol) has no anti-inflammatory activity.
4. Narcotic analgesics bind to the opiate receptors and act on the CNS pathways.
   a. Morphine preparations
      (1) Long acting over 8 to 12 hours (MS Contin, Oromorph)
      (2) Short acting—morphine sulfate or hydromorphone (Dilaudid) may be used for breakthrough pain. Relief lasts 3 to 4 hours.
      (3) Oxycodone (Tylox)—a moderately strong-acting opioid given in combination with acetaminophen or aspirin.
      (4) Propoxyphene (Darvon)—a weak short-acting opioid.

B. *Intraspinal Administration of Opiates*
1. A catheter is placed into spinal epidural or subarachnoid (intrathecal) space for the management of acute or chronic pain.
2. Catheter may be placed percutaneously and sutured in site or tunneled subcutaneously to the abdominal wall and exteriorized, or the pump system may be implanted.
3. Catheter is positioned as near as possible to the spinal segment where the pain is projected.
4. Preservative-free sterile morphine or other analgesic/local anesthetic drug is injected into the system at specified intervals.
   a. May be delivered by patient-controlled analgesia (PCA) pump.
   b. May be continuous or bolus infusions.
5. Spinally administered local anesthetics produce their effects predominantly by action on axons of spinal nerve roots; produce long-lasting pain relief with relatively low doses with little or no blunting of patient's level of responsiveness.
6. Complications include respiratory depression, urinary retention, pruritus, infection, leakage, technical problems, and development of tolerance.
7. Patient education
   a. The patient and family are taught drug administration, pump instruction, catheter and exit site care, monitoring of respiration, and recognition of respiratory depression and its treatment.
   b. Arrange for home health care nurse to visit.

Nursing Assessment and Interventions

1. Evaluate objectively the nature of the patient's pain: location, duration, quality, and impact on daily activities.
2. Use a pain intensity scale of 0 (no pain) to 10 (worst possible pain). Take careful history of prior and present medications, response, and side effects.
3. Assess relief from medications and duration of relief. (Use the same measuring scale every time).
4. Base the initial analgesic choice on the patient's report of pain.
5. Administer drugs orally whenever possible; avoid intramuscular injection.
6. Administer analgesia "around the clock" rather than PRN.
7. Convey the impression that the patient's pain is understood and that the pain can be controlled.
8. Take a careful pain history. Explore pain interventions that have been used and their effectiveness. Determine if the intensity of the pain correlates with the prescribed analgesic.
9. Reevaluate the pain frequently. The requirement for analgesia should decrease if other treatment is given, including radiation or chemotherapy.
10. Use alternative measures to relieve pain such as imaging, relaxation, and biofeedback.
11. Provide ongoing support and open communication.
12. Consider referral to a pain specialist for intractable pain.
13. Provide education.
    a. Method of administration of medications and importance of maintaining prescribed schedule
    b. Need to call health professionals if pain has increased or occurred in another area of the body
    c. Side effects of medication
       (1) Constipation—best treated prophylactically
       (2) Nausea—antiemetic therapy helpful
       (3) Tolerance—increasing doses often required to achieve the same effect. This is a normal physiologic response to opioids. Patient reports shorter duration of effect. There is no maximum opioid dose as long as side effects are tolerable.
    d. Addiction usually is not a problem to needed narcotics.

◆ COMPLICATIONS IN CANCER

Septic Shock

Septic shock is a systemic disease associated with the presence and persistence of pathogenic microorganisms or their toxins in the blood.

A. Diagnostic Evaluation
1. Culture—blood, urine, stool, sputum, central and peripheral IV lines, and any open wounds to determine source and type of infection
2. Chest x-ray—to detect underlying pneumonia
3. Arterial blood gas evaluation—decreased pH reflects acidosis
4. BUN and creatinine—elevated due to decreased circulating blood volume

5. CBC with differential—elevated WBC with shift to left

B. Management
1. Antibiotics are started immediately; broad-spectrum antibiotics are given until organism identified.
2. IV fluids and plasma expanders are used to restore circulating volume.
3. Vasopressors are administered to support blood pressure.
4. Oxygen is used to prevent tissue hypoxia.
5. Vital signs, respiratory status, urine output, and any signs of bleeding are monitored carefully.
6. Complications such as renal failure, respiratory failure, cardiac failure, metabolic acidosis, and disseminated intravascular coagulation, are treated aggressively.

Spinal Cord Compression (SCC)

Epidural spinal cord compression is pressure on the spinal cord or cauda equina nerve roots from a lesion outside the spinal dura. Associated with vertebral metastases. Common primary tumors include: breast, prostate, lung, kidney, lymphoma, and sarcoma. More than one level usually is involved.

A. Clinical Manifestations
1. Progressive back pain—median duration of pain depends on the primary tumor.
2. Pain can be local, radicular, or segmental in type. Most common is local pain over the site of compression. Constant, relentlessly progressive, made worse by recumbency. Radicular pain can be unilateral or bilateral. Segmental pain is uncommon. Usually dull, unaffected by movement, diffuse, and indicative of intrinsic cord damage.
3. Weakness and unsteadiness may be noted before changes in motor function. Progression is often rapid with foot drop and impaired ambulation. Urgent investigation and treatment are crucial to minimize risk of paraplegia. The degree of weakness and ability to walk at presentation are important clinical predictors of outcome.
4. Bowel and bladder function—loss of sphincter tone and urinary retention or incontinence. Depends on the site of compression. Constipation requires direct questioning. Associated with moderate to severe weakness.
5. Changes in sensation—paresthesia, numbness, tingling. Severity usually mirrors the severity of motor weakness. Localizing signs are variable.

B. Diagnostic Evaluation
1. Neurologic examination—early diagnosis is important.
2. X-ray of the painful site—may or may not be abnormal.
3. MRI—useful in evaluating spinal cord lesions, multiple levels. Immediately indicated if radiculopathy or myelopathy is present or x-rays are abnormal.
4. Myelogram with CT scan—to determine the precise level of involvement.

C. Management
1. Corticosteroids—reduce inflammation and swelling at site, increase neurologic function, and relieve pain.
2. Radiation to the tumor on spinal column, if applicable.
3. Immediate decompressive surgery (laminectomy) if applicable.

D. Complications
1. Respiratory impairment including pneumonia and atelectasis
2. Mobility impairment including immobility, foot drop, skin impairment, postural hypotension
3. Sensory losses creating safety concerns
4. Bladder or bowel dysfunction

E. Patient Education
1. Facilitate referral to home care services for nursing assessment, nursing intervention, and rehabilitation for residual deficits.
2. Facilitate referral to appropriate outpatient services including physical therapy, occupational therapy, and psychosocial support.
3. Provide instruction regarding safety issues for residual sensory deficits (eg, test bath water temperature, careful use of extreme hot or cold).

Hypercalcemia

Hypercalcemia is an elevated serum calcium level. Patients with tumors that frequently metastasize to the bone (lung, breast, and prostate cancer) are at increased risk for hypercalcemia. Some tumors (bronchogenic carcinoma and kidney cancer) can secrete a parathormone (PTH)-like substance that may also cause hypercalcemia.

A. Clinical Manifestations
1. Signs and symptoms may vary depending on the severity of the hypercalcemia and the onset.
2. Symptoms may be nonspecific and insidious such as nausea and vomiting, anorexia, weakness, constipation, polyuria, polydipsia, and loss of memory.
3. A very rapid and life-threatening increase in calcium may cause dehydration, renal failure, and coma.

B. Diagnostic Evaluation
1. Serum calcium level is increased.
2. Electrolyte levels, BUN, creatinine are obtained to determine hydration status and renal function.

C. Management
1. Hydration with IV normal saline (0.9% NaCl) is the initial treatment for patients with acute hypercalcemia and clinical symptoms to dilute the calcium and promote its renal excretion.
2. Pharmacotherapy
   a. Diuretics may be used to promote further diuresis and calcium excretion.
   b. Plicamycin (Mithracin) and etidronate disodium (Didronel) are useful for patients who do not respond to normal saline diuresis. Plicamycin blocks PTH and may also inhibit bone resorption.
   c. Calcitonin (Calcimar) inhibits osteoclast activity and causes hypocalcemia. It has a rapid onset of action.
   d. Oral phosphates are used for chronic hypercalcemia, which can inhibit bone resorption.
   e. Diphosphonates are used to stimulate osteoblast activity, which increases bone uptake of calcium.

D. Nursing Interventions
1. Prevent and detect hypercalcemia early.
   a. Recognize patients at risk and monitor for signs and symptoms such as nausea and vomiting, constipation, lethargy, and anorexia.

   b. Emphasize importance of mobility to minimize bone demineralization and constipation.
   c. Instruct patient on the importance of adequate hydration.
2. Administer normal saline infusions as prescribed.
3. Administer medications as prescribed.
4. Maintain accurate intake and output; observe for oliguria or anuria.
5. Take vital signs every 4 hours, especially apical pulse and blood pressure.
6. Monitor electrolyte values and renal function.
7. Assess mental status.
8. Assess cardiorespiratory status for signs of fluid overload.

Superior Vena Cava Syndrome (SVCS)

Superior vena cava syndrome is an obstruction and thrombosis of the superior vena cava by tumor or enlarged lymph node resulting in impaired venous drainage of the head, neck, arms, and thorax. Patients at risk for SVCS are primarily those with mediastinal tumors.

A. Clinical Manifestations
1. Dyspnea and "tight collar" syndrome occurring for 2 to 4 weeks before diagnosis. Facial and neck swelling is frequently described by the patient as a "tight collar" feeling.
2. Chest pain, cough, and dysphagia are present.
3. Cyanosis and edema of the head and upper extremities may be apparent. Collateral circulation with dilated chest wall veins may be visible.
4. Progressive dyspnea, orthopnea, and neck vein distention occur.
5. CNS symptoms include headache, vertigo, irritability, lethargy, and visual disturbances.

B. Diagnostic Evaluation
1. Chest x-ray to confirm SVCS
2. CT scan to determine extent of tumor and obstruction

C. Management
1. Radiation therapy, if possible, is used to reduce tumor size and relieve pressure.
2. Chemotherapy may be used in conjunction with radiation. Specific chemotherapeutic agents depend on the tumor type.
3. Surgery (rarely used due to the associated high morbidity and mortality risks).
4. Oxygen is given for relief of dyspnea; maintenance of airway.
5. Analgesics and tranquilizers are used for discomfort and anxiety.
6. Fibrinolytic and anticoagulants may be used if a thrombus is suspected or to prevent the formation of a thrombus.

D. Nursing Interventions
1. Administer oxygen as prescribed to relieve hypoxia.
2. Place patient in Fowler's position—facilitates gravity drainage and reduces facial edema.
3. Limit the patient's activity and provide a quiet environment.
4. Reassure patient that cyanotic color and facial edema will subside with treatment.

◆ PSYCHOSOCIAL COMPONENTS OF CARE

Nursing Assessment

1. Assess preillness lifestyle. How did patient solve other problems?
2. Assess for signs of anxiety and coexistence of depression: agitation/restlessness, sleep disturbances, excessive autonomic activity, weight gain or loss, mood changes.
3. What activities of daily living can the patient perform?
4. What changes in lifestyle have resulted from cancer and its treatment?
5. Ascertain the patient's perception of the disease and treatment.
6. Evaluate available social support; who is the most significant other?
7. Try to gain a sense of emotional strengths and potential problem areas.

Nursing Diagnoses

A. Anxiety related to complex disease process, treatment options, and prognosis
B. Ineffective Individual Coping related to life-altering disease process
C. Fear of Death and Dying

Nursing Interventions

A. *Reducing Anxiety*
1. Establish and sustain an unhurried approach to give the patient time to organize fears, thoughts, and feelings.
2. Allow patient to share feelings about having cancer.
3. Reflect and amplify insights and judgments; try to reduce anxiety through reflection and reorientation.
4. Recognize feelings of losing control.
5. Discuss methods of stress reduction (imagery, relaxation, biofeedback).
6. Discuss the positive aspects of treatment.
7. Encourage expression of positive emotions—emphasis on living in the here and now, greater appreciation of life, etc.
8. Reinforce effective coping behaviors.
9. Encourage patient to join a support group such as Make Today Count or Living Through Concern. Refer to local chapter of the American Cancer Society or call 1-800-ACS-2345.
10. Remain available as problems arise. Give patient telephone numbers of persons to call when needed—creates a sense of security.
11. Initiate referrals for additional rehabilitation and psychosocial services as appropriate.

B. *Promoting Effective Coping*
1. Encourage patient and family members to enroll in cancer education program.
2. Encourage patient to learn everything about treatment plan because this promotes a sense of control.
3. Provide expert physical care, while teaching patient to take over care as able.
4. Assist patient in strengthening support system (family, friends, visitors, health care staff, volunteers, support groups)—strengthens self-esteem through the experience of feeling accepted and valued.
5. Help patient readjust expectations and goals to promote ongoing adjustment.
6. Support patient in coping mechanisms chosen.

C. *Allaying Fear of Death and Dying*
1. Educate patient and family about hospice. Hospice is the provision of home or inpatient facility supportive care with minimal impact from high-technology diagnostic and therapeutic procedures. The major goals of therapy are to stabilize and control symptoms, provide adequate pain control, and provide respite for the primary caregiver. It involves an interdisciplinary team of hospice nurses, physicians, pharmacist, social worker, clergy, and volunteers. This team coordinates and supervises services 7 days a week, 24 hours a day.
2. Assess and respect the patient's wish to refuse active therapy when there is limited potential for a response to therapy.
3. Discuss the hospice philosophy with the patient and significant other(s). Identify the primary caregiver(s). Discuss the status and prognosis with the patient and family and arrive at a consensus on treatment goals.
   a. Consider treating treatable conditions that are causing symptoms or pain.
   b. Administer analgesics vigorously on a regular basis rather than PRN.
   c. Administer medications by the easiest route.
   d. Recognize that anorexia and small food volume is normal. Reassure the family members.
   e. Recognize that providing IV or nasogastric hydration may not be desirable because it may cause discomfort and prolong the dying process.
4. Facilitate emotional support for the patient. Anxiety and depression are common among patients approaching death. Tranquilizers should be used with caution in small doses. Recognize that we all die uniquely.
5. Provide bereavement support to survivors.

Selected References

American Joint Committee on Cancer (1983). *Manual for staging of cancer* (2nd ed.). Philadelphia: J. B. Lippincott.

Cancer statistics. (1995). *Cancer Journal for Clinicians, 45* (1), 8-31.

Casciapo, D. (1988). *Manual of clinical oncology* (2nd ed.). Boston: Little, Brown.

Cherny, N. & Portenoy, R. (1994). The management of cancer pain. *Cancer*

CA: A Cancer Journal for Clinicians, 44 (5), 259-304.

Groenwald, S. Frogge, M., & Yarboro, C. (1992). *Cancer nursing principles and practice* (2nd ed.). Boston: James and Bartlett.

Held, J. & Peahotu, A. (1993). Nursing care of the patient with spinal cord compression. *Oncology Nursing Forum, 20* (10), 1507–1514.

McCaffery, M. & Ferrell, B. R. (1994). How to use the new AHCPR Cancer Pain Guidelines. *AJN, 94* (7), 42–47.

U. S. Department of Health and Human Services, Agency for Health Care Policy and Research. (1994). *Management of cancer pain clinical practice guidelines*, No. 9. Washington, DC: Author.

Care of the Older Adult

Physiology

◆ NORMAL CHANGES OF AGING

There are a number of normal age-related changes that occur in all major systems of the body. These may present at different times for different people. It is important to be able to differentiate between normal and abnormal changes in elderly people, and to educate patients and families about these differences.

Vision

A. **Characteristics**
1. Decreased visual acuity
2. Decreased visual fields, and thus decreased peripheral vision
3. Decreased dark adaptation
4. Elevated minimal threshold of light perception
5. Presbyopia (farsightedness) due to decreased visual accommodation from loss of lens elasticity
6. Decreased color discrimination due to the yellowing of the lens; short wavelength colors, such as blues and greens are more difficult to see
7. Increased sensitivity to glare
8. Decreased depth perception

B. **Assessment Findings**
1. Arcus senilis—deposits of lipid around the eye, seen as a white circle around the iris; causes no visual impairments
2. Cataracts—lens thickening and decreased permeability; noted on examination with the ophthalmoscope; results in fuzziness of vision
3. Smaller pupil size
4. Complaints of decreased ability to read, discomfort from light, changes in depth perception, falls, collisions, difficulty handling small objects, difficulty with activities of daily living, and tunnel vision

C. **Nursing Considerations/Teaching Points**
1. Make sure objects are in the patient's visual field.
2. Use large lettering to label medications and any distributed written information.
3. Allow the individual more time to focus and adjust to the environment.
4. Avoid glare.
5. Use night lights to help with dark adaptation problems.
6. Use the colors red and yellow to stimulate vision.
7. Mark the edges of stairs and curbs to help with depth perception problems.

Hearing

A. **Characteristics**
1. Approximately 30% to 50% of people older than 65 have significant hearing loss.
2. Three types of hearing disorders are common in the older population.
   a. Presbycusis—progressive irreversible bilateral loss of high tone perception often associated with aging
   b. Central deafness—occurs from nerve damage within the brain (considered a pathologic rather than normal change)
   c. Conduction deafness—results from blockage or impairment of the mechanical movement in the outer or middle ear (also a pathologic condition)
3. Hearing loss in the elderly is often a combined problem. The majority of the loss is due to auditory nerve changes or deterioration of the structures of the ear. There may also be nerve damage beyond the ear. Presbycusis and central deafness can result in permanent hearing loss; conduction deafness is reversible.
4. Usual progression from high tone or high frequency loss to a general loss of both high and low tones
5. Consonants (higher pitched sounds) not heard well
6. Hearing loss increases with age and is greater in men.
7. Increased in the sound threshold (ie, greater sound needed to stimulate the older adult)
8. Decreased speech discrimination, especially with background noise
9. Cerumen impaction is a reversible, and frequently overlooked cause of a conductive hearing loss.

B. **Assessment Findings**
1. Increased volume of patient's own speech
2. Turning of head toward speaker
3. Requests of a speaker to repeat
4. Inappropriate answers, but otherwise cognitively intact
5. The person may withdraw, demonstrate a short attention span, and become frustrated, angry, and depressed.

6. Lack of response to a loud noise

C. *Nursing Considerations/Teaching Points*
1. Suggest hearing testing for further evaluation and consideration of an assistive device.
2. Face the person directly so he or she can lip read.
3. Use gestures and objects to help with verbal communication.
4. Touch the person to get his or her attention before talking.
5. Speak into the person's "good ear."
6. DON'T SHOUT. Shouting increases the tone of the voice, and elderly people are unable to hear these high tones.
7. Speak slowly and clearly.
8. Suggest amplifiers on telephones and alarms.
9. Allow the person more time to answer your questions.
10. Evaluate the person's ear canals regularly and assist with cerumen removal. Cerumen removal is facilitated by:
    a. Use of ceruminolytic agents such as Debrox, 10 drops in the affected ear twice a day for 5 days, followed by flushing the ear with warm water, or preferably an electronic irrigation device.
    b. Careful use of an ear spoon to mechanically remove cerumen.

Smell

A. *Characteristics*
1. Progressive decrease in smell as olfactory nerve fibers decrease with age
2. Discrimination of fruity odors seems to persist the longest.

B. *Assessment Finding*
1. Inability to notice unpleasant odors such as fires, body odor, or excessive perfume use
2. Decreased appetite

C. *Nursing Considerations/Teaching Points*
1. At mealtime, name food items and give the person time to think of the smell/taste of the food.
2. Suggest use of stronger spices and flavorings to stimulate smell.

Taste

A. *Characteristics*
1. Taste buds decrease with age, especially in men. People over 60 years of age have lost half of their taste buds. By age 80, only one sixth of the taste buds remain.
2. Taste buds are lost from the front to the back (ie, sweet and salty tastes are lost first, whereas bitter and sour tastes remain longer).

B. *Assessment Findings*
1. Complaints that food has no taste
2. Excessive use of sugar and salt
3. Inability to identify the foods
4. Decrease in appetite and weight loss

C. *Nursing Considerations/Teaching Points*
1. Serve food attractively, and separate different types of foods.
2. Vary the texture of foods.

3. Encourage good oral hygiene.

Kinesthetic Sense

A. *Characteristics*
1. With age, the receptors in the joints and muscles that tell us where we are in space lose their ability to function. Therefore, there is a change in balance.
2. Walking with shorter step length, less leg lift, a wider base, and tendency to lean forward
3. With age, less ability to stop a fall from occurring

B. *Assessment Findings*
1. Alterations in posture, ability to transfer, and gait
2. Complaint of dizziness

C. *Nursing Considerations/Teaching Points*
1. Position items within reach.
2. Give person more time to move.

Cardiovascular

A. *Characteristics*
1. With age, the valves of the heart become thick and rigid as a result of sclerosis and fibrosis, compounding any cardiac disease already present.
2. Blood vessels also become thick and rigid, resulting in elevated blood pressure.
3. Cardiac function is relatively unchanged with aging. Resting heart rate and heart size are not age-related.
4. Slower response to stress. Once the pulse rate is elevated it takes longer to return to baseline.
5. Decline in maximum oxygen consumption

B. *Assessment Findings*
1. Elevated blood pressure up to 160/90 is considered normal over age 65.
2. Persistent tachycardia following stress

C. *Nursing Considerations/Teaching Points*
1. Encourage regular blood pressure evaluation.
2. Encourage longer cool-down period after exercise to return to baseline cardiac function.

Pulmonary

A. *Characteristics*
1. With age, there is a weakening of the intercostal respiratory muscles, and the elastic recoil of the chest wall diminishes.
2. There is no change in total lung capacity, however residual volume and functional residual capacity increase.
3. PO_2 decreases with age due to ventilation–perfusion mismatches. However, elderly people are not hypoxic without coexistent disease.
4. There is a decrease in the mucous transport/ciliary system. Therefore, there is resulting decreased clearance of mucus and foreign bodies, including bacteria.

B. *Assessment Findings*
1. Prolonged cough, inability to raise secretions
2. Increased frequency of respiratory infections

C. *Nursing Considerations/Teaching Points*
1. Elderly people undergoing any surgical treatment need special attention paid to deep breathing exercises.
2. Teach measures to prevent pulmonary infections—avoid crowds during cold and flu season, wash hands frequently, report early signs of infection.

Immunologic

A. *Characteristics*
1. The function of T-cell lymphocytes, such as cell-mediated immunity, declines with age due to involution and atrophy of the thymus gland.
2. Decreased T-cell helper activity; increased T-cell suppressor activity
3. Declining B-cell function as a result of T-cell changes

B. *Assessment Findings*
1. More frequent infections
2. Increased incidence of many types of cancer

C. *Nursing Considerations/Teaching Points*
1. Teach people that they are at increased risk of infection, cancer, and autoimmune disease, therefore routine follow-up and screening are essential.

Neurologic

A. *Characteristics*
1. There is gradual loss in the number of neurons with age, but no major change in neurotransmitter levels.
2. Some brain tissue atrophy is normal and does not relate to cognitive impairment.
3. Decreased muscle tone, motor speed and nerve conduction velocity

B. *Assessment Findings*
1. Decreased position and vibration sense
2. Diminished reflexes, possible absent ankle jerks
3. Complaint of falls

C. *Nursing Considerations/Teaching Points*
1. Because of these changes, in combination with sensory changes, fall prevention techniques are essential to teach to elderly people.
   a. Environmental safety techniques include: nonslip surfaces, securely fastened handrails, sufficient light, glarefree lights, avoidance of low-lying objects, chairs of the proper height with armrests, skidproof strips or mats in the tub or shower, toilet and tub grab bars, elevated toilet seats.
   b. Home safety evaluations should be done on all community-dwelling elderly people to reduce the risk of falls. A home safety checklist can be obtained from the National Safety Council, 219 19th Street NW, Suite 40, Washington, DC 20036, 202-293-2270.

COMMUNITY-BASED CARE TIP:
Obtain the National Safety Council Home Safety Checklist and have home nurses or family members of the older adult fill it out before patient is discharged from hospital or extended care facility. Use the information to suggest changes in the home for safety.

Musculoskeletal

A. *Characteristics*
1. Declining muscle mass and endurance with age, although deconditioning may be an associated factor
2. Decreased bone density, less so in men than in women
3. Decreased thickness and resiliency of cartilage, with a resulting increase in the stiffness of joints

B. *Assessment Findings*
1. Muscle atrophy
2. Increased incidence of fractures
3. Complaint of joint stiffness in absence of arthritis

C. *Nursing Considerations/Teaching Points*
1. Early intervention to encourage regular exercise in the elderly population is important to prevent exacerbation of these normal changes.

Endocrine

A. *Characteristics*
1. Decreased secretion of trophic hormones from the pituitary gland
2. Blunted growth hormone release during stress
3. Elevated vasopressin (antidiuretic hormone); exaggerated response to osmotic challenge
4. Elevated levels of follicle-stimulating hormone and luteinizing hormone because of reduced end-organ response
5. Normal insulin secretion at rest with an age-related decrease in secretion in response to a glucose load; this may be a function of weight or genetic factors.

B. *Assessment Findings*
1. Usually asymptomatic

C. *Nursing Considerations/Teaching Points*
1. Encourage routine screening for elevated blood sugar.
2. Provide dietary education on well-balanced diet.

Reproductive

A. *Characteristics*
1. In women, menopause leads to decreases in the size of the ovaries and hormone production. This results in uterine involution, vaginal atrophy, and loss of breast mass.
2. In men, testosterone production and secretion decrease with age, However, serum levels may be in the low-normal range through age 80.

B. *Assessment Findings*
1. Vaginal dryness, painful intercourse
2. Atrophic vaginitis

C. *Nursing Considerations/Teaching Points*
1. Suggest the use of additional lubrication during sexual intercourse.
2. Advise sexually active older men that spermatogenesis may continue into advanced age.

Renal and Body Composition

A. *Characteristics*
1. Increased body fat and decreased lean muscle mass, even when weight remains stable

2. Decreased renal function, measured by the glomerular filtration rate, or creatinine clearance

3. Despite reduced total body creatinine due to decreased muscle mass in the older adult, serum creatinine often remains within normal range. This is because of decreased elimination of creatinine by the kidneys.

4. About 10% decline in creatinine clearance per decade after age 40; however, relatively unchanged serum creatinine

B. *Assessment Findings*
1. Usually asymptomatic

C. *Nursing Considerations/Teaching Points*
1. Be aware that although creatinine level may be within normal range, creatinine clearance may be decreased. To obtain an accurate creatinine clearance in an elderly person, the following formula should be used:
   a. (140−age)(weight[kg])/(72)(serum creatinine [mg per dL]).

2. Drugs that are cleared through the kidneys may be given in decreased dosage. Side effects and toxicity must be closely monitored.

Skin

A. *Characteristics*
1. Thinning of all three layers of the skin, epidermis, dermis and subcutaneous tissue leads to greater fragility of the skin and decreased ability of the skin to function as a barrier to external factors.
2. Fewer melanocytes and decreased tanning
3. Less efficient thermoregulation to heat because of fewer sweat glands
4. Drier skin because the decreased number of sebaceous glands results in reduced oil production
5. Other changes in aging skin include reduced sensory input, decreased elasticity, and impaired cell-related immune response.

B. *Assessment Finding*
1. Dry, irritated skin

C. *Nursing Considerations/Teaching Points*
1. Excessive use of soap, which can be drying to the skin, should be avoided.
2. Careful skin evaluation and lubrication are necessary to prevent fissures and breakdown.
3. Heat regulation needs to be controlled by proper clothing and avoidance of extreme temperatures.
4. Avoid direct application of extreme hot or cold to skin because damage may occur without feeling it.

Hematopoietic

A. *Characteristics*
1. Unchanged number of stem cells of all three cell lines; however, bone marrow cellularity is decreased by 33% during adult life.
2. Declining marrow activity, especially in response to stress, such as with blood loss or infection

B. *Assessment Finding*
1. Asymptomatic

C. *Nursing Considerations/Teaching Points*
1. Anemia and granulocytopenia are not normal consequences of aging and should be investigated.

Altered Presentation of Disease

A. *Characteristics*
1. In part due to the physiologic changes that occur with aging, the manifestations of illness in the older patient are less dramatic than in younger patients.
2. Most elderly persons have at least one chronic condition. These coexisting conditions can complicate the evaluation of new symptoms.

B. *Assessment Findings*
1. The classic indicators of disease are often absent or disorders present atypically (Table 7-1).
2. Older people are less likely to complain of new symptoms but rather attribute them to aging or existing conditions. Many elderly people minimize symptoms because of fears of hospitalization or health care costs.

C. *Nursing Considerations/Teaching Points*
1. Have a high index of suspicion for underlying illness if older adult is in pain or has behavioral changes.

Assessment

◆ FUNCTIONAL ASSESSMENT

Functional assessment is the measurement of a patient's ability to complete functional tasks and fulfill social roles, specifically addressing a person's ability to complete tasks ranging from simple self-care to higher-level activities.

Purpose

1. Functional assessment is essential in the care of the elderly because it:
   a. Offers a systematic approach to assessing elderly people for deficits that often go undetected
   b. Helps the nurse to identify problems and utilize appropriate resources
   c. Provides a way to assess progress and decline over time
   d. Helps the nurse evaluate the safety of the person's ability to live alone
2. Functional status includes the evaluation of sensory changes, ability to complete activities of daily living, instrumental activities of daily living, gait and balance problems, and elimination.

Instruments to Measure Functional Ability

1. Functional status may be assessed by several methods: self-report, direct observation, or family report. Direct observation is the method of choice, when possible.

TABLE 7-1 Atypical Presentation of Disorders in the Older Adult

Disorder	Atypical Presentation
Acute intestinal infection	1. Abdominal pain may be absent. 2. May present with acute confusional state, leukocytosis, and acidosis.
Appendicitis	1. Pain may be diffuse, not localized in right lower quadrant.
Biliary disease	1. Confusion, declining function, and other nonspecific symptoms. 2. Abnormal liver function tests may be only sign.
Congestive heart failure	1. Initially may have change in mental status and fatigue.
Hyperthyroidism	1. Apathy, palpitations, weight loss, weakness.
Hypothyroidism	1. Present with weight loss.
Myocardial infarction	1. Chest pain may be absent. 2. Syncope, dyspnea, vomiting, or confusion may be presenting symptoms.
Perforated ulcer	1. Rigidity may be absent until late.
Pneumonia	1. May present with confusion. 2. Fever and cough may be absent.
Pulmonary embolism	1. May present with change in mental status. 2. May not have fever, leukocytosis, or tachycardia.
Septicemia	1. May be afebrile.
Systemic lupus erythematosus	1. Pneumonitis, subcutaneous nodules, and discoid lesions are more common presentation. 2. Malar rash, Raynaud's phenomenon, and nephritis are less common.

2. The instrument chosen should be based on what is the specific goal or purpose for the evaluation. For example, if the focus is on basic self care and mobility, the Barthel index should be used.
3. See Tables 7-2 and 7-3 for scales measuring functional ability: Katz Index for Activities of Daily Living and Instrumental Activities of Daily Living. Use these scales to determine how independent the older adult is and repeat them periodically to compare level of functioning over time. See Selected References for reference to Barthel index.

◆ PSYCHOSOCIAL ASSESSMENT

Altered Mental Status

1. Assessment of cognitive function to detect altered mental status involves examination of memory, perception, communication, orientation, calculation, comprehension, problem solving, thought processes, language, construction abilities, abstraction, attention, aphasia, and apraxia.
2. Assessment can be facilitated by use of the Folstein Mini-Mental State Examination (Table 7-4).
   a. This scale can help to follow the elderly person's mental status over time, and assess for acute and or chronic changes.
   b. Although success on scales such as this has been associated with education and socioeconomic status, this scale continues to be used as an appropriate screening tool for abnormal cognitive function.
3. Assessment of altered mental status may elicit criteria that lead to a diagnosis of dementia. It is essential to differentiate dementia from delirium (which is treatable and reversible).

a. Delirium is abrupt in onset, disorientation occurs early, the behavior is variable hour to hour, there is a clouded, altered or changing level of consciousness, short attention span, disturbed sleep–wake cycle, and hallucinations are common.
b. Dementia has a gradual onset, the behavior is usually stable, disorientation occurs late, consciousness is not clouded, attention span generally is not reduced, day–night reversal of sleep–wake cycles can occur rather than hour-to-hour variation, and hallucinations do not occur until late.

Social Activities and Support

1. Important aspects of social function in geriatrics include social relationship (frequency, contacts, quality), social activities, social resources, and social support. This information is important to help in making decisions about care.
2. Elicit information by asking questions such as:
   a. How often do you socialize with others?
   b. With whom do you socialize?
   c. What type of activities do you get involved in?
   d. Do you enjoy socializing?
   e. Who can you call for help?
   f. Do you know of any church or community groups you can call for help?

Emotional/Affective Status

A. **Characteristics**
1. Depression may occur for the first time in older age and has been related to the many changes that occur with age:

TABLE 7-2 Activities of Daily Living

1. Bathing—Sponge bath, tub bath or shower
   0 = no assistance (gets in and out of tub by self)
   1 = uses a device to get in or out of tub but able to bathe self
   2 = requires partial assistance with bathing
   3 = full bath required (unable to bathe)
2. Dressing—includes getting clothes from closet and drawers (under and outer garments and able to use fasteners)
   0 = no assistance with getting clothes and dressing self
   1 = able to get clothes and get dressed, except for assistance with shoes
   2 = receives assistance with getting clothes or getting dressed
   3 = requires complete assistance or stays partly or completely undressed
3. Toileting—going to bathroom for bowel and urine elimination, self-cleaning and arranging clothes
   0 = requires no assistance
   1 = requires no assistance but uses device (cane, walker, wheelchair, bedpan at night, but able to empty in morning)
   2 = receives partial assistance with going to the bathroom or in cleansing or arranging clothing
   3 = receives full assistance or does not go to the bathroom
4. Transfer
   0 = moves well in and out of bed and/or chair without assistance
   1 = moves well in and out of bed and/or chair with device
   2 = moves in and out of bed and/or chair with assistance
   3 = requires full assistance
5. Continence
   0 = controls urination and bowel movements completely by self
   1 = has occasional ''accidents''
   2 = supervision helps keep bowel or urine control or is incontinent
   3 = catheter is used
6. Feeding
   0 = able to prepare foods, serve and feed self without assistance
   1 = requires help in preparation of food but is able to feed self
   2 = requires help in preparation of food, cutting of meat, buttering
   3 = receives full assistance or is fed partly or completely by tubes

_____ SCORE

Katz index for activities of daily living.
Best score is 0, most independent; worst score is 18, most dependent.
Adapted from Katz, S., Ford, A.B., Moskowitz, R. et al. (1963). Studies of illness in the aged, the index of ADL: A standardized measure of biologic and psychosocial function. *JAMA*, 185, 914–919.

a. The independence of one's children
b. The reality of retirement
c. The loss of roles, income, spouse, friends, family, homes, pets, functional ability, health, and ability to participate in leisure activities such as reading
d. Ageist messages from society supporting and encouraging the value of youth
2. Depression may also be caused by underlying illnesses, such as Parkinson's disease, and drugs such as antihypertensives, antiarthritics, and antianxiety agents.
3. Depression is often difficult to identify in the elderly because the presentation is different than in younger

people. Obtain the following information to assess for depression:
a. Complaints of insomnia, weight loss, anorexia, and constipation (vegetative symptoms)
b. Preoccupation with past life events

TABLE 7-3 Instrumental Activities of Daily Living

1. Can you use the telephone?
   0 = without help, including looking up numbers and dialing
   2 = with some help (can answer phone or dial ''0'' in emergency, but need special help in getting the number or dialing
   Why? _____
   3 = completely unable to use the telephone
2. Can you get to places out of walking distance?
   0 = without help (travels alone on buses, taxis, drives own car)
   1 = with some help in transferring on and off (device and/ or person)
   2 = with help of someone while traveling
   3 = totally dependent on specialized arrangements for travel (ie, ambulance) or doesn't travel at all
3. Can you go shopping for groceries or clothing?
   0 = without help taking care of all shopping needs (assuming had own transportation)
   1 = able to take care of all shopping needs but requires companion to help
   2 = requires assistance in preparation of shopping list as well as a companion to help with shopping
   3 = totally dependent on another person for all shopping needs
4. Can you prepare your own meals?
   0 = without assistance (plan and cook full meals for yourself)
   2 = with some assistance (can prepare some things but unable to cook a full meal)
   Why? _____
   3 = totally unable to prepare meals
5. Can you do your housework?
   0 = without assistance (scrub floor, etc.)
   2 = able to do light housekeeping but needs help with heavy work
   ie
   3 = unable to do any housework
6. Can you take your own medicine?
   0 = without assistance (correct doses, correct time)
   1 = able if someone prepares it for you
   2 = able to if someone prepares it for you and reminds you to take it
   3 = require someone to prepare and give you your medication
7. Can you handle your own money?
   0 = without assistance (able to pay bills, write checks)
   2 = able to manage day-to-day buying but need help with managing check book and paying bills
   Why? _____
   How long has this been going on? _____
   3 = requires full assistance with money management

_____ SCORE

Katz index for instrumental activities of daily living.
Best score is 0, most independent; worst score is 21, most dependent.
Adapted from Katz, S., Ford, A. B., Moskowitz, R. et al. (1963). Studies of illness in the aged. The index of ADL: A standardized measure of biologic and psychosocial function. *JAMA*, 185, 914–919.

TABLE 7-4 Folstein Mini-Mental State Examination

Maximum score	Factor
	Orientation
5	What is the (year) (season) (date) (day) (month)?
5	Where are we (state) (county) (town) (hospital) (floor)?
	Registration
3	Name three objects; allow one second to say each. Then, ask the patient to repeat the three objects after you have said them. Give one point for each correct answer. Repeat until the patient learns all three. Count trials and record number.
	Attention and calculation
5	Ask the patient to begin with 100 and count backward sevens (stop after five answers). Alternatively, spell "world" backward.
	Recall
3	Ask the patient to repeat the three objects that you previously asked him or her to remember.
	Language
2	Show the patient a pencil and a watch and ask him or her to name them.
1	Ask the patient to repeat the following: "No ifs, ands or buts."
3	Give the patient a three-stage command: "Take a paper in your right hand, fold it in half and put in on the floor."
1	Show the patient the written item "Close your eyes" and ask the patient to read and obey it.
1	Tell the patient to write a sentence.
1	Tell the patient to copy a design (complex polygon).
30	Total score possible

Scoring: 24 to 30 correct—intact cognitive function
20 to 23 correct—mild cognitive impairment
16 to 19 correct—moderate cognitive impairment
15 or less correct—severe cognitive impairment

Folstein, M. F., Folstein, S. E., & McHugh, P. R. (1975). "Mini-mental state." A practical method for grading the cognitive state of patients for the clinician. *J. Psychiatr Res*, 12(3), 189–98.

c. Decrease in concentration, memory, and decision making (dementia syndrome)
d. Other somatic complaints such as decreased appetite, musculoskeletal aches and pains, chest pain
e. History of chronic illness or other health problems
f. Current medications
4. Evaluate depression using the Brink Depression Scale as a screening tool (Table 7-5).
5. Suicide is sometimes associated with depression, with suicides being especially high in older white men. Assess for suicide risk.

B. Nursing/Patient Care Considerations
1. Treatment of depression should be given to older adults and includes drugs, psychotherapy, and, in some cases, electroconvulsive therapy.
2. Complement other therapeutic measures by providing opportunities to increase the person's self-esteem.
a. Encourage participation in activities that are meaningful.
b. Compliment the person.
c. Help the person develop a sense of mastery.
d. Encourage reminiscence of meaningful past events.
3. Help the person identify and use social supports.

Motivation in the Elderly

A. Characteristics
1. Motivation is an important variable in the elderly person's ability to recover from any disabling event, and the ability to maintain his or her highest level of wellness.
2. It is possible to evaluate a persons's motivation to comply with a given treatment plan, and adopt interventions to help to improve the elderly person's motivation.
3. Factors that influence motivation in the elderly include:
a. Needs, such as hunger
b. Past experiences, specifically with health care providers
c. Negative attitudes toward aging
d. Beliefs about independence and dependence
e. Internal factors such as sensory changes, cognitive status, and medication side effects
f. External factors such social norms (particularly if those norms conflict with treatment), time, money, and social supports

TABLE 7-5 Geriatric Depression Scale (Short Form)

Choose the best answer for how you felt over the past week.

	YES	NO
1. Are you basically satisfied with your life?	☐	☐
2. Have you dropped many of your activities and interests?	☐	☐
3. Do you feel that your life is empty?	☐	☐
4. Do you often get bored?	☐	☐
5. Are you in good spirits most of the time?	☐	☐
6. Are you afraid that something bad is going to happen to you?	☐	☐
7. Do you feel happy most of the time?	☐	☐
8. Do you often feel helpless?	☐	☐
9. Do you prefer to stay at home rather than going out and doing new things?	☐	☐
10. Do you feel you have more problems with memory than most?	☐	☐
11. Do you think it is wonderful to be alive now?	☐	☐
12. Do you feel pretty worthless the way you are now?	☐	☐
13. Do you feel full of energy?	☐	☐
14. Do you feel that your situation is hopeless?	☐	☐
15. Do you think that most people are better off than you are?	☐	☐

TOTAL SCORE _____

The following answers count one point; scores 5 indicate probable depression.

1. NO	6. YES	11. NO
2. YES	7. NO	12. YES
3. YES	8. YES	13. NO
4. YES	9. YES	14. YES
5. NO	10. YES	15. YES

Yesavage, J. A., & Brink, T. L. (1983). Development and validaton of a geriatric depression screening scale: A preliminary report. *J. Psychiatr Res*, 17, 37–49.

4. Problems in motivation due to age-related differences include:
   a. A shift from achievement motivation to conservative motivation
   b. Increasing difficulty in the establishment of rewards for elderly people, due to their many losses
   c. A tendency to see a task as being more difficult than a younger person would
   d. A tendency to become easily discouraged; the older adult may not initiate behavior as readily
   e. Greater significance placed on the meaning of a task; it must be meaningful to the elderly person
   f. Evidence that elderly people do not do well on tasks if they are asked to do them rapidly, under a time limit, or in a stressful situation
   g. Increased importance placed on the cost of participating in an activity; fear of failing can be expressed either as increased anxiety or decreased willingness to take risks.
   h. Increased need for elderly people to get approval for trying
5. The motivation equation, developed by McDaniel, can be used to evaluate motivation in the elderly.
   a. Motivation = Wants × Beliefs × Rewards/Costs
   b. Motivation can be increased by increasing the numerator and decreasing the denominator of the equation. For example, providing pain medication before exercising may decrease the cost of the behavior and increase the person's motivation to participate in exercise.

B. *Nursing/Patient Care Considerations*
1. Strategies to improve motivation include:
   a. Establish whose motives are being discussed, the patient's, the family's, or the health care provider's; involve the patient in setting the goals.
   b. Explore with the patient any indication of fear of failure.
   c. Set up the motivation equation and try to increase the numerator and/or decrease the denominator of the desired behavior (eg, establish rewards by finding out what is important to the patient, or decrease the cost of performing a certain behavior).
   d. Encourage the patient to verbally express emotional factors associated with the activity.
   e. Examine the setting for the desired behavior to occur. Is the environment too stressful, too dark, or too noisy?
   f. Attempt to use role models. Elderly role models can change ageist attitudes and stimulate patients to perform the desired behavior.
   g. Set small goals to be met either daily or each shift. This provides frequent rewards.
   h. Do not be afraid to use yourself. Research has indicated that being nice, demonstrating caring, use of humor, verbal encouragement and support can all help motivate the elderly person.

Health Maintenance

◆ PRIMARY PREVENTION

Primary prevention is the prevention of disease before it occurs. Primary prevention can be broken down into counseling, immunizations, and chemoprophylaxis.

Counseling

1. Encourage smoking cessation (see p. 12).
   a. Approximately 20% of people between age 65 and 74 and 10% of those over age 75 still smoke cigarettes.
   b. Tobacco use has been linked to heart disease; peripheral vascular disease; cerebrovascular disease; chronic obstructive pulmonary disease; cancer such as lung, bladder and esophageal malignancies; and numerous other health problems that decrease the quality of life or cause premature death.
   c. Although much damage has been done to the lungs and blood vessels by many years of smoking, elderly persons can still benefit from smoking cessation by increasing the quality of life.
2. Encourage physical activity (see p. 12).
   a. It has been stated that less than 10% of those over 65 are physically active and that almost 50% are sedentary.
   b. It has been recommended that elderly people participate in regular activity, especially aerobic activities that promote cardiovascular fitness, such as walking, cycling, or swimming.
   c. Refer to physical, occupational, or rehabilitation therapist. An individualized exercise prescription should be developed and cleared with the health care provider.
3. Identify alcohol abuse in the elderly.
   a. The consequences of alcoholism include liver disease, gastrointestinal (GI) bleeding, and motor vehicle accidents.
   b. Question elderly people about drug or alcohol abuse. Although street drug use is rare, prescription drug abuse may be occurring.
   c. Refer for counseling.
4. Evaluate and counsel on dental health.
   a. Dental problems in the elderly including missing teeth, ill-fitting dentures, periodontal disease, and decayed teeth.
   b. Dental problems often lead to poor eating habits, apathy, and fatigue.
   c. Regular dental health care should be encouraged to improve nutrition and the quality of life.

Immunizations

A. Pneumococcal Pneumonia and Influenza
1. Pneumococcal pneumonia and influenza are significant causes of mortality and morbidity in the elderly.
2. It is recommended that the pneumococcal vaccine be given at least once to all people over age 65. Some experts suggest that in high-risk groups this be repeated every 6 years.
3. Two options are available for the prevention of influenza.
   a. Annual influenza vaccine for all people over 65.
   b. Amantadine (Symmetrel) or rimantadine (Flumadine) prophylaxis is only effective against influenza A. These agents may be given for the entire flu season, or initiated at the beginning of a flu outbreak; they are also effective in ameliorating symptoms if given within 48 hours of onset of illness.

B. Tetanus-Diphtheria
1. Tetanus-diphtheria immunization is an important but frequently forgotten component of health maintenance, especially in the elderly.

   a. The fatality rate of tetanus exceeds 50% in those over age 65.
   b. Combined tetanus-diphtheria boosters should be given every 10 years.

Chemoprophylaxis

1. It has been recommended that low-dose aspirin therapy be considered for people with high blood cholesterol or other risk factors for myocardial infarction.
   a. Contraindicated if patient is at risk for GI bleeding
2. Estrogen therapy is recommended in postmenopausal women who are at risk for coronary artery disease and osteoporosis.
   a. Contraindicated if there is history of breast cancer, thrombophlebitis or undiagnosed genital bleeding

◆ SECONDARY PREVENTION

Secondary prevention is the detection of disease in an early stage, commonly referred to as screening. Most commonly considered in the elderly are screening for colorectal cancer, breast cancer and prostatic cancer, uterine cancer, and tuberculosis screening.

Screening Recommendations

1. The recommendation for bowel cancer screening is for yearly stool specimens for occult blood and sigmoidoscopy every 3 years after age 50.
2. Monthly self-breast examination, yearly breast examination by a health care provider and yearly mammography are suggested for breast cancer screening for women over age 50.
3. Yearly screening for tuberculosis via skin test is recommended for the older adult, especially if institutionalized.
4. Yearly rectal examinations and blood test for prostatic specific antigen (PSA) are recommended in older men to screen for prostatic disease.
5. Annual examination with PAP test is recommended in older women to rule out cervical or genital malignancies; after hysterectomy for noncancerous process, PAP may be done every 3 to 5 years.
6. Yearly visual screening is important to assess for visual changes and cataracts.

◆ Tertiary Prevention

Tertiary prevention addresses the treatment of established disease to avoid complications and death. The major areas of focus for the older adult are preventing the complications of immobility, and rehabilitation.

Preventing Complications of Immobility

A. Positioning
1. The goal of frequent position changes is to prevent contractures, stimulate circulation and prevent pressure sores, prevent thrombophlebitis and pulmonary embolism, promote lung expansion and prevent pneumonia, and decrease edema of the extremities. Changing position from lying to sitting several times a day can help prevent changes in the cardiovascular system known as deconditioning.

2. The recommendation is to change body position at least every 2 hours, and preferably more frequently than that in patients who have no spontaneous movement.

B. *Maintain proper body alignment*
1. Dorsal or supine position
   a. The head is in line with the spine, both laterally and anteroposteriorly.
   b. The trunk is positioned so flexion of the hips is minimized to prevent hip contracture.
   c. The arms are flexed at the elbow with the hands resting against the lateral abdomen.
   d. The legs are extended in a neutral position with the toes pointed toward the ceiling.
   e. The heels are suspended in a space between the mattress and the footboard to prevent heel pressure.
   f. Trochanter rolls are placed under the greater trochanters in the hip joint areas.
2. Side-lying or lateral position
   a. The head is in line with the spine.
   b. The body is in alignment and is not twisted.
   c. The uppermost hip joint is slightly forward and supported by a pillow in a position of slight abduction.
   d. A pillow supports the arm, which is flexed at both the elbow and shoulder joints.
3. Prone position
   a. The head is turned laterally and is in alignment with the rest of the body.
   b. The arms are abducted and externally rotated at the shoulder joint; the elbows are flexed.
   c. A small, flat support is placed under the pelvis, extending from the level of the umbilicus to the upper third of the thigh.
   d. The lower extremities remain in a neutral position.
   e. The toes are suspended over the edge of the mattress.

C. *Encourage therapeutic exercise*
1. It has been reported that there is a daily loss of 1% to 1.5% of initial strength in an immobilized older adult.
2. The goals of therapeutic exercise are to develop and retrain deficient muscles, to restore as much normal movement as possible to prevent deformity, to stimulate the functions of various organs and body systems, to build strength and endurance and to promote relaxation.
3. Perform passive range-of-motion exercise.
   a. Carried out without assistance from the patient
   b. The purpose is to retain as much joint range of motion as possible, and to maintain circulation.
   c. Move the joint smoothly through its full range of motion (Table 7-6). Do not push beyond the point of pain.
4. Perform active assistive range of motion.
   a. Carried out by the patient with the assistance of the nurse.
   b. The purpose is to encourage normal muscle function.
   c. Support the distal part and encourage the patient to take the joint actively through its range of motion.
   d. Give only the amount of assistance necessary to accomplish the action.
5. Encourage active range of motion.
   a. Accomplished by the patient without assistance.
   b. The purpose is to increase muscle strength.
   c. When possible, active exercise should be done against gravity.
   d. Encourage the patient to move the joint through the full range of motion without assistance.
   e. Ensure that the patient does not substitute another joint movement for the one intended.
   f. Other active forms of exercise include turning from side to side, turning from back to abdomen, and moving up and down in bed.
6. Assist with resistive exercise.
   a. Carried out by the patient working against resistance produced by either manual or mechanical means.
   b. The purpose is to increase muscle strength.
   c. Encourage the patient to move the joint through its range of motion while you or someone else provides slight resistance at first, and then progressively increases resistance.
   d. Weights may be used and are attached at the distal point of the involved joint.
   e. The movements should be done smoothly.
7. Teach isometric or muscle-setting exercise.
   a. Involve alternately contracting and relaxing a muscle while keeping the part in a fixed position; performed by the patient.
   b. The purpose is to maintain strength when a joint is immobilized.
   c. Teach the patient to contract or tighten the muscle as much as possible without moving the joint.
   d. The patient holds the position for several seconds, then relaxes.

Geriatric Rehabilitation

A. *Characteristics*
1. The primary goal is restoring the older adult to maximum functional level.
2. Multidisciplinary service involving input from the primary care provider; nursing personnel; physical, occupational, speech and recreational therapists; social worker; psychologist; and dietitian.
3. Rehabilitation nursing involves developing a rehabilitation philosophy of care.
   a. Patients are encouraged, and allowed sufficient time, to perform as much of their personal care as possible.
   b. Goals are set *with* the patient rather than *for* the patient.
   c. Prevention of further impairment is imperative.
   d. Focus on skin and wound care, regaining or maintaining bowel and bladder function, independent medication use, good nutritional status, psychosocial support, an appropriate activity/rest balance, and patient and family education.

B. *Nursing/Patient Care Considerations*
1. Impaired cognitive function may have an impact on the quality of rehabilitation.
   a. Assess for physical problems that may exacerbate cognitive dysfunction (eg, infection, drug side effects, metabolic or circulatory problems, or fatigue).
   b. Provide innovative measures to encourage ambulation and increased function; provide frequent verbal cues and large print reminders; focus on basic self-care abilities.
   c. Implement appropriate safety measures such as bed siderails, proper lighting, appropriate staffing, and restraints if necessary.

2. Disability has a tremendous impact on the patient's body image and requires an adjustment by the patient. Be aware of the stages of psychological reaction the patient may undergo.
   a. Period of confusion, disorganization and denial.
   b. Period of depression and/or anxiety and grief
   c. Period of adaptation and adjustment
3. Interventions in rehabilitation nursing include:
   a. Provide an atmosphere of acceptance.
   b. Identify and encourage positive coping patterns.
   c. Encourage socialization and participation in group activities.
   d. Give positive reinforcement and feedback about progress.
   e. Involve families as much as possible.

4. Family (significant other) coping may impact on rehabilitation efforts.
   a. Assist the family (significant other) to face the reality of the patient's disability.
   b. Involve the family (significant other) in decision making and in the patient's care in order for them to develop and practice the skill necessary for the patient to reach rehabilitation goals.
   c. Help extend and enlarge the family (significant other) skills by teaching problem solving, treatment needs of the patient, ways to communicate to health care providers, and the use of community resources.
   d. Assess the level of caregiver fatigue or burnout (Table 7-7).

TABLE 7-6 Range of Motion

SHOULDER

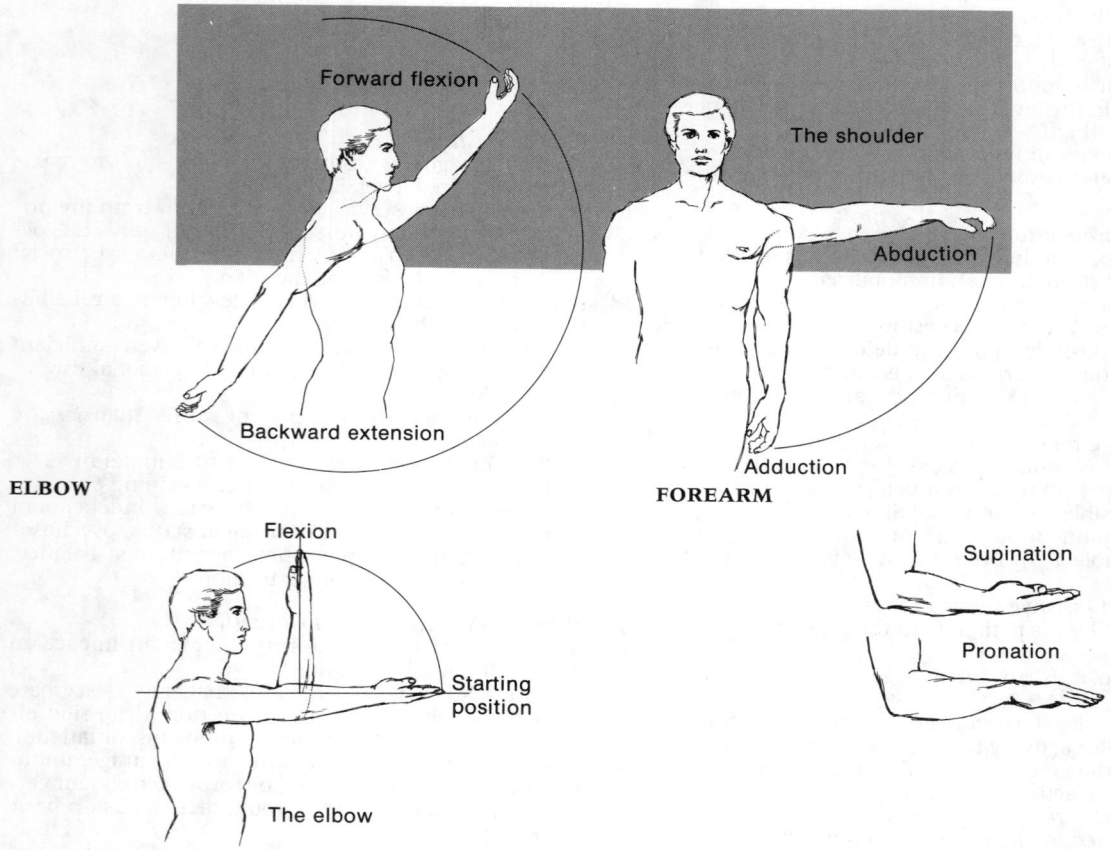

ELBOW

FOREARM

(continued)

TABLE 7-6 Range of Motion *(continued)*

WRIST

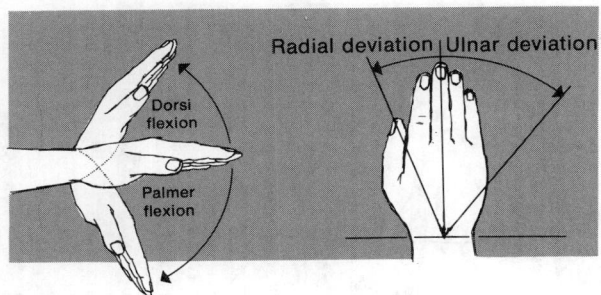

THUMB

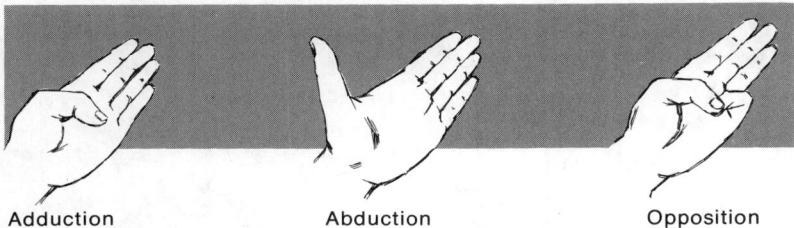

Adduction   Abduction   Opposition

FINGERS

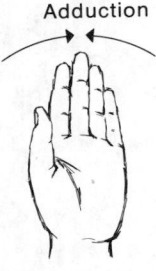
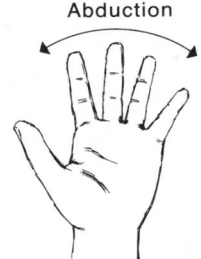
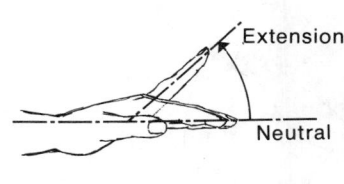

ANKLE

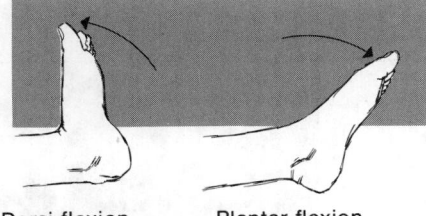

Dorsi-flexion   Plantar flexion

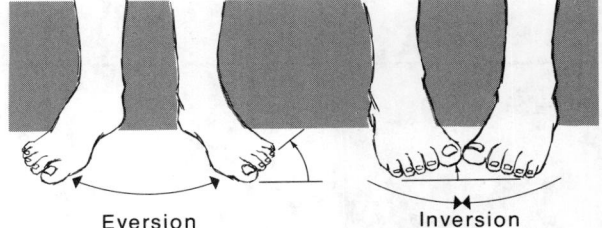

Eversion   Inversion

TOES

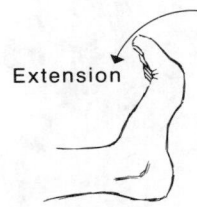
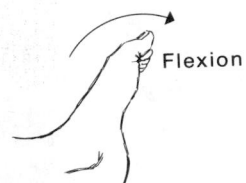

Extension   Flexion

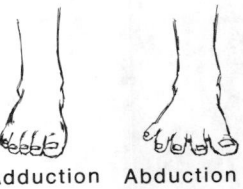

Adduction Abduction

(continued)

TABLE 7-6 Range of Motion *(continued)*

HIP

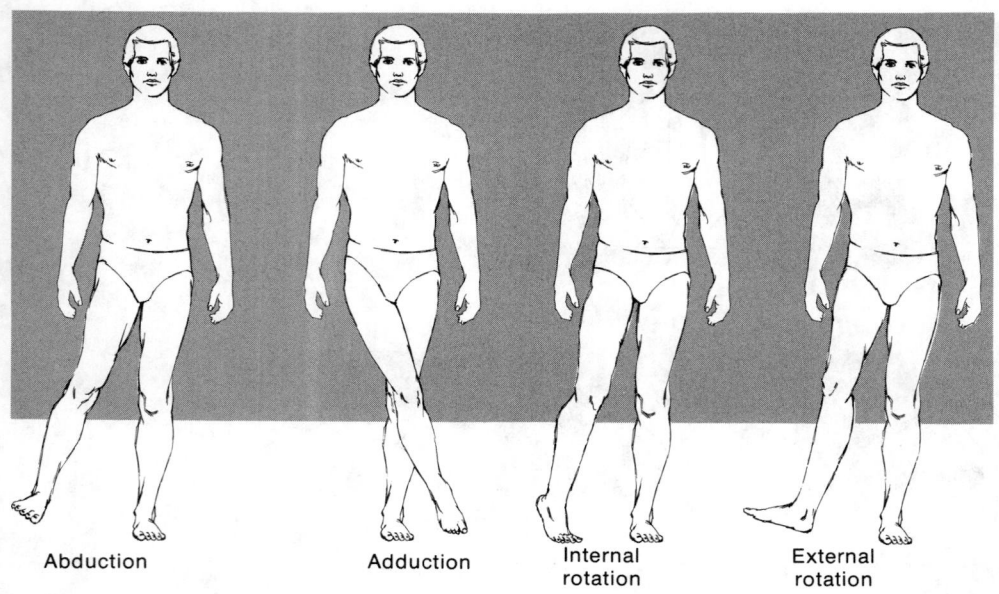

Abduction   Adduction   Internal   External
                                      rotation   rotation

KNEE

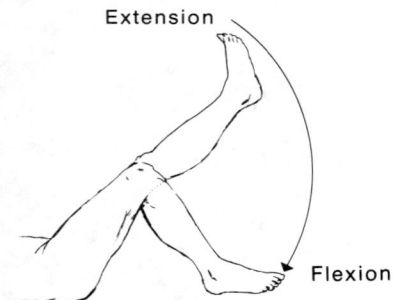

Extension

Flexion

(continued)

TABLE 7-6 Range of Motion *(continued)*

CERVICAL SPINE

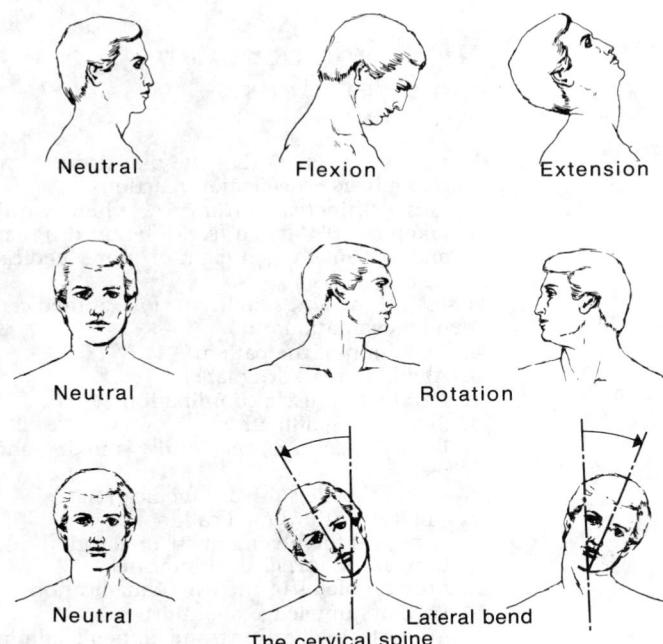

Neutral   Flexion   Extension

Neutral   Rotation

Neutral   Lateral bend

The cervical spine

TABLE 7-7 Caregiver Strain Index

Instructions given to the caregiver: I am going to read a list of things that other people have found to be difficult in caring for patients after they come home from the hospital. Would you tell me whether any of these apply to you? (Give the examples.)

Score one point for "yes" and zero for "no."

1. Sleep is disturbed (eg, because _____ is in and out of bed or wanders around at night).
2. It is inconvenient (eg, because helping takes so much time or it's a long drive over to help).
3. It is a physical strain (eg, because of lifting in and out of a chair).
4. It is confining (eg, because helping restricts free time or cannot visit).
5. There have been family adjustments (eg, because helping has disrupted routine or there has been no privacy).
6. There have been changes in personal plans (eg, had to turn down a job or could not go on vacation).
7. There have been other demands on my time (eg, from other family members).
8. There have been emotional adjustments (eg, because of severe arguments).
9. Some behavior is upsetting (eg, incontinence; _____ has trouble remembering things; _____ accuses others of taking things).
10. It is upsetting to find that _____ has changed so much from before (eg, _____ is a different person from before).
11. There have been work adjustments (eg, because of having to take time off).
12. It is a financial strain.
13. It has been completely overwhelming (eg, because of worry about _____ or concerns about how to continue to manage).

Scoring: Total score of 7 or more suggests a greater level of stress.

Robinson, B. C. (1983). Validation of a caregiver strain index. *J. Gerontol*, 38(3), 344–8. ©1983 The Gerontological Society of America.

Special Health Problems of the Older Adult

◆ ALTERED RESPONSE TO MEDICATION

Adults over age 65 consume 30% to 40% of all prescription drugs and an even higher proportion of the over-the-counter drugs consumed. Age-related changes predispose older adults to problems with medication side effects.

Etiology/Altered Physiology

A. Factors Altering Drug Responses in the Elderly
1. Drug absorption is affected by the following age-related changes:
   a. Decreased gastric acid
   b. Decreased GI motility
   c. Decreased gastric blood flow
   d. Changes in GI villi
   e. Decreased blood flow and body temperature in rectum
2. Drug distribution is affected by:
   a. Decreased body size
   b. Decreased water content in the body
   c. Increased total body fat
   d. Drugs distributed in water have a higher concentration in the elderly (eg, gentamicin [Garamycin]).
   e. Drugs distributed in fat have a wider distribution and less intense but prolonged effect (eg, phenobarbital [Luminal]).
3. Drug metabolism in the older adult:
   a. Is altered by a decrease in liver size, blood flow, enzyme activity and protein synthesis
   b. Requires more time than in younger adults. Therefore, there is increased drug activity time in drugs that are metabolized in the liver (eg, propranolol [Inderal], theophylline [Theo-Dur]).
4. Excretion of drugs is altered in older adults due to the following renal changes:
   a. Decreased renal tubular function and blood flow
   b. This causes a decrease in renal filtration and an increase in blood levels of drugs that are excreted through the kidneys (eg, cimetidine [Tagamet]).

Nursing Assessment

1. Drug toxicities are different than they are in younger people.
2. Fewer symptoms may be identified, and they may develop slower; however, the reactions may be more pronounced and further advanced once they do present.
3. Behavioral side effects are more common in elderly people because the blood–brain barrier becomes less effective; the first reaction to a drug is confusion.
4. Many potential drug side effects are not identified because they are attributed to old age; fatigue, confusion, anorexia, or indigestion as drug side effects may not be reported.

5. Allergic reactions to drugs increase with age due to a greater likelihood of earlier exposure.

Nursing/Patient Care Considerations

1. Maintain awareness that the older adult is at greater risk for adverse medication reactions.
   a. This risk increases from 6% when two drugs are taken to 50% when five different drugs are taken, and to 100% when eight or more medications are taken.
2. Assess the patient's ability to follow medication regimen by evaluation of:
   a. Cognition of the patient
   b. Ability to read drug labels
   c. Hand and muscle coordination
   d. Swallowing difficulty
   e. Lifestyle patterns, specifically smoking and alcohol use
   f. Cultural beliefs toward medication
   g. Ability to afford medication
   h. Caregiver involvement in medication administration; assess caregiver if indicated
3. Identify problems in the use of medications such as:
   a. Lack of knowledge about drugs
   b. Multiple medications and difficult administration techniques
   c. Caregiver misunderstanding of medication use
4. Appropriate interventions for safe drug use include:
   a. Obtain a complete drug history.
   b. Reinforce verbal instructions with written instructions using large print and simple wording. If necessary, use color coding rather than drug names.
   c. Write what the drug is used for and what the side effects can be.
   d. Make sure the patient or caregiver can open the medication container.
   e. Arrange medication schedules to coincide with regular activity, such as eating (if appropriate for that drug). Simplify the drug regimen as much as possible.
   f. If necessary, arrange a check-off system using a chart to ensure compliance.
   g. If possible, visibly evaluate all medications in the home, or ask patient to bring all medications for evaluation.
   h. Encourage patient to discard all old or unneeded medications, and to check expiration dates.
   i. Encourage patient to store medications in original containers and in a dry, dark place.
   j. Encourage patient to avoid over-the-counter medication without checking with the primary care provider before use.
   k. Encourage patient to report any drug side effects.
   l. Work with patient to maintain a drug regimen that follows the principles for geriatric drug use; start dosages low and go slow, use only necessary medications, titrate the dose to the patient response, simplify the regimen, and have frequent reevaluations done regarding the medication regimen.

◆ ALTERED NUTRITIONAL STATUS

Normal age-related changes, behavioral changes, and pathologic conditions may lead to malnutrition in the older adult.

Etiology/Altered Physiology

1. Changes in the oral cavity including loss of teeth, diminished saliva production, and difficulty with mastication may cause decreased food intake.
2. A decrease in gastric juice secretion with reduced pepsin hinders protein digestion, and iron, vitamin B_{12}, calcium and folic acid absorption; there are no significant changes in the small or large bowel.
3. Sensory changes involving taste and smell cause anorexia.
4. Psychosocial factors including changes in living situation, widowhood, depression, loneliness, decreased choice of food for institutionalized elderly, need to adhere to special diets, economic status, and ability to obtain and prepare food all impact on what is eaten.
5. Alcohol use interferes with the absorption of the B-complex vitamins. Additionally, alcohol is high in calories and low in nutritional value.
6. Medications can alter nutrition by directly decreasing absorption and utilization of nutrients. Indirectly, medications can result in anorexia, serostomia, dysgeusia, and early satiety.
7. Dysphagia (difficulty swallowing), which commonly occurs after cerebral vascular accident, intubation, head and neck surgery, or related to Parkinson's disease and dementia, may cause decreased food intake.

Nursing Assessment

1. Patients with dysphagia may report difficulty swallowing, difficulty managing saliva. They cough after swallowing, they sound "wet" after eating, they may have pocketing of food, they may have an absent or diminished gag reflex.
2. Protein-energy malnutrition can present with either a 10% weight loss over 6 months alone (marasmus) or weight loss with low serum albumin levels (kwashiorkor).
3. The single best predictor of a malnourished patient is a cholesterol level below 150 mg/dL.

Nursing/Patient Care Considerations

1. Educate older adult and family or significant other on basic nutritional requirements and on overcoming barriers that interfere with optimal nutrition.
   a. The Required Dietary Allowances (RDA) for healthy older adults is the same as that for younger adults, with three exceptions: decreased caloric intake, a concomitant decrease in B vitamins, and decreased iron requirements for postmenopausal women.
2. Encourage good mouth care.

3. Avoid alcohol if possible; refer for counseling if necessary and compensate for the nutritional consequences of alcohol abuse with liquid supplements, B vitamins.
4. Review all prescription and over-the-counter medications with patients, and evaluate the influence of these on nutritional status.
5. If food procurement, preparation, and enjoyment are a problem, identify community resources to offer assistance in obtaining food and community meals.
6. In institutional settings, environmental factors may influence food enjoyment. Encourage socialization when eating, and try to minimize the negative effects of disruptive people. Try to improve aesthetics.
7. To compensate for age-related changes in taste and smell, encourage use of low-sodium food additives.
8. Encourage proper body position (ie, sitting upright during mealtimes) and staying up for one-half hour after eating to help with digestion.
9. If possible, encourage five to six small meals rather than three large meals.
10. If appropriate, encourage the family to bring in food favorites for the patient.
11. Position food on the plate so that if there is visual neglect, or impairment, the patient is best able to see the food served.
12. Identify patients with dysphagia and obtain a referral to a speech therapist.
    a. Work with the speech therapist and primary health care provider to determine what consistency of food is safe for the patient to swallow. If the patient is unable to swallow thin liquids, slushes, puddings, or applesauce should be given to ensure adequate hydration.
    b. Use good compensatory techniques if indicated. These include sitting upright, tucking and turning the head, placing the food on the unaffected side of the tongue, swallow twice to clear the pharyngeal tract, tuck chin to chest and bring tongue up and back and hold breath to swallow.
    c. Write out swallowing instructions for patient and family, and educate family regarding the importance of maintaining these precautions.

◆ URINARY INCONTINENCE

Approximately 10 million Americans suffer from urinary incontinence. That includes 15% to 30% of community-dwelling elderly and 40% to 70% of institutionalized elderly. It is often not reported by elderly people because they consider it to be a normal age change, and there is a low expectation of benefit from treatment.

Etiology/Altered Physiology

1. There are four basic types of urinary incontinence:
   a. Stress—an involuntary loss of urine with increases in intraabdominal pressure. Usually caused from weakness and laxity of pelvic floor musculature, or bladder outlet weakness.
   b. Urge—involves leakage of urine because of inability to delay voiding after sensation of bladder fullness is perceived. This is associated with detrusor hyperactivity, central nervous system disorders, or local genitourinary conditions.

c. Overflow—due to a leakage of urine resulting from mechanical forces on an overdistended bladder. This results from mechanical obstruction or an acontractile bladder.

d. Functional—involves urinary leakage associated with inability to get to the toilet because of cognitive and/or physical functioning.

Nursing Assessment

1. Identify reversible causes of incontinence using the DRIP acronym.
   a. D—Delirium, especially new onset delirium
   b. R—Restricted mobility, retention
   c. I—Infection (especially sudden onset cystitis), inflammation (such as atrophic vaginitis or urethritis), impaction (fecal)
   d. P—Polyuria (from poorly controlled diabetes or diuretic treatment), pharmaceuticals (including psychotropics, anticholinergics, alpha agonists, beta agonists, calcium channel blockers, narcotics, alpha antagonists, and alcohol)
2. Evaluate lower urinary tract function.
   a. Stress maneuvers are evaluated by asking the patient, with a full bladder, to cough three times while standing. Observe for leakage of urine.
   b. Check for postvoid residual by inserting a 12 or 14 French straight catheter a few minutes after the patient voids.
   c. Evaluate bladder filling by leaving the straight catheter in place and using a 50 mL syringe to fill the bladder with sterile water. Hold the syringe approximately 15 cm above the pubic symphysis. Continue to fill the bladder in 25-mL increments until the patient feels the urge to void. Observe for involuntary bladder contractions. These contractions are detected by continuous upward movement of the column of fluid in the absence of abdominal straining.

Nursing/Patient Care Considerations

1. For stress or urge incontinence, teach Kegel (pelvic muscle) exercises.
   a. Tell the patient to first practice stopping stream of urine while voiding to identify proper contraction of the pubococcygeal muscle; contraction will result in stopping flow, relaxation allows flow.
   b. Once proper contraction is verified, advise the patient to practice contraction for 5 to 10 seconds, then relaxation of the muscle for 5 to 10 seconds in sets of 10 three times a day.
   c. The exercise can be practiced anywhere at any time because it involves contraction of an internal muscle. The abdomen should be relaxed, and no movement should be visible by doing Kegel exercises.
2. Assist with biofeedback that involves the use of bladder, rectal or vaginal pressure recordings to train patients to contract pelvic floor muscles and relax the bladder.
3. Institute a behavioral training program, using bladder records, biofeedback, and pelvic floor exercises for patients with stress or urge incontinence.

4. Other interventions include:
   a. Bladder retraining—progressive lengthening or shortening of voiding intervals to restore the normal pattern of voiding; this is useful after period of immobility or catheterization.
   b. Scheduled toileting—using a fixed toileting schedule to prevent wetting episodes for patients with urge or functional incontinence.
   c. Habit training—involves using a variable toileting schedule based on the patient's pattern of voiding; also incorporates positive reinforcement.
   d. Prompted voiding—includes regular prompts to void every 1 to 2 hours with positive reinforcement.

◆ URINARY RETENTION

Urinary retention is a common problem in the older adult, often related to neurologic or other underlying condition.

Etiology/Altered Physiology

1. Frequently encountered in the acute care setting, postcatheterization, after stroke, in diabetics due to atonic neuropathic bladder, due to fecal impaction, and males with prostatic enlargement.
2. The patient with urinary retention may void small amounts, or may be incontinent continuously due to overflow of urine.
3. Patients with urinary retention usually will have incontinence during the night.
4. Urinary retention may also be caused or aggravated by drugs with anticholinergic properties such as levodopa (Sinemet) or the tricyclic antidepressants, especially amitriptyline (Elavil).

Nursing Assessment

1. Take a complete history and perform physical examination to rule out causes of urinary retention.
2. Monitor for a distended bladder and perform postvoid catheterization; residual of greater than 300 mL of urine signals urinary retention.

Nursing/Patient Care Considerations

1. Remove fecal impaction to help patient regain bladder function.
2. If prostatic disease is suspected, appropriate referral is necessary.
3. Encourage male to use standing position and female the sitting position to facilitate urinary flow; provide privacy.
4. Evaluate medication regimen and discuss the necessity or substitution of offending medication with health care provider.
5. If no underlying condition is suspected, attempt intermittent catheterizations every 8 hours, in combination with regular voiding attempts by patient. If there is no response in 2 weeks (ie, no decrease in postvoid residuals), referral to a urologist may be necessary for medical management of the urinary retention.

◆ FECAL INCONTINENCE

Fecal incontinence is an inability to voluntarily control the passage of gas or feces. Although not as common as urinary incontinence, fecal incontinence afflicts 13% to 47% of hospitalized elders and 10% to 30% of nursing home residents. It has been noted to affect 10.9 men and 13.3 women per 1,000 older adults living at home.

Etiology/Altered Physiology

1. Fecal continence depends on normal rectal and anal sensation, rectal reservoir capacity, and internal and external sphincteric mechanisms.
2. In institutionalized elderly, fecal impaction is a primary cause of fecal incontinence due to stool leaking around a fecal mass.
3. In the noninstitutionalized elderly, fecal incontinence is often associated with dysfunction of one of the anorectal continence mechanisms such as impaired contractile strength of the sphincters, and lower rectal volume capacity. Stroke and spinal cord injuries cause loss of sensation in the rectal area.
4. Often no cause can be determined for the fecal loss, and it is believed that the incontinence may be due to a degenerative injury to the pudendal nerve.

Nursing Assessment

1. Perform a rectal examination to check for impaction or decreased rectal sphincter tone.
2. If the fecal incontinence is diarrheal in nature, stool for leukocytes, culture and sensitivity, ova and parasites, and *Clostridium difficile* evaluation may be indicated.

Nursing/Patient Care Considerations

1. If there is no infection and no impaction, it may be helpful to increase dietary fiber in an attempt to add bulk to the stool to stimulate regular defecation.
2. Antidiarrheals, such as loperamide, may be effective in managing diarrhea.
3. Once an impaction is detected and removed, aggressive attempts should be made to set up a regular bowel pattern. This includes regular toileting times set preferably after breakfast, and increased fluid and fiber intake. Laxatives should be used only as a last resort.
4. In the bedbound patient, increased fiber in the diet is contraindicated. These patients may require a bisacodyl (Dulcolax) suppository or an enema to help with rectal evacuation two to three times per week.
5. Older adults with neurogenic fecal incontinence, such as patients with spinal cord injuries, and post CVA, should have treatment to induce fecal evacuation at regularly scheduled times.
   a. A glycerin (Glyrol) or bisacodyl (Dulcolax) suppository two to three times a week before breakfast (to use the normal gastrocolic reflex that starts after the first meal of the day) may help to induce a complete rectal evacuation and decrease stool incontinence.

◆ PRESSURE SORES

Pressure sores (decubitus ulcers) are localized ulcerations of the skin or deeper structures. They most commonly result from prolonged periods of bedrest in acute or long-term care facilities (Fig. 7-1).

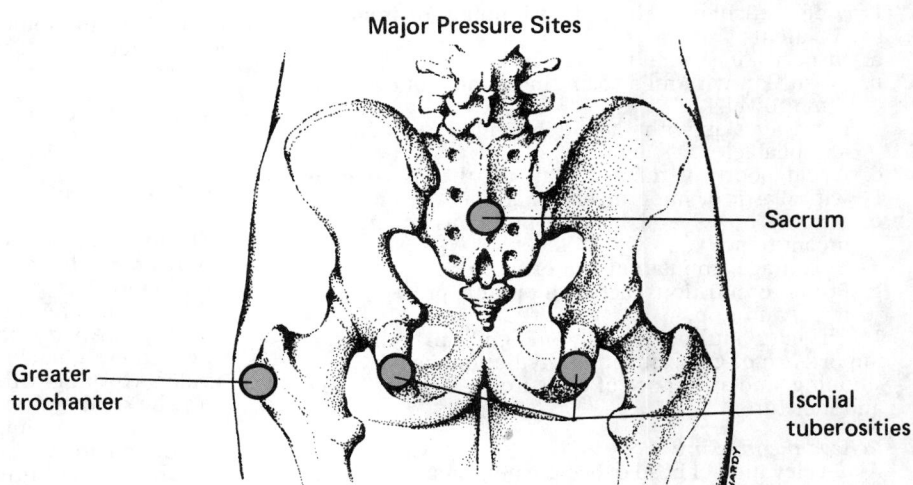

Major Pressure Sites

Sacrum

Greater trochanter

Ischial tuberosities

FIGURE 7-1 Sites of pressure sores.

Etiology/Altered Physiology

A. Factors in the development of pressure sores
1. Pressure of 70 mm Hg applied for longer than 2 hours can produce tissue destruction; healing cannot occur without relieving the pressure.
2. Friction contributes to pressure sore development by causing abrasion of the stratum corneum.
3. Shearing force, produced by sliding of adjacent surfaces, is particularly important in the partial sitting position. This force ruptures capillaries over the sacrum.
4. Moisture on the skin results in maceration of the epithelium.

B. Risk factors for pressure sores
1. Bowel or bladder incontinence
2. Malnourishment or significant weight loss
3. Edema, anemia, hypoxia, or hypotension
4. Neurologic impairment or immobility
5. Altered mental status, including delirium or dementia

Nursing Assessment

1. Assess for risk factors for pressure sore development and alter those factors, if possible.
2. Assess skin of the older adult frequently for the development of pressure sores.
3. Stage the ulcer so appropriate treatment can be started.
4. One commonly used staging system advocated by the National Pressure Ulcer Advisory Panel includes four levels:
   a. Stage one—nonblanching macule that may appear red or violet
   b. Stage two—skin breakdown as far as the dermis
   c. Stage three—skin breakdown into the subcutaneous tissue
   d. Stage four—penetrate bone, muscle or the joint

Nursing/Patient Care Considerations

A. Prevent pressure sore development
1. Provide meticulous care and positioning for immobilized patients.
   a. Inspect skin several times daily.
   b. Wash skin with mild soap, rinse, and blot dry with a soft towel.
   c. Lubricate skin with a bland lotion to keep skin soft and pliable.
   d. Avoid poorly ventilated mattress that is covered with plastic or impermeable material.
   e. Employ bowel and bladder programs to prevent incontinence.
   f. Encourage ambulation and exercise.
   g. Promote nutritious diet with optimal protein, vitamins, and iron.
2. Teach older adult and family or significant other the importance of good nutrition, hydration, activity, positioning, and avoidance of pressure, shearing, friction and moisture.

B. Relieve the pressure
1. Avoid elevation of head of bed greater than 30 degrees.
2. Reposition every 2 hours.

3. Use special devices to cushion specific areas, such as flotation rings, lamb's wool or fleece pads, egg-crate mattresses, booties, elbow pads.
4. Use an alternating pressure mattress or air fluidized bed for patients at high risk, to prevent or treat pressure sores.
5. Provide for activity and ambulation as much as possible.
6. Advise frequent shifting of weight and occasional raising of bottom off chair while sitting.

C. Clean and debride the wound
1. Use normal saline for cleaning and disinfecting wounds.
2. Apply wet-to-dry dressings or enzyme ointments for debridement as directed; or assist with surgical debridement.

D. Treat local infection
1. Open wounds are always colonized with bacteria, hence wound cultures are unneccesary unless there is evidence of systemic infection or progressive local infection such as cellulitis.
2. Apply topical antibiotics to locally infected pressure ulcer as prescribed.

E. Cover the wound with a protective dressing
1. This minimizes disruption of migrating fibroblasts and epithelial cells, and results in a moist, nutrient-rich environment for healing to occur.
   a. Polyurethane thin film dressings can be used for superficial low-exudate wounds. They are air and water permeable, but do not absorb exudate.
   b. Hydrocolloids can provide padding to wounds but can lead to maceration; they are not oxygen permeable.
   c. Polyurethane foam/membrane dressings absorb exudate and are oxygen permeable.
   d. Hydrogel dressing are multilayered and include properties of both hydrocolloids and polyurethane. (See Table 7-8 for comparison of selected occlusive dressings.)

Legal/Ethical Considerations

◆ RESTRAINT USE

Since the Nursing Home Reform Act took effect in October 1990, long-term care facilities throughout the United States have been required to follow new guidelines emphasizing individualized, less restrictive care for residents. See Procedure Guidelines 7-1.

Guidelines

1. The following are the federal requirements for the use of restraints based on the 1987 Omnibus Budget Reconciliation Act.
2. These guidelines must be met in any long-term-care facility that participates in Medicare or Medicaid. However, these guidelines are useful for health care providers working with elderly people in all settings.
   a. The resident has the right to be free from any physical restraints imposed or psychoactive drug administered for purposes of discipline or convenience and not required to treat the resident's medical symptoms.

TABLE 7-8 Comparison of Selected Occlusive Dressings

Dressing	Manufacturer	Cost*	Use	Advantages	Disadvantages
Hydrocolloid Duoderm	ConvaTec	$6.04 per 4 × 4 square	Padding under brace Stage I ulcer	Easy to apply Water impermeable No skin excoriation	Poor absorptive capacity Poor oxygen exchange Messy residue Pressure area
Polyurethane film Op-Site	Acme United Corp.	$1.27 per 4 × 4 square	Nondraining wounds	Transparent Self-adhesive Oxygen permeable	No absorptive capacity May cause excoriation Difficult to apply
Polyurethane film Tegaderm	3M	$2.00 per 4.5 × 4.5 square	Same as above	Same as above	Same as above
Polyurethane membrane Mitraflex	Calgon Vestal	$4.00 per 4 × 4 square	Skin tears Tape burns Blisters Stage II ulcers Low-moderate exudate Wounds	Good absorptive ability Good oxygen exchange Easy to apply Self-adhesive Water impermeable May debride	May cause excoriation
Polyurethane foam Epi-Lock	Calgon Vestal	$4.77 per 4 × 4 square	Same as above	Good absorptive ability Good oxygen exchange Water impermeable May debride No skin excoriation	Nonadhesive
Hydrogel Spenco Second skin	Spenco	Unable to determine cost	Superficial nondraining wounds	No skin excoriation Transparent	Difficult to apply Nonadherent Dehydrates easily
Hydrogel Bio Film	B.F. Goodrich	Unable to determine cost	Stage I-III pressure ulcers	No skin excoriation Transparent Some ability to absorb drainage Easy to apply	May require picture framing to remain in place

* Cost may vary depending on supplier and state.
Resnick, B. (1993). Wound care for the elderly. *Geriatric Nursing*, 14(1), 26–28.

b. Physical restraints are any manual method of physical or mechanical device, material, or equipment attached or adjacent to the resident's body that the person cannot remove easily, which restricts freedom of movement or access to one's body (includes leg and arm restraints, hand mitts, soft ties or vest, wheelchair safety bars and gerichairs).
c. There must be a trial of less restrictive measures unless the physical restraint is necessary to provide lifesaving treatment.
d. The resident or his or her legal representative must consent to the use of restraints.
e. Residents who are restrained should be released, exercised, toileted, and checked for skin redness every 2 hours.
f. The need for restraints should be reevaluated periodically.
g. The specific institution will have to develop policies and procedures for the appropriate use of restraints and psychoactive drugs.
h. Primary health care providers will have to write appropriate orders for restraints and/or psychoactive drugs.

3. The most frequently reported reason for nurses' use of restraints is to prevent patients from harming themselves or others. Specifically, they are used to prevent falls and prevent removal of catheters or intravenous lines.
4. Multiple studies have found that restraints actually increase the falls that occur, can result in patient strangulation, increase patient confusion, can cause pressure ulcers and nosocomial infections, can decrease functional ability, and can result in social isolation.
5. In regard to the patient's personal and social integrity, restraints have resulted in emotional responses of anger, fear, resistance, humiliation, demoralization, discomfort, resignation, and denial.

Alternative Interventions Instead of Restraints

1. Evaluate those patients who are considered to be in need of a restraint. Evaluation should include: physical function (see Functional Assessment), cognitive status

(see Mental Status Testing), elimination history, history of falls, visual impairment, blood pressure (specifically evaluating for orthostatic hypotension), and medication use.

2. Attempt to correct any problems identified in the evaluation, such as visual impairment, unsafe gait.

3. Use the evaluation to determine patients at high risk of falling (ie, those with confusion, orthostatic hypotension, multiple medication regimens, and altered gait).

4. Alternatives to restraints for patients at high risk of falling when ambulating independently include:
   a. Use of beanbag chairs, or specially designed chairs that make independent transfer difficult for the older adult
   b. Tilting the front of a chair upward by inserting a small to medium folded blanket under the anterior portion of the cushion
   c. Instituting increased exercise activities to help strengthen muscles and improve function

5. For the patient who interferes with treatment, it may be helpful to evaluate the need for the invasive treatments. When such treatments are essential, attempt the use of mittens or gloves rather than use of restraints.

6. For the patient who wanders, it may be helpful to provide an exercise program, or establish a bounded environment in which the person can ambulate freely

---

PROCEDURE GUIDELINES 7-1 ◆ Safety Guidelines for Restraint Use

EQUIPMENT   Restraint device
Full bed siderails
Siderail covers

PROCEDURE

NURSING ACTION	RATIONALE
PREPARATORY PHASE	
1. Select the least restrictive physical restraint.	1. Passive restraints such as geriatric chairs with trays are more desirable than active restraints (vests, leg, arm, wrist, hand restraints or seat belts).
2. Examine the restraint device to ensure that it is not torn or damaged, and that it works properly and is the proper size for the patient.	2. A damaged or improperly fitting restraint poses a significant safety risk because the patient could become suspended by the restraint, causing chest compression.

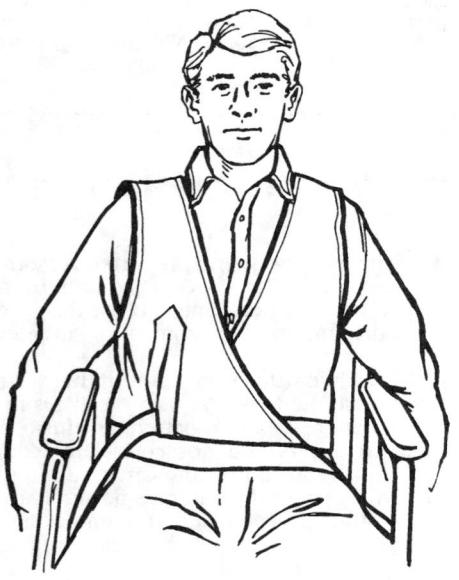 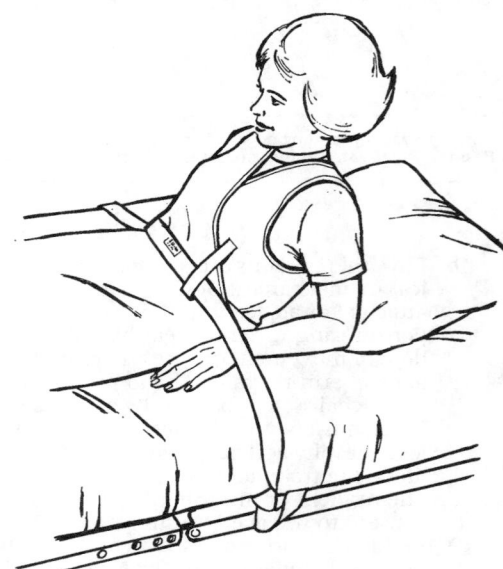

Proper position of patient restraint in wheelchair and bed. Straps of most vest-type restraints should cross in front of patient. Left: safety vest; right: budget vest.

3. If the restraint is being used in bed, make sure that full siderails can be placed in the up position. Obtain siderail covers if the patient's limbs could fit over, under, around, through, or between siderails.	3. Siderails that are only $\frac{1}{2}$ or $\frac{3}{4}$ length of the bed may allow the patient to slip partially off the bed and to become suspended in the restraint.

PROCEDURES (cont'd)	NURSING ACTION	RATIONALE

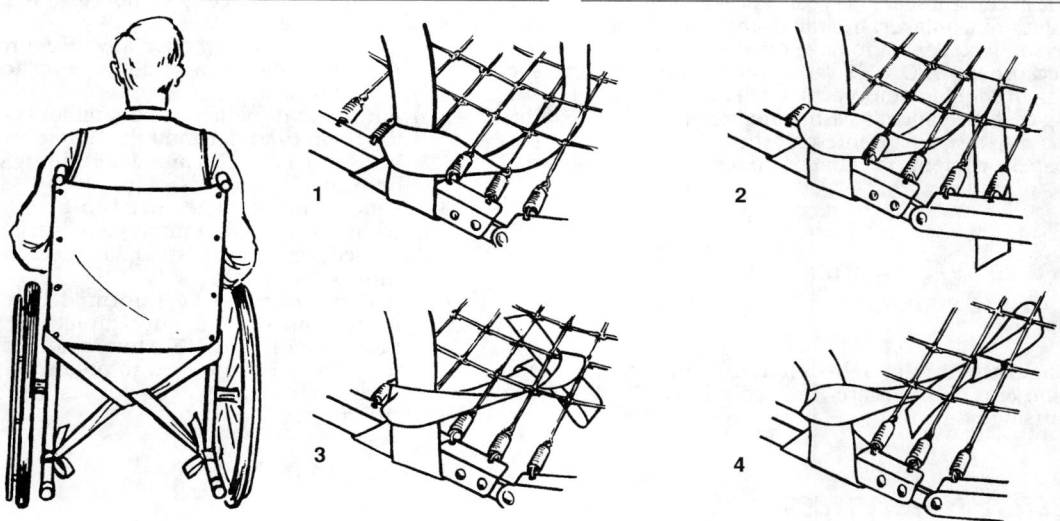

Straps should be secured out of patient reach to kick spurs of wheelchair or moveable part of bedframe.

4. Completely review manufacturer's instructions before applying the restraint.

4. Complete information can be obtained from Posey Co., 5635 Peck Rd., Arcadia, CA 91006, 800-44-POSEY.

PERFORMANCE PHASE

1. Apply the restraint with the patient positioned in the middle of the bed or sitting with hips well to the back of chair.
2. Make sure the front and back of restraint are positioned appropriately on the patient and that straps are crossed in the front, unless the vest is specifically designed with positioning slot in the back.
3. Secure straps out of patient's reach to the moveable part of a spring bedframe or wheelchair kickspurs. Use quick-release knots.

1. Proper positioning helps prevent injury or falls.
2. Crossing the straps in the back or applying a vest restraint backward may result in serious injury or death.

3. Ensures that adjustment of bed position or siderails will not interfere with restraint. Quick-release knots allow timely intervention in emergency situations.

FOLLOW-UP PHASE

1. Monitor the patient frequently once restraint is applied.

2. Use ancillary staff to sit with and try to calm agitated or restless patients whenever possible, even if restraint has been consented to.
3. Never use restraints on a toilet or commode or in a motor vehicle. Do not send restraint home with patient.

1. Will detect loosening, which may cause injury or restriction caused by the restraint.
2. Studies have shown that use of restraints only contributes to falls.
3. Restraints are specifically designed to be used with hospital beds, wheelchairs, and geriatric chairs, and by those trained in their proper use. Misuse may result in injury.

◆ ADVANCE DIRECTIVES

Based on the ethical principle of autonomy (a person's privilege of self-rule), advance directives provide a clear and detailed expression of a person's wishes for care.

Advance directives may be limited to a single situation, such as a "living will" for the terminally ill, or may address a multitude of different scenarios in detail.

Types of Advance Directives

A. Living Wills
1. Living Wills were the first and most widespread type of advance directive.
2. They were proposed as a mechanism for refusing "heroic" or unwanted medical intervention for the dying person.
3. They allow a person to state in writing that certain life-sustaining treatments should be withdrawn or withheld when that person is dying and unable to directly communicate his or her wishes.
4. The Living Will only allows for the refusal of further treatment. They are not precise in terms of directives, and focus only on the patient who is clearly terminally ill.

B. Durable Power of Attorney for Health Care (DPOA-HC)
1. This document appoints a person to act on behalf of another person, provides guidance for the proxy, and endures even when the maker is incapacitated.

2. The DPOA-HC is always a written document.
3. The document states the preferences and perhaps even the values of its maker. It outlines the types of decisions the person would want to have made on his or her behalf.
4. Because no DPOA-HC can cover all situations, the document should name a person who has the task of ensuring that the patient's wishes are honored. The proxy has the responsibility to interpret the DPOA-HC and extrapolate its contents to situations not specifically covered.

Nursing/Patient Care Considerations

1. Under the Patient Self-Determination Act, all patients who enter a Medicare- or Medicaid-certified hospital, nursing home or home health agency must:

a. Be provided with information about the state's laws and the facility's policies regarding advance directive.
b. Be asked if they have advance directives.
c. Have their advance directives placed in their medical record.

2. Education of patients and families is essential in helping them to understand the difference between Living Wills or DPOA-HC, and determining which document best suits their needs.
3. Patients and families need to be educated regarding what is involved in undergoing various life-sustaining procedures so they can make a decision regarding their future treatment.
4. Patients need to be informed that they can have more than one advance directive. That is, if a patient has a Living Will, but is not terminally ill, they need to be encouraged to obtain a DPOA-HC to ensure their health care wishes will be met in any situation.

Selected References

Carlson, R. (1991). Dysphagia: Causes and treatments in the elderly. *Geriatric Consultant, 2,* 20-24.

Frantz, R. & Gardner, S. (1994). Clinical concerns: management of dry skin. *J. Gerontol Nurs, 20 (9),* 15-19.

Geriatric Monograph 148 (1991). Kansas City, MO: American Academy of Family Physicians.

Ginter, S., & Mion, L. (1992). Falls in the nursing home: Preventable or inevitable? *J Gerontol Nurs, 18*(11), 43-49.

Goldstein, M., Hawthorne, M., Engeberg, S., McDowell, J., Burgio, K. (1992). Urinary incontinence: Why people do not seek help. *J Gerontol Nurs, 18*(4), 15-21.

MacKay, S. (1992). Durable power of attorney for health care. *Geriatric Nursing, 13*(2), 99-110.

Madson, S. (1993). Patient self-determination act: Implications for long-term care. *J Gerontol Nurs, 19*(21), 15-19.

Mahoney, F., & Barthel, D. (1965). Functional evaluation: The Barthel Index. *Maryland State Med J, 14,* 62-72.

Miller, C. (1990). *Nursing care of older adults: Theory and practice.* Glenview, IL: Scott, Foresman and Company.

Ouslander, J., Osterweil, D, & Morley, J. (1991). *Medical care in the nursing home.* New York: McGraw-Hill.

Resnick, B. (1993). Retraining the bladder after catheterization. *Am J Nurs, 93*(11), 46-50.

Resnick, B. (1993). Wound care for the elderly. *Geriatric Nursing, 14*(1), 26-28.

Resnick, B. (1991). Geriatric motivation: Clinically helping the elderly to comply. *J Gerontol Nurs, 17*(5), 17-21.

Stolley, J. (1995). Freeing your patients from restraints. *RN, 95*(2), 26-30.

Strumpf, N., Evan, L., Wagner, J., Patterson, J. (1992). Reducing physical restraints: Developing an educational program. *J Gerontol Nurs, 18*(11), 21-28.

Wolfe, S., & Schirm, V. (1992). Medication counseling for the elderly: Effects on knowledge and compliance after hospital discharge. *Geriatric Nursing, 13*(3), 134-139.

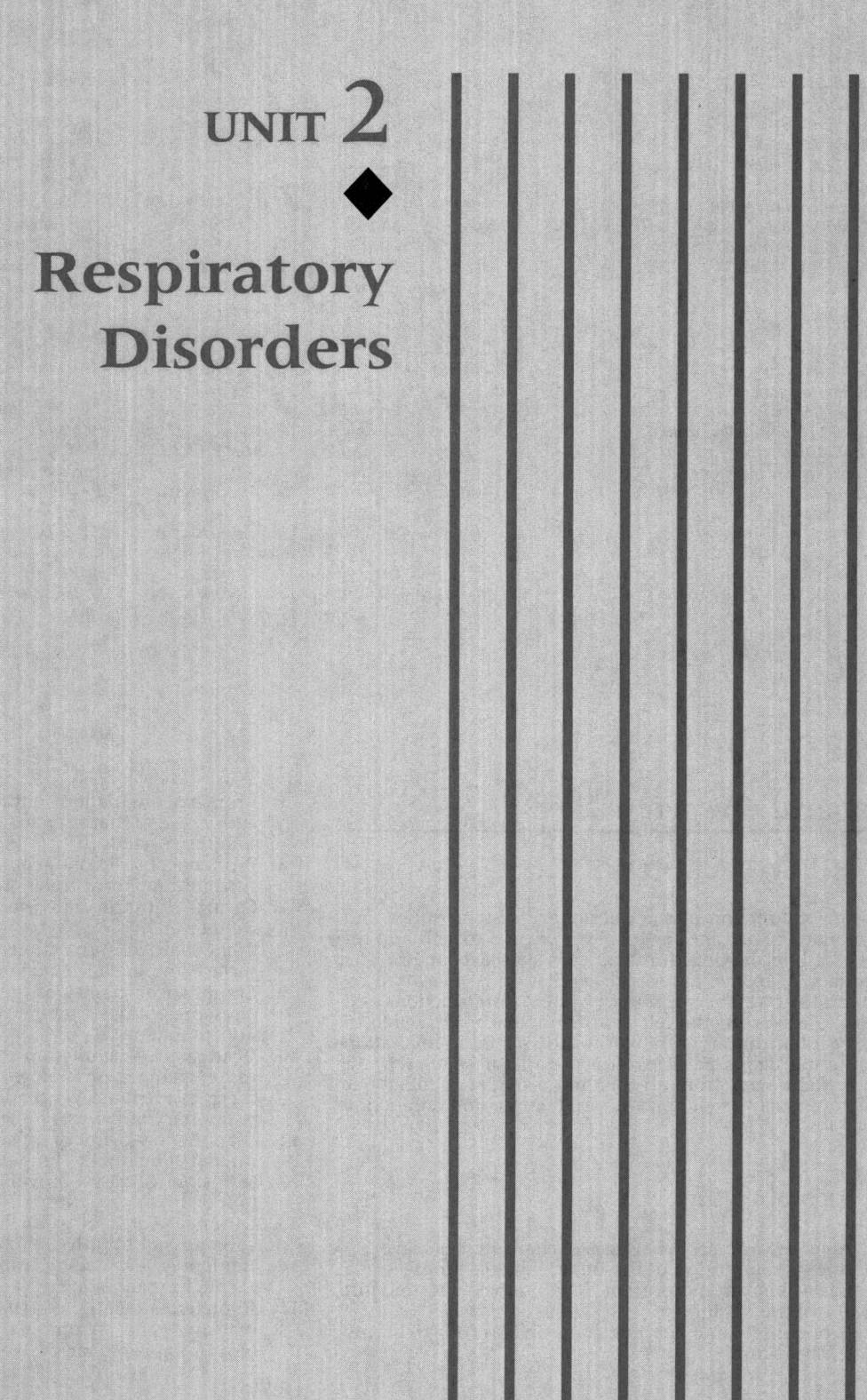

UNIT 2

◆

Respiratory
Disorders

CHAPTER 8

Respiratory Function and Therapy

General Overview

◆ RESPIRATORY FUNCTION

The major function of the pulmonary system (lungs and pulmonary circulation) is to deliver oxygen to cells and remove carbon dioxide from the cells (gas exchange). The adequacy of oxygenation and ventilation is measured by Pao_2 and $Paco_2$. The pulmonary system also functions as a blood reservoir for the left ventricle when it is needed to boost cardiac output; protector for the systemic circulation by filtering debris/particles; fluid regulator so that water can be kept away from alveoli; and provider of metabolic functions such as surfactant production and endocrine functions.

Terminology

1. Alveolus—air sac where gas exchange takes place
2. Apex—top portion of the upper lobes of lungs
3. Base—bottom portion of lower lobes, located just above the diaphragm
4. Bronchus—large airways; lung divides into right and left bronchi

5. Bronchial circulation (pulmonary circulation)—circulatory system that supplies oxygenated blood to the respiratory system
6. Bronchoconstriction—constriction of smooth muscle surrounding bronchioles
7. Carina—location of division of the right and left mainstem bronchi
8. Cilia—hairlike projections on the tracheobronchial surface lining, which aid in the movement of secretions
9. Compliance—ability of the lungs to distend (eg, emphysema—lungs very compliant; fibrosis—lungs noncompliant)
10. Dead space—ventilation that does not participate in gas exchange; physiologic dead space occurs when there is adequate ventilation but no perfusion, as in pulmonary embolus
11. Diaphragm—primary muscle used for respiration (located just below the lung bases)
12. Diffusion (of gas)—movement of gases from a higher to lower concentration
13. Dyspnea—difficulty in breathing; breathlessness; shortness of breath
14. Hemoptysis—bleeding from the lung; main symptom is coughing up blood
15. Hypoxemia—Pao_2 less than normal, which may or may not cause symptoms. Normal Pao_2 is 80 to 100 mm Hg on room air.

16. Hypoxia—insufficient oxygenation at the cellular level due to an imbalance in oxygen delivery and oxygen consumption. Usually causes symptoms reflecting decreased oxygen reaching the brain and heart.
17. Mediastinum—compartment between lungs containing lymph and vascular tissue that separates left from right lung
18. Orthopnea—shortness of breath when in reclining position
19. Paroxysmal nocturnal dyspnea (PND)—shortness of breath with sudden onset; occurs after going to sleep in recumbent position
20. Perfusion—blood flow, carrying oxygen and carbon dioxide, that passes by alveoli
21. Pleura—membrane that covers the outside of the lung (visceral pleura) and lines the thorax (parietal pleura) that creates a potential space
22. Respiration—gas exchange from air to blood and blood to body cells
23. Shunt—adequate perfusion without ventilation, as in pulmonary edema, atelectasis, chronic obstructive pulmonary disease (COPD)
24. Surfactant—substance released by cells within the lung; maintains surface tension and keeps alveoli open allowing for better gas exchange
25. Ventilation—movement of air (gases) in and out of the lungs
26. Ventilation–Perfusion (V/Q) imbalance—mismatch of ventilation and perfusion; is a cause for hypoxemia. V/Q mismatch can be due to:
    a. Blood perfusing an area of the lung where ventilation is reduced or absent
    b. Excessive amount of blood flow for the amount of ventilation present

Assessment

◆ SUBJECTIVE DATA

Explore the patient's symptoms through characterization and history taking to help anticipate needs and plan care.

Dyspnea

1. Characteristics—Is the dyspnea acute or chronic? Has it come about suddenly or gradually? Is more than one pillow required to sleep? Is the dyspnea progressive, recurrent, or paroxysmal? Walking how far leads to shortness of breath?
2. Associated factors—Is there a cough associated with the dyspnea and is it productive? What activities precipitate the shortness of breath? Does it seem to be worse when upset? Is it influenced by the time of day or seasons? Does it occur at rest or with exertion? Any fever, chills, night sweats? Any change in body weight?
3. History—Is there a family history or patient history of chronic lung disease? What is the smoking history?
4. Significance—Sudden dyspnea could indicate pulmonary embolus, pneumothorax, myocardial infarction, acute ventricular failure, or acute respiratory failure. In a postsurgical or postpartum patient, dyspnea may indicate pulmonary embolus or edema. Orthopnea can

be indicative of heart disease or COPD. If dyspnea is associated with a wheeze, consider asthma or COPD.

Chest Pain

1. Characteristics—Is the pain sharp, dull, stabbing or aching? Is it intermittent or persistent? Is the pain localized or does it radiate? If it radiates, where? How intense is the pain?
2. Associated factors—What effect do inspiration and expiration have on the pain? What factors seem to precipitate the pain?
3. History—Is there a smoking history or environmental exposure? Has the pain ever been experienced before? What was the cause? Is there a preexisting pulmonary or cardiac diagnosis?
4. Significance—Chest pain related to pulmonary causes is usually felt on the side where pathology arises, but it can be referred. Dull persistent pain may indicate carcinoma of the lung; whereas sharp stabbing pain usually arises from the pleura.

Cough

1. Characteristics—Is the cough dry, hacking, brassy, or wheezy? Is it strong or weak?
2. Associated factors—Is the cough productive? If so, what is the consistency, odor, amount and color of the sputum? Is there a particular time or event when coughing begins? Is the onset recent or gradual? Is it associated with food intake?
3. History—Has there been any environmental or occupational exposure to dust, fumes, or gases that could lead to cough? Is there a smoking history? Is the smoking current or in past? Are there past pulmonary diagnoses?
4. Significance—A dry, irritative cough may indicate viral respiratory tract infection. A cough at night should alert to potential left-sided heart failure or asthma. A morning cough with sputum might be bronchitis. A severe or changing cough should be evaluated for bronchogenic carcinoma. Consider bacterial pneumonia if sputum is rusty, and lung tumor if it is pink-tinged. A profuse pink frothy sputum would be indicative of pulmonary edema. A cough associated with food intake could indicate problems with aspiration.

Hemoptysis

1. Characteristics—Is the blood from the lungs? It could be from gastrointestinal system (hematemesis) or upper airway (epistaxis). Is it bright red and frothy? How much?
2. Associated factors—Is onset associated with certain circumstances or activities? Was the onset sudden and is it intermittent or continuous? Was there an initial sensation of tickling in the throat? Was there a salty taste, burning or bubbling sensation in the chest before bleeding?
3. History—Was there any recent chest trauma or respiratory treatment (chest percussion)?
4. Significance—Hemoptysis can be linked to pulmonary infection, lung carcinoma, abnormalities of the heart or blood vessels, pulmonary artery or vein abnormalities, or pulmonary emboli and infarction.

◆ PHYSICAL EXAMINATION

Perform a physical examination of the chest using inspection, palpation, auscultation, and percussion to determine respiratory status and differentiate primary lung problems from cardiac problems.

Key Observations

1. What is the respiratory rate, depth, and pattern? Are accessory muscles being used?
2. Is there central cyanosis indicating possible hypoxemia or cardiac disease?
3. Are the jugular veins distended? Is there peripheral edema or other signs of cardiac dysfunction?
4. Does palpation of the chest cause pain? Is chest excursion symmetric?
5. Are the lung fields clear or are there rhonchi, wheezing or crackles? Are breath sounds equal bilaterally?
6. Examine sputum or hemoptysis if available for amount, color and consistency. Does it have an acidic pH (less than 7) indicating that it is from the stomach and not the lungs?

Diagnostic Tests

◆ LABORATORY STUDIES

Arterial Blood Gas (ABG) Analysis

A. Description
1. A measurement of oxygen, carbon dioxide, as well as the pH of the blood that provides a means of assessing the adequacy of ventilation and oxygenation.
2. Also helps assess the acid–base status of the body—whether acidosis or alkalosis is present and to what degree (compensated or uncompensated).

B. Nursing/Patient Care Considerations
1. Blood can be obtained from any artery but is most often drawn from the radial, brachial, or femoral site. It can be drawn directly by arterial puncture or accessed by way of indwelling arterial catheter. (See Procedure Guidelines 8-1.)
2. If the radial artery is used, an Allen's test must be performed before the puncture to determine if collateral circulation is present.
3. Interpret ABGs by looking at the following:
   (P equals pressure)
   a. Pao_2—partial pressure of oxygen in arterial blood (greater than 95 to 100 mm Hg)
   b. $Paco_2$—partial pressure of carbon dioxide in arterial blood (35 to 45 mm Hg)
   c. Sao_2—saturation of oxygen in arterial blood (greater than 95%)
   d. pH–hydrogen ion concentration, or degree of acid–base balance (7.35 to 7.45)

Sputum Examination

A. Description
1. Sputum is obtained for evaluation of gross appearance, microscopic examination, Gram's stain, culture, and cytology.

a. The direct smear shows presence of white blood cells and intracellular (pathogenic) bacteria and extracellular (mostly nonpathogenic) bacteria.
b. The sputum culture is used to make diagnosis, determine drug sensitivity, and serve as a guide for drug treatment (ie, choice of antibiotic).
c. Cytology (exfoliative cytology) is used to identify tumor cells.

B. Nursing/Patient Care Considerations
1. Patients receiving antibiotics, steroids, and immunosuppressive agents for prolonged time may have periodic sputum examinations, because these agents may give rise to opportunistic pulmonary infections.
2. It is important that the sputum be collected correctly and that the specimen be sent to a lab immediately. Allowing it to stand in a warm room will result in overgrowth of organisms, making identification of pathogen difficult; this also alters cell morphology.
3. Sputum can be obtained by various methods:
   a. Deep breathing and coughing
      (1) Obtain early morning specimen—yields best sample of deep pulmonary secretions from all lung fields.
      (2) Have patient clear nose and throat and rinse mouth—to decrease sputum contamination.
      (3) Instruct patient to take several deep breaths, exhale, and perform a series of short coughs.
      (4) Have patient cough deeply and expectorate the sputum into a sterile container.
   b. Ultrasonic and/or heated hypertonic saline nebulization
      (1) Patient inhales through mouth slowly and deeply for 10 to 20 minutes.
      (2) Nebulization increases the moisture content of air going to lower tract; particles will condense on tracheobronchial tree and aid in expectoration.
   c. Trachea suction—aspiration of secretions through endotracheal or tracheostomy tube
   d. Bronchoscopic removal—provides sputum sampling by aspiration of secretions; brushing through a sterile catheter; bronchoalveolar lavage, and transbronchial biopsy
   e. Gastric aspiration (rarely necessary since advent of ultrasonic nebulizer)
      (1) Nasogastric tube is inserted into the stomach to siphon out swallowed pulmonary secretions.
      (2) Useful only for culture of tubercle bacilli, but not for direct examination
   f. Transtracheal aspiration (see Procedure Guidelines 8-2) involves passing a needle and then a catheter through a percutaneous puncture of the cricothyroid membrane. Transtracheal aspiration bypasses the oropharynx and avoids specimen contamination by mouth flora.

Pleural Fluid Analysis

A. Description
1. Pleural fluid is continuously produced and reabsorbed, with a thin layer of fluid normally in the pleural space. Abnormal accumulation of pleural fluid (effusion) occurs in diseases of the pleura, heart, or lymphatics. The pleural fluid is studied, along with other tests, to determine the underlying cause.

2. Obtained by aspiration (thoracentesis) or by tube thoracotomy (chest tube insertion). (See Procedure Guidelines 8-3.)

3. The fluid is examined for cell count, differential, specific gravity, cytology, protein, glucose, pH, LDH, and amylase. Pleural fluid is usually light straw colored.

B. *Nursing/Patient Care Considerations*
1. Observe and record total amount of fluid withdrawn, nature of fluid, and its color and viscosity.
2. Prepare sample of fluid and ensure transport to the laboratory.

PROCEDURE GUIDELINES 8-1 ◆ Assisting with Arterial Puncture for Blood Gas Analysis

EQUIPMENT

Commercially available blood gas kit
or
2- or 3-mL syringe
23- or 25-gauge needle
0.5 mL sodium heparin (1:1,000)

Stopper or cap
Lidocaine
Sterile germicide
Cup or plastic bag with crushed ice
Gloves

PROCEDURE

NURSING ACTION	RATIONALE
PREPARATORY PHASE	
1. Record patient's inspired oxygen concentration.	1. Changes in inspired oxygen concentration alter the change in PaO_2. Degree of hypoxemia cannot be assessed without knowing the inspired oxygen concentration.
2. Take patient's temperature.	2. May be taken into consideration when results are evaluated. Hyperthermia and hypothermia influence oxygen release from hemoglobin.
If not using a commercially available blood gas kit:	3.
3. Heparinize the 2-mL syringe.	
a. Withdraw heparin into the syringe to wet the plunger and fill dead space in the needle.	a. This action coats the interior of the syringe with heparin to prevent blood from clotting.
b. Hold syringe in an upright position and expel excess heparin and air bubbles.	b. Air in the syringe may affect measurement of PaO_2. Heparin in the syringe may affect measurement of the pH.

PERFORMANCE PHASE (BY PHYSICIAN, NURSE, OR RESPIRATORY THERAPIST WITH SPECIAL INSTRUCTION)

NURSING ACTION	RATIONALE
1. Wash hands.	
2. Don gloves.	
3. Palpate the radial, brachial or femoral artery.	3. The radial artery is the preferred site of puncture. Arterial puncture is performed on areas where a good pulse is palpable.
4. If puncturing the radial artery, perform the Allen test.	4. The Allen test is a simple method for assessing collateral circulation in the hand. Ensures circulation if radial artery thrombosis occurs.
IN THE CONSCIOUS PATIENT:	
a. Obliterate the radial and ulnar pulses simultaneously by pressing on both blood vessels at the wrist.	a. Impedes arterial blood flow into the hand.
b. Ask patient to clench and unclench fist until blanching of the skin occurs.	b. Forces blood from the hand.
c. Release pressure on ulnar artery (while still compressing radial artery). Watch for return of skin color within 15 seconds.	c. Documents that ulnar artery alone is capable of supplying blood to the hand, because radial artery is still occluded.

Note: If the ulnar does not have sufficient blood flow to supply the entire hand, another artery should be used.

IN THE UNCONSCIOUS PATIENT:
a. Obliterate the radial and ulnar pulses simultaneously at the wrist.
b. Elevate patient's hand above heart and squeeze or compress hand until blanching occurs.
c. Lower patient's hand while still compressing the radial artery (release pressure on ulnar artery) and watch for return of skin color.

(continued)

PROCEDURE GUIDELINES 8-1 ◆ Assisting with Arterial Puncture for Blood Gas Analysis *(continued)*

PROCEDURE
(cont'd)

NURSING ACTION	RATIONALE
5. For the radial side, place a small towel roll under the patient's wrist.	5. To make the artery more accessible.
6. Feel along the course of the radial artery and palpate for maximum pulsation with the middle and index fingers. Prepare the skin with germicide. The skin and subcutaneous tissues may be infiltrated with a local anesthetic agent (lidocaine).	6. The wrist should be stabilized to allow for better control of the needle.
7. The needle is at a 45- to 60-degree angle to the skin surface (see accompanying figure) and is advanced into the artery. Once the artery is punctured, arterial pressure will push up the hub of the syringe and a pulsating flow of blood will fill the syringe.	7. The arterial pressure will cause the syringe to be filled within a few seconds.

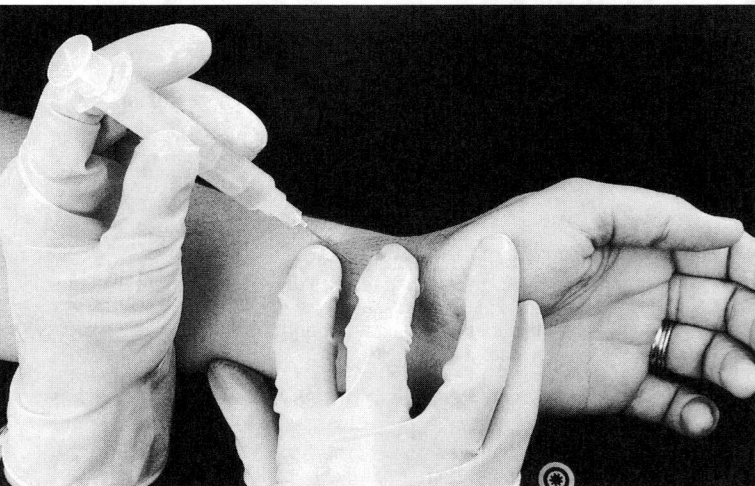

Technique of arterial puncture for blood gas analysis.

NURSING ACTION	RATIONALE
8. After blood is obtained, withdraw needle and apply firm pressure over the puncture with a dry sponge.	8. Significant bleeding can occur because of pressure in the artery.
9. Remove air bubbles from syringe and needle. Insert needle into rubber stopper.	9. Immediate capping of the needle prevents room air from mixing with the blood specimen.
10. Place the capped syringe in the container of ice.	10. Icing the syringe will prevent a clinically significant loss of O_2.
11. Maintain firm pressure on the puncture site for 5 minutes. If the patient is on anticoagulant medication, apply direct pressure over puncture site for 10 to 15 minutes and then apply a firm pressure dressing.	11. Firm pressure on the puncture site prevents further bleeding and hematoma formation.
12. For patients requiring serial monitoring of arterial blood, an arterial catheter (connected to a flush solution of heparinized saline) is inserted into the radial or femoral artery.	12. All connections must be tight to avoid disconnection and rapid blood loss. The arterial line also allows for direct blood pressure monitoring in the critically ill patient.

FOLLOW-UP PHASE

NURSING ACTION	RATIONALE
1. Send labeled, iced specimen to the laboratory immediately.	1. Blood gas analysis should be done as soon as possible, because PaO_2 and pH can change rapidly.
2. Palpate the pulse (distal to the puncture site), inspect the puncture site, and assess for cold hand, numbness, tingling, or discoloration.	2. Hematoma and arterial thrombosis are complications following this procedure.
3. Change ventilator settings, inspired oxygen concentration or type and setting of respiratory therapy equipment if indicated by the results.	3. The PaO_2 results will determine whether to maintain, increase, or decrease the F_1O_2. The PaO_2 and pH results will detect if any changes are needed in tidal volume or rate of patient's ventilator.

PROCEDURE GUIDELINES 8-2 ◆ Assisting With Transtracheal Aspiration

EQUIPMENT
Sterile transtracheal set:
 No. 14, No. 16, and No. 18 gauge needles
 Polyethylene catheter
 Syringe
 Skin preparation solutions
 Local anesthetic
 Sterile gloves; mask
 Specimen containers

Atropine
ECG monitoring equipment
Endotracheal tube
Suction apparatus with catheters
Cardiac resuscitation equipment

PROCEDURE

NURSING ACTION	RATIONALE

PREPARATORY PHASE

1. Explain the procedure and give reassurance by skilled and empathetic attention to the patient's needs. Instruct the patient to breathe quietly and to remain still.
2. Administer supplemental oxygen, as directed, during the procedure if the patient's arterial oxygen tension is below normal while the patient is breathing room air.
3. Extend the patient's neck and place a pillow under shoulders.

1. Inform the patient that the procedure will cause coughing and that there will be an unpleasant sensation of a foreign body in the lower airway.
2. This prevents worsening of hypoxemia.

3. This is the optimum position for cricothyroid puncture.

PERFORMANCE PHASE

The cricothyroid membrane is identified by palpation.

1. The skin over the cricothyroid area is cleansed and the area is infiltrated with local anesthetic.

2. A No. 14, 16, or 18 gauge needle is inserted through the cricothyroid membrane into the trachea, and a polyethylene catheter is threaded through the needle into the lower trachea. Caution the patient against swallowing or talking while the needle is introduced through the cricothyroid membrane.
3. The needle is withdrawn, leaving the catheter in place.

1. The cricothyroid membrane is less vascular and offers more safety in preventing posterior wall puncture than other areas.

3. The catheter's passage usually stimulates vigorous coughing.

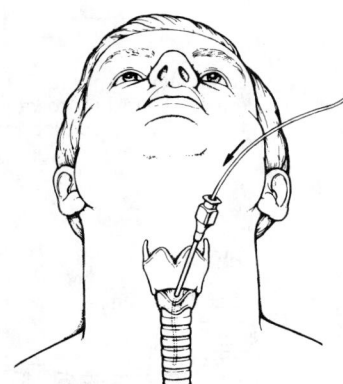

Transtracheal aspiration. After the catheter is positioned into the trachea, the needle is withdrawn leaving the catheter in place.

(continued)

PROCEDURE GUIDELINES 8-2 ◆ Assisting With Transtracheal Aspiration

(continued)

PROCEDURE (cont'd)	NURSING ACTION	RATIONALE

4. A syringe is attached to the catheter and secretions may be aspirated back into the syringe as the patient coughs. Request the patient to turn head while coughing.

4. Sterile saline (2 to 5 mL) may be injected into catheter to induce coughing, if necessary.

5. Air is removed from the syringe, and the syringe is capped or the sample is injected into an anaerobic transfer vial. The specimen is sent to the laboratory for immediate processing.

5. This ensures anaerobic conditions. Cytologic, mycobacterial, and other studies are carried out.

6. The catheter is withdrawn, and pressure is applied over the puncture site.

6. Gentle firm pressure over the site for about 5 minutes helps prevent bleeding and reduces subcutaneous emphysema.

FOLLOW-UP PHASE

1. Instruct the patient to rest quietly for about an hour.
2. Observe for the following complications: local bleeding, puncture of posterior tracheal wall, subcutaneous emphysema, vasovagal reactions, cardiac dysrhythmias.

2. Assess for hoarseness after the procedure; this may be from a submucosal tracheal hematoma, which can cause suffocation. Inform the patient that minor blood streaking of sputum almost always occurs after this procedure.

PROCEDURE GUIDELINES 8-3 ◆ Assisting the Patient Undergoing Thoracentesis

EQUIPMENT		

Thoracentesis tray (if available)
  or
Syringes: 5-, 20-, 50-mL
Needles: No. 22, No. 26, No. 16 (7.5 cm long)
Three-way stopcock and tubing
Hemostat
Biopsy needle

Germicide solution
Local anesthetic (eg, lidocaine 1%)
Sterile gauze sponges (4 × 4 and 2 × 2)
Sterile towels and drape
Sterile specimen containers
Sterile gloves

PROCEDURE	NURSING ACTION	RATIONALE

PREPARATORY PHASE

1. Ascertain in advance if chest x-ray and/or other tests have been prescribed and completed. These should be available at the bedside.

1. Localization of pleural fluid is accomplished by physical examination, chest roentgenogram, ultrasound localization, or fluoroscopic localization.

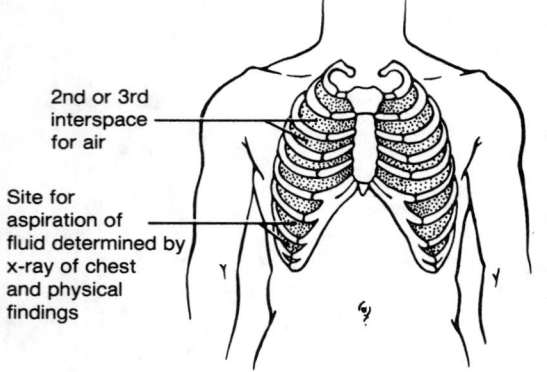

2nd or 3rd interspace for air

Site for aspiration of fluid determined by x-ray of chest and physical findings

Technique of thoracentesis.

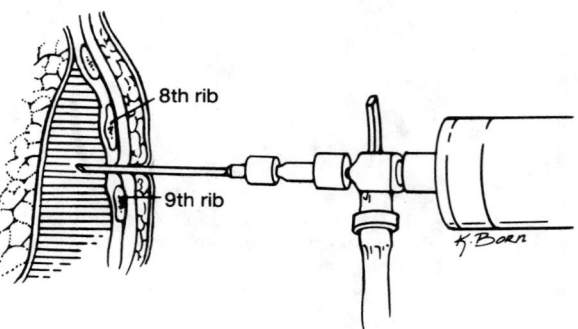

8th rib

9th rib

Site of insertion, and the needle/catheter in the pleural space

PROCEDURES (cont'd)	NURSING ACTION	RATIONALE

NURSING ACTION

2. See if consent form has been explained and signed.
3. Determine if the patient is allergic to the local anesthetic agent to be used. Give sedation if prescribed.
4. Inform the patient about the procedure and indicate how he or she can be helpful. Explain:
   a. The nature of the procedure.
   b. The importance of remaining immobile.
   c. Pressure sensations to be experienced.
   d. That no discomfort is anticipated after the procedure.
5. Make the patient comfortable with adequate supports. If possible, place upright (see accompanying figure) and help patient maintain position during procedure.

RATIONALE

4. An explanation helps orient the patient to the procedure, assists with coping and provides an opportunity to ask questions and verbalize anxiety.

5. The upright position ensures that the diaphragm is most dependent and facilitates the removal of fluid that usually localizes at the base of the chest. A comfortable position helps the patient to relax.

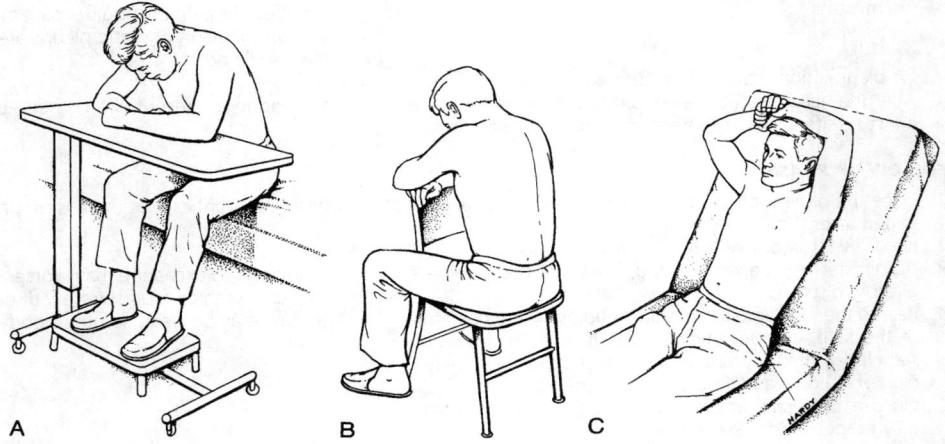

Positioning the patient for a thoracentesis. The nurse assists the patient to one of three positions, and offers comfort and support throughout the procedure. (**A**) Sitting on the edge of the bed with head and arms on and over the bed table. (**B**) Straddling a chair with arms and head resting on the back of the chair. (**C**) Lying on unaffected side with the bed elevated 30 to 45 degrees. (Suddarth, D. S. (1991). The Lippincott manual of nursing practice (5th ed.). Philadelphia: JB Lippincott.

6. Support and reassure the patient during the procedure.
   a. Prepare the patient for sensations of cold from skin germicide and for pressure and sting from infiltration of local anesthetic agent.
   b. Encourage the patient to refrain from coughing.
   c. Be prepared to monitor patient's condition throughout the procedure.

6. Sudden and unexpected movement by the patient can cause trauma to the visceral pleura with resultant trauma to the lung. A local anesthetic inhibits nerve conduction and is used to prevent pain during the procedure.

PERFORMANCE PHASE

1. The site for aspiration is determined from chest x-rays, by percussion, or by fluoroscopic or ultrasound localization. If fluid is in the pleural cavity, the thoracentesis site is determined by study of the chest x-ray and physical findings, with attention to the site of maximal dullness on percussion.
2. The procedure is done under aseptic conditions. After the skin is cleansed, the healthcare provider slowly injects a local anesthetic with a small-caliber needle into the intercostal space.

1. If air is in the pleural cavity, the thoracentesis site is usually in the 2nd or 3rd intercostal space in the midclavicular line. Air rises in the thorax because the density of air is much less than the density of liquid.

2. An intradermal wheal is raised slowly; rapid intradermal injection causes pain. The parietal pleura is very sensitive and should be well infiltrated with anesthetic before the thoracentesis needle is passed through it.

(continued)

PROCEDURE GUIDELINES 8-3 ◆ Assisting the Patient Undergoing Thoracentesis (continued)

PROCEDURES (cont'd)	NURSING ACTION	RATIONALE

3. The thoracentesis needle is advanced with the syringe attached. When the pleural space is reached, suction may be applied with the syringe.
   a. A 20-mL or 50-mL syringe with a three-way adapter (stopcock) is attached to the needle. (One end of the adapter is attached to the needle and the other to the tubing leading to a receptacle that receives the fluid being aspirated.)

   b. If a considerable quantity of fluid is to be removed, the needle is held in place on the chest wall with a small hemostat.

   c. A pleural biopsy may be performed.
4. After the needle is withdrawn, pressure is applied over the puncture site and a small sterile dressing is fixed in place.

a. When a larger quantity of fluid is withdrawn, a three-way adapter serves to keep air from entering the pleural cavity. The amount of fluid removed depends on clinical status of the patient and absence of complications during the procedure.

b. The hemostat steadies the needle on the chest wall and prevents too deep a penetration of pleural space. Sudden pleuritic pain or shoulder pain may indicate that the visceral or diaphragmatic pleura are being irritated by the needle point.

4. This is done to prevent air entry into pleural space.

FOLLOW-UP PHASE

1. Place the patient on bedrest. A chest x-ray is usually obtained after thoracentesis.
2. Record vital signs every 15 minutes for 1 hour.
3. Administer oxygen, as directed, if patient has cardiorespiratory disease.
4. Record the total amount of fluid withdrawn and the nature of the fluid, its color and viscosity. If prescribed, prepare samples of fluid for laboratory evaluation (usually bacteriology, cell count and differential, determinations of protein, glucose, LDH, specific gravity). A small amount of heparin may be needed for several of the specimen containers to prevent coagulation. A specimen container with preservative may be needed if a pleural biopsy is to obtained.
5. Evaluate the patient at intervals for increasing respirations, faintness, vertigo, tightness in the chest, uncontrollable cough, blood-tinged mucus, and rapid pulse and signs of hypoxemia.

1. Chest x-ray verifies that there is no pneumothorax.

3. Pulmonary gas exchange may worsen after thoracentesis in patients with cardiorespiratory disease.
4. The fluid may be clear, serous, bloody, or purulent.

5. Pneumothorax, tension pneumothorax, hemothorax, subcutaneous emphysema, or pyogenic infection may result from a thoracentesis.

◆ RADIOLOGY/IMAGING

Chest X-Ray (Roentgenogram)

A. Description
1. Normal pulmonary tissue is radiolucent and appears black on film. Thus, densities produced by tumors, foreign bodies, infiltrates, and so forth can be detected as lighter or white images.
2. This test shows the position of normal structures, displacement, and presence of abnormal shadows. It may reveal pathology in the lungs in the absence of symptoms.

B. Nursing/Patient Care Considerations
1. Should be taken upright if patient's condition permits. Assist technician at bedside in preparing patient for portable chest x-ray.
2. Encourage patient to take deep breath and hold breath as x-ray is taken.

3. Ensure that all jewelry or metal objects in x-ray field are removed so as not to interfere with film.

Computerized Axial Tomography (CAT, CT)

A. Description
1. An imaging method in which the lungs are scanned in successive layers by a narrow x-ray beam. A computer printout is obtained of the absorption values of the tissues in the plane that is being scanned.
2. It may be used to define pulmonary nodules or to demonstrate mediastinal abnormalities and hilar adenopathy.

B. Nursing/Patient Care Considerations
1. Describe test to patient/family and ensure consent is obtained (if required by your institution). Test takes about 30 minutes.
2. Be alert to any allergies to iodine or contrast dye that might be used during testing.

Magnetic Resonance Imaging (MRI)

A. Description
1. A type of emission tomography based on magnetizing patient tissue, generating a weak electromagnetic signal, and mapping that signal for visualization.
2. Provides contrast between various soft tissues, and contrast media not necessary.
3. It is helpful to synchronize the MRI image to the electrocardiogram in thoracic studies.

B. Nursing/Patient Care Considerations
1. Explain procedure to patient and assess ability to remain still in a closed space; sedation may be necessary.
2. Evaluate patient for magnetic implants such as pacemakers, prosthetic valves, or joints, which preclude the use of MRI.
3. Check with MRI technician about the use of equipment such as respirator or mechanical intravenous (IV) pump in MRI room.
4. Evaluate the patient for claustrophobia and teach relaxation techniques to use during test. Sedation may be necessary.

Pulmonary Angiography

A. Description
1. An imaging method used to study the pulmonary vessels and the pulmonary circulation.
2. For visualization, radiopaque medium is injected by way of a catheter in the main pulmonary artery rapidly into the vasculature of the lungs. Films are then taken in rapid succession after injection.
3. Is considered the "gold standard" for diagnosis of pulmonary embolus.

B. Nursing/Patient Care Considerations
1. Instruct patient that injection of dye may cause flushing, cough, and a warm sensation.
2. After the procedure, make sure pressure is maintained over access site and monitor pulse rate, blood pressure, and circulation distal to the injection site.

Ventilation–Perfusion (V/Q) Scan

A. Description
1. Radioisotope imaging of ventilation and blood flow to the lungs. The scintillation camera may be interfaced to a computer to record, collate, and refine date.
2. Perfusion scan is done after injection of a radioactive isotope.
   a. Measures blood perfusion through the lungs; evaluates lung function on a regional basis.
   b. Useful in perfusion (vascular) abnormalities such as pulmonary embolism.
3. Ventilation scan is done after inhalation of radioactive gas (xenon, krypton), which diffuses throughout the lungs.
   a. Useful in detecting ventilation abnormalities such as emphysema.

B. Nursing/Patient Care Considerations Explain the procedure to the patient and encourage cooperation with inhalation and brief episodes of breath holding.

◆ OTHER DIAGNOSTIC TESTS

Bronchoscopy

A. Description
1. The direct inspection and observation of the larynx, trachea, and bronchi through flexible or rigid bronchoscope.
   a. Flexible fiberoptic bronchoscope allows for more patient comfort and better visualization of smaller airways.
   b. Rigid bronchoscopy is preferred for small children and endobronchial tumor resection.
2. Has both diagnostic and therapeutic uses in pulmonary conditions. Diagnostic uses include:
   a. Collecting secretions for cytologic/bacteriologic studies.
   b. Determining location and extent of pathologic process and to obtain tissue or brush biopsy for cytologic examination or culture.
   c. Determining whether a tumor can be resected surgically.
   d. Diagnosing bleeding sites (source of hemoptysis).
3. Therapeutic uses include removal of foreign bodies or thickened secretions from tracheobronchial tree and the excision of lesions.

B. Nursing/Patient Care Considerations
1. See that an informed consent form has been signed.
2. Administer prescribed medication to reduce secretions, block the vasovagal reflex, and relieve anxiety. Give encouragement and nursing support.
3. Restrict fluid and food for 6 to 12 hours before procedure (to reduce risk of aspiration when reflexes are blocked).
4. Remove dentures, contact lenses, and other prostheses.
5. After the procedure:
   a. Monitor cardiac rhythm.
   b. Withhold cracked ice/fluids until patient demonstrates gag reflex.
   c. Monitor respiratory effort.
   d. Consider monitoring oximetry.
6. Report cyanosis, hypotension, tachycardia or dysrhythmia, hemoptysis, dyspnea, decreased breath sounds.

NURSING ALERT:
After bronchoscopy, be alert for complications: pneumothorax, dysrhythmias, and bronchospasm.

Lung Biopsy

A. Description
1. Procedures used for obtaining histologic material from the lung to aid in diagnosis. These include:
   a. Transbronchoscopic biopsy—biopsy forceps inserted through bronchoscope and specimen of lung tissue obtained.
   b. Transthoracic needle aspiration biopsy—specimen obtained through needle aspiration under fluoroscopic guidance.
   c. Open lung biopsy—specimen obtained through small anterior thoracotomy; used in making a diagnosis when other biopsy methods have not been effective or are not possible.

B. Nursing/Patient Care Considerations
1. Obtain permit for consent, if required.
2. Observe for possible complications including pneumothorax, hemorrhage (hemoptysis), and bacterial contamination of pleural space.
3. See bronchoscopy (above) or thoracic surgery (p. 201) for postprocedure care.

Pulmonary Function Tests (PFTs)

A. Description
1. Used to detect and measure abnormalities in respiratory function. Such tests include measurements of lung volumes, ventilatory function, diffusing capacity, gas exchange, lung compliance, airway resistance, and distribution of gases in the lung.
2. Ventilatory studies (spirometry) is the most common group of tests.
   a. Requires water spirometer, electronic spirometer, or wedge spirometer that plots volume against time (timed vital capacity).
   b. Patient is asked to take as deep a breath as possible and then to exhale into spirometer as completely and as forcefully as possible.
   c. Results are compared with normals for patient's age, height, and sex (Table 8-1).
   d. A reduction in the vital capacity alone may indicate a restrictive form of lung disease (disease due to increased lung stiffness).
   e. A reduction in several parameters usually indicates an obstructive flow due to bronchial obstruction or loss of lung elastic recoil.
3. Lung volumes are determined by asking the patient to inhale known concentration of inert gas such as helium or 100% oxygen and measuring concentration of

inert gas or nitrogen in exhaled air (dilution method) or by plethysmography.
   a. Yields thoracic volume (total lung capacity, plus any unventilated blebs or bullae).
   b. An increased residual volume is found in air-trapping due to obstructive lung disease.
   c. A reduction in several parameters usually indicates a restrictive form of lung disease or chest wall abnormality.
4. Diffusing capacity measures lung surface effective for the transfer of gas in the lung by having patient inhale gas containing known low concentration of carbon monoxide and measuring carbon monoxide concentration in exhaled air. Difference between inhaled and exhaled concentrations is related directly to uptake of carbon monoxide across alveolar–capillary membrane.
   a. Is reduced in parenchymal lung disease, possibly in severe anemia, and in some forms of heart disease.

B. Nursing/Patient Care Considerations Instruct patient in correct technique for completing PFTs; coach patient through test, if needed.

Pulse Oximetry

A. Description
1. Oximeters function by passing a light beam through a vascular bed, such as the finger or earlobe to determine the amount of light absorbed by oxygenated (red) and deoxygenated (blue) blood.
2. Calculates the amount of arterial blood that is saturated with oxygen (SaO_2) and displays this as a digital value.
3. Indications include:
   a. Unstable patient who may experience sudden changes in blood oxygen level.

TABLE 8-1 Pulmonary Function Tests

Term	Symbol	Description	Remarks
Vital capacity	VC	Maximum volume of air exhaled after a maximum inspiration	VC < 10–15 mL/kg suggests need for mechanical ventilation VC > 10-15 mL/kg suggests ability to wean
Forced vital capacity	FVC	Vital capacity performed with a maximally forced expiratory effort	Reduced in obstructive disease (COPD) due to air trapping Reflects airflow in large airways
Forced expiratory volume in 1 second	FEV_1	Volume of air exhaled in the first second of the performance of a FVC	Reduced in obstructive disease (COPD) due to air trapping Reflects airflow in larger airways
Ratio of FEV_1/FVC	FEV_1/FVC	FEV_1 expressed as a percentage of the FVC	Decreased in obstructive disease Normal in restrictive disease
Forced midexpiratory flow	$FEF_{25\%-75\%}$	Average flow during the middle half of the FVC	Reflects airflow in small airways Smokers may have change in this test before other symptoms develop
Peak expiratory flow rate	PEFR	Most rapid flow during a forced expiration after a maximum inspiration	Used to measure response to bronchodilators, airflow obstruction in patients with asthma
Maximal voluntary ventilation	MVV	Volume of air expired in a specified period (12 seconds) during repetitive maximal effort	An important factor in exercise tolerance

b. Evaluation of need for home oxygen therapy.
c. Need to follow the trend but need to decrease number of ABGs drawn.
4. The oxyhemoglobin dissociation curve allows for correlation between SaO_2 and PaO_2 (Fig. 8-1).
   a. Increased body temperature, acidosis and increased 2,3,DPG cause a shift in the curve to the right, thus increasing the ability of hemoglobin to release oxygen to the tissues.
   b. Decreased temperature, decreased 2,3,DPG and alkalosis cause a shift to the left, causing hemoglobin to hold on to the oxygen, reducing the amount of oxygen being released to the tissues.
5. Increased bilirubin, increased carboxyhemoglobin, low perfusion or $SaO_2 < 80\%$ may alter light absorption and interfere with results.

NURSING ALERT:
If the SaO_2 drops below 80%, the reading displayed by the oximeter may vary by ±2% from the actual SaO_2. Oximeters rely on differences in light absorption to determine SaO_2. At lower saturations, oxygenated hemoglobin appears more blue in color and is less easily distinguished from deoxygenated hemoglobin. ABG should be used in this situation.

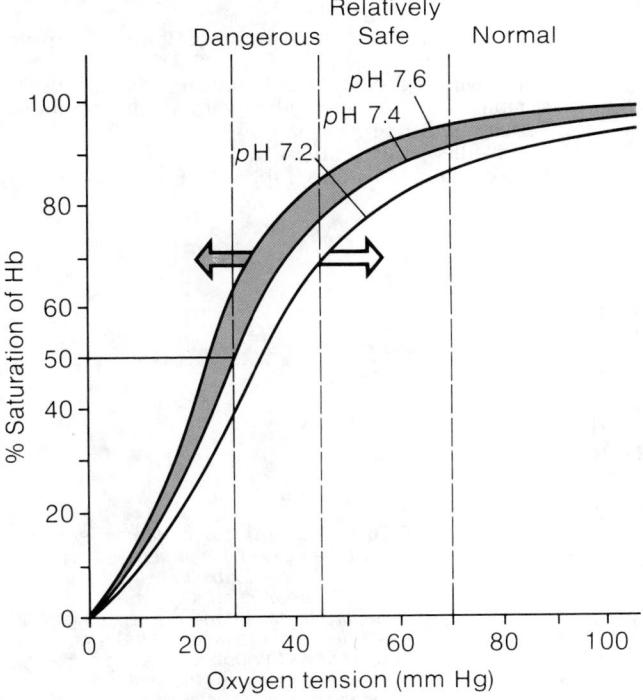

FIGURE 8-1 *Oxygen-hemoglobin dissociation curve. The oxygen can attach to the hemoglobin more easily (higher SaO_2 per PO_2) but has more trouble coming off the hemoglobin at the tissues (less tissue oxygenation). Decreased oxygen affinity (shift to the right) means that it is more difficult for the oxygen to attach to the hemoglobin (lower SaO_2 per PO_2), but it can come off at the tissues more easily. P_{50} is normally 27 mmHg. A shift to the right gives a higher P_{50}, and a shift to the left gives a lower P_{50}.*

B. *Nursing/Patient Care Considerations*
1. Assess patient's hemoglobin. (SaO_2 may not correlate well with PaO_2 if hemoglobin is not within normal limits.)
2. Remove patient's nail polish because it can affect the ability of the sensor to correctly determine oxygen saturation.
3. Correlate oximetry with ABG and then use for single reading or trending of oxygenation (does not monitor $PaCO_2$).
4. Assess site of oximetry monitoring for perfusion and rotate sensor sites on regular basis.

Capnography

A. *Description*
1. Used to determine and monitor end-tidal CO_2 ($EtCO_2$)—the amount of carbon dioxide that is expired with each breath.
2. The $EtCO_2$ is displayed as a capnogram (a waveform and numeric reading).
3. Correlates well with $PaCO_2$.
4. Being increasingly used in the critical care setting, and as a pocket-sized model in the emergency department.

B. *Nursing/Patient Care Considerations*
1. Draw ABGs initially to correlate $EtCO_2$ with $PaCO_2$.
2. Does not evaluate pH or oxygenation.
3. Effective for confirming endotracheal tube placement and for monitoring CO_2 in patients who tend to retain CO_2 (COPD).

General Procedures/Treatment Modalities

◆ ARTIFICIAL AIRWAY MANAGEMENT

Airway management may be indicated in patients with loss of consciousness, facial or oral trauma, copious respiratory secretions, respiratory distress, and the need for mechanical ventilation.

Types of Airways

1. Oropharyngeal airway—curved plastic device inserted through the mouth and positioned in the posterior pharynx to move tongue away from palate and open the airway.
   a. Usually for short-term use in the unconscious patient, or may be used along with an oral endotracheal tube.
   b. Not used if recent oral trauma, surgery, or loose teeth are present.
   c. Does not protect against aspiration.

NURSING ALERT:
Position patient on side and suction oral cavity frequently to prevent aspiration of oral secretions or vomitus when an oral airway is in place.

2. Nasopharyngeal airway—soft rubber or plastic tube inserted through nose into posterior pharynx.
   a. Facilitates frequent nasopharyngeal suctioning.
   b. Use extreme caution with patients on anticoagulants or bleeding disorders.
   c. Select size that is slightly smaller than diameter of nostril and slightly longer than distance from tip of nose to earlobe.
   d. Check nasal mucous membranes for irritation or ulceration, and clean airway with hydrogen peroxide and water.

> **NURSING ALERT:**
> Nasopharyngeal airways may obstruct sinus drainage and produce acute sinusitis. Be alert to fever and signs of pain.

3. Endotracheal tube—flexible tube inserted through the mouth or nose and into the trachea beyond the vocal cords that acts as an artificial airway.
   a. Allows for deep tracheal suction and removal of secretions.
   b. Permits mechanical ventilation.
   c. Seals off trachea so aspiration from the gastrointestinal (GI) tract cannot occur.
   d. Can be easily inserted in an emergency, but maintaining placement is more difficult so not for long-term use.
4. Tracheostomy tube—firm, curved artificial airway inserted directly into the trachea at the level of the second or third tracheal ring through a surgically made incision.
   a. Permits mechanical ventilation and facilitates secretion removal.
   b. Can be for long-term use.
   c. Bypasses upper airway defenses, increasing susceptibility to infection.

Endotracheal Tube Insertion

1. Orotracheal insertion is technically easier, because it is done under direct visualization. (See Procedure Guidelines 8-4.)
   a. Disadvantages are increased oral secretions, decreased patient comfort, difficulty with tube stabilization, and inability of patient to use lip movement as a communication means.
2. Nasotracheal insertion may be more comfortable to the patient and is easier to stabilize.
   a. Disadvantages are that blind insertion is required; possible development of pressure necrosis of the nasal airway, sinusitis, and otitis media.
3. Tube types vary according to length and inner diameter, type of cuff, and number of lumens.
   a. Usual sizes for adults are 6.0, 7.0, 8.0 and 9.0 mm.
   b. Most cuffs are high volume, low pressure, with self-sealing inflation valves; or the cuff may be of foam rubber (Fome-Cuff).
   c. Most tubes have a single lumen, however dual-lumen tubes may be used to ventilate each lung independently (Fig. 8-2).
4. May be contraindicated when glottis is obscured by vomitus, bleeding, foreign body, or trauma, or cervical spine injury or deformity.

Tracheostomy Tube Insertion

1. Tube types vary according to presence of inner cannula and presence and type of cuff (Fig. 8-3).
   a. Tubes with high-volume, low-pressure cuffs with self-sealing inflation valves; with or without inner cannula.
   b. Fenestrated tube.
   c. Foam-filled cuffs (Fome-Cuff).
   d. Speaking tracheostomy tube.

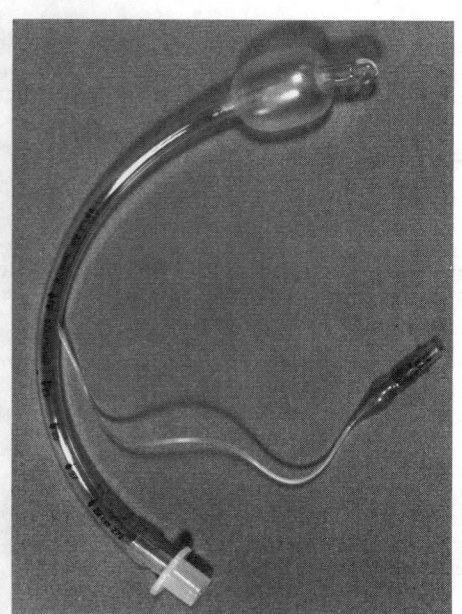

A

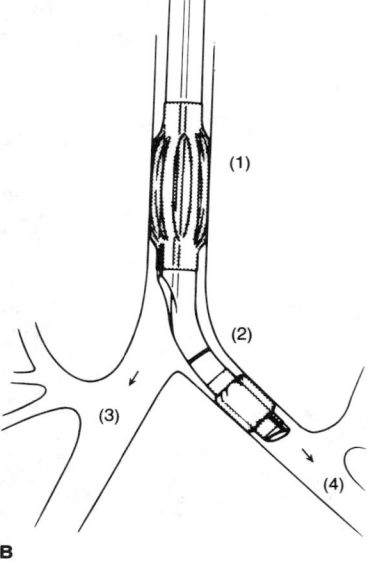

B

FIGURE 8-2 (**A**) Single lumen endotracheal tube. (**B**) Double lumen endotracheal tube. When the double lumen tube is used, two cuffs are inflated. One cuff (1) is positioned in the tracks and the second cuff (2) in the left mainstem bronchus. After inflation, air flows through an opening below the tracheal cuff (3) to the right lung and through an opening below the bronchial cuff (4) to the left lung. This permits differential ventilation of both lungs, lavage of one lung, or selective inflation of either lung during thoracic surgery. (From Marshall, B. E., Longnecker, D. E., & Fairley, H. B., (Eds.). (1988). Anesthesia for thoracic procedures, (p. 381). Boston: Blackwell Scientific Publications. Used with permission)

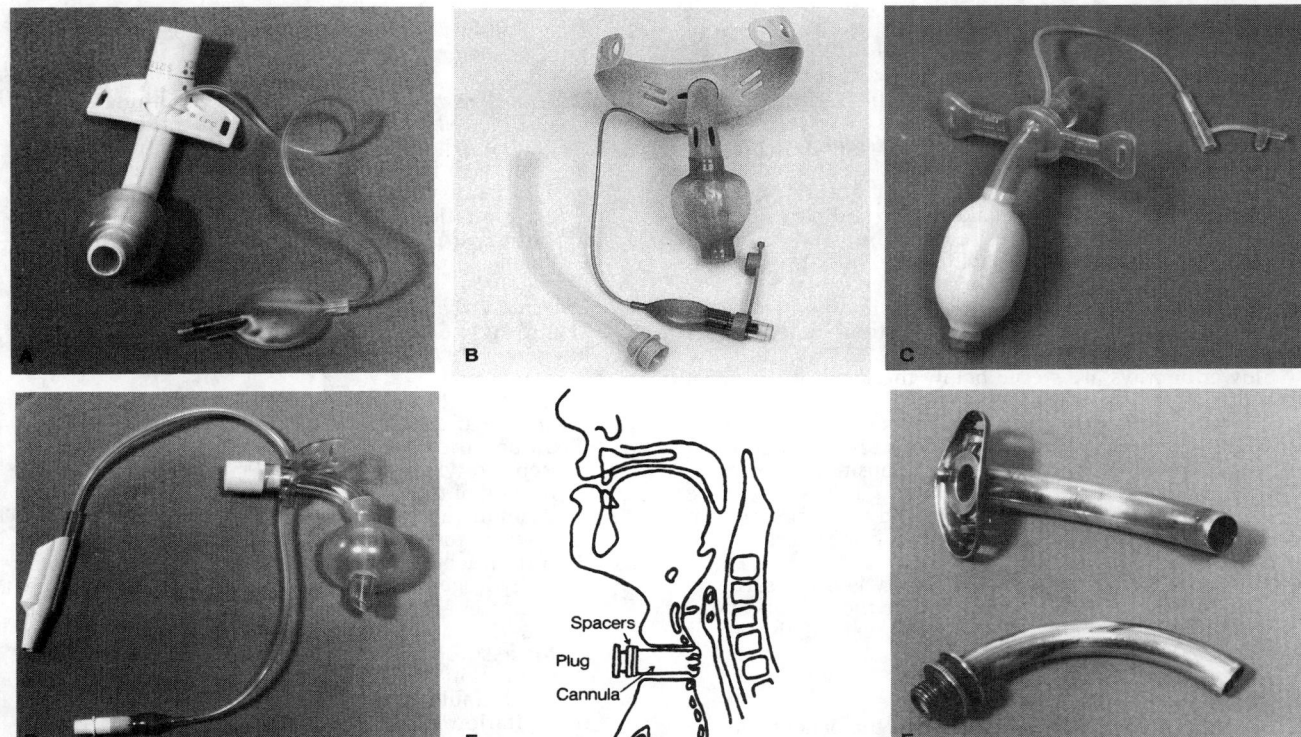

FIGURE 8-3 Types of tracheostomy tubes. (**A**) Low pressure cuff (Shiley). (**B**) Fenestrated tube (Portex). (**C**) Polyurethane foam-filled cuff (FOME-Cuff). (**D**) Pitt speaking tube (National Catheter Corporation). (**E**) Tracheal button. (**F**) Silver tube. (Photographs courtesy of Photography Department, Montefiore Hospital, Pittsburgh, PA. Line drawing from Shelly, R. W. (1981). A post-insertion protocol for management of the olympic tracheostomy button. J Neurosurg Nurs, 13(6), 296.)

e. Tracheal button.
f. Silver tube (rarely used).

2. Vary according to length and inner diameter in millimeters. Usual sizes for an adult are 6.0, 7.0, 8.0, and 9.0 mm.
3. Tracheostomy is usually planned, either as an adjunct to therapy for respiratory dysfunction or for longer term airway management when endotracheal intubation has been used for more than 14 days.
4. May be done at the bedside in an emergency when other means of creating an airway have failed. (See Procedure Guidelines 8-5.)

Indications for Endotracheal Intubation or Tracheostomy

1. Acute respiratory failure, CNS depression, neuromuscular disease, pulmonary disease, chest wall injury.
2. Upper airway obstruction (tumor, inflammation, foreign body, laryngeal spasm).
3. Anticipated upper airway obstruction from edema or soft tissue swelling due to head and neck trauma, some postoperative head and neck procedures involving the airway, facial or airway burns, decreased level of consciousness.
4. Aspiration prophylaxis.
5. Fracture of cervical vertebrae with spinal cord injury; requiring ventilatory assistance.

Complications of Endotracheal or Tracheostomy Tubes

1. Laryngeal or tracheal injury.
   a. Sore throat, hoarse voice.
   b. Glottic edema.
   c. Ulceration of tracheal mucosa.
   d. Vocal cord ulceration, granuloma, or polyps.
   e. Vocal cord paralysis.
   f. Postextubation tracheal stenosis.
   g. Tracheal dilation.
   h. Formation of tracheal-esophageal fistula.
   i. Formation of tracheal-arterial fistula.
   j. Innominate artery erosion.
2. Pulmonary infection and sepsis.
3. Dependence on artificial airway.

Nursing Care for Patients With Artificial Airways

A. General Care Measures
1. Ensure adequate ventilation and oxygenation through the use of supplemental oxygen or mechanical ventilation as indicated.

2. Assess breath sounds every 2 hours. Note evidence of ineffective secretion clearance (rhonchi, crackles), which suggests need for suctioning.
3. Provide adequate humidity when the natural humidifying pathway of the oropharynx is bypassed.
4. Provide adequate suctioning of oral secretions to prevent aspiration and decrease oral microbial colonization.
5. Use clean technique when inserting an oral or nasopharyngeal airway, and take it out and clean it with hydrogen peroxide at least every 8 hours.
6. Perform frequent oral care with soft toothbrush or swabs and antiseptic mouthwash or hydrogen peroxide.
7. Ensure that aseptic technique is maintained when inserting an endotracheal or tracheostomy tube. The artificial airway bypasses the upper airway, and the lower airways are sterile below the level of the vocal cords.
8. Elevate the patient to a semi-Fowler's or sitting position, when possible; these positions result in improved lung compliance. The patient's position, however, should be changed at least every 2 hours to ensure ventilation of all lung segments and prevent secretion stagnation. Position changes are also necessary to avoid skin breakdown.
9. If an oral or nasopharyngeal airway is used, turn the patient's head to the side to reduce the risk of aspiration (because there is no cuff to seal off the lower airway).

B. Nutritional Considerations
1. Consciousness is usually impaired in the patient with an oropharyngeal airway, so oral feeding is contraindicated.
2. To enhance comfort, remove a nasopharyngeal airway in the conscious patient during mealtime.
3. Recognize that an endotracheal tube holds the epiglottis open. Therefore, only the inflated cuff prevents the aspiration of oropharyngeal contents into the lungs. The patient must not receive oral feeding. Administer enteral tube feedings or parenteral feedings as ordered.
4. Administer oral feedings to a conscious patient with a tracheostomy, usually with the cuff inflated. The inflated cuff prevents aspiration of food contents into the lungs, but causes the tracheal wall to bulge into the esophageal lumen, and may make swallowing more difficult.
   a. Patients who are not on mechanical ventilation and are awake, alert, and able to protect the airway are candidates for eating with the cuff deflated.
   b. To assess ability to protect the airway, sit the patient upright and feed the patient colored gelatin or juice. If color from gelatin can be suctioned from the tracheostomy tube, aspiration is occurring, and the cuff must be inflated during feeding and for 1 hour afterward.

> **NURSING ALERT:** ❖❖
> Consider feeding patient early in process of intubation so nutritional status does not decline further. It is difficult to wean patients who have compromised nutritional status.

C. Cuff Maintenance
1. Endotracheal tube cuffs should be inflated continuously and deflated only during intubation, extubation, and tube repositioning.

2. Tracheostomy tube cuffs also should be inflated continuously in patients on mechanical ventilation or CPAP.
3. Tracheostomized patients who are breathing spontaneously may have the cuffs inflated continuously (in the patient with decreased level of consciousness without ability to fully protect airway), deflated continuously, or inflated only for feeding if the patient is at risk of aspiration.
4. Monitor cuff pressure every 4 hours. (See Procedure Guidelines 8-6.)

D. External Tube Site Care
1. Secure an endotracheal tube so it cannot be disrupted by the weight of ventilator or oxygen tubing or patient movement.
   a. Use strips of adhesive tape crossed around the tube and secured to tape on the patient's cheeks or around the back of patient's head.
   b. Replace when soiled or insecure or when repositioning of tube is necessary.
   c. Position tubing so traction is not applied to endotracheal tube.
2. Perform tracheostomy site care at least every 8 hours using hydrogen peroxide and water and change tracheostomy ties at least once a day. (See Procedure Guidelines 8-7.)
   a. Make sure ventilator or oxygen tubing is supported so traction is not applied to the tracheostomy tube.
3. Have available at all times at the patient's bedside a resuscitation bag, oxygen source, and mask to ventilate the patient in the event of accidental tube removal. Anticipate your course of action in such an event.
   a. Endotracheal tube—know location and assembly of reintubation equipment. Know how to contact someone immediately for reintubation.
   b. Tracheostomy—have extra tracheostomy tube, obturator, and hemostats at bedside. Be aware of reinsertion technique, if policy permits, or know how to contact someone immediately for reinserting the tube.

> **NURSING ALERT:** ❖❖
> In the event of accidental endotracheal or tracheostomy tube removal, use a bag/mask resuscitation device to ventilate the patient by mouth, while covering tracheostomy stoma. However, if the patient has complete upper airway obstruction, a gaping stoma, or a laryngectomy, mouth-to-stoma ventilation must be performed.

E. Psychological Considerations
1. Assist patient to deal with psychological aspects related to artificial airway.
2. Recognize that the patient is usually apprehensive, particularly about choking, inability to communicate verbally, inability to remove secretions, difficulty in breathing, or mechanical failure.
3. Explain the function of the equipment carefully.
4. Inform the patient and family that speaking will not be possible while the tube is in place, unless using a tracheostomy tube with a deflated cuff, a fenestrated tube, a Passey-Muir speaking valve, or a speaking tracheostomy tube.
5. Develop with the patient the best method of communication (eg, sign language, lip movement, letter boards, paper and pencil, magic slate, or coded messages).

a. Patients with tracheostomy tubes or nasal endotracheal tubes may effectively use orally operated electrolarynx devices.
b. Devise a means for the patient to get the nurse's attention when someone is not immediately available at the bedside, such as call bell, hand-operated bell, rattle, and so forth.
6. Anticipate some of the patient's questions by discussing "Is it permanent?" "Will it hurt to breathe?""Will someone be with me?"

7. Advise the patient that as condition improves a tracheostomy button may be used to plug the tracheostomy site. A tracheostomy button is a rigid cannula that is placed into the tracheostomy stoma after removal of a cuffed or uncuffed tracheostomy tube. When in proper position, the button does not extend into the tracheal lumen. The outer edge of the button is at the skin surface and the inner edge is at the anterior tracheal wall. (See Procedure Guidelines 8-8.)

(text continues on page 167)

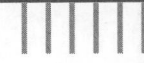

PROCEDURE GUIDELINES 8-4 ◆ Endotracheal Intubation

EQUIPMENT

Laryngoscope with curved or straight blade and working light source (Check batteries and bulb periodically.)
Endotracheal tube with low-pressure cuff and adapter to connect tube to ventilator or resuscitation bag
Stylet to guide the endotracheal tube
Oral airway (assorted sizes) or bite block to keep patient from biting into and occluding the endotracheal tube
Adhesive tape or tube fixation system
Sterile anesthetic lubricant jelly (water-soluble)
10-mL syringe
Suction source
Suction catheter and tonsil suction
Resuscitation bag and mask connected to oxygen source
Sterile towel
Gloves
Goggles or other eye protection

PROCEDURE

NURSING ACTION	RATIONALE
PREPARATORY PHASE	
1. Assess the patient's heart rate, level of consciousness, and respiratory status.	1. Provides a baseline to estimate patient's tolerance of procedure.
PERFORMANCE PHASE	
1. Remove the patient's dental bridgework and plates.	1. May interfere with insertion. Will not be able to remove easily from patient once intubated.
2. Remove headboard of bed (optional).	
3. Prepare equipment.	3.
a. Ensure function of resuscitation bag with mask and suction.	a. Patient may require ventilatory assistance during procedure. Suction should be functional, because gagging and emesis may occur during procedure.
b. Assemble the laryngoscope. Make sure the light bulb is tightly attached and functional.	
c. Select an endotracheal tube of the appropriate size (6.0 to 9.0 mm for average adult).	
d. Place the endotracheal tube on a sterile towel.	d. Although the tube will pass through the contaminated mouth or nose, the airway below the vocal cords is sterile, and efforts must be made to prevent iatrogenic contamination of the distal end of the tube and cuff. The proximal end of the tube may be handled, because it will reside in the upper airway.
e. Inflate the cuff to make sure it assumes a symmetric shape and holds volume without leakage. Then deflate maximally.	e. Malfunction of the cuff must be ascertained before tube placement occurs.
f. Lubricate the distal end of the tube liberally with the sterile anesthetic water-soluble jelly.	f. Aids in insertion.
g. Insert the stylet into the tube (if oral intubation is planned). Nasal intubation does not employ use of the stylet.	g. Stiffens the soft tube, allowing it to be more easily directed into the trachea.
4. Aspirate stomach contents if nasogastric tube is in place.	
5. If time allows, inform the patient of impending inability to talk and discuss alternate means of communication.	5. Discuss alternate means of communication.
6. If the patient is confused, it may be necessary to apply soft wrist restraints.	6. Restraint of the confused patient may be necessary to promote patient safety and maintain sterile technique.
7. Put on goggles and gloves or other eye protection system.	7. Prevents contact with patient's oral secretions.

(continued)

PROCEDURE GUIDELINES 8-4 ◆ Endotracheal Intubation *(continued)*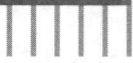

PROCEDURE (cont'd)	NURSING ACTION	RATIONALE

8. During oral intubation if cervical spine is not injured, place patient's head in a "sniffing" position (ie, extended at the junction of the neck and thorax and flexed at the junction of the spine and skull).

8. Upper airway is open maximally in this position.

9. Spray the back of the patient's throat with anaesthetic spray if time is available.

9. Will decrease gagging.

10. Ventilate and oxygenate the patient with the resuscitation bag and mask before intubation.

10. Preoxygenation decreases the likelihood of cardiac dysrhythmias or respiratory distress secondary to hypoxemia.

11. Hold the handle of the laryngoscope in the left hand and hold the patient's mouth open with the right hand by placing crossed fingers on the teeth.

11. Leverage is improved by crossing the thumb and index fingers when opening the patient's mouth (scissor-twist technique).

12. Insert the curved blade of the laryngoscope along the right side of the tongue, push the tongue to the left, and use right thumb and index finger to pull patient's lower lip away from lower teeth.

12. Rolling the lip away from teeth prevents injury by being caught between teeth and blade.

13. Lift laryngoscope forward (toward ceiling) to expose the epiglottis.

13. Do not use teeth as a fulcrum; this could lead to dental damage.

14. Lift laryngoscope upward and forward at a 45-degree angle to expose glottis and visualize vocal cords.

14. This stretches the hypoepiglottis ligament, folding the epiglottis upward and exposing the glottis.

15. As the epiglottis is lifted forward (toward ceiling), the vertical opening of the larynx between the vocal cords will come into view (see accompanying figure).

15. Do not use wrist. Use shoulder and arm to lift the epiglottis.

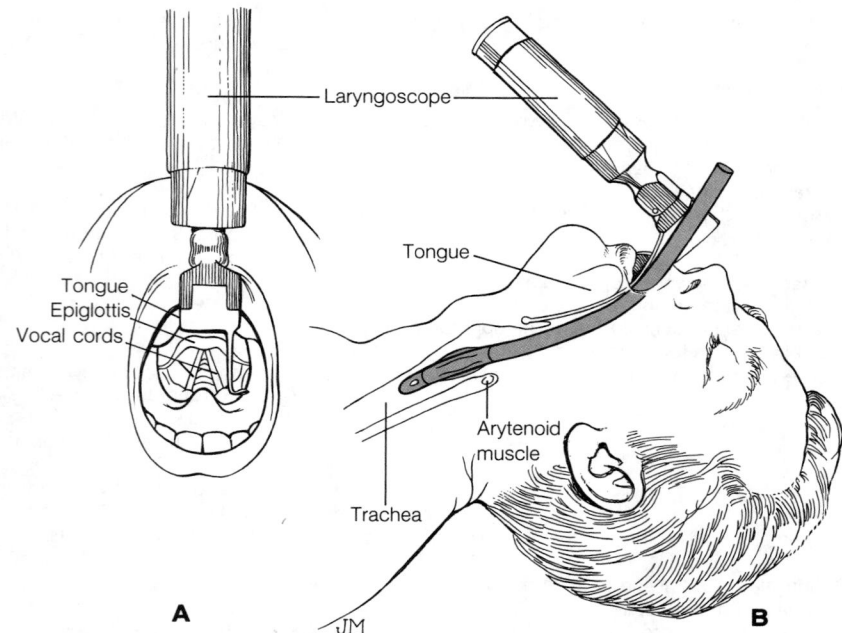

*Endotracheal intubation. (**A**) The primary glottic landmarks for tracheal intubation as visualized with proper placement of the laryngoscope. (**B**) Positioning the endotube.*

16. Once vocal cords are visualized, insert tube into the right corner of the mouth and pass the tube while keeping vocal cords in constant view.

16. Make sure you do not insert tube into esophagus; the esophageal mucosa is pink and the opening is horizontal rather than vertical.

PROCEDURE (cont'd)

NURSING ACTION	RATIONALE
17. Gently push the tube through the triangular space formed by the vocal cords and back wall of trachea.	17. If the vocal cords are in spasm (closed), wait a few seconds before passing tube.
18. Stop insertion just after the tube cuff has disappeared from view beyond the cords.	18. Advancing tube further may lead to its entry into a mainstem bronchus (usually the right bronchus) causing collapse of the unventilated lung.
19. Withdraw laryngoscope while holding endotracheal tube in place. Disassemble mask from resuscitation bag, attach bag to ET tube, and ventilate the patient.	
20. Inflate cuff with the minimal amount of air required to occlude the trachea.	20. Listen over the cuff area with a stethoscope. Occlusion occurs when no air leak is heard during ventilator inspiration or compression of the resuscitation bag.
21. Insert bite block if necessary.	21. This keeps patient from biting down on the tube and obstructing the airway.
22. Ascertain expansion of both sides of the chest by observation and auscultation of breath sounds.	22. Observation and auscultation help in determining that tube remains in position and has not slipped into the right mainstem bronchus.
23. Record distance from proximal end of tube to the point where the tube reaches the teeth.	23. This will allow for detection of any later change in tube position.
24. Secure tube to the patient's face with adhesive tape or apply a commercially available endotracheal tube stabilization device.	24. The tube must be fixed securely to ensure that it will not be dislodged. Dislodgement of a tube with an inflated cuff may result in damage to the vocal cords.
25. Obtain chest x-ray to verify tube position.	

FOLLOW-UP PHASE

1. Record tube type and size, cuff pressure, and patient tolerance of the procedure. Auscultate breath sounds every 2 hours or if signs and symptoms of respiratory distress occur. Assess ABGs after intubation if requested by the physician.

1. ABGs may be prescribed to ensure adequacy of ventilation and oxygenation. Tube displacement may result in extubation (cuff above vocal cords), tube touching carina (causing paroxysmal coughing), or intubation of a mainstem bronchus (resulting in collapse of the unventilated lung).

2. Measure cuff pressure with manometer; adjust pressure. Make adjustment in tube placement on the basis of the chest x-ray results.

2. The tube may be advanced or removed several centimeters for proper placement on the basis of the chest x-ray results.

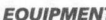

PROCEDURE GUIDELINES 8-5 ◆ **Assisting with Tracheostomy Insertion**

EQUIPMENT

Tracheostomy tube (sizes 6.0 to 9.0 mm. for most adults)
Sterile instruments: hemostat, scalpel and blade, forceps, suture material, scissors
Sterile gown and drapes, gloves
Cap and mask
Antiseptic prep solution
Gauze sponges
Shave prep kit
Sedation

Local anesthetic and syringe
Resuscitation bag and mask with oxygen source
Suction source and catheters
Syringe for cuff inflation
Respiratory support available for post-tracheostomy (mechanical ventilation, tracheal oxygen mask, CPAP, T-piece)
Goggles or other eye protection device

PROCEDURE

NURSING ACTION	RATIONALE
PREPARATORY PHASE	
1. Monitor vital signs (heart rate, respiration, blood pressure, temperature) before insertion.	1. Provides baseline for assessment of progress or complications.

(continued)

PROCEDURE GUIDELINES 8-5 ♦ Assisting with Tracheostomy Insertion
(continued)

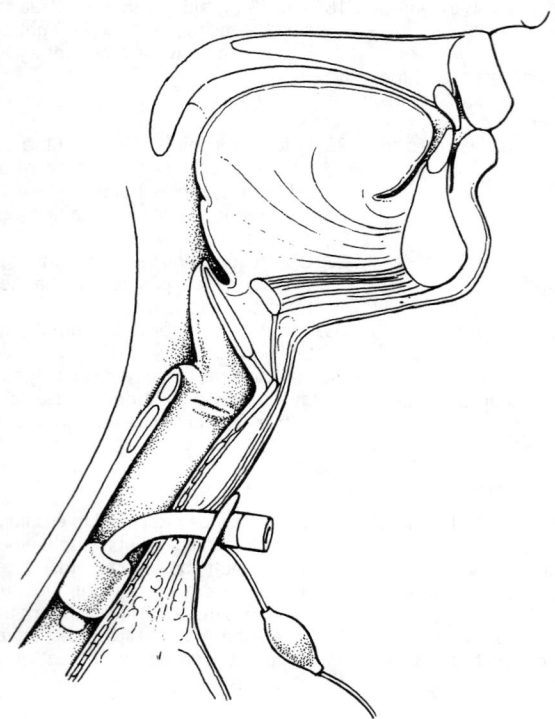

Tracheostomy tube placement.

PERFORMANCE PHASE

1. Explain the procedure to the patient. Discuss a communication system with the patient.
2. Obtain consent for operative procedure.
3. Shave neck region.

4. Assemble equipment. Using aseptic technique, inflate tracheostomy cuff and evaluate for symmetry and volume leakage. Deflate maximally.
5. Position the patient (supine with head extended, with a support under shoulders).
6. Apply soft wrist restraints if patient is confused.

7. Give medication if ordered.
8. Position light source.
9. Assist with antiseptic prep.
10. Assist with gowning and gloving.
11. Assist with sterile draping.
12. Put on goggles.

1. Apprehension about inability to talk is usually a major concern of the tracheostomized patient.

3. Hair and beard may harbor microorganisms. If beard is to be removed, inform the patient or family.
4. Ensures that the cuff is functional before tube insertion.

5. This position brings the trachea forward.

6. Restraint of the confused patient may be necessary to ensure patient safety and preservation of aseptic technique.

12. Spraying of blood or airway secretions may occur during this procedure.

PROCEDURE (cont'd)	NURSING ACTION	RATIONALE

NURSING ACTION

13. During procedure, monitor the patient's vital signs, suction as necessary, give medication as prescribed, and be prepared to administer emergency care.
14. Immediately after the tube is inserted, inflate the cuff. The chest should be auscultated for the presence of bilateral breath sounds.
15. Secure the tracheostomy tube with twill tapes or other securing device and apply dressing.
16. Apply appropriate respiratory assistive device (mechanical ventilation, tracheostomy, oxygen mask, CPAP, T-piece adapter).
17. Check the tracheostomy tube cuff pressure.
18. "Tie sutures" or "stay sutures" of 00 silk may have been placed through either side of the tracheal cartilage at the incision and brought out through the wound. Each is to be taped to the skin at a 45-degree angle laterally to the sternum.

FOLLOW-UP PHASE

1. Assess vital signs and ventilatory status; note tube size used, physician performing procedure, type, dose, and route of medications given.
2. Obtain chest x-ray.
3. Assess and chart condition of stoma:
    a. Bleeding

    b. Swelling
    c. Subcutaneous air

4. An extra tube, obturator, and hemostat should be kept at the bedside. In the event of tube dislodgement, reinsertion of a new tube may be necessary. For emergency tube insertion:
    a. Spread the wound with a hemostat or stay sutures.
    b. Insert replacement tube (containing the obturator) at an angle.
    c. Point cannula downward and insert the tube maximally.
    d. Remove the obturator.

RATIONALE

13. Bradycardia may result from vagal stimulation due to tracheal manipulation, or hypoxemia. Hypoxemia may also cause cardiac irritability.
14. Ensures ventilation of both lungs.

17. Excessive cuff pressure may cause tracheal damage.
18. Should the tracheostomy tube become dislodged, the stay sutures may be grasped and used to spread the tracheal cartilage apart, facilitating placement of the new tube.

1. Provides baseline.

2. Documents proper tube placement.
3.
    a. Some bleeding around the stoma site is not uncommon for the first few hours. Monitor and inform the physician of any increase in bleeding. Clean site aseptically when necessary. Do not change tracheostomy ties for first 24 hours, because accidental dislodgement of the tube could result when the ties are loose, and tube reinsertion through the as yet unformed stoma may be difficult or impossible to accomplish.

    c. When positive pressure respiratory assistive devices are used (mechanical ventilation, CPAP) before the wound is healed, air may be forced into the subcutaneous fat layer. This can be seen as enlargement of the neck and facial tissues and felt as crepitus or "cracking" when the skin is depressed. Report immediately.

4. The hemostat will open the airway and allow ventilation in the spontaneously breathing patient. Avoid inserting the tube horizontally, because the tube may be forced against the back wall of the trachea.

PROCEDURE GUIDELINES 8-6 ◆ Artificial Airway Cuff Maintenance

EQUIPMENT
Suction catheter
Tonsil suction
Suction source
10-mL syringe

Pressure manometer (mercury or aneroid)
Manual resuscitation bag with reservoir, connected to
100% O_2 at 10 to 15 L/min
Goggles or other eye protection device

PROCEDURE	NURSING ACTION	RATIONALE

PREPARATORY PHASE

1. Note degree of air leakage around cuff by listening over the cuff area with a stethoscope.
2. Auscultate breath sounds.

1. Provides a baseline. Air leakage is heard as a crowing sound at peak airway pressure.
2. Provides data baseline.

PERFORMANCE PHASE

1. Explain procedure to the patient.
2. Put on goggles.

1. Decreases the patient's anxiety and promotes cooperation.
2. Spraying of secretions may occur.

DEFLATING THE CUFF

1. Suction the trachea, then the oral and nasal pharynx. Then replace the catheter with a second sterile suction catheter.

2. Deflate the cuff slowly.

3. (Concomitant with step 2) Have the patient cough, or manually inflate the lungs with the resuscitation bag. Be ready to receive secretions in a tissue, or aspirate with tonsil suction.
4. Suction through the tracheostomy or endotracheal tube.

5. Provide adequate ventilation while the cuff is deflated.
   a. If the patient does not require assisted ventilation, maintain humidified oxygen as directed.
   b. If the patient requires assisted ventilation, provide manual ventilation via a resuscitation bag. Leave cuff deflated for as long as the tube repositioning requires; then reinflate.

1. Removes secretions collected above the cuff, which could be aspirated into the lungs when the cuff is deflated. Do not reenter the trachea with the same catheter used for suctioning the mouth.
2. The small test balloon at the end of the tubing remains inflated as long as the cuff at the distal end of the tube is inflated. A vacuum within the syringe is sensed when no more air can be aspirated.
3. Positive pressure in the airways may help force secretions upward and prevent aspiration of secretions.

4. Secretions that may have been present above the inflated cuff and around the exterior tube have now seeped downward. Coughing reflex may be stimulated, helping to mobilize secretions.
5.

   b. Monitor patient closely for tolerance. Loss of tidal volume or PEEP may promote hypoxemia and hypocarbia. Cuff should not be deflated for more than 30 to 45 seconds.

INFLATING A CUFF

1. No leak technique:
   a. Attach air-filled syringe to cuff injection port.
   b. Slowly inject air until no air escapes from the patient's lungs around the cuff.
   c. Note amount of air injected to provide a seal.

2. Minimal leak technique (for mechanical ventilation):

   a. Attach air-filled syringe to cuff injection port.
   b. Slowly inject air until no leak is heard at maximum peak airway pressure.
   c. Slowly remove air from cuff until a small air leak is heard at maximum peak airway pressure.
   d. Note amount of air injected.

1. Air leakage will be heard when the intra-airway pressure is most positive (maximum peak airway pressure). For the spontaneously breathing patient, air leakage will be heard on exhalation. For the patient on positive pressure ventilation, air leakage will be heard at maximum ventilator inspiration.
2. Inflates cuff at lowest possible pressure while still maintaining an adequate seal. Prevents tracheal necrosis from excessive or prolonged cuff pressure.

   c. Adjustment in tidal volume setting may be necessary to compensate for the leak.

PROCEDURE (cont'd)	NURSING ACTION	RATIONALE

3. Measurement of minimal occluding volume (see accompanying figure).

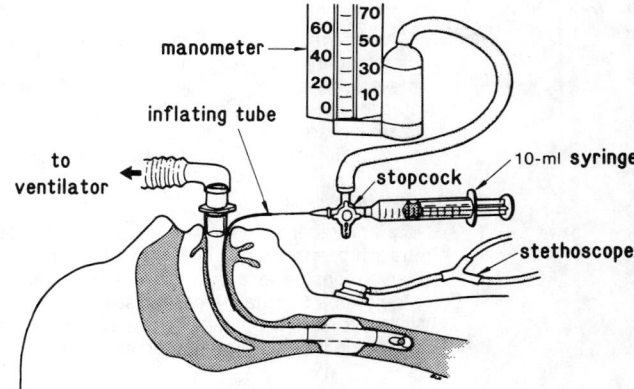

Determination of minimal occluding volume and cuff inflation pressure. A stopcock is inserted into the cuff injection port. When the stopcock is opened to the manometer, cuff pressure is registered on the manometer. An aneroid manometer can also be used. (Sills, J. (1986). An emergency cuff inflation technique. Respiratory Care, 31(3), 201.)

a. Inject sufficient air into the manometer tubing to raise the dial reading 1 cm H_2O above the zero reading.
b. Insert male port of three-way stopcock into cuff injection port. One female port of stopcock holds the air-filled syringe, and one port holds the pressure manometer.
c. Inject air into cuff until desired intracuff pressure is reached at maximum peak airway pressure.

d. Note amount of air needed to achieve the desired intracuff pressure.
e. Remove the stopcock from the injection port.

a. This "pressurizes" the tubing and prevents loss of air from the cuff to the tubing when the reading is taken.

c. Aneroid manometer measures cuff pressure in cm H_2O: A pressure of 20 to 25 cm H_2O is desired. Mercury manometer pressure should be 15 to 20 mm Hg. Pressure greater than upper limit may cause compression of tracheal vessels, resulting in decreased blood flow to tissue. Pressure less than lower limit may allow aspiration of gastric or oral secretions.

e. Most injection ports have self-sealing valves. If not, a cap or closed stopcock may be left in the injection port (clamping of the inflation tubing is discouraged, because it may result in cracking or kinking of the line permanently).

MONITORING CUFF PRESSURE

1. While the cuff is inflated, monitor cuff pressure every 4 hours. Maintain cuff pressure between 15 and 20 mm Hg or 20 and 25 cm H_2O.
2. Document the amount of air required to maintain cuff pressure at this level.

1. Excessive pressure will decrease blood flow to the tissue, resulting in tracheal necrosis. Insufficient cuff pressure predisposes to aspiration.
2. Establishes a baseline for evaluation of change in pressure.

INABILITY TO MAINTAIN A SEAL

1. Assess the degree of leakage and length of time elapsed since cuff volume was replenished.

1. If an inflated cuff leaks air within 10 minutes, assessment is necessary. Possibilities may be:
   a. Cuff positioned above the vocal cords (direct visualization necessary for repositioning).
   b. Incompetence of self-sealing valve on injection port.
   c. Tracheal dilatation (requiring larger size tube).
   d. Cuff may be ruptured, requiring a new tube.

2. Inflate the cuff to desired level.
3. Disconnect syringe (and manometer if used).
4. Assess for leakage.

(continued)

PROCEDURE GUIDELINES 8-6 ◆ Artificial Airway Cuff Maintenance
(continued)

PROCEDURE (cont'd)	NURSING ACTION	RATIONALE
	5. If leakage recurs, place three-way stopcock between syringe and injection port, inflate cuff, close stopcock. Remove syringe (and manometer if used) leaving closed stopcock in injection port.	5. Closed stopcock left in injection port acts as "plug" if self-sealing valve in incompetent.
	6. If air leak persists, tube repositioning or replacement may be necessary. Consult with appropriate personnel.	

FOLLOW-UP PHASE

1. Note and record amount of air used for adequate seal, intracuff pressure, and inability to achieve seal. Document interventions necessary to reintubate, or change tracheostomy tube to obtain a desired seal.

2. While the cuff is inflated, assess cuff pressure every 4 hours. The cuff pressure manometer is useful for this.

2. Leakage of air from the cuff or cuff injection port may occur. Assess the inflation status and adjust as needed.

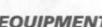

PROCEDURE GUIDELINES 8-7 ◆ Tracheostomy Care (Routine)

EQUIPMENT		
Assemble the following equipment or obtain a prepackaged tracheostomy care kit: Sterile towel Sterile gauze sponges (12) Sterile cotton swabs Sterile gloves		Hydrogen peroxide Sterile water Antiseptic solution and ointment (optional) Tracheostomy tie tapes or commercially available tracheostomy securing device Goggles or other eye protection device

PROCEDURE	NURSING ACTION	RATIONALE

PREPARATORY PHASE

1. Assess condition of stoma before tracheostomy care (redness, swelling, character of secretions, presence of purulence or bleeding).

1. The presence of skin breakdown or infection must be monitored. Culture of the site may be warranted by appearance of these signs.

PERFORMANCE PHASE

1. Suction the trachea and pharynx thoroughly before tracheostomy care.

1. Removal of secretions before tracheostomy care keeps the area clean longer.

2. Explain procedure to the patient.
3. Wash hands thoroughly.
4. Assemble equipment:
   a. Place sterile towel on patient's chest under tracheostomy site.
   b. Open 4 gauze sponges and pour hydrogen peroxide on them.
   c. Open 2 gauze sponges and pour antiseptic solution on them.
   d. Open 2 gauze sponges; keep dry.
   e. Open 2 gauze sponges and pour sterile water on them.
   f. Place tracheostomy tube tapes on field.
   g. Put on goggles and sterile gloves.

4.
   a. Provides sterile field.

   b. For removal of mucus and crust, which promotes bacterial growth.
   c. May be applied to fresh stoma or infected stoma. Not necessary for clean, healed stoma.

   g. Goggles prevent spraying of secretions into the nurse's eyes. Sterile gloves prevent contamination of the wound by nurse's hands and also protect the nurse's hands from infection.

5. Clean the external end of the tracheostomy tube with 2 gauze sponges with hydrogen peroxide; discard sponges.

5. Designate the hand you clean with as contaminated and reserve the other hand as sterile for handling sterile equipment.

PROCEDURE (cont'd)	NURSING ACTION	RATIONALE

NURSING ACTION

6. Clean the stoma area with 2 peroxide-soaked gauze sponges. Make only a single sweep with each gauze sponge before discarding.
7. Loosen and remove crust with sterile cotton swabs.
8. Repeat step 6 using the sterile water-soaked gauze sponges.
9. Repeat step 6 using dry sponges.

10. (Optional) An infected wound may be cleaned with gauze saturated with an antiseptic solution, then dried. A thin layer of antibiotic ointment may be applied to the stoma with a cotton swab.
11. Change a disposable inner cannula, touching only the external portion, and lock it securely into place. If inner cannula is reusable, remove it with your contaminated hand and clean it in hydrogen peroxide solution, using brush or pipe cleaners with your sterile hand. When clean, drop it into sterile saline solution and agitate it to rinse thoroughly with your sterile hand. Tap it gently to dry it and replace it with your sterile hand.
12. Change the tracheostomy tie tapes:
    a. Cut soiled tape while holding tube securely with other hand. Use care not to cut the pilot balloon tubing.
    b. Remove old tapes carefully.
    c. Grasp slit end of clean tape and pull it through opening on side of the tracheostomy tube.
    d. Pull other end of tape securely through the slit end of the tape.
    e. Repeat on the other side.
    f. Tie the tapes at the side of the neck in a square knot. Alternate knot from side to side each time tapes are changed.
    g. Tape should be tight enough to keep tube securely in the stoma, but loose enough to permit two fingers to fit between the tapes and the neck.

Note: If only one clinician is available, the stoma is new (<2 weeks), or the patient's condition is unstable, follow steps c through f before removing old tapes. Two sets of ties will be in place at the same time. After completing step f, cut and remove the old tapes. Also, a tracheostomy-securing device can be used instead of the tracheostomy ties.

13. Place a gauze pad between the stoma site and the tracheostomy tube to absorb secretions and prevent irritation of the stoma according to institution policy (see accompanying figure). Many clinicians feel that gauze should not be used around the stoma. In their opinion, the dressing keeps the area moist and dark, promoting stomal infection. They believe the stoma should be left open to the air and the surrounding area kept dry. A dressing is used only if secretions are draining onto subclavian or neck IV sites or chest incisions.

RATIONALE

6. Hydrogen peroxide may help loosen dry crusted secretions.

8. Ensures that all hydrogen peroxide is removed.

9. Ensures dryness of the area. Wetness promotes infection and irritation.
10. May help clear wound infection.

11. Because cannula is dirty when you remove it, use your contaminated hand. It is considered sterile once you clean it, so handle it with your sterile hand.

12.
    a. Stabilization of the tube helps prevent accidental dislodgement and keeps irritation and coughing due to tube manipulation at a minimum.

    f. To prevent irritation and rotate pressure site.

    g. Excessive tightness of tapes will compress jugular veins, decrease blood circulation to the skin under the tape, and result in discomfort for the patient.

(continued)

PROCEDURE GUIDELINES 8-7 ◆ Tracheostomy Care (Routine) *(continued)*

PROCEDURE (cont'd)	NURSING ACTION	RATIONALE

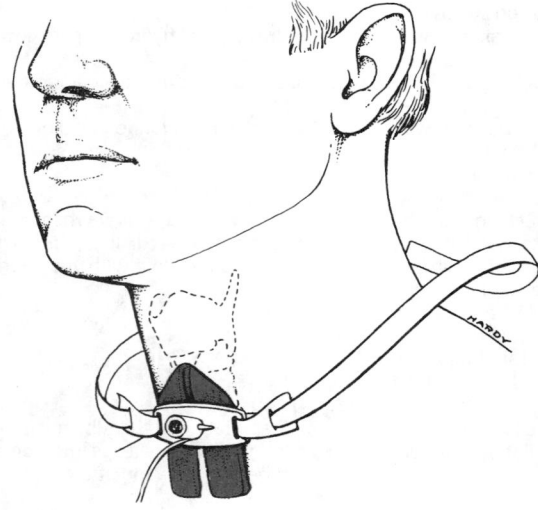

Placement of tracheostomy tube tapes and elective gauze pad.

FOLLOW-UP PHASE

1. Document procedure performance, observations of stoma (irritation, redness, edema, subcutaneous air), and character of secretions (color, purulence). Report changes in stoma appearance or secretions.
2. Cleaning of the fresh stoma should be performed every 8 hours, or more frequently if indicated by accumulation of secretions. Ties should be changed every 24 hours, or more frequently if soiled or wet.

1. Provides a baseline.

2. The area must be kept clean and dry to prevent infection or irritation of tissues.

PROCEDURE GUIDELINES 8-8 ◆ Insertion of a Tracheostomy Button

EQUIPMENT   Tracheostomy button kit (includes cannula, solid closure plug, spacers, universal adapter)
Water-soluble lubricant
Syringe for deflation of tracheostomy cuff
Replacement tracheostomy tube

PROCEDURE	NURSING ACTION	RATIONALE

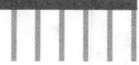

PREPARATORY PHASE

1. Assess whether patient meets criteria for use of tracheostomy button. Criteria include: able to be adequately oxygenated with nasal cannula or face mask; able to swallow and protect the airway; able to cough up secretions; and a noninfected, nonirritated tracheal stoma.
2. Determine vital signs, level of consciousness, SaO_2 or ABG.

PERFORMANCE PHASE

1. Elevate the head of the bed 45 degrees, suction the airway, deflate the tracheostomy tube cuff, and remove the tube.

1. If patient does not meet these criteria, use of tracheostomy tube as airway must be continued.

2. Provides baseline for future assessment.

1. Protects against aspiration.

PROCEDURE (cont'd)	NURSING ACTION	RATIONALE
	2. Determine the distance from anterior tracheal wall to the outer edge of the stoma (skin surface) using a probe with a right angle bend (contained in the kit).	2. Insert the angled end of the probe into the stoma, pull gently until the probe touches the anterior wall, then mark the probe at the outer edge of the stoma (skin surface).
	3. Compare the length of the tracheostomy button cannula with this measurement. If the cannula is too long, it can be sized to fit by adding spacers included into the kit.	3. Spacer rings can be slipped over the cannula to size it for individualized patient requirements.
	4. Coat the cannula with water-soluble lubricant. Ask the patient to relax and take several deep breaths. Insert the cannula into the stoma.	4. The cannula should pass easily into the stoma. If insertion is difficult, recheck cannula size. Several sizes are available.
	5. Insert the closure plug into the cannula. Ties may be used to hold the button in place until the stoma closes around the button.	5. A slight snap will be heard as the plug enters the cannula. The plug causes the proximal end of the cannula to flare, holding it in place.
	6. Remove button two times a week, clean with antibacterial soap, and replace it.	6. Periodic removal helps to keep tissue from granulating into the distal portion of the cannula.
	FOLLOW-UP PHASE	
	1. Observe immediate patient response and obtain SaO_2 or ABG after insertion. Report changes.	1. Use of the button increases dead space, which may increase work of breathing or cause a decrease in SaO_2.
	2. Determine ability of patient to cough out secretions and swallow with button in place.	2. Confirms patient will not retain secretions or be at risk for aspiration with use of this device.

◆ MOBILIZATION OF SECRETIONS

Patients with respiratory disorders or other disorders such as loss of consciousness that may impair respiratory function often require help with mobilization and removal of secretions. Increased amount and viscosity of secretions and/or inability to clear secretions through the normal cough mechanism may lead to pooling of secretions in lower airways. Pooling of secretions leads to infection and inadequate gas exchange.

Secretions should be removed by suctioning when necessary, and can be mobilized through the chest physical therapy measures of postural drainage, percussion, and vibration. Breathing exercises are done with chest physical therapy to increase the efficiency of breathing.

Nasotracheal Suctioning

1. Suctioning of the tracheobronchial tree in a patient without an artificial airway can be accomplished by inserting a suction catheter through the nares into the nasal passage, down through the oropharynx, past the glottis, and into the trachea. (See Procedure Guidelines 8-9.)
2. Contraindications include:
   a. Bleeding disorders such as disseminated intravascular coagulation , thrombocytopenia, leukemia.
   b. Laryngeal edema, laryngeal spasm.
   c. Esophageal varices.
   d. Tracheal surgery.
   e. Gastric surgery with high anastomosis.
   f. Myocardial infarction.
3. May cause trauma to the nasal passages.
   a. Do not attempt to force the catheter if resistance is met.
   b. Report if significant bleeding occurs.
4. Insert a nasal airway if repeated suctioning is necessary to protect the nasal passages from trauma.

5. Be alert for signs of laryngeal edema due to irritation and trauma. Stop if suctioning becomes difficult or if the patient develops new upper airway noise or obstruction.

Suctioning Through an Endotracheal or Tracheostomy Tube

1. Ineffective coughing may cause secretion collection in the artificial airway or tracheobronchial tree, resulting in narrowing of the airway, respiratory insufficiency and stasis of secretions.
2. Assess the need for suctioning at least every 2 hours through auscultation of the chest.
   a. Ventilation with a manual resuscitation bag will facilitate auscultation and may stimulate coughing, decreasing the need for suctioning.
3. Maintain sterile technique while suctioning. (See Procedure Guidelines 8-10.)
4. Administer supplemental 100% oxygen through the mechanical ventilator or manual resuscitation bag before, after, and between suctioning passes to prevent hypoxemia.
5. Closed system suctioning may be done with the suction catheter contained in the mechanical ventilator tubing. Ventilator disconnection is not necessary so time is saved, sterility is maintained, and risk of exposure to body fluids is eliminated.

Chest Physical Therapy

A. Breathing Exercises
1. Techniques used to compensate for respiratory deficits and conserve energy by increasing efficiency of breathing. (See Procedure Guidelines 8-11.)

2. The overall purposes for doing breathing exercises are:
   a. To relax muscles and relieve anxiety.
   b. To eliminate useless uncoordinated patterns of respiratory muscle activity.
   c. To slow the respiratory rate.
   d. To decrease the work of breathing.
3. *Diaphragmatic breathing* is used primarily to strengthen the diaphragm, which is the main muscle of respiration. It also aids in decreasing the use of accessory muscles and allows for better control over the breathing pattern, especially during stressful situations.
4. *Pursed-lip breathing* is used primarily to slow the respiratory rate and assist in emptying the lungs of retained CO_2. This technique is helpful to patients always, but especially when they feel extreme dyspnea due to exertion.
5. Breathing exercises are most helpful to patients when practiced and used on a regular basis.

B. *Percussion/Vibration*
1. Manual techniques designed to loosen secretions and promote drainage of mucus and secretions from the lungs.
2. Indicated for lung conditions that cause increased production of secretions such as bronchiectasis, empyema, cystic fibrosis, and chronic bronchitis.
3. Contraindicated in lung abscess or tumor, pneumothorax, diseases of the chest wall, lung hemorrhage, painful chest conditions, tuberculosis.
4. Percussion is movement done by striking the chest wall in a rhythmic fashion with cupped hands over the chest segment to be drained. The wrists are alternately flexed and extended so the chest is cupped or clapped in a painless manner. (See Procedure Guidelines 8-12.)
5. Vibration is the technique of applying manual compression and tremor to the chest wall during the exhalation phase of respiration.

C. *Postural Drainage*
1. Use of specific positions so the force of gravity can assist in the removal of bronchial secretions from the affected bronchioles into the bronchi and trachea by means of coughing or suctioning (Fig. 8-4).
2. The patient is positioned so the diseased area(s) are in a near vertical position, and gravity is used to assist drainage of the specific segment(s).
3. The positions assumed are determined by the location, severity, and duration of mucus obstruction.
4. The exercises are usually performed two to four times daily, before meals and at bedtime.
5. The procedure should be discontinued if tachycardia, palpitations, dyspnea, chest pain occur—may indicate hypoxemia. Discontinue if hemoptysis occurs.

NURSING ALERT:
Postural drainage and chest percussion may result in hypoxia and should only be used if secretions are believed to be present.

6. Bronchodilators, broncholytic agents, water, or saline may be nebulized and inhaled before postural drainage to reduce bronchospasm, decrease thickness of mucus and sputum, and combat edema of the bronchial walls. (See Procedure Guidelines 8-13.)
7. Ensure patient is comfortable before the procedure starts and as comfortable as possible while he or she assumes each position.
8. Auscultate the chest to determine the areas of needed drainage.
9. Encourage the patient to cough after spending the allotted time in each position.
10. Encourage diaphragmatic breathing throughout postural drainage; this helps widen airways so secretions can be drained.

(text continues on page 177)

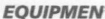

PROCEDURE GUIDELINES 8-9 ◆ Nasotracheal (NT) Suctioning

EQUIPMENT	
Assemble the following equipment or obtain a prepackaged kit:	Sterile water
Disposable curved-tipped suction catheter	Anesthetic water-soluble lubricant jelly
Sterile towel	Suction source at −80 to −120 mm Hg
Sterile disposable gloves	Resuscitation bag with face mask. Connect 100% O_2 source with flow of 10 L/min

PROCEDURE	
NURSING ACTION	**RATIONALE**

PREPARATORY PHASE

1. Monitor heart rate, respiratory rate, color, ease of respirations. If the patient is on monitor, continue monitoring heart rate or arterial blood pressure. Discontinue the suctioning and apply oxygen if heart rate decreases by 20 beats per minute or increases by 40 beats per minute, if blood pressure increases, or if cardiac dysrhythmia is noted.

1. Suctioning may cause the occurrence of:
   a. Hypoxemia—Initially resulting in tachycardia and increased blood pressure, and later causing cardiac ectopy, bradycardia, hypotension, and cyanosis.
   b. Vagal stimulation resulting in bradycardia.

PERFORMANCE PHASE

1. Ascertain that the suction apparatus is functional. Place suction tubing within easy reach.

1. The procedure must be done aseptically, because the catheter will be entering the trachea below the level of the vocal cords, and introduction of bacteria is contraindicated.

PROCEDURE (cont'd)	NURSING ACTION	RATIONALE

NURSING ACTION

2. Inform and instruct the patient regarding procedure.

    a. At a certain interval the patient will be requested to cough to open the lung passage so the catheter will go into the lungs and not into the stomach. The patient will also be encouraged to try not to swallow, because this will also cause the catheter to enter the stomach.
    b. The postoperative patient can splint the wound to make the coughing produced by NT suctioning less painful.
3. Place the patient in a semi-Fowler's or sitting position if possible.

4. Place sterile towel across the patient's chest. Squeeze small amount of sterile anesthetic water-soluble lubricant jelly onto the towel.
5. Open sterile pack containing curved-tipped suction catheter.
6. Aseptically glove both hands. Designate one hand (usually the dominant one) as "sterile" and the other hand as "contaminated."

7. Grasp sterile catheter with sterile hand.
8. Lubricate catheter with the anesthetic jelly and pass the catheter into the nostril and back into the pharynx.
9. Pass the catheter into the trachea. To do this, ask the patient to cough or say "ahh." If the patient is incapable of either, try to advance the catheter on inspiration. Asking the patient to stick out tongue, or hold tongue extended with a gauze sponge, may also help to open the airway. If a protracted amount of time is needed to position the catheter in the trachea, stop and oxygenate the patient with face mask or the resuscitation bag-mask unit at intervals. If three attempts to place the catheter are unsuccessful, request assistance.

10. Specific positioning of catheter for deep bronchial suctioning:
    a. For left bronchial suctioning, turn the patient's head to the extreme right, chin up.
    b. For right bronchial suctioning, turn the patient's head to the extreme left, chin up.

Note: The value of turning the head as an aid to entering the right or left mainstem bronchi is not accepted by all clinicians.

11. Never apply suction until catheter is in the trachea.
    a. Once correct position is ascertained, apply suction and gently rotate catheter while pulling it slightly upward. Do not remove catheter from the trachea.

12. Disconnect the catheter from the suctioning source after 5 to 10 seconds. Apply oxygen by placing a face-mask over the patient's nose, mouth, and catheter, and instruct the patient to breathe deeply.
13. Reconnect suction source. Repeat as necessary.

RATIONALE

2. A thorough explanation will decrease patient anxiety and promote patient cooperation.

3. NT suctioning should follow chest physical therapy, postural drainage, and/or ultrasonic nebulization therapy. The patient should not be suctioned after eating or after a tube feeding is given (unless absolutely necessary) to decrease the possibility of emesis and aspiration.

6. The "contaminated" hand must also be gloved to ensure that organisms in the sputum do not come in contact with the nurse's hand, possibly resulting in infection of the nurse.

8. If obstruction is met, do not force the catheter. Remove it and try the other nostril.
9. These maneuvers may aid in opening the glottis and allowing passage of the catheter into the trachea. To evaluate proper placement, listen at the catheter end for air, or feel for air movement against the cheek. An increase in intensity of breath sounds or more air movement against cheek indicates nearness to the larynx. Gagging or sudden lessening of sound means the catheter is in the hypopharynx. Draw back and advance again. The presence of the catheter in the trachea is indicated by:
    a. Sudden paroxysms of coughing.
    b. Movement of air through the catheter.
    c. Vigorous bubbling of air when the distal end of the suction catheter is placed in a cup of sterile water.
    d. Inability of the patient to speak.
10. Turning the patient's head to one side elevates the bronchial passage on the opposite side, making catheter insertion easier. Suctioning of a particular lung segment may be of value in patients with unilateral pneumonia, atelectasis, or collapse.

11.
    a. Because entry into the trachea is often difficult, less change in arterial oxygen may be caused by leaving the catheter in the trachea than by repeated insertion attempts.
12. Be sure adequate time is allowed to reoxygenate the patient, as oxygen is removed, as well as secretions, during suctioning.
13. No more than three to four suction passes should be made per suction episode.

(continued)

PROCEDURE GUIDELINES 8-9 ◆ Nasotracheal (NT) Suctioning *(continued)*

PROCEDURE (cont'd)	NURSING ACTION	RATIONALE

14. During the last suction pass, remove the catheter completely while applying suction and rotating the catheter gently. Apply oxygen when catheter is removed.

14. Never leave the catheter in the trachea after the suction procedure is concluded, because the epiglottis is splinted open and aspiration may occur.

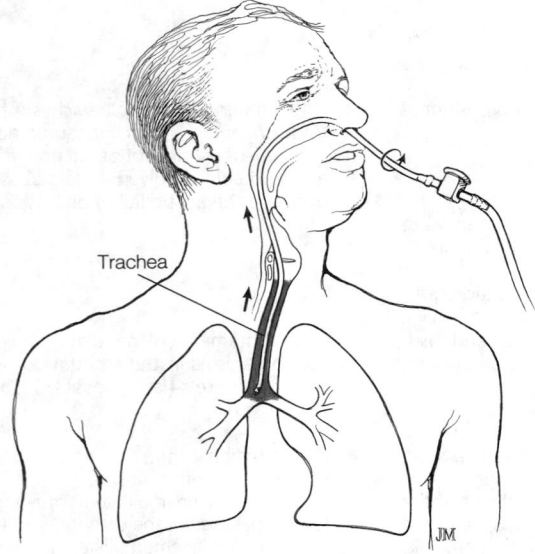

Trachea

Placement of nasotracheal tube for suctioning the tracheo-bronchial tree.

FOLLOW-UP PHASE

1. Dispose of disposable equipment
2. Measure heart rate and blood pressure. Record the patient's tolerance of procedure, type and amount of secretions removed, and complications.

2. Report any patient intolerance of procedure (changes in vital signs, bleeding, laryngospasm, upper airway noise).

PROCEDURE GUIDELINES 8-10 ◆ Sterile Tracheobronchial Suction by Way of Tracheostomy or Endotracheal Tube (Spontaneous or Mechanical Ventilation)

EQUIPMENT

Assemble the following equipment or obtain a prepackaged suctioning kit:
Sterile suction catheters—No. 14 or 16 (adult), No. 8 or 10 (child). The outer diameter of the suction catheter should be no greater than one half the inner diameter of the artificial airway.
Two sterile gloves
Sterile towel
Suction source at 80 to 120 mm Hg
Sterile water

Resuscitation bag with a reservoir connected to 100% oxygen source (if patient is on PEEP or CPAP, add positive end-expiratory pressure (PEEP) valve to exhalation valve on resuscitation bag in an amount equal to that on the ventilator or CPAP device)
Normal saline solution (in syringe or single-dose packet)
Sterile cup for water
Alcohol swabs
Sterile water-soluble lubricant jelly
Goggles or other eye protection device

PROCEDURE	NURSING ACTION	RATIONALE

PREPARATORY PHASE

1. Monitor heart rate and auscultate breath sounds. If the patient is monitored, continuously monitor heart rate and arterial blood pressure. If arterial blood gases are done routinely, know baseline values. (It is important to establish a baseline because suctioning should be discontinued and oxygen applied or manual ventilation reinstituted if, during the suction procedure, the heart rate decreases by 20 beats per minute or increases by 40 beats per minute, blood pressure drops, or cardiac dysrhythmia is noted.)

1. Suctioning may cause:
   a. Hypoxemia, initially resulting in tachycardia and increased blood pressure, progressing to cardiac ectopy, bradycardia, hypotension, and cyanosis.
   b. Vagal stimulation, which may result in bradycardia.

PERFORMANCE PHASE

1. Instruct the patient how to "splint" surgical incision, because coughing will be induced during the procedure. Explain the importance of performing the suction procedure in an aseptic manner.

1. Thorough explanation lessens patient's anxiety and promotes cooperation.

2. Assemble equipment. Check function of suction and manual resuscitation bag connected to 100% O_2 source. Put on goggles.

2. Make sure that all equipment is functional before sterile technique is instituted to prevent interruption once the procedure is begun. Use of 100% O_2 will help to prevent hypoxemia.

3. Wash hands thoroughly.
4. Open sterile towel. Place in a biblike fashion on patient's chest. Open alcohol wipes and place on corner of towel. Place small amount of sterile water-soluble jelly on towel.
5. Open sterile gloves. Place on towel.
6. Open suction catheter package.
7. If the patient is on mechanical ventilation, test to make sure disconnection of ventilator attachment may be made with one hand.
8. Don sterile gloves. Designate one hand as contaminated for disconnecting, bagging, and working the suction control. Usually the dominant hand is kept sterile and will be used to thread the suction catheter.

8. The hand designated as sterile must remain uncontaminated so organisms are not introduced into the lungs. The contaminated hand must also be gloved to prevent sputum from contacting the nurse's hand, possibly resulting in an infection of the nurse.

9. Use the sterile hand to remove carefully the suction catheter from the package, curling the catheter around the gloved fingers.
10. Connect suction source to the suction fitting of the catheter with the contaminated hand.
11. Using the contaminated hand, disconnect the patient from the ventilator, CPAP device, or other oxygen source. (Place the ventilator connector on the sterile towel and flip a corner of the towel over the connection to prevent fluid from spraying into the area.)

11. Prevents contamination of the connection.

12. Ventilate and oxygenate the patient with the resuscitator bag, compressing firmly and as completely as possible approximately four to five times (try to approximate the patient's tidal volume). This procedure is called "bagging" the patient. In the spontaneously breathing patient, coordinate manual ventilations with the patient's own inspiratory effort.

12. Ventilation before suctioning helps prevent hypoxemia. When possible, two nurses work as a team to suction. Attempting to ventilate against the patient's own respiratory efforts may result in high airway pressures, predisposing the patient to barotrauma (lung injury due to pressure).

13. Lubricate the tip of the suction catheter. Gently insert suction catheter as far as possible into the artificial airway without applying suction. Most patients will cough when the catheter touches the carina.

13. Suctioning on insertion would unnecessarily decrease oxygen in the airway.

14. Withdraw catheter 2 to 3 cm and apply suction. Quickly rotate the catheter while it is being withdrawn.

14. Failure to withdraw and rotate catheter may result in damage to tracheal mucosa. Release suction if a pulling sensation is felt.

15. Limit suction time to no more than 10 seconds. Discontinue if heart rate decreases by 20 beats per minute or increases by 40 beats per minute, or if cardiac ectopy is observed.

15. Suctioning removes oxygen as well as secretions and may also cause vagal stimulation.

(continued)

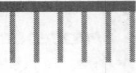

PROCEDURE GUIDELINES 8-10 ◆ Sterile Tracheobronchial Suction by Way of Tracheostomy or Endotracheal Tube (Spontaneous or Mechanical Ventilation) *(continued)*

PROCEDURE *(cont'd)*

NURSING ACTION	RATIONALE
16. Bag patient between suction passes with approximately four to five manual ventilations.	16. The oxygen removed by suctioning must be replenished before suctioning is attempted again.
17. At this point, sterile normal saline may be instilled into the trachea by way of the artificial airway if secretions are tenacious.	17. Some clinicians believe secretion removal may be facilitated with saline instillation. Others believe saline does not mix with mucus and that suctioning of the saline just instilled is the only effect produced by performing this step. It is now thought that the greatest benefit of instilling sterile normal saline is to initiate a cough.
a. Open prepackaged container and instill 3 to 5 mL normal saline into the artificial airway during spontaneous inspiration.	a. Instillation of the saline during inspiration will prevent the saline from being blown back out of the tube.
b. Bag vigorously and then suction.	b. Bagging stimulates cough and distributes saline to loosen secretions.
18. Rinse catheter between suction passes by inserting tip in cup of sterile water and applying suction.	
19. Continue making suction passes, bagging the patient between passes, until the airways are clear of accumulated secretions. No more than four suction passes should be made per suctioning episode.	19. Repeated suctioning of a patient in a short time interval predisposes to hypoxemia, as well as being tiring and traumatic to the patient.
20. Give the patient four to five "sigh" breaths with the bag.	20. Sighing is accomplished by depressing the bag slowly and completely with two hands to deliver approximately 1½ times the normal tidal volume to the patient, allowing for maximal lung expansion and prevention of atelectasis.
21. Return the patient to the ventilator or apply CPAP or other oxygen-delivery device.	
22. Suction oral secretions from the oropharynx above the artificial airway cuff.	
23. Clean elbow fitting of resuscitation bag with alcohol; cover with a sterile glove or 4 × 4.	

FOLLOW-UP PHASE

1. Note any change in vital signs or patient's intolerance to the procedure. Record amount and consistency of secretions.	1. Evaluate the effectiveness of procedure and patient response.
2. Assess need for further suctioning at least every 2 hours, or more frequently if secretions are copious.	

Note: A closed system for suctioning may be in place in the ventilator circuit that allows suctioning without removal from the ventilator.

COMMUNITY-BASED CARE TIP:
Teach caregivers to suction in the home situation using clean technique, rather than sterile. Wash hands well before suctioning and reuse catheter after rinsing it in warm water.

PROCEDURE GUIDELINES 8-11 ◆ Teaching the Patient Breathing Exercises

PROCEDURE	NURSING ACTION	RATIONALE

PREPARATORY PHASE

1. Have patient clear the nasal passages before beginning exercises.

PERFORMANCE PHASE

Instruct the patient as follows:

DIAPHRAGMATIC BREATHING

1. Place one hand on stomach just below the ribs and the other hand on the middle of the chest.
2. Breathe in slowly and deeply through the nose, letting the abdomen protrude as far as it will. The abdomen enlarges during inspiration and decreases in size during expiration.
3. Breathe out through pursed lips while contracting (tightening) the abdominal muscles. Press firmly inward and upward on the abdomen while breathing out.
4. The chest should not move; attention is directed at the abdomen, not the chest.
5. Repeat for 1 minute (followed by a rest period of 2 minutes). Work up to 10 minutes, four times daily.
6. Learn to do diaphragmatic breathing while lying, then sitting, and ultimately standing and walking.

1. This helps the patient become aware of the diaphragm and its function in breathing.
2. Slow inhalation provides ventilation and hyperinflation of the lungs.
3. Contracting the abdominal muscles assists the diaphragm in rising to empty the lungs. The hand generates pressure on the abdomen to facilitate more complete expiration.
4. Contraction of the abdominal muscles should take place during expiration.

6. Diaphragmatic breathing helps the patient breathe in a controlled manner during activities that produce dyspnea. If shortness of breath occurs, advise stopping the exercises until breathing pattern comes under control.

PURSED LIP BREATHING

1. Inhale through the nose.
2. Exhale slowly and evenly against pursed lips while contracting (tightening) the abdominal muscles. (Avoid exhaling forcefully.)

2. Pursing the lips increases intrabronchial pressure (helps maintain the bronchi in an open position) as well as intraalveolar pressure. The pursed-lips maneuver also prolongs the expiratory phase of breathing, makes it easier to empty the air in the lungs, and promotes carbon dioxide elimination.

3. Sit in a chair. Fold arms across the abdomen.
   a. Inhale through the nose.
   b. Bend over and exhale slowly through pursed lips while counting to 7.
4. While walking.
   a. Inhale while walking two steps.
   b. Exhale through pursed lips while walking four steps.

3.

   b. Leaning forward pushes the abdominal organs upward.
4. Try any similar combinations according to breathing tolerance of patient.

LOWER SIDE RIB BREATHING

1. Place hands on sides of lower ribs.
2. Inhale deeply and slowly while sides expand moving hands outward.
3. Exhale slowly through pursed lips and feel the hands and ribs move inward.
4. Rest.

LOWER BACK AND RIBS BREATHING

1. Sit in a chair. Place hands behind back; hold flat against lower ribs.
2. Inhale deeply and slowly while rib cage expands backward; the hands will move outward.
3. Keep hands in place. Blow out slowly; hands will move in.

SEGMENTAL BREATHING

1. Place hands on sides of lower ribs.
2. Inhale deeply and slowly while concentrating on moving the right hand outward by expanding the right rib cage.
3. Ensure that the right hand moves outward more than the left hand.
4. Keeping hands in place, exhale slowly, and feel the right hand and ribs moving in.
5. Repeat, concentrating on expanding left side more than the right side.
6. Rest.

PATIENT EDUCATION

Instruct patient to:

1. Always inhale through the nose. This permits filtration, humidification, and warming of air.
2. Breathe slowly in a rhythmic and relaxed manner. This permits more complete exhalation and emptying of lungs; helps overcome anxiety associated with dyspnea and decreases oxygen requirement.
3. Avoid sudden exertion.
4. Practice in several positions; air distribution and pulmonary circulation vary according to position of the chest.

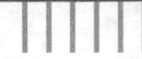

PROCEDURE GUIDELINES 8-12 ◆ Percussion (Clapping) and Vibration

EQUIPMENT
Pillows
Tilt table
Emesis basin
Sputum cup
Paper tissues

PROCEDURE	**NURSING ACTION**	**RATIONALE**

PERFORMANCE PHASE

1. Instruct the patient to use diaphragmatic breathing.

2. Position the patient in prescribed postural drainage position(s) (p. 176). The spine should be straight to promote rib cage expansion.

1. Diaphragmatic breathing helps the patient relax and helps widen airways.
2. The patient is positioned according to the area of the lung that is to be drained.

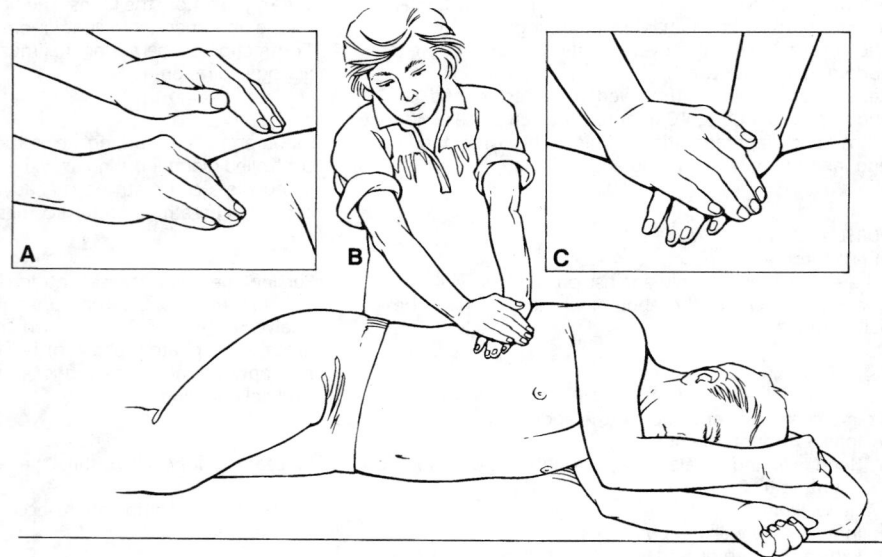

Percussion and vibration. (**A**) Proper hand positioning for percussion. (**B**) Proper technique for vibration. Note that the wrists and elbows are kept stiff and the vibrating motion is produced by the shoulder muscles. (**C**) Proper hand position for vibration.

3. Percuss (or clap) with cupped hands over the chest wall for 1 or 2 minutes from:
   a. The lower ribs to shoulders in the back.
   b. The lower ribs to top of chest in the front.
4. Avoid clapping over the spine, liver, kidneys, spleen, breast, scapula, clavicle, or sternum.
5. Instruct the patient to inhale slowly and deeply. Vibrate the chest wall as the patient exhales slowly through pursed lips.
   a. Place one hand on top of the other over affected area or place one hand on each side of the rib cage.
   b. Tense the muscles of the hands and arms while applying moderate pressure downward and vibrate hands and arms.
   c. Relieve pressure on the thorax as the patient inhales.
   d. Encourage the patient to cough, using abdominal muscles, after three or four vibrations.

3. This action helps dislodge mucous plugs and mobilize secretions toward the main bronchi and trachea. The air trapped between the operator's hand and chest wall will produce a characteristic hollow sound.
4. Percussion over these areas may cause injuries to the spine or internal organs.
5. This sets up a vibration that carries through the chest wall and helps free the mucus.

   b. This maneuver is performed in the direction in which the ribs move on expiration.

   d. Contracting the abdominal muscles while coughing increases cough effectiveness. Coughing aids in the movement and expulsion of secretions.

PROCEDURE (cont'd)	**NURSING ACTION**	**RATIONALE**
	6. Allow the patient to rest several minutes.	
	7. Listen with a stethoscope for changes in breath sounds.	7. The appearance of crackles and rhonchi indicate movement of air around mucus in the bronchi.
	8. Repeat the percussion and vibration cycle according to the patient's tolerance and clinical response; usually 15 to 30 minutes.	

PROCEDURE GUIDELINES 8-13 ♦ Administering Nebulizer Therapy (Sidestream Jet Nebulizer)

EQUIPMENT   Air compressor
Connection tubing
Nebulizer
Medication and saline solution

PROCEDURE	**NURSING ACTION**	**RATIONALE**

PREPARATORY PHASE

1. Monitor the heart rate before and after the treatment for patients using bronchodilator drugs.	1. Bronchodilators may cause tachycardia, palpitations, dizziness, nausea, or nervousness.

PERFORMANCE PHASE

1. Explain the procedure to the patient. *This therapy depends on patient effort.*	1. Proper explanation of the procedure helps to ensure the patient's cooperation and effectiveness of the treatment.
2. Place the patient in a comfortable sitting or a semi-Fowler's position.	2. Diaphragmatic excursion and lung compliance are greater in this position. This ensures maximal distribution and deposition of aerosolized particles to basilar areas of the lungs.
3. Add the prescribed amount of medication and saline to the nebulizer. Connect the tubing to the compressor and set the flow at 6 to 8 L/min.	3. A fine mist from the device should be visible.
4. Instruct the patient to exhale.	
5. Tell the patient to take in a deep breath from the mouthpiece, hold breath briefly, then exhale.	5. This encourages optimal dispersion of the medication.
6. Nose clips are sometimes used if the patient has difficulty breathing only through the mouth.	
7. Observe expansion of chest to ascertain that patient is taking deep breaths.	7. This will ensure medication is deposited below the level of the oropharynx.
8. Instruct the patient to breathe slowly and deeply until all the medication is nebulized.	8. Medication will usually be nebulized within 15 minutes at a flow of 6 to 8 L/min.
9. On completion of the treatment, encourage the patient to cough after several deep breaths.	9. The medication may dilate airways, facilitating expectoration of secretions.

FOLLOW-UP PHASE

1. Record medication used and description of secretions.	
2. Disassemble and clean nebulizer after each use. Keep this equipment in the patient's room. The equipment is changed every 24 hours.	2. Each patient has own breathing circuit (nebulizer, tubing, and mouthpiece). Through proper cleaning, sterilization, and storage of equipment, organisms can be prevented from entering the lungs.

COMMUNITY-BASED CARE TIP:
Nebulizer tubing and mouthpiece can be reused at home repeatedly. Recommend thorough rinsing with hot water after each use and periodic washing with liquid soap and hot water.

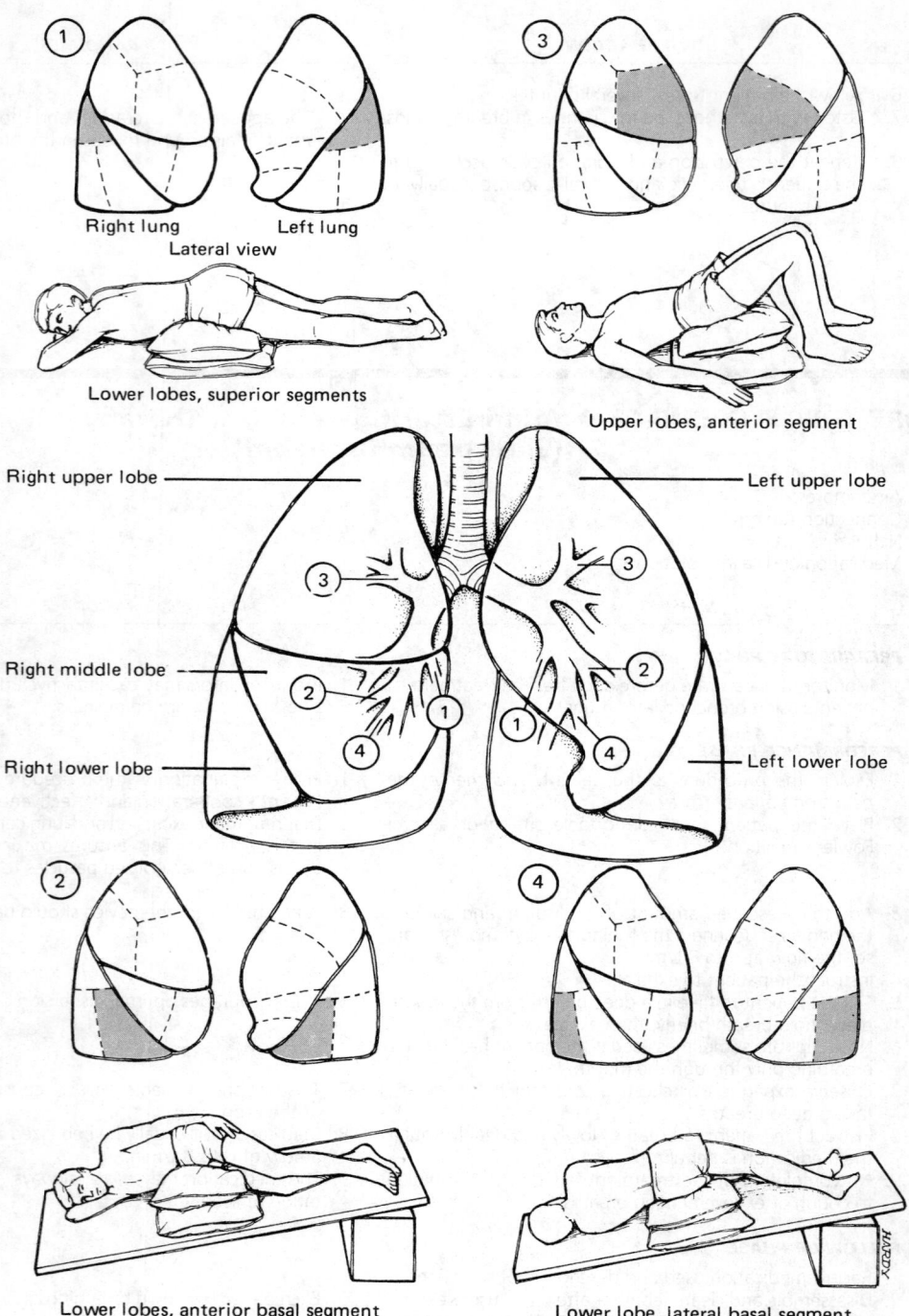

Right lung   Left lung
Lateral view
Lower lobes, superior segments

Upper lobes, anterior segment

Right upper lobe — — Left upper lobe

Right middle lobe —

Right lower lobe —

— Left lower lobe

Lower lobes, anterior basal segment

Lower lobe, lateral basal segment

FIGURE 8-4 *Postural drainage positions. Anatomic segments of the lung with four postural drainage positions. The numbers relate the position to the corresponding anatomic segment of the lung.*

◆ ADMINISTERING OXYGEN THERAPY

Oxygen is an odorless, tasteless, colorless, transparent gas that is slightly heavier than air. Oxygen can be dispensed from a cylinder, piped-in system, liquid oxygen reservoir, or oxygen concentrator. It may be administered by nasal cannula, transtracheal catheter, or various types of face masks. It may also be applied directly to the endotracheal or tracheal tube by way of a mechanical ventilator, T-piece, or manual resuscitation bag. The method selected depends on the required concentration of oxygen, desired variability in delivered oxygen concentration (none, minimal, moderate), and required ventilatory assistance (mechanical ventilator, spontaneous breathing).

Methods of Oxygen Administration

1. Nasal cannula (see Procedure Guidelines 8-14)—nasal prongs that deliver low flow of oxygen.
   a. Requires nose breathing.
   b. Cannot deliver oxygen concentrations much higher than 40%.
2. Simple face mask (see Procedure Guidelines 8-15)—mask that delivers moderate oxygen flow to nose and mouth.
   a. Delivers oxygen concentrations of 40% to 60%.
3. Venturi mask (see Procedure Guidelines 8-16)—mask with device that mixes air and oxygen to deliver constant oxygen concentration.
   a. Total gas flow at the patient's face must meet or exceed peak inspiratory flow rate. When other mask outputs do not meet inspiratory flow rate of patient, room air (drawn through mask side holes) mixes with the gas mixture provided by the face mask, lowering the inspired oxygen concentration.
   b. Venturi mask mixes a fixed flow of oxygen with a high but variable flow of air to produce a constant oxygen concentration. Oxygen enters by way of a jet (restricted opening) at a high velocity. Room air also enters and mixes with oxygen at this site. The higher the velocity (smaller the opening), the more room air is drawn into the mask.
   c. Mask output ranges from approximately 97 L/min (24%) to approximately 33 L/min (50%).
   d. Virtually eliminates rebreathing of carbon dioxide. Excess gas leaves through openings in the mask, carrying with it the expired carbon dioxide.
4. Partial rebreather mask (see Procedure Guidelines 8-17) has an inflatable bag that stores 100% oxygen.
   a. On inspiration, the patient inhales from the mask and bag; on expiration, the bag refills with oxygen and expired gases exit through perforations on both sides of the mask and some enters bag (Fig. 8-5).
   b. High concentrations of oxygen (50% to 75%) can be delivered.
5. Nonrebreathing mask (see Procedure Guidelines 8-17) has an inflatable bag to store 100% oxygen and a one-way valve between the bag and mask to prevent exhaled air from entering the bag.
   a. Has one-way valves covering one or both the exhalation ports to prevent entry of room air on inspiration.
   b. Has a flap or spring-loaded valves to permit entry of room air should the oxygen source fail or patient needs exceed the available oxygen flow.
   c. Optimally, all the patient's inspiratory volume will be provided by the mask/reservoir, allowing delivery of nearly 100% oxygen.

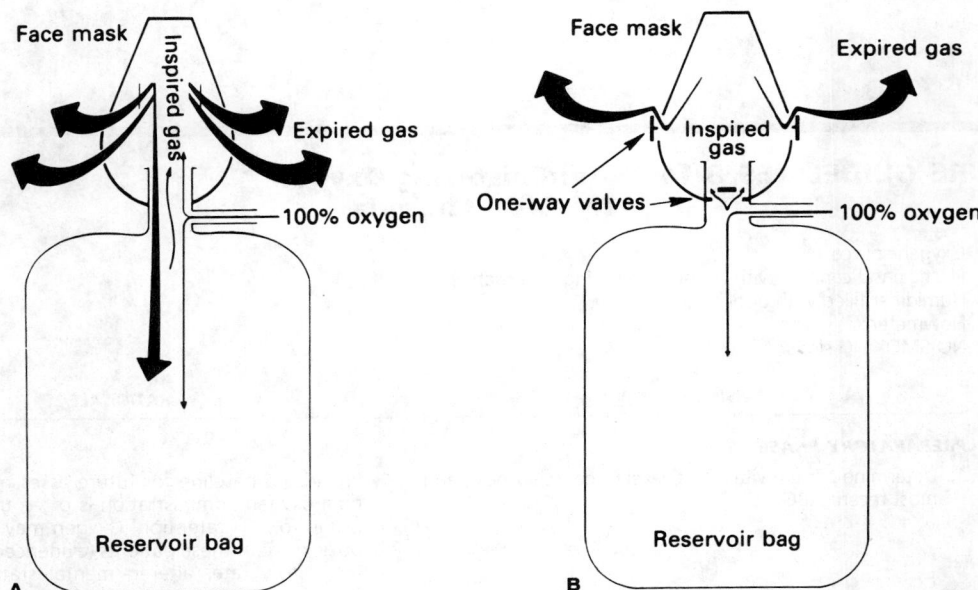

FIGURE 8-5 (**A**) Air flow diagram with partial rebreathing mask. (**B**) Air flow diagram with nonrebreathing mask. Arrows indicate direction of flow. (Burton, G. C., & Hodgkin, J. E. [Eds.], (1984). Respiratory care: A guide to practice (2nd ed.). Philadelphia: JB Lippincott.

6. Transtracheal catheter (see Procedure Guidelines 8-18)—accomplished by way of a small (8Fr) catheter inserted between the second and third tracheal cartilage.
   a. Does not interfere with talking, drinking, or eating and can be concealed under a shirt or blouse.
   b. Oxygen delivery is more efficient because all oxygen enters the lungs.
   c. Patients who meet criteria for continuous home oxygen therapy ($Pao_2 < 55$ mm Hg on room air) may use this delivery method instead of nasal cannula.
7. Continuous positive airway pressure (CPAP) mask (see Procedure Guidelines 8-19) is used to provide expiratory and inspiratory positive airway pressure in a manner similar to positive end expiratory pressure (PEEP) and without endotracheal intubation.
   a. Has an inflatable cushion and head strap designed to tightly seal the mask against the face.
   b. A PEEP valve is incorporated into the exhalation port to maintain positive pressure on exhalation.
   c. High inspiratory flow rates are needed to maintain positive pressure on inspiration.
8. T-piece (Briggs) adapter (see Procedure Guidelines 8-20) is used to administer oxygen to patient with endotracheal or tracheostomy tube who is breathing spontaneously.
   a. High concentration of humidity and oxygen delivered through wide bore tubing.
   b. Expired gases exits through open reservoir tubing.
9. Manual resuscitation bag (see Procedure Guidelines 8-21) delivers high concentration of oxygen to patient with insufficient inspiratory effort.
   a. With mask, uses upper airway by delivering oxygen to mouth and nose of patient.
   b. Without mask, adapter fits on endotracheal or tracheostomy tube.
   c. Usually used in cardiopulmonary arrest, hyperinflation during suctioning, or transport of ventilator-dependent patients.

Nursing Assessment and Interventions

1. Assess need for oxygen by observing for symptoms of hypoxia:
   a. Tachypnea.
   b. Tachycardia or dysrhythmias (premature ventricular contractions).
   c. A change in level of consciousness (symptoms of decreased cerebral oxygenation are irritability, confusion, lethargy, and coma, if untreated).
   d. Cyanosis occurs as a late sign ($Pao_2 \leq 45$ mm Hg).
   e. Labored respirations indicate severe respiratory distress.
   f. Myocardial stress—increase in heart rate and stroke volume (cardiac output) is the primary mechanism for compensation for hypoxemia or hypoxia.
2. Obtain ABGs and assess the patient's current oxygenation, ventilation, and acid–base status.
3. Administer oxygen in the appropriate concentration.
   a. Low concentration (24% to 28%)—appropriate for patients prone to retain carbon dioxide (COPD, drug overdose), who are dependent on hypoxemia (hypoxic drive) to maintain respiration. If hypoxemia is suddenly reversed, hypoxic drive may be lost and respiratory arrest may occur.
   b. High concentrations ($\geq 30\%$)—appropriate in patients not predisposed to carbon dioxide retention.
4. Monitor response to therapy by oximetry and/or ABGs.
5. Increase or decrease the inspired oxygen concentration (FiO_2), as appropriate.

All JCAHO-accredited hospitals must be smoke-free, however other health care facilities and homes where oxygen is used may allow smoking. Ensure that no smoking is conducted where oxygen is used.

(text continues on page 191)

PROCEDURE GUIDELINES 8-14 ◆ Administering Oxygen by Nasal Cannula

EQUIPMENT
Oxygen source
Plastic nasal cannula with connecting tubing (disposable)
Humidifier filled with distilled water
Flowmeter
NO SMOKING signs

PROCEDURE

NURSING ACTION	RATIONALE
PREPARATORY PHASE	
1. Determine current vital signs, level of consciousness, and most recent ABG.	1. Provides a baseline for future assessment. Nasal cannula oxygen administration is often used for patients prone to CO_2 retention. Oxygen may depress the hypoxic drive of these patients (evidenced by a decreased respiratory rate, altered mental status, and further $Paco_2$ elevation).
2. Assess risk of CO_2 retention with oxygen administration.	2. If $Paco_2$ is decreased or normal, the patient is not experiencing CO_2 retention and can use oxygen without fear of the above consequences.

| PROCEDURE (cont'd) | NURSING ACTION | RATIONALE |

PERFORMANCE PHASE

1. Post NO SMOKING signs on the patient's door and in view of patient and visitors.
2. Show the nasal cannula to the patient and explain the procedure.
3. Make sure the humidifier is filled to the appropriate mark.

    3. Humidification may not be ordered if the flow rate is ≤4 L/min.

4. Attach the connecting tube from the nasal cannula to the humidifier outlet.
5. Set flow rate at prescribed liters/minute. Feel to determine if oxygen is flowing through the tips of the cannula.

    5. Because a nasal cannula is a low-flow system (patient's tidal volume supplies part of the inspired gas), oxygen concentration will vary, depending on the patient's respiratory rate and tidal volume. Approximate oxygen concentrations delivered are:
    1 L = 24% to 25%
    2 L = 27% to 29%
    3 L = 30% to 33%
    4 L = 33% to 37%
    5 L = 36% to 41%
    6 L = 39% to 45%

NURSING ALERT:
Patients who require low, constant concentrations of oxygen and whose breathing pattern varies greatly may need to use a Venturi mask, particularly if they are carbon dioxide retainers.

6. Place the tips of the cannula in the patient's nose and adjust straps around ears for snug, comfortable fit.

    6. Inspect skin behind ears periodically for irritation or breakdown.

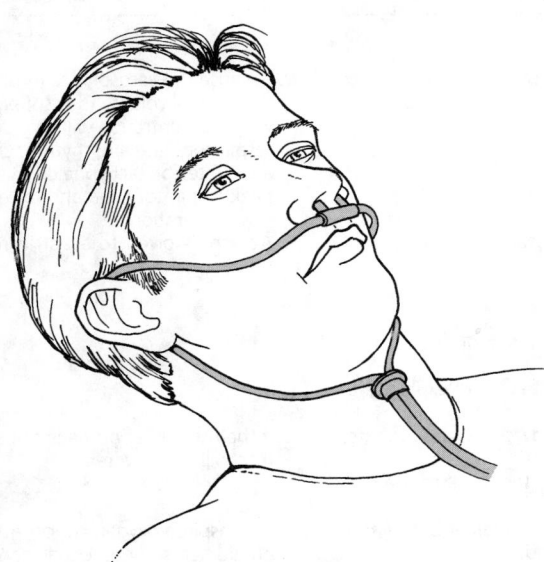

Administering oxygen by nasal cannula. Patient's inspiration consists of a mixture of supplemental oxygen supplied via the nasal cannula and room air. Oxygen concentration is variable and depends on patient's tidal volume and ventilatory pattern.

(continued)

PROCEDURE GUIDELINES 8-14 ◆ Administering Oxygen by Nasal Cannula *(continued)*

FOLLOW-UP PHASE

1. Record flow rate used and immediate patient response.

2. Assess patient's condition, ABG or SaO_2, and the functioning of equipment at regular intervals.

3. Determine patient comfort with oxygen use.

1. Note the patient's tolerance of treatment. Report any intolerance noted.
2. Depression of hypoxic drive is most likely to occur within the first hours of oxygen use. Monitoring of SaO_2 with oximetry can be substituted for ABG if the patient is not retaining CO_2.
3. Flow rates in excess of 4 L/min may cause irritation to the nasal and pharyngeal mucosa.

NURSING ALERT:
Avoid use of petroleum jelly to lubricate nares, because it may clog openings of cannula.

PROCEDURE GUIDELINES 8-15 ◆ Administering Oxygen by Simple Face Mask With/Without Aerosol

EQUIPMENT

Oxygen source
Humidifier bottle with distilled water, if high humidity is desired
Plastic aerosol mask
Large-bore tubing (high humidity) or small-bore tubing

Flowmeter
NO SMOKING signs
For heated aerosol therapy:
    Humidifier heating element

PROCEDURE

NURSING ACTION	RATIONALE

PREPARATORY PHASE

1. Determine current vital signs, level of consciousness, and SaO_2 or ABG, if patient is at risk for CO_2 retention.

2. Assess viscosity and volume of sputum produced.

1. Because the aerosol face mask is a low-flow system (patient's tidal volume may supply part of inspired gas), oxygen concentration will vary depending on the patient's respiratory rate and rhythm. Oxygen delivery may be inadequate for tachypneic patients (flow does not meet peak inspiratory demand) or excessive for patients with slow respirations.
2. Aerosol is given to assist in mobilizing retained secretions.

PERFORMANCE PHASE

1. Post NO SMOKING signs on patient's door and in view of the patient and visitors.
2. Show the aerosol mask to the patient and explain the procedure.
3. Make sure the humidifier is filled to the appropriate mark.
4. Attach the large-bore tubing from the mask to the humidifier in the heating element, if used.
5. Set desired oxygen concentration humidifier bottle and plug in the heating element, if used.

6. If the patient is tachypneic and concentration of 50% oxygen or greater is desired, two humidifiers and flowmeters should be yoked together.
7. Adjust the flow rate until the desired mist is produced (usually 10 to 12 L/min).

8. Apply the mask to the patients' face and adjust the straps so the mask fits securely.

3. If the humidifier bottle is not sufficiently full, less moisture will be delivered.

5. The inspired oxygen concentration is determined by the humidifier setting. Usual concentrations are 35% to 50%.
6. The aerosol mask is a low-flow system. Yoking two humidifiers together doubles humidifier flow but does not change the inspired oxygen concentration.
7. This ensures that the patient is receiving flow sufficient to meet inspiratory demand and maintains a constant accurate concentration of oxygen.

PROCEDURE (cont'd)	NURSING ACTION	RATIONALE

9. Drain the tubing frequently by emptying condensate into a separate receptacle, not into the humidifier. If a heating element is used, the tubing will have to be drained more often.

9. The tubing must be kept free of condensate. Condensate allowed to accumulate in the delivery tube will block flow and alter oxygen concentration. If condensate is emptied into the humidifier, bacteria may be aerosolized into the lungs.

10. If a heating element is used, check the temperature. The humidifier bottle should be warm, not hot, to touch.

10. Excessive temperatures can cause airway burns; patients with elevated temperature should be humidified with an unheated device.

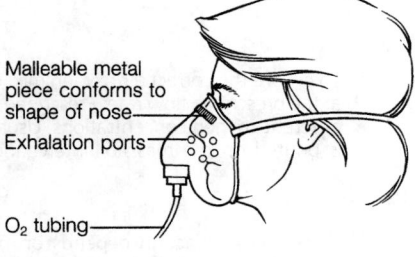

Malleable metal piece conforms to shape of nose

Exhalation ports

O_2 tubing

Simple face mask. Oxygen concentration varies with patient's tidal volume and respiratory rate.

FOLLOW-UP PHASE

1. Record FiO_2 and immediate patient response. Note the patient's tolerance of treatment. Notify the physician if intolerance occurs.

2. Assess the patient's condition and the functioning of equipment at regular intervals.

2. Assess the patient for change in mental status, diaphoresis, changes in blood pressure, and increasing heart and respiratory rates.

3. If the patient's condition changes, assess SaO_2 or ABG.

3. If the patient has a high V_E, flow from the mask may not be sufficient to meet inspiratory needs without pulling in room air. Room air will dilute the oxygen provided and lower the inspired oxygen concentration, resulting in hypoxemia. A change in mask or delivery system may be indicated.

4. Record changes in volume and tenacity of sputum produced.

4. Indicates effectiveness of humidification.

PROCEDURE GUIDELINES 8-16 ◆ Administering Oxygen by Venturi Mask (High air flow oxygen entrainment [HAFOE] system)

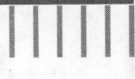

EQUIPMENT

Oxygen source
Flowmeter
Venturi mask for correct concentration (24%, 28%, 31%, 35%, 40%, 50%) or correct concentration adapter if interchangeable color-coded adapters are used

If high humidity desired:
  Compressed air source and flowmeter
  Humidifier with distilled water
  Large-bore tubing
NO SMOKING signs

PROCEDURE	NURSING ACTION	RATIONALE

PREPARATORY PHASE

1. Determine current vital signs, level of consciousness, and most recent ABG.

1. Provides a baseline for future assessment. Venturi masks are used for patients prone to CO_2 retention. Oxygen may depress the hypoxic drive of these patients (evidenced by a decreased respiratory rate, altered mental status, and further $PaCO_2$ elevation).

2. Assess risk of CO_2 retention with oxygen administration.

2. Risk is greater if the patient is experiencing an exacerbation of illness.

(continued)

PROCEDURE GUIDELINES 8-16 ◆ Administering Oxygen by Venturi Mask (High air flow oxygen entrainment [HAFOE] system) *(continued)*

PROCEDURE (cont'd)	NURSING ACTION	RATIONALE

PERFORMANCE PHASE

1. Post NO SMOKING signs on the door of the patient's room and in view of patient and visitors.
2. Show the Venturi mask to the patient and explain the procedure.
3. Connect the mask by lightweight tubing to the oxygen source.
4. Turn on the oxygen flowmeter and adjust to the prescribed rate (usually indicated on the mask). Check to see that oxygen is flowing out the vent holes in the mask.

4. To ensure the correct air/oxygen mix, oxygen must be set at the prescribed flow rate. Prescribed flow rates differ for different oxygen concentrations. Usually this information is printed on the mask or interchangeable color-coded source.

5. Place Venturi mask over the patient's nose and mouth and under the chin. Adjust elastic strap.
6. Check to make sure holes for air entry are not obstructed by the patient's bedding.
7. If high humidity is used:
   a. Connect the humidifier to a compressed air source.
   b. Attach large-bore tubing to the humidifier and connect the tubing to the fitting for high humidity at the base of the Venturi mask.

6. Proper mask function depends on mixing of sufficient amount of air and oxygen.
7. When a Venturi mask is used with high humidity, both an oxygen source and compressed air source are required. The compressed air source provides air for the air/oxygen mix. Excessive oxygen would be inspired if both tubings were connected to an oxygen source.

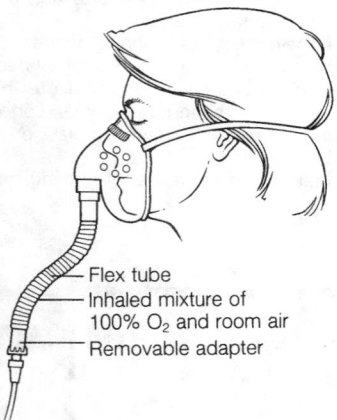

— Flex tube
— Inhaled mixture of 100% O_2 and room air
— Removable adapter

Venturi mask. Constant high concentrations of oxygen can be delivered.

FOLLOW-UP PHASE

1. Record flow rate used and immediate patient response. Note the patient's tolerance of treatment. Report if intolerance occurs.
2. If CO_2 retention is present, assess ABG every 30 minutes for 1 to 2 hours or until the Pao_2 is >50 mm Hg and the $Paco_2$ is no longer increasing. Monitor pH. Report if the pH decreases below the initial assessment value.
3. Determine patient comfort with oxygen use.

1. Depression of hypoxic drive is most likely to occur within the first hours of oxygen use.

2. A modest (5 to 10 mm Hg) increase in $Paco_2$ may occur after initiation therapy. A decreasing pH indicates failure of compensatory mechanisms. Mechanical ventilation may be required.

3. Venturi masks are best tolerated for relatively short periods because of their size and appearance. They also must be removed for eating and drinking. With improvement in patient condition, a nasal cannula may often be substituted.

PROCEDURE GUIDELINES 8-17 ◆ Administering Oxygen by Partial Rebreathing or Nonrebreathing Mask

EQUIPMENT
Oxygen source
Plastic face mask with reservoir bag and tubing
Humidifier with distilled water
Flowmeter
NO SMOKING signs

PROCEDURE

NURSING ACTION	RATIONALE
PREPARATORY PHASE	
1. Determine current vital signs, level of consciousness.	1. Provides a baseline for evaluating patient response. Typically used for short-term support of patients who require a high inspired oxygen concentration.
2. Determine most recent SaO_2 or ABG.	2. Allows objective evaluation of patient response.
PERFORMANCE PHASE	
1. Post NO SMOKING signs on the patient's door and in view of the patient and visitors.	
2. Fill humidifier with distilled water.	2. If the humidifier is not sufficiently full, less moisture will be delivered.
3. Attach tubing to outlet on humidifier.	
4. Attach flowmeter.	
5. Show the mask to the patient and explain the procedure.	
6. Flush the reservoir bag with oxygen to inflate the bag and adjust flowmeter to 6 to 10 L/min.	6. Bag serves as a reservoir, holding oxygen for patient inspiration.
7. Place the mask on the patient's face.	7. Be sure the mask fits snugly, because there must be an airtight seal between the mask and the patient's face.
8. Adjust liter flow so the rebreathing bag will not collapse during the inspiratory cycle, even during deep inspiration.	8. With a well-fitting rebreathing bag adjusted so that the patient's inhalation does not deflate the bag, inspired oxygen concentration of 60% to 90% can be achieved. Some patients may require flow rates higher than 10 L/min to ensure that the bag does not collapse on inspiration.

NURSING ALERT:
1. Adjust the flow to prevent collapse of the bag, even during deep inspiration.
2. A partial rebreathing mask does not have a one-way valve between the mask and reservoir bag. If the bag is allowed to collapse on inspiration, more exhaled air can enter the reservoir and the patient can inhale high concentrations of CO_2.
3. A nonrebreathing mask will deliver a lower concentration of O_2 if the bag is allowed to collapse on inspiration. O_2 from the bag will be diluted by room air drawn in through the side holes of the mask.

NURSING ACTION	RATIONALE
9. Stay with the patient for a time to make the patient comfortable and observe reactions.	
10. Remove mask periodically (if the patient's condition permits) to dry the face around the mask. Powder skin and massage face around the mask.	10. These actions reduce moisture accumulation under the mask. Massage of the face stimulates circulation and reduces pressure over the area.

(continued)

PROCEDURE GUIDELINES 8-17 ◆ Administering Oxygen by Partial Rebreathing or Nonrebreathing Mask
(continued)

PROCEDURE (cont'd)	NURSING ACTION	RATIONALE

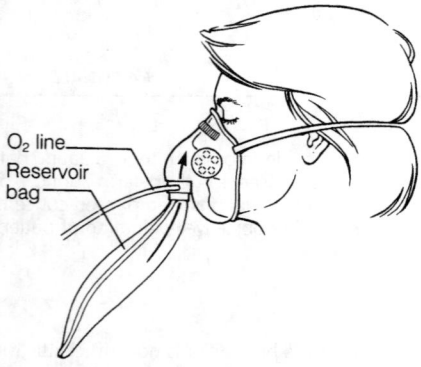

O₂ line
Reservoir bag

Partial rebreathing mask. 100% oxygen fills bag, but concentration delivered varies with respiration. Nonrebreathing mask is similar with the addition of a one-way valve that prevents expired air from entering bag and one-way flaps over exhalation ports.

FOLLOW-UP PHASE

1. Record flow rate and immediate patient response. Note the patient's tolerance of treatment. Report if intolerance occurs.
2. Observe the patient for change of condition. Assess equipment for malfunctioning and low water level in humidifier.

2. Assess the patient for change in mental status, diaphoresis, change in blood pressure, and increasing heart and respiratory rates.

NURSING ALERT:
Monitor functioning of mask to ensure that side ports of mask do not get blocked. This could lead to patient inability to exhale and may lead to suffocation.

PROCEDURE GUIDELINES 8-18 ◆ Administering Oxygen by Transtracheal Catheter

EQUIPMENT
Oxygen source
Transtracheal catheter with connecting tubing
Flowmeter
NO SMOKING signs

PROCEDURE	NURSING ACTION	RATIONALE

PREPARATORY PHASE

1. Determine current vital signs, level of consciousness, and ABG, if patient is at risk for CO_2 retention.
2. Note evidence of infection (warmth, redness, swelling at insertion site) or temperature elevation.

3. Assess catheter patency. Obstruction is indicated by a decreased SaO_2, whistling of the humidifier, high pressure in the delivery tubing, or stimulation of a cough.

1. Provides a baseline for future assessment.

2. The transtracheal catheter provides a direct communication between the skin and trachea. If the insertion site is not kept clean and dry, infection can develop.

3. Mucus can form on the end of the catheter and restrict oxygen delivery. This increases pressure in the delivery tubing and humidifier. The mucus may touch the back of the trachea, stimulating a cough.

PROCEDURE (cont'd)

NURSING ACTION	RATIONALE

PERFORMANCE PHASE

STENT PHASE

1. Post NO SMOKING signs on the patient's door and in view of the patient and visitors.
2. Instruct the patient in purpose of stent.

2. The stent is used to maintain a patent tract during the first week after catheter insertion. It facilitates tract healing and allows gradual adjustment to use of the catheter. It is not used for oxygen delivery.

3. Teach that care of stent involves daily cleaning of the site with cotton-tipped applicators and observation for signs of infection. A 4 × 4 may be placed over the stent.

3. Until the tract heals, the patient is at increased risk for infection. Because the stent is open to the trachea, mucus may be coughed from the stent.

IMMATURE TRACT (STENT IS REMOVED AND TRANSTRACHEAL CATHETER INSERTED)

1. Instruct patient in cleaning and irrigation procedure. The patient should inject one half (1.5 mL) ampule of sterile normal saline into the catheter, insert and remove the cleaning rod three times, and inject the remaining sterile normal saline two to three times a day (morning, noon, evening).

1. The catheter cannot be removed from the tract for cleaning until the tract completely heals (about 2 months). Cleaning in place helps to prevent mucus from forming on the end of the catheter and obstructing oxygen delivery.

2. Teach the patient use of the staged cough technique (ie, sit with feet on floor, pillow over abdomen, inhale three to four times in through the nose and out through the mouth, on the last exhalation cough while bending forward with pillow against abdomen.)

2. Use of this cough technique helps to increase airflow during coughing. Higher airflows help to dislodge any mucus that has formed on the outside of the catheter and cannot be removed by the cleaning technique.

3. Instruct the patient to clean the insertion site daily with cotton-tipped applicators and report signs of infection.

3. Mucus may form at the insertion site. Keeping the tract clean and dry decreases infection risk. DO NOT use hydrogen peroxide because it can dry mucous membranes.

4. Teach the patient to place two small strips of transparent tape over the chain on either side of the catheter for the first 2 weeks of catheter use.

4. This helps to keep the catheter in place during the night when the patient is sleeping. Serves as a second security system to keep the catheter from being inadvertently pulled from the tract during the initial adjustment phase.

5. Instruct the patient to replace the nasal cannula and call for instruction if the catheter is displaced from the tract or if symptoms of subcutaneous emphysema develop (swelling at insertion site, tight chain, change in voice).

5. If the catheter comes out of the tract before it is mature, reinsertion may be difficult. If the tract is not completely healed, O_2 may enter the tissues around the insertion site. The patient may need to return to the clinic for assistance in replacing the catheter or delay using it until the tract is fully healed.

MATURE TRACT (CATHETER IS REMOVED FOR CLEANING)

1. Instruct the patient in steps involved in removing the tract for cleaning. Two catheters are used. The catheter in the tract is removed and replaced with a second catheter. The catheter removed from the tract is cleaned with antibacterial soap under warm running water. It then is air-dried and stored for reuse.

1. The catheter should easily enter the tract. Practicing while looking in a mirror helps to develop skill in removing and reinserting the catheter. This step should be performed twice daily if a catheter with multiple side holes (SCOOP 2) is used. Removal daily, or less often, is necessary with a single end hole catheter (SCOOP 1).

2. Instruct the patient to report immediately signs of infection and difficulty replacing the catheter.

2. These problems are less common with a mature tract, but can still occur.

(continued)

PROCEDURE GUIDELINES 8-18 ◆ Administering Oxygen by Transtracheal Catheter *(continued)*

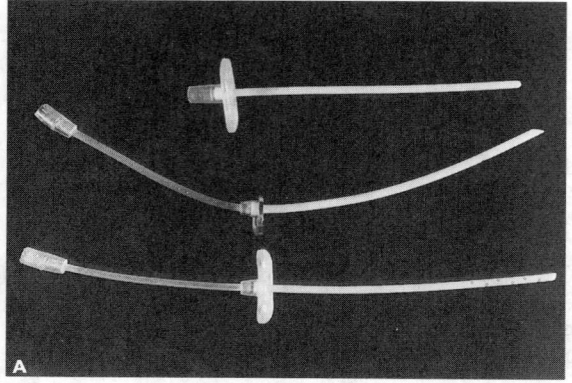
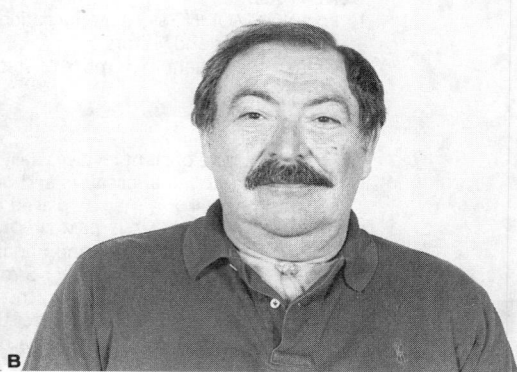
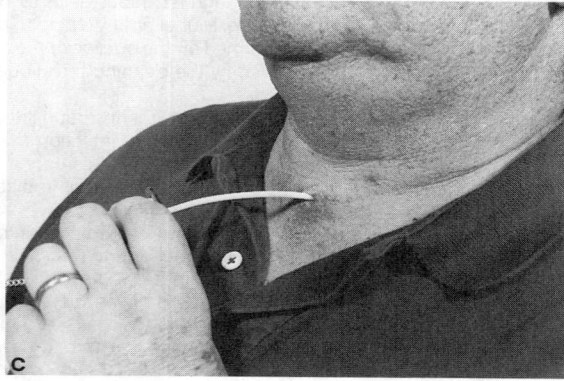
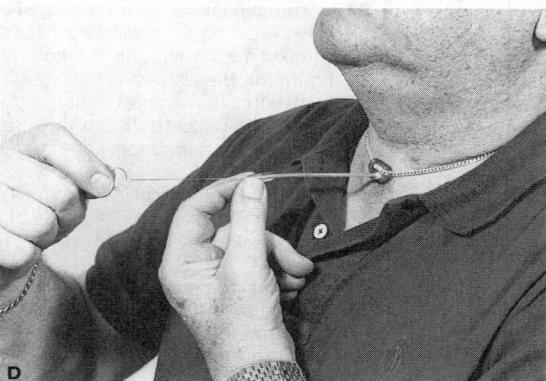

*Administering oxygen by transtracheal catheter. (**A**) Stent (upper), SCOOP 1 (middle), and SCOOP 2 (lower) catheter. (**B**) Transtracheal catheter in place. (**C**) While the tract is immature, the catheter is irrigated and cleaned two or three times a day with a cleaning rod. (**D**) When the tract is mature, the catheter can be removed from the tract for cleaning. (Courtesy of Medical Media Department, Veterans Administration Medical Center, Pittsburgh, PA.)*

PROCEDURE (cont'd)

NURSING ACTION	RATIONALE
FOLLOW-UP PHASE	
1. Record flow rate of oxygen used and patient response.	1. Transtracheal oxygen delivery is more efficient. The same SaO_2 is typically maintained at one half of the former flow rate.
2. Determine patient ability to perform care independently.	2. Repeat demonstration of care may be required before the patient masters self-care skills.
3. Ensure patient is able to demonstrate appropriate use of oxygen and attachment of oxygen to transtracheal catheter.	
4. Discuss with patient signs and symptoms of oxygen toxicity and carbon dioxide retention.	4. Too much carbon dioxide retention could lead to confusion, decreased level of consciousness or somnolence.

PROCEDURE GUIDELINES 8-19 ◆ Administering Oxygen by Continuous Positive Airway Pressure (CPAP) Mask

EQUIPMENT

Oxygen blender
Flowmeter
CPAP mask
Valve for prescribed PEEP (2.5, 5, 7.5, 10 cm H_2O)
Nebulizer with distilled water

Large-bore tubing
Nasogastric tube
Sealing pad to accommodate nasogastric tube
NO SMOKING signs

PROCEDURE

NURSING ACTION	RATIONALE

PREPARATORY PHASE

1. Assess the patient's level of consciousness and gag reflex.

2. Determine current ABGs.

1. CPAP mask may lead to aspiration unless the patient is breathing spontaneously and is able to protect the airway.
2. Document that patient meets criteria for use of this mask (normal or decreased $Paco_2$) and provides baseline to evaluate whether therapy results in CO_2 retention.

NURSING ALERT:
1. CPAP is used when patients have not responded to attempts to increase Pao_2 with other types of masks.
2. The patient will require frequent assessment to detect changes in respiratory status, cardiovascular status, and level of consciousness.
3. If the patient's level of consciousness decreases or ABGs deteriorate, intubation may be necessary.

PERFORMANCE PHASE

1. Post NO SMOKING signs on the patient's door and in view of the patient and visitors.
2. Show the mask to the patient and explain the procedure.
3. Make sure humidifier is filled to the appropriate mark.
4. Insert nasogastric tube.

4. With CPAP, the patient may swallow air, causing gastric distention or emesis. Prophylactic nasogastric suction diminishes this risk.

Note: Some clinicians do not believe a nasogastric tube is needed if the PEEP level is less than 10 cm H_2O.

5. Attach nasogastric tube adapter.
6. Set desired concentration of oxygen blender and adjust flow rate so it is sufficient to meet the patient's inspiratory demand.

5. Use of adapter may decrease air leak around the mask.
6. O_2 blenders are devices that mix air and O_2 using a proportioning valve. Concentrations of 21% to 100% may be delivered, depending on the model. Because the patient will be receiving all minute ventilation from this "closed system," it is essential that the flow rate be adequate to meet changes in the patient's breathing pattern.

7. Place the mask on the patient's face, adjust the head strap, and inflate the mask cushion to ensure a tight seal.

7. To maintain CPAP, an airtight seal is required. Head straps and the inflatable cushion help to ensure that difficult areas, such as the nose and chin, are sealed with greater comfort to the patient.

(continued)

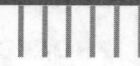

PROCEDURE GUIDELINES 8-19 ◆ Administering Oxygen by Continuous Positive Airway Pressure (CPAP) Mask

(continued)

PROCEDURE (cont'd)	NURSING ACTION	RATIONALE

8. Organize care to remove the mask as infrequently as possible.

8. If mask is removed (for coughing, suctioning), CPAP is not maintained and inspired oxygen concentrations drop.

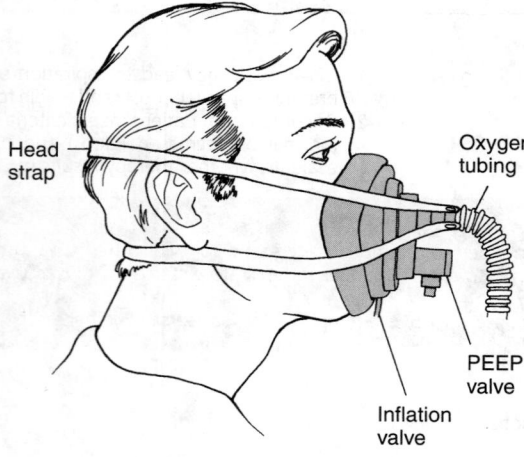

Head strap — Oxygen tubing — PEEP valve — Inflation valve

Administering oxygen by face mask with continuous positive airway pressure (CPAP).

FOLLOW-UP PHASE

1. Assess ABGs, hemodynamic status, and level of consciousness frequently.

1. Provides objective documentation of patient response. CPAP may increase work of breathing, resulting in patient tiring and inability to maintain ventilation without intubation. CPAP may also decrease venous return (PEEP effect), resulting in decreased cardiac output.

2. Immediately report any increase in Pa_{CO_2}.

2. An increase in $PaCO_2$ suggests hypoventilation, resulting from tiring of the patient or inadequate alveolar ventilation. Need for intubation and mechanical ventilation should be evaluated.

3. Assess patency of nasogastric tube at frequent intervals.
4. Assess patient comfort and functioning of the equipment frequently.

3. May become obstructed, causing gastric distention.
4. Tight fit of the mask may predispose to skin breakdown. System may develop leaks, resulting in air escaping between the patient's face and mask.

5. Record patient response. With improvement, oxygen therapy without positive airway pressure can be substituted. With deterioration, intubation and mechanical ventilation may be required. Note the patient's tolerance of treatment. Report if intolerance occurs.

5. Face mask CPAP is usually continued only for short periods (72 hours) because of patient tiring and the necessity to remove mask for suctioning and coughing.

PROCEDURE GUIDELINES 8-20 ◆ Administering Oxygen via Endotracheal and Tracheostomy Tubes With a T-Piece (Briggs) Adapter

EQUIPMENT		

EQUIPMENT

Oxygen
Oxygen blender
Flowmeter
Humidifier with distilled water (heating element may be used as described in aerosol masks)

Large-bore tubing
T-piece and reservoir tubing
NO SMOKING signs

PROCEDURE	NURSING ACTION	RATIONALE

PREPARATORY PHASE

1. Assess patient's SaO_2, hemodynamic status, and level of consciousness frequently. If patient condition changes, assess ABGs.
2. Assess viscosity and volume of sputum produced.

1. Provides baseline to assess response.

2. Aerosol is given to assist in mobilizing retained secretions.

PERFORMANCE PHASE

1. Post NO SMOKING signs on the patient's door and in view of the patient and visitors.
2. Show the T-tube to the patient and explain the procedure.
3. Make sure the humidifier is filled to the appropriate mark.

4. Attach the large-bore tubing from the T-tube to the humidifier outlet.
5. Set desired oxygen concentration of O_2 blender or humidifier bottle and plug in heating element if used.

6. Adjust the flow rate until the desired mist is produced and meets the patient's inspiratory demand.

7. Drain the tubing frequently by emptying condensate into a separate receptacle, not into the humidifier. If a heating element is used, the tubing will have to be drained more often.

8. If a heating element is used, check the temperature. The humidifier bottle should be warm, not hot, to touch.

3. If humidifier is not sufficiently full, less aerosol will be delivered.

5. O_2 blenders are devices that mix air and O_2 using a proportioning valve. Concentrations of 21% to 100% may be delivered at flows of 2 to 100 L/min, depending on the model. Used in situation when precise control is required.
6. The aerosol mist in the reservoir tubing attached to the T-tube should not be completely withdrawn on patient inspiration. If mist is withdrawn (does not extend from reservoir tubing) on inspiration, room air may be inspired and O_2 concentration decreased.
7. The tubing must be kept free of condensate. Condensate allowed to accumulate in the delivery tube will block flow and alter oxygen concentration. If condensate is emptied into the humidifier, bacteria may be aerosolized into the lungs.
8. Excessive temperatures can cause airway burns; patients with elevated temperatures will be better humidified with an unheated device.

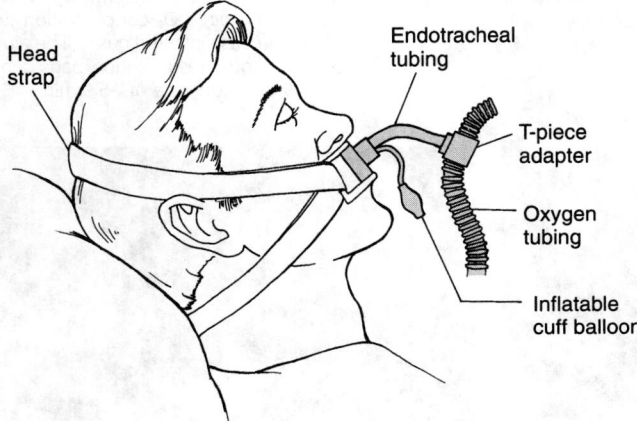

Administering oxygen via endotracheal tube with a T-piece adapter. A T-piece adapter is attached to the endotracheal tube and large-bore tubing, which serves as a source of oxygen and humidity.

FOLLOW-UP PHASE

1. Record FiO_2 and immediate patient response. Note the patient's tolerance of treatment. Report if intolerance occurs.
2. Assess the patient's condition and the functioning of equipment at regular intervals.

3. If the patient's condition changes, assess SaO_2 or ABGs and vital signs. Note changes suggesting increased work of breathing (diaphoresis, intercostal muscle retraction).

4. Record changes in volume and tenacity of sputum produced.

2. Assess the patient for change in mental status, diaphoresis, perspiration, changes in blood pressure, and increasing heart and respiratory rates.
3. If the patient is being weaned, return to the ventilator if changes suggesting inability to tolerate spontaneous ventilation occur (See Weaning the Patient from Mechanical Ventilation, p. 198).
4. Indicates effectiveness of humidification therapy.

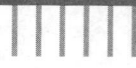

PROCEDURE GUIDELINES 8-21 ◆ Administering Oxygen by Manual Resuscitation Bag

EQUIPMENT

Oxygen source
Resuscitation bag and mask
Reservoir tubing or reservoir bag
O_2 connecting tubing

Nipple adapter to attach flowmeter to connecting tubing
Flowmeter
Gloves
Goggles or other eye protection

PROCEDURE

NURSING ACTION	RATIONALE

PREPARATORY PHASE

1. In cardiopulmonary arrest:
   a. Follow steps to establish that a cardiopulmonary arrest has occurred.

   b. Use caution not to injure or increase injury to the cervical spine when opening the airway.

2. In suctioning or transport situation; Assess patient's heart rate, level of consciousness, and respiratory status.

PERFORMANCE PHASE

1. Attach connecting tubing from flowmeter and nipple adapter to resuscitation bag.

2. Turn flowmeter to ''flush'' position.

3. Attach reservoir tubing or reservoir bag to resuscitation bag.

4. Put on goggles and gloves.

1.
   a. These steps are: establish unresponsiveness; call for help; position the patient on a firm, flat surface; open the mouth and remove vomitus or debris, if visible; assess presence of respirations with the airway open; if apneic, ventilate; palpate the carotid pulse; if absent, deliver chest compressions.
   b. If cervical spine injury is a potential, the modified jaw thrust should be used. In other situations, the head-tilt/chin-lift method can be used. These maneuvers lift the tongue off the back of the throat and, in some situations, may be all that is needed to restore breathing.

2. Provides a baseline to stimulate patient's tolerance of procedure.

1. A humidifier bottle is not used, because the high flow rates of oxygen required would force water into the tubing and clog it.

2. A high flow rate or ''flush'' position is necessary to meet the minute ventilation of the patient.

3. A high inspired O_2 concentration is required. Without a reservoir, inspired O_2 concentration will be low (28% to 56%), because inspired gas will be air/O_2 mix. With a reservoir, manual resuscitation bags can achieve a FiO_2 of >96% at a flow rate of 15 L/min.

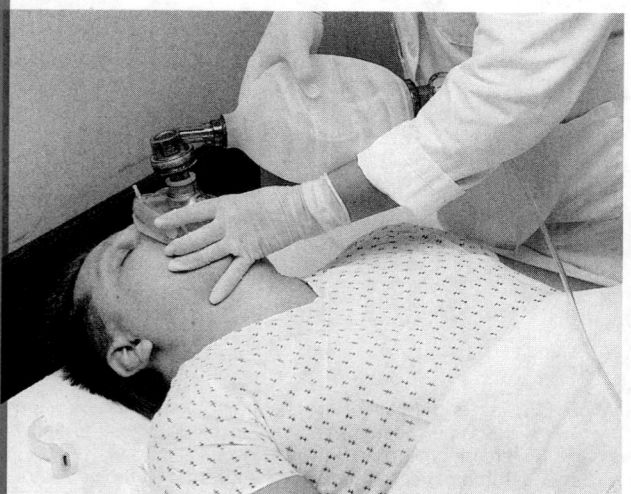 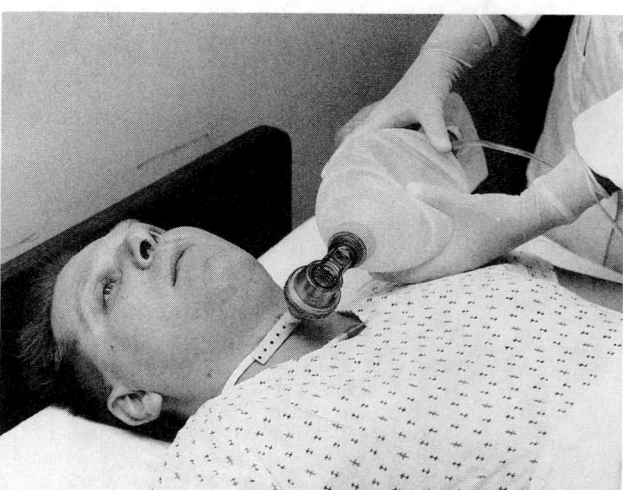

Using a manual resuscitation bag, with mask (left), or connected to an artificial airway (right).

PROCEDURE (cont'd)	NURSING ACTION	RATIONALE

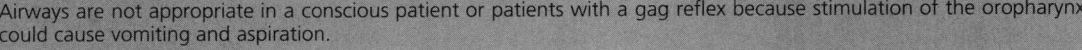

NURSING ALERT:
Ensure that good seal is maintained between face and mask so volume delivered through compression of bag is not lost.

CARDIOPULMONARY ARREST

1. If respirations are absent after the airway is open, insert an oropharyngeal airway and ventilate twice with slow, full breaths of 1 to 1.5 seconds each. Allow 2 seconds between breaths.

1. The airway helps prevent obstruction from prolapse of the tongue in an unconscious patient. If ventilation is difficult, confirm that airway is unobstructed.

NURSING ALERT:
Airways are not appropriate in a conscious patient or patients with a gag reflex because stimulation of the oropharynx could cause vomiting and aspiration.

2. Breaths will have to be quickly interposed between cardiac compressions. If the patient needs only respiratory assistance, watch for chest expansion and listen with the stethoscope to ensure adequate ventilation.
3. A rate of approximately 12 to 15 breaths per minute is used unless the patient is being given external cardiac compressions.

2. Squeeze resuscitation bag with sufficient force and at the rate necessary to maintain adequate minute ventilation.

3. Continue squeezing bag at appropriate interval until CPR is no longer required.

PREOXYGENATION AND SUCTIONING

1. If hyperinflation is being used with suctioning, ventilate the patient before and after each suctioning pass (including after the last suction pass).

1. Hyperinflation before suctioning helps prevent hypoxemia. Hyperinflation after suctioning replaces O_2 removed during the procedure and helps to prevent atelectasis. The larger tidal volumes may also assist in mobilizing secretions and promote surfactant secretion.

TRANSPORT

1. If hyperinflation is used in transport, suction patient before disconnection for transport; monitor heart and respiratory rates and level of consciousness during procedure.
2. Ventilate at rate of 12 to 15 breaths per minute.

1. Establishes a patent airway before patient is moved. Provides information for assessing tolerance of transport.

FOLLOW-UP PHASE

1. In cardiopulmonary arrest, verify return of spontaneous pulse and respirations. Initiate further support as needed.
2. In suctioning or transport, return to previous support. Note patient tolerance of procedure.

1. Establishes patient's need for definitive therapy (drugs, defibrillation, intensive care).
2. Note SaO_2, heart rate, rate and ease of respirations, arterial blood pressure (if monitored), level of consciousness. Report if intolerance occurs.

◆ MECHANICAL VENTILATION

The mechanical ventilator device functions as a substitute for the bellows action of the thoracic cage and diaphragm. The mechanical ventilator can maintain ventilation automatically for prolonged periods. It is indicated when the patient is unable to maintain safe levels of oxygen or carbon dioxide by spontaneous breathing even with the assistance of other oxygen delivery devices.

Clinical Indications

A. *Mechanical Failure of Ventilation*
1. Neuromuscular disease.
2. Central nervous system disease.
3. Central nervous system depression (drug intoxication, respiratory depressants, cardiac arrest).
4. Musculoskeletal disease.
5. Inefficiency of thoracic cage in generating pressure gradients necessary for ventilation (chest injury, thoracic malformation).

B. *Disorders of Pulmonary Gas Exchange*
1. Acute respiratory failure.
2. Chronic respiratory failure.
3. Left ventricular failure.
4. Pulmonary diseases resulting in diffusion abnormality.
5. Pulmonary diseases resulting in ventilation/perfusion mismatch.

Underlying Principles

1. Variables that control ventilation and oxygenation include:
   a. Ventilator rate—adjusted by rate setting.

b. Tidal volume (V_T)—adjusted by tidal volume setting; measured as inhaled volume.
c. Fraction inspired oxygen concentration (FiO_2)—set on ventilator or with an oxygen blender; measured with an oxygen analyzer.
d. Ventilator dead space—circuitry (tubing) common to inhalation and exhalation; tubing is calibrated.
e. PEEP—set within the ventilator or with the use of external PEEP devices; measured at the proximal airway.

2. CO_2 elimination is controlled by tidal volume, rate, and dead space.
3. Oxygen tension is controlled by oxygen concentration and PEEP (also by rate and tidal volume).
4. In most cases, the duration of inspiration should not exceed exhalation.
   a. Rate, tidal volume, gas flow in liters per minute, and inspiratory pause all control inspiratory time.
   b. Inverse inspiration:exhalation (I:E) ratio results in "stacking" of breaths or buildup of pressure within the airway. Barotrauma and decreased cardiac output can result when inverse I:E ratio is used.
5. The inspired gas must be warmed and humidified to prevent thickening of secretions and decrease in body temperature. Sterile water is warmed and humidified by way of a heated humidifier.

Types of Ventilators

A. Negative Pressure Ventilators
1. Applies negative pressure around the chest wall. This causes intra-airway pressure to become negative, thus drawing air into the lungs through the patient's nose and mouth.
2. No artificial airway is necessary; patient must be able to control and protect own airway.
3. Indicated for selected patients with respiratory neuromuscular problems, or as adjunct to weaning from positive pressure ventilation.
4. Examples are the iron lung and cuirass ventilator.

B. Positive Pressure Ventilators
During mechanical inspiration, air is actively delivered to the patient's lungs under positive pressure. Exhalation is passive. Requires use of a cuffed artificial airway.

1. Pressure limited.
   a. Terminates the inspiratory phase when a preselected airway pressure is achieved.
   b. Volume delivered depends on lung compliance.
   c. Use of volume-based alarms is recommended because any obstruction between the machine and lungs that allows a buildup of pressure in the ventilator circuitry will cause the ventilator to cycle, but the patient will receive no volume.
2. Volume limited.
   a. Terminates the inspiratory phase when a designated volume of gas is delivered into the ventilator circuit (10 to 15 mL/kg body weight—usual starting volume).
   b. Delivers the predetermined volume regardless of changing lung compliance (although airway pressures will increase as compliance decreases). Airway pressures vary from patient to patient and from breath to breath.

c. Pressure-limiting valves, which prevent excessive pressure buildup within the patient-ventilator system, are used. Without this valve, pressure could increase indefinitely and pulmonary barotrauma could result. Usually equipped with a system that alarms when selected pressure limit is exceeded and vents excess inspired air to the atmosphere.

Modes of Operation

A. Controlled Ventilation (CV)
1. Cycles automatically at rate selected by operator.
2. Provides a fixed level of ventilation, but will not cycle or have gas available in circuitry to respond to patient's own inspiratory efforts. This typically increases work of breathing for patients attempting to breathe spontaneously.
3. Possibly indicated for patients whose respiratory drive is absent.

B. Assist/Control (A/C)
1. Inspiratory cycle of ventilator is activated by the patient's voluntary inspiratory effort and delivers preset volume.
2. Ventilator also cycles at a rate predetermined by the operator. Should the patient stop breathing, or breathe so weakly that the ventilator cannot function as an assistor, this mandatory baseline rate will prevent apnea. A minimum level of minute ventilation (VE) is provided.
3. Indicated for patients who are breathing spontaneously, but who have the potential to lose their respiratory drive or muscular control of ventilation. In this mode, the patient's work of breathing is greatly reduced.

C. Intermittent Mandatory Ventilation (IMV)
1. Allows patient to breathe spontaneously through ventilator circuitry.
2. Periodically, at preselected rate and volume, cycles to give a "mandated" ventilator breath. A minimum level of ventilation is provided.
3. Gas provided for spontaneous breaths usually flows continuously through the ventilator.
4. Indicated for patients who are breathing spontaneously, but at a tidal volume and/or rate less than adequate for their needs. Allows the patient to do some of the work of breathing.
5. Can cause stacked breaths when machine breath and patient-generated breath occur concurrently.

D. Synchronized Intermittent Mandatory Ventilation (SIMV)
1. Allows patient to breathe spontaneously through the ventilator circuitry.
2. Periodically, at a preselected time, a mandatory breath is delivered. The patient may initiate the mandatory breath with own inspiratory effort, and the ventilator breath will be synchronized with the patient's efforts, or will be "assisted." If the patient does not provide inspiratory effort, the breath will still be delivered, or "controlled."
3. Gas provided for spontaneous breathing is usually delivered through a demand regulator, which is activated by the patient.

4. Indicated for patients who are breathing spontaneously, but at a tidal volume and/or rate less than adequate for their needs. Allows the patient to do some of the work of breathing.

E. *Pressure Support*
1. A positive pressure is set.
2. During spontaneous inspiration, ventilator circuitry is rapidly pressurized to the predetermined pressure and held at this pressure.
3. When the inspiratory flow rate decreases to a preset minimal level (20% to 25% or peak inspiratory flow), the positive pressure returns to baseline. The patient may exhale or complete inspiration without pressure support.
4. The patient ventilates spontaneously, establishing own rate, and inspiring the tidal volume that feels appropriate.
5. Pressure support may be used independently as a ventilatory mode or used in conjunction with CPAP or SIMV.

Special Positive Pressure Ventilation Techniques

A. *Positive End-Expiratory Pressure (PEEP)*
1. Maneuver by which pressure during mechanical ventilation is maintained above atmospheric at end of exhalation, resulting in an increased functional residual capacity. Airway pressure is therefore positive throughout the entire ventilatory cycle.
2. Purpose is to increase functional residual capacity (or the amount of air left in the lungs at the end of expiration). This aids in:
   a. Increasing the surface area of gas exchange.
   b. Preventing collapse of alveolar units and development of atelectasis.
   c. Decreasing intrapulmonary shunt.
3. Benefits
   a. Because a greater surface area for diffusion is available and shunting is reduced, it is often possible to use a lower fraction of inspired oxygen concentration (FiO_2) than otherwise would be required to obtain adequate arterial oxygen levels. This reduces the risk of oxygen toxicity in conditions such as adult respiratory distress syndrome (ARDS).
   b. Positive intra-airway pressure may be helpful in reducing the transudation of fluid from the pulmonary capillaries in situations where capillary pressure is increased (ie, left heart failure).
   c. Increased lung compliance resulting in decreased work of breathing.
4. Hazards
   a. Because the mean airway pressure is increased by PEEP, venous return is impeded. This may result in a decrease in cardiac output (especially noted in hypovolemic patients).
   b. The increased airway pressure may possibly result in alveolar rupture. The likelihood is greater in patients with noncompliant lungs. This barotrauma may result in pneumothorax, tension pneumothorax, or development of subcutaneous emphysema.
   c. The decreased venous return may cause antidiuretic hormone formation to be stimulated, resulting in decreased urine output.

5. Precautions
   a. Monitor frequently for signs and symptoms of pneumothorax (increased pulmonary artery pressure, increased size of hemithorax, decreased lung movement, hyperresonant percussion, diminished breath sounds).
   b. Monitor for signs of decreased venous return (decreased blood pressure, decreased cardiac output, decreased urine output, peripheral edema).
   c. Abrupt discontinuance of PEEP is not recommended. The patient should not be without PEEP for longer than 15 seconds. The manual resuscitation bag used for ventilation during suction procedure or patient transport should be equipped with a PEEP device. In-line suctioning may also be used so PEEP can be maintained. Some clinicians feel that loss of PEEP for short periods is not detrimental in the lower ranges (less than 10 cm H_2O). An exception might be patients with increased intracranial pressure.
   d. Intrapulmonary blood vessel pressure may increase because of compression of the vessels by increased intra-airway pressure. Therefore, central venous pressure (CVP) and pulmonary artery pressure (PAP) and pulmonary capillary wedge pressure (PCWP) may be increased. The clinician must bear this in mind when determining the clinical significance of these pressures.

B. *Continuous Positive Airway Pressure (CPAP)*
1. Also provides for positive airway pressure during all parts of a respiratory cycle, but refers to spontaneous ventilation rather than mechanical ventilation.
2. May be delivered through ventilator circuitry when ventilator rate is at "0" or may be delivered through a separate CPAP circuitry that does not require the ventilator.
3. Indicated for patients who are capable of maintaining an adequate tidal volume, but who have pathology preventing maintenance of adequate levels of tissue oxygenation.
4. CPAP has the same benefits, hazards, and precautions noted with PEEP. Mean airway pressures may be lower because of lack of mechanical ventilation breaths. This results in less risk of barotrauma and impedance of venous return.

Newer Modes of Ventilation

A. *Inverse Ratio Ventilation (IRV)*
1. I:E ratio is greater than 1 (normally inspiration is shorter than expiration).
2. Potentially used in patients who are in acute severe hypoxemic respiratory failure. Oxygenation is thought to be improved.
3. Used with heavily sedated patients.
4. Still under investigation—only used in rare cases.

B. *Noninvasive Positive Pressure Ventilation (NIPPV)*
1. Uses a nasal mask, nasal pillow, oral mask or mouthpiece attached to a standard ventilator. Delivers air through portable ventilator that is either volume-cycled or flow-cycled.
2. Used primarily in the past for patients with chronic respiratory failure associated with neuromuscular disease. Now, is being used somewhat successfully during acute exacerbations. Some patients are able to avoid invasive intubation. Other indications include weaning and postextubation respiratory decompensation.

3. Used easily in home setting—equipment is portable and relatively easy to use.

C. High-Frequency Ventilation (HFV)
1. Uses very small tidal volumes (less than dead space volume) and high frequency (ratios greater than 100).
2. Gas exchange occurs through various mechanisms, not the same as conventional ventilation (convection).
3. Types
  a. High-frequency oscillatory ventilation (HFOV)
  b. High-frequency jet ventilation (HFJV)
4. Theory is that there is decreased barotrauma by having small tidal volumes and that oxygenation is improved by constant flow of gases.
5. Has not yet proven to be significantly helpful, but is being tested in neonates (HFOV), and in adults for the treatment of ARDS (HFJV), as well as bronchopleural fistulas (HFJV).

Nursing Assessment and Interventions

1. Monitor for complications.
  a. Airway obstruction (thickened secretions, mechanical problem with artificial airway or ventilator circuitry)
  b. Tracheal damage
  c. Pulmonary infection
  d. Barotrauma (pneumothorax or tension pneumothorax)
  e. Decreased cardiac output
  f. Atelectasis
  g. Alteration in GI function (dilation, bleeding)
  h. Alteration in renal function
  i. Alteration in cognitive-perceptual status

2. Suction the patient as indicated.
  a. When secretions can be seen or sounds resulting from secretions are heard with or without the use of a stethoscope.
  b. After chest physiotherapy.
  c. After bronchodilator treatments.
  d. After a sudden rise or the "popping off" of the peak airway pressure in mechanically ventilated patients that is not due to the artificial airway or ventilator tube kinking, the patient biting the tube, the patient coughing or struggling against the ventilator, or a pneumothorax.
  e. Routine suction is not indicated, but should be based on assessment, patient's underlying condition, and chest X-ray findings.
3. Provide routine care for patient on mechanical ventilator. (See Procedure Guidelines 8-22.)
4. Assist with the weaning process, when indicated (patient gradually assumes responsibility for regulating and performing own ventilations). (See Procedure Guidelines 8-23.)
  a. Patient must have acceptable ABGs, no evidence of acute pulmonary pathology, and be hemodynamically stable.
  b. Obtain serial ABGs and/or oximetry readings, as indicated.
  c. Monitor very closely for change in pulse and blood pressure, anxiety, and increased rate of respirations.
  d. The use of anxiolytics to assist with weaning the anxious patient is controversial; they may or may not be beneficial.
5. Once weaning is successful, extubate and provide alternate means of oxygen. (See Procedure Guidelines 8-24.)
  a. Extubation will be considered when the pulmonary function parameters of tidal volume (V_T), vital capacity (VC), and negative inspiratory force (NIF) are adequate, indicating strong respiratory muscle function.

(text continues on page 201)

PROCEDURE GUIDELINES 8-22 ◆ Managing the Patient Requiring Mechanical Ventilation

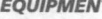

EQUIPMENT   Artificial airway
Mechanical ventilator
Ventilation circuitry
Humidifier
See manufacturer's directions for specific machine.

PROCEDURE	NURSING ACTION	RATIONALE
	PREPARATORY PHASE	
	1. Obtain baseline samples for blood gas determinations (pH, Pa_{O_2}, Pa_{CO_2}, HCO_3) and chest x-ray.	1. Baseline measurements serve as a guide in determining progress of therapy.
	PERFORMANCE PHASE	
	1. Give a brief explanation to the patient.	1. Emphasize that mechanical ventilation is a temporary measure. The patient should be prepared psychologically for weaning at the time the ventilator is first used.
	2. Establish the airway by means of a cuffed endotracheal or tracheostomy tube (see p. 157).	2. A closed system between the ventilator and patient's lower airway is necessary for positive pressure ventilation.

PROCEDURE (cont'd)	NURSING ACTION	RATIONALE

NURSING ACTION

3. Prepare the ventilator. (Respiratory therapist does this in many institutions.)
   a. Set up desired circuitry.
   b. Connect oxygen and compressed air source.
   c. Turn on power.
   d. Set tidal volume (usually 10 to 15 mL/kg body weight).
   e. Set oxygen concentration.
   f. Set ventilator sensitivity.
   g. Set rate at 12 to 14 breaths per minute (variable).

   h. Adjust flow rate (velocity of gas flow during inspiration). Usually set at 40 to 60 L/min. Is dependent on rate and tidal volume. Set to avoid inverse inspiratory:expiratory (I:E) ratio. Usual I:E ratio is 1:2.

   i. Select mode of ventilation.
   j. Check machine function—measure tidal volume, rate, I:E ratio, analyze oxygen, check all alarms.
4. Couple the patient's airway to the ventilator.

5. Assess patient for adequate chest movement and rate. Do not depend on digital rate readout of ventilator. Note peak airway pressure and PEEP. Adjust gas flow if necessary to provide safe I:E ratio.
6. Set airway pressure alarms according to patient's baseline:
   a. High pressure alarm

   b. Low pressure alarm

7. Assess frequently for change in respiratory status via ABGs, pulse oximetry, spontaneous rate, use of accessory muscles, breath sounds, and vital signs. Other means of assessing are through the use of exhaled carbon dioxide (Capnography, p. 153 or mixed venous oxygen saturation monitoring, p. 261). If change is noted, notify appropriate personnel.
8. Monitor and troubleshoot alarm conditions. Ensure appropriate ventilation at all times.

RATIONALE

d. Adjusted according to pH and $Paco_2$.

e. Adjusted according to Pao_2.

g. This setting approximates normal ventilation. These machines' settings are subject to change according to the patient's condition and response, and the ventilator type being used.
h. The slower the flow, the lower will be the peak airway pressure resulting from set volume delivery. This results in lower intrathoracic pressure and less impedance of venous return. However, a flow that is too low for the rate selected may result in inverse inspiratory:expiratory ratios.

j. Ensures safe function.
4. Be sure all connections are secure. Prevent ventilator tubing from "pulling" on artificial airway, possibly resulting in tube dislodgement or tracheal damage.
5. Ensures proper function of equipment.

6.

   a. High airway pressure or "pop off" pressure is set at about 20 cm H_2O above peak airway pressure. An alarm sounds if airway pressure selected is exceeded. Alarm activation indicates: decreased lung compliance (worsening pulmonary disease); decreased lung volume (such as pneumothorax, tension pneumothorax, hemothorax, pleural effusion); increased airway resistance (secretions, coughing, breathing out of phase with the ventilator); loss of patency of airway (mucous plug, airway spasm, biting or kinking of tube).
   b. Low airway pressure alarm set at 5 to 10 cm H_2O below peak airway pressure. Alarm activation indicates inability to build up airway pressure because of disconnection or leak, or inability to build up airway pressure because of insufficient gas flow to meet patient's inspiratory needs.

8. Priority is ventilation and oxygenation of the patient. In alarm conditions that cannot be immediately corrected, disconnect the patient from mechanical ventilation and manually ventilate with resuscitation bag.

(continued)

PROCEDURE GUIDELINES 8-22 ◆ Managing the Patient Requiring Mechanical Ventilation *(continued)*

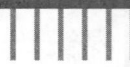

PROCEDURE (cont'd)	NURSING ACTION	RATIONALE

9. Positioning
   a. Turn patient from side to side every 2 hours, or more frequently if possible.

   b. Lateral turns of 120 degrees are desirable; from right semiprone to left semiprone.
   c. Sit the patient upright at regular intervals if possible.

9.
   a. For patients on long-term ventilation, this may result in sleep deprivation. Evolve a turning schedule best suited to a particular patient's condition.

   c. Upright posture increases lung compliance.

NURSING ALERT:
For patients in severe compromised respiratory state or who are unstable hemodynamically, consider use of specialty bed with rotational therapy. New versions may also have built-in vibration and percussion as adjunct therapy options.

10. Carry out passive range-of-motion exercises of all extremities for patients unable to do so.
11. Assess for need of suctioning at least every 2 hours.

12. Assess breath sounds every 2 hours:
    a. Listen with stethoscope to the chest from bottom to top on both sides.

    b. Determine whether breath sounds are present or absent, normal or abnormal, and whether a change has occurred.
    c. Observe the patient's diaphragmatic excursions and use of accessory muscles of respiration.
13. Humidification
    a. Check the water level in the humidification reservoir to ensure that the patient is never ventilated with dry gas. Empty the water that condenses in the delivery and exhalation tubing into a separate receptacle, not into the humidifier. Always wash hands after emptying fluid from ventilator circuitry. Humidifier must be changed every 24 hours.
14. Assess airway pressures at frequent intervals.

15. Measure delivered tidal volume and analyze oxygen concentration every 4 hours or more frequently if indicated.
16. Monitor cardiovascular function. Assess for depression.
    a. Monitor pulse rate and arterial blood pressure; intraarterial pressure monitoring may be carried out.
    b. Use Swan-Ganz catheter to monitor pulmonary capillary wedge pressure, mixed venous oxygen, and cardiac output.
17. Monitor for pulmonary infection.
    a. Aspirate tracheal secretions into a sterile container and send to laboratory for culture and sensitivity testing. This is done immediately after endotracheal intubation and in some instances on an every-other-day basis.
    b. Daily Gram's staining of secretions may also be done in some institutions.
    c. Monitor for systemic signs and symptoms of pulmonary infection (pulmonary physical examination findings, increased heart rate, increased temperature, increased WBC count).

11. Patients with artificial airways on mechanical ventilation are unable to clear secretions on their own. Suctioning may help to clear secretions and stimulate the cough reflex.
12.
    a. Auscultation of the chest is a means of assessing airway patency and ventilatory distribution. It also confirms the proper placement of the endotracheal or tracheostomy tube.

13.
    a. Water condensing in the inspiratory tubing may cause increased resistance to gas flow. This may result in increased peak airway pressures. Warm, moist tubing is a perfect breeding area for bacteria. If this water is allowed to enter the humidifier, bacteria may be aerosolized into the lungs. Emptying the tubing also prevents introduction of water into the patient's airways.
14. Monitor for changes in compliance, or onset of conditions that may cause airway pressure to increase or decrease.

16.
    a. Arterial catheterization for intraarterial pressure monitoring also provides access for ABG samples.
    b. Intermittent and continuous positive pressure ventilation may increase the pulmonary artery pressures and decrease cardiac output.
17.
    a. This technique allows for the earliest detection of infection or change in infecting organisms in the tracheobronchial tree.

PROCEDURE (cont'd)	NURSING ACTION	RATIONALE

18. Evaluate need for sedation or muscle relaxants.

18. Sedatives may be prescribed to decrease anxiety, or to relax the patient to prevent "competing" with the ventilator. At times, pharmacologically induced paralysis may be necessary to permit mechanical ventilation.

NURSING ALERT:
Never administer paralyzing agents until the patient is intubated and on mechanical ventilation. Sedatives should be prescribed in conjunction with paralyzing agents.

19. Report intake and output precisely and obtain an accurate daily weight to monitor fluid balance.

19. Positive fluid balance resulting in increase in body weight and interstitial pulmonary edema is a frequent problem in patients requiring mechanical ventilation. Prevention requires early recognition of fluid accumulation. An average adult who is dependent on parenteral nutrition can be expected to lose 0.25 kg (½ lb)/day; therefore, constant body weight indicates positive fluid balance.

20. Monitor nutritional status.

20. Patients on mechanical ventilation require inflation of artificial airway cuffs at all times. Patients with tracheostomy tubes may eat, if capable, or may require enteral feeding tubes or parenteral nourishment. Patients with endotracheal tubes are to be NPO (the tube splints the epiglottis open) and must be entirely tube fed or parenterally nourished.

21. Monitor GI function.

   a. Test all stools and gastric drainage for occult blood.

   b. Measure abdominal girth daily.

21. Mechanically ventilated patients are at risk for development of stress ulcers.

   a. Stress may cause some patients requiring mechanical ventilation to develop GI bleeding.

   b. Abdominal distention occurs frequently with respiratory failure and further hinders respiration by elevation of the diaphragm. Measurement of abdominal girth provides objective assessment of the degree of distention.

22. Provide for care and communication needs of patient with an artificial airway.

23. Provide psychological support.

   a. Assist with communication.
   b. Orient to environment and function of mechanical ventilator.
   c. Ensure that the patient has adequate rest and sleep.

23. Mechanical ventilation may result in sleep deprivation and loss of touch with surroundings and reality.

FOLLOW-UP PHASE

1. Maintain a flow sheet to record ventilation patterns, ABGs, venous chemical determinations, hemoglobin and hematocrit, status of fluid balance, weight, and assessment of the patient's condition. Notify appropriate personnel of changes in the patient's condition.
2. Change ventilator circuitry every 24 hours; assess ventilator's function every 4 hours or more frequently if problem occurs.

1. Establishes means of assessing effectiveness and progress of treatment.

2. Prevents contamination of lower airways.

PROCEDURE GUIDELINES 8-23 ◆ Weaning the Patient From Mechanical Ventilation

EQUIPMENT   Varies according to technique used
Briggs T-piece (see earlier section)
IMV or SIMV (set up in addition to ventilator or incorporated in ventilator and circuitry)
Pressure support

PROCEDURE	NURSING ACTION	RATIONALE

PREPARATORY PHASE

1. For weaning to be successful, the patient must be physiologically capable of maintaining spontaneous respirations. Assessments must ensure that:
   a. The underlying disease process is significantly reversed, as evidenced by pulmonary examination, ABGs, chest x-ray.
   b. The patient can mechanically perform ventilation. Should be able to generate a negative inspiratory force (NIF) > -20 cm H_2O, have a vital capacity (VC) 10 to 15 mL/kg; have a resting minute ventilation (V_E) < 10 L/min; and be able to double this; have a spontaneous respiratory rate of <25 breaths per minute; without significant tachycardia; not be hypotensive; have optimal hemoglobin for condition; have adequate nutritional status.

   1. Provides baseline; ensures that patient is capable of having adequate neuromuscular control to provide adequate ventilation.

2. Assess for other factors that may cause respiratory insufficiency.
   a. Acid–base abnormality
   b. Nutritional depletion
   c. Electrolyte abnormality
   d. Fever
   e. Abnormal fluid balance
   f. Hyperglycemia
   g. Infection
   h. Pain
   i. Sleep deprivation
   j. Decreased level of consciousness

   2. Weaning is difficult when these conditions are present.

3. Assess psychological readiness for weaning.

   3. Patient must be physically and psychologically ready for weaning.

PERFORMANCE PHASE

1. Ensure psychological preparation. Explain procedure and that weaning is not always successful on the initial attempt.

   1. Explaining procedure to patient will decrease patient anxiety and promote cooperation. The patient should not be discouraged if weaning is unsuccessful on the first attempt.

2. Prepare appropriate equipment.
3. Position the patient in sitting or semi-Fowler's position.
4. Pick optimal time of day, preferably early morning.
5. Perform bronchial hygiene necessary to ensure that the patient is in best condition (postural drainage, suctioning) before weaning attempt.

   3. Increase lung compliance, decreases work of breathing.
   4. The patient should be rested.
   5. The patient should be in best pulmonary condition for weaning to be successful.

T-PIECE
This system provides oxygen enrichment and humidity to a patient with an endotracheal or tracheostomy tube while allowing completely spontaneous respirations (for set-up and function see oxygen delivery section).

1. Discontinue mechanical ventilation and apply T-piece adapter.

   1. Stay with the patient during weaning time to decrease patient anxiety and monitor for tolerance of procedure.

2. Monitor the patient for factors indicating need for reinstitution of mechanical ventilation.
   a. Blood pressure increase or decrease greater than 20 mm Hg systolic or 10 mm Hg diastolic
   b. Heart rate increase of 20 beats/min or greater than 110

   2. Indicates intolerance of weaning procedure.

PROCEDURE (cont'd)	NURSING ACTION	RATIONALE

NURSING ACTION

   c. Respiratory rate increase greater that 10 breaths/min or rate greater than 30
   d. Tidal volume less than 250 to 300 mL (in adults)
   e. Appearance of new cardiac ectopy, or increase in baseline ectopy
   f. Pao_2 less than 60, $Paco_2$ greater than 55, or pH less than 7.35 (may accept lower Pao_2 and pH, and higher $Paco_2$ in patients with COPD)

3. Increase time off ventilator with each weaning attempt as the patient's condition indicates. Evaluate for toleration before moving to the next increment.
4. Institute other techniques helpful in encouraging weaning.
   a. Mental stimulation
   b. Biofeedback
   c. Participation in care
   d. Provision of rewards
   e. Contact with successfully weaned patients
5. When patient tolerates 40 to 60 min of continuous weaning, weaning increments can increase rapidly.
6. When the patient can maintain spontaneous ventilation throughout day, begin night weaning.

CPAP WEANING
1. The principles and techniques for CPAP weaning are the same as for T-piece weaning.
2. The patient breathes with CPAP at low level (2.5 to 5 cm H_2O), rather than with the T-piece, for periods that increase in length.

IMV OR SIMV WEANING
1. Set ventilator to IMV or SIMV mode.
2. Set rate interval.

3. If the patient is on continuous flow IMV circuitry, observe reservoir bag to be sure that it remains mostly inflated during all phases of ventilation.
4. If gas for the patient's spontaneous breath is delivered via a demand valve regulator, ensure that machine sensitivity is at maximum setting.
5. Evaluate for tolerance of procedure. Monitor for factors indicating need for increase or decrease of mandatory respiratory rate (see step 3 of T-piece adaptor section above). In rapid weaning, changes may be made approximately every 20 to 30 min.
6. If $Paco_2$ and pH levels remain stable, then continue to decrease mandatory rate as patient tolerates.

PRESSURE SUPPORT
1. May be beneficial adjunct to IMV or SIMV weaning.
2. The amount of pressure support (cm H_2O) provided to the airway is progressively decreased over time, allowing the patient to increase role in supporting own spontaneous ventilation.

FOLLOW-UP PHASE
1. Record at each weaning interval: heart rate, blood pressure, respiratory rate, FiO_2, ABG, pulse oximetry value, respiratory and ventilator rate (if IMV or SIMV), or length of time off ventilator (if T-piece weaning).
Note: It is not within the scope of this manual to establish criteria for the use of one weaning modality as opposed to another.

RATIONALE

3. The patient will progress as he or she becomes mentally and physically able to perform adequate spontaneous ventilation.
4. Provides motivation and positive feedback.

1. This weaning technique is preferred for patients prone to atelectasis when placed on a T-piece.

2. This determines the time interval between machine-delivered breaths, during which the patient will breathe on own.
3. The gas flow rate into the bag must be adequate to prevent the bag from collapsing during inspiration. Flow rates of 6 to 10 L/min are usually adequate.
4. Aids in decreasing work of breathing necessary to open demand valve.
5. If the patient does not tolerate the procedure, the $Paco_2$ will rise and pH will fall.

6. May be done as frequently as every 20 to 30 min with ABG monitoring, pulse oximetry, documentation of successful weaning.

1. Provides record of procedure and assessment of progress.

PROCEDURE GUIDELINES 8-24 ◆ Extubation

EQUIPMENT
Tonsil suction (surgical suction instrument)
10-mL syringe
Resuscitation bag and mask with oxygen flow
Face mask connected to large-bore tubing, humidifier, and
  oxygen source

Suction catheter
Suction source
Gloves, goggles, or other eye protection device

PROCEDURE	NURSING ACTION	RATIONALE

PREPARATORY PHASE

1. Monitor heart rate, lung expansion, and breath sounds before extubation. Record V_T, VC, NIF.
2. Assess the patient for other signs of adequate muscle power.
   a. Instruct the patient to tightly squeeze the index and middle fingers of your hand. Resistance to removal of your fingers from the patient's grasp must be demonstrated.
   b. Ask the patient to lift head from the pillow and hold for 2 to 3 seconds.

1. V_T, VC, and NIF are measured to assess respiratory muscle function and adequacy of ventilation.
2. Adequate muscle strength is necessary to ensure maintenance of a patent airway.

NURSING ALERT:
Keep in mind that patient's underlying problems must be improved or resolved before extubation is considered. Patient should also be free from infection and malnutrition.

PERFORMANCE PHASE

1. Obtain orders for extubation and postextubation oxygen therapy.
2. Explain the procedure to the patient:
   a. Artificial airway will be removed.
   b. Suctioning will occur before extubation.
   c. Deep breath should be taken on command.
   d. Instruction will be given to cough after extubation.
3. Prepare necessary equipment. Have ready for use tonsil suction, suction catheter, 10-mL syringe, bag-mask unit, and oxygen via face mask.
4. Place patient in sitting or semi-Fowler's position (unless contraindicated).
5. Put on goggles.
6. Suction endotracheal tube.
7. Suction oropharyngeal airway above the endotracheal cuff as thoroughly as possible.
8. Put on gloves. Loosen tape or endotracheal tube-securing device.
9. Extubate the patient:
   a. Ask the patient to take as deep a breath as possible (if the patient is not following commands, give a deep breath with the resuscitation bag).
   b. At peak inspiration, deflate the cuff completely and pull the tube out in the direction of the curve (out and downward).
10. Once the tube is fully removed, ask the patient to cough or exhale forcefully to remove secretions. Then suction the back of the patient's airway with the tonsil suction.

11. Evaluate immediately for any signs of airway obstruction, stridor, or difficult breathing. If the patient develops any of the above problems, attempt to ventilate the patient with the resuscitation bag and mask and prepare for reintubation. (Nebulized treatments may be ordered to avoid having to reintubate patient.)

1. Do not attempt extubation until postextubation oxygen therapy is available and functioning at the bedside.
2. Increases patient cooperation.

4. Increases lung compliance and decreases work of breathing. Facilitates coughing.
5. Spraying of airway secretions may occur.
7. Secretions not cleared from above the cuff will be aspirated when the cuff is deflated.

9.
   a. At peak inspiration, the trachea and vocal cords will dilate, allowing a less traumatic tube removal.

10. Frequently, old blood is seen in the secretions of newly extubated patients. Monitor for the appearance of bright red blood due to trauma occurring during extubation.
11. Immediate complications:
   a. Laryngospasm may develop, causing obstruction of the airway.
   b. Edema may develop at the cuff site. Signs of narrowing airway lumen are high-pitched crowing sounds, decreased air movement, and respiratory distress.

PROCEDURE (cont'd)	NURSING ACTION	RATIONALE
	FOLLOW-UP PHASE	
	1. Note patient tolerance of procedure, upper and lower airway sounds postextubation, description of secretions.	1. Establishes a baseline to assess improvement/development of complications.
	2. Observe patient closely postextubation for any signs and symptoms of airway obstruction or respiratory insufficiency.	2. Tracheal or laryngeal edema develop postextubation (a possibility for up to 24 hours). Signs and symptoms include high-pitched, crowing upper airway sounds and respiratory distress.
	3. Observe character of voice.	3. Hoarseness is a common postextubation complaint. Observe for worsening hoarseness or vocal cord paralysis.

◆ THORACIC SURGERIES (Table 8-2)

Thoracic surgeries are operative procedures performed to aid in the diagnosis and treatment of certain pulmonary conditions. Procedures include thoracotomy, lobectomy (Fig. 8-6), pneumonectomy, segmental resection, and wedge resection. These procedures may or may not require chest drainage immediately after surgery.

> **NURSING ALERT:**
> Meticulous attention must be given to the preoperative and postoperative care of patients undergoing thoracic surgery. These operations are wide in scope and represent a major stress on the cardiorespiratory system.

Preoperative Management/ Nursing Care

Goal is to maximize respiratory function to improve the outcome postoperatively and reduce risk of complications.

1. Encourage the patient to stop smoking to restore bronchial ciliary action and to reduce the amount of sputum and likelihood of postoperative atelectasis.
2. Teach an effective coughing technique.
   a. Sit upright with knees flexed and body bending slightly forward (or lie on side with hips and knees flexed if unable to sit up).
   b. Splint the incision with hands or folded towel.
   c. Take three short breaths, followed by a deep inspiration, inhaling slowly and evenly through the nose.

TABLE 8-2 Thoracic Surgery Types

Types	Descriptions	Indications
Exploratory thoracotomy	Internal view of lung • Usually posterolateral parascapular but could be anterior incision • Chest tubes after procedure	May be used to confirm carcinoma or for chest trauma (to detect source of bleeding)
Lobectomy	Lobe removal • Thoractomy incison at site of lobe removal • Chest tubes after procedure	Used when pathology is limited to one area of lung: bronchogenic carcinoma, giant emphysematous blebs, or bullae, benign tumors, metastatic malignant tumors, bronchiectasis and fungus infections
Pneumonectomy	Removal of an entire lung • Posterolateral or anterolateral thoracotomy incision • Sometimes there is a rib resection • No chest drains/tubes usually because fluid accumulation in empty space is desirable	Performed chiefly for carcinoma, but may be used for lung abscesses, bronchiectasis, or extensive tuberculosis *Note:* Right lung is more vascular than left; may cause more physiologic problems if removed
Segmentectomy (segmental resection)	Only certain segment of lung removed • Segments function as individual units	Used when pathology is very localized (ie, bronchiectasis) and when patient has preexisting cardiopulmonary compromise
Wedge resection	Small localized section of lung tissue removed—usually pie-shaped • Incision made without regard to segments • Chest tubes after procedure	Performed for random lung biopsy and small peripheral nodules

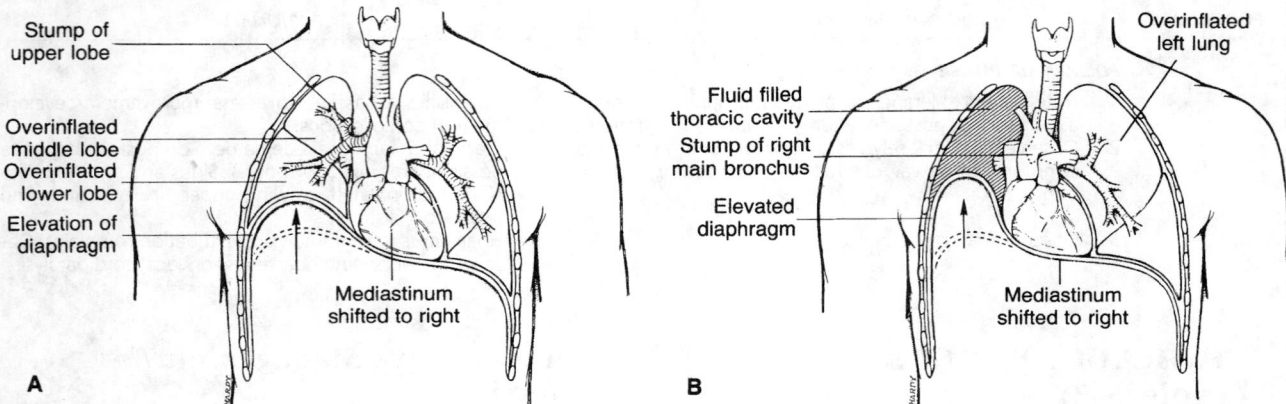

FIGURE 8-6 *Operative procedures. (A) Lobectomy. (B) Pneumonectomy.*

d. Contract abdominal muscles and cough twice forcefully with mouth open and tongue out.
e. Alternate technique—huffing and coughing—is less painful.
   (1) Take a deep diaphragmatic breath and exhale forcefully against hand; exhale in a quick distinct pant, or "huff."
3. Humidify the air to loosen secretions.
4. Administer bronchodilators to reduce bronchospasm.
5. Administer antimicrobials for infection.
6. Encourage deep breathing with the use of incentive spirometer (see Procedure Guidelines 8-25) to prevent atelectasis postoperatively.
7. Teach diaphragmatic breathing (see p. 173).
8. Carry out chest physical therapy and postural drainage to reduce pooling of lung secretions.
9. Evaluate cardiovascular status for risk and prevention of complication.
10. Encourage activity to improve exercise tolerance.
11. Administer medications and limit sodium and fluid to improve congestive heart failure, if indicated.
12. Correct anemia, dehydration, and hypoproteinemia with intravenous infusions, tube feedings, and blood transfusions as indicated.
13. Give prophylactic anticoagulant as prescribed to reduce perioperative incidence of deep vein thrombosis and pulmonary embolism.
14. Provide teaching and counseling.
    a. Orient the patient to events that will occur in the postoperative period—coughing and deep breathing, suctioning, chest tube and drainage bottles, oxygen therapy, ventilator therapy, pain control, leg exercises and range-of-motion exercises for affected shoulder.
15. Ensure that patient fully understands surgery and is emotionally prepared for it; verify that informed consent has been obtained.

Postoperative Management/ Nursing Care

1. Use mechanical ventilator until respiratory function and cardiovascular status stabilize. Assist with weaning and extubation.

2. Auscultate chest, monitor vital signs, monitor electrocardiogram (ECG), and assess respiratory rate and depth frequently.
   a. Arterial line, CVP, and pulmonary artery catheter are usually used.
3. Monitor ABGs frequently.
4. Monitor and manage chest drainage system to drain fluid, blood, clots, and air from the pleura after surgery (see p. 205). Chest drainage is usually not used after pneumonectomy, however, because it is desirable that the pleural space fill with an effusion, which eventually obliterates the space.

Complications

1. Hypoxia—watch for restlessness, tachycardia, tachypnea, and elevated blood pressure.
2. Postoperative bleeding—monitor for restlessness, anxiety, pallor, tachycardia, and hypotension.
3. Pneumonia; atelectasis.
4. Bronchopleural fistula from disruption of a bronchial suture or staple; bronchial stump leak.
   a. Observe for sudden onset of respiratory distress or cough productive of serosanguineous fluid.
   b. Position with the operative side down.
   c. Prepare for immediate chest tube insertion and/or surgical intervention.
5. Cardiac dysrhythmias (usually occurring third to fourth postoperative day); myocardial infarction or heart failure.

Nursing Diagnoses

A. Ineffective Breathing Pattern Related to Surgical Procedure
B. Risk for Fluid Volume Deficit Related to Chest Drainage and Blood Loss
C. Pain Related to Chest Incision and Presence of Chest Tubes
D. Impaired Physical Mobility of Affected Shoulder and Arm Related to Surgical Procedure and Chest Drainage

Nursing Interventions

A. *Maintaining Adequate Breathing Pattern*
1. Auscultate chest for adequacy of air movement to detect bronchospasm, consolidation.
2. Obtain ABGs and pulmonary function measurements as ordered.
3. Monitor level of consciousness and inspiratory effort closely to begin weaning from ventilator as soon as possible.
4. Suction frequently using meticulous aseptic technique.

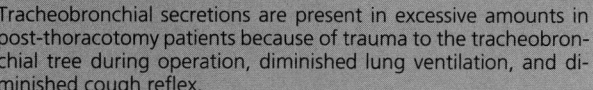

NURSING ALERT:
Tracheobronchial secretions are present in excessive amounts in post-thoracotomy patients because of trauma to the tracheobronchial tree during operation, diminished lung ventilation, and diminished cough reflex.

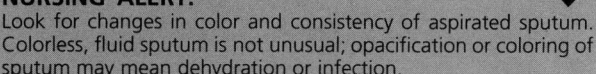

NURSING ALERT:
Look for changes in color and consistency of aspirated sputum. Colorless, fluid sputum is not unusual; opacification or coloring of sputum may mean dehydration or infection.

5. Elevate the head of the bed 30 to 40 degrees when patient is oriented and blood pressure is stabilized to improve movement of diaphragm.
6. Encourage coughing and deep breathing exercises and use of an incentive spirometer to prevent bronchospasm, retained secretions, atelectasis, and pneumonia.

B. *Stabilizing Hemodynamic Status*
1. Take blood pressure, pulse, and respiration every 15 minutes or more frequently as indicated; extend the time intervals according the patient's clinical status.
2. Monitor heart rate and rhythm by way of auscultation and ECG, because dysrhythmias are frequently seen after thoracic surgery.
3. Monitor the central venous pressure for prompt recognition of hypovolemia and for effectiveness of fluid replacement.
4. Monitor cardiac output and pulmonary artery systolic, diastolic, and wedge pressures. Watch for subtle changes, especially in the patient with underlying cardiovascular disease.
5. Assess chest tube drainage for amount and character of fluid.
   a. Chest drainage should progressively decrease after first 12 hours.
   b. Prepare for blood replacement and possible reoperation to achieve hemostasis if bleeding persists.
6. Maintain intake and output record, including chest tube drainage.
7. Monitor infusions of blood and parenteral fluids closely because patient is at risk for fluid overload if portion of pulmonary vascular system has been reduced.

C. *Achieving Adequate Pain Control*
1. Provide appropriate pain relief—pain limits chest excursions, thereby decreasing ventilation.
   a. Severity of pain varies with type of incision and with the patient's reaction to and ability to cope with pain. Usually a posterolateral incision is the most painful.

2. Give narcotics (usually by continuous IV infusion or by epidural catheter) for pain relief, as prescribed, to permit patient to breathe more deeply and cough more effectively.
   a. Avoid respiratory and CNS depression with too much narcotic; patient should be alert enough to cough.
3. Assist with intercostal nerve block or cryoanalgesia (intercostal nerve freezing) for pain control as ordered (see p. 227).
4. Position for comfort and optimal ventilation (head of bed elevated 15 to 30 degrees); this also helps residual air to rise in upper portion of pleural space, where it can be removed by the chest tube.
   a. Patients with limited respiratory reserve may not be able to turn on unoperated side, because this may limit ventilation of the operated side.
   b. Vary the position from horizontal to semierect to prevent retention of secretions in the dependent portion of the lungs.
5. Encourage splinting of incision with pillow, folded towel, or hands, while turning.
6. Teach relaxation techniques such as progressive muscle relaxation and imagery to help reduce pain.

D. *Increasing Mobility of Affected Shoulder*
1. Begin range of motion of arm and shoulder on affected side immediately to prevent ankylosis of the shoulder ("frozen" shoulder).
2. Perform exercises at time of maximal pain relief.
3. Encourage patient to actively perform exercises three to four times a day, taking care not to disrupt chest tube or IV lines.

Patient Education/Health Maintenance

1. Advise that there will be some intercostal pain for several weeks, which can be relieved by local heat and oral analgesia.
2. Advise that weakness and fatigability are common during the first 3 weeks after a thoracotomy, but exercise tolerance will improve with conditioning.
3. Suggest alternating walking and other activities with frequent short rest periods. Walk at a moderate pace and gradually extend walking time and distance.
4. Encourage continuing deep-breathing exercises for several weeks after surgery to attain full expansion of residual lung tissue.
5. Instruct on maintaining good body alignment to ensure full lung expansion.
6. Advise that chest muscles may be weaker than normal for 3 to 6 months after surgery so to avoid lifting more than 20 lb until complete healing has taken place.
7. Warn that any activity that causes undue fatigue, increased shortness of breath, or chest pain should be stopped immediately.
8. Because all or part of one lung has been removed, warn to stay away from respiratory irritants (smoke, fumes, high level of air pollution).
   a. Avoid anything that may cause spasms of coughing.
   b. Sit in nonsmoking areas in public places.
9. Encourage to have an annual influenza injection and obtain a pneumococcal pneumonia vaccine.
10. Encourage to keep follow-up visits.

Evaluation

A. Respirations 24, shallow; lungs clear; ABGs within normal limits

B. Blood pressure, CVP, and pulse stable
C. Coughing and turning independently; reports relief of pain
D. Performing active range of motion of affected arm and shoulder

---

PROCEDURE GUIDELINES 8-25 ◆ Assisting the Patient Using an Incentive Spirometer

EQUIPMENT   According to the type of device used

PROCEDURE	**NURSING ACTION**	**RATIONALE**

PREPARATORY PHASE

1. Measure the patient's normal V_T and auscultate the chest.

1. The patient's baseline is established.

PERFORMANCE PHASE

1. Explain the procedure and its purpose to the patient.

1. Optimal results are achieved when the patient is given pretreatment instruction. Preoperative instruction is also beneficial for the surgical patient.

2. Place the patient in a comfortable sitting or semi-Fowler's position.

2. Diaphragmatic excursion is greater in this position; however, if the patient is medically unable to be in this position, the exercise may be done in any position.

3. For the postoperative patient, try as much as possible to avoid discomfort with the treatment administration. Try to coordinate treatment with administration of pain-relief medications. Instruct and assist the patient with splinting of incision.

3. More likely to have best results in using incentive spirometry when patient has as little pain as possible.

4. Set the incentive spirometer V_T indicator at the desired goal the patient is to reach or exceed (500 mL is often used to start). The V_T is set according to the manufacturer's instructions.

4. The initial V_T may be prescribed, but the purpose of the device is to establish a baseline V_T and provide incentive to achieve greater volumes progressively.

5. Demonstrate the technique to the patient.

6. Instruct the patient to exhale fully.

7. Tell the patient to take in a slow, easy deep breath from the mouthpiece.

7. Noseclips are sometimes used if the patient has difficulty breathing only through mouth. This will ensure full credit for each breath measured.

8. When the desired goal is reached (lungs fully inflated), ask the patient to continue the inspiratory effort for 3 seconds, even though the patient may not actually be drawing in more air.

8. Sustaining the inspiratory effort helps to open closed alveoli.

9. Instruct the patient to remove the mouthpiece, relax and passively exhale; patient should take several normal breaths before attempting another one with the incentive spirometer.

9. Usually one incentive breath per minute minimizes patient fatigue. No more that four to five maneuvers should be performed per minute to minimize hypocarbia.

10. Continue to monitor the patient's spirometer breaths, periodically increasing the tidal volume as the patient tolerates.

11. At the conclusion of the treatment, encourage the patient to cough after a deep breath.

11. The deep lung inflation may loosen secretions and enable the patient to expectorate them.

12. Instruct the patient to take 10 sustained maximal inspiratory maneuvers per hour and note the volume on the spirometer.

12. A total of 10 sustained maximal inspiratory maneuvers per hour during waking hours is a typical order. A counter on the incentive spirometer indicates the number of breaths the patient has taken.

PROCEDURE (cont'd)	NURSING ACTION	RATIONALE

Flow incentive spirometer. Patients are instructed to inhale briskly to elevate the balls and to keep them floating as long as possible. The volume inhaled is estimated and variable.

FOLLOW-UP PHASE

1. Auscultate the chest. Chart any improvement or variation, the volume attained, effectiveness of cough, description of any secretions expectorated.

1. Note the effectiveness and patient tolerance of the treatment.

◆ CHEST DRAINAGE

Chest drainage is the insertion of a tube into the pleural space to evacuate air or fluid, to help regain negative pressure. Whenever the chest is opened, from any cause, there is loss of negative pressure, which can result in collapse of the lung. The collection of air, fluid, or other substances in the chest can compromise cardiopulmonary function and even cause collapse of the lung, because these substances take up space.

It is necessary to keep the pleural space evacuated postoperatively and to maintain negative pressure within this potential space. Therefore, during or immediately after thoracic surgery, chest tubes/catheters are positioned strategically in the pleural space, sutured to the skin, and connected to some type of drainage apparatus to remove the residual air and drainage fluid from the pleural or mediastinal space. This assists in the reexpansion of remaining lung tissue.

Chest drainage can also be used to treat spontaneous pneumothorax and pneumothorax or hemothorax caused by trauma. Sites for chest tube placement are:

1. For pneumothorax (air)—second or third interspace along midclavicular or anterior axillary line.
2. For hemothorax (fluid)—sixth or seventh lateral interspace in the midaxillary line.

Principles of Chest Drainage

1. Many types of commercial chest drainage systems are in use, most of which use the water-seal principle. The chest tube/catheter is attached to a bottle, using a one-way valve principle. Water acts as a seal and permits air and fluid to drain from the chest. However, air cannot reenter the submerged tip of the tube.
2. Chest drainage can be categorized into three types of mechanical systems (Fig. 8-7).

A. *Single-Bottle Water-Seal System*
1. The end of the drainage tube from the patient's chest is covered by a layer of water, which permits drainage of air and fluid from the pleural space, but does not allow air to move back into the chest. Functionally, drainage depends on gravity, on the mechanics of respiration, and, if desired, on suction by the addition of controlled vacuum.
2. The tube from the patient extends approximately 2.5 cm (1 inch) below the level of the water in the container. There is a vent for the escape of any air that may be leaking from the lung. The water level fluctuates as the patient breathes; it goes up when the patient inhales and down when the patient exhales.

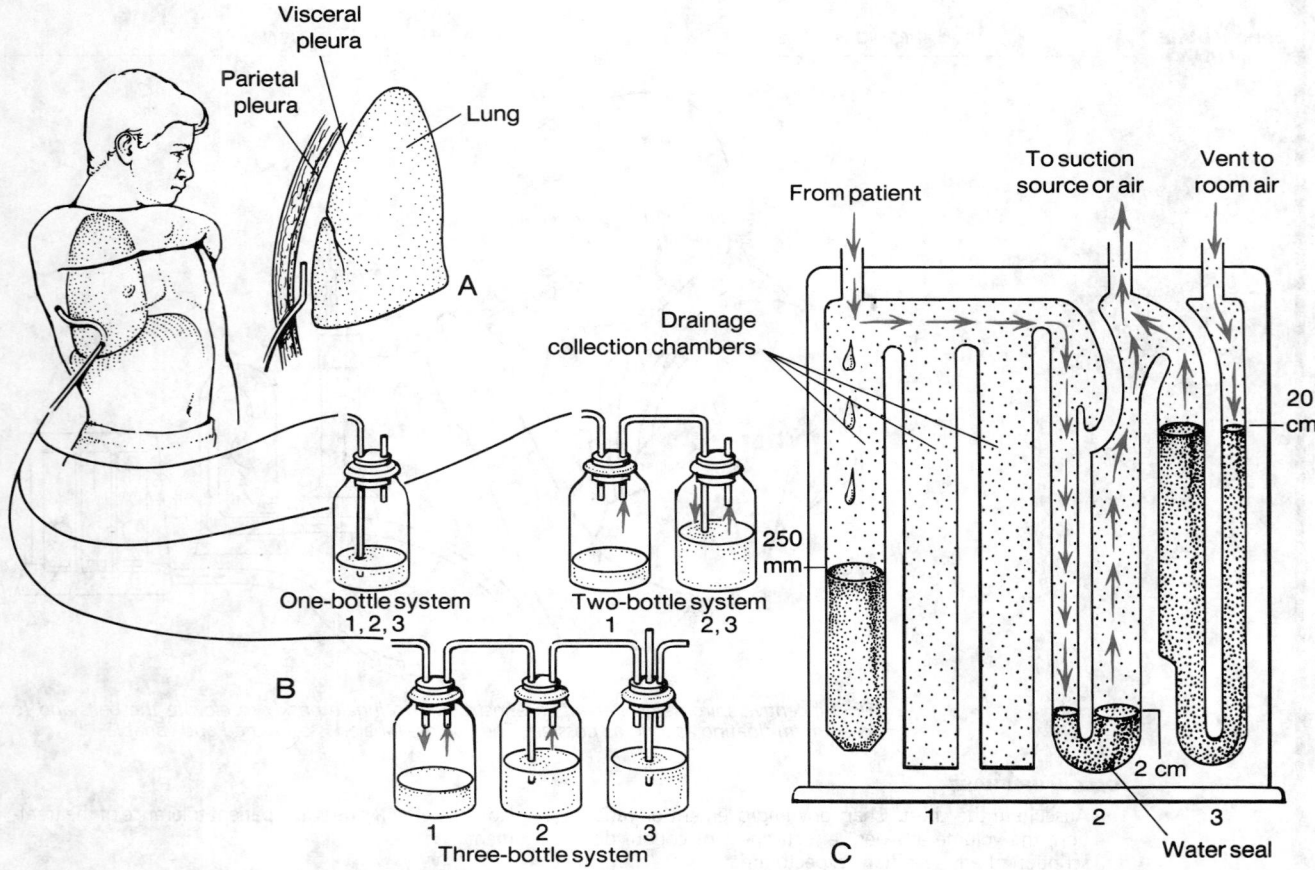

FIGURE 8-7 *Chest drainage system. (**A**) Strategic placement of a chest catheter in the pleural space. (**B**) Three types of mechanical drainage systems. (**C**) A Pleur-Evac operating system: (1) the collection chamber, (2) the water seal chamber, and (3) the suction control chamber. The Pleur-Evac is a single unit with all three bottles identified as chambers. (Brunner, L. S., & Suddarth, D. S. (1988). Textbook of medical-surgical nursing (6th ed.). Philadelphia: JB Lippincott.*

3. At the end of the drainage tube, bubbling may or may not be visible. Bubbling can mean either persistent leakage of air from the lung or other tissues or a leak in the system.

B. Two-Bottle Water-Seal System
1. The two-bottle system consists of the same water-seal chamber, plus a fluid-collection bottle.
2. Drainage is similar to that of a single unit, except that when pleural fluid drains, the underwater-seal system is not affected by the volume of the drainage.
3. Effective drainage depends on gravity or on the amount of suction added to the system. When vacuum (suction) is added to the system from a vacuum source, such as wall suction, the connection is made at the vent stem of the underwater-seal bottle.
4. The amount of suction applied to the system is regulated by the wall gauge.

C. Three-Bottle Water-Seal System
1. The three-bottle system is similar in all respects to the two-bottle system, except for the addition of a third bottle to control the amount of suction applied.
2. The amount of suction is determined by the depth to which the tip of the venting glass tube is submerged in the water.
3. In the three-bottle system (as in the other two systems), drainage depends on gravity or the amount of suction applied. The amount of suction in the three-bottle system is controlled by the manometer bottle. The mechanical suction motor or wall suction creates and maintains a negative pressure throughout the entire closed drainage system.
4. The manometer bottle regulates the amount of vacuum in the system. This bottle contains three tubes:
   a. A short tube above the water level comes from the water-seal bottle.
   b. Another short tube leads to the vacuum or suction motor, or to wall suction.

c. The third tube is a long tube that extends below the water level in the bottle and opens to the atmosphere outside the bottle. This tube regulates the amount of vacuum in the system, depending on the depth to which the tube is submerged—the usual depth is 20 cm (7.6 inches).

5. When the vacuum in the system becomes greater than the depth to which the tube is submerged, outside air is sucked into the system. This results in constant bubbling in the manometer bottle, which indicates that the system is functioning properly.

> **NURSING ALERT:** ❖
> When the motor or the wall vacuum is turned off, the drainage system should be open to the atmosphere so intrapleural air can escape from the system. This can be done by detaching the tubing from the suction port to provide a vent.

6. In the commercially available systems, the three bottles are contained in one unit and identified as "chambers" (Fig. 8-28 C). The principles remain the same for the commercially available products as they do for the glass bottle system.

Nursing/Patient Care Considerations

1. Assist with chest tube insertion. (See Procedure Guidelines 8-26.)
2. Assess patient's pain at insertion site and give medication appropriately. If patient is in pain, chest excursion and lung inflation will be hampered.
3. Maintain chest tubes to provide drainage and enhance lung reinflation. (See Procedure Guidelines 8-27.)

PROCEDURE GUIDELINES 8-26 ◆ Assisting With Chest Tube Insertion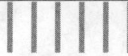

EQUIPMENT

Tube thoracostomy tray
Syringes
Needles/trocar
Basins/skin germicide
Sponges
Scalpel/sterile drape/gloves
Two large clamps

Suture material
Local anesthetic
Chest tube (appropriate size); connector
Chest drainage system—connecting tubes and tubing, collection bottles or commercial system, vacuum pump (if required)

PROCEDURE

NURSING ACTION	RATIONALE
PREPARATORY PHASE	
1. Assess patient for pneumothorax, hemothorax, presence of respiratory distress.	
2. Obtain a chest x-ray. Other means of localization of pleural fluid include ultrasound and/or fluoroscopic localization.	2. To evaluate extent of lung collapse or amount of bleeding in pleural space.
3. Assemble drainage system.	
4. Reassure the patient and explain the steps of the procedure. Tell the patient to expect a needle prick and a sensation of slight pressure during infiltration anesthesia.	4. The patient can cope by remaining immobile and doing relaxed breathing during tube insertion.
5. Position the patient as for an intercostal nerve block, or according to physician preference.	5. The tube insertion site depends on the substance to be drained, the patient's mobility, and the presence/absence of coexisting conditions.
PERFORMANCE PHASE	
NEEDLE OR INTRACATH TECHNIQUE	
1. The skin is prepared and anesthetized using local anesthetic with a short 25-gauge needle. A larger needle is used to infiltrate the subcutaneous tissue, intercostal muscles, and parietal pleura.	1. The area is anesthetized to make tube insertion and manipulation relatively painless.
2. An exploratory needle is inserted.	2. To puncture the pleura and determine the presence of air/blood in the pleural cavity.
3. The IntraCath catheter is inserted through the needle into the pleural space. The needle is removed, and the catheter is pushed several centimeters into the pleural space.	
4. The catheter is taped to the skin.	4. To prevent it from being pushed out of the chest during patient movement or lung expansion.
5. The catheter is attached to a connector/tubing and attached to a drainage system (underwater-seal or commercial system).	

(continued)

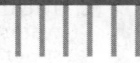

PROCEDURE GUIDELINES 8-26 ♦ Assisting With Chest Tube Insertion
(continued)

PROCEDURE (cont'd)	NURSING ACTION	RATIONALE

PROCEDURE (cont'd)

TROCAR TECHNIQUE FOR CHEST TUBE INSERTION

A trocar catheter is used for the insertion of a large-bore tube for removal of a modest to large amount of air leak or for the evacuation of serous effusion.

NURSING ACTION	RATIONALE
1. A small incision is made over the prepared, anesthetized site. Blunt dissection (with a hemostat) through the muscle planes in the interspace to the parietal pleura is performed.	1. To admit the diameter of the chest tube.
2. The trocar is directed into the pleural space, the cannula is removed, and a chest tube is inserted into the pleural space and connected to a drainage system.	2. There is a trocar catheter available equipped with an indwelling pointed rod for ease of insertion.

HEMOSTAT TECHNIQUE USING A LARGE-BORE CHEST TUBE

A large bore chest tube is used to drain blood or thick effusions from the pleural space.

NURSING ACTION	RATIONALE
1. After skin preparation and anesthetic infiltration, an incision is made through the skin and subcutaneous tissue.	1. The skin incision is usually made one interspace below proposed site of penetration of the intercostal muscles and pleura.
2. A curved hemostat is inserted into the pleural cavity and the tissue is spread with the clamp.	2. To make a tissue tract for the chest tube.
3. The tract is explored with an examining finger.	3. Digital examination helps confirm the presence of the tract and penetration of the pleural cavity.
4. The tube is held by the hemostat and directed through the opening up over the ribs and into the pleural cavity.	
5. The clamp is withdrawn and the chest tube is connected to a chest drainage system.	5. The chest tube has multiple openings at the proximal end for drainage of air/blood.
6. The tube is sutured in place and covered with a sterile dressing.	

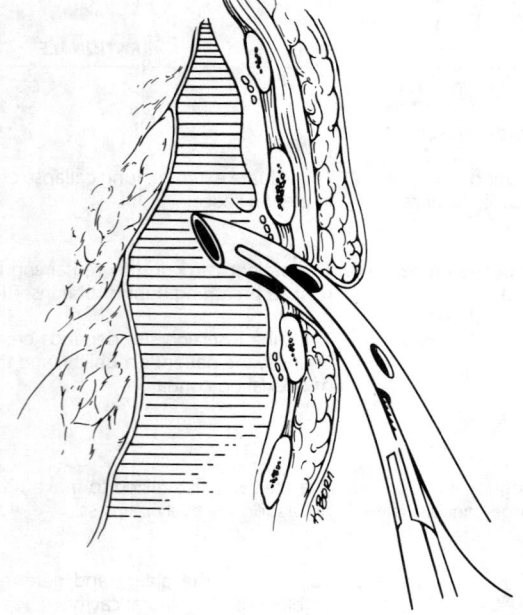

Chest tube (tube thoracostomy) inserted via hemostat technique.

FOLLOW-UP PHASE

NURSING ACTION	RATIONALE
1. Observe the drainage system for blood/air. Observe for fluctuation in the tube on respiration. (See chest drainage, p. 209.)	1. If a hemothorax is draining through a thoracostomy tube into a bottle containing sterile normal saline, the blood is available for autotransfusion.
2. Secure a follow-up chest x-ray.	2. To confirm correct chest tube placement and reexpansion of the lung.
3. Assess for bleeding, infection, leakage of air and fluid around the tube.	

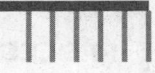

PROCEDURE GUIDELINES 8-27 ◆ Managing the Patient With Water-Seal Chest Drainage

EQUIPMENT
Closed chest drainage system
Holder for drainage system (if needed)
Vacuum motor
Sterile connector for emergency use

PROCEDURE

NURSING ACTION	RATIONALE
PERFORMANCE PHASE	
1. Attach the drainage tube from the pleural space (the patient) to the tubing that leads to a long tube with end submerged in sterile normal saline.	1. Water-seal drainage provides for the escape of air and fluid into a drainage bottle. The water acts as a seal and keeps the air from being drawn back into the pleural space.

2. Check the tube connections periodically. Tape if necessary.
  a. The tube should be approximately 2.5 cm (1 inch) below the water level.
 	
  b. The short tube is left open to the atmosphere.
	2. Tube connections are checked to ensure tight fit and patency of the tubes.
	  a. If the tube is submerged too deep below the water level, a higher intrapleural pressure is required to expel air.
	  b. Venting the short glass tube lets air escape from the bottle.

3. Mark the original fluid level with tape on the outside of the drainage bottle. Mark hourly/daily increments (date and time) at the drainage level.	3. This marking will show the amount of fluid loss and how fast fluid is collecting in the drainage bottle. It serves as a basis for blood replacement, if the fluid is blood. Grossly bloody drainage will appear in the bottle in the immediate postoperative period and, if excessive, may necessitate reoperation. Drainage usually declines progressively after the first 24 hours.
4. Make sure the tubing does not loop or interfere with the movements of the patient.	4. Fluid collecting in the dependent segment of the tubing will decrease the negative pressure applied to the catheter. Kinking, looping, or pressure on the drainage tubing can produce back pressure, thus possibly forcing drainage back into the pleural space or impeding drainage from the pleural space.
5. Encourage the patient to assume a position of comfort. Encourage good body alignment. When the patient is in a lateral position, place a rolled towel under the tubing to protect it from the weight of the patient's body. Encourage the patient to change position frequently.	5. The patient's position should be changed frequently to promote drainage and body kept in good alignment to prevent postural deformity and contractures. Proper positioning helps breathing and promotes better air exchange. Pain medication may be indicated to enhance comfort and deep breathing.
6. Put the arm and shoulder of the affected side through range-of-motion exercises several times daily. Some pain medication may be necessary.	6. Exercise helps to avoid ankylosis of the shoulder and assist in lessening postoperative pain and discomfort.
7. "Milk" the tubing in the direction of the drainage bottle as often as ordered. (Many institutions do not advocate milking because of the increased intrapleural pressure it causes.)	7. "Milking" the tubing prevents it from becoming plugged with clots of fibrin. Constant attention to maintaining the patency of the tube will facilitate prompt expansion of the lung and minimize complications.
8. Make sure there is fluctuation ("tidaling") of the fluid level in the long glass tube.	8. Fluctuation of the water level in the tube shows that there is effective communication between the pleural space and the drainage bottle; provides a valuable indication of the patency of the drainage system, and is a gauge of intrapleural pressure.

9. Fluctuations of fluid in the tubing will stop when:
  a. The lung has reexpanded.
  b. The tubing is obstructed by blood clots or fibrin.
  c. A dependent loop develops (see step 4).
  d. Suction motor or wall suction is not operating properly.	

(continued)

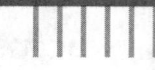

PROCEDURE GUIDELINES 8-27 ◆ Managing the Patient With Water-Seal Chest Drainage *(continued)*

PROCEDURE (cont'd)	NURSING ACTION	RATIONALE

NURSING ACTION

10. Watch for leaks of air in the drainage system as indicated by constant bubbling in the water-seal bottle.
    a. Report excessive bubbling in the water-seal change immediately.
    b. "Milking" of chest tubes in patients with air leaks should be done only if requested by surgeon.
11. Observe and report immediately signs of rapid, shallow breathing, cyanosis, pressure in the chest, subcutaneous emphysema, or symptoms of hemorrhage.

12. Encourage the patient to breathe deeply and cough at frequent intervals. If there are signs of incisional pain, adequate pain medication is indicated.

13. If the patient has to be transported to another area, place the drainage bottle below the chest level (as close to the floor as possible).
14. If the tube becomes disconnected, cut off the contaminated tips of the chest tube and tubing, insert a sterile connector in the chest tube and tubing, and reattach to the drainage system. Otherwise, do not clamp the chest tube during transport.
15. When assisting with removal of the tube:
    a. Administer pain medication 30 minutes before removal of chest tube.
    b. Instruct the patient to perform a gentle Valsalva maneuver or to breathe quietly.
    c. The chest tube is clamped and removed.
    d. Simultaneously, a small bandage is applied and made airtight with petroleum gauze covered by a 4 × 4-inch gauze and thoroughly covered and sealed with tape.

FOLLOW-UP PHASE

1. Monitor patient's pulmonary status for signs and symptoms of decompensation.

RATIONALE

10. Leaking and trapping of air in the pleural space can result in tension pneumothorax.

11. Many clinical conditions may cause these signs and symptoms, including tension pneumothorax, mediastinal shift, hemorrhage, severe incisional pain, pulmonary embolus, and cardiac tamponade. Surgical intervention may be necessary.
12. Deep breathing and coughing help to raise the intrapleural pressure, which allows emptying of any accumulation in the pleural space and removes secretions from the tracheobronchial tree so that the lung expands.
13. The drainage apparatus must be kept at a level lower than the patient's chest to prevent backflow of fluid into the pleural space.

15. The chest tube is removed as directed when the lung is reexpanded (usually 24 hours to several days). During the tube removal, avoid a large sudden inspiratory effort, which may produce a pneumothorax.

1. Patient could have reformation of pneumothorax upon removal.

Selected References

Bolton, P. J., & Kline, K. A. (1994). Understanding modes of mechanical ventilation, *American Journal of Nursing, 94*(6), 36-43.

Carroll, P. (1995). A med/surg nurses guide to mechanical ventilation. *RN, 58*(2), 26-31, 35.

Dabbs, A. D., & Olslund, L. (1994). The new alternatives to intubation, *American Journal of Nursing, 94*(8), 42-45.

Dillon, P. (1994). Reviewing respiratory assessment skills. *Nursing '94, 24*(6), 68–70.

Freichels, T. (1993). Orchestrating the care of mechanically ventilated patients, *American Journal of Nursing, 93*(10), 26-33.

Long, B., et al. (1993). *Medical surgical nursing: A nursing process approach* (3rd ed.). Mosby, St. Louis.

Mathews, P. (1995). Safely delivering a breath of fresh air. *Nursing '95, 25*(5), 66–69.

Murray, J. F., & Nadel, J. (1994). *Textbook of respiratory medicine* (2nd ed.). W. B. Saunders, Philadelphia.

Perry, A., & Potter, P. (1994). *Clinical nursing skills and techniques* (3rd ed.). Mosby, St. Louis.

Smeltzer, S. C., & Bare, B. G. (1992). *Brunner and Suddarth's textbook of medical-surgical nursing* (7th ed.). J. B. Lippincott, Philadelphia.

Stringfield, Y. N. (1993). Back to basics. Acidosis, alkalosis, and ABGs. *American Journal of Nursing, 93*(10), 26-33.

Tasota, F., et al. (1994). Assessing ABGs: Maintaining the delicate balance. *Nursing '94, 24*(5), 34-36.

Witta, K. M. (1993). When gauging respiratory status is critical. *RN, 56*(11), 40-46.

Respiratory Disorders

Acute Disorders

◆ RESPIRATORY FAILURE

Respiratory failure is an alteration in the function of the respiratory system that causes the Pao_2 to fall below 50 mm Hg (hypoxemia) or the $Paco_2$ to rise above 50 mm Hg (hypercapnia), as determined by arterial blood gas (ABG) analysis.

Classification

A. **Acute Respiratory Failure**
1. Characterized by hypoxemia (Pao_2 less than 50 mm Hg) or hypercapnia ($Paco_2$ greater than 50 mm Hg) and acidemia (pH less than 7.35).
2. Occurs rapidly, usually in minutes to hours or days.

B. **Chronic Respiratory Failure**
1. Characterized by hypoxemia (decreased Pao_2) or hypercapnia (increased $Paco_2$) with a normal pH (7.35 to 7.40).
2. Occurs over a period of months to years—allows for activation of compensatory mechanisms.

C. **Acute and Chronic Respiratory Failure**
1. Characterized by an abrupt increase in the degree of hypoxemia or hypercapnia in patients with preexisting chronic respiratory failure.
2. May occur following an acute upper respiratory infection or pneumonia, or without obvious cause.
3. Extent of deterioration is best assessed by comparing the patient's present ABGs with previous ABGs (patient "normals").

Pathophysiology/Etiology

A. **Oxygenation Failure**
Characterized by a decrease in Pao_2 and normal or decreased $Paco_2$

1. Primary problem is inability to adequately oxygenate the blood, resulting in hypoxemia.

2. Hypoxemia occurs because damage to the alveolar-capillary membrane causes leakage of fluid into the interstitial space or into the alveoli and slows or prevents movement of oxygen from the alveoli to the pulmonary capillary blood.
   a. Typically this damage is widespread, resulting in many areas of the lung being poorly ventilated or nonventilated.
   b. Consequences are severe ventilation–perfusion imbalance and shunt.
3. Hypocapnia results from hypoxemia and decreased pulmonary compliance. Fluid within the lungs makes the lung less compliant (stiffer).
   a. Change in compliance reflexively stimulates the increased ventilation.
   b. Ventilation is also increased as a response to hypoxemia.
   c. Ultimately, if treatment is unsuccessful, the $Paco_2$ will increase, and the patient will experience both an increase in $Paco_2$ and a decrease in Pao_2.
4. Etiology includes:
   a. Cardiogenic pulmonary edema (left ventricular failure; mitral stenosis)
   b. Adult respiratory distress syndrome or ARDS (shock of any etiology; infectious causes such as gram-negative sepsis, viral pneumonia, bacterial pneumonia; trauma such as fat emboli, head injury, lung contusion; aspiration of gastric fluid, near drowning; inhaled toxins such as oxygen in high concentrations, smoke, corrosive chemicals; hematologic conditions such as massive transfusions, post cardiopulmonary bypass; and metabolic disorders such as pancreatitis, uremia).

B. **Ventilatory Failure with Normal Lungs**
Characterized by a decrease in Pao_2, increase in $Paco_2$ and a decrease in pH.

1. Primary problem is insufficient respiratory center stimulation or insufficient chest wall movement, resulting in alveolar hypoventilation.
2. Hypercapnia occurs because impaired neuromuscular function or chest wall expansion limits the amount of carbon dioxide removed from the lungs.
   a. Primary problem is not the lungs. The patient's minute ventilation (tidal volume times the number of breaths per minute) is insufficient to allow normal alveolar gas exchange.

3. The CO_2 not excreted by the lungs combines with H_2O to form carbonic acid (H_2CO_3). This predisposes to acidemia and a fall in pH.
4. Hypoxemia occurs as a consequence of hypercapnia. When the $Paco_2$ rises, the Pao_2 must fall unless increased amounts of oxygen are added to the inspired air.
5. Etiology includes:
   a. Insufficient respiratory center activity (drug intoxication such as narcotic overdose, general anesthesia; vascular disorders such as cerebral vascular insufficiency, brain tumor; trauma such as head injury, increased intracranial pressure)
   b. Insufficient chest wall function (neuromuscular disease such as Guillain-Barré, myasthenia gravis, poliomyelitis; trauma to the chest wall resulting in multiple fractures; spinal cord trauma; kyphoscoliosis)

C. *Ventilatory Failure with Intrinsic Lung Disease*
Characterized by a decrease in Pao_2 and decreased pH

1. Primary problem is acute exacerbation or chronic progression of previously existing lung disease, resulting in CO_2 retention.
2. Hypercapnia occurs because damage to the lung parenchyma and/or airway obstruction limits the amount of carbon dioxide removed by the lungs.
   a. Primary problem is preexisting lung disease—usually chronic bronchitis, emphysema, or severe asthma. This limits CO_2 removal from the lungs.
3. The CO_2 not excreted by the lungs combines with H_2O to form carbonic acid (H_2CO_3). This predisposes to acidemia and a fall in pH.
4. Hypoxemia occurs as a consequence of hypercapnia. In addition, damage to the lung parenchyma and/or airway obstruction limits the amount of oxygen that enters the pulmonary capillary blood.
5. Etiology includes:
   a. Chronic obstructive pulmonary disease or COPD (chronic bronchitis, emphysema, cystic fibrosis)
   b. Severe asthma

Clinical Manifestations

1. Hypoxemia—restlessness, agitation, dyspnea, disorientation, confusion, delirium, loss of consciousness.
2. Hypercapnia—headache, somnolence, dizziness, confusion.
3. Tachypnea initially; then when no longer able to compensate, bradypnea.
4. Accessory muscle use.
5. Asynchronous respirations.

NURSING ALERT:
Obtain ABGs whenever the history or signs and symptoms suggest the patient is at risk for developing respiratory failure. Initial and subsequent values should be recorded on a flow sheet so comparisons can be made over time. Need for ABG can be decreased by using an oximeter to continuously monitor the SaO_2.

Diagnostic Evaluation

1. ABGs—show changes in Pao_2, $Paco_2$, and pH from patient's normal; or Pao_2 less than 50 mm Hg, $Paco_2$ greater than 50 mm Hg, pH less than 7.35.
2. Pulse oximetry—decreasing SaO_2.
3. End tidal CO_2 monitoring—elevated.
4. CBC, serum electrolytes, chest X-ray, urinalysis, electrocardiogram (ECG), blood and sputum cultures—to determine underlying cause and patient's condition.

Management

1. Oxygen therapy to correct the hypoxemia.
2. Chest physical therapy and hydration to mobilize secretions.
3. Bronchodilators and possibly corticosteroids to reduce bronchospasm and inflammation.
4. Diuretics for pulmonary congestion.
5. Mechanical ventilation as indicated.

Complications

1. Oxygen toxicity of prolonged high FiO_2 required.
2. Barotrauma from mechanical ventilation intervention.

Nursing Assessment

1. Note changes suggesting increased work of breathing (diaphoresis, intercostal muscle retraction) or pulmonary edema (fine, coarse crackles).
2. Assess breath sounds.
   a. Diminished or absent sounds indicate inability to ventilate the lungs sufficiently to prevent atelectasis.
   b. Crackles indicate ineffective airway clearance.
   c. Wheezing indicates bronchospasm.
   d. Rhonchi and crackles indicate ineffective secretion clearance.
3. Assess level of consciousness and ability to tolerate increased work of breathing.
   a. Confusion, rapid shallow breathing, abdominal paradox (inward movement of abdominal wall during inspiration), and intercostal retractions suggest inability to maintain adequate minute ventilation.
4. Assess for signs of hypoxemia and hypercapnia.
5. Determine vital capacity (VC), respiratory rate, minute ventilation (V_E), and negative inspiratory force (NIF) and compare with values indicating need for mechanical ventilation:
   a. VC < 10 to 15 mL/kg.
   b. Respiratory rate > 35/min.
   c. V_E > 10 L/min.
   d. NIF < −20 to −25 cm H_2O.
6. Determine ABGs and compare with previous values.
   a. If the patient cannot maintain a minute ventilation sufficient to prevent CO_2 retention, the pH will fall.
   b. Mechanical ventilation may be needed if the pH falls to < 7.30.
7. Determine hemodynamic status (blood pressure, pulmonary wedge pressure, cardiac output, SvO_2) and compare with previous values if patient on mechanical ventilation and positive end-expiratory pressure

(PEEP), which may decrease venous return, resulting in decreased cardiac output.

Nursing Diagnoses

A. Impaired gas exchange related to inadequate respiratory center activity or chest wall movement, airway obstruction, and/or fluid in lungs
B. Ineffective airway clearance related to increased or tenacious secretions

Nursing Interventions

A. *Improving Gas Exchange*
1. Administer antibiotics, cardiac medications, and diuretics as ordered for underlying disorder.
2. Administer oxygen to maintain Pao_2 of 60 mm Hg or SaO_2 > 90% using devices that provide increased oxygen concentrations (aerosol mask, partial rebreathing mask, nonrebreathing mask).
3. Monitor fluid balance by intake and output measurement, urine specific gravity, daily weight, and direct measurement of pulmonary capillary wedge pressure to detect presence of hypo/hypervolemia.
4. Provide measures to prevent atelectasis and promote chest expansion and secretion clearance, as ordered (incentive spirometer, nebulization, out of bed, head of bed elevated 30 degrees).
5. Monitor adequacy of alveolar ventilation by frequent measurement of respiratory rate, vital capacity, inspiratory force, and ABGs.
6. Compare monitored values with criteria indicating need for mechanical ventilation (see Nursing Assessment). Report and prepare to assist with intubation and initiation of mechanical ventilation, if indicated.

B. *Maintaining Airway Clearance*
1. Administer medications to increase alveolar ventilation—bronchodilators to reduce bronchospasm, corticosteroids to reduce airway inflammation.
2. Perform chest physiotherapy to remove mucus. Teach slow, pursed-lip breathing to reduce airway obstruction.
3. Administer IV fluids and mucolytics to reduce sputum viscosity.
4. If the patient becomes increasingly lethargic, cannot cough or expectorate secretions, cannot cooperate with therapy, or if pH falls below 7.30, despite use of the above therapy, report and prepare to assist with intubation and initiation of mechanical ventilation.

Patient Education/Health Maintenance

1. Instruct patient with preexisting pulmonary disease to seek early intervention for infections to prevent acute respiratory failure.
2. Teach patient about medication regimen.
3. Encourage patients at risk, especially the elderly and those with preexisting lung disease, to get yearly influenza and one-time pneumococcal pneumonia immunizations.

Evaluation

A. ABGs within patient's normal limits
B. Decreased secretions; lungs clear

◆ ADULT RESPIRATORY DISTRESS SYNDROME (ARDS)

ARDS is a clinical syndrome also called noncardiogenic pulmonary edema in which there is severe hypoxemia and decreased compliance of the lungs, which leads to both oxygenation and ventilatory failure. Mortality is 50% to 60% but is improved with early intervention.

Pathophysiology/Etiology

1. Pulmonary and/or nonpulmonary insult to the alveolar-capillary membrane causes fluid leakage into interstitial spaces.
2. Ventilation–perfusion (V/Q) mismatch caused by shunting of blood (Fig. 9-1).
3. Etiologies are numerous and can be pulmonary or nonpulmonary. These include (but are not limited to):
   a. Pneumonia, sepsis, aspiration.
   b. Shock (any cause), trauma.
   c. Metabolic, hematologic, and immunologic disorders.
   d. Inhaled agents—smoke, high concentration of oxygen, corrosive substances.
   e. Major surgery, fat or air embolism.

Clinical Manifestations

1. Severe dyspnea, use of accessory muscles.
2. Increasing requirements of oxygen therapy. Hypoxemia refractory to supplemental oxygen therapy.
3. Severe crackles and rhonchi heard on auscultation.

Diagnostic Evaluation

1. The hallmark sign for ARDS is a shunt; hypoxemia remains despite increasing oxygen therapy.
2. Decreased lung compliance; increasing pressure required to ventilate patient on mechanical ventilation.
3. Chest x-ray exhibits bilateral infiltrates.
4. Swan-Ganz readings: pulmonary artery wedge pressure > 18 mm Hg.

Management

1. The underlying cause for ARDS must be determined so appropriate treatment can be initiated.
2. Ventilatory support with PEEP will be instituted. PEEP keeps the alveoli open, thereby improving gas exchange. Therefore, a lower oxygen concentration (FiO_2) can be used to maintain satisfactory oxygenation.
3. Fluid management must be maintained. The patient may be hypovolemic due to the movement of fluid into the interstitium of the lung. Swan-Ganz monitoring and inotropic medication can be helpful.

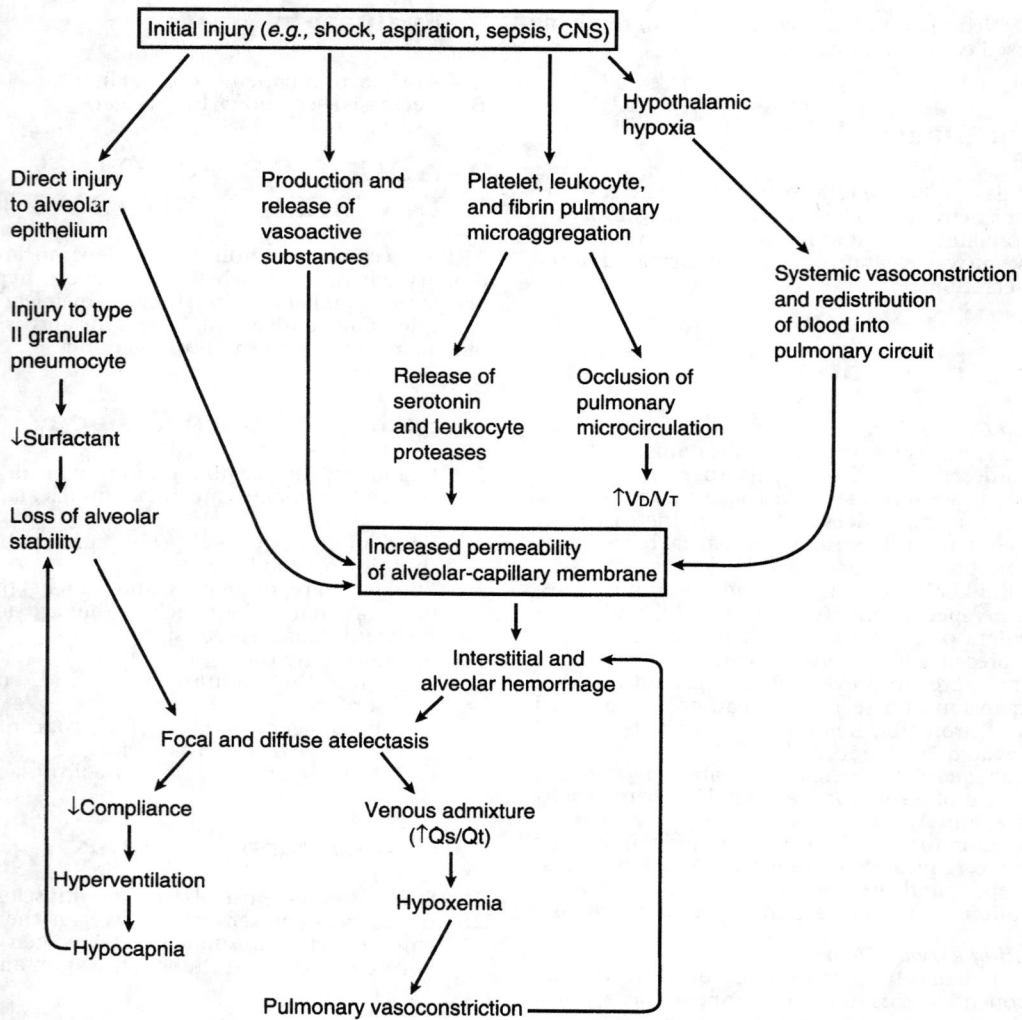

FIGURE 9-1 *Pathogenesis of ARDS. (After Burton, G. G., & Hodgkin, J. E. [Eds.]. (1984). Respiratory care: A guide to clinical practice (2nd ed.). Philadelphia: JB Lippincott.)*

4. Medications are aimed at treating the underlying cause. Corticosteroids are used infrequently due to the controversy regarding benefits of usage.
5. Adequate nutrition should be initiated early and maintained.

Complications

1. Infections such as pneumonia, sepsis.
2. Respiratory complications such as pulmonary emboli, barotrauma, oxygen toxicity, or pulmonary fibrosis.
3. Gastrointestinal complications such as stress ulcer, ileus.
4. Cardiac complications such as decreased cardiac output and dysrhythmias.
5. Renal failure, disseminated intravascular coagulation (DIC).

Nursing Interventions

Care is similar to patient with respiratory failure (p. 211) and pulmonary edema (p. 313). Also see Mechanical Ventilation, p. 191.

◆ ACUTE BRONCHITIS

Acute bronchitis is an infection of the lower respiratory tract that is generally an acute sequela to an upper respiratory tract infection.

Pathophysiology/Etiology

1. Primarily viral etiology, but may also arise from bacterial agents.

2. Airways become inflamed and irritated with increased mucous production.

Clinical Manifestations

1. Fever, tachypnea.
2. Cough, clear to purulent sputum.
3. Pleuritic chest pain, occasionally.
4. Diffuse rhonchi and crackles heard on auscultation.

Diagnostic Evaluation

1. Chest X-ray—no evidence of infiltrates or consolidation.

Management

1. Antibiotic therapy for 7 to 10 days.
2. Hydration if patient dehydrated.
3. Symptom management for fever, cough.

Nursing Assessment

1. Obtain history of upper airway infection, course of symptoms.
2. Assess severity of cough and characteristics of sputum production.
3. Auscultate chest for diffuse rhonchi and crackles as opposed to localized crackles usually heard with pneumonia.

Nursing Diagnoses

A. Ineffective Airway Clearance related to sputum production

Nursing Interventions

A. *Establishing Effective Airway Clearance*
1. Administer or teach self-administration of antibiotics as ordered.
2. Encourage mobilization of secretions, through hydration, chest physical therapy, and coughing.
3. Administer or teach self-administration of inhaled bronchodilators, if ordered to reduce bronchospasm and promote sputum expectoration.
4. Caution patients on the use of over-the-counter cough suppressants, antihistamines, and decongestants that may cause drying and retention of secretions. Cough preparations containing the mucolytic guaifenesin may be appropriate.

Patient Education/Health Maintenance

1. Instruct patient about medication regimen, including the completion of the full course of antibiotics pre-scribed and the effects of meals on the absorption of the medications.
2. Ensure that patient is aware of early signs and symptoms of acute bronchitis and to seek medical attention.
3. Advise patient that a dry cough may persist after bronchitis due to irritation of the airways. A bedside humidifier and avoidance of dry environments may help.

Evaluation

A. Coughing up clear secretions effectively

◆ PNEUMONIA

Pneumonia is an inflammatory process, involving the terminal airways and alveoli of the lung, caused by infectious agents (Table 9-1). It is classified according to its causative agent.

Pathophysiology/Etiology

1. The organism gains access to the lungs through aspiration of oropharyngeal contents, by inhalation of respiratory secretions from infected individuals, via the bloodstream, or from direct spread to the lungs from surgery or trauma.
2. Patients with bacterial pneumonia may have an underlying disease that impairs host defense; pneumonia arises from endogenous flora of the person whose resistance has been altered, or from aspiration of oropharyngeal secretions.
  a. Immunocompromised patients include those receiving corticosteroids or immunosuppressants, those with cancer, those being treated with chemotherapy or radiotherapy, those undergoing organ transplantation, alcoholics, intravenous (IV) drug abusers, and those with human immunodeficiency virus (HIV) disease and acquired immunodeficiency syndrome (AIDS).
  b. These people have an increased chance of developing overwhelming infection.
  c. Infectious agents include aerobic and anaerobic gram-negative bacilli, *Staphylococcus, Nocardia,* fungi, *Candida,* viruses such as cytomegalovirus (CMV), *Pneumocystis carinii,* reactivation of tuberculosis, and others.
3. When bacterial pneumonia occurs in a healthy person, there usually is a history of preceding viral illness.
4. Other predisposing factors include conditions interfering with normal drainage of the lung such as tumor, general anesthesia and postoperative immobility, depression of the central nervous system from drugs, neurologic disorders, or other conditions, and intubation or respiratory instrumentation.
5. Pneumonia may be divided into three groups:
  a. Community-acquired, due to a number of organisms, including *Streptococcus pneumoniae.*
  b. Hospital or nursing home acquired (nosocomial), due primarily to gram-negative bacilli and staphylococci.
  c. Pneumonia in the immunocompromised person.
6. Persons over 65 have a high mortality rate, even with appropriate antimicrobial therapy.

TABLE 9-1   Commonly Encountered Pneumonias

Type	Organism Responsible	Manifestations	Clinical Features	Treatment	Complications
Bacterial					
Streptococcal pneumonia (pneumococcal pneumonia)	*Streptococcus pneumoniae*	Sudden onset, with shaking and chills Rapidly rising fever; tachypnea Cough; with expectoration of rusty or green (purulent) sputum Pleuritic pain aggravated by cough Chest dull to percussion; crackles, bronchial breath sounds Confusion may be only presenting feature in elderly	May be history of previous respiratory infection Herpes simplex lesions often present on face or lips Usually involves one or more lobes	Cephalosporins; trimethoprim-sulfamethoxazole (Bactrim), amoxicillin clavulanate (Augmentin); macrolide antibiotics such as azithromycin (Zithromax) or clarithromycin (Biaxin)	Shock Pleural effusion Superinfections Pericarditis Otitis media
Staphylococcal pneumonia	*Staphylococcus aureus*	Often prior history of viral infection, especially influenza Insidious development of cough, with expectoration of yellow, blood-streaked mucus Onset may be sudden if patient is outside hospital Fever, pleuritic chest pain, progressive dyspnea Pulse varies; may be slow in proportion to temperature	Frequently seen in hospital setting; during influenza epidemics; in intravenous drug abuse These infections often lead to necrosis and destruction of lung tissue Treatment must be vigorous and prolonged owing to disease's tendency to destroy the lungs Organism may develop rapid drug resistance Prolonged convalescence usual	Cephalosporins; penicillinase-resistant extended-spectrum penicillins; vancomycin (Vancocin) for methicillin-resistant *S. aureus*	Effusion/pneumothorax Lung abscess Empyema Meningitis
Pneumonia due to gram-negative enteric bacilli	*Klebsiella* species; *Pseudomonas* organisms; *Escherichia coli* *Serratia, Proteus* species	Sudden onset with fever, chills, dyspnea Pleuritic chest pain and production of purulent sputum	Usually infection occurs from aspiration of pharyngeal flora into bronchioles Seen in persons with severe illness; among the more common causes of hospital-acquired pneumonia	Usually multiple-drug regimens recommended; aminoglycoside antibiotic; cephalosporins; and/or penicillinase-resistant extended-spectrum penicillin	Early necrosis of lung tissue with rapid abscess formation High mortality
Legionnaires' disease	*Legionella pneumophila*	High fever, chills, cough, chest pain, tachypnea Respiratory distress	Peak incidence in persons over 50 who are cigarette smokers and have underlying diseases that increase susceptibility to infection	Erythromycin (Eryc) or newer macrolide antibiotic	Respiratory failure

216

Disease	Causative Organism	Clinical Symptoms	Characteristics	Treatment	Complications/Prognosis
Hemophilus influenza pneumonia	*H. influenzae*	Abrupt onset of coughing, fever, chills, chest pain	May affect healthy young adults	Erythromycin (Eryc), newer macrolide antibiotic, trimethoprim-sulfamethoxazole (Bactrim)	High mortality in patients with underlying disease (cancer; COPD) Pleural effusion common
Nonbacterial Pneumonias					
Mycoplasma pneumonia or chlamydial pneumonia	*Mycoplasma pneumoniae, Chlamydia trachomatis*	Gradual onset; severe headache; irritating hacking cough producing scanty, mucoid sputum Anorexia; malaise Fever; nasal congestion; sore throat	Occurs most commonly in children and young adults, as well as in older adults in community hospital setting Rise in serum-complement-fixing antibodies to the organism	Erythromycin (Eryc); newer macrolide antibiotic; tetracycline (Tetracyn); doxycycline (Vibramycin)	Persisting cough, meningoencephalitis, polyneuritis, monoarticular arthritis, pericarditis, myocarditis
Viral pneumonia	Influenza viruses Parainfluenza viruses Respiratory syncytial viruses Rhinoviruses Adenovirus Varicella, rubella, rubeola, herpes simplex, cytomegalovirus, Epstein–Barr virus	Cough Constitutional symptoms may be pronounced (severe headache, anorexia, fever, and myalgia)	In majority of patients, influenza begins as an acute coryza; others have bronchitis, pleurisy, and so forth, whereas still others develop gastrointestinal symptoms Risk of developing influenza related to crowding and close contact of groups of individuals	Treat symptomatically Amantadine (Symmetrel) relieves symptoms Prophylactic vaccination recommended for high-risk persons (over 65; chronic cardiac or pulmonary disease, diabetes, and other metabolic disorders)	Persons with underlying disease have increased risk of complications; primary influenzal pneumonia; secondary bacterial pneumonia Bacterial superinfection Pericarditis Endocarditis
Pneumocystis carinii pneumonia	*Pneumocystis carinii*	Insidious onset Increasing dyspnea and nonproductive cough Tachypnea; progresses rapidly to intercostal retraction, nasal flaring, and cyanosis Lowering of arterial oxygen tension Chest x-ray will reveal diffuse, bilateral interstitial pneumonia	Usually seen in host whose resistance is compromised; most common opportunistic infection in AIDS Organism invades lungs of patients who have suppressed immune system (from cancer, AIDS, leukemia) or after immunosuppressive therapy for cancer, organ transplant, or collagen disease	Pentamidine methanesulfonate Trimethoprim-sulfamethoxazole (Bactrim); dapsone with trimethoprim (Trimpex); clindamycin (Cleocin) with primaquine	Patients are critically ill Prognosis guarded, because it usually is a complication of a severe underlying disorder
Fungal pneumonia	*Aspergillus fumigatus*	Fever, productive cough, chest pain, hemoptysis Chest x-ray reveals broad range of abnormalities from infiltration to consolidation, cavitation, and empyema	Frequently associated with concurrent infection by viruses, (cytomegalovirus) bacteria, and fungi Neutropenic individual most susceptible May develop *Aspergillus* as a superinfection	Amphotericin B (Fungizone); Intraconazole	High fatality rate Invades blood vessels and destroys lung tissue by direct invasion and vascular infarction

217

NURSING ALERT:
Recurring pneumonia often indicates underlying disease such as cancer of the lung or multiple myeloma.

Clinical Manifestations

(For most common forms of bacterial pneumonia.)

1. Sudden onset; shaking chill; rapidly rising fever of 39.5° to 40.5°C. (101° to 105°F)
2. Cough productive of purulent sputum.
3. Pleuritic chest pain aggravated by respiration/coughing.
4. Tachypnea accompanied by respiratory grunting, nasal flaring, use of accessory muscles of respiration.
5. Rapid, bounding pulse.

Diagnostic Evaluation

1. Chest x-ray to show presence/extent of pulmonary disease.
2. Gram's stain, culture, and sensitivity studies of sputum—may indicate offending organism.
3. Blood culture to detect bacteremia (bloodstream invasion) occurring with bacterial pneumonia.
4. Immunologic test for detecting microbial antigens in serum, sputum, and urine.

Management

1. Antimicrobial therapy—depends on laboratory identification of causative organism and sensitivity to specific antimicrobials.
2. Oxygen therapy if patient has inadequate gas exchange.

Complications

1. Pleural effusion.
2. Sustained hypotension and shock, especially in gram-negative bacterial disease, particularly in the elderly.
3. Superinfection: pericarditis, bacteremia, meningitis.
4. Delirium—this is considered a medical emergency.
5. Atelectasis—due to mucous plugs.
6. Delayed resolution.

Nursing Assessment

1. Take a careful history to help establish etiologic diagnosis.
   a. History of *recent* respiratory illness? Mode of onset?
   b. Presence of fever, chills, chest pain?
   c. Any family illness?
   d. Medications? Alcohol, tobacco, or IV drug use?
2. Observe for anxious, flushed appearance, shallow respirations, splinting of affected side, confusion, disorientation.
3. Auscultate for crackles overlying affected region, and for bronchial breath sounds when consolidation (filling of airspaces with exudate) is present.

Nursing Diagnoses

A. Impaired gas exchange related to decreased ventilation secondary to inflammation and infection involving distal airspaces
B. Ineffective airway clearance related to excessive tracheobronchial secretions
C. Pain related to inflammatory process and dyspnea

Nursing Interventions

A. *Improving Gas Exchange*
1. Observe for cyanosis, dyspnea, hypoxia, and confusion, indicating worsening condition.
2. Follow ABGs to determine oxygen need and response to oxygen therapy.
3. Administer oxygen at concentration to maintain PaO_2 at acceptable level—hypoxemia may be encountered because of abnormal ventilation–perfusion ratios in affected lung segments.
4. Avoid high concentrations of oxygen in patients with COPD; use of high oxygen concentrations may worsen alveolar ventilation by removing the patient's only remaining ventilatory drive.
5. Place patient in a fairly upright position to obtain greater lung expansion to improve aeration.

B. *Enhancing Airway Clearance*
1. Obtain freshly expectorated sputum for Gram's stain and culture, as directed. Instruct the patient as follows:
   a. Rinse mouth with water to minimize contamination by normal flora.
   b. Breathe deeply several times.
   c. Cough deeply and expectorate raised sputum into sterile container.
2. Encourage patient to cough—retained secretions interfere with gas exchange. Suction as necessary.
3. Encourage increased fluid intake, unless contraindicated, to thin mucus and promote expectoration and replace fluid losses due to fever, diaphoresis, dehydration, and dyspnea.
4. Humidify air or oxygen therapy to loosen secretions and improve ventilation.
5. Employ chest wall percussion and postural drainage when appropriate to loosen and mobilize secretions.
6. Auscultate the chest for crackles.
7. Administer cough suppressants when coughing is nonproductive, debilitating, and when coughing paroxysms cause serious hypoxemia.

C. *Relieving Pleuritic Pain*
1. Place in a comfortable position (semi-Fowler's) for resting and breathing; encourage frequent change of position to prevent pooling of secretions in lungs.
2. Demonstrate how to splint the chest while coughing.
3. Avoid suppressing a productive cough.
4. Administer prescribed analgesic agent to relieve pain. Avoid narcotics in patients with a history of COPD.

GERONTOLOGIC ALERT:
Sedatives, narcotics, and cough suppressants are generally contraindicated in the elderly, because of their tendency to suppress cough and gag reflexes and respiratory drive.

NURSING ALERT:
Restlessness, confusion, aggressiveness may be due to cerebral hypoxia. In such instances, sedatives are inappropriate.

5. Apply heat and/or cold to chest as prescribed.
6. Assist with intercostal nerve block for pain relief.
7. Encourage modified bedrest during febrile period.
8. Watch for abdominal distention or ileus, which may be due to swallowing of air during intervals of severe dyspnea. Insert a nasogastric or rectal tube as directed.

D. Monitoring for Complications
1. Remember that fatal complications may develop during the early period of antimicrobial treatment.
2. Monitor temperature, pulse, respiration, and blood pressure at regular intervals to assess the patient's response to therapy.
3. Listen to lungs and heart. Heart murmurs or friction rub may indicate acute bacterial endocarditis, pericarditis, or myocarditis.
4. Employ special nursing surveillance for patients with the following conditions:
   a. Alcoholism, COPD, immunosuppression; these persons, as well as elderly patients, may have little or no fever.
   b. Chronic bronchitis; it is difficult to detect subtle changes in condition, because the patient may have seriously compromised pulmonary function.
   c. Epilepsy—pneumonia may result from aspiration after a seizure.
   d. Delirium, which may be caused by hypoxia, meningitis, delirium tremens of alcoholism.
      (1) Prepare for lumbar puncture; meningitis may be lethal.
      (2) Ensure adequate hydration and give mild sedation.
      (3) Give oxygen.
      (4) Delirium must be controlled to prevent exhaustion and cardiac failure.
5. Assess these patients for *unusual behavior*, alterations in mental status, stupor, and congestive heart failure.
6. Assess for resistant fever or return of fever, indicating bacterial resistance to antibiotics.

Patient Education/Health Maintenance

1. Advise patient that fatigue, weakness, and depression may be prolonged after pneumonia.
2. Encourage chair rest after fever subsides; gradually increase activities to bring energy level back to preillness stage.
3. Encourage breathing exercises to clear lungs and promote full expansion and function after the fever subsides.
4. Explain that a chest x-ray is taken 4 to 6 weeks after recovery to evaluate lungs for clearing and detect any tumor or underlying cause.
5. Advise smoking cessation. Cigarette smoking destroys tracheobronchial cilial action, which is the first line of defense of lungs; also irritates mucosa of bronchi and inhibits function of alveolar scavenger cells (macrophages).
6. Advise the patient to keep up natural resistance with good nutrition, adequate rest—one episode of pneumonia may make the individual susceptible to recurring respiratory infections.
7. Instruct the patient to avoid fatigue, sudden extremes in temperature, and excessive alcohol intake, which lower resistance to pneumonia.
8. Encourage the yearly influenza immunization and immunization for *S. pneumoniae*, if indicated, a major cause of bacterial pneumonia.
9. Advise avoidance of contact with people who have upper respiratory infections for several months after pneumonia and resolves.

Evaluation

A. Cyanosis and dyspnea reduced; ABGs improved
B. Coughing effectively; absence of crackles
C. Appears more comfortable; free of pain

◆ ASPIRATION PNEUMONIA

Aspiration is the inhalation of oropharyngeal secretions and/or stomach contents into the lungs. It may produce an acute form of pneumonia.

Pathophysiology/Etiology

1. Patients at risk and factors associated with risk:
   a. Loss of protective airway reflexes (swallowing, laryngeal, cough) caused by altered state of consciousness, alcohol or drug overdose, during resuscitation procedures, seriously ill or debilitated patients, abnormalities of gag and swallowing reflexes
   b. Nasogastric tube feedings
   c. Obstetric patients—from general anesthesia, lithotomy position, delayed emptying of stomach from enlarged uterus, labor contractions
   d. Gastrointestinal (GI) conditions—hiatal hernia, intestinal obstruction, abdominal distention
   e. Prolonged endotracheal intubation/tracheostomy—can depress glottic and laryngeal reflexes from disuse
2. Effects of aspiration depend on volume and character of aspirated material
   a. Particulate matter—mechanical blockage of airways and secondary infection
   b. Anaerobic bacterial aspiration—from oropharyngeal secretions
   c. Gastric juice—destructive to alveoli and capillaries; results in outpouring of protein-rich fluids into the interstitial and intraalveolar spaces—impairs exchange of oxygen and carbon dioxide, producing hypoxemia, respiratory insufficiency and failure

Clinical Manifestations

1. Tachycardia, fever
2. Dyspnea, cough, tachypnea
3. Cyanosis
4. Crackles, rhonchi, wheezing
5. Pink, frothy sputum (may simulate acute pulmonary edema)

Diagnostic Evaluation

1. Chest x-ray—may be normal initially, with time shows consolidation and other abnormalities

Management

(Depends on the material aspirated)

1. Clearing the obstructed airway.
   a. If foreign body becomes lodged in the patient's throat, remove object with forceps.
   b. Place the patient in tilted head-down position on right side (right side more frequently affected if patient has aspirated solid particles).
   c. Suction trachea/endotracheal tube—to remove any particulate matter.
2. Laryngoscopy/bronchoscopy if patient has been asphyxiated by solid material.
3. Fluid volume replacement for correction of hypotension.
4. Antimicrobial therapy if there is evidence of superimposed bacterial infection.
5. Correction of acidosis; respiratory acidosis and metabolic acidosis indicate a severe reaction due to aspiration of gastric contents.
6. Oxygen therapy and assisted ventilation if adequate blood gas values cannot be maintained.

Complications

1. Lung abscess; empyema
2. Necrotizing pneumonia

Nursing Assessment

1. Assess for airway obstruction.
2. Assess for risk factors for aspiration.
3. Assess for development of fever, foul-smelling sputum, and development of congestion.

Nursing Diagnoses/Interventions

(Same as for pneumonia, p. 218.)

Prevention

1. Be on guard constantly and monitor patients at risk as described above.
2. Elevate head of bed for debilitated patients, for those receiving tube feedings, and for those with motor diseases of the esophagus.
3. Place patients with impaired reflexes in a lateral position.
4. Be sure that nasogastric tube is patent.
5. Give tube feedings slowly, with patient sitting up in bed.
   a. Check position of tube in stomach before feeding.
   b. Check seal of cuff of tracheostomy or endotracheal tube before feeding.

6. Keep the patients in a fasting state before anesthesia (at least 8 hours).
7. Feed patients with impaired swallowing slowly, and ensure that no food is retained in mouth after feeding.

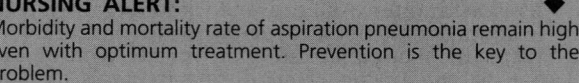

NURSING ALERT:
Morbidity and mortality rate of aspiration pneumonia remain high even with optimum treatment. Prevention is the key to the problem.

◆ PULMONARY EMBOLISM

Pulmonary embolism refers to the obstruction of one or more pulmonary arteries by a thrombus (or thrombi) originating usually in the deep veins of the legs or in the right side of the heart, which becomes dislodged and is carried to the lungs.
Pulmonary infarction—necrosis of lung tissue that can result from interference with blood supply.

Pathophysiology/Etiology

1. Obstruction, either partial or full, of pulmonary arteries, which causes decrease or absent blood flow; therefore, there is ventilation but no perfusion (ventilation–perfusion or V/Q mismatch).
2. Hemodynamic consequences:
   a. Increased pulmonary vascular resistance
   b. Increased pulmonary arterial pressure
   c. Increased right ventricular workload to maintain pulmonary blood flow
   d. Right ventricular failure
   e. Decreased cardiac output
   f. Decreased blood pressure
   g. Shock
3. Pulmonary emboli can vary in size and seriousness of consequences.
4. Predisposing factors include:
   a. Stasis; prolonged immobilization
   b. Concurrent phlebitis
   c. Previous heart (CHF; myocardial infarction) or lung disease
   d. Injury to vessel wall
   e. Coagulation disorders
   f. Metabolic, endocrine, vascular, or collagen disorders
   g. Malignancy
   h. Advancing age; estrogen therapy

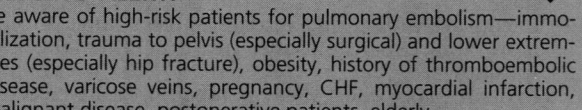

NURSING ALERT:
Be aware of high-risk patients for pulmonary embolism—immobilization, trauma to pelvis (especially surgical) and lower extremities (especially hip fracture), obesity, history of thromboembolic disease, varicose veins, pregnancy, CHF, myocardial infarction, malignant disease, postoperative patients, elderly.

Clinical Manifestations

1. *Dyspnea*, pleuritic pain, tachypnea, apprehension
   a. Chest pain with apprehension and a sense of im-

pending doom occurs when most of the pulmonary artery is obstructed.
2. Cyanosis, tachydysrhythmias, syncope, circulatory collapse and possibly death encountered in patients with massive pulmonary embolism
3. Subtle deterioration in patient's condition with no explainable cause
4. Pleural friction rub

NURSING ALERT:
Have a high index of suspicion for pulmonary embolus if there is a subtle deterioration in the patient's condition and unexplained cardiovascular and pulmonary findings.

Diagnostic Evaluation

1. ABGs—Decreased PaO$_2$ is usually found, due to perfusion abnormality of the lung.
2. Chest x-ray—Normal or possible wedge-shaped infiltrate.
3. Ventilation–perfusion (V/Q) lung scans—Perfusion scan investigates regional blood flow to determine presence of perfusion defects; ventilation scan may be done in patient with large perfusion defects.
4. Pulmonary angiogram (most definitive)—Emboli seen as "filling defects."

Management

A. Emergency Management
For massive pulmonary embolism; goal is to stabilize cardiorespiratory status

NURSING ALERT:
Massive pulmonary embolism is a medical emergency; the patient's condition tends to deteriorate rapidly. There is a profound decrease in cardiac output, with an accompanying increase in right ventricular pressure.

1. Oxygen is administered to relieve hypoxemia, respiratory distress, and cyanosis.
2. An infusion is started to open an IV route for drugs/fluids.
3. Vasopressors, inotropic agents such as dopamine (Intropin) and/or antidysrhythmic agents may be indicated to support circulation if the patient is unstable.
4. The ECG is monitored continuously for right ventricular failure, which may have a rapid onset.
5. Small doses of intravenous morphine are given to relieve anxiety, to alleviate chest discomfort (which improves ventilation), and to ease adaptation to mechanical ventilator, if this is necessary.
6. Pulmonary angiography, hemodynamic measurements, arterial blood gas determinations, and so forth, are carried out.

B. Subsequent Management
Anticoagulation and thrombolysis

1. IV heparin (Heparin)—Stops further thrombus formation and extends the clotting time of the blood; it is an anticoagulant and antithrombotic.
   a. IV loading dose usually followed by continuous pump or drip infusion or given intermittently every 4 to 6 hours.
   b. Dosage adjusted to maintain the activated partial thromboplastin time (PTT) at 1.5 to 2 times the pretreatment value (if the value was normal).
   c. Protamine sulfate may be given to neutralize heparin in event of severe bleeding.
2. Oral anticoagulation with warfarin (Coumadin) is usually used for follow-up anticoagulant therapy after heparin therapy has been established; interrupts the coagulation mechanism by interfering with the vitamin K–dependent synthesis of prothrombin and factors VII, IX, and X.
   a. Dosage is controlled by monitoring serial tests of prothrombin time; desired prothrombin time is 1.2 to 1.5 times control value.
   b. Reported as international normalized ratio (INR) of 1.2 to 1.5 by most laboratories.
   c. Anticoagulation is used to prevent new clot formation but does not dissolve previously formed clots. Thrombolytics are used to dissolve clots.

GERONTOLOGIC ALERT:
Consider the patient's age in dosing of anticoagulation therapy—usually will need a decreased dosing regimen.

3. Thrombolytic agents such as urokinase (Abbokinase) and streptokinase (Streptase) may be used in patients with massive pulmonary embolism; effective in lysing recently formed thrombi; improve circulatory and hemodynamic status. Administered IV in a loading dose followed by constant infusion.
4. Newer clot-specific thrombolytics (tissue plasminogen activator [t-PA], streptokinase activator complex, single-chain urokinase)—activate plasminogen only within thrombus itself rather than systematically; minimize occurrence of generalized fibrinolysis and subsequent bleeding.

C. Surgical Intervention
When anticoagulation is contraindicated or patient has recurrent embolization or develops serious complications from drug therapy.

1. Interruption of vena cava—Reduces channel size to prevent lower extremity emboli from reaching lungs. Accomplished by:
   a. Ligation, plication, or clipping of the inferior vena cava.
   b. Placement of transvenously inserted intraluminal filter in inferior vena cava to prevent migration of emboli (Fig. 9-2).
2. Embolectomy (removal of pulmonary embolic obstruction).

Complications

1. Bleeding as a result of treatment.
2. Respiratory failure.

Nursing Assessment

1. Take nursing history with emphasis on onset and severity of dyspnea and nature of chest pain.

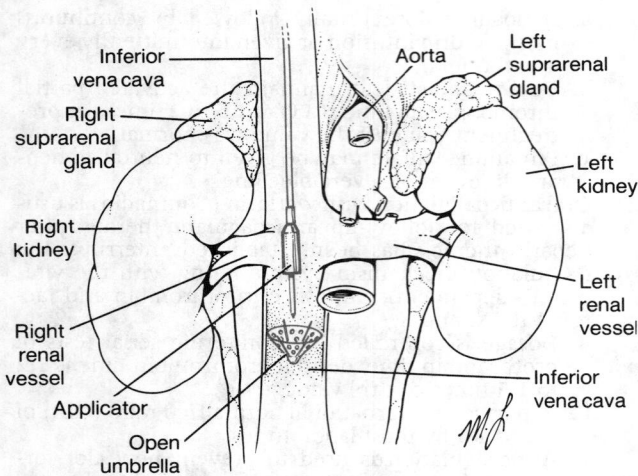

FIGURE 9-2 *Insertion of umbrella filter in inferior vena cava to prevent pulmonary embolism. Filter (compressed within an applicator catheter) is inserted through an incision in the right internal jugular vein. The applicator is withdrawn when the filter fixes itself to the wall of the inferior vena cava after ejection from the applicator.*

2. Examine the patient's legs carefully. Assess for swelling of leg, duskiness, pain on pressure over gastrocnemius muscle, pain on dorsiflexion of the foot (positive Homan's sign), which indicate thrombophlebitis as source.
3. Monitor respiratory rate—may be accelerated out of proportion to degree of fever and tachycardia.
    a. Inspect rate of inspiration to expiration.
    b. Percuss for resonance, dullness, and flatness.
    c. Auscultate for friction rub, crackles, rhonchi, and wheezing.
4. Auscultate heart; listen for splitting of second heart sound.

Nursing Diagnoses

A. Ineffective Breathing Pattern related to acute increase in alveolar dead space and possible changes in lung mechanics from embolism
B. Altered Tissue Perfusion (pulmonary) related to decreased blood circulation
C. Pain (pleuritic) related to congestion, possible pleural effusion, possible lung infarction
D. Anxiety related to dyspnea, pain, and seriousness of condition

Nursing Interventions

A. Correcting Breathing Pattern
1. Assess for hypoxia, headache, restlessness, apprehension, pallor, cyanosis, behavioral changes.
2. Monitor vital signs, ECG, oximetry, and ABG levels for adequacy of oxygenation.
3. Monitor patient's response to IV fluids/vasopressors.
4. Monitor oxygen therapy—used to relieve hypoxemia.

5. Prepare patient for assisted ventilation when hypoxemia is due to local areas of pneumoconstriction and abnormalities of ventilation–perfusion ratios.

B. Improving Tissue Perfusion
1. Closely monitor for shock—decreasing blood pressure, tachycardia, cool, clammy skin.
2. Monitor prescribed medications given to preserve right ventricular filling pressure and increase blood pressure.
3. Maintain patient on bedrest to reduce oxygen demands and risk of rebleeding.
4. Monitor urinary output hourly, because there may be reduced renal perfusion and decreased glomerular filtration.

C. Relieving Pain
1. Watch patient for signs of discomfort and pain.
2. Ascertain if pain worsens with deep breathing and coughing; listen for friction rub.
3. Give prescribed morphine (Duramorph) and monitor for pain relief and signs of respiratory depression.
4. Position with head of bed slightly elevated (unless contraindicated by shock) and with chest splinted for deep breathing and coughing.

D. Reducing Anxiety
1. Correct dyspnea and relieve physical discomfort.
2. Explain diagnostic procedures and the patient's role; correct any misconceptions.
3. Listen to the patient's concerns—attentive listening relieves anxiety and reduces emotional distress.
4. Speak calmly and slowly.
5. Do everything possible to enhance the patient's sense of control.

E. Intervening for Complications
1. Shock—From low cardiac output secondary to resistance to right ventricular outflow or to myocardial dysfunction due to ischemia.
    a. Assess for skin color changes, particularly nail beds, lips, ear lobes, and mucous membranes.
    b. Monitor blood pressure.
    c. Measure urinary output.
    d. Monitor IV infusion of isoproterenol (Isuprel) or other prescribed agents.
2. Bleeding—Related to anticoagulant or thrombolytic therapy.
    a. Assess patient for bleeding; major bleeding may occur from GI tract, brain, lungs, nose, and genitourinary (GU) tract.
    b. Perform stool guaiac test to detect occult blood loss.
    c. Monitor platelet count to detect heparin-induced thrombocytopenia.
    d. Minimize risk of bleeding by performing essential ABGs on upper extremities; apply digital compression at puncture site for 30 minutes; apply pressure dressing to previously involved sites; check site for oozing.
    e. Maintain patient on strict bedrest during thrombolytic therapy; avoid unnecessary handling.
    f. Discontinue infusion in the event of uncontrolled bleeding.

Patient Education/Health Maintenance

1. Advise patient of the possible need to continue taking anticoagulant therapy for 6 weeks up to an indefinite period.

2. Teach about signs of bleeding, especially of gums, nose, bruising, blood in urine and stools.
3. Warn against taking medications unless approved by health care provider, because many drugs interact with anticoagulants.
4. Instruct patient to tell dentist about taking an anticoagulant.
5. Warn against inactivity for prolonged periods or sitting with legs crossed to prevent recurrence.
6. Warn against sports/activities that may cause injury to legs and predispose to a thrombus.
7. Encourage wearing a Medic-Alert bracelet identifying patient as anticoagulant user.
8. Instruct to lose weight if applicable; obesity is a risk factor for women.
9. Discuss contraceptive methods with patient if applicable; female patients are advised against taking oral contraceptives.

Evaluation

A. Verbalizes less shortness of breath
B. Vital signs stable, adequate urinary output
C. Reports freedom from pain
D. Appears more relaxed; sleeping at long intervals

◆ TUBERCULOSIS

Tuberculosis is an infectious disease caused by bacteria (*Mycobacterium tuberculosis*) that are usually spread from person to person through the air. It usually infects the lung, but can occur at virtually any site in the body. The incidence of tuberculosis is on the rise, especially drug-resistant varieties. HIV-infected patients are especially at risk.

Pathophysiology/Etiology

A. *Transmission*
1. The term *mycobacterium* is descriptive of the organism, which is a bacterium that resembles a fungus. The organisms multiply slowly and are characterized as acid-fast aerobic organisms that can be killed by heat, sunshine, drying, and ultraviolet light.
2. Tuberculosis is an airborne disease transmitted by droplet nuclei, usually from within the respiratory tract of an infected person who exhales them during coughing, talking, sneezing, or singing.
3. When an uninfected susceptible person inhales the droplet-containing air, the organism is carried into the lung to the pulmonary alveoli.
4. Most people who become infected do not develop clinical illness, because the body's immune system brings the infection under control.

B. *Pathology*
1. The bacilli of tuberculosis infect the lung, forming a tubercle (lesion).
2. The tubercle
   a. May heal, leaving scar tissue.
   b. May continue as a granuloma, then heal, or be reactivated.
   c. May eventually proceed to necrosis, liquefaction, sloughing, and cavitation.

3. The initial lesion may disseminate tubercle bacilli by extension to adjacent tissues, via bloodstream, via lymphatic system, or through the bronchi.

Clinical Manifestations

Patient may be asymptomatic or may have insidious symptoms that are ignored.

1. Constitutional symptoms
   a. Fatigue, anorexia, weight loss, low-grade fever, night sweats, indigestion.
   b. Some patients have acute febrile illness, chills, generalized influenzalike symptoms.
2. Pulmonary signs and symptoms
   a. Cough (insidious onset) progressing in frequency and producing mucoid or mucopurulent sputum.
   b. Hemoptysis; chest pain; dyspnea (indicates extensive involvement).
3. Extrapulmonary tuberculosis: *Mycobacterium* can infect any organ in the body including pleurae, lymph nodes, genitourinary tract, bones/joints, peritoneum, central nervous system.

Diagnostic Evaluation

1. Sputum smear and culture—Diagnosis made by finding the acid-fast bacilli in sputum.
2. Chest x-ray to determine presence and extent of disease.
3. Tuberculin skin test (PPD or Mantoux test)—Inoculation of tubercle bacillus extract (tuberculin) into the intradermal layer of the inner aspect of the forearm (Procedure Guidelines 9-1). It is used to detect *Mycobacterium tuberculosis* infection, either past or present, active or inactive.
4. Screening tests—Multiple puncture tests such as tine test introduce either dried or liquid tuberculin into skin by puncturing the skin with an applicator.
   a. Used for screening large groups because there is no way to standardize the amount of tuberculin introduced, which does not allow precise interpretation of test results.
   b. All significant reactors to multiple puncture tests must be confirmed with the Mantoux test.

Management

(See Table 9-2.)

1. A combination of drugs to which the organisms are susceptible is given to destroy viable bacilli as rapidly as possible and to protect against the emergence of drug-resistant organisms.
2. Current recommended regimen of uncomplicated pulmonary tuberculosis is 2 months of bactericidal drugs isoniazid (INH), rifampin (Rifadin), and pyrazinamide (PYZ) followed by 4 months of isoniazid and rifampin.
3. Six months of therapy is usually effective for killing the three populations of bacilli: those rapidly dividing, those slowly dividing, and those only intermittently dividing.

TABLE 9-2 Recommended Drugs for the Initial Treatment of Tuberculosis in Adults

Drug	Dosage Forms	Daily Dose*	Twice Weekly Dose	Thrice Weekly Dose	Major Adverse Reactions
Isoniazid (INH)	Tablets: 100 mg 300 mg Syrup: 50 mg/5 mL Vials: 1 g	5 mg/kg PO or IM	15 mg/kg Maximum 900 mg	15 mg/kg Maximum 900 mg	Hepatic enzyme elevation, peripheral neuropathy, hepatitis, hypersensitivity
Rifampin (Rifadin)	Capsules: 150 mg 300 mg Syrup: formulated from capsules, 10 mg/mL	10 mg/kg PO	10 mg/kg Maximum 600 mg	10 mg/kg Maximum 600 mg	Orange discoloration of secretions and urine; nausea, vomiting, hepatitis, febrile reaction, purpura (rare)
Pyrazinamide (PYZ)	Tablets: 500 mg	15–30 mg/kg PO	50–70 mg/kg	50–70 mg/kg Maximum 3 g	Hepatotoxicity, hyperuricemia, arthralgias, skin rash, gastrointestinal upset
Streptomycin	Vials: 1 g, 4 g	15 mg/kg IM	25–30 mg/kg	25–30 mg/kg Maximum 1.5 g	Ototoxicity, nephrotoxicity
Ethambutol (Myambutol)	Tablets: 100 mg 400 mg	15–25 mg/kg PO	50 mg/kg	25–30 mg/kg	Optic neuritis (decreased red-green color discrimination, decreased visual acuity), skin rash

4. Sputum smears may be obtained every 2 weeks until they are negative; sputum cultures do not become negative for 3 to 5 months.
5. Second-line drugs such as capreomycin (Capastat), kanamycin (Kantrex), ethionamide (Trecator-SC), para-aminosalicylic acid, and cycloserine (Sandimmune) are used in patients with resistance, for retreatment, and in those with intolerance to other agents. Patients taking these drugs should be monitored by health providers experienced in their use.

Complications

1. Pleural effusion
2. Tuberculosis pneumonia
3. Other organ involvement with tuberculosis

Nursing Assessment

1. Obtain history of exposure to tuberculosis.
2. Assess for symptoms of active disease—productive cough, night sweats, afternoon temperature elevation, weight loss, pleuritic chest pain.
3. Auscultate lungs for crackles.
4. If patient is on isoniazid, assess for liver dysfunction.
   a. Question the patient about loss of appetite, fatigue, joint pain, fever, and dark urine.
   b. Monitor for fever, right upper quadrant abdominal tenderness, nausea, vomiting, rash, persistent paresthesias of hands and feet.
   c. Monitor results of periodic liver function studies.

Nursing Diagnoses

A. Ineffective Breathing Pattern related to decreased lung capacity
B. Risk for Infection Transmission related to nature of the disease and patient's symptoms
C. Altered Nutrition: less than body requirements related to poor appetite, fatigue, and productive cough
D. Noncompliance related to lack of motivation and long-term treatment

Nursing Interventions

A. *Improving Breathing Pattern*
1. Administer and teach self-administration of medications as ordered.
2. Encourage rest and avoidance of exertion.
3. Monitor breath sounds, respiratory rate, sputum production, and dyspnea.
4. Provide supplemental oxygen as ordered.

B. *Preventing Transmission of Infection*
1. Be aware that tuberculosis is transmitted by respiratory droplets or secretions.
2. Provide care for hospitalized patient in a negative pressure room to prevent respiratory droplets from leaving room when door is opened.
3. Enforce that all staff and visitors use standard dust/mist/fume masks (Class C) for any contact with patient.
4. Use high-efficiency particulate masks such as Hepafilter masks for high-risk procedures such as suctioning, bronchoscopy, or pentamadine treatments.

5. Use Universal Precautions for additional protection: gowns and gloves for any direct contact with patient, linens or articles in room, meticulous handwashing, and so forth.
6. Educate the patient to control spread of infection through secretions.
   a. Cover mouth and nose with double-ply tissue when coughing/sneezing. Do not sneeze into bare hand.
   b. Wash hands after coughing/sneezing.
   c. Dispose of tissues promptly into closed plastic bag.

C. *Improving Nutritional Status*
1. Encourage and explain the importance of eating a nutritious diet to promote healing and improve defense against infection.
2. Provide small frequent meals and liquid supplements during symptomatic period.
3. Monitor weight.
4. Administer vitamin supplements, as ordered, particularly pyridoxine (vitamin B_6) to prevent peripheral neuropathy in patients taking isoniazid.

D. *Avoiding Noncompliance*
1. Educate the patient about the etiology, transmission, and effects of tuberculosis. Stress the importance of continuing to take medicine for the prescribed time because bacilli multiply very slowly and thus can only be eradicated over a long period of time.
2. Review the side effects of the drug therapy (see Table 9-2). Question the patient specifically about common toxicities of drugs being used and emphasize immediate reporting should these occur.
3. Participate in observation of medication taking, weekly pill counts, or other programs designed to increase compliance with treatment for tuberculosis.

> **NURSING ALERT:** ❖
> Patient compliance remains a major problem in eradicating tuberculosis. Therefore, it may be helpful or necessary to have patient take medication in observed setting.

4. Investigate living conditions, availability of transportation, financial status, alcohol and drug abuse, and motivation, which may affect compliance with follow-up and treatment. Initiate referrals to a social worker for interventions in these areas.

Patient Education/Health Maintenance

1. Review possible complications: hemorrhage, pleurisy, symptoms of recurrence (persistent cough, fever, or hemoptysis).
2. Advise on avoidance of job-related exposure to excessive amounts of silicone (working in foundry, rock quarry, sand blasting), which increases chance of reactivation.
3. Encourage the patient to report at specified intervals for bacteriologic (smear) examination of sputum to monitor therapeutic response and compliance.
4. Instruct in basic hygiene practices and investigate living conditions. Crowded conditions contribute to development and spread of tuberculosis.
5. Encourage follow-up chest x-rays for rest of life to evaluate for recurrence.
6. Instruct on prophylaxis with isoniazid for persons infected with the tubercle bacillus without active disease to prevent disease from occurring, or to people at high risk of becoming infected. Prophylaxis is recommended for the following groups:
   a. Household members and other close associates of potentially infectious tuberculosis cases
   b. Newly infected persons (positive skin test within 2 years)
   c. Persons with past tuberculosis who have not received adequate therapy
   d. Persons with significant reactions to tuberculin skin test and who are in special clinical situations (silicosis, diabetes, B-cell malignancies, end-stage renal disease, severe malnutrition, immunosuppression, HIV positive)
   e. Tuberculin skin reactors under age 35 years with none of the aforementioned risk factors

Evaluation

A. Afebrile; dyspnea relieved
B. Universal precautions observed; patient disposing of respiratory secretions properly
C. Maintains body weight
D. Taking medications as prescribed

PROCEDURE GUIDELINES 9-1 ◆ Tuberculin Skin Test

EQUIPMENT Purified protein derivative (PPD) tuberculin antigen; intermediate strength
Tuberculin syringe
Short 1.25 cm (½ inch) 26- or 27-gauge steel needle
Alcohol sponge

PROCEDURE	NURSING ACTION	RATIONALE
	PREPARATORY PHASE	
	1. Determine if the patient has ever had BCG vaccine, recent viral disease, immunosuppression by disease, drugs, or steroids.	1. Any of these may cause false readings.

(continued)

PROCEDURE GUIDELINES 9-1 ◆ Tuberculin Skin Test *(continued)*

PROCEDURE (cont'd)	NURSING ACTION	RATIONALE

PERFORMANCE PHASE

1. Draw up PPD-tuberculin into tuberculin syringe.

2. Cleanse the skin of the inner aspect of forearm with alcohol. Allow to dry.
3. Stretch the skin taut.
4. Hold the tuberculin syringe close to the skin so the hub of the needle touches it as the needle is introduced, bevel up.
5. Inject the tuberculin into the superficial layer of the skin to form a wheal 6 mm to 10 mm in diameter.

FOLLOW-UP PHASE

TO READ THE TEST

1. Read the test within 48 to 72 hours when the induration is most evident.
2. Have a good light available. Flex the forearm slightly at the elbow.
3. Inspect for the presence of *induration;* inspect from a side view against the light; inspect by direct light.
4. Palpate: Lightly rub the finger across the injection site from the area of normal skin to the area of induration. Outline the diameter of induration.
5. Measure the maximum transverse diameter of induration (not erythema) in millimeters with a flexible ruler.

INTERPRETATION

1. Induration of 5 mm or more in diameter

2. Induration of 10 mm or more in diameter

3. Induration of 15 mm or more in diameter

RATIONALE

1. Follow the manufacturer's directions. Each 0.1-mL dose should contain 5 tuberculin units (TU of PPD-tuberculin). Use the antigen immediately to avoid absorption onto the plastic/glass syringe.

4. This reduces the needle angle at the skin surface and facilitates the injection of tuberculin just beneath the surface of the skin.
5. If no wheal appears (because the injection was made too deep), inject again at another site at least 5 cm (2 inches) away.

1. Tuberculin skin tests are tests of *delayed hypersensitivity.*

3. Induration refers to hardening or thickening of tissues.

4. Erythema (redness) without induration is generally considered to be of no significance.

5. The extent of induration is measured in two diameters and recorded

1. Considered positive in
   a. Persons with known HIV or unknown HIV but with risk factors for HIV
   b. Persons who have had recent contact with active tuberculosis
   c. Persons who have fibrotic changes on chest x-ray, consistent with healed TB
2. Considered positive in all persons who do not meet above criteria but who have other risk factors for tuberculosis, such as homelessness, alcoholism, malnutrition, and healthcare work.
3. Considered positive in persons who do not meet the above criteria.

◆ PLEURISY

Pleurisy is a clinical term to describe *pleuritis* (inflammation of the pleura, both parietal and visceral).

Pathophysiology/Etiology

May occur in the course of many pulmonary diseases:

1. Pneumonia (bacterial, viral)
2. Tuberculosis
3. Pulmonary infarction, embolism
4. Pulmonary abscess
5. Upper respiratory tract infection
6. Pulmonary neoplasm

Clinical Manifestations

1. Chest pain—Becomes severe, sharp, and knifelike on inspiration (pleuritic pain).
   a. May become minimal or absent when breath is held.
   b. May be localized or radiate to shoulder or abdomen.
2. Intercostal tenderness.
3. Pleural friction rub—Grating or leathery sounds heard in both phases of respiration; heard low in the axilla or over the lung base posteriorly; may be heard for only a day or so.
4. Evidence of infection; fever, malaise, increased white cell count.

Diagnostic Evaluation

1. Chest x-ray may show pleural thickening.
2. Sputum examination may indicate infectious organism.

3. Examination of pleural fluid obtained by thoracentesis for smear and culture.
4. Pleural biopsy may be necessary to rule out other conditions.

Management

1. Treatment for the underlying primary disease (pneumonia, infarction, and so forth). Inflammation usually resolves when the primary disease subsides.
2. Pain relief, using both pharmacologic and nonpharmacologic methods.
3. Intercostal nerve block may be necessary when pain causes hypoventilation (see Procedure Guidelines 9-2).

Complications

1. Severe pleural effusion.

Nursing Assessment

1. Assess patient's level of pain.
2. Observe for signs and symptoms of pleural effusion (dyspnea, pain, decreased local excursion of chest wall).
3. Auscultate lungs for pleural friction rub.

Nursing Diagnoses

A. Ineffective Breathing Pattern related to stabbing chest pain

Nursing Interventions

A. *Relieving Pain*
1. Assist patient to find comfortable position that will promote aeration; lying on affected side decreases stretching of the pleura and, therefore, the pain decreases.
2. Instruct patient in splinting chest while taking a deep breath or coughing.
3. Administer or teach self-administration of pain medications as ordered.
4. Employ nonpharmacologic interventions for pain relief such as application of heat, muscle relaxation, and imagery.
5. Assist with intercostal nerve block if indicated.

Patient Education/Health Maintenance

1. Instruct patient to seek early intervention for pulmonary diseases so pleurisy can be avoided.
2. Reassure and encourage patience because pain will subside.
3. Advise on reporting shortness of breath, which could indicate pleural effusion.

Evaluation

A. Respirations deep without pain.

PROCEDURE GUIDELINES 9-2 ◆ Assisting With an Intercostal Nerve Block

EQUIPMENT
Syringes, 10-mL Luer-Lok
Needles, No. 22 to 30 gauge
Anesthetic solution (lidocaine, bupivacaine, procaine)
Skin germicide; sterile gloves

PROCEDURE	NURSING ACTION	RATIONALE

PREPARATORY PHASE

1. Inform the patient that he or she will experience the prick of the needle and a slight sensation of pressure.
2. Position the patient as directed:
   a. Have the patient sit up, bend forward, and hug a pillow, OR
   b. Place the patient prone with pillow under chest, OR
   c. Have the patient lie on unaffected side with upper arm hanging over the side of the table.
3. Ask the patient to identify the site of pain.

    a. This posture moves the scapulae forward and out of the way.
    b. The prone position helps immobilize the patient.
    c. This pulls the scapula out of the way.

3. To determine which intercostal nerves are to be injected.

PERFORMANCE PHASE (BY THE PHYSICIAN)

1. After the skin is prepared, the lower margin of the rib is palpated and a small skin wheal is raised, using a 25- to 30-gauge needle.

1. This is infiltration anesthesia.

(continued)

PROCEDURE GUIDELINES 9-2 ◆ Assisting With an Intercostal Nerve Block
(continued)

PROCEDURE (cont'd)	NURSING ACTION	RATIONALE

2. Usually nerve blocks are done at the posterior angle of the ribs between the posterior axillary line and the spine.

3. A fine needle is advanced through the wheal and directed downward so it slips under the edge of the rib into the upper portion of the interspace.

4. The syringe (needle in place) is aspirated.

5. The local anesthetic (usually 3–5 mL) is injected into the area.

2. The posterior angle is the most prominent and accessible, and an injection at this area produces a block of the entire distal nerve.

3. The intercostal nerve runs in a groove along the under-surface of the above rib.

4. To ensure that the needle has not punctured the lung or that an intercostal vessel has been entered.

5. Usually the local anesthetic is injected above and below the painful rib to obtain complete relief of pain, as the sensory fields of intercostal nerves overlap.

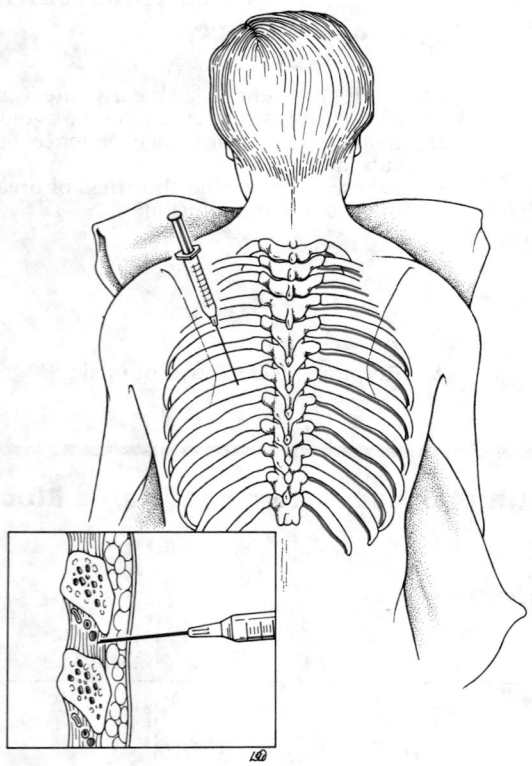

Intercostal nerve block.

FOLLOW-UP PHASE

1. Assess for relief of pain and less painful coughing.
2. Obtain a chest x-ray.
3. Complications:
   a. Intravascular injection
   b. Puncture of the lung with pneumothorax
   c. Hypotension

1. This is the expected outcome.
2. To ensure that a pneumothorax has not occurred.

◆ PLEURAL EFFUSION

Pleural effusion refers to a collection of fluid in the pleural space. It is almost always secondary to other diseases.

Pathophysiology/Etiology

1. May be either transudative or exudative.
2. Transudative effusions occur primarily in noninflammatory conditions; is an accumulation of low-protein, low cell count fluid.
3. Exudative effusions occur in an area of inflammation; is an accumulation of high-protein fluid.
4. Is a complication of:
   a. Disseminated cancer (particularly lung and breast); lymphoma.
   b. Pleuropulmonary infections (pneumonia).
   c. Congestive heart failure (CHF); cirrhosis; nephrosis.
   d. Other conditions—sarcoidosis, systemic lupus erythematosus (SLE), peritoneal dialysis, and so forth.

Clinical Manifestations

1. Dyspnea, pleuritic chest pain, cough.
2. Dullness or flatness to percussion (over areas of fluid) with decreased or absent breath sounds.

Diagnostic Evaluation

1. Chest x-ray or ultrasound to detect presence of fluid
2. Thoracentesis—Biochemical, bacteriologic, and cytologic studies of pleural fluid to indicate cause

Management

A. *General*
1. Treatment is directed at underlying cause (heart disease, infection).
2. Thoracentesis is done to remove fluid, to collect a specimen, and to relieve dyspnea.

B. *For Malignant Effusions*
1. Chest tube drainage, radiation, chemotherapy, surgical pleurodectomy, pleuroperitoneal shunt, or pleurodesis

> **NURSING ALERT:** ❖
> In malignant conditions, thoracentesis may provide only transient benefits, as effusion may reaccumulate within a few days.

2. *Pleurodesis*—production of adhesions between the parietal and visceral pleura accomplished by tube thoracostomy, pleural space drainage, and intrapleural instillation of a sclerosing agent (tetracycline)
   a. Drug introduced through tube into pleural space; tube clamped
   b. Patient is helped to assume varying positions for 3 to 5 minutes each to allow drug to spread to all surfaces of the pleura
   c. Tube is unclamped as prescribed
   d. Chest drainage continued for 24 hours or longer
   e. Resulting pleural irritation, inflammation, and fibrosis causes adhesion of the visceral and parietal surfaces when they are brought together by the negative pressure caused by chest suction.

Complications

1. Large effusion could lead to respiratory failure.

Nursing Assessment

1. Obtain history of previous pulmonary condition.
2. Assess patient for dyspnea and tachypnea.
3. Auscultate and percuss lungs for abnormalities.

Nursing Diagnoses

A. Ineffective Breathing Pattern related to collection of fluid in pleural space

Nursing Interventions

A. *Maintaining Normal Breathing Pattern*
1. Institute treatments to resolve the underlying cause, as ordered.
2. Assist with thoracentesis, if indicated (see p. 148).
3. Maintain chest drainage as needed (see p. 209).
4. Provide care after pleurodesis.
   a. Monitor for excessive pain from the sclerosing agent, which may cause hypoventilation.
   b. Administer prescribed analgesic.
   c. Assist patient undergoing instillation of intrapleural lidocaine if pain relief is not forthcoming.
   d. Administer oxygen as indicated by dyspnea.
   e. Observe patient's breathing pattern, and other vital signs, for evidence of improvement or deterioration.

Patient Education/Health Maintenance

1. Instruct patient to seek early intervention for unusual shortness of breath, especially if patient has underlying chronic lung disease.

Evaluation

A. Reports absence of shortness of breath

◆ LUNG ABSCESS

A *lung abscess* is a localized, pus-containing, necrotic lesion in the lung characterized by cavity formation.

Pathophysiology/Etiology

1. Most often occurs due to aspiration of vomitus or infected material from upper respiratory tract.

2. Secondary causes include:
   a. Aspiration of foreign body into lung.
   b. Pulmonary embolus.
   c. Trauma.
   d. Tuberculosis, necrotizing pneumonia.
   e. Bronchial obstruction (usually a tumor) causes obstruction to bronchus, leading to infection distal to the growth.
3. The right lung is involved more frequently than the left because of dependent position of the right bronchus, the less acute angle which the right main bronchus forms within the trachea, and its larger size.
4. In the initial stages, the cavity in the lung may or may not communicate with the bronchus.
5. Eventually, the cavity becomes surrounded or encapsulated by a wall of fibrous tissue, except at one or two points where the necrotic process extends until it reaches the lumen of some bronchus or pleural space and establishes a communication with the respiratory tract, the pleural cavity (bronchopleural fistula), or both.
6. The organisms most often seen are *Klebsiella pneumoniae* and *Staphylococcus aureus*.

Clinical Manifestations

1. Cough, fever and malaise from segmental pneumonitis and atelectasis.
2. Headache, anemia, weight loss, dyspnea, weakness.
3. Pleuritic chest pain from extension of suppurative pneumonitis to pleural surface.
4. Production of mucopurulent sputum, often foul-smelling; blood streaking common; may become profuse after abscess ruptures into bronchial tree.
5. Chest may be dull to percussion, decreased or absent breath sounds, intermittent pleural friction rub.

Diagnostic Evaluation

1. X-ray of chest for diagnosis and location of lesion
2. Direct bronchoscopic visualization to exclude possibility of tumor or foreign body; bronchial washings and brush biopsy may be done for cytopathologic study
3. Sputum culture and sensitivity to determine causative organism(s) and antimicrobial sensitivity

Management

1. Administration of appropriate antimicrobial agent, usually by IV route, until clinical condition improves; then oral administration.
2. Chest physical therapy and postural drainage to drain cavity.
3. Bronchoscopy to drain abscess is controversial.
4. Surgical intervention only if patient fails to respond to medical management, sustains a hemorrhage, or has a suspected tumor.
5. Nutritional management usually is a high-calorie, high-protein diet.

Complications

1. Hemoptysis from erosion of a vessel
2. Empyema, bronchopleural fistula
3. Brain abscess

Nursing Assessment

1. Examine oral cavity, because poor condition of teeth and gums increases number of anaerobes in oral cavity and could be source for infection.
2. Perform chest examination for abnormalities.
3. Monitor for foul-smelling sputum, which indicates an anaerobic pulmonary infection.
4. Review results of laboratory and x-ray findings for location of abscess and identification of causative organism.

Nursing Diagnoses

A. Ineffective Breathing Pattern related to presence of suppurative lung disease
B. Pain related to infection
C. Altered Nutrition: less than body requirements related to catabolic state from chronic infection

Nursing Interventions

A. *Minimizing Respiratory Dysfunction*
1. Monitor patient's response to antimicrobial therapy; take temperature at prescribed intervals.
2. Carry out drainage procedures to hasten resolution.
   a. Postural drainage positions to be assumed depend on location of abscess.
   b. Carry out percussion, coughing, and breathing exercises.
   c. Measure and record the volume of sputum to follow patient's clinical course.
   d. Give adequate fluids to enhance liquefying of secretions.

B. *Attaining Comfort*
1. Use nursing measures to combat generalized discomfort; oral hygiene, positions of comfort, relaxing massage.
2. Take temperature, pulse, and respirations at regular intervals to determine type of fever and monitor the severity and duration of the infectious process.
3. Encourage rest and limitation of physical activity during febrile periods.
4. Monitor chest tube functioning.

C. *Improving Nutritional Status*
1. Provide a high-protein and high-calorie diet.
2. Offer liquid supplements for additional nutritional support when anorexia limits patient's intake.
3. Monitor weight weekly.

Patient Education/Health Maintenance

1. Teach the patient that an extended course of antimicrobial therapy (4 to 8 weeks) is usually necessary; mixed infections are common and may require multiple antibiotics.
2. Encourage patient to have periodontal care, especially in presence of gingival lesions.
3. Stress importance of follow-up x-rays to monitor abscess cavity closure.

4. Remind family that patient may aspirate if weakness, confusion, alcoholism, seizures, and swallowing difficulties are present.
5. Encourage patient to assume responsibility for attaining/maintaining an optimal state of health through a planned program of nutrition, rest, and exercise.

Evaluation

A. Achieves improved respiratory function; temperature in normal range; less purulent sputum expectorated
B. Appears more comfortable; verbalizes less pain
C. Eating better; weight stable

◆ CANCER OF THE LUNG (BRONCHOGENIC CANCER)

Bronchogenic cancer refers to a malignant tumor of the lung arising within the wall or epithelial lining of the bronchus. The lung is also a common site of metastasis from cancer elsewhere in the body by way of venous circulation or lymphatic spread. Bronchogenic cancer is classified according to cell type:

Epidermoid (squamous cell)—most common
Adenocarcinoma
Small cell (oat cell) carcinoma
Large cell (undifferentiated) carcinoma

Pathophysiology/Etiology

A. *Predisposing factors*
1. Cigarette smoking—Amount, frequency, and duration of smoking have positive relationship to cancer of the lung.
2. Occupational exposure to asbestos, arsenic, chromium, nickel, iron, radioactive substances, isopropyl oil, coal tar products, petroleum oil mists alone or in combination with tobacco smoke.

> **NURSING ALERT:**
> Suspect cancer of the lung in patients who belong to a susceptible age group and who have repeated unresolved respiratory infections.

B. *Staging*
1. Refers to anatomic extent of tumor, lymph node involvement, and metastatic spread
2. Staging done by:
   a. Tissue diagnosis
   b. Lymph node biopsy
   c. Mediastinoscopy

Clinical Manifestations

Usually occur late and are related to size and location of tumor, extent of spread, and involvement of other structures

1. Cough, especially a new type or changing cough, results from bronchial irritation.
2. Dyspnea; wheezing (suggests partial bronchial obstruction)
3. Chest pain (poorly localized and aching)
4. Excessive sputum production; repeated upper respiratory infections
5. Hemoptysis
6. Malaise, fever, weight loss, fatigue, anorexia
7. Paraneoplastic syndrome—Metabolic or neurologic disturbances related to the secretion of substances by the neoplasm
8. Symptoms of metastases—Bone pain, abdominal discomfort, nausea and vomiting from liver involvement, pancytopenia from bone marrow involvement, headache from CNS metastasis
9. Usual sites of metastases—Lymph nodes, bones, liver

Diagnostic Evaluation

1. X-ray of the chest, including fluoroscopy and tomography; lung cancers may be partly or completely hidden by other structures.
2. Cytologic examination of sputum/chest fluids for malignant cells.
3. Fiberoptic bronchoscopy for observation of location and extent of tumor; for biopsy.
4. CT—Sensitive in detecting small nodules and metastatic lesions.
5. Lymph node biopsy; mediastinoscopy to establish lymphatic spread; to plan treatment.
6. Pulmonary function tests (PFTs) combined with split-function perfusion scan to determine if patient will have adequate pulmonary reserve to withstand surgical procedure.

Management

The treatment depends on the cell type, stage of disease, and the physiologic status of the patient. It includes a multidisciplinary approach that may be used separately or in combination, including:

1. Surgical resection
2. Radiotherapy
3. Chemotherapy
4. Immunotherapy

See Chapter 6 for more information on these methods.

Complications

1. Superior vena cava syndrome—Oncologic complication caused by obstruction of major blood vessels draining the head, neck, and upper torso.
2. Hypercalcemia—Commonly from bone metastases.
3. Syndrome of inappropriate antidiuretic hormone (SIADH) secretion with hyponatremia and abnormal water retention.
4. Pleural effusion.
5. Infectious complications, especially upper respiratory infections.
6. Brain metastasis; spinal cord compression.

Nursing Assessment

1. Determine onset and duration of coughing, sputum production, and the degree of dyspnea. Auscultate for breath sounds. Observe symmetry of chest during respirations.
2. Take anthropometric measurements; weigh patient; review laboratory biochemical tests; conduct appraisal of 24-hour food intake.
3. Ask about pain; location, intensity, factors influencing pain.

Nursing Diagnoses

A. Ineffective Breathing Pattern related to obstructive and restrictive respiratory processes associated with lung cancer
B. Altered Nutrition: less than body requirements related to hypermetabolic state, taste aversion, anorexia secondary to radiotherapy/chemotherapy
C. Pain related to tumor effects, invasion of adjacent structures, toxicities associated with radiotherapy/chemotherapy
D. Anxiety related to uncertain outcome and fear of recurrence

Nursing Interventions

See Chapter 6.

A. *Improving Breathing Patterns*
  1. Prepare patient physically, emotionally, and intellectually for prescribed therapeutic program.
  2. Elevate head of bed to promote gravity drainage and prevent fluid collection in upper body (from superior vena cava syndrome).
  3. Teach breathing retraining exercises to increase diaphragmatic excursion with resultant reduction in work of breathing.
  4. Give prescribed treatment for productive cough (expectorant; antimicrobial agent) to prevent thickened secretions and subsequent dyspnea.
  5. Augment the patient's ability to cough effectively.
    a. Splint chest manually with hands.
    b. Instruct patient to inspire fully and cough two to three times in one breath.
    c. Provide humidifier/vaporizer to provide moisture to loosen secretions.
  6. Support patient undergoing removal of pleural fluid (by thoracentesis or tube thoracostomy) and instillation of sclerosing agent to obliterate pleural space and prevent fluid recurrence.
  7. Administer oxygen by way of nasal cannula as prescribed.
  8. Encourage energy conservation through decreasing activities.
  9. Allow patient to sleep in a reclining chair if severely dyspneic.
  10. Recognize the anxiety associated with dyspnea; teach relaxation techniques.

B. *Improving Nutritional Status*
  1. Emphasize that nutrition is an important part of the treatment of lung cancer.
    a. Encourage small amounts of high-calorie and high-protein foods frequently, rather than three daily meals.
    b. Suggest eating major meal in the morning if rapidly becoming satiated and feeling full are problems.
    c. Ensure adequate protein intake—milk, eggs, chicken, fowl, fish, and oral nutritional supplements if patient cannot tolerate other meats.
  2. Administer or encourage prescribed vitamin supplement to avoid deficiency states, glossitis, and cheilosis.
  3. Change consistency of diet to soft or liquid if patient has esophagitis from radiation therapy.
  4. Give enteral or total parenteral nutrition for malnourished patient who is unable or unwilling to eat.

C. *Controlling Pain*
  1. Take a history of pain complaint; assess presence/absence of support system.
  2. Administer prescribed drug, usually starting with nonsteroidal antiinflammatory drugs (NSAID) and progressing to adjuvant analgesic and narcotic agents.
    a. Administer regularly to maintain pain at tolerable level.
    b. Titrate to achieve pain control.
  3. Consider alternative methods, such as cognitive and behavioral training, biofeedback, relaxation, to increase patient's sense of control.
  4. Evaluate problems of insomnia, depression, anxiety, and so forth that may be contributing to patient's pain.
  5. Initiate bowel training program, because constipation is a side effect of some analgesic/narcotic agents.
  6. Facilitate referral to pain clinic/specialist if pain becomes refractory (unyielding) to usual methods of control.

D. *Minimizing Anxiety*
  1. Realize that shock, disbelief, denial, anger, and depression are all normal reactions to the diagnosis of lung cancer.
  2. Try to have the patient express any concerns; share these concerns with health professionals.
  3. Encourage the patient to communicate feelings to significant persons in his or her life.
  4. Expect some feelings of anxiety and depression to recur during illness.
  5. Encourage the patient to keep busy and remain in the mainstream. Continue with usual activities (work, recreation, sexual) as much as possible.

Patient Education/Health Maintenance

1. Teach patient to use NSAID or other prescribed medication as necessary for pain without being overly concerned about addiction.
2. Help the patient realize that not every ache and pain is due to the results of lung cancer; some patients do not even experience pain.
3. Tell the patient that radiation therapy may be used for pain control if tumor has spread to bone.
4. Advise the patient to report any new or persistent pain; it may be due to some other cause, such as arthritis.
5. Suggest talking to a social worker about financial assistance, or other services that may be needed.

6. For additional information and support, refer to: American Cancer Society—call local chapter or 1-800-ACS-2345.

Evaluation

A. Able to perform self-care without dyspnea
B. Eating small meals four to five times a day; weight stable
C. Reports pain decreased from level 6 to level 2 with medication
D. Verbalizing anger; practicing relaxation techniques

Chronic Disorders

◆ BRONCHIECTASIS

Bronchiectasis is a chronic dilatation of the bronchi and bronchioles due to inflammation and destruction of their walls.

Pathophysiology/Etiology

1. There is damage to the bronchial wall, which leads to the buildup of thick sputum, causing obstruction.
2. Severe coughing results in the permanent dilation of the bronchial walls.
3. Usually involves the lower lobes.
4. As the process progresses, there is atelectasis and fibrosis, which lead to respiratory insufficiency.
5. Pulmonary infections, obstruction of bronchi, aspiration of foreign bodies, vomitus, or material from upper respiratory tract, and immunodeficiency are common causes.

Clinical Manifestations

1. Persistent cough with production of copious amounts of purulent sputum
2. Intermittent hemoptysis; breathlessness
3. Recurrent fever and bouts of pulmonary infection
4. Crackles and rhonchi heard over involved lobes
5. Finger clubbing

Diagnostic Evaluation

1. Chest x-ray may reveal areas of atelectasis with widespread dilatation of bronchi.
2. Sputum examination may detect offending pathogens.

Management

Goal: Prevent progression of disease.

1. Infection controlled by:
   a. Smoking cessation
   b. Prompt antimicrobial treatment of exacerbations of infection
   c. Immunization against potential pulmonary pathogens (influenza and pneumonia)
2. Bronchodilators for selected patients with increased airway hyperreactivity
3. Surgical resection (segmental resection) when conservative management fails

Complications

1. Progressive suppuration
2. Hemoptysis; major pulmonary hemorrhage
3. Emphysema; chronic respiratory insufficiency

Nursing Assessment

1. Obtain history regarding amount and characteristics of sputum produced, including hemoptysis.
2. Auscultate lungs for diffuse rhonchi and crackles.

Nursing Diagnosis

1. Ineffective Airway Clearance related to tenacious and copious secretions.

Nursing Interventions

A. *Maintaining Airway Clearance*
1. Encourage use of chest physical therapy techniques to empty the bronchi of their accumulated secretions.
   a. Assist with postural drainage positioning for involved lung segment(s) to drain the bronchiectatic areas by gravity, thus reducing degree of infection and symptoms.
   b. Employ percussion and vibration to assist in mobilizing secretions.
   c. Encourage productive coughing to help clear secretions.
2. Encourage increased intake of fluids to reduce viscosity of sputum and make expectoration easier.
3. Use vaporizer to provide humidification and keep secretions thin.

Patient Education/Health Maintenance

1. Instruct the patient to avoid noxious fumes, dusts, smoke and other pulmonary irritants.
2. Teach the patient to monitor sputum. Report if change in quantity (increase/decrease) or character occurs.
3. Instruct the patient and family about importance of pulmonary drainage.
   a. Teach drainage exercises and chest physical therapy techniques.
   b. Encourage postural drainage before rising in the morning, because sputum accumulates during night.
   c. Encourage patient to engage in physical activity throughout day to help move mucus.

4. Encourage regular dental care because copious sputum production may affect dentition.
5. Emphasize the importance of influenza and pneumonia immunizations and prompt treatment of all respiratory infections.

Evaluation

A. Decreased sputum; lungs clear after chest physical therapy

◆ CHRONIC OBSTRUCTIVE PULMONARY DISEASE (COPD)

COPD is a term that refers to a group of conditions characterized by continued increased resistance to expiratory airflow. COPD includes chronic bronchitis and pulmonary emphysema. Some clinicians consider asthma as part of COPD, but, due to its reversibility, it is considered by most to be a separate entity (see Asthma, p. 811).

Chronic bronchitis is a chronic inflammation of the lower respiratory tract characterized by excessive mucous secretion, cough, and dyspnea associated with recurring infections of the lower respiratory tract.

Pulmonary emphysema is a complex lung disease characterized by destruction of the alveoli, enlargement of distal airspaces, and a breakdown of alveolar walls. There is a slowly progressive deterioration of lung function for many years before the development of illness.

Pathophysiology/Etiology

1. Basically, the person with COPD may have (Fig. 9-3):
   a. Excessive secretion of mucus and chronic infection within the airways (bronchitis)—infection, irritation, hypersensitivity → local hyperemia → hypertrophy of mucous glands → increase in size and number of mucus-producing elements in bronchi (mucous glands and goblet cells) → inflammation and edema → narrowing and obstruction of airflow.
   b. Increase in size of air spaces distal to the terminal bronchioles, with loss of alveolar walls and elastic recoil of the lungs (emphysema).
   c. There may be an overlap of these conditions.
2. As a result of these conditions, there is a subsequent derangement of airway dynamics (eg, obstruction to airflow).

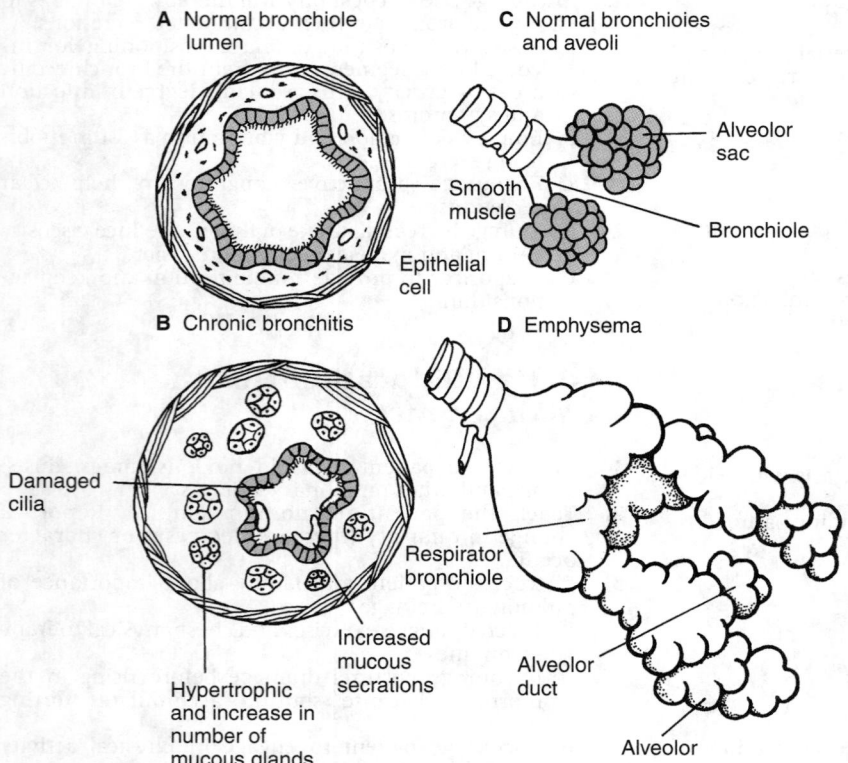

A Normal bronchiole lumen

Epithelial cell

B Chronic bronchitis

Damaged cilia

Hypertrophic and increase in number of mucous glands

Increased mucous secretions

C Normal bronchioies and aveoli

Smooth muscle

Alveolor sac

Bronchiole

D Emphysema

Respirator bronchiole

Alveolor duct

Alveolor sac

FIGURE 9-3 *Airway changes in COPD compared to normal.*

3. The etiology of COPD includes:
   a. Cigarette smoking
   b. Air pollution, occupational exposure
   c. Allergy, autoimmunity
   d. Infection
   e. Genetic predisposition, aging

Clinical Manifestations

A. *Chronic Bronchitis*
Usually insidious, developing over a period of years

1. Presence of a productive cough lasting at least 3 months a year for 2 successive years
2. Production of thick, gelatinous sputum; greater amounts produced during superimposed infections
3. Wheezing and dyspnea as disease progresses

B. *Emphysema*
Gradual in onset and steadily progressive

1. Dyspnea, decreased exercise tolerance.
2. Cough may be minimal, except with respiratory infection.
3. Sputum expectoration—Mild.
4. Increased anteroposterior diameter of chest (barrel chest).

Diagnostic Evaluation

1. PFTs demonstrate airflow obstruction—reduced FEV1, FEV1 to FVC ratio; increased residual volume to total lung capacity (TLC) ratio, possibly increased TLC (see p. 152)
2. ABGs—Decreased Pao_2, pH, and increased CO_2
3. Chest x-ray—In late stages, hyperinflation, flattened diaphragm, increased retrosternal space, decreased vascular markings, possible bullae
4. Alpha$_1$-antitrypsin assay useful in identifying genetically determined deficiency in emphysema

Management

Goal: Reverse airflow obstruction.

1. Smoking cessation.
2. Bronchodilators, of which there are two main categories (Table 9-3):
   a. Sympathomimetics such as metaproterenol (Alupent)—Given to protect against bronchospasm.
      (1) Aerosol formulations provide optimum therapy, because drug is applied directly to receptors in airways.
      (2) Bronchodilating aerosols delivered by metered-dose inhalers or hand-held or pump-driven devices.
   b. Methylxanthines such as theophylline (theodur) given orally as sustained-release formulation for chronic maintenance therapy.
3. Antimicrobial agents for episodes of respiratory infection.
4. Corticosteroids used in acute exacerbations for anti-inflammatory effect can be given by mouth, IV, or inhaler.
5. Chest physical therapy, including postural drainage, breathing retraining.
6. Low-flow oxygen therapy for patient with severe hypoxemia.
7. Pulmonary rehabilitation to reduce symptoms that limit activity.

NURSING ALERT:
Theophylline is not in favor as much as it has been in the past due to systemic side effects. More of an emphasis is now placed on the use of steroid inhalers.

Complications

1. Respiratory failure
2. Pneumonia; overwhelming respiratory infection
3. Right heart failure; dysrhythmias
4. Depression

Nursing Assessment

1. Determine smoking history, exposure history, positive family history of respiratory disease, onset of dyspnea.
2. Note amount, color, and consistency of sputum.
3. Inspect for use of accessory muscles of respiration and use of abdominal muscles during expiration; note increase of anteroposterior diameter of chest.
4. Auscultate for decreased/absent breath sounds, crackles, decreased heart sounds.

Nursing Diagnoses

A. Ineffective Airway Clearance related to bronchoconstriction, increased mucous production, ineffective cough, possible bronchopulmonary infection
B. Ineffective Breathing Pattern related to chronic airflow limitation
C. Risk for Infection related to compromised pulmonary function and defense mechanisms
D. Impaired Gas Exchange related to chronic pulmonary obstruction; ventilation–perfusion abnormalities
E. Altered Nutrition: less than body requirements related to increased work of breathing, air swallowing, medication effects
F. Activity Intolerance related to compromised pulmonary function, resulting in shortness of breath and fatigue
G. Sleep Pattern Disturbance related to hypoxemia and hypercapnia
H. Impaired Individual Coping related to the stress of living with chronic disease

NURSING ALERT:
Early in the patient's course, issues of a living will, advanced directives, and resuscitation status need to be addressed. It is better to have these discussions with the patient before crisis situations.

Nursing Interventions

A. *Improving Airway Clearance*
1. Eliminate all pulmonary irritants, particularly cigarette smoking.

TABLE 9-3 Drugs Commonly Used to Prevent or Reverse Bronchospasm

Drugs/Administration	Pharmacologic Effects	Indications	Undesired Effects	Nursing Implications
Bronchodilators				
Aminophylline (Amoline) intravenous injection	Methylxanthine compound—relaxes smooth muscle by increasing level of cyclic adenosine monophosphate	Acute exacerbation of asthma or bronchitis	CNS—irritability, restlessness, insomnia CV—palpitations, tachycardia, hypotension GI—nausea, vomiting, diarrhea	Too rapid administration can cause hypotension, extra systoles, muscle tremors. Administer at prescribed rate with an intravenous infusion pump.
Theophylline preparations (Theo-Dur) (oral)	Methylxanthine compound—relaxes muscle by increasing cyclic adenosine monophosphate	Maintenance therapy for bronchospasm	CNS—irritability, restlessness, insomnia CV—palpitations, tachycardia, hypotension GI—nausea, vomiting, diarrhea	Teach patients to take at equal intervals throughout the day. To decrease GI irritation, take with milk or crackers.
Terbutaline (Brethine) (oral, metered-dose inhaler, subcutaneous injection)	Symphathomimetic with selective beta$_2$ activity	Acute exacerbation of asthma or bronchitis (subcutaneous preparation) Maintenance therapy for bronchospasms (inhaled and oral preparation)	Nervousness, tachycardia, headache, nausea (subcutaneous preparation) Hand tremors (subcutaneous and oral preparations)	Caution patients that hand tremors may occur. Tremors decrease with prolonged oral use.
Metaproterenol (Alupent) (oral, metered-dose inhaler, inhalant solution)	Sympathomimetic with selective beta$_2$ activity	Maintenance therapy for bronchospasm	Nervousness, tachycardia, headache, nausea	Observe inhalation by patient to be certain that correct technique is used.
Albuterol (Proventil) (oral, metered-dose inhaler)	Sympathomimetic with highly selective beta$_2$ activity	Maintenance therapy for bronchospasm	Nervousness, tachycardia, headache, nausea	Observe inhalation by patient to be certain that correct techniques is used.
Pirbuterol acetate (Maxair) (metered-dose inhaler)	Sympathomimetic with selective beta$_2$ activity	Maintenance therapy for bronchospasm	Nervousness, tachycardia, headache, nausea	Observe inhalation by patient to be certain that correct technique is used.

Drug	Action	Use	Side Effects	Nursing Considerations
Salmeterol xinafoate (Serevent) (metered-dose inhaler)	Sympathomimetic with selective beta$_2$ activity	Maintenance therapy for bronchospasm, long-acting (12 h)	Nervousness, tachycardia, headache, nausea	Observe inhalation by patient to be certain that correct technique is used.
Ipratropium bromide (Atrovent) (metered-dose inhaler)	Anticholinergic	Maintenance therapy for bronchospasm	Rare. Can cause blurring of vision if sprayed into the eyes (atropine derivative)	Instruct patient to close lips around inhaler mouthpiece, close eyes during inhalation.
Corticosteroids				
Hydrocortisone/prednisone (Deltasone) (intravenous injection, oral preparation)	Potent antiinflammatory activity	Acute exacerbation of asthma or bronchitis (IV preparation) Maintenance therapy (oral preparation)	CNS—depression, euphoria GI—gastric irritation, peptic ulcer Metabolic—hypernatremia, hypokalemia	Should not be abruptly discontinued, as causes suppression of adrenal function.
Beclomethasone (Vanceril) (metered-dose inhaler)	Synthetic corticosteroid with potent antiinflammatory activity; effective only by inhalation	Asthma (alternative to use of oral steroids) COPD	Oral candidiasis Systemic side effects associated with oral steroids do not occur	Inhaled as a powder. May precipitate bronchospasm in acute exacerbation. Not used with status asthmaticus or acute asthma episodes.
Triamcinolone acetonide (Azmacort) (metered-dose inhaler)	Antiinflammatory steroid; effective only by inhalation	Asthma COPD	Oral candidiasis No systemic side effects.	Packaged with a spacer. Decreases oral deposition and oral candidiasis.
Flunisolide (AeroBid) (metered-dose inhaler)	Antiinflammatory steroid; effective only by inhalation.	Asthma COPD	Oral candidiasis No systemic side effects.	Longer-acting. May be prescribed twice a day, rather than four times a day.
Miscellaneous				
Cromolyn sodium (Intal) (solution for inhalation, powder used with special inhaler)	Inhibits release of histamine, from mast cells in the respiratory tract, *prevents* bronchospasm Not effective in acute attack; must be used for 2 to 4 weeks to show effectiveness	Maintenance therapy for asthma	Cough, bronchospasm	Should not be used with status asthmaticus or acute asthma episodes. May be given in combination with bronchodilator if administration causes bronchospasm.

a. Cessation of smoking usually results in less pulmonary irritation, sputum production, and cough.
b. Keep patient's room as dust-free as possible.
c. Add moisture (humidifier, vaporizer) to indoor environment.

2. Administer bronchodilators to control bronchospasm and assist with raising sputum.
   a. Assess for side effects—tremulousness, tachycardia, cardiac dysrhythmias, central nervous system stimulation, hypertension.
   b. Auscultate the chest after administration of aerosol bronchodilators to assess for improvement of aeration and reduction of adventitious breath sounds.
   c. Observe if patient has reduction in dyspnea.
   d. Monitor serum theophylline level, as ordered, to ensure therapeutic level and prevent toxicity.
3. Use postural drainage positions to aid in clearance of secretions, because mucopurulent secretions are responsible for airway obstruction (see p. 176).
4. Use controlled coughing (see p. 77).
5. Keep secretions liquid.
   a. Encourage high level of fluid intake (8 to 10 glasses; 2 to 2.5 L daily) within level of cardiac reserve.
   b. Give inhalations of nebulized water to humidify bronchial tree and liquefy sputum.
   c. Avoid dairy products if these increase sputum production.

B. Improving Breathing Pattern

1. Teach and supervise breathing retraining exercises to strengthen diaphragm and muscles of expiration to decrease work of breathing (see p. 172).
   a. Teach lower costal, diaphragmatic, and abdominal breathing, using a slow and relaxed breathing pattern to reduce respiratory rate and decrease energy cost of breathing.
   b. Use pursed-lip breathing at intervals and during periods of dyspnea to control rate and depth of respiration and improve respiratory muscle coordination.
2. Discuss and demonstrate relaxation exercises to reduce stress, tension, and anxiety.
3. Encourage patient to assume position of comfort to decrease dyspnea.

C. Controlling Infection

1. Recognize early manifestations of respiratory infection—increased dyspnea, fatigue; change in color, amount, and character of sputum; nervousness; irritability; low-grade fever.
2. Obtain sputum for smear and culture.
3. Administer prescribed antimicrobials to control secondary bacterial infections in the bronchial tree, thus clearing the airways.

D. Improving Gas Exchange

1. Watch for and report excessive somnolence, restlessness, aggressiveness, anxiety, or confusion; central cyanosis; and shortness of breath at rest, which frequently is caused by acute respiratory insufficiency and may signal respiratory failure.
2. Review ABGs; record values on a flow sheet so comparisons can be made over time.
3. Give low-flow oxygen as ordered to correct hypoxemia in a controlled manner and minimize CO_2 retention.

NURSING ALERT:
Normally, CO_2 levels in the blood provide a stimulus for respiration. However, in patients with COPD, chronically elevated CO_2 impairs this mechanism and low oxygen levels act as stimulus for respiration. Giving a high concentration of supplemental oxygen may remove the hypoxic drive, leading to increased hypoventilation, respiratory decompensation, and the development of a worsening respiratory acidosis.

4. Be prepared to assist with intubation and mechanical ventilation if acute respiratory failure and rapid CO_2 retention occur.

E. Improving Nutrition

1. Take nutritional history, weight, and anthropometric measurements.
2. Encourage frequent small meals if patient is dyspneic; even a small increase in abdominal contents may press on diaphragm and impede breathing.
3. Offer liquid nutritional supplements to improve caloric intake and counteract weight loss.
4. Avoid foods producing abdominal discomfort.
5. Employ good oral hygiene before meals to sharpen taste sensations.
6. Encourage pursed-lip breathing between bites if patient is very short of breath; rest after meals.
7. Give supplemental oxygen while patient is eating to relieve dyspnea, as directed.
8. Monitor body weight.

F. Increasing Activity Tolerance

1. Reemphasize the importance of graded exercise and physical conditioning programs (enhances delivery of oxygen to tissues; allows a higher level of functioning with greater comfort). This may be part of a formalized pulmonary rehabilitation program or a referral to physical or occupational therapy.
   a. Discuss walking, stationary bicycling, swimming.
   b. Encourage use of portable oxygen system for ambulation for patients with hypoxemia and marked disability.
2. Encourage patient to carry out *regular* exercise program to increase physical endurance.
3. Train patient in energy conservation techniques.

G. Improving Sleep Patterns

1. Maintain a balanced schedule of activity and rest.
2. Use nocturnal oxygen therapy when appropriate.
3. Avoid the use of sedatives that may cause respiratory depression.

H. Enhancing Coping

1. Understand that the constant shortness of breath and fatigue make the patient irritable, apprehensive, anxious, and depressed, with feelings of helplessness/hopelessness.
2. Assess the patient for reactive behaviors (anger, depression, acceptance).
3. Demonstrate a positive and interested approach to the patient.
   a. Be a good listener and show that you care.
   b. Be sensitive to patient's fears, anxiety, and depression; may provide emotional relief and insight.
4. Strengthen the patient's self-image.
5. Allow the patient to express feelings and retain (within a controlled degree) the mechanisms of denial and repression.

6. Be aware that sexual dysfunction is common in patients with COPD; encourage alternate displays of affection to loved one.
7. Support spouse/family members.

Patient Education/Health Maintenance

A. General Education
1. Give the patient a clear explanation of the disease, what to expect, how to treat and live with it. Reinforce by frequent explanations, reading material, demonstrations, and question and answer sessions.
2. Review with the patient the objectives of treatment and nursing management.
3. Work with the patient to set goals (ie, stair climbing, return to work, and so forth).

B. Avoid Exposure to Respiratory Irritants
1. Advise patient to stop smoking and avoid smoke-filled rooms.
2. Advise patient to avoid sweeping, dusting, and exposure to paint, aerosols, bleaches, and other respiratory irritants.
3. Advise patient to keep kitchen well ventilated.
4. Warn patient to stay out of extremely hot/cold weather to avoid aggravating bronchial obstruction and sputum production.
   a. Keep a warm mask or scarf over nose and mouth to warm inspired air in cold weather.
   b. Stay indoors with air conditioning when air pollution level is high.
   c. Try to avoid abrupt environmental changes.
   d. Shower in warm (not too hot or too cold) water.
5. Instruct patient to humidify indoor air in winter; maintain 30% to 50% humidity for optimal mucociliary function.
6. Suggest the use of an air cleanser to remove dust, pollen, and other particulates. This is controversial as to the benefit to the patient.

C. Prevent and Treat Respiratory Infections
1. Warn against exposure to persons with respiratory infections; a respiratory infection makes symptoms worse and can produce further irreversible damage.
2. Advise patient to avoid crowds and areas with poor ventilation.
3. Stress the importance of obtaining influenza and pneumococcal vaccines to decrease likelihood of developing these infections.
4. Teach how to recognize and report evidence of respiratory infection *promptly*—chest pain, changes in character of sputum (amount, color, or consistency), increasing difficulty in raising sputum, increasing cough/wheezing, increasing shortness of breath.
5. Instruct on taking prescribed antimicrobial at first sign of infection.
   a. Have a current prescription available.
   b. Have periodic sputum cultures when receiving long-term antimicrobial therapy.

D. Reduce Bronchial Secretions
1. Advise to maintain an adequate fluid intake (8 to 10 glasses daily); mark down the amount of liquid consumed daily.
2. Encourage use of bronchodilators only as directed.
3. Teach postural drainage exercises as prescribed.
   a. Stay in each position 5 to 15 minutes.
   b. Use controlled cough after each position.

E. Improve Airflow
1. Teach use of metered-dose inhaler properly to maximize aerosol deposition in the bronchial tree.
   a. Breathe out normally; open mouth and let mouthpiece touch lip or place inhaler 2 to 4 inches in front of mouth.
   b. Inhale slowly and activate cartridge to release spray.
   c. Pause, holding breath for about 10 seconds; exhale slowly.
2. Suggest the use of a spacer device to allow easier inhalation of bronchodilator medication to patient who cannot use inhaler effectively.

F. Breathing Exercises
1. Explain that goal is to strengthen and coordinate muscles of breathing to lessen work of breathing and help lung empty more completely.
2. Stress the importance of controlled breathing.
3. Teach diaphragmatic breathing and pursed-lip breathing for episodes of dyspnea and stress.
4. Encourage muscle toning by regular exercise.

G. General Health
1. Teach good habits of nutrition.
2. Encourage high-protein diet with adequate mineral, vitamin, and fluid intake.
3. Advise against excessive hot or cold fluids/foods that may provoke an irritating cough.
4. Advise to avoid hard-to-chew foods (causes tiring) and gas-forming foods, which cause distention and restrict diaphragmatic movement.
5. Encourage five to six small meals daily to ease shortness of breath during and after meals.
6. Suggest rest periods before and after meals if eating produces shortness of breath.
7. Advise against eating when upset/angry.
8. Warn against potassium depletion. Patients with COPD tend to have low potassium levels; also patient may be taking diuretics.
   a. Watch for weakness, numbness, tingling of fingers, leg cramps.
   b. Foods high in potassium include bananas, dried fruits, dates, figs, orange juice, grape juice, milk, peaches, potatoes, tomatoes.
9. Advise on restricting sodium, as directed.
10. Avoid carbohydrates if CO_2 is retained by patient, because it increases CO_2.
11. Use community resources (Meals on Wheels) if energy level is low.

H. Living With Shortness of Breath
1. Encourage to live within the limitations that emphysema imposes.
2. Help to relax and work at a slower pace.
3. Encourage to enroll in a pulmonary rehabilitation program where available.
4. Suggest vocational counseling to secure a sedentary job if presently in a demanding manual job.
5. Warn to avoid overfatigue, which is a factor in producing respiratory distress.
6. Advise to adjust activities according to individual fatigue patterns.
7. Advise to try to cope with emotional stress as positively as possible. Such stress triggers attacks of dyspnea.
8. Stress that existing lung function can be preserved through health supervision for rest of life.

COMMUNITY-BASED CARE TIP:
All of the above patient education can be provided in a pulmonary rehabilitation program that is offered in most communities. Studies on pulmonary rehabilitation indicate that there is no appreciable difference in lung function as a result of the program, but there is a decrease in hospital admissions, decreased length of stay, and a better sense by the patient of coping, well-being and quality of life. Contact the local American Lung Association or local hospitals for further information.

Evaluation

A. Coughing up secretions easily; decreased wheezing and crackles
B. Reports less dyspnea; effectively using pursed-lip breathing
C. No signs of superimposed respiratory infection
D. ABGs improved on low-flow oxygen
E. Tolerating small, frequent meals; weight stable
F. Reports walking longer distances without tiring
G. Reports better sleep; using low-flow oxygen at night
H. Demonstrates more effective coping; expresses feelings; seeking support group

◆ PULMONARY HEART DISEASE (COR PULMONALE)

Pulmonary heart disease is an alteration in the structure or function of the right ventricle resulting from disease affecting lung structure or function or its vasculature (except when this alteration results from disease of the left side of the heart or from congenital heart disease). Cor pulmonale refers to heart disease caused by lung disease.

Pathophysiology/Etiology

1. Condition that deprives lungs of oxygen → hypoxemia → hypercapnia → acidosis → circulatory complications → pulmonary hypertension → right heart enlargement → right heart failure.
2. Etiology includes:
   a. Pulmonary vascular disease
   b. Pulmonary embolism
   c. COPD

Clinical Manifestations

1. Increasing dyspnea and fatigue; progressive dyspnea (orthopnea, paroxysmal nocturnal dyspnea), chronic cough
2. Distended neck veins, peripheral edema, hepatomegaly
3. Bibasilar crackles and split second heart sound on auscultation of chest
4. Manifestations of carbon dioxide narcosis—headache, confusion, somnolence, coma

Diagnostic Evaluation

1. ABGs—Decreased Pao_2 and pH, increased $Paco_2$.
2. PFTs may show airway obstruction.

3. Electrocardiogram changes are consistent with right ventricular hypertrophy.
4. Chest x-ray shows right heart enlargement.

Management

Goal: Treatment of underlying lung disease and management of heart disease.

1. Long-term, low-flow oxygen to improve oxygen delivery to peripheral tissues, thus decreasing cardiac work and lessening sympathetic vasoconstriction. Liter flow individualized during activities, rest, and sleep.
2. Diuretics to lower pulmonary artery pressure (PAP) by reducing total blood volume and excess fluid in lungs.
3. Pulmonary vasodilators such as nitroprusside (Nipride); hydralazine (Apresoline); calcium channel blockers to dilate pulmonary vascular bed and reduce pulmonary vascular resistance; use is controversial.
4. Chest physical therapy, bronchodilators to improve lung function.
5. Mechanical ventilation, if patient in respiratory failure.
6. Sodium restriction to reduce edema.

Complications

1. Respiratory failure
2. Dysrhythmias

Nursing Assessment

1. Determine if patient has longstanding history of lung disease.
2. Assess degree of dyspnea and fatigue.
3. Inspect for jugular venous distention and peripheral edema.

Nursing Diagnoses

A. Impaired Gas Exchange related to excess fluid in lungs; increased pulmonary vascular resistance
B. Fluid Volume Excess related to right heart failure

Nursing Interventions

A. *Improving Gas Exchange*
1. Monitor ABG values as a guide in assessing adequacy of ventilation.
2. Use continuous low-flow oxygen as directed to reduce PAP.
3. Avoid central nervous system depressants (narcotics, hypnotics). They have depressant action on respiratory centers and mask symptoms of hypercapnia.
4. Monitor for signs of respiratory infection, because infection causes carbon dioxide retention and hypoxemia.

B. *Attaining Fluid Balance*
1. Watch alterations in electrolyte levels, especially potassium, which can lead to disturbances of cardiac rhythm.
2. Employ ECG monitoring when necessary, and monitor closely for dysrhythmias.

3. Limit physical activity until improvement is seen.
4. Restrict sodium intake based on evidence of fluid retention.

Patient Education/Health Maintenance

1. Emphasize the importance of stopping cigarette smoking; cigarette smoking is a major cause of pulmonary heart disease.
   a. Query the patient about smoking habits.
   b. Inform the patient of risks of smoking and benefits to be gained when smoking is stopped.
2. Teach the patient to recognize and treat infections immediately.
3. Inform the patient of interrelationship among infection, air pollution, and cardiopulmonary disease.
4. Explain to the patient/family that restlessness, depression, and poor sleeping, as well as irritable and angry behavior, may be characteristic; patient should improve with rise in O_2 and fall in CO_2 levels in ABG values.
5. Explain that if the patient has chronic lung disease it may be necessary to have continuous low-flow oxygen therapy at home.

Evaluation

A. Less dyspneic; ABGs improved
B. Edema reduced; no dysrhythmias

◆ OCCUPATIONAL LUNG DISEASES

Diseases of the lungs can occur in a variety of occupations as a result of exposure to organic or inorganic (mineral) dusts and noxious gases. The most common occupational lung diseases are:

Silicosis is a chronic pulmonary fibrosis caused by inhalation of silica dust.
Asbestosis is a diffuse interstitial fibrosis of the lung caused by inhalation of asbestos dust and particles.
Coal worker's pneumoconiosis (CWP; "black lung") is a variety of respiratory disease found in coal workers in which there is an accumulation of coal dust in the lungs, causing a tissue reaction in its presence.

Pathophysiology/Etiology

1. Effects of inhaling noxious particles, gases, or fumes depend on composition of inhaled substance, its antigenic (precipitating an immune response) or irritating properties, the dose inhaled, the length of time inhaled, and the host's response.
2. Exposure to inorganic dusts stimulates pulmonary interstitial fibroblasts, resulting in pulmonary interstitial fibrosis.
3. Noxious fumes may cause acute injury to alveolar wall with increasing capillary permeability and pulmonary edema.
4. Occupational lung diseases usually develop slowly (over 20 to 30 years) and are asymptomatic in the early stages.

A. **Silicosis**
1. Exposure to silica dust is encountered in almost any form of mining because the earth's crust is composed of silica and silicates (gold, coal, tin, copper mining); also stone cutting, quarrying, manufacture of abrasives, ceramics, pottery, and foundry work.
2. When silica particles (which have fibrogenic properties) are inhaled, nodular lesions are produced throughout the lungs. These nodules undergo fibrosis, enlarge, and fuse.
3. Dense masses form in the upper portion of the lungs; restrictive and obstructive lung disease results.

B. **Asbestosis**
1. Found in workers involved in manufacture, cutting, and demolition of asbestos-containing materials; there are over 4,000 known sources of asbestos fiber (asbestos mining and manufacturing, construction, roofing, demolition work, brake linings, floor tiles, paints, plastics, shipyards, insulation).
2. Asbestos fibers are inhaled and enter alveoli, which in time are obliterated by fibrous tissue that surrounds the asbestos particles.
3. Fibrous pleural thickening and pleural plaque formation produce restrictive lung disease, decrease in lung volume, diminished gas transfer, and hypoxemia with subsequent development of cor pulmonale.

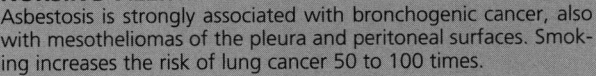

NURSING ALERT:
Asbestosis is strongly associated with bronchogenic cancer, also with mesotheliomas of the pleura and peritoneal surfaces. Smoking increases the risk of lung cancer 50 to 100 times.

C. **Coal Worker's Pneumoconiosis**
1. Dusts (coal, kaolin, mica, silica) are inhaled and deposited in the alveoli and respiratory bronchioles.
2. There is an increase of macrophages that engulf the particles and transport them to terminal bronchioles.
3. When normal clearance mechanisms no longer can handle the excessive dust load, the respiratory bronchioles and alveoli become clogged with coal dust, dying macrophages, and fibroblasts, which lead to the formation of the coal macule, the primary lesion of CWP.
4. As macules enlarge, there is dilation of the weakening bronchiole, with subsequent development of focal or centrilobular emphysema.

Clinical Manifestations

1. Chronic cough; productive in silicosis and CWP
2. Dyspnea on exertion; progressive and irreversible in asbestosis and CWP
3. Susceptibility to lower respiratory tract infections
4. Bibasilar crackles in asbestosis
5. Expectoration of varying amounts of black fluid in CWP

Diagnostic Evaluation

1. Chest x-ray—Nodules of upper lobes in silicosis and CWP; diffuse parenchymal fibrosis, especially of lower lobes, in asbestosis.
2. PFT primarily shows restrictive pattern.
3. Bronchoscopy with lavage to identify specific exposure.
4. CT, sputum examination, and lung biopsy may be needed to rule out other disorders.

Management

1. There is no specific treatment; exposure is eliminated and the patient is treated symptomatically.
2. Give prophylactic isoniazid (INH) to patient with positive tuberculin test, because silicosis is associated with high risk of tuberculosis.
3. Persuade persons who have been exposed to asbestos fibers to stop smoking to decrease risk of lung cancer.
4. Keep asbestosis worker under cancer surveillance; watch for changing cough, hemoptysis, weight loss, melena, and so forth.
5. Bronchodilators may be of some benefit if any degree of airway obstruction is present.

Complications

1. Respiratory failure
2. Lung cancer

Nursing Assessment

1. Obtain occupational exposure history. Determine length and degree of exposure.
2. Obtain history of smoking, respiratory infections, and other chronic lung disease.
3. Evaluate symptoms and auscultate lungs for crackles.

Nursing Diagnoses

A. Ineffective Breathing Pattern related to fibrotic lung tissue causing restriction
B. Impaired Gas Exchange related to fibrotic lung tissue and secretions

Nursing Interventions

A. **Improving Breathing Pattern**
1. Administer oxygen therapy as required.
2. Administer or teach self-administration of bronchodilators, as ordered.
3. Encourage smoking cessation.

B. **Promoting Gas Exchange**
1. Encourage mobilization of secretions through hydration and breathing and coughing exercises.
2. Advise on pacing activities to prevent exertion.

Patient Education/Health Maintenance

1. Provide information regarding the importance of smoking cessation as well as methods of smoking cessation.
2. Instruct patient in methods of health maintenance, such as adequate nutrition and exercise, so additional medical problems can be avoided.
3. Advise patient that compensation may be obtained for impairment related to occupational lung disease through the Workman's Compensation Act.

4. Provide information to healthy workers on prevention of occupational lung disease.
   a. Enclose toxic substances to reduce their concentration in the air.
   b. Employ engineering controls to reduce exposure.
   c. Monitor air samples.
   d. Ventilate the environment properly to reduce dust content of work atmosphere.
   e. Use protective devices such as face masks, respirators, hoods, and so forth.

Evaluation

A. Reports less dyspnea
B. Effectively mobilizes secretions

Traumatic Disorders

◆ PNEUMOTHORAX

Air in the pleural space occurring spontaneously or from trauma. In patients with chest trauma, it is usually the result of a laceration to the lung parenchyma, tracheobronchial tree, or esophagus.

The patient's clinical status depends on the rate of air leakage and size of wound. Pneumothorax is classified as:

Spontaneous pneumothorax—Sudden onset of air in the pleural space with deflation of the affected lung in the absence of trauma.
Open pneumothorax (sucking wound of chest)—Implies an opening in the chest wall large enough to allow air to pass freely in and out of thoracic cavity with each attempted respiration.
Tension pneumothorax—Buildup of air under pressure in the pleural space resulting in interference with filling of both the heart and lungs.

Pathophysiology/Etiology

1. When there is a large open hole in the chest wall, the patient will have a "steal" in ventilation of other lung.
2. A portion of the tidal volume will move back and forth through the hole in the chest wall, rather than the trachea as it normally does.
3. Spontaneous pneumothorax is usually due to rupture of a subpleural bleb.
   a. May occur secondary to chronic respiratory diseases or idiopathically.
   b. May occur in healthy people, particularly in thin, white males and those with family history of pneumothorax.

Clinical Manifestations

1. Hyperresonance; diminished breath sounds.
2. Reduced mobility of affected half of thorax.
3. Tracheal deviation away from affected side in tension pneumothorax.
4. Clinical picture of open or tension pneumothorax is one of air hunger, agitation, hypotension, and cyanosis.

5. Mild to moderate dyspnea and chest discomfort may be present with spontaneous pneumothorax.

Diagnostic Evaluation

1. Chest x-ray to confirm presence of air in pleural space.

Management

A. *Spontaneous pneumothorax*
1. Treatment is generally nonoperative if pneumothorax is not too extensive.
   a. Observe and allow for spontaneous resolution for less than 50% pneumothorax in otherwise healthy person.
   b. Needle aspiration or chest tube drainage may be necessary to achieve reexpansion of collapsed lung if greater than 50% pneumothorax.
2. Surgical intervention by pleurodesis (see p. 231) or thoracotomy with resection of apical blebs is advised for patients with recurrent spontaneous pneumothorax.

B. *Tension Pneumothorax*
1. Immediate decompression to prevent cardiovascular collapse by thoracentesis or chest tube insertion to let air escape
2. Chest tube drainage with underwater-seal suction to allow for full lung expansion and healing

C. *Open Pneumothorax*
1. Close the chest wound immediately to restore adequate ventilation and respiration.
   a. Patient is instructed to inhale and exhale gently against a closed glottis (Valsalva maneuver) as a pressure dressing (petrolatum gauze secured with elastic adhesive) is applied. This maneuver helps to expand collapsed lung.
2. Chest tube is inserted and water-seal drainage set up to permit evacuation of fluid/air and produce reexpansion of the lung.
3. Surgical intervention may be necessary to repair trauma.

Complications

1. Acute respiratory failure
2. Cardiovascular collapse with tension pneumothorax

Nursing Assessment

1. Obtain history for chronic respiratory disease, trauma, and onset of symptoms.
2. Inspect chest for reduced mobility and tracheal deviation.
3. Auscultate chest for diminished breath sounds and percuss for hyperresonance.

Nursing Diagnoses

A. Ineffective Breathing Pattern related to air in the pleural space
B. Impaired Gas Exchange related to atelectasis and collapse of lung

Nursing Interventions

A. *Achieving Effective Breathing Pattern*
1. Provide emergency care as indicated.
   a. Apply petroleum gauze to sucking chest wound (see Management, above)
   b. Assist with emergency thoracentesis or thoracostomy.
   c. Be prepared to perform cardiopulmonary resuscitation (CPR) or administer medications if cardiovascular collapse occurs.
2. Maintain patent airway; suction as needed.
3. Position upright if condition permits to allow greater chest expansion.
4. Maintain patency of chest tubes.
5. Assist patient to splint chest while turning or coughing and administer pain medications as needed.

B. *Impaired Gas Exchange Will Be Resolved*
1. Encourage patient in the use of inspiratory spirometer.
2. Monitor oximetry and ABGs to determine oxygenation.
3. Provide oxygen as needed.

Patient Education/Health Maintenance

1. Instruct patient to continue use of the inspiratory spirometer at home.
2. For patients with spontaneous pneumothorax, there is an increased chance of repeat occurrence; therefore, encourage these patients to report sudden dyspnea immediately.

Evaluation

A. Breath sounds equal bilaterally; less dyspneic
B. ABGs improved

◆ CHEST INJURIES

Chest injuries are potentially life-threatening because of 1) immediate disturbances of cardiorespiratory physiology and hemorrhage; and 2) later developments of infection, damaged lung, and thoracic cage.

Patients with chest trauma may have injuries to multiple organ systems. The patient should be examined for intraabdominal injuries, which must be treated aggressively.

Pathophysiology/Clinical Manifestations

A. *Rib Fracture*
1. Most common chest injury
2. May interfere with ventilation and may lacerate underlying lung
3. Causes pain at fracture site; painful, shallow respirations; localized tenderness and crepitus (crackling) over fracture site

B. *Hemothorax*
1. Blood in pleural space as a result of penetrating or blunt chest trauma.
2. Accompany a high percentage of chest injuries.

3. Can result in hidden blood loss.
4. Patient may be asymptomatic, dyspneic, apprehensive, or in shock.

C. Flail Chest
1. Loss of stability of chest wall as a result of multiple rib fractures, or combined rib and sternum fractures.
2. When this occurs, one portion of the chest has lost its bony connection to the rest of the rib cage.
3. During respiration, the detached part of the chest will be pulled in on inspiration and blown out on expiration (paradoxical movement).
4. Normal mechanics of breathing are impaired to a degree that seriously jeopardizes ventilation, causing dyspnea and cyanosis.
5. Generally associated with other serious chest injuries; lung contusion, lung laceration, diffuse alveolar damage.

D. Pulmonary Contusion
1. Bruise of the lung parenchyma that results in leakage of blood and edema fluid into the alveolar and interstitial spaces of the lung
2. May not be fully developed for 24 to 72 hours
3. Signs and symptoms include:
   a. Tachypnea, tachycardia
   b. Crackles on auscultation
   c. Pleuritic chest pain
   d. Copious secretions
   e. Cough—Constant, loose, rattling

E. Cardiac Tamponade
1. Compression of the heart as a result of accumulation of fluid within the pericardial space
2. Caused by penetrating injuries
3. Signs and symptoms include:
   a. Falling blood pressure
   b. Distended neck veins, elevated central venous pressure (CVP)
   c. Muffled heart sounds
   d. Pulsus paradoxus (systolic blood pressure drops and fluctuates with respiration)
   e. Dyspnea, cyanosis, shock

> **NURSING ALERT:** ◆
> A rapidly developing tamponade interferes with ventricular filling and causes impairment of circulation. Thus, there is a reduced cardiac output and poor venous return to the heart. Cardiac collapse can result. In the patient with hypovolemia due to associated injuries, the CVP may not rise, thus masking the signs of cardiac tamponade.

Management/Nursing Interventions

The goal is to restore normal cardiorespiratory function as quickly as possible. This is accomplished by performing effective resuscitation while simultaneously assessing the patient, restoring chest wall integrity, and reexpanding the lung. The order of priority is determined by the clinical status of the patient.

A. Rib Fracture
1. Give analgesics (usually non-narcotic) to assist in effective coughing and deep breathing.
2. Encourage deep breathing with strong inspiration; give local support to injured area by splinting with hands.

3. Assist with intercostal nerve block (see Procedure Guideline 9-2) to relieve pain so coughing and deep breathing may be accomplished. An *intercostal nerve block* is the injection of a local anesthetic into the area surrounding the intercostal nerves to relieve pain temporarily after rib fracture(s), chest wall injury, or thoracotomy.
4. For multiple rib fractures, epidural anesthesia may be used.

B. Hemothorax
1. Assist with thoracentesis to aspirate blood from pleural space, if being done before a chest tube insertion.
2. Assist with chest tube insertion and set up drainage system to accomplish complete and continuous removal of blood and air.
   a. Auscultate lungs and monitor for relief of dyspnea.
   b. Monitor amount of blood loss in drainage.
3. Replace volume with IV fluids or blood products.

C. Flail Chest
1. Stabilize the flail portion of the chest with hands; apply a pressure dressing and turn the patient on injured side, or place 10-lb sandbag at site of flail.
2. Thoracic epidural analgesia may be used for some patients to relieve pain and improve ventilation
3. If respiratory failure is present, prepare for immediate endotracheal intubation and mechanical ventilation—treats underlying pulmonary contusion and serves to stabilize the thoracic cage for healing of fractures, improves alveolar ventilation, and restores thoracic cage stability and intrathoracic volume by decreasing work of breathing.
4. Prepare for operative stabilization of chest wall in select patients.

D. Pulmonary Contusion
For moderate lung contusion

1. Employ mechanical ventilation to keep lungs inflated.
2. Administer diuretics to reduce edema.
3. Correct metabolic acidosis with IV sodium bicarbonate.
4. Use pulmonary artery pressure monitoring.
5. Monitor for development of pneumonia.

E. Cardiac Tamponade
For penetrating injuries

1. Assist with pericardiocentesis (see p.) to provide emergency relief and improve hemodynamic function until operation can be undertaken.
2. Prepare for emergency thoracotomy to control bleeding and to repair cardiac injury.

F. Additional Responsibilities
1. Suction as indicated through nose or mouth or endotracheal tube.
2. Prepare for tracheostomy, if indicated.
   a. Tracheostomy helps to clear tracheobronchial tree, helps the patient breathe with less effort, decreases the amount of dead air space in the respiratory tree, and helps reduce paradoxical motion.
   b. When used with mechanical ventilation, provides a closed system and stabilizes the chest.
3. Secure one or more IV lines for fluid replacement, and obtain blood for baseline studies such as hemoglobin and hematocrit.
4. Monitor serial CVP readings to prevent hypovolemia and circulatory overload.

5. Monitor ABG results to determine need for supplemental oxygen, mechanical ventilation.
6. Obtain urinary output hourly to evaluate tissue perfusion.
7. Continue to monitor thoracic drainage to provide information about rate of blood loss, whether bleeding has stopped, whether surgical intervention is necessary.
8. Institute ECG monitoring for early detection and treatment of cardiac dysrhythmias (dysrhythmias are a frequent cause of death in chest trauma).
9. Maintain ongoing surveillance for complications:
   a. Aspiration
   b. Atelectasis
   c. Pneumonia
   d. Mediastinal/subcutaneous emphysema
   e. Respiratory failure

Patient Education/Health Maintenance

1. Instruct patient in splinting techniques.
2. Ensure that patient is aware of importance of automobile seat belt use.
3. Teach patient to report signs of complications—increasing dyspnea, fever, cough.

Selected References

American Thoracic Society and Centers for Disease Control. (1994). Treatment of tuberculosis and tuberculosis infection in adults and children. *American Journal of Respiratory Critical Care Medicine, 149,* 1359-1374.

Atkins, P. J., et al. (1994). Respiratory consequences of multisystem crisis: ARDS. *Critical Care Nursing Quarterly, 16*(4), 27-38.

Cole, M. R. (1993). Correct inhaler use crucial to success of respiratory therapy. *Provider, 19*(8), 53.

Groffbach, I. (1994). The COPD patient in acute respiratory failure. *Critical Care Nurse, 14* (6), 32–40.

Johannsen, J. M. (1994). COPD: Current comprehensive care for emphysema and bronchitis. *Nurse Practitioner, 19*(1), 59-67.

Kuhn, M. A. (1994). Multiple trauma with respiratory distress. *Critical Care Nurse, 14*(2), 68-72, 77-80.

Michie, J. (1994). An introduction to lung cancer physiotherapy. 80 (12), 844–847.

Murray, J. F., & Nadel, J. (1994). *Textbook of respiratory medicine* (2nd ed.). Philadelphia: W. B. Saunders.

Perry, A., & Potter, P. (1994). *Clinical nursing skills and techniques* (3rd ed.). St. Louis: Mosby.

Poe, R. H. (1994). Theophylline: Still a reasonable choice? *Journal of Respiratory Disease, 15*(1), 19-22, 25-26, 29-30.

Shish, J., Wilson, J., & Broderick, A., et al. (1994). Asbestos-induced pleural fibrosis and impaired exercise physiology. *Chest, 105* (5), 1370–1376.

UNIT 3

◆

Cardiovascular Disease

CHAPTER 10

Cardiovascular Function and Therapy

Assessment

◆ COMMON MANIFESTATIONS OF HEART DISEASE

Chest pain is the most common manifestation among patients with cardiac disease. Other complaints include shortness of breath, palpitations, weakness or fatigue, and dizziness or syncope.

Chest Pain

A. *Characterization*
1. Nature and intensity
    a. Ask patient to describe in own words what the pain is like—dull, sharp, crushing, burning, heaviness, ache, pressure?
    b. Ask patient to rate pain relative to pain experienced in the past using a scale of 1 to 10 (10 being the most severe pain and 1 the least).
2. Onset and duration
    a. When did the pain start?
    b. How long did the pain episode last?
3. Location and radiation
    a. Ask patient to point to area where it hurts most. (Positive Levine's sign: clenched fist brought to patient's chest; indicative of diffuse visceral pain associated with unstable cardiac disease.)
    b. Ask the patient if the pain seems to travel (most commonly radiates to left arm, jaw, back and abdominal region).
4. Precipitating and relieving factors
    a. What activity was patient doing just before pain (rapid walking, exposure to cold, eating a spicy meal)?
    b. What relieves the pain (rest, medications, change of position)?
5. Associated signs/symptoms: observe for nausea, diaphoresis, dyspnea, fatigue, palpitations, disorientation.

B. *Significance*
1. Ischemia caused by an increase in demand for coronary blood flow and oxygen delivery, which exceeds available blood supply; due to coronary artery disease (angina pectoris, myocardial infarction [MI]).
2. Excruciating "shearing" pain radiating to back and flanks may indicate acute dissecting aneurysm of the aorta.
3. Sharp precordial pain (over heart area) radiating to left shoulder and upper back, aggravated by respirations—indicates acute pericarditis.

Shortness of Breath (Dyspnea)

A. *Characterization*
1. What precipitates or relieves dyspnea?
2. How many pillows does patient sleep with at night? (Several pillows is indicative of advanced heart failure.)
3. How far can patient walk or how many flights of stairs can patient climb before becoming dyspneic?
4. Determine the type of dyspnea.
    a. Exertional—Breathlessness on moderate exertion that is relieved by rest.
    b. Paroxysmal nocturnal—Sudden dypsnea at night; awakens patient with feeling of suffocation; sitting up relieves breathlessness.
    c. Orthopnea—Shortness of breath when lying down. Patient must keep head elevated with more than one pillow to minimize dyspnea.

B. *Significance*
1. It may be a sign of left ventricular failure or transient congestive heart failure.

Palpitations

A. *Characterization*
1. Do you ever feel your heart pound, beat too fast, or skip beats?

2. Do you feel dizzy or faint when you experience these sensations?
3. What brings on this sensation?
4. How long does it last?
5. What do you do to relieve these sensations?

B. Significance
1. Pounding, jumping sensations in chest usually due to tachydysrhythmias.
2. Skipped beats usually due to premature atrial or ventricular beats.

Weakness/Fatigue

A. Characterization
1. What activities can you perform without becoming tired?
2. What activities cause you to become tired?
3. Is the fatigue relieved by rest?
4. Is leg weakness accompanied by pain or swelling?

B. Significance
1. Fatigue is produced by low cardiac output. The heart is unable to provide sufficient blood to meet the increased metabolic needs of cells.
2. As heart disease advances, fatigue is precipitated by less effort.
3. Weakness or tiring of the legs may be caused by peripheral arterial or venous disease.

Dizziness and Syncope

A. Characterization
1. How many episodes of syncope/near syncope have been experienced?
2. Did a hot room, hunger, sudden position change, or pressure on your neck precipitate the episode (rules out incidents that may cause a vasovagal response)?
3. How long does dizziness last?
4. What relieves dizziness?

B. Significance
1. Syncope is a transient loss of consciousness due to a fall in cardiac output with resulting cerebral ischemia. Near syncope refers to lightheadedness, dizziness, temporary confusion.
2. Dysrhythmias related to cardiac disease may cause syncope.

◆ NURSING HISTORY

History of Present Illness

1. What other symptoms has the patient noticed?
2. long has the patient been ill? What has the course of the illness been?
3. Obtain a review of systems.

Past Medical History

A. Medical and Surgical History
1. Hypertension, diabetes mellitus, hyperlipidemia, or other chronic illnesses which cause or aggravate cardiovascular disease.

2. Past illnesses/hospitalizations: trauma to chest (possible myocardial contusion); sore throat/dental extractions (possible endocarditis); rheumatic fever (valvular dysfunction, endocarditis); thromboembolism (MI, pulmonary embolism)
3. Medications—Many cardiac drugs must be tapered off to prevent a "rebound effect"; many drugs affect heart rate and may cause orthostatic hypotension; estrogen preparations may lead to thromboembolism.

B. Family History
1. Ask if patient's family members (patients, grandparents, siblings, blood relatives) were diagnosed with coronary artery disease, hypertension, hyperlipidemia, diabetes.

C. Lifestyle
1. Assess for risk factors to cardiovascular disease such as smoking, obesity, pattern of recurrent weight gain after dieting, sedentary lifestyle, stress, alcohol consumption.

◆ PHYSICAL EXAMINATION

Vital Signs

A. Determine Heart Rate
1. Time for 1 full minute; note regularity.
2. Compare apical and radial heart rate (pulse deficit).

B. Monitor Blood Pressure
1. Take pressure in both arms and note differences (5- to 10-mm Hg difference is normal). Difference >10 may indicate subclavian steal syndrome or dissecting aortic aneurysm.
2. Determine pulse pressure (systolic pressure minus diastolic pressure) to evaluate cardiac output (30–40 mm Hg normal; less than 30 mm Hg indicates decreased cardiac output).
3. Note presence of pulsus alternans—loud sounds alternate with soft sounds with each auscultatory beat (hallmark of left ventricular failure).
4. Note presence of pulsus paradoxus—abnormal fall in blood pressure during inspirations (cardinal sign of cardiac tamponade.

C. Assess for Postural/Orthostatic Hypotension
1. Autonomic compensatory factors for upright posture are inadequate due to volume depletion, bedrest, drugs such as alpha adrenergic blockers, or neurologic disease; prompt hypotension occurs with assumption of the upright position.
2. Note changes in heart rate and blood pressure in at least two of three positions: lying, standing, sitting; allow at least 3 minutes between position changes before obtaining rate and pressure.
3. Orthostatic changes evident if blood pressure decreases by 15 mm Hg (systolic) or 5 mm Hg diastolic and/or heart rate increases 15 beats with position changes. Keep in mind that patients on beta blockers may not exhibit a compensatory increase in heart rate.

Skin and Extremities

A. Palpate for Temperature and Evidence of Diaphoresis
1. Warm/dry skin indicates adequate cardiac output.
2. Cool, clammy skin indicates compensatory vasoconstriction due to low cardiac output.

B. Observe for Cyanosis, Jaundice, and Fatty Skin Deposits (Xanthomas)
1. Cyanosis—Bluish discoloration of the skin and mucous membranes.
   a. Central cyanosis—Low oxygen saturation of arterial blood. Noted on tongue, buccal mucosa, and lips. Indicative of cardiorespiratory disease; may be evident in heart failure or pulmonary edema.
   b. Peripheral cyanosis—Reduced blood flow through extremities due to vasoconstriction. Noted on distal aspects of extremities, tip of nose, and ear lobes; due to cold exposure or obstructive peripheral vascular disease.
2. Jaundice—Yellow discoloration of sclera of eyes and/or skin; may be sign of right-sided heart failure or chronic hemolysis from prosthetic heart valve.
3. Yellow plaque (fatty deposits) evident on skin; associated with hyperlipidemia and coronary artery disease.

C. Inspect Nailbeds for Splinter Hemorrhages and Clubbing
1. Thin brown lines in nailbed are associated with endocarditis.
2. Clubbing (swollen nail base and loss of normal angle) is associated with congenital heart disease and cor pulmonale.

D. Inspect and Palpate for Edema
1. Edema is an abnormal accumulation of serous fluid in soft tissue.
2. Location of edema is influenced by gravity—Fluid collects bilaterally in lower parts of the body: sacral area (bedridden patients), ankles, and feet (ambulatory patients), and "pits" with pressure (dependent-pitting edema).
3. Weight gain occurs before clinical evidence of edema. Edema is a late sign of heart failure.
4. Describe degree of edema in terms of depth of pitting that occurs with slight pressure; mild—0 to $\frac{1}{4}$ inch, moderate—$\frac{1}{2}$ inch, severe—$\frac{3}{4}$ to 1 inch.

E. Palpate Arterial Pulses
1. Examine the pulses bilaterally; peripheral pulses should be equal.
   a. Note amplitude (fullness), which depends on pulse pressure (difference between systolic and diastolic pressures); this gives an estimate of stroke volume.
   b. Small volume pulse may be from low stroke volume and peripheral vasoconstriction (MI, shock, constrictive pericarditis, vasoconstrictive drugs).
   c. Large volume pulse produced by large stroke volume (aortic regurgitation, pregnancy, thyrotoxicosis, bradycardia, patent ductus arteriosus).
   d. Palpate carotid artery—Reveals character of pulse in the proximal aorta and provides indication of any abnormality causing disease of left ventricle.

Chest and Neck

A. General Assessment
1. Palpate the precordial area with palmar base of hand.
2. Note pulsation in apical area (fifth intercostal space—midclavicular line).
3. Pulsation (apical impulse) should be approximately 2 cm in diameter; lateral displacement of greater than 7 to 9 cm from sternal border indicates left ventricular hypertrophy.

B. Respiration
1. Note rate, depth, and respiratory pattern, use of accessory muscles.

C. Jugular Venous Pulse
1. Venous pulsation can be more easily seen than felt.
2. Identification of venous pulse permits assessment of height of venous pressure.
3. See page 31 for technique.

D. Heart Auscultation
1. Four main areas of auscultation: aortic area, pulmonary area, mitral area, and the tricuspid area.
2. Listen with diaphragm for rate and regularity of rhythm.
   a. Determine if an irregularity is related to respiratory movements.
   b. Evaluate the sequence in which an irregularity occurs.
3. During auscultation, feel the pulsation of the right carotid artery and the radial artery to assess for pulse deficit.
4. Auscultate with bell of stethoscope for an S3 gallop (may indicate ventricular failure), an S4 gallop (may be present in left ventricular hypertrophy, pulmonary or aortic stenosis, and hypertension), murmurs (indicate incompetent or stenotic valves), or pericardial friction rub (pericarditis).

Diagnostic Tests

Cardiovascular function and disease are evaluated by a variety of blood tests, ultrasound techniques, fluoroscopy and nuclear imaging studies, and electrocardiography. The ECG and its application in exercise stress testing are invaluable in the evaluation of chest pain and cardiac dysfunction.

◆ LABORATORY STUDIES

Enzyme and Isoenzyme Tests

A. Description
1. When myocardial tissue is damaged (myocardial infarction), certain cardiac enzymes are released into the bloodstream and result in elevated peripheral blood enzyme levels:
   a. Creatine kinase (CK)
   b. Lactic dehydrogenase (LDH)
   c. Aspartate aminotransferase (AST, formerly SGOT). However, these enzymes may be widely distributed in tissues and elevated in conditions not associated with MI such as damage to skeletal muscles, liver, brain, kidneys, and other organs.
2. Isoenzymes of CK and LDH can be identified by laboratory methods to reveal the specific tissue that is damaged.

B. Nursing/Patient Care Considerations
1. Ensure that enzymes are drawn in a serial pattern, usually on admission and every 6 to 24 hours until three samples are obtained; enzyme activity then is correlated to the extent of heart muscle damage.
2. Normal values, rise, and peak of enzymes following MI include:

a. CK—Rise in 12 hours; peak in 36 to 72 hours; normalize (35 to 232 IU) in 3 to 5 days.
b. LDH—Rise in 12 hours; peak in 12 to 24 hours; normalize (100 to 190 IU) in 10 days.
c. AST—Rise in 8 to 12 hours; peak in 18 to 36 hours; normalize in 3 to 4 days.
d. CK-MB—Rise in 4 to 8 hours, peak in 24 hours, normalize (less than 5 IU) in 72 hours.
e. LDH1 and LDH2—LDH2 is normally greater than LDH1, except when the heart muscle is damaged a reversal occurs; a "flipped" pattern results, with LDH1 exceeding the value of LDH2, usually within 12 to 24 hours.

> **NURSING ALERT:** ◆◆
> The greater the peak in enzyme activity and the length of time an enzyme remains at peak level correlate with serious damage of the heart muscle and a poorer prognosis for the patient.

◆ RADIOLOGY/IMAGING

Chest X-Ray

A. *Description* Shows heart size, contour, and position; reveals cardiac and pericardial calcifications and demonstrates physiologic alterations in pulmonary circulation

B. *Nursing/Patient Care Considerations*
1. Advise patient to remove all metal jewelry before having x-ray.
2. If portable chest x-ray is being done on bedridden or critically ill patient, assist with high Fowler's position during x-ray and ensure that all tubes, IV lines, and monitoring remain in place.

Myocardial Imaging

A. *Description* With the use of radionuclides and scintillation cameras, radionuclide angiograms can be used to assess left ventricular performance

1. "Hot spot" or positive imaging using technetium-99m stannous pyrophosphate is used when diagnosis of MI is unclear.
2. "Cold spot" imaging using thallium-201 can be used to rule out MI if negative. However, if positive, it cannot differentiate between old and new infarction and areas of ischemia versus infarction.
3. Radionuclide ventriculogram using technetium-99m provides measurements of right and left ventricular ejection fraction, distinguishes regional from global ventricular wall motion, and allows for subjective analysis of cardiac anatomy to detect intracardiac shunts or valvular or congenital abnormalities.

B. *Nursing/Patient Care Considerations* Advise patient that a radionuclide will be injected through a central venous, Swan-Ganz, or IV catheter or antecubital vein. Reassure the patient that the radionuclide will not cause radiation injury or affect heart function.

Angiography

A. *Description*
1. Injection of contrast medium into the vascular system (to outline the heart and blood vessels) accompanied by cineangiograms (rapidly changing films or movies on an intensified fluoroscopic screen), which record the passage of contrast medium through the vascular tree.
2. Useful for providing information regarding coronary anatomy, structural abnormalities (occlusions, defects, fistulae) or abnormal heart valve function.
3. Types of angiography, include:
   a. Selective angiocardiography—Contrast medium is injected through a catheter directly into one of the heart chambers, coronary arteries, or greater vessel.
   b. Aortography—A form of angiography that outlines the lumen of the aorta and major arteries arising from it.
   c. Coronary arteriography (most common form of selective angiocardiography)—Used as an evaluation tool before coronary artery surgery or myocardial revascularization and after surgery to evaluate graft patency. See section on cardiac catheterization page 253.
   d. Peripheral arteriography—To determine arterial patency of extremities.

B. *Nursing/Patient Care Considerations*
1. Before angiogram, keep the patient in a fasting state—To minimize danger of pulmonary aspiration should emesis occur.
2. After angiogram
   a. Record vital signs every 15 minutes × 4 (or more often as patient's condition indicates until vital signs are stable).
   b. Check for bleeding at puncture or cutdown site.
   c. Check distal extremity for normal color and intact pulses.
   d. The patient may complain of mild headache and/or discomfort in the groin or other site depending on route by which contrast medium was administered.
   e. Check for bedrest and special fluid instructions.

Echocardiography (Ultrasound Cardiography)

A. *Description*
1. A record of high-frequency sound vibrations that have been sent into the heart through the chest wall. The cardiac structures return the echoes derived from the ultrasound. The motions of the echoes are traced on an oscilloscope and recorded on film.
2. Clinical usefulness includes: demonstration of valvular and other structural deformities, detection of pericardial effusion, evaluation of prosthetic valve function, diagnosis of cardiac tumors of asymmetric thickening of interventricular septum, diagnosis of cardiomegaly (heart enlargement).
3. Types include two-dimensional and M mode.
   a. Two-dimensional echocardiography—Provides a wider view of the heart and its structures because it involves a planar ultrasound beam.

b. M-mode—Utilizes a single ultrasound beam and provides a narrow segmental view

c. The methods are complementary and are often used in conjunction.

B. **Nursing/Patient Care Considerations** Advise the patient that echocardiography is noninvasive and that no preparation is necessary.

Assist patient to cleanse chest of transducer gel after the test.

Doppler Ultrasound

1. Noninvasive method of evaluating peripheral venous patency and valvular competence and arterial patency.
2. The entire test takes about 5 to 10 minutes and no special preparation is necessary.
3. Tell the patient that a cuff is applied to the leg to detect arterial patency, and will be inflated and deflated similar to blood pressure measurement.

Plethysmography (Pulse Volume Recording [PVR])

1. A noninvasive measurement of changes in calf volume corresponding to changes in blood volume brought about by temporary venous occlusion with a high pneumatic cuff.
2. Ocular pneumoplethysmography (OPG)—Measures indirectly carotid artery blood flow; this is done by the application of pneumatic pressure on the eye to measure ophthalmic artery pressure.
3. Advise the patient that cuff inflation may cause brief discomfort, but not pain.

Oscillometry

1. Degree of arterial occlusion may be measured by an oscillometer, which measures pulse volume. One extremity may be compared with the other to evaluate arterial patency.
2. An inflatable cuff is wrapped around the extremity, and the oscillometric index is determined by inflating the cuff and reading the dial.
3. Advise patient to remain still while cuff is inflated and deflated to prevent interference with pressure readings.

Phlebography (Venography)

A. **Description** An x-ray visualization of the vascular tree after the injection of a contrast medium (Renografin) to detect venous occlusion

B. **Nursing/Patient Care Considerations**
1. Inform the patient that he or she may experience an intense burning sensation in the vessel where the solution is injected. This will last for only a few seconds.
2. Note any evidence of allergic reaction to the contrast medium; this may occur as soon as the contrast medium is injected, or it may occur after the test.
   a. Perspiring, dyspnea, nausea, vomiting

b. Rapid heart rate, numbness of extremities
c. Hives

3. Advise the patient to notify the health care provider of any signs of allergic reaction.
4. Observe injection site for signs of redness, swelling, bleeding, thrombosis.

Digital Subtraction Angiography (DSA) or Digital Intravenous Angiography

A. **Description** Radiologic technique that uses computer subtraction to display an enhanced image of the arterial system. Contrast medium is injected by way of a catheter inserted into the brachial vein, and a guidewire is threaded into the superior vena cava.

B. **Nursing/Patient Care Considerations**
1. Advise on no food intake within 2 hours of the test to prevent vomiting if there is a reaction to the contrast medium.
2. Make sure the patient will be able to hold breath and lie very still when directed.
3. Instruct the patient to increase fluid intake over next 24 hours (1,500 to 2,000 mL) to aid in excretion of contrast medium.

◆ OTHER DIAGNOSTIC TESTS

The Electrocardiogram (ECG)

A. **Basic Principles**
1. Electrical activity is generated by the cells of the heart as ions are exchanged across cell membranes.
2. Electrodes that are capable of conducting electrical activity from the heart to the ECG machine are placed at strategic positions on the extremities and chest precordium (Fig. 10-1).
3. The electrical energy sensed is then converted to a graphic display by the ECG machine. This display is referred to as the electrocardiogram.
4. A heart contraction is represented by wave forms on the ECG graph paper that are designated P, Q, R, S, and T waves.
5. Wave forms are referred to as deflections relative to an isoelectric line (a line that expresses no energy). The isoelectric line can be determined by looking at the T-to-P interval.
   a. The P wave is the first positive deflection and represents atrial depolarization.
   b. The Q wave is the first negative deflection after the P wave; the R wave is the first positive deflection after the P wave.
   c. The S wave is the negative deflection after the R wave.
   d. The QRS wave form is generally regarded as a unit and represents ventricular depolarization.
   e. The T wave follows the S wave and is joined to the QRS complex by the ST segment. The T wave represents the return of ions to the appropriate side of the cell membrane. This signifies relaxation of the muscle fibers and is referred to as repolarization of the ventricles.
   f. The QT interval is the time between the Q wave and the T wave.

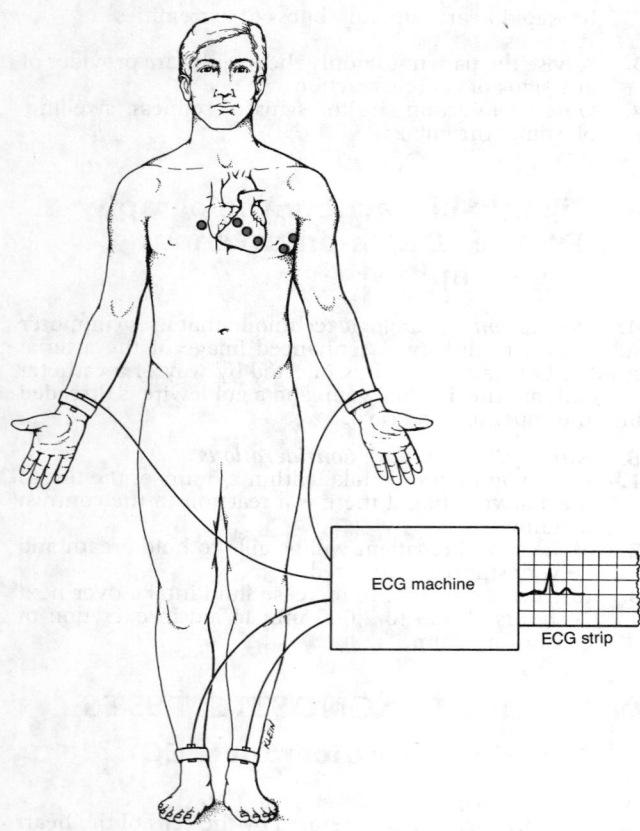

FIGURE 10-1 *Transmission of heart's impulse to a graphic display by ECG machine. The electrodes that are capable of conducting electrical activity from the heart to the ECG machine are placed at strategic positions on the extremities and chest precordium.*

B. Indications The ECG is a useful tool in the diagnosis of those conditions that may cause aberrations in the electrical activity of the heart. Examples of these conditions are as follows:

1. MI and other types of coronary artery diseases, such as angina
2. Cardiac dysrhythmias
3. Cardiac enlargement
4. Electrolyte disturbances, especially of calcium and potassium levels
5. Inflammatory diseases of the heart
6. Effects on the heart by drugs such as digitalis (Lanoxin) and tricyclic antidepressants

C. ECG Leads and Normal Wave Form Interpretation (Fig. 10-2)
1. The standard ECG consists of 12 leads (I, II, III, AVR, AVL, AVF, V1, V2, V3, V4, V5, V6).
   a. Each lead records the heart's electrical activity from a different anatomic position.
   b. Identification of specific myocardial changes on certain leads assists in defining pathologic conditions.

2. The normal amplitude of the P wave is 3 mm or less; the normal duration of the P wave is 0.04 to 0.11 seconds. P waves that exceed these measurements are considered to be a deviation from normal.
3. The PR interval is measured from the upstroke of the P wave to the QR junction and is normally between 0.12 and 0.20 seconds.
   a. The PR interval represents the time of impulse transmission from the SA node to the AV node.
   b. There is a built-in delay in time at the AV node to allow for adequate ventricular filling to maintain normal stroke volume (the amount of blood ejected with each contraction).
4. The QRS complex contains separate waves and segments, which should be evaluated separately. Normal QRS complex should be between 0.06 and 0.10 seconds.
   a. The Q wave, or first downward stroke after the P wave, is usually less than 3 mm in depth. A Q wave of significant deflection is not normally present in the healthy heart. A pathologic Q wave usually indicates an old MI.
   b. The R wave is the first positive deflection after the P wave, normally 5 to 10 mm in height. Increases and decreases in amplitude become significant in certain disease states. Ventricular hypertrophy produces very high R waves because the hypertrophied muscle requires a stronger electrical current to depolarize.
5. The S–T segment begins at the end of the S wave, the first negative deflection after the R wave, and terminates at the upstroke of the T wave.
6. The T wave represents the repolarization of myocardial fibers or provides the resting state of myocardial work; the T wave should always be present.
   a. Normally, the T wave should not exceed a 5-mm amplitude in all leads except the precordial (V1 to V6) leads, where it may be as high as 10 mm.

D. Nursing/Patient Care Considerations
1. Perform ECG or begin continuous ECG monitoring as indicated.

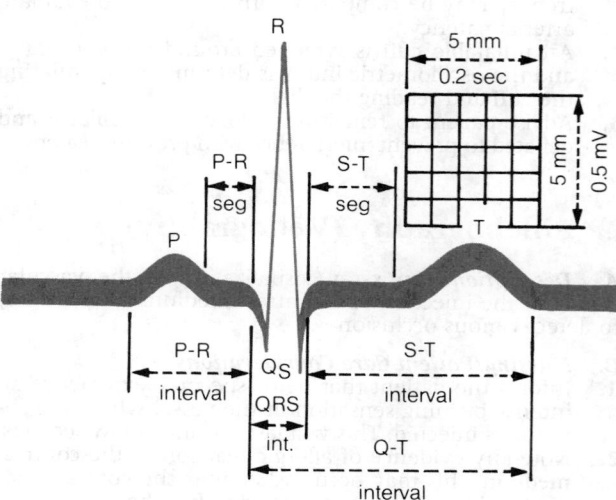

FIGURE 10-2 *Wave form analysis.*

a. Provide privacy and ask the patient to undress, exposing chest, wrists, and ankles. Assist with draping as appropriate.

b. Place leads on chest and extremities as labeled, using self-adhesive electrodes or water-soluble gel or other conductive material.

c. Instruct patient to lie still, avoiding movement, coughing, or talking while ECG is recording to avoid artifact.

d. Make sure ECG machine is plugged in and grounded, and operate according to manufacturer's directions.

e. If continuous cardiac monitoring is being done, advise patient on the parameters of mobility and not to panic if an alarm sounds.

2. Interpret ECG (Fig. 10-3). Develop a systematic approach to assist in accurate interpretation for dysrhythmias, myocardial damage, or other changes.

a. Determine the rate. Is it fast, slow, or normal?

(1) A gross determination of rate can be determined by counting the number of QRS complexes within a 6-second time interval (use the superior margin of ECG paper) and multiply the complexes by a factor of 10.
Note: One must be cautioned that this method is accurate only for rhythms that are occurring at normal intervals and should not be used for determining rate in irregular rhythms. Irregular rhythms are always counted for 1 full minute for accuracy.

(2) Another means of obtaining rate is to divide the number of large five-square blocks between each two QRS complexes into 300. Three hundred large blocks represent 1 minute on the ECG paper.
Example: In Figure 10-3, the number of large square blocks between complexes #5 and #6 equals 5, or a rate of 60.

b. Next, determine the rhythm. Is it regular, irregular, regularly irregular, or irregularly irregular?

(1) Use calipers or count blocks between QRS complexes to determine regularity.

c. Finally, examine each wave and segment for abnormality.

(1) Find the P waves. Is one present for each QRS complex? Are they absent as in junctional rhythm? Are they replaced by other wave forms? What is the configuration like? Are they identical, well-formed, or do they change shape as in atrial fibrillation or paroxysmal atrial tachycardia?

(2) Measure the PR interval. Prolonged PR interval may be a precursor to a variety of heart blocks due to drug therapy or myocardial disease.

(3) Look for pathologic Q waves, or one that is greater than 0.04 seconds in time and greater than 3 mm in depth or greater than one third the height of the R wave.

(4) Measure the QRS complex. Are they identical in configuration? Do they fall early? Does the configuration vary? Are any wide and bizarre, representing a premature ventricular contraction?

(5) Examine the S–T segments. Elevation of the S–T segment heralds a pattern of injury and usually occurs as an initial change in acute MI. S–T depression occurs in ischemic states. Calcium and potassium changes also affect the S–T segment.

(6) Look at the T wave. Is it positively or negatively deflected? Is it peaked? Inverted T waves may indicate ischemia.

(7) Measure the QT interval. The normal QT interval should be less than one half the RR interval. Prolonged QT interval may indicate digitalis toxicity, long-term quinidine (Quinaglute) or procainamide (Pronestyl) therapy, or hypomagnesemia.

Cardiac Catheterization

A. Description

1. Cardiac catheterization is a diagnostic procedure in which a catheter(s) is (are) introduced into the heart

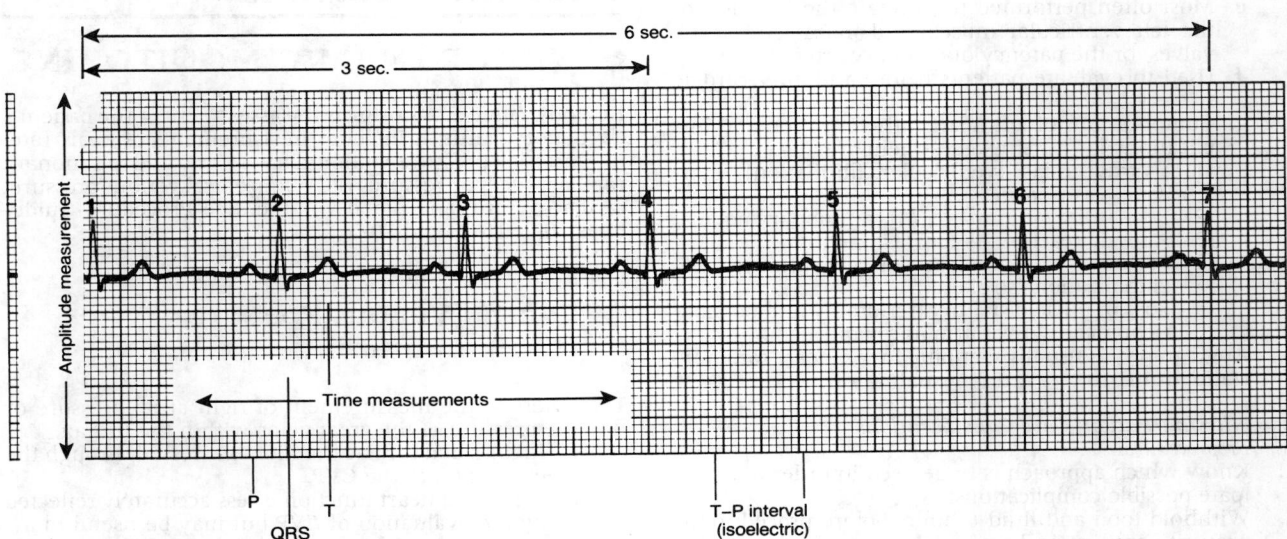

FIGURE 10-3 *Lead II normal sinus rhythm and ECG paper*

and blood vessels to 1) measure oxygen concentration, saturation, tension, and pressure in the various heart chambers; 2) detect shunts; 3) provide blood samples for analysis; and 4) determine cardiac output and pulmonary blood flow.

2. Right-heart catheterization—A radiopaque catheter is passed from an antecubital or femoral vein into the right atrium, right ventricle, and pulmonary vasculature under direct visualization with a fluoroscope.
   a. Right atrium and right ventricle pressures are measured; blood samples are taken for hematocrit and oxygen saturation.
   b. After entering the right atrium, the catheter is then passed through the tricuspid valve, and similar tests are performed on blood within the right ventricle.
   c. Finally, the catheter is passed through the pulmonic valve and as far as possible beyond that point; capillary samples are obtained and ''capillary pressures'' (wedge pressure) are recorded.
   d. Complications—Cardiac dysrhythmias, venous spasm, thrombophlebitis, infection of cutdown site, cardiac perforation, and cardiac tamponade.

3. Left-heart catheterization—Usually done by retrograde catheterization of the left ventricle or by transseptal catheterization of the left atrium.
   a. Retrograde approach—Catheter inserted under direct vision into right brachial artery and advanced under fluoroscopic control into the ascending aorta and into the left ventricle; or, catheter may be introduced percutaneously by puncture of femoral artery.
   b. Transseptal approach—Catheter is passed from the right femoral vein (percutaneously or by saphenous vein cutdown) into right atrium. A long needle is passed up through the catheter and is used to puncture the septum separating the right and left atria; needle is withdrawn and the catheter is advanced under fluoroscopic control into left ventricle.
   c. The catheter tip is placed at the coronary sinus, and contrast medium is injected directly into one or both of the coronary arteries to evaluate patency.
   d. Gives hemodynamic data—Permits flow and pressure measurements of left heart.
   e. Most often performed to evaluate the function of the left ventricular muscle and mitral and aortic valves, or the patency of coronary arteries.
   f. Used to evaluate patients before and after cardiac surgery.
   g. Complications of left heart catheterization and implications for nursing assessment are
      (1) Dysrhythmias (ventricular fibrillation), syncope, vasospasm
      (2) Pericardial tamponade, MI, pulmonary edema
      (3) Allergic reaction to contrast medium
      (4) Perforation of great vessels of heart; systemic embolization (stroke, MI)
      (5) Loss of pulse distal to arteriotomy and possible ischemia of lower arm and hand.

4. Angiography is usually combined with heart catheterization for coronary artery visualization.

B. **Nursing/Patient Care Considerations**
Preprocedure:
1. Know which approach is to be used in order to anticipate possible complications.
2. Withhold food and fluid 6 hours before procedure to prevent vomiting and aspiration.
3. Ascertain history of previous allergies.

4. Mark distal pulses for easy reference after catheterization.
5. Explain that patient will be lying on an examining table for a prolonged period and that certain sensations may be experienced:
   a. Occasional thudding sensations in the chest—from extrasystoles, particularly when the catheter is manipulated in ventricular chambers.
   b. Strong desire to cough may occur during contrast medium injection into right heart during angiography.
   c. Transient feeling of heat, particularly in the head, from injection of contrast medium.
6. Remove dentures; give prescribed medication.

Postprocedure:
1. Record the blood pressure and apical pulse every 15 minutes (or more frequently) until vital signs are stable after the procedure to discern dysrhythmias.
2. Check peripheral pulses in affected extremity (dorsalis pedis, posterior tibial pulse in the lower extremity, and radial pulse in upper extremity); evaluate extremity temperature, color, and complaints of pain, numbness, or tingling sensation to determine signs of arterial insufficiency.
3. Watch puncture (cutdown) sites for hematoma formation. Question patient about increase in pain/tenderness at site.
4. Assess for complaints of chest pain and report occurrence immediately. MI may occur and is a serious complication of cardiac catheterization.
5. See that the patient remains in bed with little movement of the involved extremity until the following morning.
6. Evaluate complaints of back pain, thigh or groin pain (may indicate retroperitoneal bleeding).
7. Be alert for signs/symptoms of vagal reaction (nausea, diaphoresis, hypotension, bradycardia); treat as directed with atropine and fluids.

General Procedure/ Treatment Modalities

◆ HEMODYNAMIC MONITORING

Hemodynamic monitoring is the assessment of the patient's circulatory status; it includes measurements of heart rate, intraarterial pressure, pulmonary artery and pulmonary capillary wedge pressures (PCWP), central venous pressure, cardiac output, and blood volume. See Procedure Guidelines 10-1, 10-2, and 10-3.

Central Venous Pressure (CVP) Monitoring

1. Refers to the measurement of right atrial pressure or the pressure of the great veins within the thorax.
   a. Right-sided cardiac function is assessed through the evaluation of the CVP.
   b. Left-sided heart function is less accurately reflected by the evaluation of CVP but may be useful in assessing chronic right and left heart failure and/or differentiating right and left ventricular infarctions.

2. Requires the threading of a catheter into a large central vein (subclavian, internal/external jugular, median basilic, or femoral). The catheter tip then is positioned in the right atrium, upper portion of the superior vena cava or the inferior vena cava (femoral approach only).
3. Purposes of CVP monitoring include:
   a. To serve as a guide for fluid replacement
   b. To monitor pressures in the right atrium and central veins
   c. To administer blood products, total parenteral nutrition, and drug therapy contraindicated for peripheral infusion
   d. To obtain venous access when peripheral vein sites are inadequate
   e. To insert a temporary pacemaker
   f. To obtain central venous blood samples

Pulmonary Artery Pressure (PAP) Monitoring

A. Purposes
1. To monitor pressures in the right atrium (CVP), right ventricle, pulmonary artery, and distal branches of the pulmonary artery (PCWP). The latter reflects the level of the pressure in the left atrium (or filling pressure in the left ventricle); thus, pressures on the left side of the heart are inferred from pressure measurement obtained on the right side of the circulation.
2. To measure cardiac output through thermodilution
3. To obtain blood for central venous oxygen saturation
4. To continuously monitor mixed venous oxygen saturation (SvO$_2$); available on special catheters
5. To provide for temporary atrial/ventricular pacing and intraatrial electrocardiography (available only on special catheters)

B. Underlying Considerations
1. Left atrial pressure is closely related to left ventricular end diastolic pressure (LVEDP—filling pressure of the left ventricle) and is therefore an indicator of left ventricular function.
2. The pulmonary artery diastolic pressure (PAD) reflects the LVEDP in patients with normal lungs and mitral valve. The PAD can be continuously monitored as an approximation of LVEDP (limits excessive balloon inflation to obtain a PCWP and subsequent risk of balloon rupture).
3. The SvO$_2$ is affected by four factors: cardiac output, hemoglobin, arterial oxygen saturation (SaO$_2$), and tissue oxygen consumption.
4. Changes in SvO$_2$ alert the clinician to changes in these factors. More rapid detection of change facilitates interventions to correct problems before significant deterioration in patient's condition occurs.
5. If the amount of oxygen supplied to the tissues is inadequate to meet demands, more oxygen will be extracted from venous blood and the SvO$_2$ will decrease. If oxygen supply exceeds demand, the SvO$_2$ will increase.

C. Methods
1. The Swan-Ganz catheter is a flow-directed, balloon-tipped, four- to five-lumen catheter that is percutaneously inserted at the bedside and allows for continuous PAP monitoring as well as periodic measurement of PCWP and other parameters.

2. The catheter is 110 cm long, marked at increments of 10 cm, and is available in varying diameters.
3. Most catheters in use incorporate thermodilution for determination of cardiac output.
4. If monitoring of SvO$_2$ is desired, a pulmonary artery catheter incorporating fiberoptics is used.
5. If temporary cardiac pacing capability is desired, a catheter with a lumen for a pacing wire may be used.
6. Catheter may be inserted under fluoroscopy or at the bedside using the hemodynamic wave form as a guide to correct position.

Cardiac Output

Cardiac output is the amount (volume) of blood ejected by the left ventricle into the aorta in 1 minute. The normal cardiac output is 4 to 8 L/min.

A. Underlying Concepts
1. Cardiac output is determined by stroke volume (SV) and heart rate (HR).
   a. HR = number of cardiac contractions per minute. The integrity of the conduction system and nervous system innervation of the heart influence functioning of this determinant.
   b. SV = amount of blood ejected from ventricle per beat. The amount of blood returning to the heart (preload), venous tone, resistance imposed on the ventricle before ejection (afterload), and the integrity of the cardiac muscle (contractility) influence the functioning of this determinant.
2. The body alters cardiac output by increases/decreases in one of both of these parameters. Cardiac output is maintained if the HR fails by an increase in SV. Likewise, a decrease in SV produces a compensatory rise in HR to keep the cardiac output normal.
3. Cardiac output will decrease if either of the determinants cannot inversely compensate for the other.
4. Cardiac output measurements are adjusted to patient size by calculating the cardiac index (CI). CI = cardiac output divided by body surface area (BSA); BSA is determined through standard charts based on individual height and weight. Normal CI is 2.5 to 4.0 L/min/m^2.

B. Assessment of Cardiac Output
Low cardiac output may be detected by:
1. Changes in mental status
2. An increase in heart rate
3. Shortness of breath
4. Cyanosis or duskiness of buccal mucosa, nailbeds, and ear lobes
5. Falling blood pressure
6. Low urine output
7. Cool, moist skin

C. Methods
1. Cardiac output is measured by a variety of techniques. In the clinical setting, it is usually measured by the thermodilution technique used in conjunction with a flow-directed balloon catheter. (Swan-Ganz catheter.)
2. The Swan-Ganz catheter is positioned in its final position in a branch of the pulmonary artery; it has a thermistor (external sensing device) situated 4 cm from the tip of the catheter, which measures the temperature of the blood that flows by it (see p. 262).

PROCEDURE GUIDELINES 10-1 ♦ Central Venous Pressure (CVP) Monitoring

EQUIPMENT

Venous pressure tray
Cutdown tray
Infusion solution/infusion set with CVP manometer
Heparin flush system/pressure bag (if transducer
   to be used)
IV pole

Arm board (for antecubital insertion)
Sterile dressing/tape
Gowns, masks, caps, and sterile gloves
ECG monitoring
Carpenter's level (for establishing zero point)

PROCEDURE

NURSING ACTION	RATIONALE
PREPARATORY PHASE	
1. Assemble equipment according to manufacturer's directions.	1. Evaluate patient's PT, PTT, CBC.
2. Explain the procedure to the patient and obtain informed consent.	2. Procedure is similar to an IV, and the patient may move in bed as desired after passage of catheter.
a. Explain to patient how to perform the Valsalva maneuver.	a. The Valsalva maneuver performed during catheter insertion and removal decreases chance of air emboli.
b. NPO 6 hours before insertion	
3. Position patient appropriately.	3. Provides for maximum visibility of veins.
a. Place in supine position.	
(1) Arm vein—extend arm and secure on armboard.	
(2) Neck veins—place patient in Trendelenburg's position. Place a small rolled towel under shoulders (subclavian approach).	Trendelenburg's position prevents chance of air emboli. Anatomic access and clinical status of the patient are considered in site selection.
4. Flush IV infusion set and manometer (measuring device) *Or,* prepare heparin flush for use with transducer.	4. Secure all connections to prevent air emboli and bleeding.
a. Attach manometer to IV pole. The zero point of the manometer should be on a level with the patient's right atrium.	a. The level of the right atrium is at the 4th intercostal space midaxillary line.
b. Calibrate/zero transducer and level port with patient's right atrium.	b. Mark midaxillary line with indelible ink for subsequent readings.
5. Place patient on ECG monitor.	5. Dysrhythmias may be noted during insertion as catheter is advanced.
INSERTION PHASE (BY PHYSICIAN)	
1. Physician dons gown, cap, and mask.	1. CVP insertion is a sterile procedure.
2. The CVP site is surgically cleansed. The physician introduces the CVP catheter percutaneously or by direct venous cutdown.	2. Patient may be asked to perform Valsalva maneuver to protect against chance of air embolus.
3. Assist patient to remain motionless during insertion.	
4. Monitor for dysrhythmias as catheter is threaded to great vein or right atrium.	
5. Connect primed IV tubing/heparin flush system to catheter and allow IV solution to flow at a minimum rate to keep vein open (25 mL maximum).	5. Catheter placement must be verified before hypertonic or blood products can be administered.
6. The catheter should be sutured in place.	6. Prevents inadvertent catheter advancement or dislodgement.
7. Place a sterile occlusive dressing over site.	
8. Obtain a chest x-ray.	8. Verify correct catheter position.
TO MEASURE THE CVP	
1. Place the patient in a position of comfort. This is the baseline position used for subsequent readings.	
2. Position the zero point of the manometer at the level of the right atrium (see accompanying figure).	2. The zero point or baseline for the manometer should be on a level with the patient's right atrium. The middle of the right atrium is the midaxillary line in the 4th intercostal space.

PROCEDURE	NURSING ACTION	RATIONALE
(cont'd)		

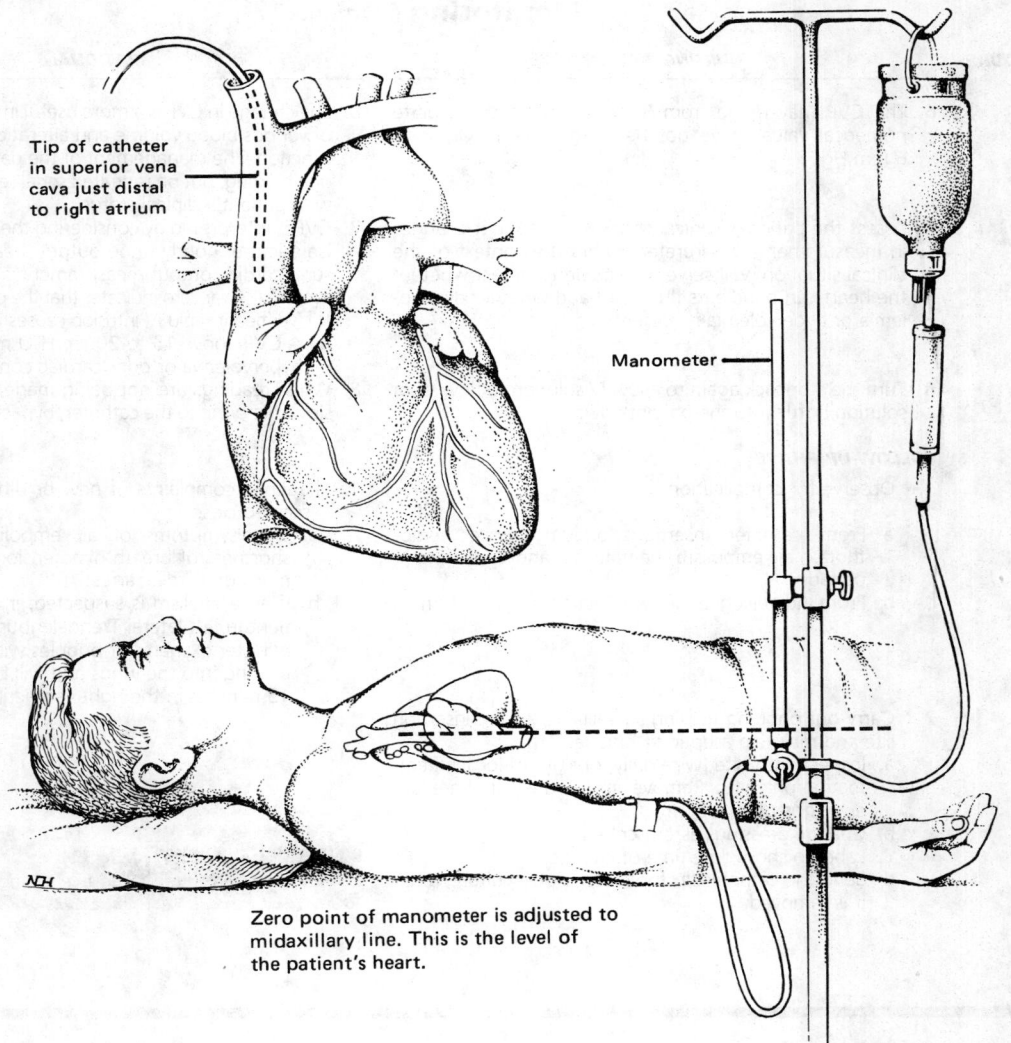

Tip of catheter in superior vena cava just distal to right atrium

Manometer

Zero point of manometer is adjusted to midaxillary line. This is the level of the patient's heart.

Central venous pressure.

3. Turn the stopcock so the IV solution flows into the manometer, filling to about the 20- to 25-cm level. Then turn stopcock so solution in manometer flows into patient.
4. Observe the fall in the height of the column of fluid in manometer. Record the level at which the solution stabilizes or stops moving downward. This is the central venous pressure. Record CVP and the position of the patient.

5. The CVP catheter may be connected to a transducer and an electrical monitor with either digital or calibrated CVP wave readout.

4. The column of fluid will fall until it meets an equal pressure (ie, the patient's central venous pressure). The CVP reading is reflected by the height of a column of fluid in the manometer when there is open communication between the catheter and the manometer. The fluid in the manometer will fluctuate slightly with the patient's respirations. This confirms that the CVP line is not obstructed by clotted blood.

(continued)

PROCEDURE GUIDELINES 10-1 ◆ Central Venous Pressure (CVP) Monitoring *(continued)*

PROCEDURE *(cont'd)*	**NURSING ACTION**	**RATIONALE**

6. The CVP may range from 5 to 12 cm H_2O. (Absolute numerical values have not been agreed on.) Or, 2 to 6 mm Hg.

7. Assess the patient's clinical condition. Frequent changes in measurements (interpreted within the context of the clinical situation) will serve as a guide to detect whether the heart can handle its fluid load and whether hypovolemia or hypervolemia is present.

8. Turn the stopcock again to allow IV solution to flow from solution bottle into the patient's veins.

FOLLOW-UP PHASE

1. Observe for complications.

   a. From catheter insertion: pneumothorax, hemothorax, air embolism, hematoma, and cardiac tamponade
   b. From indwelling catheter: infection, air embolism

2. Carry out ongoing nursing surveillance of the insertion site and maintain aseptic technique.
   a. Inspect entry site twice daily for signs of local inflammation/phlebitis. Remove immediately if there are any signs of infection.
   b. Change dressings as prescribed.
   c. Label to show date/time of change.
   d. Send the catheter tip for bacteriologic culture when it is removed.

RATIONALE

6. The change in CVP is a more useful indication of adequacy of venous blood volume and alterations of cardiovascular function. The management of the patient is not based on one reading, but on repeated serial readings in correlation with patient's clinical status.
7. CVP is interpreted by considering the patient's entire clinical picture; hourly urine output, heart rate, blood pressure, cardiac output measurements.
   a. A CVP near zero indicates that the patient is hypovolemic (verified if rapid IV infusion causes patient to improve).
   b. A CVP above 15 to 20 cm H_2O may be due to either hypervolemia or poor cardiac contractility.
8. When readings are not being made, flow is from a very slow microdrip to the catheter, bypassing the manometer.

1. Patient's complaints of new or different pain must be assessed closely.
   a. Signs/symptoms of air embolism include: severe shortness of breath hypotension, hypoxia, rumbling murmur, cardiac arrest.
   b. If air embolism is suspected, immediately place patient in left lateral Trendelenburg's position and administer oxygen. Air bubbles will be prevented from moving into the lungs and will be absorbed in 10 to 15 minutes in the right ventricular outflow tract.

NURSING ALERT:
A CVP line is a potential source of septicemia.

PROCEDURE GUIDELINES 10-2 ◆ Measuring Pulmonary Artery Pressure by Flow-Directed Balloon-Tipped Catheter (Swan-Ganz Catheter)

EQUIPMENT

Swan–Ganz catheter set
ECG, monitor and display unit with paper recorder
For SvO_2 monitoring, fiberoptic PA catheter, optical module, and microprocessor unit.
Defibrillator
Pressure transducer (disposable/reusable)
Cutdown tray
Sterile saline solution

Pressurized bag
Heparin infusion in plastic bag
Continuous flush device
Local anesthetic
Skin antiseptic
Transparent/gauze dressing
Tape

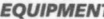

PROCEDURE	**NURSING ACTION**	**RATIONALE**

PREPARATORY PHASE (BY NURSES)

1. Explain procedure to the patient and family/significant other. Obtain informed consent.
2. Check vital signs and apply ECG electrodes.

RATIONALE

1. Explain that patient may feel the catheter moving through veins, and this is normal.

PROCEDURE (cont'd)	NURSING ACTION	RATIONALE

NURSING ACTION

3. Place patient in a position of comfort; this is the baseline position.

4. Set up equipment according to manufacturer's directives:
   a. The pulmonary artery catheter requires a transducer; recording, amplifying, and flush systems.

   b. Flush system according to manufacturer's directions.

RATIONALE

3. Note the angle of elevation if patient cannot lie flat, as subsequent pressure readings are taken from this baseline position to ensure consistency. Patient may need to be in Trendelenburg's position briefly if the jugular or subclavian vein is used.

4. a. Monitoring systems may vary greatly. The complexity of equipment requires an understanding of the equipment in use. A constant microdrip of heparin flush solution is maintained to ensure catheter patency.

   b. Flushing of the catheter system ensures patency and eliminates air bubbles.

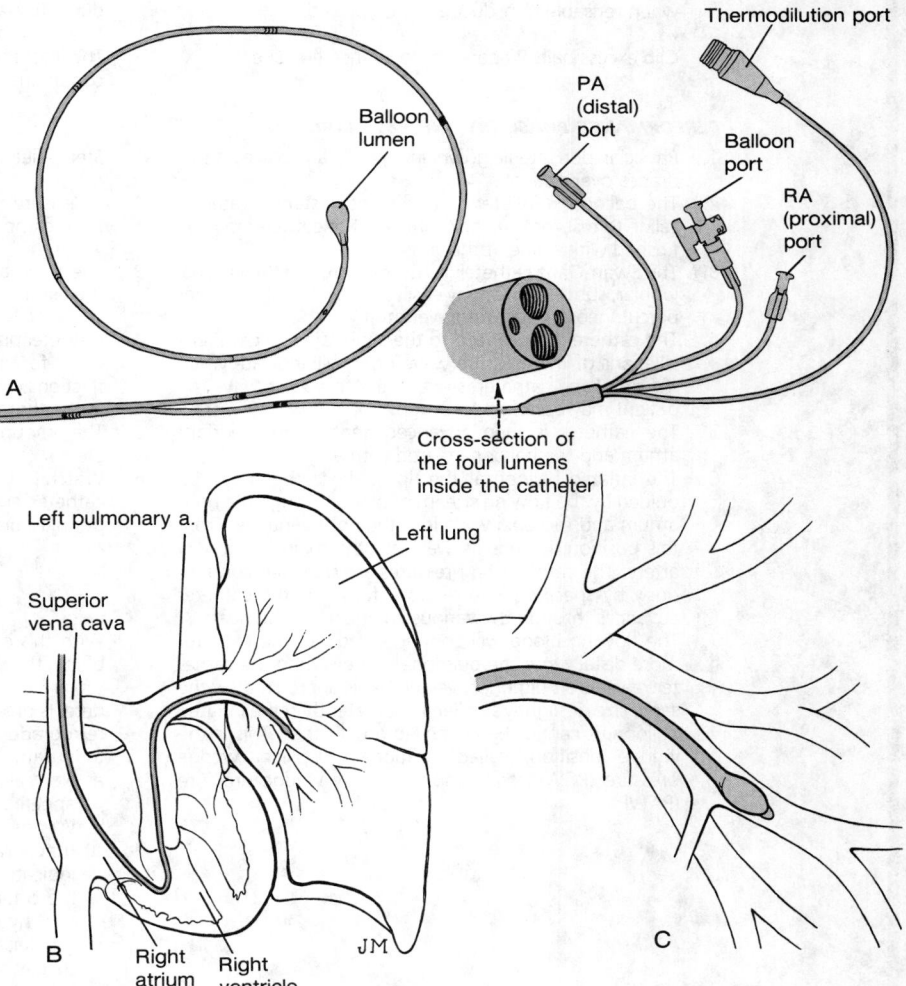

(**A**) Swan-Ganz catheter. (**B**) Location of the Swan–Ganz catheter within the heart. The catheter enters the right atrium via the superior vena cava. The balloon is then inflated, allowing the catheter to follow the blood flow through the tricuspid valve, through the right ventricle, through the pulmonic valve, and into the main pulmonary artery. Waveform and pressure readings are noted during insertion to identify location of the catheter within the heart. The balloon is deflated once the catheter is in the pulmonary artery and properly secured. (**C**) Pulmonary capillary wedge pressure (PCWP). The catheter floats into a distal branch of the pulmonary artery when the balloon is inflated, and becomes "wedged." The wedged catheter occludes blood flow from behind, and the tip of the lumen records pressures in front of the catheter. The balloon is then deflated, allowing the catheter to float back into the main pulmonary artery.

(continued)

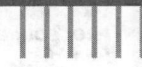

PROCEDURE GUIDELINES 10-2 ◆ Measuring Pulmonary Artery Pressure by Flow-Directed Balloon-Tipped Catheter (Swan-Ganz Catheter)
(continued)

PROCEDURE
(cont'd)

NURSING ACTION	RATIONALE
5. Adjust transducer to level of patient's right atrium (phlebostatic axis 4th intercostal space, midaxillary line) (see figure).	5. Differences between the level of the right atrium and the transducer will result in incorrect pressure readings; the phlebostatic axis is at the level of the right atrium.
6. Calibrate pressure equipment (especially important when reusable transducers are employed).	6. A known quantity of pressure is applied to the transducer (usually by mercury manometer) to ensure accurate monitoring of pressure readings.
7. Clip excess hair. Prepare skin over insertion site.	7. The catheter is inserted percutaneously under sterile conditions.

PERFORMANCE PHASE (BY THE PHYSICIAN)

NURSING ACTION	RATIONALE
1. Physician dons sterile gown and gloves, and places sterile drapes over patient.	1. Sterile field is established to prevent chance of infection.
2. The balloon is inflated with air under sterile water or saline to test for leakage (bubbles). The catheter may be flushed with saline at this time.	2. To ensure that the balloon is intact and to remove air from catheter
3. The Swan-Ganz catheter is inserted through the internal jugular, subclavian, or any easily accessible vein by either percutaneous puncture or venotomy.	3. The internal jugular vein establishes a short route into the central venous system.
4. The catheter is advanced to the superior vena cava. Oscillations of the pressure waveforms will indicate when the tip of the catheter is within the thoracic cavity. The patient may be asked to cough.	4. Catheter placement may be determined by characteristic wave forms and changes. Coughing will produce deflections in the pressure tracing when the catheter tip is in the thorax.
5. The catheter is then advanced gently into the right atrium and the balloon inflated with air.	5. The amount of air to be used is indicated on the catheter.
6. The inflated balloon at the tip of the catheter will be guided by the flowing stream of blood through the right atrium and tricuspid valve into the right ventricle. From this position, it finds its way into the main pulmonary artery. The catheter tip pressures are recorded continuously by specific pressure wave forms as the catheter advances through the various chambers of the heart.	6. Watch ECG monitor for signs of ventricular irritability as catheter enters the right ventricle. Report any signs of dysrhythmia to the physician.
7. The flowing blood will continue to direct the catheter more distally into the pulmonary tree. When the catheter reaches a pulmonary vessel that is approximately the same size or slightly smaller in diameter than the inflated balloon, it cannot be advanced any further. This is the wedge position, called pulmonary capillary wedge pressure (PCWP) or pulmonary artery wedge pressure (PAWP).	7. With the catheter in the wedge position, the balloon blocks the flow of blood from the right side of the heart toward the lungs. The sensor at the tip of the balloon detects pressures distally, which results in the sensing of retrograde left atrial pressures. The PCWP is thus equal to left atrial pressures. a. Normal PCWP is 8–12 mmHg. Optimal LV function appears to be at a wedge between 14–18 mm Hg. b. Wedge pressure is a valuable parameter of cardiac function. Filling pressures less than 8–10 mm Hg may indicate hypovolemia and in an acutely injured heart are often associated with reduction in cardiac output, hypotension, and tachycardia. Filling pressures greater than 20 mm Hg are associated with left ventricular failure, pulmonary congestion, and hypervolemia.
8. The balloon is deflated, causing the catheter to retract spontaneously into a larger pulmonary artery. This gives a continuous pulmonary artery systolic, diastolic, and mean pressure.	8. The normal systolic pulmonary pressure ranges are 20–30 mm Hg, and the diastolic pulmonary pressure ranges are 8–12 mm Hg. The normal mean pulmonary artery pressure (average pressure in pulmonary artery throughout the entire cardiac cycle) is 15–20 mm Hg.
9. The catheter is then attached to a continuous heparin flush and transducer.	9. A low-flow continuous irrigation ensures that the catheter remains patent. The transducer converts the pressure wave into an electronic wave that is displayed on the oscilloscope.

PROCEDURE (cont'd)	**NURSING ACTION**	**RATIONALE**

NURSING ACTION

10. The catheter is sutured in place and covered with a sterile dressing.
11. A chest x-ray is obtained after Swan-Ganz insertion if fluoroscopy was not used to guide insertion.

TO OBTAIN A WEDGE PRESSURE READING

1. Note amount of air to be injected into balloon, usually 1 mL. Do not introduce more air into balloon than specified.
2. Inflate the balloon slowly until the contour of the pulmonary arterial pressure changes to that of pulmonary wedge pressure. As soon as a wedge pattern is observed, no more air is introduced.
   a. Note the digital pressure recordings on the monitor (an average of pressure waves is displayed, but these waves are not taken at end expiration).
   b. Obtain a strip of the pressure tracing.

   c. Determine PCWP from strip at end expiration.
3. Deflate the balloon as soon as the pressure reading is obtained. Do not draw back with force on the syringe because too forceful a deflation may damage the balloon.

4. Record PCWP reading and amount of air needed to obtain wedge reading. Document recorded waveform by placing a strip of the waveform in patient's chart showing wedge tracing reverting to pulmonary artery waveform.

TO OBTAIN A SvO$_2$ READING:

1. Before insertion, perform a preinsertion calibration of the catheter.
2. After insertion, perform a calibration for light intensity and an in vivo calibration every 8 hours.

RATIONALE

11. To confirm catheter position and to provide a baseline for future reference

2. The transducer converts the pressure wave into an electronic wave that is displayed on a screen.

   a. PCWP should be determined at end expiration because respiratory variation of the waveform occurs due to changes in intrathoracic pressures.
   b. A calibrated oscilloscope or graph paper is needed to read pressures at end expiration.

3. Segmental lung infarction may occur if the catheter balloon is left inflated for long periods. Pulmonary capillary wedge pressure is only measured intermittently. Do not allow catheter to remain in wedge position when patient is unattended or when not directly making the measurement.
4. Overinflation of the balloon may cause a "superwedge" waveform, and data obtained will be inaccurate. Overinflation of balloon may cause balloon to lose elastic properties and rupture. The strip provides documentation that catheter was not left in wedge position.

1. This calibrates the catheter to light intensity in the environment.
2. The in vivo calibration ensures that there is minimal difference, or "drift" between the actual SvO$_2$ value and the value displayed on the monitor. The light calibration adjusts for changes in light in the environment.

NURSING ALERT:
Also perform in vivo calibration if the optical module is disconnected at the catheter junction, if calibration data are lost, or if the SvO$_2$ is ±4% of the SvO$_2$ value calculated from mixed venous values obtained from the pulmonary artery catheter.

3. Monitor SvO$_2$ at frequent intervals. Values of 60%–80% are normal.

4. If the SvO$_2$ changes ± 10% from the prior value, confirm that the change reflects a change in patient condition.

5. If the catheter is not functioning properly, initiate steps to resolve the problem.

6. If no catheter malfunction is identified, report changes to the physician, initiate therapy based on standards of care.

3. Causes of an SvO$_2$ < 60% include:
   a. Decrease in cardiac output
   b. Decrease in SaO$_2$
   c. Decrease in hemoglobin
   d. Increase in O$_2$ consumption
   Causes of an SvO$_2$ > 80% include:
   a. Increase in SaO$_2$
   b. Decrease in O$_2$ consumption
4. The value displayed may not be accurate if fibrin or a clot is obstructing the catheter tip (low-intensity signal), if the catheter is touching the vessel wall or in a wedged position (high-intensity signal), or if the catheter is no longer calibrated accurately.
5. These steps may include aspiration to determine if a clot is obstructing the catheter or notifying the physician of the need to reposition the catheter.
6. Prompt intervention can restore normal tissue oxygen delivery before untoward effects occur.

(continued)

PROCEDURE GUIDELINES 10-2 ◆ Measuring Pulmonary Artery Pressure by Flow-Directed Balloon-Tipped Catheter (Swan-Ganz Catheter)

(continued)

PROCEDURE (cont'd)	NURSING ACTION	RATIONALE

FOLLOW-UP PHASE

	NURSING ACTION	RATIONALE
1.	Inspect the insertion site daily. Look for signs of infection, swelling, and bleeding.	1. A foreign body (catheter) in the vascular system increases the risk of sepsis.
2.	Record date and time of dressing change and IV tubing change.	
3.	Assess contour of waveform frequently and compare with previous documented waveforms.	3. Catheter may move forward and become lodged in wedge position or drift back into right ventricle. Turn patient to left side and ask him to cough (may dislodge catheter from wedge position). If not dislodged, notify physician.
4.	Assess for complications: pulmonary embolism, dysrhythmias, heart block, damage to tricuspid valve, intracardiac knotting of catheter, thrombophlebitis, infection, balloon rupture, rupture of pulmonary artery.	4. Blood coming back into syringe indicates balloon rupture. Notify physician immediately.
5.	When indicated, the catheter is removed without excessive force or traction; pressure dressing is applied over the site.	5. The site should be checked periodically for bleeding.

PROCEDURE GUIDELINES 10-3 ◆ Measurement of Cardiac Output (CO) by Thermodilution Method

EQUIPMENT		
Flow-directed thermodilution catheter in place		Normal saline or D5W solution bag
CO set, which includes IV tubing		Cardiac monitor with CO computation capability or stand-alone CO computer
10-mL syringe and three-way stopcock		Temperature sensor cable

PROCEDURE	NURSING ACTION	RATIONALE
1.	Explain procedure to patient.	
2.	Connect IV solution bag and CO set maintaining aseptic technique.	2. Solution will be injected directly into the heart and must be sterile.
3.	If you do not have a prepackaged CO set, attach IV solution bag to IV tubing, connect a three-way stopcock to the end of the tubing; connect a 10-mL syringe to the middle part of the three-way stopcock.	
4.	Attach the three-way stopcock to the proximal injectate port of the thermodilution catheter. This port should be reserved solely for determination of CO. No medications.	4. The proximal injectate port should have its distal end in the right atrium. If medications are infusing in this port, they will be flushed through in bolus form when CO measurements are taken.
5.	Another three-way stopcock may be used to allow for IV solution to run at a keep open rate.	5. Once the CO set is connected, the system should remain closed.
6.	Connect temperature sensor cable to the thermistor port of the thermodilution catheter.	6. When solution is injected through catheter, it mixes with the blood in the right side of the heart and flows to the pulmonary artery where blood temperature is detected by the thermistor.
7.	Set cardiac monitor to CO computation format. If using a stand-alone CO computer, enter the temperature of the injectable solution and the code number for the size of thermodilution catheter in use (code will be located on the thermodilution catheter packaging).	7. The injectate solution should be 15–20 degrees cooler than the patient's body temperature. Room temperature injectate is usually adequate.
8.	Fill 10-mL syringe with injectate solution by turning stopcock off to patient and open to syringe and solution.	

PROCEDURE (cont'd)	NURSING ACTION	RATIONALE
	9. Turn off IV keep open solution if present.	9. Need closed system from syringe to catheter.
	10. Turn stopcock off to injectate solution and open to patient and syringe.	
	11. Press 'inject' button on the CO computer or monitor and inject 10 mL rapidly (within 4 seconds) and smoothly into the proximal port.	11. Delay will interfere with results.
	12. Wait for computation to be complete. Repeat the procedure two or three times to obtain an average.	12. Some monitors display a waveform for the injectate dispersal to evaluate the adequacy of dispersal and temperature sensing.
	13. Turn stopcock off to the syringe and injectate and allow keep open IV fluid to infuse through the proximal port.	

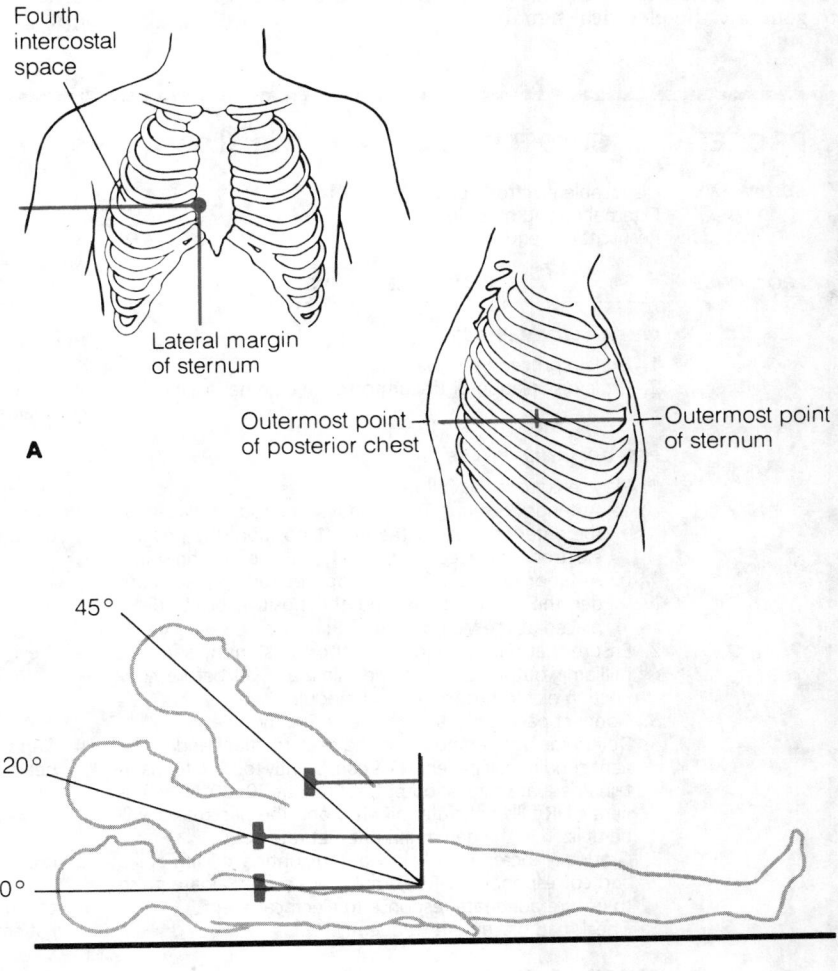

Fourth intercostal space

Lateral margin of sternum

A

Outermost point of posterior chest

Outermost point of sternum

45°

20°

0°

B

*The phlebostatic axis and the phlebostatic level. (**A**) The phlebostatic axis is the crossing of two reference lines: (1) a line from the fourth intercostal space at the point where it joins the sternum, drawn out to the side of the body beneath the axilla; (2) a line midpoint between the anterior and posterior surfaces of the chest. (**B**) The phlebostatic level is a horizontal line through the phlebostatic axis. The transducer or the zero mark on the manometer must be level with this axis for accurate measurements. As the patient moves from the flat to erect positions, the chest moves and therefore the reference level; the phlebostatic level stays horizontal through the same reference point. (After Shinn, J., et al: Heart Lung, 8[2], 324.)*

◆ CARDIAC PACING

A cardiac pacemaker is an electronic device that delivers direct stimulation to the heart. The purpose of the pacemaker is to initiate and maintain the heart rate when the heart's natural pacemaker is unable to do so. Pacing may be accomplished through a permanent implantable system; a temporary system with an external pulse generator and percutaneously threaded leads; or a transcutaneous external system with electrode pads placed over the chest. See Procedure Guidelines 10-4.

Pacemaker Design

A. Pulse Generator Contains the circuitry and batteries to generate the electrical signal

1. Pulse generators may be temporary (external) or permanently implanted (internal).
    a. Pulse generators are outside the body in temporary pacing systems and subcutaneously implanted in permanent systems.
    b. Temporary pacing systems are for short-term therapy; permanent pacing systems provide for long-term therapy.
    c. Temporary external (transcutaneous) pacemakers are used frequently during emergency situations requiring immediate cardiac pacing.
2. The pulse generator in a permanent pacing system is encapsulated in a metal can, which protects the generator from electromagnetic interferences.
3. A temporary pacing system generator is contained in a small box with dials for programming (Fig. 10-4). The external box is attached to the patient with Velcro straps.

PROCEDURE GUIDELINES 10-4 ◆ Transcutaneous Cardiac Pacing

EQUIPMENT Disposable electrode pads
External pacing module
Resuscitative equipment

PROCEDURE — NURSING ACTION	RATIONALE
PREPARATORY PHASE	
1. Explain procedure to patient	1. Allays anxiety
2. Explain sensation of discomfort with external pacing	2. Discomfort is felt with each firing, but can be relieved with analgesics.
PERFORMANCE PHASE	
1. Place electrodes as follows:	1. Electrodes must be placed so the current passes through as much of the myocardium as possible with the least distance between the pads.
a. Anterior/Posterior: The negative electrode is placed on the anterior chest at the V3-V1 position, the positive electrode is placed on the back to the left of the spine.	
b. Anterior/Anterior: the negative electrode is placed under the right clavicle and the positive electrode is placed at the V6 position.	
2. Ensure that pacing module is off or on standby and that milliamp output is set at the minimal level before connecting electrodes to external module.	2. Prevents accidental shock on connection
3. Connect pacing electrodes to external module.	
4. Determine rate setting according to instructions and/or patient condition. If patient HR is consistently too low to maintain adequate cardiac output, set rate at 70–80. If the patient's HR falls only intermittently and the pacemaker will be utilized in the demand mode, set rate at 60.	4. Can be set at a fixed rate or on demand, to pace only if heart rate falls below 60 (or other rate).
5. Gradually increase milliamp output until a pacing spike and corresponding QRS complex are seen. Palpate pulse to ensure adequate response to electrical event.	5. If using the demand mode, set the rate higher than the patient's rate to establish the correct output and capture, then return the rate to 60.
6. Check pad placement frequently.	6. Patient perspiration may cause pads to loosen or slip.
FOLLOW-UP PHASE	
1. Check vital signs at least every 15 min. while continuous pacing is employed	1. To determine if cardiac output is adequate
2. Monitor ECG continuously for pacer functioning	2. To detect malfunction (may occur due to electrode loosening)
3. Assure patient that treatment is temporary.	3. Should only be used continuously for 2 hours
4. Prepare patient for transvenous or permanent pacemaker insertion as indicated	

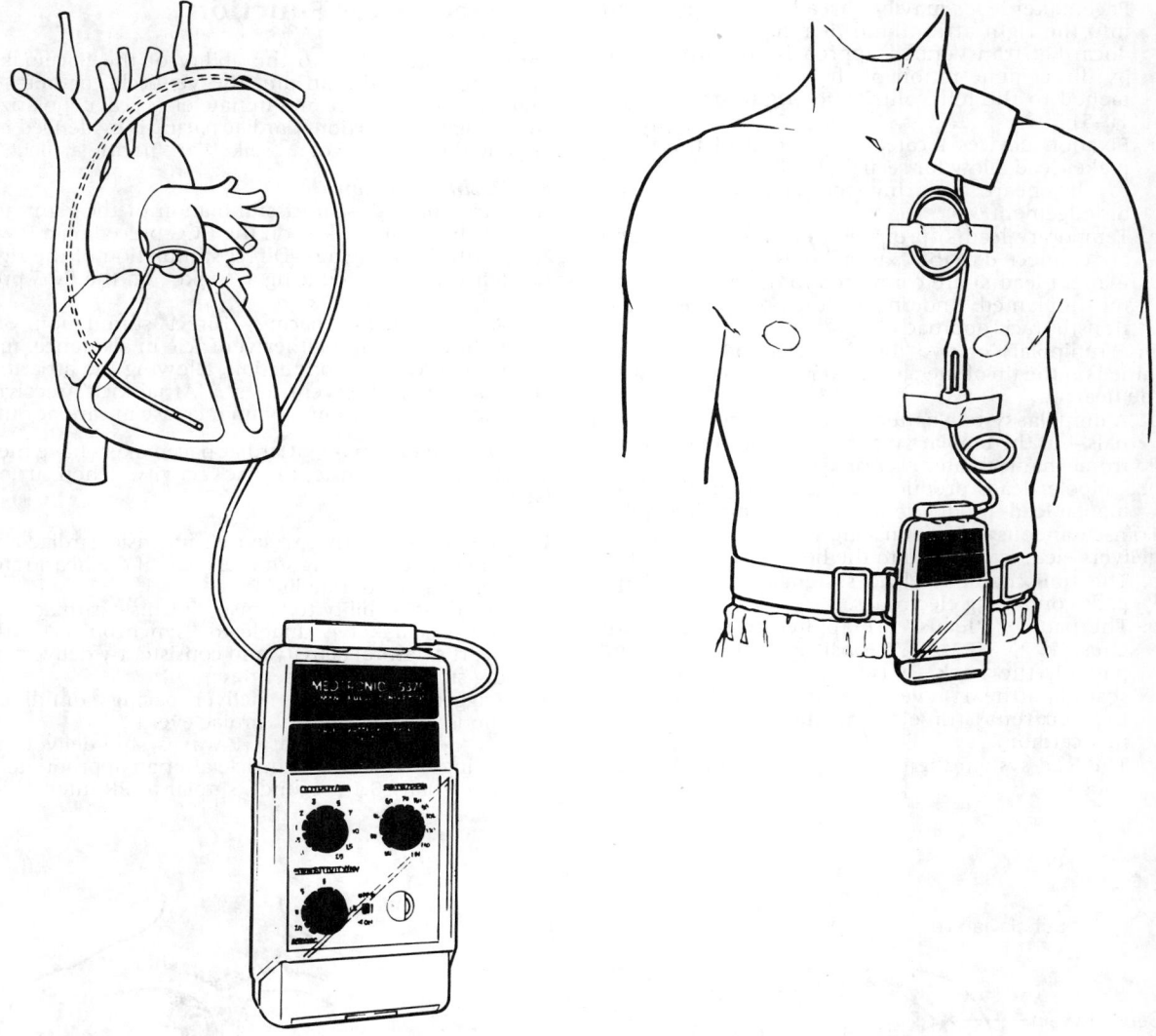

FIGURE 10-4 *Temporary transvenous pacer wire with external pulse generator. (Courtesy of MEDTRONIC, Inc.)*

a. Transcutaneous external pacing systems house the generator in a piece of equipment similar to an ECG portable monitor. Dials for programming the unit and ECG monitoring are contained in the device.

b. Electromechanical interference is more likely to occur with temporary systems.

c. Temporary pacing systems use batteries, which need replacement based on use of device. The transcutaneous system has rechargeable battery circuitry.

4. Permanent pacing systems use reliable power sources such as lithium or nuclear batteries. Lithium batteries have a projected life span of 8 to 12 years, whereas nuclear power sources, although used infrequently, offer a 20-year projected life span.

B. Pacemaker Lead Transmits the electrical signal from the pulse generator to the heart

1. One or two leads may be placed in the heart.
   a. A "single-chamber" pacemaker has one lead in either the atrial or ventricular chamber. The sensing and pacing capabilities of the pacemaker are confined to the chamber where the lead is placed.
   b. "Dual-chamber" pacemakers have two leads. One lead is in the atrium and the other lead is located in the ventricle. Pacing and sensing can occur in both heart chambers, closely "mimicking" normal heart function (physiologic pacing).

c. Pacemaker leads may be threaded through a vein into the right atrium and/or right ventricle (endocardial/transvenous approach) or introduced by direct penetration of the chest wall and attached to the left ventricle or right atrium (Fig. 10-5).

d. Fixation devices located at the end of the pacemaker lead allow for secure attachment of the lead to the heart, reducing the possibility of lead dislodgement.

e. Temporary lead(s) protrude from the incision and are connected to the external pulse generator. Permanent lead(s) are connected to the pulse generator implanted underneath the skin (epicardial/transthoracic approach).

2. One (unipolar) or two (bipolar) electrodes are contained on the tip of the pacemaker lead in contact with the heart.

a. A unipolar system better senses intrinsic cardiac signals, but the bipolar system is less affected by electromechanical interference.

b. Unipolar leads produce a large spike on the ECG; bipolar leads produce a small, almost invisible spike.

3. Transcutaneous external pacing system noninvasively delivers electrical stimuli to the heart.

a. The transcutaneous lead system consists of large pads containing electrodes.

b. The pads or "leads" are applied to the anterior chest (V2, V3, or V5 position) and a second pad on the back (between the spine and left scapula at heart level). Leads must be placed so the current travels through most of the myocardium.

c. The lead system then is connected to the external console.

Pacemaker Function

Cardiac pacing refers to the ability of the pacemaker to stimulate either the atrium, the ventricle, or both heart chambers in sequence and initiate electrical depolarization and cardiac contraction. Cardiac pacing is evidenced on the ECG by the presence of a "spike" or "pacing artifact."

A. Pacing Functions
1. Atrial pacing—Direct stimulation of the right atrium producing a "spike" on the ECG preceding a P wave
2. Ventricular pacing—Direct stimulation of the right or left ventricle producing a "spike" on the ECG preceding a QRS complex
3. Atrioventricular pacing—Direct stimulation of the right atrium and either ventricle in sequence; mimics normal cardiac conduction, allowing the atria to contract before the ventricles. ("Atrial kick" received by the ventricles allows for an increase in cardiac output.)

B. Sensing Functions   Cardiac pacemakers have the ability to "see" intrinsic cardiac activity when it occurs (sensing).

1. Demand—Ability to "sense" intrinsic cardiac activity and deliver a pacing stimulus only if the heart rate falls below a preset rate limit.
2. Fixed—No ability to "sense" intrinsic cardiac activity; the pacemaker is unable to "synchronize" with the heart's natural activity and consistently delivers a pacing stimulus at a preset rate.
3. Triggered—Ability to deliver pacing stimuli in response to "sensing" a cardiac event.
   a. "Sees" atrial activity (P waves) and delivers a pacing spike to the ventricle after an appropriate delay (usually 0.16 seconds, similar to PR interval)

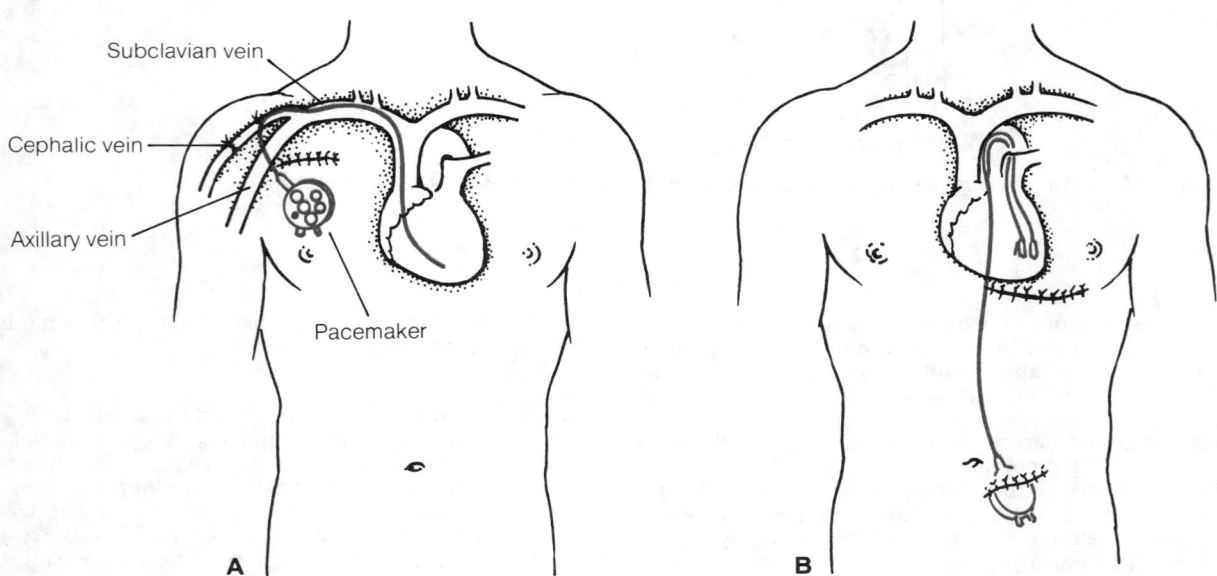

FIGURE 10-5   **(A)** The catheter is unipolar and is threaded to the apical area of the right ventricle via a major vein. **(B)** The catheter is bipolar and is passed through an opening in the chest wall and is sutured to the external surface of the left ventricle.

b. Maintains atrioventricular synchrony and increases heart rate based on increases in the body demands that occur with exercise or during stress.
c. "Physiologic" sensors are currently being developed as alternatives to "trigger" a ventricular response, as many patients have atrial dysfunction.
d. "Sensor-driven" rate-responsive pacemakers do not sense atrial activity; a triggered ventricular beat occurs when the pacemaker senses either increases in muscle activity, temperature, oxygen utilization, or changes in blood pH.

C. *Capture Function*
1. The pacemaker's ability to generate a response from the heart (contraction) after electrical stimulation is referred to as capture.
   a. "Electrical" capture is indicated by a P wave or QRS corresponding to a pacemaker spike.
   b. "Mechanical" capture of the ventricles is determined by a palpable pulse corresponding to the electrical event.

Pacemaker Codes

The Intersociety Commission for Heart Disease (ICHD) has established a five-letter code (1984) to describe the normal functioning of today's sophisticated pacemakers.

1. Letters 1, 2, 3
   a. The first letter of the code refers to the chamber paced.
   b. The second letter refers to the chamber sensed.
   c. The third letter refers to the response to sensing.
2. Letters 4 and 5
   a. The fourth and fifth letters refer to special functions of today's pacemakers.
   b. The fourth letter refers to the programmability of the pacemaker.
   c. The fifth letter refers to the various modes of operation for antitachycardic pacemakers. These pacemakers are used to control tachydysrhythmias in patients who have failed conventional drug therapy.

Clinical Indications

1. Symptomatic bradydysrhythmias
2. Symptomatic heart block
   a. Mobitz II second-degree heart block
   b. Complete heart block
   c. Bifascicular and trifascicular bundle branch blocks
3. Prophylaxis
   a. After acute MI: dysrhythmia and conduction defects
   b. Before or after cardiac surgery
   c. During diagnostic testing:
      (1) Cardiac catheterization
      (2) Electrophysiology studies
      (3) Percutaneous coronary angioplasty (PTCA)
      (4) Stress testing
      (5) Before permanent pacing
4. Tachydysrhythmias; to break rapid rhythm disturbances
   a. Supraventricular
   b. Ventricular

Nursing Assessment

Assess patient's knowledge level of procedure: nothing by mouth (NPO) before procedure; IV line insertion; performed in operating or special procedures room with fluoroscope and continuous ECG monitoring; local anesthetic to minimize discomfort; sedation.

Nursing Diagnoses

A. Decreased Cardiac Output related to potential pacemaker malfunction and dysrhythmias
B. Risk for Injury related to pneumothorax, hemothorax, bleeding, microshock, and accidental malfunction
C. Risk for Infection related to surgical implantation of pacemaker generator and/or leads
D. Anxiety related to pacemaker insertion, fear of death, lack of knowledge, and role change
E. Impaired Physical Mobility related to imposed restrictions of arm movement and bedrest
F. Pain related to surgical incision and transcutaneous external pacing stimuli
G. Disturbance in Body Image, related to pacemaker implantation

Nursing Interventions

A. *Maintaining Cardiac Output*
1. Record the following information after insertion of the pacemaker:
   a. Pacemaker manufacturer, model, and lead type
   b. Operating mode (based on ICHD code)
   c. Programmed settings: lower rate limit; upper rate limit; AV delay; pacing thresholds
   d. Patient's underlying rhythm
   e. Patient's response to procedure
2. Attach ECG electrodes for continuous monitoring of heart rate and rhythm.
   a. Set alarm limits five beats below lower rate limit and five to ten beats above upper rate limits (ensures immediate detection of pacemaker malfunction or failure).
   b. Keep alarms on at all times.
   c. Analyze ECG strip every 4 hours.
      (1) Identify presence/absence of pacing artifact.
      (2) Differentiate paced P waves and paced QRS complexes from spontaneous beats.
      (3) Measure AV delay (if pacemaker has dual chamber functions).
      (4) Determine the paced rate.
      (5) Analyze the paced rhythm for presence and consistency of capture (every pacing spike is followed by atrial and/or ventricular depolarization).
      (6) Analyze the rhythm for presence and consistency of proper sensing. (After a spontaneous beat, the pacemaker should not fire unless the interval between the spontaneous beat and the paced beat equals the lower pacing rate and/or the paced beat follows the programmed AV delay).
3. Monitor vital signs every 15 minutes until stable; then as directed.

4. Monitor urine output and level of consciousness—ensures adequate cardiac output achieved with paced rhythm.
5. Observe for the presence of dysrhythmias (ventricular ectopic activity can occur because of irritation of ventricular wall by lead wire).
   a. Monitor for competitive rhythms such as runs of atrial fibrillation or flutter, accelerated junctional or idioventricular or ventricular tachycardia.
   b. Report all dysrhythmias.
   c. Administer antidysrhythmic therapy as directed.
6. Obtain 12-lead ECG daily as directed.

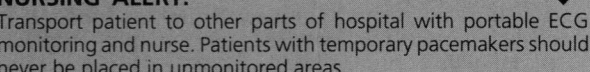

NURSING ALERT:
Transport patient to other parts of hospital with portable ECG monitoring and nurse. Patients with temporary pacemakers should never be placed in unmonitored areas.

B. Avoiding Injury
1. Note that a postinsertion chest x-ray has been taken to ensure correct lead wire position and that no fluid is in lungs.
2. Monitor for signs/symptoms of hemothorax or pneumothorax:
   a. Hemothorax—Inadvertent puncture of the subclavian vein or artery; can cause fatal hemorrhage; observe for diaphoresis, hypotension, and restlessness; immediate surgical intervention may be necessary.
   b. Pneumothorax—Inadvertent puncture of the lung; observe for acute onset of dyspnea, cyanosis, chest pain, absent breath sounds over involved lung, acute anxiety, hypotension. Prepare for chest tube insertion.
3. Evaluate continually for evidence of bleeding.
   a. Check incision site frequently for bleeding.
      (1) Apply manual pressure and pressure dressing to control bleeding.
      (2) Palpate for pulses distal to insertion site. (Swelling of tissues from bleeding may impede arterial flow.)
4. Monitor for evidence of lead migration and perforation of heart.
   a. Observe for muscle twitching and/or hiccups (may indicate chest wall or diaphragmatic pacing).
   b. Evaluate patient's complaints of chest pain (may indicate perforation of pericardial sac).
   c. Auscultate for pericardial friction rub.
   d. Observe for signs/symptoms of cardiac tamponade; distant heart sounds, distended neck veins, pulsus paradoxus.
5. Provide an electrically safe environment for patient. Stray electrical current can enter the heart through temporary pacemaker lead system and induce dysrhythmias.
   a. Protect exposed parts of electrode lead terminal in temporary pacing systems with a rubber glove. (Newer external generators have the lead terminals enclosed in a case; a rubber glove is not necessary.)
   b. Wear rubber gloves whenever touching temporary pacing leads. (Static electricity from your hands can enter the patient's body through the lead system.)
   c. Make sure all equipment is grounded with three-prong plugs inserted into a proper outlet; biomedical engineer should routinely check room to ensure safe environment.

d. Temporary epicardial pacing wires (most common after cardiac surgery) should have the terminal needles protected by a plastic tube; place tube in rubber glove to protect it from fluids or electrical current.
6. Be aware of hazards in the hospital environment that can interfere with pacemaker function or cause pacemaker failure and/or permanent pacemaker damage.
   a. Avoid use of electric razors.
   b. Avoid direct placement of defibrillator paddles over pacemaker generator; anterior placement of paddles should be 4 to 5 inches away from pacemaker; always evaluate pacemaker function after defibrillation.
   c. Electrocautery devices and transcutaneous nerve stimulators (TENS units) pose a risk.
   d. Patients with permanent pacemakers should never be exposed to magnetic resonance imaging (MRI) because the strength of the magnetic field may alter or erase pacemaker program memory.
   e. Caution must be used if patient is to receive radiation therapy; the pacemaker should be repositioned if unit lies directly in the radiation field.
7. Prevent possible accidental pacemaker malfunctions.
   a. Use clear plastic covering over external temporary generators at all times (eliminates potential manipulation of programmed settings).
   b. Secure temporary pacemaker generator to patient's chest or waist; never hang on IV pole.
   c. Transfer of patient from bed to stretcher should only be attempted with an adequate number of personnel, so that patient can remain passive; caution personnel to avoid underarm lifts.
   d. Place a sign over patient's bed alerting personnel to presence of temporary pacemaker.
   e. Evaluate transcutaneous pacing electrodes every 2 hours for secure contact to chest wall; change electrode pads as directed or if patient is diaphoretic.
      Note: Transcutaneous pacing should not be employed continuously for longer than 2 hours.
8. Monitor for electrolyte imbalances, hypoxia, and myocardial ischemia. (The amount of energy the pacemaker needs to stimulate depolarization may need adjustment if any of these are present.)

C. Preventing Infection
1. Take temperature every 4 hours; report elevations. (Suspect pacemaker system for infection source if elevation occurs.)
2. Observe incision site for signs/symptoms of local infection: redness, purulent drainage, warmth, soreness.
3. Be alert to manifestations of bacteremia. (Patients with endocardial leads are susceptible to endocarditis; see p. 301.)
4. Clean incision site as directed, using sterile technique.
5. Monitor vein through which the pacing lead wire was placed for evidence of phlebitis.
6. Evaluate patient's complaints of increasing tenderness and discomfort at incision site.
7. Administer antibiotic therapy as prescribed.

D. Relieving Anxiety
1. Offer careful explanations regarding anticipated procedures and treatments and answer the patient's questions with concise explanations.
2. Encourage the patient to use coping mechanisms to overcome anxieties—talking, crying, walking.
3. Encourage the patient to accept responsibility for care.
   a. Review plan of care with the patient.

b. Encourage the patient to make decisions regarding a daily schedule of self-care activities.

c. Engage the patient in goal setting. Establish with the patient priorities of care and time frames to accomplish goals up until discharge.

4. Monitor for unwarranted fears expressed by the patient (commonly, pacemaker failure) and provide explanations to alleviate fear. Explain to the patient life expectancy of batteries and the measures taken to check for failure (see Patient Education, below).

E. Minimizing the Effects of Immobility

1. Explain the purpose for bedrest (24 to 48 hours) and immobilization of extremity nearest to permanent or temporary pacemaker lead implant (allows for stabilization of lead in heart and prevents lead dislodgement).

2. Encourage patient to take deep breaths frequently each hour—promotes pulmonary function; caution against vigorous coughing (lead dislodgement may occur).

3. Instruct patient in dorsiflexion exercises of ankles and tightening of calf muscles. This promotes venous return and prevents venous stasis. Exercises should be done hourly.

4. Restrict movement of affected extremity.
   a. Place arm nearest to permanent pacemaker implant in sling as directed; extremity with temporary pacing wire should be immobilized and kept straight as prescribed.
   b. Instruct patient to gradually resume range of motion of extremity as directed (usually 24 hours for permanent implants); avoid over-the-head motions for approximately 5 days.
   c. Evaluate patient's arm movements to ensure normal range-of-motion progression; assist patient with passive range of motion of extremity as necessary (prevents development of shoulder stiffness caused by prolonged joint immobility); consult physical therapy as directed if stiffness and pain occur.

5. Assist patients with activities of daily living (ADLs) as appropriate.

F. Relieving Pain

1. Prepare patient for discomfort that may be experienced after pacemaker implant or initiation of transcutaneous pacing.
   a. Explain to patient that incisional pain will occur postprocedure; pain will subside after the first week, but some soreness will be experienced for up to 3 to 4 weeks.
   b. Explain to patient the potential for discomfort during transcutaneous pacing; ensure patient that the lowest energy possible will be used and analgesics will be given.

2. Administer analgesics as directed; attempt to coincide peak analgesic effect with performance of range-of-motion exercises and ADLs.

3. Offer back rubs to promote relaxation.

4. Provide patient with diversional activities.

5. Evaluate effectiveness of pain-relieving modalities.

G. Maintaining a Positive Body Image

1. Encourage the patient to express concerns regarding self-image and pacer implant.

2. Reassure the patient that sexual activity and modes of dressing will not be altered by pacemaker implantation.

3. Offer the patient the opportunity to talk to others who have had a pacemaker implantation.

4. Encourage spouse of patient or significant other to discuss concerns of self-image with the patient.

Patient Education/ Health Maintenance

A. Anatomy and Physiology of the Heart
Use diagrams to identify heart structure, conduction system, area where pacemaker is inserted, and why the pacemaker is needed.

B. Pacemaker Function

1. Give the patient the manufacturer's instructions (for particular pacemaker) and help familiarize patient with pacemaker.

2. If available, give the patient a pacemaker to hold and identify unique features of patient's pacemaker; or show patient picture of pacemaker.

3. Explain to patient the purpose and function of the component parts of the pacemaker: generator and lead system.

C. Activity

1. Reassure patient that normal activities will be able to be resumed.

2. Explain to patient that it takes about 2 months to develop full range of motion of arm (fibrosis occurs around the lead and stabilizes it in heart).

3. Specific instructions include:
   a. Instruct patient not to lift items over 3 lb or perform difficult arm maneuvers.
   b. Caution patient against excessive stretching or bending exercises.
   c. Avoid contact sports, tennis, golfing, bowling, and yardwork until resumption of these activities is permitted by physician.
   d. Caution patient not to fire rifle with it resting over pacemaker implant.
   e. Sexual activity may be resumed when desired.

4. Instruct patient to gauge activities according to sensations of moderate pain in arm or site of implant and stretching sensation in and around implant site.

D. Pacemaker Failure

1. Teach the patient to check own pulse rate at least every week for 1 full minute at rest to be certain that preset rate remains constant. (Patients may check pulse daily to ensure all is well and promote a sense of control.)

2. Teach the patient to:
   a. Report immediately any slowing of pulse greater than four to five beats per minute, or any increase in pulse rate.
   b. Report signs and symptom of dizziness, fainting, palpitation, prolonged hiccups, and chest pain to health care provider immediately. These signs are indicative of pacemaker failure.
   c. Take pulse while these feelings are being experienced.

3. Encourage the patient to wear identification bracelet and carry pacemaker identification card that lists pacemaker type, rate, healthcare provider's name, and the hospital where the pacemaker was inserted; encourage significant other to keep a card with patient's pacemaker information so someone else will have it.

E. Electromagnetic Interference
Advise the patient that improvements in pacemaker design have reduced problems of electromagnetic interference (EMI).

1. High-energy radar, television and radio transmitters, industrial arc welders, electrocautery equipment, transcutaneous nerve stimulators (TENS), large motors (cars, boats), oversized magnets (MRI equipment found at hospitals, junkyards where magnets lift cars), ultrasonic dental cleaning equipment, electric razors.
   a. Avoid direct contact and close proximity with these devices because they may affect the functioning of the pacemaker. (In many cases, no damage to the generator will occur; devices may confuse the pacemaker and readjust the settings.)
   b. Teach the patient that if dizziness or sensations of a fast heart rate occur to move 4 to 6 feet away from source and check pulse. Pulse should return to normal.
2. Antitheft devices and airport security alarms will not affect pacemaker function, although the metal may trigger the alarm. Instruct patient to show ID card.
3. Household and kitchen appliances will not affect pacemaker function. Microwave ovens are no longer a threat to pacemaker operation (old warning signs may still be near microwave ovens).

F. Care of Pacemaker Site
1. Advise patient to wear loose-fitting clothing around the area of pacemaker implantation until healing has taken place.
2. Watch for signs and symptoms of infection around generator and leads—fever, heat, pain, skin breakdown at implant site.
3. Advise patient to keep incision clean and dry. Encourage tub baths for the first 10 days after pacemaker implant rather than showers.
   a. Instruct patient not to scrub incision site or clean site with bath water.
   b. Teach patient to clean incision site with antiseptic as directed.
4. Explain to patient that healing will take approximately 3 months.
   a. Instruct patient to maintain a well-balanced diet to promote healing.

GERONTOLOGIC ALERT:
Elderly patients may experience delayed wound healing because of poor nutritional status. Evaluate nutritional intake carefully and offer a balanced diet to ensure proper healing.

5. Instruct patient to inform dentist of pacemaker so antibiotic prophylaxis can be administered before extractions or vigorous dental cleaning (prevents development of endocarditis).

G. Follow-up
1. See that the patient has a copy of ECG tracing (according to agency policy) for future comparisons. Encourage patient to have regular pacemaker checkup for monitoring function and integrity of pacemaker.

2. Transtelephonic evaluation of implanted cardiac pacemakers for battery and electrode failure is available.
3. Review medications with the patient before discharge.
4. Inform the patient that the pulse generator will have to be surgically removed for a variety of reasons (battery depletion) and replaced; improved power sources and circuitry make reoperation less frequent.
   a. Relatively simple procedure performed under local anesthesia.

Evaluation

A. Vital signs stable; pacing spikes rated on ECG tracing
B. Breath sounds noted throughout; respirations unlabored
C. Incision without drainage
D. Asking questions and participating in care
E. Exercising in bed; arm remains immobilized
F. Reports relief of pain
G. Verbalizes acceptance of pacemaker

◆ DEFIBRILLATION AND CARDIOVERSION

Defibrillation (or counter shock) is the passing of an electrical shock of short duration through the heart to terminate ventricular fibrillation or ventricular tachycardia without pulse. A defibrillator is an instrument that delivers an electric shock to the heart to convert ventricular fibrillation to normal sinus rhythm. (Defibrillators are not used to convert other abnormal and rapid cardiac rhythms.) See Procedure Guidelines 10-5.

Cardioversion is the use of defibrillation in a synchronized mode (termed synchronized cardioversion), or the timed electrical shock to the heart for the purpose of terminating certain dysrhythmias. It is timed not to hit the T wave during the cardiac cycle, because an electrical discharge during this phase may cause ventricular fibrillation. See Procedure Guidelines 10-6.

Indications

A. Defibrillation
1. Ventricular fibrillation
2. Ventricular tachycardia without a pulse

B. Synchronized Cardioversion
1. Atrial fibrillation
2. Atrial flutter
3. Supraventricular tachycardia

NURSING ALERT: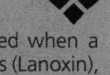
Synchronized cardioversion is generally contraindicated when a patient has been taking a significant amount of digitalis (Lanoxin), because more lethal dysrhythmias may ensue after electrical discharge.

PROCEDURE GUIDELINES 10-5 ◆ Direct Current Defibrillation for Ventricular Fibrillation

EQUIPMENT   DC defibrillator with paddles
Interface material (disposable conductive gel pads, electrode gels and pastes)
Resuscitative equipment

PROCEDURE

NURSING ACTION	RATIONALE
PERFORMANCE PHASE	
1. *Monitored patient*—if ventricular fibrillation recognized within 2 minutes, give precordial thump, assess rhythm and carotid pulse, and expose anterior chest. *Unmonitored patient*—expose anterior chest.	
2. *Unmonitored patient*—START CARDIOPULMONARY RESUSCITATION IMMEDIATELY. *Monitored patient*—if within 2 minutes of detection of ventricular fibrillation, defibrillate before initiating cardiopulmonary resuscitation. Beyond 2 minutes, START RESUSCITATION EFFORTS IMMEDIATELY.	2. This procedure should be carried out immediately after ventricular fibrillation is detected to minimize cerebral and circulatory deterioration. Cardiopulmonary resuscitation is essential before and after defibrillation to ensure blood supply to the cerebral and coronary arteries.
3. Apply interface material to the patient (gel pads) or to the paddles (gel, paste). The electrode paddles should be in firm contact with the patient's skin.	3. The interface material helps provide better conduction and prevents skin burns. Do not allow any paste on the skin between the electrodes. If the paste areas touch, the current may short circuit (severely burning the patient) and may not penetrate the heart. Saline pads are not recommended because the saline can easily drip, forming a path for the current.
4. Remove oxygen from immediate area.	4. Prevents danger of fire or explosion.
5. A second person should turn on the defibrillator to the prescribed setting. The American Heart Association recommends that initial defibrillation should be 200–300 watt-seconds of *delivered* energy. A second attempt at same level should be given if first attempt unsuccessful. A third attempt with an increase of energy level to 360 watt-seconds should be attempted. Allow only approx. 5 sec. between the successive attempts to assess rhythm and pulse.	5. The shock is measured in joules or watt-seconds (the dose is 2 joules/kg in pediatric patients based on estimated body weight). The ideal energy dose for defibrillation remains controversial.
6. Apply one electrode just to the right of the upper sternum below the clavicle and the other electrode just to the left of the cardiac apex or left nipple (see figure). About 20–25 lb of pressure is applied to paddles to ensure good contact with the patient's skin.	6. The paddles are placed so that the electrical discharge flows through as much myocardial mass as possible. If anteroposterior paddles are used, the anterior paddle is held with pressure on the middle sternum while the patient lies on the posterior paddle under the left infrascapular region. In this method the countershock more directly traverses the heart.
7. Grasp the paddles only by the insulated handles.	
8. Charge the paddles. Once paddles are charged, GIVE THE COMMAND FOR PERSONNEL TO STAND CLEAR OF THE PATIENT AND THE BED. Look quickly to make sure all are away from the patient and bed.	8. If a person touches the bed, he or she may act as a ground for the current and receive a shock, especially if there are electrolyte solutions on the floor.
9. Push the discharge buttons in both paddles simultaneously.	
10. Remove the paddles from the patient *immediately* after the shock is administered (unless monitoring leads are in the paddles).	
11. Resume cardiopulmonary resuscitation efforts until stable rhythm, spontaneous respirations, pulse, and blood pressure return.	11. After the third attempt to countershock, CPR efforts should be resumed; total delay should be no more than 5 seconds to oxygenate the patient and restore circulation.
12. Look at the ECG monitor to determine the specific therapy for the resultant electrical mechanism. Further high-energy countershocks may be necessary.	

(continued)

PROCEDURE GUIDELINES 10-5 ◆ Direct Current Defibrillation for Ventricular Fibrillation *(continued)*

PROCEDURE (cont'd)	NURSING ACTION	RATIONALE

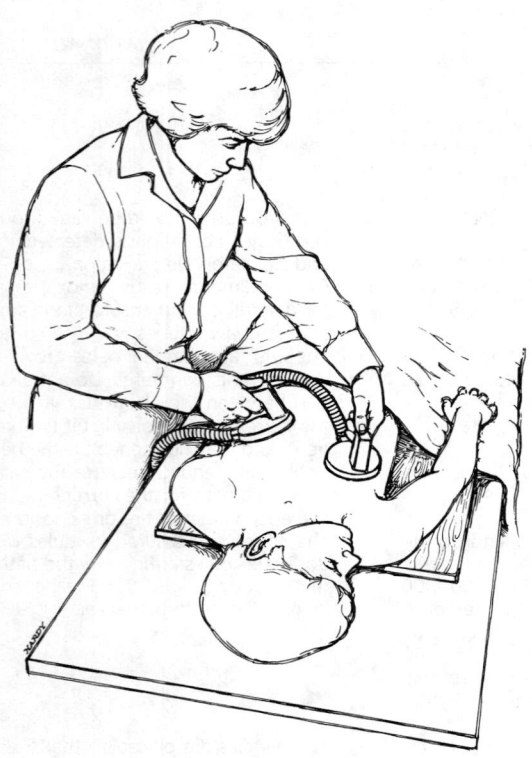

Paddle placement in ventricular defibrillation.

FOLLOW-UP PHASE

1. After the patient is defibrillated and rhythm is restored, lidocaine is usually given to prevent recurrent episodes.
2. Continue with intensive monitoring/care.

1. Any resultant dysrhythmia may require appropriate drug intervention.

PROCEDURE GUIDELINES 10-6 ◆ Synchronized Cardioversion

EQUIPMENT   Cardioverter and ECG machine
Conduction jelly or gel pads and cardiac medications
Resuscitative equipment

PROCEDURE	NURSING ACTION	RATIONALE

NURSING ACTION

1. If the procedure is elective, it is advisable to have the patient "NPO" 12 hours before the cardioversion.
   a. Reassure the patient and see that informed consent has been obtained.
   b. Make sure the patient has not been taking digitalis and that the serum potassium is normal.
2. Make sure IV line is secure.

3. Obtain a 12-lead ECG before and after cardioversion with the ECG machine. The ECG machine wires are best left on the patient, because the ECG printout is of much better quality than that of the monitor. This fact is especially important when one is trying to dissect complicated dysrhythmias.
4. a. Allow the patient to receive oxygen before and after cardioversion.
   b. Do *not* give oxygen during the procedure.

5. Place the paddles in one of the following two positions:
   a. *Anterior-posterior position*
   One paddle—left infrascapular area
   Other paddle—upper sternum at 3rd interspace
   b. *Anterior position*
   One paddle—just to right of sternum at 2nd interspace
   Other paddle—just under left nipple
6. Determine if the machine's synchronization mechanism is working before applying the paddles.
   a. The discharge should hit near the peak of the R wave.

   b. The R wave usually must be of substantial height; if it is not, adjust the gain (sensitivity) or change the lead. On many machines, the R wave must be upright before there is synchronization.
7. If using paste, apply to all of the paddle surface, but make sure there is no excess around the edges of the paddles.

   a. The paste should be rubbed into the skin very thoroughly; this allows more electricity to penetrate the body surface.
   b. Make sure paddles are clean because surface material will interfere with the flow of electricity.
   c. Apply firm pressure to the paddle.
8. If using gel pads, place pads where paddles are to be positioned.
9. Set dial for lowest level of electrical energy that can be expected to convert the dysrhythmia. Some dysrhythmias (such as atrial flutter) can be converted with very low energies, such as 25 watt-seconds (joules).
10. A short acting sedative such as midazolan (Versed) should be given if the patient is conscious.
11. After the patient is in a light sleep from the IV medication and when no one is touching the bed or patient, discharge the cardioverter. If cardioversion does not occur, proceed to a higher energy level.
12. Monitor the ECG after conversion occurs. Blood pressures should be recorded about every 15 minutes until the preshock blood pressure is reached.

RATIONALE

1. During sedation or the procedure, the patient may vomit and aspirate if the stomach is full.
   a. Do not use word "shock" because this will increase the patient's apprehension.
   b. Low potassium may precipitate postshock dysrhythmias.
2. An IV line may be necessary for administration of emergency medications.
3. An ECG is taken to ensure that the patient has not had a recent myocardial infarction (either just before or after the cardioversion).

4. a. Oxygen will help prevent unwanted dysrhythmias after cardioversion.
   b. An explosion could occur if a spark from the paddles should ignite the oxygen during the procedure.

6.
   a. If the electrical discharge hits the T wave, ventricular fibrillation may occur.
   b. Synchronization is not used for ventricular fibrillation. (The machine will not work for defibrillation if the synchronization mode is on.)

7. If there is excess paste around the paddles, the discharge may run onto the skin, causing a burn. If there is not firm contact between the paddle and skin, a burn may occur; also, electricity is lost from the heart.

8. Excessive energies may cause unnecessary discomfort to the patient.
9. This helps produce amnesia concerning the cardioversion.

11. The patient may revert to previous dysrhythmias after conversion.

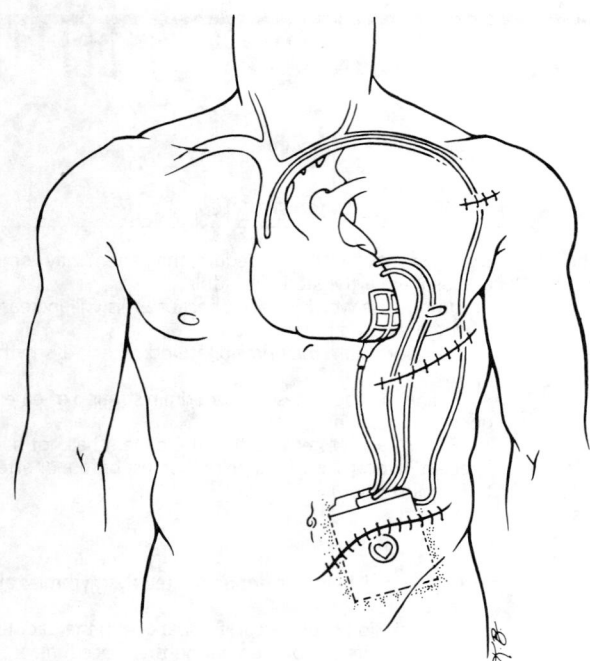

FIGURE 10-6 *Automatic implantable defibrillator.*

◆ AUTOMATIC IMPLANTABLE DEFIBRILLATOR

The automatic implantable defibrillator is a device that delivers electrical shocks directly to the heart muscle (defibrillation) in order to terminate lethal dysrhythmias: ventricular fibrillation and ventricular tachycardia (Fig. 10-6). The automatic implantable defibrillator is surgically placed by one of four approaches: lateral thoracotomy, median sternotomy (in conjunction with cardiac surgery), subxiphoid, or subintercostal.

Design

The implantable defibrillator is slightly larger than a pacemaker and consists of two component parts:
1. Pulse generator—Contains the circuitry and battery to detect dysrhythmias and generate the electrical shock. The generator is placed in a subcutaneous pocket in the upper abdominal quadrant.
   a. Battery life depends on usage. Longevity is estimated at 12 to 24 months or 100 shocks.
   b. The direct current electrical shock delivered is 25 to 32 joules.
2. Lead system—Two sets of leads are used and can be placed in various positions on or in the heart.
   a. One set of lead electrodes senses lethal dysrhythmias in the heart.
   b. The other set of lead electrodes transmits the electrical shock from the pulse generator to the heart.
3. The implantable defibrillator is noninvasively turned on and off by a doughnut-shaped magnet.

Function

Four electrical shocks are delivered in a programmed sequence:

1. The device allows 10 to 35 seconds to detect a lethal dysrhythmia, charge, and "defibrillate" the heart. The lethal dysrhythmia must meet two programmed criteria (rate and amount of time spent from the isoelectric line) to trigger the device to emit an initial electrical shock. The amount of joules necessary to convert each patient is determined during insertion and testing of the device, usually 15 to 25 joules.
2. Nontermination of the lethal dysrhythmia by the initial shock triggers the device to continue the sequence (detect, charge, and defibrillate) until a total of four or five shocks have been delivered (number of shocks depends on device model implanted).
   a. Subsequent shocks are slightly higher, at 30 to 32 joules.
   b. The total sequence lasts approximately 2 minutes.
3. Nontermination of the lethal dysrhythmia after the shock sequence signals the device to revert to the "detection" mode of operation and not to reinitiate the shocking sequence. The device will reinitiate the shocking sequence only if a rhythm other than the lethal dysrhythmia is detected and maintained for at least 35 seconds. If this criterion is met and another lethal dysrhythmia is detected, the device will cycle through the shocking sequence again.
4. Termination of a lethal dysrhythmia at any time during the shocking sequence signals the device to interrupt the sequence, return to a detection mode and reinitiate the shocking sequence if another lethal dysrhythmia is detected.

Indications

1. Failure of maximal conventional medical therapy to control ventricular fibrillation and/or ventricular tachycardia (as determined by electrophysiology studies).
2. Survival of one episode of sudden cardiac death not associated with acute MI.

Complications

1. Infection
2. Bleeding
3. Device failure
4. Pacemaker interaction
5. Constrictive pericarditis

Nursing Diagnoses

A. Anxiety related to invasive procedure and fear of death
B. Risk for Infection related to invasive procedure and implanted device
C. Decreased Cardiac Output related to surgical procedure and/or dysrhythmias
D. Ineffective Breathing Pattern related to surgical procedure and discomfort

Nursing Interventions

A. Reducing Anxiety

1. Explain to patient and family reason for implant, surgical procedure, and pre- and postprocedure management:
   a. Performed in the operating room; anesthesia required
   b. Incision location
   c. Endotracheal intubation; chest tubes
   d. Intravenous (IV) line; continuous ECG monitoring
   e. Early mobilization after procedure
   f. Cough and deep breathing exercises
   g. Management of incisional pain
   h. Turning on the device (usually 48 to 72 hours postimplantation)
2. Provide emotional support to patient and family.
   a. Encourage patient and family to verbalize fears and/or expectations of hospitalization, lifestyle adjustments, self-concept, body image, and device malfunction (misfiring/failure to fire).
   b. Reinforce to patient that daily activities will not increase the risk of the device misfiring.
   c. Explain the sensation that might be felt if the device fires and the patient is conscious. (Many patients will become unconscious before the device fires and therefore feel no sensations.) Sensations experienced in conscious patients vary, but are often described as a severe chest blow.
3. Allow patient to participate in care as much as possible.
   a. Encourage patient to dress in street clothes during hospitalization. (Loose-fitting clothes are recommended to prevent chafing/irritation at implant site.)
   b. Allow patient to look at incision site.
   c. Offer patient instructional booklets on the device.

B. Preventing Infection

1. Check temperature every 4 hours; report elevations. (Suspect defibrillator system as infection source if elevation occurs; infections commonly occur within 5 to 10 days.) Early postoperative fever may also be due to atelectasis; auscultate lungs.
2. Evaluate incision site every 4 hours; note redness, swelling, purulent/serous drainage; palpate around incision site for tenderness, warmth, and/or drainage.
3. Culture all drainage from incision.
4. Evaluate incision for tissue erosion.
5. Monitor white blood cell (WBC) count and differential.
6. Cleanse incision and change dressing as directed, using aseptic technique.
7. Encourage a high-calorie/high-protein diet to promote wound healing and decrease chance of postoperative complications.

GERONTOLOGIC ALERT:
Elderly patients may not demonstrate abnormal temperature elevations with infections and experience prolonged wound healing.

C. Maintaining Cardiac Output

1. Monitor vital signs frequently until stable.
2. Evaluate incision site for evidence of bleeding and/or hematoma.
3. Monitor chest tube drainage for excessive amount and note color.
4. Evaluate urine output.
5. Be alert to potential for dysrhythmias postoperatively. (Manipulation of heart and swelling may induce dysrhythmias 24 to 48 hours after implant.)

6. Treat dysrhythmias as directed—antidysrhythmic therapy and/or electrical countershock (standard anterior paddle placement or anterior/posterior paddle placement is recommended); correct underlying causes such as hypoxia and/or electrolyte disturbances.

NURSING ALERT:
CPR should be started immediately on any patient with an implantable defibrillator who becomes unconscious and has no pulse. A slight "buzz" sensation will be felt if the implanted device delivers a shock, but it is not harmful. Gloves may be worn to minimize the sensation.

7. Evaluate carefully all complaints of chest pain (noncardiac pain may be due to lead fracture or dislodgement; pain may be noted along wire pathways).
8. Auscultate heart sounds every 4 hours for presence of friction rub.

D. Promoting Effective Breathing Pattern

1. Ask patient to take several deep breaths every hour to expand lung fields.
2. Encourage cough and deep breathing exercises frequently; medicate with analgesics before exercises and provide a pillow for splinting.
3. Monitor use of incentive spirometer.
4. Elevate head of bed to promote adequate ventilation.
5. Auscultate lung fields every 4 hours.
6. Assist with position changes every 2 hours while on bedrest.
7. Encourage early ambulation.
8. Administer analgesics as ordered.

Patient Education/ Health Maintenance

A. Introduction to Implantable Defibrillator

1. Review anatomy of the heart with emphasis on the conduction system, using a diagram of the heart.
2. Give accurate explanations, using correct medical terminology (allows patient to interact with the healthcare team more effectively), regarding reason for device implantation, component parts of system, function of device.
   a. Use manufacturer's instructional booklet and video presentation about the device.
   b. Encourage family members to participate in education process.

B. Living With the Implantable Defibrillator

1. Instruct patient and family on actions to be taken should the device fire.
   a. Explain signs/symptoms that may be experienced if a lethal dysrhythmia occurs: palpitations, dizziness, shortness of breath, chest pain.
   b. If signs/symptoms are experienced, lie down and try to call "911" for help if alone.
   c. Family members should check for a pulse if patient becomes unconscious. CPR should be started immediately if no pulse is present and "911" has been called.
   d. Reinforce that shocks emitted from device are not harmful, and CPR should never be delayed to wait for device to complete the shocking sequence.
   e. If patient remains conscious and/or is unconscious with a pulse, family members should monitor patient during episode, continually assessing for a pulse dur-

ing shocking sequence. After the episode, follow instructions as directed by healthcare provider.
f. Keep a diary of all episodes and shocks received from device. Include date, time, and associated symptoms.
2. Explore with patient/family fears regarding failure of device, sensation associated with a shock, and injury to others if a shock occurs.
a. Sensations experienced vary but are most commonly described as a severe blow to the chest.
b. No injury will occur to others if in contact with patient during a shock; a slight shock may be felt by your partner if the device fires during sexual intercourse.
c. Battery life depends on frequency of use. The device is evaluated every 2 months for 1 year and every month thereafter.
3. Review sources of electromechanical interference that should be avoided (see p. 270).
a. The device will usually not become damaged but may be turned off due to interference.
b. A "beeping" sound may be audible if device is turned off by interferences.
c. Airport security devices and hand-held airport security devices may affect device function. These devices must be avoided. Carry Medic-alert card and show to security personnel.
d. Areas/diagnostic tests using large magnets must be avoided.
e. Notify healthcare provider if contact with sources of potential interference.
4. Notify dentist of implanted device because prophylaxis with antibiotics may be necessary before dental care.
5. Review with healthcare provider resumption of activities such as driving and sports.

C. *Other Instructions*
1. Review care of incision site (see p. 270).
2. Loose-fitting clothing should be worn until healing takes place.
3. Provide Medic-alert card; encourage carrying card at all times and obtaining a corresponding Medic-alert bracelet.
4. Reinforce how to keep diary of episodes and date of 2-month follow-up appointment.
5. Provide information to family members regarding CPR training courses.

Evaluation

A. Verbalizes understanding of device and surgical procedure

B. Afebrile; incision without drainage
C. Vital signs stable; no dysrhythmias
D. Respirations unlabored, lungs clear

◆ PERICARDIOCENTESIS

Pericardiocentesis is the puncturing of the pericardial sac to aspirate fluid. Excessive fluid within the pericardial sac can cause compression of the heart chambers, resulting in an acute decrease in cardiac output (cardiac tamponade). Fluid accumulation can occur rapidly (acute) or slowly (stable).

Acute—A rapid increase of fluid into pericardial space (as little as 200 mL) causes a marked rise in intrapericardial pressure. Emergency intervention is required to prevent severe circulatory compromise.

Stable—Slow accumulation of fluid into pericardial sac over weeks or months, causing pericardium to stretch and accommodate up to 2 L of fluid without severe increases in intrapericardial pressure. See Procedure Guidelines 10-7.

Purposes

1. To remove fluid from the pericardial sac caused by:
a. Infection
b. Malignant neoplasm or lymphoma
c. Trauma
(1) Accidental—Blunt or penetrating wounds
(2) Iatrogenic—Cardiac surgery; cardiopulmonary resuscitation; perforation of heart by catheter or transvenous pacemaker
d. Drug reactions
e. Radiation
f. MI
2. To obtain fluid for diagnosis
3. To instill certain therapeutic drugs

Sites for Pericardiocentesis

1. Subxiphoid—Needle inserted in the angle between left costal margin and xiphoid
2. Near cardiac apex, 2 cm (0.8 inch) inside left border of cardiac dullness
3. To the left of the 5th or 6th interspace at the sternal margin
4. Right side of 4th intercostal space just inside border of dullness

PROCEDURE GUIDELINES 10-7 ◆ Assisting the Patient Undergoing Pericardiocentesis

EQUIPMENT   Pericardiocentesis tray
Intracath set
Skin antiseptic
1%–2% lidocaine
Sterile gloves

ECG for monitoring purposes
Sterile ground wire—to be connected between pericardial needle and V lead of ECG (use alligator clip type connectors)
Equipment for cardiopulmonary resuscitation

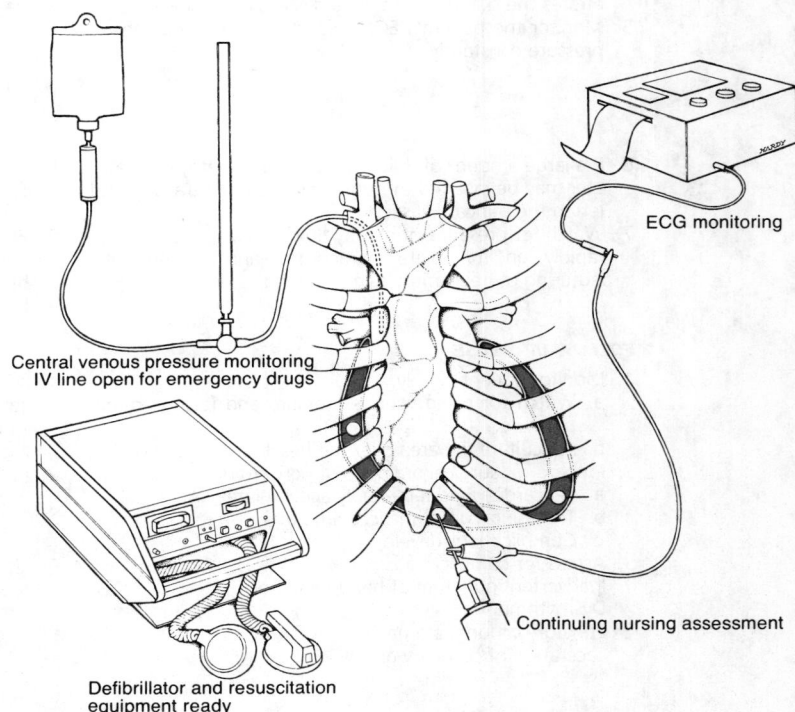

ECG monitoring

Central venous pressure monitoring
IV line open for emergency drugs

Continuing nursing assessment

Defibrillator and resuscitation equipment ready

Nursing support of the patient undergoing pericardiocentesis. (Small circles indicate sites for pericardial aspiration.)

PROCEDURE	NURSING ACTION	RATIONALE

PREPARATORY PHASE

1. Medicate the patient as prescribed.
2. Start a slow intravenous drip of saline or glucose.

3. Place the patient in a comfortable position with the head of the bed or treatment table raised to a 45-degree angle.
4. Apply the limb leads of the ECG to the patient.
5. Have defibrillator available for immediate use.
6. Have pacemaker available.
7. Open the tray using aseptic technique.

PERFORMANCE PHASE (BY PHYSICIAN)

1. The site is prepared with skin antiseptic; the area is draped with sterile towels and injected with anesthetic.
2. The pericardial aspiration needle is attached to a 50-mL syringe by a three-way stopcock. The V lead (precordial lead wire) of the ECG is attached to the hub of the aspirating needle by a sterile wire and alligator clips or clamp.

2. This preserves a route for intravenous therapy in the event of an emergency.
3. This position makes it easier to insert needle into pericardial sac.
4. The patient is monitored during the procedure by ECG.
5. In case the procedure has severe adverse effect.

2. There is danger of laceration of myocardium/coronary artery and of cardiac dysrhythmias.

(continued)

PROCEDURE GUIDELINES 10-7 ◆ Assisting the Patient Undergoing Pericardiocentesis *(continued)*

PROCEDURE (cont'd)	NURSING ACTION	RATIONALE
	3. The needle is advanced slowly until fluid is obtained.	3. Fluid is generally aspirated at a depth of 2.5–4 cm (1 to 1½ inches).
	4. When the pericardial sac has been entered, a hemostat is clamped to the needle at the chest wall just where it penetrates the skin. Pericardial fluid is aspirated slowly.	4. This prevents movement of the needle and further penetration while fluid is being removed. Aspirated fluid may be cloudy, clear, or bloody.
	5. Monitor the patient's ECG, blood pressure, and venous pressure constantly.	5. a. The ST segment rises if the point of the needle contacts the ventricle; there may be ventricular ectopic beats. b. The PR segment is elevated when the needle touches the atrium. c. Large, erratic QRS complexes indicate penetration of the myocardium.
	6. If a large amount of fluid is present, a polyethylene catheter may be inserted through a needle (an intracath) and left in the pericardial sac.	6. An indwelling catheter left in the pericardial space permits further slow drainage of fluid and prevents recurrence of cardiac tamponade.
	7. Watch for presence of bloody fluid. If blood accumulates rapidly, an immediate thoracotomy and cardiorrhaphy (suturing of heart muscle) may be indicated.	7. Bloody pericardial fluid may be due to trauma. Bloody pericardial effusion fluid does not clot readily, whereas blood obtained from inadvertent puncture of one of the heart chambers does clot.

FOLLOW-UP PHASE

1. Monitor patient closely.
   a. Watch for rising venous pressure and falling arterial pressure.
   b. Auscultate the area over the heart.
2. Prepare for surgical drainage of pericardium if:
   a. Pericardial fluid repeatedly accumulates, or
   b. The aspiration is unsuccessful, or
   c. Complications develop
3. Assess for complications:
   Inadvertent puncture of heart chamber
   Dysrhythmias
   Puncture of lung, stomach, or liver
   Laceration of coronary artery or myocardium

1. After pericardiocentesis, careful monitoring of blood pressure, venous pressure, and heart sounds will be necessary to indicate possible recurrence of tamponade; repeated aspiration is then necessary.
2. In the presence of these signs, the patient is probably experiencing cardiac tamponade.

3. Listen for decrease in intensity of heart sounds indicating recurring cardiac tamponade.

◆ PERCUTANEOUS TRANSLUMINAL CORONARY ANGIOPLASTY (PTCA)

Percutaneous transluminal coronary angioplasty is a technique used for the treatment of coronary artery disease (CAD). A balloon-tipped catheter is introduced through a guidewire into a coronary vessel with a noncalcified atheromatous lesion. The balloon of the catheter is then inflated, causing disruption of the intima and changes in the atheroma. The result is an increase in the diameter of the lumen of the coronary vessel (as judged by angiographic criteria) and improvement of blood flow below the lesion. Balloon inflation/deflation may be repeated until satisfactory results are achieved (Fig. 10-7).

Indications

Patients meeting these criteria are generally acceptable candidates for PTCA:

1. Stable angina (less than 1 year) or unstable angina (less than 6 months), despite optimal medical therapy

2. Single-vessel or multivessel disease (balloon dilatation of the most severe "culprit" lesion is initially attempted to determine if successful angioplasty can be achieved); surgery to bypass the lesion may be recommended if PTCA is unsuccessful.
3. Proximal, accessible noncalcified lesions; midvessel lesions may also be attempted with success.
4. Suitable candidate for heart surgery and has consented to heart surgery as an alternative treatment
5. Evolving MI (may be in combination with thrombolytic therapy) and obstructed coronary bypass grafts

Contraindications

1. Patients with left main coronary artery disease
2. Patients with severe left ventricular dysfunction

Complications

1. Coronary occlusion, coronary dissection, MI, coronary artery spasm, and prolonged angina may necessitate immediate coronary artery bypass graft surgery. A cardiac surgical team must be on standby during all PTCA procedures.

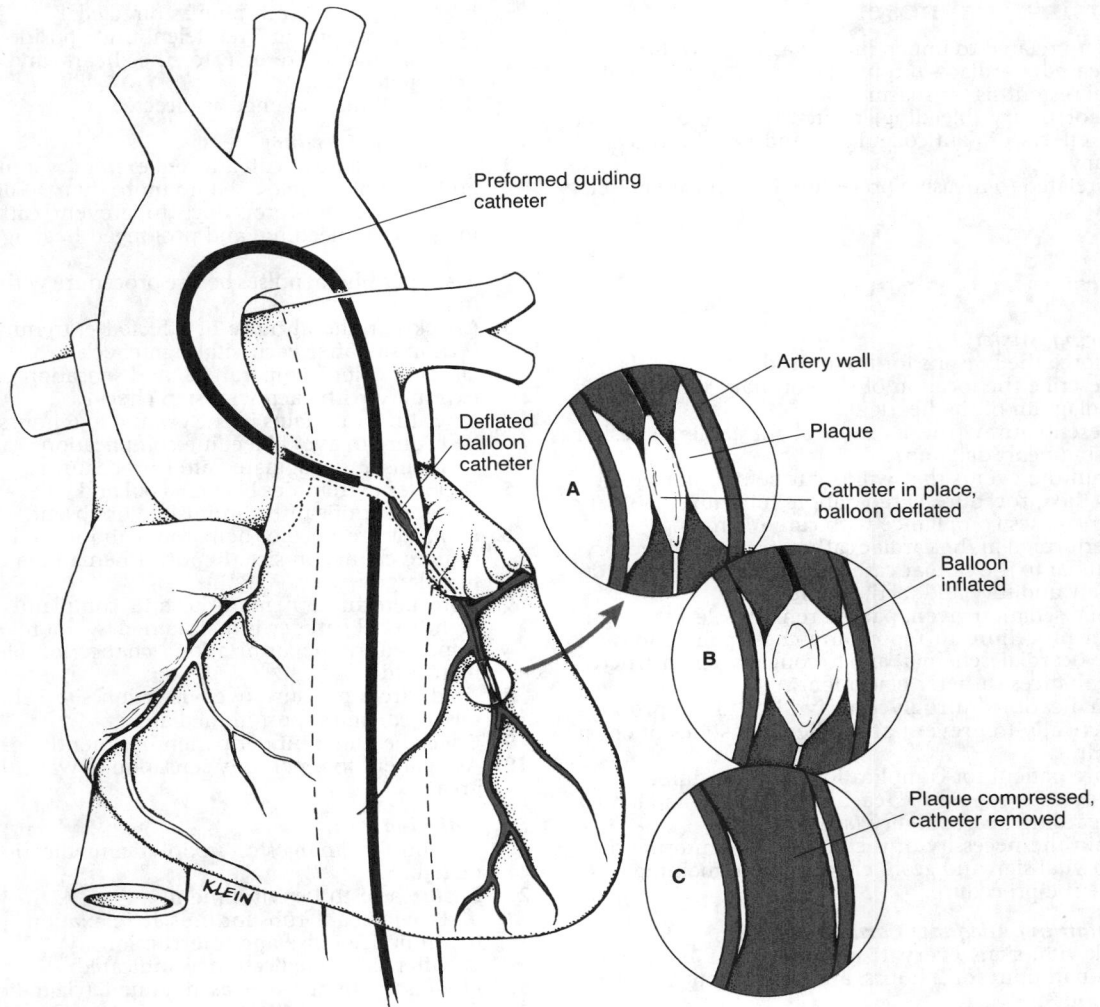

FIGURE 10-7 *Percutaneous transluminal coronary angioplasty. (**A**) The balloon-tipped catheter is passed into the affected coronary artery. (**B**) The balloon is then rapidly inflated and deflated with controlled pressure. (**C**) The balloon disrupts the intima and causes changes in the atheroma, resulting in an increase in the diameter of the lumen of the vessel and improvement of blood flow. (Redrawn after Purcell, J. A., & Giffin, P. A. (1981). Percutaneous transluminal coronary angioplasty. Am J Nurs, 9, 1620–1626.)*

2. PTCA is associated with a restenosis rate of 30% to 40%. Restenosis may occur acutely (within 24 hours) or within 6 months. A second angioplasty may be performed with improved long-term results.

Recent Advances

1. Laser-assisted balloon angioplasty
   a. A laser light is directed by a percutaneously inserted flexible fiberoptic catheter and is able to "vaporize" atheromatous lesions in the coronary vessels.
   b. Balloon angioplasty of the vessel may then be performed.
   c. This new technique may minimize damage to the intimal lining, open diseased vessels more effec-

tively, prevent early and long-term restenosis, and expand the use to calcified, unusual lesions and total occlusions.

2. Atherectomy
   a. A burr-tipped high-speed rotating catheter is inserted percutaneously into a coronary vessel and "drills" through the atheromatous lesion, changing it to microscopic debris.
   b. This new technique may open diseased vessels more effectively, especially in patients who have coronary lesions not amenable to standard angioplasty.

3. Intracoronary stenting
   a. A tiny coil or diamond mesh tubular device (stent) is placed in the coronary artery immediately after successful balloon angioplasty.
   b. The stent remains in the vessel to prevent restenosis.

Nursing Diagnoses

A. Anxiety related to impending invasive procedure
B. Decreased Cardiac Output related to dysrhythmias, vessel restenosis, or spasm
C. Risk for Injury (bleeding) related to femoral catheter and effect of anticoagulant and/or thrombolytic therapy
D. Pain related to invasive procedure or myocardial ischemia

Nursing Interventions

A. *Reducing Anxiety*
1. Reinforce the reasons for the procedure.
   a. Describe the location of the coronary vessels using a diagram of the heart.
   b. Describe/draw the location of the patient's lesion using heart diagram.
2. Explain the events that will occur before, during, and after the procedure. Preparation minimizes anxiety and increases compliance with care regimen.
   a. Performed in the cardiac catheterization laboratory; similar to the cardiac catheterization procedure. Review auditory and tactile stimuli.
   b. Mild sedation given; patient remains alert throughout procedure to report any chest pain (indicates myocardial ischemia) and to cough when instructed (enhances catheter placement).
   c. Medication (nitroglycerin) will be given prophylactically to prevent and relieve episodes of chest pain.
3. Prepare patient for complications of procedure.
   a. Provide preoperative teaching to patient and family regarding heart surgery (see p. 283).
4. Explain the necessity of the IV, ECG monitoring, frequent vital sign and groin checks, and remaining NPO before the procedure.

B. *Maintaining Adequate Cardiac Output*
1. Check vital signs every 15 minutes for 1 hour, then every half hour for 2 hours, and subsequently every 1 to 2 hours.
2. Continually evaluate for signs/symptoms of restenosis.
   a. Emphasize importance of reporting any chest discomfort or jaw, back, arm pain and/or nausea, abdominal distress.
   b. Take ECG for all complaints suspicious of possible myocardial ischemia.
   c. Administer oxygen and vasodilator therapy for pain as directed.
   d. Obtain CPK and isoenzymes as directed.
   e. Keep patient NPO if prolonged chest pain occurs (patient may return to catheterization laboratory).
3. Evaluate fluid and electrolyte balance.
   a. Record intake and output.
   b. Encourage fluid intake to prevent dehydration. Contrast medium used during procedure causes diuresis.
   c. Observe for dysrhythmias possibly related to potassium imbalance. Excessive diuresis causes potassium depletion.
   d. Administer potassium supplement as prescribed.
4. Be alert to potential of vasovagal reaction during removal of groin catheter.
   a. Observe for bradycardia, hypotension, diaphoresis, nausea.

b. Administer IV atropine as directed.
c. Place patient in Trendelenburg's position to promote blood return to the heart and improve hypotension.
d. Give fluid challenge as directed.

C. *Preventing Bleeding*
1. Maintain bedrest with affected extremity immobilized, and head of bed elevated no more than 30 degrees 12 to 24 hours postprocedure to prevent catheter dislodgement, bleeding, and prolonged healing of vessel lining.
2. Mark peripheral pulses before procedure with indelible ink.
3. Check peripheral pulse of affected extremity and insertion site after each vital sign check.
4. Observe color, temperature, and sensation of affected extremity with each vital sign check.
   a. Catheter remains in the groin 4 to 6 hours postprocedure to avoid bleeding complications (patient remains anticoagulated after procedure).
5. Report if extremities become cool and pale, and pulses become significantly diminished or absent.
6. Look for presence of hematoma and mark hematoma to note change in size. Report if hematoma continues to enlarge.
7. Note petechiae, hematuria, and complaints of flank pain (vessel patency is maintained by not reversing intraprocedure heparinization; chance of bleeding is increased).
8. Hold direct pressure over insertion site if bleeding is observed, and report immediately.
9. Check bed linen under patient frequently for blood.
10. Ask patient to report any sensation of warmth at groin area.

D. *Relieving Pain*
1. Administer analgesics/anxiolytic medication as directed.
2. Ensure a restful environment.
   a. Provide back rubs for muscle relaxation.
   b. Minimize noise and interruptions.
   c. Offer sleep medication as indicated.
3. Progress patient's diet as tolerated (clear liquids/full liquid diet until catheters removed); assist patient with meals.

Patient Education/ Health Maintenance

Instruct patient as follows:

1. Modification of cardiac risk factors as means of controlling progression of coronary artery disease
2. Name of medications, action, dosage, and side effects
   a. Common medications prevent clot formation (aspirin, dipyridamole [Persantine]); increase blood flow to heart (isosorbide dinitrate [Isordil]); or slow heart rate/decrease chest pain (propranolol [Inderal]); increase blood flow and prevent coronary artery spasm (diltiazem [Cardizem]); (nifedipine [Procardia]).
   b. Dates and importance of follow-up tests—exercise ECG, thallium-201 perfusion imaging. Symptoms for which patient should seek medical attention—side effects of medications, chest pain, or weight increases greater than 5 lb.

(1) Stenosis can recur within 6 months. Second angioplasty is usually successful for more than 1 year.
(2) Chest pain unrelieved with nitroglycerin and persisting longer than 15 minutes after rest is significant.

Evaluation

A. Verbalizes understanding of procedure
B. Vital signs stable; urine output adequate
C. No bleeding or hematoma at insertion site
D. Verbalizes relief of pain

◆ INTRAAORTIC BALLOON PUMP (IABP) COUNTERPULSATION

Counterpulsation is a method of assisting the failing heart and circulation by mechanical support. The mechanism of counterpulsation therapy is opposite to the normal pumping action of the heart; counterpulsation devices pump while the heart muscle relaxes (diastole) and relax when the heart muscle contracts (systole).

A. *Intraaortic Balloon Pump (Fig. 10-8)*
A balloon catheter is introduced into the femoral artery percutaneously or surgically, threaded to the descending thoracic aorta, and positioned distal to the subclavian artery.

1. The balloon catheter is attached to an external console, allowing for inflation/deflation of the balloon with gas such as carbon dioxide.
2. The external console integrates the inflation/deflation sequence with the mechanical events of the cardiac cycle (systole/diastole) by "triggering" gas delivery in synchronization with the patient's ECG and "timing" the duration of inflation and point of deflation in conjunction with the patient's arterial pressure waveform.

B. *Counterpulsation With IABP*
1. Eases the workload of a damaged heart by increasing coronary blood flow (diastolic augmentation) and decreasing the resistance in the arterial tree against which the heart must pump (afterload reduction).
2. This results in an increase in cardiac output and a reduction in myocardial oxygen requirements.
3. The balloon is inflated at the onset of diastole; this results in an increase in diastolic pressure (diastolic augmentation), which increases blood flow through the coronary arteries.
4. The balloon is deflated just before the onset of systole, facilitating the emptying of blood from the left ventricle.
5. Clinical uses
  a. Treatment of cardiogenic shock after MI
  b. Low cardiac output states—After open heart surgery; life-threatening dysrhythmias
  c. High cardiac output states—Sepsis, hemorrhage
  d. Myocardial ischemia unresponsive to medical therapy and external counterpulsation pressure

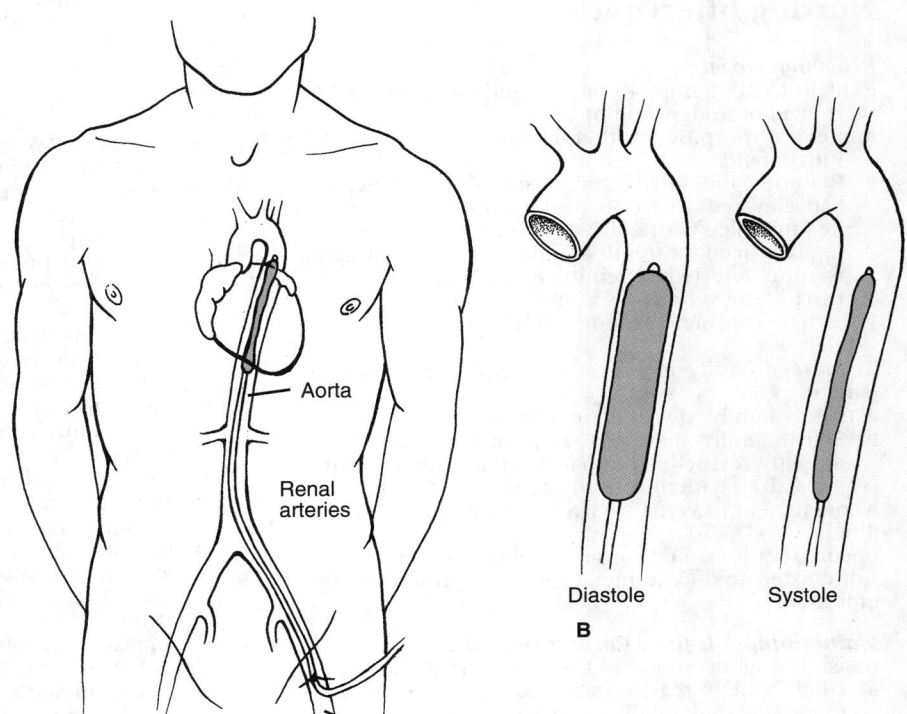

FIGURE 10-8 *Counterpulsation.* (**A**) *Introduction of the intra-aortic balloon catheter via the femoral artery.* (**B**) *The intra-aortic balloon pump augments diastole, resulting in increased perfusion of the coronary arteries and myocardium and a decrease in the left ventricular work load.*

Aorta

Renal arteries

Femoral artery

Diastole

Systole

B

A

Contraindications

1. Aortic valve insufficiency
2. Aortic aneurysm and/or dissection
3. Severe aortoiliac disease

Complications

1. Ischemia of limb distal to insertion site
2. Impairment of cerebral circulation due to balloon migration occluding the subclavian artery or by embolus
3. Impairment of renal circulation due to balloon malposition or embolus
4. Dissection of the aorta
5. Thrombocytopenia
6. Septicemia
7. Infection at insertion site
8. Hemorrhage due to anticoagulation

Nursing Diagnoses

A. Anxiety related to invasive procedure, critical illness, and environment
B. Decreased Cardiac Output related to myocardial ischemia and/or mechanical intervention
C. Altered Tissue Perfusion related to foreign body in aorta
D. Impaired Skin Integrity related to decreased mobility

Nursing Interventions

A. *Relieving Anxiety*
1. Explain IABP therapy to patient and family geared to their level of understanding.
   a. Review purpose of therapy and how the IABP functions.
   b. Reinforce mobility restrictions: supine with head of bed elevated 15 to 30 degrees, no movement or flexing of leg with IABP catheter.
   c. Explain need for frequent monitoring of vital signs, rhythm, affected extremity, and pulses.
   d. Discuss the sounds associated with functioning external console: balloon inflation/deflation and alarms.
2. Encourage family members to participate in care of patient.
   a. Allow family to visit patient frequently.
   b. Solicit family members' assistance in reinforcing mobility restrictions to patient and notifying nursing staff of patient comfort needs.
3. Allow patient to verbalize fears regarding therapy and illness.
4. Ensure that informed consent is obtained.
5. Administer anxiolytic medications as prescribed and indicated.

B. *Maintaining Adequate Cardiac Output*
1. Assist during insertion of IABP catheter.
   a. Offer patient reassurance and comfort measures (patient is only mildly sedated).
   b. Ensure strict aseptic environment during insertion.

c. Establish ECG monitoring, choosing the lead with the largest R wave (external console senses R wave of ECG to trigger gas delivery) and without artifact (integration of the patient's cardiac cycle with the inflation/deflation balloon sequence depends on a continuous clear ECG tracing).
   d. Record date, time, and the patient's tolerance to procedure.
2. Start IABP immediately after insertion, as directed; review manufacturer's manual for IABP equipment in use.
   a. Adjust the duration of balloon inflation/deflation by the arterial waveform, inflation is "timed" to begin at the dicrotic notch of the arterial waveform, and deflation occurs before the next systole.
   b. Compare the patient's arterial pressure waveform with/without balloon augmentation to evaluate effectiveness of therapy. Note difference in patient's end diastolic pressure and balloon-assisted end diastolic pressure (the balloon-assisted end diastolic pressure should be lower, indicating a reduction in afterload).
   c. Monitor hemodynamic parameters with Swan-Ganz catheter (see p. 258). Record mean arterial pressure, CVP, PAP, PCWP, and cardiac output to evaluate overall effectiveness of therapy. Perform hemodynamic calculations to evaluate SVR and left ventricular stroke work (LVSW).
3. Monitor vital signs every 15 to 30 minutes for 4 to 9 hours then hourly, if stable.
4. Monitor neurologic status at least every 2 hours.
5. Monitor urine output from indwelling catheter every hour.
6. Maintain accurate intake/output.
7. Report chest pain immediately.
8. Treat dysrhythmias as directed.
9. Check for blood oozing around IABP catheter every hour for 8 hours, then every 4 hours (anticoagulation therapy is used to prevent thrombus formation); apply direct pressure and report bleeding.

C. *Maintaining Adequate Tissue Perfusion*
1. Evaluate for ischemia of extremity with IABP catheter.
   a. Mark pulses with indelible ink to facilitate checks.
   b. Monitor peripheral pulses (dorsalis pedis, posterior tibial, popliteal, and left radial) for rhythm, character, and pulse quality every 15 minutes for 1 hour, then every 30 minutes for 1 hour, and then hourly.
   c. Use Doppler device for pulses difficult to palpate and to auscultate for bruits/hums.
   d. Observe skin temperature, color, sensation, and movement of affected extremity. Dusky, cool, mottled, painful, numb/tingling extremity indicates ischemia.
2. Observe for possible indications of thromboemboli.
   a. Note decreases in urine output after initiation of therapy—may indicate renal artery emboli.
   b. Perform neurologic checks every hour to evaluate for cerebral emboli.
   c. Auscultate bowel sounds to detect evidence of ischemia.
3. Recognize early signs/symptoms of compartment syndrome. Increased pressure in tissue reduces blood flow.
   a. Note complaints of pain, pressure, and numbness of affected extremity induced by passive stretching.
   b. Palpate affected extremity for swelling and tension.

c. Monitor CPK values. Highly elevated CPKs may indicate compartment syndrome.

4. Keep head of bed elevated 15 to 30 degrees if tolerated to prevent upward migration of catheter.

D. *Maintaining Skin Integrity*
1. Assess skin frequently for signs of redness or breakdown.
2. Place patient on specialty mattress or bed designed to prevent pressure sores (preferably before balloon insertion).
3. Pad bony prominences.
4. Implement passive range-of-motion exercises with exception of extremity with IABP catheter.
5. Turn patient from side to side as a unit every 2 hours. Patients are usually debilitated and prone to pressure sores.

Evaluation

A. Patient states activity restrictions and rationale
B. BP and cardiac output readings improved
C. Peripheral pulses strong; extremities warm and nailbeds pink
D. No skin redness or breakdown

◆ HEART SURGERY

Open heart surgery is most commonly performed for coronary artery disease, valvular dysfunction, and congenital heart defects. The procedure requires temporary cardiopulmonary bypass (blood is diverted from the heart and the lungs and mechanically oxygenated and circulated) to provide a dry, bloodless field during the operation.

Types of Heart Surgery

1. Coronary artery bypass surgery
   a. A graft (leg and arm veins) is anastomosed to the aorta, and the other end of the graft is secured to a distal portion of a coronary vessel.
   b. The graft ''bypasses'' the obstructive lesion in the vessel, and adequate blood flow is restored to the heart muscle supplied by the artery.
   c. Multiple grafts can be placed to bypass lesions, and the internal mammary artery may also be used for grafts.
2. Valvular surgery
   a. Prosthetic or biologic valves are placed in the heart as definitive therapy for incompetent heart valves.
   b. Valve replacement can be done in conjunction with coronary artery bypass surgery.
3. Congenital heart surgery
   a. Defects of the heart can be surgically repaired and reconstructed.
   b. Temporary cardiopulmonary bypass is not always required.

Preoperative Management/ Nursing Care

1. Review of patient's condition to determine status of pulmonary, renal, hepatic, hematologic, and metabolic systems

   a. Cardiac history; history of cardiac dysrhythmias
   b. Pulmonary health. Patients with COPD may require prolonged postoperative respiratory support.
   c. Depression—Can produce a serious postoperative depressive state and can affect postoperative morbidity and mortality.
   d. Present alcohol intake; smoking history
2. Obtain preoperative laboratory studies.
   a. Complete blood count; serum electrolytes; lipid profile; and nose, throat, sputum, and urine cultures
   b. Antibody screen
   c. Preoperative coagulation survey (platelet count, prothrombin time, partial thromboplastin time)—Extracorporeal circulation will affect certain coagulation factors.
   d. Renal and hepatic function tests
3. Evaluate medication regimen. These patients are usually on multiple drugs.
   a. Digitalis—May be receiving large doses to improve myocardial contractility; may be stopped several days before surgery to avoid digitoxic dysrhythmias from cardiopulmonary bypass.
   b. Diuretics—Assess for potassium depletion and volume depletion; give potassium supplement to replenish body stores. May be omitted several days preoperatively to avoid electrolyte imbalance and consequent dysrhythmias postoperatively.
   c. Beta-adrenergic blockers (propranolol [Inderal])—Usually continued
   d. Psychotropic drugs (diazepam [Valium]; chlordiazepoxide [Librium])—Postoperative withdrawal may cause extreme agitation.
   e. Antihypertensives (reserpine [Serapsil])—Omitted as far in advance of procedure as possible to allow norepinephrine repletion.
   f. Alcohol—Sudden withdrawal may produce delirium.
   g. Anticoagulant drugs—Discontinued several days before operation to allow coagulation mechanism to return to normal.
   h. Corticosteroids—If taken within the year before surgery, may be given supplemental doses to cover stress of surgery.
   i. Prophylactic antibiotics may be given preoperatively.
   j. Drug sensitivities or allergies are noted.
4. Improve underlying pulmonary disease and respiratory function to reduce risk of complications.
   a. Encourage patient to stop smoking.
   b. Treat infection and pulmonary vascular congestion.

GERONTOLOGIC ALERT:
Elderly and debilitated patients are at greater risk for postoperative respiratory complications.

5. Prepare the patient for events in the postoperative period.
   a. Take the patient and family on tour of ICU. This lessens anxiety about being in ICU.
      (1) Introduce the patient to staff personnel who will be caring for him or her.
      (2) Give family a schedule of visiting hours and times for phone contact.

b. Teach chest physical therapy procedures to optimize pulmonary function.
   (1) Have the patient practice with incentive spirometer.
   (2) Show and practice diaphragmatic breathing techniques.
   (3) Have the patient practice effective coughing, leg exercises.
c. Prepare patient for presence of monitors, chest tubes, IVs, blood transfusion, endotracheal tube, nasogastric tube, pacing wires, arterial line, indwelling catheter.
   (1) Explain to the patient that two chest tubes will be inserted below incision into chest cavity for drainage and maintenance of negative pressure.
   (2) Explain to the patient that endotracheal tube will prevent speaking, but communication will be possible through writing until tube is removed (usually within 24 hours).
   (3) Explain to the patient that diet will consist of liquids until 24 hours after surgery.
   (4) Explain to the patient that monitoring equipment and IV lines will restrict movement, and nursing staff will position the patient comfortably every 2 hours and as necessary.
d. Discuss with the patient the need to monitor vital signs frequently and the likelihood of frequent disturbances of the patient's rest.
e. Discuss pain management with the patient; assure the patient that analgesics will be administered as necessary to control pain.
f. Tell the patient that both hands may be loosely restrained for a number of hours after surgery to eliminate possibility of pulling out tubes and IV lines inadvertently.
6. Evaluate the patient's emotional state and try to reduce anxieties. Patients undergoing heart surgery are more anxious and fearful than other surgical patients. (Moderate anxiety assists patient to cope with stresses of surgery. Low anxiety level may indicate that the patient is in denial. High anxiety may impair the patient's ability to learn and listen.)
   a. Offer support and help patient and family mobilize positive coping mechanisms.
   b. Answer questions and allay fears and misconceptions.
7. Surgical preparation:
   a. Shave anterior and lateral surfaces of trunk and neck; shave entire body down to ankles (for coronary bypass).
   b. Shower/bathe with Betadine soap.
   c. Give sedative before going to the operating room.

Potential Complications

1. Cardiac dysrhythmias frequently occur after heart surgery.
   a. Premature ventricular contractions occur most frequently after aortic valve replacement and coronary bypass surgery. May be treated with pacing, lidocaine (Xylocaine), potassium.
   b. Atrial arrhythmias also occur after valvular surgery.
   c. Dysrhythmias also apt to occur with ischemia, hypoxia, alterations in serum potassium, edema, bleeding, acid–base or electrolyte disturbances, digitalis toxicity, myocardial failure.

2. Cardiac tamponade results from bleeding into the pericardial sac or accumulation of fluids in the sac, which compresses the heart and prevents adequate filling of the ventricles.
3. MI
4. Cardiac failure (low output syndrome)
5. Persistent bleeding from cardiac incision, tissue fragility, trauma to tissues, clotting defects; blood clotting disturbances usually transitory after cardiopulmonary bypass; however, a significant platelet deficiency may be present.
6. Hypovolemia
7. Renal insufficiency or failure. Renal injury may be caused by deficient perfusion, hemolysis, low cardiac output before and after open-heart surgery; use of vasopressor agents to increase blood pressure.
8. Hypotension may be caused by inadequate cardiac contractility and reduction in blood volume or by mechanical ventilation (when the patient "fights" the ventilator, or PEEP is used), all of which can produce a reduction in cardiac output.
9. Embolization may result from injury to the intima of the blood vessels, dislodgement of a clot from a damaged valve, venous stasis aggravated by certain dysrhythmias, loosening of mural thrombi, and coagulation problems.
   a. Common embolic sites are lungs, coronary arteries, mesentery, extremities, kidneys, spleen, and brain.
10. Postpericardiotomy syndrome—A group of symptoms occurring after cardiac and pericardial trauma and MI
    a. Cause is not certain; may be from anticardiac antibodies, viral etiology, or other cause.
    b. Manifestations—Fever, malaise, arthralgias, dyspnea, pericardial effusion, pleural effusion, friction rub
11. Postperfusion syndrome—Diffuse syndrome characterized by fever, splenomegaly, lymphocytosis
12. Febrile complications—Probably from body's reaction to tissue trauma or accumulation of blood and serum in pleural and pericardial spaces
13. Hepatitis

Postoperative Management/ Nursing Care

1. Ensure adequate oxygenation in early postoperative period; respiratory insufficiency is common after open-heart surgery.
   a. Assisted or controlled ventilation (see p. 191) is employed. Respiratory support is used during first 24 hours to provide airway in the event of cardiac arrest, to decrease work of heart, and to maintain effective ventilation.
   b. Chest x-ray taken immediately after surgery and daily thereafter to evaluate state of lung expansion and to detect atelectasis; to demonstrate heart size and contour, confirm placement of central line, endotracheal tube, and chest drains.
2. Employ hemodynamic monitoring during immediate postoperative period, for cardiovascular and respiratory status and fluid and electrolyte balance to prevent complications or to recognize them as early as possible.
3. Monitor drainage of mediastinal and pleural chest tubes.
4. Monitor fluid and electrolyte balance closely. Adequate circulating blood volume is necessary for optimal cellular activity; metabolic acidosis and electrolyte imbalance can occur after use of pump oxygenator.

a. Hypokalemia (low potassium level) may be caused by inadequate intake, diuretics, vomiting, excessive nasogastric drainage, stress from surgery.

b. Hyperkalemia (high potassium level) may be caused by increased intake, red cell breakdown from the pump, acidosis, renal insufficiency, tissue necrosis, and adrenal cortical insufficiency.

c. Hyponatremia (low sodium) may be due to reduction of total body sodium or to an increased water intake, causing a dilution of body sodium.

d. Hypocalcemia (low calcium level) may be due to alkalosis (which reduces the amount of Ca^{++} in the extracellular fluid) and multiple blood transfusions.

e. Hypercalcemia (high calcium level) may cause dysrhythmias imitating those caused by digitalis toxicity.

5. Administer postoperative medications.
   a. Aspirin daily as MI prophylaxis
   b. Analgesics
   c. Antihypertensives or antidysrhythmics restarted if needed
6. Monitor for complications.
7. Institute cardiac pacing if indicated by way of temporary pacing wires from incision.
   a. Valvular and some other surgeries cause swelling in AV nodal area, requiring pacing.
   b. If stable, pacing wires are discontinued within 48 hours.

Nursing Diagnoses

A. Anxiety related to fear of unknown, fear of death, and fear of pain
B. Impaired Gas Exchange related to alveolar capillary membrane changes, immobility, altered blood flow
C. Decreased Cardiac Output, related to mechanical factors: decreased preload and impaired contractility
D. Risk for Fluid Volume Deficit and Electrolyte Imbalance related to physiologic effects of heart–lung machine
E. Pain related to sternotomy and leg incisions
F. Sensory/Perceptual Alterations related to intensive care environment, sleep deprivation, inability to speak, and immobility

Nursing Interventions

A. *Minimizing Anxiety*
1. Orient the patient to surroundings as soon as awakens from surgical procedure. Tell the patient that operation is over, location, the time of day, and your name.
2. Allow family members to visit the patient as soon as condition stabilizes. Encourage family members to talk to and touch the patient. (Family members may be overwhelmed by critical care environment.)
3. As the patient becomes more alert, explain purpose of all the equipment in environment. Continually orient the patient to time and place.
4. Administer anxiolytics as directed.

B. *Promoting Adequate Gas Exchange*
1. Frequently check function of mechanical ventilator, patient's respiratory effort, and ABGs.
2. Check endotracheal tube placement.
3. Auscultate chest for breath sounds. Crackles indicate pulmonary congestion; decreased or absent breath sounds indicate pneumothorax.

4. Sedate patient adequately to help tolerate endotracheal tube and cope with ventilatory sensations.
5. Use chest physiotherapy for patients with lung congestion to prevent retention of secretions and atelectasis.
6. Promote coughing, deep breathing, and turning to keep airway patent, prevent atelectasis, and facilitate lung expansion.
7. Suction tracheobronchial secretions carefully. Prolonged suctioning leads to hypoxia and possible cardiac arrest.
8. Restrict fluids (per request) for first few days. There is danger of pulmonary congestion from excessive fluid intake.
9. Assist with weaning process and extubation (see p. 198) when indicated.

C. *Maintaining Adequate Cardiac Output*
1. Monitor cardiovascular status to determine effectiveness of cardiac output. Serial readings of blood pressure by way of intraarterial line, heart rate, CVP, and left atrial or PAP from monitor modules are observed, correlated with the patient's condition, and recorded.
   a. Monitor arterial pressure every 15 minutes until stable and as directed thereafter.
   b. Measure left atrial pressure or pulmonary artery wedge pressure to determine the left ventricular end-diastolic volume.
   c. Take CVP readings.
2. Check urine output every 1/2 to 1 hour (from indwelling catheter).
3. Observe buccal mucosa, nailbeds, lips, ear lobes, and extremities for duskiness/cyanosis—signs of low cardiac output.
4. Feel the skin; cool, moist skin reveals lowered cardiac output. Note temperature and color of extremities.
5. Monitor neurologic status.
   a. Observe for symptoms of hypoxia—restlessness, headache, confusion, dyspnea, hypotension, and cyanosis.
   b. Note the patient's neurologic status hourly in terms of level of responsiveness, response to verbal commands and painful stimuli, pupillary size and reaction to light, and movement of extremities; hand-grasp ability.
   c. Monitor for and treat postoperative convulsive seizures.

D. *Maintaining Adequate Fluid Volume*
1. Administer IV fluids as ordered but limit if signs of fluid overloading occur.
2. Keep intake and output flow sheet as a method of determining positive or negative fluid balance and the patient's fluid requirements.
   a. IV fluids (including flush solutions through arterial and venous lines) are considered intake.
   b. Measure postoperative chest drainage—should not exceed 200 mL/h for first 4 to 6 hours.
3. Be alert to changes in serum electrolytes.
   a. Hypokalemia may cause dysrhythmias, digitalis toxicity, metabolic alkalosis, weakened myocardium, cardiac arrest.
      (1) Watch for specific ECG changes.
      (2) Give IV potassium replacement as directed.
   b. Hyperkalemia may cause mental confusion, restlessness, nausea, weakness, and paresthesia of extremities.

(1) Be prepared to administer an ion-exchange resin, sodium polystyrene sulfonate (Kayexalate), which binds the potassium.

c. Hyponatremia may cause weakness, fatigue, confusion, convulsions, and coma.

d. Hypocalcemia may cause numbness and tingling in the fingertips, toes, ear, and nose, carpopedal spasm, muscle cramps, and tetany.
   (1) Give replacement therapy as directed.

e. Hypercalcemia may cause digitalis toxicity.
   (1) Institute treatment as directed. This condition may lead to asystole and death.

E. *Relieving Pain*

1. Examine sternotomy incision and leg dressings.
2. Record nature, type, location, and duration of pain. Pain and anxiety increase pulse rate, oxygen consumption, and cardiac work.
3. Differentiate between incisional pain and anginal pain.
4. Report restlessness and apprehension not corrected by analgesics—may be from hypoxia or a low-output state.
5. Administer medication as often as prescribed or monitor constant infusion to reduce amount of pain and to aid the patient in performing deep breathing and coughing exercises more effectively.
6. Assist patient to position of comfort.
7. Encourage early mobilization.

F. *Promoting Perceptual and Psychological Orientation*

1. Watch for symptoms of postcardiotomy delirium (may appear after brief lucid period).
   a. Signs and symptoms include delirium (impairment of orientation, memory, intellectual function, judgment), transient perceptual distortions, visual and auditory hallucinations, disorientation, and paranoid delusions.
   b. Symptoms may be related to sleep deprivation, increased sensory input, disorientation to night and day, prolonged inability to speak because of endotracheal intubation, age, and preoperative cardiac status.
2. Keep the patient oriented to time and place; notify the patient of procedures and expectations of cooperation. Give repeated explanations of what is happening.
3. Encourage family to come in at regular times—helps the patient regain sense of reality.
4. Plan care to allow rest periods, day–night pattern, and uninterrupted sleep.
5. Encourage mobility as soon as possible. Keep environment as free as possible of excessive auditory and sensory input. Prevent bodily injury.
6. Reassure the patient and family that psychiatric disorders after cardiac surgery are usually transient.
7. Remove the patient from ICU as soon as possible. Allow patient to talk about event of psychotic episode—helps deal with and assimilate experience.

G. *Other Nursing Responsibilities: Avoiding Complications*

1. Dysrhythmias
   a. Monitor ECG continuously.
   b. Treat dysrhythmias immediately because they may lead to a decreased cardiac output.
   c. Evaluate cause of dysrhythmias: inadequate oxygenation, electrolyte imbalance, MI, mechanical irritation (ie, pacing wires, invasive lines, chest tubes).

2. Cardiac tamponade
   a. Assess for signs of tamponade—arterial hypotension, rising CVP, rising left atrial pressure, muffled heart sounds, weak, thready pulse, neck vein distention, falling urinary output.
   b. Check for diminished amount of drainage in the chest-collection bottle; may indicate that fluid is accumulating elsewhere.
   c. Prepare for pericardiocentesis (see p. 276).

3. MI
   a. Check cardiac enzymes daily. Elevations may indicate MI.
   b. Symptoms may be masked by the usual postoperative discomfort.
      (1) Watch for decreased cardiac output in the presence of normal circulating volume and filling pressure.
      (2) Obtain serial ECGs and isoenzymes to determine extent of myocardial injury.
      (3) Assess pain to differentiate myocardial pain from incisional pain.
   c. Treatment is individualized. Postoperative activity level may be reduced to allow heart adequate time for healing.

4. Embolization
   a. Initiate preventive measures such as antiembolic stockings; omit pressure on popliteal space (leg crossing, raising knee gatch); start passive and active exercises.
   b. Assess respiratory and mental status as described above.
   c. Maintain integrity of all invasive lines.

5. Bleeding
   a. Watch for steady and continuous drainage of blood.
   b. Assess for arterial hypotension, low CVP, increasing pulse rate, and low left atrial and pulmonary artery wedge pressures.
   c. Prepare to administer blood products, IV solutions or protamine sulfate or vitamin K (AquaMEPHYTON)
   d. Prepare for potential return to surgery for bleeding persisting (over 300 mL/h) for 2 hours.

6. Fever/infection
   a. Control higher degrees of fever by use of hypothermia mattress.
   b. Evaluate for atelectasis, pleural effusion, or pneumonia if fever persists. (The most common cause of early postoperative fever [within 24 hours] is atelectasis.)
   c. Evaluate for urinary tract infection/wound infection.
   d. Bear in mind the possibility of infective endocarditis if fever persists.
   e. Draw blood for culture to rule out endocarditis.

7. Renal insufficiency
   a. Measure urine volume; less than 20 mL/h can indicate decreased renal function.
   b. Carry out specific gravity tests to determine kidneys' ability to concentrate urine in renal tubules.
   c. Watch BUN and serum creatinine levels, as well as urine and serum electrolyte levels.
   d. Give rapid-acting diuretics and/or inotropic drugs (dopamine [Intropin], dobutamine [Dobutrex]) to increase cardiac output and renal blood flow.
   e. Prepare the patient for peritoneal dialysis or hemodialysis if indicated. (Renal insufficiency may produce serious cardiac dysrhythmias.)

Patient Education/ Health Maintenance

Note: Specific guidelines will vary slightly between institutions and healthcare providers. Check hospital policy and orders.

1. Instruct about activities.
   a. Increase activities gradually within limits. Avoid strenuous activities until after exercise stress testing.
   b. Take short rest periods.
   c. Avoid lifting more than 20 lb.
   d. Participate in activities that do not cause pain or discomfort.
   e. Increase walking time and distance each day.
   f. Stairs (one to two times daily) the first week; increase as tolerated.
   g. Avoid large crowds at first.
   h. Avoid driving until after first postoperative checkup. At this time, check with healthcare provider.
   i. Resumption of sexual relations parallels ability to participate in other activities. Usually may resume sexual activities 2 weeks after surgery. Avoid if tired or after heavy meal. Consult healthcare provider if chest discomfort, difficult breathing, or palpitations occur and last longer than 15 minutes after intercourse.
   j. Return to work after first postoperative checkup, as advised by healthcare provider.
   k. Expect some chest discomfort.
2. Advise about diet.
   a. Some patients are placed on minimum salt restriction (eg, no salt added at table); cholesterol may be limited.
   b. Weigh daily and report weight gain of more than 5 lb per week.
3. Teach about medications.
   a. Label all medications; give purposes and side effects.
   b. Patients with prosthetic valves may continue warfarin (Coumadin) regimen indefinitely. Explain bleeding precautions.
4. Advise patients with prosthetic valves:
   a. Pregnancy is usually discouraged.
   b. Need for antibiotic coverage before dental and surgical procedures.
   c. Patients on anticoagulants should watch for bleeding and should avoid use of aspirin (and many other drugs)—interferes with action of warfarin.
5. Advise the patient to carry an identification card stating cardiac condition and medications being taken.
6. Encourage compliance with rehabilitation and exercise program after exercise stress testing.
7. Inform the patient whom to contact (and how) in case of an emergency.
8. See also Patient Education After MI, page 297, and Patient Education, Infective Endocarditis, page 304.
9. Explore community support groups: American Heart Association, Mended Hearts Society.

Evaluation

A. Verbalizes understanding of surgical procedure, reduction in fear
B. Extubated 24 hours postoperative; spontaneous unlabored respirations 14 to 18 per minute
C. Blood pressure and heart rate stable; adequate urine output
D. Serum electrolytes within normal range
E. Verbalizes reduced pain
F. Oriented to time and place; no hallucinations
G. No bleeding noted; afebrile; ECGs shows normal sinus rhythm

Selected References

Apple-Hardin, S.(1992). The role of the nurse in noninvasive temporary pacing. *Critical Care Nurse, 12*(3), 10-21.

Brown, L. M., & Brown, A. S. (1994). Transesophageal echocardiography: Implications for the critical care nurse. *Critical Care Nurse, 14*(3), 55-59.

Conover, M. B. (1991). *Understanding electrocardopgraphy* (6th ed.). St. Louis: CU Mosby.

Darling, E. (1994). Overview of electrophysiologic testing. *Critical Care Nursing Clinics of North America, 6*(1), 1-14.

Hochrein, M., & Sohl, L. (1992). Heart smart: A guide to cardiac test. *American Journal of Nursing, 92*(12), 22-25.

Hodgins, C., & Sorenson, G. (1994). Directional coronary athrectomy: A new treatment for coronary artery disease. *Critical Care Nurse, 14*(1), 61-66.

Hudak, C. M., et al. (1994). *Critical care nursing: A holistic approach* (6th ed.). Philadelphia: J.B. Lippincott.

Gaw-Ens, B. (1994). Informational support for families Immediately after CABG surgery. *Critical Care Nurse, 14*(1). 41-50.

Gortner, S., Dirks, J., & Wolfe, M. (1992). The road to recovery for elders after CABG. *American Journal of Nursing, 92*(8), 44-49.

Kinney, M., et al. (1991). *AACN's clinical reference for critical care nursing* (3rd ed.). New York: McGraw-Hill.

Kohles, M., Donaho, B., & Finney, C. (Eds.). (1992). *The nursing clinics of North America, 27*(1), 141-283. Philadelphia: W.B. Saunders.

Millar, S., Sampson, L., & Soukup, Sr., M. (1985). *AACN procedure manual for critical care.* Philadelphia: W.B. Saunders.

Moser, S., Crawford, D., & Thomas, A. (1993). Updated care guidelines for patients with automatic implantable cardioverterdefibrillators. *Critical Care Nurse, 12*(2), 62-71.

Pettney, L., & Leflar-Dileva, K. (1994). Preparing for cardiomyoplasty: A new horizon in cardiac surgery. *Dimensions of Critical Care Nursing, 13*(5), 226-236.

Recker, D. (1994). Patient perception of preoperative cardiac surgical teaching done pre and post admission. *Critical Care Nurse, 14*(1), 52-58.

Saver, C. (1994). Decoding the ACLS algorithms. *American Journal of Nursing, 94*(1), 26-36.

Sirovatka, B. (1993). The implantable cardioverter defibrillator: Patient and family education. *Dimensions of Critical Care Nursing. 12*(6), 328-334.

Smith, M. A. (1994). Noninvasive hemodynamic monitoring with thoracic electrical bioimpedence. *Critical Care Nurse, 14*(3), 56-59.

Thompson, E. (1993). Transesophageal echocardiography: A new window on the heart and great vessels. *Critical Care Nurse, 13*(3), 55-66.

CHAPTER 11 ◆

Cardiac Disorders

Cardiac Disorders

◆ CORONARY ARTERY DISEASE

Coronary artery disease (CAD) is characterized by the accumulation of fatty deposits along the innermost layer of the coronary arteries. The fatty deposits may develop in childhood and progressively enlarge and thicken throughout the life span. The enlarged lesion (atheroma/plaque) can cause a critical narrowing (75% occlusion) of the coronary artery lumen, resulting in a decrease in coronary blood flow and an inadequate supply of oxygen to the heart muscle.

Pathophysiology/Etiology

1. The most widely accepted cause of CAD is the accumulation of lipids (mainly cholesterol) and fibrous materials (smooth muscle cells) within the coronary artery lumen.
   a. Increased blood levels of low-density lipoprotein (LDL—known as the "bad" cholesterol because it transports cholesterol to body tissues) irritate and damage the inner layer of the coronary vessels.
   b. LDL enters the vessel after damaging the protective barrier, accumulates, and forms fatty streaks.
      (1) Fatty streaks are yellow, flat, and cause no significant coronary artery obstruction.
      (2) These lesions develop frequently between the ages of 8 and 18 years.
   c. Smooth muscle cells (from the middle layer of the coronary artery) move to the inner layer to engulf the fatty substance, produce fibrous tissue, and stimulate calcium deposition.
2. This cycle continues, resulting in the transformation of the fatty streak into a fibrous plaque, and eventually a "complicated" CAD lesion evolves.
   a. A complicated lesion develops as small blood vessels grow into the fibrous plaque and the core of the lesion enlarges and calcifies.
   b. The complicated lesion can cause significant coronary obstruction by hemorrhage and ulceration of the plaque.
3. Risk Factors
   a. The three major risk factors include high blood cholesterol levels, hypertension, and cigarette smoking.
   b. Unmodifiable risk factors include age, male sex, race, and family history of CAD.
   c. Other risk factors include diabetes mellitus, obesity, sedentary lifestyle, stress, and Type A personality.

Clinical Manifestations

A. Stable (Effort) Angina Pectoris Chest pain precipitated by physical exertion or emotional stress; increased oxygen demands are placed on the heart muscle, but the ability of the coronary artery to deliver blood to the muscle is impaired because of obstruction by a significant coronary lesion (75% narrowing of the vessel). Rest and nitroglycerin relieve the pain

1. *Character*—substernal chest pain, pressure, heaviness, or discomfort. Other sensations include a squeezing, aching, burning, choking, strangling, and/or cramping pain.
   a. Pain may be mild or severe and typically presents with a gradual buildup of discomfort and subsequent gradual fading away.
   b. May produce numbness or weakness in arms, wrists, or hands.
   c. Associated symptoms include diaphoresis, nausea, indigestion, dyspnea, tachycardia, and increase in blood pressure.
2. *Location*—behind middle or upper third of sternum; the patient generally will make a fist over the site of the pain (positive Levine sign; indicates diffuse deep visceral pain), rather than point to it with his or her finger.
3. *Radiation*—usually radiates to neck, jaw, shoulders, arms, hands, and posterior intrascapular area. Pain occurs more commonly on the left side than the right.
4. *Duration*—usually lasts 1 to 5 minutes after stopping activity; nitroglycerin relieves pain within 1 minute.
5. *Other precipitating factors*—exposure to hot or cold weather, eating a heavy meal, and sexual intercourse increase the workload of the heart and therefore increase oxygen demand.

B. Unstable (Preinfarction) Angina Pectoris Chest pain occurring at rest; no increase in oxygen demand is placed on the heart muscle, but an acute lack of blood flow to the muscle occurs because of coronary artery spasm aggravated by the presence of an enlarged plaque or hemorrhage/ulceration of a complicated lesion. Critical narrowing of the vessel lumen occurs abruptly in either instance
1. A change in frequency, duration, and intensity of stable angina symptoms is indicative of progression to unstable angina.

2. Unstable angina pain lasts longer than 10 minutes, is unrelieved by rest or sublingual nitroglycerin, and mimics signs and symptoms of impending myocardial infarction (see MI, p. 292).

> **NURSING ALERT:**
> Unstable angina can cause sudden death or result in a myocardial infarction. Early recognition and treatment are imperative to prevent complications.

C. Silent Ischemia The absence of chest pain with documented evidence of an imbalance between myocardial oxygen supply and demand (ST depression of 1 mm or more) as determined by ECG, exercise stress test, or ambulatory (Holter) ECG monitoring

1. Silent ischemia most commonly occurs in the early morning hours (6:00 AM–10:00 AM).
2. Arousal causes an increase in sympathetic stimulation and blood viscosity, and coronary vessel tone increase in the morning, causing silent ischemic episodes.

Diagnostic Evaluation

1. *Characteristic chest pain* and clinical history
2. *Nitroglycerin test*—relief of pain with nitroglycerin
3. *ECG stress testing*—progressive increases of speed and elevation of walking on a treadmill increase the workload of the heart. ST and T wave changes occur if myocardial ischemia is induced.
4. *Radionuclide imaging*—a radioisotope, thallium 201, injected during exercise is imaged by camera. Low uptake of the isotope by heart muscle indicates regions of ischemia induced by exercise. Images taken during rest show a reversal of ischemia in those regions affected.
5. *Radionuclide ventriculography* (gated blood pool scanning)—red blood cells tagged with a radioisotope are imaged by camera during exercise and at rest. Wall motion abnormalities of the heart can be detected and ejection fraction estimated.
6. *Cardiac catheterization*—coronary angiography performed during the procedure determines the presence, location, and extent of coronary lesions.

Management

A. Drug Therapy
Antianginal medications (nitrates, beta blockers, calcium channel blockers) are used to maintain a balance between oxygen supply and demand. Reduction of the work load of the heart decreases oxygen demand and consumption. Coronary vessel relaxation promotes blood flow to the heart muscle, thereby increasing oxygen supply.

1. *Nitrates*—cause generalized vasodilation throughout the body.
   a. Nitrates can be administered orally, sublingually, transdermally, or IV and provide short- or long-lasting effects.
   b. Short-acting nitrates provide immediate relief of acute anginal attacks or prophylaxis if taken prior to activity.
   c. Long-acting nitrates prevent anginal episodes and/or reduce severity and frequency of attacks.
2. *Beta blockers*—inhibit sympathetic stimulation of receptors that are located in the conduction system of the heart and in heart muscle.
   a. Some beta blockers inhibit sympathetic stimulation of receptors in the lungs as well as the heart ("non-selective" beta blockers); vasoconstriction of the large airways in the lung occurs; generally contraindicated for patients with chronic obstructive lung disease.
   b. "Cardioselective" beta blockers (in recommended drug ranges) affect only the heart and can be used safely in patients with lung disease.
3. *Calcium channel blockers*—inhibit the movement of calcium within the heart muscle and coronary vessels; promote vasodilation and prevent/control coronary artery spasm.
4. *Antilipid medications*—decrease blood cholesterol and triglyceride levels in patients with elevated levels.

B. Percutaneous Transluminal Angioplasty
1. A balloon-tipped catheter is placed in a coronary vessel narrowed by plaque.
2. The balloon is inflated and deflated to stretch the vessel wall and flatten the lesion (see PTCA, p. 278).
3. Blood flows freely through the unclogged vessel to the heart.

C. Intracoronary Athrectomy
1. A blade-tipped catheter is guided into a coronary vessel to the site of the plaque.
2. Depending on the type of blade, the plaque is either cut, shaved, or pulverized, and then removed.
3. Requires a larger catheter introduction sheath so its use is limited to larger vessels.

D. Coronary Artery Bypass Surgery
1. A graft is surgically attached to the aorta, and the other end of the graft is attached to a distal portion of a coronary vessel.
2. Bypasses obstructive lesions in the vessel and returns adequate blood flow to the heart muscle supplied by the artery (see Heart Surgery, p. 283).

E. Lifestyle Modification
1. Cessation of smoking
2. Control of high blood pressure
3. Lowering of blood cholesterol level

Complications

1. Sudden death due to lethal dysrhythmias
2. Congestive heart failure
3. MI

Nursing Assessment

1. Ask patient to describe anginal attacks.
   a. When do attacks tend to occur? Following a meal? After engaging in certain activities? After physical activities in general? After visits of family/others?
   b. Where is the pain located? Does it radiate?
   c. Was the onset of pain sudden? Gradual?
   d. How long did it last—seconds? minutes? hours?
   e. Was the pain steady and unwavering in quality?

f. Is the discomfort accompanied by other symptoms? Sweating? Lightheadedness? Nausea? Palpitations? Shortness of breath?
g. How is the pain relieved? How long does it take for pain relief?
2. Obtain a baseline 12-lead ECG.
3. Assess patient's and family's knowledge of disease.
4. Identify patient's and family's level of anxiety and use of appropriate coping mechanisms.
5. Gather information regarding the patient's cardiac risk factors.
6. Evaluate patient's medical history for conditions that may influence choice of drug therapy (diabetes, heart failure, previous myocardial infarction, obstructive lung disease).
7. Identify factors that may contribute to noncompliance with prescribed drug therapy.
8. Review renal/hepatic studies and complete blood count.
9. Discuss with patient current activity levels. (Effectiveness of antianginal drug therapy is evaluated by patient's ability to attain higher activity levels.)
10. Discuss patient beliefs regarding modification of risk factors and willingness to change.

Nursing Diagnoses

A. Pain related to an imbalance in oxygen supply and demand
B. Decreased Cardiac Output related to reduced preload, afterload, contractility, and heart rate secondary to hemodynamic effects of drug therapy
C. Anxiety related to chest pain, uncertain prognosis, and threatening environment

Nursing Interventions

A. Relieving Pain
1. Determine intensity of patient's angina.
a. Ask patient to compare the pain with other pain experienced in the past, and on a scale of 1 (lowest) to 10 (highest), rate current pain.
b. Observe for other signs and symptoms: diaphoresis, shortness of breath, protective body posture, dusky facial color, and/or changes in level of consciousness.
2. Place patient in comfortable position.
3. Administer oxygen if prescribed.
4. Obtain blood pressure, apical heart rate, and respiratory rate.
5. Obtain a 12-lead ECG as directed.
6. Administer antianginal medication as prescribed.
7. Report findings to health care providers.
8. Monitor for relief of pain and note duration of anginal episode.
9. Take vital signs every 5 to 10 minutes until angina pain subsides.
10. Monitor for progression of stable angina to unstable angina: increase in frequency and intensity of pain, pain occurring at rest or at low levels of exertion, pain lasting longer than 15 minutes.
11. Determine level of activity that precipitated anginal episode.
12. Identify specific activities patient may engage in that are below the level at which anginal pain occurs.

13. Reinforce the importance of notifying nursing staff whenever angina pain is experienced.

B. Maintaining Cardiac Output
1. Monitor carefully the patient's response to drug therapy.
a. Take blood pressure and heart rate in a sitting and lying position on initiation of long-term therapy (provides baseline data to evaluate for orthostatic hypotension that may occur with drug therapy).
b. Recheck vital signs as indicated by onset of action of drug and at time of drug's peak effect.
c. Note changes in blood pressure of more than 10 mm Hg and changes in heart rate of more than 10 beats.
d. Note patient complaints of headache (especially with use of nitrates) and dizziness.
(1) Administer or teach self-administration of analgesics as directed for headache.
(2) Encourage supine position for dizziness (usually associated with a decrease in blood pressure; preload is enhanced by this mechanism, thereby increasing blood pressure).
e. Institute continuous ECG monitoring or obtain 12-lead ECG as directed.
(1) Interpret rhythm strip every 4 hours for patients on continuous monitoring (beta blockers and calcium channel blockers can cause significant bradycardia and various degrees of heart block).
f. Evaluate for development of heart failure (beta blockers and some calcium channel blockers decrease contractility, thus increasing the likelihood of heart failure).
(1) Obtain serial weights.
(2) Auscultate lung fields for crackles.
(3) Monitor for the presence of edema.
2. Be sure to remove previous nitrate patch or paste before applying new paste or pad (prevents hypotension).
3. Be alert to adverse reaction related to abrupt discontinuation of beta blocker and calcium channel blocker therapy. These drugs must be tapered to prevent a "rebound phenomenon": tachycardia, increase in chest pain, hypertension.
4. Report all untoward drug effects to health care provider.

C. Decreasing Anxiety
1. Explain to the patient and family reasons for hospitalization, diagnostic tests, and therapies administered.
2. Encourage the patient to verbalize fears and concerns regarding illness through frequent conversations—conveys to the patient a willingness to listen.
3. Answer the patient's questions with concise explanations.
4. Administer medications to relieve patient anxiety as directed. Sedatives and tranquilizers—may be used to prevent attacks precipitated by aggravation, excitement, or tension.
5. Explain to the patient the importance of anxiety reduction to assist in control of angina. (Anxiety and fear put an increased stress on the heart, requiring the heart to use more oxygen.) Teach relaxation techniques.
6. Discuss measures to be taken when an anginal episode occurs. (Preparing patient decreases anxiety and allows patient to accurately describe angina.)
a. Review the questions that will be asked during anginal episodes.

b. Review the interventions that will be employed to relieve anginal attacks.

Patient Education/Health Maintenance

A. Instruct Patient and Family About CAD
1. Review the chambers of the heart and the coronary artery system, using a diagram of the heart.
2. Show patient a diagram of a clogged artery; explain how the blockage occurs; point out on the diagram the location of the patient's lesions.
3. Explain what angina is (a warning sign from the heart that there is not enough blood and oxygen because of the blocked artery or spasm).
4. Review specific risk factors that affect CAD development and progression; highlight those risk factors that can be modified and controlled to reduce risk.
5. Discuss the signs and symptoms of angina, precipitating factors, and treatment for attacks. Stress to patient the importance of treating angina symptoms at once.
6. Distinguish for patient the different signs and symptoms associated with stable angina versus preinfarction angina.

B. Identify Suitable Activity Level to Prevent Angina
Advise the patient on the following:

1. Participate in a normal daily program of activities that do not produce chest discomfort, shortness of breath, and undue fatigue. Begin regular exercise regimen as directed by health care provider.
2. Avoid activities known to cause anginal pain—sudden exertion, walking against the wind, extremes of temperature, high altitude, emotionally stressful situations; these may accelerate heart rate, raise blood pressure, and increase cardiac work.
3. Refrain from engaging in physical activity for 2 hours after meals. Rest after each meal if possible.
4. Do not undertake activities requiring heavy effort (eg, carrying heavy objects).
5. Try to avoid cold weather if possible; dress warmly and walk more slowly. Wear scarf over nose and mouth when in cold air.
6. Reduce weight, if necessary, to reduce cardiac load.

C. Instruct About Appropriate Use of Medications and Side Effects
1. Carry nitroglycerin at all times.
   a. Nitroglycerin is volatile and is inactivated by heat, moisture, air, light, and time.
   b. Keep nitroglycerin in original dark glass container, tightly closed to prevent absorption of drug by other pills or pillbox.
   c. Nitroglycerin should cause a slight burning or stinging sensation under the tongue when it is potent.
2. Place nitroglycerin under tongue at first sign of chest discomfort.
   a. Stop all effort or activity; sit, and take nitroglycerin tablet—relief should be obtained in a few minutes.
   b. Bite the tablet between front teeth and slip under tongue to dissolve if quick action is desired.
   c. Repeat dosage in a few minutes for total of 3 tablets if relief is not obtained.

d. Keep a record of number of tablets taken to evaluate any change in anginal pattern.
e. Take nitroglycerin prophylactically to avoid pain known to occur with certain activities.

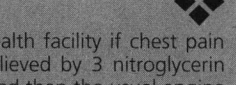
NURSING ALERT:
Instruct patient to go to the nearest health facility if chest pain persists more than 15 minutes, is unrelieved by 3 nitroglycerin tablets, or is more intense and widespread than the usual angina episodes. (Patient should not drive self.)

3. Demonstrate for patient how to administer nitroglycerin paste correctly.
   a. Place paste on calibrated strip.
   b. Remove previous paste on skin by wiping gently with tissue.
   c. Rotate site of administration to avoid skin irritation.
   d. Apply paste to skin; use plastic wrap to protect clothing if not provided on strip.
   e. Have patient return demonstration.
4. Instruct patient on administration of transdermal nitroglycerin patches.
   a. Remove previous patch; wipe area with tissue to remove any residual medication.
   b. Apply patch to a clean dry nonhairy area of body.
   c. Rotate administration sites.
   d. Instruct patient not to remove patch for swimming or bathing.
5. Teach about side effects of other medications.
   a. Constipation—verapamil (Calan)
   b. Ankle edema—nifedipine (Procardia)
   c. Heart failure (shortness of breath, weight gain, edema)—beta or calcium channel blockers
   d. Dizziness—vasodilators, antihypertensives

COMMUNITY-BASED CARE TIP:
Ensure that patient has enough medication until next follow-up appointment or trip to the pharmacy. Warn against abrupt withdrawal of beta or calcium channel blockers to prevent rebound effect.

D. Counsel on Risk Factors and Lifestyle Changes
1. Inform patient of methods of stress reduction such as biofeedback and relaxation techniques.
2. Review information on low-fat/low-cholesterol diet with patient.
   a. Suggest to patient available cookbooks (American Heart Association) that may assist in planning and preparing foods.
   b. Have dietitian visit patient to design a menu plan.
3. Inform patient of available cardiac rehabilitation programs that offer structured classes on exercise, smoking cessation, and weight control.
4. Avoid excessive caffeine intake (coffee, cola drinks) that can increase the heart rate and produce angina.
5. Do not use "diet pills," nasal decongestants, or any over-the-counter medications that can increase the heart rate or stimulate high blood pressure.
6. Avoid the use of alcohol or drink only in moderation (alcohol can increase hypotensive side effects of drugs).

7. Encourage follow-up visits for control of diabetes and hypertension.

Evaluation

A. Verbalizes relief of pain
B. Blood pressure and heart rate stable
C. Verbalizes lessening anxiety, ability to cope

◆ MYOCARDIAL INFARCTION

Myocardial infarction (MI) refers to a dynamic process by which one or more regions of the heart muscle experience a severe and prolonged decrease in oxygen supply because of insufficient coronary blood flow; subsequently, necrosis or "death" to the myocardial tissue occurs. The onset of the myocardial infarction process may be sudden or gradual and the progression of the event to completion takes approximately 3 to 6 hours.

Pathophysiology/Etiology

1. Acute coronary thrombosis (partial or total)—associated with 90% of MIs.
   a. Severe coronary artery disease (greater than 70% narrowing of the artery) precipitates thrombus formation.
   b. Intramural hemorrhage into atheromatous plaques causes the lesion to enlarge and occlude the vessel; dissecting hemorrhage can also occur.
   c. The plaque ruptures into the vessel lumen and a thrombus forms on top of the ulcerated lesion, with resultant vessel occlusion.
2. Other etiologic factors include: coronary artery spasm, coronary artery embolism, infectious diseases causing arterial inflammation, hypoxia, anemia, and severe exertion or stress on the heart in the presence of significant coronary artery disease (ie, surgical procedures or shoveling snow).
3. Different degrees of damage occur to the heart muscle (Fig. 11-1):
   a. *Zone of necrosis*—death to the heart muscle caused by extensive and complete oxygen deprivation; irreversible damage
   b. *Zone of injury*—region of the heart muscle surrounding the area of necrosis; inflamed and injured, but still viable if adequate oxygenation can be restored
   c. *Zone of ischemia*—region of the heart muscle surrounding the area of injury, which is ischemic and viable; not endangered unless extension of the infarction occurs.
4. According to the layers of the heart muscle involved, MIs can be classified as:
   a. Transmural (Q wave) infarction—area of necrosis occurs throughout the entire thickness of the heart muscle.
   b. Subendocardial (nontransmural/non-Q) infarction—area of necrosis is confined to the innermost layer of the heart lining the chambers.

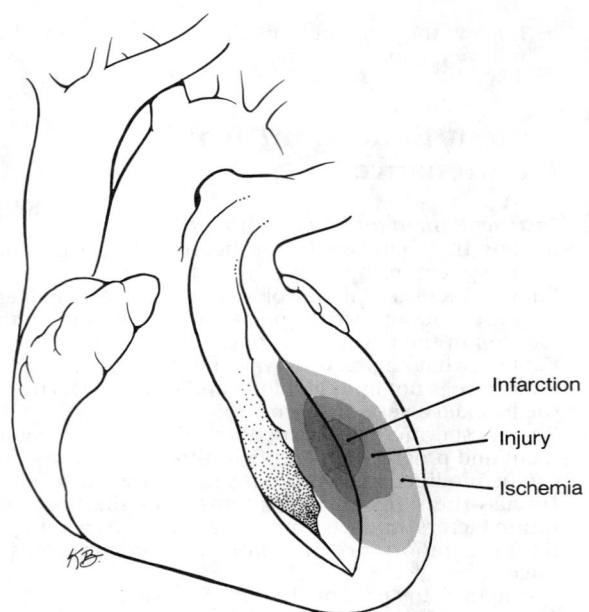

FIGURE 11-1 *Different degrees of damage occur to the heart muscle after a myocardial infarction. The diagram shows the zones of necrosis, injury, and ischemia.*

NURSING ALERT:
Patients with subendocardial infarctions should be considered as having an uncompleted MI; monitor carefully for signs and symptoms of extension of heart muscle damage.

5. Location of MI is identified as the location of the damaged heart muscle within the left ventricle: inferior, anterior, lateral, and posterior.
   a. Left ventricle is the most common and dangerous location for an MI, as it is the main pumping chamber of the heart.
   b. Right ventricular infarctions commonly occur in conjunction with damage to the inferior and/or posterior wall of the left ventricle.
6. Region of the heart muscle that becomes damaged—determined by the coronary artery that becomes obstructed (Fig. 11-2).
7. The amount of heart muscle damage and the location of the MI—determines prognosis.

Clinical Manifestations

1. Chest pain
   a. Severe, diffuse steady substernal pain of a crushing and squeezing nature
   b. Not relieved by rest or sublingual vasodilator therapy, but requires narcotics
   c. May radiate to the arms (commonly the left), shoulders, neck, back, and/or jaw
   d. Continues for more than 15 minutes
   e. May produce anxiety and fear, resulting in an increase in heart rate, blood pressure, and respiratory rate

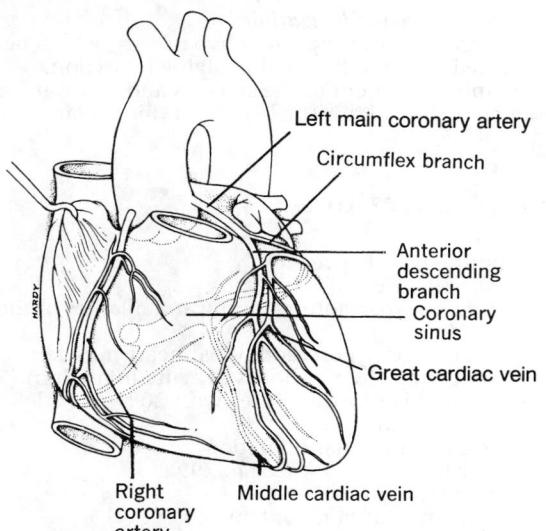

FIGURE 11-2 *Diagram of the coronary arteries arising from the aorta and encircling the heart. Some of the coronary veins also are shown. (Chaffee, E. E., & Greisheimer, E. M.* Basic physiology and anatomy. *Philadelphia: JB Lippincott.)*

2. Diaphoresis, cool clammy skin, facial pallor
3. Hypertension or hypotension
4. Bradycardia or tachycardia
5. Premature ventricular and/or atrial beats
6. Palpitations, severe anxiety, dyspnea
7. Disorientation, confusion, restlessness
8. Fainting, marked weakness
9. Nausea, vomiting, hiccups
10. Atypical symptoms: epigastric or abdominal distress, dull aching or tingling sensations, shortness of breath, extreme fatigue

NURSING ALERT:
Many patients do not have symptoms; these are "silent myocardial infarctions." Nevertheless, there still is resultant damage to the heart.

GERONTOLOGIC ALERT:
Elderly patients are more likely to experience silent MIs or have atypical symptoms: hypotension, low body temperature, vague complaints of discomfort, mild perspiration, strokelike symptoms, dizziness, change in sensorium.

Diagnostic Evaluation

A. **ECG Changes**
1. Generally occur within 2 to 12 hours, but may take 72 to 96 hours
2. Necrotic, injured, and ischemic tissue alter ventricular depolarization and repolarization.
   a. ST segment depression and T wave inversion indicate a pattern of ischemia.

b. ST elevation indicates an injury pattern
c. Q waves (Fig. 11-3) indicate tissue necrosis and are permanent. A pathologic Q wave is one that is greater than 3 mm in depth or greater than one-third the height of the R wave.

NURSING ALERT:
A normal ECG does not rule out the possibility of infarction, as ECG changes can be subtle and obscured by underlying conditions (bundle branch blocks, electrolyte disturbances).

B. **Elevation of Serum Enzymes and Isoenzymes**
1. Enzymes are drawn in a serial pattern, usually on admission and every 6 to 24 hours until three samples are obtained; enzyme activity then is correlated to the extent of heart muscle damage (see p. 249).
2. Enzymes commonly evaluated include creatinine kinase (CK), lactic dehydrogenase (LDH), and aspartate aminotransferase (AST).
3. CK and LDH can be broken down further into isoenzymes, which are more organ-specific.
   a. CK-MB is specific to heart muscle and thus the most sensitive enzyme for determining heart muscle damage.
   b. LDH1 and LDH2 are specific to heart muscle and thus elevated.

C. **Other Findings**
1. White blood cell count and sedimentation rate elevate due to inflammatory process associated with the damaged heart muscle.
2. Radionuclide imaging allows recognition of areas of decreased perfusion.
3. Positron emission tomography determines the presence of reversible heart muscle injury and irreversible or necrotic tissue; extent to which the injured heart muscle has responded to treatment also can be determined.

Management

Therapy is aimed at the protection of ischemic and injured heart tissue to preserve muscle function, reduce the infarct size, and prevent death. Innovative modalities provide early restoration of coronary blood flow, and the use of phar-

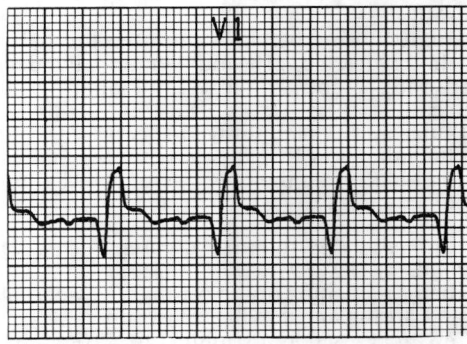

FIGURE 11-3 *Abnormal Q wave.*

macologic agents improve oxygen supply and demand, reduce and/or prevent dysrhythmias, and inhibit the progression of coronary artery disease.

A. Oxygen Therapy
Improves oxygenation to ischemic heart muscle.

B. Pain Control
Endogenous catecholamine release during pain imposes an increased workload on the heart muscle, thus causing an increase in oxygen demand.

1. *Opiate analgesic therapy*
   a. Morphine is used to relieve pain, improve cardiac hemodynamics by reducing preload and afterload, and to provide anxiety relief.
   b. Meperidine (Demerol) is useful for pain management in those patients allergic to morphine or sensitive to respiratory depression.
2. *Vasodilator therapy*
   a. Nitroglycerin (sublingual, IV, paste) promotes venous (low-dose) and arterial (high-dose) relaxation as well as relaxation of coronary vessels and prevention of coronary spasm.
   b. Myocardial oxygen demand is reduced with subsequent pain relief.
   c. Persistent chest pain requires IV nitroglycerin.
3. *Anxiolytic therapy*
   a. Benzodiazepines are used with analgesics when anxiety complicates chest pain and its relief.

C. Pharmacologic Therapy
1. Thrombolytic agents such as tissue plasminogen activator (Activase), steptokinase (Streptase), and urokinase (Abbokinase), reestablish blood flow in coronary vessels by dissolving obstructing thrombus.
   a. No effect on the underlying stenosis that precipitated the thrombus to form.
   b. Administered IV or intracoronary.
2. Anticoagulation therapy is useful as an adjunct to thrombolytic therapy. Also used in situations of prolonged bedrest, pulmonary embolism, deep vein thrombosis, mural thrombi, cardiogenic shock, and patients with atrial fibrillation.
3. Beta-adrenergic blocking agents improve oxygen supply and demand, decrease sympathetic stimulation to the heart, promote blood flow in the small vessels of the heart, and have antidysrhythmic effects.
   a. Appears to lower mortality and decrease chance of reinfarction and sudden death post-MI.
4. Antidysrhythmic therapy—lidocaine (Xylocaine) decreases ventricular irritability, which commonly occurs post-MI.
5. Calcium channel blockers improve the balance between oxygen supply and demand by decreasing heart rate, blood pressure, and dilating coronary vessels.
   a. Diltiazem has been shown to decrease the incidence of reinfarction in patients with non–Q-wave MIs and is currently the only calcium blocker proven to be beneficial.

D. Percutaneous Transluminal Coronary Angioplasty (PTCA)
1. Mechanical opening of the coronary vessel can be performed during an evolving infarction.
2. PTCA can be used as an adjunct to thrombolytic therapy (see PTCA, p. 278).

E. Surgical Revascularization
1. Emergency coronary artery bypass surgery can be performed within 6 hours of evolving infarction.
2. Definite treatment of the stenosis and less scar formation on the heart is the benefit of this therapy.

Complications

1. Rhythm disturbances
2. Cardiac failure
   a. Infarct expansion (thinning and dilation of the necrotic zone)
   b. Infarct extension (additional heart muscle necrosis occurring after 24 hours of acute infarction).
   c. Congestive heart failure (with 20%–35% left ventricle damage)
   d. Right ventricular infarction
   e. Cardiogenic shock (see p. 299)
   f. Reinfarction
   g. Ischemic cardiomyopathy
3. Cardiac rupture
4. Papillary muscle rupture
5. Ventricular mural thrombus
6. Thromboemboli
7. Ventricular aneurysm
8. Cardiac tamponade
9. Pericarditis (2–3 days post-MI)
10. Psychiatric problems—depression, personality changes

Nursing Assessment

1. Gather information regarding the patient's chest pain:
   a. Nature and intensity—describe the pain in patient's own words and compare it with pain experienced in the past.
   b. Onset and duration—exact time pain occurred, as well as the time pain relieved or diminished (if applicable).
   c. Location and radiation—point to the area where the pain is located and to other areas where the pain seems to travel.
   d. Precipitating and aggravating factors—describe the activity performed just prior to the onset of pain and if any maneuvers and/or medications alleviated the pain.
2. Question patient about other symptoms experienced associated with the pain. Observe patient for diaphoresis, facial pallor, dyspnea, guarding behaviors, rigid body posture, extreme weakness, confusion.
3. Evaluate cognitive, behavioral, and emotional status.
4. Question patient regarding prior health status with emphasis on current medications, allergies (opiate analgesics, iodine, shellfish), recent trauma or surgery, aspirin ingestion, peptic ulcers, fainting spells, drug and alcohol use.
5. Analyze information for contraindications for thrombolytic therapy and/or PTCA.
6. Gather information on presence or absence of cardiac risk factors.
7. Identify patient's social support system and potential caregiver(s).
8. Identify significant other's reaction to the crisis situation.

Nursing Diagnoses

Also see Nursing Care Plan 11-1.

A. Pain related to an imbalance in oxygen supply and demand
B. Anxiety related to chest pain, fear of death, threatening environment
C. Decreased Cardiac Output related to impaired contractility.
D. Activity Intolerance related to insufficient oxygenation to perform activities of daily living (ADL), deconditioning effects of bedrest
E. Risk for Injury (bleeding) related to dissolution of protective clots
F. Altered Tissue Perfusion (myocardial): related to coronary restenosis, extension of infarction
G. Ineffective Individual Coping related to threats to self-esteem, disruption of sleep–rest pattern, lack of significant support system, and loss of control

Nursing Interventions

A. *Reducing Pain*
1. Handle patient carefully while providing initial care, starting IV infusion, obtaining baseline vital signs, and attaching electrodes for continuous ECG monitoring.
2. Administer oxygen by nasal cannula if prescribed and encourage patient to take deep breaths—may decrease incidence of dysrhythmias by allowing the heart to be less ischemic and less irritable; may reduce infarct size, decrease anxiety, and resolve chest pain.
3. Offer support and reassurance to patient that relief of pain is a priority.
4. Administer sublingual nitroglycerin as directed; recheck blood pressure (BP), heart rate (HR), and respiratory rate prior to administering nitrate therapy and 10 to 15 minutes after dose.
5. Administer narcotics as prescribed (morphine [Duramorph] or meperidine [Demerol])—decreases sympathetic activity and reduces heart rate, respirations, blood pressure, muscle tension, and anxiety.
   a. Use caution in administering narcotics to patients with chronic obstructive pulmonary disease, hypotension, dehydration, and to the elderly.
   b. Be alert that meperidine can have a vagolytic effect and cause tachycardia, thus increasing myocardial oxygen demands.

> **GERONTOLOGIC ALERT:**
> Elderly patients are extremely susceptible to respiratory depression in response to narcotics. Analgesic agents with less profound effects on the respiratory center should be used. Anxiolytic agents also should be used with caution.

6. Obtain baseline vital signs prior to giving agents and 10 to 15 minutes after each dose. Place patient in a supine position during administration to minimize hypotension.
7. Give IV nitroglycerin as prescribed. Monitor BP continuously with automatic blood pressure machine or intra-arterially or every 5 minutes with auscultatory method while titrating for pain relief.

> **NURSING ALERT:**
> Intravenous administration is the preferred route for analgesic medication, as intramuscular injections can cause elevations in serum enzymes, resulting in an incorrect diagnosis of myocardial infarction.

8. Review with patient frequently the importance of reporting any chest pain, discomfort, and/or epigastric distress without delay.

B. *Alleviating Anxiety*
1. Explain equipment, procedures, and need for frequent assessment to patient and significant others.
2. Discuss with patient and family member the anticipated nursing and medical regimen.
   a. Explain visiting hours and need to limit number of visitors at one time.
   b. Offer family members preferred times to phone unit to check on patient's status.
3. Observe for autonomic signs of anxiety such as increases in heart rate, BP, respiratory rate, tremulousness.
4. Administer antianxiety agents as prescribed.
   a. Explain to patient the reason for sedation: undue anxiety can make the heart more irritable and require more oxygen.
   b. Assure patient that the goal of sedation is to promote comfort and therefore should be requested if anxious, excitable, or "jittery" feelings occur.
   c. Observe for adverse effects of sedation such as lethargy, confusion, and/or increased agitation.
5. Maintain consistency of care with one or two nurses regularly assisting patient, especially if severe anxiety is present.
6. Offer back massage to promote relaxation, decrease muscle tension, and improve skin integrity.

C. *Maintaining Hemodynamic Stability*
1. Monitor BP every 2 hours or as directed—hypertension increases afterload of the heart, elevating oxygen demand; hypotension causes reduced coronary and tissue perfusion.
2. Monitor respirations and lung fields every 2 to 4 hours or as prescribed.
   a. Auscultate for normal and abnormal breath sounds (crackles may indicate left ventricular failure; diffuse crackles indicate pulmonary edema).

> **NURSING ALERT:**
> Auscultation of clear lungs in the presence of cool, clammy skin, jugular venous distension, and hypotension may indicate right ventricular infarction.

   b. Observe for dyspnea, tachypnea, frothy pink sputum, orthopnea—may indicate left ventricular failure, pulmonary embolus, pulmonary edema.
3. Evaluate heart rate and heart sounds every 2 to 4 hours or as directed.
   a. Compare apical heart rate with radial pulse rate and determine the pulse deficit.
   b. Auscultate heart for the presence of a third heart sound (failing ventricle), fourth heart sound (stiffening ventricular muscle due to MI), friction rub (pericarditis), murmurs (valvular and papillary muscle dysfunction, intraventricular septal rupture).

4. Note presence of jugular venous distention and liver engorgement.
   a. Estimate right atrial pressure by determining jugular venous pressure.
   b. Observe for hepatojugular reflux.
5. Evaluate the major arterial pulses (weak pulse and/or presence of pulsus alternans indicates decreased cardiac output; irregularity results from dysrhythmias).
6. Take body temperature every 4 hours or as directed (most patients develop an increase in temperature within 24–48 hours due to tissue necrosis).
7. Observe for presence of edema.
8. Monitor skin color and temperature (cool, clammy skin and pallor associated with vasoconstriction secondary to decreased cardiac output).
9. Be alert to change in mental status such as confusion, restlessness, disorientation.
10. Employ hemodynamic monitoring as indicated.
11. Evaluate urine output (30 mL/hr)—decrease in volume reflects a decrease in renal blood flow.
12. Monitor for life-threatening dysrhythmias (common within 24 hours following infarctions).
    a. Be vigilant for occurrence of any type of premature ventricular beats—may predict ventricular fibrillation or ventricular tachycardia.
    b. Anticipate possibility of reperfusion dysrhythmias following thrombolytic therapy.
    c. Correct dysrhythmias immediately as directed. Lidocaine (Xylocaine) may be given prophylactically to protect against ventricular fibrillation and ventricular tachycardia.

D. Increasing Activity Tolerance
1. Promote rest with early gradual increase in mobilization—prevents deconditioning, which occurs with bedrest.
   a. Minimize environmental noise.
   b. Provide a comfortable environmental temperature.
   c. Avoid unnecessary interruptions and procedures.
   d. Structure routine care measures to include rest periods after activity.
   e. Discuss with patient and family members the purpose of limited activity and visitors—to help the heart heal by lowering heart rate and blood pressure to maintain cardiac workload at lowest level and decrease oxygen consumption.
   f. Promote restful diversional activities for patient (reading, listening to music, drawing, crossword puzzles, crafts).
   g. Encourage frequent position changes while in bed.
2. Assist patient with prescribed activities.
   a. Assist patient to rise slowly from a supine position to minimize orthostatic hypotension.
   b. Encourage passive and active range-of-motion exercise as directed while on bedrest.
   c. Measure the length and width of the unit so that patients can gradually increase their activity levels with specific guidelines (walk one width [150 ft.] of the unit).
   d. Elevate patient's feet when out of bed in chair to promote venous return.
   e. Implement a step-by-step program for progressive activity as directed.

E. Preventing Bleeding
1. Take vital signs every 15 minutes during infusion of thrombolytic agent and then hourly.

2. Observe for presence of hematomas or skin breakdown, especially in potential pressure areas such as the sacrum, back, elbows, ankles.
3. Be alert to verbal complaints of back pain indicative of possible retroperitoneal bleeding.
4. Observe all puncture sites every 15 minutes during infusion of thrombolytic therapy and then hourly for bleeding.
5. Apply manual pressure to venous or arterial sites if bleeding occurs. Use pressure dressings for coverage of all access sites.
6. Observe for blood in stool, emesis, urine, and sputum.
7. Minimize venipunctures and arterial punctures; use heparin lock for blood sampling and medication administration.
8. Avoid intramuscular injections.
9. Caution patient about vigorous tooth brushing, hair combing, or shaving.
10. Avoid trauma to patient by minimizing frequent handling of patient.
11. Monitor lab work: prothrombin time (PT), partial thromboplastin time (PTT), hematocrit (Hct), and hemoglobin (Hgb).
12. Check for current blood type and crossmatch.
13. Administer antacids as directed to prevent stress ulcers.
14. Implement emergency interventions as directed in the event of bleeding: fluid, volume expanders, blood products.
15. Monitor for changes in mental status and headache.
16. Avoid vigorous oral suctioning.
17. Avoid use of automatic BP device above puncture sites or hematoma. Use care in taking BP; use arm not being used for thrombolytic therapy.

F. Maintaining Tissue Perfusion
1. Observe for persistent and/or recurrence of signs and symptoms of ischemia: chest pain, diaphoresis, hypotension—may indicate extension of MI and/or reocclusion of coronary vessel.
2. Report immediately.
3. Administer oxygen as directed.
4. Record a 12-lead ECG.
5. Prepare patient for possible emergency procedure(s): cardiac catheterization, bypass surgery, PTCA, thrombolytic therapy.

G. Strengthening Coping Abilities
1. Listen carefully to patient and family members to ascertain their cognitive appraisals of stressors and threats.
2. Assist patient to establish a positive attitude toward illness and progress adaptively through the grieving process.
3. Manipulate environment to promote restful sleep by maintaining patient's usual sleep patterns.
4. Be alert to signs and symptoms of sleep deprivation—irritability, disorientation, hallucinations, diminished pain tolerance, aggressiveness.
5. Minimize possible adverse emotional response to transfer from the intensive care unit to the intermediate care unit:
   a. Introduce the admitting nurse from the intermediate care unit to the patient before transfer.
   b. Plan for the intermediate care nurse to answer questions the patient may have and to inform patient what to expect relative to physical layout of unit, nursing routines, and visiting hours.

Patient Education/Health Maintenance

Goals are to restore patient to optimal physiologic, psychological, social, and work level; aid in restoring confidence and self-esteem; develop patient's self-monitoring skills and assist in managing cardiac problems; modify risk factors.

1. Inform the patient and family member about what has happened to heart.
   a. Explain basic cardiac anatomy and physiology
   b. Identify the difference between angina and MI.
   c. Describe how the heart heals and that healing is not complete for 6 to 8 weeks following attack.
   d. Discuss what the patient can do to assist in the recovery process and reduce the chance of future heart attacks.
2. Instruct patient on how to judge the body's response to activity.
   a. Introduce the concept that different activities require varied expenditures of oxygen.
   b. Emphasize the importance of rest and relaxation alternating with activity.
   c. Instruct patient how to take pulse prior to and after activity, as well as guidelines for the acceptable increases in heart rate that should occur.
   d. Review signs and symptoms indicative of a poor response to increased activity levels: chest pain, extreme fatigue, shortness of breath.
3. Design an individualized activity progression program for patient as directed.
   a. Determine activity levels appropriate for patient as prescribed and by predischarge low-level exercise stress test.
   b. Encourage patient and family member to list activities they enjoy and would like to resume.
   c. Establish the energy expenditure of each activity (ie, which are most demanding on the heart) and rank activities from lowest to highest.
   d. Instruct patient to move from one activity to another after the heart has been able to manage the previous workload as determined by signs and symptoms and pulse rate.
   e. Give patient specific activity guidelines and explain activity guidelines will be reevaluated after heart heals:
      (1) Walk daily, gradually increasing distance and time as prescribed.
      (2) Avoid activities that tense muscles, such as weight lifting, lifting heavy objects, isometric exercises, pushing and/or pulling heavy loads.
      (3) Avoid working with arms overhead.
      (4) Gradually return to work.
      (5) Avoid extremes in temperature.
      (6) Do not rush, avoid tenseness.
   f. Tell patient that sexual relations may be resumed on advice of health care provider, usually after exercise tolerance is assessed.
      (1) If patient can walk briskly or climb two flights of stairs, can usually resume sexual activity with familiar partner; resumption of sexual activity parallels resumption of usual activities.
      (2) Sexual activity should be avoided after eating a heavy meal, after drinking alcohol, or when tired.
   g. Advise getting at least 7 hours of sleep each night and take 20- to 30-minute rest periods twice a day.
   h. Advise limiting visitors to 3 to 4 daily for 15 to 30 minutes and shorten phone conversations.
4. Advise eating 3 to 4 small meals per day rather than large heavy meals. Rest 1 hour after meals.
5. Advise limiting caffeine and alcohol intake.
6. Driving a car must be cleared with health care provider at a follow-up visit.
7. Teach patient about medication regimen and side effects.
8. Instruct the patient to notify the health care provider when the following symptoms appear:
   a. Chest pressure or pain not relieved in 15 minutes by nitroglycerin or rest
   b. Shortness of breath
   c. Unusual fatigue
   d. Swelling of feet and ankles
   e. Fainting, dizziness
   f. Very slow or rapid heart beat
9. Assist patient to reduce risk of another MI by risk factor modification.
   a. Explain to patient the major risk factors that can increase chances for having another MI: smoking, high blood cholesterol levels, and hypertension. Related risk factors include obesity, family history, diabetes, stress, and lack of exercise.
   b. Instruct patient in strategies to modify risk factors.
10. For additional information and support refer to: The American Heart, Lung, and Blood Institute; Public Inquiries and Reports Office, Building 31; Besthesda, MD 20205.

NURSING CARE PLAN 11-1 ◆ *Caring for a Patient With Acute MI*

Mr. M. is a 60-year-old male admitted to your unit with a diagnosis of an acute inferior wall MI. From your assessment and knowledge of acute MI, you develop your plan of care.

Subjective data: Mr. M. is complaining of severe crushing chest pain unrelieved by rest which has lasted for 2 hours. The pain is substernal and does not radiate. He tells you that he smokes 2 packs of cigarettes per day, is a manager at an electronics firm, and that his father died at age 59 from a heart attack.

Objective data: Vital signs: Pulse 110 and irregular, BP 90/68, respirations 28. His cardiac monitor shows sinus tachycardia with frequent PVCs and his 12-lead ECG shows ST elevation in leads II, III, and AVF. He has no significant Q waves at this time. His heart sound are normal except for the irregularity, and his lungs are clear. He is pale, diaphoretic, and holding his chest.

(continued)

NURSING CARE PLAN 11-1 ◆ *Caring for a Patient With Acute MI* (continued)

NURSING DIAGNOSIS: Pain related to an imbalance in oxygen supply and demand

GOAL: Pain will be reduced.

NURSING INTERVENTIONS	RATIONALE	EVALUATION
1. Position Mr. M. in bed in semi-Fowler's position.	1. This allows for rest and adequate chest excursion, to increase available oxygen, and to decrease cardiac work.	1. Resting in semi-Fowler's position
2. Administer oxygen via nasal cannula at 4 L/min.	2. To increase oxygen supply. May decrease pain and PVCs.	2. Color improved and verbalizes decreased pain.
3. Administer nitroglycerine and morphine based on vital signs and pain relief.	3. Both medications will help to alleviate pain by decreasing venous return to the heart, thereby decreasing cardiac work. Morphine will also help to decrease the patient's sensation of pain.	3. Verbalizes decreased pain.
4. Monitor BP closely, via noninvasive BP monitor.	4. Both of the above medications may decrease the BP as both will decrease venous return. Intra arterial blood pressure monitoring may be used if condition warrants.	4. BP remains stable.
5. Attach electrodes for continuous bedside cardiac monitor. Monitor heart rate and rhythm frequently.	5. Increases in heart rate may indicate pain, anxiety, hypotension. Decreases in heart rate may indicate heart blocks. Dysrhythmias are common during the initial stages of an acute MI.	5. Heart rate within normal limits.
6. Administer and monitor thrombolytic therapy.	6. May help to relieve the coronary occlusion.	6. Blood flow restored as evidenced by decreased pain and no further ECG changes.
7. Monitor for signs of bleeding, avoid unnecessary venous or arterial punctures.	7. Thrombolytics cause clot lysis, may cause bleeding.	7. No signs of bleeding.

NURSING DIAGNOSIS: Decreased cardiac output related to decreased cardiac contractility and dysrhythmias

GOAL: Cardiac output will improve.

NURSING INTERVENTIONS	RATIONALE	EVALUATION
1. Administer IV fluids as ordered.	1. IV fluid may be necessary to compensate for the decreased venous return caused by nitrates and morphine.	1. BP improved.

NURSING INTERVENTIONS	RATIONALE	EVALUATION
2. Monitor closely for signs of developing left ventricular failure, ie, auscultate lung sounds for crackles and heart sounds for S₃.	2. Left ventricular failure may develop as a result of the decreased myocardial contractility and/or the administration of excess IV fluids.	2. Lungs clear and heart sounds normal.
3. Monitor urine output hourly.	3. A decrease in urine output may indicate a decrease in renal blood flow.	3. Urine output greater than 30 mL per hour.

(continued)

NURSING CARE PLAN 11-1 ◆ Caring for a Patient With Acute MI (continued)

NURSING INTERVENTIONS	RATIONALE	EVALUATION
4. Monitor mental status.	4. A change in mental status may indicate a decrease in cardiac output.	4. Remains alert and oriented.
5. Employ hemodynamic monitoring: CVP and pulmonary artery pressures via a pulmonary artery catheter; calculate cardiac index and systemic vascular resistance.	5. These parameters will help to guide fluid volume administration, vasoactive drug administration, and assess cardiac performance.	5. CVP, PAP, PCWP, CI, and SVR remain within normal limits.
6. Interpret rhythm strip at least every 4 hours, more frequently as condition warrants. Administer antiarrhythmics, if indicated.	6. Dysrhythmias such as PVCs result in a decreased stroke volume and less coronary artery filling time. Frequent monitoring, especially during the first few hours of an acute MI and during thrombolytic therapy administration is necessary to prevent/treat lethal dysrhythmias.	6. PVCs decreasing in frequency.
7. Administer vasopressors; titrate to BP response.	7. Administration of vasopressors in the setting of acute MI is controversial in that they may cause an increase in systemic vascular resistance which increases cardiac work.	7. BP improved without worsening chest pain or ECG changes.

NURSING DIAGNOSIS: Anxiety related to chest pain, fear of death, threatening environment, invasive therapies, and uncertain prognosis

GOAL: Anxiety will be alleviated.

NURSING INTERVENTIONS	RATIONALE	EVALUATION
1. Explain equipment, procedures and need for frequent assessment to Mr. M. and his family. Discuss visiting hours and the need to allow for rest.	1. Aids in decreasing anxiety due to threatening environment.	1. Mr. M. and family verbalize understanding of plan of care. Plan for visiting established.
2. Observe for autonomic signs/symptoms of anxiety, ie, increased heart rate, BP, and respiratory rate.	2. Anxiety is associated with an increase in sympathetic activity which increases cardiac work.	2. No autonomic signs of anxiety.
3. Administer diazepam (Valium).	3. May aid in limiting Mr. M.'s anxiety.	3. Verbalizes decrease in anxiety after medication.
4. Offer back massage.	4. Touch and massage may promote relaxation.	4. Verbalizes decrease in tension after massage.
5. Maintain continuity of care.	5. Consistency of routine and staff promotes trust and confidence.	5. Cooperative with care and talkative with staff.

◆ CARDIOGENIC SHOCK

Cardiogenic shock occurs when the heart muscle loses its contractile power. Extensive damage of the left ventricle (40% or greater) due to myocardial infarction commonly initiates a perpetuating "shock cycle."

Pathophysiology/Etiology

1. Impaired contractility causes a marked reduction in cardiac output.
2. Decreased cardiac output results in a lack of blood and oxygen to the heart as well as other vital organs (brain and kidneys).

3. Lack of blood and oxygen to the heart muscle results in continued damage to the muscle, a further decline in contractile power, and a continued inability of the heart to provide blood and oxygen to vital organs.
4. End-stage cardiomyopathy, severe valvular dysfunction, and ventricular aneurysm also can precipitate cardiogenic shock.

Clinical Manifestations

1. Confusion, restlessness, mental lethargy (due to poor perfusion of brain)
2. Low systolic pressure (80 mm Hg or 30 mm Hg less than previous levels)
3. Oliguria—urine output less than 30 mL per hour for at least 2 hours—due to decreased perfusion of kidneys
4. Cold, clammy skin (blood is shunted from the peripheral circulation to perfuse vital organs)
5. Weak, thready peripheral pulses, fatigue, hypotension—due to inadequate cardiac output
6. Dyspnea, tachypnea, cyanosis (increased left ventricular pressures result in elevation of left atrial and pulmonary pressures, causing pulmonary congestion)
7. Dysrhythmias (due to lack of oxygen to heart muscle) and sinus tachycardiac as a compensatory mechanism for a decreased cardiac output)
8. Chest pain (due to lack of oxygen and blood to heart muscle)

Diagnostic Evaluation

1. Altered hemodynamic parameters (PCWP 18 mm Hg or greater, cardiac index less than 2.2, systemic vascular resistance elevation).
2. Chest x-ray—pulmonary vascular congestion.
3. Abnormal lab values—elevated blood urea nitrogen (BUN) and creatinine, elevated liver enzymes.

Management

A. *Pharmacologic Therapy*
1. Cardiac glycosides (digoxin, [Lanoxin]) and positive inotropic drugs (dopamine [Intropin], dobutamine [Dobutrex], amrinone [Inocor]) stimulate cardiac contractility.
2. Vasodilator therapy
   a. Decreases the workload of the heart by reducing venous return and lessening the resistance against which the heart pumps (preload and afterload reduction)
   b. Cardiac output improves, left ventricular pressures and pulmonary congestion decrease, and myocardial oxygen consumption is reduced.
3. Vasopressor therapy is controversial as it may increase systemic vascular resistance.
4. Diuretic therapy
   a. Decreases total body fluid volume
   b. Relieves systemic and pulmonary congestion

B. *Counterpulsation Therapy (see p. 281)*
1. Improves blood flow to the heart muscle and reduces myocardial oxygen needs
2. Results in improved cardiac output and preservation of viable heart tissue

C. *Cardiopulmonary Bypass (see p. 283)*
D. *Left Ventricular Assist Device (LVAD)*
E. *Emergency Cardiac Surgery (see p. 283)*
1. Bypass graft
2. Heart transplantation

Complications

1. Neurological Impairment
2. Acute respiratory distress syndrome (ARDS)
3. Renal failure
4. Multiorgan dysfunction syndrome
5. Death

Nursing Assessment

1. Identify patients at risk for development of cardiogenic shock.
2. Assess for early signs and symptoms indicative of shock:
   a. Restlessness, confusion, or change in mental status
   b. Increasing heart rate
   c. Decreasing pulse pressure (indicates impaired cardiac output)
   d. Presence of pulsus alternans (indicates left heart failure)
   e. Decreasing urine output, weakness, fatigue
3. Observe for presence of central and peripheral cyanosis.
4. Observe for development of edema.
5. Identify signs and symptoms indicative of extension of myocardial infarction—recurrence of chest pain, diaphoresis.
6. Identify patient's and significant other's reaction to crisis situation.

Nursing Diagnoses

A. Decreased Cardiac Output related to impaired contractility due to extensive heart muscle damage
B. Impaired Gas Exchange related to pulmonary congestion due to elevated left ventricular pressures
C. Altered Tissue Perfusion (renal, cerebral, cardiopulmonary, gastrointestinal, and peripheral) related to decreased blood flow
D. Anxiety related to intensive care environment and threat of death

Nursing Interventions

A. *Improving Cardiac Output*
1. Establish continuous ECG monitoring to detect dysrhythmias, which increase myocardial oxygen consumption.
2. Monitor hemodynamic parameters continually with Swan–Ganz catheter (see p. 258) to evaluate effectiveness of implemented therapy.
   a. Obtain PAP, PCWP, and CO readings as indicated.
   b. Calculate the cardiac index (CI; cardiac output relative to body size) and systemic vascular resistance (SVR; measurement of afterload).

c. Cautiously titrate vasoactive drug therapy according to hemodynamic parameters.
   (1) Be alert to adverse responses to drug therapy; dopamine (Intropin) may cause increases in heart rate; vasodilators nitroglycerin (Tridil) and nitroprusside (Nipridel) may worsen hypotension; digoxin (Lanoxin) may result in dysrhythmias from toxicity; diuretics may cause hyponatremia, hypokalemia, and hypovolemia.
   (2) Administer vasoactive drug therapy through central venous access (peripheral tissue necrosis can occur if peripheral IV access infiltrates, and peripheral drug distribution may be lessened from vasoconstriction).
3. Monitor blood pressure and mean arterial pressure (MAP) with intra-arterial line (cuff pressures are difficult to ascertain and may be inaccurate) every 30 minutes and every 5 minutes during active titration of vasoactive drug therapy.
4. Maintain MAP greater than 60 mm Hg (blood flow through coronary vessels is inadequate with a MAP less than 60 mm Hg).
5. Measure and record urine output every hour from indwelling catheter and fluid intake.
6. Obtain daily weights.
7. Evaluate serum electrolytes for hyponatremia and hypokalemia.
8. Be alert to incidence of chest pain (indicates myocardial ischemia and may further extend heart damage).
   a. Report immediately.
   b. Obtain a 12-lead ECG recording.
   c. Anticipate use of counterpulsation therapy.

B. *Improving Oxygenation*
1. Monitor rate and rhythm of respirations every hour.
2. Auscultate lung fields for abnormal sounds (coarse crackles indicate severe pulmonary congestion) every hour; notify health care provider.
3. Evaluate arterial blood gases (ABGs).
4. Administer oxygen therapy to increase oxygen tension and improve hypoxia.
5. Elevate head of bed 20 to 30 degrees as tolerated (may worsen hypotension) to facilitate lung expansion.
6. Reposition patient frequently to promote ventilation and maintain skin integrity.
7. Observe for frothy pink-tinged sputum and cough (may indicate pulmonary edema); report immediately.

C. *Maintaining Tissue Perfusion*
1. Perform a neurologic check every hour, using the Glasgow Coma Scale.
2. Report changes immediately.
3. Obtain BUN and creatinine blood levels to evaluate renal function.
4. Auscultate for bowel sounds every 2 hours.
5. Evaluate character, rate, rhythm, and quality of arterial pulses every 2 hours.
6. Monitor temperature every 2 to 4 hours.
7. Employ sheepskin foot and elbow protectors to prevent skin breakdown.

D. *Relieving Anxiety*
1. Explain equipment and rationale for therapy to patient and family. Increasing knowledge assists in alleviating fear and anxiety.
2. Encourage patient to verbalize fears concerning diagnosis and prognosis.
3. Explain sensations patient will experience prior to procedures and routine care measures.
4. Offer reassurance and encouragement.
5. Provide for periods of uninterrupted rest and sleep.
6. Assist patient to maintain as much control as possible over environment and care.
   a. Develop a schedule for routine care measures and rest periods with patient.
   b. Ensure that a calendar and clock are in view of patient.

Patient Education/Health Maintenance

1. Teach patients on digoxin (Lanoxin) the importance of taking their medication as prescribed; taking pulse before daily dose; and reporting for periodic blood levels.
2. Teach signs of impending heart failure—increasing edema, shortness of breath, decreasing urine output, decreasing blood pressure, increasing pulse—and tell patient to notify health care provider immediately.
3. See specific measures for myocardial infarction, p. 297, cardiomyopathy, p. 310, and valvular disease, p. 317.

Evaluation

A. CO greater than 4 liters/minute; CI greater than 2.2, PCWP less than 18 mm Hg
B. Respirations unlabored and regular; normal breath sounds throughout lung fields
C. Normal sensorium; urine output adequate; skin warm and dry
D. Verbalizes lessened anxiety and fear

◆ INFECTIVE ENDOCARDITIS

Infective endocarditis (IE) (bacterial endocarditis) is an infection of the inner lining of the heart caused by direct invasion of bacteria or other organisms leading to deformity of the valve leaflets.

Pathophysiology/Etiology

1. When the inner lining of the heart (endocardium) becomes inflamed, a fibrin clot (vegetation) forms.
2. The fibrin clot may become colonized by pathogens during transient episodes of bacteremia resulting from invasive procedures (venous/arterial cannulation, dental work causing gingival bleeding, GI tract surgery, liver biopsy, sigmoidoscopy, etc.), indwelling catheters, urinary tract infections, and wound/skin infections.
3. Platelets and fibrin surround the invading microorganisms, forming a protective covering and causing the infected vegetation to enlarge.
   a. The enlarged vegetation (the basic lesion of endocarditis) can deform, thicken, stiffen, and scar the free margins of valve leaflets, as well as the fibrous ring (annulus) supporting the valve.
   b. The vegetation(s) may also travel to various organs/tissues (spleen, kidney, coronary artery, brain, and lungs) and obstruct blood flow.

c. The "protective covering" surrounding the vegetation makes it difficult for white blood cells and antimicrobial agents to infiltrate and destroy the infected lesion.

4. Causal organisms include:
   a. Bacteria
      (1) *Streptococcus viridans*—bacteremia occurs after dental work or upper respiratory infection.
      (2) *Staphylococcus aureus*—bacteremia occurs after cardiac surgery or parenteral drug abuse.
      (3) *Enterococci* (penicillin-resistant group D streptococci)—bacteremia usually occurs in elderly patients (over age 60) with genitourinary tract infection.
   b. Fungi (*Candida albicans, Aspergillus*)
   c. Rickettsiae

5. Infective endocarditis may develop on a heart valve already injured by rheumatic fever, congenital defects, on abnormally vascularized valves, normal heart valves, and mechanical/biological heart valves.

6. Infective endocarditis may be acute or subacute, depending on the microorganisms involved. Acute IE manifests rapidly with danger of intractable heart failure and occurs more commonly on normal heart valves.

7. Subacute IE manifests a prolonged chronic course with a lesser chance of complications and occurs more commonly on damaged or defective valves.

8. Infective endocarditis may follow cardiac surgery, especially when prosthetic heart valves are used. Foreign bodies such as pacemakers, patches, grafts, and dialysis shunts predispose to infection.

9. High incidence among drug abusers, in whom the disease mainly affects normal valves, usually the tricuspid.

10. Hospitalized patients with indwelling catheters, those on prolonged intravenous therapy or prolonged antibiotic therapy, and those on immunosuppressive drugs or steroids may develop fungal endocarditis.

11. Relapse due to metastatic infection is possible, usually within the first 2 months after completion of antibiotic regimen.

Clinical Manifestations

Severity of manifestations depends on invading microorganism.

A. *General Manifestations*
1. Fever, chills, sweats (fever may be absent in elderly or in patients with uremia)
2. Anorexia, weight loss, weakness
3. Cough, back and joint pain (especially in patients over age 60)
4. Splenomegaly

B. *Skin and Nail Manifestations*
1. Petechiae—conjunctiva, mucous membranes
2. Splinter hemorrhages in nail beds
3. Osler's nodes—painful red nodes on pads of fingers and toes; usually late sign of infection and found with a subacute infection
4. Janeway's lesions—light pink macules on palms or soles, nontender, may change to light tan within several days, fade in 1 to 2 weeks. Usually an early sign of endocardial infection.

C. *Heart Manifestations*
1. New pathologic or changing murmur—no murmur with other signs and symptoms may indicate right heart infection

2. Tachycardia—related to decreased cardiac output

D. *Central Nervous System Manifestations*
1. Localized headaches
2. Transient cerebral ischemia
3. Altered mental status, aphasia
4. Hemiplegia
5. Cortical sensory loss
6. Roth's spots on fundi

E. *Pulmonary Manifestations*
1. Usually occur with right-sided heart involvement
2. Pneumonitis, pleuritis, pulmonary edema, pulmonary infiltrates

F. *Embolic Phenomena*
1. Lung—hemoptysis, chest pain, shortness of breath
2. Kidney—hematuria
3. Spleen—pain in upper left quadrant of abdomen radiating to left shoulder
4. Heart—myocardial infarction
5. Brain—sudden blindness, paralysis, brain abscess, meningitis
6. Blood vessels—mycotic aneurysms
7. Abdomen—melena, acute pain

Diagnostic Evaluation

Varied clinical manifestations and similarities to other diseases make early diagnosis of IE difficult.

1. Blood cultures—at least two positive serial blood cultures isolating bacteria or fungi
2. Elevated sedimentation rate, tests indicative of anemia, mild leukocytosis, urine abnormalities indicating nephrosis
3. ECG—usually normal
4. Echocardiography—identification of vegetations and assessment of location and size of lesions

Management

1. Antimicrobial therapy based on sensitivity of causative agent; penicillin G (Megacillin), nafcillin (Unipen), vancomycin (Vancocin), gentamicin (Garamycin), rifampin alone or in combination for 4 to 6 weeks. Bactericidal serum levels of selected antibiotics are monitored by titering it against the causative organism; if serum lacks adequate bactericidal activity, more antibiotic or a different antibiotic is given.
2. Audiogram obtained before antibiotic regimen initiated
3. Urine cultures obtained after 48 hours to assess efficacy of drug therapy
4. Repeat blood cultures obtained after 48 hours to assess efficacy of drug therapy
5. Close follow-up by cardiologist
6. Supplemental nutrition
7. Surgical intervention for:
   a. Acute destructive valvular lesion—excision of infected valves or removal of prosthetic valve
   b. Hemodynamic impairment
   c. Recurrent emboli
   d. Infection that cannot be eliminated with antimicrobial therapy
   e. Drainage of abscess or empyema—for patient with localized abscess or empyema
   f. Repair of peripheral or cerebral mycotic aneurysm

Complications

1. Severe heart failure due to valvular insufficiency
2. Uncontrolled/refractory infection
3. Embolic episodes (ischemia or necrosis of extremities and organs)
4. Conduction disturbances

Nursing Assessment

1. Identify factors that may predispose to endocarditis, such as rheumatic heart disease, congenital heart defects, idiopathic hypertrophic subaortic stenosis (IHSS), IV drug abuse, prosthetic heart valves, aortic or mitral stenosis, previous history of endocarditis.
2. Determine onset of signs and symptoms of endocarditis (early treatment of infection improves prognosis).
3. Identify potential incidents that may have precipitated a transient bacteremia capable of causing endocarditis.
4. Obtain blood cultures, complete blood count, renal and hepatic studies, and a baseline 12-lead ECG.
5. Assess patient for allergies, with special emphasis on untoward reactions to antibiotic therapy.
6. Note if patient is currently on antibiotic therapy (may affect blood culture results).
7. Identify patient's and family's level of anxiety and use of appropriate coping mechanisms.

Nursing Diagnoses

A. Decreased Cardiac Output related to structural factors (incompetent valves)
B. Altered Tissue Perfusion (renal, cerebral, cardiopulmonary, gastrointestinal, and peripheral) related to interruption of blood flow
C. Hyperthermia related to illness, potential dehydration, and aggressive antibiotic therapy
D. Altered Nutrition (less than body requirements) related to anorexia
E. Anxiety related to acute illness and hospitalization

Nursing Interventions

A. *Maintaining Adequate Cardiac Output*
1. Auscultate heart to detect new murmur or change in existing murmur; presence of gallop.
2. Monitor blood pressure and pulse.
   a. Note presence of pulsus alternans (indicative of left heart failure).
   b. Evaluate pulse pressure (30–40 mm Hg normal; indicates adequate cardiac output).
3. Evaluate jugular venous distention.
4. Record intake and output.
5. Record daily weight.
6. Auscultate lung fields for evidence of crackles (rales).

B. *Maintaining Tissue Perfusion*
1. Observe the patient for altered mentation, hemoptysis, hematuria, aphasia, loss of muscle strength, complaints of pain.
2. Observe for splinter hemorrhages of nailbeds, Osler's nodes, and Janeway's lesions.

3. Notify health care provider of observed changes in the patient's status.
4. Position patient frequently to prevent skin breakdown and pulmonary complications associated with bedrest.

C. *Maintaining Normothermia*
1. Observe basic principles of asepsis, good handwashing techniques, and continuity of patient care by primary nurse.
2. Employ meticulous IV care for long-term antibiotic therapy.
   a. Note the date of needle or cannula insertion on nursing care plan.
   b. Rotate IV site every 72 hours or if site becomes tender, reddened, infiltrated, or has purulent drainage.
   c. Change gauze or transparent dressing every 24 hours to prevent infection.
3. Administer parenteral antibiotic therapy as directed.
   a. Develop chart for rotation of sites for intramuscular administration of antibiotic therapy.
   b. Observe for untoward reaction to antibiotic therapy (severe respiratory distress, rash, itching, fever).
   c. Observe for side effects of long-term antibiotic therapy—ototoxicity, renal failure.
4. Monitor temperature every 2 to 4 hours.
   a. Document results on graph.
   b. Note increases in heart rate and/or respirations with elevated temperatures.
   c. Provide cooling measures such as alcohol or tepid water sponge bath and/or cooling blanket as directed.
   d. Provide blankets and temperature-controlled comfortable environment if patient has shaking chills; change bed linens as necessary.
   e. Administer analgesic medications as directed.
5. Observe patient for a general "sense of well-being" within 5 to 7 days after initiation of therapy.
6. Monitor laboratory values—hematocrit, BUN, creatinine, WBC, antibiotic levels, blood cultures.
7. Promote adequate hydration, as diaphoresis and increased metabolic rate may cause dehydration.
   a. Encourage oral fluid intake.
   b. Administer IV fluids as directed.
   c. Observe skin turgor and mucous membranes.

D. *Improving Nutritional Status*
1. Assess the patient's daily caloric intake.
2. Discuss food preferences with the patient.
3. Consult with a dietitian regarding nutritional needs of patient and food preferences.
4. Encourage small meals and snacks throughout the day.
5. Record daily caloric intake and weight.
6. Educate family members about the patient's caloric needs.
7. Encourage family members to assist the patient with meals and bring in the patient's favorite foods.

E. *Reducing Anxiety*
1. Encourage the patient to verbalize fears regarding illness and hospitalization.
2. Explain all procedures to patient before initiation.
3. Offer the patient literature, if available, about his or her disease.
4. Encourage diversional activities for the patient such as television, reading, and interaction with other patients.
5. Encourage family members to interact with the patient as frequently as possible.

Patient Education/Health Maintenance

A. *For Patients at Risk for Infective Endocarditis*
1. Discuss anatomy of heart and changes that occur during endocarditis, using diagrams of the heart.
2. Give the patient written literature on early signs and symptoms of disease; review these with the patient.
3. Discuss with individual the mode of entry of infection.
4. Indicate that antibiotic prophylaxis is recommended for persons with:
   a. Congenital heart defects, prosthetic/biologic heart valves, IHSS
   b. Past history of endocarditis·
   c. Mitral valve prolapse with insufficiency
   d. Rheumatic heart disease and valvular dysfunction
   e. Undergoing procedures most likely to cause bacteremia (dental procedures causing gingival bleeding, surgery on or instrumentation of GI tract, and certain genitourinary procedures, etc.).
5. Identify individual steps necessary to prevent infection.
   a. Good oral hygiene, regular tooth brushing, and flossing
   b. Notification to health care personnel of any history of congenital heart disease or valvular disease.
   c. Discuss importance of carrying emergency identification with information of medical history at all times.
   d. Take temperature if infection is suspected and notify health care provider of elevation.
   e. Educate persons at risk to look for and treat signs and symptoms of illness indicating bacteremia—injuries, sore throats, furuncles, etc.
6. Provide patient with American Heart Association Bacterial Endocarditis wallet card outlining recommended antibiotic prophylaxis for procedures (obtain at local American Heart Association chapter).
7. Encourage susceptible individuals to receive pneumococcal and influenza vaccines.
   a. Teach that vaccines reduce the risk of severe infections that could precipitate heart failure.
8. Teach women in childbearing years the risks of using IUDs for birth control (source of infection) and that antibiotic therapy is not necessary for individuals having normal deliveries.

B. *For Individuals Who Have Had Endocarditis Regarding Possible Relapse*
1. Discuss importance of keeping follow-up appointments after hospital discharge (infection can recur in 1–2 months).
2. Review the tests that will be performed after hospital discharge—blood cultures, physical examination.
3. Teach individual to inspect soles of feet for Janeway's lesions (indicative of possible relapse).
4. Contact social worker to assist the patient with financial planning and home discharge arrangements if applicable.

Evaluation

A. Blood pressure stable; no changed in murmur; no gallop noted
B. No change in level of consciousness (LOC), strength, or neurologic function
C. Normal temperature, negative blood cultures, normal WBC count, BUN, and creatinine, no hearing impairments
D. Increased daily caloric intake tolerated well
E. Verbalizes decrease in anxiety

◆ RHEUMATIC ENDOCARDITIS (RHEUMATIC HEART DISEASE)

Rheumatic endocarditis is damage done to the heart, particularly the valves, resulting in valve leakage (regurgitation) and/or obstruction (narrowing or stenosis). There are associated compensatory changes in the size of the heart's chambers and the thickness of chamber walls.

Pathophysiology/Etiology

1. *Rheumatic fever* is a sequela to group A streptococcal infection. It is a preventable disease through the detection and adequate treatment of streptococcal pharyngitis.
2. Symptoms of streptococcal pharyngitis
   a. Sudden onset of sore throat; throat reddened with exudate
   b. Swollen, tender lymph nodes at angle of jaw
   c. Headache and fever 38.9°–40° C. (101°–104° F.)
   d. Abdominal pain (children)

NURSING ALERT:
Some cases of streptococcal throat infection are relatively asymptomatic.

Clinical Manifestations

1. Polyarthritis; warm and swollen joints
2. Carditis
3. Chorea (irregular, jerky, involuntary, unpredictable muscular movements)
4. Erythema marginatum (wavy, thin red-line rash on trunk and extremities)
5. Subcutaneous nodules
6. Fever
7. Prolonged PR interval demonstrated by ECG
8. Heart murmurs; pleural and pericardial rubs

Diagnostic Evaluation

1. Throat culture—to determine presence of streptococcal organisms
2. Increased sedimentation rate; WBC count and differential and C-reactive protein—increase during acute phase of infection
3. Elevated antistreptolysin titer

Management

1. Antimicrobial therapy—to eradicate involved organism
2. Rest—to maintain optimal cardiac function
3. Salicylates—to control fever and pain
4. Prevention of recurrent episodes

Complications

1. Valvular heart disease
2. Cardiomyopathy
3. Congestive heart failure

Nursing Assessment

1. Ask patient about symptoms of fever or throat or joint pain.
2. Ask patient about chest pain, dyspnea, fatigue
3. Observe for skin lesions or rash on trunk and extremities.
4. Palpate for firm, nontender movable nodules near tendons of joints.
5. Auscultate heart sounds for murmurs and/or rubs.

Nursing Diagnoses

A. Hyperthermia related to disease process
B. Decreased Cardiac Output related to decreased cardiac contractility
C. Activity Intolerance related to joint pain and easy fatiguability

Nursing Interventions

A. *Reducing Fever*
1. Administer penicillin therapy as prescribed to eradicate hemolytic streptococcus; an erythromycin preparation may be used if the patient is allergic to penicillin.
2. Give salicylates as prescribed to suppress rheumatic activity by controlling toxic manifestations, to reduce fever, and to relieve joint pain.
3. Assess for effectiveness of drug therapy.
   a. Take and record temperature every 3 hours.
   b. Evaluate the patient's comfort level every 3 hours.

B. *Maintaining Adequate Cardiac Output*
1. Assess for signs and symptoms of acute rheumatic carditis.
   a. Be alert to the patient's complaints of chest pain, palpitations, and/or precordial "tightness."
   b. Monitor for tachycardia (usually persistent when the patient sleeps) or bradycardia.
   c. Be alert to development of second-degree heart block or Wenckebach's syndrome (acute rheumatic carditis causes PR interval prolongation).
2. Auscultate heart sounds every 4 hours.
   a. Document presence of murmur or pericardial friction rub
   b. Document extra heart sounds (S_3 gallop, S_4 gallop).
3. See discussion on rheumatic fever in children, Chapter 43.

4. Monitor for development of chronic rheumatic endocarditis which may include valvular disease and congestive heart failure.

C. *Maintaining Activity*
1. Maintain bedrest for duration of fever or if signs of active carditis are present.
2. Provide range-of-motion exercise program.
3. Provide diversional activities that prevent exertion.
4. Discuss need for tutorial services with parents to help child keep up with school work.

Patient Education/Health Maintenance

A. *Preventing Recurrence*
1. Counsel the patient to maintain good nutrition.
2. Counsel the patient on hygienic practices.
   a. Discuss proper hand-washing, disposal of tissues, laundering of handkerchiefs (decrease chance of exposure to microbes).
   b. Discuss importance of using patient's own toothbrush, soap, and washcloths when living in group situations.
3. Counsel the patient on importance of receiving adequate rest.
4. Counsel the patient to seek treatment immediately should sore throat occur.
   a. Explore with patient his or her ability to pay for medical treatment. If appropriate, contact social services for the patient. (Financial difficulties may inhibit the patient from seeking early treatment of symptoms.)

B. *Other Points*
1. Instruct the patient to use prophylactic penicillin therapy before undergoing surgery of genitourinary tract, lower GI tract, and respiratory tract.
2. See Patient Education, Endocarditis, page 304.

Evaluation

A. Afebrile
B. Denies chest pain; normal sinus rhythm
C. Bedrest maintained while febrile

◆ MYOCARDITIS

Myocarditis is an inflammatory process involving the myocardium.

Pathophysiology/Etiology

1. Focal or diffuse inflammation of the myocardium, may be acute or chronic
2. May follow infectious process—viral (particularly coxsackie group B, and may develop after influenza A or B, herpes simplex), bacterial, mycotic, parasitic, protozoal, rickettsial, and spirochetal infections
3. May be associated with chemotherapy (esp. doxorubicin [Adriamycin]), or immunosuppressive therapy.

4. Conditions such as sarcoidosis and collagen diseases may lead to myocarditis.

Clinical Manifestations

1. Symptoms depend on type of infection, degree of myocardial damage, capacity of myocardium to recover, and host resistance. Can be acute or chronic and occur at any age. Symptoms may be minor and go unnoticed.
  a. Fatigue and dyspnea
  b. Palpitations
  c. Occasional precordial discomfort
2. Cardiac enlargement.
3. Abnormal heart sounds: murmur, S_3 or S_4, or friction rubs.
4. Signs of congestive heart failure, ie, pulsus alternans, dyspnea, crackles.
5. Fever with tachycardia.

Diagnostic Evaluation

1. Transient ECG changes—ST segment flattened, T wave inversion, conduction defects, extrasystoles, supraventricular and ventricular ectopic beats
2. Elevated WBC count and sedimentation rate
3. Chest x-ray—may show heart enlargement and lung congestion
4. Elevated antibody titers (antistreptolysin-O [ASO titer] as in rheumatic fever)
5. Stool and throat cultures isolating bacteria or a virus
6. Endomyocardial biopsy for definitive diagnosis

Management

Treatment objectives are targeted toward management of complications.

1. Diuretic and digoxin (Lanoxin) therapy for congestive heart failure and atrial fibrillation
2. Antidysrhythmic therapy (usually quinidine [Quinaglute] or procainamide [Pronestyl])
3. Strict bedrest to promote healing of damaged myocardium
4. Antimicrobial therapy if causative bacteria is isolated

Complications

1. Congestive heart failure
2. Cardiomyopathy

Nursing Assessment

1. Assess for fatigue, palpitations, fever, dyspnea, and chest pain.
2. Auscultate heart sounds
3. Evaluate history for precipitating factors.

Nursing Diagnoses

A. Hyperthermia related to inflammatory/infectious process

B. Decreased Cardiac Output related to decreased cardiac contractility and dysrhythmias
C. Activity Intolerance related to impaired cardiac performance and febrile illness

Nursing Interventions

A. *Reducing Fever*
1. Administer antipyretics as directed.
2. Check temperature every 4 hours.
3. Administer antibiotics as directed.

B. *Maintaining Cardiac Output*
1. Evaluate for clinical evidence that disease is subsiding—monitor pulse, auscultate for abnormal heart sounds (murmur or change in existing murmur), check temperature, auscultate lung fields, monitor respirations.
2. Record daily intake and output.
3. Record weight daily.
4. Check for peripheral edema.
5. Elevate head of bed, if necessary, to enhance respiration.
6. Treat the symptoms of congestive heart failure as prescribed (see p. 311).

> **NURSING ALERT:**
> Patients with myocarditis may be sensitive to digitalis—assess for toxic signs and symptoms such as anorexia, nausea, fatigue, weakness, yellow-green halos around visual images, prolonged PR interval.

7. Evaluate the patient's pulse and apical rate for signs of tachycardia and gallop rhythm—indications that congestive heart failure is recurring.
8. Evaluate for evidences of dysrhythmias—*patients with myocarditis are prone to develop dysrhythmias.*
  a. Institute continuous cardiac monitoring if evidence of a dysrhythmia develops.
  b. Have equipment for resuscitation, cardiac defibrillation, and cardiac pacing available in the event of life-threatening dysrhythmia.

C. *Reducing Fatigue*
1. Ensure bedrest to reduce heart rate, stroke volume, blood pressure, and heart contractility; also helps to decrease residual damage and complications of myocarditis, and promotes healing.
  a. Prolonged bedrest may be required—until there is reduction in heart size and improvement of function.
2. Provide diversional activities for patient.
3. Allow the patient to use bedside commode rather than bedpan (reduces cardiovascular workload).
4. Discuss with the patient activities that can be continued after discharge.
  a. Discuss the need to modify activities in the immediate future.
  b. Explore with the patient lifestyle modifications and discuss adequacy of self-concept.

Patient Education/Health Maintenance

Instruct the patient as follows:

1. There is usually some residual heart enlargement; physical activity may be *slowly* increased; begin with

chair rest for increasing periods; follow with walking in the room and then outdoors.
2. Report any symptom involving rapidly beating heart.
3. Avoid competitive sports, alcohol, and other myocardial toxins (doxorubicin [Adriamycin]).
4. Pregnancy is not advisable for women with cardiomyopathies associated with myocarditis.
5. Prevent infectious diseases with appropriate immunizations.
6. Encourage family members to support the patient and learn about the illness.

Evaluation

A. Afebrile
B. BP and heart rate stable; no dysrhythmias noted
C. Bedrest maintained

◆ PERICARDITIS

Pericarditis is an inflammation of the pericardium, the membranous sac enveloping the heart. It is often a manifestation of a more generalized disease.

Pericardial effusion is an outpouring of fluid into the pericardial cavity seen in pericarditis.

Constrictive pericarditis is a condition in which a chronic inflammatory thickening of the pericardium compresses the heart so that it is unable to fill normally during diastole.

Pathophysiology/Etiology

1. Acute idiopathic pericarditis is the most common and typical form; etiology unknown
2. Other causes include:
   a. Infection
      (1) Viral (influenza; coxsackievirus)
      (2) Bacterial—staphylococcus, meningococcus, streptococcus, pneumococcus, gonococcus, *Mycobacterium tuberculosis*
      (3) Fungal
      (4) Parasitic
   b. Connective tissue disorders (lupus erythematosus, periarteritis nodosa)
   c. Myocardial infarction; early, 24 to 72 hours; or late, 1 week to 2 years (Dressler's syndrome)
   d. Malignant disease; thoracic irradiation
   e. Chest trauma, heart surgery, including pacemaker implantation
   f. Drug induced (procainamide [Pronestyl]; phenytoin [Dilantin])

Clinical Manifestations

1. Pain in anterior chest, aggravated by thoracic motion—may vary from mild to sharp and severe; located in precordial area (may be felt beneath clavicle, neck, scapular region)—may be relieved by leaning forward.
2. Pericardial friction rub—scratchy, grating, or creaking sound occurring in the presence of pericardial inflammation
3. Dyspnea—from compression of heart and surrounding thoracic structures

4. Fever, sweating, chills—due to inflammation of pericardium
5. Dysrhythmias

Diagnostic Evaluation

1. Echocardiogram—most sensitive method for detecting pericardial effusion
2. Chest x-ray—may show heart enlargement
3. ECG—to evaluate for myocardial infarction
4. WBC and differential elevations indicating infection
5. Antinuclear antibody serologic tests elevated in lupus erythematosus
6. PPD test positive in for tuberculosis; ASO titers—elevated if rheumatic fever is present
7. Pericardiocentesis—for examination of pericardial fluid for etiologic diagnosis
8. BUN—to evaluate for uremia

Management

The objectives of treatment are targeted toward determining the etiology of the problem, administering pharmacologic therapy for specified etiology, when known, and being alert to the possible complication of cardiac tamponade.

1. Bacterial pericarditis—penicillin or other antimicrobial agents
2. Rheumatic fever—procaine penicillin (Duracillin), prednisone (Orasone)
3. Tuberculosis—antituberculosis chemotherapy (see p. 224)
4. Fungal pericarditis—amphotericin B (Fungizone)
5. Systemic lupus erythematosus— steroids
6. Renal pericarditis—dialysis, indomethacin (Indocin), biochemical control of end-stage renal disease
7. Neoplastic pericarditis—intrapericardial instillation of chemotherapy; radiotherapy
8. Postmyocardial infarction syndrome—bedrest, aspirin, prednisone
9. Postpericardiotomy syndrome (after open-heart surgery)—treat symptomatically
10. Emergency pericardiocentesis if cardiac tamponade develops
11. Partial pericardiectomy (pericardial "window") or total pericardiectomy for recurrent constrictive pericarditis

Complications

1. Cardiac tamponade
2. Congestive heart failure
3. Hemopericardium (especially patients post-MI receiving anticoagulants)

Nursing Assessment

1. Evaluate Complaint of Chest Pain.
   a. Ask the patient if pain is aggravated by breathing, turning in bed, twisting body, coughing, yawning, or swallowing.
   b. Elevate head of bed; position pillow on over-the-bed table so that the patient can lean on it.

c. Assess if above intervention relieves the patient's chest pain (associated pleuritic pain of pericarditis is usually relieved by sitting up and/or leaning forward).

d. Be alert to the patient's medical diagnoses when assessing pain. Postmyocardial infarction patients may experience a dull, crushing pain radiating to neck, arm, and shoulders, mimicking an extension of infarction.

2. Auscultate heart sounds.
   a. Listen for friction rub by asking patient to hold breath briefly.
   b. Listen to the heart with patient in different positions.
3. Evaluate history for precipitating factors.

Nursing Diagnoses

A. *Chest Pain related to pericardial inflammation*

B. *Decreased Cardiac Output related to impaired ventricular expansion*

Nursing Interventions

A. *Reducing Discomfort*
1. Give prescribed drug regimen for pain and symptomatic relief.
   a. Nonsteroidal anti-inflammatory drugs (NSAIDs) suppress inflammatory symptoms of acute pericarditis
   b. Corticosteroids—for more severe symptoms
2. Relieve anxiety of the patient and family by explaining the difference between pain of pericarditis and pain of recurrent myocardial infarction. (Patients may fear extension of myocardial tissue damage.)
3. Explain to the patient and family that pericarditis does not indicate further heart damage.
4. Encourage the patient to remain on bedrest when chest pain, fever, and friction rub occur.
5. Assist patient to position of comfort.

B. *Maintaining Cardiac Output*

> **NURSING ALERT:** ◆
> Normal pericardial sac contains less than 25 to 30 mL of fluid; pericardial fluid may accumulate slowly without noticeable symptoms. However, a rapidly developing effusion can produce serious hemodynamic alterations.

1. Assess heart rate, rhythm, BP, respirations at least hourly in the acute phase.
2. Assess for signs of cardiac tamponade increased heart rate, decreased BP, presence of paradoxical pulse, distended neck veins, restlessness, muffled heart sounds.
3. Prepare for emergency pericardiocentesis or surgery. Keep pericardiocentesis tray at bedside. (see p. 276).
4. Assess for signs of congestive heart failure (see p. 310).
5. Monitor closely for the development of dysrhythmias.

Patient Education/Health Maintenance

1. Teach patient the etiology of pericarditis.
2. Instruct patient about signs and symptoms of pericarditis and the need for long-term medication therapy to help relieve symptoms.

3. Review all medications with the patient—purpose, side effects, dosage, and special precautions.

Evaluation

A. Patient verbalizes relief of pain
B. BP and heart rate stable; no dysrhythmias; no friction rub

◆ CARDIOMYOPATHY

Cardiomyopathy refers to any disease of the heart muscle. In primary cardiomyopathy the cause of the disorder is unknown; in secondary cardiomyopathy the cause of the disorder is known or suspected (coronary artery disease can cause ischemic cardiomyopathy).

The cardiomyopathies are categorized into three major groups (dilated, hypertrophic, restrictive) to delineate the variations in structural and functional abnormalities that can occur.

Pathophysiology/Etiology

A. *Dilated Cardiomyopathy*
1. Both the right and left ventricle enlarge (dilate) significantly, causing a decrease in the ability of the heart to pump blood efficiently to the body.
2. Blood remaining in the ventricles after contraction causes increases in ventricular, atrial, and pulmonary pressures.
3. The increased pressures continue to diminish the ability of the heart to pump blood to the body, and heart failure occurs.
4. Alcohol abuse, chemotherapy, chemical agents, pregnancy (third trimester, postpartum), and infections can cause dilated cardiomyopathy.

B. *Hypertrophic Cardiomyopathy (HCM)*
1. HCM is primarily due to the abnormal thickening of the ventricular septum of the heart.
2. The thickening of the heart muscle commonly occurs asymmetrically (septum is proportionately thicker than the other ventricular walls), but also may occur symmetrically (septum and the ventricular free wall both become equally thickened).
3. The ultrastructure of the heart is also disrupted by patches of myocardial fibrosis, disorganization of myocardial fibers, and abnormalities of the coronary microvasculature.
4. The thickened heart muscle and ultrastructure disruption change the shape, size, and distensibility of the ventricular cavity and alter the normal thickness and functioning of the mitral valve; as a result, the heart's ability to relax and contract normally is impaired.
   a. Muscle stiffness impairs the filling of the ventricle with blood during relaxation.
   b. Forceful contractions eject blood from the heart too rapidly, causing abnormal pressure gradients; mechanical narrowing of the passage by which the blood leaves the heart also may occur, acutely obstructing blood flow to the body.
5. HCM is a genetically transmitted disorder.

C. *Restrictive Cardiomyopathy*
1. The heart muscle becomes infiltrated by various substances, resulting in severe fibrosis.

2. The heart muscle becomes stiff and nondistensible, impairing the ability of the ventricle to fill with blood adequately.
3. Amyloidosis and hemochromatosis (excess iron deposition) may cause restrictive cardiomyopathy.

Clinical Manifestations

1. Exertional dyspnea
2. Chest pain
3. Signs of congestive heart failure (see p. 310).
4. Pulmonary edema (see p. 313).
5. Dysrhythmias (frequent atrial/ventricular ectopic beats, sinus, atrial, and ventricular tachycardia).
6. Pericardial effusions (with restrictive cardiomyopathy).

Diagnostic Evaluation

1. Chest x-ray (cardiomegaly)
2. ECG—may show dysrhythmia
3. Echocardiogram detects abnormalities of heart wall movements.
4. 24-hour Holter monitoring to detect dysrhythmias.
5. Radionuclide imaging to assess ventricular function.
6. Cardiac catheterization may help determine cause.

Management

The goal of therapy is to maximize ventricular function and prevent complications.

A. Dilated Cardiomyopathy
1. Effective management of heart failure by conventional therapy (see p. 311).
2. Oral anticoagulants may be instituted to prevent thrombus and pulmonary embolus.
3. Heart transplantation must be considered in the terminal disease phase.

> **NURSING ALERT:**
> Patients with dilated cardiomyopathy are susceptible to digoxin toxicity. Monitor patient carefully for evidence of nausea, vomiting, yellow vision, and dysrhythmias.

B. Hypertrophic Cardiomyopathy
1. *Beta-adrenergic blockers*—reduce the force of the heart muscle's contraction, diminish obstructive pressure gradients, and decrease oxygen requirements. Propranolol (Inderal) is the agent of choice.
2. *Calcium channel blockers*—primarily improve the heart's ability to relax, but also have an effect on reducing the force of the heart muscle's contraction, thereby providing symptom relief. Verapamil (Calan) is the agent of choice and is implemented after failure of beta-adrenergic agents to control symptoms.
3. *Antidysrhythmic therapy*—amiodarone (Cordarone) is the agent of choice to prophylactically prevent lethal dysrhythmias.
4. *Myotomy and myectomy*—surgical resection of a portion of the septum to reduce muscle thickness and provide symptom relief.

5. *Device implantation*—Pacemakers and automatic internal defibrillators may be implanted to treat severe bradycardias and lethal tachycardias.

> **NURSING ALERT:**
> Chest pain experienced by HCM patients is managed by rest and elevation of the feet (improves venous return to the heart). Vasodilator therapy (nitroglycerin) may worsen chest pain by decreasing venous return to the heart and further increasing obstruction of blood flow from the heart; agents that increase contractility of the heart muscle (dopamine, dobutamine) should also be avoided or used with extreme caution.

C. Restrictive Cardiomyopathy
1. Therapy is palliative unless specific underlying process is established.
2. Heart failure can be controlled with fluid restriction and diuretic therapy.
3. Digoxin (Lanoxin) is beneficial for controlling atrial fibrillation.
4. Oral anticoagulants are instituted to prevent emboli.

Complications

1. Mural thrombus (due to blood stasis in ventricles with dilated cardiomyopathy)
2. Severe heart failure
3. Sudden cardiac death
4. Pulmonary embolism

Nursing Assessment

1. Evaluate the patient's chief complaint which may include the following: fever, syncope, general aches, fatigue, palpitations, dyspnea.
2. Evaluate etiologic factors such as alcohol abuse, pregnancy, recent infection, or history of endocrine disorders.
3. Assess for positive family history.
4. Auscultate lung sounds for crackles (pulmonary edema) decreased sounds (pleural effusion).
5. Assess heart size and auscultate for abnormal sounds.
6. Evaluate cardiac rhythm and ECG for evidence of atrial or ventricular enlargement and infarction.

Nursing Diagnoses

A. Decreased Cardiac Output related to decreased ventricular function and/or dysrhythmias
B. Anxiety related to fear of death and hospitalization
C. Fatigue related to disease process

Nursing Interventions

A. Improving Cardiac Output
1. Monitor heart rate, rhythm, temperature, and respiratory rate at least every 4 hours.
2. Evaluate CVP, pulmonary artery and pulmonary capillary wedge pressures via a pulmonary artery catheter to assess progress and effect of drug therapy.

3. Calculate cardiac output, cardiac index, and systemic vascular resistance.
4. Observe for changes in cardiac output such as: decreased BP, change in mental status, decreased urine output.
5. Administer pharmacologic support as directed and observe for changes in hemodynamic and clinical status.
6. Administer medications to control or eradicate dysrhythmias as directed.
7. Administer anticoagulants as directed especially for patients in atrial fibrillation.
   a. Monitor coagulation studies.
   b. Observe for evidence of bleeding.

B. *Relieving Anxiety*
1. Explain all procedures and treatments.
2. Inform patient and visitors of visiting hours and policy and whom to contact for information.
3. Orient patient to unit, purpose of equipment, and plan of care.
4. Encourage questions and voicing of fears and concerns.

C. *Reducing Fatigue*
1. Ensure that patient and visitors understand the importance of rest.
2. Assist patient in identifying stressors and reducing their effect. (Especially important for patients with hypertrophic cardiomyopathy as stress worsens the outflow obstruction.)
3. Provide uninterrupted periods and assist with ambulation as ordered.
4. Teach the use of diversional activities and relaxation techniques to relieve tension.

Patient Education/Health Maintenance

1. Teach about medications such as digoxin (Lanoxin).
   a. Take daily after taking pulse; notify health care provider if pulse below 60 (or other specified rate).
   b. Report signs of digitalis toxicity—anorexia, nausea, vomiting, yellow vision.
   c. Follow-up for periodic blood levels.
2. Advise low sodium diet. Teach how to read labels.
3. Advise reporting signs of heart failure: weight gain, edema, shortness of breath, increased fatigue.
4. Ensure that family members know cardiopulmonary resuscitation (CPR) because sudden cardiac arrest is possible.

Evaluation

A. BP and hemodynamic parameters stable; urine output adequate; alert
B. Asking questions and cooperating with care
C. Resting at intervals

◆ CONGESTIVE HEART FAILURE

Congestive heart failure is a clinical syndrome that results from the heart's inability to pump the amount of oxygenated blood necessary to meet the metabolic requirements of the body.

Pathophysiology/Etiology

1. Cardiac compensatory mechanisms (increases in heart rate, vasoconstriction, heart enlargement) occur to assist the failing heart.
   a. These mechanisms are able to "compensate" for the heart's inability to pump effectively and maintain sufficient blood flow to organs and tissue at rest.
   b. Physiologic stressors that increase the workload of the heart (exercise, infection) may cause these mechanisms to fail and precipitate the "clinical syndrome" associated with a failing heart (elevated ventricular/atrial pressures, sodium and water retention, decreased cardiac output, circulatory and pulmonary congestion).
   c. The compensatory mechanisms themselves may hasten the onset of failure as they increase afterload and cardiac work.
2. Caused by disorders of heart muscle resulting in decreased contractile properties of the heart; coronary heart disease leading to myocardial infarction; hypertension; valvular heart disease; congenital heart disease; cardiomyopathies; dysrhythmias.
3. Other causes include:
   a. Pulmonary embolism; chronic lung disease
   b. Hemorrhage and anemia
   c. Anesthesia and surgery
   d. Transfusions or infusions
   e. Increased body demands (fever, infection, pregnancy, arteriovenous fistula)
   f. Drug-induced
   g. Physical and emotional stress
   h. Excessive sodium intake

Clinical Manifestations

Initially there may be isolated left ventricular failure, but in time, the right ventricle fails because of the additional workload. Combined left and right ventricular failure is common.

A. *Left-sided Heart Failure (Forward Failure)*
1. Congestion occurs mainly in the lungs from backing up of blood into pulmonary veins and capillaries
   a. Shortness of breath, dyspnea on exertion, paroxysmal nocturnal dyspnea (due to reabsorption of dependent edema that has developed during day), orthopnea, pulmonary edema
   b. Cough—may be dry, unproductive; often occurs at night
2. Fatigability—from low cardiac output, nocturia, insomnia, dyspnea, catabolic effect of chronic failure
3. Insomnia, restlessness
4. Tachycardia—S_3 ventricular gallop

B. *Right-sided Heart Failure (Backward Failure)*
Signs and symptoms of elevated pressures and congestion in systemic veins and capillaries:

1. Edema of ankles; unexplained weight gain (pitting edema is obvious only after retention of at least 4.5 kg [10 pounds] of fluid).
2. Liver congestion—may produce upper abdominal pain
3. Distended neck veins
4. Abnormal fluid in body cavities (pleural space, abdominal cavity)

5. Anorexia and nausea—from hepatic and visceral engorgement
6. Nocturia—diuresis occurs at night with rest and improved cardiac output
7. Weakness

C. *Cardiovascular Findings in Both Types*
1. Cardiomegaly (enlargement of the heart)—detected by physical examination and chest x-ray
2. Ventricular gallop—evident on auscultation; ECG
3. Rapid heart rate
4. Development of pulsus alternans (alternation in strength of beat)

Diagnostic Evaluation

1. ECG may show ventricular hypertrophy, strain
2. Echocardiography may show ventricular hypertrophy, dilation of chambers, abnormal wall motion
3. Chest x-ray—may show cardiomegaly, pleural effusion, and vascular congestion
4. ABG studies—may show hypoxemia due to pulmonary vascular congesion
5. Liver function studies—may be altered because of hepatic congestion

Management

Treatment is directed at eliminating excessive accumulation of body water, increasing the force and efficiency of myocardial contraction and reducing the workload of the heart. These goals are achieved through promoting rest and administering pharmacologic agents.

A. *Diuretics*
1. Eliminate excess body water and decrease ventricular pressures
2. A low-sodium diet and fluid restriction complement this therapy
3. Some diuretics may have slight venodilator properties.

B. *Positive Inotropic Agents*
1. Increase the heart's ability to pump more effectively by improving the contractile force of the muscle
2. Digoxin (Lanoxin) may only be effective in severe cases of failure
3. Dopamine (Intropin) also improves renal blood flow in low dose range
4. Dobutamine (Dobutrex)
5. Amrinone (Inocor) is a potent vasodilators.

C. *Vasodilator Therapy*
1. Decreases the workload of the heart by dilating peripheral vessels.
2. By relaxing capacitance vessels (veins and venules), vasodilators reduce ventricular filling pressures (preload) and volumes.
3. By relaxing resistance vessels (arterioles), vasodilators can reduce impedance to left ventricular ejection and improve stroke volume.
4. Vasodilators used in congestive heart failure:
   a. Nitrates such as nitroglycerin (Tridil), isosorbide dinitrate (Isordil), nitroglycerin ointment (Nitrobid)—predominantly dilate systemic veins
   b. Hydralazine (Apresoline)—predominantly affects arterioles; reduces arteriolar tone
   c. Prazosin (Minipress)—balanced effects on both arterial and venous circulation
   d. Sodium nitroprusside (Nipride)—predominantly affects arterioles
   e. Morphine sulfate (Duramorph)—decreases venous return, decreases pain and anxiety and thus cardiac work.

D. *Angiotensin-Converting Enzyme Inhibitors (ACE Inhibitors)*
1. Inhibit the adverse effects of angiotensin II (potent vasoconstrictor)
2. Decreases left ventricular afterload with a subsequent decrease in heart rate associated with heart failure, thereby reducing the workload of the heart and increasing cardiac output
3. Captopril (Capoten) and enalapril (Vasotec) are commonly used.

E. *Heart Transplantation*
Used in advanced heart failure.

Complications

1. Intractable or refractory heart failure—patient becomes progressively refractory to therapy (does not yield to treatment)
2. Cardiac dysrhythmias
3. Myocardial failure
4. Digitalis toxicity—from decreased renal function, potassium depletion, etc.
5. Pulmonary infarction; pneumonia; emboli

Nursing Assessment

1. Obtain history of symptoms, limits of activity, and response to rest.
2. Assess peripheral arterial pulses; note quality, character; assess heart, and blood pressure rhythm and rate.
3. Inspect/palpate precordium for lateral displacement of point of maximum impulse.
4. Identify sleeping patterns and sleep aids commonly used by patient.

Nursing Diagnoses

A. Decreased Cardiac Output related to impaired contractility and increased preload/afterload
B. Impaired Gas Exchange related to alveolar edema due to elevated ventricular pressures
C. Fluid Volume Excess related to sodium and water retention
D. Activity Intolerance related to oxygen supply and demand imbalance

Nursing Interventions

A. *Maintaining Adequate Cardiac Output*
1. Place patient at physical and emotional rest to reduce work of heart.
   a. Provide rest in semirecumbent position or in armchair in air-conditioned environment—reduces work of heart, increases heart reserve, reduces blood pressure, decreases work of respiratory mus-

cles and oxygen utilization, improves efficiency of heart contraction; recumbency promotes diuresis by improving renal perfusion.

   b. Provide bedside commode—to reduce work of getting to bathroom and for defecation.

   c. Provide for psychological rest—emotional stress produces vasoconstriction, elevates arterial pressure, and speeds the heart.

      (1) Promote physical comfort.

      (2) Avoid situations that tend to promote anxiety/agitation.

      (3) Offer careful explanations and answers to the patient's questions.

2. Evaluate frequently for progression of left ventricular failure. Take frequent blood pressure readings.

   a. Observe for lowering of systolic pressure.

   b. Note narrowing of pulse pressure.

   c. Note alternations in strong and weak pulsations (pulsus alternans).

3. Auscultate heart sounds frequently.

   a. Note presence of S_3 or S_4 gallop (S_3 gallop is a significant indicator of congestive heart failure).

   b. Monitor for premature ventricular beats.

4. Observe for signs and symptoms of reduced peripheral tissue perfusion: cool temperature of skin, facial pallor, poor capillary refill of nailbeds.

5. Administer pharmacotherapy as directed.

6. Monitor clinical response of patient with respect to relief of symptoms (lessening dyspnea and orthopnea, decrease in crackles, relief of peripheral edema).

NURSING ALERT:
Watch for sudden unexpected hypotension, which can cause myocardial ischemia and decrease perfusion to vital organs.

B. *Improving Oxygenation*

1. Raise head of bed 20 to 30 cm (8–10 in)—reduces venous return to heart and lungs; alleviates pulmonary congestion.

   a. Support lower arms with pillows—to eliminate pull of their weight on shoulder muscles.

   b. Sit orthopneic patient on side of bed with feet supported by a chair, head and arms resting on an over-the-bed table, and lumbosacral area supported with pillows.

2. Auscultate lung fields every 4 hours for crackles and wheezes in dependent lung fields (fluid accumulates in areas affected by gravity).

   a. Mark with water-soluble ink the level on the patient's back where adventitious breath sounds are heard.

   b. Use markings for comparative assessment during changes in tours of duty with other nursing personnel.

3. Observe for increased rate of respirations (could be indicative of falling arterial pH).

4. Observe for Cheyne–Stokes respirations (may occur in elderly because of a decrease in cerebral perfusion stimulating a neurogenic response).

5. Position the patient every 2 hours (or encourage the patient to change position frequently)—to help prevent atelectasis and pneumonia.

6. Encourage deep-breathing exercises every 1 to 2 hours—to avoid atelectasis.

7. Offer small, frequent feedings—to avoid excessive gastric filling and abdominal distention with subsequent elevation of diaphragm that causes decrease in lung capacity.

8. Administer oxygen as directed.

C. *Restoring Fluid Balance*

1. Administer prescribed diuretic as ordered.

2. Give diuretic early in the morning—nighttime diuresis disturbs sleep.

3. Keep input and output record—the patient may lose large volume of fluid after a single dose of diuretic.

4. Weigh the patient daily—to determine if edema is being controlled: weight loss should not exceed 0.45 to 0.9 kg (1–2 lb/day).

5. Assess for weakness, malaise, muscle cramps—diuretic therapy may produce hypovolemia and electrolyte depletion, namely *hypokalemia*. Hypokalemia may cause weakening of cardiac contractions and may precipitate digitalis toxicity in the form of dysrhythmias.

6. Give oral potassium as prescribed.

7. Watch for problems associated with diuretic therapy including: disorders of hyperuricemia, volume depletion, and hyponatremia, magnesium depletion, hyperglycemia, and diabetes mellitus.

8. Watch for signs of bladder distention in the elderly male with prostatic hyperplasia.

9. Observe for symptoms of electrolyte depletion—lassitude, apathy, mental confusion, anorexia, decreasing urinary output, azotemia.

10. Limit intravenous fluid administration through use of heparin lock (allows for periodic drug administration without increasing excessive fluid intake).

11. Monitor for pitting edema of lower extremities and sacral area.

   a. Use "egg crate" mattress and sheepskin to prevent pressure sores (poor blood flow and edema increase susceptibility).

12. Observe for the complications of bedrest—pressure sores (especially in edematous patients), phlebothrombosis, pulmonary embolism.

13. Be alert to complaints of right upper quadrant abdominal pain, poor appetite, nausea, and abdominal distention (may indicate hepatic and visceral engorgement).

14. Monitor the patient's diet. Diet may be limited in sodium—to prevent, control, or eliminate edema; may also be limited in calories.

15. Caution patients to avoid added salt in food and foods with high sodium content.

D. *Improving Activity Tolerance*

1. Increase the patient's activities gradually. Alter or modify the patient's activities—to keep within the limits of his cardiac reserve.

   a. Assist the patient with self-care activities early in the day (fatigue sets in as day progresses).

   b. Be alert to complaints of chest pain or skeletal pain during or after activities.

2. Observe the pulse, symptoms, and behavioral response to increased activity.

   a. Monitor the patient's heart rate during self-care activities.

   b. Allow heart rate to decrease to preactivity level before initiating a new activity.

      (1) Note time lapse between cessation of activity and decrease in heart rate (decreased stroke volume causes immediate rise in heart rate).

      (2) Document time lapse and revise patient care plan as appropriate (progressive increase in

time lapse may be indicative of increased left ventricular failure).
3. Relieve nighttime anxiety and provide for rest and sleep—patients with congestive heart failure have a tendency to be restless at night because of cerebral hypoxia with superimposed nitrogen retention.
   a. Give appropriate sedation—to relieve insomnia and restlessness.

Patient Education/Health Maintenance

1. Explain the disease process to the patient; the term "failure" may have terrifying implications.
   a. Explain the pumping action of the heart—"to move blood through the body to provide nutrients and aid in the removal of waste material."
   b. Explain the difference between "heart attack" and congestive heart failure.
2. Teach the signs and symptoms of recurrence. Watch for:
   a. Gain in weight—report weight gain of more than 2 to 3 pounds (0.9–1.4 kg) in a few days. Weigh at same time daily to detect any tendency toward fluid retention.
   b. Swelling of ankles, feet, or abdomen
   c. Persistent cough
   d. Tiredness; loss of appetite
   e. Frequent urination at night
3. Review medication regimen.
   a. Label all medications.
   b. Give written instructions concerning pharmacologic therapy.
   c. Make sure the patient has a check-off system that will show that he/she has taken medications.
   d. Teach the patient to take and record pulse rate and blood pressure.
   e. Inform the patient of the signs and symptoms of adverse drug effects.
   f. If the patient is taking oral potassium solution, it may be diluted with juice and taken after a meal.
   g. Tell the patient to weigh self daily and log weight if on diuretic therapy.
4. Review activity program. Instruct the patient as follows:
   a. Increase walking and other activities gradually, provided they do not cause fatigue and dyspnea.
   b. In general, continue at whatever activity level can be maintained without the appearance of symptoms.
   c. Avoid excesses in eating and drinking.
   d. Undertake a weight reduction program until optimal weight is reached.
   e. Avoid extremes in heat and cold—which increase the work of the heart; air conditioning may be essential in a hot, humid environment.
   f. Keep *regular* appointment with health care provider or clinic.
5. Restrict sodium as directed.
   a. Give patient a booklet containing sodium content of common foods from local chapter of American Heart Association.
   b. Give patient a written diet plan with lists of permitted and restricted foods.
   c. Advise patient to look at all labels to ascertain sodium content (antacids, laxatives, cough remedies, etc.).

d. Teach the patient to rinse the mouth well after using tooth cleansers and mouthwashes—some of these contain large amounts of sodium. Water softeners are to be avoided.
e. Teach the patient that sodium is present in alkalizers, cough remedies, laxatives, pain relievers, estrogens, and other drugs.
f. Encourage use of flavorings, spices, herbs, and lemon juice.
g. Avoid salt substitutes in the presence of renal disease.

Evaluation

A. Normal blood pressure and heart rate
B. Respiratory rate 16 to 20, ABGs within normal limits, no signs of crackles or wheezes in lung fields
C. Weight decrease of 1 pound (2.2 kg) daily, no pitting edema of lower extremities and sacral area
D. Heart rate within normal limits, rests between activities

◆ ACUTE PULMONARY EDEMA

Acute pulmonary edema refers to the presence of excess fluid in the lung, either in the interstitial spaces or in the alveoli.

Pathophysiology/Etiology

1. The presence of fluid in the alveoli impedes gas exchange, especially oxygen movement into pulmonary capillaries.
2. May be caused by:
   a. Heart disease—acute left ventricular failure, myocardial infarction, aortic stenosis, severe mitral valve disease, hypertension, congestive heart failure
   b. Circulatory overload—transfusions and infusions
   c. Drug hypersensitivity; allergy; poisoning
   d. Lung injuries—smoke inhalation, shock lung, pulmonary embolism, or infarct
   e. Central nervous system injuries—stroke, head trauma
   f. Infection and fever—infectious pneumonia (viral, bacterial, parasitic)
   g. Postcardioversion, postanesthesia, postcardiopulmonary bypass
   h. Narcotic overdose

Clinical Manifestations

1. Coughing and restlessness during sleep (premonitory symptoms)
2. Extreme dyspnea and orthopnea—patient usually uses accessory muscles of respiration with retraction of intercostal spaces and supraclavicular areas
3. Cough with varying amounts of white- or pink-tinged frothy sputum
4. Extreme anxiety and panic
5. Noisy breathing—inspiratory and expiratory wheezing and bubbling sounds
6. Cyanosis with profuse perspiration
7. Distended neck veins
8. Tachycardia

9. Precordial pain (if pulmonary edema secondary to myocardial infarction)

Diagnostic Evaluation

1. Chest x-ray—shows interstitial edema
2. Echocardiogram to detect valvular disease
3. Measurement of pulmonary artery wedge pressure by Swan–Ganz catheter (differentiates etiology of pulmonary edema—cardiogenic or altered alveolar–capillary membrane)
4. Blood cultures in suspected infection—may be positive
5. Cardiac enzymes in suspected myocardial infarction—may be elevated

Management

1. The immediate objective of treatment is to improve oxygenation and reduce pulmonary congestion.
2. Identification and correction of precipitating factors and underlying conditions is then necessary to prevent recurrence.
3. Increasing oxygen tension (oxygen therapy), reducing fluid volume (diuretics, vasodilators), improving the heart's ability to pump effectively (glycosides, beta agonists), and decreasing anxiety guide therapeutic interventions.
4. *Oxygen therapy*—high concentrations of oxygen are used to combat hypoxemia. Intubation and ventilatory support may be necessary to improve hypoxemia and prevent hypercarbia.
5. *Morphine sulfate (Duramorph)*—reduces anxiety, promotes venous pooling of blood in the periphery, and reduces resistance against which the heart must pump.
6. *Vasodilator therapy* (nitroglycerin [Tridil] and nitroprusside [Nipride])—reduces the amount of blood returning to the heart and resistance against which the heart must pump.
7. *Diuretic therapy* (furosemide [Lasix], ethacrynic acid [Edecrin])—reduces blood volume and pulmonary congestion by producing prompt diuresis.
8. *Contractility enhancement therapy* (digoxin [Lanoxin], dopamine [Intropin], and aminophylline [Amoline]).
   a. Improves the ability of the heart muscle to pump more effectively, allowing for complete emptying of blood from the ventricle and a subsequent decrease in fluid backing up into the lungs.
   b. Aminophylline also prevents bronchospasm associated with pulmonary congestion.

Complications

1. Dysrhythmias
2. Respiratory failure

Nursing Assessment

1. Be alert to development of a new nonproductive cough.
2. Assess for signs and symptoms of hypoxia: restlessness, confusion, headache.
3. Auscultate lung fields frequently.

   a. Note inspiratory and expiratory wheezes, rhonchi, moist fine crackles appearing initially in lung bases and extending upward.
4. Auscultate for extra heart sounds.
   a. Note presence of third heart sound (may be difficult to hear because of respiratory sounds).
5. Identify precipitating factors that place patient at risk for development of pulmonary edema.

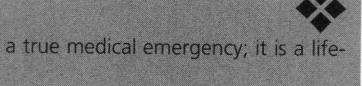

NURSING ALERT:
Acute pulmonary edema is a true medical emergency; it is a life-threatening condition.

Nursing Diagnoses

A. Impaired Gas Exchange related to excess fluid in the lungs
B. Anxiety related to sensation of suffocation and fear

Nursing Interventions

A. *Improving Oxygenation*
1. Give oxygen in high concentration—to relieve hypoxia and dyspnea.
2. *Take steps to reduce venous return to the heart.*
   a. Place patient in upright position; head and shoulders up, feet and legs hanging down—to favor pooling of blood in dependent portions of body by gravitational forces; to decrease venous return.
3. Give morphine in small titrated intermittent doses (IV) as directed.
   a. Morphine is *not* given if pulmonary edema is caused by stroke or occurs in the presence of chronic pulmonary disease or cardiogenic shock.
   b. Watch for excessive respiratory depression.
   c. Monitor blood pressure, as morphine may intensify hypotension.
   d. Have morphine antagonist available—naloxone hydrochloride (Narcan).
4. Give injections of diuretic IV.
   a. Insert an indwelling catheter—large urinary volume will accumulate rapidly.
   b. *Watch for falling blood pressure, increasing heart rate, and decreasing urinary output—indications that the total circulation is not tolerating diuresis and that hypovolemia may develop.*
   c. Check electrolyte levels, as potassium loss may be significant.
   d. Watch for signs of urinary obstruction in men with prostatic hyperplasia.
5. Administer vasodilator if patient fails to respond to therapy.
   a. Monitor by measuring pulmonary artery pressure and cardiac output.
6. Administer aminophylline (Amoline) if ordered.
   a. Monitor blood levels of drug.
   b. Evaluate for side effects of drug—ventricular dysrhythmias, hypotension, headache.
7. Administer cardiac glycosides as ordered.
8. Assist with cardioversion if indicated (pulmonary edema precipitates tachycardias).
9. Give appropriate drugs for severe, sustained hypertension.

10. Continually evaluate the patient's response to therapy. Reevaluate lung fields and cardiac status (see Assessment).

B. Decreasing Anxiety
1. Stay with the patient and display a confident attitude—the presence of another person is therapeutic, because the acute anxiety of the patient may tend to intensify the severity of patient's condition. (Arterial vasoconstriction diminishes as anxiety is relieved.)
2. Explain to the patient in a calm manner all therapies administered and the reason for their use.
   a. Give brief explanations related to goal of therapies (ie, "Morphine will help you relax and ease the work of breathing.").
   b. Explain to the patient importance of wearing oxygen mask. Assure the patient that mask will not increase sensation of suffocation.
3. Inform the patient and family of progress toward resolution of pulmonary edema.
4. Allow time for the patient and family to voice concerns and fears.

Patient Education/Health Maintenance

During convalescence, instruct the patient as follows to prevent recurrences of pulmonary edema:

1. Remind patient of early symptoms before onset of acute pulmonary edema; these should be reported promptly.
2. If coughing develops (a wet cough), sit with legs dangling over side of bed.
3. See Patient Education, Congestive Heart Failure, page 313.

Evaluation

A. Unlabored respirations at 14 to 18 times per minute, lungs clear on auscultation
B. Appears calm; rests comfortably

◆ ACQUIRED VALVULAR DISEASE OF THE HEART

The function of normal heart valves is to maintain the forward flow of blood from the atria to the ventricles and from the ventricles to the great vessels.

Valvular damage may interfere with valvular function by stenosis or by impaired closure that allows backward leakage of blood (valvular insufficiency, regurgitation, or incompetence).

Pathophysiology/Etiology

A. Mitral Stenosis
1. *Mitral stenosis* is the progressive thickening and contracture of valve cusps with narrowing of the orifice and progressive obstruction to blood flow.

2. Acute rheumatic valvulitis has "glued" the mitral valve flaps (commissures) together, thus shortening the chordae tendinae, so that the flap edges are pulled down, greatly narrowing the mitral orifice.
3. The left atrium has difficulty in emptying itself through the narrow orifice into the left ventricle; therefore, it dilates and hypertrophies. Pulmonary circulation becomes congested.
4. As a result of the abnormally high pulmonary arterial pressure that must be maintained, the right ventricle is subjected to a pressure overload and may eventually fail.

B. Mitral Insufficiency
1. Mitral insufficiency (regurgitation) is incomplete closure of the mitral valve during systole, allowing blood to flow back into the left atrium.
2. Left atrial pressures increase.
3. Left ventricular hypertrophy may develop due to inefficient emptying.
4. May be due to valve distortion or shortening or damage to chordae tendenal or papillary muscles caused by mitral valve prolapse, chronic rheumatic heart disease, postinfarction mitral regurgitation, infective endocarditis, and penetrating and nonpenetrating trauma.

C. Aortic Stenosis
1. Aortic stenosis is a narrowing of the orifice between the left ventricle and the aorta.
2. The obstruction to the aortic outflow places a pressure load on the left ventricle that results in hypertrophy and failure.
3. Left atrial pressure increases.
4. Pulmonary vascular pressure increases which may eventually lead to right ventricular failure.
5. May be caused by congenital anomalies, calcification, or rheumatic fever.

D. Aortic Insufficiency
1. Valve flaps fail to completely seal the aortic orifice during diastole and thus permit backflow of blood from the aorta into the left ventricle.
2. The left ventricle increases the force of contraction to maintain an adequate cardiac output often resulting in hypertrophy.
3. The low aortic diastolic pressures result in decreased coronary artery perfusion.
4. May be caused by rheumatic endocarditis, infective endocarditis, or congenital malformation, Marfan's syndrome, Ehler–Danlos syndrome, systemic lupus erythematosus, or by diseases that cause dilation or tearing of the ascending aorta (syphilitic disease, rheumatoid spondylitis, dissecting aneurysm).

E. Tricuspid Stenosis
1. Tricuspid stenosis is restriction of the tricuspid valve orifice due to commissural fusion and fibrosis.
2. Usually follows rheumatic fever and is commonly associated with diseases of the mitral valve.

F. Tricuspid Insufficiency (Regurgitation)
1. Tricuspid insufficiency allows the regurgitation of blood from the right ventricle into the right atrium during ventricular systole.
2. Common cause is dilation of right ventricle or rheumatic fever.

Clinical Manifestations

1. Fatigue, weakness
2. Dyspnea, cough, orthopnea, nocturnal dyspnea
3. Murmur
   a. Mitral stenosis—increased first heart sound, opening snap, and low-pitched rumbling diastolic murmur heard at the apex
   b. Mitral insufficiency—soft first heart sound and a blowing pansystolic murmur heard at the apex and transmitted to the axilla (characteristic of mild regurgitation due to papillary muscle dysfunction of mitral prolapse)
   c. Aortic stenosis—loud, rough systolic murmur over aortic area; often associated with a palpable thrill
   d. Aortic insufficiency—high-pitched blowing decrescendo diastolic murmur audible along the left sternal edge
   e. Tricuspid stenosis—similar to those of rheumatic mitral disease; blowing diastolic murmur along left sternal border
   f. Tricuspid insufficiency—pansystolic murmur in tricuspid area
4. Dysrhythmias, palpitations
5. Hemoptysis (from pulmonary hypertension) and hoarseness (from compression of left recurrent laryngeal nerve) in mitral stenosis.
6. Low blood pressure, dizziness, syncope, angina, and symptoms of CHF in aortic stenosis.
7. Arterial pulsations visible and palpable over precordium and visible in neck; widened pulse pressure; and water-hammer (Corrigan's) pulse (pulse strikes palpating finger with a quick, sharp stroke and then suddenly collapses) in aortic insufficiency
8. Symptoms of right-sided heart failure—edema, ascites, hepatomegaly—in tricuspid stenosis and insufficiency.

Diagnostic Evaluation

1. ECG—may show dysrhythmias
2. Echocardiography—show abnormalities of valve structure and function and chamber size and thickness.
3. Chest x-ray—may show cardiomegaly and pulmonary vascular congestion.
4. Cardiac catheterization and angiocardiography—to confirm diagnosis and determine severity.

Management

A. Medical Therapy
1. Antibiotic prophylaxis for endocarditis before invasive procedures—indicated in most cases
2. Treatment of heart failure—diuretics, sodium restriction, vasodilators, cardiac glycosides, etc. as indicated

B. Surgical Intervention
See p. 283 for care of the patient undergoing heart surgery.

1. For mitral stenosis:
   a. Closed mitral valvotomy—introduction of a dilator through the mitral valve to split its commissures
   b. Open mitral valvotomy—direct incision of the commissures
   c. Mitral valve replacement
   d. Balloon valvuloplasty—a balloon-tipped catheter is percutaneously inserted, threaded to the affected valve, and positioned across the narrowed orifice. The balloon is inflated/deflated, causing a "cracking" of the calcified commisures and enlargement of the valve orifice.
2. For mitral insufficiency—mitral valve replacement or annuloplasty (retailoring of the valve ring)
3. For aortic stenosis or insufficiency:
   a. Replacement of aortic valve with prosthetic or tissue valves.
   b. Balloon valvuloplasty (aortic stenosis)
4. For tricuspid stenosis or insufficiency—valvuloplasty or replacement may be done at time of surgical intervention for associated rheumatic mitral or aortic disease

Complications

1. Congestive heart failure
2. Possible right-sided heart failure
3. Dysrhythmias

Nursing Assessment

A. Mitral Stenosis
1. Auscultate for accentuated first heart sound, usually accompanied with an "opening snap" (due to sudden tensing of valve leaflets) at apex with diaphragm of stethoscope.
2. Place the patient in left lateral recumbent position. With bell of stethoscope at apex, auscultate for a low-pitched diastolic murmur (rumbling murmur). Note duration of murmur (long duration is indicative of significant stenosis).

B. Mitral Insufficiency
1. Auscultate for diminished first heart sound.
2. Auscultate for systolic murmur (prominent finding), commencing immediately after first heart sound at apex, and note radiation of sound to axilla and left intrascapular area.
3. Mild insufficiency may produce a pansystolic murmur (little connection between severity of mitral insufficiency and intensity of murmur auscultated).

C. Aortic Stenosis
1. Auscultate for prominent fourth heart sound and possible paradoxical splitting of second heart sound (suggestive of associated left ventricular dysfunction). First heart sound is normal.
2. Auscultate for a midsystolic murmur at the base of the heart (heard best) and at the apex of heart. Note harsh and rasping quality at base of heart and a higher pitch at apex of heart.

D. Aortic Insufficiency
1. Auscultate for soft first heart sound.
2. Place the patient in sitting position leaning forward.
3. Place diaphragm of stethoscope along left sternal border at the third and fourth intercostal space and then along the right sternal border. Auscultate for a high-pitched diastolic murmur. To increase audibility of murmur, ask the patient to hold breath at end of deep expiration. Re-auscultate for murmur.

E. Tricuspid Stenosis
1. Auscultate for a blowing diastolic murmur at the lower left sternal border (increases with inspiration).

F. Tricuspid Insufficiency
1. Auscultate for a third heart sound (may be accentuated by inspiration).
2. Auscultate for a pansystolic murmur in the parasternal region at the fourth intercostal space. Murmur is usually high-pitched.

Nursing Diagnosis

A. Decreased Cardiac Output related to altered preload, afterload or contractility
B. Activity Intolerance related to reduced oxygen supply
C. Ineffective Individual Coping related to acute/chronic illness.

Nursing Interventions

A. Maintaining Adequate Cardiac Output
1. Assess frequently for change in existing murmur or new murmur.
2. Assess for signs of left and/or right ventricular failure.
3. Monitor and treat dysrhythmias as ordered.
4. Prepare the patient for surgical intervention, see p. 283.

B. Improving Tolerance
1. Maintain bedrest while symptoms of congestive heart failure are present.
2. Allow patient to rest between interventions.
3. Begin activities gradually, ie, chair sitting for brief periods.
4. Assist or perform hygiene needs for patient to reserve strength for ambulation.

B. Strengthening Coping Abilities
1. Instruct the patient regarding specific valvular dysfunction, possible etiology, and therapies implemented to relieve symptoms.
   a. Include family members in discussions with the patient.
   b. Stress the importance of adapting lifestyle to cope with illness.

2. Discuss with the patient surgical intervention as the treatment modality, if applicable.
3. Assess the patient's use of appropriate coping mechanisms to deal with illness.
4. Refer the patient to appropriate counseling services, if indicated (vocational, social work, cardiac rehabilitation).

Patient Education/Health Maintenance

1. Review activity restriction/schedule with patient and family.
2. Instruct patient to report signs of impending or worsening heart failure: dyspnea, cough, increased fatigue, ankle swelling.
3. Review sodium and/or fluid restrictions.
4. Review medications: purpose, action, schedule and side effects.
5. See Patient Education, Congestive Heart Failure, page 313; Infective Endocarditis, page 304; and Rheumatic Endocarditis, page 305.

Evaluation

A. Blood pressure and heart rate within normal limits
B. Tolerating chair sitting for 15 minutes every 2 hours
C. Discussing ways to cope with lifestyle/activity changes

◆ CARDIAC DYSRHYTHMIAS

Cardiac dysrthythmias are disturbances in regular heart rate and/or rhythm due to change in electrical conduction or automaticity. Dysrhythmias may arise from the SA node (sinus bradycardia or tachycardia) or anywhere within the atria or ventricles (known as ectopy or ectopic beats). Some may be benign and asymptomatic, while other dysrhythmias are life-threatening.

Dysrhythmias may be detected by change in pulse, abnormality on auscultation of heart rate, or ECG abnormality. Continuous cardiac monitoring is indicated for potentially life-threatening dysrhythmias.

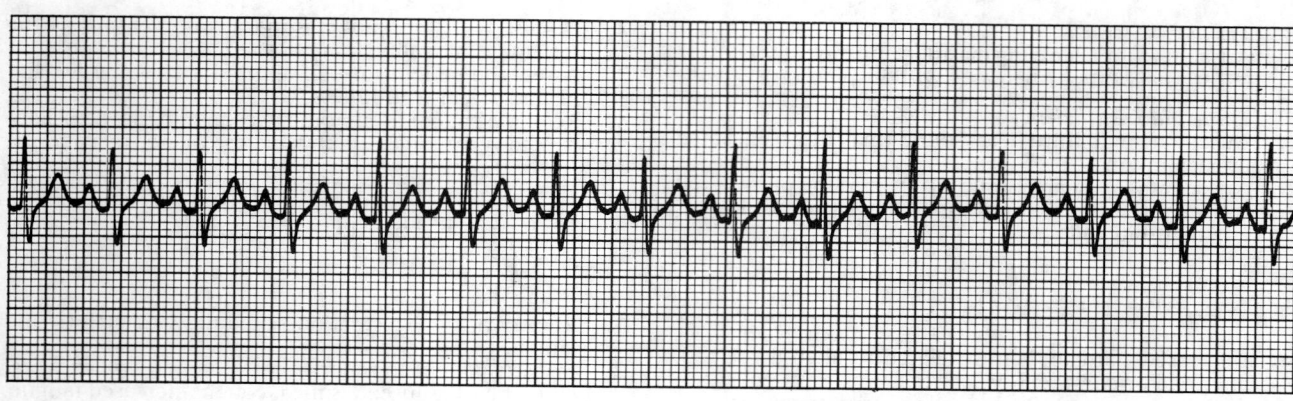

FIGURE 11-4 *Sinus tachycardia.*

Sinus Tachycardia (Fig. 11-4)

A. *Etiology*
1. Sympathetic nerve fibers, which act to speed up excitation of the SA node, are stimulated by underlying causes such as: anxiety, exercise, fever, shock, drugs, altered metabolic states (such as hyperthyroidism), or electrolyte disturbances.
2. The wave of impulse is transmitted through the normal conduction pathways; the rate of sinus stimulation is simply greater than normal (rate exceeds 100 beats per minute).

B. *Analysis*
Rate—130
Rhythm—R-R intervals are regular

P wave—present for each QRS complex, normal configuration, and each P wave is identical
P-R interval—falls between 0.12 and 02.0, or 0.16 seconds
QRS complex—normal in appearance, one follows each P wave
QRS interval—0.06 seconds
T wave—follows each QRS complex and is positively conducted

C. *Management*
1. Treatment is directed toward elimination of the cause, rather than the dysrhythmia.
2. Urgency is dependent on the effect of rapid heart rate on coronary artery filling time to prevent cardiac ischemia.

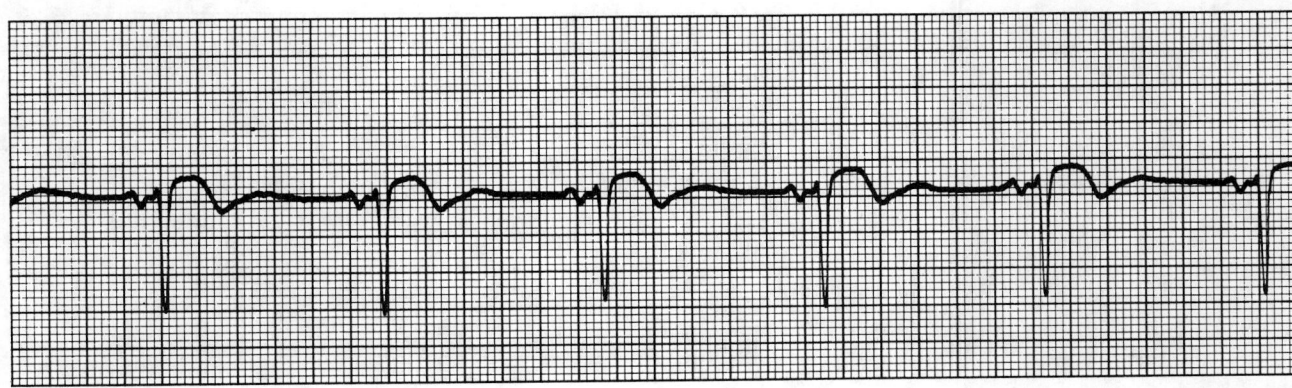

FIGURE 11-5 *Sinus bradycardia.*

Sinus Bradycardia (Fig. 11-5)

A. Etiology
1. The parasympathetic fibers (vagal tone) are stimulated and cause the sinus node to slow.
2. Underlying causes
   a. Can be expected in the well-trained athlete
   b. Drugs
   c. Altered metabolic states, such as hypothyroidism
   d. The process of aging, which causes increasing fibrotic tissue and scarring of the SA node.
   e. Certain cardiac diseases, such as acute MI (especially inferior wall MI)
3. The wave of impulse is transmitted through the normal conduction pathways; the rate of sinus stimulation is simply less than normal (less than 60 beats per minute).

B. Analysis
Rate—55
Rhythm—R-R interval is regular
P wave—present for each QRS complex, normal configuration, and each P wave is identical
P-R interval—falls between 0.12 and 0.20, or 0.18
QRS—normal in appearance, one follows each P wave
QRS interval—0.06
T wave—follows each QRS and is positively conducted

C. Management
1. The urgency of treatment is dependent on the effect of the slow rate on maintenance of cardiac output.
2. Atropine 0.5 mg. IV push blocks vagal stimulation to the SA node and therefore accelerates heart rate.
3. If the bradycardia persists, a pacemaker may be required.

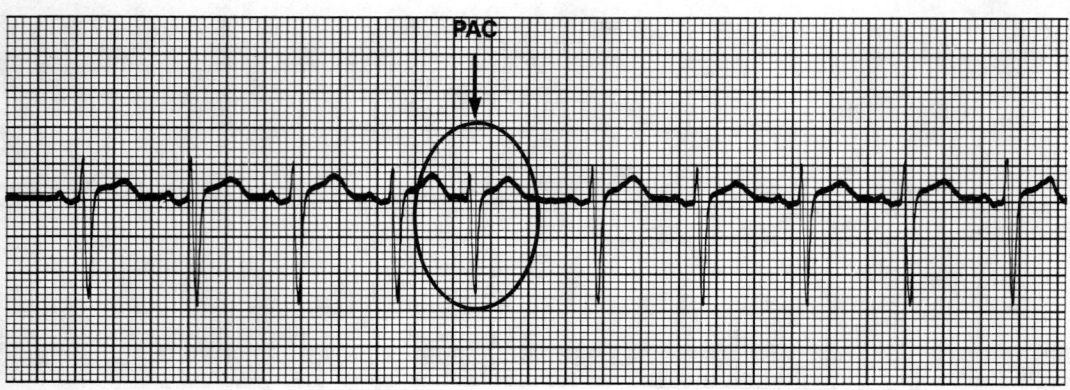

FIGURE 11-6 *Normal sinus rhythm with premature atrial contraction.*

Premature Atrial Contraction (PAC) (Fig. 11-6)

A. Etiology
1. May occur in the healthy or diseased heart. Is of no particular significance in the healthy heart. In the diseased heart, it may represent ischemia and a resultant irritability in the atria.
2. The PAC may increase in frequency and be the precursor of more serious dysrhythmias in the diseased heart.
3. The wave of impulse of the PAC originates within the atria and outside the sinus node.
4. Because the impulse originates within the atria, the P wave will be present, but it will be different in appearance as compared with those beats originating within the sinus node.
5. The impulse traverses the remainder of the conduction system in a normal pattern; thus the QRS complex is identical in configuration to the normal sinus beats.

B. Analysis
Rate—may be slow or fast
Rhythm—will be irregular; this is caused by the early occurrence of the PAC.
P wave—will be present for each normal QRS complex; the P wave of the premature contraction will be distorted in shape.
P-R interval—may be normal but can also be shortened, depending on where in the atria the impulse originated. The closer the site of atrial impulse formation to the AV node, the shorter the P-R interval will be.
QRS complex—within normal limits because all conduction below the atria is normal.
T wave—normally conducted.

C. Management
1. Generally requires no treatment.
2. PACs should be monitored for increasing frequency.

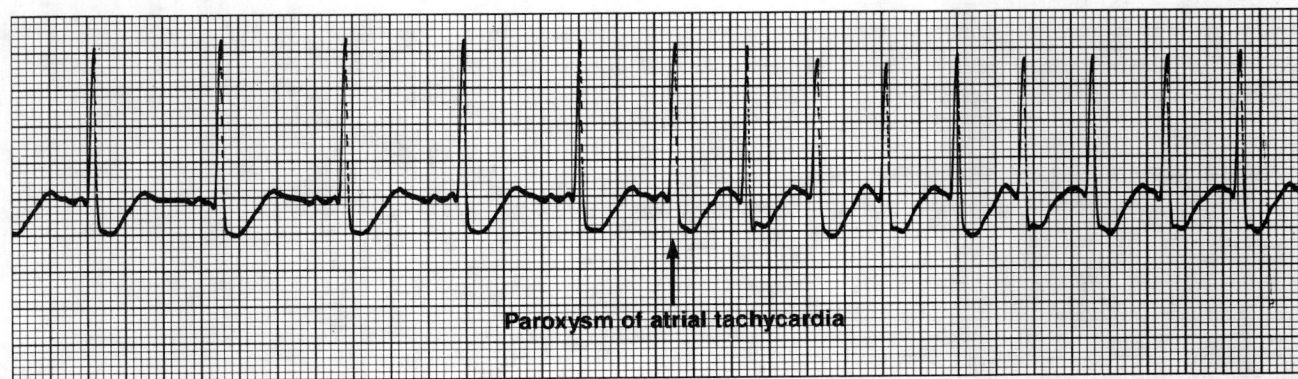

FIGURE 11-7 *Paroxysmal atrial tachycardia.*

Paroxysmal Atrial Tachycardia (PAT) (Fig. 11-7)

A. *Etiology*
1. Causes include:
   a. Syndromes of accelerated pathways (eg, Wolff-Parkinson-White syndrome)
   b. Syndrome of mitral valve prolapse
   c. Ischemic coronary artery diseases
   d. Excessive use of alcohol, cigarettes, caffeine
   e. Drugs —digoxin (Lanoxin) is a frequent cause
2. An ectopic atrial focus captures the rhythm of the heart and is stimulated at a very rapid rate; the impulse is conducted normally through the conduction system so that the QRS complex usually appears within normal limits.
3. The rate is often so rapid that P waves are not obvious but may be "buried" in the preceding T wave.

B. *Analysis of PAT*
Rate—between 150 and 250 beats per minute
Rhythm—regular
P waves—are present before each QRS complex; however, the faster the rate, the more difficult it becomes to visualize P waves. The P waves can frequently be measured with calipers by observing the varying configuration of the preceding T waves
P-R interval—usually not measureable
QRS complex—will appear normal in configuration and within 0.06 to 0.10 seconds

T waves—will be distorted in appearance as a result of P waves being buried in them.

C. *Management*
1. Treatment is directed to first slowing the rate and second, reverting the dysrhythmia to a normal sinus rhythm.
2. Reducing the rate may be accomplished by having the patient perform a Valsalva maneuver. This stimulates the vagus nerve to slow the heart.
   a. A Valsalva maneuver may be done by having the patient gag or "bear down" as though attempting to have a bowel movement.
   b. The health care provider may choose to perform carotid massage.
3. Adenosine (Adenocard) is the drug of choice for PAT associated with hypotension, chest pain, or shortness of breath.
   a. The initial dose is 6 mg rapid IV push followed by 12 mg. If no response in 1 to 2 minutes, a third bolus of 12 mg may be needed.
   b. Has a very short half-life and is therefore eliminated quickly.
4. Beta-adrenergic blockers such as esmolol (Brevibloc) may be used.
5. The calcium channel blocking agents (eg, verapamil [Calan]) are effective in reverting this dysrhythmia. Beware of hypotension especially in the volume-depleted patient.
6. If drug therapy is ineffective, elective cardioversion can be used.

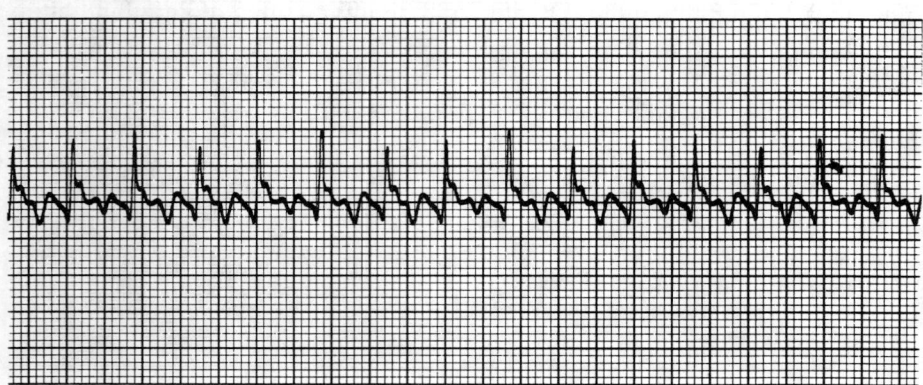

FIGURE 11-8 *Atrial flutter.*

Atrial Flutter (Fig. 11-8)

A. Etiology
1. Occurs with atrial stretching or enlargement (as atrio-ventricular valvular disease), myocardial infarction, and congestive heart failure.
2. An ectopic atrial focus captures the rhythm in atrial flutter and fires at an extremely rapid rate (200–400) with regularity.
3. Conduction of the impulse through the conduction system is normal; thus the QRS complex is unaffected.
4. An important feature of this dysrhythmia is that the AV node sets up a therapeutic block, which disallows some impulse transmission.
   a. This can produce a varying block or a fixed block; ie, sometimes the AV node will transmit every second flutter wave, producing a 2:1 block, or the rhythm can be 3:1 or 4:1.
   b. If the AV node conducted 1:1 then the outcome would be a ventricular rate of about 300/min. This would rapidly deteriorate.

B. Analysis
Rate—atrial rate between 250 and 400 beats per minute; ventricular rate will depend on degree of block

Rhythm—regular or irregular, depending on kind of block (eg, 2:1, 3:1, or a combination)
P wave—not present; instead, it is replaced by a sawtoothed pattern that is produced by the rapid firing of the atrial focus. these waves are also referred to as "F" waves.
P-R interval—not measurable
QRS complex—normal configuration and normal conduction time
T wave—present but may be obscured by flutter waves

C. Management
1. The urgency of treatment depends on the ventricular response rate and resultant symptoms. Too rapid or slow a rate will decrease cardiac output.
2. A calcium channel blocker such as diltiazem (Cardizem) may be used to slow AV nodal conduction. Use with caution in the patient with CHF, hypotension, or concomitant beta-blocker therapy.
3. Digitalis and quinidine preparations may be used.
4. A beta-adrenergic blocking drug such as esmolol (Brevibloc) or propranolol (Inderal) may also be used.
5. If drug therapy is unsuccessful, atrial flutter will often respond to cardioversion. Small doses of electrical current are often successful.

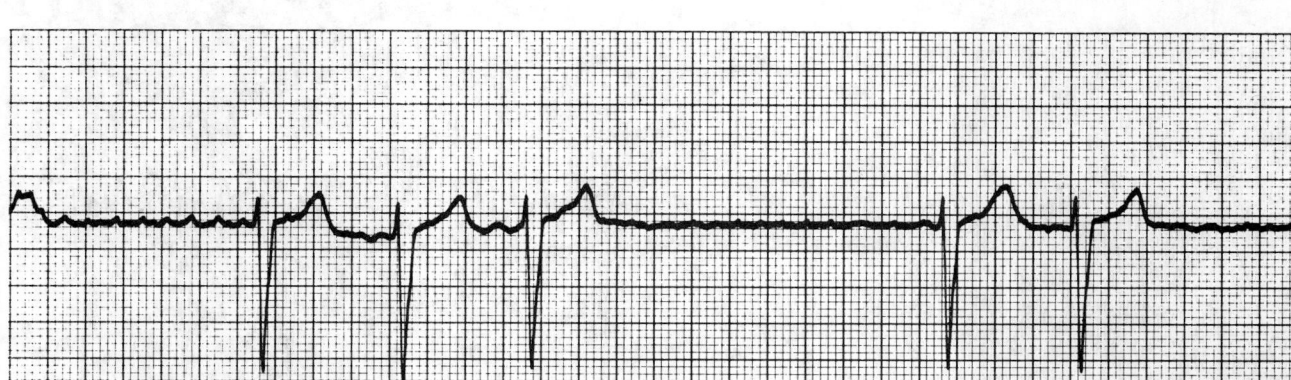

FIGURE 11-9 *Atrial fibrillation with slow ventricular response (controlled).*

Atrial Fibrillation (Fig. 11-9)

A. *Etiology*
1. Fibrotic changes associated with the aging process, acute MI, valvular diseases, and digitalis preparations may cause atrial fibrillation.
2. Multiple atrial foci fire impulses at rapid and disorganized rates.
3. The atria are not depolarized effectively; hence, there are no well-formed P waves.
4. Instead, the baseline between QRS complexes is filled with a "wiggly" line that is described as fine or coarse.
5. If the atrial rate is rapid enough, the line will appear almost flat. The atria are said to be firing at rates of between 300 and 500 times per minute.
6. The conduction of a QRS complex is so random that the rhythm is extremely irregular.
7. Atrial fibrillation may be described as controlled if the ventricular response is 100 beats per minute or less; the dysrhythmia is uncontrolled if the rate is above 150 beats per minute.

B. *Analysis*
Rate—atrial fibrillation is usually immeasurable because fibrillatory waves replace P waves; ventricular rate may vary from bradycardia to tachycardia
Rhythm—classically described as an "irregular irregularity"
P wave—replaced by fibrillatory waves, sometimes called "little f" waves
P-R interval—immeasurable
QRS complex—a normally conducted complex
T wave—normally conducted

C. *Management*
1. Controlled atrial fibrillation of long-standing duration requires no treatment as long as the patient is experiencing no untoward effects. Most cardiologists agree that reversion of long-standing atrial fibrillation is hazardous because of the potential for a thrombus to be dislodged from the atria at the time of reversion.
2. Uncontrolled atrial fibrillation (ventricular responses of 100 beats per minute or greater) is treated with digitalis preparations. If the atrial fibrillation is of recent onset, the cardiologist may choose to revert the rhythm to a sinus rhythm.
3. Atrial fibrillation is treated with electrical cardioversion if the patient is unstable.
4. The beta-adrenergic blocking drugs or calcium ion antagonists may also be used if digitalis and quinidine prove ineffective.
5. Adenosine (Adenocard) may be used to assist in diagnosing the rhythm.

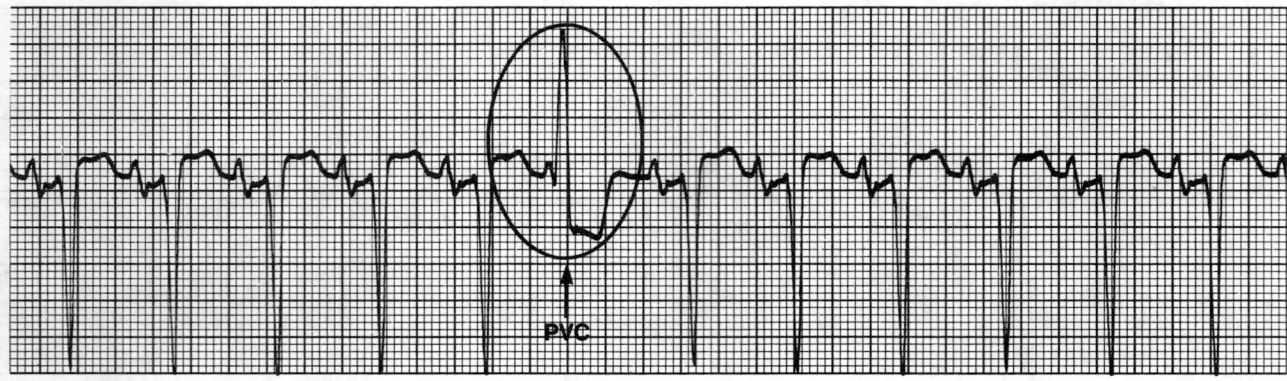

FIGURE 11-10 *Normal sinus rhythm with premature ventricular contraction.*

Premature Ventricular Contraction (PVC) (Fig. 11-10)

A. Etiology
1. May be caused by acute MI, other forms of heart disease, pulmonary diseases, electrolyte disturbances, metabolic instability, and drug abuse.
2. The wave of impulse originates from an ectopic focus (foci) within the ventricles at a rate faster than the next normally occurring beat.
3. Because the normal conduction pathway is bypassed, the configuration of the PVC is wider than normal and is distorted in appearance.
4. PVCs may occur in regular sequence with normal rhythm—every other beat (bigeminy), every 3rd beat (trigeminy, etc.) (Fig. 11-11).

B. Analysis
Rate—may be slow or fast
Rhythm—will be irregular because of the premature firing of the ventricular ectopic focus.

P wave—will be absent, because the impulse originates in the ventricle, bypassing the atria and AV node.
P-R interval—immeasurable
QRS complex—will be widened greater than 0.12 seconds, bizarre in appearance when compared with normal QRS complex. The QRS of a PVC is often referred to as having a "sore thumb" appearance.
T wave—the T wave of the PVC is usually deflected opposite to the QRS

C. Management
1. PVCs are usually the precursors of more serious ventricular dysrhythmias. The following conditions involving PVCs require prompt and vigorous treatment:
   a. PVCs occurring at a rate exceeding 6 per minute.
   b. Occur as 2 or more consecutively
   c. PVCs fall on the peak or down slope of the T wave (period of vulnerability).
   d. Are of varying configurations, indicating a multiplicity of foci.
2. The standard treatment of PVCs is with lidocaine hydrochloride (Xylocaine) by IV push.

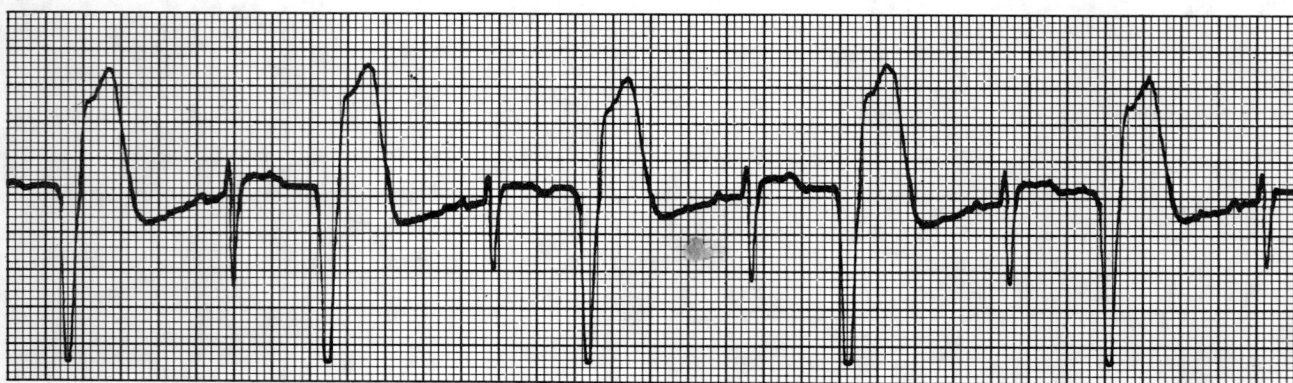

FIGURE 11-11 *Ventricular bigeminy.*

a. For effective treatment of PVCs, it is important to raise the serum level of lidocaine as rapidly as possible without causing toxic effects.

b. An initial bolus of 1 to 15 mg/kg may be administered.

c. If the dysrhythmia continues to "break through," another 1 mg/kg bolus may be given within 15 minutes.

d. The bolus should be followed by a continuous IV infusion of lidocaine 2 gm/500 mL D5W at 1 to 4 mg/minute.

3. Be alert to the development of confusion, slurring of speech, and diminished mentation, as lidocaine toxicity affects the central nervous system. Should these symptoms appear, slowing the lidocaine may cause them to abate.

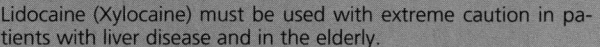

NURSING ALERT:
Lidocaine (Xylocaine) must be used with extreme caution in patients with liver disease and in the elderly.

4. If ventricular ectopy occurs concomitantly with a bradycardia, use lidocaine with caution, if at all. The ectopy may be compensation for the bradycardia. If lidocaine abolishes compensatory beats, the cardiac output may be seriously compromised, to the patient's detriment.

5. If ventricular premature beats occur in conjunction with a bradydysrhythmia, atropine may be chosen to accelerate the heart rate and eliminate the need for ectopic beats.

6. Atropine should be used with caution in the acute MI. The injured myocardium may not be able to tolerate the accelerated rate.

7. If lidocaine proves to be ineffective in controlling PVCs, procainamide (Pronestyl) may be given (IV push), followed by a continuous drip. The average bolus dose is 300 mg. Procainamide may cause hypotension.

8. If lidocaine and procainamide prove ineffective, either alone or in combination therapy, bretylium tosylate (Bretylol) may be used. Bretylium is administered in a continuous infusion.

9. Magnesium sulfate may be used, especially in patients with acute MI. It may be given as 1 gm IV over 5 minutes to 24 hours depending on the urgency of the situation.

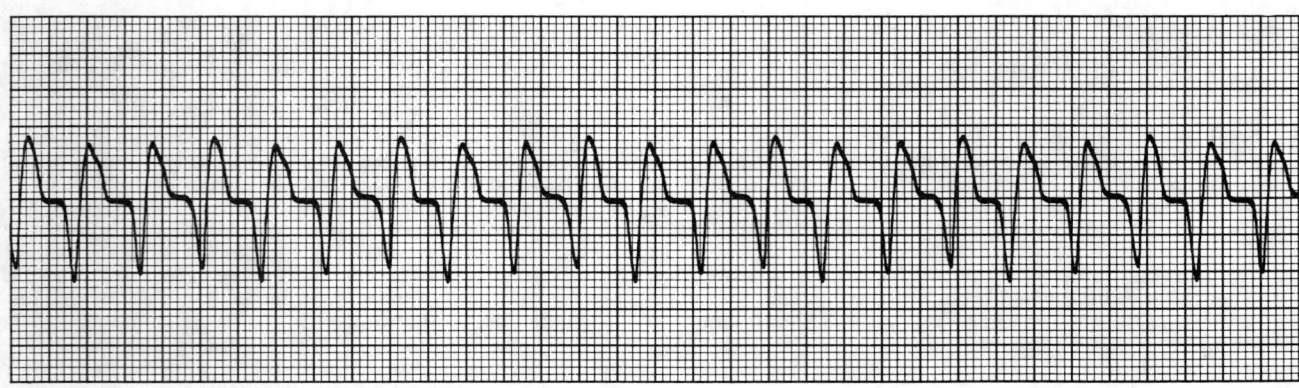

FIGURE 11-12 Ventricular tachycardia.

Ventricular Tachycardia (Fig. 11-12)

A. Etiology
1. Occurs in:
   a. Acute MI
   b. Syndromes of accelerated rhythm that deteriorate (eg, Wolff-Parkinson-White syndrome).
   c. Metabolic acidosis, especially lactic acidosis
   d. Electrolyte disturbances
   e. Toxicity to certain drugs, such as digoxin (Lanoxin) or isoproterenol (Isuprel)
2. A life-threatening dysrhythmia that originates from an irritable focus within the ventricle at a rapid rate.
3. Because the ventricles are capable of an inherent rate of 40 beats per minute or less, a ventricular rhythm at a rate of 100 beats per minute may be considered tachycardia.

B. Analysis
Rate—usually between 140 and 220 beats per minute
Rhythm—usually regular but may be irregular
P wave—not present
P-R interval—immeasurable
QRS complex—broad, bizarre in configuration, widened greater than 0.12 seconds
T wave—usually deflected opposite to the QRS complex.

C. Management
1. If the patient is alert and not hemodynamically decompensating, lidocaine hydrochloride (Xylocaine) is administered as a bolus. This is followed by a continuous lidocaine infusion.
2. If the event is witnessed and the patient is unconscious, administer a precordial blow.
3. If the patient loses consciousness and pulse, immediate defibrillation is indicated.

NURSING ALERT:
Ventricular tachycardia is life-threatening, and its presentation calls for immediate intervention by the nurse.

4. If the patient remains alert and drug therapy is not working, then synchronized cardioversion is applied. The purpose of cardioversion is to abolish all cardiac rhythm and allow the normal pacemaker the opportunity to capture the rhythm.
5. In some cases, ventricular tachycardia may be refractory to drug therapy. Nonpharmacologic treatments such as endocardial resection, aneurysmectomy, antitachycardia pacemakers, cryoblation, automatic internal defibrillators, and catheter ablation are alternative treatment modalities.
6. An atypical form of ventricular tachycardia, referred to as polymorphous ventricular tachycardia or tordsades de pointes, can result as a consequence of quinidine (Quinaglute) therapy. It is important differentiate this atypical form because its therapy differs from that of the more typical ventricular tachycardia.
   a. Torsades de pointes is characterized by a Q-T interval prolonged to greater than 0.60 seconds, varying R-R intervals, and polymorphous QRS complexes.
   b. The treatment of choice is administration of magnesium sulfate 1 gm IV over 5 to 60 minutes.
   c. If the patient loses consciousness and pulse, defibrillate.
   d. Ventricular pacing to override the ventricular rate and hence capture the rhythm is also an acceptable treatment.
   e. Lidocaine and procainamide (Pronestyl) are avoided, because their effect is to prolong the Q-T interval.

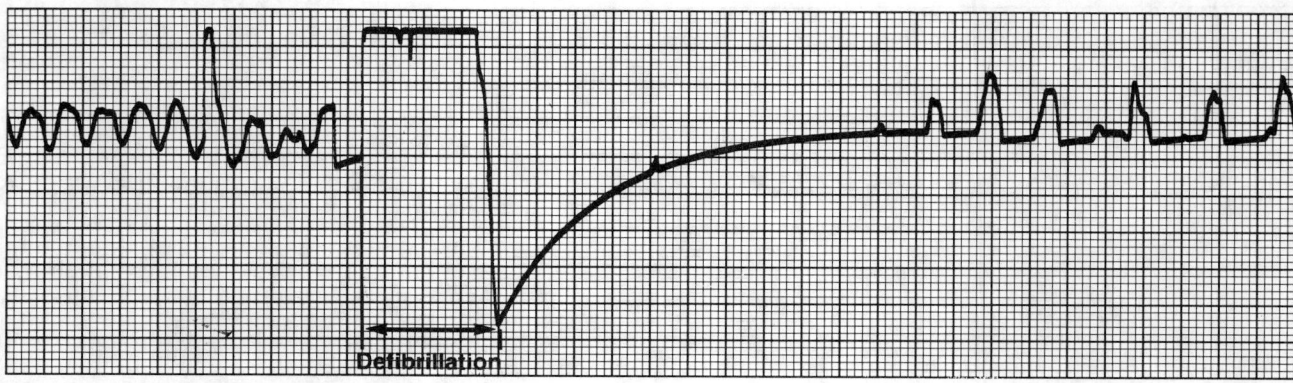

FIGURE 11-13 *Ventricular fibrillation with defibrillation.*

Ventricular Fibrillation (Fig. 11-13)

A. Etiology
1. Occurs in acute MI, acidosis, electrolyte disturbances, and other deteriorating ventricular rhythms.
2. The ventricles are firing chaotically at rates that exceed 300 beats per minute and so do not allow for effective impulse conduction.
3. Cardiac output ceases, and the patient loses pulse, blood pressure, and consciousness.
4. Clinical death occurs and must be reversed immediately, or the patient will succumb.

B. Analysis
Rate—immeasurable because of absence of well-formed QRS complexes
Rhythm—chaotic
P wave—not present
QRS complex—bizarre, chaotic, no definite contour
T wave—not apparent

C. Management
1. The only treatment for ventricular fibrillation is immediate defibrillation. Defibrillate at 200 watts/second, then 200 to 300, then 360; pause only to check rhythm and pulse quickly between these defibrillations. Epinephrine may make the fibrillation more vulnerable to defibrillation.
2. If the third shock is unsuccessful, begin CPR and administer epinephrine (Adrenalin) 1 mg IV push.
3. Unsuccessful defibrillation may be a result of lactic acidosis.
4. Check adequacy of CPR.

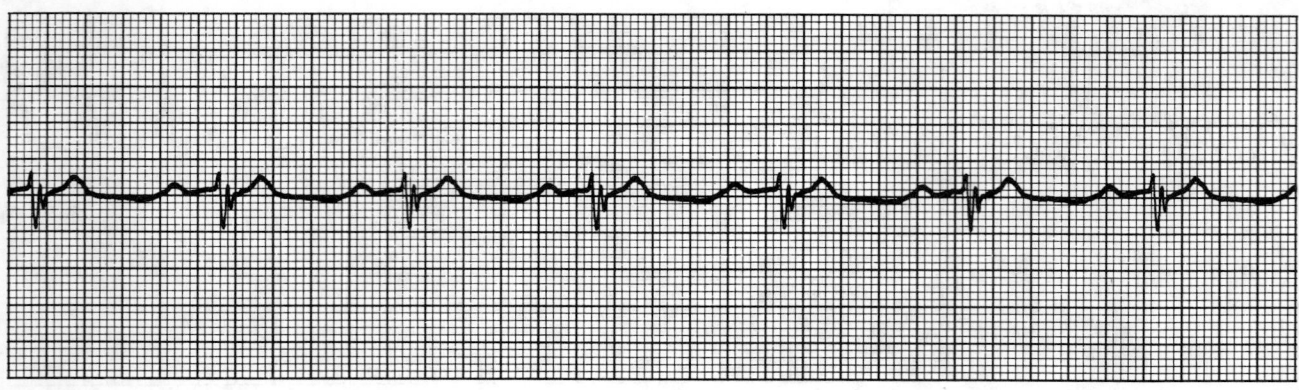

FIGURE 11-14 First-degree AV block.

Atrioventricular (AV) Block

A. Etiology
1. May be caused by ischemia or inferior wall MI, digitalis toxicity, hypothyroidism, or Stokes–Adams syndrome.
2. Impaired tissue at the level of the AV node prevents the timely passage of the wave of impulse through the conduction system.
3. In first-degree AV block, the impulse is transmitted normally, but it is delayed longer at the level of the AV node. The P-R interval exceeds 0.20 seconds.
4. In second-degree AV block, there is no relationship between the atrial activity recorded on the monitor and the ventricular activity. Both chambers are discharging impulses, but activity of the atria and activity of the ventricles bear no relationship to each other.

B. Analysis
1. First Degree AV Block (Fig. 11-14)
    Rate—usually normal but may be slow
    Rhythm—regular
    P wave—present for each QRS complex, identical in configuration
    P-R interval—prolonged to greater than 0.20 seconds
    QRS complex—normal in appearance and between 0.06 and 0.10 seconds
    T wave—normally conducted

2. Second-degree AV block (Fig. 11-15)
    Rate—usually normal
    Rhythm—may be regular or irregular
    P wave—present but some may not be followed by a QRS complex. A ratio of 2, 3, or 4 P waves to 1 QRS complex may exist.
    P-R interval—varies in Mobitz I (Wenchenbac), usually lengthens until one is nonconducted; constant in Mobitz II, but not all Ps conducted.
3. Third-Degree AV Block (complete heart block) (Fig. 11-16)
    Rate—atrial rate is measured independently of the ventricular rate. The ventricular rate is usually very slow.
    Rhythm—each independent rhythm will be regular, but they will bear no relationship to each other.
    P wave—present but no consistent relationship with the QRS
    P-R interval—not really measurable
    QRS complex—dependent on the escape mechanism, ie, AV nodal will have normal QRS, ventricular will be wide and the rate will be slower.

C. Management
Like that of other dysrhythmias, the treatment of heart blocks depends on the effect the rate is having on cardiac output.

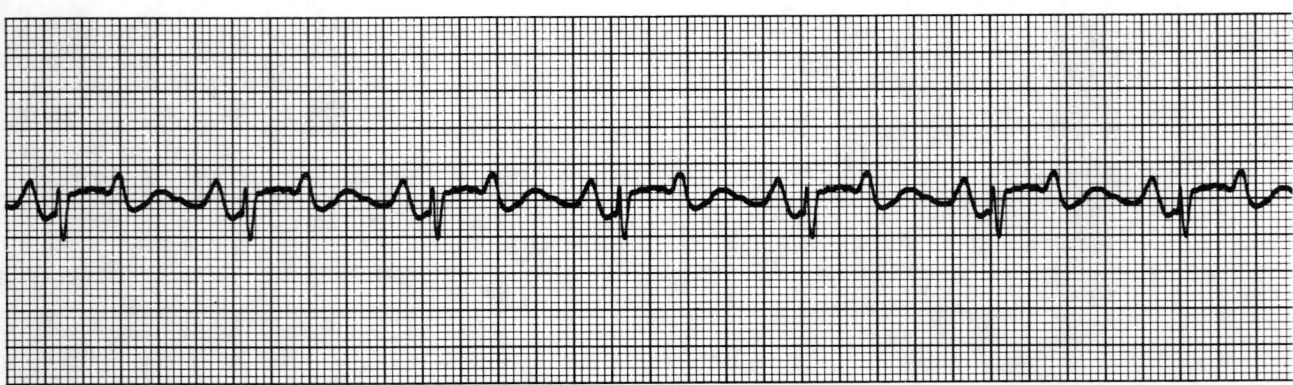

FIGURE 11-15 Second-degree AV block (Mobitz I).

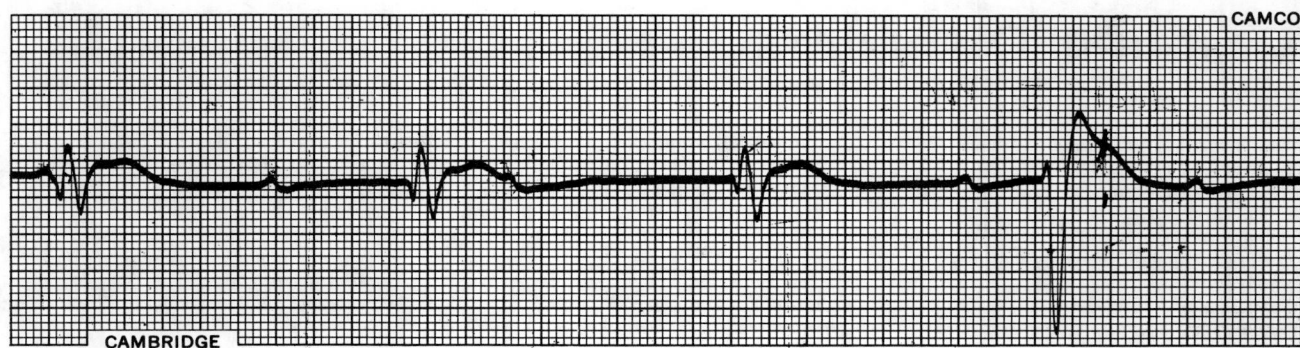

FIGURE 11-16 *Third-degree AV block.*

1. First-degree AV block usually requires no treatment.
2. Second-degree AV block may require treatment if the ventricular rate falls too low to maintain effective cardiac output.
3. Third-degree AV block may require treatment of choice when intervention is called for.
4. Transcutaneous pacing should be employed in the emergent situation.

5. Atropine may be given while awaiting the pacemaker, but it must be remembered that the effect of atropine is to block vagal tone, and the vagus acts on the sinus node. Because the AV node is the culprit in heart block, atropine may not be helpful.

Selected References

Alspach, J., ed. (1991). *Core curriculum for critical care nursing* (4th ed.). Philadelphia: W.B. Saunders.

Aragon, D., & Martin, M. (1993). What you should know about thrombolytic therapy for acute MI. *American Journal of Nursing, 93*(9), 24-31.

Dossey, B., Guzzetta, C., & Vanderstaay-Kenner, C. (1992). *Critical care nursing: Body mind spirit* (3rd ed.). Philadelphia: J.B. Lippincott.

Guyton, A. (1991). *Textbook of medical physiology* (8th ed.). Philadelphia: W.B. Saunders.

Hadley, S., & Saarmann, L. (1991). Lipid physiology and nutritional considerations in coronary heart disease. *Critical Care Nurse, 11*(10), 28-35.

Matrisciano, L. (1992). Unstable angina: An overview. *Critical Care Nurse, 12*(8), 38-40.

Morton, P.G. (1994). Update on new antiarrhythmic drugs. *Critical Care Nursing Clinics of North America, 6*(1), 69-84.

O'Neal, P. (1994). How to spot early signs of cardiogenic shock. *American Journal of Nursing, 94*(5), 36-41.

Porterfield, L., & Porterfield, J. (1993). Digitalis toxicity: A common occurrence. *Critical Care Nurse, 13*(6), 40-43.

Snelson, C., Cline, B., & Luby, C. Infective endocarditis: A challenging diagnosis. *Dimensions of Critical Care Nursing, 12*(1), 4-16.

Thompson, J., McFarland, G., Hirsch, J., & Tuclar, S. (1993). *Mosby's clinical nursing* (3rd ed.). Philadelphia: C.V. Mosby.

Witherell, C. (1994). Cardiac rhythm control devices. *Critical Care Nursing Clinics of North America, 6*(1), 85-101.

Wright, J., Shelton, B. (1993). *Desk Reference for Critical Care Nursing.* Boston: Jones & Bartlett Publishers.

CHAPTER 12 ◆

Vascular Disorders

Management of Vascular Disorders

◆ ANTICOAGULANT THERAPY

Anticoagulant therapy is the administration of medications to achieve the following:

- Disrupt the blood's natural clotting mechanism.
- Prevent formation of a thrombus in postoperative patients.
- Intercept the extension of a thrombus once it has formed.

Types of anticoagulants include coumarin derivatives such as warfarin sodium (Coumadin), given orally, and heparin sodium (Heparin), given parenterally. A new low molecular weight heparin, enoxa pararin (Lovenox) is being given prophylactically following total hip replacement. The benefits are more steady bioavailability, longer half-life, and less platelet inhibition than standard heparin. Anticoagulants may be contraindicated or used with extreme caution in conditions that may lead to bleeding, in patients who may have poor follow-up, and in patients with hepatic and renal insufficiency (Procedure Guidelines 12-1.)

Clinical Indications

1. Venous thrombosis—because of the danger of extension and the danger of emboli
2. Pulmonary embolism—prophylactically, if patient is known to be suspect; also indicated during recovery phase to prevent further clot formation
3. Patient susceptible to embolism—such as a surgical patient who has rheumatic heart disease, one who has had valve surgery
4. Coronary occlusion with myocardial infarction (MI)
5. Stroke caused by emboli or cerebral thrombi—to reduce sludging of blood; useful in prevention and treatment of strokes

> **NURSING ALERT:**
> Anticoagulation may not be prescribed preoperatively because of fear of increasing possibility of hemorrhage during operation. Mini-doses of heparin may be prescribed.

Nursing Interventions

A. **Administering Anticoagulants**
1. Administer heparin by subcutaneous injection (see p. 331) or intravenously (IV) through a continuous infusion or heparin lock.
   a. Use a continuous infusion pump.
   b. Check frequently to ensure that system is working properly: exact dosage, no leaks, no kinks.
2. Check patient's weight because dosage is calculated on the basis of weight.
3. Double check strength and dosage of heparin, especially when giving a high dose.
4. Administer coumarin derivative orally after checking most recent clotting studies and ensuring proper dosage.
5. Be aware that heparin may be continued for 4 to 5 days after oral anticoagulant is started due to delayed onset of therapeutic effectiveness with oral anticoagulants.

B. **Monitoring Clotting Profile**
1. Be sure clotting profiles are obtained before treatment is initiated, to detect hidden bleeding tendencies.
2. Obtain partial thromboplastin time (PTT) or prothrombin time (PT) daily, or as ordered, and check results before giving next dose of anticoagulant. Dosage may be adjusted to achieve desired elevation of these levels.
   a. PTT monitors heparin therapy—ratio of patient's PTT to control should be 1.5 to 2 (ratio of patient's PTT to control).
   b. PT monitors oral anticoagulant therapy—international normalized ratio (INR) should be greater than 2.0 to 2.5 based on condition being treated.
3. Evaluate results of hematocrit, hemoglobin, and platelet studies periodically or if bleeding is suspected.
4. Be aware of the following with regard to sensitivity to coumarin derivatives and obtain a PT as ordered:

May be intensified by
Antibiotics
Mineral oil
Quinidine
Salicylates
Tolbutamide (Orinase)

May be decreased by
Antacids
Barbiturates
Oral contraceptives
Adrenal corticosteroids

> **NURSING ALERT:** ❖
> Drug interactions can alter the effect of anticoagulants. Review the effect of other medications the patient may be taking during anticoagulant therapy.

C. **Preventing Bleeding**
1. Follow precautions to prevent bleeding.
  a. Handle patient carefully while turning and positioning.
  c. Maintain pressure on IV, blood draw sites for at least 5 minutes. Apply ice if patient is prone to bruising.
  d. Assist with ambulation to prevent falls.
2. Observe carefully for any possible signs of bleeding and report immediately so that anticoagulant dosage may be reviewed and altered if necessary:
  a. Urine—note evidence of hematuria; use test strip to detect microhematuria.
  b. Stool—check for tarry color; use test cards for occult blood.
  c. Emesis basin following tooth brushing—note any pink or bloody return.
  d. Inspect skin carefully for any bruising.
3. Have on hand the antidotes to anticoagulants being used:
  a. Heparin—protamine sulfate
  b. Warfarin—phytonadione (vitamin K_1, Aquamephyton)

> **NURSING ALERT:** ❖
> There is risk of bleeding in any patient receiving anticoagulants.

Patient Education/Health Maintenance

1. Instruct patient about taking anticoagulant.
  a. Follow instructions carefully and take medications exactly as prescribed.
  b. Take medications at the same time each day and do not stop taking them even if symptoms are not present.
  c. Wear a bracelet or carry a card indicating that anticoagulants are being taken; include name, address, and telephone number of health care provider.
2. Advise the patient to notify the health care provider:
  a. In case of accident, infection, or other significant illness that may affect blood clotting
  b. If surgical care by another health care provider or dentist is needed, inform other provider that anticoagulants are being taken.
  c. If a dose of anticoagulant is forgotten, do not take extra pills to make up for a skipped dose.
  d. In case of diarrhea, upset stomach, high fever
3. Advise the patient to avoid:
  a. Taking any other medications without first checking with health care provider, particularly:
    (1) Vitamins
    (2) Aspirin
    (3) Mineral oil
    (4) Cold medicines
    (5) Antibiotics
    (6) Phenylbutazone (Butazolidin)
  b. Excessive use of alcohol because alcohol may affect clotting ability; check on acceptable limits for social drinking.
  c. Participation in activities in which there is high risk of injury
  d. Foods that may cause diarrhea or upset stomach
4. Instruct the patient to be alert for these warning signs:
  a. Excessive bleeding that does not stop quickly (such as following shaving, a small cut, teeth brushing with gum injury, nose bleed)
  b. Excessive menstrual bleeding
  c. Skin discoloration or bruises that appear suddenly
  d. Black or bloody bowel movements; for questionable stool discoloration, test for occult blood
  e. Blood in urine
  f. Faintness, dizziness, or unusual weakness
5. Stress the importance of close follow-up and compliance with periodic laboratory work for blood clotting profiles.

PROCEDURE GUIDELINES 12-1 ◆ Subcutaneous Injection of Heparin

PURPOSE   When prolonged therapy is indicated, heparin may be given subcutaneously into fatty tissues.

EQUIPMENT   1- or 2-mL syringe or disposable tuberculin syringe
Fine sharp needle, no. 27, 1.6-cm (⅝ in.) long (or premeasured Tubex cartridge-needle unit)
Skin antiseptic

CONSIDERATIONS   1. Most convenient sites are along lower abdominal fat pad—to avoid inadvertent intramuscular injection and hematoma formation.
  a. A common location site is the fatty area anterior to either iliac crest.
  b. Avoid injection sites within 5 cm (2 in.) of the umbilicus because of possibility of entering a larger blood vessel.
2. Areas where subcutaneous layer is thin should be avoided.

(continued)

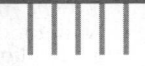
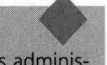

PROCEDURE GUIDELINES 12-1 ◆ Subcutaneous Injection of Heparin
(continued)

GERONTOLOGIC ALERT:
The aging individual begins to lose subcutaneous fat padding. Examine patient for best site for subcutaneous administration of heparin.

PROCEDURE	NURSING ACTION	RATIONALE

PERFORMANCE PHASE

1. Sponge the area gently with alcohol. Do not rub!

2. Attempt to stretch skin out, using palm of left hand. Some prefer to (gently) pick up a well-defined fold of skin.

3. Holding the shaft of the syringe in dart fashion, insert needle directly through the skin at a right angle just into the subcutaneous fatty layer.
4. Move right hand into position to direct plunger.
   a. Do not move needle tip once it is inserted.
   b. Do not pull back plunger for testing.

5. Firmly push plunger down as far as it will go.
6. When injection has been made, withdraw needle gently at the same angle at which it entered, releasing skin roll on withdrawal of needle.
7. Press an alcohol sponge to the site for a few seconds.

FOLLOW-UP CARE

1. *Do not rub the area. Instruct patient not to rub area.*
2. *Site of injection*
   a. Change site of injection each time heparin is administered.
   b. A chart can be marked with time, date, and measured dosage so that rotation of sites can be ensured.

Note: Low-dose heparin may be used to prevent deep vein thrombosis postoperatively.

RATIONALE

1. Rubbing or pinching skin might initiate damage to the tissue; heparin would aggravate any bleeding.
2. Try to empty blood vessels in local area to lessen likelihood of their being pierced by needle—with subsequent hematoma formation.

4. Aspiration in a forcible manner can damage small blood vessels and frequently lead to bleeding and hematoma formation, especially in the presence of high local concentration of heparin.
5. This ensures administration of total dose of heparin.
6. To minimize tissue damage.

7. To minimize oozing or bleeding.

1. Rubbing would increase the likelihood of bleeding.

◆ THROMBOLYTIC THERAPY

Thrombolytic therapy is administration of thrombolytic agents to dissolve any formed thrombus and inhibit the body's hemostatic function. Thrombolytic agents are available for parenteral use only. Commonly used thrombolytics include:

- Streptokinase (Streptase)
- Urokinase (Abbokinase)
- Tissue plasminogen activator (tPA, Activase)

Thrombolytic therapy is contraindicated in conditions that may lead to bleeding and should only be given in a controlled setting such as a cardiac catheterization laboratory or an intensive care unit. Thrombolytic therapy for deep vein thrombosis, however, may be given on step-down units or medical/surgical floors.

Clinical Indications

1. Acute MI from coronary thrombosis
2. Pulmonary embolus
3. Occlusion of peripheral arteries
4. Deep vein thrombosis

Nursing Interventions

1. Monitor clotting profiles; these are essential before the initiation of treatment to disclose any bleeding tendencies and to serve as a baseline for assessment of drug efficacy.
2. Observe for signs of bleeding and report immediately.
   a. Have typed and crossmatched blood on hold in case bleeding is severe.
   b. Have aminocaproic acid (Amicar) on hand to treat bleeding.

3. Monitor for allergic reaction. A small number of patients (less than 5%) may experience an allergic reaction.
   a. Observe the patient for the onset of a new rash, fever, and chills.
   b. Report any suspected allergic reaction immediately.
   c. Administer corticosteroids, if ordered, to treat reaction.
4. Monitor electrocardiogram (ECG) for arrhythmias after reperfusion if thrombolytic therapy is being used for coronary thrombus.
5. Frequently assess color, warmth, and sensation of extremity if therapy is being used for peripheral arterial occlusion.

◆ CARE OF THE PATIENT UNDERGOING VASCULAR SURGERY

Vascular surgery may involve operations of the arteries, veins, or lymphatic system. Surgery may be performed on an urgent basis, as in embolectomy for acute arterial embolism, or electively for vein ligation and stripping for varicose veins after conservative management fails. Other surgeries include thrombectomy and vena caval filter insertion for venous problems and arterial bypass grafting (aortoiliac, aortofemoral, and femoropopliteal), endarterectomy, and percutaneous transluminal angioplasty (PCTA) for arterial problems.

Preoperative Management/ Nursing Care

1. Nutritional status is assessed and improved preoperatively to aid in wound healing postoperatively.
2. Chronic skin and tissue changes are assessed preoperatively and impairment is minimized through protection of the affected part(s), treatment with antibiotics, and proper positioning to enhance circulation (elevated for venous and lymphatic problems, level or slightly dependent for arterial problems).
3. Additional health conditions such as heart disease, diabetes mellitus, chronic lung disease, and hypertension are fully evaluated and management adjusted to decrease operative risks.
4. Risk factors for vascular disease such as smoking, obesity, and sedentary lifestyle are reviewed and patient teaching begun to prevent recurrence/progression of vascular disorder.
5. The patient is prepared emotionally and physically for surgery, with teaching focusing on positioning in bed, exercises and activity expected to be followed postoperatively, frequent checks of circulation and wound, and prevention of complications such as bleeding, infection, and neurovascular compromise.

Postoperative Management/ Nursing Care

1. Bed rest may be maintained for 24 hours to reduce swelling and the risk of bleeding.
2. Extremity(s) is positioned straight and supported to prevent trauma and promote circulation.
3. Anticoagulation may be continued, but increases chance of bleeding following surgery.
4. Hydration, nutrition, and oxygenation are promoted to ensure wound healing.
5. If revascularization involves a graft, the donor site is protected and assessed, as well.

Nursing Diagnoses

A. Altered Tissue Perfusion (peripheral) related to underlying vascular disorder, postoperative swelling, and bandages
B. Risk for infection related to surgical incision and impaired circulation
C. Pain related to surgical incision and swelling
D. Impaired physical mobility related to pain and imposed restrictions

Nursing Interventions

A. *Promoting Tissue Perfusion*
1. Maintain dressing or compression bandages as directed.
2. Monitor for bleeding through dressing—reinforce and notify surgeon as indicated.
3. Monitor for hematoma formation beneath skin—increased pain and swelling. Apply pressure and ice and notify surgeon.
4. Measure vital signs frequently for tachycardia and hypotension, which may indicate hemorrhage.
5. Perform frequent neurovascular checks to involved extremity. Check warmth, color, capillary refill, sensation, movement, and pulses; compare to other side.
6. Position as directed, usually legs elevated and fully supported for venous and lymphatic disorders; flat and straight for arterial disorders.

B. *Preventing Infection*
1. Maintain IV infusion or heparin lock for antibiotic administration as ordered.
2. Check incision site for drainage, warmth, and erythema, which indicate infection.
3. Monitor temperature for elevation.

C. *Relieving Pain*
1. Assess pain level and administer analgesic as ordered.
2. Position for comfort using pillows for support.
3. Watch for side effects of narcotics such as hypotension, respiratory depression, nausea and vomiting, and constipation.
4. Time pain medication before activity.

D. *Minimizing Immobility*
1. Encourage isometric and range-of-motion exercises while on bed rest.
   a. Exercise affected extremity by pushing foot into footboard, making a fist, or simply contracting muscles without movement.
   b. Perform full range of motion of other extremities.
2. Encourage ambulation as soon as allowed.
   a. Avoid dangling legs because of possible compression against the back of bed or chair.
   b. Avoid long periods of sitting or standing.
   c. Encourage short periods of walking every 2 hours.

Patient Teaching/Health Maintenance

1. Teach care of incision at home. Ensure that patient has proper supplies.
2. Instruct on wearing of elastic stockings as ordered.
3. Teach signs of infection, graft failure, or worsening circulatory problem that should be reported.
4. Refer for additional support to overcome obesity or smoking.
5. Review any medications, especially anticoagulants (see p. 331).
6. Ensure the patient knows when and where to follow-up.

Evaluation

A. Extremity with good color, capillary refill, and pulses; warm and sensitive to touch; moving adequately
B. No signs of infection
C. Reports adequate pain control
D. Ambulating for 10 minutes every 2 hours without difficulty

Conditions of Veins

◆ THROMBOPHLEBITIS, PHLEBOTHROMBOSIS, DEEP VEIN THROMBOSIS

Note: While the terms do not necessarily represent identical pathologies, for clinical purposes they are used interchangeably when discussing the same process.

Thrombophlebitis is a condition in which a clot forms in a vein secondary to phlebitis or because of partial obstruction of the vein.

Phlebothrombosis is the formation of a thrombus or thrombi in a vein; in general, the clotting is related to 1) stasis, 2) abnormality of the walls of the vein(s), and 3) abnormality of clotting mechanism. Deep veins of the lower extremities are most commonly involved.

Deep vein thrombosis (DVT) is the thrombosis of deep rather than superficial veins. Two serious complications are pulmonary embolism and postphlebitic syndrome.

Phlebitis is an inflammation in the wall of a vein. The term is used clinically to indicate a superficial and localized condition that can be treated with application of heat.

Pathophysiology/Etiology

A. *General Points*
1. Three antecedent factors are believed to play a significant role in the development of venous thromboses: 1) stasis of blood, 2) injury to the vessel wall, and 3) altered blood coagulation (Virchow's triad).
2. Usually two of the three factors occur before thrombosis develops.

B. *Thrombosis-Related Situations*
1. Venous stasis—following operations, childbirth, or bed rest for any prolonged illness
2. Prolonged sitting or as a complication of varicose veins
3. Injury (bruise) to a vein; may result from direct trauma to veins from IV injections, indwelling catheters
4. Extension of an infection of tissues surrounding the vessel
5. Continuous pressure of a tumor, aneurysm, or excessive weight gain in pregnancy
6. Unusual activity in a person who has been sedentary
7. Hypercoagulability associated with malignant disease, blood dyscrasias

C. *High-Risk Factors*
1. Malignancy
2. Previous venous insufficiency
3. Conditions causing prolonged bed rest—MI, congestive heart failure (CHF), sepsis, traction
4. Leg trauma—fractures, cast, joint replacements
5. General surgery—over 40 years of age
6. Obesity, smoking

Clinical Manifestations

1. Clinical features vary with site and length of affected vein.
2. DVT may occur asymptomatically or may produce severe pain, fevers, chills, malaise, and swelling and cyanosis of affected arm or leg.
3. Superficial thrombophlebitis produces visible and palpable signs such as heat, pain, swelling, erythema, tenderness, and induration along the length of the affected vein.
4. Extensive vein involvement may cause lymphadenitis.

Diagnostic Evaluation

1. Phlebography (venography)—an x-ray visualization of the vascular tree after the injection of a contrast medium (Renografin); shows obstruction
2. Impedance plethysmography (IPG)—A noninvasive measurement of changes in calf volume corresponding to changes in blood volume brought about by temporary venous occlusion with a high pneumatic cuff. Electrodes measure electrical impedance as cuff is deflated. Slow decrease in impedance indicates diminished blood flow associated with a thrombus.
3. Fibrinogen I 125 uptake test—an invasive radioactive test in which labeled fibrinogen, given before a thrombus forms, will be concentrated in the area of clot formation. Formation of clots may be detected with serial scanning and by comparing one leg with the other. This is the most sensitive method to screen for acute calf vein thrombosis.
4. Doppler flow studies—used with duplex scanning to demonstrate a three-dimensional view of venous segments. When a segment won't compress, indicates presence of a clot. Serial tests are done.

Management

Goals: To prevent propagation of the thrombus and reduce the risk of pulmonary embolus; to prevent recurrent thromboemboli

A. Anticoagulation—for documented cases of DVT to prevent embolization. Heparin is given IV initially, followed by 3 to 6 months of oral anticoagulant therapy (see p. 330).

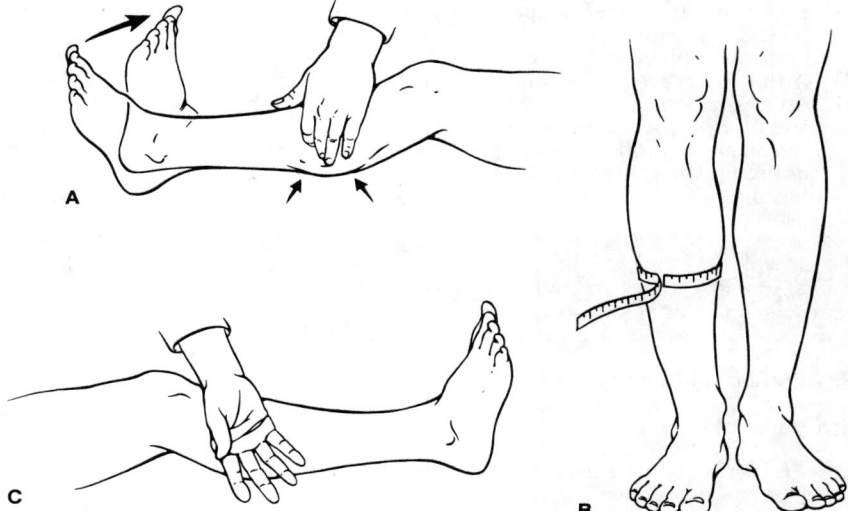

FIGURE 12-1 *Nursing assessment for deep vein thrombosis. (**A**) Pain and tenderness in the calf of the affected extremity, especially on dorsiflexion of the foot (Homan's sign). (**B**) The affected extremity may have a larger circumference than the unaffected extremity caused by edema. (**C**) The affected extremity will be warm to touch compared to the unaffected extremity.*

B. Thrombolytic therapy—may be used in life- or limb-threatening situations; not used more frequently due to risk of bleeding.

C. Nonpharmacologic therapies—for superficial thrombophlebitis and as an adjunct to anticoagulation with DVT

1. Dry heat
   a. Warm water bottles
   b. Heat cradle (thermostatically controlled or regulated with electric bulbs)
   c. Ultrasound (acoustic vibration with frequencies beyond human ear perception)
2. Moist heat
   a. Hydrotherapy
   b. Whirlpool bath
   c. Warm compresses
3. Pressure gradient therapy to promote vasodilatation (compression devices and garments)
   a. Electrically or pneumatically controlled boots or sleeves
   b. Elastic garments
4. Bed rest to prevent muscle contraction with walking that may dislodge clot

D. Surgery

1. Placement of a filter into the inferior vena cava to prevent pulmonary embolism in a patient who cannot tolerate prolonged anticoagulant therapy
2. Thrombectomy may be necessary for severely compromised venous drainage of the extremity.
3. See page 333 for surgical care.

Complications

1. Pulmonary embolism
2. Postphlebitic syndrome

Nursing Assessment

1. Obtain history of risk factors for thrombophlebitis.
2. Note symmetry or asymmetry of legs.
   a. Measure and record leg circumferences daily (Procedure Guidelines 12-2).
3. Observe for evidence of venous distention or edema, puffiness, stretched skin, hardness to touch.
4. Examine for signs of obstruction due to occluding thrombus—swelling, particularly in loose connective tissue or popliteal space, ankle, or suprapubic area.
5. Hand-test extremities for temperature variations—use dorsum (back) of same hand; first compare ankles, then move to the calf and up to the knee.
6. Assess for calf pain, which may be aggravated when foot is dorsiflexed with the knee flexed (Homan's sign) (Fig. 12-1). Unfortunately, this sign is nonspecific and has a low sensitivity for detecting thrombophlebitis.

Nursing Diagnoses

A. Pain related to decreased venous blood flow
B. Risk for Injury (bleeding) related to anticoagulant therapy
C. Impaired Physical Mobility related to pain and imposed treatment

Nursing Interventions

A. *Relieving Pain*
1. Elevate legs as directed to promote venous drainage and reduce swelling.
2. Apply warm compresses or heating pad as directed to promote circulation and reduce pain.

a. Ensure that water temperature is not too hot.
b. Cover plastic water bottle or heating pad with towel before applying to skin.
3. Administer acetaminophen (Tylenol), codeine, or other analgesic as prescribed and as needed. Avoid the use of aspirin (or aspirin-containing drugs) and non-steroidal anti-inflammatory drugs (NSAIDS) during anticoagulant therapy to prevent further risk of bleeding.

> **NURSING ALERT:**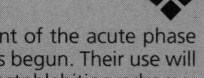
> Avoid massaging or rubbing calf because of the danger of breaking up the clot, which can then circulate as an embolus.

B. Preventing Bleeding
See page 779 for nursing interventions for patients on anticoagulant therapy.

C. Preventing Other Hazards of Immobility
1. Prevent venous stasis by proper positioning in bed.
   a. Support full length of legs when they are to be elevated (Fig. 12-2).
   b. Prevent bony prominence of one leg from pressing on soft tissue of other leg (in side-lying position, place a soft pillow between legs).
   c. Avoid hyperflexion at knee as in jackknife position (head up, knees up, pelvis and legs down); this promotes stasis in pelvis and extremities.
2. Initiate active exercises, unless contraindicated, in which case use passive exercises.
   a. If the patient is on bed rest:
      (1) Simulate walking if lying on back—5 minutes every 2 hours.
      (2) Simulate bicycle pedaling if lying on side—5 minutes every 2 hours.
   b. If contraindicated, resort to passive exercises—5 minutes every 2 hours.
3. Encourage adequate fluid intake, frequent changes of position, and effective coughing and deep-breathing exercises.
4. Be alert for signs of pulmonary embolism—chest pain, dyspnea, and apprehension, and report immediately.

5. After the acute phase (5–7 days), apply elastic stockings, as directed (Fig. 12-3). Remove twice daily and check for skin changes and calf tenderness.
6. Encourage ambulation when allowed (usually after 5–7 days, when clot has fully adhered to vessel wall).
   a. If permissible, have the patient sit up and move to side of bed in sitting position. Provide a foot support (stool or chair)—dangling of feet is not desirable because pressure may be exerted against popliteal vessels and may obstruct blood flow.
   b. If the patient is permitted out of bed, encourage walking 10 minutes each hour.
   c. Discourage crossing of legs and long periods of sitting because compression of vessels can restrict blood flow.

Patient Education/Health Maintenance

1. Teach patient signs of recurrent thrombophlebitis and pulmonary embolism to report immediately.
2. Provide thorough instructions about anticoagulant therapy (see p. 331).
3. Teach patient to promote circulation and prevent stasis by applying elastic hose at home.

> **NURSING ALERT:**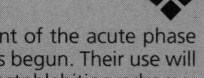
> Elastic hose have no role in the management of the acute phase of DVT but are of value once ambulation has begun. Their use will minimize or delay the development of the postphlebitic syndrome.

4. Advise against straining or any maneuver that increases venous pressure in the leg. Eliminate the necessity to strain at stool by increasing fiber and fluids in the diet.
5. Warn patient of hazards of smoking and obesity: nicotine constricts veins, decreasing venous blood flow. Extra pounds increase pressure on leg veins. Arrange consultation with dietitian, if necessary.

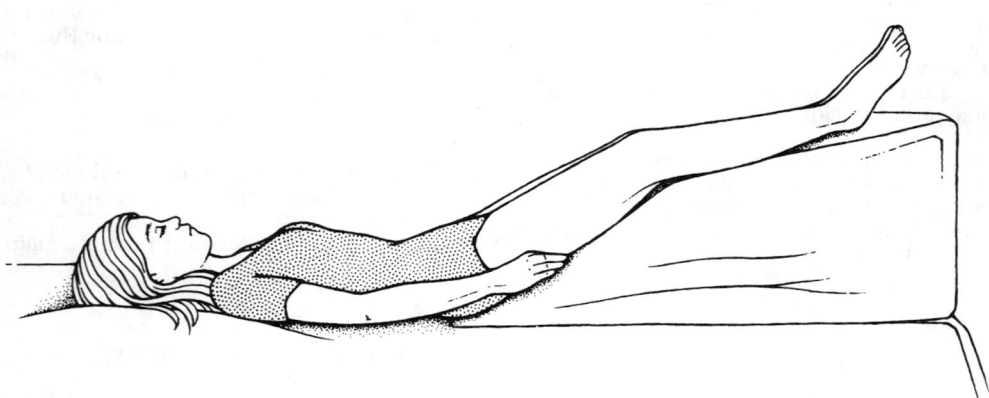

FIGURE 12-2 *This leg elevator is of foam construction with a removable cotton cover that may be machine washed. It is clamped to the lower end of the mattress. This position is anatomically correct and provides adequate support to all parts of the leg. Edema and stasis of the lower extremities can be controlled. (Courtesy of Jobst)*

Put on supports early in the morning, before swelling occurs.

Always begin with supports "inside-out" . . . as they are when you receive them.

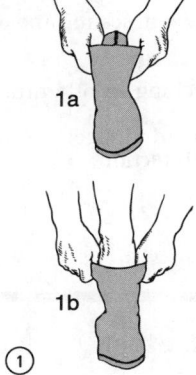
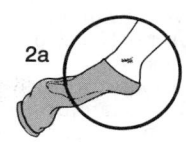
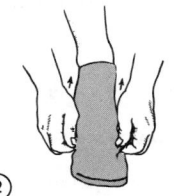
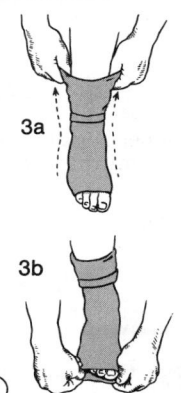
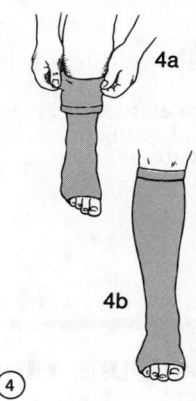

Sit with feet in easy reach. Support must be "inside out," with its foot inverted back to heel. Seam faces down (sketch 1a). Grasp each side firmly and pull onto foot (sketch 1b).

Pull past midpoint of heel (sketch 2a), so support will not slip back. Then, reach just beyond toes and grasp fabric between fingers and start pulling over foot. Pull from sides . . . never by seams.

Pull all the way up past ankle (sketch 3a). Seat heel in place. Pull foot portion of support out toward tips of toes (sketch 3b) to set fabric evenly on foot. Allow to settle back normally.

Using short (2 inches at a time) snappy pulls (sketch 4a) pull support up to point it was measured to end (sketch 4b). Smooth evenly down leg. **Never allow top to roll or turn down.**

FIGURE 12-3 Method of applying supporting hose. (Courtesy of Jobst).

COMMUNITY-BASED CARE TIP:
Practice preventive measures for bedridden patients who are prone to develop thrombosis:
1. Have the patient lie in bed in the slightly reversed Trendelenburg position because it is better for the veins to be full of blood than empty.
2. Place a footboard across the foot of the bed.
3. Instruct the patient to press the balls of the feet against the footboard, as if rising up on toes.
4. Then have the patient relax the foot.
5. Request that the patient do this 5 to 10 times each hour.

Evaluation

A. Patient verbalizes reduced pain.
B. No bleeding is observed.
C. Normal respiratory status is maintained.

◆ CHRONIC VENOUS INSUFFICIENCY (POSTPHLEBITIC SYNDROME)

Postphlebitic syndrome is a form of chronic venous stasis; it may be a residual effect of phlebitis. It results from chronic occlusion of the veins or destruction of the valves.

Pathophysiology/Etiology

1. Smaller vessels have dilated because main channel for returning blood from the leg to the heart was blocked by a thrombus.

2. Valves of diseased veins can no longer prevent back-flow, thereby → chronic venous stasis → swelling and edema → superficial varicose veins.
3. Lower leg becomes discolored because of venous stasis and pigmentation ulceration (postphlebitis).
4. Most commonly involves iliac and femoral veins and occasionally saphenous vein

Clinical Manifestations

1. Chronic edema; worse while legs dependent
2. Intractable induration, discoloration, pain, ulceration; the medial malleolus is the most common site.

Diagnostic Evaluation and Management

1. Noninvasive screening—Doppler, plethysmography—shows obstruction and valve incompetency.
2. Best treatment is prevention of phlebitis and constant use of compression if phlebitis has occurred.
3. After this syndrome has developed, only palliative and symptomatic treatment is possible because the damage is irreparable.

Complications

1. Stasis ulcers
2. Cellulitis
3. Recurrent thrombosis

Nursing Interventions/ Patient Education

Instruct the patient as follows:

1. Wear elastic stockings to prevent edema.
2. Avoid sitting or standing for long periods of time.
3. Elevate legs on a chair for 5 minutes every 2 hours.

4. Elevate legs above level of head by lying down two to three times daily.
5. Raise foot of bed 15 to 20 cm (6–8 in.) at night to allow venous drainage by gravity.
6. Apply bland, oily lotions to prevent scaling and dryness of skin.
7. Avoid constricting bandages.
8. Prevent injury, bruising, scratching, or other trauma to skin of leg and foot.
9. Be alert for signs of ulceration, drainage, warmth, erythema, and pain, indicating infection.

PROCEDURE GUIDELINES 12-2 ◆ Obtaining Leg Measurements to Detect Early Swelling

PURPOSE   To obtain leg measurements for detection and monitoring of thrombophlebitis

EQUIPMENT   Flexible tape measure in centimeters/inches
Black felt-tip pen

PROCEDURE

NURSING ACTION	RATIONALE
PREPARATORY PHASE	
1. Instruct patient to lie in dorsal recumbent position.	
PERFORMANCE PHASE	
1. On admission of the patient, measure the circumference of the ankle, calf, and thigh.	1. This will provide baseline data.
2. Obtain measurements at the widest part of the ankle, calf, and thigh.	2. To provide a consistent anatomic place of measurement; some clinics have a predetermined starting point, such as 15 or 20 cm from the knee cap.
3. Mark the leg with a black felt-tip pen where measurement taken.	3. To promote accuracy of measurements
4. Thereafter, when measuring, place the measuring tape on the marked line.	
5. Repeat measurements taken on admission the next morning before any patient activity.	5. Otherwise, later measurements may give a false reading because of gravitational edema.
6. Thereafter, obtain measurements at the same time of day weekly unless there is evidence of swelling, in which case it is done daily.	6. Weekly—to detect swelling Daily—to monitor swelling and its response to treatment
7. Record measurements:	

Leg Measurements
Date:
Time:

	Right			Left	
Ankle _____		cm/in.	Ankle _____		cm/in.
Calf _____		cm/in.	Calf _____		cm/in.
Thigh _____		cm./in.	Thigh _____		cm./in.

8. Compare measurements:

   a. Check one leg with the other.

   b. Check each leg with baseline data.

SIGNIFICANT FINDINGS:
1.5 cm (males) difference between legs or compared with baseline
1.2 cm (females) difference between legs or compared with baseline

◆ STASIS ULCERS

Stasis ulcer is an excavation of the skin surface produced by sloughing of inflammatory necrotic tissue, usually caused by vascular insufficiency in the lower extremity.

Pathophysiology/Etiology

1. Stasis ulcer results from inadequate oxygen and other nutrients to the tissues because of edema and decreased circulation.
2. Secondary bacterial infection occurs because of decreased circulation that limits the body's response to infection.
3. Postphlebitic syndrome and stasis are responsible for most leg ulcers.

Clinical Manifestations

Severity of symptoms depends on the extent and duration of vascular insufficiency.

1. Open sore that is inflamed
2. Drainage may be present or the area may be covered by a dark crust.
3. Patient may complain of swelling, heaviness, aching, and fatigue.
4. Edema and pigmentation around ulcer

> **GERONTOLOGIC ALERT:**
> The occurrence of stasis ulcers is increasing, especially in the aging population.

Diagnostic Evaluation

1. Noninvasive tests such plethysmography and venous Doppler may show impeded blood flow and incompetent valves.
2. Wound cultures will identify microorganisms if infected.

Management

A. Removing Devitalized Tissue
1. Necrotic material is flushed out with cleansing agents to dissolve slough. These agents are chemically or naturally derived enzymes that are proteolytic or fibrinolytic.
2. Surgical excision of slough—if necrotic tissue is loose, this procedure can be done without anesthesia; if the tissue is adherent, anesthesia will be required.

B. Stimulating Formation of Granulation Tissue
1. Dressing of choice
   a. Nonadherent so removal is painless and does not damage newly forming tissue
   b. Highly absorbent
   c. Safe, nontoxic
   d. Sterile, accessible, and inexpensive

2. Application of compression over dressings generally through the use of bandages or elastic stockings. In some circumstances, inflatable pneumatic leggings may be appropriate.
3. Unna's boot, an effective treatment of choice, is an example of a combined dressing and compression bandage.
4. Bed rest with leg elevation
5. Systemic drug therapy
   a. No single agent affects ulcer healing.
   b. Diuretic therapy for edema reduction may improve capillary circulation.
6. Application of skin grafts
   a. Skin grafts are used for ulcers that will not heal.
   b. They are not recommended for first-line treatment.

C. Preventing Recurrence
1. Ligation of the saphenofemoral or saphenopopliteal vessels with stripping
2. Ligation of the lower leg communicating veins
3. Deep vein bypass or reconstruction
4. Injection compression sclerotherapy
5. See page 333 for surgical care.

Complications

1. Infection
2. Sepsis

Nursing Assessment

1. Observe appearance and temperature of the skin.
2. Note location and appearance of ulcer.
3. Determine presence and quality of all peripheral pulses. Use Doppler if needed.
4. Observe for drainage and signs of infection.

Nursing Diagnoses

A. Impaired Tissue Integrity related to stasis ulcer

B. Pain related to stasis ulcer

Nursing Interventions

A. Restoring Tissue Integrity
1. Elevate affected extremity to decrease edema.
2. Place cotton between toes to prevent pressure on a toe ulcer.
3. Provide overbed cradle to protect leg from pressure of bed linens.
4. Consider air-fluidized bed to provide pressure relief.
5. Administer prescribed antibiotics.
6. Apply wet to dry dressings, chemical beads or ointments, and topical antibiotics as ordered.
7. Apply Unna's boot to affected lower extremity as ordered.

B. Reducing Pain
1. Administer prescribed analgesics, such as NSAIDs, to reduce pain and inflammation.

2. Medicate 30 to 45 minutes before a dressing change.
3. Encourage short periods of ambulation after pain medication is given.

Patient Education/Health Maintenance

1. Stress the importance of following explicitly the recommendations of the health care provider.
2. Explain the hazards of trying other remedies without professional advice.
3. Indicate that the treatment may be long but that patience is an important aspect.
4. Encourage maintenance of healthy tissue when the ulcer is healed by continuing with the safeguards practiced before because breakdown of healthy tissue frequently occurs.
5. Encourage participation in physical therapy and a regular exercise program.
6. Encourage weight control and proper dietary intake to ensure adequate amounts of protein and vitamins.
7. Teach patient the correct method of dressing changes.

COMMUNITY-BASED CARE TIPS:
1. Discuss resources in community for obtaining necessary dressing change supplies.
2. Assess the patient's ability to obtain supplies and perform dressing changes at home. Include other persons in teaching and use community resources as indicated.

Evaluation

A. Skin is normal color and temperature, nontender, nonswollen and demonstrates new epithelium.
B. Patient verbalizes only minimal discomfort with dressing changes.

◆ VARICOSE VEINS

Primary varicose veins—bilateral dilatation and elongation of saphenous veins; deeper veins are normal. As the condition progresses, because of hydrostatic pressure and vein weakness, the vein walls become distended, with asymmetrical dilatation, and some of the valves become incompetent. The process is irreversible. *Secondary varicose veins* result from obstruction of deep veins.

Telangectasias (spider veins) are dilated superficial capillaries, arterioles, and venules. They may be cosmetically unattractive but do not pose a threat to circulation.

Pathophysiology/Etiology

1. Dilatation of the vein prevents the valve cusps from meeting; this results in increased back-up pressure, which is passed into the next lower segment of the vein. The combination of vein dilatation and valve incompetence produces the varicosity (Fig. 12-4).

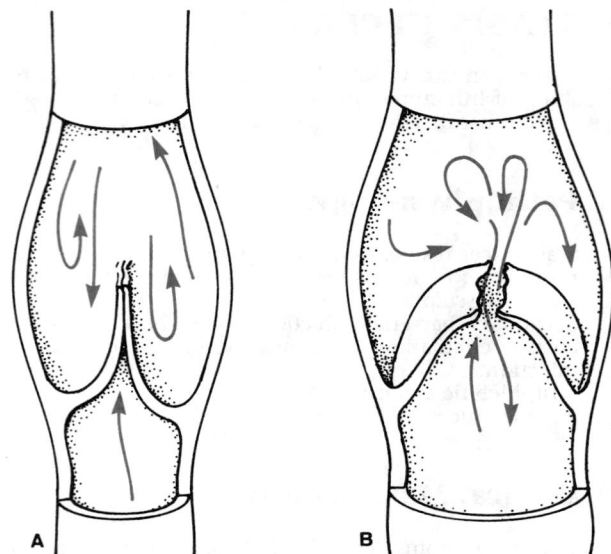

FIGURE 12-4 *Valve incompetence develops as dilatation of a vessel prevents effective approximation of valve cusps. (A) Closed venous valve. (B) Incompetent venous valve.*

2. Varicosities may occur elsewhere in the body (esophageal and hemorrhoidal veins) when flow or pressure is abnormally high.
3. Predisposing factors
   a. Hereditary weakness of vein wall or valves
   b. Long-standing distention of veins brought about by pregnancy, obesity, or prolonged standing
   c. Old age—loss of tissue elasticity

Clinical Manifestations

1. Disfigurement due to large, discolored, tortuous leg veins
2. Easy leg fatigue, cramps in leg, heavy feeling, increased pain during menstruation, nocturnal muscle cramps

Diagnostic Evaluation

1. Walking tourniquet test—to demonstrate presence or absence of valvular incompetence of communicating veins
   a. A tourniquet is snugly fastened around the lower extremity just above the highest noted varicosities.
   b. The patient is directed to walk briskly for 2 minutes.
   c. Failure of varicosities to empty suggests valvular incompetence of communicating veins distal to tourniquet.
2. Photoplethysmography—a noninvasive technique to observe venous flow hemodynamics by noting changes in the blood content of the skin; used to detect incompetence in valves located inside the vein
3. Doppler ultrasound—can detect accurately and rapidly the presence or absence of venous reflux in deep or superficial vessels

4. Venous outflow and reflux plethysmography—able to detect deep venous occlusion
5. Ascending and descending venography—an invasive technique that can also demonstrate venous occlusion and patterns of collateral flow. This test is expensive; it may not be required if a careful history, physical examination, and laboratory testing are done.

Management

1. Conservative therapies such as encouraging weight loss if appropriate and avoiding activities that cause venous stasis by obstructing venous flow
2. Surgery may be considered for ulceration, bleeding, and cosmetic purposes in selected patients, if patency of deep veins is ensured.
3. Surgical procedures—a single method or combination of methods is tailored to meet the needs of the individual:
   a. Sclerosing injection—not used as frequently today; may be combined with ligation or limited to treatment of isolated varicosities. The affected vessel may be sclerosed by injecting sodium tetradecyl sulfate or similar sclerosing agent. Compression bandage is then applied without interruption for 6 weeks; inflamed endothelial surfaces adhere by direct contact.
   b. Multiple vein ligation
   c. Ligation and stripping of the greater and lesser saphenous systems. This is the most effective procedure.
   d. Laser therapy

Complications

1. Hemorrhage due to the weakening of the vein wall and pressure on it
2. Skin infection and breakdown, producing ulcers (rare in primary varices)

Nursing Assessment

1. Inspect for dilated tortuous vessel.
2. Perform the manual compression test to determine severity of varicose vein.
   a. With the fingertips of one hand, feel the dilated vein.
   b. With your other hand, compress firmly at least 20 cm (8 in.) higher on the leg.
   c. Feel for an impulse transmitted toward your lower hand.
   d. Competent saphenous valves should block the impulse. If you feel the impulse, the patient has varicose veins with incompetent valves.
3. Assess for any ulceration, chronic venous insufficiency, or signs of infection.

Nursing Diagnoses

A. Impaired Tissue Integrity related to chronic changes and postoperative inflammation
B. *Pain related to surgical incisions, inflammation*

Nursing Interventions

A. *Promoting Tissue Integrity Postoperatively*
1. Maintain elastic compression bandages from toes to groin. Monitor neurovascular status of feet (color, warmth, capillary refill, sensation, pulses) to prevent compromise from swelling.
2. Elevate legs about 30°, providing support for the entire leg. Ensure that knee gatch is positioned for straight incline.
3. Monitor for signs of bleeding; especially the first 24 hours.
   a. Blood soaked through bandages
   b. Increased pain, hematoma formation
   c. Hypotension and tachycardia
4. If incisional bleeding occurs, elevate the leg above the level of the heart, apply pressure over the site, and notify the surgeon.
5. Be alert for complaints of pain over bony prominences of the foot and ankle; if the elastic bandage is too tight, loosen it—later, have it reapplied.
6. Maintain IV infusion for fluids and antibiotics as ordered.
7. After removal of compression bandages (about 7 days postoperatively), observe or teach patient to observe for signs of cellulitis or incisional infection.
8. Encourage use of elastic stockings for several weeks to months following surgery.

B. *Relieving Pain*
1. Administer analgesics as prescribed.
2. Encourage mostly bed rest the first day with legs elevated. The second day, encourage ambulation for 5 to 10 minutes every 2 hours.
3. Advise that, when ambulatory, avoid prolonged standing or sitting or crossing or dangling legs to prevent obstruction.

Patient Education/Health Maintenance

A. *Postoperative Instructions*
Instruct the patient to:

1. Wear pressure bandages or elastic stockings as prescribed—usually 3 to 4 weeks after surgery.
2. Elevate legs about 30° and provide adequate support for entire leg.
3. Take analgesics for pain as ordered.
4. Report signs such as sensory loss, calf pain, or fever to the health care provider.
5. Avoid dangling of legs.
6. Walk as able.
7. Note that complaints of patchy numbness can be expected but should disappear in less than a year.
8. Follow conservative management instructions (below) to prevent recurrence.

B. Conservative Management
Instruct the patient to:

1. Avoid activities that cause venous stasis by obstructing venous flow.
    a. Wearing tight garters, tight girdle
    b. Sitting or standing for prolonged periods of time
    c. Crossing the legs at knees for prolonged periods while sitting (reduces circulation by 15%)
2. Control excessive weight gain.
3. Wear firm elastic support as prescribed, from toe to thigh when in upright position.
    a. Put elastic stockings on in bed before getting up.
    b. Waist-high elastic support hose are available and may be useful.
4. Elevate foot of bed 15 to 20 cm (6–8 in.) for night sleeping.
5. Avoid injuring legs.

Evaluation

A. Skin is normal color and temperature, nontender, nonswollen, and intact.
B. Patient is actively moving extremity; verbalizes reduced pain.

Conditions of the Arteries

◆ ARTERIOSCLEROSIS AND ATHEROSCLEROSIS

Arteriosclerosis is an arterial disease manifested by a loss of elasticity and a hardening of the vessel wall.

Atherosclerosis is the most common type of arteriosclerosis, manifested by the formation of atheromas (patchy lipoidal degeneration of the intima).

Pathophysiology/Etiology

1. Etiology thought to be reaction-to-injury theory
    a. Endothelial cell injury causes increased platelet and monocyte aggregation to site of injury.
    b. Smooth muscle cells migrate and proliferate.
    c. Matrix of collagen and elastic fibers form.
2. Atherosclerotic lesions are two types: fatty streaks and fibrous plaques (Fig. 12-5).
3. Risk factors include heredity, increasing age, male gender, cigarette smoking, hypertension, elevated blood cholesterol levels, diabetes mellitus, obesity, physical inactivity, and stress.

Clinical Manifestations

1. May affect entire vascular system or one segment of the vascular tree
2. Symptoms are based on area affected.
    a. Brain—cerebroarteriosclerosis
    b. Heart—coronary artery disease
    c. Gastrointestinal tract—aneurysms eroding into the bowel
    d. Kidneys—renal artery stenosis
    e. Extremities—propensity for emboli
3. Decreased pulses; bruits

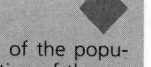

GERONTOLOGIC ALERT:
Atherosclerotic cardiovascular disease afflicts 80% of the population over age 65 and is the most common condition of the arterial system in the elderly.

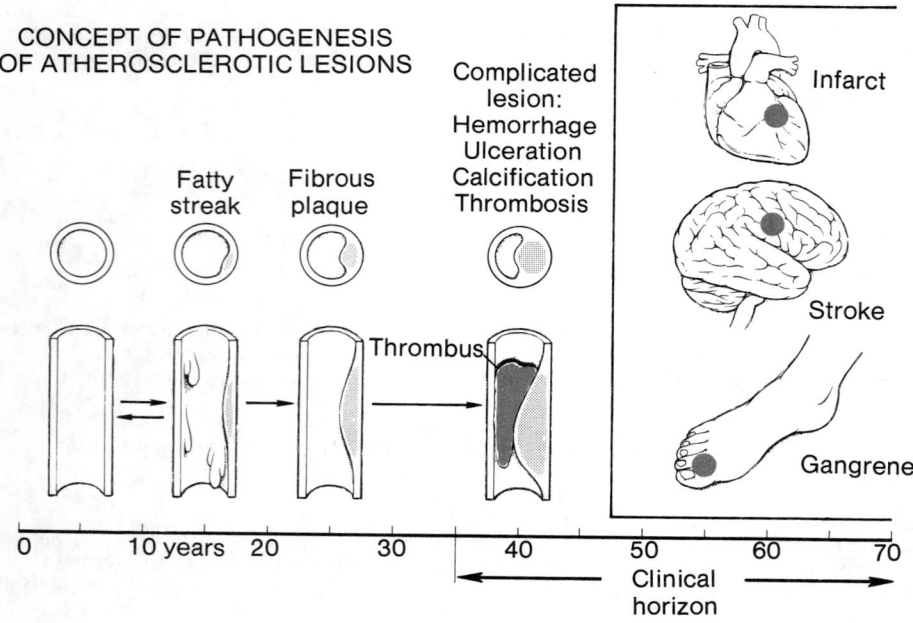

FIGURE 12-5 *Schematic concept of the progression of atherosclerosis. Fatty streaks constitute one of the earliest lesions of atherosclerosis. Many fatty streaks regress, whereas others progress to fibrous plaques and eventually to atheromata. These may then become complicated by hemorrhage, ulceration, calcification, or thrombosis and may produce complications. (Adapted from Hurst J. W., Logue R. B. The Heart. (1990). New York: McGraw–Hill.)*

Diagnostic Evaluation

Specific to body system affected:

1. Arteriography of involved area may show stenosis and increased collateral circulation.
2. ECG, echocardiogram, Holter monitoring, exercise stress testing, myocardial imaging, and cardiac catheterization may be done to evaluate coronary artery disease.

Management

A. *Medical Management*
1. Modification of risk factors
2. Specific treatment for end-organ dysfunction—see cerebrovascular insufficiency, page 376; angina, page 288; occlusive arterial disease, below.

B. *Surgical Management*
1. Percutaneous transluminal angioplasty (PCTA) to relieve arterial stenosis when lesions are accessible, as in superficial femoral and iliac arteries, through the use of special inflatable balloon catheters.
2. Laser angioplasty—amplified light waves are transmitted by fiberoptic catheters. Laser beam heats the tip of a percutaneous catheter and vaporizes the atherosclerotic plaque.
3. Rotational atherectomy—high-speed rotary cutter that removes lesions by abrading plaque. Benefits of this therapy are minimal damage to the normal endothelium and low incidence of complications.
4. Operative reconstruction of involved vessels

Complications

1. Cardiac
   a. Coronary atherosclerosis
   b. Angina
   c. Acute MI
2. Cerebrovascular disease
   a. Transient ischemic attacks
   b. Stroke
3. Atherosclerosis of the aorta—aneurysms
4. Atherosclerotic lesions of extremities—may lead to gangrene
5. Renal artery stenosis—renal insufficiency

Nursing Interventions/ Patient Education

Attention is directed to reducing risk factors by avoiding tension, reducing excess weight, giving up cigarette smoking, controlling diabetes, and adjusting diet to reduce cholesterol intake.

◆ OCCLUSIVE ARTERIAL DISEASE

Occlusive arterial disease is a form of arteriosclerosis in which the vascular system of the legs becomes blocked. Chronic occlusive arterial disease occurs much more frequently than does acute (which is the sudden and complete blocking of a vessel by a thrombus or embolus).

Pathophysiology/Etiology

A. *Arteriosclerosis Obliterans*
1. Occurs at bifurcations of a vessel
2. Aortoiliac, femoropopliteal, and popliteal-tibial vessels most common sites

B. *Thromboangiitis Obliterans (Buerger's Disease)*
1. An occlusion caused by inflammation and thrombosis
2. Thrombi originate in left side of heart as a consequence of atrial fibrillation or mitral stenosis.
3. Thrombogenesis also occurs at site of atherosclerotic plaque. Arterial occlusion obstructs blood flow to the distal extremity.

Clinical Manifestations

Symptoms appear gradually:

1. Intermittent claudication
2. Coldness of extremity
3. Color change—pallor
4. Decrease in size of leg
5. Tingling, numbness of toes
6. Later—pain, even when leg is at rest; occurs at night, requiring patients to get out of bed to walk to relieve pain
7. Cramplike, excruciating pain in calf muscles
8. Ulcers of toes and feet develop

Diagnostic Evaluation

1. Vascular physical examination, including brachial and ankle systolic pressures, before and after exercise; an increase in pressure after exercise indicates an absence of hemodynamically significant arterial disease
2. Doppler ultrasound—increased velocity of flow through a stenotic vessel, or no flow with total occlusion
3. Segmental plethysmography—decreased pressure
4. Angiography—to confirm occlusion

Management

Goals:

- To preserve the extremity
- To relieve intermittent claudication

1. Conservative treatment to manage intermittent claudication includes walking, weight reduction, no smoking, and control of other conditions such as hypertension and diabetes mellitus.
2. Treatment with pentoxifylline (Trental) to improve blood flow by increasing erythrocyte flexibility and lowering blood viscosity

3. Where conservative measures clearly are not enough, constructive arterial surgery (endarterectomy, arterial bypass grafting, or a combination) may be required.
4. PCTA may be used alone or with reconstructive surgery for dilatation of localized noncalcified segments of narrowed arteries.
5. Microvascular surgery may be required for small artery occlusive disease.
6. See page 333 for surgical care.

Complications

1. Ulceration with slow healing
2. Gangrene, sepsis

3. Severe occlusion may necessitate limb or partial limb amputation.

Nursing Assessment

1. Observe extremity for color, sensation and temperature. Compare bilaterally for differences.
2. Palpate pulses (Fig. 12-6) and record; auscultate for bruits.
3. Inspect nails for thickening and opacity; inspect skin for shiny, atrophic, hairless, and dry appearance, reflecting chronic changes.
4. Assess for pain, even when leg is at rest.
5. Assess for ulcers of toes and feet.

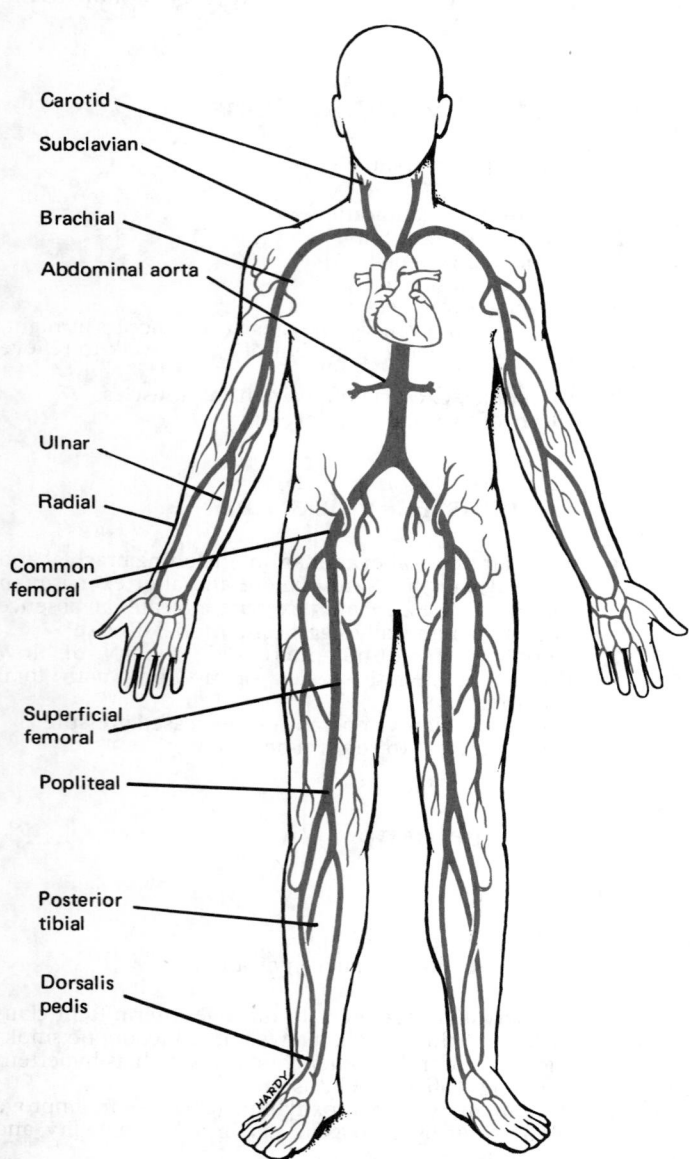

Carotid
Subclavian
Brachial
Abdominal aorta
Ulnar
Radial
Common femoral
Superficial femoral
Popliteal
Posterior tibial
Dorsalis pedis

FIGURE 12-6 *Salient points in evaluating peripheral arterial insufficiency. Reduced or absent femoral pulses indicate aortoiliac disease. Absent popliteal pulses indicate superficial femoral occlusion. Pulse deficits in one extremity, with normal pulses in contralateral extremity, suggest acute arterial embolus. Absent pedal pulses indicate tibioperoneal artery involvement.*

Nursing Diagnoses

A. Altered Tissue Perfusion (peripheral) related to decreased arterial blood flow
B. Risk for Injury related to sensorimotor deficits
C. Risk for Infection related to decreased arterial flow

Nursing Interventions

Also see Arterial Embolism.

A. Promoting Tissue Perfusion
1. Inspect and identify new ulcerations or extension of existing ulcerations.
2. Provide and encourage well-balanced diet to enhance sound healing.
3. Encourage walking or performance of range-of-motion exercises to increase blood flow.
4. Teach Buerger-Allen exercises—exercises by which gravity alternately fills and empties the blood vessels (Fig. 12-7).
   a. Begin with the patient lying flat in bed. Elevate legs to above level of heart—2 minutes or until blanching occurs.
   b. Allow legs to be dependent; exercise feet—3 minutes or until legs are pink.
   c. Instruct the patient to lie flat—5 minutes.
   d. Repeat a, b, and c five times; do entire set three times a day.
5. Administer or teach self-administration of pain medication to achieve comfort level conducive to ambulation.

B. Preventing Injury
1. Encourage patient to wear protective footwear such as rubber-soled slippers or shoes with closed, wide toebox when out of bed.
2. Avoid adhesive tape on affected skin.
3. Perform and teach foot care, including washing and carefully drying and inspecting feet daily.

C. Preventing Infection
1. Apply lanolin or petrolatum to lower extremities to prevent drying and cracking of skin.
2. Encourage patient to wear clean hose daily; woolen socks for winter, cotton for summer.
3. Teach patient to:
   a. Trim toenails straight across after soaking the feet in warm water.
   b. Place wisps of cotton under corner of great toenail if there is a tendency toward ingrown toenails.
   c. Have a podiatrist cut corns and calluses; do not use corn pads or strong medications.
4. Teach patient signs to report:
   a. Redness, swelling, irritation, blistering
   b. Itching, burning—athlete's foot
   c. Bruises, cuts, unusual appearance of skin

Patient Education/Health Maintenance

1. Teach patient the importance of walking to improve circulation.
2. Instruct patient not to sit or stand in one position for long periods of time.
3. Teach patient methods to promote vasodilation by keeping extremity warm, ceasing smoking, and stopping use of other vasoconstricting substances such as caffeine.
4. Instruct patient to avoid tight-fitting elastic-topped socks and not to cross legs when sitting or lying.

Evaluation

A. No new ulcer formation
B. Verbalizes importance of wearing protective shoes and washing and inspecting feet daily
C. No signs of infection of lower extremities

◆ ARTERIAL EMBOLISM

Arterial emboli are clots floating in arterial blood that may cause complete arterial obstruction. The clinical picture is different from that of a venous occlusion (Table 12-1).

Pathophysiology/Etiology

1. Most commonly originate in the heart as a result of atrial fibrillation, MI, or CHF (about 85%)
2. Arteriosclerosis may cause roughening or ulceration of atheromatous plaques, which can lead to emboli.
3. May also be associated with immobility, anemia, and dehydration
4. Emboli tend to lodge at bifurcations and atherosclerotic narrowings.

Clinical Manifestations

1. The patient may be asymptomatic.
2. The patient may experience acute pain and loss of sensory and motor function due to emboli blocking the artery and associated vasomotor reflex.

TABLE 12-1 Assessment of Acute Arterial Occlusion Versus Deep Vein Thrombosis

Factor	Acute Arterial Occlusion	Deep Vein Thrombosis
Onset	Sudden	Gradual
Color	Pale; later—mottled, cyanotic	Slightly cyanotic; rubescent
Skin temperature	Cold	Warm
Leg size—diameter	May be reduced from normal	Enlarged
Superficial veins	Collapsed	Appear enlarged and prominent
Arterial pulsation	Pulse deficit noted	Normal and palpable (except in marked edema)
Effect of elevating leg	Condition worsens	Condition improves

POSITION 1
Place legs on a pillow-cushioned chair for one minute to drain blood.

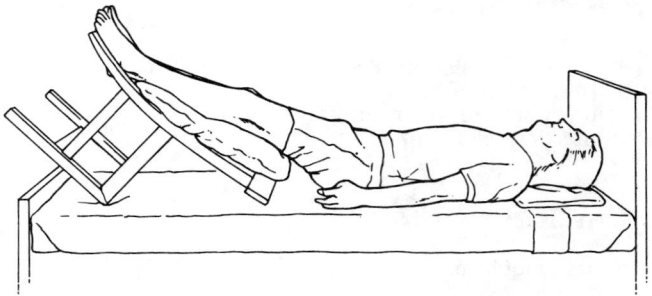

POSITION 2
Hold each of these stretching positions for 30 seconds to enhance blood return.

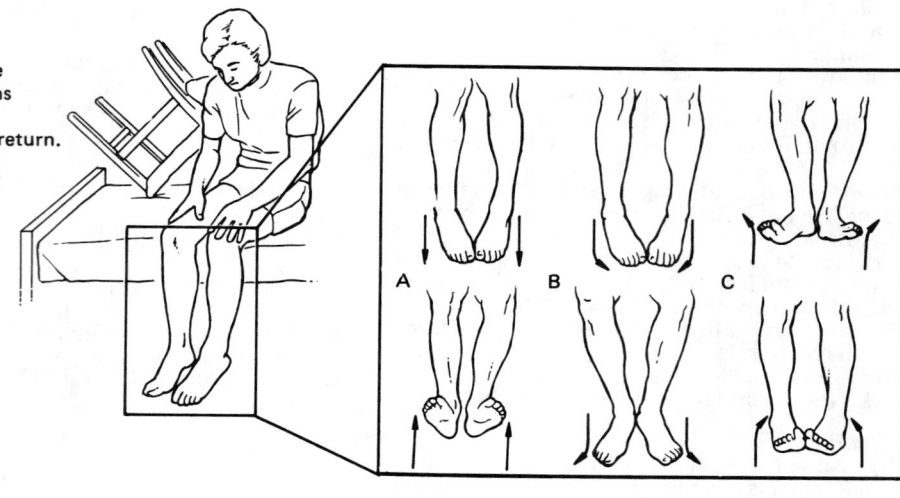

POSITION 3
Lie flat on back, with legs straight. Hold position for one minute.

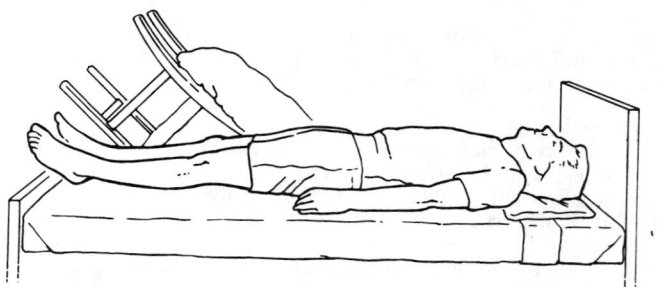

FIGURE 12-7 *Buerger-Allen exercises. Do exercise series 6 times, 4 times a day. (Forshee T, Minckley B. Lumbar sympathectomy. RN. 1976;39[2].)*

a. Paralysis of part
b. Anesthesia of part
c. Pallor and coldness

Diagnostic Evaluation

1. Doppler ultrasonography, segmental limb pressure, and pulse volume recordings—may indicate decreased flow.
2. Radionuclide scan—may identify clot.
3. Arteriography—confirms diagnosis.

4. Digital subtraction angiography and magnetic resonance imaging (MRI) may be done for cerebral embolization.

Management

1. Bed rest
2. Drug therapy—anticoagulants (see p. 330), thrombolytics (see p. 332)
3. Treatment of shock

4. Surgery—embolectomy (Fig. 12-8) must be performed within 6 to 10 hours to prevent muscle necrosis and loss of extremity.

NURSING ALERT:
Arterial embolization of a large artery, such as the iliac, that has major systemic effects is life-threatening and requires emergency operative intervention.

Complications

1. Irreversible ischemia and loss of extremity
2. Shock (if large artery occluded)

Nursing Assessment

1. Assess for acute, severe pain.
2. Assess for gradual loss of sensory and motor function.
3. Check for aggravation of pain by movement of and pressure on the extremity.
4. Palpate for loss of distal pulses.
5. Inspect for pale, mottled, and numb extremity.
6. Inspect for collapse of superficial veins due to decreased blood flow to the extremity.
7. Inspect for sharp line of color and temperature demarcation. This may occur distal to the site of occlusion as a result of ischemia.

Nursing Diagnoses

A. Risk for Injury related to sensorimotor deficits
B. Altered Tissue Perfusion (peripheral) related to lack of blood flow by clot
C. Risk for Infection related to surgery

Nursing Interventions

A. Preventing Injury to Extremity
1. Protect extremity by keeping it at or below the body's horizontal plane.
2. Protect leg from hard surfaces and tight or heavy surfaces and tight or heavy overlying bed linens.
3. Handle extremity gently and prevent pressure or friction while repositioning.
4. Administer pain medications as ordered.

B. Promoting Tissue Perfusion
1. Administer heparin IV to reduce tendency of emboli to form or expand (useful in smaller arteries).
2. Administer thrombolytic therapy IV to dissolve clot as ordered.
3. Monitor patient for signs of bleeding (gums, urine, stool).
4. Monitor PT and PTT.
5. Prepare the patient for surgery (see p. 333).
6. Postoperatively, promote movement of extremity to stimulate circulation and prevent stasis.

C. Preventing Infection
1. Postoperatively, check surgical wound for bleeding, swelling, erythema, and discharge.
2. Maintain IV infusion or venous access device to administer IV antibiotics if indicated.

3. Continue to monitor the patient for tachycardia, fever, pain, erythema, warmth, swelling, and drainage at incision site.

Patient Education/Health Maintenance

1. Teach prevention techniques such as daily aerobic activity, observation for skin breakdown, and prevention of injury.
2. Teach patient the medical regimen and importance of taking prescribed medications such as oral anticoagulants to prevent reembolization (see p. 331).
3. Encourage patient to report symptoms of arterial occlusion—paralysis, numbness, tingling, pallor, and coldness of extremity.

Evaluation

A. Extremity protected and positioned below level of heart
B. Limb has normal color, sensation, movement, and temperature.
C. No signs of infection

◆ VASOSPASTIC DISORDER (RAYNAUD'S PHENOMENON)

Raynaud's phenomenon is a general term to describe a condition in which there is an increased or unusual sensitivity to cold or emotional factors, occurring primarily in the hands.

Pathophysiology/Etiology

1. The condition is a form of intermittent arteriolar vasoconstriction that results in coldness, pain and pallor of fingertips, toes, or tip of the nose
2. The cause is unknown although many patients with the disease seem to have immunologic disorders.
3. Episodes may be triggered by emotional factors or by unusual sensitivity to cold.
4. Most common in women between ages 16 and 40 and seen much more frequently in cold climates and during the winter months

Clinical Manifestations

1. Intermittent arteriolar vasoconstriction resulting in coldness, pain, pallor
2. Involvement of the fingers appears to be asymmetric; thumbs are less often involved.
3. Characteristic color changes: white-blue-red
   a. White—blanching, dead-white appearance if spasm is severe
   b. Blue—cyanotic, relatively stagnant blood flow
   c. Red—a reactive hyperemia on rewarming
4. Occasionally, there is ulceration of the fingertips.

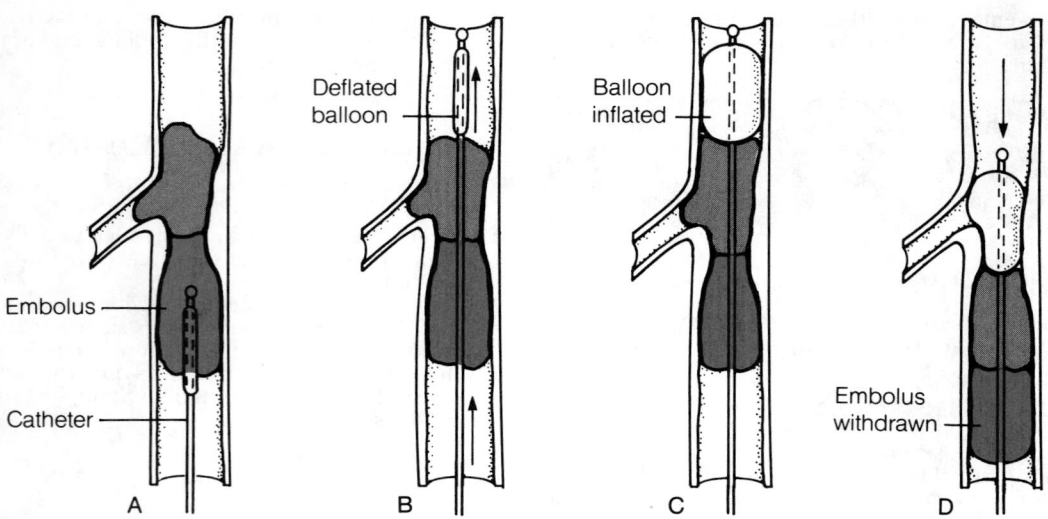

FIGURE 12-8 *Extracting an embolus from a vessel can be done with the use of a Fogarty embolectomy catheter. The catheter with a soft deflated balloon near the tip is threaded through the artery via an arteriotomy. (A and B) It is passed through the embolus and its thrombus; (C) it is then inflated. (D) A steady pull downward withdraws the embolus along with the catheter.*

Diagnostic Evaluation

1. Clinical symptoms must last at least 2 years to confirm the diagnosis.
2. Tests to rule out secondary disease processes such as chronic arterial occlusive or connective tissue disease may be done.

Management

1. Avoidance of trigger/aggravating factors
2. Calcium channel blockers are frequently used to prevent or reduce vasospasm.
3. Nitroglycerin or sympatholytics such as reserpine (Serpasil), guanethidine (Ismelin), or prasozin (Minipress) may be helpful for some.
   a. Side effects such as headache, dizziness, orthostatic hypotension may be prohibitive.
4. Antiplatelet agents such as aspirin or dipyridamole (Persantine) may be given to prevent total occlusion.
5. Sympathectomy—removal of the sympathetic ganglia or division of their branches may offer some improvement.

Complications

1. Chronic disease may cause atrophy of skin and muscles.
2. Ulceration and gangrene (rare)

Nursing Assessment

1. Perform thorough history and review of systems for clues to underlying disorder.

2. Assess for blanching of digits when exposed to cold. Color turns cyanotic, then red with normal temperature.
3. Note whether warmth brings about symptom relief.

Nursing Diagnoses

A. Sensory Alterations (tactile) related to vasospastic process
B. Pain related to hyperemic stage

Nursing Interventions

A. *Minimizing Sensory Alteration*
1. Assist patient in avoiding exposure to cold; for example, use gloves to handle cold items (water pitcher, refrigerated items).
2. Encourage patient to stop smoking.
3. Help patient to understand need for avoidance of stressful situations.
4. Offer patient options for stress management.
5. Administer and teach patient about drug therapy.
   a. Need to take drugs every day to prevent or minimize symptoms.
   b. Follow orthostatic hypotension precaution if on sympatholytics.
6. Advise patient that episode may be terminated by placing hands (or feet) in warm water.

B. *Relieving Pain*
1. Explain to patient that pain may be experienced when spasm is relieved—hyperemic phase.
2. Administer or teach self-administration of analgesics.

3. Reassure patient that pain is temporary; persistent pain, ulceration, or signs of infection should be reported.

Patient Education/Health Maintenance

1. Avoid whatever provokes vasoconstriction of vessels of hands.
2. Prevent injury to hands, which can aggravate vasoconstriction and lead to ulceration.
3. Minimize exposure to cold because this precipitates a reaction.
4. Wear warm clothing—boots, gloves, and hooded jackets—when going out in cold weather.
  a. Turn heat on in automobile during travel.
  b. Shop in heated stores; avoid unheated buildings.
  c. Avoid getting wet.
5. Avoid placing hands in cold water, the freezer, or the refrigerator unless protective gloves are worn.
6. Use extra precautions to avoid injuries to fingers and hands from needle sticks and knife cuts.

Evaluation

1. Wears gloves while handling cold items
2. Reports decreased length of painful phase with episodes

◆ ANEURYSM

Aneurysm is a distention of an artery brought about by a weakening/destruction of the media of the arterial wall. It tends to enlarge, thereby producing serious complications by compressing surrounding structures or rupturing, causing a fatal hemorrhage. Aneurysm of the aorta commonly occurs. In dissecting aortic aneurysm there is a tear in the intima of the aorta; as a result of pressure, blood splits the wall and may produce a large hematoma or may continue to rip the wall.

Peripheral vessel aneurysms may involve the renal artery, subclavian artery, popliteal artery (knee), or any major artery. These produce a pulsating mass and may cause pain or pressure on surrounding structures.

Pathophysiology/Etiology

1. Medial degeneration is the mechanism for aneurysm formation. Medial degeneration occurs as a normal part of the aging process, in hypertension, and as a complication of Marfan syndrome known as Erdheim's cystic medial necrosis.
2. The ascending aorta and the aortic arch are the sites of greatest hemodynamic stress and also are the most common sites of arterial dissection.
3. Contributing factors include:
  a. Local infection, pyogenic or fungal (mycotic aneurysm)
  b. Congenital weakness of vessels
  c. Arteriosclerosis
  d. Syphilis
  e. Trauma

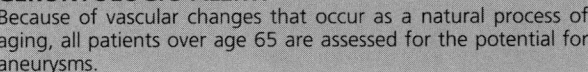

GERONTOLOGIC ALERT:
Because of vascular changes that occur as a natural process of aging, all patients over age 65 are assessed for the potential for aneurysms.

4. Morphologically, aneurysms may be classified as follows:
  a. Saccular—distention of a vessel projecting from one side
  b. Fusiform—distention of the whole artery (i.e., entire circumference is involved)
  c. Dissecting—hemorrhagic or intramural hematoma, separating the medial layers of the aortic wall

Clinical Manifestations

A. Aneurysm of the Thoracoabdominal Aorta
(Lower descending thoracic aorta and upper abdominal aorta)

1. At first no symptoms; later symptoms may come from CHF or a pulsating tumor mass in the chest.
2. Pain and pressure symptoms
  a. Constant, boring pain because of pressure
  b. Intermittent and neuralgic pain because of impingement on nerves
3. Dyspnea, causing pressure against trachea
4. Cough, often paroxysmal and brassy in sound
5. Hoarseness, voice weakness, or complete aphonia, resulting from pressure against recurrent laryngeal nerve
6. Dysphagia due to impingement on esophagus
7. Edema of chest wall—infrequent
8. Dilated superficial veins on chest
9. Cyanosis because of vein compression of chest vessels
10. Ipsilateral dilatation of pupils due to pressure against cervical sympathetic chain
11. Pulse difference in two wrists if aneurysm interferes with circulation in left subclavian artery
12. Abnormal pulsation apparent on chest wall—due to erosion of aneurysm through rib cage—in syphilis

B. Abdominal Aneurysm
1. Many of these patients are asymptomatic; most are men (9:1).
2. Abdominal pain is most common; persistent or intermittent—often localized in middle or lower abdomen to the left of midline.
3. Low back pain
4. Feeling of an abdominal pulsating mass, palpated as a thrill, auscultated as a bruit (Fig. 12-9)
5. Hypertension; blood pressure in arm greater than thigh

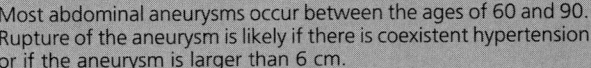

GERONTOLOGIC ALERT:
Most abdominal aneurysms occur between the ages of 60 and 90. Rupture of the aneurysm is likely if there is coexistent hypertension or if the aneurysm is larger than 6 cm.

Diagnostic Evaluation

1. Abdominal or chest x-ray may show calcification that outlines aneurysm.

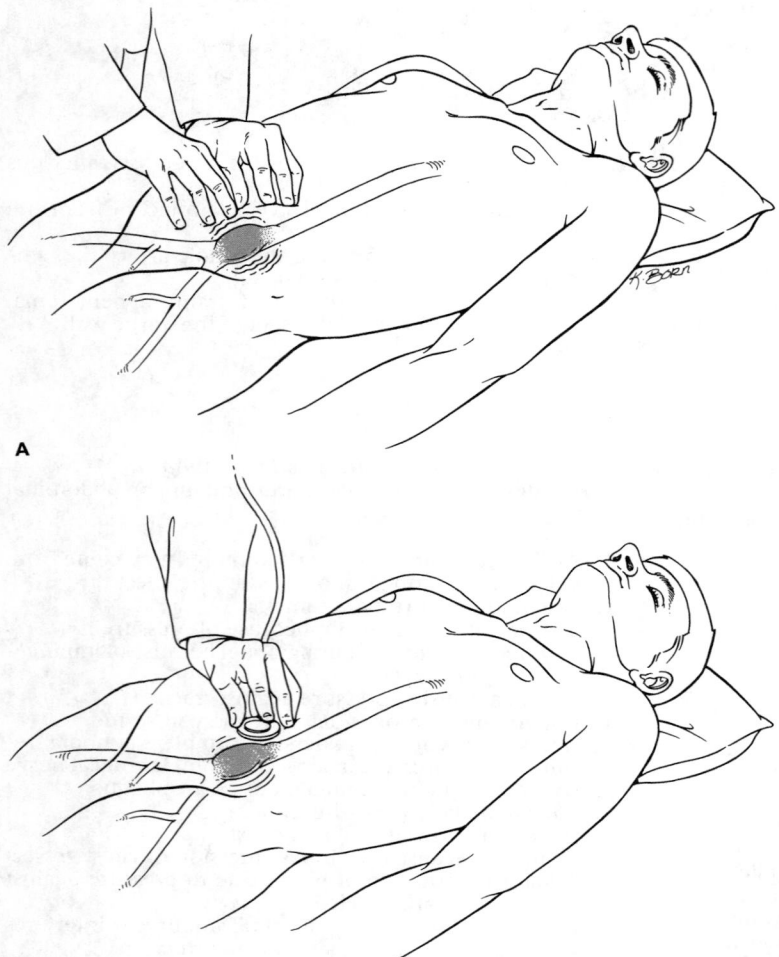

A

B

FIGURE 12-9 *Palpating and auscultating for an abdominal aortic aneurysm. (**A**) Hand applied over the aorta will feel a pulsatile rumbling referred to as a thrill (likened to the purring of a cat). (**B**) The bell of stethoscope applied over the aorta will produce a murmurlike sound called a bruit.*

2. Computed tomography (CT) scanning and ultrasonography are used to detect and monitor size of aneurysm.
3. Aortography allows visualization of aneurysm and vessel.

Management

1. May follow small aneurysms (4 cm or less) with CT scanning or ultrasound every 6 months and aggressively control blood pressure.
2. The prognosis is poor for untreated patients as aneurysm enlarges.
3. Surgery—remove aneurysm and restore vascular continuity with bypass graft.
   a. Aortic arch aneurysms are the most difficult to treat.
   b. Complications of surgery include arterial occlusion, graft hemorrhage, infection, ischemic colon, and impotence.

Complications

1. Fatal hemorrhage
2. Paraplegia due to interruption of anterior spinal artery
3. Abdominal ischemia
4. Stroke or cardiac tamponade

Nursing Assessment

1. In patient with thoracoabdominal aortic aneurysm, be alert for sudden onset of sharp, ripping or tearing pain located in anterior chest, epigastric area, shoulders, or back indicating acute dissection or rupture.
2. In patients with abdominal aortic aneurysm, assess for pain and intense low back pain caused by rapid expansion. Be alert for syncope, tachycardia, and hypotension, which may be followed by fatal hemorrhage due to rupture.

Nursing Diagnoses

A. Altered Tissue Perfusion (vital organs) related to aneurysm rupture or dissection
B. Risk for Infection related to surgery
C. Pain related to pressure of aneurysm on nerves and postoperatively

Nursing Interventions

A. *Maintaining Perfusion of Vital Organs*
1. Assess for signs and symptoms of pressure caused by aneurysm or dissection.
2. Prepare patient for diagnostic studies or surgery as indicated.
3. Monitor vital signs continuously postoperatively.
4. Check extremities for sensation, temperature, pulses, color, capillary refill, and petechiae to monitor for arterial occlusion.
5. Monitor for bleeding from the wound grid for signs of hemorrhage—hypotension, tachycardia, pallor, diaphoresis.
6. Monitor urinary output hourly.
7. Maintain IV infusion to administer medications to control blood pressure and provide fluids postoperatively.
8. Position patient to enhance circulation.
   a. Keep head of bed elevated no more than 45° for first 3 days postoperatively.
   b. Warn patient not to cross legs or sit for long periods.

B. *Preventing Infection*
1. Monitor temperature and incision for signs of infection.
2. Administer antibiotics, if ordered.

C. *Relieving Pain*
1. Administer pain medication as ordered or monitor patient-controlled analgesia.
2. Keep head of bed elevated no more than 45° for the first 3 days postoperatively to prevent pressure on repair and graft site.
3. Administer nasogastric decompression for ileus following surgery, until bowel sounds return.
4. Measure abdominal girth or limb girth (of graft site) daily.
5. Monitor for watery, bloody diarrhea, which indicates ischemic bowel due to reduced perfusion during surgery.
6. Monitor for signs and symptoms of spinal cord ischemia—pain, numbness, parasthesias, weakness.

Patient Education/Health Maintenance

1. Teach patient about medications to control blood pressure and the importance of taking them.
2. Discuss disease process and signs and symptoms of expanding aneurysm or impending rupture or rupture to be reported.
3. For postsurgical patients, discuss warning signs of postoperative complications (fever, inflammation of operative site, bleeding, and swelling).
4. Encourage adequate balanced intake for wound healing.

5. Encourage patient to maintain an exercise schedule postoperatively.

Evaluation

A. Tissue normal color, sensation and temperature; nontender, nonswollen and intact
B. Afebrile, no signs of infection
C. Reports control of pain with medication

◆ HYPERTENSION

Hypertension (high blood pressure) is a disease of vascular regulation in which the mechanisms that control arterial pressure within the normal range are altered. Predominant mechanisms of control are the central nervous system (CNS), the renal pressor system (renin-angiotensin-aldosterone system), and extracellular fluid volume. Why these mechanisms fail is not known. The basic explanation is that blood pressure is elevated when there is increased cardiac output plus increased peripheral vascular resistance.

Pathophysiology/Etiology

A. *Primary or Essential Hypertension*
(Approximately 90% of patients with hypertension)

1. When the diastolic pressure is 90 mm Hg or higher and other causes of hypertension are absent, the condition is said to be *primary hypertension*. More specifically, an individual is considered hypertensive when the average of three or more blood pressure readings taken at rest several days apart exceeds the upper limits of the following table:
2. Cause of essential hypertension is unknown; however, there are several areas of investigation:
   a. Hyperactivity of sympathetic vasoconstricting nerves
   b. Presence of blood component containing a vasoconstrictor that acts on smooth muscle, sensitizing it to constrictor substances
   c. Increased cardiac output, followed by arteriole constriction
   d. Prostaglandins affect regulatory mechanisms, which include the renin-angiotensin system, renal sodium and water excretion, and vascular smooth muscle tone.
   e. Familial (genetic) tendency
3. Terminology to describe hypertension:
   a. *Labile*—intermittently elevated blood pressure

Classification of Hypertension

Classification	Diastolic Pressure (mm Hg)	Percentage of Individuals
Mild	90–104	70%
Moderate	105–114	20%
Severe	115	10%

b. *Accelerated*—sudden and severe escalation in arterial pressure, producing many symptoms and vascular damage

c. *Resistant*—hypertension that is not responsive to usual treatment

B. Secondary Hypertension
(Occurs in approximately 5% to 10% of patients with hypertension)

1. Follows other pathology
2. Renal pathology—may lead to hypertension
   a. Congenital anomalies, pyelonephritis, renal artery obstruction, acute and chronic glomerulonephritis
   b. Reduced blood flow to kidney (such as atherosclerotic plaque)—release of renin. Renin reacts with serum protein in liver (α_2-globulin) → angiotensin I; this plus angiotensin-converting enzyme (ACE) → angiotensin II → leads to increased blood pressure.
3. Coarctation of aorta (stenosis of aorta)—blood flow to upper extremities is greater than flow to lower extremities—hypertension of upper part of body.
4. Endocrine disturbances
   a. Pheochromocytoma—a tumor of the adrenal gland that causes release of epinephrine and norepinephrine and a rise in blood pressure
   b. Adrenal cortex tumors lead to an increase in aldosterone secretion and an elevated blood pressure.
   c. Cushing's syndrome leads to an increase in adrenocortical steroids and hypertension.
   d. Hyperthyroidism

C. Accelerated Hypertension—A Hypertensive Crisis
Blood pressure elevates very rapidly, threatening one or more of the target organs: brain, kidney, heart (see p. 357).

Prevalence and Risk Factors

1. Hypertension is one of the most prevalent chronic diseases for which treatment is available; however, most patients with hypertension are untreated.
2. There are no symptoms; thus, it is termed "the silent killer."
3. Increase in incidence is associated with the following risk factors:
   a. Age—between 30 and 70
   b. Race—African American
   c. Birth control pills
   d. Overweight
   e. Family history
   f. Smoking
   g. Sedentary lifestyle
   h. Stress
   i. Diabetes mellitus

Clinical Manifestations

1. Usually asymptomatic
2. May cause headache, dizziness, blurred vision when greatly elevated
3. Blood pressure readings as stated in table, above

Diagnostic Evaluation

1. ECG—to determine effects of hypertension on the heart (left ventricular hypertrophy, ischemia) or presence of underlying heart disease
2. Chest x-ray—may show cardiomegaly
3. Proteinuria, elevated serum blood urea nitrogen (BUN) and creatinine levels—indicate kidney disease as a cause or effect of hypertension
4. Serum potassium—decreased in primary hyperaldosteronism; elevated in Cushing's syndrome, both causes of secondary hypertension
5. Urine for catecholamines—increased in pheochromocytoma
6. Renal scan to detect renal vascular diseases

Management

A. Lifestyle Modifications
1. Lose weight, if more than 10% above ideal weight.
2. Limit alcohol, no more than 1 oz ethanol daily
3. Get regular aerobic exercise 3 times per week.
4. Cut sodium intake to less than 2 g per day
5. Include recommended daily allowances of potassium, calcium and magnesium in diet.
6. Stop smoking.
7. Reduce dietary saturated fat and cholesterol.
8. If, despite lifestyle changes, the blood pressure remains at or above 140/90 mm Hg over 3 to 6 months, drug therapy should be initiated.

B. Drug Therapy
See Table 12-2.

1. Considerations in selecting therapy include:
   a. Race—African Americans respond well to diuretic therapy; whites respond well to ACE inhibitors.
   b. Age—some side effects may not be tolerated well by elderly persons.
   c. Concommitant diseases and therapies—some agents also treat migraines, benign prostatic hyperplasia, CHF.
   d. Quality of life impact—tolerance of side effects
   e. Economic considerations—newer agents very expensive
   f. Doses per day—may be compliance problem
2. Agents include:
   a. Diuretics—lower blood pressure by promoting urinary excretion of water and sodium to lower blood volume
   b. β Blockers—adrenergic inhibitors that lower blood pressure by slowing the heart and reducing cardiac output as well as release of renin from the kidneys
   c. α-Receptor blockers—lower blood pressure by dilating peripheral blood vessels and lowering peripheral vascular resistance
   d. Angiotensin—converting enzyme (ACE) inhibitors—lower blood pressure by blocking the enzyme that converts angiotensin I to the potent vasoconstrictor angiotensin II. These drugs also raise the level of bradykinin, a potent vasodilator and lower aldosterone levels.
   e. Calcium antagonists (calcium channel blockers)—stop the movement of calcium into the cells; relax smooth muscle, which causes vasodilation; and inhibit reabsorption of sodium in the renal tubules

TABLE 12-2   Pharmacotherapy for Hypertension

Adverse Effects	Drug Interactions	Other Nursing Considerations

DIURETICS
Thiazides and related sulfonamides, including chlorthalidone (Hygroton, Thalitone), hydrochlorothiazide (Esidrex, Hydrodiuril, others), and metolazone (Diulo, Zaroxolyn)

Adverse Effects	Drug Interactions	Other Nursing Considerations
Hypokalemia Hypomagnesemia Hyponatremia Hyperuricemia Hypercalcemia Hyperglycemia Hypercholesterolemia Hypertriglyceridemia Sexual dysfunction	Antihypertensive effect may be reduced when combined with cholestyramine, (Cholybar, Questran, Questran Light), colestipol (Colestid), or NSAIDs. Because diuretics cause hypokalemia, they increase the risk of digitalis toxicity and cardiac arrhythmias. Combined with the loop diuretic furosemide, thiazides can produce excessive diuresis in patients with renal impairment. These drugs can raise serum lithium levels.	Correct hypomagnesemia before giving potassium to treat hypokalemia. Encourage patients to restrict daily sodium intake and eat foods high in potassium. Gout patients may need higher doses of medication that reduces serum uric acid. Monitor levels of low-density lipoportein cholesterol and triglycerides. Watch lab reports for abnormalities in electrolyte levels. Ask the patient to report muscle weakness, cramps, and fatigue. Monitor kidney function by checking BUN and serum creatinine levels.

Loop diuretics: bumetanide (Bumex), ethacrynic acid (Edecrin), and furosemide (Lasix, Myrosemide)

Adverse Effects	Drug Interactions	Other Nursing Considerations
Same as for thiazides, except no hypercalcemia Ototoxicity	These drugs have many of the same interactions seen with thiazide diuretics. Aminoglycoside antibiotics increase the ototoxic effects of these drugs. Loop diuretics decrease the anticoagulant effect of heparin.	Watch patients for signs and symptoms of dehydration, potassium depletion, and acid base imbalance. Consider these drugs for patients in chronic renal failure. To monitor for ototoxic effects, ask the patient if he has experienced any hearing problem.

Potassium-sparing diuretics: amiloride (Midamor), spironolactone (Aldactone), and triamterene (Dyrenium)

Adverse Effects	Drug Interactions	Other Nursing Considerations
Hyperkalemia, especially in patients with renal failure With spironolactone, painful breast swelling and diminished libido in men, and menstrual irregularities in women With triamterene, risk of renal calculi	Patients also treated with an ACE inhibitor, NSAID, or captopril may develop hyperkalemia. Spironolactone can increase serum digoxin to toxic levels.	Monitor serum potassium and electrolyte levels. Assess heart rate and rhythm for irregularities.

ADRENERGIC INHIBITORS
β Blockers, including atenolol (Tenormin), metoprolol (Lopressor), and propranolol (Inderal)

Adverse Effects	Drug Interactions	Other Nursing Considerations
Bronchospasm, fatigue, insomnia May aggravate peripheral arterial insufficiency. Depression of cardiac contractility can exacerbate CHF. In diabetics, masking of symptoms of hypoglycemia With the exception of intrinsic sympathomimetic activity (ISA) drugs, β blockers interfere with lipid metabolism. This leads to hypertriglyceridemia and a decrease in HDL cholesterol.	NSAIDs, rifampin (Rifadin, Rimactine), nicotine, and phenobarbital can decrease the effectiveness of these drugs. Cimetidine (Tagamet) increases serum levels of these drugs, enhancing the antihypertensive effects. Calcium channel blockers can increase depressant effects on cardiac function.	All β blockers are contraindicated in patients with CHF or advanced degrees of heart block. If β blockers must be used in patients with respiratory problems, they must be cardioselective. Use with caution in patients with peripheral vascular disease. Monitor the patient's heart rate to detect bradycardia. Warn patients with ischemic heart disease not to discontinue therapy abruptly. Check lab reports for changes in lipid levels, especially in diabetic patients.

α-β Blocker: labetalol (Normodyne, Trandate)

Adverse Effects	Drug Interactions	Other Nursing Considerations
Bronchospasm Orthostatic hypotension May aggravate peripheral vascular insufficiency.	Glutethimide (Doriglute) decreases the effect of this drug as it is more readily broken down by the liver. Halothane (Fluothane) and nitroglycerine increase the drug's side effect of hypotension. Patients on this drug who also take tricyclic antidepressants may experience tremors.	Contraindicated in patients with asthma, chronic obstructive pulmonary disease, CHF, or advanced degrees of heart block. Advise patients to rise slowly from a lying or sitting position.

(continued)

TABLE 12-2 Pharmacotherapy for Hypertension *(continued)*

Adverse Effects	Drug Interactions	Other Nursing Considerations
α_1-Receptor blockers: doxazosin (Cardura), prazosin (Minipress), and terazosin (Hytrin)		
Orthostatic hypotension, syncope, weakness, palpitations, headache Sexual dysfunction	Diuretics increase the chance of orthostatic hypotension. Sympathomimetics and NSAIDs, especially indomethacin (Indocid), may reduce the antihypertensive effect of these drugs.	Advise patients to rise slowly from a lying or sitting position. Tell patients to take their first dose at bedtime.
ACE INHIBITORS **including captopril (Capoten), enalapril (Vasotec), and lisinopril (Prinivil, Zestril)**		
Cough Hypersensitivity reaction with rash and angioneurotic edema Hyperkalemia, especially in patients with renal insufficiency Hypotension, particularly in patients also taking diuretics Reversible renal failure in patients with renal artery stenosis, cardiac failure, or volume depletion Impaired sense of taste	NSAIDs and antacids may decrease these drugs' ability to control blood pressure. When combined with these drugs, diuretics may deplete blood volume too vigorously and cause excessive hypotension. Hyperkalemia may occur when patients also take potassium supplements, potassium-sparing diuretics, or NSAIDs. These drugs can increase serum lithium levels.	Observe patients for rash, swelling, and other symptoms of hypersensitivity. Make sure diuretic therapy has been temporarily discontinued before patient starts taking an ACE inhibitor. Monitor electrolytes for any rise in potassium levels. Advise patients to get up slowly from a sitting or lying positon. Check lab reports for a rise in BUN or serum creatinine, indicating the beginning of renal failure. Contraindicated in second and third trimesters of pregnancy.
CALCIUM ANTAGONISTS **including diltiazem (Cardizem), nicardipine (Cardene), nifedipine (Procardia), and verapamil (Calan, Isoptin)**		
Headache, dizziness, peripheral edema, tachycardia, gingival hyperplasia	The antihypertensive effects of some of these drugs may be reduced when taken with rifampin, carbamazepine (Epitol, Tegretol), phenobarbital, or phenytoin. Cimetidine may increase the pharmacologic effects of these drugs. Verapamil and diltiazem increase serum levels and the toxicity of digoxin and carbamazepine. Verapamil may increase serum levels of prazosin, quinidine, and theophylline.	Use cautiously in patients with CHF because these drugs may aggravate angina and myocardial ischemia. Use cautiously in patients taking digitalis or β blockers. Monitor the patient's heart rate, watching for additive effects of other cardiodepressant drugs. Monitor blood pressure during dosage adjustment to avoid hypotension.
CENTRALLY ACTING ALPHA$_2$-AGONISTS **clonidine (Catapres), guanabenz (Wytensin), guanfacine (Tenex), and methyldopa (Aldomet)**		
Drowsiness, sedation, dry mouth, fatigue Orthostatic dizziness	Rebound hypertension may occur with abrupt discontinuation, particularly in cases of prior administration of high doses or continuation of concomitant beta blocker therapy. Alcohol and CNS depressants can increase drowsiness.	Methyldopa may cause liver damage, fever, and Coombs-positive hemolytic anemia. Observe patients for drug-induced mood changes. Patients using the clonidine patch may experience localized skin irritation, redness, and itching.
PERIPHERAL ACTING ADRENERGIC ANTAGONISTS **guanadrel (Hylorel), guanethidine (Ismelin), and reserpine (Serpaline, other rauwolfia alkaloids)**		
Diarrhea, as well as orthostatic and exercise-induced hypotension, can be severe with guanadrel and guanethidine. Lethargy, nasal congestion, and depression occur more often with rauwolfia alkaloids.	Tricyclic antidepressants, phenothiazines, monoamine oxidase inhibitors, and over-the-counter cold and diet medications may reduce the effectiveness of these drugs. β blockers taken with these drugs may increase orthostatic hypotension or bradycardia.	Instruct the patient to rise slowly because of orthostatic hypotension. Increased gastrointestinal motility and secretion make these drugs a poor choice for a patient with an active peptic ulcer. Avoid giving rauwolfia alkaloids to patients with a history of mental depression.

(continued)

TABLE 12-2 Pharmacotherapy for Hypertension *(continued)*

Adverse Effects	Drug Interactions	Other Nursing Considerations
DIRECT VASODILATORS		
Hydralazine (Apresoline) and minoxidil (Loniten)		
Headache, tachycardia, fluid retention	NSAIDs, especially indomethacin, may reduce the antihypertensive effect of vasodilators.	Do not give to patients with coronary artery disease and mitral valvular rheumatic heart disease.
Excesive localized hair growth with minoxidil	Concurrent use with diazoxide (Hyperstat), guanethidine, or nitrates can cause a severe hypotensive effect.	Use with caution in patients with renal impairment.
		May cause or aggrevate pleural and pericardial effusions.
		Watch for symptoms of lupus syndrome, including fever and swollen, painful joints.

Soloman J. Hypertension: the new drug therapies. *RN.* 1994;57(1);26–33.
Source: The Fifth Report of the Joint National Committee on Detection, Evaluation, and Treatment of High Blood Pressure.

3. If hypertension is not controlled with the first drug within 1 to 3 months, three options can be considered:
   a. If the patient has faithfully taken the drug and not developed any side effects, the dose of the drug may be increased.
   b. If the patient has had adverse effects, another class of drugs can be substituted.
   c. A second drug from another class could be added. If adding the second agent lowers the pressure, the first agent can be slowly withdrawn.
4. The best management of hypertension is to use the fewest drugs at the lowest doses while encouraging the patient to maintain lifestyle changes. After blood pressure has been under control for at least a year, a slow progressive decline in drug therapy can be attempted.
5. If the desired blood pressure is still not achieved with the addition of a second drug, a third agent or a diuretic or both (if not already prescribed) could be added. These supplemental agents include:
   a. Centrally acting α_2-agonists—lower blood pressure by diminishing sympathetic outflow from the brain thereby lowering peripheral resistance.
   b. Peripheral adrenergic antagonists—inhibit peripheral adrenergic release of vasoconstricting catecholamines, such as norepinephrine.
   c. Direct vasodilators—direct smooth muscle relaxants that primarily dilate arteries and arterioles

Complications

See Figure 12-10.

1. Angina pectoris or MI due to decreased coronary perfusion
2. Left ventricular hypertrophy and CHF due to consistently elevated aortic pressure
3. Renal failure due to thickening of renal vessels and diminished perfusion to the glomerulus
4. Stroke or cerebral hemorrhage due to cerebral ischemia and arteriosclerosis
5. Retinopathy
6. Accelerated hypertension (see p. 357)

Nursing Assessment

A. Nursing History
Query the patient with regard to the following:

1. Family history of high blood pressure
2. Previous episodes of high blood pressure
3. Excessive salt intake
4. Lipid abnormalities
5. Smoking (cigarette)
6. Episodes of headache, weakness, muscle cramp, tingling, palpitations, sweating, visual disturbances
7. Medication that could elevate blood pressure:
   a. Oral contraceptives, steroids
   b. NSAIDs
   c. Nasal decongestants, appetite suppressants, tricyclic antidepressants
8. Other disease processes such as gout or diabetes, asthma, peptic ulcer

B. Physical Examination
1. Auscultate heart rate and palpate peripheral pulses; determine respirations.
2. If skilled in doing so, perform funduscopic examination of the eyes for the purpose of noting vascular changes. Look for edema, spasm, and hemorrhage of the eye vessels.
3. Examine the heart for a shift of the point of maximal impulse to the left, which occurs in heart enlargement.
4. Auscultate for bruits over peripheral arteries to determine the presence of atherosclerosis, which may be manifested as obstructed blood flow.
5. Determine mentation status by asking patient about memory, ability to concentrate, and ability to perform simple mathematic calculations.

C. Blood Pressure Determination
1. Measure the blood pressure of the patient under the same conditions each time.
2. Avoid taking blood pressure readings immediately after stressful or taxing situations.
3. Place the patient in a position of comfort.

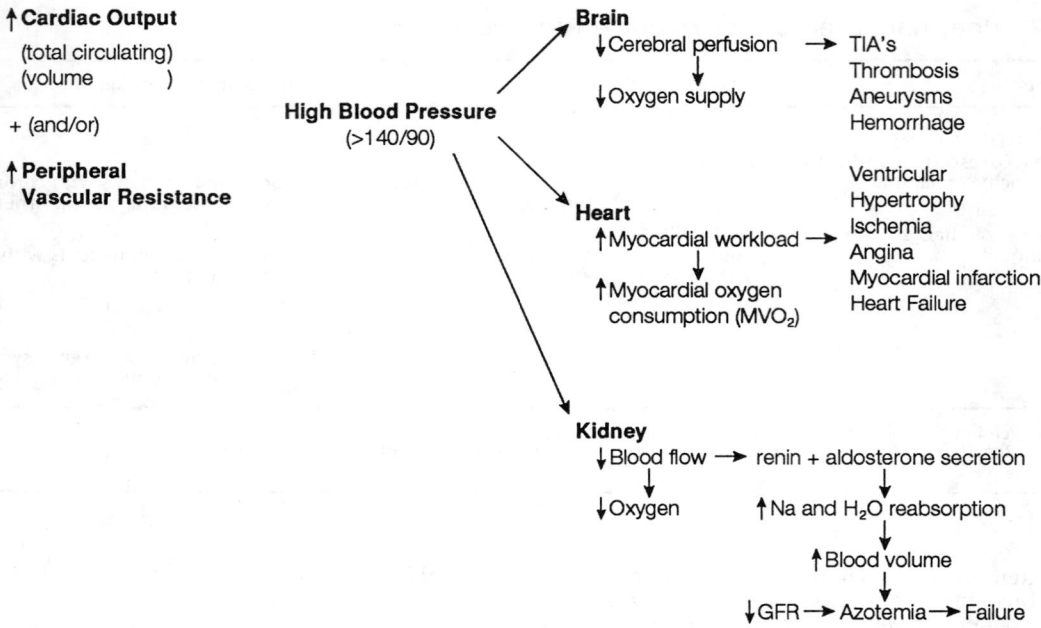

FIGURE 12-10 *Determinants and clinical effects of high blood pressure. GFR, glomerular filtration rate; TIA, transient ischemic attack*

4. Support the bared arm; avoid constriction of arm by a rolled sleeve.
5. Use a blood pressure cuff of the correct size (Table 12-3).
   a. It is recommended that the width of the cuff be 20% greater than the width of the measured extremity.
   b. The length should be sufficient to encircle the measured extremity.
   c. The average dimensions for an adult cuff are 13 cm wide by 24 cm long.
6. Be aware that falsely elevated blood pressures may be obtained with a cuff that is too narrow; falsely low readings may be obtained with a cuff that is too wide.
7. Auscultate and record precisely the systolic and diastolic pressures based on Korotkoff sounds.
   a. Systolic—the pressure within the cuff indicated by the level of the mercury column at the moment when the first clear, rhythmic pulsatile sound is heard (phase 1)
   b. First diastolic—the pressure within the cuff indicated by the level of the mercury column at the moment when the sound becomes muffled (phase 4)
   c. Second diastolic—the pressure within the cuff at the moment the sound disappears, that is, the onset of silence (phase 5)
   d. Phases 2 and 3 are less distinct sounds produced between systolic and first diastolic and are not identified clinically nor recorded.

NURSING ALERT:
The finding of an isolated elevated blood pressure does not necessarily indicate hypertension. However, the patient should be regarded at risk for high blood pressure until further assessment through history taking and diagnostic testing either confirms or denies the diagnosis.

Nursing Diagnoses

A. Knowledge Deficit regarding the relationship between the treatment regimen and control of the disease process
B. Ineffective Management of Therapeutic Regimen related to medication side effects and difficult lifestyle adjustments

Nursing Interventions/ Patient Education

A. *Providing Basic Education*
1. Explain the meaning of high blood pressure, risk factors, and their influences on the cardiovascular, cerebral, and renal systems.
2. Stress that there can never be total cure, only control of essential hypertension; emphasize the consequences of uncontrolled hypertension.
3. Stress the fact that there may be no correlation between high blood pressure and symptoms; the patient cannot tell by the way he or she feels whether blood pressure is normal or elevated.
4. Have the patient recognize that hypertension is chronic and requires persistent therapy and periodic evaluation; effective treatment improves life expectancy; therefore, follow-up health care visits are mandatory.
5. Present a coordinated and complementary plan of guidance.
   a. Inform the patient of the meaning of the various diagnostic and therapeutic activities to minimize anxiety and to obtain cooperation.

TABLE 12-3 Recommended Bladder Dimensions for Blood Pressure Cuffs

Arm Circumference at Midpoint* (cm)	Cuff Type	Bladder Width (cm)	Bladder Length (cm)
5–7.5	Newborn	3	5
7.5–13	Infant	5	8
13–20	Child	8	13
24–32	Adult	13	24
32–42	Wide adult	17	32
42–50†	Thigh	20	42

* Midpoint of arm is defined as half the distance from acromion to olecranon. Use nonstretchable metal tape.
† In persons with very large limbs, indirect blood pressure should be measured in leg or forearm.
From Recommendations for Human Blood Pressure Determination by Sphygmomanometers, American Heart Association, 1987.

b. Solicit the assistance of the patient's spouse/family/friend—provide information regarding the total treatment plan.
c. Be aware of the dietary plan developed for this particular patient.
6. Explain the pharmacologic control of hypertension.
   a. Explain that the drugs used for effective control of elevated blood pressure will likely produce side effects.
   b. Warn the patient of the possibility that hypotension may occur after the intake of certain drugs.
      (1) Instruct the patient to get up slowly to offset the feeling of dizziness.
      (2) Encourage the patient to lie down immediately if feels faint.
   c. Alert the patient to expect effects such as nasal congestion, asthenia (loss of strength), anorexia (loss of appetite), and orthostatic hypotension (dizziness on changing position).
   d. Inform the patient that the goal of treatment is to control blood pressure, reduce the possibility of complications, and use the minimum number of drugs with lowest dosage necessary to accomplish this.
7. Educate the patient to be aware of toxic manifestations and report them so that adjustments can be made in individual pharmacotherapy.
   a. Note that dosages are individualized; therefore, they may need to be adjusted because it is often impossible to predict reactions.
   b. Remember that certain circumstances produce vasodilation—a hot bath, hot weather, febrile illness, consumption of alcohol.
   c. Be aware that blood pressure is decreased when circulating blood volume is reduced—dehydration, diarrhea, hemorrhage.
   d. Consider the presence of edema as a reportable symptom, particularly when guanethidine is taken; these medications are less effective in the presence of edema.

GERONTOLOGIC ALERT:
The multiple drugs required to control blood pressure may be difficult for the elderly patient to comprehend. The names of drugs are frequently difficult for the patient to pronounce. Color coding of medication bottles with an accompanying color-coded time of administration chart is one way to assist the patient in remembering when to take medications. Elderly patients are also more sensitive to therapeutic levels of drugs and may demonstrate side effects while on an otherwise average dosage. They may be more sensitive to postural hypotension and should be cautioned to change positions with great care.

B. **Encouraging Self-Management**
1. Enlist the patient's cooperation in redirecting lifestyle in keeping with the guidelines of therapy.
   a. Present a written instructional program to fit individual requirements.
   b. Reassure the patient when encouragement is needed; the modifications required must appear meaningful.
   c. Encourage patient in adapting and adjusting activities in line with the prescribed therapeutic regimen.
2. Develop a plan of instruction to be practiced by the patient at home.
   a. Instruct the patient regarding proper method of taking blood pressure at home and at work if health care provider so desires. Inform patient of the readings that are to be reported.
   b. Plan the patient's medication schedule so that the many medications are given at proper and convenient times; set up a daily checklist on which the patient can record the medication taken.
   c. Determine recommended dietary plans.

Evaluation

A. Demonstrates increased knowledge about high blood pressure, medication effects, and prescribed therapeutic activities
B. Adheres to therapeutic regimen by limiting sodium intake, exercising, conscientiously taking medications, and keeping follow-up appointments

◆ ACCELERATED HYPERTENSION

Accelerated hypertension occurs when the blood pressure elevates extremely rapidly, threatening one or more of the target organs: brain, kidney, heart.

Pathophysiology

1. Elevated diastolic pressure → strain on arterial wall → thickening and calcification of arterial media (sclerosis) → narrowed blood vessel lumen.
2. Sclerosis of vessels → increased wall permeability → deposits placed on intima and media of vessels → cerebral, myocardial, or renal eschemia.

Clinical Manifestations

1. Brain effects
   a. Encephalopathy
   b. Stroke
   c. Progressive headache, stupor, seizures
2. Kidney effects
   a. Blood flow decreased, vasoconstriction
   b. BUN elevated
   c. Plasma renin activity increased
   d. Urine specific gravity lowered
   e. Proteinuria
3. Heart effects
   a. Left ventricular failure
   b. Acute MI

Management

Goal

- To lower blood pressure to reduce the probability of permanent damage to a target organ: brain, heart, kidney

1. If diastolic blood pressure exceeds 115 to 130 mm Hg, hospitalization is recommended.
2. Immediate treatment if the following are present:
   a. Seizures
   b. Abnormal neurologic signs
   c. Severe occipital headache
   d. Pulmonary edema
3. The patient is hemodynamically monitored in the intensive care unit.
4. Antihypertensive agents are administered parenterally. Agents include:
   a. Vasodilators such as sodium nitroprusside (Nipride), nitroglycerin (Tridil), diazoxide (Hyperstat), or hydralazine (Apresoline)
   b. Adrenergic inhibitors such as phentolamine (Regitine), labetalol (Normodyne), and methyldopa (Aldomet)
   c. The calcium antagonist nifedipine (Adalat) may also be used.
5. Diuretics may be administered to maintain a sodium diuresis when the arterial pressure falls.
6. Vasopressor agents should be available if the blood pressure responds too vigorously to antihypertensive agents.

Nursing Interventions

1. Record blood pressure frequently or monitor blood pressure via intraarterial line or electronically controlled cuff. Some drugs necessitate the taking of blood pressure readings every 5 minutes or more frequently while titrating drug therapies.

NURSING ALERT:
The blood pressure should be reduced gradually and wide pressure variations avoided because the patient's usual range may not be tolerated.

2. Monitor for side effects of medications—headache, tachycardia, orthostatic hypotension.
3. Measure urine output accurately.
4. Observe for hypokalemia, especially if patient is placed on diuretic therapy. Monitor for ventricular dysrhythmias.
5. Observe for CNS complications.
   a. Note signs of confusion, irritability, lethargy, and disorientation.
   b. Listen for complaints of headache, difficulty with vision.
   c. Check for evidence of nausea or vomiting.
   d. Be alert for signs of seizure activity. Provide a safe environment—padded side rails. Keep bed in lowest position.
6. Reduce activity and provide quiet environment.
7. Monitor ECG continuously.
8. Maintain constant vigilance until blood pressure is decreased and stable; then begin hypertension teaching program.

Lymphatic Disorders

The lymphatic system is a network of vessels and nodes that are interrelated with the circulatory system. It removes tissue fluid from intercellular spaces and protects the body from bacterial invasion. Lymph nodes are located along the course of the lymphatic vessels and filter lymph before it is returned to the bloodstream.

◆ LYMPHEDEMA AND LYMPHANGITIS

Lymphedema is a swelling of the tissues (particularly in the dependent position), produced by an obstruction to the lymph flow in an extremity.

Lymphangitis is an acute inflammation of lymphatic channels, which most commonly arises from a focus of infection in an extremity.

Pathophysiology/Etiology

A. *Lymphedema*
1. Classified as primary (congenital malformations) or secondary (acquired obstruction)
2. Swelling in the extremities occurs due to an increased quantity of lymph fluid that results from an obstruction of lymphatics.
3. Obstruction may be in both the lymph nodes and lymphatic vessels.
4. It may be associated with radical mastectomy, varicose veins, chronic phlebitis, and elephantiasis.

B. *Lymphangitis*
1. Arises most commonly from infection in an extremity
2. The characteristic red streak extending up an arm or leg from the infected wound outlines the course of the lymphatics as they drain.
3. Recurrent lymphangitis is often associated with lymphedema.

Clinical Manifestations

1. Edema may be massive and is often firm in lymphedema.
2. Lymphangitis
   a. Displays characteristic red streaks that extend up an arm or leg from an infection that is not localized and that can lead to septicemia
   b. Produces general symptoms—high fever, chills
   c. Produces local symptoms—local pain, tenderness, swelling along involved lymphatics
   d. Produces local lymph node symptoms—enlarged, red, tender (acute lymphadenitis)
   e. Produces an abscess—necrotic, pus-producing (suppurative lymphadenitis)

Diagnostic Evaluation

1. Lymphangiography—outlines lymphatic system
2. Lymphoscintigraphy—reliable alternative to lymphangiography using radioactive colloid material—detects obstruction or inflammation

Management

A. *Lymphedema*
1. Strict bed rest with leg elevation
2. Active and passive exercises
3. External compression devices
4. Elastic stockings (when ambulatory)
5. Diuretics (controversial)
6. Surgery
   a. Excision of affected subcutaneous tissue and fascia with skin grafting
   b. Transfer of superficial lymphatics to deep lymphatic system by buried dermal flap
   c. Complications include flap necrosis, hematoma, abscess under flap, cellulitis.
   d. See pages 72–98 for surgical care.

B. *Lymphangitis*
1. Administer antibiotic agents because causative organisms usually are streptococci and staphylococci.
2. Treat affected part by rest, elevation, and the application of hot, moist dressings.
3. Incise and drain if necrosis and abscess formation occur.

Complications

1. Abscess formation (rare with lymphangitis)
2. Firm, nonpitting lymphedema unresponsive to treatment (congenital lymphedema called lymphedema praecox)
3. Elephantiasis secondary to parasite (*Filaria*)—chronic fibrosis of subcutaneous tissue and chronic swelling of the extremity
4. Septicemia

Nursing Assessment

1. Assess extremity for edema and inflammation.
   a. Palpate edema to evaluate its quality (soft and pitting, or firm and nonpitting).
   b. Note any areas of abscess formation (suppurative lymphadenitis).
2. Watch for signs of fever and chills.

Nursing Diagnoses

A. Risk for Impaired Skin Integrity related to edema and/or inflammation
B. Pain related to incising and/or surgery

Nursing Interventions

A. *Maintaining Skin Integrity*
1. Apply elastic bandages or stockings (after acute attack with lymphangitis).
2. Advise the patient to rest frequently with affected part elevated each joint higher than the preceding one.
3. Administer diuretics as prescribed to control excess fluid.
4. Give antibiotics as prescribed.
5. Recommend isometric exercises with extremity elevated.
6. Suggest moderate sodium restriction in diet.
7. Observe postoperatively for signs of infection.

B. *Relieving Pain Postoperatively*
1. Encourage comfortable position and immobilization of affected area.
2. Administer or teach patient to administer analgesics as prescribed; monitor for side effects.
3. Use bed cradle to relieve pressure from bed covers.

Patient Education/Health Maintenance

1. Encourage use of elastic bandage or stocking. May need for several months to prevent long-term edema.
2. Advise patient to avoid trauma to extremity.
3. Advise patient to practice good hygiene to avoid superimposed infections.

Evaluation

A. Skin is normal color and temperature, nontender, nonswollen and intact.
B. Patient verbalizes no pain on actively moving extremity.

Selected References

Bright, L. & Georgi, S. (1992). Peripheral vascular disease: is it arterial or venous? *Am J Nurs 95* (9), 34-43

Byers, J. F. & Goshorn, J. (1995). How to manage diuretic therapy. *Am J Nurs 95*(2), 38-43.

Deglin, J. H. & Deglin, S. (1992). Hypertension: current trends and choices in pharmacotherapeutics. *AACN Clinical Issues in Critical Care Nursing (92)*3, 507.

Fahey, V. (1994). *Vascular Nursing.* 2nd ed. Philadelphia: WB Saunders.

Fellows, E. (1995). Abdominal aortic aneurysm; warning flags to watch for. *AJN 95* (5), 26–32.

Fletcher, A. E. & Bulpitt, C. J. (1992). How far should blood pressure be lowered? *N Engl J Med 326*(4), 251.

Hickey, A. (1994). Catching deep vein thrombosis in time. *Nursing '94 24* (10), 34–41.

Hurst, J. W., ed. (1990). *The Heart.* 7th ed. New York: McGraw-Hill.

Johannsen, J. (1993). Update: guidelines for treating hypertension. *Am J Nurs (93)*3, 42-49.

Joint National Committee on Detection, Evaluation and Treatment of High Blood Pressure. *1992 Report.* Bethesda, MD: National Heart, Lung and Blood Institute. US Dept of Health and Human Services, NIH publication.

Long, B. & Phipps, W. (1993). *Medical-Surgical Nursing.* St. Louis: CV Mosby.

Loscalzo, J., Creager, M., et al., eds. (1992). *Vascular Medicine.* Boston: Little, Brown.

Soloman, J. (1994). Hypertension: the new drug therapies. *RN 57*(1), 26-33

Thelan, L. A. & Davie, J. (1994). *Critical Care Nursing.* St. Louis: CV Mosby.

Underhill, S. (1989). *Cardiac Nursing.* 2nd ed. Philadelphia: JB Lippincott.

Young, J., Graor, R., Olin, J., et al. (1991). *Peripheral Vascular Diseases.* St. Louis: Mosby-Year Book.

CHAPTER 13 ◆

Neurologic Disorders

Assessment

Common manifestations of neurologic dysfunction include motor, sensory, autonomic, and cognitive deficits. By exploring these symptoms, obtaining pertinent history, and performing a thorough neurologic exam, you will better understand the underlying neurologic disorder and be able to plan care. See Chapter 3, p. 48 for neurologic exam techniques.

Diagnostic Tests

◆ RADIOLOGY/IMAGING

A variety of radiologic and imaging studies can be performed to evaluate structure and function of the brain, spinal cord, and other parts of the nervous system. Whereas the computed tomography (CT) and magnetic resonance imaging (MRI) scans are widely used for many neurologic disorders, many new tests and new applications of older tests are being developed.

Positron Emission Tomography (PET) Scan

A. Description
A PET scan is a computer-based imaging technique that permits study of the brain's metabolism and function; displays pictures of metabolic and biochemical activity within the brain, such as thinking, speaking, and hearing. Can be combined with cerebral angiography.

B. Nursing/Patient Care Considerations
1. Explain that this procedure requires inhalation of a radioactive gas or injection with a radioactive substance that emits positively charged particles.
2. Reassure the patient that radiation exposure is minimal, and electrical shocks will not be felt from the "charged" particles.
3. Tell the patient the image is created when the negative particles found in the body combine with the positive particles of the imaging substance.

Single Photon Emission Computed Tomography (SPECT)

A. Description
SPECT is a three-dimensional imaging technique using nuclear medicine procedures that employ radionuclides and instruments that emit and detect single photons; useful in localizing and sizing stroke and identifying seizure foci.

B. Nursing/Patient Care Considerations
Tell patient that a contrast medium will be injected; reassure patient that radiation exposure is minimal.

Cerebral Angiography

A. Description
1. An x-ray study of the cerebral circulation after injection of contrast material into a selected artery. Used to determine position of arteries, intracranial lesions, abnormal vasculature, or to add specificity to the CT scan.
2. A variation of cerebral angiography, digital subtraction angiography uses computerized techniques to subtract electronically surrounding bony and soft tissue structures to give an unobstructed picture of blood vessels.

B. *Nursing/Patient Care Considerations*
1. Omit the meal before the test, although clear liquids may be taken.
2. Mark pedal peripheral pulses.
3. Explain that a catheter will be placed in the femoral artery (the brachial artery may also be used) and threaded into the required cerebral vessel.
4. Tell the patient that incisional discomfort and sensation of warmth in the face and metallic taste should be expected; sedation may be used.
5. Check with the patient for allergies to contrast material, shellfish, or iodine.
6. After the angiography:
   a. Check the patient frequently for neurologic sequelae, such as motor or sensory alterations, deterioration in level of consciousness, speech disturbances, dysrhythmias, or blood pressure fluctuations.
   b. Check the puncture site for development of a hematoma.
   c. Evaluate peripheral pulses—change may indicate occlusion.
   d. Note color and temperature of involved extremity.

Myelography

A. *Description*
1. An x-ray of the spinal subarachnoid space after injection of an opaque medium or air through a spinal puncture; outlines the spinal arachnoid space and shows distortion of the spinal cord or dural sac by tumor, cysts, herniated intravertebral disks, or other lesions.
2. After injection, the head of the table is tilted down, and the course of the contrast material is observed.

B. *Nursing/Patient Care Considerations*
1. Omit the meal before the procedure.
2. Administer sedative before the procedure as prescribed.
3. Explain that the medium often results in a headache due to central nervous system (CNS) irritation by the chemical.
   a. If the patient has received Metazamide (a water-based contrast medium), elevate the head of the bed 15 to 30 degrees to reduce the upward dispersion of the medium.
   b. If Pantopaque (an oil-based contrast medium) is used, instruct the patient to lie in a recumbent position for 12 to 24 hours to reduce cerebrospinal fluid (CSF) leakage and decrease headache.
4. Encourage the patient to drink liberal quantities of fluid for rehydration and replacement of CSF.
5. Assess neurologic and vital signs; note motor and sensory deviations from baseline.
6. Check patient's ability to void.
7. Watch for fever, photophobia, stiff neck, or other signs of chemical or bacterial meningitis.

Brain Scan

A. *Description*
Intravenous (IV) injection of a radiopharmaceutical substance traced by the scanner that prints out a picture. Radioactive uptake is increased at the site of cellular membrane disruption/pathology.

B. *Nursing/Patient Care Considerations*
Explain to the patient that no discomfort will be felt during this procedure.

Magnetic Source Imaging (MSI)

A. *Description*
1. Currently the only technology that provides locational information about brain function without injection of isotopes, attachment of electrodes, or other types of invasive procedures. Uses biomagnetic field produced by electrical currents of active neurons to determine brain function.
2. Data recorded by a biomagnetometer.

B. *Nursing/Patient Care Considerations*
1. Remove all metal from patient; report any metal implants.
2. Change patient into clothing without metal clasps, etc.
3. Explain that dental work may need to be demagnetized.
4. Tell the patient washable markings will be penned on his or her head for reference points.

Cerebral Blood Flow Studies

A. *Description*
Injection or inhalation of a radioisotope or nitrous oxide, which is absorbed by the brain. The information is read by 16 to 32 probes placed on the head and analyzed by a computer. Provides regional or overall data regarding cerebral blood flow. Normal blood flow is 50 to 55 mL flow/100 g of cerebral tissue/minute.

B. *Nursing/Patient Care Considerations*
Reassure the patient that this is a relatively noninvasive procedure and requires cooperation only during the inhalation or injection process.

Intracarotid Amytal Procedure (WADA Test)

A. *Description*
1. A technique used to assess language dominance and memory function before ablative surgery for epilepsy.
2. The patient undergoes a cerebral angiography to visualize the cerebral vasculature, and a catheter is placed into the internal carotid artery. Once the catheter is positioned, a short-acting barbiturate is injected (sodium amobarbital [Amytal]) to anesthetize the cerebral hemisphere to mimic the proposed surgery.
3. Electroencephalogram (EEG) and clinical symptoms are used to determine effectiveness. The patient is then tested for language and memory. Drug effects wear off in 2 to 12 minutes.

B. *Nursing/Patient Care Considerations*
1. Perform preoperative teaching as for a cerebral angiography.
2. Instruct the patient to be NPO after 8 p.m. the night before the test.
3. Reassure the patient that any speech alterations will be temporary.

◆ OTHER DIAGNOSTIC TESTS

Other diagnostic tests include lumbar puncture, which accesses information about the CNS through direct contact with the CSF; a variety of tests that measure electrical impulses in portions of the nervous system; and neuropsychologic evaluation.

Lumbar Puncture

A. Description
1. A needle is inserted into lumbar subarachnoid space and CSF is withdrawn for diagnostic and therapeutic purposes.
2. Purposes
   a. To obtain CSF for examination (microbiologic, serologic, cytologic, or chemical analysis).
   b. To measure and relieve cerebrospinal pressure.
   c. To determine the presence or absence of blood in the spinal fluid.
   d. To detect spinal subarachnoid block.
   e. To administer antibiotics and cancer chemotherapy intrathecally in certain cases.

B. Nursing/Patient Care Considerations
See Procedure Guidelines 13-1.

Electroencephalography (EEG)

A. Description
1. A recording of electrical activity that is generated in the brain by means of electrodes applied on the scalp surface (or microelectrodes placed on or within the brain tissue). Provides physiologic assessment of cerebral activity for diagnosis of epilepsy, coma, organic brain syndrome, sleep disorders, and brain death.
2. For a baseline study, the patient lies quietly with eyes closed. For activation procedures, done to elicit abnormal electrical discharges, the patient is asked to hyperventilate for 3 to 4 minutes and then look into a bright flashing light for photic stimulation.
3. Special pharyngeal electrodes (inserted through the nose) and sphenoidal electrodes (inserted transcutaneously) or invasive recording with electrodes placed internally through burr holes or stereotactically may be done to clarify epileptogenic foci.

B. Nursing/Patient Care Considerations
1. For routine EEG, tranquilizers and stimulants should be held for 24 to 48 hours before the study.
2. Meals should be taken as usual to avoid changes secondary to low blood glucose levels.
3. Reassure the patient that electrical shocks will not be experienced.

Magnetoencephalogram (MEG)

A. Description
A magnetoencephalogram uses a magnetometer to measure the location, depth, orientation, and polarity of spike field strength. Used in determination of epileptogenic focus.

B. Nursing/Patient Care Considerations
1. Remove all metal.

2. Demagnetize dental work.
3. Reassure the patient that nothing will be felt.

Evoked Potentials

A. Description
1. These electrophysiologic studies involve changes and response in brain activity recorded from scalp electrodes that are elicited by the introduction of external visual, auditory, or somatosensory stimuli.
   a. For visually evoked responses, the patient looks at visual stimuli, such as lights or patterns; EEG electrodes are placed over the occiput and record the transmission time from the retina to the occiput.
   b. Auditory-evoked responses use sound, such as clicks, and the transmission time up the brain stem into the cortex is measured.
   c. Somatosensory-evoked response uses stimuli applied to peripheral nerves; transmission time up the spinal cord to the sensory cortex is measured.

B. Nursing/Patient Care Considerations
Explain that the procedure will not be painful, nor will the patient experience any feelings of electric shock.

Electromyography (EMG)

A. Description
Electromyography is a technique involving metal electrodes and an amplifier and oscilloscope to study electrical activity arising from muscles at rest and muscles that are contracted. Useful in determination of neuromuscular disease.

B. Nursing/Patient Care Considerations
Explain that some degree of discomfort from the needles may be experienced.

Nerve Conduction Tests (NCTs)

A. Description
Tests are performed by stimulating a peripheral nerve at several points along its course and recording the muscle action potential or the sensory action potential that results.

B. Nursing/Patient Care Considerations
Tell the patient some discomfort may be experienced by the external stimulation and uncontrolled muscle activity.

Neuropsychologic Evaluation

A. Description
This is a series of tests that evaluate the different cognitive behavioral functions of the brain. This evaluation can assist identification of the area of damage to the brain and provide a baseline of cognitive functions to which the efficacy of interventions (medical and surgical) can be evaluated.

B. Nursing/Patient Care Considerations
1. Reassure the patient that this is not a test to see if he or she is "crazy." Explain that it evaluates the ability to remember, calculate numbers, and perform abstract reasoning. A full examination is a 4- to 6-hour process depending on the patient's ability to concentrate.
2. Anticipate fatigue and frustration after the examination.

Stereotaxis

A. *Description*

Stereotactic surgery involves use of three-dimensional co-ordinates derived from the relationship of special frames to the target area. Allows for precise targeting of deep brain lesions for biopsy or surgery. Minimizes tissue trauma to surrounding cerebral areas. Can also be used for aspiration of intracranial hematomas, abscesses, and cystic lesion.

B. *Nursing/Patient Care Considerations*
1. Explain to the patient that although the stereotactic surgery penetrates the skull, it does not penetrate the brain.
2. Tell the patient that a CT scan will help pinpoint the exact surgical site and that the position of the electrode or microinstrument will be checked by x-ray or CT scan before the procedure begins.
3. Keep patient NPO before the procedure.
4. Administer analgesics for headaches as ordered.

Polysomnography (PSG)

A. *Description*

A noninvasive all-night sleep study that measures character of sleep, simultaneously monitoring EEG, cardiac and respiratory function, and movements during sleep.

B. *Nursing/Patient Care Considerations*
1. Explain that the electrodes placed on the scalp, chest, extremities, and face will be uncomfortable but do not deliver electrical current.
2. Reassure the patient that the technician will be in the next room.
3. Tell the patient to wear comfortable nightwear.

Multisleep Latency Test (MSLT)

A. *Description*

This is a sleep study performed during the day. It consists of four "napping" periods of 20 to 35 minutes, during which time the patient lies down on a bed in a darkened room and is allowed to fall asleep.

B. *Nursing/Patient Care Considerations*
1. Explain the time and duration of the naps.
2. Reassure the patient that he or she will be free to move about between naps.
3. Tell the patient to wear comfortable clothing and to bring reading or other materials for use between naps.

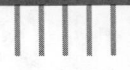

PROCEDURE GUIDELINES 13-1 ◆ Assisting the Patient Undergoing a Lumbar Puncture

EQUIPMENT	Sterile lumbar puncture set	Skin antiseptic
	Sterile gloves	Band-Aid
	Xylocaine 1%–2%	

PROCEDURE	NURSING ACTION	RATIONALE
	PREPARATORY PHASE	
	1. Before procedure, the patient should empty bladder and bowel.	1. To enhance comfort.
	2. Give a step-by-step summary of the procedure. *For Lying Position:* see accompanying figure.	2. Reassures the patient and gains cooperation.

(continued)

PROCEDURE GUIDELINES 13-1 ◆ Assisting the Patient Undergoing a Lumbar Puncture *(continued)*

PROCEDURE
(cont'd)

NURSING ACTION

RATIONALE

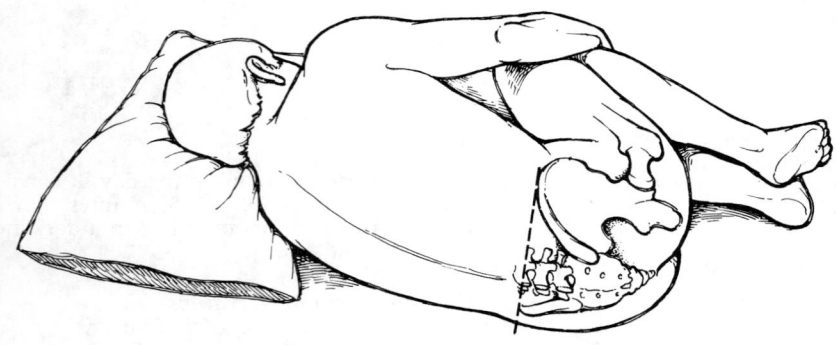

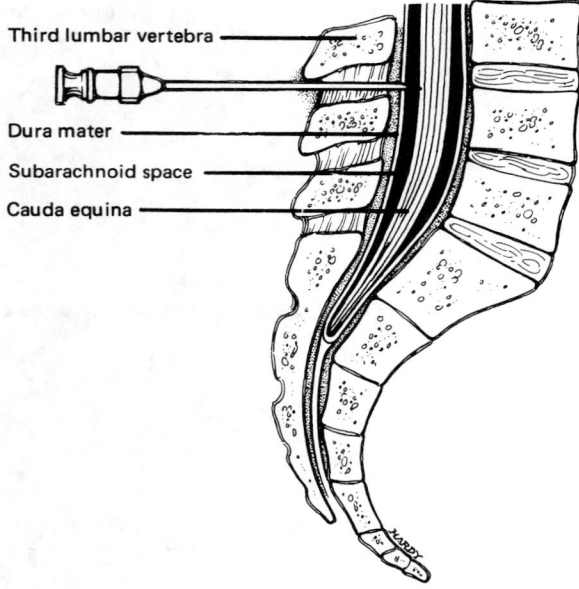

Third lumbar vertebra

Dura mater

Subarachnoid space

Cauda equina

Technique of lumbar puncture.

3. Position the patient on side with a small pillow under head and a pillow between legs. Patient should be lying on a firm surface.
4. Instruct the patient to arch the lumbar segment of back and draw knees up to abdomen, chin to chest, clasping knees with hands.
5. Assist the patient in maintaining this position by supporting behind the knees and neck. Assist the patient to maintain the posture throughout the examination.
For Sitting Position:
6. Have the patient straddle a straight-back chair (facing the back) and rest head against arms, which are folded on the back of the chair.

3. The spine is maintained in a horizontal position. The pillow between the legs prevents the upper leg from rolling forward.
4. This posture offers maximal widening of the interspinous spaces and affords easier entry into the subarachnoid space.
5. Supporting the patient helps prevent sudden movements, which can produce a traumatic (bloody) tap and thus impede correct diagnosis.

6. In obese patients and those who have difficulty in assuming an arched side-lying position, this posture may allow more accurate identification of the spinous processes and interspaces.

PROCEDURE (cont'd)	NURSING ACTION	RATIONALE

PERFORMANCE PHASE (BY THE PHYSICIAN)

1. The skin is prepared with antiseptic solution, and the skin and subcutaneous spaces are infiltrated with local anesthetic agent.
2. A spinal puncture needle is introduced at the L3–L4 interspace. The needle is advanced until the "give" of the ligamentum flavum is felt and the needle enters the subarachnoid space. The manometer is attached to the spinal puncture needle.
3. After the needle enters the subarachnoid space, help the patient to slowly straighten legs.
4. Instruct the patient to breathe quietly (not to hold breath or strain) and not to talk.
5. The initial pressure reading is obtained by measuring the level of the fluid column after it comes to rest.
6. About 2–3 ml of spinal fluid is placed in each of three test tubes for observation, comparison, and laboratory analysis.

1. To reduce risk of contamination and decrease pain.
2. L3–L4 interspace is *below* the level of the spinal cord.
3. This maneuver prevents a false increase in intraspinal pressure. Muscle tension and compression of the abdomen give falsely high pressures.
4. Hyperventilation may lower a truly elevated pressure. Talking can elevate CSF pressure.
5. With respiration there is normally some fluctuation of spinal fluid in the manometer. Normal range of spinal fluid pressure with the patient in the lateral recumbent position is 70–200 mm H_2O.
6. Spinal fluid should be clear and colorless. Bloody spinal fluid may indicate cerebral contusion, laceration, subarachnoid hemorrhage, or a traumatic tap.

LUMBAR MANOMETRIC TEST (QUECKENSTEDT TEST)

1. A blood pressure cuff is placed around the patient's neck and inflated to a pressure of 20 mm. Hg (or an assistant compresses jugular vein or veins for 10 seconds).

This test is made when a spinal subarachnoid block is suspected (tumor; vertebral fracture or dislocation). In normal persons there is a rapid rise in pressure of CSF in response to jugular compression with rapid return to normal when the compression is released. If the pressure fails to rise or rises and falls slowly, there is evidence of a block due to a lesion's compressing the spinal subarachnoid pathways. This test is not done if an intracranial lesion is suspected.

2. Pressure readings are made at 10-second intervals.
3. After the needle is withdrawn, a Band-Aid is applied to the puncture site.

FOLLOW-UP PHASE

1. After the procedure, the patient is asked to remain prone (on abdomen) for about 3 hours.

1. This allows the tissue surfaces along the needle track to come together to prevent cerebrospinal fluid leakage.

General Procedures/ Treatment Modalities

◆ NURSING MANAGEMENT OF THE PATIENT WITH AN ALTERED STATE OF CONSCIOUSNESS

Unconsciousness is a condition in which there is a depression of cerebral function ranging from stupor to coma. Coma may be defined as no eye opening on stimulation, absence of comprehensible speech, and failure to obey commands. Altered state of consciousness may be caused by hypoxemia and a variety of neurologic and metabolic disorders. Diagnostic evaluation and management depend on the suspected or confirmed underlying cause.

Nursing Assessment

1. Assess the patient's level of responsiveness (arousal and awareness).
   a. Responds to command or stimulation (press pen against side of patient's nail bed for stimulation)
   b. Eye opening
   c. Verbal responses
   d. Motor responses
2. Assess motor function for strength and symmetry.
3. Record the patient's exact reactions. Use Glasgow coma scale for documentation (Table 13-1).
4. Test brain stem reflexes to assess for brain stem dysfunction.
   a. Pupil size, symmetry, and reaction to light.
   b. Reflex eye movements elicited to head turning (oculocephalic response) or testing of oculovestibular response (calorics) by medical staff.
5. Check respiratory rate and pattern (normal, Kussmaul's, Cheyne-Stokes, apneic).
6. Check swallowing reflexes and deep tendon reflexes.

TABLE 13-1 The Glasgow Coma Scale (GCS)

Parameter	Finding	Score
Eye opening	Spontaneously	4
	To speech	3
	To pain	2
	Do not open	1
Best verbal response	Oriented	5
	Confused	4
	Inappropriate speech	3
	Unintelligible speech	2
	No verbalization	1
Best motor response	Obeys command	6
	Localizes pain	5
	Withdraws from pain	4
	Abnormal flexion	3
	Abnormal extension	2
	No motor response	1

Interpretation: best score = 15; worst score = 3; 7 or less generally indicates coma; changes from baseline are most important.

7. Examine head for signs of trauma, and mouth, nose, and ears for evidence of blood and CSF.
8. Monitor any change in neurologic status over time.

Nursing Diagnoses

A. Ineffective Airway Clearance related to upper airway obstruction by tongue and soft tissues; inability to clear respiratory secretions
B. Risk for Fluid Volume Deficit related to inability to ingest fluids, dehydration from osmotic therapy (when used to reduce intracranial pressure)
C. Altered Oral Mucous Membranes related to mouth breathing, absence of pharyngeal reflex, inability to ingest fluid
D. Risk for Impaired Skin Integrity related to immobility or restlessness
E. Impaired Tissue Integrity of Cornea related to diminished/absent corneal reflex
F. Hypothermia related to damage to hypothalamic center
G. Altered Urinary Elimination (Incontinence or Retention) related to unconscious state
H. Bowel Incontinence related to unconscious state

Nursing Interventions

A. *Maintaining an Effective Airway*
1. Place the patient in a three-fourths prone or semiprone or lateral position—prevents the tongue from obstructing the airway, encourages drainage of respiratory secretions, and promotes oxygen and carbon dioxide exchange.
2. Keep the airway free of secretions with efficient suctioning—in the absence of the cough and swallowing reflexes, secretions rapidly accumulate in the posterior pharynx and upper trachea and can lead to fatal respiratory complications.

a. Insert oral airway if tongue is paralyzed or is obstructing the airway—an obstructed airway increases intracranial pressure. This is considered a short-term measure.
b. Prepare for insertion of cuffed endotracheal tube to protect the airway from aspiration and to allow efficient removal of tracheobronchial secretions.
c. See p. 170 for technique of tracheal suctioning.
d. Use oxygen therapy as prescribed to deliver oxygenated blood to the central nervous system.

B. *Attaining and Maintaining Fluid and Electrolyte Balance*
1. Monitor prescribed IV fluids carefully, because a large volume of fluid may aggravate cerebral edema.
2. Alternatively, use hyperalimentation or nasogastric feedings.
3. Measure urinary output and specific gravity.
4. Evaluate pulses (radial, carotid, apical, and pedal); measure blood pressure—these parameters are a measure of circulatory adequacy/inadequacy.
5. Maintain circulation; support the blood pressure and treat life-threatening cardiac dysrhythmias.

C. *Maintaining Healthy Oral Mucous Membranes*
1. Remove dentures. Inspect patient's mouth for dryness, inflammation, and the presence of crusting.
2. Cleanse the mouth with prescribed solution every 2 hours—to prevent parotitis (inflammation of parotid gland).
3. Apply lip emollient to prevent angular stomatitis and cheilitis.

D. *Maintaining Skin Integrity*
1. Keep the skin clean, dry, and free of pressure—comatose patients are susceptible to the formation of pressure sores.
2. Clip the patient's nails to prevent excoriation.
3. Turn the patient from side to side on a regular schedule—relieves pressure areas and helps clear lungs by mobilizing secretions; turning also provides kinesthetic (sensation of movement), proprioceptive (awareness of position), and vestibular (equilibrium) stimulation.
4. Reposition carefully after turning to prevent ischemic necrosis over pressure areas and pressure on nerves that can lead to compression neuropathies.
5. Put all extremities through range-of-motion exercises at least four times daily; contracture deformities develop early in unconscious patients.

E. *Maintaining Corneal Integrity*
1. Protect the eyes from corneal irritation—the cornea functions as a shield. If the eyes remain open for long periods, corneal drying, irritation, and ulceration are likely to result.
a. Make sure the patient's eye is not rubbing against bedding if blinking and corneal reflexes are absent.
b. Inspect the size of the pupils and condition of eyes with a flashlight.
c. Remove contact lenses if worn.
d. Irrigate eyes with sterile prescribed solution to remove discharge and debris.
e. Instill prescribed ophthalmic ointment in each eye—prevents glazing and corneal ulceration.
f. Instill artificial tears as prescribed.
2. Prepare for temporary tarsorrhaphy (suturing of eyelids in closed position) if unconscious state is prolonged.

F. *Reducing Fever*

1. Look for possible sites of infections (respiratory, CNS, urinary tract, wound) when fever is present in an unconscious patient.
2. Control persistent elevations of temperature—increased metabolic demands will overburden brain circulation and oxygenation, resulting in cerebral deterioration.
   a. Cool room to 18.3°C. (65°F.). However, an older patient requires a warmer temperature.
   b. Remove bedding over the patient except light sheet or loincloth.
   c. Use cool-water sponging and an electric fan blowing over the patient to increase surface cooling.
   d. Consider use of hypothermia blanket if hyperthermia is of neurogenic origin. Esophageal or other core temperature is monitored continuously.

G. *Promoting Urinary Elimination*

1. Palpate over the patient's bladder at intervals to detect urinary retention and an overdistended bladder.
2. Insert an indwelling urethral catheter for short-term management.
3. Use intermittent bladder catheterization for distention as soon as possible—to minimize risk of infection.
4. Monitor for fever and cloudy urine; inspect the urethral orifice for suppurative drainage.
5. Initiate a bladder training program (p.133) as soon as consciousness is regained.

H. *Promoting Bowel Function*

1. Observe for constipation—from immobility and lack of dietary fiber.
   a. Stool softener may be prescribed and given with tube feeding.
   b. Glycerin suppository may be prescribed to stimulate bowel emptying.
2. Monitor for diarrhea—from infection, antibiotics, hyperosmolar fluids, and fecal impaction.
   a. Perform a rectal examination if fecal impaction is suspected.
   b. Use commercial fecal collection bags and meticulous skin care if patient has fecal incontinence.
3. Auscultate for bowel sounds; measure the girth of the abdomen with a tape measure to detect abdominal distention.
4. Palpate lower abdomen for distention.

Family Education and Support

1. Develop a supportive and trusting relationship with the family or significant other(s).
2. Provide information and frequent updates on patient's condition and progress.
3. Involve them in routine care and teach procedures that they can perform at home.
4. Demonstrate and teach methods of sensory stimulation to be used frequently.
   a. Use physical touch and reassuring voice tone.
   b. Talk in meaningful way even when patient does not seem to respond.
   c. Orient patient periodically to person, time, and place.
5. Encourage adequate room lighting to prevent hallucinations for the semiconscious patient.
6. Teach family to recognize and report unusual restlessness that could indicate cerebral hypoxia or metabolic imbalance.
7. Enlist help of social worker, home health agency, or other resources to assist family with such issues as financial concerns, need for medical equipment in home, and respite care.

Evaluation

A. Maintains clear airway; coughs up secretions
B. Absence of signs of dehydration
C. Intact, pink mucous membranes
D. No skin breakdown or erythema
E. Absence of trauma to cornea
F. Core temperature within normal limits
G. Catheterized at intervals for clear urine
H. Daily bowel movement stimulated with glycerin suppository

◆ NURSING MANAGEMENT OF THE PATIENT WITH INCREASING INTRACRANIAL PRESSURE

Intracranial pressure (ICP) is the pressure/volume relationship between the cranium and the contents within the cranial vault. The volume within the cranium consists of blood, brain tissue, and CSF. The pressure relationship of these elements constantly adjusts to achieve an acceptable "steady state" or equilibrium between the components of the intracranial system. Status of the ICP is reflected by the cerebral spinal fluid.

Increased ICP is defined as CSF pressure greater than 15 mm Hg. Factors that influence the ability of the body to achieve this steady state include systemic blood pressure, ventilation and oxygenation, metabolic rate and oxygen consumption (fever, shivering, activity), regional cerebral vasospasm, and oxygen saturation/hematocrit. Inability to maintain a steady state, resulting in increased ICP, can result from head injury, cerebral edema, abscess and infection, lesions, intracranial surgery, and radiation therapy. Increased ICP constitutes an emergency and requires prompt treatment.

Intracranial pressure can be monitored by means of an intraventricular catheter, a subarachnoid screw or bolt, or an epidural pressure-recording device.

Clinical Manifestations and Nursing Assessment

A. *Change in Level of Consciousness*
Caused by cerebral pressure.

1. The level of consciousness or responsiveness is the most important measure of the patient's condition.
2. Look for lethargy, delay in response to verbal suggestions, and slowing of speech.
3. Watch for sudden changes in condition—quietness to restlessness, orientation to confusion, increasing drowsiness, stupor, coma.
4. Progressive deterioration is a serious sign that may necessitate immediate surgical intervention.

B. *Changes in Vital Signs*
Caused by pressure on brain stem.

1. Rising blood pressure or widening pulse pressure (the difference between systolic and diastolic blood pressure).
2. Pulse changes—bradycardia changing to tachycardia as ICP rises.
3. Respiratory irregularities; tachypnea (early sign of increased ICP); slowing of rate with lengthening periods of apnea; Cheyne-Stokes or Kussmaul's breathing.
4. Moderately elevated temperature.

C. *Pupillary Changes*
Caused by pressure on optic and oculomotor nerves.

1. Inspect the pupils with a flashlight to evaluate size, configuration, and reaction to light. Compare both eyes for similarities, differences.
2. Evaluate gaze to determine if it is conjugate (paired, working together) or if eye movements are abnormal.
3. Evaluate ability of eyes to abduct and adduct.
4. Inspect the retina and optic nerve for hemorrhage and papilledema.

D. *Other Changes*
1. Headache—increasing in intensity; aggravated by movement/straining.
2. Vomiting—recurrent with little or no nausea; may be projectile.
3. Subtle changes—restlessness, headache, forced breathing, purposeless movements, and mental cloudiness.

Management/Nursing Interventions

NURSING ALERT:
Increased ICP is a true medical emergency and requires prompt treatment.

1. Establish and maintain airway, breathing, and circulation.
2. Administer osmotic diuretics such as mannitol (Osmitrol) or urea (Ureaphil), as ordered, to remove water and fluid from areas of brain with an intact blood–brain barrier.
   a. Insert an indwelling urinary catheter for management of diuresis.
3. Administer steroids such as dexamethasone (Decadron), as ordered, to reduce edema surrounding brain tumor, if present.
4. Assist with hyperventilation with a volume ventilator to cause respiratory alkalosis, which causes cerebral vasoconstriction and decreases cerebral blood volume and results in reduced ICP.
5. Monitor effects of neuromuscular paralyzing agents, such as pancurmonium (Pavulon), which may be given along with mechanical ventilation to prevent sudden changes in ICP due to coughing, straining, or fighting the ventilator.
6. Treat fever as requested, because fever increases cerebral blood flow and cerebral blood volume; acute increases in ICP occur with fever spikes.

7. Administer high-dose barbiturates and other anesthetic agents, as ordered, to induce comatose state and suppress brain metabolism, which in turn reduces cerebral blood flow and ICP.
   a. Be alert to the high level of nursing support required.
   b. Monitor ICP, EEG, arterial pressure, and serum barbiturate levels as indicated.
8. Avoid positions or activities that may increase ICP, including turning the patient's head, prone position, flexion of the neck.
   a. Minimize suctioning or other stimuli that precipitously increase ICP.
   b. Keep head of bed elevated 30 degrees to reduce jugular venous pressure and decrease ICP.
9. Use ICP monitoring when ordered for sustained increased ICP (above 20 mm Hg persisting 15 minutes or more or if there is a significant shift in pressure).

Continuous Intracranial Pressure Monitoring

See Procedure Guidelines 13-2.

A. *Monitoring Systems*
1. Intraventricular catheter—inserted into lateral ventricle using a drill or burr hole opening; connected to fluid-filled transducer, which converts mechanical pressure to electrical impulses and waveform; allows for ventricular drainage.
2. Subarachnoid screw (bolt)—hollow screw inserted into subarachnoid space beneath skull and dura through drill hole; also connected to pressure transducer system.
3. Epidural sensor—inserted beneath skull but not through dura, so does not measure pressure directly; fiberoptic cable is connected directly to monitor.

B. *Waveforms*
1. Intracranial pressure fluctuates, creating three distinct waveforms.
2. Plateau or A waves are characterized by rapid increases and decreases of pressure with recurring elevations of 15 to 50 mm Hg or higher and may last 2 to 15 minutes.
   a. A waves are clinically significant.
   b. May be accompanied by transient symptoms of headache, nausea, decreased consciousness.
3. B waves are of shorter duration and smaller amplitude than A waves and are not clinically significant unless they occur frequently; then they may precede A waves.
4. C waves are small, rhythmic oscillations that are not clinically significant but fluctuate with changes in blood pressure.

C. *Nursing Interventions*
1. Note the pattern of waveforms and any sustained elevation of pressure above 15 mm Hg.
2. Note what stimuli cause increased pressure, such as bathing, suctioning, repositioning.
3. Watch for developing or increasing frequency of plateau waves. Report these and begin measures to lower increased ICP as described above.

PROCEDURE GUIDELINES 13-2 ◆ Intracranial Pressure Monitoring (ICP)

EQUIPMENT

Sterile gloves
Airway
Ambu Bag
ICP Monitoring system (intraventricular, subarachnoid, epidural)

IV pole or standard on which to mount the system
IV solutions as ordered
IV high pressure tubing
Burr hole tray for insertion or as needed
Topical anesthetic

PROCEDURE

NURSING ACTION	RATIONALE
PREPARATORY PHASE	
1. Explain the need for extensive, continuous assessment and appropriate nursing intervention to the family and patient.	1. Explanations will decrease anxiety, allow patient and family a sense of control, and encourage compliance with procedure.
2. Gather and assemble equipment. Flush lines with ordered solution according to manufacturer's directions.	2. Availability of equipment will enhance success of procedure.
3. Calibrate equipment according to directions.	3. Accurate interpretation of ICP values and wave patterns will depend on appropriate baseline function.
4. Perform neurologic assessment.	4. Patient baseline must be established to determine changes and guide therapy.
5. Administer light sedation/analgesia if patient is agitated.	5. Procedure is invasive and injury may result with excessive patient movement.
PERFORMANCE PHASE	
1. Establish head of bed at 30 degrees.	1. Facilitates venous drainage decreasing intracranial volume and prevents collapse of the ventricles if ventricular placement.
2. Shave and cleanse the operative site.	2. Removes bacteria from the site, reducing the risk of infection.
3. Establish the sterile field.	3. A sterile field reduces the risk of infection.
4. Assist with burr hole and placement of intracranial monitoring system.	4. Direct monitoring of intracranial pressure allows for early detection of decompensation and management of complications.
5. Connect monitoring catheter to transducer/monitoring equipment according to directions.	5. Allows for conduction of intracranial and cerebral perfusion pressures to the interpretive component of the system.
6. Observe numerical readings and wave patterns. Adjust characteristics to obtain optimal visual reading.	6. Changes in baseline readings indicate alterations in intracranial pressure or problems with the mechanics of the monitoring system.

(continued)

PROCEDURE GUIDELINES 13-2 ◆ Intracranial Pressure Monitoring (ICP)
(continued)

PROCEDURE (cont'd)	NURSING ACTION	RATIONALE

A. Normal ICP waveform

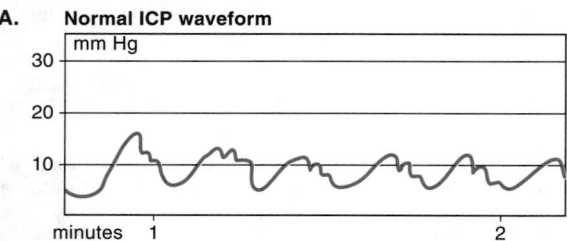

B. A waves (plateau waves)

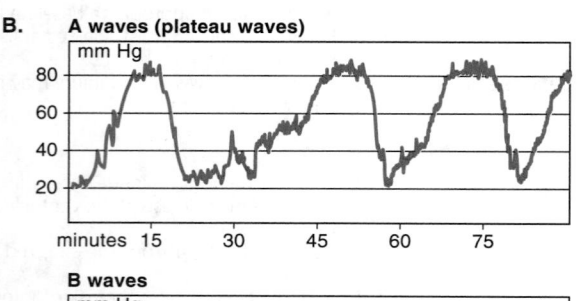

B waves

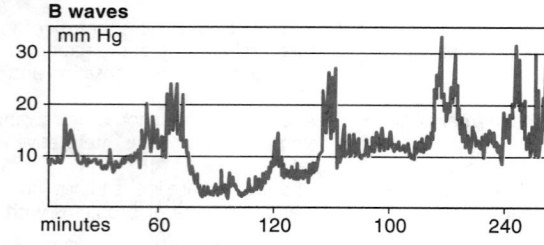

C waves

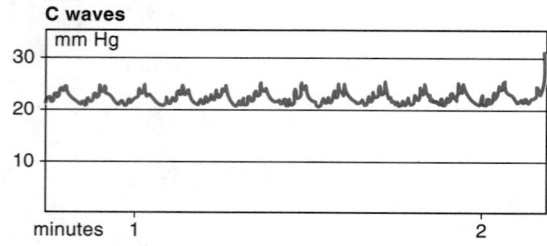

A. Normal waveform. B. A waves (plateau waves), B waves, and C waves.

7. Cover the catheter insertion site with a sterile dressing. Observe for possible CSF drainage depending on the placement of the catheter.
8. Adjust alarm system according to ordered parameters.

7. The skull and meninges have been penetrated leaving the patient at risk for infection.
8. Alarms should be on at all times to alert the nurse away from the bedside of ongoing adverse changes.

FOLLOW-UP PHASE

1. Frequently assess the patient and the system to ascertain neurologic status and patency of the system.
2. Irrigate the system using sterile technique according to policy or p.r.n. as indicated to maintain patency.

1. Manipulation of the system may inadvertently close the system, leaving the patient without benefit of monitoring.
2. Irrigation helps maintain the patency of the system.

PROCEDURE (cont'd)	NURSING ACTION	RATIONALE
	3. Report dampened wave forms, and have 1 cc of normal saline available for irrigation if indicated.	3. The tip of the catheter may have migrated against the ventricular wall or cerebral tissue depending on location, or ventricular collapse may be imminent. Irrigation is done by the healthcare provider in this case.
	4. Assess head dressing for CSF drainage. Change dressing according to policy.	4. Because of its high glucose content, CSF is an excellent media for bacterial growth.
	5. Adjust the height of the transducer of the system to the level of the patient's ventricles (inner canthus of eye and tip of ear) with every position change for accurate readings.	5. Position of the transducer in relation to the ventricles will influence the accuracy of the readings because of fluid gradient pressures.

◆ NURSING MANAGEMENT OF THE PATIENT UNDERGOING INTRACRANIAL SURGERY

Craniotomy is the surgical opening of the skull to gain access to intracranial structures to remove a tumor, relieve IICP, evacuate a blood clot, stop hemorrhage, or remove epileptogenic tissue (Fig.13-1). Surgical approach may be supratentorial (above the tentorium or dural covering that divides the cerebrum from cerebellum) or infratentorial (below the tentorium, including the brain stem). Craniotomy may be performed by means of burr holes (made with a drill or hand tools) or by making a bony flap.

Craniectomy is excision of a portion of the skull. Cranioplasty is repair of a cranial defect by means of a plastic or metal plate. Transphenoidal surgery is an approach that gains access to the pituitary gland through the nasal cavity and sphenoidal sinus (discussed in Chapter 22, Endocrine Disorders, p. 703).

Preoperative Management/ Nursing Care

1. Reinforce surgeon's explanation of diagnostic findings, procedure, expectations.
2. Assist the patient with the presurgical shampoo with an antimicrobial agent; explain the extent of head shave.
3. Administer steroids to reduce cerebral edema.
4. Administer anticonvulsants to reduce risk of seizures.
5. Explain the use of intraoperative antibiotics to reduce risk of infection and urinary catheterization to assess urinary volume during operative period.
6. A hyperosmolar agent (mannitol [Osmitrol]) and a diuretic (furosemide [Lasix]) may be administered immediately preoperatively if needed to reduce cerebral edema.
7. Evaluate and record the patient's neurologic baseline and vital signs for postoperative comparison.
8. Explain the immediate postoperative care and where the physician will contact the family after surgery.
9. Support the patient with neurologic deficits.

Postoperative Management/ Nursing Care

1. Assess respiratory status by monitoring rate, depth, and pattern of respirations. Maintain a patent airway.
2. Monitor vital signs and neurologic status. Use Glasgow coma scale (see p. 368). Document findings.
3. Manage arterial and central venous pressure or Swan-Ganz lines for accurate manipulation of blood pressure and fluid status.
4. Administer pharmacologic agents, as prescribed, to control ICP according to procedure for increased ICP.
5. Control incisional and headache pain with codeine and acetaminophen, as prescribed.
6. Anticipate the use of postoperative anticonvulsants for patients undergoing supratentorial craniotomy. Place the patient on back or unoperative side with a pillow beneath patient's head.
7. After an infratentorial operation, keep the patient on side and off back with only a small firm pillow under patient's head.
8. Prepare for CT if patient's status deteriorates.
9. Provide oral fluids after swallow reflex and bowel sounds have returned. Weigh daily, monitoring intake and output.
10. Monitor the patient for signs of infection, checking craniotomy site, ventricular drainage, nuchal rigidity, or presence of CSF.
11. Use measures to reduce periorbital edema, such as cold compresses or moist tea bags. Apply lubricant to eyelids.

Potential Complications

1. Intracranial hemorrhage/hematoma
2. Cerebral edema
3. Infections (eg, postoperative meningitis, pulmonary, wound)
4. Seizures
5. Cranial nerve dysfunction

Nursing Diagnoses

A. Impaired Cerebral Tissue Perfusion due to increased ICP
B. Risk for Aspiration related to decreased swallow reflex and postsurgical positioning

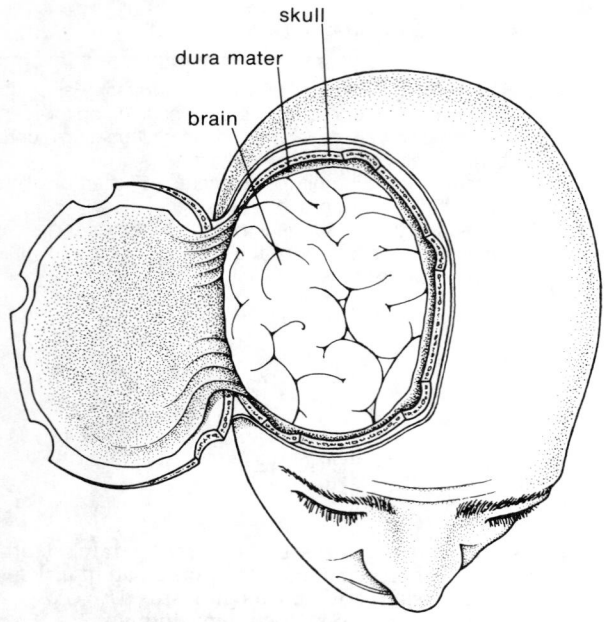

skull

dura mater

brain

FIGURE 13-1 *Craniotomy.*

C. Risk for Infection related to invasive procedure.
D. Pain related to physiologic changes produced due to invasive procedure
E. Constipation related to use of narcotic medication and immobility

Nursing Interventions

A. *Maintaining Intracranial Pressure Within Normal Range*
1. Closely monitor level of consciousness, vital signs, pupillary response, and ICP, if indicated.
2. Teach patient to avoid activities that can raise ICP, such as excessive flexion or rotation of the head and Valsalva's maneuver (coughing, straining at stool).
3. Administer corticosteroids and other medications as prescribed to reduce ICP.

B. *Preventing Aspiration*
1. Offer fluids only when patient is alert and swallow reflex has returned.
2. Have suction equipment available at bedside. Suction only if necessary and do so carefully to prevent rise in ICP.
3. Elevate head of bed to maximum of order and patient comfort.

C. *Preventing Nosocomial Infections*
1. Use sterile technique for dressing changes, catheter care, and ventricular drain management.
2. Be aware of patients at higher risk of infection—those undergoing lengthy operations, those with ventricular drains left in longer than 72 hours, and those with operations of the third ventricle.
3. Assess surgical site for redness, tenderness, and drainage.

4. Watch for leakage of CSF, which increases the danger of meningitis.
　　a. Watch for sudden discharge of fluid from wound; massive leak requires surgical repair.
　　b. Warn against coughing, sneezing, or nose blowing, which may aggravate CSF leakage.
　　c. Assess for moderate elevation of temperature and neck rigidity.
　　d. Note patency of ventricular catheter system.
5. Institute measures to prevent respiratory or urinary tract infection postoperatively (see p. 77).

D. *Relieving Pain*
1. Medicate patient according to assessment findings.
2. Elevate head of bed per procedure protocol to relieve headache.
3. Provide distractive measures for pain management.
4. Darken room if patient is photophobic.

E. *Avoiding Constipation*
1. Encourage fluids when patient able to manage liquids.
2. Ambulate patient as soon as possible.
3. Change to nonnarcotic agents for pain control as soon as possible.

Evaluation

A. Easily arousable to verbal stimulation, vital signs stable, pupils equal and reactive, no vomiting
B. Gag reflex present; breath sounds clear
C. Afebrile without signs of infection
D. Verbalization of decreased pain
E. Passed soft stool

Cranial Nerve Disorders

◆ BELL'S PALSY

An acute peripheral facial paralysis involving the seventh cranial nerve (facial) unilaterally. Also known as idiopathic facial paralysis.

Pathophysiology/Etiology

1. Etiology is unknown. Possible causes include viral infection, vascular ischemia, autoimmune disease.
2. Most patients experience an upper respiratory infection 1 to 3 weeks before onset of symptoms.
3. Recurrence in patients with history of Bell's palsy or diabetes.

Clinical Manifestations

1. Paralysis of facial muscles; can affect speech, distort face.
2. Involvement of all branches of facial nerve: facial numbness, diminished taste, numbness of tongue, decreased blink reflex, inability to close eye, painful sensations.

Diagnostic Evaluation

1. Physical examination for evaluation of seventh cranial nerve function and corneal sensation.
2. Electrophysiologic testing, specifically sensory nerve action potentials to evaluate nerve function.

Management

1. Physical therapy to maintain muscle tone.
2. Corticosteroid therapy to decrease inflammation.
3. Surgery to decompress facial nerve and correct eyelid deformities, and protection of the eye.
4. Nonsteroidal anti-inflammatory drugs to relieve pain.

Complications

1. Corneal ulceration
2. Impairment of vision

> **NURSING ALERT:**
> Keratitis (inflammation of the cornea) is a major threat to a patient with Bell's palsy. Protect the cornea if eye does not close.

Nursing Assessment

1. Test motor and sensory components of facial nerve including the face, tongue, and eye.
2. Assess patient's ability to close eye, eat, drink, and speak clearly.

Nursing Diagnosis

A. Impaired Tissue Integrity related to loss of protective eye closure
B. Pain related to physiologic alterations of disorder

Nursing Interventions

A. Protecting Corneal Integrity
1. Administer or teach patient to administer artificial tears and ophthalmic ointment as prescribed.
2. Patch eye to keep shut at night as directed.
3. Advise patient to report eye pain immediately.
4. Inspect eye for redness or discharge.

B. *Relieving Pain*
1. Administer or teach patient to administer corticosteroids to reduce inflammation and nonnarcotic analgesics to relieve pain.
2. Teach patient to apply moist heat to face and perform facial massage.

Patient Education/ Health Maintenance

1. Instruct the patient to wear wrap-around sunglasses to decrease normal evaporation from the eye from sun and wind, to avoid eye irritants, and to increase environmental humidity.
2. Instruct the patient in use of ophthalmic ointment, proper methods of lid closure, and patching of the eye.
3. Demonstrate facial exercises (eg, raise eyebrows, squeeze eyes shut, purse lips) and stress their importance to prevent muscle atrophy.

Evaluation

A. Cornea without redness, pain, or discharge
B. Patient reports adequate pain control

◆ TRIGEMINAL NEURALGIA (TIC DOULOUREUX)

A neurologic condition of the fifth cranial nerve (trigeminal) characterized by sudden paroxysm of sharp stabbing pain (Fig. 13-2).

Pathophysiology/Etiology

1. Unknown cause
2. Degenerative, compressive, or viral causes suspected

Clinical Manifestations

1. Sudden, severe episodes of pain that end abruptly, lasting less than 30 to 60 seconds.
2. Attacks precipitated by activities, such as touching the face, talking, chewing, and yawning, that place pressure on the terminal end of the branch affected.

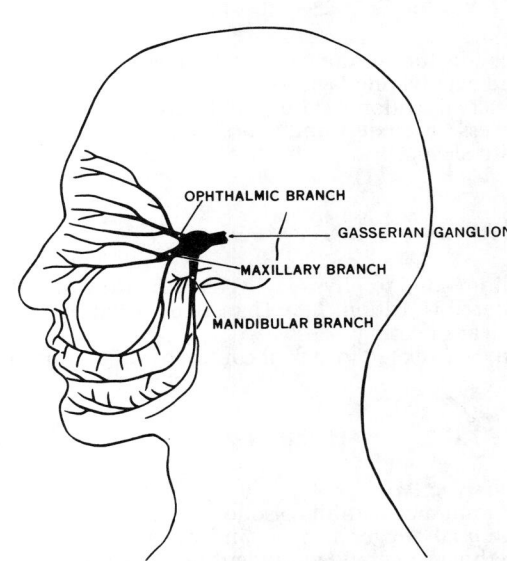

FIGURE 13-2 *The main divisions of the trigeminal nerve are ophthalmic, maxillary, and mandibular. Sensory root fibers arise in the gasserian ganglion.*

Diagnostic Evaluation

1. History of characteristic symptoms and pattern.
2. CT, MRI, skull x-rays to rule out other disorders.

Management

A. Pharmacologic
Use of carbemazepine (Tegratol), imipramine (Tofranil), phenytoin (Dilantin), baclofen (Lioresal), or divalproex (Depakote).

B. Surgical
1. Alcohol or phenol block—pain may recur several months after injection.
2. Percutaneous radiofrequency trigeminal gangliolysis—low voltage stimulation of nerve by electrode inserted through foramen ovale; sensory function destroyed but attempt to preserve motor function; may cause decreased corneal sensation, parasthesias, jaw weakness.
3. Microvascular decompression of trigeminal nerve—intracranial procedure; see page 373 for nursing care.
4. Rhizotomy (transection of nerve root at gasserian ganglion)—causes complete loss of sensation; other complications include burning, stinging, discomfort in and around eye, herpetic lesions of face, keratitis, and corneal ulceration.

Complications

1. Anorexia and weight loss
2. Dehydration

Nursing Assessment

1. Take history of the pain, including duration, severity, and aggravating factors.
2. Assess nutritional status and hydration.
3. Assess for anxiety and depression, including problems with sleep, social interaction, coping ability.

Nursing Diagnoses

A. Pain related to physiologic changes of the disorder
B. Altered Nutrition: Less Than Body Requirements due to fear of eating
C. Anxiety related to lack of control over painful episodes

Nursing Interventions

A. Relieving Pain
1. To minimize painful episodes, review with the patient potential trigger factors, and develop individualized methods of coping with identified triggers.
2. Encourage the patient to take medication regularly.
3. Help the patient maintain a method of communication without causing pain from talking.

B. Maintaining Adequate Nutrition
1. To maximize nutritional intake, instruct the patient to take foods and fluids at room temperature and to chew on the unaffected side.
2. Have the patient consult with the dietitian for appropriate meal texture and composition.
3. Encourage small, frequent meals to avoid fatigue and pain.
4. Advise nutritional supplements if indicated.

B. Reducing Anxiety
1. Support patient through treatment trials.
2. Teach relaxation exercises, such as relaxation breathing, progressive muscle relaxation, and imagery to relieve tension.

Patient Education/ Health Maintenance

1. Educate the surgical patient regarding self-care after denervation procedures.
   a. Instill eye drops every 4 hours for loss of corneal sensation.
   b. Instruct patient to chew on unaffected side to avoid biting tongue, lips, and inside of mouth.
   c. Have patient do jaw opening exercises as directed.
2. Instruct patient to maintain regular dental checkups, because pain will not be felt with caries.

Evaluation

A. Patient verbalizes reduced pain
B. Weight maintained
C. Patient verbalizes decreased anxiety

Cerebrovascular Disease

◆ CEREBROVASCULAR INSUFFICIENCY

Cerebrovascular insufficiency is an interruption or inadequate blood flow to an area of the brain resulting in transient or permanent neurologic dysfunction.

Pathophysiology/Etiology

1. Cerebrovascular insufficiency is caused by atherosclerotic plaque or thrombosis, increased Pco_2, decreased Po_2, decreased blood viscosity, hyperthermia/hypothermia, increased ICP.
2. Carotid arteries, major intracranial vessels, or microcirculation may be affected.
3. Cardiac causes of emboli include atrial fibrillation, mitral valve prolapse, infectious endocarditis, and prosthetic heart valve.
4. Event may be classified as transient ischemic attack (TIA)—transient episode of cerebral dysfunction with associated clinical manifestations lasting usually minutes to an hour, possibly up to 24 hours.

5. Symptoms persisting longer than 24 hours are classified as stroke.

Clinical Manifestations of Transient Ischemic Attacks

1. History of intermittent neurologic deficit sudden in onset, with maximal deficit within 5 minutes and lasting less than 24 hours.
2. Carotid system involvement: amaurosis fugax, homonymous hemianopia, unilateral weakness, unilateral numbness/paresthesias, aphasia, dysarthria.
3. Vertebrobasilar system involvement: vertigo, bilateral homonymous hemianopia, diplopia, weakness that is bilateral or alternates sides, dysarthria, dysphagia, ataxia, perioral numbness.
4. Carotid bruit.

Diagnostic Evaluation

1. Cerebral angiography, carotid angiography, oculoplethysmography, Doppler ultrasound—all provide information about carotid and intracranial circulation.
2. Prothrombin time if anticoagulation is considered.
3. MRI may be done to rule out stroke.
4. Transesophageal echocardiography to rule out emboli from heart.

Management

1. Platelet aggregation inhibitors, such as aspirin and ticlopidine (Ticlid), to reduce risk of stroke.
2. Surgical intervention to increase blood flow to brain—carotid endarterectomy, extracranial/intracranial anastomosis, or angioplasty.
3. Reduction of other risk factors to prevent stroke, such as control of blood pressure, diabetes, and hyperlipidemia and smoking cessation.
4. Anticoagulation for patients who continue to have symptoms despite antiplatelet therapy and those with major source of cardiac emboli.

Complications

1. Complete ischemic stroke

Nursing Assessment

1. Obtain history of possible TIA; hypertensive and diabetic control; hyperlipidemia; cardiovascular disease, such as atrial fibrillation; smoking.
2. Perform physical exam, including neurologic, cardiac, and circulatory systems; be sure to listen for carotid bruit.

Nursing Diagnoses

A. Altered Cerebral Tissue Perfusion related to underlying atherosclerosis
B. Pain related to surgical procedure

Nursing Interventions

A. *Improving Cerebral Perfusion*
1. Teach patient signs and symptoms of TIA and need to notify health care provider immediately.
2. Administer or teach self-administration of anticoagulants, antihypertensives, and other medication, monitoring for side effects and therapeutic effect.
3. Prepare patient for surgical intervention as indicated (carotid endarterectomy or extracranial–intracranial anastomosis).

B. *Relieving Pain and Providing Care Following Carotid Endarterectomy*
For postoperative extracranial–intracranial care, see Nursing Management of the Patient Undergoing Intracranial Surgery, page 373.

1. After surgery, closely monitor vital signs and administer medication as prescribed to avoid hypotension (which can cause cerebral ischemia) or hypertension (which may precipitate cerebral hemorrhage).
2. Perform frequent neurologic checks, including pupil size, equality and reaction; handgrip and plantar flexion strength; sensation; mental status; and speech. Notify the health care provider of any deficits immediately.
3. Monitor for hoarseness, impaired gag reflex, or difficulty swallowing and facial weakness, which indicate cranial nerve injury.
4. Keep head in neutral position to relieve stress on surgical site; monitor drainage.
5. Keep tracheostomy tube at bedside and assess for stridor; hematoma formation can cause airway obstruction.
6. Observe operative area closely for swelling; mild swelling is expected, but if hematoma formation is suspected, prepare patient for immediate surgery.
7. Medicate for pain and avoid agitation or sudden changes in position, which could affect blood pressure.
8. Elevate head of bed when vital signs are stable.

> **NURSING ALERT:**
> Extracranial–intracranial anastomosis is used for focal areas of ischemia. Pressure over the anastomosis of the superior temporal artery (extracranial) and the middle cerebral artery (intracranial) can result in rupture or ischemia of the site. If the patient wears glasses, remove the bow on the operative side to avoid this possible pressure point.

Patient Education/ Health Maintenance

1. Encourage patient receiving anticoagulants to comply with follow-up monitoring of prothrombin time and/or partial thromboplastin time and to report any signs of bleeding. Encourage the use of electric razors and toothbrushes.

2. Provide information on smoking cessation, low-fat/low-cholesterol diet, birth control alternatives, and exercise, and stress the need to change lifestyle to halt cerebrovascular disease and prevent stroke.

Evaluation

A. Patient is alert without neurologic deficits
B. Respirations unlabored, vital signs stable, no swelling of neck; reports relief of pain

◆ CEREBROVASCULAR ACCIDENT/STROKE

Stroke or cerebrovascular accident is the onset and persistence of neurologic dysfunction lasting longer than 24 hours and resulting from disruption of blood supply to the brain and indicates infarction rather than ischemia.

Pathophysiology/Etiology

1. Partial or complete occlusion of a cerebral blood vessel resulting from cerebral thrombosis (due to arteriosclerosis) or embolism.
2. Ischemia related to decreased blood flow to an area of the brain secondary to systemic disease, such as cardiac or metabolic disease.
3. Hemorrhage occurring outside the dura (extradural), beneath the dura mater (subdural), in the subarachnoid space (subarachnoid), or within the brain substance (intracerebral).
4. Risk factors include hypertension, TIAs, heart disease, elevated cholesterol, diabetes mellitus, obesity, carotid stenosis, polycythemia, cigarette smoking.

Clinical Manifestations

Clinical manifestations vary depending on the vessel affected and the cerebral territories it perfuses. Symptoms are usually multiple.

1. Sudden, severe headache
2. Numbness (paresthesia), weakness (paresis), or loss of motor ability (plegia) on one side of the body
3. Difficulty in swallowing (dysphagia)
4. Aphasia
5. Visual difficulties, including loss of half of a visual field, double vision.
6. Altered cognitive abilities and psychologic affect

Diagnostic Evaluation

1. Carotid ultrasound—to detect carotid stenosis.
2. CT—to determine cause and location of stroke.
3. Cerebral angiography—to determine extent of cerebrovascular insufficiency.
4. PET, MRI may be done to localize ischemic damage.

Management

A. **Acute Treatment**
1. Support of vital functions—maintain airway, breathing, oxygenation, circulation.
2. Reperfusion and hemodilution with volume expanders (dextran or pentastarch); thrombolytic therapy with tissue plasminogen activator (t-PA, Activase) or urokinase (Abbokinase); vasodilation with nimodipine (Nimotop).
3. Management of increased ICP (see p. 369).
4. Diuretic treatment to reduce cerebral edema, which peaks 3 to 5 days after infarction.
5. Calcium channel blockers to reduce blood pressure and prevent cerebral vasospasm.

B. **Subsequent Treatment**
1. Anticoagulation after hemorrhage is ruled out.
2. Antiplatelet agents such as ticlopidine (Ticlid) or aspirin.
3. Antispasmodic agents for spastic paralysis.
4. Physical therapy and rehabilitation program.
5. Treatment of poststroke depression with antidepressants.

Complications

1. Aspiration pneumonia
2. Spasticity, contractures
3. Deep-vein thrombosis; pulmonary embolism
4. Poststroke depression
5. Brain stem herniation

Nursing Assessment

1. Maintain neurologic flow sheet during acute phase.
2. Assess for voluntary or involuntary movements, tone of muscles, presence of deep tendon reflexes (reflex return signals end of flaccid period and return of muscle tone).
3. Also assess mental status, cranial nerve function, sensation/proprioception, bladder control.
4. Monitor bowel and bladder function.
5. Monitor effectiveness of anticoagulation therapy.
6. Frequently assess level of function and psychosocial response to condition.

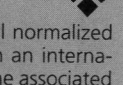

NURSING ALERT:
Prothrombin time levels are reported in international normalized ratios (INR). Anticoagulants are adjusted to maintain an international normalized ratio at 2.0 to prevent stroke and the associated complication of intracranial and subdural hemorrhage. Report international normalized ratios that are elevated to reduce the risk of bleeding or decreased levels to adjust therapy to be more effective.

Nursing Diagnoses

A. Risk for Injury related to neurologic deficits
B. Impaired Physical Mobility related to motor deficits
C. Altered Thought Processes related to brain damage

D. Impaired Verbal Communication related to brain injury

E. Self-care Deficit (bathing, dressing, toileting) related to hemiparesis/paralysis

F. Altered Nutrition: Less Than Body Requirements, related to impaired self-feeding, chewing, swallowing

G. Altered Urinary Elimination related to motor/sensory deficits

H. Altered Family Process related to catastrophic illness, cognitive and behavioral sequelae of stroke, and caregiving burden

Nursing Interventions

A. *Preventing Falls and Other Injuries*

1. Maintain bed rest during acute phase (48 to 72 hours after onset of stroke) with head of bed slightly elevated and side rails in place.

2. Administer oxygen as ordered during acute phase to maximize cerebral oxygenation.

3. Frequently assess respiratory status, vital signs, heart rate and rhythm, and urinary output to maintain and support vital functions.

4. When patient becomes more alert after acute phase, maintain frequent vigilance and interactions aimed at orienting, assessing, and meeting the needs of the patient.

5. Try to allay confusion and agitation with calm reassurance and presence.

B. *Preventing Complications of Immobility*

1. Use a foot board during flaccid period after stroke to keep foot dorsiflexed; avoid its use after spasticity develops.

2. Avoid excessive pressure on ball of foot after spasticity develops.

3. Do not allow top bedding to pull affected foot into plantar flexion.

4. Maintain functional position of all extremities.

   a. Apply splints and braces as needed—volar splint to support functional position of wrist, sling to prevent shoulder subluxation of flaccid arm, high-top sneaker for ankle and foot support. Splints support flaccid extremities and can also be used on spastic extremities to decrease stretch stimulation and reduce spasticity.

   b. Apply a trochanter roll from the crest of the ilium to the midthigh to prevent external rotation of the hip.

   c. Place a pillow in the axilla of the affected side when there is limited external rotation to keep arm away from chest and prevent adduction of the affected shoulder.

   d. Place the affected upper extremity slightly flexed on pillow supports with each joint positioned higher than the preceding one to prevent edema and resultant fibrosis; alternate elbow extension.

   e. Place the hand in slight supination with fingers slightly flexed.

   f. Place the patient in a prone position for 15 to 30 minutes daily and avoid sitting up in chair for long periods to prevent knee and hip flexion contractures.

5. Exercise the affected extremities passively through range of motion four to five times daily to maintain joint mobility and enhance circulation; encourage active range-of-motion exercise as able (see p. 128).

COMMUNITY-BASED CARE TIP:
Hemiplegic deformities resulting from stroke commonly include "frozen" shoulder; adduction and internal rotation of arm with flexion of elbow, wrist and fingers; external rotation of the hip with flexion of the knee and plantar flexion of the ankle. Instruct the patient and family in range-of-motion exercises. Reinforce that these muscle and ligament deformities resulting from stroke can be prevented with daily stretching and strengthening exercises.

6. Teach patient to use unaffected extremity to move affected one.

7. Prepare for ambulation cautiously.

   a. Check for orthostatic hypotension.

   b. Graduate the patient from a reclining position to head elevated, and dangle legs at the bedside before transferring out of bed or ambulating; assess sitting balance in bed.

   c. Assess the patient for excessive exertion.

   d. Have patient wear walking shoes.

   e. Assess standing balance and and have patient practice standing.

   f. Help patient begin walking as soon as standing balance is achieved; ensure safety with a patient waist belt.

C. *Optimizing Cognitive Abilities*

1. Be aware of patient's cognitive alterations and adjust interaction and environment accordingly.

2. Participate in cognitive retraining program—reality orientation, visual imagery, cueing procedures—as outlined by occupational or rehabilitation therapist.

3. Use pictures of family members, clock, calendar; post schedule of daily activities where patient can see.

4. Focus on patient's strengths and give positive feedback.

D. *Facilitating Communication*

1. Speak slowly, using visual cues and gestures; be consistent and repeat as necessary.

2. Give plenty of time for response, and reinforce correct responses.

3. Minimize distractions.

4. Use alternative methods of communication other than verbal.

E. *Fostering Independence*

1. Teach patient to use nonaffected side for activities of daily living (ADLs) but not to neglect affected side.

2. Adjust the environment (eg, call light, tray) to side of awareness if spatial neglect or visual field cuts are present; approach patient from uninvolved side.

3. Teach the patient to scan environment if visual deficits are present.

4. Encourage family to provide clothing that is a size larger than the patient wears, with front closures, Velcro, and stretch fabric; teach patient to dress while sitting to maintain balance.

5. Ensure that personal care items, urinal, commode, etc., are nearby and that patient obtains assistance with transfers and other activities as needed.

F. *Promoting Adequate Oral Intake*

1. Help patient relearn swallowing sequence.

   a. Have patient attempt to suck on gloved finger to strengthen oral musculature.

   b. Place ice on tongue and encourage sucking.

   c. Progress to popsicle and soft foods.

BOX 13-1 *Aphasia*

Aphasia is an acquired disorder of communication resulting from brain damage due to stroke, head injury, brain tumors, or brain cysts. It may involve impairment of the ability to speak, understand the speech of others, read, write, calculate, and understand gestures. The majority of aphasic individuals have difficulty with expression and comprehension to varying degrees. Fatigue will have adverse effect on speech.

To enhance your communication with the aphasic patient, keep the environment simple and relaxed, minimize distractions, and use multiple sensory channels. Refer the family to: American Speech-Language-Hearing Association, 10801 Rockville Pike, Rockville, MD 20852.

Aphasia Syndromes

Fluent aphasia: patient retains verbal fluency but may have difficulty in understanding speech.
a. Wernicke's aphasia; patient speaks readily but speech lacks clear content, information, and direction; jargon frequently used.
b. Anomic or amnesic aphasia: speech is almost normal, but marred by word-finding difficulty.
c. Conduction aphasia; comprehension of language is good but has difficulty repeating spoken material.

Nonfluent aphasia: speech is sparse and produced slowly and with effort and poor articulation; usually has a relative preservation of auditory comprehension.

Global aphasia; severe disruption of all aspects of communication (verbal speech, written, reading, understanding).

Specific Nursing Interventions

Speak at your normal rate and volume: the patient is not hard of hearing.
Allow plenty of time to answer.
Do not ask questions that require complex answers.
Rote phrases can be spontaneous.
Provide pad and pen if the patient prefers and is able to write.
Avoid forcing speech.
Watch the patient for clues and gestures if his or her speech is jargon; make neutral statements.
Allow plenty of time for response.
Ask for minimal word response.
Encourage patient to speak slowly.
Expect frustration and anger at inability to communicate.
Keep environment simple.
Use gestures as well as language.
Allow patient to manipulate objects for additional sensory input.

---

d. Make sure soft or pureed diet is provided, based on ability to chew.
2. Encourage small, frequent meals and allow plenty of time.
3. Remind patient to chew on unaffected side.
4. Inspect mouth for food collection or injury and encourage frequent oral hygiene.
5. Teach the family how to assist the patient with meals to facilitate chewing and swallowing.
   a. Reduce environmental distractions to improve patient concentration.
   b. Provide oral care before eating to improve aesthetics and afterward to remove food debris.
   c. Position the patient so he or she is sitting with 90 degrees of flexion at the hips and 45 degrees of flexion at the neck. Use pillows behind the back and along the weak side to achieve correct position.
   d. Maintain position for 30 to 45 minutes after the meals to prevent regurgitation and aspiration.

G. Attaining Bladder Control
1. Perform intermittent or indwelling bladder catheterization during acute stage.
2. Establish regular schedule of voiding—every 2 to 3 hours—once bladder tone returns.
3. Assist with standing or sitting to void (especially males).
4. See page 133 for bladder retraining program details.

H. Strengthening Family Coping
1. Encourage the family to maintain outside interests.

2. Teach stress management techniques, such as relaxation exercises, use of community and church support networks.
3. Encourage participation in support group for family of stroke victim and respite program or other available resources in area.
4. Involve as many family and friends in care as possible.
5. Provide information about stroke and expected outcome.

Patient Education/ Health Maintenance

1. Teach the patient and family to adapt home environment for safety and ease of use.
2. Instruct patient in need for rest periods throughout day.
3. Reassure the family that it is common for poststroke patients to experience emotional lability and depression; treatment can be given.
4. Encourage consistency in the environment without distraction.
5. Assist family to obtain self-help aids for the patient.
6. Instruct the family in management of aphasia (Box 13-1).
7. Refer the patient and family for more information and support to agencies such as: The National Stroke Association; 1420 Ogden Street; Denver, CO 80218; 303-839-1992.

Evaluation

A. No falls, vital signs stable
B. Body alignment maintained, no contractures
C. Oriented to person, place, and time
D. Communicates appropriately
E. Brushing teeth, putting on shirt and pants independently
F. Feeds self two thirds of meal
G. Voiding on commode at 2-hour intervals
H. Family seeking help and assistance from others

◆ RUPTURE OF INTRACRANIAL ANEURYSM OR ARTERIOVENOUS MALFORMATION (AVM)

An intracranial aneurysm is the saccular dilation of the wall of a cerebral artery due to congenital absence of the muscle layer of the vessel. Consistent blood flow against the weakened area results in growth of the aneurysm and thinning of the vessel wall. Rupture of the aneurysm leads to hemorrhage within the subarachnoid space, which produces symptoms of a hemorrhagic stroke.

An AVM is a tangle of abnormal arteries and veins in which the normal capillary bed is absent. Because of the back flow pressure, a fistula develops, resulting in vascular dilatation and chronic hypoperfusion. Approximately 50% of patients with AVMs present with hemorrhage.

The Hunt–Hess grading scale is used to determine prognosis and timing of surgical intervention for both aneurysm and AVM rupture. Studies show surgery is more effective if done before vasospasm occurs.

  0: Unruptured aneurysm; asymptomatic discovery
  I: Asymptomatic rupture or minimal headache or stiff neck, no fixed deficit
 II: Moderate to severe headache, nuchal rigidity, no other neurologic deficits other than cranial nerve palsy
 III: Drowsiness, confusion, or mild focal deficit
 IV: Stupor, moderate to severe hemiparesis, possible early decerebrate rigidity
 V: Deep coma, decerebrate rigidity

Etiology/Pathophysiology

1. Cause unknown or related to atherosclerosis, intracranial AVM, hypertensive vascular disease, head trauma.
2. May become symptomatic due to pressure of enlarging aneurysm on nearby cranial nerves or brain tissue.
3. Rupture and hemorrhage into subarachnoid space may cause increased ICP and ischemia.
4. Vasospasm may occur 4 to 12 days after rupture, causing ischemia and infarction.
5. Rebleeding may occur due to lysis of clot.

Clinical Manifestations

1. Sudden onset of severe headache, nausea, photophobia, but no neurologic deficits; may be a "warning bleed" caused by leaking of aneurysm or rupture of the AVM.
2. May present with loss of consciousness and severe deficits if massive bleed.

3. Other signs and symptoms include visual disturbances, dizziness, nuchal rigidity, hemiparesis, papilledema.

Diagnostic Evaluation

1. CT, MRI of the head to determine presence of blood in subarachnoid space, rule out other lesions.
2. Lumbar puncture—shows blood and elevated opening pressure.
3. Cerebral angiography—to detect presence and location of aneurysm and provide information about vasospasm.

Management

1. Management of increased ICP with osmotic diuretics such as mannitol (Osmitrol).
2. Antifibrinolytic therapy with aminocaproic acid (Amicar) to inhibit clot lysis and prevent additional bleeding.
3. Management of systemic hypertension with nitroprusside (Nipride) and close monitoring to prevent precipitous drop in blood pressure, aggravating ischemia.
4. Prevention of vasospasm with calcium channel blockers such as verapamil (Isoptin) and plasma expanders.
5. Prophylactic seizure management with phenytoin (Dilantin) and phenobarbital (Luminal).
6. Surgical interventions to prevent further bleeding.
   a. Clipping or ligation of the aneurysm/AVM.
   b. Strengthening the wall by wrapping if inaccessible to clipping or ligation.
   c. Embolization with particles (AVM) or balloon angioplasty (aneurysm).
   d. See page 373 for care of craniotomy patient.

Complications

1. Rebleeding—highest incidence in first 3 weeks
2. Cerebral vasospasm
3. Hydrocephalus
4. Seizures

Nursing Assessment

1. Obtain baseline neurologic assessment and monitor for decreasing level of consciousness, focal neurologic deficits—may signal vasospasm.
2. Assess vital signs and pupillary changes frequently for development of increased ICP.
3. Assess for increasing headache—could signal rebleeding.

Nursing Diagnoses

A. Risk for Injury related to seizures and potential rebleeding
B. Altered Cerebral Perfusion related to disease process
C. Pain secondary to presence of cerebral hemorrhage
D. Anxiety related to treatment, intracranial surgery

Nursing Interventions

A. *Modifying Activity to Prevent Complications*
1. Medicate patient as ordered during periods of extreme agitation.
2. Institute seizure precautions by providing padded side rails, suction equipment, padded tongue blade, and oral airway at the bedside.
3. Institute subarachnoid precautions:
   a. Maintain absolute bed rest with head elevated 15 to 30 degrees to reduce cerebral edema.
   b. Maintain quiet, tranquil environment with low lighting, no noise, and no unnecessary activity to prevent photophobia, agitation, and pain.
   c. Provide physical care, such as bathing and feeding.
   d. Restrict visitors to only immediate family or significant other who has been counselled to ensure tranquility.
   e. Encourage the awake patient to avoid activities that increase blood pressure or ICP; Valsalva's maneuver for position changing, straining, sneezing, acute flexion/rotation of the neck, cigarette smoking.
   f. Teach the awake patient to exhale through mouth during defecation to reduce strain; administer stool softeners as ordered.
   g. Avoid caffeinated beverages.

B. *Maintaining Cerebral Perfusion*
1. Frequently monitor neurologic status based on condition, including level of consciousness, pupillary reaction, motor and sensory function, cranial nerve function, speech, presence of headache.
2. Document findings and report changes; subtle change in level of consciousness, such as drowsiness and speech slurring, may be first sign of deterioration.
3. See page 367 for care of patients with altered state of consciousness.

C. *Reducing Pain*
1. Assess level of pain and pain relief; report any increase in headache.
2. Administer analgesics as prescribed; if narcotic being given with sedative, monitor for CNS depression, decreased respirations, decreased blood pressure.
3. Encourage distraction with soft music and other measures that will promote calm.

D. *Reducing Anxiety*
1. Use reassurance and therapeutic conversation to relieve fear and anxiety.
2. Inform the patient regarding all treatment modalities.
3. Prepare patient and family for surgery (see p. 373).
4. Encourage discussion of risks/benefits with the surgeon.

Patient Education/ Health Maintenance

1. Educate the patient to the risk of rebleed, which is highest within first 3 weeks of rupture, but may remain for rest of life.
2. Educate the patient to activities to avoid to prevent sudden increased pressure, such as heavy lifting and straining.
3. Encourage lifelong medical follow-up and immediate attention if severe headache develops.

4. Teach patient and family how to deal with permanent neurologic deficits and ensure that they obtain rehabilitation referral.

Evaluation

A. Quiet environment maintained; vital signs stable
B. Neurologic parameters stable
C. Patient verbalizes decreased pain
D. Patient and family able to state reason for surgery, possible risks

Infectious Disorders

◆ MENINGITIS

Meningitis is the inflammation of the meninges, or membranes lining the brain and spinal cord.

Pathophysiology/Etiology

1. Usually secondary to other bacterial infection, such as sinusitis, otitis media, pneumonia, endocarditis, or osteomyelitis
2. Common bacterial organisms include *Neisseria meningitidis* (meningococcal meningitis), *Haemophilus influenzae*, and *Streptococcus pneumoniae*.
3. Aseptic meningitis is caused by a virus or noninfectious insult, such as blood in the subarachnoid space.

Clinical Manifestations

1. Headache, backache
2. Petechial or purpuric rash with meningococcal meningitis
3. Fever and leukocytosis
4. Change in patient's mental status
5. Photophobia
6. Nuchal rigidity, positive Brudzinski's and Kernig's signs

Diagnostic Evaluation

1. Complete blood count with differential—elevated white blood cell count, neutrophils.
2. Blood cultures—may indicate organism.
3. Lumbar puncture with CSF cultures—elevated cell count, may indicate organism.
4. MRI/CT with and without contrast—to rule out other disorders.

Management

1. Antibiotics in large doses IV to allow adequate amount to cross blood–brain barrier: penicillins, cephalosporins, vancomycin (Vancocin).
2. Steroids and osmotic diuretics to reduce cerebral edema.

Complications

1. Seizures, increased ICP
2. Syndrome of inappropriate antidiuretic hormone secretion

Nursing Assessment

1. Obtain history of recent infection, such as upper respiratory infection.
2. Assess neurologic status and vital signs.
3. Evaluate for signs of meningeal irritation—Brudzinski's and Kernig's signs (Fig. 13-3).

Nursing Diagnosis

A. Hyperthermia related to infectious process and cerebral edema

B. Risk for Fluid Volume Deficit related to fever and decreased intake
C. Altered Cerebral Tissue Perfusion related to infectious process and cerebral edema
D. Pain related to meningeal irritation

Nursing Interventions

A. *Reducing Fever*
1. Administer antibiotics on time to maintain optimal blood levels.
2. Monitor temperature frequently or continuously and administer antipyretics as ordered.
3. Institute other cooling measures, such as use of a hypothermia blanket, as indicated.

B. *Maintaining Fluid Balance*
1. Administer IV fluids as ordered, preventing fluid overload, which may worsen cerebral edema.

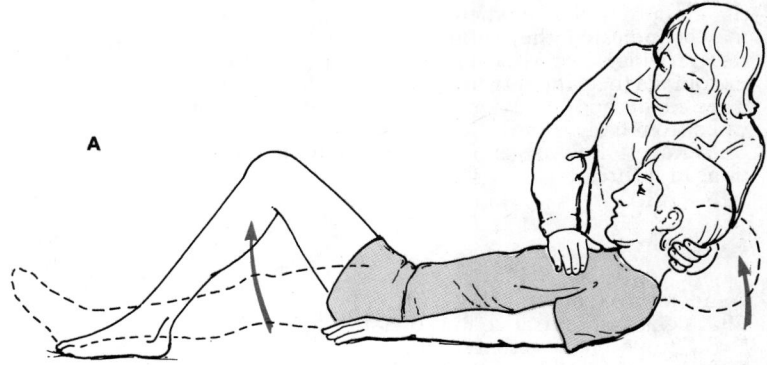

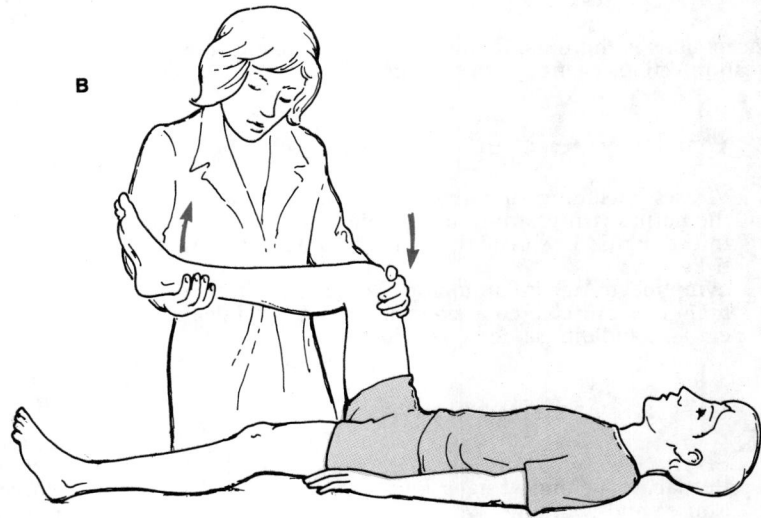

FIGURE 13-3 *Signs of meningeal irritation include nuchal rigidity, a positive Brudzinski's and Kernig's signs. To elicit Brudzinski's sign; place the patient supine and flex the head upward. Resulting flexion of both hips, knees, and ankles with neck flexion indicate meningeal irritation. To test for the Kernig's sign, once again place the patient supine. Keeping one leg straight, flex the other hip and knee to a bent knee to form a 90 degree angle. Slowly extend the lower leg. This places a stretch on the meninges, resulting in pain and spasm of the hamstring muscle. Resistance to further extension can be felt.*

2. Monitor intake and output closely.
3. Monitor central venous pressure frequently.

C. *Enhancing Cerebral Perfusion*
1. Assess level of consciousness, vital signs, and neurologic parameters frequently.
2. Maintain quiet, calm environment to prevent agitation, which may cause increased ICP.
3. Notify the health care provider of increasing temperature, decreasing level of consciousness, onset of seizures, or altered respirations, which signal deterioration.

D. *Reducing Pain*
1. Administer analgesics as ordered; monitor for response and adverse reactions. Narcotics should be avoided to prevent interference in assessment of level of consciousness.
2. Darken the room if photophobia is present.
3. Assist with position of comfort for neck stiffness and turn patient slowly and carefully with head and neck in alignment.

Patient Education/ Health Maintenance

1. Advise close contacts of the patient with meningitis that prophylactic treatment with rifampin (Rifadin) may be indicated; they should check with their health care providers or the local public health department.
2. Encourage the patient to follow medication regimen as directed, because infectious agent must be fully eradicated from body.
3. Encourage follow-up and prompt attention to infections in future.

Evaluation

A. Temperature remains below 101°F (38.3°C)
B. Vital signs and central venous pressure stable
C. Easily arousable to verbal stimuli
D. Verbalizes relief of headache

◆ ENCEPHALITIS

Encephalitis is the inflammation of cerebral tissue caused by an infectious agent or other toxin.

Etiology/Altered Physiology

1. Viruses, including rabies virus, the enteroviruses, and the herpes viruses are common infectious agents.
2. Infection may be spread through infected mosquitos or ticks.
3. Lymphocyte-rich inflammatory exudates infiltrate the brain and cause cerebral edema, basal ganglia degeneration, and diffuse nerve cell destruction.

Clinical Manifestations

1. Fever
2. Headache, meningeal signs
3. Nausea and vomiting

4. Confusion and change in level of consciousness
5. Seizures
6. Subacute or chronic presentation in some forms of encephalitis

Diagnostic Evaluation

1. Lumbar puncture with evaluation of CSF—increased cell count
2. CT and EEG may show abnormalities
3. MRI/CT—detect diffuse inflammation

Management

1. Acyclovir (Zovirax) given IV if caused by *Herpes simplex* virus
2. Anticonvulsants to prevent and treat seizures
3. Glucocorticosteroids to reduce cerebral edema
4. Sedatives and analgesics
5. Supportive care

Complications

1. Coma
2. Frequently fatal

Nursing Assessment

1. Obtain history from family or patient of recent infection, insect bite, animal bite.
2. Perform neurologic assessment, including level of consciousness, personality changes, and meningeal signs.

Nursing Diagnoses

A. Risk for Injury related to seizures and cerebral edema
B. Altered Cerebral Tissue Perfusion related to disease process
C. Hyperthermia related to infectious process

Nursing Interventions

A. *Preventing Injury*
1. Maintain quiet environment and provide care gently, avoiding overactivity and agitation, which may cause increased ICP.
2. Maintain seizure precautions with side rails padded, airway and suction equipment at bedside.
3. Administer medications as ordered, monitor response and adverse reactions.

B. *Promoting Cerebral Perfusion*
1. Monitor neurologic status closely. Watch for subtle changes, such as behavior or personality changes, weakness, or cranial nerve involvement. Notify health care provider.
2. Reorient patient frequently.
3. Provide supportive care if coma develops; may last several weeks.

4. Encourage significant others to interact with patient even while in coma and to participate in care to promote rehabilitation.

C. *Relieving Fever*
1. Monitor temperature and vital signs frequently.
2. Administer antipyretics and other cooling measures as indicated.
3. Monitor fluid intake and output and provide fluid replacement through IV lines as needed.
4. Be alert to signs of other coexisting infections, such as urinary tract infection or pneumonia, and notify health care provider so cultures can be obtained and treatment started.

Patient Education/ Health Maintenance

1. Explain the effects of the disease process and the rationale for care.
2. Reassure significant others based on patient's prognosis.
3. Encourage follow-up for evaluation of deficits and rehabilitation potential.
4. Educate others about the signs and symptoms of encephalitis if epidemic is suspected.
5. Encourage rabies prophylaxis whenever bite by unvaccinated animal is obtained.

Evaluation

A. Lungs clear, no injury after seizure
B. Drowsy but arousable to verbal stimuli
C. Temperature below 100°F (37.8°C), urine output adequate

◆ BRAIN ABSCESS

Brain abscess is a free or encapsulted collection of infectious material of brain parenchyma itself, between the dura and the arachnoid linings (subdural empyema) or between the dura and the skull (cranial epidural abscess).

Etiology/Pathophysiology

1. May be caused by local extension of sinus, middle ear, or mastoid infection; hematogenous spread of lung or endocardial infection; or direct invasion of the brain through trauma or surgery.
2. Frequently occur in frontal or temporal lobes or cerebellum.
3. Microabscesses may be caused by fungal infections, particularly in immunosuppressed patients.

Clinical Manifestations

1. Headache, worse in morning, and persistent over time
2. Nausea, vomiting
3. Drowsiness, confusion
4. Seizures
5. Focal signs, such as weakness of an extremity or decreased vision

Diagnostic Evaluation

1. CT, MRI—to locate site(s) of abscess and follow evolution and resolution of suppurative process
2. Cultures from suspected source of infection—to identify organism and sensitivity to antimicrobials
3. Brain biopsy may be necessary—to confirm diagnosis and determine suitable treatment

Management

1. Antimicrobial therapy in large IV doses to reduce infectivity of the abscess before surgery or as sole treatment of multiple abscesses
2. Surgical intervention—aspiration through burr hole or with stereotactic equipment, or excision by craniotomy
3. Glucocorticosteroids and osmotic diuretics to reduce cerebral edema
4. Anticonvulsants

Complications

1. Permanent neurologic deficits, such as seizure disorders, visual defects, hemiparesis, and cranial nerve palsies.
2. Relapse is common.

Nursing Assessment

1. Obtain history of previous infection, immunosuppression, headache, and related symptoms.
2. Perform neurologic assessment, including cranial nerve evaluation, motor, and cognitive status.

Nursing Diagnoses

A. Pain related to cerebral mass
B. Altered Thought Processes related to disease process
C. Sensory-Perceptual Alteration (Visual) related to cerebral mass
D. Anxiety related to surgery, prognosis, and relapse

Nursing Interventions

A. *Relieving Pain*
1. Administer pain medications as ordered.
2. Provide comfort measures, such as quiet environment, positioning with head sightly elevated, and assistance with hygiene needs.
3. Provide passive relaxation techniques, such as soft music and backrubs.

B. *Promoting Thought Processes*
1. Frequently monitor vital signs, level of consciousness, orientation, and seizure activity.
2. Report changes to health care provider; could signal increasing cerebral edema.
3. Administer medications as ordered, noting response and adverse reactions.

4. Prepare patient for repeated diagnostic tests to evaluate response to therapy and timing of surgery.

C. *Minimizing Visual Deficit*
1. Maintain a safe environment with side rails up, call light within reach, and frequent observation.
2. Evaluate other cranial nerve function and report changes.
3. Refer for occupational therapy if visual deficit appears permanent.

D. *Reducing Anxiety*
1. Prepare patient and family for surgery when indicated.
   a. Encourage discussion with surgeon to understand risks, benefits of the procedure.
   b. Explain nursing care. (See care related to craniotomy, p. 373.)

Patient Education/ Health Maintenance

1. Encourage follow-up to ensure adequate treatment.
2. Encourage rehabilitation to overcome permanent deficits.
3. Advise prompt attention to infections in the future, particularly ear and sinus infections and dental abscesses.

Evaluation

A. Patient verbalizes reduced pain
B. Oriented to person, place, and time; following simple commands
C. Visual acuity reduced, other cranial nerves intact

Degenerative Disorders

◆ PARKINSON'S DISEASE

Parkinson's disease is a progressive neurologic disease affecting the brain centers responsible for control and regulation of movement.

Pathophysiology/Etiology

1. A deficiency of dopamine in the substantia nigra of the brain is thought to be responsible for the symptoms of parkinsonism.
2. Underlying etiology may be related to a virus, genetic susceptibility, toxicity, or other unknown cause.

Clinical Manifestations

1. Bradykinesia (slowness of movement), loss of spontaneous movement
2. Resting tremor of 4 to 5 Hz
3. Rigidity in performance of all movements
4. Autonomic disorders—sleeplessness, salivation, sweating, orthostatic hypotension
5. Depression, dementia
6. Masklike facies

Diagnostic Evaluation

Observation of clinical symptoms; may do imaging studies to rule out other disorders.

Management

1. Anticholinergics to reduce transmission of cholinergic pathways, which are thought to be overactive when dopamine is deficient.
2. Amantadine (Symmetrel), which is thought to increase release of dopamine in the brain.
3. Levodopa, a dopamine precursor, combined with carbidopa, a decarboxylase inhibitor, to inhibit destruction of L-dopa in the bloodstream, making more available to the brain. The combination is levodopacarbidopa (Sinemet).
4. Bromocriptine (Parlodel), a dopaminergic agonist that activates dopamine receptors in the brain.
5. Use of the monoamine oxidase inhibitor deprenyl (Eldepryl) to delay the onset of disability and need for levodopa therapy.

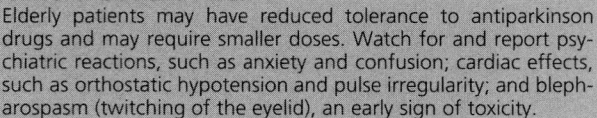

GERONTOLOGIC ALERT:
Elderly patients may have reduced tolerance to antiparkinson drugs and may require smaller doses. Watch for and report psychiatric reactions, such as anxiety and confusion; cardiac effects, such as orthostatic hypotension and pulse irregularity; and blepharospasm (twitching of the eyelid), an early sign of toxicity.

Complications

1. Dementia
2. Aspiration
3. Injury from falls

Nursing Assessment

1. Obtain history of symptoms and their effect on functioning.
2. Assess cranial nerves, cerebellar function (coordination), motor function.
3. Observe gait and performance of activities.
4. Assess speech for clarity and pace.
5. Assess for signs of depression.

Nursing Diagnoses

A. Impaired Physical Mobility related to bradykinesia, rigidity, and tremor
B. Altered Nutritional Status, Less Than Body Requirements related to motor difficulties with feeding, chewing, and swallowing
C. Impaired Verbal Communication related to decreased speech volume and facial muscle involvement
D. Constipation related to diminished motor function and inactivity
E. Ineffective Individual Coping related to physical limitations and loss of independence

Nursing Interventions

A. *Improving Mobility*
1. Encourage the patient in daily exercise, such as walking, riding a stationary bike, swimming, or gardening.
2. Advise the patient to do stretching and postural exercises as outlined by physical therapist.
3. Encourage the patient to take warm baths and receive massages to help relax muscles.
4. Instruct the patient to take frequent rest periods to overcome fatigue and frustration.
5. Teach postural exercises and walking techniques to offset shuffling gait and tendency to lean forward.
   a. Instruct patient to use a broad-based gait.
   b. Have patient make a conscious effort to swing arms, raise the feet while walking, use a heel–toe gait, and increase the width of stride.
   c. Tell patient to practice walking to marching music or sound of ticking metronome—provides sensory reinforcement.

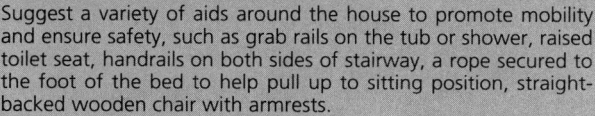

COMMUNITY-BASED CARE TIP:
Suggest a variety of aids around the house to promote mobility and ensure safety, such as grab rails on the tub or shower, raised toilet seat, handrails on both sides of stairway, a rope secured to the foot of the bed to help pull up to sitting position, straight-backed wooden chair with armrests.

B. *Optimizing Nutritional Status*
1. Teach patient to think through the sequence of swallowing—close lips with teeth together; lift tongue up with food on it; then move tongue back and swallow while tilting head forward.
2. Instruct patient to chew deliberately and slowly, using both sides of mouth.
3. Tell patient to make conscious effort to control accumulation of saliva by holding head upright and swallowing periodically.
4. Have patient use secure, stabilized dishes and eating utensils.
5. Suggest smaller meals and additional snacks.
6. Monitor weight.

C. *Maximizing Communication Ability*
1. Encourage compliance with medication regimen.
2. Suggest referral to speech therapist.
3. Teach patient facial exercises and breathing methods to obtain appropriate pronunciation, volume, and intonation.
   a. Take a deep breath before speaking to increase the volume of sound and number of words spoken with each breath.
   b. Exaggerate pronunciation and speak in short sentences; read aloud in front of a mirror or into a tape recorder to monitor progress.
   c. Exercise facial muscles by smiling, frowning, grimacing, and puckering.

D. *Preventing Constipation*
1. Encourage foods with moderate fiber content—whole grains, fruits, and vegetables.
2. Increase water intake.
3. Obtain a raised toilet seat to encourage normal position.
4. Encourage patient to follow regular bowel routine.

E. *Strengthening Coping Ability*
1. Help the patient establish realistic goals and outline ways to achieve goals.
2. Provide emotional support and encouragement.
3. Encourage use of all resources, such as therapists, primary care provider, social worker, social support network.
4. Encourage open communication, discussion of feelings, and exchange of information about Parkinson's disease.
5. Have patient take active role in activity planning and evaluation of treatment plan.

Patient Education/ Health Maintenance

1. Instruct the patient to avoid sedatives, unless specifically prescribed, which have additive effect with other medications and to avoid vitamin B preparations, and vitamin-fortified foods that can reverse effects of medication.
2. Instruct the patient in medication regimen and adverse reactions, such as orthostatic hypotension, dry mouth, dystonia, muscle twitching, urinary retention, impaired glucose tolerance, anemia, and elevated liver function tests.
3. Encourage follow-up and monitoring for diabetes, glaucoma, hepatotoxicity, and anemia while undergoing drug therapy.
4. Teach patient ambulation cues to avoid "freezing" in place and possibly avoid falls by doing one of the following:
   a. Raise head, raise toes, then rock from one foot to another while bending knees slightly.
   b. Raise arms in a sudden short motion.
   c. Take a small step backward, then start forward.
   d. Step sideways, then start forward.
5. Instruct the family not to pull patient during episodes of "freezing," which increases the problem and may cause falling.
6. Refer the patient to such agencies as: The United Parkinson's Foundation; 360 West Superior Street; Chicago, IL 60620; 312-664-2344

Evaluation

A. Attending physical therapy sessions, doing facial exercises 10 minutes twice a day
B. Eating three small meals and two snacks, no weight loss
C. Annunciation clear, speaking in 4 to 5 words per breath
D. Passing soft stool every day
E. Asking questions about Parkinson's, obtaining help from son or daughter

◆ MULTIPLE SCLEROSIS

Multiple sclerosis is a chronic disease of the CNS characterized by occurrence of small patches of demyelination of the white matter of the optic nerve, brain, and spinal cord.

Pathophysiology/Etiology

1. Demyelination refers to the destruction of the myelin, the fatty and protein material that covers certain nerve fibers in the brain and spinal cord.
2. Demyelination results in disordered transmission of nerve impulses.
3. Inflammatory changes lead to scarring of the affected nerve fibers.
4. Cause unknown but possibly related to autoimmune dysfunction, genetic susceptibility, or an infectious process.
5. More prevalent in the northern latitudes and among Caucasians.

Clinical Manifestations

Lesions can occur anywhere within the white matter of the CNS. Symptoms reflect the location of the area of demyelination.

1. Fatigue and weakness
2. Abnormal reflexes—absent or exaggerated
3. Visual disturbances—impaired and double vision, nystagmus
4. Motor dysfunction—weakness, tremor, incoordination
5. Sensory disturbances—paresthesias, impaired deep sensation, impaired vibratory and position sense
6. Impaired speech—slurring, scanning (dysarthria)
7. Urinary dysfunction—hesitancy, frequency, urgency, retention, incontinence
8. Neurobehavioral syndromes—depression, cognitive impairment, emotional lability

Diagnostic Evaluation

1. Electrophoresis study of CSF; abnormal IgG antibody appears in CSF.
2. MRI visualizes small plaques scattered throughout white matter of CNS.
3. Visual, auditory, and somatosensory evoked potentials—slowed conduction is evidence of demyelination.

Management

Treatment is aimed at relieving symptoms and helping the patient function.

A. *Acute Attacks*
1. Corticosteroids or adrenocorticotrophic hormone are used to decrease inflammation, shorten duration of relapse or exacerbation.
2. Immunosuppressive agents may stabilize the course of the disease.
3. Beta-interferon (Betaseron) is being used for treatment of rapidly progressing symptoms in some persons.

B. *Chronic Symptom Management*
1. Treatment of spasticity with agents such as baclofen (Lioresal), dantrolene (Dantrium), diazepam (Valium); physical therapy; nerve blocks and surgical intervention.

2. Control of fatigue with amantadine (Symmetrel).
3. Treatment of depression with antidepressant drugs and counseling.
4. Bladder management with anticholinergics, intermittent catheterization for drainage.
5. Bowel management with stool softeners, bulk laxative, suppositories.
6. Rehabilitation management with physical therapy, occupational therapy.
7. Control dystonia with carbamazepine (Tegratol).
8. Management of pain syndromes with carbamazepine (Tegratol), phenytoin (Dilantin), perphenazine with amitriptyline (Triavil).

Complications

1. Respiratory dysfunction
2. Infections; bladder, respiratory, sepsis
3. Complications from immobility

Nursing Assessment

1. Observe motor strength, coordination, and gait.
2. Perform cranial nerve assessment.
3. Evaluate elimination function.
4. Explore coping, effect on activity and sexual function, emotional adjustment.

Nursing Diagnoses

A. Impaired Physical Mobility related to muscle weakness, spasticity, and incoordination
B. Fatigue related to disease process and stress of coping
C. Sensory-Perceptual Alteration (Tactile, Kinesthetic, Visual) related to disease process
D. Altered Urinary Elimination related to disease process
E. Altered Family Processes related to inability to fulfill expected roles
F. Sexual Dysfunction related to disease process

Nursing Interventions

A. *Promoting Motor Function*
1. Perform muscle stretching and strengthening exercises daily or teach patient or family to perform, using stretch-hold-relax routine to minimize spasticity and prevent contractures.
2. Apply ice packs before stretching to reduce spasticity.
3. Tell patient to avoid muscle fatigue by stopping activity just short of fatigue and take frequent rest periods.
4. Encourage ambulation and activity and teach patient how to use such devices as braces, canes, and walkers when necessary.
5. Inform the patient to avoid sudden changes in position, which may cause fall due to loss of position sense, and to walk with a wide-based gait.
6. Encourage frequent change in position while immobilized to prevent contractures; sleeping prone will minimize flexor spasm of hips and knees.

B. *Minimizing Fatigue*
1. Help patient and family understand that fatigue is an integral part of multiple sclerosis.

2. Plan ahead and prioritize activities. Take brief rest periods throughout the day.
3. Avoid overheating, overexertion, and infection.
4. Encourage energy conservation techniques, such as sitting to perform activity, limiting trips up and down stairs, pulling or pushing rather than lifting.
5. Help patient develop healthy lifestyle with balanced diet, rest, exercise, and relaxation.

C. *Optimizing Sensory Function*
1. Suggest use of an eyepatch or frosted lens (alternate eyes) for patients with double vision.
2. Encourage ophthalmologic consultation to maximize vision.
3. Provide a safe environment for patient with any sensory alteration.
   a. Orient patient to the environment and keep arrangement of furniture and personal articles constant.
   b. Make sure floor is free of obstacles, loose rugs, or slippery areas.
   c. Teach the use of all senses to maintain awareness of environment.

D. *Maintaining Urinary Elimination*
1. Ensure adequate fluid intake to help prevent infection and stone formation.
2. Assess for urinary retention, catheterize for residual urine as indicated.
3. Teach patient to report signs of urinary tract infection immediately.
4. Set up bladder training program to reduce incontinence.
   a. Encourage fluids every 2 hours.
   b. Follow regular schedule of voiding, every 1 to 2 hours, lengthening as tolerated.
   c. Restrict fluid volume and salty foods 1 to 2 hours before bedtime.
5. See page 133 for more information on urinary retention and incontinence.

E. *Normalizing Family Processes*
1. Encourage verbalization of feelings of each family member.
2. Encourage counseling and use of church or community resources.
3. Suggest dividing up household duties, child-care responsibilities to prevent strain on one individual.
4. Explore adaptation of some roles so that patient can still function in family unit.

F. *Promoting Sexual Function*
1. Encourage open communication between partners.
2. Discuss birth control options if appropriate.
3. Suggest sexual activity when patient is most rested.
4. Suggest consultation with sexual therapist to help obtain greater sexual satisfaction.

Patient Education/ Health Maintenance

1. Encourage the patient to maintain previous activities, although at a lowered level of intensity.
2. Teach the patient to respect fatigue and avoid physical overexertion and emotional stress; remind patient that activity tolerance may vary from day to day.

3. Advise the patient to avoid exposure to heat and cold or infectious agents.
4. Encourage nutritious diet that is high in fiber to promote health and good bowel elimination.
5. Advise the patient that some medications may accentuate weakness such as some antibiotics, muscle relaxants, antiarrhythmics and antihypertensives, antipsychotics, oral contraceptives, and antihistamines; check with health care provider before taking any new medications.
6. Teach the patient receiving beta-interferon (Betaseron) to expect side effects of flulike symptoms, fever, asthenia, chills, myalgias, sweating, and local reaction at the injection site. Liver function test elevation and neutropenia may also occur. Side effects may persist for up to 6 months of treatment before subsiding.
7. Instruct the patient receiving Betaseron in self-injection technique.
8. Refer the patient/family to such agencies as: The National Multiple Sclerosis Society; 733 Third Avenue; New York, NY 10017; 212-986-3240.

Evaluation

A. Performing exercises correctly without spasm
B. Resting at intervals, tolerating activity well
C. Moving about in environment without injury
D. Voiding every 2 hours, two episodes incontinence
E. Family sharing care, discussing feelings
F. Patient reports satisfaction with sexual activity.

◆ ALZHEIMER'S DISEASE

A degenerative disorder characterized by dementia with progressive impairment in memory, cognitive function, language, judgment, and self-care ability.

Pathophysiology/Etiology

1. Gross pathophysiologic changes include cortical atrophy, enlarged ventricles, and basal ganglia wasting.
2. Microscopically, changes occur in the proteins of the nerve cells of the cerebral cortex and lead to accumulation of neurofibrillary tangles and neuritic plaques (deposits of protein and altered cell structures on the interneuronal junctions).
3. Biochemically, neurotransmitter systems are impaired.
4. Cause unknown, but there appears to be a genetic predisposition.
5. Viruses, environmental toxins, and previous head injury may also play a role.

Clinical Manifestations

1. Stage I—poor short-term memory, mildly impaired remote recall, impaired visuospatial skills, mild language impairment, indifference, occasional irritability.
2. Stage II—severe memory impairment, spatial disorientation, fluent aphasia, inability to make calculations, indifference, irritability, apraxia, delusions, restlessness, pacing.

3. Stage III—very poor cognitive function, rigidity of the extremities and flexion posture, urinary and fecal incontinence.

Diagnostic Evaluation

1. MRI, CT, and other tests to rule out treatable forms of dementia.
2. Neuropsychologic evaluation to establish clinical criteria for diagnosis.
3. Laboratory tests to rule out metabolic disorders.

Management

Management is for symptom relief only. No curative treatment exists.

1. Chlorpromazine (Thorazine) and haloperidol (Haldol) may control agitation and hallucinations.
2. Tacrine (Cognex) is thought to improve cognitive functioning and quality of life.

NURSING ALERT:
Acute catastrophic reactions, characterized by agitation or insomnia, occur in the patient with Alzheimer's disease when the coping mechanisms fail. This may be precipitated by the strange environment of the hospital. Behavior may be managed by haloperidol (Haldol) 2 to 5 mg PO or IM; lorazepam (Ativan) 5 mg PO or 1 mg IM; nortriptyline (Pamelor) or trazodone (Desyrel) if accompanied by depression; antihistamines; chloral hydrate (Noctec); and maintenance of a simple, quiet, softly lit environment.

COMMUNITY-BASED CARE TIP:
Episodes of catastrophic reactions and insomnia can be managed at home by the use of soft background music (white noise); having the patient wear a wander-guard alarm, and providing repetitive stimulation, such as music and rocking.

Complications

1. Infections; respiratory, urinary tract.
2. Injury due to lack of insight, hallucinations, and confusion.
3. Malnutrition due to inattention to mealtime and hunger or lack of ability to prepare meals.

Nursing Assessment

1. Perform cognitive assessment for orientation, insight, abstract thinking, and memory.
2. Evaluate nutrition and hydration; check weight, skin turgor, meal habits.
3. Assess motor ability, strength, muscle tone, and flexibility.

Nursing Diagnoses

A. Altered Thought Processes related to physiologic changes of the disease
B. Risk for Injury due to loss of cognitive abilities
C. Impaired Social Interaction related to decreased ability to understand environment
D. Sleep Pattern Disturbance secondary to disease process
E. Altered Nutrition (Less Than Body Requirements) related to memory loss and altered planning abilities
F. Caregiver role strain related to physical needs and behavioral manifestations of the disease process

Nursing Interventions

A. *Improving Cognitive Response*
1. Simplify the environment: decrease noise and social interaction to a level tolerable for the patient.
2. Maintain a strict routine, decrease the number of choices available to the patient, use pictures to identify activities.
3. Post large calendar and clock in patient's view and orient frequently to time, person, and place.
4. Use lists and written instructions as reminders to daily activities.
5. Maintain consistency in interactions and introduce new people slowly.

B. *Preventing Injury*
1. Try to avoid restraints but maintain observation of the patient as necessary.
2. Provide for adequate lighting to avoid misinterpretation of the environment.
3. Remove unneeded furniture and equipment from the room.
4. Provide identification tag and/or Medic Alert bracelet.
5. Make sure patient has nonslip shoes or slippers that are easy to put on.

COMMUNITY-BASED CARE TIP:
Remind family members of possible dangers around the house as patient becomes less responsible for behavior. Encourage them to turn down the temperature of the hot water heater, remove dials from stove and other electrical appliances, remove matches and lighters, and safely store away tools and other potentially dangerous items.

C. *Maintaining Socialization*
1. Encourage the family to interact at a level meaningful to the patient.
2. Instruct the family that their presence is helpful even though actual interaction with the patient may be limited.
3. Ask the family to bring objects meaningful to the patient.

D. *Ensuring Adequate Rest*
1. Administer antipsychotics to manage agitation.
2. Provide periods of physical exercise to expend energy.
3. Support normal sleep habits and bedtime ritual.
   a. Keep regular bedtime.
   b. Have patient change into pajamas at bedtime.
   c. Allow desired bedtime activity, such as snack, warm noncaffeinated beverage, listening to music, or prayer.

4. Maintain quiet, relaxing environment to avoid confusion and agitation.

E. *Maintaining Optimal Nutrition*
1. Provide foods familiar to the patient.
2. Provide small, frequent meals with snacks.
3. Make finger foods available to the patient.
4. Provide foods high in calories and fiber.
5. Encourage fluids.
6. Ensure that dentures are well fitting and that dental care is maintained.
7. Weigh patient weekly.

F. *Supporting Caregiver*
1. Encourage caregiver to discuss feelings.
2. Encourage caregiver to maintain own health and emotional well-being.
3. Stress the need for relaxation time or respite care periodically.
4. Assist the caregiver in finding resources, such as community or church groups, social service programs, or hospital-based support groups.
5. Assess caregiver's level of stress and refer for counseling as needed.
6. Support decision to place patient in a nursing facility.

Patient Education/ Health Maintenance

1. Encourage activities that provide physical exercise and repetitive movement but that require little thought, such as dancing, painting, doing laundry, or vacuuming.
2. Teach patient and family to eliminate stimulants, such as caffeine, from diet.
3. Discuss with the family the need to organize finances and to make advanced directive decisions and guardianship arrangements before they are needed to allow the patient input into the process.
4. For additional information, refer families to such agencies as: The Alzheimer's Association; 919 North Michigan Avenue, Suite 1000; Chicago, IL 60611; 800-272-3900.

Evaluation

A. Participating in ADL without confusion or agitation
B. No injury reported
C. Interacting with family
D. Sleeping 6 hours at night with 1 hour rest period twice a day
E. Eating three small meals, two to three snacks; no weight loss
F. Caregiver reports using respite care twice a week

◆ AMYOTROPHIC LATERAL SCLEROSIS (ALS)

Amyotrophic lateral sclerosis , also known as Lou Gehrig's disease, is an incapacitating disease that results in progressive weakness accompanied by other lower motor neuron signs, such as atrophy or fasciculations.

Pathophysiology/Etiology

1. Degeneration of upper motor neurons (nerves leading from the brain to medulla or spinal cord) and lower motor neurons (nerves leading from the spinal cord to the muscles of the body).
2. Results in progressive loss of voluntary muscle contraction and functional capacity.
3. Cause is unknown.
4. Usually affects men in the fifth or sixth decade of life.

Clinical Manifestations

1. Progressive weakness and wasting of muscles of arms, trunk, and legs.
2. Fasciculations and signs of spasticity.
3. Progressive difficulty swallowing (drooling, regurgitation of liquids through nose), speaking (nasal and unintelligible), and, ultimately, breathing.

Diagnostic Evaluation

1. Electromyography to evaluate denervation and muscle atrophy.
2. Nerve conduction study to evaluate nerve pathways.
3. Pulmonary function tests to evaluate respiratory function.
4. Barium swallow to evaluate ability to achieve various phases of swallow.
5. MRI, CT—to rule out other disorders.
6. Laboratory tests: creatine kinase, heavy metal screen, thyroid function tests, CSF evaluation to rule out other causes of muscle weakness.

Management

No specific treatment available to arrest or alter course of the disease.

1. Baclofen (Lioresal) to control spasticity
2. Diazepam (Valium) to control fasciculations
3. Antidepressants, sleep medications
4. Feeding gastrostomy
5. Mechanical ventilation eventually becomes necessary

Complications

1. Respiratory failure
2. Aspiration pneumonia
3. Cardiopulmonary arrest

Nursing Assessment

1. Evaluate respiratory function; rate, depth, tidal volume.
2. Perform cranial nerve assessment, particularly gag reflex and swallowing.
3. Assess voluntary motor function and strength.

Nursing Diagnoses

A. Ineffective Breathing Pattern related to respiratory muscle weakness
B. Impaired Physical Mobility related to disease process
C. Altered Nutrition (Less Than Body Requirements) related to inability to swallow
D. Fatigue related to denervation of muscles
E. Social Isolation related to fatigability and decreased communication skills
F. Risk for Infection related to inability to clear airway

Nursing Interventions

A. Maintaining Respiration
1. Monitor vital capacity frequently. Document pattern and report any decrease below patient's baseline.
2. Position patient upright, suction upper airway, and perform chest physical therapy to enhance respiratory function.
3. Encourage use of incentive spirometer to exercise respiratory muscles.
4. Assess for signs of hypoxia, such as tachypnea, hypopnea, restlessness, poor sleep, and excessive fatigue.
5. Obtain arterial blood gases as ordered.
6. Establish the wishes of the patient in terms of life-support measures; obtain copy of living will for chart if applicable.
7. Assist with intubation, tracheostomy, and mechanical ventilation when indicated (see Chapter 8, p. 142).
8. Provide suctioning and routine care of a patient with artificial airway and mechanical ventilation.

B. Optimizing Mobility
1. Encourage the patient to continue usual activities as long as possible, but modify exertion to avoid fatigue.
2. Encourage physical therapy exercises to strengthen unaffected muscles and perform range-of-motion exercises to prevent contractures.
3. Encourage energy-conservation techniques.
4. Obtain assistive devices as needed to help patient maintain independence, such as special feeding devices, remote controls, and a motorized wheelchair.

C. Meeting Nutritional Requirements
1. Provide high-calorie, small, frequent feedings.
2. Provide meals that are of a texture the patient can handle; semisolid food is usually easiest to swallow.
   a. Avoid easily aspirated, pureed, and mucous-producing foods (eg, milk).
   b. Try warm or cold foods that stimulate temperature receptors in mouth and may help in swallowing.
   c. Do not wash down solids with fluids—may cause choking and aspiration.
3. Allow patient to make own food selection.
4. Provide assistive devices for self-feeding when possible.
5. Make mealtime a pleasant experience in a bright room, with quiet company so the patient may concentrate on eating and avoid undue embarrassment.
6. Examine oral cavity for food debris before and after meals and assess swallowing function and buildup of saliva.
7. Encourage rest periods before meals to alleviate muscle fatigue.
8. Place patient upright for meals with neck flexed to partially protect the airway.
9. Instruct patient to take a breath before swallowing, hold breath to swallow, exhale or cough after swallow, and swallow again.
10. Tell patient to avoid talking while eating.
11. Suggest gastrostomy or other alternate feeding methods when appropriate.

D. Minimizing Fatigue
1. Encourage activity alternating with frequent naps.
2. Encourage patient to accomplish most important activities early in day.
3. Consult with occupational therapist about energy-conservation techniques in performing ADLs.

E. Maintaining Social Interaction
1. Use mechanical speech aids or communication board.
2. Use an environmental control board.
3. Eye movements/blinks may be the last voluntary movement; develop a code system to serve as a communication method.
4. Because standard call lights cannot be activated by the severely debilitated ALS patient, provide some type of constant monitoring and surveillance to meet patient's needs.
5. Allow patient to select which social activities are meaningful.
6. Refer to counselor or psychologist for coping with communication barriers and inevitability of losses.

F. Preventing Aspiration and Infection
1. Consult with speech therapist for techniques and devices to assist swallowing.
2. Discourage bed rest to prevent pulmonary stasis.
3. Perform chest physiotherapy as tolerated.
4. Monitor for fever and tachycardia and obtain sputum, urine, and other cultures as indicated.

Patient Education/ Health Maintenance

1. Stress the importance of maintaining physical exercise.
2. Review with the patient and family proper eating mechanics to avoid fatigue and aspiration.
3. Inform the patient of right to make decisions regarding a living will if he or she decides against artificial ventilation.
4. Encourage the family to seek support and respite care.
5. Remind the family that the patient with ALS maintains full alertness, sensory function, and intelligence. Encourage them to maintain interaction, socialization, and stimulation.
6. Refer the patient/family to agencies such as: The Amyotrophic Lateral Sclerosis Association; 21021 Ventura Boulevard, Suite 321; Woodland Hills, CA 91364 800-782-4747.

Evaluation

A. Respirations 28, shallow, unlabored at rest
B. Feeding self with assistive utensils
C. Tolerating small, frequent feedings without aspiration
D. Napping twice a day for 1 to 2 hours
E. Communicating needs effectively to staff and family
F. No signs of respiratory or urinary infection

Neuromuscular Disorders

◆ GUILLAIN-BARRÉ SYNDROME (POLYRADICULONEURITIS)

Guillain-Barré syndrome is an acute inflammatory demyelinating polyneuropathy of the peripheral sensory and motor nerves and nerve roots.

Pathophysiology/Etiology

1. Believed to be an autoimmune disorder.
2. Viral infection, immunization, or other event may trigger the autoimmune response.
3. Cell-mediated immune reaction is aimed at peripheral nerves, causing demyelination and possibly axonal degeneration.

Clinical Manifestations

1. Paresthesias.
2. Acute onset of symmetrical progressive muscle weakness; most often beginning in the legs and ascending to involve the trunk, upper extremities, and facial muscles. Paralysis may develop.
3. Difficulty with swallowing, speech, and chewing due to cranial nerve involvement.
4. Decreased or absent deep tendon reflexes, position and vibratory perception.
5. Autonomic dysfunction (increased heart rate and postural hypotension).
6. Decreased vital capacity, depth of respirations, and breath sounds.
7. Occasionally spasm and fasciculations of muscles.
8. May be paresthesias, dysthesias.

Diagnostic Evaluation

1. CSF examination—low blood cell count, high protein.
2. Electrophysiologic studies—NCT shows decreased conduction velocity of peripheral nerves.

Management

1. Plasmapheresis produces temporary reduction of circulating antibodies.
2. Electrocardiography monitoring and treatment of cardiac dysrhythmias.
3. Analgesics and muscle relaxants as needed.
4. Intubation and mechanical ventilation if respiratory paralysis develops.

Complications

1. Respiratory failure
2. Cardiac dysrhythmias
3. Complications of immobility and paralysis

Nursing Assessment

1. Assess pain level due to muscle spasms and paresthesias.
2. Assess respiratory status closely to determine hypoventilation due to weakness.
3. Perform cranial nerve assessment, especially ninth cranial nerve for gag reflex.
4. Assess motor strength.

Nursing Diagnoses

A. Ineffective Breathing Pattern related to weakness/paralysis of respiratory muscles
B. Impaired Physical Mobility related to paralysis
C. Impaired Verbal Communication related to intubation, cranial nerve dysfunction
D. Altered Nutrition, Less Than Body Requirements, related to cranial nerve dysfunction
E. Pain related to disease pathology
F. Anxiety related to communication difficulties and deteriorating physical condition

Nursing Interventions

A. *Maintaining Respiration*
1. Monitor respiratory status through vital capacity measurements, rate and depth of respirations, breath sounds.
2. Monitor level of weakness as it ascends toward respiratory muscles.
3. Watch for breathlessness while talking, a sign of respiratory fatigue.
4. Maintain calm environment and position patient with head of bed elevated to provide for maximum chest excursion.
5. Avoid narcotics and sedatives that may depress respirations.
6. Monitor the patient for signs of impending respiratory failure; heart rate above 120 or below 70 beats/minute; respiratory rate above 30/minute; prepare to intubate.

B. *Avoiding Complications of Immobility*
1. Position patient correctly and provide range-of-motion exercises (see p. 128).
2. Encourage physical and occupational therapy exercises to regain strength during rehabilitative period.
3. Assess for complications, such as contractures, pressure sores, edema of lower extremities, and constipation.
4. Provide assistive devices as needed, such as cane or wheelchair, for patient to take home.

C. *Promoting Adequate Nutrition*
1. Auscultate for bowel sounds; hold enteral feedings if bowel sounds are absent to prevent gastric distention.
2. Assess chewing and swallowing ability by testing fifth and ninth cranial nerves; if function is inadequate, provide alternate feeding.
3. During rehabilitation period, encourage a well-balanced, nutritious diet in small, frequent feedings with vitamin supplement if indicated.

D. *Maintaining Communication*
1. Develop a communication system with patient who cannot speak.

2. Have frequent contact with patient and provide explanation and reassurance, remembering that patient is fully conscious.
3. Provide some type of patient call system.
4. Encourage speech therapy during rehabilitation phase.

E. *Relieving Pain*
1. Administer analgesics as required; monitor for adverse reactions, such as hypotension, nausea and vomiting, and respiratory depression.
2. Provide adjunct pain management therapies, such as therapeutic touch, massage, diversion, imagery.
3. Provide explanations to relieve anxiety, which augments pain.
4. Turn the patient frequently to relieve painful pressure areas.

F. *Reducing Anxiety*
1. Get to know the patient and build a trusting relationship.
2. Discuss fears and concerns while verbal communication is possible.
3. Reassure patient that recovery is probable.
4. Use relaxation techniques, such as listening to soft music.
5. Provide choices in care and give patient a sense of control.
6. Enlist the support of significant others.

Patient Education/ Health Maintenance

1. Advise patient and family that acute phase lasts 1 to 4 weeks, then patient stabilizes and rehabilitation can begin; however, convalescence may be lengthy, from 3 months to 2 years.
2. Instruct patient in breathing exercises or use of incentive spirometer to reestablish normal patterns.
3. Teach patient to wear good supportive and protective shoes while out of bed to prevent injuries due to weakness and paresthesias.
4. Instruct patient to check feet routinely for injuries, because trauma may go unnoticed due to sensory changes.
5. Reinforce maintenance of normal weight; additional weight will further stress the motor abilities.
6. Encourage the use of scheduled rest periods to avoid overfatigue.
7. Refer the patient/family to agencies such as: The Guillain-Barré Syndrome Foundation International; PO Box 262; Wynnewood, PA 19096; 610-667-0131.

Evaluation

A. Respirations 24, deep, unlabored
B. Providing assistive range-of-motion exercises every 2 hours; no pressure sores or edema present
C. Gag reflex present, eating small meals without aspiration
D. Using short phrases and head nodding to communicate effectively
E. Patient verbalizes decreased pain
F. Patient verbalizes reduced anxiety

◆ MYASTHENIA GRAVIS

Myasthenia gravis is a disorder affecting the neuromuscular transmission of impulses in the voluntary muscles of the body.

Pathophysiology/Etiology

1. Reduction of acetylcholine receptors at neuromuscular junctions brought about by an autoimmune attack; thought to be antibody mediated.
2. Unknown cause.
3. An acute myasthenic crisis may result from natural deterioration, emotional upset, upper respiratory infection, surgery, trauma, or adrenocorticotrophic hormone therapy.
4. Cholinergic crisis can result from overmedication with anticholinergic drugs, which release too much acetylcholine at the neuromuscular junction.
5. Brittle crisis occurs when the receptors at the neuromuscular junction become insensitive to anticholinesterase medication.

Clinical Manifestations

1. Extreme muscular weakness and easy fatigability.
2. Visual disturbances; diplopia and ptosis from ocular weakness.
3. Masklike facial expression from involvement of facial muscles.
4. Dysarthria and dysphagia from weakness of laryngeal and pharyngeal muscles.
5. Impending crisis:
   a. Sudden respiratory distress
   b. Signs of dysphagia, dysarthria, ptosis, and diplopia
   c. Tachycardia, anxiety
   d. Rapidly increasing weakness of extremities and trunk

Diagnostic Evaluation

1. Serum test for acetylcholine receptor antibodies—positive in up to 90% of patients.
2. Edrophonium (Tensilon) test—IV injection relieves symptoms temporarily.
3. Electrophysiologic testing—reveals decremental response to repetitive nerve stimulation.
4. CT scan for thymoma or thymus hyperplasia thought to initiate the autoimmune response.

Management

1. Anticholinesterase drugs such as neostigmine (Prostigmin) and pyridostigmine (Mestinon, Regonol) to enhance neuromuscular transmission.
2. Immunosuppressive drugs such as prednisone (Orasone) and azathioprine (Imuran).
3. Plasmapheresis to temporarily remove antibodies from the blood.
4. Thymectomy for those individuals with tumor or hyperplasia of the thymus gland.

5. Interventions for crisis:
   a. Endophonium (Tensilon) to differentiate crisis and treat myasthenic crisis; temporarily worsens cholinergic crisis, unpredictable results with brittle crisis
   b. Ventilatory support
   c. Plasmapheresis
   d. Neostigmine (Prostigmin) IV for myasthenic crisis
   e. Withdraw anticholinergic medications, give atropine to reduce excessive secretions for cholinergic crisis

Complications

1. Aspiration
2. Complications of decreased physical mobility
3. Respiratory failure

Nursing Assessment

1. Assess cranial nerve function, motor fatigability with repetitive activity, and speech.
2. Assess respiratory status and vital capacity measurements.

Nursing Diagnoses

A. Fatigue related to disease process
B. Risk of Aspiration related to muscle weakness of face and tongue
C. Social Isolation related to diminished speech capabilities and increased secretions

Nursing Interventions

A. *Minimizing Fatigue*
1. Administer medications so that their peak effect coincides with meals or essential activities.
2. Assist the patient in developing realistic activity schedule.
3. Provide an eyepatch and alternate eyes for the patient with diplopia to allow safe participation in activity.
4. Allow for rest periods throughout the day.
5. Obtain assistive devices to help patient perform ADLs despite weakness.

> **NURSING ALERT:** ❖
> Many medications can accentuate the weakness experienced by the patient with myasthenia, including some antibiotics, antiarrhythmics, local and general anesthetics, muscle relaxants, and analgesics. Assess function after administering any new drug and report deterioration in condition.

B. *Preventing Aspiration*
1. Teach patient to position head in a slightly flexed position to protect airway during eating.
2. Have suction available that patient can operate.
3. Administer IV fluids and nasogastric tube feedings to patient in crisis or with impaired swallowing; elevate head of bed after feeding.

4. Suction the patient frequently if on a mechanical ventilator; assess breath sounds, and check chest x-ray reports, because aspiration is a common problem.

C. *Maintaining Social Interactions*
1. Encourage patient to use an alternate communication method, such as flash cards or a letter board, if speech is affected.
2. Teach patient to tilt head, and carry a handkerchief to manage secretions in public.
3. Show the patient how to cup chin in hands during speech to support lower jaw and assist with speech.

Patient Education/ Health Maintenance

1. Instruct the patient and family regarding the symptoms of crisis.
2. Teach the patient and family regarding the use of home suction.
3. Review the peak times of medications and how to schedule activity for best results.
4. Stress the importance of scheduled rest periods before fatigue develops.
5. Teach the patient ways to prevent crisis and aggravation of symptoms.
   a. Avoid exposure to colds, and other infections.
   b. Avoid excessive heat and cold.
   c. Inform the dentist of condition, because use of procaine (Novocain) is not well tolerated.
   d. Avoid emotional upset.
6. Encourage patient to wear a Medic Alert bracelet.
7. Refer patient and family to agencies such as: The Myasthenia Gravis Foundation, Inc.; 61 Gramercy Park North; New York, NY 10010; 212-533-7005.

Evaluation

A. Bathing and dressing without fatigue
B. Suctioning own secretions, lungs clear
C. Visiting with friends

◆ MUSCULAR DYSTROPHY

A group of genetically determined, progressive, degenerative myopathies affecting a variety of muscle groups.

Pathophysiology/Etiology

1. Inherited, may be X-linked.
2. Genetic coding defect causes abnormal muscle development and function.

Clinical Manifestations

Progressive muscular weakness (Table 13-2).

Diagnostic Evaluation

1. NCT and EMG show abnormalities.
2. Serum creatinine kinase (CK)—elevated.
3. Muscle biopsy—for definitive diagnosis.

TABLE 13-2 Clinical Manifestations of Muscular Dystrophies

Disorder	Genetics	Onset	Clinical Manifestations
Duchenne's muscular dystrophy	Autosomal recessive (X-linked)	3–6 years	Progressive weakness and atrophy of iliopsoas, gluteal, and quadriceps muscles; pseudohypertrophy of the calves; waddling gait, difficulty walking and climbing stairs; later, weakening of pretibial, pectoral girdle, and upper limbs; heart abnormalities; death due to pulmonary infections before 20 years
			Etiology: genetic defect in which gene coding for "dystrophin" is absent
Becker's muscular dystrophy	X-linked	11 years	Similar to Duchenne's dystrophy except that course is more benign; dystrophin is abnormal
Emery-Dreifuss syndrome	X-linked	Childhood-adulthood	Upper arm and pectoral girdle weakness; distal muscles spared; severe cardiomyopathy
Facioscapulohumeral dystrophy	Autosomal dominant	6–20 years	Inability to raise arms over head, close eyes firmly, and purse the lips; scapular winging; "Popeye" effect of arms (forearms large and upper arm slim)
Limb-girdle (scapulohumeral and pelvifemoral) dystrophy	X-linked; autosomal recessive		Facial muscles spared; absence of pseudohypertrophy of the calves
Progressive external ophthalmoplegia	Familial	Childhood	Ptosis and ophthalmoparesis without strabismus or diplopia
Oculopharyngeal dystrophy	Autosomal dominant	40–50 years	Bilateral ptosis and dysphagia
Myotonic dystrophy	Autosomal dominant; genetically linked to a marker on chromosome 19 with high penetrance	Third decade	Weakness of levator palpebrae, facial, masseter, pharyngeal, laryngeal muscles, sternomastoid (weakness results in "swan neck" deformity), forearm, hand, pretibial, and cardiac muscles; myotonia of muscles: can bring out with forced eyelid closure or clenching the fist
			Changes in nonmuscular tissues: frontal baldness, blue-green cataracts, testicular atrophy, increased insulin response to glucose
Congenital myotonic dystrophy		Birth	Profound hypotonia, facial diplegia, ptosis, tented upper lip and open jaw; difficulty in sucking and swallowing and respiratory distress
Late-onset distal muscular dystrophy (Milhorat and Wolff: Welander)	Autosomal dominant	Middle adult	Weakness and wasting of muscles of hands, forearms, and lower legs

From: Kelley WN (ed.) Essentials of Internal Medicine. Philadelphia: JB Lippincott, 1994.

Management

1. No specific treatment, but such medications as antiarrhythmics, anticonvulsants, and corticosteroids may be used to control manifestations.
2. Surgical tendon releasing to treat contractures.
3. Physical therapy to preserve function.

Complications

1. Infections (pulmonary, urinary, systemic)
2. Cardiac dysrhythmias
3. Respiratory insufficiency
4. Depression

Nursing Assessment

1. Assess muscle strength.
2. Determine respiratory status.
3. Evaluate ADL skills.

Nursing Diagnoses

A. Ineffective Breathing Pattern related to muscle weakness
B. Impaired Physical Mobility related to disease process
C. Decreased Cardiac Output related to cardiac muscle involvement
D. Impaired Swallowing related to muscle weakness
E. Diversional Activity Deficit related to weakness

Nursing Interventions

A. Maintaining Breathing Pattern
1. Encourage upright positioning to provide for maximum chest excursion.
2. Encourage energy-conservation techniques and avoidance of exertion.
3. Teach deep-breathing exercises to strengthen respiratory muscles.
4. Assess rate, depth, and pattern of respirations; listen to breath sounds; and report any change in condition
5. Note results of arterial blood gases, sputum cultures, and chest x-rays.
6. Encourage coughing and deep breathing or perform chest physiotherapy as indicated.

B. Preserving Optimal Motor Function
1. Refer to physical therapy for stretching and strengthening exercise to optimize remaining motor function.
2. Perform range-of-motion exercises to preserve mobility and prevent atrophy.
3. Schedule activity with consideration to energy highs throughout the day.
4. Consult with occupational therapist for assistive devices to maintain independence.
5. Apply braces and splints to prevent contractures.

C. Improving Cardiac Output
1. Monitor vital signs, cardiac rhythm, and signs of congestive heart failure, such as edema, adventitious breath sounds, and weight gain.
2. Monitor intake and output and maintain IV or oral fluid intake as ordered.

D. Monitoring Swallowing Function
1. Assess cranial nerve function for swallowing (gag reflex) and chewing.
2. Provide a diet that the patient can handle; blenderizing food may be necessary.
3. Encourage eating in upright position without talking and in small, more frequent meals.
4. Administer alternate enteral feeding if gag reflex is diminished.

E. Encouraging Diversional Activities
1. Encourage diversional activities that prevent overexertion and frustration, but discourage long periods of bed rest and inactivity, such as TV watching.
2. If upper extremities are mostly affected, suggest walking or riding a stationary bike; if lower extremities are mostly affected, encourage use of a wheelchair to promote mobility and performing simple crafts.
3. Discuss patient's interests and assist with preferred activities.
4. Investigate with the patient various methods of stress management to deal with frustration.
5. Administer analgesics and antidepressants as ordered to facilitate participation in activities.

Patient Education/ Health Maintenance

1. Encourage genetic counseling if indicated to determine options of family planning.
2. Instruct the patient and family in range-of-motion exercises, pulmonary care, and methods of transfer and locomotion.
3. Refer to community respite and counseling services.
4. Stress the importance of fluids to decrease risk of urinary/pulmonary infection.
5. Advise patient or family to report signs of respiratory infection immediately to obtain treatment and prevent congestive heart failure.
6. Refer patient/family to agencies such as: The Muscular Dystrophy Association; 3300 East Sunrise Drive; Tuscon, AZ 85718; 520-529-2000.

Evaluation

A. Respirations unlabored and deep with clear breath sounds
B. Ambulating unassisted, no contractures noted
C. Vital signs stable, no edema
D. Tolerating small blenderized feedings without aspiration
E. Out of bed most of day, doing puzzles, playing games

Trauma

◆ HEAD INJURY

Head injury, also known as brain injury, is the disruption of normal brain function due to trauma-related injury resulting in compromised neurologic function; classified as mild (Glasgow Coma Scale [GCS] 13-15 with loss of consciousness 0 to 15 minutes), moderate (GCS 9-12 with loss of consciousness for up to 6 hours), or severe (GCS 3-8 with loss of consciousness greater than 6 hours). May cause focal or diffuse symptoms. Also see Chapter 33, page 946, for emergency management of head injury.

Pathophysiology/Etiology

1. Types of brain injuries include concussion, cerebral contusion, brain stem contusion, epidural hematoma, subdural hematoma, and skull fracture.
2. Caused by blunt or penetrating injury.
3. Neurologic deficits result from shearing of white matter, ischemia and mass effect from hemorrhage, and cerebral edema of surrounding brain tissue.

Clinical Manifestations

1. Disturbances in consciousness: confusion to coma
2. Headache, vertigo
3. Agitation, restlessness
4. Respiratory irregularities
5. Cognitive deficits
6. Pupillary abnormalities
7. Sudden onset of neurologic deficit

Diagnostic Evaluation

1. CT scan to identify and localize lesions, edema, bleeding.
2. Skull and cervical spine films to identify fracture, displacement.

3. Neuropsychologic tests during rehabilitation phase to determine cognitive deficits.

Management

1. Management of increased ICP.
2. Antibiotics to prevent infection with open skull fractures or penetrating wounds.
3. Surgery for evacuation of intracranial hematomas, debridement of penetrating wounds, elevation of skull fractures, or repair of CSF leaks.

Complications

1. Infections; systemic (respiratory, urinary), neurologic (meningitis, ventriculitis).
2. Increased ICP, hydrocephalus.
3. Posttraumatic seizure disorder.
4. Permanent neurologic deficits: cognitive, motor, sensory, speech.
5. Neurobehavioral alterations; impulsivity, uninhibited aggression, emotional lability.

Nursing Assessment

1. Monitor for signs of increased ICP—altered level of consciousness, abnormal pupil responses, vomiting, increased pulse pressure, bradycardia, hyperthermia.
2. Observe for CSF leakage.
3. Note contusions about eyes and ears.
4. Perform cranial nerve, motor, sensory, and reflex assessment.

NURSING ALERT:
Regard every patient who has a brain injury as having a potential spinal cord injury. A significant number of patients are under the influence of alcohol at the time of injury, which may mask the nature and severity of the injury.

Nursing Diagnoses

A. Altered Cerebral Tissue Perfusion related to increased ICP
B. Ineffective Breathing Pattern related to increased ICP or brain stem injury
C. Altered Nutrition, Less Than Body Requirements related to compromised neurologic function and stress of injury
D. Altered Thought Processes related to physiology of injury
E. Risk for Injury related to altered thought processes
F. Ineffective Family Coping related to unpredictability of outcome

Nursing Interventions

A. *Maintaining Adequate Cerebral Perfusion*
1. Maintain a patent airway.

2. Monitor ICP (see p. 371).
3. Monitor results of serial serum and urine electrolyte and osmolality studies to maintain the level of dehydration ordered to reduce cerebral edema.
4. Restrict fluid intake if needed to avoid increased ICP.
5. Monitor central venous pressure or Swan-Ganz measurements to guide fluid replacement.
6. Administer IV solutions slowly to avoid overhydration and cerebral edema.
7. Insert urethral catheter to measure urinary output.

B. *Maintaining Respiration*
1. Monitor respiratory rate, depth, and pattern of respirations; report any abnormal pattern, such as Cheyne-Stokes respirations or periods of apnea.
2. Assist with intubation and ventilatory assistance if needed.
3. Turn patient every 2 hours and assist with coughing and deep breathing.
4. Suction patient as needed, however, hyperventilate the patient before suctioning to prevent hypoxia.

C. *Meeting Nutritional Needs*
1. Provide nasogastric feedings once bowel sounds have returned if patient is unable to swallow; elevate the head of the bed after feedings and check residuals to prevent aspiration. Feed the patient as soon as possible after a head injury and administer H_2 blocking agents to prevent gastric ulceration and hemorrhage from gastric acid hypersecretion.
2. Consult with dietitian to provide the increased calories and nitrogen requirement resulting from the metabolic changes of brain injury

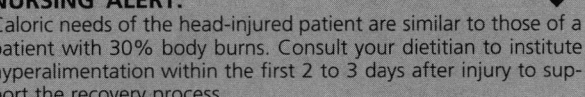

NURSING ALERT:
Caloric needs of the head-injured patient are similar to those of a patient with 30% body burns. Consult your dietitian to institute hyperalimentation within the first 2 to 3 days after injury to support the recovery process.

3. Administer IV hyperalimentation as ordered.
4. During rehabilitation, recognize the dysphagic patient and encourage oral feeding of soft or pureed foods in an unhurried manner. Refer to speech or physical therapist as indicated for feeding difficulties.

D. *Promoting Cognitive Function*
1. Provide stimulation of all sensory avenues.
2. Observe patient for fatigue or restlessness from overstimulation.
3. Use meaningful stimulation.
4. Involve family in sensory stimulation program.
5. Provide frequent concrete orientation information.
6. Refer patient for cognitive retraining if appropriate.

E. *Preventing Injury*
1. Instruct the family regarding the behavioral phases of recovery from brain injury, such as restlessness and combativeness.
2. Investigate for physical sources of restlessness, such as uncomfortable position, signs of urinary tract infection, or pressure sore development.
3. Reassure patient and family during periods of agitation and irrational behavior.
4. Pad side rails, and wrap hands in mitts if patient is agitated. Maintain constant vigilance and avoid restraints if possible.

5. Keep environmental stimuli to a minimum.
6. Provide adequate light if patient is hallucinating.
7. Perform passive range-of-motion exercises to release muscle tension from inactivity.
8. Avoid sedatives to avoid medication induced-confusion and altered states of cognition.

F. Strengthening Family Coping
1. Refer family to community support services, such as respite care.
2. Assist the family members to establish stress management techniques that can be integrated into their lifestyle, such as ventilation of feelings, use of respite care, relaxation techniques.
3. Consult with social worker or psychologist to assist the family in adjusting to patient's permanent neurologic deficits.
4. Help the family assist the patient to recognize current progress and not focus on limitations.

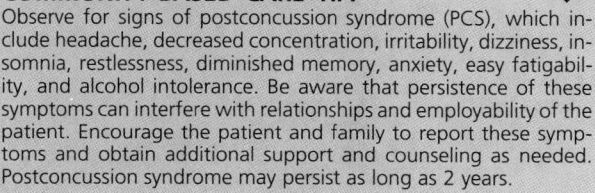

COMMUNITY-BASED CARE TIP:
Observe for signs of postconcussion syndrome (PCS), which include headache, decreased concentration, irritability, dizziness, insomnia, restlessness, diminished memory, anxiety, easy fatigability, and alcohol intolerance. Be aware that persistence of these symptoms can interfere with relationships and employability of the patient. Encourage the patient and family to report these symptoms and obtain additional support and counseling as needed. Postconcussion syndrome may persist as long as 2 years.

Patient Education/ Health Maintenance

1. Review with the family the signs of increased ICP.
2. Reinforce the lability of cognitive, language, and physical functioning of the person with brain injury and the lengthy recovery period.
3. Teach the family therapeutic use of touch, massage, and music to calm the agitated patient.
4. Refer the patient/family to agencies such as: National Head Injury Foundation; Suite 100, 1776 Massachusetts Avenue NW; Washington, DC 20036; 202-296-6443.

Evaluation

A. ICP stable
B. Respirations 24, regular
C. Tube feedings tolerated well without residual
D. Oriented to person, place, and time
E. Less agitated; side rails maintained
F. Family reports using respite care

◆ SPINAL CORD INJURY

Spinal cord injury is a traumatic injury to the spinal cord that may vary from a mild cord concussion with transient numbness to immediate and permanent quadriplegia. The most common sites are the cervical areas C-5, C-6, and C-7 and the junction of the thoracic and lumbar vertebrae; T-12, L-1. Injury to the spinal cord may result in loss of function below the level of cord injury.

Also see Chapter 33, page 947, for emergency management of spinal cord injury.

Pathophysiology/Etiology

1. Extent of injury varies from transient concussion or contusion to laceration and compression to complete transection of the cord.
2. Interruption of function is due to ischemia, edema, and hemorrhage that lead to an irreversible cycle.
3. Caused by mechanical displacement of the vertebral column through trauma that impinges on the spinal cord and or its nerve roots.

Clinical Manifestations

Clinical manifestations vary and are dependent on the location and severity of cord damage. In general, complete transection causes all loss of function below the level of the lesion (Fig. 13-4), and incomplete cord damage results in a variety of regional deficits (Table 13-3).

Diagnostic Evaluation

1. X-ray of spinal column to include open mouth studies for adequate visualization of C-1 and C-2.
2. MRI of spine—to detect soft tissue injury, hemorrhage, edema, bony injury.
3. Electrophysiologic monitoring to determine function of neural pathways.

Management

Requires a multidisciplinary approach because of multiple systems involvement and injuries.

A. Immediate Posttrauma (less than 1 hour)
1. Immobilization should include head, body, and hips.
2. Methylprednisolone (Solu-Medrol) IV except if patient is allergic or pregnant.

B. Acute Phase (1 to 24 hours)
1. Maintenance of pulmonary and cardiovascular stability.
   a. Intubation and mechanical ventilation if needed.
   b. Diaphragmatic pacing with electrical stimulation.
2. Ensure perfusion of spinal cord with restoration of blood pressure.
   a. Administration of naloxone (Narcan) and local cooling of the cord.
   b. Continue methylprednisolone infusion.
   c. Foley inserted.

C. Subacute Phase (within 1 week)
1. H2 receptor blockers to prevent gastric irritation and hemorrhage.
2. Small doses of heparin to reduce risk of thrombophlebitis and pulmonary emboli.
3. Hyperalimentation to retard negative nitrogen balance.
4. Stabilize vertebral column and ligamentous injuries through traction or surgical intervention (Fig. 13-5).

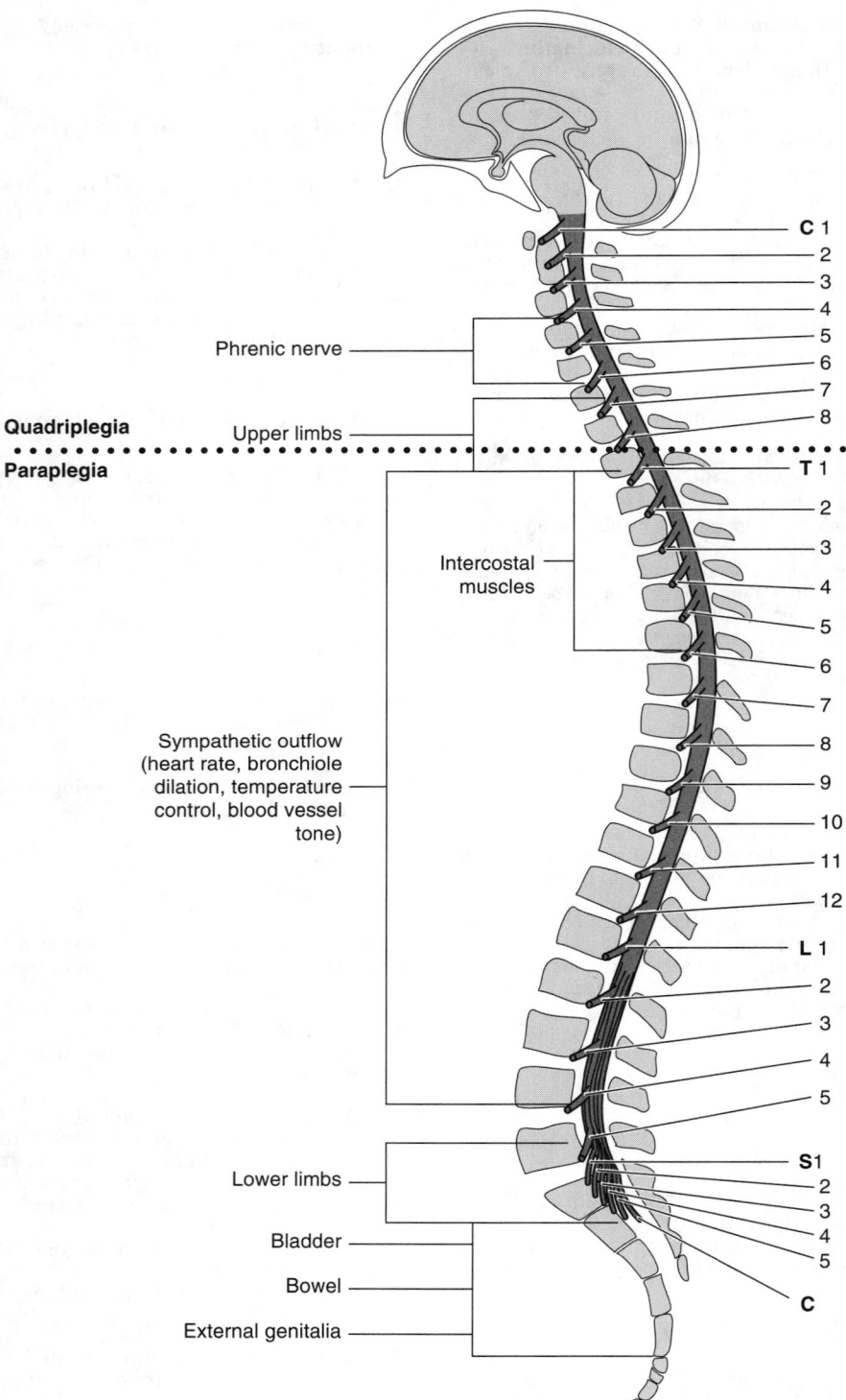

FIGURE 13-4 Levels of spinal cord innervation.

TABLE 13-3 Incomplete Cord Syndromes

Lesion	Mechanism of Injury	Preserved	Impaired
Anterior cord syndrome (dorsal columns of the spinal cord are spared)	Flexion	Light touch Vibratory sensation Proprioception	Motor function Pain and temperature sensation
Posterior cord syndrome (anterior columns of the cord are spared)	Extension	Motor function Pain and temperature sensation	Light touch Vibratory sensation Proprioception
Central cord syndrome (central gray matter of the cord is injured)	Flexion or extension	Motor function of lower extremities	Motor function of upper extremities
Brown-Séquard syndrome (hemisection of the cord)	Penetrating trauma	Contralateral—pain and temperature sensation Ipsilateral—movement, light touch, proprioception	Contralateral—movement, light touch, proprioception Ipsilateral—pain and temperature

(Neff J., Kidd P. [1993]. *Trauma Nursing: The Art and Science.* Chicago: Mosby.)

D. Chronic Phase (beyond 1 week)
Rehabilitation to include medical support, physical therapy, urologic evaluation, occupational therapy.

Complications

1. Spinal shock noted by loss of all reflex, motor, sensory and autonomic activity below the level of the lesion
2. Respiratory insufficiency
3. Cardiac arrest
4. Thromboembolic complications
5. Infections—respiratory, urinary, pressure sores, sepsis
6. Autonomic dysreflexia—exaggerated autonomic responses to stimuli below the level of the lesion in patients with lesions at or above T-6

Nursing Assessment

1. Perform frequent motor and sensory function assessment of trunk and extremities—extent of deficits may widen due to edema and hemorrhage.
2. Assess vital signs to determine degree of autonomic dysfunction.
3. Assess rectal sphincter tone to determine bowel and bladder function.
4. Perform psychosocial assessment to evaluate motivation, support network, financial or other problems.
5. Assess for indicators of powerlessness, including verbal expression of no control over situation, depression, nonparticipation, dependence on others, passivity.

Nursing Diagnoses

A. Ineffective Breathing Pattern related to paralysis of respiratory muscles or diaphragm
B. Impaired Physical Mobility related to motor dysfunction
C. Risk for Impaired Skin Integrity related to immobility
D. Urinary Retention related to inability to void spontaneously
E. Constipation related to lack of bowel control
F. Risk for Injury related to autonomic dysfunction
G. Powerlessness related to loss of function, long rehabilitation

Nursing Interventions

A. **Attaining an Adequate Breathing Pattern**
1. For patients with high-level lesions, continuously monitor respirations and maintain a patent airway. Be prepared to intubate if respiratory fatigue or arrest occur.
2. Frequently assess cough and vital capacity. Teach effective coughing if able (Box 13-2).
3. Provide adequate fluids and humidification of inspired air to loosen secretions.
4. Suction as needed; observe vagal response (bradycardia—should be temporary).
5. When appropriate, implement chest physiotherapy regimen to assist pulmonary drainage and prevent infection.
6. Monitor results of arterial blood gases, chest x-ray, and sputum cultures.

B. **Avoiding Complications of Immobility**
1. Transfer the patient to a turning table or rotating bed when stable.
2. Position patient in proper alignment.
3. Perform range-of-motion exercises to prevent contractures and maintain rehabilitation potential.
4. Monitor blood pressure with position change in the patient with lesions above midthoracic area to prevent orthostatic hypotension.
5. Encourage physical therapy and practicing of exercises as tolerated.
6. Encourage weight-bearing activity to prevent osteoporosis and risk of kidney stones.
7. Apply elastic support hose and administer anticoagulants as ordered to reduce the risk of thrombophlebitis.

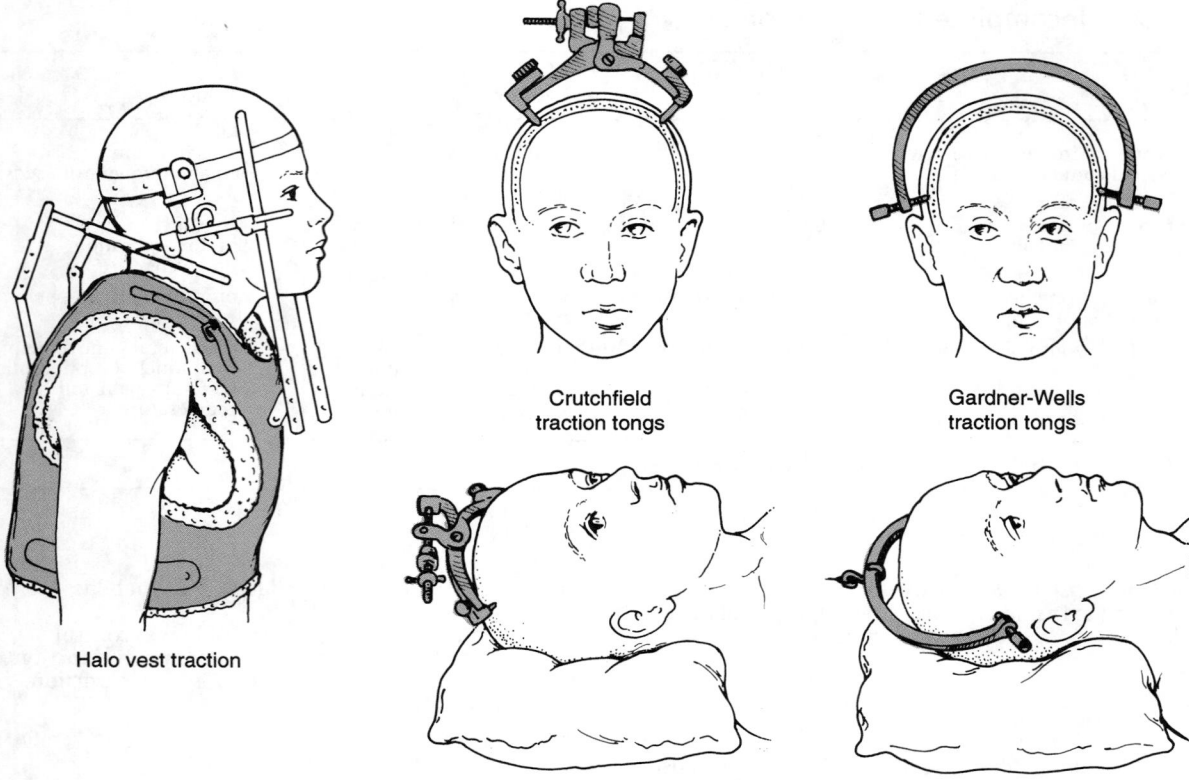

Crutchfield
traction tongs

Gardner-Wells
traction tongs

Halo vest traction

Cervical spine injuries are managed with immediate immobilization, early reduction, and stabilization of the vertebral column. Cervical traction with either skeletal tongs or a halo-vest device accomplishes these goals.

A. Skeletal Tongs

1. Crutchfield and Vinke tongs require predrilled holes in the skull under local anesthesia; Gardner-Wells and Heifitz tongs do not.
2. Weight is added to traction gradually to accomplish reduction of vertebral fracture, then enough weight is kept to maintain vertebral alignment.
3. Make sure that tongs are several inches from the head of the bed and weights hang freely.
4. To care for a patient in skeletal tongs, inspect tong sites for signs of infection; shave hair around sites as needed; cleanse the sites with povidone-iodine (Betadine) solution or other antiseptic; and check back of head for signs of pressure and massage the head periodically without moving neck.

B. Halo-Vest Devices

1. A halo ring is fixed to the skull by 4 pins and connected to a removable vest by a metal frame.

2. The halo ring may initially be connected to bed traction or may be applied after tongs are removed; the vest is used to attain mobility.
3. To care for a patient in a vest, inspect skin under the vest; encourage position changes frequently, including the prone position to relieve pressure; wash and dry skin well through side openings; avoid using powder under vest, which causes friction and possibly pressure sores; turn the patient and vest as a unit; and make sure a vest wrench is taped to the front of the vest for quick release if CPR is required.
4. To provide halo care, cleanse pin sites daily and observe for redness, drainage, and tenderness; observe for loosening of pins and stabilize the patient's head while notifying surgeon if pin becomes detached; provide assistance with activities, because the patient is top heavy and cannot scan the environment easily; and provide emotional support to help patient adjust to bizarre appearance.

FIGURE **13-5** *Cervical traction.*

C. *Protecting Skin Integrity*

1. Pay special attention to pressure points when repositioning patient.
2. Inspect for pressure sore development every 2 hours when turning patient, including the back of head, ears, heels, and elbows.
3. Keep skin clean and dry and well lubricated.

D. *Promoting Urinary Elimination*

1. Use intermittent catheterization rather than an indwelling catheter as soon as possible to minimize risk of infection; however, avoid overdistention of the bladder.
2. If reflex voiding is present, monitor for urinary retention by percussing the suprapubic area for dullness or catheterizing for residual urine after voiding.

BOX 13-2 *Performing the Quad Cough*

Many patients with incomplete or low cervical transection of the spinal cord have an impairment of the diaphragmatic and intercostal muscles. The result is a weak or ineffective cough. To increase the mechanical effectiveness of the patient's cough, perform or teach the following procedure to a significant other:

1. Place the patient in supine, low semi-Fowler's position.
2. Place the heels of your hands, one on top of the other, in the center of the abdomen, above the navel and below tip of the sternum (similar to position used for obstructed airway in an unconscious patient).
3. Have the patient hyperventilate and exhale once or twice, on your instruction. Allow your hands to move with the patient.
4. At the next breath, on your instruction, have the patient take a deep breath and cough while exhaling. As patient coughs, thrust your hands forward and down (similar to obstructed airway maneuver) to add power to the diaphragm activity.
5. Allow one or two normal breaths and repeat the procedure once or twice more. Nursing Alert: Avoid excessive depth of your thrust maneuver to prevent injury.

3. Monitor intake and output.
4. Increase fluid intake to prevent infection.
5. Train the patient in reflex voiding by encouraging fluids at 2-hour intervals during the day and applying pressure to suprapubic area one-half hour later in attempt to void. Avoid fluids in the evening to prevent dribbling and overdistention at night.

E. Promoting Bowel Activity
1. Assess bowel sounds and note abdominal distention. Paralytic ileus is common immediately after injury.
2. Initiate nasogastric suction if necessary.
3. Encourage intake of high-calorie, high-protein, and high-fiber diet when bowel sounds return and food is tolerated.
4. Assess for loose stool oozing from rectum and perform rectal exam to check for fecal impaction; remove fecal matter if necessary.
5. Institute a bowel program as early as possible.
   a. Have the patient attempt to defecate at same time every day, usually after a meal.
   b. Help stimulate defecation by inserting a glycerin suppository into rectum.
   c. Have patient assume a sitting position and lean forward to increase intraabdominal pressure.

F. Controlling Autonomic Dysreflexia
1. Protect the patient from possible stimuli for autonomic dysreflexia.
   a. Bowel or bladder distention caused by fecal impaction, urinary retention, or a kinked indwelling catheter.
   b. Abnormal skin stimulation, such as lying on wrinkled sheets, hot or cold stimulation, or pain from constricting clothing.
   c. Distention or contraction of visceral organs such as gastric distention or emptying an overdistended bladder too fast.
   d. Infection, especially of the urinary tract.

2. Be alert to signs of autonomic dysreflexia, such as pounding headache, profuse sweating, nasal congestion, piloerection (goosebumps), bradycardia, and severe hypertension.
3. If autonomic dysreflexia does occur, immediately place the patient in a sitting position to help lower the blood pressure and diminish ICP.
4. Remove possible causative stimuli.
5. Administer antihypertensive medication as ordered.
6. Monitor blood pressure every 3 to 5 minutes until return to normal.

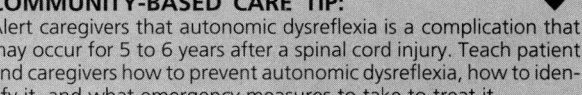

COMMUNITY-BASED CARE TIP:
Alert caregivers that autonomic dysreflexia is a complication that may occur for 5 to 6 years after a spinal cord injury. Teach patient and caregivers how to prevent autonomic dysreflexia, how to identify it, and what emergency measures to take to treat it.

G. Empowering Patient
1. Explain all procedures to the patient. Answer any questions.
2. Allow patient to make modifications to treatment plan when possible.
3. Schedule procedures and planning sessions when patient is rested and experiencing decreased anxiety.
4. Praise patient for accomplishments; minimize deficits.
5. Discuss stress management techniques, such as relaxation therapy, counseling, and problem solving.
6. Identify motivating factors and priorities with the patient.

Patient Education/ Health Maintenance

1. Teach patient and family about the physiology of nerve transmission and how spinal injury has affected normal function.
2. Reinforce that rehabilitation is lengthy and involves compliance with therapy to increase function.
3. Explain that spasticity may develop 2 weeks to 3 months after injury and may interfere with routine care and ADLs. Spasticity should be managed by:
   a. Maintaining calm, stress-free environment.
   b. Allowing plenty of time for activities such as positioning and transferring.
   c. Performing joint range-of-motion exercises with slow, smooth movements.
   d. Avoiding temperature extremes.
   e. Administering muscle relaxants such as diazepam (Valium), baclofen (Lioresal), and dantrolene (Dantrium) as prescribed.
4. Teach patient to protect skin from pressure sore development by frequent repositioning while in bed, weight-shifting and lift-offs every 15 minutes while in a wheelchair, and avoidance of shear forces and friction.
5. Teach inspection of skin daily for development of pressure sores, using a mirror if necessary.
6. Encourage sexual counseling, if indicated, to promote satisfaction in personal relationships.
   a. Women with spinal cord injuries experience little sensation during sexual intercourse, but fertility and ability to bear children are usually not affected.
   b. Men with spinal cord injuries may consider implantation of a penile prosthesis to obtain an erection.

Evaluation

A. Respirations adequate, arterial blood gases within normal limits
B. Repositioning hourly, no orthostatic changes
C. No evidence of pressure sores
D. Reflex voiding without retention
E. Passed soft stool following glycerin suppository
F. No episodes of autonomic dysreflexia
G. Patient verbalizes feeling of control over condition

◆ PERIPHERAL NERVE INJURY

Peripheral nerve injuries result from laceration, contusion, stretch, missile, crush, or penetration type of forces. Mechanisms of injury include gunshot and stab wounds, falls, and car accidents. Partial amputation may occur. Nerve injuries are classified according to the Sunderland system, which helps determine the need for surgery:

Grade	Description	Surgery
I	Loss of axonal conduction	No
II	Loss of axonal continuity	No
III	Loss of axonal and endoneural continuity	Yes if severe
IV	Loss of perineural continuity & fascial disruption	Yes; graft if needed
V	Loss of continuity of entire nerve trunk	Yes; graft usually needed

Pathophysiology/Etiology

1. Axonal changes are complete within 48 hours of injury. By the 4th day, conduction is lost.
2. Peripheral nerves respond to mild injury by local demyelination that can produce a conduction block of sensory or motor function. Deficits are reversible.
3. More severe injuries produce axonal interruption, wallerian degeneration resulting in distal axonal and myelin loss, and empty endoneural tubes.
4. Axonal and wallerian degeneration are completed by approximately 2 weeks after injury.
5. The rate of axon regeneration is approximately 1 mm/day. Muscle must be reinnervated within 18 months of injury for functional outcome. Sensory function can return years after injury. Lesions of the upper trunk generally have a better regeneration prognosis than injuries of the lower trunk because of the shorter distance to the endoneural tube to be covered by the regenerating cells.

Clinical Manifestations

1. Flaccid paralysis
2. Absence of deep tendon reflexes
3. Atonic/hypotonic muscles
4. Progressive muscle atrophy
5. Fasciculations peak 2 to 3 weeks after injury
6. Trophic changes: skin is warm and dry 3 weeks after injury, then becomes cold and cyanotic with loss of hair, brittle fingernails, and ulceration development

7. Causalgia (chronic pain syndrome)
8. Specifics to area affected:
   a. Radial nerve injury—weakness in extension, possible wrist drop, inability to grasp objects/make a fist, impaired sensation over posterior forearm and dorsum of the hand
   b. Brachial plexus—difficulty in abduction of shoulder, weakness with supination and flexion of the forearm (upper trunk) or extension of the forearm (middle trunk) or paralysis and atrophy of small muscles of the hand (lower trunk)
   c. Median and ulnar nerve injuries—sensory (median nerve) and motor (ulnar) loss of function in the hand (pronation, opposition of thumb, paralysis of finer flexor muscles)
   d. Femoral—weakness of knee and hip extension, atrophy of quadriceps, absence of knee jerk, loss of sensation of anterior aspect of the thigh
   e. Common peroneal—footdrop, sensory loss on dorsum of foot, difficulty with eversion
   f. Sciatic—footdrop, pain across gluteus and thigh, loss of knee flexion, weakness/paralysis of muscles below knee

Diagnostic Evaluation

1. EMG—to detect if muscle is innervated
2. Tinel's sign (tapping the axons of the regenerating nerve produces a paraesthesia in the normal distribution of the nerve) to determine rate of axonal regeneration

Management

1. Debridement and surgical anastomosis if indicated.
2. Dextran to decrease intravascular thrombus formation in the affected extremity.
3. Corticosteroids to decrease swelling (or an osmotic diuretic if severe).
4. Splinting, casting depending on accompanying tissue trauma.

Complications

1. Infection
2. Compartment syndrome
3. Loss of anastomosis

Nursing Assessment

1. Perform frequent neurovascular checks of the affected extremity (sensation, motor function, pulses, temperature, capillary refill, degree of swelling).
2. Assess degree of pain.
3. Test reflexes of affected extremity.

Nursing Diagnoses

A. Sensory/Perceptual Alteration (Tactile) related to injury
B. Pain related to injury
C. Risk for Infection secondary to tissue disruption

Nursing Interventions

A. *Optimizing Sensory and Motor Function*
1. Administer corticosteroids and diuretics as ordered to decrease swelling and development of compartment syndrome.
2. Keep extremity elevated to promote venous drainage.
3. Perform neurovascular check to evaluate status of injury.
   a. Incorporate Tinel's sign into assessment.
   b. Report any changes in condition.

B. *Promoting Comfort*
1. Administer and teach self-administration of analgesics as ordered.
2. Elevate extremity.
3. Avoid exposure of denerved areas to temperature extremes.
4. Apply such devices as splints and slings as ordered.
5. Maintain mobility with range-of-motion exercises. Perform gently and after administration of analgesics.

C. *Preventing Infection*
1. Assess wound and dressing frequently for erythema, warmth, swelling, odor, and drainage.
2. Monitor temperature with vital signs for hyperthermia and tachycardia indicating infection.
3. Encourage deep-breathing exercises and ambulation to prevent pulmonary complications.

Patient Education/ Health Maintenance

1. Teach management of wound and dressing.
2. Review analgesia schedule and need for elevation of injured area.
3. Teach exercises for involved area.
4. Suggest assistive devices to promote independence.
5. Stress the importance of complying with long-term rehabilitation, physical therapy, and follow-up evaluations.

Evaluation

A. Stable neurovascular status
B. Patient reports adequate relief of pain
C. Wound/surgical site is free of erythema, drainage, odor

Central Nervous System Tumors

◆ BRAIN TUMORS

A brain tumor is a localized intracranial neoplasm that occupies space within the skull and tends to cause a rise in ICP.

Pathophysiology/Etiology

1. May originate in the CNS or metastasize from tumors elsewhere in the body.

2. May be benign or malignant; all produce effects of space-occupying lesion (edema, increased ICP). Malignancy may be related not to cell type or invasiveness, but rather to location and inoperability.
3. May arise from any tissue of the CNS.
   a. Astrocytoma—arising from connective tissue of the brain (astrocytes); highly invasive, poorly margined; Grades 1 and 2.
   b. Glioblastoma—Grade 3 and 4 astrocytomas.
   c. Oligodendrogliomas—arise from the frontal and temporal lobes of the cerebrum.
   d. Colloid cysts—develop within lateral or third ventricles.
   e. Meningioma—arising from linings of the brain.
   f. Acoustic neuroma—develops in or on the eighth cranial nerve.
   g. Metastatic lesions—commonly from lung and breast cancer, usually multiple and unresectable.
   h. Tumors of the ductless glands—pituitary or pineal.
   i. Hemangioma—angioma from blood vessels of the brain.
   j. Congenital tumors

Clinical Manifestations

Depend on tumor location and biologic nature of the tumor. If the tumor is in a noneloquent area of the brain or slow growing, specific symptoms may not develop until the late stages of the process. Instead, the tumor may produce generalized symptoms related to the increasing size of the tumor and the expanding area of cerebral edema surrounding the margins of the tumor. This is referred to as the "mass" effect of the tumor.

1. Generalized symptoms (due to increased ICP)—headache (especially in the morning), vomiting, papilledema, malaise, altered cognition and consciousness.
2. Focal neurologic deficits (related to region of tumor):
   a. Parietal area—motor or sensory alterations, speech and memory disturbances, visuospatial deficits.
   b. Frontal lobe—personality changes, contralateral motor weakness, Broca's aphasia.
   c. Temporal area—memory disturbances, auditory hallucinations, Wernicke's aphasia, complex partial seizures, visual field deficits.
   d. Occipital area—visual agnosia and visual field deficits
   e. Cerebellar area—coordination, gait, and balance disturbances.
   f. Brain stem—dysphagia, incontinence, cardiovascular instability, cranial nerve dysfunction.
   g. Hypothalamus—loss of temperature control, diabetes insipidus.
   h. Pituitary/sella turcica—visual field deficits, amenorrhea, galactorrhea, impotence, cushingoid symptoms.
3. Referred symptoms (related to the vasogenic edema of the tumor presence)—usually present symptoms of ischemia of region distal to the actual lesion.

Diagnostic Evaluation

1. CT/MRI scan—shows tumor, edema, shift of structures due to mass effect.
2. EEG—detects locus of irritability.

3. Stereotactic biopsy/surgery—needed for definitive diagnosis, cell type.

Management

Effectiveness of treatment depends on tumor type and location, capsulation, or infiltrative status. Tumors in vital areas, such as the brain stem, or nonencapsulated and infiltrating tumors may not be surgically accessible, and treatment may produce severe neurologic deficits (blindness, paralysis, mental impairment). Treatment is usually multimodal.

1. Surgery, including stereotaxic resection, with preceding corticosteroid and anticonvulsant therapy.
2. Radiation therapy.
  a. Whole brain after scalp incision heals; may cause brain edema and delayed necrosis.
  b. Brachytherapy—can use radioisotopes implanted directly into tumor to permit high doses.
3. Chemotherapy with single or combination drug therapy; may require autologous bone marrow transplantation (aspirated before chemotherapy and reinfused afterward to treat bone marrow depression).
4. Laser resection (CO_2 or Nd:YAG).
5. Ultrasonic aspiration

Complications

1. Increased ICP and brain herniation.
2. Neurologic deficits from expanding tumor or treatment.

Nursing Assessment

1. Assess vital signs and signs of increased ICP (see p. 369).
2. Assess cranial nerves.
3. Assess behavior, affect, mental status.

Nursing Diagnoses

A. Pain related to brain mass, surgical intervention
B. Risk for Injury related to altered level of consciousness, possible seizures, and sensory and motor deficits
C. Anxiety related to diagnosis, surgery, radiation, and/or chemotherapy

Nursing Interventions

A. *Relieving Pain*
1. Provide analgesics as ordered and required.
2. Maintain the head of the bed at 15 to 30 degrees to reduce cerebral venous congestion.
3. Provide a darkened room or sunglasses if the patient is photophobic.
4. Maintain a quiet environment to increase patient's pain tolerance.
5. Provide scheduled rest periods to help patient recuperate from stress of pain.

6. Instruct the patient to lie with the operative side up.
7. Alter diet as tolerated if patient has pain on chewing.

B. *Preventing Injury*
1. Report any signs of increased ICP or worsening condition immediately.
2. Pad the side rails of the bed to prevent injury if seizures occur.
3. Maintain availability of medications for management of status epilepticus (see p. 410).
4. If the patient is dysphagic or unconscious, elevate the head of the bed 15 to 30 degrees and position patient's head to the side to prevent aspiration.
5. If dysphagic, position the patient upright and instruct in sequenced swallowing to maintain feeding function.
6. Maintain oxygen and suction at the bedside in case of aspiration.
7. For the patient with visual field deficits, place materials in visual field.
8. Teach the patient with hemianopsia to scan to the "other side" and place weak extremities in safe position when moving in bed or chair.
9. Provide appropriate care and teaching for patient receiving chemotherapy (see p. 102).
10. Provide appropriate care and teaching for the patient receiving radiation (see p. 111).
11. Provide routine postoperative care for the patient undergoing craniotomy (see p. 373).

C. *Minimizing Anxiety*
1. Provide a safe environment in which the patient may verbalize anxieties.
2. Answer questions and provide written information.
3. Include the patient/family in all treatment options and scheduling.
4. Introduce stress management techniques.
5. Assess the patient's usual coping behaviors and provide support in these areas.
6. Consult with social worker for community resources.

Patient Education/ Health Maintenance

1. Explain the side effects of treatment.
2. Encourage close follow-up after diagnosis and treatment.
3. Explain the importance of continuing corticosteroids and how to manage side effects, such as weight gain and hyperglycemia.
4. Encourage the use of community resources for physical and psychological support, such as transportation to medical appointments, financial assistance, respite care.
5. Refer the patient/family to: The American Brain Tumor Society; 3725 North Talman Avenue; Chicago, IL 60618.

Evaluation

A. Patient reports satisfactory comfort level
B. No injuries reported
C. Patient and family verbalize understanding of treatment and available resources

◆ TUMORS OF THE SPINAL CORD AND CANAL

Tumors of the spinal cord and canal may be extradural (existing outside the dural membranes) and of metastatic origin; intradural–extramedullary (within the subarachnoid space), including meningiomas and schwannomas; or intramedullary (within the spinal cord), including astrocytomas, ependymomas, and oligodendrogliomas.

Pathophysiology/Etiology

1. Cause for abnormal cell growth is unknown.
2. Extradural tumors spread to the vertebral bodies.
3. Spinal cord and/or nerve compression results.

Clinical Manifestations

Depends on location and type of tumor.

1. Pain that is localized or radiates
2. Weakness of extremity with abnormal reflexes
3. Sensory changes
4. Bladder dysfunction

Diagnostic Evaluation

1. MRI—shows tumor
2. Myelography—may be performed before surgery

Management

1. Surgical excision of tumor, if possible.
2. Laminectomy and decompression if tumor cannot be excised, followed by radiation.

Complications

1. Spinal cord infarction
2. Persistent tumor
3. Hydrocephalus
4. Infection

Nursing Assessment

1. Perform motor and sensory components of the neurologic exam.
2. Assess pain.
3. Assess autonomic nervous system relative to level of lesion—pupillary responses, vital signs, bowel and bladder function.

Nursing Diagnoses

A. Anxiety related to surgery and outcome
B. Pain related to nerve compression
C. Sensory/Perceptual Alteration (Tactile, Kinesthetic) related to nerve compression
D. Altered Urinary Elimination related spinal cord compression

Nursing Interventions

A. *Relieving Anxiety*
1. Provide a safe environment for patient to verbalize anxieties.
2. Provide explanations regarding all procedures. Answer all questions.
3. Refer to cancer and spinal cord lesion support groups as needed.
4. Provide the patient/family with written information regarding disease process and medical interventions.
5. Reduce environment stimulation.
6. Promote periods of rest to enhance coping skills.
7. Involve the family in distraction techniques.
8. Provide options in care when possible.

B. *Relieving Pain*
1. Administer analgesics as needed and as ordered.
2. Instruct the patient in the use of patient control analgesia, if available.
3. Instruct the patient in relaxation techniques, such as deep breathing, distraction, imagery.
4. Position patient off surgical site postoperatively.

C. *Compensating for Sensory Alterations*
1. Reassure patient that degree of sensory/motor impairment may decrease during the postoperative recovery period as the amount of surgical edema decreases.
2. Instruct the patient with sensory loss to visually scan the extremity during use to avoid injury related to lack of tactile input.
3. Instruct the patient with painful paresthesias in appropriate use of ice, exercise, or rest.
4. Assess the patient with sensory and motor alterations and refer to physical therapy for assistance with ADLs, ambulation.

D. *Achieving Urinary Continence*
1. Assess the urinary elimination pattern of the patient.
2. Instruct the patient in the therapeutic intake of fluid volume and relationship to elimination.
3. Instruct the patient in an appropriate means of urinary continence control, such as self-catheterization, diapers, Credé's massage.
4. Monitor intake and output.
5. Assess for urinary retention by percussing the bladder for dullness and/or catheterizing for residual after voiding.

E. *Additional Postoperative Care*
1. Provide routine postoperative care to prevent complications.
2. Monitor surgical site for bleeding, CSF drainage, signs of infection.
3. Keep surgical dressing clean and dry.
4. Cleanse surgical site as ordered.
5. Pad the bed rails and chair if the patient experiences numbness or paresthesias, to prevent injury.
6. Support the weak/paralytic extremity in a functional position.

Patient Education/ Health Maintenance

1. Encourage the patient with motor impairment to use adaptive devices.
2. Demonstrate proper positioning and transfer techniques.
3. Instruct the patient with sensory losses about dangers of extreme temperatures and the need for adequate foot protection at all times.

Evaluation

A. Asking questions, seeking support group
B. Reports that pain is relieved
C. Patient is integrating management of neurologic deficits into lifestyle
D. Voiding at intervals without residual

Other Disorders

◆ SEIZURE DISORDERS

Seizures (also known as epileptic seizures and, if recurrent, epilepsy) are thought to result from disturbances in the cells of the brain that cause them to give off abnormal, recurrent, uncontrolled electrical discharges.

Pathophysiology/Etiology

A. *Altered Physiology*
1. The pathophysiology of seizures is unknown. It is known, however, that the brain has certain metabolic needs for oxygen and glucose. Neurons also have certain permeability gradients and voltage gradients that are affected by changes in the chemical and humoral environment.
2. Factors that change the permeability of the cell population (ischemia, hemorrhage) and ion concentration (Na+, K+) can produce neurons that are hyperexcitable and demonstrate hypersynchrony, producing an abnormal discharge.

B. *Classification*
Seizures are classified by the origin of the seizure activity and associated clinical manifestations.

1. Anything the brain can do as a normal function, it can do as seizure behavior.
2. Simple partial seizures can have motor, somatosensory, psychic or autonomic symptoms **without** impairment of consciousness.
3. Complex partial seizures have an **impairment** (but not a loss) of consciousness with simple partial features, automatisms, or impairment of consciousness only.
4. Generalized seizures have a loss of consciousness with convulsive or nonconvulsive behaviors.
5. Simple partial seizures can progress to complex partial seizures, and complex partial seizures can secondarily become generalized.

6. Nonepileptogenic behaviors can emulate seizures but have a psychogenic rather than organic origin.

C. *Cause*
The cause may be unknown or due to one of the following:

1. Trauma to head or brain resulting in scar tissue or cerebral atrophy
2. Tumors
3. Cranial surgery
4. Metabolic disorders (hypocalcemia, hypoglycemia/ hyperglycemia, hyponatremia, anoxia)
5. Drug toxicity, such as theophylline (Theo-dur), lidocaine (Xylocaine), penicillin
6. CNS infection
7. Circulatory disorders
8. Drug withdrawal states (alcohol, barbiturates)
9. Congenital neurodegenerative disorders

Clinical Manifestations

Related to area of the brain involved in the seizure activity. May range from single abnormal sensations, aberrant motor activity, altered consciousness/personality to loss of consciousness and convulsive movements.

1. Impaired consciousness.
2. Disturbed muscle tone or movement.
3. Disturbances of behavior, mood, sensation, or perception.
4. Disturbances of autonomic functions.

Diagnostic Evaluation

1. EEG with or without video monitoring—locates epileptic focus, spread, intensity, and duration; helps classify seizure type.
2. MRI, CT scan—to identify lesion that may be cause of seizure.
3. SPECT or PET scan or MSI—additional tests to identify seizure foci.
4. Neuropsychological studies—to evaluate for behavioral disturbances.

Management

1. Pharmacotherapy: drug selected according to seizure type (Table 13-4).
2. Biofeedback: useful in the patient with reliable auras.
3. Surgery: resective and palliative operations (temporal lobectomy, extratemporal resection, corpus callosotomy, hemispherectomy).
4. Psychotherapy

Complications

1. Status epilepticus.
2. Injuries due to falls.

Nursing Assessment

1. Obtain seizure history, including prodromal signs and symptoms, seizure behavior, postictal state, history of status epilepticus.

TABLE 13-4 Antiepileptic Medications

Drug/Dosage/Indications	Adverse Reactions	Patient Teaching
Clonazepam (Klonipin): generalized seizures such as absence, atonic, myoclonic; PO up to 20 mg/day, increase 0.5 mg over 3-day period	Dose-related: visual disturbances, ataxia, cognitive impairment. Idiosyncratic: rash, hirsuitism, vivid dreams.	Take with meals. Avoid driving. Avoid alcohol ingestion.
Carbamazepine (Tegretol): partial and generalized seizures; give PO up to 1,600 mg/day in divided doses or to clinical toxicity	Dose-related: blurred vision, dizziness, visual disturbances, ataxia lethargy. Idiosyncratic: skin rash, hepatic dysfunction (bleeding, dark urine), leukopenia, aplastic anemia.	Dose-related effects may diminish. Take PO with food. Must comply with ordered lab studies. Available in chewable tablets, if preferred. Drug induces own metabolizing enzymes, effectiveness of dose may decrease within 3–6 weeks.
Ethosuximide (Zarontin): generalized seizures initially 1,000 mg/day in divided doses; increase by 250 mg every 4–7 days to 1.5 gm	Dose-related: GI upset, sedation, unsteadiness. Idiosyncratic: skin rash, psychotic behaviors.	Take with food, milk to decrease GI upset. Use hard candy, gum to prevent dry mouth.
Felbamate (Felbatol): partial and generalized seizures: 2,400–3,600 mg/day in divided doses	Dose-related: decrease appetite, weight loss, GI upset. Idiosyncratic: sleep disturbances.	Take with food, milk.
Gabapentin (Nuerontin): for partial and generalized seizures: PO 900–1,800 mg/day in divided doses	Dose-related: somnolence, dizziness, fatigue, and nystagmus. Idiosyncratic: hypotension, rash, hematuria.	Avoid working around machinery or driving if somnolence is experienced
Phenytoin (Dilantin): partial and generalized seizures, IV 900 mg–1.5 g run at 50 mg/min, if previously on phenytoin 100–300 mg same rate. PO 300 mg/day in divided doses	Dose-related: nystagmus, ataxia, visual changes, seizure exacerbation, slurred speech. Idiosyncratic: aplastic anemia, rash, Steven-Johnson syndrome.	Urine may turn pink. Good oral hygiene is necessary (brushing and flossing) to prevent gingival hyperplasia.
Primidone (Mysoline): partial seizures, PO 250 mg/day up to 2 gm/day in divided doses	Dose-related: visual disturbances, sedation. Idiosyncratic: thrombocytopenia, lymphadenopathy, hallucinations.	Do not withdraw medication without first consulting health care provider.
Valproic acid (Depakene, Depakote): partial and generalized seizures, PO initially 15 mg/kg/day, add 5–10 mg/kg/day, up to 60 mg/kg/day in divided doses	Dose-related: GI upset, tremor, increased liver enzymes, hyperammonemia, somnolence, thrombocytopenia. Idiosyncratic: hepatic failure, pancreatitis.	Do not dilute elixir with carbonated beverages. Avoid driving. Take with food.

2. Document the following about seizure activity:
   a. Circumstances before attack, such as visual, auditory, olfactory, or tactile stimuli; emotional or psychological disturbances; sleep; hyperventilation.
   b. Description of movement, including where movement or stiffness started; type of movement and parts involved; progression of movement; whether beginning of seizure was witnessed.
   c. Position of the eyes and head; size of pupils.
   d. Presence of automatisms, such as lip smacking or repeated swallowing.
   e. Incontinence of urine or feces.
   f. Duration of each phase of the attack.
   g. Presence of unconsciousness and its duration.
   h. Behavior after attack, including inability to speak, any weakness or paralysis, sleep.
3. Psychosocial effect of seizures.
4. History of drug or alcohol abuse.
5. Compliance and medication-taking strategies.

NURSING ALERT:
Noncompliance with medication taking as well as toxicity of antiepileptic medications can increase seizure frequency. Obtain drug levels before implementing medication changes.

Nursing Diagnoses

A. Altered Cerebral Tissue Perfusion related to seizure activity
B. Risk for Injury related to seizure activity

C. Ineffective Individual Coping related to psychosocial and economic consequences of epilepsy

Nursing Interventions

A. Maintaining Cerebral Tissue Perfusion
1. Maintain a patent airway until patient is fully awake after a seizure.
2. Provide oxygen during the seizure if color change occurs.
3. Stress the importance of taking medications regularly.
4. Monitor serum levels for therapeutic range of medications.
5. Monitor patient for toxic side effects of medications.
6. Monitor platelet and liver functions for toxicity due to medications.

B. Preventing Injury
1. Provide a safe environment by padding side rails and removing clutter.
2. Place the bed in a low position.
3. Do not restrain the patient during a seizure.
4. Do not put anything in the patient's mouth during a seizure.
5. Place the patient on side during a seizure to prevent aspiration
6. Protect the patient's head during a seizure.
7. Stay with the patient who is ambulating or who is in a confused state during seizure.
8. Provide a helmet to the patient who falls during seizure.
9. Manage the patient in status epilepticus (Box 13-3).

C. Strengthening Coping
1. Consult with social worker for community resources for vocational rehabilitation, counselors, support groups.
2. Teach stress reduction techniques that will fit into patient's lifestyle.
3. Initiate appropriate consultation for management of behaviors related to personality disorders, brain damage secondary to chronic epilepsy.
4. Answer questions related to use of computerized video EEG monitoring and surgery for epilepsy management.

Patient Education/ Health Maintenance

1. Encourage the patient to determine existence of trigger factors for seizures, for example, skipped meals, lack of sleep, emotional stress.
2. Remind the patient of the importance of following medication regimen.
3. Tell the patient to avoid alcohol, because it interferes with metabolism of antiepileptic medications.
4. Encourage the patient and family to discuss feelings and attitudes about epilepsy.
5. Encourage patient to wear a Medic Alert card or bracelet.
6. Encourage a moderate lifestyle that includes exercise, mental activity, and nutritional diet.
7. For the surgical candidate, reinforce instructions related to surgical outcome of the specific surgical approach (temporal lobectomy, corpus callosotomy, hemispherectomy, and extratemporal resection).

BOX 13-3 Emergency Management of Status Epilepticus

Status epilepticus (acute, prolonged, repetitive seizure activity) is a series of generalized seizures without return to consciousness between attacks. The term has been broadened to include continuous clinical and/or electrical seizures lasting at least 5 minutes, even without impairment of consciousness.

Status epilepticus is considered a serious neurologic emergency. It has a high mortality and morbidity rate (permanent brain damage; severe neurologic deficits).

Factors that precipitate status epilepticus include medication withdrawal, fever, metabolic or environmental stresses, alcohol withdrawal, sleep deprivation, etc., in patient with preexisting seizure disorder.

Interventions
1. Establish an airway and maintain blood pressure.
2. Obtain blood studies for glucose, blood urea nitrogen, electrolytes, and anticonvulsant drug levels to determine metabolic abnormalities and serve as a guide for maintenance of biochemical homeostasis.
3. Administer oxygen—there is some respiratory arrest at height of each seizure, which may produce venous congestion and hypoxia of brain.
4. Establish IV lines and keep open for blood sampling, drug administration, and infusion of fluids.
5. Administer intravenous anticonvulsant (lorazepam [Ativan], phenytoin [Dilantin]) give *slowly* to ensure effective brain tissue and serum concentrations.
   a. Additional anticonvulsants given as directed—effects of lorazepam are of short duration.
   b. Anticonvulsant drug levels monitored regularly.
6. Monitor the patient continuously; depression of respiration and blood pressure induced by drug therapy may be delayed.
7. Use mechanical ventilation as needed.
8. If initial treatment is unsuccessful, general anesthesia may be required.
9. Assist with search for precipitating factors.
   a. Monitor vital and neurologic signs on a continuing basis.
   b. Use electroencephalographic monitoring to determine nature and abolition (after diazepam administration) of epileptic activity.
   c. Determine (from family member) if there is a history of epilepsy, alcohol/drug use, trauma, recent infection.

---

8. Refer the patient/family to: The Epilepsy Foundation of America; 4351 Garden City Drive; Landover, Maryland 20785; 800-492-2523.

Evaluation

A. Taking medication as ordered, drug level within normal range
B. No injuries observed
C. Reports using support services and stress management techniques

◆ NARCOLEPSY

Narcolepsy is a syndrome characterized by excessive day-time somnolence, cataplexy, hypnagogic hallucinations, and disturbed nocturnal sleep. Onset is usually between ages 15 and 25.

Pathophysiology/Etiology

1. Cause of narcolepsy is controversial.
2. Thought to be a disorder of the rapid eye movement sleep cycle, during which the inhibitory and excitatory mechanisms function abnormally.
3. Although considered a hypersomnia disorder, the person does not experience excessive amounts of sleep in a 24-hour period.

Clinical Manifestations

1. Excessive daytime sleepiness is the most common symptom, may not be recognized by the patient.
2. Patient may complain of inability to focus vision or thought process rather than a feeling of sleepiness.
3. Cataplexy—sudden, temporary loss of muscle tone and inability to move a body part or the entire body.
   a. May be frightening because patient is fully awake.
   b. Usually triggered by heightened emotional states (anger, laughter).
4. Hypnagogic hallucinations occur just before falling asleep.
   a. Visual, but may also involve the auditory system.
   b. Sensory hallucinations may also occur.
5. Nocturnal sleep disturbance—occurs $2^1/_2$ to 3 hours after falling asleep.
   a. After being awake for 45 to 60 minutes, the patient will fall back to sleep for another $2^1/_2$ to 3 hours and then awaken again.
   b. This is believed to be the source of the daytime somnolence.

Diagnostic Evaluation

1. Polysomnograph—abnormal
2. Multisleep Latency Test—decreased latency

Management

1. Mutual goal setting, because not everyone derives benefit from treatment.
2. Nondrug therapy: short naps (10 to 20 minutes twice daily), caffeinated beverages, exercise, and avoidance of heavy meals
3. Stimulants: pemoline (Cylert), methylphenidate (Ritalin), dextroamphetamine (Dexedrine), methamphetamine (Desoxyn)
4. Antidepressants for cataplexy; protriptyline (Vivactil), desipramine (Norpramin), fluozetine (Prozac)

Complications

1. Injury related to falling asleep.
2. Psychosocial problems and disturbed relationships.

Nursing Assessment

1. Obtain history of sleep and activity pattern.
2. Assess emotional status and social interactions.

Nursing Diagnoses

A. Sleep Pattern Disturbance related to disease process
B. Fatigue related to disrupted nighttime sleep
C. Ineffective Individual Coping related to interference with activity

Nursing Interventions

A. *Promoting Normal Sleep–Wake Cycle*
1. Review daily schedule to determine periods of sleep and cataplexy.
2. Help patient establish nondrug therapies (exercise, diet) that will fit into lifestyle.
3. Administer or teach self-administration of prescribed medications.
   a. Advise of side effects of amphetamines, such as nervousness, irritability, tremors, and GI upset.
   b. Warn patient to take only as prescribed and to not increase dosage because of addiction and overdosage potential.

B. *Reducing Fatigue*
1. Schedule 10- to 20-minute rest periods two to three times/day.
   a. Help patient incorporate naps into lifestyle.
2. Encourage patient to incorporate small amounts of caffeinated beverages at intervals, and smaller, more frequent meals rather than large, heavy meals during the day to maintain energy.
3. Plan diversional activities and relaxation during fatigued periods.

C. *Strengthening Coping*
1. Encourage active participation in selection of treatment modalities.
2. Assist patient in identifying trigger factors of worsening symptoms.
3. Teach problem-solving strategy to promote sense of control over activities and symptoms during the day.
4. Review patient coping mechanisms and reinforce positive ones.
5. Encourage use of support groups and community resources.

Patient Education/ Health Maintenance

1. Review the normal sleep cycle and the pathophysiology of narcolepsy.

2. Stress the importance of nonpharmacologic measures as an adjunct to treatment.
3. Inform the patient of rights of employment conditions under the American Disabilities Act.

Evaluation

A. Patient complying with medication regimen
B. Reports working without undue fatigue
C. Identifying trigger factors

◆ HEADACHE SYNDROMES

Headaches are one of the most common human ailments. Pain in the head is a symptom of underlying pathology. More than one type of headache may occur simultaneously, for example, pain of a vascular or sinus headache along with muscle contraction headache.

Pathophysiology/Etiology

1. Muscle contraction/tension.
   a. Due to irritation of sensitive nerve endings in the head, jaw, and neck from prolonged muscle contraction.
   b. Often related to poor posture, prolonged or abnormal postures, clenching teeth.
2. Familial predisposition (vascular headaches—migraine and cluster).
   a. Thought to be the result of serotonin abnormalities.
   b. Initial constriction, then dilation of intracranial and extracranial arteries.
   c. Migraines occur in 10% of Americans.
   d. Cluster headaches occur mostly in men.
3. Infection (sinusitis).
4. Inflammation (temporal arteritis)—usually over age 50.
5. Toxins.

Clinical Manifestations

1. Tension: pain and pressure in the back of the head and neck, across forehead, bitemporal areas; dull, persistent ache; tender spots of head or neck.
2. Migraine: sensory, motor, or mood alterations precede headache; gradual onset of severe unilateral, throbbing headache, may become bilateral.
   a. With classic migraine, characteristic aura may include scintillating scotoma, hemianopia, and paresthesias; usually lasts less than a day.
   b. With common migraine, nausea, vomiting, and photophobia may accompany headache; may last more than 1 day and leaves the individual fatigued.
   c. May be triggered in women by hormonal fluctuations (menses, pregnancy).
3. Cluster headache: pain is severe, unilateral, and always occurs on the same side and occurs suddenly at the same time of day, possibly at night.
   a. Occurs in clusters of 2 to 8 weeks followed by headache-free periods.

b. Associated with unilateral excessive tearing, redness of the eye, facial swelling, flushing, and sweating.
   c. Attacks last 20 minutes to 2 hours. Several attacks may occur in 1 day.
4. Sinus headache: pain is usually felt over sinus areas, above eyes, along the side of the nose, and behind ears.
   a. May be accompanied by fever, nasal drainage, erythema, swelling and tenderness of the sinus areas with acute sinusitis.
5. Temporal arteritis: unilateral or bilateral pain, particularly severe at night, with tender temporal arteries.

Diagnostic Evaluation

1. Skull/sinus films to rule out lesions, sinusitis.
2. CT/MRI scan to rule out lesions, hemorrhage.
3. Estimated sedimentation rate (ESR) and other blood studies to help determine inflammatory process with temporal arteritis.

Treatment

A. Pharmacologic Treatment
Medications are intended to reduce the frequency, severity, and duration of the headache. Effectiveness of medication is individualized. Some persons may need a combination of medications.

1. Aspirin, acetaminophen, and nonsteroidal anti-inflammatory drugs for mild-to-moderate pain of tension, sinus, or mild vascular headaches.
2. Some drugs may abort vascular headaches if taken at the onset, including methysergide (Sansert), a serotonin antagonist; ergotamine (Ergostat), a vasoconstrictor; or sumatriptan (Imitrex), a 5HT agonist.
3. Inhalation of 100% oxygen may abort a cluster headache.
4. Some drugs may be used continuously as prophylactic treatment for recurrent migraines, including beta-blockers, calcium channel blockers, and tricyclic antidepressants.
5. Antihistamines and decongestants may be effective for sinus headaches.
6. Corticosteroids may be used for temporal arteritis.
7. Occasionally, narcotic analgesics, muscle relaxants, and antianxiety agents may be needed for severe pain.

B. Nonpharmacologic Management
1. Relaxation techniques.
2. Biofeedback.
3. Avoidance of tyramine-containing foods to prevent migraines.
4. Rest in a quiet, dark room.

Complications

1. Usually none.

Nursing Assessment

1. Obtain a history of related symptoms, triggering factors, degree of pain, and medications used.
2. Perform a complete neurologic examination to detect any focal deficits of signs of increased ICP that indicate tumor or hemorrhage.
3. Assess coping mechanisms and emotional status.

Nursing Diagnoses

A. Pain related to headache
B. Ineffective Individual Coping related to chronic and/or disabling pain

Nursing Interventions

A. Controlling Pain
1. Reduce environmental stimuli: light, noise, movement.
2. Suggest light massage to tight muscles in neck, scalp, back for tension headaches.
3. Apply warm, moist heat to areas of muscle tension.
4. Encourage patient to lie down and attempt to sleep.
5. Teach progressive muscle relaxation to treat and prevent tension headaches.
   a. Alternately tense and relax each group of muscles for a count of five, starting with the forehead and working downward to the feet.
   b. Try to maintain state of relaxation of each muscle group until whole body feels relaxed.
   c. Relaxation of just head and neck may also be helpful if time is limited.
6. Teach patient the cause of headache and proper use of medication.
7. Encourage adequate rest once headache is relieved to recover from fatigue of the pain.

B. *Promoting Positive Coping*
1. Encourage patient to become aware of triggering factors and early symptoms of headache, so headache can be prevented or promptly treated.
2. Encourage adequate nutrition, rest and relaxation, and avoidance of stress and overexertion to better cope with headaches.
3. Implement problem solving to help patient manage problems that arise in social or work situations related to headaches.
4. Review coping mechanisms and strengthen positive ones.

Patient Education/ Health Maintenance

1. Teach proper administration of medication.
   a. Self-injection of sumatriptan (Imitrex), given subcutaneously with autoinjector.
   b. Inhalation of ergotamine (Ergostat) through metered-dose inhaler.
2. Teach side effects of medications.
   a. GI upset, gastritis, and possible ulcer formation with nonsteroidal anti-inflammatory drugs—take with food.
   b. Numbness, coldness, paresthesias, and pain of extremities with ergot derivatives—report to health care provider.
   c. Chest pain, wheezing, flushing with sumatriptan (Imitrex)—report to health care provider.
   d. Hypotension with beta blockers and calcium channel blockers—arise slowly, do not exceed prescribed dosage, do not discontinue beta blockers abruptly.
3. Advise avoidance of alcohol, which can worsen headaches.
4. Teach about foods that are high in tyramine that may trigger migraines—aged cheese, red wine, liver.

Evaluation

A. Patient reports fewer, less severe headaches
B. Describes use of positive coping mechanisms

◆ HERNIATED INTERVERTEBRAL DISK (RUPTURED DISK)

Herniation of the intervertebral disk is a protrusion of the nucleus of the disk into the annulus (fibrous ring around the disk) with subsequent nerve compression. The herniation may occur in any portion of the vertebral column (Fig. 13-6).

Pathophysiology/Etiology

1. The intervertebral disk is a cartilaginous plate made up of gelatinous material in the center, known as the nucleus pulposus, and is encapsulated in the fibrous annulus.
2. Degeneration (aging), trauma, and congenital predisposition may lead to herniation of the nucleus through the annulus.

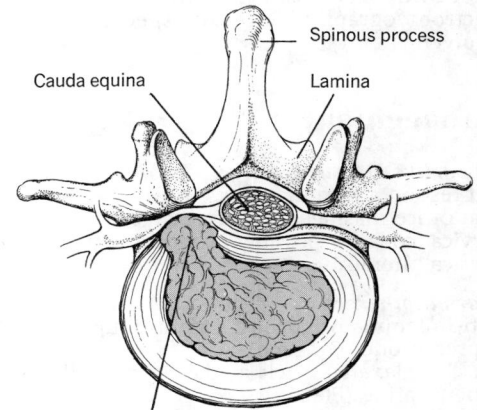

FIGURE 13-6 *Ruptured vertebral disk. (Chaffee EE and Greisheimer EM. Basic Physiology and Anatomy, 3rd ed. Philadelphia, JB Lippincott.)*

3. The herniation compresses the spinal nerve root on one side and with further degeneration of the disk may eventually produce pressure on the spinal cord.

4. This sequence may take months to years, producing acute and chronic symptoms.

Clinical Manifestations

Depend on location, size, rate of development, and effect on surrounding structures.

A. *Cervical*
1. Pain and stiffness in the neck, top of shoulders, and region of the scapula.
2. Pain in upper extremities and head.
3. Paresthesias and numbness of upper extremities.
4. Weakness of upper extremities.

B. *Lumbar*
1. Low back pain with varying degrees of sensory and motor dysfunction.
2. Pain radiating from the low back into the buttocks and down the leg.
3. Postural deformity of the lumbar spine.
4. Positive straight-leg raise test: pain occurs in leg below the knee when leg raised from a supine position.
5. Weakness and asymmetric reflexes.
6. Sensory loss.

> **NURSING ALERT:** ❖
> Cauda equina syndrome is an emergency caused by compression of the cauda equina area of the spinal cord. Symptoms include bowel, bladder, or sexual dysfunction or saddle area numbness. It must be recognized early and compression relieved to prevent permanent loss of these functions.

Diagnostic Evaluation

1. Myelogram—demonstrates herniation and pressure on spinal cord or nerve roots.
2. CT or MRI—demonstrates herniation.
3. Electromyography—localizes specific spinal nerve involvement.

Management

A. *Supportive Measures*
1. Bed rest on a firm mattress.
2. Heat or ice massage to affected area.
3. Cervical collar or possibly cervical traction.
4. Physical therapy.

B. *Pharmacotherapy*
1. Anti-inflammatory drugs, such as ibuprofen (Motrin) or prednisone (Orasone).
2. Muscle relaxants, such as diazepam (Valium) or cyclobenzaprine (Flexeril).
3. Analgesics, narcotics may be necessary during acute phase.

C. *Surgical Intervention*
1. May be done if there is progression of neurologic deficit or failure to improve with conservative management.

2. Surgical procedures include diskectomy, laminectomy, spinal fusion, microdiskectomy, and percutaneous diskectomy.

D. *Chemonucleolysis*
1. For lumbar disc herniation.
2. Injection of chymopapain (Chymodiactin) into herniated disk that produces loss of water and proteoglycans from the disk, reducing the size of the disk and subsequent pressure on the nerve root.

Complications

1. Permanent neurologic dysfunction (weakness, numbness).

Nursing Assessment

1. Perform repeated assessments of motor function, sensation, and reflexes to determine progression of condition.
2. Assess level at which straight-leg raise test is positive; generally radiation of pain below knee at 45 degrees of elevation is considered positive for nerve root involvement; positive at lesser elevation may indicate worsening condition.
3. Assess pain level on scale of 1 to 10.

Nursing Diagnoses

A. Pain related to area of compression
B. Impaired Physical Mobility related to pain and disease physiology

Nursing Interventions

A. Minimizing Pain
1. Administer or teach self-administration of anti-inflammatory drugs as prescribed and with food or antacid to prevent GI upset.
2. Administer or teach self-administration of prescribed muscle relaxant; observe safety, because drowsiness may result.
3. Administer or teach self-administration of analgesics as prescribed; be prepared for sedation.
4. Use bedboards under mattress and maintain bed rest except for short trips to bathroom; maintain supine or low-Fowler's position or side-lying position with slight knee flexion and pillow between knees.
5. Apply moist heat to affected area of back as desired.
6. Encourage relaxation techniques, such as imagery and progressive muscle relaxation.

B. *Maintaining Mobility*
1. Encourage range-of-motion exercises while in bed.
2. Properly fit and use a cervical collar (if appropriate to level of injury).
3. Apply a back brace or cervical skin traction, if ordered.
4. Inspect skin several times a day, especially under stabilization devices, for redness and evidence of pressure sore development.

5. Provide massage and good skin care to pressure-prone areas.
6. Assist patient with activities at bedside and discourage lifting or straining of any kind.
7. Encourage compliance with physical therapy treatments and activity restrictions as ordered.

> **COMMUNITY-BASED CARE TIP:**
> If cervical skin traction is ordered for home use, teach the patient how to apply the chin strap and head halter. The weight should hang freely over a the back of a chair or doorknob near the head of the bed. Make sure that the patient maintains proper alignment of the neck and removes traction before moving the head.

Care of the Patient Having Disk Surgery

A. *Preparing the Patient for Surgery*
1. Educate patient about surgical procedure.
   a. Procedure is generally short.
   b. Small incision will be made on back or neck; second incision will be on hip if bone graft is taken from iliac crest for spinal fusion.
   c. Routine postoperative care will include frequent assessment of vital signs and neurologic function, frequent turning and deep breathing, pain control, and ambulation on the first postoperative day.
2. Document baseline neurologic assessment to compare to after surgery.
3. Explain your actions to patient as you shave operative area, administer preoperative medications, and perform any other preoperative order.

B. *Preventing Complications Postoperatively*
1. Monitor vital signs and surgical dressing frequently, because hemorrhage is a possible complication.
2. Assess movement and sensation of extremities, report any new deficit.
3. Administer analgesics and steroid medications to control pain from incision and swelling around nerve roots and spinal cord due to surgery.
4. Maintain cervical collar if ordered.
5. Log-roll patient to reposition frequently and encourage coughing and deep breathing.
6. Position for comfort with small pillow under head (but avoid extreme neck flexion) and pillow under knees to take pressure off lower back.
7. Provide fluids as soon as gag reflex and bowel sounds are noted.
8. Assess for hoarseness, indicating that cervical surgery has resulted in recurrent laryngeal nerve injury; may cause ineffective cough.

9. Watch for dysphagia due to edema of the esophagus and provide blenderized diet.
10. Ensure that patient voids after surgery; report urinary retention.
11. Encourage ambulation as soon possible by having patient lie on side close to edge of bed and push up with arms while swinging legs toward floor in one motion; alternate walking with bed rest, discourage sitting.
12. Report any sudden reappearance of radicular pain (may indicate nerve root compression from slipping of bone graft or collapsing of disk space) or burning back pain radiating to buttocks (may indicate arachnoiditis).

Patient Education/ Health Maintenance

1. Teach patient the importance of complying with bed rest, use of cervical collar, and other conservative measures to try to reduce inflammation and heal disk herniation.
2. Tell patient who has had a cervical disk herniation to avoid extreme flexion, extension, or rotation of the neck and to keep the head in neutral position during sleep.
3. Encourage the patient with a lumbar disk herniation to remain on bed rest at home with ambulation to the bathroom only until inflammation and pain are sufficiently reduced; then ambulation can be increased, but lifting and sitting are discouraged.
4. Encourage patient to do stretching and strengthening exercises of extremities and abdomen after acute symptoms have subsided. The back can be gently stretched by lying on the back and bringing the knees up toward the chest.
5. Teach the patient about proper body mechanics and the use of leg and abdominal muscles rather than the back. Knees should be bent on lifting and load carried close to midtrunk.
6. Encourage follow-up with physical therapy as indicated for reconditioning and work hardening.
7. Tell patient to avoid the prone position, long car rides, and sitting in a soft chair.
8. Instruct the patient to report any changes in neurologic function or recurrence of radicular pain.
9. Encourage good nutrition, avoidance of obesity, and proper rest to reduce risk of recurrence.

Evaluation

A. Patient verbalizes reduced pain.
B. Immobilization maintained with stable assessment.

Selected References

Ahern G.L., Herring A.M., & Tackenberg, J. (1993). The association of multiple personality and temprolimbic epilepsy. *Archives of Neurology*, (50), 1020–1028.

Ahern, G.L., Labiner, D.M., Hutzler, R., Osburn, C., Herring, A.M., & Tackenberg, J.N. Quantitative analysis of the EEG in the intracarotid procedures. *EEG and Clinical Neurophysiology*, 12(3), 285–290.

Appollonio, A., Grafman, J., Clark, K., Nichelli, P., Jeffiro, T., & Hallett M.

(1994). Implicit and explicit memory in patients with Parkinson's disease with and without dementia. *Archives of Neurology 51*(4), 359–367.

Arbour, R. (1994). Laser and ultrasound technology in aggressive management of central nervous system tumors. *Journal of Neuroscience Nursing, 26*(1), 30–35.

Arnold, S.E., Hyman, B., & VanHoesen, G. (1994). Neuropathologic changes of the temporal pole in Alzheimer's disease and Pick's disease. *Archives of Neurology, 51*(2), 145–150.

Awad, I., Magdineo, M., & Schubert, A. (1994). Intracranial hypertension after resection of cerebral arteriovenous malformation. *Stroke, 25*(3),

Dilario, C., Faherty, B., & Manteuffel, B. (1992). Self-efficacy and social support in self-management of epilepsy. *Western Journal of Nursing Research, 14*(3), 292–306.

Dow, K.H., & Hilderly, L.J. *Nursing care in radiation oncology.* Philadelphia: W.B. Saunders, 1992.

Fearon, M. & Rusy, K. (1994). Transcranial doppler: Advanced technology for assessing hemodynamics. *Dimensions in Critical Care Nursing 13*(5), 241–248.

Godbole, K., Berbilglia, V., & Goddard, L. The head injured patient: Caloric needs, clinical progress and nursing priorities. *Journal of Neuroscience Nursing, 23*(5), 199.

Gotman, J., Bouwer, M., & Jones-Gotman, M. (1993). Intracranial EEG study of brain structures affected by internal carotid injection of amobarbital. *Neurology, 42,* 2136–2143.

Hickey, J. V. *The clinical practice of neurological and neurosurgical nursing.* Philadelphia: J.B. Lippincott, 1993.

Hodges, K., & Mussman, L. (1991). Surgical management of intractable seizure disorder. *Journal of Neuroscience Nursing, 23*(20), 93–100.

Hoffert, M. J. (1994). Treatment of migraine: A new era. *American Family Physician, 49*(3), 633–638.

Huston, C. J., & Boelman, R. (1995). Emergency! Autonomic dysreflexia. *AJN 95*(6):55

Hydo, B. (1995). Designing an effective clinical pathway for stroke patients. *AJN, 95*(3), 44–50.

Irle, E., Peper, M., Wowra, B., & Kunze, S. (1994). Mood changes after surgery for tumors of the cerebral cortex. *Archives of Neurology, 51*(2), 164–176.

Johnson, R.T., & Griffin, J.W. (1993). Current therapy in neurologic disease (4th ed.). St. Louis: BC Decker/Mosby.

Kalia, K.K., & Yonas, H. (1993). An aggressive approach to massive middle cerebral artery infarction. *Archives of Neurology, 50*(12), 1293–1300.

McDonald, E., Wiedenfeld, F.A., Hillel, A., Carpenter, C.L., & Walter, R. (1994). Survival in amyotrophic lateral sclerosis: The role of psychological factors. *Archives of Neurology, 51*(1), 17–26.

Parker, C. D. (1995). Emergency! Fast action for subarachnoid hemorrhage. *AJN, 95*(1), 47.

Pizzuti, A., Friedman, D.L., & Caskey, C.T. (1993). The myotonic dystrophy gene. *Archives of Neurology, 50*(11), 1173–1179.

Richmond, T., Metcalf, J., Daly, M., & Kish, J. (1992). Powerlessness in acute spinal cord injury patients. *Journal of Neuroscience Nursing, 24*(3), 146–152.

Shellenbarger, T. & Stover, J. (1995). ALS demands diligent nursing care. *RN, 58*(3), 30–35.

Wereman, N.M. (1990). Adaptation to multiple sclerosis: The role of social support, functional disability and perceived uncertainty. *Nursing Research, 39*(5), 294–299.

Wylie, E. (Ed.). (1993). *The treatment of epilepsy: Principles and practice.* Philadelphia: Lea and Febiger.

Eye Disorders

Introductory Information

◆ DEFINITION OF TERMS

A.   Vision   Passage of rays of light from an object through the cornea, aqueous humor, lens, and vitreous humor to the retina, and its appreciation in the cerebral cortex.

B.   Emmetropia   *Normal* vision: rays of light coming from an object at a distance of 6 m (20 ft) or more are brought to focus on the retina by the lens (Fig. 14-1A).

C.   Ametropia   *Abnormal* vision.

1.   Myopia—nearsightedness: rays of light coming from an object at a distance of 6 m (20 ft) or more are brought to a focus in front of the retina (see Figure 14-1B).
2.   Hyperopia—farsightedness: rays of light coming from an object at a distance of 6 m (20 ft) or more are brought to a focus in back of the retina (see Figure 14-1C).

D.   Accommodation   Focusing apparatus of the eye adjusts to objects at different distances by means of increasing the convexity of the lens (brought about by contraction of the ciliary muscles).

E.   Presbyopia   The elasticity of the lens decreases with increasing age; an emmetropic person with presbyopia will read the paper at arms' length and will require prescription lenses to correct the problem.

F.   Astigmatism   Uneven curvature of the cornea causing the patient to be unable to focus horizontal and vertical rays of light on the retina at the same time.

Common Abbreviations

OD (oculus dexter) or RE—right eye
OS (oculus sinister) or LE—left eye
OU (oculus unitas)—both eyes
IOP—intraocular pressure
IOL—intraocular lens
EOL—extraocular lens

Eye Care Specialists

A.   Ophthalmologist   Medical doctor specializing in diagnosis and treatment of the eye. Ophthalmology specialists may focus their practice to a specific part of the eye or disorder, such as a cornea specialist or glaucoma specialist.

B.   Optometrist   Doctor of optometry who can examine, diagnose, and manage visual problems and diseases of the eye.

C.   Optician   Fits, adjusts, and gives eyeglasses or other devices on the written prescription of an ophthalmologist or optometrist.

D.   Ocularist   Technician who makes ophthalmic prostheses.

Assessment

◆ SUBJECTIVE DATA

Subjective data for eye assessment include complaints of altered vision or other symptoms, associated lifestyle and other factors, and recent and past health history.

Presenting Symptoms

1.   Any blurred vision, double vision, loss of vision, or a portion of the visual field?
2.   Is there pain, headache, foreign body sensation (scratchy, something in the eye), photophobia, redness, itchiness, or lacrimation?

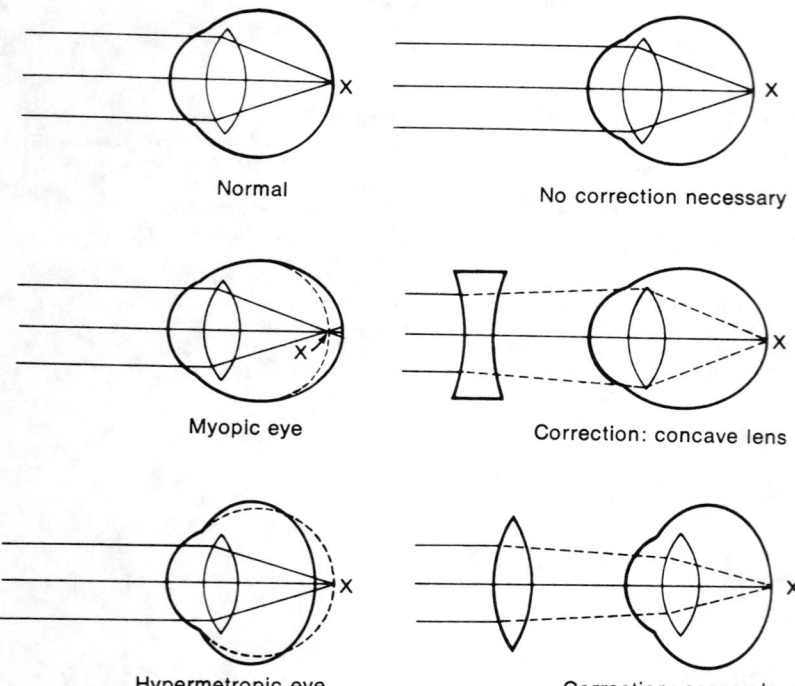

Normal

No correction necessary

Myopic eye

Correction: concave lens

Hypermetropic eye

Correction: convex lens

FIGURE 14-1 *Normal vision and refractory errors.*

Associated Factors

1. Does the patient wear contact lenses or glasses?
2. What is the patient's occupation and common sports activities?
3. How long have there been symptoms?
4. What treatments has the patient tried?

History

1. Eye injury or accident.
2. Recent infection, such as an upper respiratory infection.
3. Ocular history, such as previous injury, surgery, or use of medication.
4. Medical history, such as diabetes, hypertension, arthritis, or allergies.

◆ OCULAR EXAMINATION

Note: Every patient who seeks medical attention for an eye complaint should have their visual acuity tested.

External Examination

Includes examination of the eye and accessory organs without the aid of special apparatus.

A. **Visual Acuity**   Snellen Chart and other methods.

1. Each eye is tested separately, with and without glasses.
2. Letters and objects are of a size that can be seen by the normal eye at a distance of 6 m (20 ft) from the chart.
3. Letters appear in rows and are arranged so that the normal eye can see them at distances of 9, 12, 15 m (30, 40, 50 ft), etc.
4. A person who can identify letters of the size 6 at 6 m (20 at 20 feet) is said to have 6/6 (20/20) vision.
5. Additionally, if vision is less than 6/60 (20/200), tests may be recorded as follows:
   Counting fingers (C.F.) at —— m (feet).
   Hand motion (H.M.)—ability to detect hand movement at a certain distance:
   Light perception and projection (L.P. & P.)
   Light perception only (L.P.)
   No light perception (N.L.P.)
6. Formula for converting meters to feet:

$$\begin{array}{cc} \text{m.} & \text{ft.} \end{array}$$

$$6/6 + 3 = 20/20 + 10$$

Example: 6/6 = 20/20
6/9 = 20/30
6/60 = 20/200

B. **Visual Fields**
To determine function of optic pathways.

1. Equipment—light source and test objects.
2. Peripheral field—useful in detecting decreased peripheral vision in one or both eyes.

a. Patient is seated 18 to 24 in. in front of the tester.
b. The left eye is covered while the patient focuses with the right eye on a spot about 1 ft from the eye.
c. A test object is brought in from the side at 15-degree intervals, through complete 360 degrees.
d. The patient signals when he or she sees the test object and again when the object disappears through the 360 degrees.

C. Color Vision Tests

These tests are done to determine the person's ability to perceive primary colors and shades of colors; it is particularly significant for persons whose occupation requires discerning colors, such as artists, interior decorators, transportation workers, surgeons, nurses.

1. Equipment
   a. Polychromatic plates: these are dots of primary colors printed on a background of similar dots in a confusion of colors.
   b. Individual colored disks: each disk is matched to its next closest color.
2. Procedure
   a. Various polychromatic plates are presented to the patient under specified illumination.
   b. The patterns may be letters or numbers that the normal eye can perceive instantly, but that are confusing to the person with a perception defect.
3. Outcome
   a. Color-blindness—person is unable to perceive the figures.
   b. Red-green blindness—8% of males, 0.4% of females.
   c. Blue-yellow blindness—extremely rare.

D. Refraction

Refraction is a clinical measurement of the error of focus in an eye.

1. Usually this is accomplished by instilling a medication with cycloplegic and mydriatic properties into the conjunctiva of the eye. Tropicamide (Mydriacyl) or cyclopentolate (Cyclogyl) are two such medicines that cause ciliary muscle relaxation, pupil dilation (mydriasis), and lowered accommodative power (cycloplegia).
2. The refractive state of the eye can be determined as follows:
   a. Objectively—through retinoscopy.
   b. Subjectively—trial of lenses to arrive at the best visual image.

Note: In certain eye clinics, an autorefractor may provide automatic refraction of a person's eyes as he or she sits in front of this special instrument. Findings are computed directly onto a printout sheet.

Internal Examination

A. Ophthalmoscopic Examination

1. Direct ophthalmoscopy—uses a strong light reflected into the interior of the eye through an instrument called an ophthalmoscope.
2. Indirect ophthalmoscopy—allows the examiner to obtain a stereoscopic view of the retina. Light source is from a head-mounted light. The examiner views the retina through a convex lens held in front of the eye and a viewing device on the head mount. The image appears inverted. This method of examination allows the examiner to use binocular vision with depth perception and wider viewing field.

A.

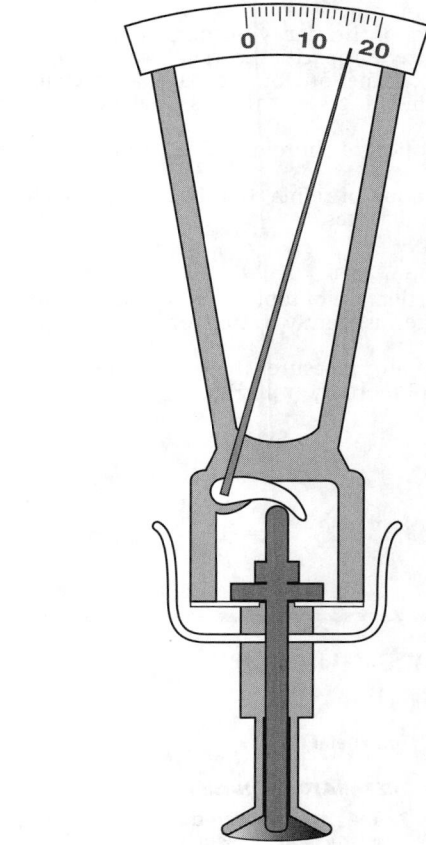

B.

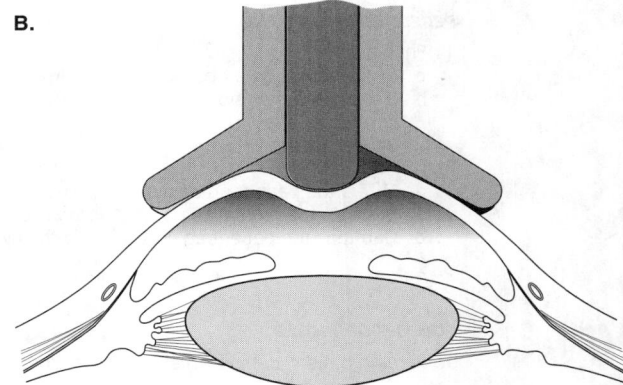

FIGURE 14-2 **(A)** *Schiøtz tonometer in which the plunger, in black, measures the ease of indentation of cornea.* **(B)** *Indentation of the anesthetized cornea by the plunger of the tonometer in order to measure ocular tension. (Newell Frank W. Ophthalmology: Principles and Concepts. ed. 4. St. Louis, CV Mosby)*

3. Clinical Significance
   a. Detection of the clarity of the media, that is, cataracts, vitreous opacities, corneal scars.
   b. Close examination for the pathologic changes in retinal blood vessels, that is, diabetes or hypertension.
   c. Examination of choroid, that is, tumors or inflammation.
   d. Examination of retina, that is, retinal detachment, scars, or diabetes.

B. *Tonometry*
1. Schiotz's tonometry
   a. After instillation of topical anesthesia, the Schiotz's tonometer is gently rested on the eyeball (Fig. 14-2).
   b. The indicator measures the ocular tension in millimeters of mercury (mm Hg).

   c. Normal tension is approximately 11 to 22 mm Hg.
2. Applanation tonometry
   a. This is the most effective measuring method for determining intraocular pressure; however, it requires a biomicroscope and a trained interpreter.
   b. After instillation of topical anesthesia, the cornea is flattened by a known amount (3.14 mm).
   c. The pressure necessary to produce this flattening is equal to the intraocular pressure, counterbalancing the tonometer.
3. Air applanation tonometry—This requires no topical anesthesia and measures tension by sensing deformation of the cornea in reaction to a puff of pressurized air.
4. Clinical significance
   a. Measurement of intraocular tension or pressure (Procedure Guidelines 14-1).

PROCEDURE GUIDELINES 14-1 ◆ Assisting the Patient Undergoing Tonometry

EQUIPMENT   Tonometer

PROCEDURE   **PREPARATORY PHASE**

1. The patient is placed in a tilt-type chair, tilted back, and instructed to look upward.

NURSING ACTION	RATIONALE

PERFORMANCE PHASE
1. Physician:
  a. Instills a drop of proparacaine 0.5% in each eye.
  b. Places a sterile tonometer gently on the center of the cornea for a few seconds.
  c. Repeats for second eye.
2. Nurse:
  a. Offers the patient an absorbent tissue.
  b. Instructs the patient to pat the *closed* eyes dry.
  c. Cautions the patient against rubbing the eyes.
	a. This will produce corneal anesthesia within a minute.
	b. Pressure from the eyeball will be transferred to the sensitive measuring indicator.
	
	c. The cornea is still anesthetized; painful abrasions can result from the natural tendency to rub the eyes because of the unusual numb sensation.

FOLLOW-UP PHASE

1. Remind patient to have an eye-pressure check at least every 2 years if pressure is normal.

Diagnostic Tests

◆ RADIOLOGY/IMAGING

There are several imaging studies beyond the basic eye examination that may be done to further evaluate eye disease.

Fluorescein Angiography

1. Introduction of sodium fluorescein intravenously (IV) or by mouth (PO). Ophthalmoscopy using a blue filter may be done and/or photographs of the ocular fundus may be obtained.
2. Provides information concerning vascular obstructions, microaneurysms, abnormal capillary permeability, and defects in retinal pigment permeability.

Ultrasonography

Sound waves are used in the diagnosis of intraocular and orbital lesions. Two types of ultrasonography are used in ophthalmoscopy:

1. A-scan—uses stationary transducers to measure the distance between changes in acoustic density. This is used to differentiate benign and malignant tumors and to measure the length of the eye to determine the power of an intraocular lens.
2. B-scan—moves linearly across the eye; increases in acoustic density are shown as an intensification on the line of the scan that presents a picture of the eye and the orbit.

General Procedures/ Treatment Modalities

◆ INSTILLATION OF MEDICATIONS

Refer to Procedure Guidelines 14-2.
Ophthalmic medications may be used for diagnostic and therapeutic purposes:

1. To dilate or contract the pupil.
2. To relieve pain and discomfort.
3. To act as an antiseptic in cleansing the eye.
4. To combat infection; to relieve inflammation.

See Table 14-1 for ophthalmic pharmacologic agents.

PROCEDURE GUIDELINES 14-2 ◆ Instillation of Medications

EQUIPMENT   Sterile solution or medication (most containers have accompanying dropper).
Small gauze squares or cotton balls.

PROCEDURE   **PREPARATORY PHASE**
1. Inform the patient of the need and reason for instilling drops.
2. Allow the patient to sit with head tilted backward or to lie in a supine position.

PERFORMANCE PHASE

NURSING ACTION	RATIONALE
1. Check the patient's name.	1. For proper patient identification.
2. Check physician's directives and bottle, vial, or tube for correct medication.	2. To avoid medication error.
3. Check physician's directives designating eye requiring drops. O.D. (oculus dexter)—right eye O.S. (oculus sinister)—left eye O.U. (oculus uterque)—both eyes	
4. Wash hands prior to instilling medication.	4. To prevent transfer of microorganisms to patient.
5. Remove cap from container and place on clean surface.	5. To prevent contamination of lid.
6. If eyedropper is used, fill eyedropper with medication but prevent medication from flowing back into bulb end.	6. Loose particles of rubber from bulb end may slip into medication.
7. Using forefinger, pull lower lid down gently (see Fig. A).	7. To expose inner surface of lid and cul-de-sac.
8. Instruct patient to look upward (see Fig. B)	8. Prevents medication from hitting sensitive cornea.
9. Drop medication into center of lower lid (cul-de-sac).	
10. Instruct patient to close eyes slowly but not to squeeze or rub them (Fig. C). Open eye (Fig. D).	10. Squeezing or rubbing would express medication from eye; closing allows medication to be distributed evenly over eye.

(continued)

PROCEDURE GUIDELINES 14-2 ◆ Instillation of Medications *(continued)*

PROCEDURE *(cont'd)*	NURSING ACTION	RATIONALE

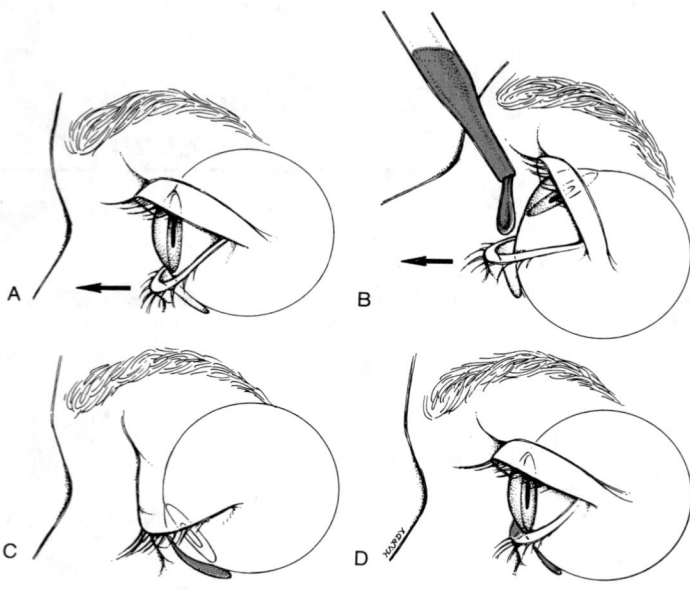

Instillation of ocular medications.

11. Wipe off excess solution with gauze or cotton balls.	11. Prevents possible skin irritation.
12. Wash hands after instilling medication.	12. Prevents transfer of microorganisms to self or other patients.

FOLLOW-UP PHASE

Record time, type, strength, and amount of medication and the eye into which medication was instilled.

PATIENT EDUCATION: SELF-INSTILLATION OF MEDICATION

1. Tilt head back.	1. Places eye and lower lid in a horizontal plane.
2. Using forefinger, pull lower lid down.	2. Exposes inner surface of lower lid.
3. With other hand, hold dropper or container horizontally and facing top of head.	3. Positions dropper or container above receiving lid.
4. Look up and instill medication onto lower lid per instructions (ie one drop). Continue with steps 10–12 above.	4. Prevents medication from hitting sensitive cornea.

Note: Eye ointment: Ointment from tube is gently squeezed as a ribbon of medication along inner lower lid with care taken not to touch eye with end of tube.
Eye Drops: Wait 5 minutes between each medication.

TABLE 14-1 Ophthalmic Pharmacologic Agents*

Pharmacology/Action	Products
1. *Sympathomimetics:* Used in the treatment of glaucoma. Immediate effect is decrease in production of aqueous humor. Long-term effect is an increase in outflow facility. May be used in combination with miotics, beta-blockers, carbonic anhydrase inhibitors, or hyperosmotic agents.	Epinephrine Epifrin, Glaucon Epitrate, Propine
2. *Miotics, direct-acting:* Cholinergic agents that affect the muscarinic receptors of the eye; results include miosis and contraction of the ciliary muscle. In narrow-angle glaucoma, miosis opens the angle to improve aqueous outflow. Contraction of the ciliary muscle enhances the outflow of aqueous humor by indirect action of the trabecular network—the exact mechanism is unknown. Primary use of miotics is in glaucoma but can be used to counter the effects of cycloplegics/mydriatics	Acetylcholine (Miochol) Carbachol (Isocarbachol, Niostat) Pilocarpine (Pilocar)
3. *Miotics, cholinesterase inhibitors:* Inhibit the enzyme cholinesterase, causing an increase in the activity of the acetylcholine already present in the body. Causes intense miosis and contraction of the ciliary muscle. Decrease in intraocular pressure that is seen is a result of increased outflow of aqueous humor. Used for treatment of open-angle glaucoma, conditions where the outflow of aqueous is obstructed; postiridectomy problems; and accommodative esotropia (inward deviation of one eye).	Demecarin bromide (Humorsol) Isoflurophate (Floropryl) Physostigmine (IsoptoEserine)
4. *Beta-adrenergic-blocking agents:* Act on the beta receptors of the adrenergic nervous system. Two types of beta sites: B_1 and B_2. B_1 site primarily the myocardium resulting in ↓ heart rate and cardiac output. B_2 primarily bronchial and vascular smooth muscle resulting in bronchoconstriction, decreased blood pressure. There are two types of ophthalmic beta-blockers: cardioselective blocker (betaxolol) acts only on B_1 sites and may on rare occasions cause cardiac effects if absorbed systemically. All other nonselective blockers act on B_1 and B_2 sites and cause significant cardiac and pulmonary effects if absorbed systemically. Used for treatment of increased intraocular pressure by decreasing the formation of aqueous humor and causing a slight increase in the outflow facility.	Betaxolol (Betoptic) Levubunolol (Betagan) Timolol (Timoptic) Carteolol (Ocupress)
5. *Carbonic anhydrase inhibitors:* Acts to inhibit the action of carbonic anhydrase. Suppression of this enzyme results in a decreased production of aqueous humor. Used in combination regime to treat glaucoma and postoperative rise in IOP.	Acetazolamide (Diamox) Methazolamide (Neptazane)
6. *Osmotic diuretics:* Osmotic agents used for reduction of IOP in acute attack of glaucoma or before ocular surgery where preoperative reduction of IOP is indicated.	Mannitol (Osmitrol) Glycerin (Glycerol) Phenylephrine (Ak-Dilate, Mydfrin)
7. *Mydriatics:* Agents that result in dilation of the pupil, vasoconstriction, and an increase in the outflow of aqueous humor. Used for pupillary dilatation for surgery and examination.	
8. *Cycloplegic mydriatics:* Block the reaction of the sphincter muscle of the iris and the muscle of the ciliary body to cholinergic stimulation resulting in dilatation of the pupil (mydriasis) and paralyses of accommodation (cycloplegia). Used in conditions requiring pupil to be dilated and kept from accommodation.	Atropine Homatropine (Ak-Homatropine) Scopolamine (Isopto-Hyoscine) Cyclopentolate (Cyclogel) Tropicamide (Mydriacyl)
9. *Ophthalmic anti-infectives:* Used for treatment of ophthalmic infections. Commercial products intended for treatment of superficial ocular problems, such as conjunctivitis, blepharitis. Extemporaneous (compounded) drops are used for more serious topical infections, ie, corneal ulcer, endophthalmitis (intraocular infection).	*Antibiotics:* Bacitracin (Ak-Tracin) Chloramphenicol (Chloroptic) Erythromycin (Ilosone) Gentamycin (Garamycin) Neomycin/polymixin/bacitracin (Neosporin) Tobramycin (Tobramycin) *Antifungal:* Amphotericin B (Fungizone) Fluconazole Natamycin (Natcyn) *Antiviral:* Trifluridine (Viroptic) Vidarabine (Vira A)
10. *Local anesthetics:* Block the transmission of nerve impulses. Used topically to provide local anesthetic for tests, such as tonometry and for procedures of short duration. Injections used in ophthalmology for retrobulbar blocks.	*Topical:* Proparacaine (Ophthaine) Tetracaine (Pontocain) *Injection:* Lidocaine
11. *Ophthalmic anti-inflammatories—Steroid:* Mostly corticosteroids. Used topically to relieve pain, photophobia, as well as suppressing other inflammatory processes of the conjunctiva, cornea, lid and interior segment of the globe.	Dexamethasone (Maxidrex, Decadron) Flurometholone (FML) Prednisolone Acetate (Predforte, Econopred Plus)

(continued)

TABLE 14-1 Ophthalmic Pharmacologic Agents* *(continued)*

Pharmacology/Action	Products
12. *Nonsteroidal anti-inflammatory drugs* (NSAIDS): Act by inhibiting an enzyme involved in the synthesis of prostaglandins which are key in the body's response to inflammation. These drugs are analgesics and anti-inflammatories.	Diclofenac Sodium (Voltaren) Flurbiprofen (Ocufen) Ketorolac (Acular) Suprofen (Profenal)
13. *Anti-allergy medications:* There are a number of different types of drugs in this category, including antihistamine, mast cell stabilizers, NSAID anesthetic, and astringents.	*Antihistamines:* Pheniramine Pyrilamine Antazoline *Mast cell stabilizer:* Cromolyn *Astringent:* Zinc sulfate

* All pharmacological agents should be reviewed from a drug handbook prior to administration for contraindications, adverse reactions, and cautions. IOP: intraocular pressure.

◆ IRRIGATION OF THE EYE

Refer to Procedure Guidelines 14-3.
    Ocular irrigation is often necessary for the following:
1. To remove secretions from the conjunctival sac.
2. To treat infections.
3. To relieve itching.
4. To irrigate chemicals or foreign bodies from the eyes.
5. To provide moisture on the surface of the eyes of an unconscious patient.

PROCEDURE GUIDELINES 14-3 ◆ Irrigating the Eye (Conjunctival Irrigation)

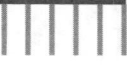

STERILE EQUIPMENT
An eyedropper, asepto bulb syringe, or plastic bottle with prescribed solution depending on the extent of irrigation needed.
For copious use, ie, chemical burns: sterile normal saline or prescribed solution and IV set-up with attached tubing.

PROCEDURE   *PREPARATORY PHASE*
1. Verify that you have the right patient.
2. The patient may sit or lie in a supine position.
3. Instruct the patient to tilt head toward the side of the affected eye.

NURSING ACTION	*RATIONALE*
1. Wash eyelashes and lids with prescribed solution at room temperature; a curved basin should be placed on the affected side of the face to catch the outflow.	1. Any materials on the lids and lashes can be washed off before exposing conjuctiva.
2. Evert the lower conjunctival sac. (If feasible, have the patient pull down lower lid with index finger).	2. Exposes inner surfaces of lower lid and conjunctival sac (involves the patient and gives a sense of control).
3. Instruct the patient to look up; avoid touching eye with equipment.	3. Prevents injury to the sensitive cornea.
4. Allow irrigating fluid to flow from the inner canthus to the outer canthus along the conjunctival sac.	4. Prevents solution from flowing toward the lacimal sac, duct, and nose, possibly transmitting infection.

PROCEDURE (cont'd)	NURSING ACTION	RATIONALE

NURSING ACTION

5. Use only enough force to flush secretions from conjunctiva. (Allow patient to hold curved basin near the eye to catch fluid.)
6. Occasionally have patient close eyes.

FOLLOW-UP PHASE

1. Pat eye dry and dry the patient's face with a soft cloth.
2. Record kind and amount of fluid used as well as its effectiveness.

RATIONALE

5. Prevents eye injury (involves the patient in the treatment).

6. Allows upper lid to meet lower lid with the possibility of dislodging additional particles.

1. Provides comfort.
2. Provides documentation for nursing actions.

◆ APPLICATION OF DRESSING OR PATCH

Refer to Procedure Guidelines 14-4.
One or both eyes may need shielding for the following:

1. To keep an eye at rest, thereby promoting healing.
2. To prevent the patient from touching eye.
3. To absorb secretions.
4. To protect the eye.
5. To control or lessen edema.

PROCEDURE GUIDELINES 14-4 ◆ Application of an Eye Patch, Eye Shield, and Pressure Dressings to the Eye

EQUIPMENT Eye covering to be used, transparent or adhesive tape, rubber glove, scissors, water

PROCEDURE	NURSING ACTION	RATIONALE

NURSING ACTION

Eye Patch

1. Instruct patient to close both eyes.
2. Place patch over the affected eye.
3. Secure the patch with three or more strips of transparent tape diagonally from midforehead to below the ear.
4. For unconscious patient, moisten the eye patch.

EYE SHIELD (PLASTIC OR METAL)

1. Apply over dressings or directly over the undressed eye, fastening with two strips of transparent tape.

2. For metal eye shields, a guard can be placed around flanged edges before use:
   a. Cut 1.2–2.5-cm (½–1-in.) strip from a rubber glove finger.
   b. Stretch it around perimeter of shield.

RATIONALE

1. It is difficult to close only the affected eye.

3. Transparent tape is easy to remove—use hypoallergenic tape if patient has allergies to tape.
4. Dry patch can irritate cornea.

1. Used primarily to protect the eye. Place tape on outer edges of shield so as not to obstruct vision through holes in shield.
2. Protects skin from metal.

   a. Covers metal edges of shield or guard.

   b. Two such pieces add cushioning and provide comfort.

(continued)

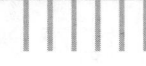

PROCEDURE GUIDELINES 14-4 ◆ Application of an Eye Patch, Eye Shield, and Pressure Dressings to the Eye
(continued)

PROCEDURE (cont'd)	NURSING ACTION	RATIONALE

PRESSURE DRESSINGS

NURSING ACTION	RATIONALE
1. Prepare 8–10 adhesive strips by cutting 2.5-cm (1-in.) adhesive tape in 35-cm (9-in.) lengths. Stretch tape (3M) may also be used.	1. Warming the tape may improve its adhesiveness.
2. Apply two eye patches to the affected eye.	2. Provides pressure dressing bulk.
3. Apply strips from forehead above unpatched eye across dressings to the cheek bone (maxillary prominence).	3. To secure dressing and apply pressure while permitting freedom of movement of the head.

NURSING ALERT:
Prolonged use of pressure dressings may cause increased temperature in the interior of the covered eye because they act as a moisture chamber. Pressure dressings, also, may need to be removed periodically for a short time so that air can freely circulate over cornea.

Note: Check for patient allergies before applying rubber strip tape to guard or to skin.

◆ REMOVING A PARTICLE FROM THE EYE

Refer to Procedure Guidelines 14-5.

Typically, removing a foreign body from the eye is an uncomplicated first-aid measure. However, if the object appears to be embedded, medical intervention is required, that is, local anesthetic, antibiotic therapy, and clinical expertise in using other instruments. The cornea should be evaluated for abrasion from the foreign body (Fig. 14-3).

PROCEDURE GUIDELINES 14-5 ◆ Removing a Particle From the Eye

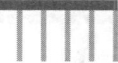

EQUIPMENT	
Local anesthesia	Cotton applicator sticks or tongue blades
Hand lens	Irrigating saline
Sterile fluorescein strips	Antibiotic solution

PROCEDURE — NURSING ACTION	RATIONALE
1. As patient looks upward, evert lower lid to expose the conjunctival sac (see Fig. A).	1. Dust particles are often washed downward by the upper lid.
2. With small cotton applicator dipped in saline, gently remove particle.	2. Wipe gently across lid—inner to outer aspect. Use hand magnifying lens if necessary.
3. If offending particle is not found, proceed to examine upper lid.	
4. Have the patient look downward while you stand in front of patient.	4. Serves as a safety measure since cornea is away from area of activity.
5. Encourage the patient to relax; move slowly and reassure patient that you will not hurt him or her.	5. Relaxation prevents squeezing the lids shut, a maneuver that contracts the obicularis muscle, making eversion of lid impossible.
6. Place cotton applicator stick or tongue blade horizontally on outer surface of upper lid. Apply pressure about 1 cm. above lid margin (see figure).	6. Because the upper tarsal plate extends 10–12 mm above the lid margin, pressure must be applied at least 1 cm above the lid margin for easy eversion of lid.
7. Grasp upper eyelashes with fingers of other hand and pull the upper lid outward and upward over cotton applicator (see figure).	7. Particles may be washed under the lid; visual exposure assists in detection. Eyelid will remain everted by itself.
8. Use fluorescein strip to detect corneal abrasion.	8. Green stain will so indicate if abrasion is present.

PROCEDURE (cont'd)	NURSING ACTION	RATIONALE

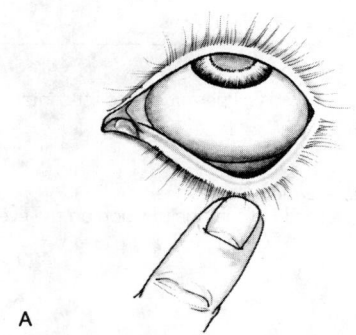 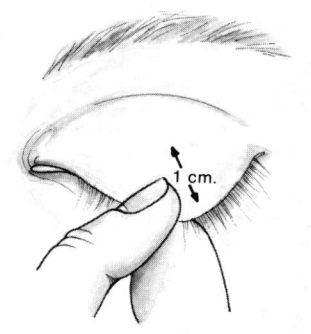 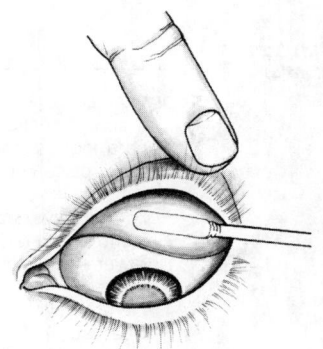

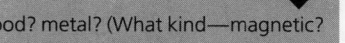

A   B   C

*Examining the eye for a foreign particle. (**A**) Evert lower lid. (**B** and **C**) Evert upper lid.*

NURSING ALERT:
It is very important to take a patient history. Determine the nature of the particle—wood? metal? (What kind—magnetic? copper?) Was it projectile?
    If particle cannot be removed by the method described above, it may have become imbedded in lens or vitreous, in which case an ophthalmologist is required immediately.

◆ REMOVING CONTACT LENSES/PROSTHESIS

Refer to Procedure Guidelines 14-6.
    Because most contact lenses are designed to be worn while awake, if a person is injured and incapacitated because of an accident, sickness, or other cause, the lenses should be removed.

Considerations

1. If the injured person is unconscious or unable to remove lenses, an optometrist or ophthalmologist is called.

2. If professional help is not available and the lenses must be removed, determine the type of lens.
    a. Soft corneal lenses are widely used. The diameter covers the cornea plus a portion of the sclera of the eye. More than 75% of wearers in the United States wear soft contacts.
    b. Rigid or gas-permeable lenses are usually smaller than the cornea of the eye, although some are made to extend beyond the cornea onto the sclera of the eye.
3. Do not remove lenses if the iris is not visible on opening the eyelids; await the arrival of an optometrist or ophthalmologist. If patient is to be transported, note that contacts are in the eyes. (Write out the message and tape it to the patient or send with transporter.)

PROCEDURE GUIDELINES 14-6 ◆ Removing Contact Lenses/Prosthesis

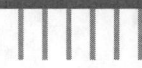

EQUIPMENT   containers, marker, labels, normal saline, eye suction cup

PROCEDURE   **PREPARATORY PHASE**
Because the patient will undoubtedly be in the recumbent position, it is acceptable to remove the lens while he or she is in this position.
Wash your hands thoroughly.

PERFORMANCE PHASE

(continued)

PROCEDURE GUIDELINES 14-6 ◆ Removing Contact Lenses/Prosthesis
(continued)

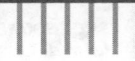

PROCEDURE (cont'd)	NURSING ACTION	RATIONALE

CORNEAL LENS (HARD TYPE)

1. If an eye suction cup is available (as in Emergency Department), simply separate eyelids to expose lens fully; then, place cup over lens and apply slight pressure to cup.
2. For right eye, stand on right side of patient.
3. Lightly place left thumb on upper eyelid; right thumb on lower eyelid close to the edge and parallel with lids (see figure).
4. Gently pull lids apart and observe if contact lens is visible (see figure). If contact lens is not visible, wait for an experienced practitioner.
5. If contact lens is visible, it should slide with the movement of the eyelids while thumbs are still kept at the edges of the eyelids.
6. Gently open the lids wider beyond the edge of the lens and maintain this position.
7. Press gently downward with right thumb on eyeball (see figure).
8. Gently slide the eyelids and thumbs together (see figure).

RATIONALE

1. The suction produced will permit cup to lift contact lens from cornea.

2. Hands will have easier access to eye.
3. Thumbs are placed in a leverage position on the eyelids.

7. This should cause the contact lens to tip up on the edge.

8. This should allow the contact lens to slide out between the lids where it can be taken off.

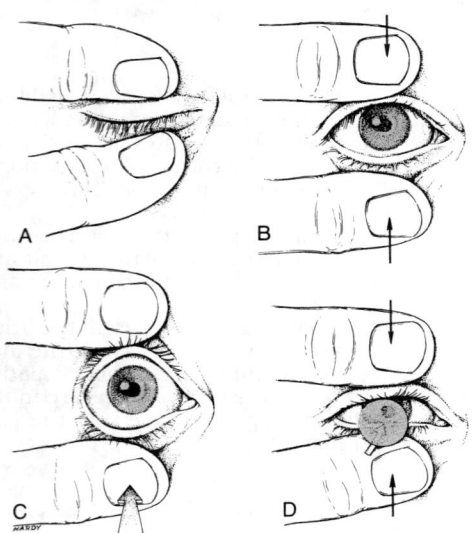

Removing a corneal contact lens.

9. FORCE SHOULD NOT BE USED!
10. If contact lens can be seen but cannot be removed, gently slide it to the white sclera.
11. For left eye, move to left side of patient and repeat procedure.

9. Cornea may be irreparably damaged.

PROCEDURE (cont'd)	NURSING ACTION	RATIONALE

SOFT CONTACT LENSES
May be removed by gently grasping and pinching contact lens between thumb and forefinger. An ophthalmologist can be called to remove lenses if the patient is unable to do so. Also note, if a contact lens cannot be removed with relative ease, discontinue efforts and wait for the ophthalmologist to remove it.

DISPOSITION OF LENSES

1. When lenses are found and removed, place in a case or bottle; label "right" and "left."
2. Store in normal saline solution.

1. Since right and left lenses are often different, storing them with proper labels will be appreciated.
2. This prevents drying and soft lenses must be kept moist.

Note: Extended-wear contacts or disposable contacts worn for more than 1 week may precipitate corneal damage.

◆ OCULAR SURGERY

Follow this nursing process overview for any patient having ocular surgery. Specific nursing interventions are listed in the next section for particular types of surgical procedures.

Nursing Assessment

1. Collect subjective and objective data during examination.
2. Ascertain sequence in which symptoms occurred.
3. Assess patient's mobility and self-care ability.
4. Assess visual and other sensory impairments.
5. Gather data regarding usual support systems used by patient. Is family near? Do friends visit regularly?
6. Review patient's daily schedule.
7. Record pertinent data in patient's record.

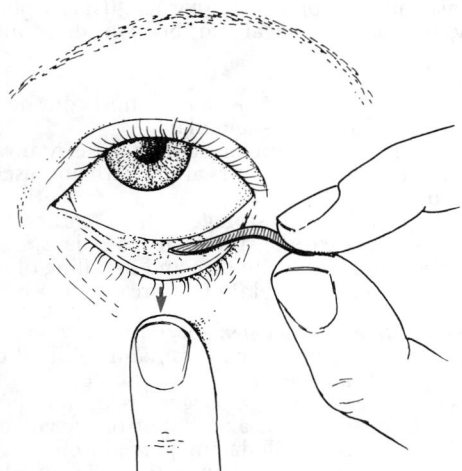

FIGURE 14-3 *Staining cornea with fluorescein strip.*
1. *After telling the patient what you plan to do, wet the distal end of a fluorescein strip with sterile normal saline solution (use sterile, individually wrapped fluorescein strip).*
2. *Pull lower eyelid down; gently touch the inner segment of the lower lid with the strip: a green stain will coat area of abrasion.*
3. *Have the patient blink several times to distribute the fluorescein dye.*
4. *The eye is now ready for examination.*

Nursing Diagnoses

A. Knowledge Deficit of postoperative expectations and continuing care
B. Risk for Injury related to altered vision
C. Sensory/Perceptual Alterations (Visual) related to disease, trauma, or postoperative eye condition
D. Fear of blindness related to altered vision
E. Self-care deficits related to reduced or altered vision

Nursing Interventions

A. *Preparing for Surgery*
1. Explain to the patient preoperative orders as well as postoperative expectations. (These will be specific for each type of surgery or health care provider.)
   a. Specific position in bed may be maintained for a few hours, for example, patient may lie on unoperated side.
   b. Small pillow may be used while patient is in supine position.
2. Instruct patient to wash hair the evening before surgery; long hair of female patients should be arranged so that it is off the face.
3. Check agency surgical policy regarding skin preparation. Patients may be requested to shower with antibacterial soap the evening before or morning of surgery.
4. Check that operative permit is correct and signed with specified eye having surgery noted.
5. Remove dentures, contact lenses, or artificial eye and any metal before patient goes to the operating room. (Wedding band can usually be taped in place.)
6. Inform patient if any eye bandages are necessary postoperatively.
7. Administer any preoperative medications, analgesics, or tranquilizers as prescribed.
8. Position side rails (up) after administering any medications and place call bell next to patient.
9. Be available to answer any questions the patient may have relating to the surgery or postoperative period. ◆

NURSING ALERT:
For eye patients requiring bed rest (ie, after keratoplasty, injury, retinal detachment surgery), measures should be taken to prevent pulmonary and/or circulatory complications. This may include passive range-of-motion exercises, antiembolism stockings, and special positioning.

B. Preventing Injury Postsurgery

1. Position the patient as permitted for specific surgery.
2. Position side rails (up) to offer patient a sense of security.
3. Place call bell next to patient; have patient call the nurse rather than risk increased intraocular pressure from the stress and strain of attempting to be self-sufficient.
4. Instruct caregivers to tell the patient when they enter and leave the room.
5. Avoid activities such as combing hair that will disturb the patient's head or cause tension on sutures or operative site.

C. Compensating for Altered Vision

1. Orient patient to any new environment—room arrangement and/or people.
2. Encourage self-care within the patient's limits.
3. Supervise attempts of patient to feed himself or herself and in other self-care activities.

D. Reducing Fear

1. Recognize that dependence on sight is exaggerated when one faces diminished or loss of sight.
2. Recognize that individual patient's concern of surgical outcome may be manifested differently, for example, fear, depression, tension, resentment, anger, or rejection.
3. Encourage the patient to express feelings.
4. Demonstrate interest and understanding.
5. Reassure the patient that rehabilitative programs and personnel are available.

E. Increasing Self-Care Activities

1. Provide diversional and occupational therapy to keep the patient occupied mentally within the limits of decreased vision.
2. Provide rest periods as necessary.
3. Provide adequate diet and fluids to promote proper elimination and decreased straining.
4. Discourage patient from smoking, reading, and self-shaving for safety reasons.
5. Caution the patient against rubbing eyes or wiping them with soiled tissues.
6. Instruct patient to wear dark glasses if eyes are light-sensitive.
7. Maintain safe environment—doors should be completely open or closed, floors kept clear of articles.

Patient Education/Health Maintenance

1. Advise patient to consult ophthalmologist before undertaking diversional or recreational therapy that may be fatiguing to the eyes—no reading; television in moderation.
2. Emphasize that lights should not be too bright or glaring.
3. Inform the patient before he or she leaves the hospital regarding medications, eyeglasses, follow-up visits.
4. Instruct the patient and family on instillation of eye medications and proper cleansing of eyes.
   a. Instillation of eye drops.
   b. Application of an eye shield.
5. Inform the patient of talking books, records, tapes, and machines available from most public libraries without charge.

6. Initiate follow-up visits with ophthalmologist.
7. Check the following with patient/family before discharge:
   a. Is a return appointment date with health care provider confirmed?
   b. Are patient's medications properly identified and labeled? Does the patient and family member know how to use the prescribed medications?
   c. Does the patient understand the restrictions placed on him/her and the reasons for them?
   d. Does patient/family know what signs/symptoms must be reported to health care provider between appointments (ie, pain, temperature above 101°F, discharge)?

Evaluation

A. Demonstrates improved vision in accordance with expectations of the surgery
B. Appears relaxed and positive concerning outcome of surgery
C. Manages self-care with minimal assistance
D. Describes precautions that must be taken as safety measures, carries cane to prevent possible falls
E. Identifies symptoms that may occur if complications develop and the appropriate action to be taken for each symptom

◆ TYPES OF SURGICAL PROCEDURES

Corneal Transplantation (Keratoplasty)

A. Description

The transplantation of a donor cornea, usually obtained at autopsy, to repair a corneal scar, burn, or deformity.

1. Types of grafts
   a. Full-thickness (6.5–8 mm)—most common.
   b. Partial-thickness—lamellar.
2. Fresh cornea is the preferred tissue; it is removed from the donor within 12 hours after death and used within 24 hours.
3. Special solutions for storage of fresh cornea are available that may extend storage up to 3 days.
4. Cryopreservation is the care and handling of a corneal graft by freezing to retain its transparency.

B. Preoperative Management/Nursing Care

1. Discuss psychological, cultural, and spiritual concerns with patient and health care personnel.
2. Advise patient that the surgery is usually performed under local anesthesia and that he or she will be awake and must remain still during procedure.
3. Cleanse the face thoroughly with antibacterial solution as ordered.
4. Administer preoperative medications as ordered.

C. Postoperative Management/Nursing Care

1. Assess for:
   a. Anxiety—healing may be slow.
   b. Security of the eye patch—patch helps protect the eye from injury and loss of aqueous humor.

    c. Level of discomfort—pain may be symptomatic of complication.
    d. Bowel and bladder habits—to prevent straining or urinary retention.
    e. Activity—avoid activities that increase intraocular pressure (sneezing, coughing, quick movement of the head).
2. Administer medications as prescribed, (i.e., pain medication, steroid eye drops).
3. Prevent infection—use aseptic technique with medication administration and dressing change.
4. Instruct patient to avoid touching dressing and eyes.

D. *Potential Complications:*
1. Hemorrhage
2. Graft dislocation
3. Infection
4. Postoperative glaucoma
5. Graft rejection—may occur 10 to 14 days postoperatively
6. Signs and symptoms include:
    a. Decreased vision
    b. Ocular irritation
    c. Corneal edema
    d. Red sclera

E. *Patient Education/Health Maintenance*
1. Teach patient signs of graft rejection occurring about 10 to 14 days postoperatively.
2. Instruct patient to monitor eye daily for graft rejection. Recommend assessment be done same time daily for comparison.
3. Teach patient that vision varies and that functional vision does not return until sutures are removed.
4. Emphasize the importance of follow-up visits.

Radial Keratotomy

A. *Description*
Procedure designed to provide correction of myopia (nearsightedness). The cornea is anesthetized topically, and under a microscope, the surgeon marks the visual axis. Eight to 16 radial incisions are made into the corneal surface to flatten it. This permits images to fall on the retina instead of in front of it.

B. *Preoperative Management/Nursing Care*
1. Instruct patient that face will be cleansed with an antiseptic solution.
2. Advise patient that draping of face will occur.
3. Explain that the procedure is quick, however, the patient needs to remain very still.
4. Administer preoperative medications as ordered.

C. *Postoperative Management/Nursing Care*
1. Irrigate eye and instill medication.
2. Patch the eye for 24 hours to protect eye.
3. Assess pain, which may be considerable, and medicate as ordered.
4. Assess level of visual acuity with eye patched.
5. Instruct patient not to rub eye to minimize corneal damage.

D. *Patient Education/Health Maintenance*
1. Reassure that postoperative photophobia is common but subsides within 6 weeks.
2. Recommend wearing sunglasses to reduce the discomfort of bright light.

3. Reinforce safety measures, because the patient's vision may fluctuate.
4. Instruct the patient to protect the affected eye from soap and flowing water while bathing.
5. Instruct female patients to avoid wearing eye makeup to minimize irritation.

Vitrectomy

A. *Description*
This procedure is performed for conditions such as unresolved hemorrhage with diabetic retinopathy, intraocular foreign body, and vitroretinal adhesions. It involves the removal of all or part of the vitreous humor, the transparent, gelatin-like substance behind the lens. As the vitreous is removed, saline is infused to replace the vitreous. At the end of the procedure, gas, air, or silicone oil may be introduced into the eye to keep the retina in place.

B. *Preoperative Management/Nursing Care*
1. Provide explanations of procedures.
2. Explain that outcomes vary.
3. Assess patient's visual acuity and level of function.
4. Give preoperative medication as ordered.

C. *Postoperative Management/Nursing Care*
1. Place pressure patch on one or both eyes after surgical closure.
2. Assist with activities to ensure patient safety.
3. Apply cold compresses to control edema and associated discomfort.
4. Restrict activity to bed rest with bathroom privileges.
5. Medicate for pain, nausea, and vomiting, as indicated.
6. Monitor vital signs and blood work, for example, patients with diabetes must have frequent monitoring of glucose levels and presence of ketones.
7. Monitor for activities that cause increasing intraocular pressure (eg, sneezing, coughing, straining, bending).
8. Instill eye medications as ordered.
9. Properly position patient—if the patient was injected with air during surgery, he or she will remain face down to keep the air/gas bubble over the retina. If not, a semi-Fowler's position is appropriate to keep the visual axis clear.
10. Evaluate drainage—a moderate amount is to be expected for about two postoperative days. Unusual amounts of color should be reported immediately.
11. Encourage patience, because the patient will be anxious to witness immediate improvement in vision.

Enucleation

A. *Description*
Complete removal of the eyeball, usually performed due to trauma, infection, tumor, or prevention of sympathetic ophthalmia. At surgery, the eye is removed by opening the conjunctiva and extraocular muscles, severing the optic nerve, and removing the eyeball. A ball implant is then covered by the muscles and maintains the contour of the eye. The conjunctiva is then closed and a plastic conformer is placed to maintain the integrity of the eyelid.

B. *Preoperative Management/Nursing Care*
1. Review the procedure with patient and family members.
2. Describe postoperative expectations in detail.

3. Provide teaching in care of enucleated eye and prosthesis:
   a. Inspecting eye and lid.
   b. Instilling medication.
   c. Irrigating site to remove mucous.
   d. Removing the prosthesis (See Procedure Guidelines 14-6).
   e. Using aseptic technique when performing procedures.
      Note: Ensure that teaching begins preoperatively.
4. Assess fear and anxiety associated with loss of body part.
5. Advise patient and family of support systems available, and make appropriate referrals.
6. Prepare the patient for surgery and give preoperative medications as ordered.

C. *Postoperative Management/Nursing Care*
1. Instill medications, usually antibiotic and steroid ointments, to prevent infection.
2. Apply pressure/ice dressings as ordered to reduce swelling.
3. Irrigate conformer area to reduce mucous.
4. Cleanse eyelid to reduce chance of infection.
5. Assist patient in adjusting to body image change.
6. Assist patient in adjusting to monocular vision—especially with loss of peripheral vision and depth perception.
7. Review that in 4 to 6 weeks after surgery, the patient will receive an ocular prosthesis (artificial eye).

D. *Complications*
1. Hemorrhage
2. Infection
3. Implant extrusion

Common Eye Disorders

◆ CATARACT

Clouding or opacity of the crystalline lens.

Pathophysiology/Etiology

1. Senile cataract—commonly occurs with aging.
2. Congenital cataract—occurs at birth.
3. Traumatic cataract—occurs after injury.
4. Aphakia—absence of creptalline lens.

Clinical Manifestations

1. Blurred or distorted vision.
2. Glare from bright lights.
3. Gradual and painless loss of vision.
4. Previously dark pupil may appear milky or white.

Diagnostic Evaluation

1. Slit-lamp examination—to provide magnification.
2. Tonometry—to determine IOP.
3. Direct and indirect ophthalmoscopy.

4. Ocular examination.
5. Perimetry—to determine the scope of the visual field.

Management

A. *General*
1. Surgical removal of the lens is indicated.
2. A patient with one cataract can usually manage without surgery.
3. If cataract occurs in both eyes, surgery is recommended when vision in the better eye causes problems in daily activities. Surgery is done on only one eye at a time.
4. Cataract surgery is usually done under local anesthesia. Preoperative medications produce decreased response to pain and lessened motor activity (neuroleptanalgesia). Oral medications are given to reduce intraocular pressure.
5. Intraocular lens (IOL) implants are usually implanted at the time of cataract extraction.
6. In some instances, after lens extraction and the healing process, the patient may be fitted with appropriate eyeglasses or contact lenses to correct refraction.

B. *Surgical Procedures*
1. Two types of extractions:
   a. Intracapsular extraction—the lens as well as the capsule are removed through a small incision.
   b. Extracapsular extraction—the lens capsule is incised, and the nucleus, cortex, and anterior capsule are extracted.
      (1) The posterior capsule is left in place and is usually the base to which an IOL is implanted.
      (2) A conservative procedure of choice, simple to perform, is done, usually under local anesthesia.
2. Two types of procedures for extraction are:
   a. Cryosurgery—a special technique in which a pencil-like instrument with a metal tip is supercooled ($-35°C$), then is touched to the exposed lens, freezing to it so that the lens is easily lifted out.
   b. Phacoemulsification—the mechanical breaking up (emulsifying) of the lens by a hollow needle vibrating at ultrasonic speed. This action is coupled with irrigation and aspiration of the emulsified particles from the anterior chamber.

C. *Intraocular Lens Implantation*
1. The implantation of a synthetic lens (intraocular lens) is designed for distance vision; the patient may wear prescription glasses for reading and near vision.
   a. Intraocular lens implant is an alternative to sight correction with glasses or contact lenses for the aphakic (absence of lens) patient.
   b. Sophisticated calculations are required to determine the prescription for the lens.
   c. Numerous types of intraocular lens are available. Designs and materials change as new developments occur. Extended-wear contact lenses may replace intraocular lens.
2. Advantages of intraocular lens include the following:
   a. Provides an alternative for the person who cannot wear cataract glasses or contact lenses.
   b. Cannot be lost or misplaced like conventional glasses.
3. Complications (specific to implantation):
   a. Pain from inflammation of various eye structures—usually controlled by nonsteroidal anti-inflammatory drugs, but systemic antibiotics and immunosuppression may be required.

b. Rosy vision (glare) due to keeping pupil from full constriction; excessive light enters pupil, causing a dazzling of macula (minute corneal opacity).
c. Degeneration of the cornea.
d. Malpositioning or dislocation of lens.

Nursing Assessment

A. Preoperative
1. Assess knowledge level regarding procedure.
2. Assess level of fear and anxiety.
3. Determine visual limitations.

B. Postoperative
1. Assess pain level.
   a. Sudden onset—may be due to ruptured vessel or suture and may lead to hemorrhage.
   b. Severe pain—accompanied by nausea and vomiting; may be caused by intraocular pressure.
2. Assess visual acuity in unoperated eye.
3. Assess patient's ability to ambulate.
4. Assess patient's level of independence.

Nursing Diagnoses

A. Sensory/Perceptual Alteration related to cataracts
B. Pain related to surgical complications

Nursing Interventions

A. Preparing the Patient for Surgery
1. Orient patient and explain procedures and plan of care to decrease anxiety.
2. Instruct patient not to touch eyes to decrease contamination.
3. Obtain conjunctival cultures, if requested, using aseptic technique.
4. Administer preoperative medications as ordered to promote comfort.

B. Preventing Complications Postoperatively
1. Medicate for pain as prescribed to promote comfort.
2. Administer medication to control nausea and vomiting.
3. Notify health care provider of sudden pain associated with restlessness and increased pulse rate.
4. Caution patient against coughing or sneezing to prevent increased IOP.
5. Advise patient against rapid movement or bending from the waist to minimize IOP.
6. Allow patient to ambulate as soon as possible and to resume independent activities.
7. Encourage patient to wear shield at night to protect operated eye from injury while sleeping.

Patient Education/ Health Maintenance

A. Promoting Independence
1. Advise patient to increase activities gradually or as directed by health care provider. Most patients can re-sume normal activity the day after the procedure. However, there may be restrictions.
2. Caution against activities that cause patient to strain, for example, lifting heavy objects, straining at defecation.
3. Instruct patient and family in proper use of medications.

B. Adjusting to Visual Change
1. Tell patient to apply plastic shield over the eye at night to avoid accidental injury during sleep.
2. Inform about fitting for temporary corrective lenses for the first 6 weeks.
   a. Prescription for permanent lenses will be determined 6 to 12 weeks after surgery for intracapsular extraction.
   b. Prescription for contact lenses will be determined about 3 to 6 weeks after phacoemulsification.
   c. Encourage patient to use dark glasses after eye dressings are removed to provide comfort.

C. Adjusting to the Eyeglasses
1. Stress the importance of patience in the coming weeks of adjustment—it is easy to become frustrated.
2. Tell patient that if glasses are to be worn, they will cause the perceived image to be about one-third larger than that seen by the patient before cataract formation. (Glass is usually heavier and thicker than the more expensive plastic cataract eyeglass lenses.)
   Note: The patient can use only one eye at a time with glasses, if only one eye is operated for cataract, because the operated eye has a 30% increase in image size and the unoperated eye still has normal-sized images, which cannot be superimposed.
3. Instruct the patient to look through the center of the corrective glasses and to turn head when looking to the side, because peripheral vision is markedly distorted.
4. It is necessary to relearn space judgment—walking, using stairs, reaching for articles on the table (such as a cup of coffee), pouring liquids.
5. Use handrails while walking.

D. Becoming Familiar With Contact Lenses
Teach the patient that:

1. With contact lenses, magnification is only about 5% to 10%; peripheral vision is not distorted.
2. Both eyes may be used together, because the image difference between an aphakic eye with a contact lens and the unoperated eye is only 8% to 10%. Space judgment presents little difficulty.
3. If the patient has difficulty applying lenses, has a tremor of the hands, or has general hygienic problems that could cause soiling and infection, there may be complications. These patients are not prime candidates for contact lenses.

E. Becoming Familiar With Intraocular Lens
1. Teach patient that with an intraocular lens, magnification problems are negligible. Both the operated eye and the unoperated eye can work together after cataract surgery with lens implantation.
2. Advise that no eyeglasses may be required for distance but may be needed for reading and writing.
3. Caution against straining of any type. Bend knees only if necessary to reach for something on the floor.
4. Recommend sponge bathing. Avoid getting soap in the eyes.

5. Advise avoidance of tilting head forward when washing hair; tilt head slightly backward. Vigorous shaking of the head is avoided.

F. *Administering Eye Medications*
1. Teach patient how to instill eye medications as directed.
2. Advise to bring all eye medications to ophthalmologist appointment to permit adjustments in dosage and medications. What will not be used can then be discarded to prevent confusion.

Evaluation

A. Vision maximized and distortions or limitations in vision described by patient.
B. Independent activities demonstrated.

◆ ACUTE (ANGLE CLOSURE) GLAUCOMA

A condition in which an obstruction occurs within the trabecular meshwork and the canal of Schlemm. Intraocular pressure is normal when the anterior chamber angle is open, and glaucoma occurs when a significant portion of that angle is closed. Glaucoma is associated with progressive visual field loss and eventual blindness if allowed to progress.

Clinical Manifestations

1. Severe pain in and around eyes due to increased ocular pressure (often above 75 mm Hg); transitory attacks.
2. Rainbow of color around lights.
3. Vision becomes cloudy and blurred.
4. Pupil dilates; nausea and vomiting may occur.
5. Although onset may have initial subclinical symptoms, severity of symptoms may progress to include systemic disturbances; (gastrointestinal, sinus, neurologic, and dental problems).

> **NURSING ALERT:**
> This type of glaucoma is a medical emergency and requires immediate treatment. Untreated, it can result in blindness in less than a week.

Diagnostic Evaluation

1. Tonometry—elevated IOP.
2. Ocular examination may reveal a pale optic disk.
3. Gonioscopy (using special instrument called gonioscope) to study the angle of the anterior chamber of the eye.
> *Note:* Because of the relative ease of developing glaucoma, unless a person older than age 40 years has a complete physical examination periodically, including measurement of eye pressure (tonometry), the disease may not be discovered until it is considerably advanced. Early detection and treatment will prevent loss of eyesight.

> **NURSING ALERT:**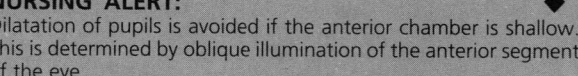
> Dilatation of pupils is avoided if the anterior chamber is shallow. This is determined by oblique illumination of the anterior segment of the eye.

Management

1. Emergency pharmacotherapy is initiated to decrease eye pressure before surgery.
2. Medications are prescribed at the discretion of the ophthalmologist according to the patient's condition and needs.
3. Medication classifications prescribed include:
  a. Parasympathomimetic drugs used as miotic drugs—pupil contracts; iris is drawn away from cornea; aqueous humor may drain through lymph spaces (meshwork) into canal of Schlemm.
  b. Sympathomimetic drugs—decrease aqueous humor production rate.
  c. Carbonic anhydrase inhibitor—restricts action of enzyme that is necessary to produce aqueous humor.
  d. Beta-blockers—nonselective—may reduce production of aqueous humor or may facilitate outflow of aqueous humor.
  e. Hyperosmotic agents—increase blood osmolarity.
4. Surgery is indicated if:
  a. Intraocular pressure is not maintained within normal limits by medical regimen.
  b. There is progressive visual field loss with optic nerve damage.
5. Types of surgery include:
  a. Peripheral iridectomy—excision of a small portion of the iris whereby aqueous humor can bypass pupil; treatment of choice.
  b. Trabeculectomy—partial-thickness scleral resection with small part of trabecular meshwork removed and iridectomy. Necessary if peripheral anterior adhesions (synechiae) have developed due to repeated glaucoma attacks.

Nursing Assessment

1. Evaluate patient for any of the clinical manifestations.
2. Assess patient's level of anxiety and knowledge base.

Nursing Diagnoses

A. Pain related to increased IOP
B. Fear related to pain and potential loss of vision

Nursing Interventions

A. *Relieving Pain*
1. Notify health care provider immediately.
2. Administer medications as directed.
3. Explain to patient that the goal of treatment is to reduce IOP as quickly as possible.
4. Explain procedures to patient.

5. Reassure patient that with reduction in IOP, pain and other signs and symptoms should subside.

B. *Relieving Fear*
1. Provide reassurance and calm presence to reduce anxiety and fear.
2. Prepare patient for surgery, if necessary.

Patient Education/ Health Maintenance

1. Instruct patient in use of medications.
2. Remind patient to keep follow-up appointments.
3. Teach patient that glaucoma is not cured but controlled.
4. Instruct patient to seek immediate medical attention if signs and symptoms of increased intraocular pressure return.
5. Advise patient to notify all health care providers of condition and medications and to avoid use of medications that may increase IOP such as corticosteroids and anticholinergics (such as antihistamines).

Evaluation

A. Patient states that pain is decreased
B. Patient describes treatment regimen and verbalizes reduced fear

◆ CHRONIC (OPEN-ANGLE) GLAUCOMA

Most common form of glaucoma, usually beginning around age 40 to 45 with clinical symptoms appearing as late as age 60 to 65. IOP becomes elevated due to microscopic obstruction of the trabecular meshwork.

Clinical Manifestations

1. Mild, bilateral discomfort (tired feeling in eyes, foggy vision).
2. Slowly developing impairment of peripheral vision—central vision unimpaired.
3. Progressive loss of visual field.
4. Halos present around lights with increased ocular pressure.

Diagnostic Evaluation

1. Tonometry—to evaluate for increased IOP.
2. Ocular examination—to check for clipping and atrophy of the optic disk.

Management

1. Often treated with a combination of miotic and carbonic anhydrase inhibitors.
2. Remission may occur; however, there is no cure. The patient should continue to see health care provider at 3- to 6-month intervals for control of IOP.

3. If medical treatment is not successful, surgery may be required, but is delayed as long as possible.
4. Types of surgery include:
   a. Laser trabeculoplasty
      (1) An outpatient procedure, treatment of choice if increased ocular pressure unresponsive to medical regimen only.
      (2) As many as 100 superficial surface burns are placed evenly at junction of pigmented and nonpigmented trabeculum meshwork for 360 degrees in anesthetized eye, which allows increased outflow of aqueous humor.
      (3) Maximum decrease in IOP is achieved in 2 to 3 months, but IOP may rise again in 1 to 2 years.
   b. Iridencleisis—an opening is created between anterior chamber and space beneath the conjunctiva; this bypasses the blocked meshwork, and aqueous humor is absorbed into conjunctival tissues.
   c. Cyclodiathermy or cyclocryotherapy—the ciliary body's function of secreting aqueous humor is decreased by damaging the body with high-frequency electrical current or supercooled probe applied to the surface of the eye over the ciliary body.
   d. Corneoscleral trephine (rarely done)—a permanent opening at the junction of the cornea and sclera is made through the anterior chamber so aqueous humor can drain.

Nursing Assessment

1. Evaluate patient for any of the listed clinical manifestations.
2. Assess patient's knowledge of disease process.
3. Assess level of anxiety related to diagnosis of glaucoma.

Nursing Diagnoses

A. Knowledge Deficit of glaucoma and surgical procedure

Nursing Interventions

Glaucoma and cataracts, at times, are accompanying disorders. Preoperative interventions are similar. See Cataracts, page 432.

A. *Providing Postoperative Care*
1. Be aware that patient with glaucoma may be ambulatory quicker than patient with cataracts, and specific interventions depend on the type of surgery performed.
2. Elevate head of bed to promote drainage of aqueous humor after a trabeculectomy.
3. Administer medications (steroids and cycloplegics) as prescribed after peripheral iridectomy to decrease inflammation and to dilate the pupil.

Patient Education/ Health Maintenance

1. The patient must remember that glaucoma cannot be cured, but it can be controlled.

(text continues on page 447)

TABLE 14-2 Other Eye Disorders

Disease	Description	Cause and Etiology	Signs and Symptoms	Diagnosis and Medical Management	Nursing Management
Problems associated with refraction					
Astigmatism	Abnormal curvature of the cornea	Uneven curvature of the cornea causing the patient to be unable to focus horizontal and vertical rays on the retina at the same time	Blurred vision Eye strain	Corrected with glasses or hard contact lenses (Correction— Cylinder lens)	*Nsg Dx:* Sensory/Perceptual Alteration (Visual) *Nsg Assessment:* 1. Eye examination to determine signs and symptoms. 2. Assess knowledge of treatment. 3. Assess for compliance to treatments. *Nsg Interventions:* 1. Assist with eye exam. *Pt Education:* 1. Instruct patient in proper use and care of eye glasses and/or contact lenses. 2. Inform patient about surgical interventions (see Radial Keratotomy).
Hyperopia	Farsightedness	Rays of light coming from an object at a distance of 6 m (20 ft) or more are brought into focus in back of the retina	Blurred vision (distance) Headaches Eye strain	Correction with glasses or contact lenses (Correction—Convex lens)	
Myopia	Nearsightedness	Rays of light coming from an object at a distance of 6 m (20 ft) or more are brought into focus in front of the retina	Blurred vision Headaches Eye strain	Correction with glasses or contact lenses (Correction— Concave lens) Radial keratotomy	

Problems associated with the eyelid

Condition	Description	Cause	Signs/Symptoms	Rx/Dx	Nursing Care
Blepharitis	Infection of the eye lid	Bacteria Virus	Crusted eyelids Redness Irritation Mucopurulent secretion	Dx: Culture Rx: Antibiotic drops or ointment	*Nsg Dx:* Risk for Infection related to disease process *Nsg Assessment:* 1. Assess for signs and symptoms of infection. 2. Assess for duration of signs and symptoms. 3. Assess for cause. 4. Assess visual acuity. *Nsg Interventions:* 1. Assist with eye exam. 2. Obtain culture if ordered. 3. Administer medication as ordered. 4. Assist with surgical procedure. *Pt. Ed.:* 1. Instruct pt in administration of medication. 2. Instruct pt in aseptic technique. 3. Instruct pt in safety measures with decreased visual acuity due to medication or patching.
Chalazion	Infection of the meibomian gland	Bacteria *Streptococcus* *Staphylococcus*	Pain Redness Swelling (under eye lid) Foreign body sensation	*Rx:* Warm soaks Ointment Drops Incision and drainage of chalazion may be required	
Hordeolum	Infection of the eyelash follicle	Bacteria *Staphylococcus*	Redness Pain White pustule at eyelash Foreign body sensation	*Rx:* Warm soak Ointment Drops Do not squeeze the pustule—may introduce contents into eye	
Ptosis	Drooping of the eyelid	Systemic disease Myasthenia gravis Nerve palsy Trauma Aging	Difficulty with vision	*Rx:* Treat underlying disease Surgery-Blephroplasty Ptosis crutches	

(continued)

TABLE 14-2 Other Eye Disorders *(continued)*

Disease	Description	Cause and Etiology	Signs and Symptoms	Diagnosis and Medical Management	Nursing Management
Problems associated with conjunctiva					
Conjunctivitis	Inflammation or infection of the conjunctiva	Allergens Bacteria Chlamydia Fungus Trauma—physical or chemical Virus	Photobia Redness Pain Swelling Lacrimation Lids frequently crusted and stuck on awakening	*Dx:* Culture *Rx:* Note: Severe conjunctivitis should be treated promptly to prevent inward spread Drops Ointment Treatment dependent on causative organism	*Nsg Dx:* Pain *Nsg Assessment:* 1. Assess for signs and symptoms of infection. 2. Assess visual acuity. 3. Assess for level of discomfort. *Nsg Intervention:* 1. Assist with eye exam. 2. Administer medications as ordered. *Pt Ed.:* 1. Instruct pt in aseptic technique. 2. Encourage pt to take medication for entire length of prescription. 3. Encourage the use of warm compresses. 4. Review safety measures with decreased visual acuity.
Subconjunctival hemorrhage	Bleeding in the conjunctiva	Breakage of small blood vessel due to sneezing, Coughing trauma, spontaneous	Red eye	May be sign of systemic problem (eg. hypertension) Vision should be tested No definitive treatment	
Problems associated with extraocular muscles	See chapter 53				
Problems associated with the cornea					
Corneal abrasion	Loss of epithelial layers of the cornea	Inadvertent contact with object, ie, fingernail, tree branch, edge of paper. Overwearing contact lens	Pain Lacrimation Photophobia Redness Swelling Inability to open eye	*Dx:* Made through fluorocein stain and slit lamp exam. *Rx:* **MEDICAL EMERGENCY** Drops Ointment Patching—may or may not be used * Cornea usually heals within 24–48 hours	*Nsg Dx:* Sensory/Perceptual Alterations (Visual) *Nsg Assessment:* Assess for: signs and symptoms. Assess for cause of problem. Assess for level of discomfort, visual acuity, level of cooperation and compliance with treatment.

Nursing Intervention:
1. Assist with eye exam.
2. Eye medication as ordered.
3. Continuous observe for level of discomfort and treat as directed.
4. Evaluate for signs of sleep deprivation with frequency of eye medication.
5. Assist family to develop a treatment regime they will be able to comply with.
6. Preop and postop nursing intervention as required. See specific procedures.

Pt Ed.:
1. Instruct pt and family in importance of strict compliance to eye medication regimen.
2. Teach patient about proper technique for contact lens wearing.
3. Explain surgical intervention to pt and family.
4. Instruct pt in safely with decreased visual acuity due to medication, patching, and disease.
5. Instruct patient in critical importance of continuous medical follow up as directed.
6. Instruct pt on use of protective devices, ie, patches and shields.

| Corneal Dystrophy | Disorder involving the epithelium and basement membrane Erosion of layers of corneal tissue | Unknown Heredity Trauma | Pain Foreign body sensation Lacrimation * Dystrophy usually bilateral | Dx: Fluorocein stain and slit-lamp exam Rx: Diet Medication Pressure patch Soft contact lenses Surgery * Almost never causes loss of vision |

(continued)

TABLE 14-2 Other Eye Disorders (continued)

Disease	Description	Cause and Etiology	Signs and Symptoms	Diagnosis and Medical Management	Nursing Management
Corneal ulcer (keratitis)	Inflammation of the cornea accompanied by loss of substance	Improper use of contact lens Infection due to: Bacteria Virus Foreign body Improperly treated corneal abrasion Systemic disease	Pain (severe) Photophobia Lacrimation Redness Complications: Iritis Prolapse of iris Corneal scarring Blindness * Endophthalmitis— inflammation of the internal eye	*Dx:* Fluorocin stain and slit-lamp exam Culture for causative organism *Rx:* **MEDICAL EMERGENCY** IV antibiotics Topical drops Steroids * May require administering drop q5–15 minutes around the clock for several days	*Nsg Dx:* Risk for infection related to inflammation and drug therapy *Nsg Assessment:* 1. Review history of present illness. 2. Assess for signs of systemic disease. 3. Assess signs and symptoms of inflammation/infection. 4. Assess for level of discomfort. 5. Assess visual acuity. *Nsg Intervention:* 1. Assist with eye exam. 2. Administer eye medications as directed.
Keraticonus	Corneal irregularity produces protrusion of the cornea in a cone shape	Unknown	Decreased visual acuity	*Rx:* Glasses Contact lenses Surgery—keratoplasty	
Problems associated with the sclera					
Episcleritis	Inflammation of the fascial coat of the eye, which lies between the conjunctiva and sclera	Unknown	Decreased visual acuity Lacrimation Pain Photophobia	*Rx:* None—Self-limiting * May use steroids and antiinflammatory agents	

				Patient Ed:
Scleritis	Acute inflammatory process involving the outer coat of the eye	May be due to chronic systemic inflammation	Redness, Swelling of lid, Lacrimation, Pain, Photophobia	*Rx:* Systemic anti-inflammatory drugs, Steroids *May be a symptom of systemic disease	1. Instruct in administration of eye medications. 2. Review signs and symptoms of infections. 3. Instruct in importance of maintaining aseptic technique. 4. Review safety measures to be used in presence of decreased visual acuity due to inflammation and medication.
Problems with uveal tract Iritis/uveitis	Inflammation of the uveal tract Anterior—anterior iritis Intermedial—pars planitis Posterior uvea— different forms of choriod retinitis	May be an acute disease (iritis) Associated with chronic systemic disease Unknown cause	Pain, Photophobia, Lacrimation, Redness, Swelling, Hypopyon (pus in anterior chamber)	*Rx:* Corticosteroids Anti-inflammatory agents *Treatment of systemic disease	
Sympathetic ophthalmia	Severe granulomatous bilateral uveitis	Surgical or traumatic perforation of the uveal tract	Pain, Loss of vision	*Rx:* Enucleation of the blind, traumatically injured eye See Enucleation	
Problems associated with the vitreous Vitreous hemorrhage	Bleeding into the vitreous	Trauma Diabetic retinopathy Posterior vitreous detachment Retinal tear and detachment Intraocular lens Unknown cause	Loss of vision	*Rx:* Photocoagulation Cryotherapy Scleral buckle Vitrectomy *Treatment depends on finding specific cause	See vitrectomy

(continued)

TABLE 14-2 Other Eye Disorders (continued)

Disease	Description	Cause and Etiology	Signs and Symptoms	Diagnosis and Medical Management	Nursing Management
Problems associated with the retina					
Central retinal artery occlusion	Occlusion of the central artery of the retina	Arterial spasm Emboli Thrombus	Sudden loss of vision in affected eye * Brief slowing of retinal blood flow or lowering of retinal blood pressure may cause transient loss of vision called amaurosis fugax	*Rx:* **MEDICAL EMERGENCY** Treatment related to: Cause Duration Retinal damage Trendelenburg position Carbogen (95% O_2–5% CO_2) Medication	*Nsg Dx:* Sensory/Perceptual Alterations (Visual) *Nsg assessment:* 1. Review history of present illness. 2. Assess signs and symptoms of disease. 3. Assess vital signs. 4. Assess visual acuity. *Nsg Intervention:* 1. Assist with eye exam. 2. Administer medications. 3. Continuously evaluate vital signs with use of carbogen). 4. Administer carbogen q50 minutes out of every hour as ordered. 5. Position patient as ordered—Trendelenburg with detached retina. 6. Facilitate patients immobilization if ordered with detached retina. 7. Assist patient ADL if bilateral patching ordered. *Pt. Ed.:* 1. Discuss low vision aids available. 2. Discuss surgical intervention—see specific surgery this chapter. 3. Review pts need to comply with treatment. 4. Discuss importance of continuous follow up care.
Macular degeneration (senile)	Progressive degeneration of the macula of the retina and choroid	Unknown May have familial tendency Generally affects people over 65 * Leading cause of blindness in elderly	Loss of central vision Blurred wavy distorted vision Yellowish spots seen on retina Dome-shaped retina may be seen Bilateral	*Dx:* Direct/indirect ophthalmoscopy Fundoscopic exam *Rx:* No treatment Laser may help	

Condition	Description	Etiology	Signs/Symptoms	Diagnosis/Treatment	Nursing
Retinal detachment	Separation of the sensory retina from the pigmented epithelium	Spontaneous Trauma Systemic disease (eg, diabetes) Tumors (eg, melanoma) Myopia Cataract extraction	Flashing lights Black spots/floaters Veil or curtain overriding visual field Loss peripheral vision Poor vision upon waking that improves throughout the day	*Dx:* Topography Direct/indirect ophthalmoscopy Slit-lamp exam *Rx:* **MEDICAL EMERGENCY** Surgery Scleral buckle Vitrectomy Cryoplexy Laser photocoagulation No treatment	
Cytomegalovirus (CMV) retinitis	See chapter 27				
Diabetic retinopathy	See Chapter 23				
Retinitis pigmentosa	See Chapter 53				
Eye trauma *Blunt* Contusion	Bruising of tissue around the eye may be accompanied by injury to parts of the eye	Trauma, ie, fist, ball	Swelling and discoloration of the tissue Bleeding into the tissue and structures of the eye	*Dx:* Tests must determine if injury to parts of eye and systemic trauma *Rx:* To reduce swelling Pain management dependent on structures involved	*Nsg Dx:* Risk for Injury related to trauma *Nsg Assessment:* 1. History of present illness. 2. Assessment of signs and symptoms. 3. Assess level of discomfort. 4. Vital signs. 5. Neurological assessment. 6. Contributing medical history. 7. Level of compliance to treatment. 8. Visual acuity *Nursing Interventions:* 1. Continuous eye irrigation (see procedure). 2. Assist with eye examination. 3. Maintain bed rest. 4. Assist with preop and postcare (see specific procedures this chapter). 5. Medicate as ordered. 6. Monitor VS and neurologic assessment. 7. Patching as ordered (see procedure).

(continued)

TABLE 14-2 Other Eye Disorders *(continued)*

Disease	Description	Cause and Etiology	Signs and Symptoms	Diagnosis and Medical Management	Nursing Management
					8. Monitor for signs of infection. 9. Maintain safe environment with decreased visual acuity due to trauma or treatment. 10. Provide psychological support. *PT Education:* 1. Medication administration. 2. Use of patch or shield. 3. Teach patient signs and symptoms to watch for with infection. 4. Teach about surgical procedure. 5. Safety with decreased visual acuity. 6. Importance of follow-up care. 7. Attempt to prevent future trauma, ie, protective eyewear.
Hyphema	Presence of blood in the anterior chamber	Trauma	Pain Blood in anterior chamber Increased intraocular pressure	*Rx:* Usually spontaneous recovery Anterior chamber filled with blood Bed rest Eye shield Interior chamber paracenthesis	
Orbital Fracture	Fracture and dislocation of walls of the orbit, orbital margins, or both	Trauma	Signs and symptoms of head injury Rhinorhea Contusion Diplopia Signs and symptoms associated with bone fragments pressing on structures	*Dx:* Xray, CT *Rx:* May heal on own if no displacement or infringement on other structures Surgery	

Foreign body	Foreign body may occur on: Cornea—25% all ocular injuries Conjunctiva Intraocular particles penetrate sclera, cornea, globe	Trauma, eg, eyelash, flying metal, sand/dirt, wood chips	Severe pain Lacrimation Foreign body sensation Photophobia Redness Swelling * Wood and plant foreign body may cause severe infection within hours	*Rx:* **MEDICAL EMERGENCY** Removal of FB through irrigation Cotton-tip applicator magnet Treatment of intra-ocular FB depends on Size Magnetic properties Tissue reaction Location Surgical removal
Laceration/ perforation	Cutting or penetration of tissue may occur Eyelid Conjunctiva Cornea Sclera Globe	Trauma, eg, scratch, dog bite, paper cut, knife	Pain Bleeding Lacrimation Photophobia	*Rx:* **MEDICAL EMERGENCY** Surgical repair— method of repair depends on severity of injury Antibiotics—topically and systemically
Ruptured globe	Concussive injury to globe with tears in the ocular coats usually the sclera	Trauma eg, high velocity ballistic missiles (bullet), sharp penetrating objects	Pain Altered intraocular pressure Limitation of gaze in field of rupture Hyphema Hemorrhage (poor prognostic sign)	*Dx:* CT Ultrasound *Rx:* **MEDICAL EMERGENCY** Surgical repair Vitrectomy Scleral buckle Antibiotics Steroids Enucleation
Burns, chemical	Burn caused by alkali or acid agent	eg, lye cleaning agents, acid	Pain Burning Lacrimation Photophobia	*Rx:* **MEDICAL EMERGENCY** Copius irrigation till pH is 7 Severe scarring may require keratoplasty Antibiotics * Determine causative agent
Burns, thermal	Usually burn to eye lids—may be first-, second-, or third-degree	Fire Intense heat	Pain Burned skin Blisters	*Rx:* First aid—apply sterile dressings Pain control Leave fluid blebs intact Suture eyelids together to protect eye Skin grafting with severe second and third degree burns

(continued)

TABLE 14-2 Other Eye Disorders *(continued)*

Disease	Description	Cause and Etiology	Signs and Symptoms	Diagnosis and Medical Management	Nursing Management
Burns, ultraviolet	UVA—produces suntan—transmitted by cornea absorbed by lens UVB—Produces sunburn—absorbed by cornea and lens UVE—Absorbed by ozone, emitted by welding equipment, germicidal lamps, lasers and absorbed by the cornea	Excessive exposure to sunlight, eg, sunlamp, snow blindness, welding	Pain Foreign body sensation Lacrimation Photophobia * Symptoms occur sometime after exposure	*Rx:* Pain relief Condition self-limiting	
Ocular Tumors Melanoma	Most common intraocular tumor Originates in outer layers of choroid and spreads in the choroid between sclera and Bruch membrane	Develop from preexisting benign melanoma diagnosed as nevi	Signs and symptoms of retinal detachment Loss of visual field in area of tumor Glaucoma	*Dx:* Ultrasound CT Biopsy *Rx:* Exact treatment not known Small tumors monitored every 6 months Tumor resection Radiation therapy Enucleation	*Nsg Dx:* 1. Body Image Disturbance related to enucleation. 2. Risk for Injury related to radiation 3. Sensory/Perceptual Alterations (Visual) * See enucleation, p. 431 and chapter 6, p. 99.

Nsg: nursing; Dx: diagnosis; Pt: patient; Rx: treatment; Ed: education; CT: computed tomography; q: every; ADLs: activities of daily living.

2. Remind the patient that periodic eye checkups are essential, because pressure changes may occur.
3. Alert patient to avoid, if possible, circumstances that may increase IOP:
   a. Upper respiratory infections.
   b. Emotional upsets—worry, fear, anger.
   c. Exertion, such as snow shoveling, pushing, heavy lifting.
4. Recommend the following:
   a. Continuous daily use of eye medications as prescribed.
   b. Moderate use of the eyes.
   c. Exercise in moderation to maintain general well-being.
   d. Unrestricted fluid intake: alcohol and coffee may be permitted unless they are noted to cause increased intraocular pressure in the particular patient.
   e. Maintenance of regular bowel habits to decrease straining.
   f. Wearing a medical identification tag indicating the patient has glaucoma.

Evaluation

A. Verbalizes restrictions and limitations; demonstrates proper instillation of ophthalmic medications

◆ RETINAL DETACHMENT

Detachment of the retina (rods and cones) from the pigmented epithelium of the retina.

Pathophysiology/Etiology

1. Spontaneous due to degenerative changes in the retina or vitreous.
2. Trauma, inflammation or other problems.
3. Occurs most commonly in patients older than age 40.

Clinical Manifestations

1. Retinal detachment may occur slowly or rapidly.
2. The patient complains of flashes of light or blurred, "sooty" vision due to stimulation of the retina by vitreous pull.
3. The patient notes sensation of particles moving in line of vision. (Normally, most persons can see floating filaments when looking at a light background.)
4. Delineated areas of vision may be blank; there is no pain.
5. A sensation of a veil-like coating coming down, coming up, or coming sideways in front of the eye may be present.
   a. This veil-like coating, or shadow is often misinterpreted as a drooping eyelid or elevated cheek.
   b. Straight-ahead vision may remain good in early stages.
6. Unless the retinal holes are sealed, the retina will progressively detach, and ultimately there will be a loss of central vision as well as peripheral vision leading to legal blindness.

Diagnostic Evaluation

1. Patient history may indicate trauma.
2. Binocular ophthalmoscopy shows gray or opaque retina. The retina is normally transparent.

Management

A. **General**
1. Sedation, bed rest, and eye patch may be used to restrict eye movements
2. Surgical intervention.
3. Return of visual acuity with a reattached retina depends on:
   a. Amount of retina detached before surgery.
   b. Whether the macula was detached.
   c. Length of time the retina was detached.
   d. Amount of external distortion caused by the scleral buckle.
   e. Possible macular damage as a result of diathermy of cryocoagulation.

B. **Surgical Procedures**
1. Photocoagulation—a light beam (either laser or xenon arc) is passed through the pupil, causing a small burn and producing an exudate between the pigment epithelium and retina.
2. Electrodiathermy—an electrode needle is passed through the sclera to allow subretinal fluid to escape. An exudate forms from the pigment epithelium and adheres to the retina.
3. Cryosurgery or retinal cryopexy—a supercooled probe is touched to the sclera, causing minimal damage; as a result of scarring, the pigment epithelium adheres to the retina.
4. Scleral buckling—a technique whereby the sclera is shortened to allow a buckling to occur, which forces the pigment epithelium closer to the retina.

C. **Complications**
1. Glaucoma
2. Infection
   Note: Surgical reattachment is successful approximately 90% to 95% of the time. If retina remains attached 2 months postoperatively, condition likely to be corrected and unlikely to reoccur.

Nursing Assessment

A. **Preoperative**
1. Assess level of anxiety and fear.
2. Assess knowledge level regarding procedures.
3. Determine visual limitations and obtain visual description from patient, for example, shadowing.

B. **Postoperative**
1. Assess pain level.
2. Assess visual acuity if unoperated eye not patched.
3. Determine patient's ability to ambulate and assume independent activities as tolerated.

Nursing Diagnoses

A. Fear related to visual deficit and surgical outcome
B. Risk for Infection related to eye surgery

Nursing Interventions

A. Preparing the Patient for Surgery
1. Instruct patient to remain quiet in prescribed position. (Detached area of retina remains in dependent position.)
2. Patch both eyes.
3. Wash face with antibacterial solution.
4. Instruct patient not to touch eyes.
5. Administer preoperative medications as ordered.

B. Preventing Complications Postoperatively
1. Caution patient to avoid bumping head.
2. Encourage patient not to cough or sneeze or to perform activities that will increase IOP.
3. Assist patient with activities as needed.
4. Encourage ambulation and independence.
5. Administer medications for pain, nausea, and vomiting as prescribed.
6. Provide sedate, diversional activities such as radio, audio books.

Patient Education/ Health Maintenance

1. Encourage self-care at discharge, if done in an unhurried manner. (Avoid falls, jerks, bumps, or accidental injury.)
2. Instruct patient in following:
   a. Rapid eye movements should be avoided for several weeks.
   b. Driving is restricted.

(1) Within 3 weeks, light activities may be pursued.
(2) Within 6 weeks, heavier activities and athletics are possible. Define such activities for the patient.
   c. Avoid straining and bending head below the waist.
   d. Use meticulous cleanliness in giving eye medications.
   e. Apply a clean, warm, moist washcloth to eyes and eyelids several times a day for 10 minutes to provide soothing and relaxing comfort.
   f. Symptoms that indicate a recurrence of the detachment: floating spots, flashing light, progressive shadows. Recommend that the patient contact health care provider if they occur.
3. Advise patient to follow up. The first follow-up visit to the ophthalmologist should occur in 2 weeks, with other visits scheduled thereafter.

Evaluation

A. Patient verbalizes understanding of surgery and restrictions
B. Patient following activity restrictions

◆ OTHER EYE DISORDERS

See Table 14-2, page 436.

Selected References

Albert, D.M., & Jakobiec, F.A. (1994). *Principles and practices of ophthalmology.* Philadelphia: W.B. Saunders.

Bartley, G. B. & Liesegang, T. J. (1992). Essentials of ophthalmology. Philadelphia: J. B. Lippincott.

Boyd-Monk, H., & Steinmetz, C.G. III. (1987). *Nursing care of the eye.*

Norwalk, CT: Appleton & Lange.

Goldberg, S. (1993). *Ophthalmology made ridiculously simple.* Miami: Med Masters.

Newell, F.W. (1992). *Ophthalmology principles and concepts* (7th ed.). St. Louis: Mosby.

Note: For further information regarding eye disorders and resources, contact: Wilmer Eye Institite at Johns Hopkins Hospital; 600 North Wolfe Street; Baltimore, MD 21287-9255.

Ear, Nose, and Throat Disorders

Assessment

◆ HISTORY

Obtaining a history, including the patient's signs and symptoms, current health patterns, and previous illnesses, will help in identifying ear, nose, and throat (ENT) problems and an appropriate plan of care.

Key Signs and Symptoms

1. Pain of mouth or throat
   a. Is it acute or chronic?
   b. Is it worse on chewing or swallowing?
   c. Is it associated with poor dentition, cough, fever, tickle in throat, or any other symptoms?
2. Headache
   a. Is it generalized or localized to sinus areas?
   b. Is it associated with congestion and postnasal drip?
3. Sore throat—Is it accompanied by swollen glands and high fever or congestion and postnasal drip?
4. Nasal congestion—Is it chronic, or accompanied by fever and purulent drainage?
5. Hoarseness
   a. Is it related to infection or voice abuse?
   b. Is it recurrent or chronic?
6. Earache—Is it worsened by manipulation of the auricle or is it a deep throbbing pain?
7. Hearing loss—Was it sudden or gradual in onset?
8. Dizziness—Is the patient lightheaded or experiencing vertigo (as if the room or self is spinning)?

Current Health Patterns

1. Inquire about nutrition, dental care, normal mouth care habits, dental caries, use of partial or full dentures, stress-related grinding, clenching or clamping of teeth.

2. Ask about consumption of alcohol, smoking, use of a pipe, and smokeless tobacco.
3. Determine personal hygiene in regard to ears. Are cotton swabs or other objects used for cleaning?
4. Is there any loud noise exposure?
5. Does the patient frequently strain voice through talking, singing, or shouting?
6. What medications is the patient taking? Have antibiotics been used? For how long?

Previous Illnesses

1. Is there a history of allergies?
2. Is there any immunosuppressive illness, such as diabetes mellitus, cancer, human immunodeficiency virus (HIV) infection?
3. Has there been any trauma?
4. Is there a history of rhinitis, sinusitis, or ear infections?
5. Is there a family history of any ENT problems or cancer?

◆ PHYSICAL EXAMINATION

Assessment of the Mouth

1. Remove dentures, if present.
2. Inspect mouth.
   a. Observe the lips for color, moisture, ulcers, lumps, localized discoloration, and cracking.
   b. Inspect the tongue for smoothness, moisture, condition of papillae, and color; note the presence of redness, swelling, lesions, or cracks (a thin white coat is normal). Note any deviation or tremor when the tongue is moved.
   c. Observe the palate and note any redness, fissures, cracks, abnormal coloring, or nodules.
   d. Inspect the gums and number of teeth: note any missing, cracked, or discolored teeth; note obvious caries and local irritations; observe the gingiva for color, retraction, evidence of bleeding, or edema.

e. Observe tooth-brushing and flossing technique, if possible.
3. Palpate.
   a. With a tongue blade, depress the tongue and note the symmetry of the uvula when the soft palate rises as the patient says "ah"; note discoloration, enlargement, exudate, ulceration of the posterior pharynx.
   b. Wearing gloves, palpate the outer lips, the gingiva, the buccal mucosa, and the floor of the mouth for lesions, masses, or tenderness.
4. Palpate the temporomandibular joint (TMJ) while patient opens and closes mouth. Note crepitus, tenderness, or spasm.

Assessment of Nose and Sinuses

1. Inspect for swelling, discoloration, deformity.
2. Have patient tilt head backward and use flashlight and nasal speculum (if available) to assess for alignment of septum, edema, drainage, and patency of nasal passages.
3. Inspect, palpate, and percuss the frontal and maxillary sinuses for tenderness or inflammation.
4. Observe retropharynx for evidence of postnasal drip.

Assessment of the Ears

1. Examine unaffected ear first in patient with ear pain. If gentleness is demonstrated during examination of good ear, patient is more likely to submit to examination of painful ear.
2. Inspect and palpate external ear for swelling, warmth, and tenderness on manipulation of auricle or tragus.
3. Perform otoscopic examination for presence of foreign body, inflammation, drainage, or tympanic membrane perforation, as indicated.
4. Assess hearing through the use of a tuning fork. Tuning fork tests (Weber's and Rinne tests) are used only for screening purposes (see Table 15-1).
   a. Weber's (lateralization) test—Place base of lightly vibrating tuning fork on top of patient's head or in middle of forehead; ask where patient hears it, one or both sides
   b. Rinne test—Place base of lightly vibrating tuning fork on mastoid process until patient can no longer hear it; then quickly place vibrating fork near the ear canal and ask if patient can still hear it

Diagnostic Tests

◆ AUDIOMETRY

Audiometry is measurement of hearing. These tests are usually done by an audiologist to confirm hearing loss.

Pure-Tone Audiometry

A. *Test Principles*
1. Sound stimulus consists of a pure (musical) tone presented in a variety of intensities and/or frequencies.

TABLE 15-1 Tuning Fork Tests

Ear Condition	Weber's Test	Rinne Test
Normal, no hearing loss	No shifting of sounds laterally	Sound perceived longer by *air* conduction
Conductive loss	Shifting of sounds to poorer ear	Sound perceived as long or longer by *bone* conduction
Sensorineural loss	Shifting of sounds to better ear	Sound perceived longer by *air* conduction

2. The louder the tone required for the patient to hear it, the greater the hearing loss.
3. Air conduction and bone conduction are tested by using ear phones and vibrating oscillator, respectively.
4. Noise level must be carefully controlled, usually by using acoustically shielded (soundproof) booth.
5. An audiogram is the plotted results of the test.
6. Evaluation of the audiogram includes:
   a. Normal human ear perception—20 to 20,000 cps (Hz).
   b. Frequencies significant for speech range—500 to 2,000 cps (Hz).
   c. Hearing is normally most astute near 1,000 cps.

B. *Examples of Hearing Impairment on an Audiogram*
1. Conductive hearing loss
   a. A problem in the outer and middle ear may result in reduced sensitivity to tones received by air conduction.
   b. If the inner ear is unimpaired, bone conduction will be within normal range.
2. Sensorineural hearing loss
   a. A weakening of sound produced in some portion of the sensorineural mechanism (eg, inner ear) results in reduced thresholds for air conduction.
   b. Usually it also causes a reduction in bone conduction.
3. Mixed hearing loss
   a. Weakening of sound in some portion of the sensorineural mechanism results in reduced bone conduction and air conduction.
   b. When there is also a lesion in the external auditory canal or middle ear, there will be additional weakening in thresholds for air conduction.

Speech Audiometry

A. *Speech Reception Threshold*
1. This is the softest hearing threshold level at which a person can correctly repeat approximately 50% of very familiar two-syllable words.
2. This test provides only a gross estimate of the patient's ability to recognize and respond to speech.

B. *Speech Discrimination Score*
1. This is a suprathreshold measure of speech discrimination.
2. The tester presents phonetically balanced monosyllabic words, which the patient is asked to repeat.
3. The percentage of correct responses is the speech discrimination score.

C. *Acoustic Impedance Evaluation*
1. This is an objective measurement (does not require direct patient response) relating to the function of the peripheral auditory mechanism.
2. A battery of acoustic impedance testing may be done.
3. Helps determine middle ear function in middle ear disorders, seventh or eighth cranial nerve disorders, or eustachian tube dysfunction.

General Procedures/Treatment Modalities

◆ NASAL SURGERY

Submucous resection of the septum is an operation in which cartilaginous and/or osseous portions of the septum that lie between the flaps of the mucous membrane and perichondrium are removed or straightened—to establish an adequate partition between the right and left nasal cavities in order to provide a clear nasal airway.

Nasal septal reconstruction involves resection or removal of cartilaginous (or bony) septum followed by reconstruction of all parts of the septum that may produce nasal airway obstruction. Reduction of fracture of nose or stabilization of maxillofacial fracture may be done secondary to trauma. Rhinoplasty involves changing the nose's external appearance.

Caldwell-Luc procedure provides for removal of diseased mucosal lining of maxillary sinus combined with development of nasal-antral window. Incision made along upper gumline above canine teeth. Other sinus procedures include nasal-antral window, ethmoidectomy (internal or external), and endoscopic surgery.

Preoperative Management/Nursing Care

1. If a fracture or trauma has occurred, raise head of bed to promote drainage, lessen edema, and make patient more comfortable.
2. Apply intermittent cold compresses and administer pain medications.
3. Administer antibiotics to reduce bacterial colonization of nose and sinuses.
4. Tell the patient that a pressure sensation may be felt in the nasal area during surgery if done under local anesthetic.
5. Describe to the patient the use of nasal packing to effect hemostasis and the appearance of facial or periorbital ecchymosis (bruising) that may be present and that it will gradually subside.

Postoperative Management/ Nursing Care

1. Goal is to promote comfort and prevent complications.
2. Administer antibiotics to prevent infection.
3. Monitor closely for bleeding, which may cause aspiration.
4. Maintain airway; position to facilitate breathing.

Complications

1. Hematoma/hemorrhage
2. Local infection—contaminated nasal packing is an excellent culture medium for pathogens
3. Aspiration
4. Pressure necrosis (from packing)

Nursing Diagnoses

A. Ineffective Breathing Pattern related to nasal packing and swelling
B. Risk for aspiration related to bleeding, inability to blow nose

Nursing Interventions

A. *Facilitating Breathing*
1. Keep head elevated (three to four pillows) day and night to keep swelling down.
2. Apply cold compresses or ice packs intermittently for 24 hours—to lessen edema and discoloration and to promote comfort.
3. Advise patient that packing will be removed 48 hours after surgery.
4. Encourage the use of a humidifier to relieve crusting of nasal mucosa and prevent irritation from dryness.
5. Encourage relaxation techniques and deep-breathing exercises for anxiety associated with nasal passages being blocked.
6. Administer frequent mouth care, because the patient is forced to breathe through the mouth; use flexible straw to sip mouthwash for rinsing purposes.

B. *Preventing Aspiration*
1. Monitor closely for bleeding; check for increased swallowing, blood dripping down back of throat (use flashlight and tongue blade).
2. Change the gauze pad under the nose as it becomes soaked with blood; bleeding should gradually decrease.
3. After Caldwell-Luc procedure, provide cold compresses over lip to help reduce swelling.
4. Check other external dressings for saturation.
5. Notify surgeon if bleeding increases.
6. Reassure the patient about the sucking sound that will be experienced on swallowing; the nasal packing prevents air from moving through the nose, and a partial vacuum is created in the throat during swallowing.
7. Instruct the patient not to blow nose but to blot secretions with tissue.

Patient Education/Health Maintenance

1. Encourage patient to use a vaporizer—helps relieve crusting of nasal mucosa from dryness.
2. Remind patient that sneezing, straining, and nose blowing increase venous pressure and can result in bleeding/hematoma.
3. Advise patient that if unable to control sneezing, keep the mouth open while sneezing.
4. Tell patient not to remove adherent crusts; they will separate by themselves from underlying tissue.

5. Instruct to avoid environmental irritants, especially smoke.
6. After Caldwell-Luc procedure or rhinoplasty, advise patient that numbness in operative area may be present for several weeks to months.
7. Instruct patient to avoid strenuous activity and trauma to nose; the motion of bony fragments (after fracture) within soft tissue will produce laceration and bleeding.
8. Tell patient that if a nasal splint is present, avoid getting it wet; do not attempt to remove it.
9. Advise patient that postoperative follow-up may need to continue for 6 to 12 months to monitor for excess callous formation or cosmetic deformity.

Evaluation

A. Mouth breathing without difficulty
B. No bleeding noted

◆ EAR SURGERY

Ear surgery may involve the tympanic membrane, the middle ear cavity, the mastoid, or the labyrinth. It may be done for perforation of the eardrum, to facilitate drainage and remove diseased tissue in cases of infection, to relieve vertigo, or to treat hearing loss.

Types of Surgery

1. Myringotomy—incision into tympanic membrane for possible drainage tube insertion.
2. Tympanoplasty—reconstruction of diseased or deformed middle ear components (Table 15-2).
   a. Type I (myringoplasty)—purpose is to close perforation by placing a graft over it in order to create a closed middle ear section, which in turn will improve hearing.
   Perforation is closed using one of the following:
   (1) Fascia from temporal muscle.
   (2) Vein grafts from hand or forearm.
   (3) Epithelium from auditory canal (eustachian tube).
   b. Type II–V—suitable replacement (polyethylene, stainless steel wire, bone, cartilage) is used to maintain continuity of conduction sound pathway. The necessity of a two-stage procedure is determined.
   (1) First stage—eradication of all diseased tissues; area is cleaned out to achieve a dry, healed middle ear.
   (2) Second stage—performed 2 to 3 months after first stage; reconstruction, using grafts.
3. Mastoidectomy—removal of mastoid process of temporal bone.
   a. Simple—performed through the ear with a tympanoplasty (closed approach).
   b. Modified or radical—wide excision of the mastoid and diseased middle ear contents through an occipital incision (open).
4. Stapedectomy—removal of footplate of stapes and insertion of a graft or prosthesis.
5. Labyrinthectomy—destruction of the labyrinth (inner ear) through the middle ear and aspiration of the endolabyrinth.
6. Endolymphatic decompression and shunt—release of pressure on the endolymphatic system in the labyrinth and creation of a shunt for fluid to the subarachnoid space or the mastoid
7. Cochlear implant—implantation of electronic device that bypasses cochlea and stimulates auditory nerve

Preoperative Management/Nursing Care

1. Hearing function is fully evaluated.
2. Antibiotics are given to treat infection.
3. The patient is prepared emotionally for the effects of surgery.

TABLE 15-2 Types of Tympanoplasty

Type	Tympanic Membrane	Ossicles	Repair Process
	Middle Ear Damage		
I	Perforated	Normal	Close perforation—myringoplasty
II	Perforated	Erosion of malleus and/or incus	Close perforation; graft against incus or whatever remains of malleus
III	Tympanic membrane destroyed or widely perforated	Rest of ossicular chain destroyed but stapes are intact and mobile	Grafts implanted to contact the normal stapes Tympanostapedopexy
IV	Tympanic membrane destroyed or widely perforated	Ossicular chain destroyed. Head, neck, and crura of stapes destroyed. Stapes footplate mobile	Expose mobile stapes footplate—graft implanted. Air pocket between graft and round window provides protection The cavum minor operation
V	Tympanic membrane destroyed or widely perforated	Ossicular chain destroyed. Head, neck, and crura of stapes destroyed. Stapes footplate fixed	Make opening in horizontal semicircular canal; graft seals off middle ear to give sound protection for round window Tympanoplasty and fenestration of lateral semicircular canal

4. Careful assessment for signs of acute infection is performed, which may delay surgery.

Postoperative Management/ Nursing Care

1. Antibiotics may be continued to prevent local and central nervous system (CNS) infection.
2. Bed rest may be maintained for the first 24 hours or longer to decrease symptoms of nausea and vertigo (if the inner ear was disturbed) or to prevent disruption of prosthesis.
3. Analgesics, antiemetics, and antihistamines are given as needed.
4. The patient is positioned to promote drainage but maintain some immobility.
5. Packing may be removed up to 6 days postoperatively if prosthesis or graft procedure.
6. Hearing will be reevaluated after edema has subsided and healing has occurred.

Complications

1. Infection—local, CNS (meningitis, brain abscess)
2. Hearing loss
3. Facial nerve paralysis

Nursing Diagnoses

A. Pain related to surgical incision and swelling
B. Risk for Infection related to local CNS infection
C. Risk for Injury related to vertigo

Nursing Interventions

A. *Relieving Pain*
1. Administer or teach self-administration of analgesic as indicated postoperatively.
2. Tell patient to expect pain to subside within first few hours with simple procedures or within first day or two with major procedures.
3. Position for comfort following the instructions from the surgeon.
   a. On side with surgical ear upward to maintain graft position and immobility.
   b. Lying on side with surgical ear down to promote drainage from ear canal.
   c. Position of patient preference.
4. Elevate head of bed to reduce swelling and pressure.
5. Advise patient to avoid sudden movement. Use pillows for support.

B. *Preventing Infection*
1. Reinforce external dressings as needed until after first changed by surgeon, then change when saturated to prevent bacterial growth in damp dressings.
2. Loosely pack cotton or gauze in ear canal as indicated, without causing increased pressure.
3. Do not probe or insert anything into ear canal.
4. Administer or teach self-administration of antibiotics as prescribed. Do not use eardrops unless specifically ordered postoperatively.

5. Wash hands before any ear care and instruct patient not to touch ear.
6. Take care not to get dressing or ear wet.
7. Advise patient not to blow nose, which could cause nasopharyngeal secretions to be forced up eustachian tube into middle ear.
8. Report and teach patient to report any increased pain, fever, ear inflammation, or drainage, indicating local infection.
9. Be alert for headache, fever, stiff neck, or altered level of consciousness, which may indicate CNS infection.

C. *Ensuring Safety*
1. Be aware that dizziness or vertigo may occur for the first several days postoperatively.
2. Maintain side rails up while patient is in bed.
3. Assist patient on ambulating for the first time after surgery and as needed thereafter.
4. Encourage the patient to move slowly, because sudden movements may exacerbate vertigo.
5. Administer or teach self-administration of antiemetics and antihistamines as ordered and as needed; watch for sedation.
6. Instruct the patient not to blow nose, cough, lean forward, or perform Valsalva's maneuver to prevent disruption of graft or prosthesis; aggravate vertigo; or force bacteria up the eustachian tube. If coughing or blowing nose are necessary, do so with open mouth to relieve pressure.

Patient Education/Health Maintenance

1. Advise the patient that there may be a temporary hearing loss for a few weeks after surgery because of tissue edema, packing, etc. The effects of a hearing restoring operation will not be known for several weeks, and additional rehabilitation may be necessary to optimize results.
2. Advise patient to protect ear, perform dressing changes, or place loose cotton in outer ear as indicated. Replace cotton twice daily or sooner if saturated by drainage.
3. Encourage follow-up for packing removal as directed.
4. Instruct the patient to avoid sudden pressure changes in the ear.
   a. Do not blow nose.
   b. Do not fly in a small plane.
   c. Do not dive.
5. Advise against smoking.
6. Tell patient to protect ears when going outdoors for the first week.
7. Tell patient to avoid getting ear wet until completely healed.
8. Tell patient to avoid crowds or exposure to colds so that upper respiratory infection is prevented.
9. Instruct patient of signs and symptoms of complications to report.
   a. Return of tinnitus
   b. Vertigo
   c. Fluctuations of hearing ability
   d. Fever, headache, ear inflammation, increased pain, stiff neck
   e. Facial drooping or numbness
10. Advise patient that facial nerve paralysis may be temporary and to increase fluid intake through a straw during this time.

Evaluation

A. Verbalizes relief of pain
B. No signs of infection
C. Ambulating without difficulty

Conditions of the Mouth and Jaw

◆ CANDIDIASIS

Candidiasis is a fungal infection commonly caused by *Candida albicans,* usually occurring in the mouth and pharynx, but can become a source of systemic dissemination, particularly in high-risk persons.

Pathophysiology/Etiology

1. Immunosuppression from disease states or treatment regimens (eg, HIV infection, corticosteroids).
2. Altered oral environment from loss of epithelial layer, antibiotic therapy, preexisting infections, poor oral hygiene or nutritional status, denture wearers.

Clinical Manifestations

1. Oral discomfort, burning, altered taste, erythema
2. Possible pseudomembranous form (thrush) with adherent white plaques, which can be wiped off
3. Possible spread to the esophagus

Diagnostic Evaluation

1. Microbiologic studies of the plaques—show characteristic hyphae; positive culture for *C. albicans*
2. Occasionally, biopsy of lesions may be necessary to rule out leukoplakia (premalignant plaques)

Management

1. Topical antifungal agents in oral rinses, tablets, creams, or vaginal tablets (e.g., nystatin [Mycostatin])
2. Systemic treatment is indicated if topical agents fail; fluconazole (Diflucan), ketoconazole (Nizoral), or amphotericin B (Fungizone)
3. Analgesics for severe pain

Complications

1. Candidal infection throughout the gastrointestinal tract
2. *Candida* sepsis

Nursing Assessment

1. Assess extent of lesions and inflammation in mouth as well as any chest discomfort indicating spread to esophagus.
2. Assess level of pain.
3. Assess nutritional status and effect of pain on oral intake.
4. Obtain history for risk factors for *Candida* infection.

Nursing Diagnoses

A. Altered Nutrition: Less Than Body Requirements related to oral discomfort
B. Knowledge Deficit related to antifungal therapy

Nursing Interventions

A. *Attaining Adequate Nutrition*
1. Administer analgesics as prescribed $\frac{1}{2}$ to 1 hour before meals.
2. Provide soft foods, soothing liquids; avoid temperature extremes.
3. Encourage saline rinses with lukewarm water or loosen encrustations with dilute hydrogen peroxide mouth rinses, followed by water rinses, as prescribed.
4. Provide gentle suctioning if pain becomes so severe that patient cannot handle secretions, and provide intravenous fluids.

B. *Ensuring Adequate Therapy*
1. Administer antifungal agents as prescribed. Observe patient for proper use of topical preparation.
   a. Ensure that mouth is clean and free of food debris before administering drug.
   b. For oral suspensions, tell patient to swish and hold in mouth for at least 5 minutes before swallowing or suck vaginal or oral tablets as directed.
2. Observe for signs and symptoms of systemic drug side effects: nausea, vomiting, diarrhea; renal, bone marrow, cardiovascular, hepatic or neurologic toxicities.
3. Explain the importance of continuing therapy for duration prescribed, usually at least 3 weeks.

Patient Education/Health Maintenance

1. Instruct high-risk patients on daily oral examination and signs and symptoms to observe.
2. Teach patient to avoid highly seasoned foods, extremes in temperature, alcoholic beverages, and smoking, all of which irritate the oral mucosa.
3. Encourage good oral hygiene.

Evaluation

A. Adequate intake of liquids and soft foods
B. Swishes oral suspension for 5 minutes before swallowing

◆ TEMPOROMANDIBULAR JOINT (TMJ) SYNDROME

Temporomandibular joint syndrome is a disorder of the temporomandibular joint structures or surrounding muscles, causing pain, muscle spasm, and changes in jaw movement.

Pathophysiology/Etiology

1. Malocclusion (uneven closure of the teeth)
2. Joint diseases—rheumatoid or osteoarthritis; lupus erythematosus, ankylosing spondylitis
3. Trauma

4. Teeth clenching or bruxism (teeth grinding)
5. Poor posture and its effect on the cervical spine
6. Psychological factors and tension—can induce or exacerbate symptoms
7. Above factors result in inflammation and muscle spasm of TMJ

Clinical Manifestations

1. Pain at the joint, temples, mandible, or masticatory muscles—worsens with jaw movement. Referred muscle spasm of the neck, trapezius, and sternocleidomastoid muscle causes discomfort.
2. Clicking or crepitus—from grating or popping of the joint.
3. Limitation of movement, dislocation, or jaw locking.
4. Headaches, earaches, or tinnitus.

Diagnostic Evaluation

1. X-rays of the head and neck—usually normal.
2. Occlusal analysis—evaluates for malocclusion of the jaw and teeth in a bite position.
3. Computed tomography (CT) and magnetic resonance imaging—usually normal unless underlying degenerative changes, fracture, or neoplasm of jaw or cervical spine.
4. Mandibular kinesiograph to assess the degree of jaw dysfunction.

Management

1. Therapeutic nightguard or splint—to realign malocclusion or joint disk and to optimize muscle relaxation.
2. Moist heat or ultrasound (deep-heat) therapy—to enhance analgesia and muscle relaxation and to promote local tissue metabolism.
3. Transcutaneous electrical nerve stimulation (TENS)—reduces muscle spasm of head, neck, and back and reduces pain.
4. Pharmacotherapy: analgesics and nonsteroidal anti-inflammatory drugs.
5. Arthroscopy—investigational procedure to visualize joint, reposition disk, lyse adhesions, or debride joint.
   a. Reserved for conditions not improved by medical management.
   b. Complications: seventh cranial nerve damage with facial paralysis and paresis; perforation of the external auditory canal; piercing of the middle cranial fossa.
6. Surgery—to remove the disk or reshape bony prominences.
   a. Complications: malocclusion, seventh cranial nerve damage, infection.

Nursing Interventions/Patient Teaching

1. Assess the character, frequency, location, and duration of pain. Evaluate what triggers and relieves the pain. Determine how effective previous treatments have been.
2. Explore the effect of the disorder on the patient's lifestyle, especially eating habits.

3. Instruct the patient on the indications, dosages, and side effects of analgesics and anti-inflammatory medications.
4. Teach the patient proper use of heat therapies. Cold applications may be preferred by some patients to reduce pain and spasm.
5. Encourage the patient to perform active mouth opening, protrusion, and lateral movement exercises of the jaw for 5 minutes, four to five times per day, as prescribed to stretch muscles and reduce spasm.
6. Discuss the use of a therapeutic nightguard or splint as directed.
7. Encourage the use of soft food and liquid supplements during times of acute pain exacerbated by eating. Advise reduction of foods that require excessive chewing, such as raw vegetables, tough meat, nuts. Discourage gum chewing.
8. Explore tension-reducing modalities with the patient, especially progressive muscle relaxation to reduce muscle tension and spasm.
9. Encourage follow-up with dentist, oral surgeon, ENT specialist, or other caregiver as indicated.

◆ MAXILLOFACIAL AND MANDIBULAR FRACTURES

Fractures of the maxillofacial bones or mandible may occur as the result of industrial, athletic, and vehicular accidents; violent acts; and falls.

Pathophysiology/Etiology

1. Mandibular fractures frequently occur due to blow to the chin.
2. Maxillofacial fractures usually occur due to blow to the cheek or face.
3. May be nondisplaced or displaced, usually closed, and includes soft tissue injury.
4. May also occur as part of planned surgical reconstruction for jaw problems.

Clinical Manifestations

1. Malocclusion, asymmetry, abnormal mobility, crepitus (grating sound with movement), pain, or tenderness
2. Tissue injury: swelling; ecchymosis; bleeding

Diagnostic Evaluation

1. X-rays: posterioanterior; oblique; occlusal; panorex—show fracture and possible displacement
2. CT scan—evaluate extent of complicated injuries

Management

1. Maintenance of adequate respiratory functioning; may include oxygen support, endotracheal intubation, or tracheostomy. See Chapter 33, Emergency Nursing.

2. Control of bleeding; usually accomplished with direct pressure.
3. Reduction of the fracture—usually closed reduction.
4. Immobilization—dependent on location, type, and severity of the fracture.
  a. Barton's bandage with a Kling or stockinette bandage.
  b. Interdental fixation with rubberbands or wiring.
  c. Intermaxillary fixation with rubberbands or wiring.
  d. Interosseous fixation with open reduction.
5. Maintenance of adequate nutritional intake with liquid or soft diet—to maintain immobilization of fracture site.
6. Pain control to promote comfort.
7. Prevention of infection with antibiotics in the presence of positive cultures.

Complications

1. Airway obstruction
2. Aspiration
3. Infection
4. Disfigurement

Nursing Assessment

1. Obtain description of injury and review chart and diagnostic tests for extent of injury.
2. Continually assess respiratory status.
3. Assess level of pain.

Nursing Diagnoses

A. Risk for aspiration related to immobilization of jaw
B. Altered Nutrition: Less Than Body Requirements related to pain, injury, and immobilization
C. Pain related to injury and surgical intervention
D. Body Image Disturbance related to disfigurement of injury

Nursing Interventions

A. *Preventing Aspiration*
1. Maintain effective airway.
  a. Elevate head of bed 30 to 45 degrees, or position leaning over a bedside stand to reduce edema and improve handling of secretions.
  b. Ensure readily accessible suctioning equipment; teach patient oral and nasal suctioning; position on side or upright during suctioning.
  c. Administer antiemetics as prescribed for nausea and vomiting to prevent aspiration.
  d. Make sure wire cutters or scissors are present for immediate removal of the wires or rubberbands if the airway becomes obstructed. (Vertical rubberbands or wires should be cut.)
  e. Ensure that a method for calling the nurse (call bell) is within easy access to the patient at all times in case of emergency.
2. Monitor blood pressure, pulse, respirations, and temperature to note early onset of infection or aspiration.

B. *Maintaining Nutritional Status*
1. Administer fluids as prescribed; place straw against teeth or through any gaps in the teeth—teeth may initially be sensitive to hot and cold.
2. Position in upright position before, during, and for 45 to 60 minutes after all feedings.
3. Evaluate ongoing nutritional and hydration status; weight; intake, output, and specific gravity; laboratory values—24-hour urea nitrogen, transferrin level, electrolytes, and albumin.
4. Advance to blenderized diet as tolerated.
5. Make environment as pleasant as possible to enhance appetite—remove all sources of odor, decrease interruptions, position comfortably.

C. *Increasing Comfort*
1. Administer liquid or a suspension of analgesics as prescribed—avoid narcotics, which may cause nausea and vomiting.
2. Administer diazepam (Valium) as prescribed to reduce anxiety and control reflex muscle spasm.
3. Apply paraffin wax to the ends of wire fixation devices to decrease irritation to the gums and oral mucosa.
4. Apply petrolatum jelly to the lips to decrease dryness and prevent cracking.

D. *Strengthening Body Image*
1. Provide firm reassurance regarding progress to reduce anxiety and allay fears.
2. Avoid unrealistic promises in relation to scars or disfigurement.
3. Allow the patient to choose the first time for looking in the mirror.
4. Provide privacy as requested—the patient may be sensitive to appearance.

E. *Other Nursing Responsibilities*
1. Provide mouth care every 2 hours while awake for the first several days, then four to six times per day.
2. Initially provide mouth care with warm normal saline mouth swishes.
3. As diet is progressed, remove collected debris with a pressurized water stream cleaner (Water Pik) and encourage the patient to brush teeth with a soft, child-sized toothbrush.
4. Observe facial injuries for swelling, erythema, pain, or warmth to detect onset of infection.
5. Change facial dressings as needed to prevent soiling with secretions, food, or drainage, which may promote bacterial growth.

Patient Education/Health Maintenance

1. Encourage adequate nutrition—inform the patient and family that foods can be blenderized and thinned with juices or broths to a consistency that can be taken through a straw.
2. Explore with the patient options for maintaining proper oral care; encourage the patient to practice the options of choice.
3. Discuss the use of antiemetic medications to prevent nausea and vomiting, stressing the complications this could cause.
4. Make sure the patient has wire cutters or scissors and knows how to use them should airway obstruction occur.
5. Encourage follow-up health care visits.

Evaluation

A. No evidence of aspiration
B. Tolerating fluids through straw
C. Verbalizes relief of pain
D. Views self in mirror; notices improvement in appearance

Problems of the Nose, Throat, and Sinuses

◆ RHINITIS

Rhinitis is an inflammation of the mucous membrane of the nose, often producing excessive nasal secretions and obstruction.

Pathophysiology/Etiology

Types of rhinitis include:

1. Allergic—IgE-mediated response causing release of vasoactive substances from mast cells (see page 807).
2. Infectious—viral (common cold) and bacterial (purulent).
3. Drug-induced (rebound rhinitis; rhinitis medicamentosus)—caused by excessive use of topical nasal decongestants.
4. Nonallergic, noninfectious (vasomotor rhinitis)—unexplained autonomic nasal dysfunction as a result of overactivity of the parasympathetic nerve supply to the mucous membranes of the nose and paranasal sinuses.

Clinical Manifestations

1. Hypersecretion; wet running/dripping nose or postnasal drip
2. Nasal obstruction symptoms: nasal congestion, pressure, or stuffiness
3. Headache

Management

1. Treatment of underlying cause
  a. Allergy—antihistamines (see page 807)
  b. Infection—antibiotics
2. Topical decongestants (for short-term use); systemic decongestants

> **NURSING ALERT:**
> Severe rebound nasal obstruction may occur with overuse of topical decongestants. Stress the importance of only using for 2 to 3 days as directed.

3. Intranasal corticosteroids—preferred treatment in vasomotor rhinitis; may be used in other types

Nursing Interventions/Patient Education

1. Avoid irritating inhalants, especially smoke, aerosols, noxious fumes.
2. Do not overuse topical nasal sprays/drops.
3. Do not blow nose too frequently or too hard; doing so may cause infection to spread, sinuses to become infected, and an eardrum to be perforated.
4. Blow through both nostrils at the same time to equalize pressure.
5. Side effect of systemic decongestants is stimulation of sympathetic nervous system—insomnia, nervousness, palpitations.
6. Intranasal corticosteroids do not cause significant systemic absorption in usual doses, but occasionally may cause pharyngeal fungal infections.

◆ EPISTAXIS

Epistaxis refers to nosebleed or hemorrhage from the nose. It most commonly originates in the anterior portion of the nasal cavity. Posterior nasal bleeding usually originates from the turbinates or lateral nasal wall.

Pathophysiology/Etiology

1. Local causes:
  a. Dryness leading to crust formation—bleeding occurs with removal of crusts by nose picking, rubbing, or blowing.
  b. Trauma—direct blows.
2. Systemic causes are less common: hypertension, arteriosclerosis, renal disease, bleeding disorders (most common systemic cause).
3. Majority of nose bleeds are anterior; posterior bleeds are more difficult to control.

Diagnostic Evaluation

1. Inspection with nasal speculum to determine site of bleeding. Important to determine which side bled first.
2. Laboratory evaluation to exclude blood dyscrasias.

Management

Depends on severity and source of bleeding in nasal cavity.

1. Patient is placed in an upright posture, leaning forward to reduce venous pressure and instructed to breathe gently through the mouth to prevent swallowing of blood.
2. With anterior bleeds, patient is instructed to compress the soft part of nasal tip with index finger and thumb for 5 to 10 minutes to maintain pressure on the nasal septum.
3. A cotton pledget soaked with a vasoconstricting agent may be inserted into each nostril and pressure applied if bleeding is not controlled by compression alone. After 5 to 10 minutes, the cotton is removed, and the site of bleeding is identified.

4. The blood vessel may be cauterized.
5. If bleeding continues or posterior bleeding is initially identified, packing may be layered into nasal cavity and the nasopharynx or balloon tamponade may be required to apply pressure over a larger area.

NURSING ALERT:
Monitor the patient for a vasovagal episode during insertion of nasal packing.

---

6. Surgical ligation of vessels may be required.

Complications

1. Rhinitis; maxillary and frontal sinusitis; hemotympanum; otitis media.

Nursing Interventions/Patient Education

1. Monitor vital signs and assist with control of bleeding.
2. Be aware that packing is uncomfortable and painful and may be in place for 2 to 5 days.
3. Monitor patient with posterior packing for hypoxia (from aspiration of blood, sedation, and preexisting pulmonary dysfunction).
4. Monitor for respiratory difficulty or obstruction—secondary to slippage of packing or balloon, swelling of palate, relaxation of tongue.
5. Instruct the patient as follows for self-management of minor bleeding episodes:
   a. Sit up and lean forward while compressing the soft part (tip) of nose between index finger and thumb.
   b. If bleeding continues, moisten a small piece of cotton with vasoconstricting nose drops (phenylephrine hydrochloride [Neo-Synephrine] or oxymetazoline hydrochloride [Afrin]) and place inside nose. Press against bleeding site 5 to 10 minutes.
6. Instruct patient to avoid blowing or picking nose after a nosebleed.

7. Advise patients prone to nosebleeds to:
   a. Apply a lubricant to nasal septum twice daily to reduce dryness.
   b. Use a humidifier if environmental air is dry.

◆ SINUSITIS

Sinusitis is an inflammation of the mucous membranes of one or more paranasal sinuses (Fig. 15-1). It is usually precipitated by congestion from a viral upper respiratory infection and/or nasal allergy. Obstruction of the sinus ostia (resulting from mucosal swelling and/or mechanical obstruction) leads to retention of secretions and is the usual precursor to sinusitis.

Acute Sinusitis

A. *Clinical Manifestations*
1. Pain; stabbing or aching, over the infected sinus
   a. Frontal sinusitis—pain in forehead intensified by bending forward
   b. Maxillary sinusitis—aching pain in facial region and from inner canthus of the eye to the teeth
   c. Ethmoid sinusitis—frontal or orbital headache
   d. Sphenoid sinusitis—headache referred to top of head and deep to the eyes
2. Nasal congestion and discharge; may or may not be present
3. Anosmia (lack of smell): inspired or expired air cannot reach the olfactory groove
4. Red and edematous nasal mucosa

B. *Diagnostic Evaluation*
1. Sinus x-rays show air-fluid level, thickening of sinus mucous membranes.
2. Antral puncture and lavage—provides culture material to identify infectious organism; also a therapeutic modality to clear sinus of bacteria, fluid, and inflammatory cells.

C. *Management*
Goal: To improve ostial patency.

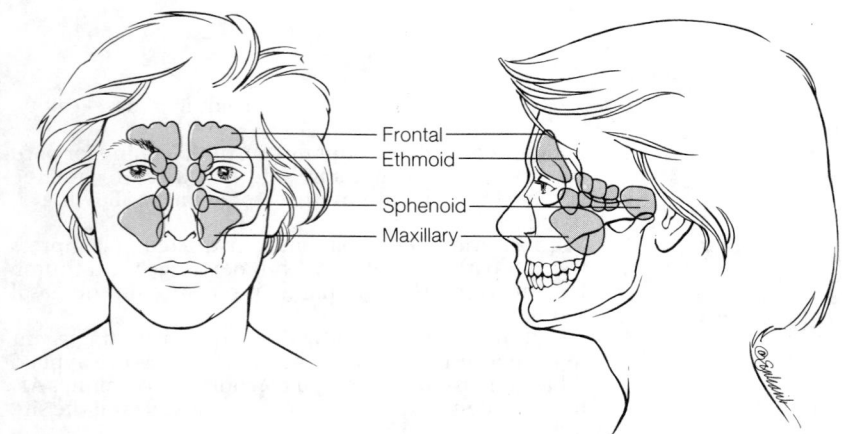

Frontal
Ethmoid
Sphenoid
Maxillary

FIGURE 15-1 *Paranasal sinuses.*

1. Topical decongestant spray or drops or systemic decongestants for mucosal shrinkage to encourage drainage from sinus. Topical therapy should be limited to no more than three successive days of use.
2. Antibiotic (trimethoprim-sulfamethoxazole [Bactrim], cephalosporins, or macrolide antibiotics) for purulent sinusitis.
3. Analgesics—pain may be significant.
4. Warm compresses; cool vapor humidity for comfort and to promote drainage.

D. Complications
Depend on anatomic location of sinus involved.

1. Extension of infection to the orbital contents and eyelids.

> **NURSING ALERT:**
> Watch for lid edema, edema of ocular conjunctiva, drooping lid, limitation of extraocular motion, visual loss. May indicate orbital cellulitis, which necessitates immediate treatment.

2. Bone infection (osteomyelitis) may spread by direct extension or through blood vessels. Frontal bone commonly affected.
3. Central nervous system complications include meningitis, subdural and epidural purulent drainage, brain abscess, cavernous sinus thrombosis (acute thrombophlebitis originating from an infection in an area having venous drainage to cavernous sinus).

Nursing Interventions/Patient Education

1. Advise patient to promptly seek medical attention for acute sinus infection to prevent chronic sinus disease.
2. Discourage swimming/diving, which may cause contaminated water to be forced into a sinus, usually the frontal sinus.
3. Stress the importance of complying with antibiotic therapy: 2 to 3 weeks usually necessary.
4. Advise patient with asthma that sinusitis has been associated with exacerbation of asthma symptoms; patient should be alert for increased wheezing, chest tightness, or cough and seek treatment.

Chronic Sinusitis

Chronic sinusitis is a suppurative inflammation of the sinuses with chronic irreversible change in the mucosa and sinus bony area.

A. Clinical Manifestations
1. Persistent nasal obstruction; chronic nasal discharge, clear or purulent when infected
2. Cough—produced by constant dripping of discharge back into nasopharynx
3. Feeling of facial fullness/pressure
4. Headache, more noticeable in the morning; fatigue

B. Diagnostic Evaluation
1. Sinus x-rays may show complete opacification of affected sinus(es).

2. Endoscopy of nose with CT imaging—reveals mucosal changes.

C. Management
1. Topical or systemic decongestants or topical corticosteroids to promote drainage.
2. Antibiotics for infection.
3. Surgical interventions (when conservative treatment is unsuccessful).
   a. Endoscopic sinus surgery—endoscopic removal of diseased tissue from affected sinus; used to treat chronic sinusitis of maxillary, ethmoid, and frontal sinuses
   b. Nasal antrostomy (nasal-antral window)—surgical placement of an opening under inferior turbinate to provide aeration of the antrum and to permit exit for purulent materials.
   c. For nursing care, see page 451.

C. Nursing Interventions/Patient Education
1. Advise patient to seek treatment for worsening of symptoms, including increase in pain or drainage.
2. Stress the importance of complying with therapy to promote drainage, treat infection to control chronic process.

◆ SPECIFIC INFECTIONS OF THE UPPER RESPIRATORY TRACT
Viral Infections (Common Cold)

Common cold (coryza) refers to a syndrome related to inflammation of the cells of the respiratory epithelium by any group of respiratory viruses.

A. Etiology
Rhinoviruses (account for 50% of common colds; more than 100 serotypes), adenoviruses; myxoviruses; paramyxoviruses, coronaviruses

B. Clinical Manifestations
Occur within 72 hours after viral inoculation.

1. Sneezing, scratchy sore throat, headache
2. Sensation of chilliness
3. Symptoms of nasal discharge (initially clear, then yellow and thickened) and obstruction
4. Cough

C. Complications
1. Persons with asthma or chronic bronchitis may experience worsening of symptoms of chronic obstructive pulmonary disease.
2. Persistence of purulent nasal discharge after 14 days may indicate bacterial sinusitis.

D. Management
1. No single specific treatment.
2. Symptomatic treatment includes:
   a. Aspirin or acetaminophen (Tylenol) to relieve systemic symptoms; does not shorten duration of infection.
   b. Cold-water vaporization of immediate environment.
   c. Decongestants, cough suppressants.

E. Nursing Interventions/Patient Education
The following measures are intended to support body defenses and reduce susceptibility:

1. Observe careful hand washing to avoid person-to-person spread of virus-contaminated secretions.
2. Use humidity measures indoors during winter months.
3. Minimize alcohol intake.
4. Avoid inhaling irritating substances: smoke, chemicals, dust, sprays.
5. Use health-enhancing behaviors, including good nutrition, regular exercise, adequate sleep, and positive coping strategies.

Herpes Simplex Infection (Type 1)

Also known as cold sores or fever blisters. The herpes simplex virus (type 1) is a DNA virus most often associated with lip and oral lesions (herpes labialis). (Genital herpes is usually caused by herpes simplex virus, type 2.)

A. Pathophysiology/Etiology
1. After a primary infection, it is thought that the herpes simplex virus remains latent in the neural ganglia and is activated by some stimulus that triggers the migration of the virus to the oral epithelium, resulting in lesions commonly called a "cold sore" or "fever blister."
2. Recurrent herpes labialis may be precipitated by exposure to sunlight, fatigue, hormonal changes, gastrointestinal disturbances, fever, and oral trauma (eg, dental procedures).

B. Clinical Manifestations
1. Prodromal period: tingling, soreness, burning, sensation, or swelling in area where lesions will develop
2. Small vesicles appear, frequently in the mucocutaneous junction of the lips or adjacent skin
3. Vesicles rupture: ulcerations fuse together and form larger weeping ulcers; lesions heal spontaneously in 7 to 14 days

C. Management
1. Acyclovir (Zovirax) may be useful for immunocomprised patients. Intravenous and oral forms are more effective than topical form.
2. Topical anesthetic, lidocaine (Xylocaine), or dyclonine (Dyclone) may provide relief of painful lesions when applied to affected areas.
3. Applications of drying lotions/liquids may help dry lesions.

D. Nursing Interventions/Patient Education
1. Advise adequate rest and nutrition and prevention of sunburn and illness to prevent outbreak.
2. Advise patient that virus is transmitted through close contact, so avoid kissing and sharing food, cups, and utensils during outbreak.
3. Recommend good hand washing and hygiene to prevent spread.

Streptococcal Pharyngitis

Streptococcal pharyngitis is an acute bacterial infection of the throat caused by group A beta-hemolytic streptococci.

A. Clinical Manifestations
1. Abrupt onset of sore throat; fever above 38.2°C (101°F)
2. Throat pain aggravated by swallowing

3. Pharynx appears reddened with edema of uvula; tonsils enlarged and reddened; pharynx and tonsils may be covered with exudate
4. Swollen, palpable, and tender cervical lymph nodes

B. Diagnostic Evaluation
1. White blood cells—leukocytosis
2. Throat culture for bacteriologic diagnosis to determine presence/absence of streptococci.
3. Rapid streptococcal antigen detection tests—detect a streptococci from throat swab within 5 minutes; false-negative rate is significant

C. Management
1. Penicillin V (Pen VK) orally for 10 days or benzathine penicillin G (Bicillin) in a single intramuscular dose—early antibiotic treatment appears to shorten duration of symptoms and prevents rheumatic fever.
2. Erythromycin (Eryc)—for patient who is allergic to penicillin.
3. Other antibiotics such as cephalosporins and quinolones may be used.

D. Complications
1. Acute rheumatic fever
2. Peritonsillar abscess/cellulitis
3. Acute glomerulonephritis
4. Scarlet fever
5. Sinusitis, otitis media, mastoiditis

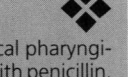

NURSING ALERT:
Acute rheumatic fever, a complication of streptococcal pharyngitis, can be prevented if patient is treated adequately with penicillin. Unfortunately, there is no evidence that antibiotic therapy will prevent acute glomerulonephritis.

D. Nursing Intervention/Patient Education
1. Advise patient to have any sore throat with fever evaluated, especially in the absence of cold symptoms.
2. Encourage compliance with full course of antibiotic therapy, despite feeling better in several days, to prevent complications.
3. Advise lukewarm saline gargles and use of antipyretic/analgesics as directed to promote comfort.
4. Encourage bed rest with increased fluid intake during fever.

Ear Disorders

◆ HEARING PROBLEMS

Problems with hearing rank high as a health disability.

Classification of Hearing Loss

1. Conductive loss—a hearing loss due to an impairment of the outer or middle ear or both. If causative problem cannot be corrected, a hearing aid may help.
2. Sensorineural (perceptive) loss—a hearing loss due to disease of the inner ear or nerve pathways; sensitivity to and discrimination of sounds are impaired. Hearing aids usually are helpful.
3. Combined hearing loss—a combination of the above.

4. Psychogenic hearing loss—usually a manifestation of an emotional disturbance and unrelated to evident structural changes in the hearing mechanisms. Loss is often total, but without physical basis; thus, the patient may suddenly recover.

Presbycusis

A progressive, bilaterally perceptive hearing loss of older individuals, usually involving high frequencies, that occurs with the aging process.

1. There is no effective medical or surgical treatment.
2. The patient should be counseled by an otologist in collaboration with an audiologist.
3. Helpful aids should be considered, such as a telephone amplifier, radio and television earphone attachments, buzzers instead of doorbell.
4. Understanding and help from family members are important.

Otosclerosis

Otosclerosis is a pathologic condition in which there is formation of new spongy bone in the labyrinth, fixation of the stapes, and prevention of sound transmission through the ossicles to the inner fluids, resulting in deafness.

A. Incidence
1. Cause is unknown.
2. Occurs more commonly in women than in men.
3. Has a familial tendency.

B. Clinical Manifestations
1. Young adult presents a history of slow, progressive hearing loss of soft, spoken tones, with no middle ear infection.
2. A frequent complaint is tinnitus; both ears may be affected equally.
3. History reveals gradual hearing loss.
4. Audiometry findings substantiate hearing loss.
5. Bone conduction is much better than air conduction.

C. Management
1. No known medical treatment exists for this form of deafness, but amplification with a hearing aid may be helpful.
2. Surgery—stapedectomy.
   a. The removal of otosclerotic lesions at the footplate of stapes and the creation of a tissue implant with prosthesis to maintain suitable conduction.
   b. To perform such delicate surgery, the otologic binocular microscope is used.

Cochlear Implant

A cochlear implant is a device that emits auditory signals for profoundly deaf individuals. The single-electrode system bypasses the damaged cochlear system and stimulates the remaining auditory nerve fibers. This results in the perception of sound.

A. Classification
Cochlear implants may be classified according to the following categories.

1. Location of electrodes
   a. Intracochlear (Fig. 15-2)
   b. Extracochlear

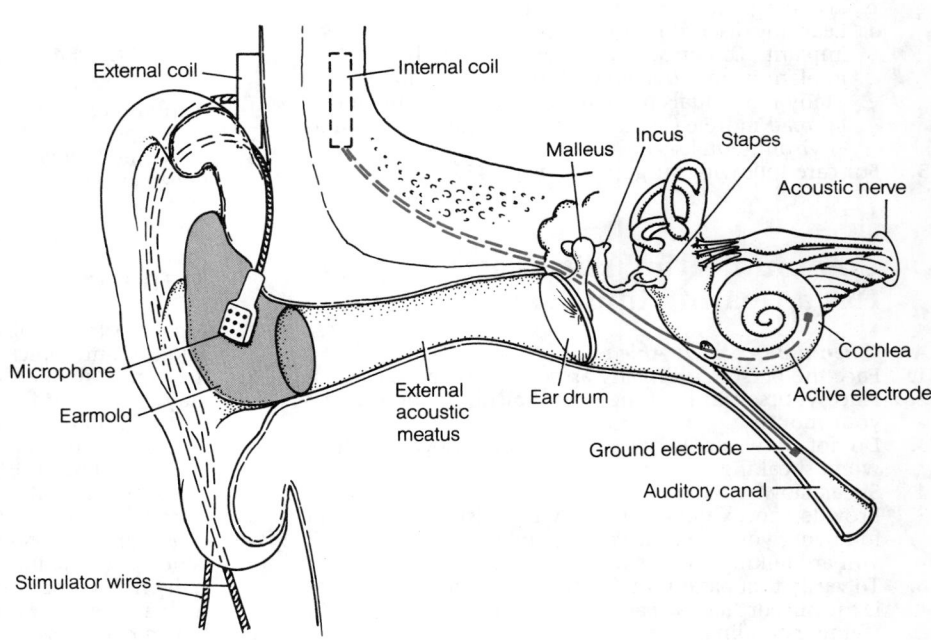

FIGURE 15-2 *Cochlear implant.*

2. Transmission of signals
   a. Single channel
   b. Multichannel
3. Features of speech signal
   a. Feature extraction—only certain features are transmitted.
   b. Nonfeature-specific—input signal is transmitted without extracting speech cues.
4. Types of electrodes
   a. Monopolar
   b. Bipolar
5. Method of stimulation
   a. Continuous
   b. Pulsatile

B. *Patient Criteria*
There are no standardized criteria for patient selection. Some data that are considered include:

1. Total hearing loss with no significant benefit from hearing aid.
2. Results of audiologic test show average hearing sensitivity at 500, 1,000, 2,000 Hz to be no better than 90 to 100 dB hearing loss in either ear.
3. Zero percent correct on speech recognition.
4. Physically healthy, with adult-onset deafness. (Some surgery is being done on infants and children.)
5. No evidence of brain impairment, psychoses, or mental retardation.
6. Reasonable expectations and optimism—motivation must be present.

C. *Nursing Interventions*
1. Encourage the prospective patient to visit with someone who is currently using an implant to learn the positive and negative results of a cochlear implant.
2. Explain the rehabilitation process—usually begins 2 months postsurgery. Included are:
   a. Adjustment of controls.
   b. Operation and maintenance of stimulator unit.
   c. Listening critically and learning lip reading.
   d. Learning discrimination of sounds through cochlear implant. Understanding speech through cochlear implant is not possible with this device alone.
   e. Many individuals trained with such an implant can lip read more easily and can distinguish voices and environmental sounds.
3. For care following surgery, see page 452.

Communicating With a Person Who Has a Hearing Impairment

A. *When the Person Is Able to Lip Read*
1. Face the person as directly as possible when speaking.
2. Place yourself in good light so that he or she can see your mouth.
3. Do not chew, smoke, or have anything in your mouth when speaking.
4. Speak slowly and enunciate distinctly.
5. Provide contextual clues that will assist the person in following your speech. For example, point to a tray if you are talking about the food on it.
6. To verify that patient understands your message, write it for him or her to read (ie, if you doubt that patient is understanding you).

B. *When It Is Difficult to Understand the Person*
1. Pay attention when the person speaks; facial and physical gestures may help you understand what person is saying.
2. Exchange conversation with person when it is possible to anticipate replies—this is particularly helpful in your initial contact with person and may help you become familiar with speech peculiarities.
3. Anticipate context of speech to assist in interpreting what person is saying.
4. If unable to understand person, resort to writing or include in your conversation someone who does understand; request that person repeat that which is not understood.

C. *Organizations That Help the Hearing Impaired*
1. Alexander Graham Bell Association for the Deaf; 3417 Volta Place NW; Washington, DC 20007; (202) 337-5220.
2. American Speech-Language-Hearing Association; 10801 Rockville Pike; Rockville, MD 20852; (301) 897-5700.
3. National Association of the Deaf; 814 Thayer Avenue; Silver Springs, MD 20910; (301) 587-1788.

◆ OTITIS EXTERNA

Otitis externa is an inflammation of the external ear canal that may occur 2 to 3 days after swimming and diving (swimmer's ear).

Pathophysiology/Etiology

1. Bacterial causes, usually *Pseudomonas, Proteus vulgaris,* streptococci, and *Staphylococcus aureus.*
2. Fungal infection with *Aspergillus niger, Candida albicans.*
3. Dermatologic conditions such as seborrhea and psoriasis, stagnant water in ear canal, and trauma to canal from cleaning ears may predispose to infection.

Clinical Manifestations

1. Pain; increased by manipulation of auricle or tragus
2. Fever; periauricular lymphadenopathy
3. Foul-smelling white to purulent drainage
4. Red, swollen ear canal with discharge on otoscopic exam

Management

1. Alcohol (dries moisture), acetic acid solution (restores acidity), and topical antibiotics (curb infection).
2. If canal is swollen and tender, topical corticosteroids may decrease inflammation and swelling.
3. If acute inflammation and closure of the ear canal prevent drops from saturating canal, a wick may need to be inserted by an ENT specialist so that drops will gain access to walls of entire ear canal.
4. Burow's solution (aluminum acetate solution) may decrease drainage caused by eczema.
5. When acute pain and swelling have subsided, a specially trained person can remove debris from ear canal with an applicator or by irrigation or suction.
6. Warm compresses and analgesics may be needed.

Nursing Interventions/Patient Education

1. Demonstrate proper application of eardrops.
   a. Lie or sit with head tilted to side and affected ear up.
   b. Pull auricle upward and outward and instill four drops or amount prescribed.
   c. Maintain position for 5 minutes to ensure proper saturation.
   d. Do not put cotton in ear, because cotton will soak up drops and impair contact with canal.
2. Advise that external otitis can be prevented or minimized by thoroughly drying the ear canal after coming into contact with water or moist environment.
3. Tell patient to use eardrops after swimming to assist in preventing swimmer's ear. Usually these solutions contain:
   a. Alcohol and glycerol to reduce moisture.
   b. Boric acid or acetic acid (vinegar) to limit growth of microorganisms and maintain normal acidity of the ear canal.
4. Advise the use of properly fitting earplugs for recurrent cases.
5. Teach proper ear hygiene—clean auricle and outer canal with washcloth only, do not insert anything smaller than finger wrapped in washcloth in ear canal.

NURSING ALERT:
Use of cotton-tipped applicators to dry the canal or remove earwax should be avoided because:
1. Cerumen may be forced against the tympanic membrane.
2. The canal lining may be abraded, making it more susceptible to infection.
3. Cerumen that coats and protects the canal may be removed.

◆ IMPACTED CERUMEN AND FOREIGN BODIES

Accumulated cerumen (earwax) may become impacted due to use of cotton swabs to clean ears and may be a problem for some people. Foreign bodies may be lodged in ear canal intentionally or accidentally by patient or other person (usually in children), or patient may be completely unaware, as in insect obstruction.

Etiology/Clinical Manifestations

1. Cerumen usually builds up over period of time, causing slightly decreased hearing acuity and feeling that ear(s) is plugged.
   a. May be underlying seborrhea or other dermatologic condition that causes flaking of skin that mixes with cerumen and becomes obstructive.
   b. Cerumen may be pushed back over tympanic membrane by action of cotton swab.
   c. Patient may instill cerumenolytic, which actually makes condition worse by softening cerumen and causing it to coalesce into larger clump.
2. Insect may fly or crawl into ear, causing initial low rumbling sound; later, feeling that ear is plugged and decreased hearing acuity.
3. Pain, fever, and drainage may occur as otitis externa develops.

Management

1. Accumulated cerumen (earwax) does not have to be removed unless it becomes impacted and interferes with hearing. May be removed by irrigating ear canal. See Procedure Guidelines 15-1.
2. Foreign bodies may be removed by instrumentation or irrigation.
   a. Insects—treat by instilling oil drops to smother insect, which then can be removed by health professional.
   b. Vegetable foreign bodies (eg, peas)—irrigation is contraindicated because vegetable matter absorbs water, which would further wedge it in the canal.
3. Unskilled persons should not attempt to remove a foreign body because:
   a. It may be forced into bony portion of the canal.
   b. The canal skin may be damaged.
   c. The eardrum may be perforated.
4. Removal should be done skillfully with instruments; if the victim is very young, general anesthesia is required.

NURSING ALERT:
Do not instill anything into external canal if eardrum may be perforated.

Nursing Interventions/Patient Education

1. Teach proper ear hygiene, especially not putting anything in ears.
2. Explain the normal protective function of cerumen.
3. If patient has problem with cerumen buildup and has been advised by health care provider to use a cerumenolytic periodically, ensure that patient is getting cerumen out of ear before more medication is instilled. A bulb syringe may be used by the patient at home to help remove softened cerumen.
4. Advise patient to report any fever, pain, drainage, or persistent hearing impairment.

COMMUNITY-BASED CARE TIP:
Hearing loss in the elderly may simply be due to impacted cerumen. Cerumen becomes thicker in the elderly, making impaction more likely. Perform otoscopic exam in the nursing home or community to check for impacted cerumen and check with health care provider to see if ear irrigation is indicated.

PROCEDURE GUIDELINES 15-1 ◆ Irrigating the External Auditory Canal

PURPOSES
1. To remove discharge from the canal.
2. To facilitate removal of cerumen or foreign body.

NURSING ALERT:
Ask if patient has a history of draining ears or has ever had a perforation or other complications from a previous ear irrigation. If the reply is "yes," check with the health care provider before proceeding with the irrigation.

EQUIPMENT AND SOLUTIONS
Kind and amount of solution desired (usually warm water)
Ear syringe or irrigating container with tubing, clamp, and catheter
Protective towels
Cotton balls and cotton-tipped applicators
Solution bowl and emesis basin
Bag for disposable items

PROCEDURE

PREPARATORY PHASE
1. After explaining procedure to the patient, place in a position of sitting or lying with head tilted forward and toward affected ear.
2. Position protective towels.

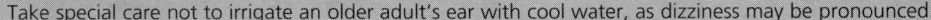

NURSING ACTION	RATIONALE

PERFORMANCE PHASE

1. Use a cotton applicator to remove any discharge on outer ear.
2. Place basin close to the patient's head and under the ear.
3. Test temperature of solution. It should be comfortable to the inner aspect of wrist area.

1. To prevent carrying discharge deeper into canal.
2. To provide a receptacle to receive irrigating solution.
3. Solutions that are hot or cold are most uncomfortable and may initiate a feeling of dizziness.

GERONTOLOGIC ALERT:
Take special care not to irrigate an older adult's ear with cool water, as dizziness may be pronounced.

4. Ascertain whether impaction is due to a foreign hydroscopic (attracts or absorbs moisture) body before proceeding.
5. Gently pull the outer ear upward and backward (adult) or downward and outward (child).
6. Place tip of syringe or irrigating catheter at opening of ear; gently direct stream of fluid against sides of canal.
7. If an irrigating container is used, elevate only high enough to remove secretions or no more than 15 cm (6 in.) above patient's ear.
8. Observe for signs of pain or dizziness.
9. If irrigating does not dislodge the wax, instill several drops of prescribed glycerin, carbamide peroxide (Debrox), or other solutions as directed 2 or 3 times daily for 2–3 days.

4. If water contacts such a substance, it may cause it to swell and produce intense pain.
5. To straighten the ear canal (see figure)
6. To decrease direct force of irrigation against eardrum and possibility of rupturing it.
7. To provide safe and effective pressure of fluid; if height is more than 15 cm (6 in.), pressure will be too great and may damage tissue.
8. Discontinue treatment if they occur.
9. To soften and loosen impaction.

PROCEDURE (cont'd)	NURSING ACTION	RATIONALE

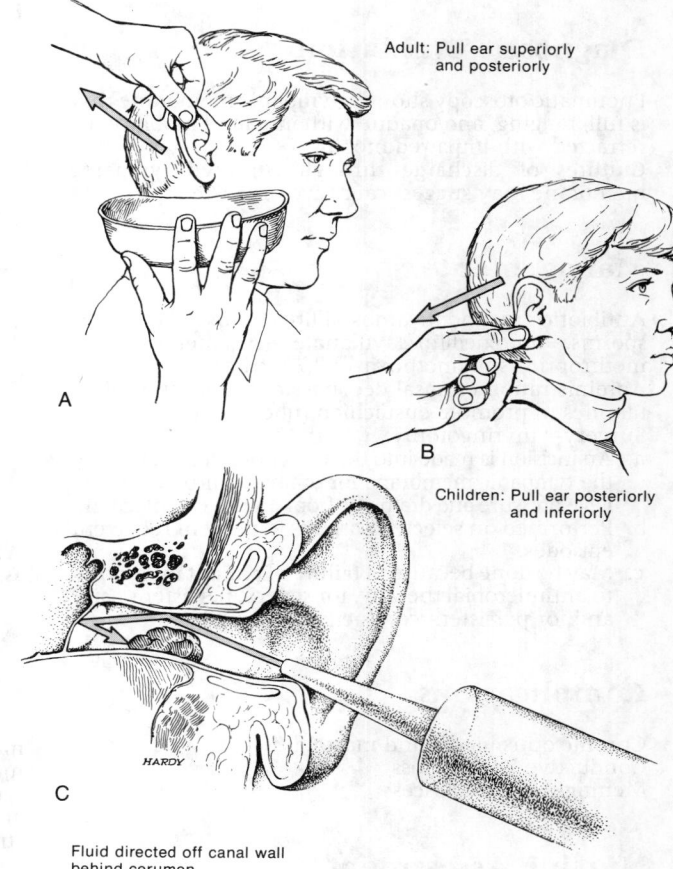

Adult: Pull ear superiorly and posteriorly

Children: Pull ear posteriorly and inferiorly

HARDY

Fluid directed off canal wall behind cerumen

*Ear irrigation. (**A**) The external auditory canal in the adult can best be exposed by pulling the earlobe upward and backward. (**B**) The same exposure can be achieved in the child by gently pulling the auricle of the ear downward and backward. (**C**) An enlarged diagram showing the direction of irrigating fluid against the side of the canal. NOTE: This is more effective in dislodging cerumen than if the flow of solution were directed straight into the canal.*

FOLLOW-UP PHASE

1. Dry external ear.
2. Remove soiled equipment and make the patient comfortable.
3. Patient should lie on irrigated (affected) side for a few minutes after procedure to allow any remaining solution to drain out.
4. Record time of irrigation, kind and amount of solution, nature of return flow, and effect of treatment.

◆ ACUTE OTITIS MEDIA

Acute otitis media is an inflammation/infection of the middle ear caused by the entrance of pathogenic organisms, with rapid onset of signs and symptoms. It is a major problem in children, but may occur at any age.

Pathophysiology/Etiology

1. Pathogenic organisms gain entry into the normally sterile middle ear, usually through a dysfunctional eustachian tube (suppurative otitis media).
2. Organisms include *Streptococcus pneumoniae, Haemophilus influenzae, Branhamella catarrhalis,* and *Staphylococcus aureus.*
3. In serous (secretory) otitis media, no purulent infection occurs, but blockage of the eustachian tube causes negative pressure and transudation of fluid from blood vessels and development of effusion in the middle ear.

Clinical Manifestations

1. Pain is usually the first symptom.
2. Fever may rise to 40 to 40.6°C (104 to 105°F).
3. Purulent drainage (otorrhea) is present if tympanic membrane is perforated.
4. Irritability may be noted in the young person.
5. Headache, hearing loss, anorexia, nausea, and vomiting may be present.

6. History may reveal prior upper respiratory infection, allergies, immunologic defect, or head injury (fractured skull).

Diagnostic Evaluation

1. Pneumatic otoscopy shows a tympanic membrane that is full, bulging, and opaque with impaired mobility (or retracted with impaired mobility).
2. Cultures of discharge through ruptured tympanic membrane may suggest causative organism.

Management

1. Antibiotic treatment: amoxicillin (Amoxil), cephalosporins, amoxicillin/clavulanate (Augmentin), trimethroprim-sulfamethoxazole (Bactrim).
2. Administration of nasal decongestants and/or antihistamines to promote eustachian tube drainage.
3. Surgery—myringotomy.
   a. An incision is made into the posterior inferior aspect of the tympanic membrane for draining purposes (to relieve pressure and drain pus from middle ear infection).
   b. Performed on selected patients to prevent recurrent episodes.
   c. May be done because of failure of patient to respond to antimicrobial therapy, for severe, persistent pain, and for persistent conductive hearing loss.

Complications

1. Chronic otitis media and mastoiditis
2. Conductive hearing loss
3. Meningitis, brain abscess

Nursing Assessment

1. Obtain history of upper respiratory infection, previous ear infections, allergies, and progression of symptoms.
2. Assess fever and level of pain.
3. Obtain baseline hearing evaluation, if indicated.

Nursing Diagnoses

A. Pain related to inflammation and increased middle ear pressure
B. Risk for infection following myringotomy

Nursing Interventions

A. *Relieving Pain*
1. Administer or teach self-administration of aspirin and other analgesics as prescribed. (Sedation is usually avoided because it may interfere with early detection of intracranial complications.)
2. Administer or teach self-administration of antibiotics, as prescribed.
3. Encourage the use of local warm compresses to promote comfort and help resolve infectious process.

4. Be alert for such symptoms as headache, slow pulse, vomiting, and vertigo, which may be significant for sequelae that involve the mastoid or even the brain.

B. *Preventing Infection Postoperatively* See Ear Surgery, page 452

Patient Education/Health Maintenance

1. Instruct the patient on activities that are to be avoided until tympanic membrane heals (swimming, shampooing hair, showering).
2. Advise the patient of hygienic practices that will prevent tympanic membrane injury (eg, avoid ear picking, inserting toothpick in ear to relieve itch).
3. Instruct patient of any symptoms that indicate recurrence (discomfort, pain, dizziness).
4. Teach patients with serous otitis to take decongestants as directed and to perform Valsalva's maneuver several times a day to help open the eustachian tube.

Evaluation

A. Patient verbalizes relief of pain at follow-up visit
B. Minimal drainage from ear

◆ CHRONIC OTITIS MEDIA AND MASTOIDITIS

Chronic otitis media and mastoiditis is a chronic inflammation of the middle ear and mastoid lasting more than 3 months from initial onset, accompanied by a nonintact tympanic membrane and discharge. It may be caused by an antibiotic-resistant organism or a particularly virulent strain of organism.

Pathophysiology/Etiology

1. The accumulation of pus under pressure in the middle ear cavity results in necrosis of tissue and extension of infection into the mastoid cells.
2. Chronic systemic disease and immunosuppression are risk factors.

Clinical Manifestations

1. Painless or dull ache and tenderness of mastoid.
2. Otorrhea may be odorless or foul smelling.
3. Vertigo and pain may be present if CNS complications have occurred.
4. History will indicate several episodes of acute otitis media, possible rupture of tympanic membrane.
5. Fever and postauricular erythema and edema.

Diagnostic Evaluation

1. Air conductive hearing loss is present through audiometric tests.

2. X-rays may note mastoid pathology, for example, cholesteatoma (soft ball of dead skin cells that erodes surrounding vital structures) or haziness of mastoid cells.

Management

Note: If advanced chronic ear disease is left untreated, inner ear and life-threatening CNS complications may develop because of erosion of surrounding structures.

A. *Medical Therapy*
1. Antibiotic and steroid eardrops may control infection and inflammation, but once mastoiditis develops, parenteral antibiotic therapy is necessary.
2. Frequent removal of epithelial debris and purulent drainage may protect tissue from damage.

B. *Surgical Interventions*
1. Indicated when cholesteatoma is present.
2. Indicated when there is pain, profound deafness, dizziness, sudden facial paralysis, or stiff neck (may lead to meningitis or brain abscess).
3. Types of procedures
  a. Simple mastoidectomy—removal of diseased bone and insertion of a drain; indicated when there is persistent infection and signs of intracranial complications.
  b. Radical mastoidectomy—removal of posterior wall of ear canal, remnants of the tympanic membrane, and the malleous and incus.
  c. Posteroanterior mastoidectomy—combines simple mastoidectomy with tympanoplasty (reconstruction of middle ear structures).

Complications

1. CNS infection
2. Postoperatively: facial nerve paralysis, bleeding, vertigo

Nursing Assessment

1. Assess for history of ear infection and treatment compliance.
2. Assess for ear drainage, patency of tympanic membrane.
3. Assess for hearing loss.
4. Palpate for mastoid tenderness.

Nursing Diagnoses

Also see Ear Surgery, page 452.
A. Pain related to infectious process, surgery
B. Risk for Infection related to complication of disease process, surgery
C. Sensory/Perceptual Alteration (Auditory) related to effects of disease process and surgery

Nursing Interventions

A. *Promoting Comfort*
1. Provide for relief of pain postoperatively.
  a. Give aspirin or other analgesic as prescribed.
  b. Apply cold compresses to area.
  c. Position for comfort—may be specific to type of surgery or surgeon's preference.
2. Postoperatively, administer sedatives cautiously for restlessness.

B. *Preventing Spread of Infection*
1. Assist with dressing changes, because area is packed with gauze for drainage—this may be done daily or every other day; packing is removed on third or fourth day.
2. Observe for signs of local infection.
3. Administer or teach patient to administer prescribed antibiotics.
4. Be alert for spread of infection to brain—unusual rise in temperature, chills, stiff neck, nausea and vomiting (meningeal signs).

C. *Monitoring for Sensory Alterations*
1. Note status of hearing.
  a. If stapes has been removed or dislodged, then hearing is lost.
  b. If stapes or cochlea has not been removed or disturbed, then hearing will probably be regained; a hearing aid may be required.
2. Warn patient that transient vertigo and nausea may be present after radical mastoidectomy due to inner ear disturbance. Ensure safety measures.
3. Be alert for unilateral facial drooping or numbness due to facial nerve injury.

Patient Education/Health Maintenance

1. Teach patient dressing changes and to continue antibiotic therapy as ordered.
2. Advise of complications and what to report.
3. Stress the importance of follow-up hearing evaluations.

Evaluation

A. Reports that pain is relieved
B. No signs of local or CNS infection
C. To be evaluated for hearing aid; vertigo minimal

◆ MENIERE'S DISEASE

Meniere's disease (endolymphatic hydrops) is a chronic disease that involves the inner ear and causes a triad of symptoms: vertigo, hearing loss, and tinnitus.

Pathophysiology/Etiology

1. Cause is unknown.
2. Fluid distention of the endolymphatic spaces of the labyrinth destroy cochlear hair cells.
3. Occurs most frequently between age 30 and 60.

Clinical Manifestations

1. Sudden attacks occur, in which patient feels that the room is spinning around (vertigo); may last 10 minutes to several hours.
2. Dizziness, tinnitus, and reduced hearing occur on involved side.

3. Headache, nausea, vomiting, and incoordination are present.
4. Sudden motion of the head may precipitate vomiting.
5. History often reveals ear trouble, vasomotor rhinitis, and allergies.
6. The most comfortable position for the patient is lying down.
7. Irritability; other personality changes.
8. After multiple attacks, tinnitus or impaired hearing may be present.

Diagnostic Evaluation

1. Caloric test/electronystagmography.
   a. Useful in differentiating Meniere's syndrome from intracranial lesion.
   b. Fluid, above or below body temperature, is instilled into the auditory canal.
   c. Results
      (1) Normal patient—complains of dizziness.
      (2) Patient with acoustic neuroma—no reaction.
      (3) Patient with Meniere's disease—severe attack as above.
2. Audiogram shows sensorineural hearing loss.
3. CT, magnetic resonance imaging to rule out tumor.

Management

A. Medical
1. Patient can be asked to keep a diary noting presence of aural symptoms (eg, tinnitus, distorted hearing) when episodes of vertigo occur—may help diagnose which ear is involved and if surgery will be needed.
2. Administration of the vestibular suppressant and diuretic acetazolamide (Diamox) when attacks are infrequent to decrease symptoms.
3. Streptomycin (intramuscularly) may be given to selectively destroy vestibular apparatus if vertigo is uncontrollable.
4. Administration of antihistamines such as dimenhydrinate (Dramamine) or meclizine (Ativert); diazepam (Valium) may also be used.
5. Antiemetics to reduce nausea, vomiting, and vertigo.

B. Surgical
1. Conservative—simple endolymphatic sac decompression or endolymphatic subarachnoid or mastoid shunt to relieve symptoms without destroying function.
2. Destructive surgery.
   a. Labyrinthectomy—recommended if the patient experiences progressive hearing loss and severe vertigo attacks so normal tasks cannot be performed; results in total deafness of affected ear.
   b. Vestibular nerve section—neurosurgical suboccipital approach to the cerebellopontine angle for intracranial vestibular nerve neurectomy.

Complications

1. Irreversible hearing loss
2. Disability and social isolation due to vertigo and hearing loss

Nursing Assessment

1. Assess for frequency and severity of attacks.
2. Provide screening hearing tests.
3. Evaluate effect on patient's life.

Nursing Diagnoses

A. Risk for Injury related to sudden attacks of vertigo
B. Social Isolation related to fear of attack and hearing loss

Nursing Interventions

For care related to labyrinth surgery, see page 452.

A. Ensuring Safety
1. Help patient recognize aura so that patient has time to prepare for an attack.
2. Encourage patient to lie down during attack, in safe place, and lie still.
3. Put side rails up on bed if in hospital.
4. Have patient close eyes if this lessens symptoms.
5. Inform patient that the dizziness may last for varying lengths of time. Maintain safety precautions until attack is complete.

B. Minimizing Feelings of Isolation
1. Provide encouragement and understanding.
2. Assist patient to identify specific triggers to control attacks.
   a. Remind the patient to move slowly, because jerking or making sudden movements may precipitate an attack.
   b. Avoid noises and glaring, bright lights, which may initiate an attack.
   c. Eliminate smoking and the intake of coffee, tea, alcohol, and stimulating drugs—due to vasoconstriction effects.
   d. Control environmental factors and personal habits that may cause stress or fatigue.
   e. If there is a tendency to allergic reactions to foods, eliminate those foods from the diet.
3. Adhere to periodic use of diuretics, as prescribed, to relieve feeling of fullness in the ear, vertigo, and tinnitus.
4. Teach patient to be aware of other sensory cues from the environment—visual, olfactory, tactile—if hearing is affected.

Patient Education/Health Maintenance

1. Teach about medication therapy, including side effects of antihistamines—drowsiness, dry mouth.
2. Advise sodium restriction as adjunct to acetazolamide therapy.
3. Advise patient to keep a log of attacks, triggers, and severity of symptoms.
4. Encourage follow-up hearing evaluations and provide information about surgical care if planned.

Evaluation

A. Patient lying down with side rails up and eyes closed during attack; resolved without injury
B. Identified caffeine, bright lights, and stress as triggering factors; verbalizes desire to eliminate these factors

Malignant Disorders

◆ CANCER OF THE ORAL CAVITY

Cancer of the oral cavity may arise from the lips, buccal mucosa, gums, hard palate, floor of the mouth, salivary glands, and anterior two-thirds of the tongue.

Pathophysiology/Etiology

1. Most prevalent in men ages 50 to 70 years; approximately 90% are squamous cell carcinoma.
2. High risk factors: use of tobacco and alcohol (particularly in combination), use of smokeless tobacco (snuff), pipe smoking, and chronic sun exposure.
3. Overall 5-year survival rate is 30% to 40%, depending on the stage of disease at diagnosis.

Clinical Manifestations

1. Often asymptomatic in early stages.
2. Mucosal erythroplasia—red inflammatory or erythroplastic mucosal changes; appears smooth, granular, and minimally elevated, with or without a white component (leukoplakia), persisting longer than 14 days.
3. Cancer of the lip—presence of a lesion that fails to heal.
4. Cancer of the tongue—swelling, ulceration, areas of tenderness or bleeding, abnormal texture, or limited movement of the tongue.
5. Floor-of-the-mouth cancer—red, slightly elevated, mucosal lesion with ill-defined borders, leukoplakia, indurated, ulceration, or wartlike growth.
6. More advanced stages characterized by ulceration, bleeding, pain, induration, and/or cervical lymphadenopathy.

Diagnostic Evaluation

1. Careful inspection of the oral cavity with indirect mirror examination of pharynx.
2. Staining of the oral lesion with toluidine blue—the lesion stains dark blue after rinsing with acetic acid (normal tissue does not absorb stain).
3. Excisional biopsy of suspected tissue.
4. Radiologic studies: chest x-ray to determine local invasiveness and metastasis.

Management

(Selection of treatment depends on size and site of lesion and how extensively surrounding tissues are involved.)

1. Small lesions can be removed by wide excision or can be treated with radiotherapy or interstitial irradiation.
2. Large lesions may be excised widely or treated by radical neck dissection for extensive lymphatic involvement, followed by external irradiation to decrease recurrence rate but maintain appearance.
3. Radiation therapy can be palliative, providing it has not been given previously.
4. Chemotherapy of previously untreated patients with locally advanced tumors has shown high response rates in clinical trials.

Complications

1. Second primary cancers of the larynx, hypopharynx, esophagus, and lungs.
2. Secondary to treatment:
   a. Surgery: transient salivary outflow obstruction, infection, voice changes, fistula formation, loss of swallowing, cosmetic defects.
   b. Radiation: temporary loss of taste, xerostomia, radiation caries, osteoradionecrosis.

Nursing Assessment

1. Obtain complete history, noting risk factors such as smoking and alcohol use.
2. Question the patient regarding changes in swallowing, smell or taste, salivation, discomfort when eating, sore throat, foul breath odor.
3. Note the quality of voice patterns and odor of breath.
4. Inspect the oral cavity: erythema, red velvety areas; white patches; bleeding; swelling; record the size, location, and description.
5. Palpate the cervical lymph nodes for size, firmness, or tenderness.

Nursing Diagnoses

A. Pain related to malignant infiltration, lesion(s), difficulty swallowing, surgery, radiation therapy
B. Altered Nutrition (Less Than Body Requirements) related to pain, difficulty in chewing or swallowing, history of alcohol abuse
C. Body Image Disturbance related to changes in facial contour, cosmetic defect from surgery

Nursing Interventions

Also see page 470 if radical neck dissection has been performed.

A. Achieving an Acceptable Level of Comfort
1. Provide systemic analgesics or analgesic gargles as prescribed.
2. If the patient can tolerate it, provide mouth care with soft toothbrush and flossing between teeth.

3. If patient cannot tolerate brushing and flossing:
    a. Gently lavage oral cavity with a catheter inserted between the patient's cheek and gums with warm water or mouthwash.
    b. Use power water spray to clean inaccessible areas if patient's comfort allows.
4. Encourage use of mouthwashes that do not contain alcohol—may irritate the gums.
5. Provide management of excessive salivation and mouth odors:
    a. Insert a gauze wick in corner of mouth; place basin conveniently to catch drooling; replace frequently—to absorb and direct excess saliva.
    b. Suction secretions with a soft rubber catheter as needed; instruct patient on suctioning methods.
6. Provide management of decreased salivation if necessary.
    a. Encourage intake of fluids, if not contraindicated.
    b. Instruct the patient to avoid dry, bulky, and irritating foods.
    c. Offer lemon lozenges or chewing gum to stimulate salivation.
7. Maintain a clean and odor-free environment by removing soiled dressings, tissues and gauzes, and providing room deodorants.

B. *Improving Nutritional Status*
1. Handle feeding problems in one or a combination of the following ways, as ordered:
    a. Intravenously.
    b. Nasogastric tube feedings or gastrostomy tube feedings.
    c. Orally; serve meals high in protein and vitamin content, low in acidity and salt.
2. Provide mouth care before and after eating.
3. Allow the patient to have meals in privacy if so desired.
4. Offer easily chewed foods; mash or blenderize if necessary.
5. Add herbs or sweeteners to enhance flavor.
6. If swallowing difficulties persist, see Procedure Guidelines 16-7, page 509; or consult the occupational or speech therapist.
7. Monitor weight, intake and output, and laboratory tests, such as blood urea nitrogen, creatinine, albumin, and total proteins.

C. *Improving Body Image*
1. Assess the patient's reaction to condition.
    a. Evaluate the patient's apprehension and offer emotional support.
    b. Correct any misinformation.
    c. Determine therapeutic plan of care for the patient's rehabilitation.
2. Recognize that face and neck surgery can be disfiguring and the patient often is embarrassed, withdrawn, and depressed.
3. Assist the patient in caring for personal appearance.
4. Observe closely for indications of the patient's needs, which may be communicated in other ways, such as acting out or withdrawn behavior.
5. Allow verbalization of fears, anger, distaste with body changes in a nondefensive manner.
6. Communicate acceptance of appearance in an honest manner.
7. Encourage the patient's family and friends to visit so that patient is aware that others care about him or her.
8. Provide diversional activities.

Patient Education/Health Maintenance

1. Repeat the details of good mouth care and cleanliness of dressings.
2. Emphasize adequate nutrition—proper consistency, proper seasoning, and right temperature. Suggest the use of a blender if necessary.
3. If suctioning is required, instruct as to method, type of equipment, and where it can be obtained.
4. Provide detailed instructions to the patient and a family member on incisional care.
5. Review signs of obstruction, hemorrhage, infection, and depression and what to do about them if they are evident.
6. Refer to a speech–language pathologist, if indicated.
7. Encourage cessation of high-risk behaviors: smoking, alcohol consumption, use of smokeless tobacco, pipe smoking.
8. Emphasize the need for routine follow-up examinations.

Evaluation

A. Reports adequate comfort levels; is pain free; handles secretions adequately
B. Achieves adequate nutritional status; able to eat prescribed diet
C. Verbalizes acceptance of body image; demonstrates behaviors that reflect self-esteem (ie, shaves, dresses, applies make-up)

◆ RADICAL NECK DISSECTION FOR HEAD AND NECK MALIGNANCY

Radical neck dissection, which may be indicated for head and neck cancer, refers to a group of malignant tumors that may occur at one or more anatomic locations in the upper respiratory and digestive tract. Specific sites include ear, nasopharynx, nose and paranasal sinuses, palate, oral cavity, larynx, hypopharynx, and thyroid gland. Most are squamous cell carcinomas. Local extension to adjacent muscle, bone, and vital structures often occurs before detection, and metastasis to cervical lymph nodes is common.

Surgical Procedures

1. Resection of lesion is the primary intervention.
2. Radical neck dissection—removal of all tissue under the skin from the ramus of the jaw down to the clavicle; from midline back to the angle of the jaw. This includes sternocleidomastoid muscle, other smaller muscles, jugular vein in the neck.
3. Modified (functional) radical neck dissection—removal of lymph nodes only.
4. Concomitant hemilaryngectomy or total laryngectomy may be necessary.
5. Often followed by postoperative radiation therapy. In some instances where resection is impossible, radical radiation therapy is the sole treatment for head and neck malignancy.

6. Surgical reconstruction may be performed with a rotational flap, skin graft, or free flap to promote healing and improve aesthetics.

Preoperative Management/Nursing Care

1. Interventions to improve nutritional status preoperatively include nutritional supplements, hyperalimentation, alcohol withdrawal, and counseling.
2. Patient's general health status is evaluated, and underlying conditions, such as cirrhosis and obstructive pulmonary or cardiovascular disease, are identified and treated, if possible.
3. Patient is evaluated for level of understanding of disease process, treatment regimen, and follow-up care.
4. Emotional preparation for major surgery, long rehabilitation, and change in body image is provided.

Postoperative Management/ Nursing Care

1. A major goal of postoperative management is protection of the airway. After the patient has fully recovered from anesthesia, the endotracheal tube is removed (unless respiratory compromise occurs).
2. The patient is closely monitored for hemorrhage. Wound drainage through portable suction should not exceed 120 mL on the first postoperative day, then decrease.
3. Prophylactic antibiotics are given to prevent infection because of extensive incision, lymph node resection, and close proximity to oral secretions.
4. Oral nutritional supplements, enteral feedings, or hyperalimentation is provided until oral intake is adequate and nutritional status is improved.

Complications

1. Surgery: salivary incontinence, malocclusion, unintelligible speech, difficulty eating or swallowing, unacceptable deformity
2. Radiation:
   a. Early: radiation mucositis, erythema, desquamation, dysphagia, secondary infection, oral pain
   b. Long-term: atrophy, fibrosis, salivary dryness, hoarseness, difficulty swallowing, bone pain, osteonecrosis, pathologic fractures, limitation of movement

Nursing Diagnoses

A. Ineffective Breathing Pattern related to laryngeal edema, secretions, presence of a tracheostomy
B. Risk for Infection related to surgery, proximity of secretions to suture line, postoperative radiation
C. Altered Nutrition (Less Than Body Requirements) related to anorexia, inability to swallow, pain on swallowing
D. Impaired Verbal Communication related to laryngeal edema, laryngectomy, tracheostomy
E. Body Image Disturbance related to surgical therapy, radiation changes

Nursing Interventions

A. **Maintaining Effective Breathing Pattern**
1. Place the patient in Fowler's position.
2. Observe for signs of respiratory embarrassment, such as dyspnea, cyanosis, edema, hoarseness, or dysphagia.
3. Provide supplemental oxygen by face mask if necessary; if tracheostomy is present, provide oxygen by collar or T-piece, providing adequate humidification.
4. Auscultate for decreased breath sounds, crackles, wheezes; auscultate over the trachea in the immediate postoperative period to assess for stridor indicative of edema.
5. Encourage deep breathing and coughing.
6. Assist the patient in assuming a sitting position to bring up secretions (support the patient's neck with the nurse's hands).
7. Suction secretions orally or aseptically through a tracheostomy if patient is unable to cough them up.

B. **Preventing Infection**
1. Assess vital signs for indication of infection: increased heart rate, elevation of temperature.
2. Inspect wound for hemorrhage, drainage, or tracheal constriction; reinforce dressings as needed.
3. Inspect incision for signs of infection: redness; warmth; swelling; drainage.
4. If portable suction is used, expect approximately 80 to 120 mL of serosanguineous secretions to be drawn off during the first postoperative day; this diminishes with each day.
5. Aseptically cleanse skin area around drain exit, using saline or prescribed solution.
6. Ensure that the incision site remains clean and dry; cleanse away any secretions immediately.

C. **Improving Nutrition**
1. Postoperatively provide intravenous fluids and hyperalimentation, tube feedings through nasogastric tube or gastrostomy tube, or oral feedings as soon as swallowing is established.
2. Provide mouth care before and after meals.
3. Assess for excessive or decreased salivation, which may impair swallowing.
4. Ensure that emergency suctioning and airway equipment is available at the bedside during meals in the event of choking or aspiration.
5. Position patient in an upright position, supporting shoulders and neck with pillows if necessary.
6. Inquire if the patient would prefer privacy during meals.
7. Provide an environment that is clean and free of interruptions and odor.
8. Assist with oral intake, providing easily chewed foods. Mash or blenderize meals if necessary.

D. **Improving Ability to Communicate**
1. If tracheostomy or laryngectomy has been performed, provide alternative methods of communication (letter board, chalk and slate, paper and pencil). If writing is a problem, it may be due to denervation of the trapezius muscle.
2. Allow adequate time for patient to communicate.
3. Place call bell and other articles that patient may need within easy access.
4. Recognize that patient may have difficulty nodding "yes" or "no" because of neck dissection.

5. Provide support and encouragement during communication attempts, recognizing that this patient often is depressed and frustrated even during limited communication.
6. Refer patient to speech–language pathologist if indicated.

E. Strengthening Body Image
1. Respect the patient's desire for privacy treatments, dressing changes, and feedings.
2. Inform visitors of appearance before they see patient so that their expressions do not cause patient to be upset.
3. Provide frequent aeration of the room and use deodorants to prevent unpleasant odors.
4. Observe for lower facial paralysis, because this may indicate facial nerve injury.
5. Watch for shoulder dysfunction, which may follow resection of spinal accessory nerves.
   a. Use postoperative muscle exercises and muscle reeducation.
   b. Work with the patient to obtain good functional range of motion.
6. Talk with the surgeon and patient about decisions on future cosmetic surgery or in the use of a prosthetic device.
7. Encourage the patient to verbalize concerns and feelings.
   a. Consult the health care provider to determine the nature and extent of explanation and prognosis that has been given to the patient.
   b. Encourage the patient to seek confirmation of personal philosophy and religious beliefs, because this may provide answers.
   c. Accentuate the positive.
   d. Encourage the patient to participate in the plan of care.
   e. Recognize that a great effort has to be made in behavior modification to change a lifestyle that included alcohol consumption and cigarette smoking. It is difficult to do.

Patient Education/Health Maintenance

A. Exercises
Instruct the patient and family regarding exercises to prevent limited range of motion and discomfort (Fig. 15-3).

1. Perform exercises morning and evening. Initially, exercises are done only once; then the number is increased by one each day until each exercise is done 10 times.
2. After each exercise, the patient is instructed to relax.
3. For neck:
   a. Gently rotate head to each side as far as possible.
   b. Tilt head to the right side as far as possible; repeat for left side.
   c. Drop chin to chest and then raise chin as high as possible.
4. For shoulder:
   a. Standing beside bed, place hand from unoperated side on bed for support.
   b. Gradually swing arm on operated side up and back as far as is comfortable for the patient.
   c. Each day, work toward finishing a complete circle.

B. Follow-up Visits
Emphasize the need for frequent follow-up visits and completion of radiation therapy if prescribed

C. For Permanent Tracheostomy
If patient has a permanent tracheostomy or laryngectomy, instruct the patient and family regarding:

1. Need for humidification.
2. Protection measures.
3. Activities to avoid that may cause aspiration.
4. Referral for speech–language pathologist, social worker to meet ongoing communication needs.

Evaluation

A. Maintains adequate breathing pattern; absence of dyspnea, shortness of breath; is able to handle secretions
B. Is free of signs and symptoms of infection; vital signs stable; incision is clean, dry, without redness or drainage
C. Is adequately hydrated, maintains stable nutritional status, is able to tolerate diet without choking or aspiration
D. Able to communicate and make needs known
E. Discusses concerns regarding condition; verbalizes positive aspects of self

◆ CANCER OF THE LARYNX

Cancer of the larynx is a malignant growth of the vocal cords (intrinsic) or any portion of the larynx (extrinsic). When treated early, the likelihood of cure is great.

Pathophysiology/Etiology

1. Occurs predominantly in men older than 60.
2. Most patients have a history of smoking; those with supraglottic laryngeal cancer frequently have a history of smoking and a high alcohol intake. Other risk factors include vocal straining, chronic laryngitis, industrial exposure, nutritional deficiency, and family predisposition.
3. In North America, about two-thirds of carcinomas of the larynx arise in the glottis, almost one-third arise in the supraglottic region, and about 3% arise in the subglottic region of the larynx.
4. When limited to the vocal cords (intrinsic), spread is slow because of lessened blood supply.
5. When cancer involves the epiglottis (extrinsic), cancer spreads more rapidly because of abundant supply of blood and lymph and soon involves the lymph nodes of the neck.

Clinical Manifestations

(Depend on tumor location; sequence in appearance related to pattern and extent of tumor growth.) (Fig. 15-4)

A. Supraglottic Cancer
1. Tickling sensation in throat
2. Dryness and fullness (lump) in throat

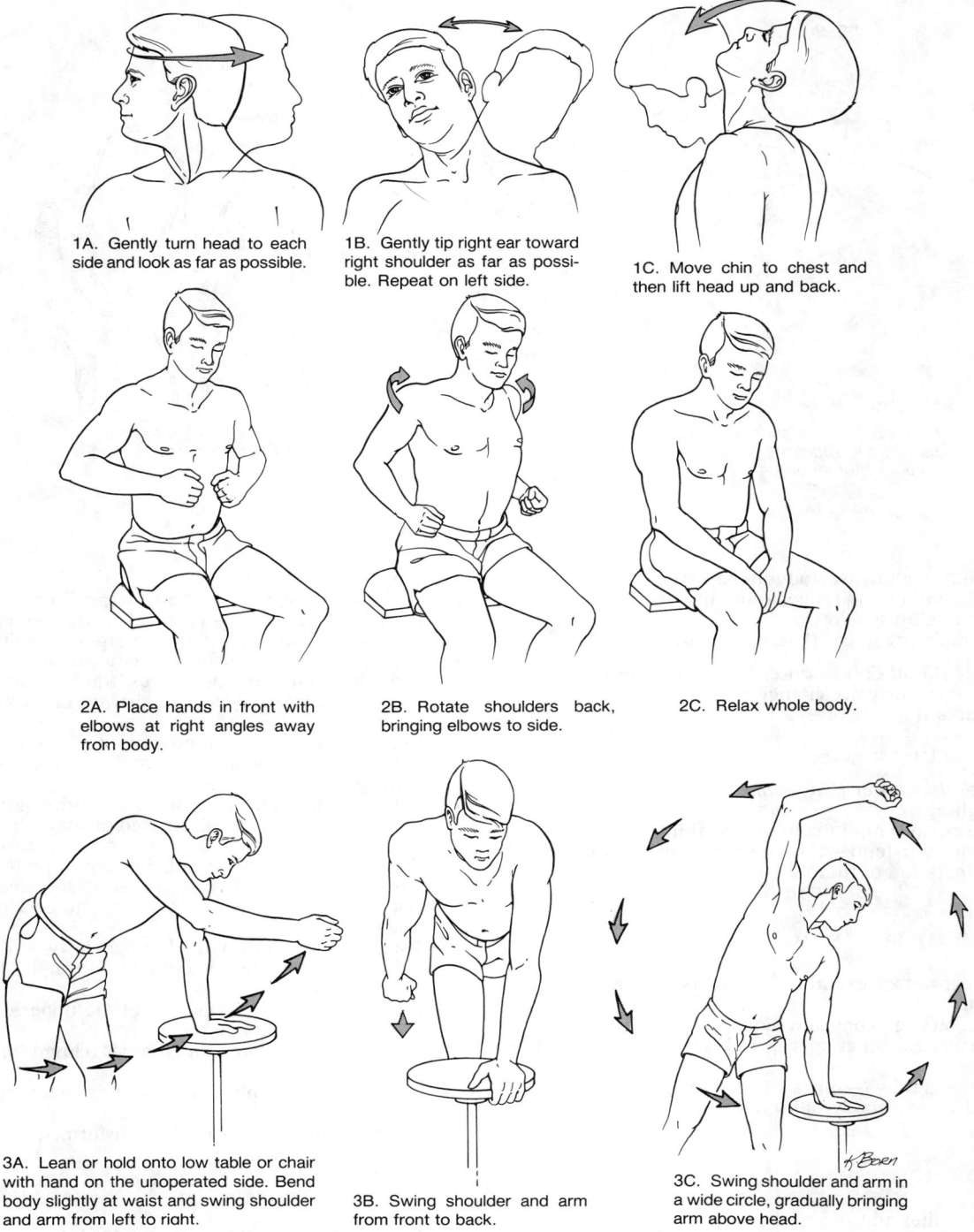

FIGURE 15-3 *Rehabilitation exercises after head and neck surgery to regain maximum shoulder function and neck motion.*

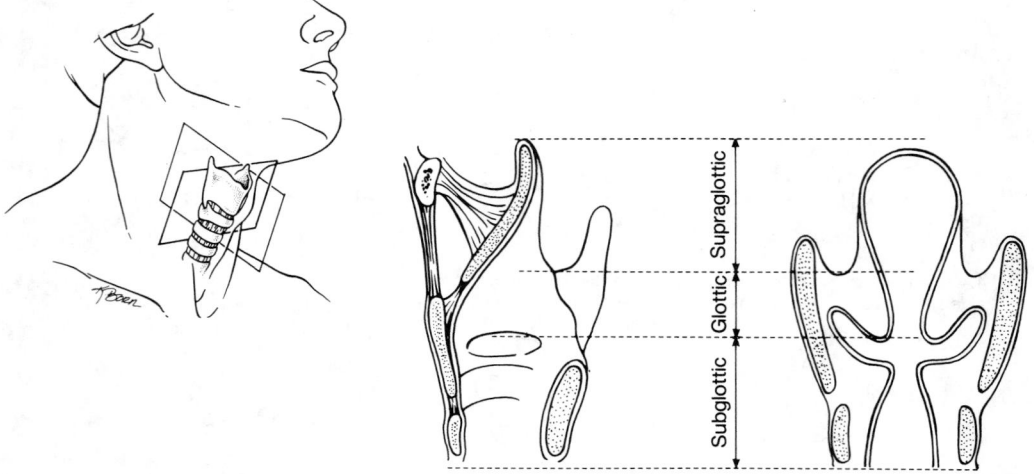

FIGURE 15-4 *Manifestations of cancer of the larynx. The larynx is divided into three regions: supraglottic, glottic, and subglottic. Clinical manifestations of cancer of the larynx depend on the tumor location and extent of tumor growth.*

3. Painful swallowing (odynophagia)—associated with invasion of extralaryngeal musculature
4. Coughing on swallowing
5. Pain radiating to ear (late symptom)

B. *Glottic (Vocal Cord) Cancer (Most Common)*
1. Hoarseness or voice change
2. Aphonia (loss of voice)
3. Dyspnea
4. Pain (in later stages)

C. *Subglottic Cancer (Uncommon)*
1. Coughing
2. Short periods of difficulty in breathing
3. Hemoptysis; fetid odor—results from ulceration and disintegration of tumor

Diagnostic Evaluation

1. Indirect mirror examination of larynx—may indicate lesion.
2. Direct laryngoscopy and biopsy to identify lesion.
3. CT scan and other special radiologic tests—to detect tumor.
4. Laryngography—contrast study of larynx to define blood vessels and lymph nodes.

Management

Depends on sites and stages of cancer.

A. *Endoscopic Removal of Early Malignancy*

B. *Radiation*
1. Singly or in combination with surgery.
2. Complications of radiation: edema of larynx, soft tissue and cartilage necrosis, chondritis (inflammation of cartilage).

C. *Surgery*
1. Carbon dioxide laser for early-stage disease.
2. Partial laryngectomy—removal of small lesion on true cord, along with a substantial margin of healthy tissue.
3. Supraglottic laryngectomy—removal of hyoid bone, epiglottis, and false vocal cords; tracheostomy may be done to maintain adequate airway; radical neck dissection may be done.
4. Hemilaryngectomy—removal of one true vocal cord, false cord, one-half of thyroid cartilage, arytenoid cartilage.
5. Total laryngectomy—removal of entire larynx (epiglottis, false or true cords, cricoid cartilage, hyoid bone; two or three tracheal rings are usually removed when there is extrinsic cancer of the larynx [extension beyond the vocal cords]). A radical neck dissection may also be done because of metastasis to cervical lymph nodes.
6. Total laryngectomy with laryngoplasty—voice rehabilitation may be attempted through the Asai operation.
   a. A dermal tube is made from the upper end of the tracheal into the hypopharynx.
   b. The tracheostomy opening is closed off with a finger.
   c. The patient expires air up the dermal tube into the pharyngeal cavity.
   d. The sound produced is transformed into almost normal speech.

Complications

1. Salivary fistula—may develop after any surgical procedure that involves entering the pharynx or esophagus.
   a. Monitor for saliva collecting beneath the skin flaps or leaking through suture line or drain site.

b. Management: Nasogastric tube feeding, meticulous local wound care with frequent dressing changes, promotion of drainage.
2. Hemorrhage (carotid artery rupture) or hematoma formation.
   a. A major postoperative complication such as skin necrosis or salivary fistula usually precedes carotid artery rupture.
   b. Management: Immediate wound exploration in operating room.
3. Stomal stenosis.
4. Aspiration.
5. Long-Term Complications
   a. Chest infections (from repeated aspiration).
   b. Recurrence of cancer in stoma

Preoperative Nursing Interventions

A. Preparing for Total Laryngectomy
1. Collaborate with the surgeon in preparing the patient; interpret and amplify what surgeon and speech–language pathologist have explained.
2. Inform patient that breathing will occur through an opening (tracheostoma) in the neck.
3. Apprise patient of the fact that speech will be altered by surgery.
   a. Expect reactions of anxiety and depression, because the psychosocial effects of voice loss are substantial.
   b. Practice a means of communication (pad and pencil, sign language, pictures, word cards, artificial larynx) that can be used until speech therapy begins.
   c. Arrange for patient to be visited by laryngectomee (one who has had larynx removed) for hope and encouragement.
   d. Inform patient of available community services.
4. Provide information about alternate modes of communication.
   a. Artificial larynx, using either neck or intraoral placement. Electrolarynx—provides communication assistance in early postoperative period or later to those unable to learn alternate method.
   b. Tracheoesophageal puncture with voice prosthesis. Puncture made between posterior wall of tracheostoma and underlying esophagus; a one-way valved voice prosthesis inserted through tracheoesophageal puncture that allows patient to shunt pulmonary air into esophagus for voice production (Fig. 15-5).
   c. Esophageal speech—accomplished by training patient to force air down the esophagus and release it in a controlled manner.
   d. Surgical reconstructive procedures to restore voice.

Nursing Assessment

1. Ask about smoking history, alcohol intake, drug history, chronic illnesses.
2. Take a nutrition history and 24-hour food intake recall, review results of laboratory test, weigh the patient.
3. Observe ability to swallow.
4. Review recommendations of speech–language pathologist and social worker.
5. Assess for independence, self-assuredness, and willingness to try new things; these are strengths on which to build.

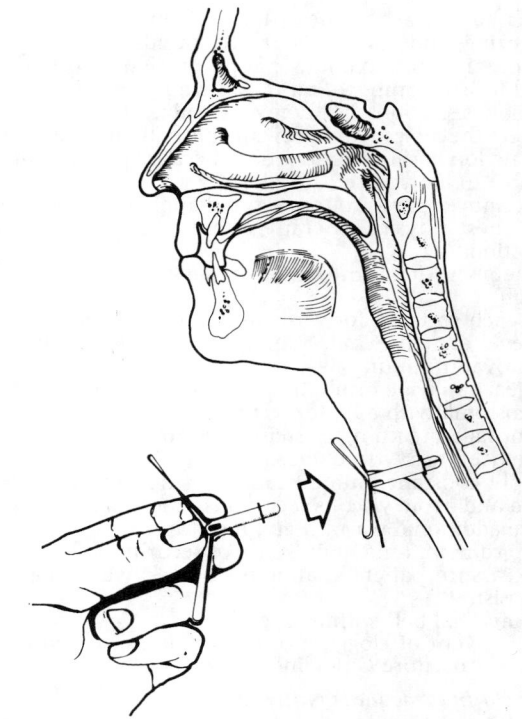

FIGURE 15-5 *Tracheoesophageal puncture for communication after laryngectomy. A one-way valved voice prosthesis can be placed in a surgically created tracheal-esophageal fistula to allow pulmonary air to be shunted into the esophagus for esophageal voice production. (From DeLisa JA. Rehabilitation Medicine: Principles and Practice. Philadelphia, JB Lippincott, 1988)*

6. Assess reality of patient's expectations.
7. Find out about patient's social support system.

Nursing Diagnoses

A. Ineffective Breathing Pattern related to presence of artificial airway, accumulation of secretions, inability to cough secondary to surgical procedure
B. Altered Nutrition (Less Than Body Requirements) related to impaired swallowing secondary to surgical alteration of pharynx and larynx; laryngeal edema and pain; radiation-induced mucositis
C. Impaired Verbal Communication related to surgery/ absence of larynx; presence of artificial airway
D. Knowledge Deficit of stoma care and living with effects of laryngectomy

Postoperative Nursing Interventions

A. Improving Breathing Pattern
1. Monitor for signs of difficult breathing: suprasternal and intercostal retractions, tachypnea, dyspnea, tachycardia, changes in sensorium.

2. Auscultate trachea/chest for evidence of stridor, wheezing, and absence of breath sounds.
3. Be sure that the patient uses a specific signal to indicate need for suctioning; enter on nursing care plan.
4. Suction secretions as they accumulate to clean and protect the airway and prevent subsequent aspiration.
   a. Suction nasal secretions also, because patient is unable to blow nose.
   b. Remove crusts from nares and apply ointment.
5. Use chest physical therapy as necessary to remove secretions.
6. Remember that postoperative patient is unable to cough:
   a. Teach to bend forward until stoma is below lung level and to exhale rapidly—aids in secretion removal from lungs.
   b. Teach to wipe resultant secretions away from tracheostoma with a handkerchief.
7. Encourage breathing exercises, because most patients have been heavy smokers.
8. Supply constant humidification to moisten tracheostoma and avoid viscous secretions; tracheal air will require additional warmth and moisture.
9. Keep calm and maintain sense of security.
   a. Reassure patient that someone is always near to assist.
   b. Have call bell within reach.
10. In the event of clogging or obstruction of the stoma, follow Procedure Guidelines 15-2.

B. *Facilitating Adequate Nutrition*
1. Monitor intravenous fluids during first few postoperative days.
2. Administer fluids and nutrients by nasogastric or esophagostomy tube.
   a. Tube feedings started after bowel sounds are heard and continued until sufficient healing of pharynx has occurred (10 to 12 days) and patient is ready to resume oral feedings.
   b. Avoid manipulating nasogastric tube as it is resting on/near suture line.
   c. Cleanse nostrils and lubricate with water-soluble lubricant.
   d. Cleanse crust on outside of tube.
   e. Pay attention to oral hygiene, with regular tooth brushing and prescribed antiseptic mouthwashes.
3. Encourage patient to relearn swallowing.
   a. Ensure quiet environment, because relearning how to swallow causes frustration and requires concentration. Have standby suction available.
   b. Place patient in sitting position, leaning slightly forward—allows larynx to move forward and hypopharynx to partially open.
   c. Explain that the epiglottis normally prevents fluid/food from entering larynx during swallowing.
4. Teach technique for swallowing:
   a. Inhale before swallowing, swallow, cough gently while exhaling, and reswallow.
   b. This ensures adequate air in lungs to cough out any food that has passed into the unguarded laryngeal region, thus preventing aspiration.

C. *Providing Alternative Communication*
1. Advise patient to communicate by writing until voice work can begin with speech–language pathologist.
2. Discourage forced whispering, which increases pharyngeal tension.
3. Reassure that speech therapy will begin as soon as patient can swallow comfortably.

4. Encourage patient to join local laryngectomy support group (Lost Chord Club, New Voice Club)—gives opportunity to practice new speech and serves as a bridge between therapy and return to social life.

D. *Providing Information About Laryngectomy*
1. Usually a laryngectomy or tracheostomy tube is worn until stoma heals (1 to 2 months); patient then starts gradual process of leaving tube out 1 hour at a time.
2. Demonstrate procedure for cleaning and changing tube.
   a. See page 164 for tracheostomy tube care.
   b. Place gauze dressing under tube to absorb secretions as prescribed. Change when it becomes soiled to prevent skin irritation and odor.
   c. Encourage patient to practice changing tracheostomy tie tapes.
3. Tracheostoma care: Teach patient to:
   a. Wash hands before touching stoma to prevent infection.
   b. Wet washcloth with warm water; wring dry and gently wipe stoma. Do not use soap, tissues, or cotton balls, because these may enter airway.
   c. Apply petrolatum around exterior of stoma to prevent skin irritation.
   d. Report excessive redness, swelling, purulent secretions, or bleeding.
4. Stoma cover
   a. Stoma cover is necessary to filter air and increase humidity of air; also necessary for hygienic purposes.
   b. Stoma cover can be crocheted or made of cotton cloth.
   c. For men: Ascot or turtleneck sweaters may be worn. When a regular shirt is worn, the second button from the top can be sewed over the buttonhole as though it were fastened—this leaves a wide opening through which a handkerchief can be inserted when coughing.
   d. For women: A variety of fashionable scarves, jewelry, high-neck dresses, and turtleneck sweaters can be worn.
5. Bowel care: Discuss high-fiber diet and use of stool softener, because patient with tracheostoma is usually not able to hold breath to "bear down" for bowel movement.

Patient Education/Health Maintenance

Teach the patient the following:

1. Provide humidification at home; use pans of water in the rooms, a humidifier, or cool-mist vaporizer, especially in bedroom.
2. Avoid cold air; cover tracheostoma with thin layer of foam rubber or other cover to warm and humidify air.
3. Drink fluids liberally (2 to 3 liters) to help liquefy secretions.
4. Always keep stoma covered for hygienic management of secretions and to keep dust/foreign matter from entering trachea.
5. Place a protective shield over stoma:
   a. Before bathing, showering, or shampooing hair and while getting a haircut or shaving
   b. Use an electric razor instead of blade, because shaving cream can irritate.
   c. Swimming is not recommended.

6. Expect some loss of smell and impairment of taste sensation.
7. Check with health care provider before taking any medication, because many drugs tend to dry the mucous membranes of the stoma.
8. Seek immediate attention for the following: pain, difficulty in breathing or swallowing, appearance of pus or blood-streaked sputum.

Evaluation

A. Breathing quietly; no evidence of noisy secretions
B. Swallowing soft foods; maintaining weight
C. Able to make needs known; speech therapy has started
D. Able to manage tracheostomal care; has made provisions for home humidification and tracheostomal supplies

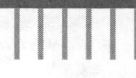

PROCEDURE GUIDELINES 15-2 ◆ Emergency First Aid for the Laryngectomee

EQUIPMENT (IF AVAILABLE)

Suction equipment
Sterile disposable catheter
#14-16 Fr. (adult)
#8-10 Fr. (child)

Sterile gloves
Sterile saline
Portable mask and bag

PROCEDURE FOR TOTAL NECK BREATHER

One who breathes ONLY through the neck opening
1. There is no connection between lungs and nose or mouth.
2. A tracheostomy or laryngectomy tube may or may not be in the neck opening.

NURSING ALERT:
No air can get through to lungs of a total laryngectomee when stoma is clogged.

NURSING ACTION	*RATIONALE*
1. PLACE PATIENT ON BACK, on a firm surface, head straight, chin up. Bare the neck down to the sternum.	1. Access to the laryngeal stoma and observation of thoracic movement are facilitated.
2. Position a blanket or any article of clothing under the shoulders.	2. This promotes extension of the neck area, permitting access.
3. Make a rapid assessment of the situation:	3.
a. Is victim wearing a tracheostomy or laryngectomy tube?	a. In a laryngectomee, tube removal cannot cause immediate danger.
b. Has patient been operated on recently?	b. If so, tracheostomy tube cannot be removed.
c. Check for tracheal obstruction. Clean stomal opening of mucus and encrusted matter.	c. Mucus, etc. may account for obstruction. Use a clean cloth or handkerchief—never tissue.
4. START MOUTH-TO-NECK BREATHING PROMPTLY: Position yourself at side of victim. Place your mouth and lips tightly over neck opening or around the tracheal tube if the person is wearing one.	4. SECONDS COUNT Do not remove the tube.
5. If suction equipment is available, insert a soft rubber tube 7.5–12.5 cm (3–5 in.) into opening for a few seconds.	5. A partially open airway transporting air to the victim is infinitely better than a clean airway that does not supply air at this crucial time.
6. Blow in a sufficient amount of air to see chest rise; then release and allow chest to fall.	
7. For the first 5 seconds, repeat every 1–2 seconds; then slow down to a steady pace of every 4–5 seconds (12–20 times per minute).	
8. Continue until spontaneous breathing returns.	

FOLLOW-UP PHASE

1. When spontaneous breathing occurs, provide oxygen from a portable supply.
2. If breathing fails again, resume mouth-to-neck breathing.

(continued)

PROCEDURE GUIDELINES 15-2 ◆ Emergency First Aid for the Laryngectomee *(continued)*

PROCEDURE (cont'd)	NURSING ACTION	RATIONALE
	3. You can also use mechanical resuscitation with the rubber or plastic inflatable bag and mask combination.	3. Attach baby-sized mask; be sure there is a tight seal against neck opening. Because a tight seal is difficult to maintain and because pressure of the mask on the major blood vessels of the neck may interfere with blood supply to the brain, mouth-to-neck breathing is safer and better.
	4. Watch the chest rise	
	5. Observe the patient constantly.	

PROCEDURE FOR PARTIAL NECK BREATHER

One who breathes MAINLY through the neck opening.
1. A connection between the lungs and the nose and mouth still exists.
2. The larynx may or may not be present.
3. A tracheostomy or laryngectomy tube may or may not be in the neck opening.

NURSING ALERT:
With mouth-to-neck breathing, FAILURE OF THE CHEST TO RISE is reliable proof that the patient is a partial neck breather. The rescuer may hear or feel air escaping from the victim's nose or mouth, but it is not getting into the lungs.

1. a. Immediately place the palm of your hand (the one nearest to the patient's head) over the lips and mouth. b. Pinch the nose shut between your third and fourth fingers. c. Place your thumb in the soft space under the chin and firmly press upward and backward.	1. This will close the area between the trachea and throat and at the same time raise the base of the tongue against the palate and pharynx.
2. Remove the patient's dentures.	2. To ensure better lip closure and effective underchin thumb closure
3. Now mouth-to-neck breathing will fill the lungs and the chest will rise.	

Selected References

Alberti, P.W., Ginsberg, I.A., Goode, R.L., & White, T.P. (1992). New reasons for hope in hearing loss. *Patient Care, 26*(6): 75–78.

Bingham, B., Hawke, M., & Kwok, P. (1992). *Atlas of clinical otolaryngology.* St. Louis: Mosby-Yearbook.

Bolger, W.E., & Kennedy, D.W. (1992). Changing concepts in chronic sinusitis. *Hospital Practice, 27*(9A): 20–22.

Donald, P.J., Gluckman, J.L., & Rice, D.H. (1995). *The sinuses.* New York: Raven Press.

English, G.M. (1993). Sinusitis: Strategies to cope with acute infection. *Consultant, 33*(4): 118–120.

Erber, N.P. (1994). Communicating with elders: Effects of amplification. *Journal of Gerontological Nursing, 20*(10): 6–10.

Farrior, J.B. (1994). Sudden hearing loss. *Emergency Medicine, 26*(2): 60–62.

Haugen, J.R., & Ramlo, J.H. (1994). Serious complications of acute sinusitis, Part 2. *Postgraduate Medicine, 93*(1): 115.

Lee, K.J. (Ed.) (1995). *Essential otolaryngology: Head and neck surgery* (6th ed.). Norwalk, CT: Appleton & Lange.

Miller, W.E. (1992). The role of the outpatient nurse in endoscopic sinus surgery. *ORL Head and Neck Nursing 10*(3): 20–24.

Powell, M.A. (1993). Adult sinusitis. *Journal of the American Academy of Nurse Practitioners, 5*(4): 179–180.

Sataloff, R.T., & Sataloff, J. (1993). *Hearing loss.* New York: Marcel Dekker, Inc.

Sawyer, D.L., & Bruya, M.A. (1990). Care of the patient having radical neck surgery or permanent laryngostomy: A nursing diagnostic approach. *Focus on Critical Care, 17*(2): 166–173.

Smeltzer, C.D. (1993). Primary care screening and evaluation of hearing loss. *Nurse Practitioner, 18*(8): 50–58.

Taylor, K.S. (1993). Geriatric hearing loss: Management strategies for nurses. *Geriatric Nursing, 14*(2): 74–76.

Webber-Jones, J. (1992). Doomed to deafness? *American Journal of Nursing, 92*(11): 37–39.

◆

Gastrointestinal and Nutritional Disorders

CHAPTER 16 ◆

Gastrointestinal Disorders

General Overview

The gastrointestinal (GI) system comprises the alimentary canal and its accessory organs, beginning at the mouth; extending through the pharynx, esophagus, stomach, small intestine, colon, rectum, and anal canal; and ending at the anus.

The GI system is responsible for the following essential bodily functions: ingestion and propulsion of food, mechanical and chemical digestion of food, absorption of nutrients into the bloodstream, and the storage and elimination of waste products from the body through feces.

Assessment

◆ SUBJECTIVE DATA

A comprehensive health history should be obtained to elicit subjective data related to major manifestations of GI problems. Common manifestations include nutritional problems, abdominal pain, indigestion, nausea and vomiting, diarrhea, constipation, and dysphagia.

Nutritional Problems

1. Characteristics—What is your normal 24-hour food intake? What is your usual weight? Has there been a recent weight gain or loss? If a recent weight change, how many pounds? How is your appetite?

2. Associated factors—Explore other factors that may influence weight changes: food preferences; family/individual routines associated with eating; cultural and religious values; psychological factors, such as depression, anxiety, stress; physical factors, such as activity level, health status, dental problems, allergies; access/transportation to grocery stores; eating habits, self-imposed dietary restrictions; body image; nutritional knowledge.

3. History—Any history of eating disorders? Any family history of ulcer disease, GI cancer, inflammatory bowel disease, obesity?

Abdominal Pain

1. Characteristics—Can you describe the pain (sharp, dull, superficial, or deep)? Is the pain intermittent or continuous? Can you point to where the pain is located? What makes the pain better, worse?

2. Associated factors—Are there other symptoms associated with the pain: fever, nausea, vomiting, diarrhea, constipation, anorexia, weight loss, dyspepsia?

3. History—Any family history of GI cancer, ulcer disease, inflammatory bowel disease? Any previous history of tumors, malignancy, or ulcers?

Indigestion (Dyspepsia)

1. Characteristics—Have you experienced any of the following symptoms: a feeling of fullness, heartburn, excessive belching, flatus, nausea, a bad taste, mild or severe pain?

Sandra Nettina: *The Lippincott Manual of Nursing Practice*, 6th ed. © 1996 Lippincott-Raven Publishers

How is your appetite? If pain or tenderness, where is it located? Does the pain radiate to any other areas? What precipitating factors are associated with the pain? What makes the symptoms better, worse? Are the symptoms associated with food intake? If associated with food, the amount and type?

2. Associated factors—Is there nausea, vomiting, or diarrhea? Is there a history of alcohol or aspirin use?
3. History—Any family history of cancer, inflammatory bowel disease? Any history of bowel obstruction? Any previous abdominal surgeries?

Nausea/Vomiting

A. *Characteristics*
1. Is the nausea or vomiting associated with certain stimuli, such as specific foods, odors, activity, or a certain time of day? Does it occur before or after food intake? How many times a day does vomiting occur? What specific fluids/foods can be tolerated when vomiting occurs? What is the amount, color, odor and consistency of the vomitus? (Table 16-1).
2. Associated factors—Is there fever, headache, dizziness, weakness, diarrhea? Any weight loss?
3. History—Any history of gallbladder disease? Ulcer disease? Gastrointestinal cancer?

Diarrhea

1. Characteristics—What is the frequency, consistency, color, quantity and odor of stools? Is there blood, mucus, pus, or food particles in the stools? Does this represent a change in bowel habits? Is there nocturnal diarrhea? What makes the diarrhea worse, better? Any associated weight loss?
2. Associated factors—Any fever, nausea, vomiting, abdominal pain, abdominal distention, flatus, cramping, urgency with straining? Is the patient taking antibiotics? Has there been any recent travel to foreign countries? Is the patient experiencing emotional stress or anxiety?
3. History—Any history of colon cancer, ulcerative colitis, Crohn's disease, malabsorption syndrome?

Constipation

1. Characteristics—What is the frequency, consistency, color of the stools? Is this a change in bowel habits? If a change, has this been gradual or sudden? What is the size of the stools? Have there been dietary changes? Is there blood or mucus in the stools?
2. Associated factors—Are there periods of diarrhea? Is there abdominal pain or distention? Is the patient experiencing stress? Is there a change in activity level? Does the patient have a regular time for defecation? Does the patient use antacids containing calcium or an anticholinergic?
3. History—Any family history of colorectal cancer? Any history of depression or metabolic disorders, such as hypothyroidism or hypercalcemia?

TABLE 16-1 **Nature of Vomitus**

Color/Taste/Consistency	Possible Source
Yellowish or greenish	May contain bile
	Medication—senna
Bright red (arterial)	Hemorrhage, peptic ulcer
Dark red (venous)	Hemorrhage, esophageal or gastric varices
"Coffee grounds"	Digested blood from slowly bleeding gastric or duodenal ulcer
Undigested food	Gastric tumor
	Ulcer, obstruction
"Bitter" taste	Bile
"Sour" or "acid"	Gastric contents
Fecal components	Intestinal obstruction

Dysphagia

1. Characteristics—Is the onset acute or gradual? Is the problem with swallowing intermittent or continuous? Is this associated with solid foods, liquids, or both?
2. Associated factors—Is there any regurgitation, heartburn, chest or back pain, weight loss? Any hoarseness, change in voice, or sore throat?
3. History—Is there a family history of esophageal cancer? Is there a history of stroke, palsy, or any other neurologic conditions? Is there a history of alcohol or tobacco intake?

◆ PHYSICAL EXAMINATION

When performing a physical exam of the abdomen, include the following: inspection of the abdomen, auscultation of all four abdominal quadrants, percussion for tympany or dullness, light and deep palpation.

> **NURSING ALERT:**
> Auscultation should be performed before percussion and palpation, which may stimulate bowel sounds. Deep palpation in noted areas of tenderness or pain should be performed last.

Key Findings

1. Tenting of the skin when skin is rolled between thumb and index finger. Tenting may indicate dehydration.
2. Mouth lesions, missing teeth, swollen or bleeding gums may contribute to weight loss and nutritional deficiencies.
3. Body weight may indicate obesity or such problems as anorexia nervosa or malignancy.
4. Palpable mass—may indicate an enlarged organ, inflammation, malignancy, hernia.
5. Rebound tenderness, guarding, and rigidity may indicate appendicitis, cholecystitis, peritonitis, pancreatitis, duodenal ulcer.
6. Protuberant or bulging abdomen or flanks—can indicate ascites.

7. Distention and absence of bowel sounds may indicate intestinal obstruction.

Characteristics of Stool

1. The appearance of blood in stool may be characteristic of its source.
   a. Upper GI bleeding—tarry black (melena).
   b. Lower GI bleeding—bright red blood.
   c. Lower rectal or anal bleeding—blood streaking on surface of stool or on toilet paper.
2. Other characteristics of stool may indicate a particular GI problem.
   a. Bulky, greasy, foamy, foul smelling, gray with silvery sheen—steatorrhea (fatty stool).
   b. Light gray "clay-colored" (due to absence of bile pigments, acholic)—biliary obstruction.
   c. Mucus or pus visible—chronic ulcerative colitis, shigellosis.
   d. Small, dry, rocky-hard masses—constipation, obstruction.
   e. Marble-sized stool pellets—spastic colon syndrome.

Diagnostic Tests

◆ LABORATORY TESTS

Laboratory tests for GI disorders include stool testing for blood (Hemoccult), other stool tests, and a variety of blood tests, such as hematocrit and hemoglobin for monitoring GI bleeding.

Hemoccult Guaiac Slide Test (Hemoquant, Hemoccult II)

A. Description
Commercially available guaiac-impregnated slides present a simple, inexpensive, and aesthetically acceptable method of testing feces for blood.

B. Nursing/Patient Care Considerations
Advise on desired patient preparation for test. Common practices are listed below:

1. Diet should be high-residue for 48 to 72 hours before specimen is collected.
2. Similar diet is followed for next 3 days:
   a. Vegetables—particularly lettuce, spinach, and corn; cooked and raw
   b. Fruits—particularly prunes, grapes, plums, and apples
   c. Any product that is "all bran" for daily cereal
3. Any foods that cause severe diarrhea or severe abdominal pain are to be avoided.

C. Procedure
1. A wooden applicator is used to apply a stool specimen to the slide (for 3 successive days). Three samples are taken because of the possibility of intermittent bleeding and false-negative results.
2. Slides inside a packet can be brought or mailed to the health care provider or lab.

3. When hydrogen peroxide (denatured alcohol-stabilizing mixture) is added to samples, any blood cells present liberate their hemoglobin, and a bluish ring appears on the electrophoretic paper. Read precisely at 30 seconds.
4. A single positive test is an indication for further diagnostic research for GI lesions. False-positive results occur in about 10% of tests. Test may become false-negative in 10% of specimens tested 4 or more days after streaking on paper.

Stool Specimen

A. Description The stool is examined for its amount, consistency, and color. Normal color varies from light to dark brown, but various foods and medications may affect stool color. Special tests may be made for fecal urobilinogen, fat nitrogen, food residue, and other substances. Fecal leukocytes are tested by Wright's stain, and stool cultures are obtained to identify bacteria, virus, or ova and parasites.

B. Nursing/Patient Care Considerations
1. Use a tongue blade to place a small amount of stool in a disposable waxed container.
2. Save a sample of any fecal material if it is unusual in appearance, contains worms or blood, is blood-streaked, has unusual color or much mucus.
3. Send specimens to be examined for parasites to the laboratory immediately so that the parasites may be observed under microscope while viable, fresh, and warm.
4. Test for occult blood or to confirm grossly visible melena or blood—Hemoccult guaiac slide test.
5. Consider that barium, bismuth, mineral oil, and antibiotics may alter the results.

◆ RADIOLOGY/ IMAGING STUDIES

Upper Gastrointestinal Series and Small-Bowel Series

A. Description
1. Upper GI series and small-bowel series are fluoroscopic x-ray examinations of the esophagus, stomach, and small intestine after the patient ingests barium sulfate.
2. As the barium passes through the GI tract, fluoroscopy outlines the GI mucosa and organs.
3. Spot films record significant findings.
4. Double contrast studies administer barium first followed by a radiolucent substance, such as air, to produce a thin layer of barium to coat the mucosa. This allows for better visualization of any type of lesion.

B. Nursing/Patient Care Considerations
1. Explain procedure to patient.
2. Instruct patient to maintain low-residue diet for 2 to 3 days before test and a clear liquid dinner the night before the procedure.
3. Emphasize nothing by mouth after midnight before the test.
4. Encourage to avoid smoking before the test.
5. Explain that the health care provider may prescribe all narcotics and anticholinergics to be held 24 hours, before the test because they interfere with small intestine motility. Other medications may be taken with sips of water, if ordered.

6. Tell the patient that he or she will be instructed at various times throughout the procedure to drink the barium (480 to 600 mL).
7. Explain that a cathartic will be prescribed after the procedure to facilitate expulsion of barium.
8. Instruct the patient that stool will be light in color for the next 2 to 3 days from the barium.
9. Instruct patient to notify health care provider if he or she has not passed the barium in 2 to 3 days, because retention of the barium may cause obstruction or fecal impaction.
10. Note that water-soluble iodinated contrast agent (such as Gastrografin) may be used for a patient with a suspected perforation or colonic obstruction. Barium is toxic to the body if it leaks into the peritoneum with perforation. It can also worsen an obstruction, thus is not used if an obstruction is suspected.

Barium Enema

A. *Description*
1. Fluoroscopic x-ray examination visualizing the entire large intestine is administered after the patient is given an enema of barium sulfate.
2. Can visualize structural changes, such as tumors, polyps, diverticula, fistulas, obstructions, and ulcerative colitis.
3. Air may be introduced after the barium to provide a double contrast study.

B. *Nursing/Patient Care Considerations*
1. Explain to the patient:
   a. What the x-ray procedure involves.
   b. That proper preparation provides a more accurate view of the tract and that preparations may vary.
   c. That it is important to retain the barium so that all surfaces of the tract are coated with opaque solution.
2. Instruct the patient on the objective of having the large intestine as clear of fecal material as possible:
   a. The patient may be given a low-residue diet 1 to 3 days before the examination.
   b. The day before examination, intake may be limited to clear liquids.
   c. The day before the examination, a cathartic may be prescribed.
   d. The evening before and on the morning of the examination, a cleansing enema may be given. Food and fluids are restricted before the examination.
3. Encourage the patient to eat after the examination, because he or she has been fasting and is undoubtedly hungry.
4. Prepare the patient for an enema or cathartic after the barium enema, and describe its importance in evacuating the barium and preventing impaction.
5. Advise the patient that barium may cause light-colored stools for several days after the procedure.

Ultrasonography (Ultrasound)

A. *Description*
1. A noninvasive test that focuses high-frequency sound waves over an abdominal organ to obtain an image of the structure.

2. Ultrasound can detect small abdominal masses, fluid-filled cysts, gallstones, dilated bile ducts, ascites, and vascular abnormalities.

B. *Nursing/Patient Care Considerations*
1. Prepare the patient before the procedure with a special diet, laxative, or other medication to cleanse the bowel and decrease gas.
2. Change position of patient, as indicated, for better visualization of certain organs.

Computed Tomography (CT Scan)

A. *Description*
1. An x-ray technique that provides excellent anatomic definition and is used to detect tumors, cysts, and abscesses.
2. The CT can also detect dilated bile ducts, pancreatic inflammation, and some gallstones.
3. Can identify changes in intestinal wall thickness and mesenteric abnormalities.
4. Ultrasound and CT can be used to perform guided needle aspiration of fluid or cells from lesions anywhere in the abdomen. The fluid or cells are then sent for laboratory tests (such as cytology or culture).

B. *Nursing/Patient Care Considerations*
1. Instruct the patient that fasting for 4 hours before the procedure and an enema or cathartic may be necessary. This is to cleanse the bowel for better visualization.
2. Ask the patient if she is pregnant. If yes, do not proceed with scan and notify health care provider.
3. Ask if there are known allergies to iodine or contrast media. A contrast medium may be given intravenously (IV) to provide better visualization of body parts. If allergic, notify the technician and health care provider immediately.
4. Instruct the patient to report symptoms of itching or shortness of breath if receiving contrast media, and observe patient closely.

◆ ENDOSCOPIC PROCEDURES

Endoscopy is the use of a flexible tube (the fiberoptic endoscope) to visualize the GI tract and to perform certain diagnostic and therapeutic procedures. Images are produced through a video screen or telescopic eyepiece. The tip of the endoscope moves in four directions, allowing for wide-angle visualization. The endoscope can be inserted through the rectum or mouth, depending on which portion of the GI tract is to be viewed.

Endoscopes contain multipurpose channels that allow for air insufflation, irrigation, fluid aspiration, and the passage of special instruments. These instruments include biopsy forceps, cytology brushes, needles, wire baskets, laser probes, and electrocautery snares.

Endoscopic functions other than visualization include biopsy or cytology of lesions, removal of foreign objects or polyps, control of internal bleeding, and opening of strictures.

Esophagogastroduodenoscopy (EGD)

A. *Description*
1. Visualization of the esophagus, stomach, and duodenum.

2. EGD can be used to diagnose hemorrhage, malignancy, ulcers, and gastritis.

3. Instruments passed through the scope can be used to perform a biopsy or cytologic study, remove polyps or foreign bodies, control bleeding, or open strictures.

B. Nursing/Patient Care Considerations

1. Explain the following to the patient:

a. The procedure that is to be performed. If done as an outpatient, advise that someone must accompany the patient to drive home, because the patient will be sedated.

b. Nothing by mouth for 8 to 12 hours before the procedure to prevent aspiration and allow for complete visualization of the stomach.

c. Removal of dentures and partial plates to facilitate passing the scope and preventing injury.

2. Inform the health care provider of any known allergies and current medications. Medications may be held until after the test is completed.

3. Obtain prior x-rays and send with the patient.

4. Describe what will occur during and after the procedure:

a. The throat will be anesthetized with a spray or gargle.

b. An IV sedative will be administered.

c. The patient will be positioned on the left side with a towel or basin at the mouth to catch secretions.

d. A plastic mouthpiece will be used to help relax the jaw and protect the endoscope. Emphasize that this will not interfere with breathing.

e. The patient may be asked to swallow once while the endoscope is being advanced. Then the patient should not swallow, talk, or move tongue. Secretions should drain from the side of the mouth and the mouth may be suctioned.

f. Air is inserted during the procedure to permit better visualization of the GI tract. Most of the air is re-moved at the end of the procedure. The patient may feel bloated, burp, or pass flatus from remaining air.

g. Keep patient on nothing-by-mouth (NPO) protocol until patient is alert and gag reflex has returned.

h. May resume regular diet after gag reflex returns and tolerating fluids.

i. May experience a sore throat for 24 to 36 hours after the procedure. When the gag reflex has returned, throat lozenges or warm saline gargles may be prescribed for comfort.

5. Monitor vital signs every 30 minutes for 3 to 4 hours and keep the side rails up until the patient is fully alert.

6. Monitor the patient for abdominal or chest pain, cervical pain, dyspnea, fever, hematemesis, melena, dysphagia, light-headedness, or a firm distended abdomen. These may indicate complications.

7. Instruct the patient on the above listed signs and symptoms and advise to report immediately should any occur, even after discharge.

8. Possible complications include perforation of the esophagus or stomach, pulmonary aspiration, and hemorrhage.

Proctosigmoidoscopy and Colonoscopy

1. Proctosigmoidoscopy is the visualization of the anal canal, rectum, and sigmoid colon through a fiberoptic sigmoidoscope. See Procedure Guidelines 16-1: Assisting With a Proctosigmoidoscopy.

2. Colonoscopy is the visualization of the entire large intestine, sigmoid colon, rectum, and anal canal.

3. Sigmoidoscopy or colonoscopy can be used to diagnose malignancy, polyps, inflammation, or strictures.

4. Lower GI endoscopy can be used to perform biopsy, remove foreign objects, or obtain specimen for culture or cytology.

PROCEDURE GUIDELINES 16-1 ◆ Assisting With a Proctosigmoidoscopy

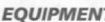

EQUIPMENT

Fleet-type enema—used at least 1 hour before the sigmoidoscopy
Oral laxative
Water-soluble lubricant
Sigmoidoscope
Biopsy forceps
Culture swab
Long applicator sticks (cotton)
Drapes or sheets

Specimen bottles containing 10% formalin
Culture tubes
4 × 4 gauze sponges
Cytology brush
Glass eyepiece to fit on scope during insufflation of air
Disposable gloves for preliminary digital examination
Suction machine
Microscopic slides with fixative or 95% ethyl alcohol
Specimen labels

NURSING ALERT:
1. Emergency resuscitation equipment needs to be available, because the vagus nerve is often stimulated and can potentiate a vagal reaction (pallor, diaphoresis, dizziness, weakness, unconsciousness, decrease in blood pressure and pulse rate, sometimes causing these vital signs to be unobtainable).
2. If giving enemas before the procedure, do not advance the tube too high into the colon, and administer the fluid slowly. If rectal bleeding or abdominal pain occur, stop at once and call the physician.

PREPARATORY Inform the health care provider of any known allergies and current medications. Certain medications, such as
PHASE anticoagulants, may be held before the test.
Obtain prior x-rays and studies and send with the patient.

PROCEDURE	*NURSING ACTION*	*RATIONALE*

1. Record baseline vital signs. Leave the blood pressure cuff in place. An automatic blood pressure machine may be used; however, a manual cuff is preferred in the event the patient has a vagal reaction (see Nursing Alert above).
2. Have the patient assume the knee-chest or Sims' lateral position.
   a. Knee-chest position
   (1) Knees are spread comfortably apart
   (2) Thighs are perpendicular to table
   (3) Feet are extended over the edge
   (4) Head is turned sideways to right (head shares pillow with chest)
   (5) Left arm is flexed to side of chest
   (6) Right arm may rest above head
   b. Sims' lateral position

   (1) Place patient on left side with left leg partially flexed at hip and knees; right leg should be fully flexed.
   (2) Pelvis to be perpendicular to table
3. Drape the patient so that only perineum is visible.

4. Explain to the patient to take slow deep breaths as the physician examines the rectum by digital examination.

5. Warm sigmoidoscope in tap water or sterilizer to slightly above body temperature; lubricate tip of scope.

6. Physician spreads buttocks and anal margins with left hand and inserts instrument with right hand (or vice versa). Have the patient breathe deeply.
7. Nurse encourages relaxation and explains each step in advance.
8. Physician may use a glass eyepiece over viewing end of scope; an insufflation bulb and tubing are attached. A small quantity of air may be pumped into the bowel. Tell patient as the air moves down the bowel he may experience flatulence. This is normal.
9. Examination of the sigmoid, rectum, and mucosa are done while the scope is being removed. If a rigid scope is used, passage of a large cotton swab through the scope may be done to remove blood, mucus, and feces. If a flexible scope is used, only suction is necessary to clear the field. Turn suction to lowest setting initially.
10. Passage of biopsy forceps, cytology brush, or culture swab through the scope is done to collect specimens.

RATIONALE
1. Monitoring of the blood pressure and pulse throughout the procedure will be necessary.

2. The position used depends on physician preference, patient condition, and nature of examining table (or bed).
   a. This position permits the sigmoid to hang forward, diminishing the angle at the rectosigmoid junction.

   b. Used for elderly, ill, or arthritic patients or those who are reluctant to assume the knee–chest position.

3. A disposable large sheet with a circular opening is practical. This will minimize embarrassment.
4. The physician is examining for tenderness, mucus, blood fistula, inflammation, ulceration, and feces. The digital examination also indicates the direction of the anal canal, its patency, and the presence of any abnormality; it promotes anal relaxation and helps to lubricate the orifice.
5. A cold scope would cause discomfort and promote contraction rather than relaxation of perianal muscles. Water-soluble lubricant permits easier passage of scope. It also minimizes the urge to defecate at tube insertion.
6. Keep instrument out of view of patient. Breathing slowly and deeply will help relax abdominal muscles and minimize cramping.
7. Reassuring the patient promotes relaxation.
8. The purpose of inflating lower bowel with air is to expand the area viewed so that vision is not obstructed by mucosal folds and to facilitate passage into the sigmoid colon.
9. This clears the field of vision.

10. Specimens will be placed in 10% formalin and labeled. A specimen for cytology is placed in a container of 95% ethyl alcohol or affixed to a microscopic slide with slide fixative. Specimens for cultures will be sent in specimen tubes.

(continued)

PROCEDURE GUIDELINES 16-1 ◆ Assisting With a Proctosigmoidoscopy
(continued)

PROCEDURE (cont'd)	NURSING ACTION	RATIONALE
	11. Relay to the physician any expressions or complaints of pain by the patient.	11. Tenderness and pain may be experienced by the patient with a history of abdominal surgery; procedure may have to be terminated in order not to risk perforation.
	FOLLOW-UP PHASE	
	1. On withdrawal of scope, assist patient into gradually assuming a relaxed position.	1. To promote comfort.
	2. Wipe perianal area	2. Prevent soilage of garments.
	3. If disposable scope is used, rinse and discard in proper receptacle. Reusable scopes are properly cleaned with solution and water, per protocol. Sterilizable parts are sterilized before scope is stored	3. Prevents contamination and infection.
	4. Record the procedure, preparation of the patient, reaction of the patient, and patient's vital signs	
	5. Label all specimens immediately and send to the laboratory	5. Minimize error; allow fresh samples for evaluation.
	6. Observe the patient for complications: hemorrhage (increased pulse, decreased blood pressure, weakness, pallor, rectal bleeding, and possible abdominal pain), perforation (sudden, severe abdominal pain), fever, malaise, changes in vital signs, bloody or mucoid rectal drainage, and possible abdominal distention	
	7. Instruct the patient on these signs and symptoms and advise to notify health care provider immediately should they occur, even after discharge.	7. Prevent risk of complications.

General Procedures/Treatment Modalities

◆ RELIEVING CONSTIPATION AND FECAL IMPACTION

A common procedure to relieve constipation or evacuate the lower bowel is an enema, the installation of a solution into the rectum and sigmoid colon. See Procedure Guidelines 16-2: Administering an Enema.

Fecal impaction may cause constipation or small amounts of diarrhea or liquid fecal seepage around the obstructing impaction. Impaction may be removed manually to promote bowel elimination (Fig. 16-1).

Purposes of Enema Administration

1. Bowel preparation for diagnostic tests or surgery to empty the bowel of fecal content.
2. Delivery of medication into the colon (such as enemas containing neomycin to decrease the bowel's bacteria count or a kayexalate enema to decrease the serum potassium level).
3. To soften the stool (oil-retention enemas).
4. To relieve gas (tidal, milk and molasses, or Fleet's enemas).
5. Promote defecation and evacuate feces from the colon for patients with constipation or an impaction.

Indications and Contraindications of Fecal Impaction Removal

1. Consider manual removal of fecal impaction in the following patients at risk:
   a. Elderly persons with chronic constipation, insufficient hydration, or who are inactive.
   b. Orthopedic patients who have been in traction or in body casts.
   c. Patients who just undergone rectal surgery or when barium has not been adequately removed after radiologic examination.
   d. Patients with neurologic or psychotic disorders.
2. Fecal impaction can occur with a descending/sigmoid colostomy. The fingers may be used to break up feces through the stoma, followed by cleansing irrigation.
3. Manual removal of fecal impaction can stimulate the vagus nerve and cause syncope and tachycardia. It is contraindicated in the following conditions:
   a. Pregnancy.
   b. After genitourinary, rectal, perineal, abdominal, or gynecologic surgery.
   c. Myocardial infarction, coronary insufficiency, pulmonary embolus, congestive heart failure, heart block.
   d. Gastrointestinal or vaginal bleeding.
   e. Blood dyscrasias, bleeding disorders.
   f. Hemorrhoids, fissures, and rectal polyps.

PROCEDURE GUIDELINES 16-2 ◆ Administering an Enema

EQUIPMENT
Prepackaged enema or enema container
Disposable gloves
Water-soluble jelly
Waterproof pad
Bath blanket

Bedpan or commode
Washcloth and towel
Basin
Toilet tissue

PREPARATORY PHASE

NURSING ACTION	RATIONALE
1. Assess the patient's bowel habits (last BM, laxative usage, bowel patterns) and physical condition (hemorrhoids, mobility, external sphincter control).	1. Enema should not be given if there is a suspicion of appendicitis or bowel obstruction.
2. Provide for privacy, and explain procedure to patient.	2. Provides comfort.

PROCEDURE

NURSING ACTION	RATIONALE
1. Wash hands	1. Promotes hygiene
2. Place patient on left side with right knee flexed (Sims' position). Place waterproof pad underneath patient and cover with bath blanket.	2. Allows for enema solution to flow by gravity along the natural curve of the sigmoid colon and rectum.
3. Place bedpan or bedside commode in position for patients that cannot ambulate to the toilet or who may have difficulty with sphincter control.	3. Allows for easy accessibility.
4. Remove plastic cover over tubing and lubricate tip of enema tubing 3–4 in. (7.5–10 cm) unless prepackaged (tip is already lubricated). Even prepackaged enema may need more lubricant.	4. Prevents trauma and eases application.
5. Apply disposable gloves.	
6. Separate buttocks and locate rectum.	
7. Instruct patient that you will be inserting tubing and to take slow, deep breaths.	7. Allows for patient relaxation and readiness.
8. Insert tubing 3–4 in. for adult patients.	8. Prevents tissue trauma of rectum.
9. Slowly instill the solution using a clamp and the height of the container to adjust flow rate if using an enema bag and tubing. For high enemas, raise enema container 12–18 in. above anus; for low enemas, 12 in. If using a prepackaged enema, slowly squeeze the container until all solution is instilled.	9. Rapid infusion can cause colon distention and cramping. Container elevated past 12–18 in. and controller on tubing not regulated contribute to rapid infusion.
10. Lower container or clamp tubing if patient complains of cramping.	
11. Withdraw rectal tubing after all enema solution has been instilled or until clear (usually not more than three enemas).	11. "Until clear" means until results do not contain fecal matter and are clear.
12. Instruct patient to hold solution as long as possible and that a feeling of distention may be felt.	12. Promotes better results.
13. Discard supplies in the appropriate trash receptacle.	13. Maintains hygiene, minimizes patient embarrassment
14. Assist patient on the bedpan or to the bedside commode or toilet when urge to defecate occurs.	
15. Observe enema return for amount, fecal content. Instruct patient not to flush toilet until the nurse has seen the results.	

NURSING ALERT:
Enemas should not be given routinely to treat constipation, because they disrupt normal defecation reflexes and the patient becomes dependent.

FOLLOW-UP PHASE

1. Document the type of enema given, volume and results on the appropriate chart forms.
2. Assess and document presence or absence of abdominal distention after enema was given.
3. Assist the patient with washing perineum and rectal area, if indicated; may also need a clean gown or linen change.

◆ NASOGASTRIC/ NASOINTESTINAL INTUBATION

Nasogastric intubation refers to the insertion of a tube through the nasopharynx into the stomach. See Procedure Guidelines 16-3.

Nasointestinal intubation is performed by inserting a small-bore weighted tube that is carried via peristalsis into the duodenum or jejunum. It is primarily used for administering feedings and maintaining nutritional intake. See Procedure Guidelines 16-4: Nasointestinal Intubation.

Purposes of Nasogastric Intubation

1. Remove fluids and gas from stomach (decompression).
2. Prevent or relieve nausea and vomiting after surgery or traumatic events by decompressing the stomach.
3. Determine the amount of pressure and motor activity in the GI tract (diagnostic studies).
4. Irrigate the stomach for active bleeding or poisoning.
5. Treat mechanical obstruction.
6. Administer medications and feeding (gavage) directly into the GI tract.
7. Obtain a specimen of gastric contents for laboratory studies when pyloric or intestinal obstruction is suspected.

PROCEDURE GUIDELINES 16-3 ◆ Nasogastric Intubation and Removal

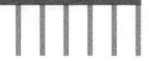

EQUIPMENT

Nasogastric tube—usually Levin or double-lumen Salem sump tube
Water-soluble lubricant
Suction equipment
Clamp for tubing
Towel, tissues, and emesis basin
Glass of water and straw
Tincture of benzoin

Hypoallergenic tape: ½" and 1"
Bio-occlusive transparent dressing
Irrigating set with 20-ml syringe or a 50-ml catheter-tip syringe
Stethoscope
Tongue blade
Penlight
Disposable gloves
Normal saline

FOLLOW-UP EQUIPMENT

Lip pomade
Mouth hygiene materials

INSERTION PROCEDURE

PREPARATORY PHASE

1. Ask the patient if he or she has ever had nasal surgery, trauma, or a deviated septum.
2. Explain procedure to the patient and tell how mouth breathing, panting, and swallowing will help in passing the tube.
3. Place the patient in a sitting or high-Fowler's position; place a towel across chest.
4. Determine with the patient what sign he or she might use, such as raising the index finger, to indicate "wait a few moments" because of gagging or discomfort.
5. Remove dentures; place emesis basin and tissues within the patient's reach.
6. Inspect the tube for defects; look for partially closed holes or rough edges.
7. Place rubber tubing in ice-chilled water for a few minutes to make the tube firmer. Plastic tubing may already be firm enough; if too stiff, dip in warm water.
8. Determine the length of the tube needed to reach the stomach by placing the end of the tube at the tip of the patient's nose. Then extend it to the earlobe and down to the xiphoid process (see figure). Mark this distance with hypoallergenic tape. (Measurement range for the average-size adult is 55–66 cm [22–26 in.].)
9. Have the patient blow nose to clear nostrils.
10. Inspect the nostrils with a penlight, observing for any obstruction. Occlude each nostril and have the patient breathe. This will help determine which nostril is more patent.
11. Wash your hands. Put on disposable gloves.

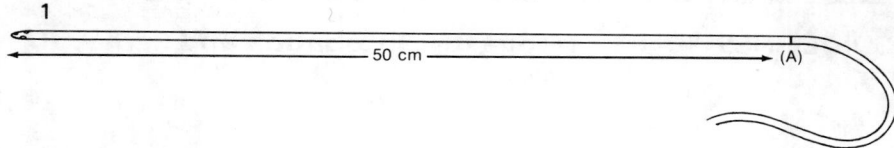

1. Mark the nasogastric tube at a point 50 cm. from the distal tip; call this point 'A'.

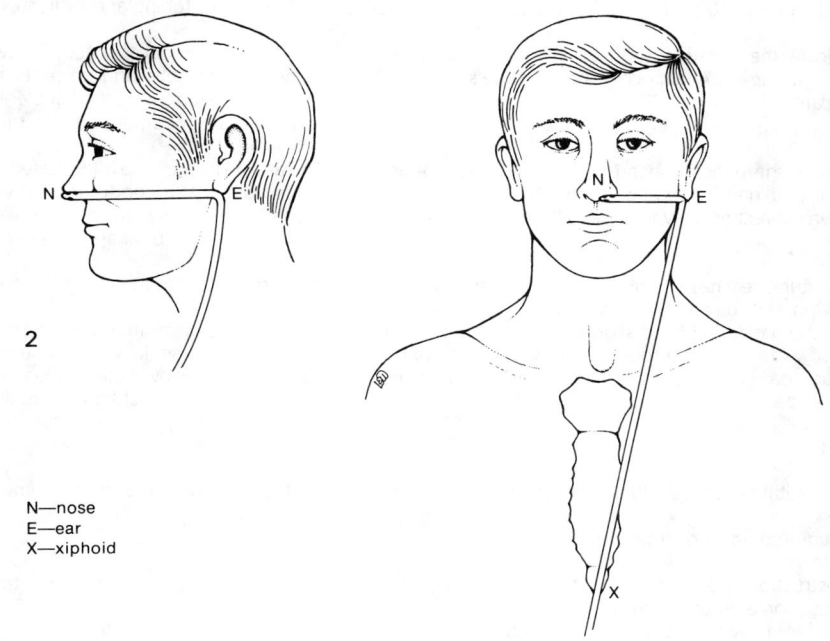

N—nose
E—ear
X—xiphoid

2. Have the patient sit in a neutral position with head facing forward. Place the distal tip of the tubing at the tip of the patient's nose (N); extend tube to the tragus (tip) of his ear (E), and then extend the tube straight down to the tip of his xiphoid (X). Mark this point 'B' on the tubing.

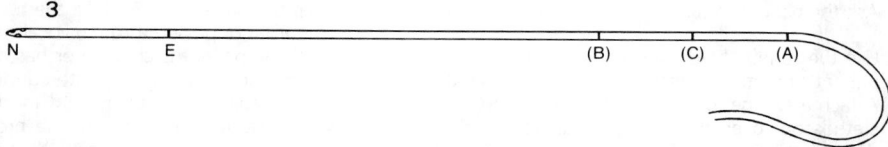

3. To locate point C on the tube, find the midpoint between points A and B. The nasogastric tube is passed to point C to ensure optimum placement in the stomach.

The above diagram and steps (1, 2, 3) indicate how far a nasogastric tube is passed for optimal placement in the stomach. (Hanson RL. Predictive criteria for length of nasogastric tube insertion for tube feeding. J Parenteral Enteral Nutr 1979 May–Jun; 3[3]:160–163)

(continued)

PROCEDURE GUIDELINES 16-3 ◆ Nasogastric Intubation and Removal
(continued)

INSERTION PROCEDURE (cont'd)

NURSING ACTION	RATIONALE
1. Coil the first 7–10 cm (3–4 in.) of the tube around your fingers.	1. This curves tubing and facilitates tube passage.
2. Lubricate the coiled portion of the tube with water-soluble lubricant. Avoid occluding the tube's holes with lubricant.	2. Lubrication reduces friction between the mucous membranes and tube and prevents injury to the nasal passages. Using a water-soluble lubricant prevents oil-aspiration pneumonia if the tube accidently slips into trachea.
3. Tilt back the patient's head before inserting tube into nostril and gently pass tube into the posterior nasopharynx, directing downward and backward toward the ear.	3. Passage of the tube is facilitated by following the natural contours of the body. The slower the advancement of the tube at this point, the less likelihood of putting pressure on the turbinates, which could cause pain and bleeding.
4. When tube reaches the pharynx, the patient may gag; allow patient to rest for a few moments.	4. Gag reflex is triggered by the presence of the tube.
5. Have the patient tilt head slightly forward. Offer several sips of water sipped through a straw or permit patient to suck on ice chips, unless contraindicated. Advance tube as patient swallows.	5. Flexed head position partially occludes the airway and the tube is less likely to enter trachea. Swallowing closes the epiglottis over the trachea and facilitates passage of tube into the esophagus. Actually, once the tube passes the cricopharyngeal sphincter into the esophagus, it can be slowly and steadily advanced even if the patient does not swallow.
6. Gently rotate the tube 180 degrees to redirect the curve.	6. This prevents the tube from entering the patient's mouth.
7. Continue to advance tube gently each time the patient swallows.	
8. If obstruction appears to prevent tube from passing, do not use force. Rotating tube gently may help. If unsuccessful, remove tube and try other nostril.	8. Avoid discomfort and trauma to patient.
9. If there are signs of distress such as gasping, coughing, or cyanosis, immediately remove tube.	9. May have entered the trachea.
10. Continue to advance the tube when the patient swallows, until the tape mark reaches the patient's nostril.	10. This is the reference point where the tube was measured.
11. To check whether the tube is in the stomach:	11.
a. Ask the patient to talk	a. If the patient cannot talk, the tube may be coiled in throat or passed through vocal cords.
b. Use the tongue blade and penlight to examine the patient's mouth—especially an unconscious patient.	b. If the patient is choking or has difficulty breathing, the tube has probably entered the trachea.
c. Attach a syringe to the end of the NG tube. Place a stethoscope over the left upper quadrant of the abdomen and inject 10–20 cc of air while auscultating the abdomen.	c. Air can be detected by a "whooshing" sound entering stomach rather than the bronchus. If belching occurs, the tube is probably in the esophagus.
d. Aspirate contents of stomach with a 50-ml catheter tip syringe. If stomach contents cannot be aspirated, place the patient on left side and advance the tube 2.5–5 cm (1–2 in.) and try again.	d. Aspirated stomach contents indicate that the tube is in the stomach.
	e. X-rays may be done to confirm tube placement.
12. After tube is passed and the correct placement is confirmed, attach the tube to suction or clamp the tube.	12. Clamping can be done using a clamp, plastic plug, or folding the tube over and slipping the bend into the tube end.
13. Apply tincture of benzoin to the area where the tape is placed.	13. This helps make the tube adhere, especially with diaphoretic patients.
14. Anchor tube with:	14. Prevents the patient's vision from being disturbed; prevents tubing from rubbing against nasal mucosa. This will ensure tape being secure.
a. Hypoallergenic tape; split lengthwise and only halfway, attach unsplit end of tape to nose and cross split ends around tubing. Apply another piece of tape to bridge of nose.	
b. Bio-occlusive transparent dressing where it exits the nose.	

INSERTION PROCEDURE (cont'd)	NURSING ACTION	RATIONALE

15. Anchor the tubing to the patient's gown. Use a rubber band to make a slip-knot to anchor the tubing to the patient's gown. Secure the rubber band to the patient's gown using a safety pin.
16. Clamp the tube until the purpose for inserting the tube takes place.
17. Attach the tube to suction equipment if prescribed.
18. Assure the patient that most discomfort he or she feels will lessen as he or she gets used to the tube.
19. Irrigate the tube at regular intervals with small volumes of prescribed fluid.
    a. If the tube is a Salem sump, it will require periodic placing of 10–20 ml of air through the vent port (blue port).
    b. Check the tube patency by placing the vent port next to your ear.

20. Cleanse nares and provide mouth care every shift.
21. Apply petrolatum to nostrils as needed and assess for skin irritation or breakdown.
22. Keep head of bed elevated at least 30 degrees.
23. Record the time, type, and size of tube inserted. Document placement checks after each assessment, along with amount, color, consistency of drainage.

15. To permit mobility of patient. This prevents tugging on the tube when the patient moves.

16. See #12.

19. NURSING ALERT:
All enteric tubes must be irrigated with small volumes of fluid and at regular intervals to ensure patency.

a. A soft hissing sound is heard if the tube is patent.
b. If the port hangs downward and the tube backs up, stomach contents will spill over the patient.

20. To promote patient comfort and decrease risk of infection.
21. To keep tissue soft and prevent crusting and skin breakdown.
22. To minimize gastroesophageal reflux.
23. To ensure proper tube and placement at all times, and assest in evaluation of tube effectiveness.

NURSING ALERT:
If the patient has a nasal condition that prevents insertion through the nose, the tube is passed through the mouth. Remove dentures, slide the tube over the tongue, and proceed the same way as a nasal intubation. Make sure to coil the end of the tube and direct it downward at the pharynx.

OTHER NURSING/PATIENT CARE CONSIDERATIONS

1. If the patient is unconscious, advance the tube between respirations to make sure it does not enter the trachea. You will need to stroke the unconscious patient's neck to facilitate passage of the tube down the esophagus.
2. Watch for cyanosis while passing the tube in an unconscious patient. Cyanosis indicates the tube has entered the trachea.
3. Never place the end of the tube in a container of fluid while checking for placement. If the tube is in the trachea, the patient could inhale the water.
4. Do not tape the tube to the forehead: it can cause necrosis of the nostril.
5. a. Sucralfate (Carafate) may be ordered after NG tube insertion to provide a protective barrier against gastric acids, pepsin & bile. After administering carafate, clamp tube for 1/2 hour, then unclamp & reconnect to suction (if ordered).
   b. Clotrimazole (Mycelex) may be ordered as prophylactic treatment for *candida albicans*.
6. Pain or vomiting after the tube is inserted indicates tube obstruction or incorrect placement.
7. The air vent on the Salem sump tube should not be used for irrigation
8. If the air vent (Salem sump tube) is draining fluid or is not drawing air, instill 20 cc of air through the vent.
9. Irrigate the NG tube every 2 hours unless otherwise ordered.
10. If the NG tube is not draining, the nurse should reposition tube by advancing or withdrawing it slightly (with a physician's order). After repositioning, always check for placement.
11. Recognize the complications when the tube is in for prolonged periods: nasal erosion, sinusitis, esophagitis, esophagotracheal fistula, gastric ulceration, and pulmonary and oral infections (see figure).

(continued)

PROCEDURE GUIDELINES 16-3 ◆ Nasogastric Intubation and Removal
(continued)

Anatomical sites

- Sinus area
- Auditory canal
- Nasopharynx
- Oropharynx
- Larynx
- Esophagus
- Trachea
- Endotrachea
- Bronchus
- Lung
- Stomach

Nasogastric tube

Endotracheal tube

Tracheotomy

Potential for infection
Otitis media
Sinusitis
Pharyngitis
Laryngitis
Tracheitis
Bronchitis
Esophagitis
Pneumonitis
Gastritis

All along the upper respiratory tract and upper digestive system, there is the potential for abnormal areas of colonization (infection) when various tubes are in place (i.e., tracheostomy, nasogastric or endotracheal tube). In addition, there is the potential for aspiration of secretions that may cause bronchitis and/or pneumonitis.

12. Notify the health care provider of any continuous problems.

REMOVAL PROCEDURE

PREPARATORY PHASE

1. Be certain that gastric or small bowel drainage is not excessive in volume.
2. Ensure, by auscultation, that audible peristalsis is present.
3. Determine whether the patient is passing flatus; this indicates peristalsis.
4. There is a physician's order for removal.

REMOVING NASOGASTRIC TUBING

NURSING ACTION	RATIONALE
1. Place a towel across the patient's chest and inform him or her that the tube is to be withdrawn.	1. No doubt, the patient will be happy to have progressed to this stage.
2. Apply disposable gloves	2. Provides protection from contaminated body fluids
3. Turn off suction, disconnect and clamp tube.	3. Prevents fluids from leaking from tube
4. Remove the tape from the patient's nose.	
5. Instruct the patient to take a deep breath and hold it.	5. This maneuver closes the epiglottis.

**REMOVAL
PROCEDURE
(cont'd)**

NURSING ACTION	*RATIONALE*
6. Slowly but evenly withdraw tubing and cover it with a towel as it emerges. (As the tube reaches the nasopharynx, you can pull quickly.)	6. Covering the tubing helps dispel patient's nausea.
7. Provide the patient with materials for oral care and lubricant for nasal dryness.	7. Mouthwash and a nasal lubricant will be appreciated by the patient.
8. Dispose of equipment in appropriate receptacle.	
9. Document time of tube removal and the patient's reaction.	
10. Document tube removal and color, consistency, and amount of drainage in suction canister.	
11. Continue to monitor the patient for signs of GI difficulties.	11. Recurrence of nausea or vomiting may require reinsertion of nasogastric tubing. Changes in vital signs may suggest infection.

PROCEDURE GUIDELINES 16-4 ◆ Nasointestinal Intubation (Small-Bore Feeding Tubes)

EQUIPMENT
1. Type of tube ordered by health care provider
2. 30 cc or 60 cc luer-lock or tip syringe
3. Water-solubie lubricant
4. Tape, rubber band, clamp, safety pin
5. Glass of water
6. Stethoscope.

PROCEDURE   *PREPARATORY AND PERFORMANCE PHASE*

> **NURSING ALERT:**
> All tubes and endoscopes should be routinely pretested for patency and function before passage.

HEALTH CARE PROVIDER ACTION/NURSE ASSISTED	*RATIONALE*
1. Tube Preparation:	
a. Do not ice plastic tubes	a. Become too stiff to work with
b. Inject 10 cc of water into the tube	b. Aides in insertion
c. Insert guidewire or stylet into tube, making sure it is positioned snugly against tube.	c. Prevents trauma
d. Dip weighted tip into glass of water	d. Activates lubricant
2. Similar to passing a short nasogastric tube and taping to patient (see Procedure Guidelines, 16-3).	
3. After the tube enters the stomach, it passes by peristalsis and gravity into the small intestine.	3. This will assist in advancing the tubing to and through the pylorus; tilting to the right is helpful.
a. Change patient's position from Fowler's to a position in which the patient is leaning forward	
4. Obtain an x-ray of the abdomen after tube insertion	4. Confirms placement.
5. Stylet should remain in place until position is confirmed.	

NURSING/PATIENT CARE CONSIDERATIONS

1. Be aware of risk of aspiration in an unconscious patient.
2. Instruct patient on complications associated with tube feedings, such as nausea, vomiting, diarrhea.

◆ CARING FOR THE PATIENT UNDERGOING GASTROINTESTINAL SURGERY

Types of Procedures

A. *Gastric Surgeries*
1. Total gastrectomy—complete excision of the stomach with esophageal–jejunal anastomosis.
2. Subtotal or partial gastrectomy—a portion of the stomach excised:
   a. Billroth I procedure—gastric remnant anastomosed to the duodenum.
   b. Billroth II procedure—gastric remnant anastomosed to the jejunum.
3. Gastrostomy (Janeway or Spivak)—rectangular stomach flap created into abdominal stoma, used for intermittent tube feedings.

COMMUNITY-BASED CARE TIP:
A person who has undergone a total gastrectomy needs lifelong parenteral administration of vitamin B_{12} to prevent pernicious anemia.

B. *Hernia Surgeries*
1. Herniorrhaphy—surgical repair of a hernia with suturing of the abdominal wall.
2. Hernioplasty—reconstructive hernia repair with mesh sewn over the defect for reinforcement.

C. *Bowel Surgeries*
1. Appendectomy—excision of the vermiform appendix.
2. Bowel resection—segmental excision of small and/or large bowels with various outcomes:
   a. Anastomosis of proximal and distal ends of bowel.
   b. Anastomosis of proximal and distal ends of bowel with temporary diverting loop ostomy.
   c. Both ends of bowel exteriorized to the abdominal wall with proximal ostomy and distal mucous fistula.
   d. Hartmann's procedure—proximal bowel end as ostomy; distal end of large bowel oversewn inside abdomen as Hartmann's pouch.
3. Low-anterior resection—subtotal resection of the rectum with colorectal or coloanal anastomosis.
4. Abdominoperineal resection—a combined abdominal and perineal approach for removal of the rectum, including anus, resulting in a permanent colostomy.
5. Subtotal colectomy—partial removal of the large bowel or colon.
6. Total colectomy—complete removal of the large bowel or colon with various outcomes:
   a. Ileorectal anastomosis—colon removal with ileum anastomosed to rectum.
   b. Proctocolectomy—colon removal including the rectum and anus, resulting in a permanent ileostomy.
   c. Ileal reservoir—anal anastomosis. Colon removal, subtotal proctectomy, possible distal rectal mucosectomy, creation of pelvic reservoir from two, three, or four loops of ileum with anastomosis with anal canal. Usually a temporary loop ileostomy is performed as fecal diversion to protect the reservoir

and the ileal–anal anastomosis. After takedown of temporary loop ileostomy (2 to 3 months postoperatively), the reservoir is used to store feces and patient eliminates under voluntary control.
   d. Kock or Barnett continent internal reservoir procedures—creation of a continent small bowel reservoir (after proctocolectomy) connected to an abdominal stoma for routine intubation to remove feces. Continence is provided through the creation of nipple valve.
7. Roux-en-Y jejunostomy—jejunum severed with distal end exteriorized as permanent stoma for intermittent tube feedings; proximal end reanastomosed to GI tract distal to stoma to reestablish pathway.

D. *Laparoscopic Surgery*
1. Gastrointestinal surgical procedures are increasingly being assisted by the use of a laparoscope, either partially or totally. The laparoscope is usually inserted through a 1-cm umbilical incision with additional trocars used for visualization and assistance. Dissection is performed with endocautery, scissors, or laser.
2. Advantages may include reduction in postoperative pain, shorter hospital and recuperative periods, cost effectiveness, and improved cosmetic outcome.
3. Contraindications may include obesity, internal adhesions, and bowel obstruction with distention.
4. Cholecystectomies and appendectomies are routinely done through laparoscopy; other GI surgeries, including ostomies and bowel resections, are increasingly being done through this surgical approach.

Preoperative Management/ Nursing Care

1. Explain all diagnostic tests and procedures to promote cooperation and relaxation.
2. Describe the reason for and type of surgical procedure as well as postoperative care (i.e., IV, patient-controlled analgesia pump, nasogastric (NG) tube, surgical drains, incision care, possibility of ostomy).
3. Explain the rationale for deep breathing, and teach the patient how to turn, cough, deep-breathe, use the incentive spirometer, and splint the incision. These measures will minimize postoperative complications.
4. Administer IV fluids or total parenteral nutrition (TPN) before surgery, as ordered, to improve fluid and electrolyte balance and nutritional status.
5. Monitor intake and output.
6. Send blood samples, as ordered, for preoperative laboratory studies, and monitor results.
7. Inform that bowel cleansing will be initiated 1 to 2 days before surgery for better visualization. Preparation may include diet modifications, such as liquid or low residue, oral laxatives, suppositories, enemas, or polyethylene glycoelectrolyte solution (CoLyte, GoLYTELY).
8. Administer antibiotics, as ordered, to decrease the bacterial growth in the colon.
9. Coordinate consultation with the enterostomal therapy nurse if patient is scheduled for an ostomy to initiate early understanding and management of postoperative care.
10. Explain that patient may not have anything by mouth after midnight the night before surgery. Medications may be withheld, if ordered. This will keep the GI tract clear.

Postoperative Management/ Nursing Care

See also Table 16-2.

1. Complete a physical assessment at least once per shift, or more frequently, as indicated.
   a. Monitor vital signs for signs of infection and shock—fever, hypotension, tachycardia.
   b. Monitor intake and output for signs of imbalance, dehydration, and shock. Include all drains in evaluating intake and output.
   c. Assess abdomen for increased pain, distention, rigidity, and rebound tenderness, because these may indicate postoperative complications. Report abnormal findings.
   d. Expect diminished or absent bowel sounds in the immediate postoperative phase.
   e. Evaluate dressing and incision. Check for purulent or bloody drainage, odor, and unusual tenderness or redness at incision site, which may indicate bleeding or infection.
   f. Evaluate for passing of flatus or feces.
   g. Monitor for nausea and vomiting. Note the presence of fecal smell or material in vomitus, because it may indicate an obstruction.
3. Monitor lab values and assess patient for signs and symptoms of electrolyte imbalance.
4. Maintain wound drains, IVs, and all other catheters. Assess sites for signs of infection or infiltration.
5. Maintain NG tube, if ordered. To maintain patency of NG tube, the tube may be irrigated with 30 cc of normal saline solution (NSS) every 2 hours and as needed. If there are large amounts of NG output, IV replacement may be necessary.

NURSING ALERT:
Due to the type of abdominal surgery and location of the suture line, the health care provider may order not to irrigate or manipulate the NG tube.

---

6. Apply antiembolism stockings. Subcutaneous heparin may also be ordered to prevent embolus.
7. Encourage and assist patient with turning, coughing, deep breathing, and incentive spirometry every 2 hours. Assist patient to dangle at bedside the night of surgery and attempt ambulation the first postoperative day, unless ordered otherwise.
8. Instruct patient on use of patient-controlled analgesia for pain control, or provide other analgesics, as ordered, to promote comfort.
9. Change wound dressing every day or as needed, maintaining aseptic technique.
10. Advance diet as ordered, after presence of bowel sounds indicates GI tract has regained motility. After 1 to 2 days of NPO postoperatively, the usual diet progression is ice chips, sips of water, clear liquids, full liquids, or soft or regular diet.
11. Teach dietary habits to include fiber, avoid gas-producing foods, and maintain adequate fluid intake.
12. Reinforce teaching and assist with ostomy care.
13. Administer medications, as ordered, which may include a stool softener or laxative when bowel function has returned.

Potential Complications

1. Paralytic ileus or obstruction
2. Peritonitis or sepsis
3. Anastomotic leakage, which may result in peritonitis

Nursing Diagnoses

A. Pain related to surgical incision
B. Altered Nutrition, Less Than Body Requirements, related to dietary modifications following surgery
C. Impaired Skin Integrity related to surgical incision
D. Constipation related to surgery
E. Risk for Infection related to surgical incision
F. Fluid Volume Deficit related to surgical procedure
G. Altered Health Maintenance, related to lack of knowledge of surgical procedure and postoperative care

Nursing Interventions

A. *Promoting Comfort*
1. Assess pain location, intensity, and characteristics, and ensure they are appropriate for postoperative stage.
2. Administer prescribed pain medications and provide instructions if using a patient-controlled analgesia pump, to keep patient comfortable.
3. Assess the effectiveness of the pain medications. If ordered, promethazine (Phenergan) can potentiate the effectiveness of pain medication.
4. Encourage the patient to change positions frequently and to splint incision when turning, coughing, or deep breathing to minimize discomfort.

B. *Improving Nutritional Status*
1. Monitor intake and output every 8 hours, or more frequently if indicated, to maintain fluid balance.
2. Advance diet as tolerated.
3. Weigh patient daily to ensure adequate calorie intake.
4. Provide snacks or high-protein, high-calorie supplements and assist in menu selection, if needed.
5. Instruct patient to avoid gas-producing foods, and encourage ambulation.

C. *Improving Skin Integrity*
1. Assess wound for signs of erythema, swelling, and purulent drainage, which may indicate infection.
2. Change surgical dressing every 24 hours and as needed to protect skin from drainage and decrease risk of infection.
3. Apply gauze on skin to protect against leaking from drains or stomas.
4. Turn patient frequently or encourage position changes to prevent skin breakdown at pressure areas.

D. *Promoting Bowel Elimination*
1. Assess for presence of bowel sounds to evaluate return of bowel function.
2. Ask the patient if passing flatus rectally; also indicative of return of bowel function.
3. Evaluate for abdominal distention, nausea, or vomiting, which may indicate obstruction.
4. Monitor stool for frequency, amount, and consistency.
5. Administer stool softener or laxative, as ordered, to promote comfort with elimination.

TABLE 16-2 Critical Pathway* for Elective Small- and Large-Bowel Surgery (Courtesy of St. Luke's Hospital, Jacksonville, Florida)

	Pre-Admission	Pre-Op	Post-Op	Level 1	Level 2	Level 3	Level 4	Level 5
Laboratory	CBC UA Chem 7 (opt) UCG/Beta HCG	PT/PTT if on anticoagulants Type and screen (opt)		CBC (opt) Chem 7 (opt)				Complete Staging Form
Radiology	CXR							
Diagnostic Cardiology	ECG (Case Specific)							
Respiratory			Incentive Spirometer Q1 Hour WA Aerosal (opt) →————————————————————→ (to Level 4)					
Medication/IVs		IV Hydration PO Antibiotics Home Medication Evaluation	Perioperative ATB Sub Q Heparin (if at risk) PCA/Epidural or other analgesia	TPN (opt) Reglan (opt) Antiemetics (opt)		IV to Hep Lock → PO Pain Meds D/C PCA		
Treatment	Pre-op Evaluations with special attention to: ☐ Contact risk ☐ Medication ☐ Diabetes ☐ Steroid ☐ Aspirin ☐ Anticoagulants	Bowel Prep/Enemas Enterostomal Therapy Consult (opt)	Maintain drains Maintain NG (opt) Maintain Foley Antiembolism stockings (PAS) I & O Daily Weights	Enterostomal Consult Wound Care →		D/C Drains Clamp N/G → D/C NG (Level 4) D/C Foley D/C PAS: Change to TEDS		Oncology consult if needed Independent Stomal Care

Activity	MOS SF 36 Survey†	Assess Ambulation	Dangle Feet at Bedside	Sit in chair / Ambulate with assistance	Phy. Therapy (opt) Ambulate × 4	Ambulate × 6	Ambulate independently →
Nutrition	Nutrition Screen Calorie/Protein Supplements (if indicated)	NPO after MN	Nutrition screening within 48 hr / NPO →	NPO/Ice Chips →	Nutrition (opt) Assessment	Clear Liquids →	Advance Diet Consult for Food Preferences (opt) →
Elimination							
Education/Teaching	Ostomy teaching (opt) / Incentive Spirometer / PCA use-other pain management / Activity expectations / Dietary Schedule / Splinting/coughing; leg exercises		Incentive Spirometer → / Pain Management → / Splinting/coughing; leg exercises →	Ostomy Teaching (opt) → / Walking Schedule → / Dietary Schedule →			
Discharge Planning	Social Service evaluation / Assess home situation, need for referral		Assess discharge needs →				Referral needs assessed / Medical equipment needs / Discharge Meds / ECF Transfer Form

ATB: antibiotic; CBC: complete blood count; CXR: chest x-ray; ECF: extended care facility; ECG: electrocradiogram; HCG: human chorionic gonadotropins; Hep: heparin; I&O: intake and output; IV: intravenous; MN: midnight; NG: nasogastric; Opt: optional; PAS: passive antiembolism stockings; PCA: patient-controlled analgesic; PO: by mouth; PT: prothrombin time; PTT: partial thromboplastin time; Q1: hourly; SF: short form functional status; SubQ: subcutaneous; TPN: total parenteral nutrition; UA: urinalysis; UCG: urinary chorionic gonadotropins; WA: while awake

* The Clinical Pathway established for this procedure does not replace the exercise of independent clinical judgment on the part of the physician treating the individual patient.

NOTE: THIS IS NOT A PHYSICIAN ORDER

† MOS SF 36 Survey—standard form used to assess functional ability. © 1992 with permission by Medical Outcomes Trust Inc., Boston, MA.

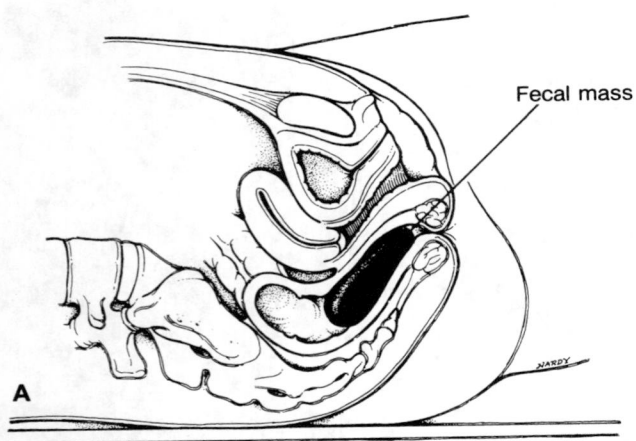

Fecal mass

A

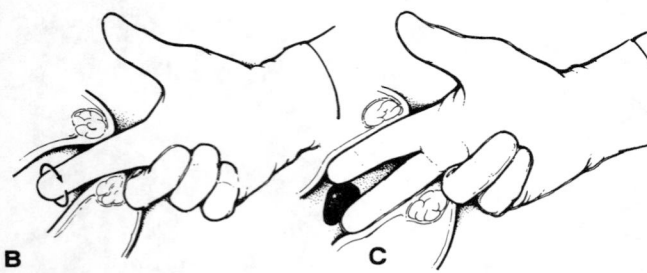

B   **C**

FIGURE 16-1 *Fecal impaction.* **(A)** *Note shaded area inside rectal sphincter—this indicates fecal impaction.* **(B)** *By gently stimulating the rectal wall with a gloved index finger and using a circular motion, it is possible to loosen fecal material.* **(C)** *It may be necessary to gently insert two fingers in an attempt to crush the fecal mass. A scissorlike motion is used.*

6. Encourage diet with adequate fiber and fluid content for natural laxative effect.
7. Encourage and assist with ambulation to promote peristalsis.

E. **Preventing Infection**
1. Monitor temperature every shift or as ordered, and review previous readings to recognize early increases.
2. Change surgical dressings every 24 hours or more frequently, as indicated. Maintain aseptic technique to avoid contamination.
3. Monitor wound for signs and symptoms of infection, such as redness, swelling, purulent drainage, odor, and pain.
4. Obtain a wound culture, as ordered.
5. Monitor patient with a Foley catheter for signs and symptoms of urinary tract infection, such as concentrated, cloudy urine; hematuria; fever. If Foley discontinued, monitor for the above plus complaints of burning and frequency.
6. Assist patient in washing perineum daily and as needed if incontinence is present, for increased comfort and hygiene.
7. Assess breath sounds and monitor for crackles.
8. Instruct patient to turn, cough, deep-breathe, and use incentive spirometer every 2 hours to minimize complications.

9. Encourage early ambulation to initiate bowel function and reduce risk of embolus.
10. Administer antibiotics, as ordered, to maintain constant blood level.

F. **Maintaining Fluid Volume**
1. Monitor intake and output every 8 hours, or more frequently, if ordered, to assess recent status. Include amount of wound drainage from dressing changes and drains that may be in place.
2. Assess patient for signs of dehydration—flushed, dry skin; tenting of skin; oliguria; tachycardia, hypotension and rapid respirations; increase in hematocrit, blood urea nitrogen, electrolytes; fever; weight loss.
3. Monitor lab results and report abnormal findings.
4. Assess patient for signs of electrolyte imbalance—nausea, vomiting; cardiac dysrhythmia, tremor, seizures, anorexia, malaise, weakness, irregular pulse; changes in behavior, mental status.
5. Weigh daily to ensure adequate caloric intake.
6. Administer parenteral fluids, enteral feedings, and blood products as ordered to maintain volume during period of decreased oral intake.

Patient Education/ Health Maintenance

1. Review signs and symptoms of wound infection, so that early intervention may be instituted.
2. Explain signs and symptoms of other postoperative complications to report—elevated temperature, nausea or vomiting, abdominal distention, changes in bowel function and stool consistency.
3. Instruct patient regarding wound care or ostomy care if applicable to promote healing and self-confidence.
4. Instruct patient on turning, coughing, deep breathing, use of incentive spirometer, ambulation. Discuss their purpose and continued importance during the recovery period.
5. Review dietary changes, such as increased fiber content and fluid intake, and their importance in improving bowel function.
6. Instruct patient on prescribed medications to encourage compliance and understanding of management.
7. Assess the need for home health follow-up and initiate the appropriate referrals if indicated.

Evaluation

A. Demonstrates increased comfort
B. Maintains weight; tolerates diet
C. Incision healing; no evidence of further skin breakdown
D. Passing flatus and stool; ambulating
E. No evidence of infection
F. Vital signs stable, fluid and electrolytes in balance, no weight loss
G. Verbalizes increased knowledge regarding surgery and postoperative care

◆ CARE OF A PATIENT UNDERGOING OSTOMY SURGERY

Types of Ostomies

A. **Colostomy**
See Figure 16-2.

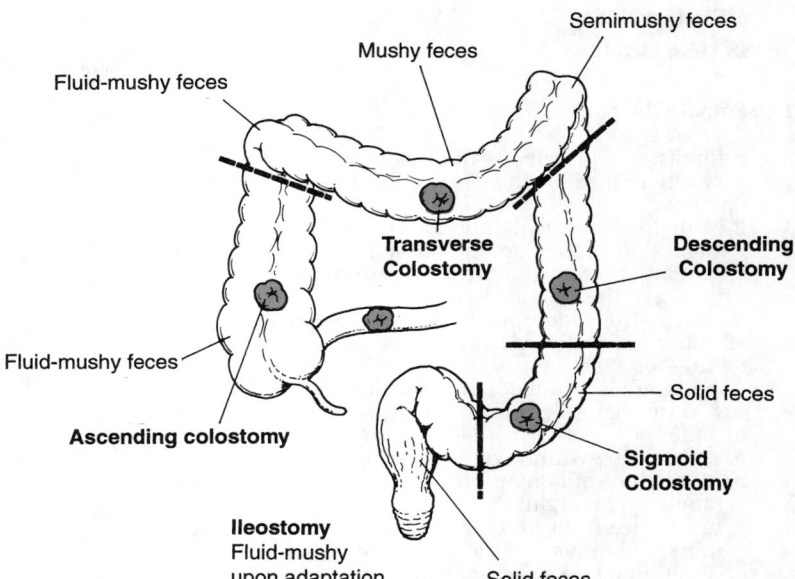

FIGURE 16-2 *A diagrammatic representation of the placement of fecal ostomies and nature of discharge at these sites.*

1. A surgically created opening between the colon and the abdominal wall to allow fecal elimination. It may be a temporary or permanent diversion.
2. Colostomy may be placed in any segment of the large intestine (colon), which will influence the nature of fecal discharge. Transverse and descending/sigmoid colostomies are the most common types.
3. Colostomies may be performed as part of abdominoperineal resection for rectal cancer; fecal diversion for unresectable cancer; temporary measure to protect an anastomosis; treatment of diverticulitis, trauma, ischemic bowel, Crohn's disease.

B. Ileostomy
1. A surgically created opening between the ileum of the small intestine and the abdominal wall to allow fecal elimination.
2. An ileostomy is usually placed in the terminal part of the ileum of the small bowel and is often brought out through the right lower quadrant of the abdomen. Stool from an ileostomy drains frequently (average, 4 to 5 times/day) and contains proteolytic enzymes, which can be harmful to skin.
3. Diagnoses which may require a temporary or permanent ileostomy include ulcerative colitis, Crohn's disease, familial polyposis, congenital defects, and trauma.

Characteristics of Stomas

1. A stoma is that part of the intestine (small or large) that is brought above the abdominal wall and that becomes the outlet for discharge of intestinal contents. It is often used interchangeably with the word "ostomy."
2. Normal stomal characteristics: pink-red, moist, bleeds slightly when rubbed, no feeling to touch, stool functions involuntary, and postoperative swelling gradually decreases over several months.

3. Stoma classifications:
   a. End stoma—after bowel is divided, the proximal bowel is exteriorized to abdominal wall, everted (which exposes mucosal lining), and sutured to dermis or subcutaneous tissue. There is only one opening that drains stool. The distal bowel is either surgically removed or sutured closed within abdominal cavity.
   b. Double barrel stoma—after bowel is divided, the proximal and distal ends of bowel are exteriorized to abdominal wall, everted, and sutured to the dermis or subcutaneous tissue. If the stomas are brought up next to each other requiring them to be pouched together, they are referred to as a double barrel stoma; if the stomas are apart to be pouched separately, they may be referred to as end stoma (proximal), which drains stool, and a mucous fistula (distal) which drains mucus. This type of stoma is usually temporary.
   c. Loop stoma—a bowel loop is brought to the abdominal wall through an incision and stabilized temporarily with a rod, catheter, or a skin or fascial bridge. The anterior wall of bowel is opened surgically or by electrocautery to expose the proximal and distal openings. The posterior wall of bowel remains intact and separates the functioning proximal opening and the nonfunctioning distal opening. This type of stoma is usually temporary.
4. Enterostomal therapy
   a. Enterostomal therapy is a nursing specialty in the care of patients with wounds, ostomies, and continence problems. These nurses play a vital role in the rehabilitation of patients with ostomies and related problems.
   b. The Wound Ostomy and Continence Nurses Society (WOCN), 2755 Bristol Street #110, Costa Mesa, CA 92626, has an official publication called the Journal of WOCN published monthly by Mosby, 11830 Westline Industrial Drive, St. Louis, MO 63146-3318.

Preoperative Management/ Nursing Care

1. Prepare the patient for general abdominal surgery (see page 494).
2. Administer replacement fluid as ordered before surgery due to possible increased output during the postoperative phase.
3. Provide low-residue diet before NPO status.
4. Explain that the abdomen will be marked by the enterostomal therapist or surgeon to ensure proper positioning of the stoma.
   Note: The abdominal location of the stoma is usually determined by anatomic location of bowel segment—for example, a sigmoid colostomy is ideally located in left lower abdominal quadrant.
   Other considerations when selecting a stoma include:
   a. Positioning within rectus muscle.
   b. Avoidance of bony prominences, such as iliac crest and costal margin.
   c. Clearance from umbilicus, scars, and deep creases, observed in lying, sitting, and standing positions.
   d. Positioning on a flat pouching surface.
   e. Avoidance of beltline when possible.
   f. Positioning within patient's visibility to optimize independent ostomy care.
5. Support the patient and family with the many psychosocial considerations of ostomy surgery.

Postoperative Management/ Nursing Care

1. Administer general abdominal surgery care (see page 494).
2. Assess stoma every shift for color and record findings:
   a. Normal color—pink-red
   b. Dusky—dark red; purplish hue (ischemic sign)
   c. Necrotic—brown or black; may be dry (health care provider notified to determine extent of necrosis)
3. Apply pouching system with $\frac{1}{8}$-in. clearance to prevent stomal constriction, which contributes to edema (Box 16-1).
4. Check for abdominal distention, which reduces blood flow to stoma through mesenteric tension.
5. Evaluate and empty drains and ostomy bag frequently to promote patency and maintain seal.
6. Monitor intake and output with extreme accuracy, because output may remain high during early postoperative period.
7. Suction and irrigate NG tube frequently, as ordered, to relieve pressure and decrease gastric contents.
8. Offer continued support to patient and family.

Complications

1. Mucocutaneous separation (between skin and stoma)
2. Stomal ischemia
3. Stomal stricture or stenosis
4. Stomal prolapse

BOX 16-1 *Fecal Ostomy Pouching Systems*

1. Pouching systems are varied according to manufacturer and patient needs. Systems are classified as one-piece or two-piece and disposable or reusable. A disposable one-piece pouch is commonly used with backing as adhesive tape, skin barrier, or both. A disposable two-piece system consists of a skin barrier wafer with or without a tape border and a pouch. Disposable systems are popular and are discarded after one use. Reusable systems are declining in use and are made of heavier material, allowing use for weeks to months. They require the use of double-backed adhesive disks, cement and/or belt to provide a seal.
2. Pouching systems are available in precut sizes and cut-to-fit options as well as with a flat backing versus degrees of convexity. Convex pouching systems are used with flush or retracted stomas to increase stomal protrusion and reduce undermining of feces.
3. Fecal pouches are available in closed-end and drainable styles. Drainable pouches require the use of a tail closure and may be used more than once. Closed-end pouches may contain a built-in filter to release gas and require no tail closure. A closed-end pouch is discarded after one use. Pouch selection depends on the patient's preference or ability to manipulate and the volume and frequency of fecal output.
4. Many accessory products are available to assist in the management of a fecal ostomy. They include skin sealants, skin barrier powders, pastes and washers, adhesive removers, tapes, belts, and pouch covers.
5. The goal is to change a pouching system on a routine basis to prevent leakage. Usually this is every 3–7 days but may vary per individual needs. Routine changes allow for examination of the peristomal skin for breakdown. Schedule the change when the bowel is least active, usually early morning before breakfast, 2–4 hours after a meal, or before bedtime. At times, the pouching system may need to be changed immediately if leakage is imminent, itching or burning of peristomal skin is present, odor is detected with a closed system, or the wafer is dissolving.

5. Peristomal hernia
6. Peristomal skin breakdown

Nursing Diagnoses

A. Knowledge Deficit related to surgical procedures and ostomy management
B. Body Image Disturbance related to change in structure, function, and appearance
C. Anxiety related to loss of bowel control and autonomy
D. Impaired Skin Integrity related to irritation of peristomal skin by drainage and equipment
E. Altered Nutrition, Less Than Body Requirements, related to increased output and inadequate intake
F. Sexual Dysfunction related to altered body structure

Nursing Interventions

A. Educating the Patient
1. Review the surgical procedure with patient and discuss the information that the surgeon and other providers have given. Clarify any misunderstandings.
2. Avoid overwhelming the patient with information.
3. Include family in discussions, when appropriate.
4. Use available educational materials, including pictures and drawings, if patient is receptive.
5. Involve the enterostomal therapist in ostomy teaching, and reinforce information, including lifestyle modifications.
6. Use a team approach; the need for information may come from many disciplines.
7. Assess patient's response to teaching. If patient not interested, provide alternative times for teaching and review.
8. Consider the psychosocial issues of the patient and their effect on learning.

B. Promoting a Positive Self-Image
1. Encourage the patient to verbalize feelings about the surgical outcome.
2. Provide support during initial viewing of the stoma, and encourage patient to touch the area.
3. Encourage spouse or significant other to view the stoma.
4. Arrange a visit by a United Ostomy Association ostomy visitor if the patient desires. This is preferably done preoperatively.
5. Offer counseling, as necessary, and encourage patient to use normal support systems, such as family, church, community groups.

C. Reducing Anxiety
1. Provide information regarding expected outcomes, such as the type and consistency of bowel function.
2. Introduce gradual steps toward achieving independent ostomy management. Have the patient:
   a. First observe stoma, pouch change, and emptying procedure. See Procedure Guidelines 16-5: Changing a Two-Piece Drainable Fecal Pouching System.
   b. Learn tail closure application and removal.
   c. Empty pouch by cuffing tail and using tail closure.
   d. Assist with pouching system change until independent.
      Note: Some patients may have decreased vision or dexterity and require additional assistance and encouragement.
3. Teach colostomy irrigation procedure, if appropriate. See Procedure Guidelines 16-6: Irrigating a Colostomy.
   a. Review that irrigating involves inserting an enema into a descending or sigmoid colostomy.
   b. Reinforce its purposes of cleansing the colon and stimulating the colon to move at a desired time regularly to regain control of fecal elimination.
      Note: Colostomy irrigation may also be performed to empty the colon of its contents (feces, gas, mucus) before a diagnostic procedure or surgery and to cleanse the colon after fecal impaction removal or with constipation.
4. Acknowledge that it is normal to have negative feelings toward ostomy surgery; empathize with patient.
5. Describe behaviors to attain a sense of control, such as resuming activities of daily living.

D. Maintaining Skin Integrity
1. Select a pouching system based on type of ostomy and condition of stoma and skin. See Box 16-1.
2. Empty pouch when one-third to one-half full to avoid overfilling, which interferes with pouch seal.
   a. Remove tail closure from pouch tail.
   b. Cuff bottom of pouch tail.
   c. Drain stool from pouch.
   d. Clean pouch tail with toilet tissue or wipe (may rinse pouch if desired).
   e. Uncuff pouch and reapply tail closure.
3. Treat peristomal skin breakdown as needed:
   a. Dust skin breakdown with skin barrier powder.
   b. Seal powder with water or skin sealant.
   c. Allow skin to dry before applying a pouching system.

E. Maximizing Nutritional Intake
1. Review dietary habits with patient to determine patterns, preferences, and bowel irritants.
2. Advise the patient to avoid foods that stimulate elimination, such as nuts, seeds, and certain fruits.
3. Recommend consistency in dietary habits as well as moderation.
4. Coordinate consult with nutritionist, as needed.
5. Weigh daily; monitor vital signs and electrolytes to determine patient's nutritional status.

F. Achieving Sexual Well-Being
1. Encourage patient and significant other to express feelings about the ostomy.
2. Discuss ways to conceal pouch during intimacy, if desired: pouch covers, special ostomy underwear. May briefly use small-capacity pouch (minipouch or cap).
3. Recommend different positions for sexual activity to decrease stoma friction and skin irritation.
4. Review when appropriate that an ostomy in a woman does not prevent a successful pregnancy.
5. Recommend counseling as needed.

Patient Education/ Health Maintenance

A. Skin Care
1. Review techniques for treating peristomal breakdown.
2. Encourage trying other products when encountering an allergic reaction.
3. Teach patient to notify health care provider of continuous problems.

B. Odor Control
1. Encourage good pouch hygiene through rinsing, keeping pouch tail free of stool, airing of reusable pouches, discarding pouches when unable to remove odor.
2. Recommend the use of pouch deodorants, room deodorizers, and oral deodorizers, such as bismuth subgallate (Devrom) or parsley.
3. Emphasize the avoidance of pin holes in pouch.

C. Gas Control
1. Suggest avoidance of straws, excessive talking while eating, chewing gum, and smoking to reduce swallowed air.
2. Inform about gas-forming foods, such as beans and cabbage, and eliminate when appropriate. It takes about 6 hours for gas to travel from mouth to colostomy.

3. Recommend using arm over stoma to muffle gas sounds.

D. *Activities of Daily Living*
1. Advise resumption of normal bathing habits (tub or shower) with or without pouching system on.
2. Suggest waterproof tape on edges of pouching system, because it may help with bathing or swimming.
3. Notify that clothing modifications are usually minimal. Girdles and pantyhose can be worn.
4. Suggest carrying an ostomy supply kit during work or travel in case of an emergency.
5. Remind the patient with an ostomy that participation in sports is possible, however, caution must be exercised with contact sports. During vigorous sports, a belt or binder may provide extra security.
6. Inform the patient about the United Ostomy Association, a self-help group for ostomates and other interested persons. The national headquarters is located at United Ostomy Association, Inc., 36 Executive Park, Suite 120, Irvine, CA 92714-6744. Their official publication is the *Ostomy Quarterly*, published quarterly with membership. Encourage participation in a local chapter. Many publish a local newsletter, conduct monthly meetings, and provide trained ostomy visitors on request by health care professionals.

7. Inform the patient that many manufacturers of ostomy supplies offer free booklets covering a wide variety of ostomy-related topics.
8. Encourage continuous contact with the patient's team of providers.

Evaluation

A. Demonstrates knowledge and positive attitude toward ostomy surgery and management
B. Expresses concerns and fears about changes in body image; tolerates seeing and touching stoma
C. Demonstrates independent pouch changing, irrigates colostomy, describes capabilities in activities
D. Describes signs of peristomal skin breakdown, cleanses skin independently, no evidence of skin irritation
E. Discusses diet modifications, avoids certain foods and fruits
F. Relates fears of sexuality, discusses alternative positions and pouches, involves significant other in discussion, states consideration or participation in counseling

Esophageal Disorders

Esophageal varices are covered in Chapter 17, page 547.

PROCEDURE GUIDELINES 16-5 ◆ Changing a Two-Piece Drainable Fecal Pouching System

EQUIPMENT   Duplicate wafer and pouch
Tail closure
Washcloth and towel
Mild non-oily soap (optional)
Accessory products prescribed for patient

NURSING ACTION	RATIONALE
PREPARATORY PHASE	
1. Explain the details of this activity.	1. Encourages patient understanding and participation to learn self-care.
2. Gather equipment and place within easy reach.	2. Minimizes distractions and fosters organization.
3. Have the patient assume a relaxed position and provide privacy. The best position may be sitting, reclining, or standing.	3. Patient must see stoma site to learn care.
PERFORMANCE PHASE	
1. To remove pouching system	
a. Wear nonsterile gloves.	a. Maintain universal precautions.
b. Push down gently on skin while lifting up on the wafer (ostomy adhesive remover may be used).	b. Minimize skin trauma.
c. Discard soiled pouch and wafer in odorproof plastic bag. Save tail closure for reuse.	c. Removes room odor and maintains universal precautions.
2. To cleanse skin:	
a. Use toilet tissue to remove feces from stoma and skin if needed.	a. Stoma may function during the change.
b. Cleanse stoma and peristomal skin with soft cloth and water, soap optional. The patient may shower with or without pouching system in place. Clip or shave peristomal hair if appropriate.	b. Minimizes skin breakdown and promotes hygiene.
c. Rinse and dry skin thoroughly after cleansing. It is normal for the stoma to bleed slightly during cleansing and drying.	c. Removes residue, which may interfere with adhesion of wafer.

PROCEDURE (cont'd)	NURSING ACTION	RATIONALE

3. To apply wafer:
   a. Use measuring guide or stomal pattern to determine stoma size.
   b. Trace correct size pattern onto back of wafer and cut to nearly stoma size. It is acceptable to cut $1/16$–$1/8$ in. larger than stoma.
   c. Apply a line of skin barrier paste around stoma or on lip of wafer opening. Allow to set according to manufacturer's instructions. (Other barrier may be used in place of paste, such as strips or washer, because some patients are allergic to the alcohol in paste.)
   d. Remove paper backing(s) from the wafer, center opening over stoma, and press wafer down onto peristomal skin.
4. Snap pouch onto the flange of the wafer according to manufacturer's directions (see accompanying figure).

a. This step is omitted when stomal shrinkage is complete, about 2 months postop.
b. Avoids wafer rubbing stoma; omit this step if the wafer is precut.

c. Extra skin protection is imperative for ileostomy and right-sided colostomy. A left-sided colostomy may not need secondary barrier because formed stool is less harmful to skin. Paste acts as "caulking" to prevent undermining of feces.
d. Ensures adherence.

4. If attached properly, there will be no leakage or odor.

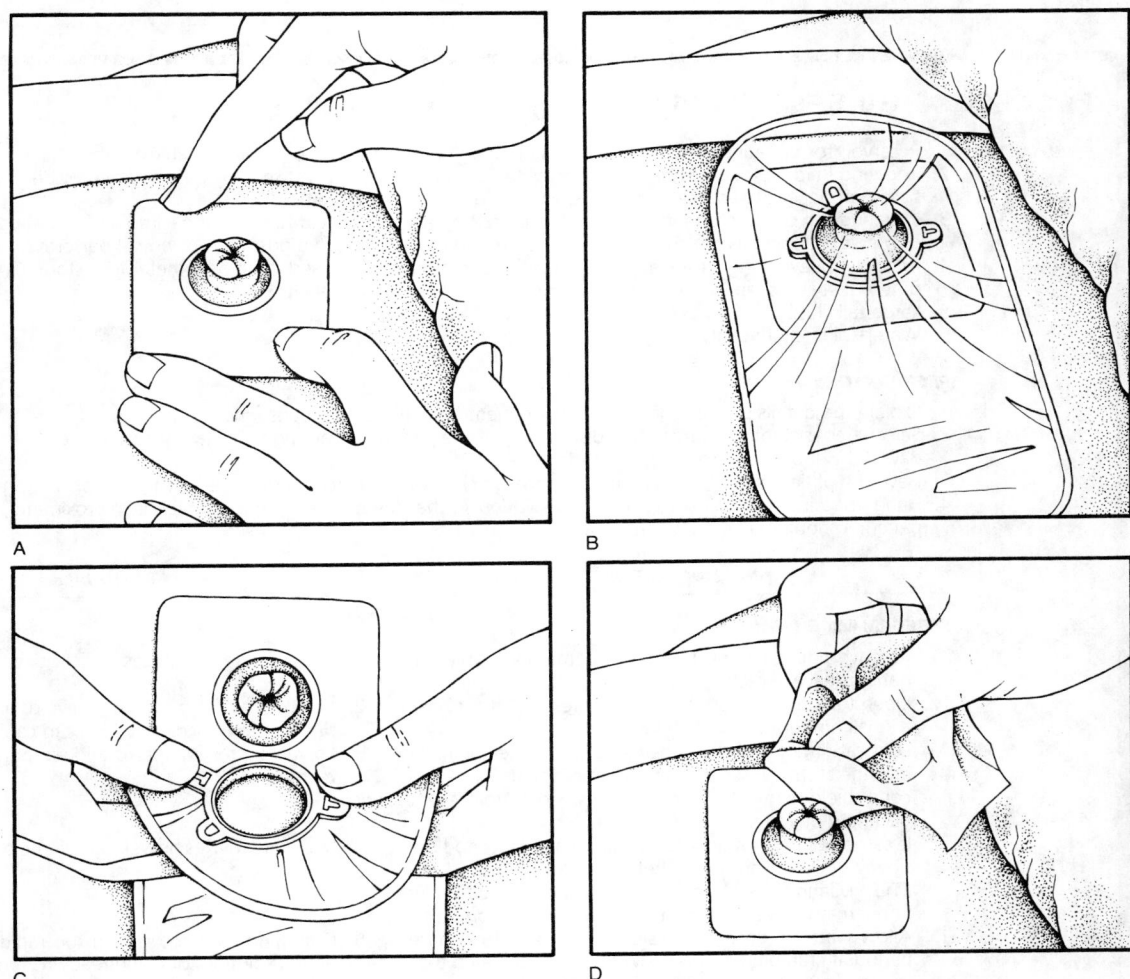

(A) A wafer with flange (1 $1/2$", 1 $3/4$", 2 $1/4$", 2 $3/4$", 4") is applied after cleaning and drying of peristomal skin. *(B)* A transparent or opaque drainable pouch is positioned over stoma at desired angle. *(C)* Pouch may be removed without removal of wafer. *(D)* Stoma may be assessed without removing wafer. (Adapted by permission from Convatec, A Bristol-Myers, Squibb Company.)

5. Apply tail closure to pouch tail.

5. Proper closure controls odor.

(continued)

PROCEDURE GUIDELINES 16-5 ◆ Changing a Two-Piece Drainable Fecal Pouching System *(continued)*

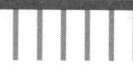

PROCEDURE (cont'd)	NURSING ACTION	RATIONALE

FOLLOW-UP PHASE

1. Dispose of plastic bag with waste materials.	
2. Clean drainable pouch with soap and water, if appropriate. Drainable pouches may be reused several times.	2. Controls odor; reduces cost.
3. A commercial deodorant can be placed in the pouch to reduce odor.	
4. Gas can be released from the pouch by releasing the tail closure or by snapping off an area on the pouch flange. Never make a pinhole in the pouch to release gas.	4. Destroys the odorproof seal.

PROCEDURE GUIDELINES 16-6 ◆ Irrigating a Colostomy

EQUIPMENT

1. Reservoir for irrigating fluids; irrigator bag or enema bag if irrigator bag not available.
2. Irrigating fluid: 500–1,500 ml lukewarm water or other solution prescribed by health care provider. (Volume is titrated based on patient tolerance and results; average amount is 1,000 ml).
3. Irrigating tip: cone tip or soft rubber catheter #22 or #24 with shield to prevent backflow of irrigating solution. (Use only if cone not available. The cone is the preferred method to avoid possibility of bowel perforation.)
4. Irrigation sleeve (long large-capacity bag with opening at top to insert cone or catheter into stoma). Available in different styles: snap-on, self-adhering to skin, or held in place by belt.
5. Large tail closure.
6. Water-soluble lubricant.

PREPARATORY PHASE

1. Explain the details of the procedure to the patient and answer any questions.
2. Select a consistent time, free from distractions. If the patient is learning to irrigate for bowel control, choose the time of day that will best fit into the patient's lifestyle.
3. Have the patient sit in front of the commode on chair or on the commode itself, providing privacy and comfort.
4. Hang irrigating reservoir with prescribed solution so that the bottom of the reservoir is approximately at the level of the patient's shoulder and above the stoma.

NURSING ACTION	RATIONALE

PERFORMANCE PHASE

1. Remove pouch or covering from stoma and apply irrigation sleeve, directing the open tail into the commode.	1. Allows water and feces to flow directly into commode.
2. Open tubing clamp on the irrigating reservoir to release a small amount of solution into the commode.	2. Removes air from the setup; avoids air from being introduced into the colon, which can cause crampy pain.
3. Lubricate the tip of the cone/catheter and gently insert into the stoma. Insert catheter no more than 3 in. Hold cone/shield gently, but firmly, against stoma to prevent backflow of water.	3. Prevents intestinal perforation and irritation of mucous membranes.
4. If catheter does not advance easily, allow water to flow slowly while advancing catheter. NEVER FORCE CATHETER. Dilating the stoma with lubricated gloved pinky finger may be necessary to direct cone/catheter properly.	4. Slow rate relaxes bowel to facilitate passage of catheter.
5. Allow water to enter colon slowly over a 5–10 minute period. If cramping occurs, slow flow rate or clamp tubing to allow cramping to subside. If cramping does not subside, remove cone/catheter to release contents.	5. Cramping may occur from too rapid flow, cold water, excess solution, or colon ready to function.
6. Hold cone/shield in place 10 seconds after water is instilled, then gently remove cone/catheter from stoma.	6. Discourages premature evacuation of fluid.
7. As feces and water flows down sleeve, periodically rinse sleeve with water. Allow 10–15 minutes for most of the returns, then dry sleeve tail and apply tail closure.	

PROCEDURE (cont'd)	NURSING ACTION	RATIONALE

8. Leave sleeve in place for approximately 20 more minutes while patient gets up and moves around.
9. When returns are complete, clean stomal area with mild soap and water; pat dry; reapply pouch or covering over stoma.

8. Ambulation stimulates peristalsis and completion of irrigation return.
9. Cleanliness and dryness promote comfort.

FOLLOW-UP PHASE

1. Clean equipment with soap and water; dry and store in well-ventilated area.
2. If applicable, the patient should use a pouch until the colostomy is sufficiently controlled.

1. This will control odor and mildew prolonging the life of equipment.
2. It may take several months to establish control. The patient can then use minipouch, stoma cap, or gauze covering as desired.

OTHER NURSING/PATIENT CARE CONSIDERATIONS

1. It is a patient preference whether colostomy irrigations are attempted for control. Irrigation may occur every day or every other day depending on bowel pattern. It usually takes 1–2 months to establish control. Patients with a preoperative history of regular, formed bowel movements are more likely to realize success.
2. Disadvantages to the colostomy irrigation approach for control include:
   a. It is a time-consuming procedure requiring consistency, which may not fit into a patient's lifestyle.
   b. Bowel dependency can occur with the irrigation as the stimulus for evacuation of bowel movements.
3. Only a patient with a descending or sigmoid colostomy is an irrigation candidate for fecal control. A colostomy more proximal than descending has too liquid and higher volume of fecal output to be managed through irrigation.

COMMUNITY-BASED CARE TIP:
If a patient discontinues colostomy irrigations after months or years of performance, due to illness, hospitalization, or preference, a bulk laxative or other stimulant may be routinely necessary to maintain regular bowel function.

◆ ESOPHAGITIS

Esophagitis is an acute or chronic inflammation of the esophagus. Severity of symptoms may be unrelated to the degree of esophageal tissue damage.

Pathophysiology/Etiology

1. Gastroesophageal reflux associated with an incompetent lower esophageal sphincter—gastric contents reflux (flow backward) through the lower esophageal sphincter into the esophagus (most common cause).
2. Can be the result of impaired gastric emptying from gastroparesis or partial gastric outlet obstruction.
3. The acidity of gastric content and amount of time in contact with esophageal mucosa is related to the degree of mucosal damage.
4. Infections—fungal (*Candida*); viral (herpes simplex or cytomegalovirus).
5. Chemical—alkali or acid.
6. Trauma—swallowing foreign body.
7. Medications—nonsteroidal anti-inflammatory drugs (NSAIDs), potassium chloride pills, quinidine, and antibiotics.
8. Mechanical obstruction—esophageal cancer, peptic stricture, or Schatzki's ring.
9. Prolonged NG intubation.
10. After gastric or duodenal surgery.
11. Repeated vomiting (common in persons with bulimia).
12. Motility disorders—achalasia, scleroderma, esophageal spasm.

Clinical Manifestations

1. Gastroesophageal reflux—heartburn, most often occurring 30 to 60 minutes after meals and with reclining positions. Complaints of spontaneous reflux (regurgitation) of sour or bitter gastric contents into the mouth. Dysphagia is a less common symptom.
2. Infectious esophagitis—dysphagia (difficulty or discomfort in swallowing) and odynophagia (sharp substernal pain on swallowing) may limit oral intake. May have substernal chest pain. Oral thrush may occur with 50% of patients with candidal esophagitis. Oral ulcers are common with herpes simplex esophagitis.
3. Chemical esophagitis—severe burning, chest pain, gagging, dysphagia, and drooling. Stridor and wheezing occur with aspiration.
4. Pill-induced esophagitis—severe retrosternal chest pain, odynophagia, dysphagia. Symptoms may begin several hours after swallowing a pill.
5. Mechanical lesions—dysphagia occurring with solids; chronic heartburn.
6. Motility disorders—dysphagia occurring with solids or liquids, chronic heartburn. May present with chest pain.

Diagnostic Evaluation

1. Endoscopy can visualize inflammation, lesions, strictures, or erosions; procedure can also dilate strictures.
2. Biopsy can be performed to identify tissue.
3. Cineradiographic esophagogram—identifies mass lesions, strictures, and abnormalities in peristalsis and esophageal clearing.

4. Esophageal manometry measures esophageal sphincter.
5. Acid perfusion test; onset of symptoms after ingestion of dilute hydrochloric acid and saline is considered positive.
6. Ambulatory 24-hour pH monitoring may be done. Determines the amount of gastroesophageal acid reflux.
7. Barium esophagography—use of barium with radiographic studies to diagnose mechanical and motility disorders.

Management

Management depends on the cause of esophagitis.

A. Lifestyle Changes
1. Head of bed raised 15 to 20 cm (6–8 in).
2. Do not lie down for 3 hours after eating—time frame for greatest reflux
3. Bland diet—avoid garlic, onion, alcohol, fatty foods, chocolate, coffee (even decaffeinated), citrus juices, colas, and tomato products.
4. Avoid overeating—causes lower esophageal sphincter relaxation.
5. No tight-fitting clothes or smoking.
6. Weight control.

B. Drug Therapy
1. Antacids—reduce gastric acidity. Use on an as-needed basis. Provide symptomatic relief but do not heal esophageal lesions.
2. Histamine-2(H_2) receptor antagonists—ranitidine (Zantac), cimetidine (Tagamet), famotidine (Pepcid); decrease gastric acid secretions. Provide symptomatic relief. May require lifelong therapy. Patients diagnosed with erosive esophagitis require higher doses.
3. Proton pump inhibitors—omeprazole (Prilosec); used for patients with erosive esophagitis that do not respond to H_2 receptor antagonists.
4. Prokinetic agents—cisapride (Propulsid), metoclopramide (Reglan), bethanechol (Urecholine); raise the lower esophageal sphincter pressure and improve gastric emptying.
5. Antifungals—used for candidal esophagitis. Topical agents include nystatin, clotrimazole (Lotrimin, Mycelex); oral agents such as ketoconazole (Nizoral) and fluconazole (Diflucan) may be used, or IV amphotericin B (Fungizone) or IV fluconazole.
6. Antivirals—ganciclovir (Cytovene) is used for cytomegalovirus. Herpetic esophagitis may be treated with acyclovir (Zovirax).
7. Sucralfate (Carafate) may be prescribed with H_2 blockers for pill-induced esophagitis. It provides a protective coating against gastric acids (dosed 2 hours apart to prevent decreased absorption of H_2 blocker).

C. Surgery
May be indicated for patients who do not respond to other approaches or who are noncompliant. Procedures include:
1. Fundoplication for reflux to throat—severe stricture.
2. Combined with vagotomy-pyloroplasty if associated with gastroduodenal ulcer.
3. Stricture may need to be resected, and an esophagogastrostomy may be required.

D. Dilatation Therapy
1. For strictures, dilatation therapy may be initiated; this may be done several times.

NURSING ALERT:
With chemical esophagitis—maintain airway, give IV fluids and analgesics. Nasogastric lavage and oral antidotes are not used due to risk of causing further damage. Surgery may be indicated.

Complications

1. Stricture formation
2. Ulceration of the esophagus, with or without fistula formation
3. Aspiration, may be complicated by pneumonia
4. Development of Barrett's esophagus—presence of columnar epithelium above the gastroesophageal junction associated with adenocarcinoma of the esophagus; related to chronic reflux induced injury

Nursing Interventions/ Patient Education

1. Teach the patient about prescribed medications, side effects, and when to notify the health care provider.
2. Inform the patient regarding medications that may exacerbate symptoms.
3. Advise the patient to sit or stand when taking any solid medication (pills, capsules): emphasize the need to follow the drug with at least 100 mL of liquid.
4. Emphasize to the patient and family what foods and activities to avoid: fatty foods, garlic, onions, alcohol, coffee and chocolate; straining, bending over, tight-fitting clothes, smoking.
5. Encourage the patient to sleep with the head of the bed elevated (not pillow elevation).
6. Encourage a weight-reduction program if the patient is overweight—to decrease intraabdominal pressure.

NURSING ALERT:
Anticholinergics may further impair functioning of the lower esophageal sphincter, allowing reflux; antihistamines, antidepressants, antihypertensives, antispasmodics, and some neuroleptics and antiparkinson drugs decrease saliva production, which may decrease acid clearance from the esophagus.

◆ HIATAL HERNIA

A hiatal hernia is a protrusion of a portion of the stomach through the hiatus of the diaphragm and into the thoracic cavity. There are two types of hiatal hernias:

1. Sliding hernia—the stomach and gastroesophageal junction slip up into the chest (most common).
2. Paraesophageal hernia (rolling hernia)—part of the greater curvature of the stomach rolls through the diaphragmatic defect.

Pathophysiology/Etiology

1. Muscle weakening due to aging or other conditions, such as esophageal carcinoma or trauma, or following certain surgical procedures.

Clinical Manifestations

1. May be asymptomatic
2. Heartburn (with or without regurgitation of gastric contents into the mouth)
3. Dysphagia; chest pain

Diagnostic Evaluation

1. Barium study of the esophagus outlines hernia.
2. Endoscopic examination visualizes defect.

Management

1. Elevation of head of bed (15–20 cm [6–8 in]) to reduce nighttime reflux.
2. Antacid therapy—to neutralize gastric acid.
3. Histamine-2 receptor antagonist (cimetidine, ranitidine)—if patient has esophagitis.
4. Surgical repair of hernia if symptoms are severe.

Complications

1. Incarceration of the portion of the stomach in the chest—constricts the blood supply.

Nursing Interventions/ Patient Education

1. Instruct patient on the prevention of reflux of gastric contents into esophagus by:
   a. Eating smaller meals.
   b. Avoiding stimulation of gastric secretions by omitting caffeine and alcohol.
   c. Refraining from smoking.
   d. Avoiding fatty foods—promote reflux and delay gastric emptying.
   e. Refraining from lying down for at least 1 hour after meals.
   f. Losing weight, if obese.
   g. Avoiding bending from the waist and/or wearing tight-fitting clothes.
2. Advise patient to report to health care facility immediately for the onset of acute chest pain—may indicate incarceration of a large paraesophageal hernia.

◆ ESOPHAGEAL TRAUMA AND PERFORATIONS

Esophageal trauma or perforations are injuries to the esophagus caused by external or internal insult.

Pathophysiology/Etiology

1. External—stab or bullet wounds, crush injuries, blunt trauma.
2. Internal
   a. Swallowed foreign objects (coins, pins, bones, dental appliances, caustic poisons).
   b. Spontaneous or postemetic rupture—usually in the presence of underlying esophageal disease (reflux, hiatal hernia).
   c. Mallory-Weiss syndrome—nonpenetrating mucosa tear at the gastroesophageal junction. Caused by an increase in transabdominal pressure from lifting, vomiting, or retching. A predisposing condition is alcoholism.

Clinical Manifestations

1. Pain at the site of injury or impaction, aggravated by swallowing; chest pain, may be severe
2. Dysphagia or odynophagia
3. Persistent foreign object sensation
4. Subcutaneous emphysema and crepitus of face, neck, or upper thorax—noted in cervical, thoracic, and esophageal perforations
5. Temperature elevation occurring within 24 hours
6. Blood-stained saliva or excessive salivation
7. Hematemesis; previous history of vomiting or retching—Mallory-Weiss syndrome
8. Respiratory difficulty if there is pressure on the tracheobronchial tree from injury or edema

Diagnostic Evaluation

1. History of recent esophageal trauma.
2. Chest x-ray to look for foreign body.
3. Esophagogram to outline trauma.
4. Endoscopy to directly visualize trauma

Management

1. Maintenance of adequate respiratory functioning; may require oxygen support or endotracheal intubation—to ensure an open airway in the presence of edema of the neck.
2. Replacement of fluids. May need blood transfusion. Bleeding may stop spontaneously; if not, endoscopic hemostatic therapy or surgery is indicated.
3. Restoration of the continuity of the esophagus by removing the cause.
4. For external wound injury—emergency first-aid wound care and surgical repair if indicated.
5. For swallowed foreign bodies:
   a. Barium swallow determines location of foreign body; usually removed through endoscopy.
   b. Some patients with a history of food impaction may be treated with a spasmolytic, such as IV glucagon.
6. For chemical ingestion:
   a. If lye or other caustic or organic solvent was swallowed, do NOT try to induce vomiting.
   b. Treat with IV fluids and analgesics.
   c. A gastrostomy may be performed, either as a temporary or a permanent means of feeding the patient.
   d. Resulting strictures may be relieved by dilating the narrow esophagus.
   e. Reconstructive surgery may be necessary to create a new passageway for food between pharynx and stomach.

Complications

1. Airway occlusion
2. Shock
3. Perforation with mediastinitis or pleural effusion
4. Stricture formation
5. Abscess or fistula formation

Nursing Assessment

1. Assess the following to determine status of patient:
   a. Vital signs
   b. Respiratory status
   c. Intake and output
   d. Bleeding
   e. Ability to swallow—choking, gagging.
2. Monitor the patient for hypovolemic shock.

Nursing Diagnoses

A. Fluid Volume Deficit related to blood loss from injury
B. Altered Nutrition, Less Than Body Requirements, related to esophageal injury
C. Ineffective Breathing Pattern related to pain and trauma
D. Pain related to injury

Nursing Interventions

A. *Maintaining Fluid Volume*
1. Administer IV fluids and blood transfusion for volume replacement, if indicated.
2. Monitor intake and output. Urine output should be greater than 30 cc/hour.
3. Monitor lab results (electrolytes, hemoglobin, and hematocrit) and report abnormal findings.

B. *Maintaining Nutritional Status*
1. Monitor daily weights and skin turgor.
2. Administer parenteral hyperalimentation as prescribed—to prevent gastric reflux into the esophagus, which may occur with enteral feedings.
3. Encourage progression of diet through NG, esophagostomy, or oral feedings once esophagoscopy or esophagogram reveals healing of the esophagus.
4. Continue to monitor intake and output.

C. *Maintaining Respiratory Function*
1. Auscultate the lungs and trachea for stridor, crackles, or wheezes. Assess respiratory rate, depth, use of accessory muscles, and skin color.
2. Position patient in semi-Fowler's position to facilitate breathing and reduce neck edema.
3. Monitor vital signs frequently for signs and symptoms of shock and infection.
4. Administer oxygen as prescribed.
5. Have emergency airway equipment at bedside.

D. *Reducing Pain*
1. Administer analgesics as prescribed—intravenous analgesia may be required to control pain and allow the esophagus to rest.
2. Provide reassurance and support.
3. Assess and record pain relief.
4. Evaluate for symptoms that may indicate spillage of digestive contents into the mediastinum, pleura, or abdominal cavity—sudden onset of acute pain.

Patient Education/ Health Maintenance

1. Instruct the patient on the indications and side effects of analgesics.
2. Inform the patient on the signs and symptoms to report on possible complications: increase in severity or nature of pain; difficulty breathing or swallowing.
3. See Procedures Guidelines 16-7: Teaching the Patient With Dysphagia How to Swallow. This assists the patient who has difficulty swallowing after injury or surgical correction of the oropharynx or upper esophagus (also helpful with neurologic deficit; stroke).
4. Teach the patient about tests or surgical procedures that may be performed.

Evaluation

A. Fluid volume is maintained. Hypovolemic shock is prevented/ treated.
B. Nutritional status is maintained; intake sufficient; diet progressing, if possible
C. Respiratory function is maintained; vital signs stable; lungs clear
D. Demonstrates increased comfort

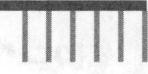

PROCEDURE GUIDELINES 16-7 ◆ Teaching the Patient With Dysphagia How to Swallow

EQUIPMENT

suction
oxygen
face mask
selected foods
glass with straw

PROCEDURE	NURSING ACTION	RATIONALE

PREPARATION

1. Explain to the patient that you plan to work with him or her in developing an effective swallow.

2. Ensure that emergency equipment is available at the bedside—suction, oxygen, face mask.
3. Place the patient in an upright sitting position in a chair or support with pillows in high-Fowler's position if unable to get out of bed—for about 20 minutes before and 45–60 minutes after meals.
4. Provide mouth care before meals. Suction the patient if secretions are present. If the patient's mouth is dry, provide a lemon wedge or pickle to suck on.
5. Prepare an environment that is pleasant, peaceful, and without interruptions. Remove distracters, such as TV, radio.

FOOD AND FLUID SELECTION

6. Foods should be chosen that hold some shape; moist enough to prevent crumbling but dry enough to hold a bolus shape—casseroles, custards, scrambled eggs.
7. Mugs and glasses with spouts or a straw should be used for liquids.
8. Avoid sticky foods—peanut butter, chocolate, milk, ice cream.
9. Dry foods can be moistened with margarine, gravy, or broths. If liquids are a problem, juices can be thickened with sherbets.
10. Avoid tepid or room temperature foods.

INSTRUCTIONS DURING MEALS

11. Have patient position head in the midline and forward, chin pointed toward chest.

12. Instruct the patient to smell the food before each bite; hold each bite for a few seconds; hold lips together firmly; concentrate on swallowing; then swallow.
13. If the patient has an increase in saliva during the meal, instruct the patient to collect the saliva with the tongue and consciously swallow it between bites throughout the meal.
14. If the patient complains of a dry mouth during meals, instruct the patient to move the tongue in a circular fashion against the insides of the cheeks.
15. Caution the patient against talking during the meal or with the mouth full of food.

RATIONALE

1. The patient's cooperation, concentration, and directed participation are essential to the success of this learning experience.
2. For use in the event that the patient chokes, vomits, or aspirates
3. This will allow time to adjust and relax in this position before meals; allows gravity to assist the swallowing procedure during meals; helps prevent reflux or regurgitation after meals.
4. This will increase patient's ability to taste and enjoy the sensation of eating.

5. Patient must be able to concentrate on the process of swallowing in a relaxed manner.

6. Foods that crumble may be aspirated when they fall apart; foods that are too moist may be drooled through the lips.
7. These utensils help prevent liquids from leaking out of corners of patient's mouth.
8. These foods stimulate thick mucos and will make swallowing more difficult.
9. Foods need to be of a consistency that will hold a bolus form until swallowed.

10. Hot and cold foods are thought to maximally stimulate receptors that activate swallowing mechanism.

11. Improves ability to consciously swallow without food falling down the posterior pharynx. Support patient's forehead with a hand if the patient lacks neck control.
12. Concentrating on each step before swallowing will increase the effectiveness of the swallow.

13. This will help prevent aspiration of saliva between mouthfuls.

14. This will help stimulate salivation.

15. Talking or laughing during eating is a common cause of airway obstruction.

(continued)

PROCEDURE GUIDELINES 16-7 ◆ Teaching the Patient With Dysphagia How to Swallow (continued)

PROCEDURE (cont'd)	NURSING ACTION	RATIONALE

FOLLOW-UP CARE

16. Provide mouth care after meals.
17. Record the amount of intake, the patient's taste and food preferences, progress, and any special tactics that were effective in helping the swallowing process.
18. Encourage family members to participate in the patient's feeding program.

16. Food particles may collect in the mouth or cheeks.
17. Progress notes will assist in moving toward self-care.

18. This will help provide continuity on discharge.

FEEDING THE PATIENT WITH AN AFFECTED SIDE OF THE MOUTH (FACIAL PARALYSIS, HEMIPLEGIA)

1. Turn the patient to the unaffected side.

2. Place food on the unaffected side of mouth rather than in the middle of the mouth.
3. Encourage the patient to form a bolus by moving the food around the mouth with the tongue.

1. This helps prevent food from falling down the weaker/paralyzed part of the oral cavity, a possible cause of aspiration.
2. Permits food to be managed more effectively.

3. This assists in placing food in a proper position for swallowing, rather than permitting food to collect near the cheek.

◆ MOTILITY DISORDERS OF THE ESOPHAGUS

Pathophysiology/Etiology

1. Primary motility disorders include achalasia, diffuse esophageal spasm, and those of nonspecific origin.
   a. Achalasia refers to excessive resting tone of the lower esophageal sphincter (LES), incomplete relaxation of the lower esophageal sphincter with swallowing, and failure of normal peristalsis in the lower two thirds of the esophagus. The pathology is related to defective innervation of the myenteric plexus innervating the involuntary muscles of the esophagus.
   b. Diffuse esophageal spasm is a motor disorder in which high-amplitude, nonpropulsive, nonperistaltic tertiary contractions (a form of aperistalsis) are present. LES functioning is frequently normal.
2. Secondary motility disorders may be caused by neuromuscular, GI, endocrine, or connective tissue disorders.

Clinical Manifestations

1. Achalasia
   a. Gradual onset of dysphagia with solids and liquids.
   b. Substernal discomfort or a feeling of fullness.
   c. Regurgitation of undigested food during a meal or within several hours after a meal.
   d. Weight loss.
2. Diffuse esophageal spasm.
   a. Intermittent dysphagia for solids or liquids—does not progress to continuous dysphagia.
   b. Stress large volume of food and hot or cold liquids may aggravate symptoms.
   c. Anterior chest pain

3. Secondary motility disorders.
   a. Symptoms of esophagitis from gastroesophageal reflux.

Diagnostic Evaluations

1. Achalasia.
   a. Chest x-ray, which may show an enlarged, fluid-filled esophagus.
   b. Barium esophagography showing dilation, decreased or absence of peristalsis, decreased emptying and a "bird beak" narrowing of the distal esophagus.
   c. Esophageal manometry to confirm the diagnoses suspected.
   d. Endoscopic ultrasound or a chest CT for suspected tumor.
2. Diffuse esophageal spasm.
   a. Barium esophagography showing simultaneous contractions of the esophagus having a "corkscrew" or "rosary bead" appearance.
   b. Esophageal manometry showing intermittent contractions with episodes of normal peristalsis.
3. Other motility disorders.
   a. Diagnostic workup may include barium esophagography or manometry.

Management

1. Achalasia
   a. Drug therapy using calcium channel blockers, such as nifedipine (Procardin), to reduce the LES pressure. This type of treatment is usually best for patients presenting with mild symptoms and a nondilated esophagus or patients who are medically unstable to undergo invasive therapies.

b. Esophageal dilation using a balloon-tipped catheter is the preferred treatment for most patients.

c. Surgical therapy (Heller's myotomy of the lower esophageal sphincter) may be used on patients who do not respond to balloon dilation. This surgery requires a laparotomy or thoracotomy or may be done through a thoracoscope.

2. Diffuse esophageal spasm.
   a. Drug therapy using nitrates and calcium channel blockers is the primary treatment.
   b. Dilation may provide some symptoms relief.
   c. Surgical myotomy is used rarely for patients with a debilitating disorder who are able to withstand a surgical procedure.

3. Other motility disorders:
   a. Treatment of the gastroesophageal reflux.
   b. Dilation may be required for peptic stricture.

Complications

1. Malnutrition
2. Pneumonia, lung abscess, bronchiectasis from nocturnal regurgitation causing aspiration
3. Esophagitis
4. Perforation from dilation procedure
5. Peptic stricture or Barrett's esophagus from severe erosive esophagitis

Nursing Assessment

1. Assess for difficulty with swallowing, vomiting, weight loss, chest pain associated with eating.
2. Inquire as to what facilitates passage of food, such as position changes, use of liquids.

Nursing Diagnoses

A. Altered Nutrition, Less Than Body Requirements, related to dysphagia
B. Pain related to heartburn or surgical procedure

Nursing Interventions

A. *Improving Nutritional Status*
1. Direct patient to eat sitting in an upright position; eat slowly and chew food thoroughly.
2. Avoid food and beverages that precipitate symptoms.
3. Suggest that the patient sleep with head elevated to avoid reflux or aspiration.
4. Provide a bland diet and tell the patient to avoid alcohol as well as spicy, very hot, and very cold foods, to minimize symptoms.
5. Eliminate sources of tension as a precipitating factor producing stress during mealtime.
6. Administer pharmacologic agents as prescribed.

B. *Promoting Comfort*
1. Assess patient for discomfort, chest pain, regurgitation, and cough. If surgical procedure was performed, assess for incisional pain.

2. Provide appropriate postoperative care. Incisional approach determines nature of postoperative care; thus, an incision through chest implies nursing care similar to that given to a patient with a thoracotomy (see p. 201).
3. Administer analgesics as ordered.
4. Assess for effectiveness of pain medication.

Patient Education/Health Maintenance

1. Encourage lifestyle activity changes similar to those for patients with reflux (see page 507).
2. See Procedure Guidelines 16-7: Teaching the Patient With Dysphagia How to Swallow (page 509).
3. Provide information on drugs to avoid, i.e., anticholinergics.
4. Advise patients to avoid medications with anticholinergic properties (such as antihistamines), which increase lower esophageal sphincter pressure.
5. Provide information on all diagnostic procedures or surgery performed.

Evaluation

A. Demonstrates proper positioning for eating; describes dietary habits that minimize symptoms; compliant with medications regimen
B. Demonstrates improved comfort
C. Verbalizes how to take medications and potential side effects

◆ ESOPHAGEAL DIVERTICULUM

An esophageal diverticulum is an outpouching of the esophageal wall, usually in the cervical posterior side, secondary to an obstructive or inflammatory process.

Pathophysiology/Etiology

1. Zenker's diverticulum—protrusion of pharyngeal mucosa at the pharyngoesophageal junction between the interior pharyngeal constrictor and cricopharyngeal muscle.
2. Mid or Distal Esophageal diverticula may develop above strictures or may be secondary to motility disorders.

Clinical Manifestations

A. *Zenker's Diverticulum*
1. Difficulty in swallowing, fullness in neck, throat discomfort, a feeling that food stops before it reaches the stomach, and regurgitation of undigested food.
2. Belching, gurgling, or nocturnal coughing brought about by diverticulum becoming filled with food or liquid, which is regurgitated and may irritate the trachea.
3. Halitosis and foul taste in mouth caused by food decomposing in a pouch (diverticulum).
4. Weight loss due to nutritional depletion.

GERONTOLGIC ALERT:
Hoarseness, asthma, and pneumonitis may be the only signs in the very elderly.

B. Mid or Distal Esophageal Diverticula
1. Generally no symptoms.

Diagnostic Evaluation

1. Barium esophagogram outlines diverticulum.
2. Endoscopy is not indicated and may be dangerous due to the possibility of rupture.

Management

A. Zenker's Diverticula
1. Small diverticula may not be treated, but the underlying cause is treated with dilatation or myotomy.
2. A transverse cervical diverticulectomy or diverticuloplexy with suspension and cricopharyngeal myotomy may be done.
   a. Caution is taken to avoid injury to common carotid artery and internal jugular vein.
   b. Sac is dissected free and then excised flush with esophageal wall.

B. Mid or Distal Esophageal Diverticula
1. Underlying primary condition must be treated.

Complications

1. Aspiration pneumonia
2. Malnutrition
3. Lung abscess

Nursing Assessment

1. Obtain history of dysphagia, coughing, throat discomfort, choking, regurgitation of food.
2. Evaluate for halitosis.
3. Determine what measures assist the patient with food intake; what foods/fluids the patient is able to tolerate.
4. Evaluate weight loss and dietary habits.

Nursing Diagnoses

A. Altered Nutrition, Less Than Body Requirements, related to dysphagia
B. Pain related to symptoms and surgical procedure

Nursing Interventions

A. Improving Nutritional Status
1. Provide frequent, small meals, which are better tolerated.
2. Elevate head of bed for 2 hours after eating.

3. Monitor intake and output.
4. Weigh daily.

B. Maintaining Comfort and Preventing Complications
1. Preoperatively, or if the condition is nonoperative, implement nursing interventions similar to those for esophagitis.
2. Postoperatively, wound care is similar to that of other surgical incisions of the same anatomic position, for example, thoracotomy (p. 201) or neck surgery.
3. Administer appropriate pain medications and assess effectiveness.
4. Patient may need oral suctioning to control drooling.
5. Maintain NG tube if in place.
   a. Irrigate tube as ordered.
   b. Do not manipulate NG tube due to location of tube and suture line.

Patient Education/Health Maintenance

1. Instruct patient regarding treatment of esophagitis caused by gastroesophageal reflux (page 506).
2. Instruct patient on importance of good oral hygiene.

Evaluation

A. Tolerates oral feedings; maintains weight or shows gradual increase
B. Demonstrates improved comfort

◆ CANCER OF THE ESOPHAGUS

Malignant lesions of the esophagus occur in four types worldwide: squamous cell, adenocarcinoma, carcinosarcoma, and sarcoma.

Pathophysiology/Etiology

A. Incidence
1. Incidence of adenocarcinoma of the distal and middle third of the esophagus appears to be increasing in the Western world.
2. Squamous cell carcinoma, most often originating in the upper half of the esophagus, appears to have an equal incidence to adenocarcinoma.
3. Highest rate in the United States occurs in men, who are usually older than age of 60; more common in nonwhite males.

B. Associated Factors
Cause is unknown, but has been associated with:

1. Barrett's esophagus
2. Achalasia
3. Chronic use of alcohol and tobacco (squamous cell carcinoma)
4. Genetic predisposition—nonwhite male population
5. Ingestion of caustic substances (such as lye), which cause esophageal strictures
6. Other head and neck cancers

Clinical Manifestations

1. Dysphagia is the usual presenting symptom, although it is a late sign by which time there often is regional or systemic involvement
2. Mild, atypical chest pain associated with eating precedes dysphagia, but is rarely significant enough for the patient to seek health care
3. Pain on swallowing (odynophagia)
4. Progressive weight loss
5. Hoarseness (if laryngeal involvement)
6. Lymphadenopathy (supraclavicular or cervical) or hepatomegaly with metastatic involvement
7. Later symptoms—hiccups, respiratory difficulty, foul breath, regurgitation of food and saliva

Diagnostic Evaluation

1. Chest x-ray may show adenopathy; mediastinal, widening, metastasis; or a tracheoesophageal fistula.
2. Endoscopy with cytology and biopsy.
3. Barium esophagram may show polypoid, infiltrative, or ulcerative lesion requiring biopsy.
4. CT may be helpful in delineating the extent of the tumor as well as in identifying presence of adjacent tissue invasion and metastases.

Management

1. The goal of treatment may be cure or palliation, depending on the staging of the tumor and the patient's overall condition in relation to nutritional, cardiovascular, pulmonary, and functional status.
2. The wide variability in treatment reflects the overall poor results from any one approach.
3. Surgery
   a. Lesions of the middle and lower esophagus are excised with use of the thoracotomy approach with esophagogastrectomy or colon interposition (section of colon is used to replace the excised portion of the esophagus).
   b. Lesions of the cervical esophagus are excised with a bilateral neck dissection and esophagogastrectomy; laryngectomy and thyroidectomy may be necessary.
   c. A two-step approach may be selected when resection with a cervical esophagostomy and feeding gastrostomy are performed initially; subsequent reconstructive surgery is performed.
4. Radiation, chemotherapy, or their combination; combination therapy appears to have better results.
5. Palliative treatment of dysphagia through dilation done by endoscopy or laser therapy.
6. The goal of palliative treatment is to reduce the complications of the tumor to improve quality of life. Any one or a combination of the aforementioned therapies can be used for palliative treatment.

Complications

1. Preoperatively: malnutrition, aspiration pneumonitis; hemorrhage; sepsis; tracheoesophageal fistula

2. Postoperatively: dumping syndrome, nutritional deficiencies, reflux esophagitis, anastomosis leakage

Nursing Assessment

1. Obtain history of symptoms, such as dysphagia, pain, cough, hoarseness.
2. Evaluate for weight loss and dietary changes.
3. Examine for lymphadenopathy.

Nursing Diagnoses

A. Altered Nutrition, Less Than Body Requirements, related to disease process and treatment
B. Risk for infection related to chronic disease, invasive procedures and treatment

Nursing Interventions

A. *Improving Nutritional and Fluid Status*
1. Provide the preoperative patient with a high-protein, high-calorie diet. Nutritional supplements may be indicated. Total parenteral nutrition may be ordered if unable to take foods/fluids orally.
2. Postoperatively, administer IV fluids as prescribed: initially the patient may require large volumes if extensive excision of lymph nodes was performed. Total parenteral nutrition may be ordered.
3. Assess for bowel sounds; administer fluids per NG tube, as prescribed.
4. Encourage patient in advancing diet from liquids to soft foods.
5. Remind patient to remain in upright position for approximately 2 hours after eating to promote digestion.
6. Provide mouth care for patient comfort and hygiene.

B. *Monitoring for Complications*
1. Monitor blood pressure, pulse, respiration, and temperature to note early onset of hemorrhage, infection, dysrhythmias, aspiration, or anastomosis leakage.
2. Observe drainage from incision and/or chest tube for bleeding or purulence.
3. Administer oxygen as prescribed to facilitate tissue oxygenation.

C. *Patient Education/Health Maintenance*
1. Encourage the patient to avoid overeating, take small bites, chew food well; avoid chunks of meat and stringy raw vegetables and fruit.
2. Depending on type of surgery, frequent small meals may be better tolerated.
3. Encourage rest postoperatively and advancing activities as tolerated.
4. Instruct patient regarding signs and symptoms of complications to report: nausea, vomiting, elevated temperature, cough, difficulty swallowing.

Evaluation

A. Maintains nutritional status: weight gain; good skin turgor; eating small, frequent meals if possible
B. No evidence of complications

Gastroduodenal Disorders

◆ GASTROINTESTINAL BLEEDING

Note: GI bleeding is not just a gastroduodenal disorder, but may occur anywhere along the alimentary tract. Bleeding is a symptom of an upper or lower GI disorder. It may be obvious in emesis or stool, or it may be occult (hidden).

Pathophysiology/Etiology

1. Trauma anywhere along the GI tract
2. Erosions or ulcers
3. Rupture of an enlarged vein, such as a varicosity (esophageal or gastric varices)
4. Inflammation, such as esophagitis (caused by acid or bile), gastritis, inflammatory bowel disease (chronic ulcerative colitis, Crohn's disease), and bacterial infection
5. Irritation of mucous membrane due to certain drugs, such as alcohol and aspirin-containing compounds
6. Diverticulosis
7. Neoplasms
8. Vascular lesions or disorders, such as bowel ischemia, aortoenteric fistula
9. Mallory-Weiss syndrome
10. Anal disorders, such as hemorrhoids or fissure

Clinical Manifestations

A. Characteristics of Blood
1. Bright red—vomited from high in esophagus (hematemesis): from rectum or distal colon (coating stool)
2. Mixed with dark red—higher up in colon and small intestine: mixed with stool
3. Shades of black ("coffee ground")—esophagus, stomach, and duodenum: vomitus from these areas
4. Tarry stool (melena)—occurs in patient who accumulates excessive blood in the stomach

B. Signs and Symptoms of Bleeding
1. Massive bleeding
   a. Acute, bright red hematemesis or large amount of melena with clots in the stool
   b. Rapid pulse, drop in blood pressure, hypovolemia, and shock
2. Subacute bleeding
   a. Intermittent melena or coffee-ground emesis
   b. Hypotension
   c. Weakness, dizziness.
3. Chronic bleeding
   a. Intermittent appearance of blood
   b. Increased weakness, paleness, or shortness of breath
   c. Occult blood

Diagnostic Evaluation

1. It is not difficult to diagnose bleeding, but it may be difficult to locate the source of bleeding.
2. History—change in bowel pattern, presence of pain or tenderness, recent intake of food and what kind (red beets?), alcohol consumption, drugs such as aspirin or steroids.
3. Complete blood count, including coagulation studies, may show decreased hematocrit and hemoglobin; abnormal prothrombin time.
4. Endoscopy—for direct visualization of mucosa.
5. Imaging—may detect etiology of bleeding.
6. Test of stool for occult blood.

Management

A. Based on Etiology
1. If aspirin is the cause, eliminate aspirin and treat bleeding.
2. If ulcer is the cause, an anti-ulcer drug is prescribed along with lifestyle change and dietary change.
3. If cancer is the cause, tumor to be removed.

B. Emergency Intervention
1. Patient remains on NPO status.
2. Intravenous lines and oxygen therapy initiated.
3. If life-threatening bleeding occurs, treat shock, administer blood replacement.

C. Nasogastric Intubation
1. Short tube such as Levin's, Salem sump, or Ewald may be used for stomach irrigation using saline. It is controversial whether this remains a therapeutic measure or has become more of a diagnostic one.

D. Other Measures
1. Electrocoagulation and photocoagulation (laser) may be the treatment of choice. Instillation of topical thrombin to clot blood at the site of bleeding may be used as adjuvant therapy.

NURSING ALERT:
Because of the action of topical thrombin, it is used only on the surface of bleeding tissue and never is injected into the blood vessels, where intravascular clotting could occur.

2. Endoscopy used in conjunction with management measures as well as in diagnostic evaluation.
3. Pharmacotherapy depends on cause; can include histamine blockers as either continuous IV or bolus infusion to block the acid-secreting action of histamine, and a cytoprotective agent such as sucralfate (Carafate).
4. Surgery is indicated when more conservative measures fail.

Complications

1. Hemorrhage
2. Shock
3. Death

Nursing Assessment

1. Obtain history regarding:
   a. Change in bowel patterns or hemorrhoids.
   b. Change in color of stools (dark black, red, or streaked with blood).
   c. Alcohol consumption.
   d. Medications, such as aspirin, antibiotics, anticoagulants.
   e. Hematemesis.

2. Obtain vital signs and weight.
3. Evaluate for presence of abdominal pain or tenderness; rectal pain.
4. Assess for any active bleeding.
5. Test for occult blood, if indicated.

Nursing Diagnoses

A. Fluid Volume Deficit related to blood loss
B. Altered Nutrition, Less Than Body Requirements, related to nausea, vomiting, diarrhea

Nursing Interventions

A. *Attaining Normal Fluid Volume*
1. Maintain NG tube and NPO status to rest GI tract and evaluate bleeding.
2. Monitor intake and output every 4 hours or more frequently as indicated, to evaluate fluid status.
3. Monitor vital signs every 4 hours or more frequently as needed.
4. Observe for changes indicating shock, such as tachycardia, hypotension, increased respirations, decreased urine output, change in mental status.
5. Administer IV fluids and blood products as ordered to maintain volume.

B. *Attaining Balanced Nutritional Status*
1. Weigh daily to monitor caloric status.
2. Administer IV fluids, TPN if ordered to promote hydration and nutrition while on PO restrictions.
3. Begin liquids when patient is no longer NPO. Advance diet as tolerated. Diet should be high caloric, high protein. Frequent, small feedings may be indicated.
4. Offer snacks; high protein supplements

Patient Education/Health Maintenance

1. Discuss the cause and treatment of GI bleeding with patient.
2. Instruct patient regarding signs and symptoms of GI bleeding: melena, emesis that is bright red or "coffee ground" color, rectal bleeding, weakness, fatigue, shortness of breath.
3. Instruct patient on how to test stool or emesis for occult blood, if applicable.

Evaluation

A. Fluid volume is maintained; hypovolemic shock is prevented
B. Nutritional status is maintained; body weight is maintained or increased

◆ PEPTIC ULCER DISEASE

A peptic ulcer is a lesion in the mucosa of the lower esophagus, stomach, pylorus or duodenum (Fig. 16-3).

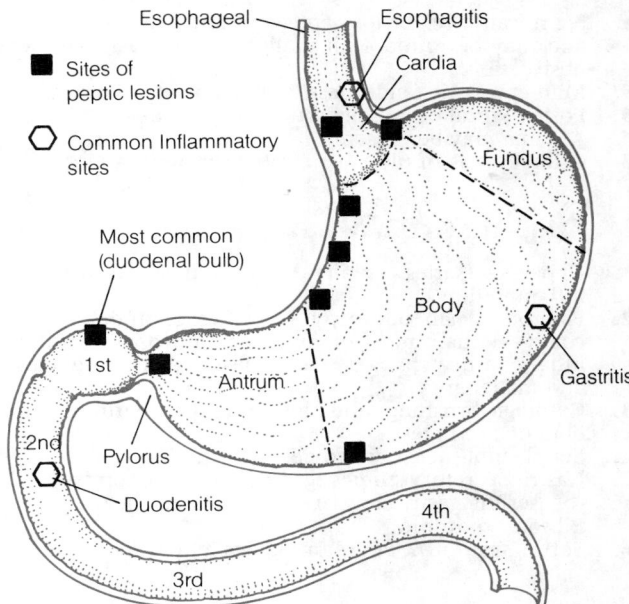

FIGURE 16-3 *The stomach is divided on the basis of its physiologic functions into two main portions. The proximal two thirds, the fundic gland area, acts as a receptacle for ingested food and secretes acid and pepsin. The distal third, the pyloric gland area, mixes and propels food into the duodenum and produces the hormone gastrin. "Peptic" lesions may occur in the esophagus (esophagitis), stomach (gastritis), or duodenum (duodenitis). Note peptic ulcer sites and common inflammatory sites.*

Pathophysiology/Etiology

1. *Helicobacter pylori* infection—exact mechanism is unclear.
2. Nonsteroidal anti-inflammatory drug (NSAID)–induced ulcers.
   a. The risk of gastric ulcers is much greater than duodenal ulcers.
   b. Aspirin is the most ulcerogenic NSAID.
3. Hypersecretion of acid:
   a. Believed to be caused by an overactive vagus nerve, which stimulates the release of gastrin.
   b. Methylxanthines (tea, coffee, cola, and chocolate) and smoking may also increase gastric acidity
   c. Found in disorders such as Zollinger-Ellison syndrome (multiple peptic ulcers).
4. Genetic predisposition and stress appear to be controversial factors.

Clinical Manifestations

1. Pain occurring in the epigastric area radiating to the back. Present in 80% to 90% of the patients. Pain may be described as dull, aching, gnawing. Nocturnal pain may also be present.
2. Pain may increase when the stomach is empty, approximately $\frac{1}{2}$ to 2 hours after eating. Patients may report relief from pain after eating or taking antacids (common with duodenal ulcers).
3. Nausea and anorexia (gastric ulcers).

4. Significant weight loss and vomiting are uncommon and may be found with malignancy or gastric outlet obstruction.
5. Mild epigastric tenderness with deep palpation.
6. Positive fecal occult blood may be present.
7. Anemia may be present.
8. Leukocytosis (if ulcer penetration or perforation).

Diagnostic Evaluation

1. Upper GI series usually outlines ulcer or area of inflammation
2. Fiberoptic panendoscopy (esophagogastroduodenoscopy)—visualization of duodenal mucosa; identifies inflammatory changes, ulcers, lesions, bleeding sites, and malignancy.
3. Cytologic brushings and biopsies may be performed to obtained samples.
4. Serial stool specimens to detect occult blood
5. Gastric secretory studies (gastric acid secretion test and the serum gastric level test)—elevated in Zollinger-Ellison syndrome
6. Serum test for *H. pylori* antibodies may be positive.

Management

A. Specific Pharmacotherapy
1. H$_2$ receptor antagonists, such as cimetidine (Tagamet), ranitidine (Zantac), famotidine (Pepcid)—inhibit action of histamine on the H$_2$ receptors of the parietal cells, thus reducing gastric acid output and concentration.
2. Antisecretory or proton pump inhibitor drug omeprazole (Prilosec)—inhibits the production of hydrochloric acid in the stomach. Heals ulcers quickly (in 4 to 8 weeks).
3. Cytoprotective drug sucralfate (Carafate)—adheres to and protects the ulcer surface by forming a protective barrier against acid, bile, pepsin.
4. Acid-neutralizing agents (antacids)—provide additional relief of symptoms. Not used alone as treatment.
5. Antisecretory and cytoprotective drug misoprostol (Cytotec)—prostoglandin analogue inhibits hydrochloric acid production in the stomach.
6. Antidiarrheal agent bismuth subsalicylate (Pepto-Bismol)—has antibacterial action against *H. pylori* and enhances mucosal protection through bicarbonate and prostaglandin production.
7. Antibiotics such as tetracycline and metronidazole (Flagyl) used with bismuth as "triple therapy" to eradicate *H. pylori*.
8. For NSAID ulcers—discontinue NSAID and treat as mentioned above. If NSAID is restarted, administer with misoprostol.

B. Dietary Measures
1. Well-balanced diet, high fiber content, meals at regular intervals.
2. Avoid caffeine, colas, and alcohol.
3. Avoid smoking—decreases healing rate and increases recurrence.

C. Surgery Indicated in emergency situations for uncontrolled bleeding or bleeding that developed despite chronic drug maintenance therapy (Fig. 16-4)
1. Gastrojejunostomy and vagotomy

a. The jejunum is anastomosed to the stomach to provide a second outlet of gastric contents.
b. The severed vagus nerve reduces secretions and movements of the stomach.
2. Antrectomy and vagotomy
a. The resected portion includes a small cuff of duodenum, the pylorus, and the antrum (about one half of the stomach).
b. The stump of the duodenum is closed by suture and the side of the jejunum is anastomosed to the cut end of the stomach.
3. Subtotal gastrectomy
a. The resected portion includes a small cuff of the duodenum, pylorus, and from two thirds to three quarters of the stomach.
b. The duodenum or side of the jejunum is anastomosed to the remaining portion of the stomach.
4. Vagotomy and pyloroplasty
a. A longitudinal incision is made in the pylorus, and it is closed transversely to permit the muscle to relax and to establish an enlarged outlet.
b. This compensates for the impaired gastric emptying produced by the vagotomy.

Complications

1. GI hemorrhage
2. Ulcer perforation
3. Gastric outlet obstruction

Nursing Assessment

1. Determine location, character, radiation of pain, factors aggravating or relieving pain, how long it lasts, when it occurs.
2. Ask about eating patterns, regularity, types of food, eating circumstances.
3. Take a social history of alcohol consumption and smoking.
4. Ask about medications (especially aspirin, anti-inflammatory drugs, or steroids).
5. Determine if GI bleeding has been experienced.
6. Take vital signs, including lying, standing, and sitting blood pressures and pulses, to determine if orthostasis is present due to bleeding.

Nursing Diagnoses

A. Fluid Volume Deficit related to hemorrhage
B. Pain related to epigastric distress secondary to hypersecretion of acid, mucosal erosion, or perforation
C. Diarrhea related to GI bleeding or antacid therapy
D. Altered Nutrition, Less Than Body Requirements, related to the disease process
E. Knowledge Deficit related to physical, dietary, and pharmacologic treatment of disease.

Nursing Interventions

A. Avoiding Fluid Volume Deficit
1. Monitor intake and output continuously to determine fluid volume status.
2. Observe stools for occult blood.

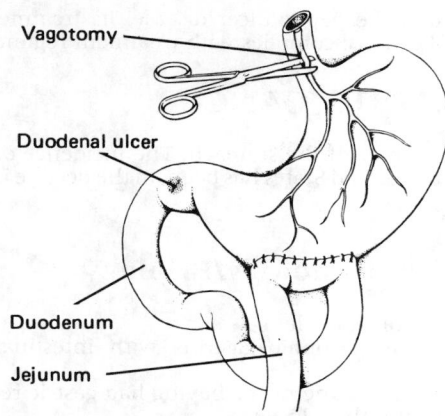

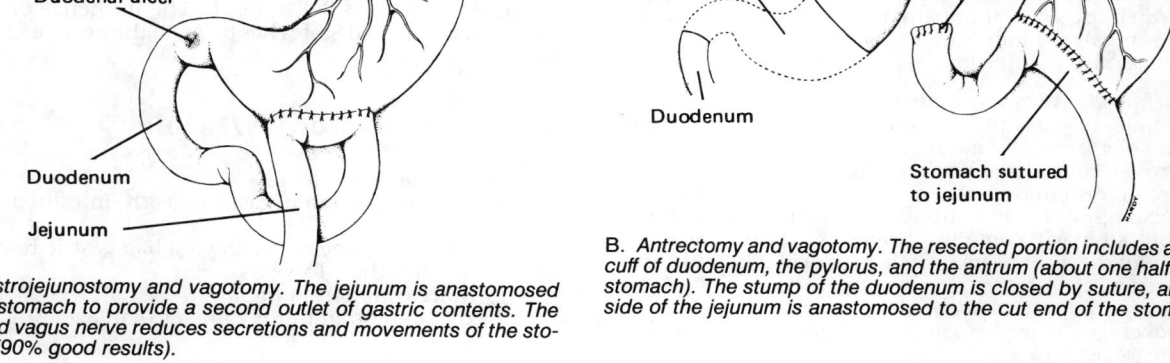

A. *Gastrojejunostomy and vagotomy. The jejunum is anastomosed to the stomach to provide a second outlet of gastric contents. The severed vagus nerve reduces secretions and movements of the stomach (90% good results).*

B. *Antrectomy and vagotomy. The resected portion includes a small cuff of duodenum, the pylorus, and the antrum (about one half of the stomach). The stump of the duodenum is closed by suture, and the side of the jejunum is anastomosed to the cut end of the stomach.*

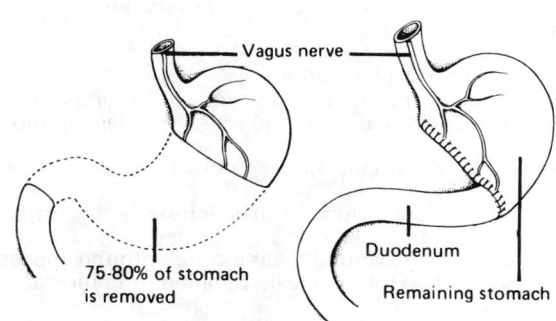

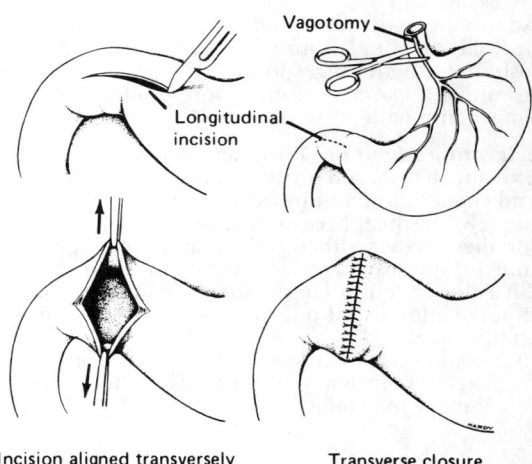

C. *Subtotal gastrectomy. The resected portion includes a small cuff of the duodenum, the pylorus, and from two thirds to three quarters of the stomach. The duodenum or side of the jejunum is anastomosed to the remaining portion of the stomach.*

D. *Vagotomy and pyloroplasty. A longitudinal incision is made in the pylorus, and it is closed transversely to permit the muscle to relax and to establish an enlarged outlet. This compensates for the impaired gastric emptying produced by vagotomy.*

FIGURE 16-4 Surgical procedures for peptic ulcer.

3. Monitor hemoglobin and hematocrit and electrolytes.
4. Administer prescribed IV fluids and blood replacement, as prescribed.
5. Insert an NG tube as prescribed and monitor the tube drainage for signs of visible and occult blood.
6. Administer medications through the NG tube to neutralize acidity, as prescribed.
7. Prepare patient for saline lavage, as ordered.
8. Observe the patient for an increase in pulse and a decrease in blood pressure (signs of shock).
9. Prepare the patient for angiography or surgery to determine or stop the source of bleeding.

B. *Achieving Pain Relief*
1. Administer prescribed medication.

2. Encourage bed rest to reduce physical activity and to separate patient from usual environment if pain continues.
3. Provide small, frequent meals to prevent gastric distention if not NPO.
4. Teach the patient that caffeine, alcoholic beverages, and nicotine may increase gastric acidity and promote erosion of the gastric mucosa.
5. Advise the patient about the irritating effects on the gastric mucosa of certain drugs, such as aspirin, NSAIDs, and certain antibiotics.

C. *Decreasing Diarrhea*
1. Monitor patient's elimination patterns to determine effects of medications.

2. Monitor vital signs and watch for signs of hypovolemia. Persistent diarrhea may be a sign of bleeding.
3. Restrict foods and fluids that promote diarrhea: raw vegetables, fruits, whole grain cereals, carbonated drinks.
4. Administer antidiarrheal medication as prescribed.
5. Watch for signs of impaired skin integrity (erythema, soreness) around anus to promote comfort and decrease risk of infection.

D. Achieving Adequate Nutrition
1. Eliminate foods that cause pain or distress; otherwise, the diet is usually not restricted.
2. Provide small, frequent feedings on time. This will decrease distention and the release of gastrin. Frequent feedings also help neutralize gastric secretions and dilute stomach contents. However, eating small, frequent meals or snacks can lead to acid rebound, which occurs 2 to 4 hours after eating.
3. Advise the patient to avoid coffee and other caffeinated beverages as well as carbonated drinks; these may increase acid.
4. Advise the patient to avoid extremely hot or cold food or fluids, to chew thoroughly, and to eat in a leisurely fashion for better digestion.
5. Administer parenteral nutrition if bleeding is prolonged and patient is emaciated, as ordered.

E. Educating About the Treatment Regimen
1. Explain all tests and procedures to increase knowledge and cooperation; minimize anxiety.
2. Review the health care provider's recommendations for diet, activity, medication, and treatment. Allow time for questions, and clarify any misunderstandings.
3. Give the patient a chart listing medications, dosages, times of administration, and desired effects to promote compliance.
4. Instruct the patient to notify health care provider immediately if there is any evidence of bleeding, tarry stools, or dizziness; may indicate an acute bleeding episode.

Patient Education/Health Maintenance

Teach the patient the following:

1. Modify lifestyle to include health practices that will prevent recurrences of ulcer pain and bleeding.
2. Plan for rest periods and avoid or learn to cope with stressful situations; avoid fatigue.
3. Avoid specific foods known to cause the individual patient distress and pain.
4. Recognize signs of potential problems (midepigastric pain). Reinstitute anti-ulcer medication if necessary.
5. Take antacids 1 hour after meals, at bedtime, and when needed. Warn the patient that antacids may cause changes in bowel habits.
6. Do not take H_2 receptor antagonists at the same time as sucralfate. This reduces the therapeutic effects of the drugs.

Evaluation

A. Vital signs stable; intake and output equal
B. Demonstrates improved comfort
C. Decreased frequency of stools
D. Eating several meals a day; reports no loss of weight

E. Can describe peptic ulcer disease, its treatment, and complications; complies with treatment regimen

◆ GASTRIC CANCER

Malignant tumor of the stomach: The incidence of gastric cancer in the United States has been on the decline in recent years.

Pathophysiology/Etiology

1. Risk factors include:
   a. Chronic atrophic gastritis with intestinal metaplasia.
   b. Pernicious anemia or having had gastric resections (greater than 15 years).
   c. More common in men.
   d. Uncommon in those younger than age 40.

Clinical Manifestations

A. Early Manifestations
(Most often patient presents with same symptoms as gastric ulcer; later, on evaluation, the lesion is found to be malignant.)

1. Progressive loss of appetite
2. Noticeable change in or appearance of GI symptoms— gastric fullness (early satiety), dyspepsia lasting more than 4 weeks
3. Blood (usually occult) in the stools
4. Vomiting
   a. May indicate pyloric obstruction or cardiac-orifice obstruction
   b. Occasionally, vomiting has a coffee-ground appearance because of slow leaks of blood from ulceration of the cancer

B. Later Manifestations
1. Pain, often induced by eating and relieved by vomiting
2. Weight loss, loss of strength, anemia, metastasis (usually to liver), hemorrhage, obstruction

Diagnostic Evaluation

1. History—weight loss and loss of strength over several months.
2. Upper GI radiography in conjunction with fiberoptic endoscopy—affords visualization and provides means for obtaining tissue samples for histologic and cytologic review.
3. Imaging, such as bone or liver scan—may determine extent of disease.

Management

1. The only successful treatment of gastric cancer is surgical removal. Gastric resection is surgical removal of part of the stomach.
2. If tumor is localized to stomach and can be removed, chances are still poor that the patient can be cured.

3. If tumor has spread beyond the area that can be excised surgically, cure cannot be accomplished.
  a. Palliative surgery such as subtotal gastrectomy with or without gastroenterostomy may be performed to maintain continuity of the GI tract.
  b. Surgery may be combined with chemotherapy to provide palliation and prolong life.

Complications

1. If surgery is performed, there may be a risk of hemorrhage or infection.
2. Metastasis and death.

Nursing Assessment

1. Assess for loss of appetite, weight loss, GI symptoms (gastric fullness, dyspepsia, vomiting).
2. Evaluate for pain, noting characteristics.
3. Check stool for occult blood.
4. Monitor complete blood count—assess for anemia.

Nursing Diagnoses

A. Pain related to disease process or surgery
B. Altered Nutrition, Less Than Body Requirements, related to malignancy and treatment
C. Fluid Volume Deficit and other complications related to surgery and impaired gastric tissue function

Nursing Interventions

A. *Promoting Comfort and Wound Healing*
1. Frequently turn the patient and encourage deep breathing to prevent vascular and pulmonary complications and promote comfort.
2. Institute NG suction to remove fluids and gas in the stomach and prevent painful distention.
3. Provide conscientious mouth care to prevent mouth dryness and ulceration.
4. Administer parenteral antibiotics, as ordered, to prevent infection.
5. See that the patient has nothing by mouth until prescribed (to promote gastric wound healing).
6. Administer analgesics as ordered.

B. *Attaining Adequate Nutritional Status*
1. Administer parenteral nutrition, if ordered.
2. Follow prescribed diet progressions.
  a. Give fluids by mouth when audible bowel signs are present.
  b. Increase fluids according to the patient's tolerance.
  c. Offer a diet with vitamin supplements when the patient's condition permits.
  d. Avoid high-carbohydrate foods, such as milk, that may trigger dumping syndrome (see below).
3. Give protein and vitamin supplements to foster wound repair and tissue building.

C. *Preventing Shock and other Complications*
1. Shock and hemorrhage
  a. Evaluate status of blood pressure, pulse, and respiration.
  b. Observe the patient for evidence of apathy, apprehension, air hunger, pallor, or clammy skin.
  c. Check the dressings and suction canister frequently for evidence of bleeding.
  d. Administer IV infusions and blood replacement as prescribed.
2. Cardiopulmonary complications
  a. Encourage the patient to cough and take deep breaths to promote ventilatory exchange and enhance circulation.
  b. Assist the patient to turn and move, thereby mobilizing secretions.
  c. Promote ambulation as prescribed to increase respiratory exchange.
3. Thrombosis and embolism
  a. Initiate a plan of self-care activities to promote circulation.
  b. Encourage early ambulation to stimulate circulation.
  c. Prevent venous stasis by use of elastic stockings if indicated.
  d. Check for tight dressings or binder that might restrict circulation.
4. Dumping syndrome—a complex reaction that may occur because of excessively rapid emptying of gastric contents. Manifestations include nausea, weakness, perspiration, palpitation, some syncope, and possibly diarrhea. Instruct the patient as follows:
  a. Eat small, frequent meals rather than three large meals.
  b. Suggest a diet high in protein and fat and low in carbohydrates, and avoid meals high in sugars, milk, chocolate, salt.
  c. Reduce fluids with meals, but take them between meals.
  d. Take anticholinergic medication before meals (if prescribed) to lessen GI activity.
  e. Relax when eating; eat slowly and regularly.
  f. Take a rest after meals.
5. Phytobezoar formation (formation of a gastric concretion composed of vegetable matter)
  a. Avoid fibrous foods, such as citrus fruits (skins and seeds), because they tend to form phytobezoars.
    (1) After a gastric resection, the remaining gastric tissue is not able to disintegrate and digest fibrous foods.
    (2) This undigested fiber congeals to form masses that become coated by mucus secretions of the stomach.
  b. Stress the importance of adequate chewing.

Patient Education/ Health Maintenance

1. Emphasize the importance of coping with stressful situations. Provide information on support groups.
2. Review nutritional requirements and regimen with the patient.
3. Stress the importance of vitamin B_{12} supplements after gastrectomy to prevent surgically induced pernicious anemia.
4. Encourage follow-up visits with the health care provider.
5. Recommend annual blood studies and medical check-ups for any evidence of pernicious anemia or other problems.
6. Instruct on measures to prevent dumping syndrome.

Evaluation

A. Demonstrates improved comfort
B. Body weight is maintained or increased
C. Vital signs stable; no evidence of complications

Intestinal Conditions

◆ APPENDICITIS

Appendicitis is inflammation of the vermiform appendix caused by an obstruction of the intestinal lumen from infection, stricture, fecal mass, foreign body, or tumor.

Pathophysiology/Etiology

1. Obstruction is followed by edema, infection, and ischemia.
2. As intraluminal tension develops, necrosis and perforation usually occur.
3. Appendicitis can affect any age group, but is most common in males 10 to 30 years old.

Clinical Manifestations

1. Generalized or localized abdominal pain in the epigastric or periumbilical areas and the upper right abdomen. Within 2 to 12 hours, the pain localizes in the right lower quadrant and intensity increases.
2. Anorexia, moderate malaise, mild fever, nausea and vomiting.
3. Usually constipation occurs; occasionally diarrhea.
4. Rebound tenderness, involuntary guarding.

Diagnostic Evaluation

1. Physical examination consistent with clinical manifestations.
2. White blood cell (WBC) count reveals moderate leukocytosis (10,000 to 16,000/mm) with shift to the left (increased neutrophils).
3. Urinalysis to rule out urinary disorders.
4. Abdominal x-ray may visualize shadow consistent with fecalith in appendix.
5. Pelvic sonogram can visualize appendix and rule out ovarian cyst.

> **NURSING ALERT:**
> Be aware of vague symptoms with the elderly; milder pain, less pronounced fever, and leukocytosis with shift to the left on differential.

Management

1. Surgery
   a. Simple appendectomy or laparoscopic appendectomy.

b. Preoperatively maintain bed rest, NPO status, IV hydration, possible antibiotic prophylaxis, and analgesia.

Complications

1. Perforation (in 95% of cases)
2. Abscess
3. Peritonitis

Nursing Assessment

1. Obtain history for location and extent of pain.
2. Auscultate for presence of bowel sounds; peristalsis may be absent or diminished.
3. On palpation of the abdomen, assess for tenderness anywhere in the right lower quadrant, but often localized over McBurney's point (point just below midpoint of line between umbilicus and iliac crest on the right side). Assess for rebound tenderness in the right lower quadrant as well as referred rebound when palpating the left lower quadrant.
4. Assess for positive psoas sign by having the patient attempt to raise the right thigh against the pressure of your hand placed over the right knee. Inflammation of the psoas muscle in acute appendicitis will increase abdominal pain with this maneuver.
5. Assess for positive obturator sign by flexing the patient's right hip and knee and rotating the leg internally. Hypogastric pain with this maneuver indicates inflammation of the obturator muscle.

Nursing Diagnoses

A. Pain related to inflamed appendix
B. Risk for Infection related to perforation

Nursing Interventions

Preoperative nursing care is listed; for postoperative care, see Care of the Patient Undergoing Gastrointestinal Surgery, page 494.

A. *Relieving Pain*
1. Monitor pain level, including location, intensity, pattern.
2. Assist patient to more comfortable positions, such as semi-Fowler's and knees up.
3. Restrict activity that may aggravate pain, such as coughing and ambulation.
4. Apply ice bag to abdomen for comfort.
5. Give analgesics only as ordered after diagnosis is determined.
6. Avoid indiscriminant palpation of the abdomen to avoid increasing the patient's discomfort.

> **NURSING ALERT:**
> Do not give antipyretics to mask fever and do not administer cathartics, because they may cause rupture.

B. *Preventing Infection*
1. Monitor frequently for signs and symptoms of worsening condition indicating perforation, abscess, or peritonitis: increasing severity of pain, tenderness, rigidity, distention, ileus, fever, malaise, tachycardia.
2. Administer antibiotics as ordered.
3. Promptly prepare patient for surgery.

Evaluation

A. Verbalizes increased comfort with positioning and analgesics
B. Afebrile; no rigidity or distention

◆ PERITONITIS

Peritonitis is a generalized or localized inflammation of the peritoneum, the membrane lining the abdominal cavity and covering visceral organs.

Pathophysiology/Etiology

A. ***Primary Peritonitis***   Acute, diffuse, relatively rare

1. Occurs primarily in young females; often due to pathogenic bacteria (streptococci, pneumococci, gonococci) introduced through uterine tubes or through hematogenous spread.
2. In patients with nephrosis or cirrhosis, the offending organism is most often *Eschericia coli.*

B. ***Secondary Peritonitis***   Contamination by GI secretions.

1. Complication of appendicitis, diverticulitis, peptic ulceration, biliary tract disease, colon inflammation, volvulus, strangulated obstruction, abdominal neoplasm.
2. May occur after abdominal trauma: gunshot wound, stab wound, blunt trauma from motor vehicle accident.
3. Postoperative complication
   a. May occur after intraoperative intestinal spillage.
   b. Compromised patients are vulnerable (those with diabetes, malignancy, malnutrition, or receiving steroid therapy).

Clinical Manifestations

1. Initially, local type of abdominal pain tends to become constant, diffuse, and more intense.
2. Abdomen becomes extremely tender and muscles become rigid: rebound tenderness and ileus may be present; patient lies very still, usually with legs drawn up.
3. Percussion—resonance and tympany due to paralytic ileus; loss of liver dullness may indicate free air in abdomen.
4. Auscultation—decreased bowel sounds.
5. Nausea and vomiting often occur; peristalsis diminishes; anorexia is present.
6. Elevation of temperature and pulse as well as leukocytosis.
7. Fever; thirst; oliguria; dry, swollen tongue; signs of dehydration.

8. Weakness, pallor, diaphoresis, and cold skin are a result of the loss of fluid, electrolytes, and protein into the abdomen.
9. Hypotension and hypokalemia may occur.
10. Shallow respirations may result from abdominal distention and upward displacement of the diaphragm.
    Note: With generalized peritonitis, large volumes of fluid may be lost into abdominal cavity (can account for losses to 5 L/day).

Diagnostic Evaluation

1. WBC to show leukocytosis (leukopenia if severe).
2. Arterial blood gases—may show metabolic acidosis with respiratory compensation.
3. Urinalysis—may indicate urinary tract problems as primary source.
4. Peritoneal aspiration (paracentesis)—to demonstrate blood, pus, bile, bacteria (gram staining), amylase.
5. Abdominal x-rays—may show gas and fluid collection in small and large intestines, generalized dilatation.
6. CT of abdomen—may reveal abscess formation.
7. Laparotomy—to identify the underlying cause.

Management

1. Treatment of inflammatory conditions preoperatively and postoperatively with antibiotic therapy—may prevent peritonitis. Broad-spectrum antibiotic therapy to cover aerobic and anaerobic organisms is initial treatment, followed by specific antibiotic therapy after culture and sensitivity results.
2. Bed rest, NPO status.
3. Parenteral replacement of fluid and electrolytes.
4. Analgesics for pain; antiemetics for nausea and vomiting.
5. Nasogastric intubation to decompress the bowel.
6. Possibly rectal tube to facilitate passage of gas.
7. Operative procedures to close perforations, remove infection source (i.e., inflamed organ, neurotic tissue), drain abscesses, and lavage peritoneal cavity.
8. Abdominal paracentesis may be done to remove accumulating fluid.

Complications

1. Intraabdominal abscess formation (ie, pelvic subphrenic space)
2. Septicemia

Nursing Assessment

1. Assess for abdominal distention and tenderness, guarding, rebound, hypoactive or absent bowel sounds to determine bowel function.
2. Observe for signs of shock—tachycardia and hypotension.
3. Monitor vital signs, arterial blood gases, complete blood count, electrolytes, and central venous pressure to monitor hemodynamic status and assess for complications.

Nursing Diagnoses

A. Pain related to peritoneal inflammation
B. Fluid Volume Deficit related to vomiting and interstitial fluid shift
C. Altered Nutrition, Less Than Body Requirements, related to GI symptomatology

Nursing Interventions

A. Achieving Pain Relief
1. Place the patient in semi-Fowler's position before surgery to enable less painful breathing.
2. After surgery, place the patient in Fowler's position to promote drainage by gravity.
3. Provide analgesics as prescribed.

B. Maintaining Fluid/Electrolyte Volume
1. Keep patient NPO to reduce peristalsis.
2. Provide IV fluids to establish adequate fluid intake and to promote adequate urinary output, as prescribed.
3. Record accurately intake and output, including the measurement of vomitus and NG drainage.
4. Minimize nausea, vomiting, and distention by use of NG suction, antiemetics.
5. Monitor for signs of hypovolemia: dry mucous membranes, oliguria, postural hypotension, tachycardia, diminished skin turgor.

C. Achieving Adequate Nutrition
1. Administer TPN, as ordered, to maintain positive nitrogen balance until patient can resume oral diet.
2. Reduce parenteral fluids and give oral food and fluids per order, when the following occur:
   a. Temperature and pulse return to normal.
   b. Abdomen becomes soft.
   c. Peristaltic sounds return (determined by abdominal auscultation).
   d. Flatus is passed and patient has bowel movements.

Patient Education/ Health Maintenance

1. Teach patient and family how to care for open wounds and drain sites, if appropriate.
2. Assess the need for home care nursing to assist with wound care and assess healing; refer as necessary.

Evaluation

A. Minimal analgesics needed; abdomen soft, nontender, and no distention
B. Balanced intake and output, no evidence of dehydration or electrolyte imbalances
C. Bowel sounds present; tolerating soft diet

◆ CROHN'S DISEASE

Crohn's disease is a chronic idiopathic inflammatory disease that can affect any part of the alimentary canal, usually the small and large intestines. It is predominantly a transmural disease of the bowel wall. Other names for this disease include regional enteritis, granulomatous colitis, transmural colitis, ileitis, ileocolitis.

Pathophysiology/Etiology

1. Etiology unknown for this disease. Theories include:
   a. Viral and bacterial organisms
   b. Immunologic disturbances
   c. Psychosomatic illness
   d. Dietary factors (chemical food additives, heavy metals, low fiber)
2. Affects both sexes equally.
3. Appears more often in Jewish persons of Eastern European origin.
4. A familial tendency exists.
5. May occur at any age, but occurs mostly in those between 15 and 35 years of age.
6. Intestinal tissue thickens, first by edema and later by formation of scar tissues and granulomas.
7. At times, skip lesions occur with normal intestine in between.
8. This condition interferes with the ability of the intestine to transport the contents of upper intestine through the constricted lumen; this causes crampy pains after meals.
9. Inflammation and ulcers form in the lining membrane, producing a constant irritating discharge.
10. For some patients, the inflamed intestine may perforate and form intraabdominal and anal abscesses.

Clinical Manifestations

These are characterized by exacerbations and remissions—may be abrupt or insidious:

1. Crampy pain after meals: this causes the patient to eat in small amounts or even to avoid eating, which then results in malnutrition, weight loss, and possible anemia (hypochromic or macrocytic).
2. Chronic diarrhea due to irritating discharge; usual consistency is soft or semiliquid. Bloody stools or steatorrhea (fatty stools) may occur.
3. Milk products and chemically or mechanically irritating food may aggravate the problem.
4. Malabsorption syndrome may occur due to protein breakdown.
5. Low-grade fever occurs if abscesses are present.
6. Lymphadenitis occurs in mesenteric nodes.
7. Abdominal tenderness occurs, especially in right lower quadrant; may simulate acute appendicitis.

Diagnostic Evaluation

1. Upper GI barium studies—classic "string sign" is noted at terminal ileum, which suggests a constriction of a segment of intestine.
2. Barium enema to permit visualization of lesions of large intestine and terminal ileum.
3. Proctosigmoidoscopy to note ulceration; biopsy.
4. Laboratory findings show increased WBC and erythrocyte sedimentation rate; decreased potassium, magnesium, calcium, and hemoglobin.

Management

A. General Treatment
1. During exacerbation, parenteral hyperalimentation is instituted to maintain nutrition while allowing the bowel to rest.
2. During remission, regular balanced diet to maintain ideal body weight.

B. Drug Therapy
There is no known cure for this disease; it is primarily treated with medications
1. Sulfasalazine (Azulfidine)—goal is to inhibit inflammatory process; effective only for colonic disease.
2. Mesalamine (Rowasa)—usually given by enema or suppository and only effective in colon; mechanism unclear, but seems to have topical rather than systemic effect.
3. Corticosteroids—to reduce inflammation; given PO or IV depending on severity of disease.
4. Mercaptopurine (Purinethol)—may allow for reduction of steroid dosage.
5. Metronidazole (Flagyl)—antimicrobial, may be indicated for perianal disease; fistula formation.
6. Antidiarrheal agents to control diarrhea related to malabsorption of bile salts.

C. Surgery
Indicated only for the complications of Crohn's disease. Approximately 70% of Crohn's disease patients will eventually require one or more operations for obstruction, fistulae, fissures, abscesses, toxic megacolon, hemorrhage or perforation. Because the goal is palliation, minimal resection, and stricturoplasty preserve bowel
Other surgical options include:

1. Bowel resection with anastomosis
2. Partial colectomy; temporary end ileostomy and Hartmann's pouch, or ileorectal anastomosis (spares rectum)
3. Total proctocolectomy with end ileostomy for severe disease in colon and rectum. See page 498 for care of the ostomy patient.
4. Koch pouch and ileal reservoir–anal anastomosis are contraindicated in Crohn's disease, because disease can develop within the pouches.

Complications

1. Stricture and fistulae formation (ischiorectal, perianal—even to bladder or vagina)
2. Hemorrhage, bowel perforation, mechanical intestinal obstruction
3. Incidence of colorectal cancer is higher in these patients

Nursing Assessment

1. Assess frequency and consistency of stools to evaluate volume losses and effectiveness of therapy.
2. Have the patient describe the location, severity, and onset of abdominal cramping or pain.
3. Ask the patient if there has been recent weight loss and weigh daily to monitor changes.
4. Have the patient describe types of foods eaten to elicit dietary exacerbations.

Nursing Diagnoses

A. Altered Nutrition, Less Than Body Requirements, related to postprandial pain
B. Fluid Volume Deficit related to diarrhea
C. Pain related to the inflammatory disease of the small intestine
D. Ineffective Individual Coping related to feelings of rejection and embarrassment

Nursing Interventions

A. Achieving Adequate Nutritional Balance
1. Monitor diet that is low in residue, fiber, and fat and high in calories, protein, and carbohydrates, with vitamin supplements (especially vitamin K). Prepare for hyperalimentation if the patient is debilitated.
2. Monitor weight daily.
3. Provide small, frequent feedings to prevent distention of the gastric pouch.
4. Have patient participate in meal planning to encourage compliance and increase knowledge.

B. Maintaining Fluid and Electrolyte Balance
1. Monitor intake and output.
2. Provide fluids as prescribed to maintain hydration (1,000 mL/24 hours is minimum intake to meet body fluid needs).
3. Monitor stool frequency and consistency.
4. Monitor electrolytes, especially potassium. Monitor acid–base balance, because diarrhea can lead to metabolic acidosis.
5. Watch for cardiac dysrhythmias and muscle weakness due to loss of electrolytes.

C. Controlling Pain
1. Administer antimicrobials and sulfonamides for control of inflammatory process, as prescribed.
2. Observe and record changes in pain—frequency, location, characteristics, precipitating events, and duration.
3. Monitor for distention, increased temperature, hypotension, and rectal bleeding—all signs of obstruction due to the inflammation.
4. Clean rectal area and apply ointments as necessary to decrease discomfort from skin breakdown.
5. Prepare patient for surgery if response to conservative medical and pharmacotherapy is unsatisfactory.
   a. Surgery intended to relieve segmental obstruction. The involved segment may be resected with anastomosis; bypass procedures may be done.
   b. Surgery is determined specifically for each patient.
   c. Recurrence of the disease is possible after surgery.

D. Providing Psychosocial Support
1. Offer understanding, concern, and encouragement—this person is often embarrassed about frequent and malodorous stools and often is fearful of eating.
2. Facilitate supportive counseling, if appropriate.
3. Encourage patient's usual support persons to be involved in management of the disease.

Evaluation

A. Improved nutritional intake; weight stable
B. Adequate fluid intake; no evidence of dehydration; electrolyte levels within normal limits
C. Demonstrates relief of pain
D. Verbalizes improved attitude toward ways to live with the disease

◆ ABDOMINAL HERNIAS

A hernia is a protrusion of an organ, tissue, or structure through the wall of the cavity in which it is normally contained. It is often called a "rupture."

Pathophysiology/Etiology

A. Causes
1. Results from congenital or acquired weakness (traumatic injury, aging) of the abdominal wall.
2. May result from increased intraabdominal pressure due to heavy lifting, obesity, pregnancy, straining, coughing, or proximity to tumor.

B. Classification By Site
1. Inguinal—hernia into the inguinal canal (more common in males).
   a. Indirect inguinal hernia—due to a weakness of the abdominal wall at the point through which the spermatic cord emerges in the male and the round ligament in the female. Through this opening the hernia extends down the inguinal canal and often into the scrotum or the labia.
   b. Direct inguinal—passes through the posterior inguinal wall; more difficult to repair than indirect inguinal hernia
2. Femoral—hernia into the femoral canal, appearing below the inguinal ligament (Poupart's ligament), that is, below the groin.
3. Umbilical—protrusion of part of the intestine at the umbilicus due to failure of umbilical orifice to close. Occurs most often in obese women, in children, and in patients with increased intraabdominal pressure from cirrhosis and ascites.
4. Ventral or incisional—hernia through the abdominal wall because of weakness in abdominal wall; may occur after impaired healing of incision due to infection, drainage, etc.
5. Parastomal—hernia through the fascial defect around a stoma and into the subcutaneous tissue.

C. Classification By Severity
1. Reducible—the protruding mass can be placed back into abdominal cavity.
2. Irreducible—the protruding mass cannot be moved back into the abdomen.
3. Incarcerated—an irreducible hernia in which the intestinal flow is completely obstructed.
4. Strangulated—an irreducible hernia in which the blood and intestinal flow are completely obstructed; develops when the loop of intestine in the sac becomes twisted or swollen and a constriction is produced at the neck of the sac.

Clinical Manifestations

1. Bulging over herniated area when patient stands or strains, and disappears when supine.
2. Hernia tends to increase in size and recurs with intraabdominal pressure.
3. Strangulated hernia presents with pain, vomiting, swelling of hernial sac, lower abdominal signs of peritoneal irritation, fever.

Diagnostic Evaluation

Based on clinical manifestations.

1. Abdominal x-rays—reveal abnormally high levels of gas in the bowel.
2. Laboratory studies (complete blood count, electrolytes)—may show hemoconcentration (increased hematocrit), dehydration (increased or decreased sodium), and increased WBC.

Management

1. Mechanical (reducible hernia only)
   a. A truss is an appliance with a pad and belt that is held snugly over a hernia to prevent abdominal contents from entering the hernial sac. Does not cure a hernia; used only when patient is not a surgical candidate.
   b. Parastomal hernia is often managed with a hernia support belt with Velcro and is placed around an ostomy pouching system (similar to a truss).
2. Surgical—recommended to correct hernia before strangulation occurs, which then becomes an emergency situation.
   a. Herniorrhaphy—removal of hernial sac; contents replaced into the abdomen; layers of muscle and fascia sutured. Laparoscopic herniorrhaphy is a possibility; often performed on outpatient basis.
   b. Hernioplasty involves reinforcement of suturing (often with mesh) for extensive hernia repair.
   c. Strangulated hernia requires resection of ischemic bowel in addition to repair of hernia.
3. Complications
   a. Bowel obstruction

Nursing Assessment

1. Ask patient if hernia is enlarging and uncomfortable.
2. Determine if patient is exhibiting signs and symptoms of strangulation, such as distention, fever, nausea, and vomiting.

Nursing Diagnoses

A. Pain related to bulging hernia (mechanical)
B. Pain related to surgical procedure
C. Risk for Infection related to emergency procedure for strangulated or incarcerated hernia

Nursing Interventions

A. Achieving Comfort
1. Fit patient with truss or belt when hernia is reduced, if ordered.
2. Trendelenburg's position may reduce pressure on hernia, when appropriate.
3. Emphasize to patient to wear truss under clothing and to apply before getting out of bed when hernia is reduced.

4. Evaluate for signs and symptoms of hernial incarceration or stangulation.

5. Insert NG tube, if ordered, to relieve pressure on herniated sac.

B. *Relieving Pain Postoperatively*

1. Have the patient splint the incision site with hand or pillow when coughing to lessen pain and protect site from increased intraabdominal pressure.

2. Administer analgesics, as ordered.

3. Teach about bed rest, intermittent ice packs, and scrotal elevation as measures used to reduce scrotal edema or swelling after repair of an inguinal hernia.

4. Encourage ambulation as soon as permitted.

5. Advise patient that difficulty in urinating is common after surgery; promote elimination to avoid discomfort, and catheterize if necessary.

C. *Preventing Infection*

1. Check dressing for drainage and incision for redness and swelling.

2. Monitor for other signs/symptoms of infection: fever, chills, malaise, diaphoresis.

3. Administer antibiotics, if appropriate.

Patient Education/ Health Maintenance

1. Advise that pain and scrotal swelling may be present for 24 to 48 hours after repair of an inguinal hernia.
    a. Apply ice intermittently.
    b. Elevate scrotum and use scrotal support.
    c. Take medication prescribed to relieve discomfort.

2. Teach to monitor self for signs of infection: pain, drainage from incision, temperature elevation. Also report continued difficulty in voiding.

3. Inform that heavy lifting should be avoided for 4 to 6 weeks. Athletics and extremes of exertion are to be avoided for 8 to 12 weeks postoperatively, per provider instructions.

Evaluation

A. Hernia effectively reduced with truss or belt; patient comfortable; no signs of infection

B. Minimal analgesics needed; no swelling present; ambulating

C. Afebrile; clean, dry wound

◆ ULCERATIVE COLITIS

Ulcerative colitis is a chronic idiopathic inflammatory disease of the mucosa and, less frequently, the submucosa of the colon and rectum.

Pathophysiology/Etiology

1. The exact cause of ulcerative colitis is unknown. Possible theories include:
    a. Viral or bacterial organisms
    b. Immunologic disorders
    c. Psychosomatic disorders
    d. Allergy to substances that release inflammatory histamine
    e. Enzyme overproduction that ulcerates mucous membranes
    f. Family history of disease

2. Most common in young adulthood and middle life, peak incidence at 20 to 40 years of age

3. Almost equal between sexes (slightly more in females)

4. More prevalent among people of the Jewish religion

Clinical Manifestations

1. Diarrhea (may be bloody or contain pus and mucus), tenesmus (painful straining), sense of urgency, and cramping

2. Multiple crypt abscesses of intestinal mucosa that may become necrotic and lead to ulceration

3. Increased bowel sounds; abdomen may appear flat, but as condition continues, abdomen may appear distended

4. There often is weight loss, fever, dehydration, hypokalemia, anorexia, nausea and vomiting, iron-deficiency anemia, and cachexia (general lack of nutrition and wasting with chronic disease)

5. Abdominal pain

6. The disease usually begins in the rectum and sigmoid and spreads upward, eventually involving the entire colon. Anal area may be excoriated and reddened; left lower abdomen may be tender on palpation.

7. There is a tendency for the patient to experience remissions and exacerbations.

8. Very high frequency of secondary and often multiple colon cancer

Diagnostic Evaluation

1. Stool examination to rule out bacillary or amebic dysentery; fecal analysis positive for blood during active disease.

2. Complete blood count—hemoglobin and hematocrit may be low due to bleeding, WBC may be increased; increased prothrombin time possible.

3. Flexible proctosigmoidoscopy and/or colonscopy with biopsy confirms diagnosis.

4. Barium enema x-ray to assess extent of disease and detect pseudopolyps, carcinoma, and strictures.

5. Decreased serum levels of potassium, magnesium, and albumin may be present.

Management

A. *General Measures*

1. Bed rest, IV fluid replacement, clear liquid diet.

2. For patients with severe dehydration and excessive diarrhea, hyperalimentation is recommended to rest the intestinal tract and restore nitrogen balance.

3. Treatment of anemia—iron supplements for chronic bleeding, blood replacement for massive bleeding.

B. *Drug Therapy*

1. Sulfasalazine (Azulfidine)—mainstay drug for acute and maintenance therapy. Dose-related side effects include vomiting, anorexia, headache, skin discoloration, dyspepsia, and lowered sperm count.

2. Oral salicylates, such as mesalamine (Pentasa), olsalazine (Dipentum)—appear to be as effective as sulfasalazine.
   a. Nephrotoxicity can occur with mesalamine; diarrhea with olsalazine.
3. Mesalamine enema available for proctosigmoiditis; suppository for proctitis.
4. Corticosteroids—primary agent used in the management of inflammatory disease
   a. Prednisolone (Delta-Cortef)—IV, to induce remission of acute severe disease.
   b. Prednisone (Orasone)—orally, for moderate to severe disease.
   c. Hydrocortisone (Cortef)—enema used for proctitis and left-sided colitis.
5. Antidiarrheal medications may be prescribed to control diarrhea, rectal urgency and cramping, abdominal pain; their use is not routine.

C. **Surgical Measures**
1. Surgery is recommended when patient fails to respond to medical therapy, if clinical status is worsening, for severe hemorrhage, or for signs of toxic megacolon.
2. Surgical procedures include:
   a. Subtotal colectomy and ileostomy and Hartmann's pouch
   b. Total proctocolectomy with end-ileostomy
   c. Total colectomy with continent ileostomy (Kock or BCIR)
   d. Total colectomy with ileal reservoir–anal anastomosis (Fig. 16-5).
3. The surgical goal is to remove entire colon and rectum to cure patient of ulcerative colitis.

Complications

1. Perforation, hemorrhage, toxic megacolon
2. Abscess formation, stricture, anal fistula
3. Malnutrition, anemia, electrolyte imbalance
4. Skin lesions (erythema nodosum, pyoderma gangrenosum)
5. Arthritis, ankylosing spondylitis
6. Colon malignancy
7. Liver disease
8. Eye lesions (uveitis, conjunctivitis)

Nursing Assessment

1. Review nursing history for patterns of fatigue and overwork, tension, family problems that may exacerbate symptoms.
2. Assess food habits that may have a bearing on triggering symptoms (milk intake may be a problem).
3. Determine number and consistency of bowel movements, any rectal bleeding present
4. Listen for hyperactive bowel sounds, assess weight.

Nursing Diagnoses

A. Pain related to disease process

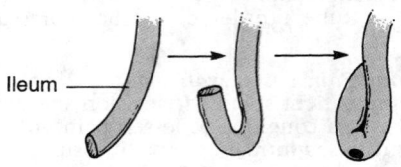

Making the internal pouch

Ileum

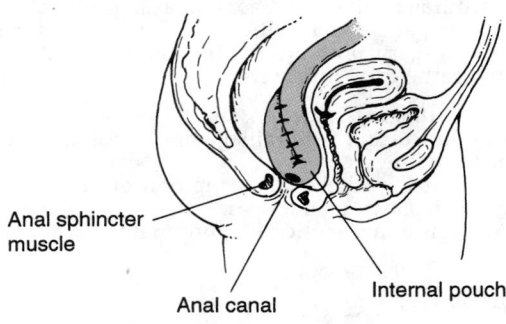

Ileal resevoir to anal anastomosis

Anal sphincter muscle

Anal canal

Internal pouch

FIGURE 16-5 *Ileal reservoir-anal anastamosis. This reservoir is constructed of two loops of small intestine forming a J configuration (J pouch).*

B. Altered Nutrition, Less Than Body Requirements, related to diarrhea, nausea, and vomiting
C. Fluid Volume Deficit related to diarrhea and loss of fluid and electrolytes
D. Risk for Infection related to disease process, surgical procedures
E. Ineffective Individual Coping related to fatigue, feeling of helplessness, and lack of support system

Nursing Interventions

A. **Promoting Comfort**
1. Follow prescribed treatment of reducing or eliminating food and fluid and instituting parenteral feeding or low-residue diets to rest the intestinal tract.
2. Give sedatives and tranquilizers, as prescribed, not only to provide general rest, but also to slow peristalsis.
3. Be aware of the possibility of pressure sores because of malnourishment and enforced inactivity, especially if patient is thin.
   a. Cleanse the skin gently after each bowel movement.
   b. Apply a protective emollient, such as petrolatum jelly, skin sealant, or moisture-barrier ointment.
4. Relieve painful rectal spasms (produced by frequent diarrheal stools) with anodyne suppositories, as prescribed.
5. Report any evidence of sudden abdominal distention—may indicate toxic megacolon.
6. Reduce physical activity to a minimum or provide frequent rest periods.
7. Provide commode or bathroom next to bed, because urgency of movements may be a problem.

B. *Achieving Nutritional and Fluid Requirements*
  1. Maintain acutely ill patient on parenteral replacement of vitamins, fluids, and electrolytes (potassium), as prescribed.
  2. When resuming oral fluids and foods, select those that are nonirritating to the mucosa (mechanically, thermally, and chemically). If this fails, an elemental diet may be prescribed to provide low residue to rest the lower intestinal tract.
  3. Avoid dairy products if patient is lactose intolerant.
  4. Provide a well-balanced, low-residue, high-protein diet to correct malnutrition.
  5. Determine which foods agree with this patient and which do not. Modify diet plan accordingly.
  6. Bolster with supplemental vitamin therapy, including vitamins C, B complex, and K, as prescribed.
  7. Avoid cold fluids, because they increase intestinal motility.
  8. Administer prescribed electrolytes (especially potassium), which have been lost in diarrheal episodes.
  9. Administer prescribed medications for symptomatic relief of diarrhea.
  10. Discourage smoking, because it also increases intestinal motility.
  11. Maintain accurate intake and output records.
  12. Weigh daily; rapid increase or decrease may relate to fluid imbalance.
  13. Monitor serum electrolytes and report any abnormalities.
  14. Observe for decreased skin turgor, dry skin, oliguria, decreased temperature, weakness, increased hemoglobin, hematocrit, blood urea nitrogen, and specific gravity, which all are signs of fluid loss leading to dehydration.

C. *Minimizing Infection and Complications*
  1. Give antibacterial drugs as prescribed.
  2. Administer corticosteroids as prescribed.
  3. Provide conscientious skin care, because excoriation is common after severe diarrhea.
  4. For severe proctitis, instill rectal steroids as prescribed to produce a remission of symptoms.
  5. Administer prescribed therapy to correct existing anemia.
  6. Observe for signs of colonic perforation and hemorrhage—abdominal rigidity, distention, hypotension, tachycardia.

D. *Providing Supportive Care*
  1. Recognize psychological needs of the patient:
     a. Fear, anxiety, and discouragement accompany diarrhea.
     b. Hypersensitivity may be evident.
  2. Acknowledge patient's complaints.
  3. Encourage the patient to talk; listen and offer psychological support.
  4. Answer questions about the permanent or temporary ileostomy, if appropriate.
  5. Initiate patient education about living with chronic disease.
     a. Done on a long-range basis.
     b. Patient should participate in the evaluation and planning of care.
  6. For information and educational brochures, contact the National Foundation for Ileitis and Colitis, 444 Park Avenue South, New York, NY 10016.
  7. Plan all aspects of care in patient conferences so that a team effort promotes the nursing process and ensures continuity of care, communication, and periodic evaluation.

  8. Work with the family in helping to understand the patient.
  9. Refer for psychological counseling, as needed.

Patient Education/ Health Maintenance

  1. Teach patient about chronic aspects of ulcerative colitis and each component of care prescribed.
  2. Encourage self-care in monitoring symptoms, seeking annual checkup, and maintaining health.
  3. Alert patient to possible postoperative problems with skin care, aesthetic difficulties, and surgical revisions.
  4. Inform patients that any early indications of relapse, such as bleeding or increased diarrhea, should be reported immediately so that steroid treatment may be initiated.
  5. If the patient has an ileostomy, facilitate referral to local chapter of the United Ostomy Association.
  6. Encourage patient to become a resource person for others undergoing similar procedure.

Evaluation

A. Reports lessening of pain; functions well with minimal analgesics
B. Demonstrates improved food and fluid intake; avoids roughage intake
C. Diarrhea is controlled. Fluid and electrolyte balance is maintained.
D. Absence of complications
E. Shows improved psychological outlook; participates in counseling, if desired; uses support systems.

◆ DIVERTICULAR DISEASE

Diverticular disease consists of prediverticular disease, diverticulosis, and diverticulitis. A diverticulum is a pouch or saccular dilatation of the colon wall. Diverticulosis is a condition exhibiting multiple diverticula. Diverticulitis is an inflammation of one or more diverticula.

Pathophysiology/Etiology

A. *Prediverticular Disease*
  1. Characterized as a weakening and degeneration of the colonic musculature. The muscle thickening narrows the bowel lumen, whereby increasing intraluminal pressure results.
  2. No diverticula are yet formed.

B. *Diverticulosis*
  1. Marks the formation of diverticula, which are herniations of the mucosal and submucosal layers of the colon developing at weak points where nutrient blood vessels penetrate the colon wall (Fig. 16-6).
  2. Causes for diverticular disease are unclear, but data suggest excessive intraluminal pressure plays a key role. A contributing factor may be a low-residue diet, which reduces fecal residue, narrows the bowel lumen, and leads to higher pressure intraabdominally during defecation.

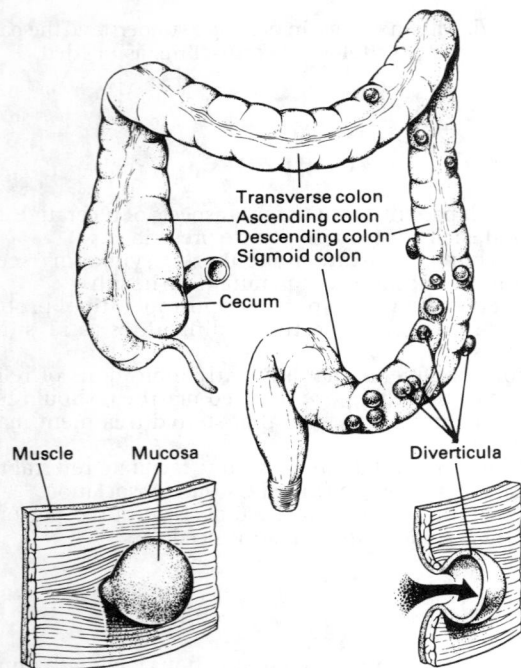

FIGURE 16-6 *Diverticula are most common in the sigmoid colon; they diminish in number and size as the colon approaches the cecum. Diverticula are rarely found in the rectum.*

3. Diverticulosis occurs most often in persons older than age 60.

C. *Diverticulitis*
1. Results when one or more diverticula become inflamed and usually perforate the thin diverticular wall, which consists of mucosal and serosal layers. The inflammation may be caused by a combination of a fecalith plug and accumulating bacteria.
2. If diverticulum perforates, local abscess or peritonitis may occur.
3. Uninflamed or minimally inflamed diverticula may erode adjacent arterial branches causing acute massive rectal bleeding.
4. It is estimated that some persons with diverticulosis will develop diverticulitis.

Clinical Manifestations

A. *Prediverticular Disease*
1. May be asymptomatic
2. Intermittent or chronic abdominal pain; worsening after eating or before bowel movements
3. Constipation and/or diarrhea

B. *Diverticulosis*
1. May be asymptomatic
2. Crampy abdominal pain
3. Bowel irregularity—constipation and/or diarrhea
4. Periodic abdominal distention
5. Sudden massive hemorrhage may be first symptom

C. *Diverticulitis*
1. Mild
   a. Bouts of soreness, mild lower abdominal cramps
   b. Bowel irregularity, constipation, and diarrhea
   c. Mild nausea, gas, low-grade fever, and leukocytosis
2. Severe acute diverticulitis
   a. Crampy pain in lower left quadrant of abdomen
   b. Low-grade fever, chills, leukocytosis
   c. Ruptured diverticula produce abscesses or peritonitis with abdominal rigidity; signs of shock and sepsis (hypotension, chills, high fever). Near a blood vessel, a rupture may cause massive hemorrhage.
   d. Sometimes, fistulae form with the bladder, the adjacent small bowel, the vagina, and the perianal area or skin.
   e. Sepsis may spread through portal vein to liver, causing liver abscesses.
   f. Chronic diverticulitis may cause adhesions that narrow the bowel's opening and can cause partial or complete bowel obstruction.
   g. Urinary frequency and dysuria are associated with bladder involvement in the inflammatory process.

Diagnostic Evaluation

1. Laboratory studies: WBC may show leukocytosis with shift to the left; hemoglobin/hematocrit may be low with chronic or acute bleeding.
2. Flat film of abdomen, ultrasonography/CT scan—free air under diaphragm with perforation into the abdominal cavity.
3. Sigmoidoscopy, possibly colonoscopy—to rule out carcinoma.
4. Barium enema (after infection subsides)—may visualize diverticular sacs, narrowing of colonic lumen, partial or complete obstruction, or fistulae.

NURSING ALERT:
In patients with acute diverticulitis, a barium enema may rupture the bowel.

Management

A. *Prediverticular Disease*
1. High-fiber diet.
2. Bran therapy or psyllium hydrophilic mucilloid (Metamucil) prescribed to counteract tendency toward constipation.

B. *Diverticulosis*
1. High-fiber diet with possible avoidance of large seeds or nuts, which may clog diverticular sac.
2. Bran therapy, psyllium preparation, or stool softeners, such as docusate sodium (Colace), to avoid constipation.
3. Intestinal diverticulosis with pain usually responds to a liquid or low-residue diet and stool softeners to relieve symptoms, minimize irritation, and reduce progression to diverticulitis.

C. *Diverticulitis*
1. Medical Management
   a. Bed rest, liquid or low-residue diet, stool softeners.
   b. Broad-spectrum antibiotic.

c. Medications to control pain and muscle spasms.

d. Blood transfusions may be needed during massive bleeding episodes. Vasopressin (Pitressin) may be used to control bleeding.

e. NPO, IV therapy, NG placement if signs/symptoms of peritonitis or massive bleed.

2. Surgical management—if there is little response to medical treatment or if complications such as hemorrhage, obstruction, or perforation occur, surgery is necessary.

a. Segment of intestine involved with diverticula is resected: two ends reanastomosed to maintain continuity.

b. Temporary colostomy is sometimes performed to divert fecal stream with continuity restored in later second-state procedure.

Complications

1. Hemorrhage from colonic diverticula, usually in the right colon
2. Bowel obstruction
3. Fistula formation
4. Septicemia

Nursing Assessment

Evaluation focuses on clinical manifestations:

1. Have patient describe amount of fiber and fluid intake per day and past and present bowel patterns. Any constipation, diarrhea, or alternating of both?
2. Ask if experiencing abdominal cramping or pain, bloody stools, or stool/gas passage from vagina or in urine.
3. Watch for signs and symptoms of peritonitis: increasing abdominal pain, guarding, rebound tenderness, abdominal distention, nausea/vomiting.
4. Monitor vital signs: temperature may be elevated, tachycardia and hypotension may indicate peritonitis/massive bleed.

Nursing Diagnoses

A. Pain related to intestinal discomfort, diarrhea, and/or constipation
B. Altered Nutrition, Less Than Body Requirements, related to diarrhea, fluid and electrolyte loss, nausea, and vomiting
C. Constipation or diarrhea, related to the disease process
D. Knowledge Deficit of the relationship between diet and diverticular disease

Nursing Interventions

A. *Achieving Pain Relief*
1. Observe for signs and location of pain, type, and severity, and intervene when appropriate.
a. Administer nonopiate analgesics as prescribed (opiates may mask signs of perforation).
b. Administer anticholinergics as prescribed to decrease colon spasm.
2. Auscultate bowel sounds to monitor bowel motility.

3. Palpate abdomen to determine rigidity or tenderness due to perforation or peritonitis.

B. *Maintaining Adequate Nutrition*
1. Follow prescribed diet that is high in soft residue and low in sugar.
a. Provide lists of these foods to enhance familiarity with proper dietary control.
b. Emphasize that proper food intake influences how well the intestinal tract functions.
2. Inform patient that bran products will add bulk to the stool and can be taken with milk or sprinkled over cereal.
3. Monitor intake and output and weight daily to determine caloric status.

C. *Promoting Normal Bowel Elimination*
1. Advise patient to establish regular bowel habits to promote regular and complete evacuation.
2. Observe color, consistency, and frequency of stools and record.
3. Encourage fluids if constipated to promote bowel stimulation.
4. Provide high-residue diet to provide bulk and more consistency to the stool.

D. *Increasing Understanding of Disease*
1. Explain the disease process to the patient and its relationship to diet.
2. Have the patient continue periodic medical supervision and follow-up; report problems and untoward symptoms.
3. Refer to nutritionist, as needed.

Evaluation

A. Expresses relief of pain and has a decrease in symptoms
B. Consumes a prescribed diet and can relate what foods to include or avoid
C. Reports near-normal bowel function; no diarrhea or constipation
D. Delineates the general nature of diverticulosis and can list dietary regimen that helps or aggravates the condition.

◆ INTESTINAL OBSTRUCTION

Intestinal obstruction is an interruption in the normal flow of intestinal contents along the intestinal tract.

The block may occur in the small or large intestine, may be complete or incomplete, may be mechanical or paralytic, and may or may not compromise the vascular supply. Obstruction most frequently occurs in the very young and the very old.

Types and Causes

A. *Mechanical* A physical block to passage of intestinal contents without disturbing blood supply of bowel. High small-bowel (jejunal) or low small-bowel (ileal) occurs four times more frequently than colonic obstruction.

1. Extrinsic—adhesions from surgery, hernia, volvulus (loop of intestine that has twisted).

2. Intrinsic—hematoma, tumor, intussusception (telescoping of intestinal wall into itself), stricture or stenosis.
3. Intraluminal—foreign body, fecal or barium impaction, polyp.
    Note: In postoperative patients, approximately 90% of mechanical obstructions are due to adhesions. In nonsurgical patients, hernia (most often inguinal) is the most common cause of mechanical obstruction.

B. *Paralytic (Adynamic, Neurogenic) Ileus*
1. Peristalsis is ineffective (diminished motor activity perhaps because of toxic or traumatic disturbance of the autonomic nervous system).
2. There is no physical obstruction and no interrupted blood supply.
3. Disappears spontaneously after 2 to 3 days.
4. Causes include:
    a. Spinal cord injuries; vertebral fractures.
    b. Postoperatively after any abdominal surgery.
    c. Peritonitis, pneumonia.
    d. Wound dehiscence (breakdown).
    e. Gastrointestinal tract surgery.

C. *Strangulation*
Obstruction compromises blood supply, leading to gangrene of the intestinal wall. Caused by prolonged mechanical obstruction.

Altered Physiology

1. Results in increased peristalsis, distention by fluid and gas, and increased bacterial growth proximal to obstruction. The intestine empties distally.
2. Increased secretions into the intestine are associated with diminution in the bowel's absorptive capacity.
3. The accumulation of gases, secretions, and oral intake above the obstruction causes increasing intraluminal pressure.
4. Venous pressure in the affected area increases, and circulatory stasis and edema result.
5. Bowel necrosis may occur because of anoxia and compression of the terminal branches of the mesenteric artery.
6. Bacteria and toxins pass across the intestinal membranes into the abdominal cavity, thereby leading to peritonitis.
7. "Closed-loop" obstruction is a condition in which the intestinal segment is occluded at both ends, preventing either the downward passage or the regurgitation of intestinal contents.

Clinical Manifestations

Fever, peritoneal irritation, increased white blood cell count, toxicity, and shock may develop with all types of intestinal obstruction.

1. Simple mechanical—high small-bowel: colic (cramps), mid- to upper abdomen, some distention, early bilious vomiting, increased bowel sounds (high-pitched tinkling heard at brief intervals), minimal diffuse tenderness

2. Simple mechanical—low small-bowel: significant colic (cramps), midabdominal, considerable distention, vomiting slight or absent, later feculent, increased bowel sounds and "hush" sounds, minimal diffuse tenderness
3. Simple mechanical—colon cramps (mid- to lower abdomen), later-appearing distention, then vomiting may develop (feculent), increase in bowel sounds, minimal diffuse tenderness.
4. Partial chronic mechanical obstruction—may occur with granulomatous bowel in Crohn's disease. Symptoms are cramping, abdominal pain, mild distention, and diarrhea.
5. Strangulation symptoms are initially those of mechanical obstruction, but later progress rapidly—pain is severe, continuous, and localized. There is moderate distention, persistent vomiting, usually decreased bowel sounds and marked localized tenderness. Stools or vomitus become melenous or bloody or contain occult blood.

Diagnostic Evaluation

1. X-rays—abdominal films show the presence and location of intestinal gas or fluid.
2. Barium enema shows a distended, air-filled colon or a closed loop of the sigmoid.
3. Laboratory results show decreased sodium, potassium, and chloride levels due to vomiting; elevated WBC counts with necrosis, strangulation, or peritonitis; increased serum amylase levels from irritation of the pancreas by the bowel loop.

Management

1. Correction of fluid and electrolyte imbalances.
    a. Sodium, potassium, blood component therapy.
    b. Ringer's lactate to correct interstitial fluid deficit.
    c. Dextrose/water to correct intracellular fluid deficit.
2. Long-tube decompression of intestine proximal to the blockage site; the tube can be passed more effectively with the patient lying on right side.
3. Treatment of shock and peritonitis.
4. Hyperalimentation may be necessary to correct protein deficiency from chronic obstruction, paralytic ileus, or infection.
5. Analgesics and sedatives, but not opiates because they inhibit GI motility.
6. Antibiotics for peritonitis.
7. Surgery consists of relieving obstruction through bowel resection. Options include:
    a. End to end anastomosis
    b. Double barrel ostomy if end to end anastomosis too risky
    c. Loop colostomy to divert fecal stream and decompress bowel, with bowel resection to be done as second procedure (see Care of the Patient Undergoing Ostomy Surgery, p. 498).

Complications

1. Dehydration due to loss of water, sodium, and chloride
2. Peritonitis

3. Shock due to loss of electrolytes and dehydration
4. Death due to shock

Nursing Assessment

1. Describe the nature and location of the patient's pain, the presence of distention, the absence of flatus or defecation in the nursing history.
2. Monitor and record bowel sounds in all four quadrants.

> **GERONTOLOGIC ALERT:**
> Watch for air-fluid lock syndrome in elderly, who often remain in the recumbent position for extended periods.
> 1. Fluid collects in dependent bowel loops.
> 2. Peristalsis is too weak to push fluid "uphill."
> 3. Obstruction primarily occurs in the large bowel.

3. Conduct frequent checks of the patient's level of responsiveness; decreasing responsiveness may offer a clue to an increasing electrolyte imbalance or impending shock.

Nursing Diagnoses

A. Pain related to obstruction, distention, and strangulation
B. Risk for Fluid volume deficit related to impaired fluid intake, vomiting, and diarrhea from intestinal obstruction
C. Diarrhea related to obstruction
D. Ineffective Breathing Pattern related to abdominal distention, interfering with normal lung expansion
E. Anxiety related to complications and severity of illness
F. Fear of death related to life-threatening symptoms of intestinal obstruction

Nursing Interventions

A. **Achieving Pain Relief**
1. Administer prescribed analgesics.
2. Provide supportive care during nasoenteral intubation, because this will help relieve discomfort.
3. To relieve air-fluid lock syndrome, turn the patient from supine to prone position every 10 minutes until enough flatus is passed to decompress the abdomen. A rectal tube may help.

B. **Maintaining Electrolyte and Fluid Balance**
1. Measure and record all intake and output.
2. Administer IV fluids, hyperalimentation, and blood as prescribed.
3. Monitor electrolytes, urinalysis, hemoglobin, and blood cell counts and report any abnormalities.
4. Minimize those factors that would enhance gastric secretions to prevent fluid loss (through NG suction); avoid conversation about meals and eliminate meals being served within patient's range of seeing or smelling.
5. Monitor urinary output to assess renal function and to detect urinary retention due to bladder compressions by the distended intestine.

6. Monitor vital signs; a drop in blood pressure may indicate decreased circulatory volume due to blood loss from strangulated hernia.
7. Postoperative nursing interventions: For an enterostomy, connect tube to drainage bottle at bedside; expect considerable amount of fecal drainage during the first 12 to 15 hours (500 to 1,000 mL).
   a. Observe drainage equipment frequently for patency.
   b. If there is difficulty with drainage, it may be necessary to inject 15 mL of warm saline solution into the enterostomy tube every 2 to 4 hours, with approval of health care provider.
   c. Protect skin around enterostomy tube with a skin sealant or barrier preparation.
8. Follow additional postoperative management, page 495.

C. **Maintaining Normal Bowel Elimination**
1. Save all stools to test for occult blood.
2. Maintain adequate fluid balance.
3. Record amount and consistency of stools.
4. Maintain NG or Miller-Abbott tube as prescribed to decompress bowel.

D. **Maintaining Proper Lung Ventilation**
1. Keep the patient in Fowler's position to promote ventilation and relieve abdominal distention.
2. Monitor arterial blood gases for oxygenation levels.

E. **Preventing Complications**
1. Prevent infarction by carefully assessing the patient's status; pain that increases in intensity or becomes localized or continuous may herald strangulation.
2. Detect early signs of peritonitis, such as rigidity and tenderness, in an effort to minimize this complication.
3. Avoid enemas.
   a. An enema may distort an x-ray picture by introducing gas into the tract distal to the obstruction.
   b. An enema may make a partial obstruction worse.
4. Observe for signs of shock—pallor, tachycardia, hypotension.
5. Watch for signs of:
   a. Metabolic alkalosis (slow, shallow respirations, changes in sensorium, tetany)
   b. Metabolic acidosis (disorientation; deep, rapid breathing; weakness; and shortness of breath on exertion).

F. **Relieving Fears**
1. Recognize the patient's concerns and initiate measure to secure patient's cooperation and confidence in the staff.
2. Ascertain the patient's specific fears and provide therapeutic responses.
3. Encourage presence of support person.
4. Offer counseling, if desired.

Evaluation

A. Experiences minimal pain
B. Urine output adequate; vital signs stable
C. Demonstrates relief of bowel obstruction—passes flatus, has first bowel movement
D. Demonstrates improved breathing ability
E. No signs of complications
F. Appears relaxed and reports feeling better

Anorectal Conditions

◆ COLORECTAL CANCER

Colorectal cancer refers to malignancies of the colon and rectum. This type is the second most common visceral cancer in the United States. Colorectal tumors are nearly always adenocarcinomas. Lymphoma, carcinoid, melanoma, and sarcomas account for only 5% of colorectal lesions.

Pathophysiology/Etiology

1. Risk factors include:
   a. Age—risk increases sharply after age 50
   b. Previous history of resected colorectal cancer
   c. Family history of colorectal cancer
   d. Polyposis syndromes
      (1) Villous polyps, adenomatous polyps carry malignant potential (especially large ones) and are routinely removed during colonoscopy.
      (2) Familial adenomatous polyposis (FAP) (also referred to as Gardner's syndrome) is an inherited condition characterized by multiple adenomatous polyps of the colon, in which cancer will inevitably develop in all affected individuals.
      (3) Turcot syndrome—an inherited condition characterized by adenomatous polyps and the coexistence of a central nervous system malignant tumor, such as glioblastoma.
   e. Chronic ulcerative colitis—increasing risk after 10-year history.
   f. Crohn's disease—less risk than with chronic ulcerative colitis
   g. Incidence is higher in industrialized countries and lower in underdeveloped countries. Reason unclear but may be related to diet.
   h. A high-fat diet, including red meat and low fiber content, is generally accepted as a contributing factor to colorectal cancer. Fiber appears to provide protection by increasing stool bulk, shortening intestinal transit time, and altering colonic flora.
   i. Immunodeficiency disease
2. Colorectal lesions occur most frequently in the rectum and sigmoid areas; however, it appears there is a trend toward increasing frequency of right-sided lesions.
3. Most adenocarcinomas are ulcerative in appearance. A left-sided lesion tends to be annular and cicatricial; a right-sided lesion tends to be a cauliflower-like mass that protrudes into the bowel lumen.
4. A lesion starts in the mucosal layers of the colonic wall and eventually penetrates the wall and invades surrounding structures and organs (bladder, prostate, ureters, vagina). Cancer spreads by direct invasion, lymphatic spread, and through the bloodstream. The liver and lungs are the most common metastatic sites.

Clinical Manifestations

Colorectal cancer is often asymptomatic. If present, symptomatology varies according to the location of the lesion and the extent of involvement:

1. Right-sided lesions—change in bowel habits, usually diarrhea; vague abdominal discomfort; black tarry stools, anemia, weakness, weight loss, palpable mass in right lower quadrant.
2. Left-sided lesions—change in bowel habits, often increasing constipation with bouts of diarrhea due to partial obstruction; bright red blood in stool; cramping pain; weight loss, anemia; palpable mass.
3. Rectal lesions—change in bowel habits with possibly urgent need to defecate, alternating constipation and diarrhea, and narrowed caliber of stool; bright red blood in stool; feeling of incomplete evacuation; rectal fullness progressing to dull constant ache.

Diagnostic Evaluation

1. Digital rectal examination detects 15% of lesions
2. Endoscopy (fiberoptic sigmoidoscopy/colonoscopy)—two thirds of all colon and rectal cancers can be seen and biopsies performed with proctoscope alone.
3. Stool examination for blood (hemoccult)—often reveals evidence of carcinoma when the patient is otherwise asymptomatic.
4. Intravenous pyelography and possible cystoscopy may be indicated to assess whether malignancy has spread locally to involve ureter or bladder.
5. Carcinoembryonic antigen (CEA)—cannot be used for early diagnosis, but it can detect metastasis or recurrence.
6. CT scan of liver, lung, and brain may reveal metastatic disease.

Management

A. Blood Replacement Administration of whole blood or packed red blood cells if severe anemia exists

B. Surgical Options
1. Wide segmental bowel resection of tumor, including regional lymph nodes and blood vessels (right hemicolectomy, transverse colectomy, left hemicolectomy, sigmoid resection)
2. Low anterior resection for upper rectal lesions—possible temporary diversion loop colostomy while rectal anastomosis heals; second procedure for takedown of colostomy
3. Abdominoperineal resection with permanent end colostomy for lower rectal lesions when adequate margins cannot be obtained or there is involvement of anal sphincters. Due to improved stapling devices used deep in the pelvis, abdominoperineal resection accounts for fewer than 5% of most colorectal resections.
4. Temporary loop colostomy to decompress bowel and divert fecal stream, followed by later bowel resection, anastomosis, and takedown of colostomy.
5. Diverting colostomy or ileostomy as palliation for obstructing, unresectable tumor.
6. More extensive surgery involving the removal of other organs if cancer has spread, such as bladder, uterus, and small intestine.
7. Total protocolectomy or ileal reservoir—anal anastomosis procedure for patients with FAP and chronic ulcerative colitis before cancer is confirmed.

C. Radiation Therapy
1. May use preoperatively to improve resectability of the tumor.
2. May use postoperatively as adjuvant therapy to treat residual disease.

D. Chemotherapy
1. May use as adjuvant therapy to improve survival time.
2. May use for residual disease, recurrence of disease, unresectable tumors, and metastatic disease.
3. Drug combinations may include 5-fluorouracil (Adrucil) plus mitomycin C (Mutamycin); 5-fluorouracil plus levamisole; and 5-fluorouracil plus leucovorin (Wellcovorin).

Complications

1. Obstruction
2. Hemorrhage
3. Anemia

Nursing Assessment

Focus on clinical manifestations/risk factors:

1. Interview patient regarding dietary habits and family and medical history to identify risk factors.
2. Question the patient regarding symptomatology of colorectal cancer, changes in bowel habits, rectal bleeding, tarry stools, abdominal discomfort, weight loss, weakness, and anemia.
3. Palpate abdomen for tenderness (usually not tender), presence of mass.
4. Test stool for occult blood.

Nursing Diagnoses

A. Altered Nutrition, Less Than Body Requirements, related to malignancy effects and weight loss
B. Constipation and/or Diarrhea related to change in bowel lumen
C. Pain related to malignancy, inflammation, and possible intestinal obstruction
D. Fatigue related to anemia, radiation, chemotherapy, and metastatic disease
E. Fear related to diagnosis, prognosis, potential for complications

Nursing Interventions

A. Achieving Adequate Nutrition
1. Meet the patient's nutritional needs by serving a high-calorie, low-residue diet for several days before surgery, if condition permits.
2. Observe and record fluid losses, such as may be sustained by vomiting and diarrhea.
3. Maintain hydration through IV therapy and record urinary output. Metabolic tissue needs are increased and more fluids are needed to eliminate waste products.
4. Serve smaller meals spaced throughout the day to maintain adequate calorie and protein intake if not NPO.

5. Encourage patient to participate in meal planning to promote compliance.
6. Adjust diet before and after treatments, such as chemotherapy or radiation. Serve clear liquids, bland diet, or NPO, as prescribed.
7. Instruct patient to take prescribed antiemetic as needed, especially if receiving chemotherapy.

B. Relieving Constipation or Diarrhea
1. Monitor amount, consistency, frequency, and color of stool.
2. For constipation, use laxatives or enemas as needed, and encourage exercise and adequate fluid/fiber intake to promote bowel motility.
3. For diarrhea, encourage adequate fluid intake to prevent fluid volume deficit and electrolyte imbalance.
4. For diarrhea related to radiation or chemotherapy, administer antidiarrheal medications and discuss foods that may slow transit time of bowel, such as bananas, rice, peanut butter and pasta.

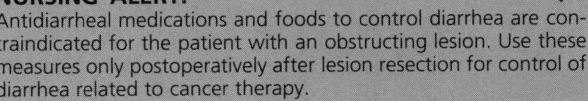

NURSING ALERT:
Antidiarrheal medications and foods to control diarrhea are contraindicated for the patient with an obstructing lesion. Use these measures only postoperatively after lesion resection for control of diarrhea related to cancer therapy.

C. Relieving Pain
1. Assess type and severity of pain and administer analgesics as needed for pain.
2. Evaluate effectiveness of analgesic regimen.
3. Investigate different approaches, such as relaxation techniques, repositioning, imaging, laughter, music, reading, and touch for control or relief of pain.

D. Maintaining Energy Level
1. Institute an individualized activity plan after assessing patient's activity level and tolerance, noting shortness of breath or tachycardia.
2. Allow for frequent rest periods to regain energy.
3. Administer blood products, as ordered, if fatigue is related to severe anemia.

E. Minimizing Fear
1. Encourage patient and family to express feelings and fears together and separately.
2. Acknowledge that it is normal to have negative feelings toward cancer, surgery, colostomy, and treatment options.
3. Provide information and answer questions regarding disease process, treatment modalities, and complications. Offer diverse educational materials, such as brochures, videotapes.
4. Refer patient and family to the American Cancer Society for information about cancer support groups and classes.
5. Refer for counseling, if desired.

Patient Education/ Health Maintenance

1. Provide detailed information or resources about treatment modalities of radiation and chemotherapy.

2. Teach and demonstrate to patient and/or family the skills necessary for colostomy management, which may include colostomy irrigation. The enterostomal therapy nurse can provide formal education in this area.
3. Initiate a home care nursing referral to assist with wound care and management of treatment side effects and to continue teaching colostomy care.

Evaluation

A. Exhibits weight gain and improves nutritional status by adequate dietary intake.
B. Has regular soft bowel movements.
C. Minimal pain, controlled with analgesics; attempts other techniques.
D. Able to perform activities of daily living with adequate amounts of energy; no shortness of breath on exertion.
E. Sleeping normally; able to discuss feelings and fears related to surgery, prognosis, and treatment options.

◆ HEMORRHOIDS

Hemorrhoids are vascular masses in the lower rectum or anus that have become loosened from connective tissue as a result of congestion in the veins of the hemorrhoidal plexus; external hemorrhoids appear outside the external sphincter, whereas internal hemorrhoids appear above the internal sphincter. When blood within the hemorrhoids becomes clotted due to obstruction, the hemorrhoids are referred to as thrombosed.

Pathophysiology/Etiology

1. Predisposing factors include:
   a. Pregnancy, prolonged sitting/standing
   b. Straining at stool, chronic constipation/diarrhea
   c. Anal infection, rectal surgery or episiotomy
   d. Hereditary factor, alcoholism
   e. Portal hypertension (cirrhosis)
   f. Coughing; sneezing; vomiting
   g. Loss of muscle tone due to old age
   h. Anal intercourse
2. Increased intraabdominal pressure causes engorgement in the vascular tissue lining the anal canal.
3. Loosening of vessels from surrounding connective tissue occurs with protrusion or prolapse into anal canal.

Clinical Manifestations

1. Sensation of incomplete fecal evacuation
2. Visible (if external) and palpable mass
3. Constipation, anal itching
4. Bleeding during defecation, bright red blood on stool due to injury of mucosa covering hemorrhoid
5. Infection or ulceration, mucus discharge
6. Pain noted more in external hemorrhoids
7. Sudden rectal pain due to thrombosis in external hemorrhoids

Diagnostic Evaluation

1. History and visualization by external examination and the use of an anoscope or proctoscope
2. Barium enema or sigmoidoscopy, to rule out more serious colonic lesions causing rectal bleeding

Management

Asymptomatic hemorrhoids require no treatment.

A. *Medical*
1. Bowel habits should be regulated with nonirritating stool softeners and high-fiber diet to keep stools soft.
2. Frequent warm sitz baths to ease pain and combat swelling.
3. Insertion of soothing anal suppository 2 to 3 times daily.
4. Application of witch hazel compresses for comfort.
5. Control of itching by improved anal hygiene measures and control of moisture.
6. Do not use topical anesthetics chronically on hemorrhoids or fissures, because they often produce hypersensitivity (allergic) perianal skin rashes with severe itching.
7. Manual reduction of external hemorrhoids if prolapsed.
8. Injection of sclerosing solutions to produce scar tissue and decrease prolapse.
9. Cryodestruction—freezing of hemorrhoids.
   a. Reported to be less painful.
   b. Some patients have a foul-smelling discharge for about a week to 10 days after cryosurgery.

B. *Surgical*
1. Surgery may be indicated when the following conditions exist:
   a. Prolonged bleeding
   b. Disabling pain
   c. Intolerable itching
   d. General unrelieved discomfort
2. Ligation with a rubber band is treatment of choice.
   a. A large anoscope is used; the apex of the internal hemorrhoid is grasped and drawn through a double-sleeved cylinder.
   b. An elastic band is loaded on the inner cylinder and released by a trigger device so that the band encircles the base of the hemorrhoid.
   c. After a period of time, the hemorrhoid sloughs away.
3. Dilatation—dilatation of the anal canal and lower rectum under general anesthesia is another treatment.
   a. This procedure is not advocated for patients whose main complaints are prolapse or incontinence.
   b. It also is not recommended for aging patients with weak sphincters.
4. Incision and removal of clot from acutely thrombosed hemorrhoid.
5. Hemorrhoidectomy—excision of internal/external hemorrhoids.

Complications

1. Hemorrhage, anemia
2. Incontinence
3. Prolapse and strangulation

Nursing Interventions/ Patient Education

1. After thrombosis or surgery, assist with frequent positioning, using pillow support for comfort.
2. Provide analgesics, warm sitz baths, or warm compresses to reduce pain and inflammation.
3. Apply witch hazel dressing to perianal area or anal creams or suppositories, if ordered, to relieve discomfort.
4. Observe anal area postoperatively for drainage and bleeding; report if excessive.
5. Administer stool softener/laxative to assist with bowel movements soon after surgery, to reduce risk of stricture.
6. Encourage regular exercise, high-fiber diet, and adequate fluid intake (8 to 10 glasses/day) to avoid straining and constipation.
7. Discourage regular use of laxatives—firm, soft stools dilate the anal canal, decreasing stricture formation.
8. Determine patient's normal bowel habits and identify predisposing factors in order to educate patient about changes necessary to prevent recurrence of symptoms.

◆ OTHER CONDITIONS OF THE ANORECTUM

See Table 16-3.

TABLE 16-3 Anorectal Disorders

Condition	Etiology	Clinical Manisfestations	Management	Nursing Considerations
Fissure Linear laceration of anal epithelium	1. Constipated stools may tear anal lining 2. Perineum strain during childbirth	Acute pain during and after bowel movement; spotting of bright red blood with stool; possibly spasm of anal canal	1. Promotion of regular, soft-bowel movements through bran, psyllium, stool softeners, suppositories. 2. Local application of silver nitrate or gentian violet solution. 3. Fissurectomy	1. Assist with warm sitz baths and local application of anesthetic ointment to reduce pain. 2. Instruct to eat high-fiber foods and drink fluids to prevent constipation.
Abscess Localized area of pus from inflammation of anorectal tissue	1. Infection develops from abrasion from foreign object, such as enema tip or fishbone 2. Acute phase of anal fistula, suspect Crohn's disease	Painful, reddened bulge or swelling near anus; pain increases with sitting; pus may drain.	1. Incision and drainage of purulent drainage 2. Warm sitz baths	1. Wound assessment 2. Pain medications as needed 3. Alert for passage of bowel movements, postoperatively.
Fistula Abnormal tubelike passage from skin near anus into anal canal.	1. Often preceded by anal abscess 2. May be associated with inflammatory bowel disease, cancer, or foreign body.	Purulent drainage from opening; itching and pain.	1. Fistulotomy 2. Fistulectomy 3. Bowel rest to allow fistula to heal; possible fecal diversion temporarily	1. Wound assessment 2. Pain medications as needed 3. Alert for passage of bowel movement postoperatively.
Anal Condylomas (warts)	1. Infectious papillomas probably sexually transmitted papovavirus 2. Must be differentiated from condylomata lata caused by syphilis	1. Thrive in moist, macerated surfaces, as with purulent drainage 2. Often recurs.	1. Conservative application of liquid nitrogen or 25% podophyllum resin intincture of Benzoin to lesions— washed off after 2–4 h 2. Electrofulguration	1. Encourage good anal hygiene and frequent use of talc dusting powder 2. Schedule follow-up visits to assess area periodically for recurrence.
Proctitis Acute or chronic inflammation of rectal mucosa.	1. Common organisms causing infection include *Neisseria gonorrhoeae*, chlamydiae, herpes virus, syphilis.	1. Anorectal pain; purulent or bloody discharge; constipation; tenesmus. 2. Often seen in homosexual men.	Treatment specific to isolated organism.	Explain rectal procedures and assist with examination and treatment.

(continued)

TABLE 16-3 **Anorectal Disorders** *(continued)*

Condition	Etiology	Clinical Manisfestations	Management	Nursing Considerations
Stricture Narrowing of the anorectal lumen, preventing dilation of sphincter.	1. Usually results from scarring after anorectal surgery (ie hemorrhoidectomy) or inflammation. 2. Status postradiation to pelvic area	1. Constipation, ribbon stools, pain with passage of bowel movements; may not completely evacuate stools, and itching.	1. Treatment of cause of inflammation 2. Dilation by digital, instrumentation or balloon methods. 3. If stenosis severe, may need plastic surgery to anal canal	1. Prevention of stenosis after anal surgery is facilitated by good anal hygiene, warm sitz baths, and dilation. 2. Postoperative care includes stool softeners, warm sitz baths, and wound care.
Rectal prolapse Mucosal membrane protrudes through anus	1. The support structures are weakened (sphincters and muscles) leading to rectal intussusception. 2. Conditions may include neurologic disorders, chronic diseases, aging.	1. Associated with constipation and straining; rectal fullness; bloody diarrhea; rectal ulcer secondary to intussusuception.	1. Treatment depends on underlying cause. 2. Sclerosing agent injection may fix rectum in place 3. Surgery may include sphincter repair or resection of prolapsed tissue.	1. Diet/Fluid instructions to avoid constipation. 2. Teach perineum-strengthening exercises.

Selected References

Beart, R. W. (1994, September 21). Colorectal cancer therapy: What's new? *WOCN J, 21*(9) 175-177.

Doughty, D. (1994). What you need to know about inflammatory bowel disease. *AJN, 94*(7), 24–30.

Doughty, D. B., & Jackson, D. B. (1993). *Gastrointestinal disorders.* St. Louis: Mosby-Year Book.

Fitzgerald, M. & Berg-Gulcher, C. (1995). Diagnosis and treatment of *Helicobactor pylori* infection in peptic ulcer disease. *Journal of the American Academy of Nurse Practitioners, 7*(5), 233–235.

Hampton, B. G., & Bryant, R. A. (1992). *Ostomies and continent diversions.* St. Louis: Mosby-Year Book.

Hastings, G. E., & Weber, R. J. (1993). Inflammatory bowel disease: Part I. Clinical features and diagnosis. *American Family Physician, 47*(3), 598-608.

Hastings, G. E., & Weber, R. J. (1993). Inflammatory bowel disease: Part II. Medical and surgical management. *American Family Physician, 47*(4), 811-818.

Juss, L. (1993, September). Acute abdominal pain: Revealing the source. *Nursing 93, 23*(9), 34-41.

McGinnis, C. & Matson, S.W. (1994). How to manage patients with a roux-en-y jejunostomy. *AJN, 94*(2), 43–45.

Price, A.L., & Rubio, P.A. (1994). Laparoscopic colorectal surgery: A challenge for ET nurses. *WOCN J, 21*(5), 179-182.

Renkes, J. (1993). GI endoscopy. *Nursing 93,* 50-55.

Surratt, S., et al. (1993). Troubleshooting a sump tube. *American Journal of Nursing, 94*(1), 42-47.

Turney, L. et al. (1994). *Current medical diagnosis and treatment.* Norwalk, CT: Appleton & Lange.

CHAPTER 17

Hepatic, Biliary, and Pancreatic Disorders

Assessment

◆ ASSESSMENT OF ACCESSORY ORGAN DYSFUNCTION

The liver, gallbladder and its bile ducts, and the pancreas are called accessory glands in the gastrointestinal (GI) system. Their function is to aid in digestion through the delivery of enzymes to the small intestine. The liver plays additional roles in detoxification of chemicals and the synthesis and storage of important nutrients. The pancreas also functions as an endocrine gland, discussed in Chapter 23, p. 736.

Major liver, biliary, and pancreatic problems can be differentiated by characterization of manifestations and through history taking and physical examination.

Common Manifestations

1. Jaundice—Is there yellow color of sclerae and skin, pruritus, dark tea-colored urine, white or clay-colored stools (steatorrhea)?
2. Any dyspepsia, anorexia, nausea, vomiting, right upper quadrant or epigastric pain, or pain radiating to back or shoulder blade? What is the relationship of pain to eating?
3. Has there been any fatigue, malaise, loss of vigor and strength, easy bruising, or weight loss?
4. Any fever, chills, headache, myalgias, arthralgias, photophobia?

History

1. Have there been any recent blood transfusions? Are there any known blood disorders?
2. Has there been any contact with a person with an infection, such as infectious hepatitis? Any new unprotected sexual activity or ingestion of potentially contaminated food, water, milk, or shellfish?
3. Has there been any drug or chemical toxicity, such as carbon tetrachloride, chloroform, phosphorus, arsenicals, ethanol, halothane (Fluothane), isoniazid (INH), or acetaminophen (Tylenol)? Have any *Amanita* mushrooms been ingested recently? Are certain medications being taken, such as phenothiazine derivatives, perphenazine (Trilafon), sulfonamides, antidiabetic drugs, propylthiouracil (PTU), monoamine oxidase inhibitors, methyldopa (Aldomet) or aminobenzoic acid (PreSun sunscreen)?
4. Any history of nonsterile needle puncture?
5. Does medical history include gallstone(s), hepatitis, tumor, pancreatitis, Wilson's disease, Budd-Chiari syndrome, liver surgery, or transplantation?
6. Any family history of gallstones?
7. How much alcohol, if any, is or has been ingested over the years?

Physical Examination Findings

1. Skin—Any yellow sclerae or skin? Any rashes or scratches on body from severe scratching due to pruritus? Any signs of bruising or petechiae on body, palmar erythema, or overt bleeding?
2. Abdomen—Any tenderness or liver enlargement in the right upper quadrant? Any ascites?
3. Peripheral vascular—Any edema or telangiectasia?
4. Neurologic—What is the level of consciousness? Any asterixis (flapping tremor elicited when the arms are extended and wrists dorsiflexed) present?

Diagnostic Tests

◆ LABORATORY TESTS

See Table 17-1, Liver Diagnostic Studies.

A. Description A tumor antigen found in serum used as a marker for pancreatic cancer

B. Nursing/Patient Care Considerations
1. Tell patient a blood test will be taken and the results will be ready in 1 to 3 days.
2. It is not a screening test for pancreatic cancer; it is a better measure of recurrence after treatment.

TABLE 17-1   Liver Diagnostic Studies

Test and Purpose	Normal	Clinical and Nursing Significance
Bile Formation and Secretion		
1. *Serum bilirubin (van den Bergh's reaction)* Measures bilirubin in the blood; this determines the ability of the liver to take up, conjugate, and excrete bilirubin. Bilirubin is a product of the breakdown of hemoglobin.		
Direct (conjugated)—soluble in water	0–5.1 μmol/L	Abnormal in biliary and liver disease, causing jaundice clinically
Indirect (unconjugated)—insoluble in water	0–14 μmol/L	Abnormal in hemolysis and in functional disorders of uptake or conjugation.
Total serum bilirubin	1.7–20.5 μmol/L	
2. *Urine bilirubin* Not normally found in urine, but if direct serum bilirubin is elevated, some spills into urine.	None (0)	Mahogany-colored urine; when specimen is shaken, yellow tinted foam can be observed. Confirm with Ictotest tablet or Dipstick. If phenazopyridine (Pyridium) is being taken, there may be a false-positive bilirubin result. (Mark laboratory slip if this medication is being taken)
3. *Urobilinogen* Formed in small intestine by action of bacteria on bilirubin. Related to amount of bilirubin excreted into bile.	Urine urobilinogen up to 0.09–4.23 μmol/24 hr. Fecal urobilinogen 0.068–0.34 mmol/24 hr.	Urine specimen is collected over 2-hr period afer lunch. Place specimen in dark brown container and send it to laboratory immediately to prevent decomposition. If the patient is receiving antimicrobials, mark laboratory slip to this effect, as production of urobilinogen can be falsely reduced.
Protein Studies		
1. *Albumin and globulin measurement* Is of greater significance than total protein measurement		As one increases, the other decreases; hence,
Albumin—produced by liver cells	35–55 g/L	Albumin ↓ cirrhosis chronic hepatitis

Globulin—produced in lymph nodes, spleen, and bone marrow and Kupffer's cells of liver	15–30 g/L	Globulin ↑ cirrhosis
		     chronic obstructive jaundice
		     viral hepatitis

Total serum protein	60–80 g/L	
2. *Prothrombin time (PT)* Prothrombin and other clotting factors are manufactured in the liver; its rate is influenced by the supply of vitamin K.	100% of control	Prothrombin time may be prolonged in liver disease, in which case it will not return to normal with vitamin K. It may also be prolonged in malabsorption of fat and fat-soluble vitamins, in which case it will return to normal with vitamin K.
Fat Metabolism		
1. *Cholesterol* It is possible to measure lipid metabolism by determining serum cholesterol levels.	3.90–6.50 mmol/L Esters = 60% of total	Serum cholesterol level is decreased in parenchymal liver disease. Serum lipid level is increased in biliary obstruction.
Liver Detoxification		
1. *Serum alkaline phosphatase* Because bile disposes this enzyme, any impairment of liver cell excretory function will cause an elevation. In cholestasis or obstruction, increased synthesis of enzyme causes very high levels in blood.	20–90 U/L at 30°C	*Abnormalities:* The level is elevated to more than 3 times normal in obstructive jaundice, intrahepatic cholestasis, liver metastasis, or granulomas. Also elevated in osteoblastic diseases, Paget's disease, and hyperparathyroidism.
Enzyme Production		
Aspartate aminotransferase or AST (formerly SGOT)	4.8–19 U/L	An elevation in these enzymes indicates liver cell damage.
Alanine aminotransferase or ALT (formerly SGPT)	2.4–7 U/L	**Note:** Opiates may also cause a rise in AST and ALT.
Lactic dehydrogenase (LDH)	80–192 U/L	Aspirin may cause an increase or decrease in AST and ALT.
Gamma glutamyl transpeptidase (GGT)	0–30 U/L at 30°C	Enzyme found in liver, kidney, heart, pancreas, spleen, brain. An elevation confirms hepatic involvement in the presence of an elevated alkaline phosphatase.

(continued)

TABLE 17-1 Liver Diagnostic Studies *(continued)*

Test and Purpose	Normal	Clinical and Nursing Significance
Ammonia (serum)	11.1–67.0 μmol/L	Ammonia levels rise when the liver is unable to convert it to urea.
Bile acids radioimmunoassay (after cholecystokinin stimulation)		Elevated serum bile acids are seen in the presence of hepatic diseases.
Total	35.0–148.0 mmol/L	
Chenodeoxycholic acid	10.0–61.4 mmol/L	
Cholic acid	6.8–81.0 mmol/L	
Deoxycholic acid	2.0–18.0 mmol/L	
Lithocholic acid	0.8–2.0 mmol/L	

SGOT: serum glutamic oxaloacetic transaminase; SGPT: serum glutamic pyruvic transaminase.

◆ RADIOLOGY/IMAGING

Hepatobiliary Scan

A. Description   A noninvasive nuclear medicine study (also referred to as an HIDA scan based on isotope used) using radioactive materials to aid in the diagnoses of hepatobiliary disorders, such as common bile duct obstruction, acute and chronic cholecystitis, bile leaks, biliary dyskinesia, biliary atresia, and liver transplant function.

B. Nursing/Patient Care Considerations
1. The patient should have nothing by mouth (NPO) at least 4 hours before the procedure.
2. If possible, no opiates should be administered for at least 4 hours before the procedure.
3. Tell the patient that scan time may be up to 4 hours, and additional images may need to be taken up to 24 hours later.

Oral Cholecystography

A. Description   Oral iodide-containing contrast medium excreted by the liver and concentrated in the gallbladder is administered to assist in the radiographic examination of the gallbladder to detect gallstones and to assess the ability of the gallbladder to fill, concentrate its contents, contract, and empty.

B. Nursing/Patient Care Considerations
1. Assess for any allergies to iodine, seafood, or contrast media.
2. Administer or teach self-administration of contrast medium 10 to 12 hours before the x-ray study, usually the evening before.
3. Instruct patient to remain NPO after taking the contrast medium to prevent contraction and emptying of the gallbladder.
4. Explain that a repeat study may be necessary if the gallbladder is not visualized on the first attempt.
5. Should not be performed on obviously jaundiced patients, because the liver cannot excrete the dye into the gallbladder.

Endoscopic Retrograde Cholangiopancreatography (ERCP)

A. Description
1. Endoscopic visualization of the common bile, pancreatic, and hepatic ducts with a flexible fiberoptic endoscope inserted into the esophagus to the duodenum.
2. The common bile duct and pancreatic duct are cannulated and contrast medium is injected into the ducts, permitting visualization and radiographic evaluation.
3. Done to detect extrahepatic biliary obstruction, such as stones, tumors of the bile duct, strictures or injuries to the bile duct, and sclerosing cholangitis; intrahepatic biliary obstruction caused by stones or tumor; and pancreatic disease, such as pancreatitis, pseudocyst, or tumor.
4. May be combined with a therapeutic biliary or pancreatic procedure, such as endoscopic sphincterotomy, biliary and pancreatic stents, tissue biopsy or fluid cytology, or retrieval of retained gallstones.

B. Nursing/Patient Care Considerations
Preprocedure

1. Assess for any allergies to iodine, seafood, or contrast media.
2. Ensure that patient remains NPO since midnight before the study.
3. Ensure that dentures are removed; instruct patient to gargle and swallow topical anesthetic to decrease gag reflex, as ordered.
4. Verify that patient has a signed informed consent before sedation is given.
5. Establish intravenous (IV) access.
6. Administer antibiotic prophylaxis as ordered.

Postprocedure

1. Monitor and document vital signs.
2. Observe for and report abdominal distention and signs of possible pancreatitis, including chills, fever, pain, vomiting, tachycardia.
3. Maintain NPO status until gag reflex returns.
   a. Check for gag reflex by applying gentle pressure on a tongue depressor placed on the back of the tongue.

Percutaneous Transhepatic Cholangiography (PTC)

A. *Description*
1. Fluoroscopic examination of the intrahepatic and extrahepatic biliary ducts after injection of contrast medium into the biliary tree through percutaneous needle injection.
2. Helps to distinguish obstructive jaundice caused by liver disease from that due to biliary obstruction, such as from a tumor, metal clips, injury to the common bile duct, stones within the bile ducts, or sclerosing cholangitis.
3. A biliary catheter may be left in place to drain the biliary tree, called percutaneous transhepatic biliary drainage (PTBD). This relieves jaundice, decreases pruritus, improves nutritional status, allows easy access into the biliary tree for further procedures, and can be used as an anatomic landmark and stent at the time of surgery.

B. *Nursing/Patient Care Considerations*
Preprocedure

1. Assess for any allergies to iodine, seafood, or contrast media to determine need to be premedicated with antihistamines and steroids to prevent reaction.
2. Instruct on remaining NPO or having clear liquids from the midnight before the procedure.
3. Verify that patient has a signed informed consent before sedatives are given.
4. Establish IV line.
5. Administer antibiotic prophylaxis as ordered.

Postprocedure

1. Monitor and document vital signs and assess puncture site for bleeding, hematoma, or bile leakage.
2. Check for and report signs of peritonitis from bile leaking into the abdomen: fever, chills, abdominal pain and tenderness, and distention.
3. Continue antibiotic prophylaxis per protocol.
4. If the patient has a PTBD, monitor catheter exit site for bleeding or bile drainage and monitor drainage in bile bag for color, amount, and consistency. The drainage initially may have some blood mixed with bile but should clear within a few hours.
   a. Report frank blood and/or blood clots that appear in the bile bag.
   b. Large amounts of bile drainage may require fluid replacement.
   c. Maintain patency and security of biliary catheter; perform routine care and dressing at catheter exit site.
   d. Perform routine flushing of catheter as per order.

> **NURSING ALERT:**
> Do not aspirate from a PTBD catheter, because this draws bacteria from the bowel back through the liver and may cause cholangitis (infection in the biliary tree).

   e. Cap off end of biliary catheter to allow internal drainage of bile, if indicated.
   f. Teach patient the care and flushing of biliary catheter and signs of complications, if indicated.

◆ OTHER DIAGNOSTIC TESTS
Liver Biopsy

A. *Description* Sampling of liver tissue through needle aspiration to establish a diagnosis of liver disease through histologic study

B. *Nursing/Patient Care Considerations*
Preprocedure

1. Ensure that prothrombin time is within normal limits.
2. Verify informed consent.
3. Establish baseline vital signs.
4. Tell patient that cooperation in holding breath for about 10 seconds during the procedure is important to obtain biopsy without damaging the diaphragm.

Postprocedure

1. Position patient on right side with pillow supporting lower rib cage for several hours.
2. Check vital signs and observe biopsy site frequently for bleeding or drainage.
3. Report increasing pulse, decreasing blood pressure, increasing pain, and apprehension, which may indicate hemorrhage.

General Procedures/ Treatment Modalities

◆ CHOLECYSTECTOMY

Cholecystectomy is the surgical removal of the gallbladder for acute and chronic cholecystitis. It is one of the most frequent surgical procedures, with more than 600,000 performed each year in the United States. The procedure may be done through open laparotomy (gallbladder removed after making an abdominal incision) or laparoscopy (gallbladder removed from a small opening just above the umbilicus by the use of a laparoscope for viewing). During laparoscopy, three other small punctures are made in the abdomen to place other special instruments used to assist in removal and manipulation of the gallbladder. The organs in the abdomen can be viewed through the laparoscope as well as on a television monitor through a camera attached to the laparoscope.

If the patient is scheduled for a laparoscopic cholecystectomy, consent may also be obtained for a traditional open cholecystectomy, in case the gallbladder is not accessible through the laparoscopic technique. Following cholecystectomy, bile ducts will eventually dilate to accommodate the volume of bile once held by the gallbladder to aid in the digestion of fats.

Preoperative Management/ Nursing Care

1. Determine if the patient knows reason for cholecystectomy, what the procedure involves, and what to expect postoperatively.

2. Patient must remain NPO from midnight the night before surgery and void before surgery.
3. Administer IV fluids before surgery to improve hydration status if the patient has been vomiting.
4. Administer antibiotics for acute cholecystitis, as ordered.

Postoperative Management/ Nursing Care

1. Postoperatively, assess for:
  a. Vital signs, level of consciousness
  b. Level of pain
  c. Wound appearance and T-tube drainage (if present)
  d. Intake and output
2. Promote ambulation to prevent thromboembolus, facilitate voiding, and stimulate peristalsis.
3. Be alert for potential complications of incisional infection, hemorrhage, and bile duct injury.

Nursing Diagnoses

A. Pain related to surgical procedure
B. Risk for Infection related to surgical procedure
C. Impaired Skin Integrity related to surgical procedure
D. Altered Nutrition: Less Than Body Requirements related to surgical procedure and T-tube placement

Nursing Interventions

A. *Relieving Pain*
1. Assess pain location, level, and characteristics.
2. Administer prescribed pain medications or monitor patient-controlled analgesia.
3. Encourage splinting of incision when moving.
4. Encourage ambulation as soon as prescribed to decrease flatus and abdominal distention and promote bowel motility.
5. Instruct patient that usual activities can usually be resumed within 10 days after laparoscopic cholecystectomy or within 6 weeks of open cholecystectomy.
  a. Sexual activity may be resumed when pain has abated.
  b. Obtain specific instructions on heavy lifting, strenuous activity, showers and tub baths, and driving from the surgeon.

B. *Preventing Infection*
1. Assess wound dressings for any increased or purulent drainage.
2. Assess T-tube site for any drainage, and note amount, color, and odor.
3. Assess bile drainage from T-tube into bile bag;
  a. Report any increase or decrease in drainage.
  b. Maintain T-tube patency and security.
4. Report right upper quadrant pain, abdominal distention, fever, chills, or jaundice (due to bile duct injury).
5. Administer antibiotics as prescribed.
6. Encourage use of incentive spirometer, coughing and deep breathing, and ambulation to decrease risk of pulmonary infection.

C. *Maintaining Skin Integrity*
1. Assess wounds for healing.
2. Perform wound care as prescribed.
3. Assess for adequate hydration.

4. Tell the patient to keep the incision or wound sites dry for 5 to 7 days and to report any signs of redness, pain, or drainage.

D. *Providing Adequate Nutrition*
1. Assess for nausea and vomiting and administer antiemetics as prescribed.
2. Discontinue suction of nasogastric tube (if used) and monitor for bowel sounds.
3. Encourage fluid intake and advance to regular diet as tolerated.
4. Administer replacement fluids for bile drainage from T-tube if indicated.
5. Clamp T-tube when indicated and assess tolerance of food and color of stools.

Evaluation

A. Verbalizes decreased pain
B. Absence of fever and signs of infection
C. Wound healing without drainage
D. Tolerating fluids and small solid feedings

Hepatic Disorders

Functions of the liver include:

- Storage of vitamins A, B, D; iron; and copper.
- Synthesis of plasma proteins, including albumin and globulins
- Synthesis of the clotting factors vitamin K and prothrombin
- Storage of glycogen and synthesis of glucose from other nutrients (gluconeogenesis)
- Break down of fatty acids for energy
- Production of bile
- Detoxification and excretion of waste products

◆ HEPATITIS

Hepatitis is a viral infection of the liver associated with a broad spectrum of clinical manifestations from asymptomatic infection through icteric hepatitis to hepatic necrosis. Five types of hepatitis virus have been identified.

Pathophysiology/Etiology

A. *Type A Hepatitis (HAV)*
1. Hepatitis A is caused by an RNA virus of the enterovirus family.
2. Mode of transmission is primarily fecal–oral, usually through the ingestion of food or liquids infected with the virus.
  a. Prevalent in underdeveloped countries or in instances of overcrowding and poor sanitation.
  b. Infected food handler can spread the disease, and people can contract it by consuming water or shellfish from contaminated waters.
  c. Commonly spread by person-to-person contact and rarely by blood transfusion.

3. Incubation period is 3 to 5 weeks, with the average being 4 weeks.
4. Occurrence is worldwide, usually among children and young adults.
5. Mortality is 0% to 1%, with recovery the rule.

B. Type B Hepatitis (HBV)
1. Hepatitis B is a double-shelled particle containing DNA. This particle is composed of the following:
   a. HBcAg—hepatitis B core antigen (antigenic material in an inner core).
   b. HBsAg—hepatitis B surface antigen (antigenic material in an outer coat).
   c. HBeAg—an independent protein circulating in the blood.
2. Each antigen elicits a specific antibody:
   a. anti-HBc—persists during the acute phase of illness; may indicate continuing hepatitis B virus in the liver.
   b. anti-HBs—detected during late convalescence; usually indicates recovery and development of immunity.
   c. anti-HBe—usually signifies reduced infectiousness.
3. Significance:
   a. HBcAg—found only in liver cells, not serum.
   b. HBsAg—usually detected transiently in blood of 80% to 90% of infected persons; may be noted in blood for months or years, indicating that the patient has acute or chronic hepatitis B or is a carrier.
   c. HBeAg—if absent, the patient is an asymptomatic carrier. If present, it indicates highly infectious period of acute, active hepatitis. If it persists, indicates progression to chronic state.
3. Mode of transmission is primarily through blood (percutaneous and permucosal route).
   a. Oral route through saliva or through breast-feeding.
   b. Sexual activity through blood, semen, saliva, or vaginal secretions.
   c. Male homosexuals are at high risk.
4. Incubation period is 2 to 5 months.
5. Occurrence is for all ages, but mostly affects young adults worldwide.
6. Mortality can be as high as 10%, with another 10% of patients progressing to carrier status or developing chronic hepatitis. It is the main cause of cirrhosis and hepatocellular carcinoma worldwide.

C. Type C Hepatitis (HCV)
1. Formerly called non-A, non-B hepatitis.
2. Mode of transmission in most cases is through blood or blood product transfusion, usually from commercial or paid blood donors.
   a. Found among IV drug users and renal dialysis patients and personnel.
   b. Can be transmitted through sexual intercourse.
   c. There are cases of HCV in the general population with no identifiable mode of transmission.
3. Incubation period varies from 1 week to several months.
4. Occurs in all age groups.
   a. Most common form of posttransfusion hepatitis.
   b. May be seen sporadically or in epidemic proportions.

D. Type D Hepatitis (HDV, Delta Hepatitis)
1. Hepatitis D virus is a defective RNA agent that appears to replicate only in the presence of the hepatitis B virus. It requires the presence of HBsAg to replicate.

a. Occurs along with HBV or may superinfect a chronic HBV carrier.
   b. It cannot outlast a hepatitis B infection.
   c. May be acute or chronic.
2. Mode of transmission and incubation are the same as for HBV.
3. Occurrence in the United States is primarily among IV drug abusers or multiply-transfused patients. The highest incidence exists in the Mediterranean, Middle East, and South America.
4. Mortality—causes about 50% of fulminant hepatitis, which has an extremely high mortality rate.

E. Type E Hepatitis (HEV)
1. A recently identified nonenveloped single-strand RNA virus.
2. Mode of transmission is fecal–oral, but because this virus is inconsistently shed in feces, detection is difficult.
3. Incubation is the same as for HAV.
4. Occurrence is primarily in India, Africa, Asia, and Central America, but may be found in recent travelers to these areas.
   a. More common in young adults and more severe in pregnant women.

Clinical Manifestations

A. Type A Hepatitis
1. May have no symptoms.
2. Prodromal symptoms: fatigue, anorexia, malaise, headache, low-grade fever, nausea, and vomiting.
   a. Highly contagious during this period, usually 2 weeks before the onset of jaundice.
3. Icteric phase: jaundice, tea-colored urine, clay-colored stools, and right upper quadrant tenderness.
4. Symptoms may be mild in children; adults are more likely to have severe symptoms and a prolonged course of disease.

B. Type B Hepatitis
1. Symptom onset usually more insidious and prolonged compared with HAV.
2. May be asymptomatic.
3. One week to 2 months of prodromal symptoms: fatigue, anorexia, transient fever, abdominal discomfort, nausea and vomiting, headache.
4. Extrahepatic manifestations may include: myalgias, photophobia, arthritis, angioedema, urticaria, maculopapular eruptions, skin rashes, vasculitis.
5. Jaundice in icteric phase.
6. May in rare cases progress to fulminant hepatic failure, also called fulminant hepatitis.
7. May become chronic active or chronic persistent (asymptomatic) hepatitis.

C. Type C Hepatitis
1. Similar to those associated with HBV but often less severe.
2. Symptoms usually occur 6 to 7 weeks after transfusion.
3. Approximately 50% develop chronic liver disease and at least 20% progress to cirrhosis.

D. Type D Hepatitis
1. Similar to HBV but more severe.
2. With superinfection of chronic HBV carriers, causes sudden worsening of condition and rapid progression of cirrhosis.

Diagnostic Evaluation

1. Elevated serum transferase levels (aspartate transaminase [AST], alanine transaminase [ALT]) for all forms of hepatitis.
2. Radioimmunoassays that reveal the presence of IgM antibodies to hepatitis virus in the acute phase of HAV.
3. Radioimmunoassays to include: HBsAg, anti-HBc, anti-HBsAg detected in various stages of HBV (Fig. 17-1).
4. Hepatitis C antibody—may not be detected for 3 to 6 month after onset of HCV illness; antigen tests for HCV are being developed that will confirm diagnosis sooner.
5. Anti-delta antibodies in the presence of HBsAg for HDV or the detection of IgM in acute disease and IgG in chronic disease.
6. Hepatitis E antigen (with HCV ruled out).
7. Liver biopsy to detect chronic active disease, progression, and response to therapy.

Management

All types of hepatitis:

1. Rest according to patient's level of fatigue.
2. Therapeutic measures to control dyspeptic symptoms and malaise.
3. Hospitalization for protracted nausea and vomiting or life-threatening complications.
4. Small, frequent feedings of a high-caloric, low-fat diet; proteins are restricted when the liver cannot metabolize protein by-products, as demonstrated by symptoms.
5. Vitamin K injected subcutaneously if prothrombin time is prolonged.
6. Intravenous fluid and electrolyte replacement as indicated.
7. Administration of antiemetic for nausea.
8. After jaundice has cleared, gradual increase in physical activity. This may require many months.

For HCV patients:

1. Long-term interferon (Betaseron) therapy may produce at least temporary remission.

Complications

1. Dehydration, hypokalemia
2. Chronic "carrier" hepatitis or chronic active hepatitis
3. Cholestatic hepatitis
4. Fulminant hepatitis (liver transplantation may be necessary)
5. HBV carriers have a higher risk of developing hepatocellular carcinoma

Nursing Assessment

1. Assess for systemic and liver-related symptoms.
2. Obtain history, such as IV drug use, sexual activity, travel, and ingestion of possible contaminated food or water to assess for any mode of transmission of the virus.

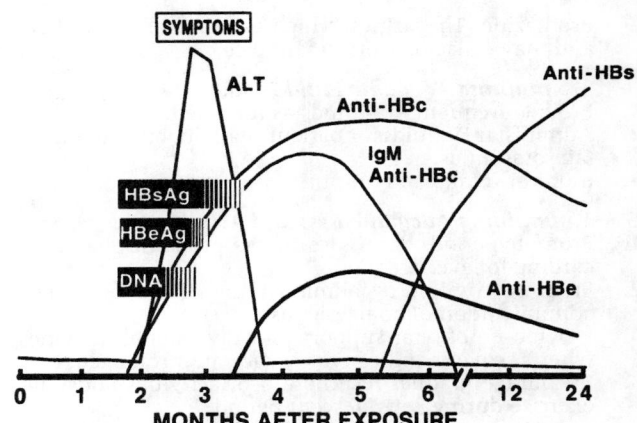

FIGURE 17-1 *Time course for clinical, laboratory, and virologic features of acute hepatitis B infection. ALT: alanine aminotransferase; anti-HBc: antibody to hepatitis B core antigen; anti-HBe: antibody to hepatitis Be antigen; anti-HBs: antibody to hepatitis B surface antigen; HBeAs: hepatitis Be antigen; HBsAg: hepatitis B surface antigen. (Perrillo RP, Regenstein FG. Viral and immune hepatitis. In: Kelley WN, ed. Textbook of internal medicine. 2nd ed. Philadelphia: JB Lippincott, 1992:553)*

3. Assess size and shape of liver to detect enlargement or characteristics of cirrhosis.
4. Obtain vital signs, including temperature.

Nursing Diagnoses

For all patients:

A. Altered Nutrition: Less Than Body Requirements related to effects of liver dysfunction
B. Fluid Volume Deficit related to nausea and/or vomiting
C. Activity Intolerance related to anorexia and liver dysfunction
D. Risk for Infection transmission related to communicable disease

For HBV patients:

A. Risk for Injury related to coagulopathy due to impaired liver function
B. Altered Thought Processes related to encephalopathy due to impaired liver function

Nursing Interventions

A. *Maintaining Adequate Nutrition*
1. Encourage frequent small feedings of high-calorie, low-fat diet. Avoid large quantities of protein during acute phase of illness.
2. Encourage eating meals in a sitting position to decrease pressure on the liver.
3. Encourage pleasing meals in an environment with minimal noxious stimuli (odors, noise, interruptions).
4. Administer or teach self-administration of antiemetics as prescribed. Avoid phenothiazines, such as chlor-

promazine (Thorazine), which have a cholestatic effect and may cause or worsen jaundice.

B. *Maintaining Adequate Fluid Intake*
1. Provide frequent oral fluids as tolerated.
2. Administer IV fluids for patients with inability to maintain oral fluids.
3. Monitor intake and output.

C. *Maintaining Adequate Rest and Activity*
1. Promote periods of rest during symptomatic phase, according to level of fatigue.
2. Promote comfort by administering or teaching self-administration of analgesics as prescribed.
3. Provide emotional support and diversional activities when recovery and convalescence are prolonged.
4. Encourage gradual resumption of activities and mild exercise during convalescent period.

D. *Ensuring Prevention of Disease Transmission*
1. Educate patient about disease and disease transmission.
2. Emphasize the self-limiting nature of most forms of hepatitis but the need for follow-up of liver function tests.
3. Stress importance of proper public and home sanitation and proper preparation and dispensation of foods.
4. Encourage specific protection for close contacts.
   a. Immune globulin (Gammar) as soon as possible to household contacts of HAV patients.
   b. Hepatitis B immune globulin as soon as possible to blood or body fluid contacts of HBV patients, followed by HBV vaccine series.
5. Explain precautions to patient and family about transmission and prevention of transmission to others.
   a. Good hand washing and hygiene after using bathroom.
   b. Avoidance of sexual activity (especially for HBV) until free of HBsAg.
   c. Avoidance of sharing needles, eating utensils, and toothbrushes to prevent blood or body fluid contact (especially for HBV).
6. Report all cases of hepatitis to public health officials.

E. *Preventing and Controlling Bleeding*
1. Monitor and teach patient to monitor and report any signs of bleeding.
2. Monitor prothrombin time and administer vitamin K as ordered.
3. Avoid trauma that may cause bruising, limit invasive procedures, if possible, and maintain adequate pressure on needle stick sites.

F. *Monitoring Thought Processes*
1. Monitor for signs of encephalopathy—lethargy and somnolence with mild confusion and personality changes, such as excessive sexual or aggressive activity, loss of usual inhibitions. Lethargy may alternate with excitability, euphoria, or unruly behavior.
2. Monitor for worsening of condition, from stupor to coma; assess for asterixis, the irregular flapping of the forcibly dorsiflexed outstretched hands.
3. Maintain calm, quiet environment and reorient patient as needed.

Patient Education/ Health Maintenance

1. Identify individuals or groups at high risk, such as IV drug abusers or their sexual contacts and those living in crowded conditions with potentially poor hygiene or sanitation, and teach them proper hygiene, waste disposal, food preparation, use of condoms, not to share needles, and other preventative measures.
2. Encourage vaccination for HBV with series of three shots (at birth, 1, and 6 months) for high-risk individuals, such as health care workers or institutionalized persons.
3. Instruct all patients who have received a blood transfusion to refrain from donating blood for 6 months (the incubation period of HBV). After hepatitis infection, blood should never be given if patient is a hepatitis B carrier or was infected with hepatitis C.
4. Stress the need to follow precautions with blood and secretions until the patient is deemed free of HBsAg.
5. Explain to HBV carriers that their blood and secretions will remain infectious.

Evaluation

A. Tolerating small carbohydrate feedings
B. No vomiting, tolerating fluids
C. Maintaining self-care and light ambulation
D. Family members seeking active immunization
E. No signs of bleeding
F. Lethargic but oriented, no tremor

◆ HEPATIC CIRRHOSIS

Cirrhosis of the liver is characterized by scarring. It is a chronic disease in which there has been diffuse destruction and fibrotic regeneration of hepatic cells. As necrotic tissue is replaced by fibrotic tissue, normal liver structure and vasculature is altered, impairing blood and lymph flow, resulting in hepatic insufficiency and portal hypertension.

Pathophysiology/Etiology

1. Laënnec's cirrhosis (macronodular)
   a. Fibrosis—mainly around central veins and portal areas.
   b. Most common cirrhosis due to chronic alcoholism and malnutrition.
2. Postnecrotic cirrhosis (micronodular).
   a. Broad bands of scar tissue.
   b. Due to previous acute viral hepatitis or drug-induced massive hepatic necrosis.
3. Biliary cirrhosis
   a. Scarring around bile ducts and lobes of the liver.
   b. Results from chronic biliary obstruction and infection (cholangitis).
   c. Much rarer than Laënnec's and postnecrotic cirrhosis

Clinical Manifestations

1. Onset is insidious; may take years to develop.
2. Early complaints include fatigue, anorexia, edema of the ankles in the evening, epistaxis and bleeding gums, and weight loss.
3. Later complaints are due to chronic failure of the liver and obstruction of portal circulation.
   a. Chronic dyspepsia, constipation or diarrhea.

b. Esophageal varices, dilated cutaneous veins around the umbilicus (caput medusa), internal hemorrhoids, ascites, splenomegaly, and pancytopenia.

c. Plasma albumin is reduced, leading to edema and contributing to ascites.

d. Anemia and poor nutrition lead to fatigue and weakness, wasting, and depression.

e. Deterioration of mental function from lethargy to delirium to coma and eventual death.

f. Estrogen–androgen imbalance cause spider angiomata and palmar erythema; menstrual irregularities in females; testicular and prostatic atrophy, gynecomastia, loss of libido, and impotence in males.

5. Bleeding tendencies, such as nosebleeds, easy bruising, hematemesis, or profuse hemorrhage from stomach and esophageal varices.

Diagnostic Evaluation

1. Liver biopsy detects destruction and fibrosis of hepatic tissue.
2. Liver scan shows abnormal thickening and a liver mass.
3. Computed tomography (CT) scan determines the size of the liver and its irregular nodular surface.
4. Esophagoscopy to determine the presence of esophageal varices.
5. Paracentesis to examine ascitic fluid for cell, protein, and bacterial counts.
6. PTC differentiates extrahepatic from intrahepatic obstructive jaundice.
7. Laparoscopy, along with liver biopsy, permits direct visualization of the liver.
8. Serum liver function tests are elevated.

Management

1. Minimize further deterioration of liver function through the withdrawal of toxic substances, alcohol, and drugs.
2. Correction of nutritional deficiencies with vitamins and nutritional supplements and a high-calorie and moderate- to high-protein diet.
3. Treatment of ascites and fluid and electrolyte imbalances.
   a. Restrict sodium and water intake, depending on amount of fluid retention.
   b. Bed rest to aid in diuresis.
   c. Diuretic therapy, frequently with spironolactone (Aldactone), a potassium-sparing diuretic that inhibits the action of aldosterone on the kidneys.
   d. Abdominal paracentesis—to remove fluid and relieve symptoms (see Procedure Guidelines 17-1); ascitic fluid may be ultrafiltrated and reinfused through a central venous access.
   e. Administration of albumin to maintain osmotic pressure.
4. Peritoneovenous shunt may be performed in patients whose ascites is resistant to other forms of treatment.
   a. Complications include bacterial infections, shunt obstruction, and intravascular coagulopathies.
5. Symptomatic relief measures, such as pain medication and antiemetics.

6. Treatment of other problems associated with liver failure.
   a. Administration of lactulose (Cephulac), neomycin (Myciguent) for hepatic encephalopathy.
7. Orthotopic liver transplantation may be necessary.

Complications

1. Hyponatremia and water retention
2. Bleeding esophageal varices
3. Coagulopathies
4. Spontaneous bacterial peritonitis
5. Hepatic encephalopathy, which may be precipitated by the use of sedatives, high-protein diet, sepsis, or electrolyte imbalance

Nursing Assessment

1. Obtain history of any precipitating factors, such as alcohol abuse, hepatitis, or biliary disease. Establish present pattern of alcohol intake.
2. Assess mental status through interview and interaction with the patient.
3. Perform abdominal examination, assessing for ascites (Fig. 17-2).
4. Observe for any bleeding.
5. Assess daily weight and abdominal girth measurements.

Nursing Diagnoses

A. Activity Intolerance related to fatigue, general debility, and discomfort
B. Altered Nutrition: Less Than Body Requirements, related to anorexia and GI disturbances
C. Impaired Skin Integrity related to edema, jaundice, and compromised immunologic status
D. Risk for Injury related to altered clotting mechanisms
E. Altered Thought Processes related to deterioration of liver function and increased serum ammonia level

Nursing Interventions

A. *Promoting Activity Tolerance*
1. Encourage alternating periods of rest and ambulation.
2. Maintain some periods of bed rest with legs elevated to mobilize edema and ascites.
3. Encourage and assist with gradually increasing periods of exercise.

B. *Improving Nutritional Status*
1. Encourage patient to eat high-calorie, moderate-protein meals and supplementary feedings.
2. Suggest small, frequent feedings and attractive meals in an aesthetically pleasing setting at mealtime.
3. Encourage oral hygiene before meals.
4. Administer or teach self-administration of medication for nausea, vomiting, diarrhea, or constipation.

C. *Protecting Skin Integrity*
1. Note and record degree of jaundice of skin and sclerae along with scratches on the body.

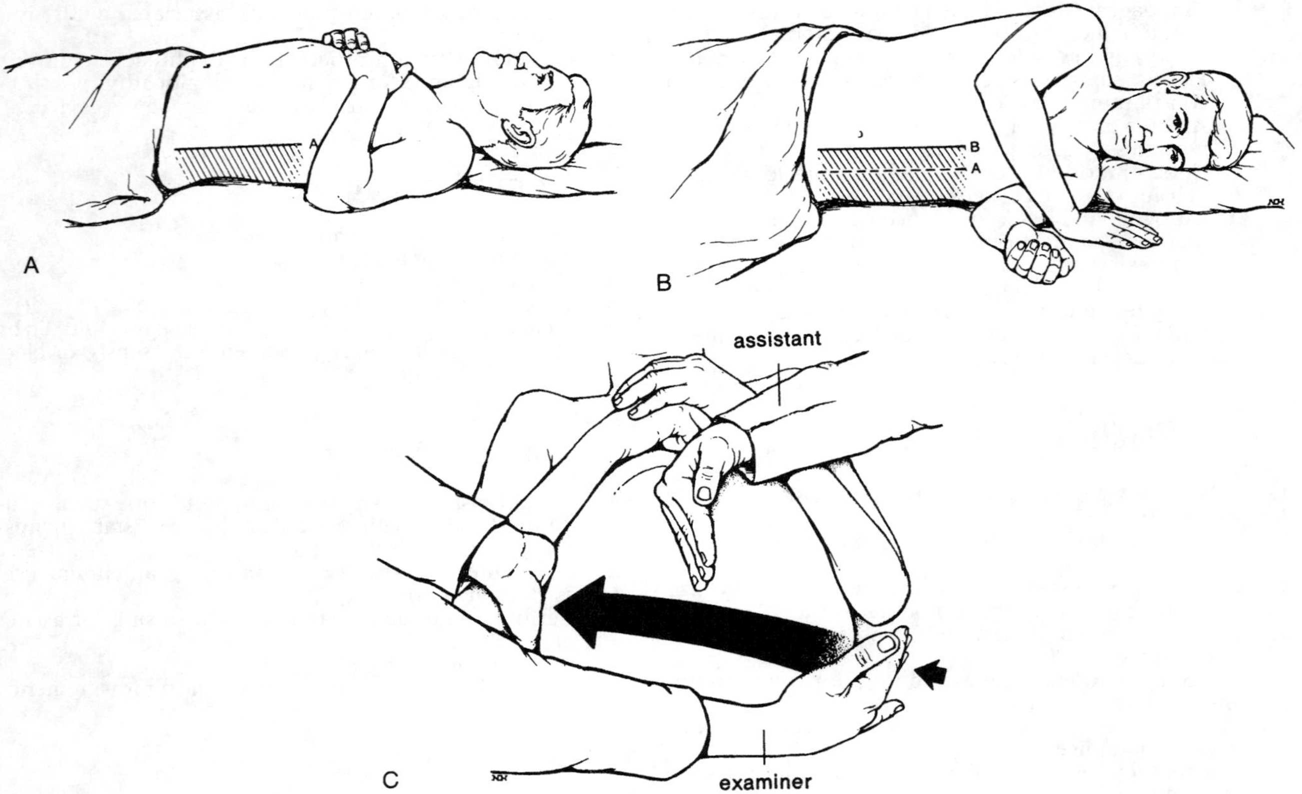

A

B

assistant

C

examiner

FIGURE 17-2   *Assessing for ascites.* **(A)** *To percuss for shifting dullness, each flank is percussed with the patient in a supine position. If fluid is present, dullness is noted at each flank. The most medial limits of the dullness should be marked as indicated in* **A.** *The patient should then be shifted to the side.* **(B)** *Note what happens to the area of dullness if fluid is present.* **(C)** *To detect the presence of a fluid wave, the examiner places one hand alongside each flank. A second person then places a hand, ulnar side down, along the patient's midline and applies light pressure. The examiner then strikes one flank sharply with one hand, while the other hand remains in place to detect any signs of a fluid impulse. The assistant's hand dampens any wave impulses traveling through the abdominal wall. (Copyright 1974, American Journal of Nursing Company. Reproduced with permission from American Journal of Nursing 1974, Sep; 74[9].)*

2. Encourage frequent skin care, bathing without soap, and massage with emollient lotions.
3. Advise patient to keep fingernails short.

D.   *Preventing Injury Through Bleeding*
1. Observe stools and emesis for color, consistency, and amount, and test each one for occult blood.
2. Be alert for symptoms of anxiety, epigastric fullness, weakness, and restlessness, which may indicate GI bleeding.
3. Observe for external bleeding: ecchymosis, leaking needle stick sites, epistaxis, petechiae, and bleeding gums.
4. Keep patient quiet and limit activity if signs of bleeding exhibited.
5. Administer vitamin K (AquaMEPHYTON) as prescribed.
6. Stay in constant attendance during episodes of bleeding.
7. Institute and teach measures to prevent trauma:
   a. Maintain safe environment
   b. Gentle blowing of nose
   c. Use of soft toothbrush

8. Encourage intake of foods with high vitamin C content.
9. Use small-gauge needles for injections, and maintain pressure over site until bleeding stopped.

E.   *Promoting Improved Thought Processes*
1. Restrict high-protein loads while serum ammonia is high to prevent hepatic encephalopathy. Monitor ammonia levels.
2. Protect from sepsis through good hand washing and prompt recognition and management of infection.
3. Monitor fluid intake and output and serum electrolyte levels to prevent dehydration and hypokalemia (may occur with the use of diuretics), which may precipitate hepatic coma.
4. Keep environment warm and limit visitors.
5. Pad the side rails of the bed and provide careful nursing surveillance to ensure patient's safety.
6. Assess level of consciousness and frequently reorient as needed.

NURSING ALERT:
Avoid the use of narcotics, sedatives, and barbiturates in the restless patient to prevent precipitation of hepatic coma.

7. Administer lactulose (Cephulac) or neomycin (Myciguent) through a retention enema or nasogastric tube, as ordered, for elevated ammonia levels and decreasing level of consciousness.

Patient Education/ Health Maintenance

1. Stress the necessity of giving up alcohol completely.
2. Urge acceptance of assistance from a substance abuse program.
3. Provide written dietary instructions.

4. Encourage daily weighing for self-monitoring of fluid retention or depletion.
5. Discuss side effects of diuretic therapy.
6. Emphasize the importance of rest, a sensible lifestyle, and an adequate, well-balanced diet.
7. Involve the person closest to the patient, because recovery often is not easy and relapses are common.
8. Stress the importance of continued follow-up for laboratory tests and evaluation by a health care provider.

Evaluation

A. Ambulating for 10 minutes each hour
B. Tolerating small, frequent feedings
C. Skin without breakdown or scratches
D. No bleeding or bruising; stool negative for occult blood
E. Patient drowsy but easily aroused, oriented

PROCEDURE GUIDELINES 17-1 ◆ Assisting With Abdominal Paracentesis

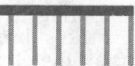

EQUIPMENT	Sterile paracentesis tray and gloves Local anesthetic Drape or cotton blankets	Collection bottle (vacuum bottle) Skin preparation tray with antiseptic Specimen bottles and laboratory forms

PROCEDURE	NURSING ACTION	RATIONALE

PREPARATORY PHASE

1. Explain procedure to the patient.	1. This may reduce the patient's fear and anxiety.
2. Record the patient's vital signs.	2. Provides baseline values for later comparison.
3. Have the patient void before treatment is begun. See that consent form has been signed.	3. This will lessen the danger of accidentally piercing the bladder with the needle or trocar.
4. Position the patient in Fowler's position with back, arms, and feet supported (sitting on the side of the bed is a frequently used position).	4. The patient is more comfortable, and a steady position can be maintained.
5. Drape the patient with sheet exposing abdomen.	5. Minimizes exposure of patient and keeps patient warm.

PERFORMANCE PHASE

1. Assist in preparing skin with antiseptic solution.	1. This is considered a minor surgical procedure, requiring aseptic precautions.
2. Open sterile tray and package of sterile gloves; provide anesthetic solution.	
3. Have collection bottle and tubing available.	
4. Assess pulse and respiratory status frequently during procedure; watch for pallor, cyanosis, or syncope (faintness).	4. Preliminary indications of shock must be watched for. Keep emergency drugs available.
5. Physician administers local anesthesia and introduces needle or trocar.	
6. Needle or trocar is connected to tubing and vacuum bottle or syringe; fluid is slowly drained from peritoneal cavity.	6. Drainage is usually limited to 1–2 L to relieve acute symptoms and minimize risk of hypovolemia and shock.
7. Apply dressing when needle is withdrawn.	7. Elasticized adhesive patch is effective, serving as waterproof adhering dressing.

(continued)

PROCEDURE GUIDELINES 17-1 ◆ Assisting With Abdominal Paracentesis
(continued)

PROCEDURE (cont'd)	NURSING ACTION	RATIONALE

FOLLOW-UP PHASE

1. Assist the patient to a comfortable position after treatment.
2. Record amount and characteristics of fluid removed, number of specimens sent to laboratory, the patient's condition during treatment.
3. Check blood pressure and vital signs every half hour for 2 hours, every hour for 4 hours, and every 4 hours for 24 hours.

   3. Close observation will detect poor circulatory adjustment and possible development of shock.

4. Usually, a dressing is sufficient; however, if the trocar wound appears large, the physician may close the incision with sutures.
5. Watch for leakage or scrotal edema after paracentesis.

   5. If seen, report at once.

◆ BLEEDING ESOPHAGEAL VARICES

Esophageal varices are dilated tortuous veins usually found in the submucosa of the lower esophagus; however, they may develop higher in the esophagus or extend into the stomach.

Pathophysiology/Etiology

1. Nearly always due to portal hypertension, which may result from obstruction of the portal venous circulation and cirrhosis of the liver.
   a. Because of increased obstruction of the portal vein, venous blood from the intestinal tract and spleen seeks an outlet through collateral circulation, which creates new pathways of return to the right atrium and causes an increased strain on the vessels in the submucosal layer of the lower esophagus and upper part of the stomach.
   b. These collateral vessels are tortuous and fragile and bleed easily.
2. Other causes of varices are abnormalities of the circulation in the splenic vein or superior vena cava and hepatic venothrombosis.
3. Mortality rate is high due to further deterioration of liver function to hepatic coma and complications, such as aspiration pneumonia, sepsis, and renal failure.

Clinical Manifestations

1. Hematemesis—vomiting of bright red blood
2. Melena—passage of black, tarry stools
3. Bright red rectal bleeding from hypermotility of the bowel
4. Blood loss may be sudden and massive, causing shock

Diagnostic Evaluation

1. Upper GI endoscopy to identify the cause and site of bleeding.
2. Serum liver function tests, including ammonia level—elevated.

Management

A. Emergency Treatment
1. Restoration of circulation blood volume with blood and IV fluids.
2. Vasopressin (Pitressin) IV to reduce portal pressure by decreasing splanchnic blood flow and to increase clotting and hemostasis.
   a. Complications include hypertension, bradycardia, esophageal ulceration or perforation, aspiration pneumonitis, worsening variceal hemorrhage, water intoxication, cardiac ischemia in patients with preexisting cardiac disease.
3. Iced saline gastric lavage to remove blood from the GI tract, to produce vasoconstriction of the esophageal and gastric blood vessels, and to enhance visualization for endoscopic examination.
4. Esophageal balloon tamponade, whereby balloons are inflated in the distal esophagus and the proximal stomach to collapse the varices and induce hemostasis (see Procedure Guidelines 17-2).
   a. Complications include esophageal necrosis, perforation, aspiration, asphyxiation, and stricture.

B. Nonurgent Treatment
1. Endoscopic sclerotherapy
   a. A sclerosing agent is injected directly into the varix with a flexible fiberoptic endoscope to promote thrombosis and sclerosis of bleeding sites.
   b. To control bleeding and reduce the frequency of subsequent variceal hemorrhages, but repeated treatments may be required.

c. May be used as prophylactic measure to treat varices before bleeding has occurred.

d. Complications include esophageal ulceration, stricture, and perforation.

2. Administration of parenteral feedings to allow the esophagus to rest.

3. Surgical ligation of varices to tie off blood vessels at the site of bleeding.

4. Esophageal transection and devascularization that separates bleeding site from portal system.

5. Surgical interventions to lower portal pressure by shunting blood around the liver—care is similar to abdominal surgery (see p. 494) complicated by severe cirrhotic liver (p. 544).

a. Portal-systemic (portacaval) shunt: portal vein is anastomosed to the inferior vena cava to reduce variceal blood flow and pressure.

b. Splenorenal shunt: a shunt is made between the splenic vein and the left renal vein after splenectomy; this is done when the portal vein cannot be used because of thrombosis or for other reasons.

c. Interposition mesocaval shunt: superior mesenteric vein is grafted to the inferior vena cava.

Complications

1. Exsanguination or recurrent hemorrhage
2. Portal systemic encephalopathy

Nursing Assessment

1. Monitor vital signs and respiratory function.
2. Assess level of consciousness and for impending signs of liver failure.

Nursing Diagnoses

A. Altered Tissue Perfusion related to GI bleeding
B. Risk for Aspiration related to GI bleeding and intubation
C. Anxiety related to fear of unknown procedures and consequences of GI bleeding

Nursing Interventions

A. *Maintaining Adequate Tissue Perfusion*
1. Assess blood pressure, heart rate, skin condition, and urine output for signs of hypovolemia and shock.
2. Monitor patient frequently having vasopressin infusion for complications: hypertension, bradycardia, abdominal cramps, chest pain, or water intoxication.
3. Observe patient for straining, gagging, or vomiting; these increase pressure in the portal system and increase risk of further bleeding.
4. Check all GI secretions and feces for occult and frank blood.
5. Monitor infusion of blood products.
6. Administer vitamin K (AquaMEPHYTON) as prescribed.

B. *Preventing Aspiration*
1. Assess respirations and monitor oxygen saturation of blood.
2. Note and report occurrence of signs of obstructed airway or ruptured esophagus from the esophageal balloon: changes in skin color, respirations, breath sounds, level of consciousness, or vital signs; presence of chest pain.
3. Check location and inflation of esophageal balloon; maintain traction on tubes if applicable.
4. Have scissors readily available. Cut tubing and remove esophageal balloon immediately if the patient develops acute respiratory distress.
5. Keep head of bed elevated to avoid gastric regurgitation and aspiration of gastric contents.
6. When using the Sengstaken-Blakemore esophageal balloon tube, ensure removal of secretions above the esophageal balloon: position nasogastric tube in the esophagus for suctioning purposes; or provide intermittent oropharyngeal suctioning.
7. Inspect nares for skin irritation; cleanse and lubricate frequently to prevent bleeding.

C. *Reducing Anxiety and Fear*
1. Provide care in a concerned, nonjudgmental manner.
2. Explain all procedures to the patient.
3. Remain with the patient or maintain close observation and place call bell within patient's reach.
4. Work swiftly and confidently, not hurriedly and anxiously.
5. Provide alternate means of communication if tubes or other equipment interfere with the patient's ability to talk.
6. Use touch and other tactile stimuli to provide reassurance to the patient.
7. Use protective restraints to prevent dislodging of tubes in confused, combative patient.

Patient Education/ Health Maintenance

1. Discuss signs and symptoms of recurrent bleeding and the need to seek emergency medical treatment if these occur.
2. Instruct the patient to avoid behaviors that increase portal system pressure: straining, gagging, Valsalva's maneuver.
3. Instruct the patient in the effects of high-protein diets and alcohol consumption in causing further complications.
4. Encourage the patient to abstain from alcohol consumption; discuss support organizations, such as Alcoholic Anonymous.

Evaluation

A. Blood pressure stable, urine output adequate
B. Airway maintained without aspiration
C. Patient cooperative and indicates understanding of treatment

PROCEDURE GUIDELINES 17-2 ◆ Using Balloon Tamponade to Control Esophageal Bleeding (Sengstaken-Blakemore Tube Method, Minnesota Tube Method)

EQUIPMENT

Esophageal balloon (Sengstaken-Blakemore or Minnesota)
Basin with cracked ice
Clamps for tubing
Water-soluble lubricant
Syringe (50 ml with catheter tip)
Towel and emesis basin

Glass of water and straw
Adhesive tape
Device to apply traction (eg, football helmet)
Large scissors (for emergency deflation)
Manometer (to measure balloon pressure)

PROCEDURE **PREPARATORY PHASE**

1. Provide support and reassure the patient that this procedure will help to control bleeding.
2. Explain procedure to the patient and explain how breathing through the mouth and swallowing can help in passing the tube. (See accompanying figure.)
3. Elevate head of bed slightly, unless the patient is in shock.

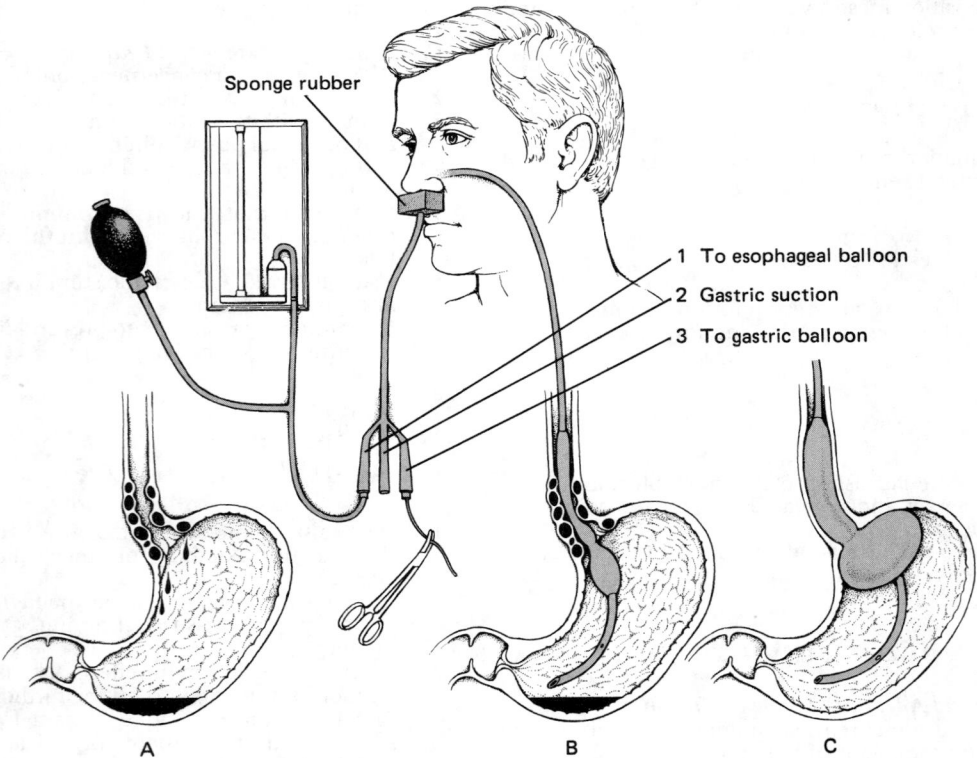

Sponge rubber

1 To esophageal balloon
2 Gastric suction
3 To gastric balloon

A   B   C

*Esophageal varices and their treatment by a compressing balloon tube (Sengstaken-Blakemore). (**A**) Dilated veins of the lower esophagus. (**B**) The tube is in place in the stomach and the lower esophagus but is not inflated. (**C**) Inflation of the tube causing compression of the veins. It may be necessary to pass an additional tube through the other nostril to aspirate. Note: The Minnesota four-lumen esophagogastric tamponade tube has an additional outlet for aspiration of the esophagus.*

PROCEDURE (cont'd)	NURSING ACTION	RATIONALE

PERFORMANCE PHASE

1. Check balloons by trial inflation to detect leaks.

2. Chill the tube, then lubricate it before the physician passes it via mouth or nose (preferable).
3. Provide the patient with a few sips of water.
4. After the tube has entered the stomach, verify its placement by irrigating the gastric tube with air while auscultating over the stomach.
5. After obtaining an x-ray film of the lower chest and upper abdomen to verify placement in the stomach, inflate gastric balloon (200–250 ml) with air and gently pull tube back to seat balloon against gastroesophageal junction.
6. Clamp gastric balloon; mark tube location at nares.

7. Apply gentle traction to the balloon tube and secure it with a foam rubber cube at the nares or tape it to the faceguard of a football helmet.
8. Attach Y connector to esophageal balloon opening. Attach syringe to one arm of the Y connector and manometer to the other. Inflate esophageal balloon to 25–35 mm Hg. Clamp esophageal balloon.
9. Apply suction to gastric aspiration opening. Irrigate at least hourly.

10. **[If using Senstaken-Blakemore tube]**
Insert a nasogastric tube, positioning it above the esophageal balloon and attach to suction.

[If using a Minnesota tube]
Attach fourth port, esophageal suction port, to suction.
11. Label each port.
12. Tape scissors to head of bed.

RATIONALE

1. This is best done under water because it is easier to see escaping air bubbles.
2. Chilling makes the tube more firm and lubrication lessens friction.
3. This will help pass the tube more easily.
4. It is imperative to be certain that the tube is in the stomach so that the gastric tube is not inflated in the esophagus.
5. This is to exert force against the cardia.

6. This prevents air leakage and tube migration. The mark on the tube allows for easy visualization of movement of the tube.
7. This prevents the tube from migrating with peristalsis and assists in exerting proper pressure.
8. Maintains enough pressure to tamponade bleeding while preventing esophageal necrosis.

9. Suctioning and irrigating the tube can remove old blood from the stomach and prevent hepatic encephalopathy; allows monitoring of bleeding status.

To suction saliva accumulated above the esophageal balloon, which may be aspirated, and to check for bleeding above the esophageal balloon

11. To prevent accidental deflation or irrigation.
12. Airway occlusion may occur if the esophageal balloon is pulled into the hypopharynx. If this occurs, the esophageal balloon tube must be cut and removed immediately.

NURSING RESPONSIBILITIES

1. Maintain *constant* vigilance while balloons are inflated in the patient.
2. Keep balloon pressures at required level to control bleeding. (Clamps help to maintain pressure.)
3. Observe and record vital signs; monitor color and amount of nasogastric lavage fluid (subtracting lavage input) for evidence of bleeding.
4. Be alert for chest pain—may indicate injury or rupture of esophagus.
5. Irrigate suction tube as prescribed; observe and record nature and color of aspirated material.
6. Keep head of bed elevated to avoid gastric regurgitation and to diminish nausea and a sensation of gagging.
7. Maintain nutritional and electrolyte levels parenterally.
8. Maintain nasogastric suction or suction to esophageal suction port to aspirate any collected saliva.
9. Note nature of breathing; if counterweight pulls the tube into oropharynx, the patient may be asphyxiated.

NURSING ALERT:
Keep a pair of scissors taped to the head of the bed. In the event of *acute respiratory distress,* use the scissors to cut across tubing (to deflate both balloons) and remove tubing.

Note: This procedure should be reserved for patients who are known, without a doubt, to be bleeding from esophageal varices and in whom all forms of conservative therapy have failed.

◆ LIVER CANCER

Cancer of the liver or hepatocellular carcinoma is a primary cancer of the liver and is relatively uncommon in the United States. It is, however, one of the most common malignancies in the world, particularly in Africa and Asia. Cholangiocarcinoma is a primary malignant tumor of the bile ducts, which can be intrahepatic or extrahepatic. This type of cancer is uncommon in the United States but is more frequently seen in Asia. These two types of cancer are often combined for reporting purposes and make the incidence data harder to interpret.

Cancer of the liver may also be a metastasis from a primary site, which is found in about one-half of all late cancer cases. Malignant tumors are likely to reach the liver by way of the portal system or the lymphatic channels or by direct extension from an abdominal tumor.

Pathophysiology/Etiology

1. Incidence of primary cancer of the liver is increasing in the United States in the younger population and in females.
2. Cirrhosis, hepatitis B virus, and hepatitis C virus have been implicated in its etiology.
3. Rarer associated causes are hemachromatosis; alpha 1-antitrypsin deficiency; aflatoxins; chemical toxins, such as vinyl chloride and Thorotrast; carcinogens in herbal medicines; nitrosamines; and ingestion of hormones, as in oral contraceptives.
4. Arises in normal tissue as a discrete tumor or in end-stage cirrhosis in a multinodular pattern.

Clinical Manifestations

1. Depends on the state of the liver in which it arises; without cirrhosis and with good liver function, carcinoma of the liver may grow to huge proportions before becoming symptomatic, but in a cirrhotic patient, the lack of hepatic reserve usually leads to a more rapid course.
2. Most common presenting symptom is right upper quadrant abdominal pain, usually dull or aching, and may radiate to the right shoulder.
3. A right upper quadrant mass, weight loss, abdominal distention with ascites, fatigue, anorexia, malaise, and unexplained fever.
4. Jaundice is present only in a minority of patients at diagnosis in primary cancer of the liver. In cholangiocarcinoma, the presenting symptom is usually obstructive jaundice.
5. If there is portal vein obstruction, ascites and esophageal varices occurs.

Diagnostic Evaluation

1. Increased levels of serum bilirubin, alkaline phosphatase, and liver enzymes
2. Alpha-fetoprotein (AFP) is the principal tumor marker for hepatocellular carcinoma and is elevated in 70% to 95% of patients with the disease.
3. Ultrasonography and CT along with magnetic resonance imaging (MRI) are the most useful noninvasive tests to detect liver cancer and assess if the tumor can be surgically removed.
4. Arteriography is necessary to determine the resectability of any tumor of the liver.
5. Percutaneous needle biopsy or biopsy assisted by ultrasonography may be done.
6. Laparoscopy with liver biopsy may be performed.

Management

A. Nonsurgical treatment Varying degrees of success with chemotherapy and radiation. These therapies may prolong survival and improve the patient's quality of life by reducing pain, but the overall effect is palliative

1. Liver cancer is radiosensitive, but treatment is restricted by the limited radiation tolerance of the normal liver.
2. Radiation therapy can help reduce pain and discomfort.
3. Chemotherapy is used as an adjuvant therapy after surgical resection of liver cancer.
   a. Systemic chemotherapy is the only treatment applicable once the cancer has spread outside the liver.
   b. Regional infusion chemotherapy by implantable pump has been used to deliver a high concentration of chemotherapy directly to the liver through the hepatic artery.
4. Hyperthermia has been used to treat hepatic metastases.
5. Hepatic artery occlusion and embolization with the use of chemotherapeutic agents is another possible method.
6. Immunotherapy is under investigation.
7. PTBD is used to drain obstructed biliary ducts in patients with inoperable tumors or in patients considered poor surgical risks.
8. Percutaneous or endoscopic placement of internal stents may also palliate a patient with obstructed bile ducts with a terminal diagnosis.

B. Surgical treatment Surgery is the best treatment but is only feasible in 25% of cases

1. Surgery is an option only after the extent of tumor and hepatic reserve have been considered
2. Surgical resection may be along anatomic divisions of the liver or nonanatomic resections.
3. Freezing hepatic tumors by cryosurgery is a new modality that preserves normal liver.
4. Liver transplantation has been performed to treat liver tumors, but results have been poor due to the high rate of recurrent primary liver malignancy. It is now recommended that the patient be treated before and after transplantation with chemotherapy and radiation therapy.
5. Care of the patient after liver surgery is similar to general abdominal surgery (see p. 494).

Complications

1. Malnutrition, biliary obstruction with jaundice
2. Fulminant liver failure, metastasis

Nursing Assessment

1. Obtain history of hepatitis, alcoholic liver disease and cirrhosis, exposure to toxins or other potential causes.
2. Assess for signs and symptoms of malnutrition, including recent weight loss, loss of strength, anorexia, and anemia.
3. Assess for abdominal pain, any right shoulder pain, along with enlargement of the liver.
4. Assess for fever, jaundice, ascites, or bleeding.
5. Note any change in mental status as precipitating hepatic encephalopathy.

Nursing Diagnoses

A. Pain related to growth of tumor
B. Altered Nutrition: Less Than Body Requirements, related to anorexia
C. Fluid Volume Excess related to ascites and edema formation

Nursing Interventions

A. *Controlling Pain*
1. Administer pharmacologic agents as ordered to control pain, considering metabolism through a liver with decreased function.
   a. Use caution not to administer doses more frequently than prescribed.
   b. Monitor for signs of drug toxicity.
2. Provide nonpharmacologic methods of pain relief, such as massage and guided imagery.
3. Position patient for comfort—usually in semi-Fowler's position.
4. Assess patient's response to pain control measures.

B. *Improving Nutritional Status*
1. Encourage patient to eat small meals and supplementary feedings, such as Ensure.
2. Assess and report changes in factors affecting nutritional needs: increased body temperature, pain, signs of infection, stress level. Encourage additional calories as tolerated.
3. Monitor weekly weight changes.

C. *Relieving Excess Fluid Volume*
1. Monitor vital signs and record accurate intake and output of fluid.
2. Restrict sodium and fluid intake as prescribed.
3. Administer diuretics and replacement potassium as prescribed.
4. Administer albumin and protein supplements as prescribed to draw fluid from interstitial to intravascular space.
5. Measure and record abdominal girth daily.
6. Weigh daily, watching for increases that indicate more fluid retention.
7. Monitor laboratory values pertinent to liver function.

Patient Education/Health Maintenance

1. Instruct patient and family on preparation for surgery, reinforce and clarify surgical procedure proposed, and review postoperative instructions.
2. Instruct patient and family on nonsurgical treatment, if appropriate.
3. Explore options for pain management.
4. Inform patient of signs and symptoms of complications.
5. Instruct patient in continued surveillance for recurrence.
6. Instruct patient and family in care of any tubes or drains.

Evaluation

A. Verbalizes reduced pain
B. Tolerating small feedings; no weight loss
C. Abdominal girth decreased; urine output greater than intake

◆ FULMINANT LIVER FAILURE

Fulminant liver failure is acute necrosis of the liver cells in the absence of preexisting liver disease, resulting in the inability of the liver to perform its many functions.

Pathophysiology/Etiology

1. Viral hepatitis is the most common cause.
2. Poisons, chemicals, and drugs such as acetaminophen (Tylenol), tetracycline (Tetracyn), isoniazid (INH), halogenated anesthetics, monoamine oxidase inhibitors, valproate (Depakene), amiodarone (Cordarone), methyldopa (Aldomet), and *Amanita* mushrooms may cause liver toxicity.
3. Ischemia and hypoxia due to hepatic vascular occlusion, hypovolemic shock, acute circulatory failure, septic shock, heat stroke may be causes.
4. Miscellaneous causes include hepatic vein obstruction, Budd-Chiari syndrome, acute fatty liver of pregnancy, partial hepatectomy, complication of liver transplantation.
5. Progression of hepatocellular injury and necrosis is rapid, with development of hepatic encephalopathy within 8 weeks of onset of disease.
6. Mortality rate is high, 60% to 85%, despite intensive treatment.

Clinical Manifestations

1. Malaise, anorexia, nausea, vomiting, fatigue
2. Jaundice, especially mucous membranes
3. Urine is tea-colored and frothy when shaken
4. Pruritus caused by bile salts deposited on skin
5. Steatorrhea and diarrhea due to decreased fat absorption
6. Peripheral edema as the fluid moves from the intravascular to the interstitial spaces, secondary to hypoproteinemia
7. Ascites from hypoproteinemia and/or portal hypertension
8. Easy bruising, petechiae, overt bleeding due to clotting deficiency
9. Altered levels of consciousness, ranging from irritability and confusion to stupor, somnolence, and coma
10. Change in deep tendon reflexes—initially hyperactive; become flaccid

11. Fetor hepaticus—breath odor of acetone
12. Portal systemic encephalopathy, also known as hepatic coma or hepatic encephalopathy, can occur in conjunction with cerebral edema
13. Cerebral edema is often the cause of death due to brain stem herniation or respiratory arrest

Diagnostic Evaluation

1. Prolonged prothrombin time, decreased platelet count
2. Elevated ammonia, amino acid, and mercaptan levels
3. Hypoglycemia or hyperglycemia
4. Dilutional hyponatremia or hypernatremia, hypokalemia, hypocalcemia, and hypomagnesemia

Management

1. Oral or rectal administration of lactulose (Cephulac) to minimize formation of ammonia and other nitrogenous by-products in the bowel.
2. Rectal administration of neomycin (Myciguent) to suppress urea-splitting enteric bacteria in the bowel and decrease ammonia formation.
3. Low-molecular-weight dextran or albumin followed by a potassium-sparing diuretic (spironolactone) to enhance fluid shift from interstitial back to intravascular spaces.
4. Pancreatic enzymes, if diarrhea and steatorrhea are present, to permit better tolerance of diet.
5. Mannitol (Osmitrol) IV for management of cerebral edema when indicated.
6. Cholestyramine (Questran) to promote fecal excretion of bile salts to decrease itching.
7. Antacids and histamine-2 (H_2) antagonists to reduce the risk of bleeding from stress ulcers.
8. Restriction of dietary protein and sodium while maintaining adequate caloric intake with diet or hypertonic dextrose solutions.
9. Supplemental vitamins (A, B complex, C, and K) and folate.
10. Infusion of fresh-frozen plasma to maintain prothrombin time; cryoprecipitate as needed.
11. Additional medical interventions, depending on the patient's condition, may include: hemodialysis, hemofiltration, hemoperfusion, or plasmapheresis.
12. Liver transplantation has become the treatment of choice.

Complications

1. Acute respiratory failure
2. Infections and sepsis
3. Cardiac dysfunction, hypotension
4. Hepatorenal failure
5. Hemorrhage

Nursing Assessment

1. Obtain history of exposure to drugs, chemicals, or toxins; exposure to infectious hepatitis; and course of illness.

2. Assess respiratory status, breath, level of consciousness, and vital signs.
3. Assess for ascites, edema, jaundice, bleeding, asterixis, presence or absence of reflexes.
4. Assess results of arterial blood gas evaluations, electrolytes, prothrombin time, and hemoglobin and hematocrit determinations.

Nursing Diagnoses

A. Fluid Volume Deficit related to hypoproteinemia, peripheral edema, ascites
B. Ineffective Breathing Pattern related to anemia and decreased lung expansion from ascites
C. Altered Nutrition: Less Than Body Requirements, related to GI side effects and decreased absorption storage, and metabolism of nutrients
D. Risk for Impaired Skin Integrity related to malnutrition, deposition of bile salts, peripheral edema, decreased activity
E. Risk for Infection related to altered immune response
F. Risk for Injury related to encephalopathy

Nursing Interventions

A. *Maintaining Adequate Fluid Volume*
1. Monitor vital signs frequently.
2. Weigh patient daily and keep an accurate intake and output record; record frequency and characteristics of stool.
3. Measure and record abdominal girth daily.
4. Assess and record the presence of peripheral edema.
5. Restrict sodium and fluids; replace electrolytes as directed.
6. Administer low-molecular-weight dextran or albumin and diuretics as prescribed.
7. Assess for any signs and symptoms of hemorrhage or bleeding.

B. *Improving Respiratory Status*
1. Monitor respiratory rate, depth, use of accessory muscles, nasal flaring, and breath sounds.
2. Evaluate results of arterial blood gases and hemoglobin and hematocrit evaluations.
3. Elevate head of the bed to lower diaphragm and decrease respiratory effort.
4. Turn frequently to prevent stasis of secretions.
5. Administer oxygen therapy as directed.

C. *Improving Nutritional Status*
1. Enlist a nutrition specialist to help evaluate nutritional status and needs.
2. Encourage the patient to eat in a sitting position to decrease abdominal tenderness and feeling of fullness.
3. Provide small, frequent meals or dietary supplements to conserve the patient's energy.
4. Provide mouth care if the patient has bleeding gums or fetor hepaticus.
5. Restrict sodium intake and protein based on ammonia levels and symptoms of encephalopathy.
6. Provide enteral and parenteral feedings as needed.

D. *Maintaining Skin Integrity*
1. Inspect skin for any alteration in integrity.
2. Provide good skin care.
3. Bathe without soap and apply soothing lotions.

4. Keep the patient's fingernails short to prevent scratching from pruritus.
5. Administer medications as prescribed for pruritus.
6. Assess for signs of bleeding from broken areas on the skin.
7. Turn the patient frequently to prevent pressure sores.
8. Avoid trauma and friction to the skin.

E. *Preventing Infection*
1. Be alert for signs of infection, such as fever, cloudy urine, abnormal breath sounds.
2. Use good hand washing and aseptic technique when caring for any break in the skin or mucous membranes.
3. Restrict visits with anyone who may have an infection.
4. Encourage the patient to try and not scratch itching skin.

F. *Preventing Injury*
1. Maintain close observation, side rails, and nurse call system.
2. Assist with ambulation as needed and avoid obstructions to prevent falls.
3. Have well-lit room and frequently reorient patient.
4. Observe for subtle changes in behavior (such as unkempt appearance), worsening of sample of handwriting, and change in sleeping pattern to detect worsening encephalopathy.

Patient Education/Health Maintenance

1. Teach patient and family to notify health care provider of increased abdominal discomfort, bleeding, increased edema or ascites, hallucinations, or lapses in consciousness.
2. Instruct to avoid activities that increase the risk of bleeding: scratching, falling, forceful nose blowing, aggressive tooth brushing, use of straight-edged razor.
3. Advise on limiting activities when fatigued and use of frequent rest periods.
4. Maintain close follow-up for laboratory testing and evaluation by health care provider.

Evaluation

A. Blood pressure stable, urine output adequate
B. Respirations unlabored
C. Tolerating 3 to 4 small feedings a day
D. Skin intact without abrasions
E. No fever or signs of infection
F. No falls

Biliary Disorders

The gallbladder stores and concentrates bile produced by the liver. The hormone cholecystokinin, secreted by the small intestine, stimulates contraction of the gallbladder and relaxation of the sphincter of Oddi for delivery of bile into the small intestine.

Bile aids function in fat emulsification (breakdown); absorption of fatty acids, cholesterol, and other lipids from the small intestine; and excretion of conjugated bilirubin from the liver.

◆ CHOLELITHIASIS, CHOLECYSTITIS, CHOLEDOCHOLITHIASIS

Cholelithiasis is the presence of stones in the gallbladder. Cholecystitis is inflammation of the gallbladder (may be acute or chronic). Choledocholithiasis is the presence of stones in the common bile duct.

Pathophysiology/Etiology

A. *Cholelithiasis*
1. Stones occur when cholesterol supersaturates the bile in the gallbladder and precipitates out of the bile. The cholesterol-saturated bile predisposes to the formation of gallstones and acts as an irritant, producing inflammatory changes in the gallbladder.
   a. Cholesterol stones are the most common type of gallstones found in the United States.
   b. Four times more women than men develop cholesterol stones.
   c. Women are usually older than 40 years of age, multiparous, and obese.
   d. Stone formation increases in users of contraceptives, estrogens, and cholesterol-lowering drugs, which are known to increase biliary cholesterol saturation.
   e. Bile acid malabsorption, genetic predisposition, and rapid weight loss are also risk factors for cholesterol gallstones.
2. Pigment stones occur when free bilirubin combines with calcium.
   a. Found in patients with cirrhosis, hemolysis, and infections in the biliary tree.
   b. These stones cannot be dissolved.
3. An estimated 25 million people in the United States have gallstones, with 1 million new cases discovered each year.
   a. Incidence of stone formation increases with age due to increased hepatic secretion of cholesterol and decreased bile acid synthesis.
   b. Increased risk in patients with malabsorption of bile salts with GI disease, bile fistula, gallstone ileus, carcinoma of the gallbladder, or in those who have had ileal resection or bypass.

B. *Cholecystitis*
1. Acute cholecystitis is an acute infection of the gallbladder.
   a. If the gallbladder is filled with pus, there is empyema of the gallbladder.
2. Most cases are caused by gallstone obstruction of the cystic duct, causing edema, inflammation, and bacterial invasion. This is called calculous cholecystitis.
3. Acalculous cholecystitis is acute gallbladder inflammation in the absence of obstruction by gallstones.
   a. Occurs after major surgical procedures, severe trauma, or burns.
4. Chronic cholecystitis occurs when the gallbladder becomes thickened, rigid, and fibrotic and functions poorly.
   a. Results from repeated attacks of cholecystitis, presence of calculi, or chronic irritation.

Clinical Manifestations

1. Gallstones that remain in the gallbladder are usually asymptomatic.
2. Biliary colic can be caused by the presence of gallstones.
   a. Steady, severe aching pain or sensation of pressure in the epigastrium or right upper quadrant, which may radiate to the right scapular area or right shoulder.
   b. Begins suddenly and persists for 1 to 3 hours until the stone falls back into the gallbladder or is passed through the cystic duct.
3. Acute cholecystitis causes biliary colic pain that persists more than 4 hours and increases with movement, including respirations.
   a. Also causes nausea and vomiting, low-grade fever, and jaundice (with stones or inflammation in the common bile duct).
   b. Right upper quadrant guarding and Murphy's sign (inability to take a deep inspiration when examiner's fingers are pressed below the hepatic margin) are present.
4. Chronic cholecystitis causes heartburn, flatulence, and indigestion.
   a. Repeated attacks of symptoms may occur resembling acute cholecystitis.

Diagnostic Evaluation

1. Oral cholecystography, ultrasonography, and hepatobiliary (HIDA) scan may visualize stones or inflammation.
2. ERCP and PTC to visualize location of stones and obstruction.
3. Elevated conjugated bilirubin due to obstruction.

Management

1. Supportive management includes: rest, IV fluids, nasogastric suction, pain management, and antibiotics (in the presence of a positive culture).
2. Surgical management.
   a. Cholecystectomy, open or laparoscopic (p. 540).
   b. Intraoperative cholangiography and choledochoscopy for common bile duct exploration.
   c. Placement of a T-tube in the common bile duct to decompress the biliary tree and allow access into the biliary tree postoperatively.
3. Oral therapy with chenodeoxycholic acid (CDCA), ursodeoxycholic acid (Actigall), or a combination of both to decrease the size of existing cholesterol stones or dissolve small ones.
   a. Indicated for patients at high risk for surgery because of age or systemic disease.
   b. Major adverse effects include diarrhea, abnormal liver function tests, increases in serum cholesterol.
4. Direct contact therapy where a local cholelitholytic agent is infused directly into the gallbladder through a percutaneous transhepatic catheter.
   a. Indicated for symptomatic, high-risk patients whose gallbladder can be visualized on oral cholecystography.
   b. Side effects include pain from the catheter, nausea, transient elevations of liver function tests and white blood count.

5. Intracorporeal lithotripsy is used to fragment stones in the gallbladder or common bile duct by ultrasound, pulsed laser, or hydraulic lithotripsy applied through an endoscope directly to the stones. The stone fragments are removed by irrigation and aspiration. A cholecystectomy may then be performed.

Complications

1. Cholangitis
2. Necrosis, empyema, or perforation of the gallbladder
3. Biliary fistula through the duodenum
4. Gallstone ileus
5. Adenocarcinoma of the gallbladder

Nursing Assessment

1. Obtain history and demographic data that may indicate risk factors for biliary disease.
2. Assess patient's pain for location, description, intensity, relieving and exacerbating factors.
3. Assess for signs of dehydration: dry mucous membranes, poor skin turgor, low urine output with elevated specific gravity.
4. Monitor temperature and white blood count for indications of infection or perforation.

Nursing Diagnosis

A. Pain related to biliary colic or stone obstruction
B. Fluid Volume Deficit related to nausea and vomiting and decreased intake

Nursing Interventions

A. *Relieving Pain*
1. Assess pain location, severity, and characteristics.
2. Administer medications or monitor patient-controlled analgesia to control pain.
3. Assist in attaining position of comfort; maintain bed rest during acute illness.

B. *Restoring Normal Fluid Volume*
1. Administer IV fluids and electrolytes as prescribed.
2. Administer antiemetics as prescribed to decrease nausea and vomiting.
3. Maintain nasogastric decompression until nausea and vomiting subside.
4. Begin food and fluids as tolerated, after acute symptoms subside or postoperatively.
5. Observe and record amount of T-tube drainage, if applicable.

Patient Education/ Health Maintenance

1. Instruct patient in care of any tubes or catheters that may be in place at discharge.
   a. Observe for bleeding or drainage around insertion site.

b. Replace gauze dressing when it becomes wet or soiled.

c. Report any change in drainage.

2. Review postoperative discharge instructions for activity, diet, medications, and postoperative follow-up.

3. Emphasize symptoms of complications to be reported; pain, fever, jaundice, unusual drainage.

4. Encourage follow-up for further treatment as indicated.

Evaluation

A. Patient verbalizes reduced pain level

B. Tolerating oral fluids, urine output adequate

Pancreatic Disorders

The pancreas secretes pancreatic hormones, including amylase and lipase, through the pancreatic duct when stimulated by cholecystokinin and secretin to aid in digestion of carbohydrates and fat in the small intestine.

◆ ACUTE PANCREATITIS

Acute pancreatitis is an inflammation of the pancreas, ranging from mild edema to extensive hemorrhage, resulting from a variety of insults to the pancreas. The structure and function of the pancreas usually return to normal after the acute attack.

Pathophysiology/Etiology

1. Excessive alcohol consumption is the most common cause in the United States.

2. Also commonly caused by biliary tract disease, such as cholelithiasis, acute and chronic cholecystitis.

3. Less common causes are bacterial or viral infection, blunt abdominal trauma, peptic ulcer disease, ischemic vascular disease, hyperlipidemia, hypercalcemia; the use of corticosteroids, thiazide diuretics, and oral contraceptives; surgery on or near the pancreas or after instrumentation of the pancreatic duct; tumors of the pancreas or ampulla; and a small incidence of hereditary pancreatitis.

4. Mortality is high (10%) because of shock, anoxia, hypotension, or fluid and electrolyte imbalances.

5. Attacks may result in complete recovery, may recur without permanent damage, or may progress to chronic pancreatitis.

6. Autodigestion of all or part of the pancreas is involved, but the exact mechanism is not completely understood.

Clinical Manifestations

(Depends on severity of pancreatic damage.)

1. Abdominal pain, usually constant, midepigastric or periumbilical, radiating to the back or flank

2. Nausea and vomiting

3. Low-grade fever

4. Involuntary abdominal guarding, epigastric tenderness to deep palpation, and reduced or absent bowel sounds

5. Dry mucous membranes; hypotension; cold, clammy skin; cyanosis; and tachycardia, which may reflect mild to moderate dehydration from vomiting or capillary leak syndrome (third space loss)

6. Shock may be the presenting manifestation in severe episodes, along with respiratory distress and acute renal failure

7. Purplish discoloration of the flanks (Grey Turner's sign) or of the periumbilical area (Cullen's sign) occurs in extensive hemorrhagic necrosis

Diagnostic Evaluation

1. Serum amylase, lipase, glucose, bilirubin, alkaline phosphatase, lactic dehydrogenase (LDH), AST, ALT, potassium, and cholesterol may be elevated

2. Serum albumin, calcium, sodium, magnesium, and possibly potassium—low due to dehydration, vomiting, and the binding of calcium in areas of fat necrosis

3. Abdominal x-ray—pancreatic calcification or peripancreatic gas pattern of a pancreatic abscess

4. Ultrasonography and CT—also determine pancreatic changes

5. Chest x-ray—for detection of pulmonary complications

Management

Depending on severity of episode, the management focuses on alleviation of symptoms and support of the patient to prevent complications.

1. Restoration of circulating blood volume with IV crystalloid or colloid solutions or blood products.

2. Maintenance of adequate oxygenation reduced by pain, anxiety, acidosis, abdominal pressure, or pleural effusions.

3. Pain control to alleviate pain and anxiety, which increases pancreatic secretions.

4. Rest of the GI tract

a. Withhold oral feedings to decrease pancreatic secretions.

b. Nasogastric intubation and suction to relieve gastric stasis, distention, and ileus.

5. Maintenance of alkaline gastric pH with H_2 antagonists and antacids to suppress acid drive of pancreatic secretions and prevent stress ulcer complications of acute illness.

6. Treatment of malnutrition with parenteral feedings, as needed.

7. Pharmacotherapy

a. Electrolyte replacements as needed.

b. Sodium bicarbonate to reverse metabolic acidosis.

c. Regular insulin to treat hyperglycemia.

d. Antibiotic therapy in the presence of infection or sepsis.

8. Surgical intervention if complications occur.

a. Incision and drainage of infection and pseudocysts.

b. Debridement or pancreatectomy to remove necrotic pancreatic tissue.

c. Cholecystectomy for gallstone pancreatitis.

Complications

1. Pancreatic abscess or pseudocyst
2. Pulmonary infiltrates, pleural effusion, adult respiratory distress syndrome
3. Hemorrhage with hypovolemic shock
4. Sepsis, acute renal failure

Nursing Assessment

1. Obtain history of gallbladder disease, alcohol use, and GI distress, including nausea and vomiting, diarrhea, and passage of stools containing fat.
2. Assess characteristics of abdominal pain.
3. Assess nutritional and fluid status.
4. Assess respiratory rate and pattern and breath sounds.

Nursing Diagnoses

A. Pain related to disease process
B. Fluid Volume Deficit related to vomiting, restricted intake, fever, and fluid shifts
C. Ineffective Breathing Pattern related to severe pain and pulmonary complications

Nursing Interventions

A. *Controlling Pain*
1. Administer narcotic analgesics as ordered to control pain. Monitor for hypotension and respiratory depression.
2. Assist patient to a comfortable position.
3. Maintain NPO status to decrease pancreatic enzyme secretion.
4. Maintain patency of nasogastric suction to remove gastric secretions and to relieve abdominal distention, if indicated.
5. Provide frequent oral hygiene and care.
6. Administer antacids followed by clamping of nasogastric tube. Check gastric aspirate pH after tube is clamped for 30 minutes.
7. Report any increase in severity of pain, which may indicate hemorrhage of the pancreas, rupture of a pseudocyst, or the dosage of the analgesic may be inadequate.

B. *Restoring Adequate Fluid Balance*
1. Monitor and record vital signs, skin color and temperature, and urinary and nasogastric output.
2. Monitor intake and output and weigh daily.

GERONTOLOGIC ALERT:
The incidence of severe, systemic complications of pancreatitis increases with age. Monitor kidney function and respiratory status closely in the elderly.

3. Evaluate laboratory data for hemoglobin, hematocrit, albumin, calcium, potassium, sodium, and magnesium levels and administer replacements as prescribed.
4. Observe and measure abdominal girth if ascites as suspected.

5. Report any trend in decreasing blood pressure or urine output or rising pulse, because this may indicate hypovolemia and shock or renal failure.

C. *Improving Respiratory Function*
1. Assess respiratory rate and rhythm, effort, oxygen saturation, and breath sounds frequently.
2. Position in upright or semi-Fowler's position to enhance diaphragmatic excursion.
3. Administer oxygen supplementation as prescribed to maintain adequate oxygen levels.
4. Report signs of respiratory distress immediately.
5. Instruct patient in coughing and deep breathing to improve respiratory function.

Patient Education/ Health Maintenance

1. Instruct patient to gradually resume a low-fat diet.
2. Instruct patient to increase activity gradually, providing for daily rest periods.
3. Reinforce information about disease process and precipitating factors. Stress that subsequent bouts of acute pancreatitis destroy more and more of the pancreas and cause additional complications.
4. If the pancreatitis is a result of alcohol abuse, the patient needs to be reminded of the importance of eliminating all alcohol; advise on Alcoholics Anonymous or other substance abuse counseling.

Evaluation

A. Verbalizes reduced pain level
B. Blood pressure stable; urine output adequate
C. Respirations unlabored; breath sounds clear

◆ CHRONIC PANCREATITIS

Chronic pancreatitis is defined as the persistence of pancreatic cellular damage after acute inflammation and decreased pancreatic exocrine function.

Pathophysiology/Etiology

1. Alcohol abuse is the most common cause; less common causes are hyperparathyroidism, hereditary pancreatitis, malnutrition, and trauma to the pancreas
2. With chronic inflammation there is destruction of the secreting cells of the pancreas, causing maldigestion and malabsorption of protein and fat and possibly diabetes mellitus if islet cells have been affected.
3. As cells are replaced by fibrous tissue, obstruction of the pancreatic and common bile ducts and duodenum may result.

Clinical Manifestations

1. Pain is usually located in the epigastrium or left upper quadrant, often radiating to the back; similar to that

observed in acute pancreatitis, but more constant and occurring at unpredictable intervals. As the disease progresses, recurring attacks of pain will be more severe, more frequent, and of longer duration.

2. Weight loss.
3. Malabsorption and steatorrhea occur late in course
4. Diabetes mellitus

Diagnostic Evaluation

1. Amylase and lipase—elevated but may not be grossly abnormal
2. Bilirubin and alkaline phosphatase—elevated if biliary obstruction occurs
    a. Secretin and cholecystokinin stimulatory tests—abnormal
    b. Fecal fat analysis—determines need for pancreatic enzyme replacement
3. CT or ultrasonography—identifies pancreatic structural changes, such as calcifications, masses, ductal irregularities, enlargement, and cysts
4. ERCP—defines ductal anatomy and localizes complications, such as pancreatic pseudocysts and ductal disruptions

Management

1. Pain management
2. Correction of nutritional deficiencies
3. Pancreatic enzyme replacement
4. Treatment of diabetes
5. Surgical interventions to reduce pain, restore drainage of pancreatic secretions, correct structural abnormalities, and manage complications. Care is similar to the patient undergoing abdominal surgery (p. 494).
    a. Pancreaticojejunostomy—side-to-side anastomosis of pancreatic duct to jejunum to drain pancreatic secretions into jejunum
    b. Revision of sphincter of ampulla of Vater
    c. Drainage of pancreatic cyst into stomach
    d. Resection or removal of pancreas (pancreatectomy)
    e. Autotransplantation of islet cells

Complications

1. Pancreatic pseudocyst
2. Pancreatic ascites and pleural effusions
3. Gastrointestinal hemorrhage
4. Biliary tract obstruction

Nursing Assessment

1. Assess level of abdominal pain.
2. Assess nutritional status.
3. Assess for signs and symptoms of diabetes.
4. Assess current level of alcohol intake and motivation and resources available to abstain from drinking.

Nursing Diagnoses

A. Pain related to chronic insult to pancreas
B. Altered nutrition, Less Than Body Requirements related to fear of eating, malabsorption, and glucose intolerance
C. Anxiety related to surgical intervention

Nursing Interventions

A. *Controlling Pain*
1. Assess and record the character, location, frequency, and duration of pain.
2. Determine precipitating and alleviating factors of the patient's pain.
3. Explore the effect of pain on the patient's lifestyle and eating habits.
4. Administer or teach self-administration of analgesics (frequently narcotics) as ordered to control pain.
5. Use nonpharmacologic methods along with pain medications to promote relaxation, such as distraction, imagery, and progressive muscle relaxation.
6. Assess response to pain control measures, and refer to chronic pain management clinic, if indicated.

B. *Improving Nutritional Status*
1. Assess nutritional status, history of weight loss, and dietary habits, including alcohol intake.
2. Administer pancreatic enzyme replacement with meals, as prescribed.
3. Administer antacids and/or H_2 receptor antagonists to prevent neutralization of enzyme supplements, as indicated.
4. Monitor intake and output and daily weight.
5. Assess for GI discomfort with meals and character of stools.
6. Monitor blood glucose levels and teach balanced, low concentrated-carbohydrate diet and insulin therapy as indicated.

> **NURSING ALERT:**
> Warn patient that dangerous hypoglycemic reaction may result from use of insulin while still drinking and skipping meals.

7. Identify foods that aggravate symptoms and teach low-fat diet.

C. *Relieving Anxiety About Surgical Intervention*
1. Describe planned surgical intervention and the expected results.
    a. Decreased pain
    b. Ability to eat better and improve general condition
2. Prepare patient for side effects/complications of surgery.
    a. Total pancreatectomy will cause permanent diabetes mellitus and dependence on insulin along with severe malabsorption and the need for lifelong pancreatic enzyme replacement.
    b. Malnutrition and debility make patient more at risk for poor healing and complications of surgery.
3. Assist patient to prepare for surgery by encouraging abstinence of alcohol and intake of nutritional and vitamin supplements.

4. Encourage patient to enlist help of support network and strengthen appropriate coping mechanisms.
5. After surgery, provide meticulous care to prevent infection, promote wound healing, and prevent routine complications of surgery (see p. 85).

Patient Education/ Health Maintenance

1. Instruct the patient regarding use of analgesics to prevent overdose or dependence.
2. Instruct on proper administration of pancreatic enzyme replacement.
   a. Take just before or during meals.
   b. May be enteric coated, so do not crush or chew tablets; powder may be obtained if difficulty swallowing tablets.
   c. Take with antacid or take H_2 antagonist as directed to prevent pancreatic enzyme from being destroyed by gastric acid secretions.
3. Advise patient to monitor number and characteristics of stools; report increased stools or food intolerance.
4. Teach blood glucose monitoring, if applicable, and urge follow-up to monitor progression of condition.
5. Stress that no treatment will be effective if alcohol consumption is continued.

Evaluation

A. Verbalizes reduced pain level
B. Weight gain noted
C. Verbalizes understanding of effects of surgical procedure

◆ PANCREATIC CANCER

Cancer of the pancreas may arise in the head (70%) or body and tail (30%) of the pancreas. Adenocarcinoma of ductal epithelium is the most common (80%) cell type. Pancreatic cancer is the fourth leading cause of cancer deaths.

Pathophysiology/Etiology

1. Incidence is increasing.
2. Usually occurs between the ages of 60 and 80.
3. Smoking, prolonged exposure to industrial chemicals, high-fat diet, excessive alcohol intake, diabetes mellitus, and chronic pancreatitis are considered risk factors.
4. Obstruction of bile flow may occur with tumors to the head of the pancreas due to pressure on the common bile duct.
5. Obstruction of pancreatic duct produces pain and exocrine dysfunction.
6. Islet cell tumors (rare) produce hyperinsulinism.

Clinical Manifestations

1. Symptoms are often vague and nonspecific, preventing early detection

2. Weight loss, pain, anorexia, nausea, vomiting, and weakness occur
3. Pain usually occurs in the upper abdomen and is gnawing or boring and may radiate to the back
   a. Pain is often worse at night, and patients tend to lie with legs drawn up or bend over while walking
   b. Pain becomes more localized, severe, and unremitting as the disease progresses
4. Early satiety and a feeling of bloating after eating may occur
5. Biliary obstruction produces jaundice, tea-colored urine, clay-colored stools, and pruritus
6. Depression and lethargy are common

Diagnostic Evaluation

1. Ultrasonography and CT—detect tumors larger than 2 cm.
2. ERCP—allows biopsy or aspiration for cytology to confirm diagnosis.
3. Liver function tests elevated; coagulation studies prolonged.
4. Carcinoembryonic antigen (CEA) and CA 19-9—may be elevated.
5. Percutaneous needle aspiration or biopsy through ultrasonography.
6. Angiography may be performed to assess for any vascular involvement.

Management

The goal of treatment may be cure or palliation, depending on the staging of the tumor. Most cases are usually too far advanced for cure. Longer palliation is now being achieved.

A. *Surgery*
1. Whipple's procedure (pancreatoduodenectomy) is the removal of the head of the pancreas, distal portion of the common bile duct including the gallbladder, duodenum, and the distal stomach with anastomosis of the remaining pancreas, stomach, and common bile duct to the jejunum (Fig. 17-3).
   a. Stomach and pylorus may be preserved—pylorus-preserving Whipple's procedure.
   b. Done for carcinoma of the head of the pancreas, periampullary area, chronic pancreatitis of the head of the pancreas, and trauma.
2. Total pancreatectomy including a splenectomy may be performed for diffuse tumor throughout the pancreas.
3. Distal pancreatectomy is the removal of the distal pancreas and spleen for tumors localized in the body and tail.
4. Palliative bypass of the bile duct (choledochojejunostomy or cholecystojejunostomy) and/or stomach (gastrojejunostomy) for unresectable tumors of the pancreas.
5. Care is similar to that of patient undergoing abdominal surgery (see p. 494).

B. *Other Measures*
1. Chemotherapy may be used in combination with radiation therapy for resectable and unresectable tumors with and without surgery.
2. Radiation therapy may be used alone palliatively or as adjuvant to surgery.

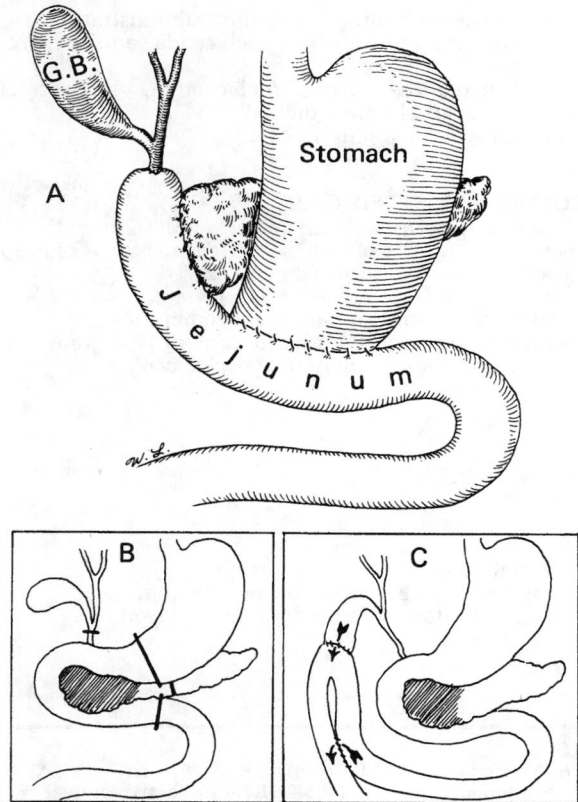

FIGURE 17-3 *Pancreatoduodenectomy (Whipple's procedure or resection).* **(A)** *End result of resection of the carcinoma of the head of the pancreas or the ampulla of Vater. The common duct is sutured to the end of the jejunum, and the remaining portion of the pancreas and the end of the stomach are sutured to the side of the jejunum.* **(B)** *Lines indicate removal of head of pancreas, duodenum, adjacent stomach, and distal segment of common bile duct.* **(C)** *Cholecystojejunostomy is an alternative procedure if a tumor of the head of the pancreas is inoperable. Bile flows into the intestine through the anastomosis of the jejunum and gallbladder.*

    a. External beam irradiation for local control, reduction of pain, and to palliate obstruction.
    b. Intraoperative radiation therapy has been successful in some centers for palliation.
3. Endoscopic or percutaneous stent placement for relief of biliary obstruction.
4. Chemical splanchnicectomy is injection of alcohol into the celiac axis nerves to denervate the nerves in the area of the pancreas for pain relief
    a. May be performed intraoperatively or percutaneously under CT guidance.
5. Clinical investigations combining various treatments are aimed at improving the prognosis of pancreatic cancer.

Complications

1. Biliary, gastric, and duodenal obstruction
2. Metastases

Nursing Assessment

1. Obtain history for risk factors, pain, and symptoms of pancreatic dysfunction.
2. Assess nutritional status, including diet history, anorexia, weight loss, nausea and vomiting, steatorrhea, skin turgor.
3. Evaluate laboratory results for alterations in glucose, pancreatic enzymes, liver function, and coagulation studies.
4. Assess psychosocial status to determine presence of depression, usual coping strategies, support systems, and experience with past serious illness.

Nursing Diagnoses

A. Pain related to nonresectable pancreatic tumor or surgical incision
B. Altered Nutrition: Less Than Body Requirements, related to disease process and/or surgical intervention
C. Fluid Volume Deficit related to hypoproteinemia, leakage at anastomosis, or hemorrhage
D. Impaired Tissue Integrity related to malnutrition, surgical incisions, and pancreatic or bile drainage

Nursing Interventions

A. *Controlling Pain*
1. Administer narcotics as ordered or monitor patient-controlled analgesia.
2. Teach relaxation techniques, such as relaxation breathing, progressive muscle relaxation, and imagery, as adjuncts for pain relief.
3. Assist with frequent turning and comfortable positioning.
4. Administer adjuvant medications, such as antidepressants and antipruritics, as prescribed.
5. Assess patient's response to pain control measures and consider consultation with hospice service for pain control if tumor is nonresectable.

B. *Improving Nutritional Status*
1. Administer parenteral nutrition as prescribed preoperatively and postoperatively.
2. Maintain nasogastric decompression and measure and record gastric output.
3. Monitor serum glucose level for hyperglycemia or hypoglycemia.
4. Progress diet slowly when oral intake is tolerated; observe for nausea, vomiting, and gastric distention.
5. Administer high-protein, high-carbohydrate diet with vitamin supplements and pancreatic enzymes as prescribed.
6. Weigh daily.

C. *Attaining Adequate Fluid Volume*
1. Monitor vital signs and record accurate intake and output of fluid.
2. Evaluate serum albumin levels and replace as prescribed.
3. Evaluate laboratory values for hyponatremia, hypochloremia, and metabolic alkalosis; replace electrolytes as prescribed.
4. Administer fluid replacement as indicated.

5. Report change in vital signs or increased pain, which may indicate hemorrhage or leak from anastomosis.

D. *Maintaining Tissue Integrity*
1. Observe skin for jaundice, breakdown, irritation, or excoriation.
2. Administer antipruritics, provide frequent skin care without soap and with thorough rinsing, apply emollient lotions, keep fingernails short to prevent scratching.
3. Inspect skin around drains for irritation and protect skin from leakage of fluids from drains and tubes.
4. Inspect surgical dressings and incision for bleeding, drainage, or signs of infection.
5. Prevent tension on suture lines of anastomoses by monitoring for abdominal distention and maintaining patency of surgically placed tubes and drains.
6. Maintain aseptic technique in handling wound dressings and drainage of all secretions.

Patient Education/Health Maintenance

1. Instruct patient and family on self-care measures for pancreatic insufficiency.

a. Glucose monitoring, insulin administration, signs and symptoms of hypoglycemia and hyperglycemia.
b. Pancreatic enzyme replacement, high-protein, high-carbohydrate diet.
2. Teach wound and drain care.

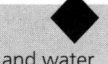

COMMUNITY-BASED CARE TIP:
Skin around drainage tubes can be washed with soap and water, dried well, and then protected by generous application of petroleum jelly or zinc oxide before dressing applied.

3. Explore options for pain management.
4. Coordinate referral for home care for IV therapy, post-operative management, or hospice care.

Evaluation

A. Verbalizes reduced pain
B. Weight stable
C. Vital signs stable; urine output adequate
D. Incision intact without drainage or bleeding

Selected References

Ahlgren, J. D., & MacDonald, J. S. (Eds.). (1992). *Gastrointestinal oncology.* Philadelphia: Lippincott.

Bayless, T. M. (Ed.). (1994). *Current therapy in gastroenterology and liver disease.* St. Louis: Mosby.

Blumgart, L. H. (Ed.). (1994). *Surgery of the liver and biliary tract* (2nd ed.). Edinburgh: Churchill Livingstone.

Burnett, D. A.,. & Rikkers, L. F. (1990). Nonoperative emergency treatment of variceal bleeding. *Surgical Clinics of North America, 70*(2), 291-306.

Butler, R. W. (1994). Managing the complications of cirrhosis. *AJN, 94*(3), 46-49.

Dusheiko, G. M. (1994). Rolling review—the pathogenesis, diagnosis and management of viral hepatitis. *Alimentary Pharmacology & Therapeutics, 8*(2), 229-253.

Fernandez-del Castillo, C., & Warshaw, A. L. (1994). Pancreatic carcinoma. *Current Opinion in Gastroenterology, 10,* 507-512.

Go, V. W. L., Dimagno, E. P., Gardner, J. D., Lebenthal, E., Reber, H. A., & Scheele, G. A. (Eds.). (1993). *The pancreas biology, pathobiology, and disease* (2nd ed.). New York: Raven Press.

Imrie, C. W. (1994). Acute pancreatitis. *Current Opinion in Gastroenterology, 10,* 496-501.

Jackson, M. M. & Rymer, T. E. (1994) Viral hepatitis: Anatomy of a diagnosis. *AJN, 94*(1), 43-48.

Korc, M., & Schmiegel, W. (1994). Chronic pancreatitis. *Current Opinion in Gastroenterology, 10,* 502-506.

Lisanti, P. & Talotta, D. (1994). An overview of viral hepatitis: A through E. *AORN Journal, 59*(5), 997-1005.

McCormick, P. A., & Burroughs, A. K. (1994). Relation between liver pathology and prognosis in patients with portal hypertension. *World Journal of Surgery, 18*(2), 171-175.

Murr, M. M., Sarr, M. G., Oishi, A. J., & van Heerden, J. A. (1994). Pancreatic Cancer. *CA A Cancer Journal for Clinicians, 44*(5), 304-318.

Schaffner, M. (1994). *Manual of gastrointestinal procedures* (3rd ed.). Baltimore: Williams & Wilkins.

Winchester, C. B., Dhekne, R. D., Moore, W. H., & Murphy, P. H. (1994). Clinical applications of nuclear medicine in gastroenterology. *Gastroenterology Nursing, 17*(1), 20-26.

Zuckerman, A. J. (1993). Viral hepatitis. *Transfusion Medicine, 3*(1), 7-19.

CHAPTER 18

Nutritional Disorders

General Considerations

◆ NUTRITION OVERVIEW

Knowledge of nutrients and the basic principles of nutrition has become increasingly important in the role of patient teaching for disease prevention and health promotion. The four basic food groups and their placement on a pyramid serves as a guide to basic, healthy nutrition.

Key Principles

1. Nutrients, including carbohydrates, fats, proteins, vitamins, and minerals have specific functions and roles within the body, and work together to provide energy, regulate metabolic processes, and synthesize tissue.
2. Nutrition influences all body systems both favorably and unfavorably. Examples of unfavorable effects include the link between cholesterol and heart disease or salt intake and high blood pressure. Favorable effects are many, such as the association of fiber intake to gastrointestinal (GI) function and the role of antioxidant vitamins, such as A, C, and E, and cancer.
3. Nutritional needs vary in response to metabolic changes, age, sex, growth periods, stress (trauma, disease, pregnancy, lactation), and physical condition.
4. Dietary and vitamin supplements may be needed depending on disease states, dietary intake, and other factors.
5. The types of foods eaten and eating patterns are developed over a lifetime and are determined by psychosocial, cultural, religious, and economic influences.
6. The nurse works in collaboration with the dietitian or nutritionist to promote optimum nutrition for each patient.

Basic Food Groups and Food Pyramid

1. Developed in 1958, the four basic food groups are grains, vegetables and fruits, meat, and milk. A fifth

group is considered when looking at fat in the diet. A well-balanced diet consists of foods from each group.
2. In response to growing scientific knowledge regarding the linkage of diet and disease, the United States Department of Agriculture developed the Food Guide Pyramid (Fig. 18-1). It reflects an increased emphasis on carbohydrates in the form of grains, fruits, and vegetables as primary food sources, with a decreased emphasis on meats, milk, and fats.
3. In addition, seven basic dietary guidelines have been developed to promote sound eating habits and optimal health. They are:
   a. Eat a variety of foods.
   b. Maintain a healthy weight.
   c. Choose a diet low in fat, saturated fat, and cholesterol.
   d. Choose a diet with plenty of vegetables, fruits, and grains.
   e. Use sugar in moderation.
   f. Use salt and sodium in moderation.
   g. Drink alcoholic beverages in moderation.

◆ NUTRITIONAL ASSESSMENT

There are many methods to assess the type and amount of food consumed, including a 24-hour recall of foods eaten over the previous day, a food diary kept by the patient for several days, and a food frequency questionnaire that reflects food intake patterns.

In addition to these specific tools, the following information is useful to determine nutritional patterns and status.

Key History Points

1. General background information—name, age, sex, family composition, socioeconomic status, occupation
2. General health status and any chronic conditions, including diabetes and associated dietary restrictions
3. Cultural/religious factors influencing dietary patterns
4. Family history of diseases, including diabetes and obesity
5. Current medications
6. Food habits
   a. Typical daily intake, including meal frequency, meal timing, meal location
   b. Snacking patterns

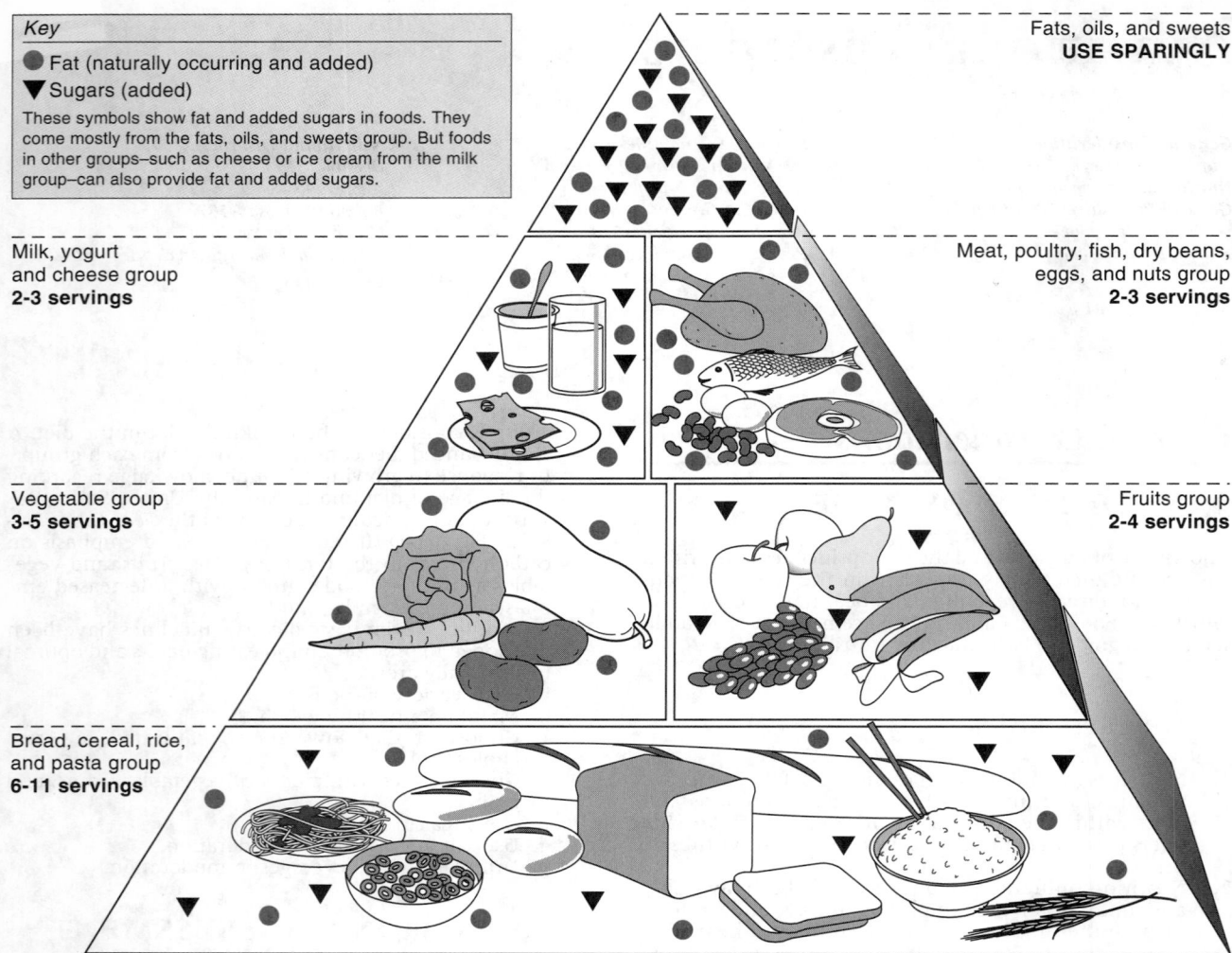

Key

● Fat (naturally occurring and added)

▼ Sugars (added)

These symbols show fat and added sugars in foods. They come mostly from the fats, oils, and sweets group. But foods in other groups—such as cheese or ice cream from the milk group—can also provide fat and added sugars.

Fats, oils, and sweets
USE SPARINGLY

Milk, yogurt
and cheese group
2-3 servings

Meat, poultry, fish, dry beans,
eggs, and nuts group
2-3 servings

Vegetable group
3-5 servings

Fruits group
2-4 servings

Bread, cereal, rice,
and pasta group
6-11 servings

FIGURE 18-1 The Food Guide Pyramid

c. Food intolerance or dislikes
d. Nutritional supplements, including vitamins, drinks, and food
e. Alcohol consumption
f. Use of specific diets/dietary restrictions
7. Food purchase and preparation
a. Who purchases and prepares food and where food is purchased
b. Facilities for food storage and preparation
c. Factors influencing the types of food purchased
8. Nutritionally related problems
a. General well-being, energy level
b. Weight change over the past 6 months
c. Difficulty chewing or swallowing, use of dentures
d. Change in sense of taste or smell
e. Presence of eructation, flatulence, nausea, vomiting, diarrhea, constipation, or abdominal pain or swelling and relation to food intake
f. Bowel habits

Physical Examination/ Anthropometrics

1. Perform a systematic physical examination, observing for a wide variety of physical findings associated with nutritional status.
a. Listless, apathetic
b. Poor muscle tone
c. Dull, brittle hair; may be thin or sparse, easily plucked
d. Rough, dry, scaly skin
e. Cheilosis (fissures at angles of mouth)
f. Stomatitis (inflammation of mouth)
g. Inflammation and easy bleeding of gums
h. Glossitis (inflammation of tongue)
i. Dental caries and poor dentition
j. Spoon-shaped, brittle, ridged nails
k. Skeletal deformities, such as bowlegs

2. Perform anthropometry as indicated. (Anthropometry comes from the word anthropology and is the science that studies the size, weight, and proportions of the human body to determine body fat mass and nutritional status.)

3. Types of anthropometric measurements include height and weight, skin-fold thickness, and circumferential tests.

4. Height and weight are determined on patient admission and later used as a baseline for comparisons in nutritional status (Table 18-1).
   a. Height is the distance from the patient's feet to the top of the head.
   b. Weight is the measure of total body energy stores.
   c. Weight should be measured using a consistent and reliable scale and at a consistent time.
   d. Weight loss of more than 10% of body weight over 6 months is considered clinically significant and may be associated with physiologic abnormalities and increased mortality.
   e. Body mass index is the ratio of weight in kilograms and height in meters. Normal range is 20 to 25 kg/m^2.

5. Skin-fold thickness provides an estimate of body fat based on the amount of fat in subcutaneous tissue (Fig. 18-2).
   a. Triceps skin-fold thickness
      (1) At the midpoint of the nondominant upper arm, grasp skin and subcutaneous fat, pulling it away from the underlying muscle, and place the caliper jaws over the skin-fold flap.
      (2) Take the reading within 2 to 3 seconds and without using excessive pressure.
      (3) Repeat the reading twice and take an average of the three readings to increase accuracy.

   b. Subscapular skin-fold thickness
      (1) Grasp the skin and subcutan... low the inferior boarder of th... measure with calipers as noted...

6. Circumferential tests provide inform... amount of skeletal muscle and adipose t...
   a. Mid–upper arm circumference—an ... esti-mate of the body's muscle mass
      (1) Place a tape measure around the midpoint of the nondominant upper arm and secure it snugly.
      (2) To calculate, multiply the triceps skin fold by 3.14 and subtract the product from the mid–upper arm circumference.
      (3) Adult standards are 16.5 mm for women and 12.5 mm for men.

Diagnostic Tests

1. Serum albumin—Albumin is responsible for maintaining blood volume and serum and electrolyte balance. A decrease in nutritional status may result in a drop in albumin synthesis.

2. Hemoglobin—Decreased amounts are related to iron deficiency anemia.

3. Serum transferrin—Responsible for binding iron to plasma and transporting it to the bone marrow. Reduced levels are found in catabolic states and some chronic diseases.

4. Twenty-four hour urine creatinine—An increase in this measure indicates increased tissue breakdown.

5. Twenty-four hour urea nitrogen—This test can be used to determine nitrogen balance.

TABLE 18-1 Height–Weight Tables

Men					Women				
Height		Small Frame	Medium Frame	Large Frame	Height		Small Frame	Medium Frame	Large Frame
Feet	Inches				Feet	Inches			
5	2	128–134	131–141	138–150	4	10	102–111	109–121	118–131
5	3	130–136	133–143	140–153	4	11	103–113	111–123	120–134
5	4	132–138	135–145	142–156	5	0	104–115	113–126	122–137
5	5	134–140	137–148	144–160	5	1	106–118	115–129	125–140
5	6	136–142	139–151	146–164	5	2	108–121	118–132	128–143
5	7	138–145	142–154	149–168	5	3	111–124	121–135	131–147
5	8	140–148	145–157	152–172	5	4	114–127	124–138	134–151
5	9	142–151	148–160	155–176	5	5	117–130	127–141	137–155
5	10	144–154	151–163	158–180	5	6	120–133	130–144	140–159
5	11	146–157	154–166	161–184	5	7	123–136	133–147	143–163
6	0	149–160	157–170	164–188	5	8	126–139	136–150	146–167
6	1	152–164	160–174	168–192	5	9	129–142	139–153	149–170
6	2	155–168	164–178	172–197	5	10	132–145	142–156	152–173
6	3	158–172	167–182	176–202	5	11	135–148	145–159	155–176
6	4	162–176	171–187	181–207	6	0	138–151	148–162	158–179

Weight according to frame (ages 25–59) for men wearing indoor clothing weighing 5 lbs., shoes with 1-in. heels; for women, indoor clothing weighing 3 lbs., shoes with 1-in. heels.
(Courtesy Metropolitan Life Insurance Company).

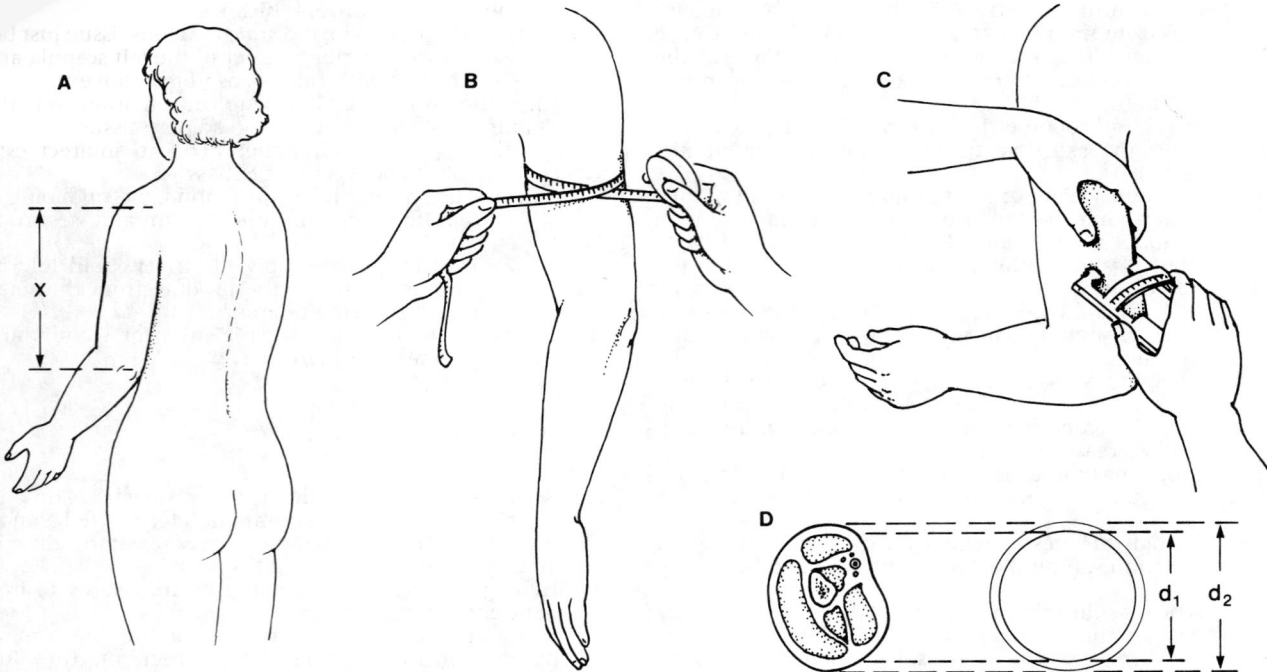

FIGURE 18-2 *Anthropometric measurements. Proper positioning of the patient is required:* **(A)** *for measuring the mid-upper arm,* **(B)** *to determine mid upper-arm circumference (MAC); this position is also used to measure* **(C)** *the triceps skinfold (TSF) thickness which is measured with a caliper;* **(D)** *shows the relation between d_1 (MAMC)—mid-upper arm muscle circumference and d_2 (MAC—mid-upper arm circumference). Mid-upper arm muscle circumference is a significant measurement in determining protein-calorie malnutrition. Formula for calculation: MAMC = MAC − (0.314 × TSF). (Adapted from Blackburn GL and Harvey KB. Nutritional assessment as a routine in clinical medicine. Postgrad Med 1982 May; 71(5):51.)*

General Procedures/ Treatment Modalities

◆ ENTERAL FEEDING

(See Procedure Guidelines 18-1: Administration of Enteral [Tube] Feedings: Intermittent or Continuous.)

Administration of nutrients directly into the stomach, duodenum, or jejunum through a tube is more physiologically beneficial and cost-effective than parenteral feeding. Enteral feeding carries less risk of infection than parenteral feeding and maintains a functional GI tract by preventing mucosal atrophy and biliary and pancreatic dysfunction. Enteral therapy is appropriate for patients with at least a minimally functional GI tract but who are unable to take nutrition by mouth.

Enteral therapy has become increasingly used as more commercially available enteral formula have been developed and long-term enteral feeding tubes have become safer and more easily inserted.

Clinical Indications

1. Increased metabolic needs—trauma, burns, cancer
2. Coma
3. Head/neck surgery
4. Malabsorption
5. Obstruction of esophagus or oropharynx
6. Severe anorexia nervosa
7. Recurrent aspiration

Sites of Tube Insertion

A. Short-Term Nutritional Support
1. Nasogastric—tube passed through the nose or mouth (orogastric) into the stomach and secured in place.
2. Nasoduodenal or nasojejunal—tube passed through the nose into duodenum or jejunum and secured in place.

B. Long-Term Nutritional Support
1. Gastrostomy—insertion of a tube either surgically or through a percutaneous endoscopic procedure into the stomach.
2. Gastrostomy button—small device inserted through gastrostomy stoma to allow for long-term feeding with minimal effect on body image.
3. Jejunostomy—insertion of a tube directly into the jejunum either surgically or through a percutaneous endoscopic procedure.
   a. Jejunostomy feedings are generally by continuous infusion using a volume control infuser.

Types of Tubes

1. Large-bore nasogastric polyurethane Levine tube—size 12 to 18F; used very short-term.
2. Small-bore nasogastric tube—made of polyurethane, silicone, or polyvinyl chloride with a tungsten-weighted tip at distal end; size 6 to 12F and 30 to 36 inches long.
3. Nasointestinal tube—made of silicone, polyurethane, or polyvinyl chloride with tungsten-weighted tip; size 6 to 12F and 40 to 60 inches long.
4. Gastrostomy tube—Foley or mushroom catheter type made of silicone, polyurethane, polyvinyl chloride, or latex; a balloon on the distal end to stabilize tube may be used and ranges in size from 5 to 30 mL capacity.
5. Gastrostomy button—silicone; size ranging from 18 to 28F and 1 in. long; useful for person wanting minimal alteration in body image.
6. Jejunostomy tube—size ranging from 5 to 14F with or without a balloon (a balloon may obstruct lumen of jejunum).

Delivery Systems for Feeding Solution

1. Intermittent or continuous infusion of feeding solution by gravity is accomplished by hanging container of feeding solution from an intravenous (IV) pole and adjusting delivery rate by flow regulator.
2. Continuous feeding by controller feeding pump allows uniform flow, particularly of viscous solutions.
3. Bolus feeding involves enteral formula poured into barrel of a large (60-mL) syringe attached to a feeding tube and allowed to infuse by gravity.

NURSING ALERT:
Bolus feeding may precipitate dumping syndrome, particularly if given into the small intestine.

Complications

(See Table 18-2.)

PROCEDURE GUIDELINES 18-1 ◆ Administration of Enteral (Tube) Feedings: Intermittent or Continuous

EQUIPMENT

Tube feeding formula
Graduated containers
30–60 ml catheter-tipped syringe
Water
Stethoscope

pH strip
Gavage feeding bag (optional)
For continuous tube feeding:
Tube feeding bag and tubing and volume control infuser

PROCEDURE

NURSING ACTION	RATIONALE
PREPARATORY PHASE	
1. Remove formula from refrigerator and allow to come to room temperature.	1. Use prepared dietary formulas within 24 hours.
2. Explain procedure to patient.	
3. Wash hands.	3. Prevent bacterial contamination of formula.
4. Protect patient from spillage.	
5. Shake formula container.	5. Shaking prevents separation of formula.
6. Elevate head of bed 30–45 degrees.	6. Prevents aspiration.
7. Using the catheter-tipped syringe, inject 20–30 cc of air while listening with a stethoscope positioned at the epigastric area (for nasogastric tubes). For nasointestinal tubes, 20 cc of air may be injected, but auscultation site may be displaced laterally and inferiorly.	7. Auscultation of a ''whooshing'' or bubbling sound assists in confirmation of proper tube placement. Should the patient burp immediately after injection of air, suspect esophageal placement of tube.
8. Aspirate stomach contents.	8. If residual gastric contents exceed 100 cc for intermittent tube feedings or greater than 1.5 times the hourly rate for continuous tube feeding, hold feeding and notify health care provider. No residual will be obtained with intestinal placement.
9. Measure pH of residual.	9. pH of gastric contents should be between 1 and 6. Intestinal pH may be over 6. Respiratory tract secretions usually measure over 6.
10. If residual is within normal limits, return gastric contents to stomach through syringe using gravity to assist flow.	10. Returning gastric contents to stomach prevents acid–base and electrolyte imbalance.
PERFORMANCE PHASE	
1. For intermittent tube feeding, attach barrel of catheter-tipped syringe to pinched-off feeding tube.	1. Pinching off the feeding tube prevents air from entering the stomach and causing distention.
2. Fill catheter-tipped syringe with formula and allow fluid to flow in by gravity.	2. The rate of flow is regulated by raising or lowering the syringe.

(continued)

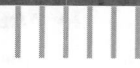

PROCEDURE GUIDELINES 18-1 ◆ Administration of Enteral (Tube) Feedings: Intermittent or Continuous
(continued)

PROCEDURE (cont'd)	NURSING ACTION	RATIONALE

PERFORMANCE PHASE

3. Pour additional formula into barrel of syringe when it is three-quarters empty.

3. Prevents air from entering stomach.

4. After administering the prescribed amount of formula, flush tubing with at least 30 cc of water.

4. Prevents clogging of feeding tube.

5. If using a gavage bag for intermittent feeding, fill bag with prescribed amount of feeding, purge feeding bag tubing of air, attach distal end to feeding tube, and regulate to run in over 10–20 min.

6. For continuous tube feeding, fill bag with 4 hours of tube feeding, flush tubing, attach to volume control infuser according to manufacturer's instructions, attach distal end to feeding tube, and start. Flush with 30–60 cc of water every 4 hours after first checking residual.

6. Prevents bacterial contamination. Maintains tube patency.

7. After intermittent feeding is completed, cover end of feeding tube with plug or clamp.

7. Prevents leakage.

FOLLOW-UP PHASE

1. Rinse equipment with warm water, and dry. Replace every 24 hours or per agency policy.

1. Limits bacterial contamination.

2. Maintain head of bed elevation for 30–60 min. after feeding is completed. If continuous feeding, maintain head elevation continuously.

2. Prevents aspiration.

3. Document type and amount of feeding, amount of water given, and patient tolerance of procedure.

4. Monitor breath sounds, bowel sounds, gastric distention, diarrhea or constipation, intake and output, daily weight, and serum chemistry results.

4. Evaluates for aspiration, effect on gastrointestinal system, and therapeutic effect of feedings.

PATIENT EDUCATION

1. Instruct patient to notify nurse if experiencing sensation of fullness, nausea, or vomiting.

1. May indicate intolerance of feeding.

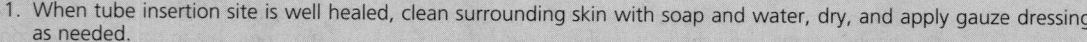

COMMUNITY-BASED CARE TIP:
Teach patient/family:
1. Technique for administration of tube feeding as outlined above.
2. Signs and symptoms of potential complications.
3. Need to assess tube placement and residual before each feeding.
4. Principles of medical asepsis, including careful hand washing, refrigeration of formula, cleaning of equipment with soap and water followed by thorough drying between feedings.

GASTROSTOMY OR JEJUNOSTOMY CARE

1. Special care of ostomy tube insertion site should include:
   a. Cleaning around tube with prescribed cleansing solution every shift and as needed.
   b. Applying sterile 4×4 gauze pad and taping in place.
   c. Applying skin barrier should peristomal skin become excoriated.
   d. Taping of tube to skin or skin barrier with hypoallergenic tape.

COMMUNITY-BASED CARE TIP:
Teach patient/family:
1. When tube insertion site is well healed, clean surrounding skin with soap and water, dry, and apply gauze dressing as needed.
2. Report signs of leakage around tube, signs of peristomal skin irritation.

TABLE 18-2 Complications of Enteral Feeding
and Treatment

Complications	Causes	Interventions
Tube displacement	Tube migration into esophagus	Observe for eructation of air when injecting air to test for tube placement in stomach. Aspirate for gastric contents; if none is obtained, suspect esophageal placement. Advance tube and auscultate for "whooshing" sound of air entering stomach as well as aspiration of gastric contents.
	Tube placement into respiratory tract	Observe for gagging, dyspnea, inability to speak, coughing when tube insertion attempted. Aspirate for gastric contents; if pH greater than 6, suspect respiratory tract placement. Obtain chest x-ray.* Withdraw tube and attempt reinsertion with patient's head flexed forward.*
Tube obstruction	Tube kinking Tube clogging	Obtain chest x-ray to confirm and withdraw and reinsert new tube.* Flush tube every 4 hours with 30 cc of water and after administration of intermittent feeding and medication administration. Administer medications in liquid form if possible. Crush medications finely.
Vomiting	Tube migration into esophagus	See interventions for tube migration above.
	Decreased absorption	Auscultate for decreased bowel sounds, observe for abdominal distention. Consider decreasing amount of tube feeding, change type of feeding to one requiring less digestive effort and a lower fat content.* Consider administration on a continuous basis.* Consider placement of a small-bore, weighted-tip nasointestinal tube.*
	Rapid rate of infusion	Administer no faster than 200–300 cc over 10–20 minutes. Consider administration on a continuous basis.*
	Excessive infusion of air	If giving a bolus feeding, pinch tubing off when refilling syringe with formula. If giving continuous feeding, make certain bag does not empty before closing off tubing.
	Patient position	Maintain patient at 30–45 degree angle of head elevation during and 30–60 minutes after feeding. If administering continuous feeding, maintain head elevation at all times.
Diarrhea	Drug therapy	Evaluate drug regimen for possible causes of drug-induced diarrhea from antibiotics, elixirs with high omolarity, H_2 blockers, magnesium-containing antacids.
	Hypoalbuminemia High osmolarity of formula	Check serum albumin levels. Administer formula requiring less digestion.* Begin administration of formula at slow rate.* Consider continuous feeding rather than intermittent.* Consider diluting formula with water and gradually increasing concentration.*
	Lactose intolerance Bacterial contamination of formula	Administer lactose-free formula.* Change administration set daily or per agency protocol. Maintain strict medical asepsis, including careful hand washing before administration of formula. Allow formula to hang no longer than 8 hours.
	Rapid infusion rate	Administer slowly; consider continuous rather than intermittent infusion.*
Constipation	Lack of fiber Decreased fluid intake Drug therapy	Administer formula with fiber.* Increase intake of water.* Evaluate drug regimin for possible cause, including aluminum-containing antacids.
Hyperglycemia	High caloric density formula (1.5–2 kcal/ ml)	Monitor serum glucose, assess for dehydration due to hyperosmotic diuresis; observe for symptoms of hyperglycemia, including polyuria, polydipsia. Change formula to lower calorie content.* Administer insulin.* Observe for hypercapnea (increased respirations, elevated Pco_2).
Electrolyte imbalance Hypernatremia	Dehydration	Assess for signs and symptoms of dehydration (I&O, daily weights, skin turgor, blood urea nitrogen, central venous pressure, tachycardia, hypotension). Rehydrate with D5W and/or hypotonic saline solutions.*
Hyponatremia	Overhydration	Observe for signs and symptoms of hypervolemia (shortness of breath, rales, I&O, daily weight, peripheral edema, elevated CVP). Observe for signs and symptoms of hyponatremia (lethargy, headaches, mental status change, nausea, vomiting, abdominal cramping). Replace sodium, administer diuretics, restrict fluids.*

(continued)

TABLE 18-2 Complications of Enteral Feeding and Treatment
(continued)

Complications	Causes	Interventions
Hyperkalemia	Metabolic acidosis/renal insufficiency	Observe for signs and symptoms of hyperkalemia (dysrhythmias, nausea, diarrhea, muscle weakness). Treat underlying cause. Administer exchange resin, glucose, and insulin.*
Hypokalemia	Diarrhea	See interventions for diarrhea. If severe, replace potassium.*

H_2: histamine; I&O: intake and output; CVP: central venous pressure.
* Obtain orders from health care provider.

◆ PARENTERAL NUTRITION

(See Procedure Guidelines 18-2: Administration of Total Nutrient Admixture [TNA].)
Parenteral nutrition is the introduction of nutrients, including amino acids, lipids, carbohydrates, vitamins, minerals, and water, through a venous access device (VAD) directly into the intravascular fluid to promote anabolism.

Clinical Indications

1. Patient unable to tolerate enteral nutrition due to:
   a. Paralytic ileus
   b. Intestinal obstruction
   c. Acute pancreatitis
   d. Malabsorption
   e. Persistent vomiting
   f. Severe diarrhea
   g. Fistula
   h. Inflammatory bowel disease
2. Hypermetabolic states for which enteral therapy is either not possible or inadequate.
   a. Burns
   b. Trauma
   c. Sepsis

Methods of Parenteral Nutrition

A. Total Nutrient Admixture (TNA)
1. Given through a central vein, often into the superior vena cava, this parenteral formula combines carbohydrates in the form of a concentrated (20%–70%) dextrose solution; proteins in the form of amino acids; lipids in the form of an emulsion (10%–20%), including triglycerides, egg phospholipids, glycerol, and water; and vitamins and minerals.
2. Central TNA is indicted for patients requiring parenteral feeding for 7 or more days.

B. Peripheral Parenteral Nutrition (PPN)
1. Given through a peripheral vein, this parenteral formula combines a lesser concentrated glucose solution with amino acids, vitamins, minerals, and lipids.

2. Unlike TNA given centrally, peripheral parenteral nutrition provides fewer calories, and generally a larger percentage of calories is supplied by lipids rather than by carbohydrates.
3. Indicated for patients requiring parenteral nutrition for fewer than 7 days.

C. Total Parenteral Nutrition (TPN)
1. Combines glucose, amino acids, vitamins, and minerals and may be given centrally or peripherally depending on the glucose concentration.
2. If lipids are needed, they are given intermittently through same or separate IV line.

D. Fat Emulsion (Lipids)
1. Ten percent or 20% emulsion composed of triglycerides, egg phospholipids, glycerol, and water.
2. May be give centrally or peripherally.

Delivery Systems for Parenteral Nutrition

1. Central venous access
   a. Insertion of long-term VADs, such as Hickman, Broviac, or Groshung catheters.
   b. Peripherally inserted central catheters (PICC lines) may be used.
   c. If multilumen, these VADs can allow for concomitant administration of TNA and other solutions, including medications or blood, each running through a separate lumen.
2. Peripheral IV access
   a. Insertion of an angiocatheter.
   b. Midline catheters of longer length and with the ability to remain in place for longer than 3 days.
3. Delivery of parenteral nutrition should always be controlled by a volume control infuser.
4. Filters should be used whenever possible.
   a. A 0.22-micron filter may be used for TPN (without added fat emulsion).
   b. A 1.2-micron filter may be used for TNA or fat emulsion.

Complications

(See Table 18-3.)

TABLE 18-3   Complications of Administration of Total Nutrient
Admixture (TNA) and Treatment

Complication	Causes	Interventions
Sepsis	High glucose content of fluid. Venous access device contamination.	Monitor temperature, WBC count, insertion site for signs and symptoms of infection. Maintain strict surgical asepsis when changing dressing and tubing. Consider decreasing glucose content of fluid.* Consider removal of venous access device with replacement in alternate site.* If blood cultures positive, consider institution of antibiotic therapy.*
Electrolyte imbalance	Iatrogenic. Effect of underlying diseases, ie, fistula, diarrhea, vomiting.	Monitor electrolyte levels at least every 2–3 days. Monitor signs and symptoms of electrolyte imbalance. Treat underlying cause.* Change concentration of electrolytes in TNA as necessary to address blood levels.*
Hyperglycemia	High glucose content of fluid. Insufficient insulin secretion.	Monitor blood glucose frequently. Decrease glucose content of fluid if possible.* Administer exogenous insulin per addition to TNA, subcutaneously or through a separate intravenous drip.*
Hypoglycemia	Abrupt discontinuation of TNA administered through a central vessel.	After discontinuation of centrally administered TNA, start $D_{10}W$ at the same rate.*
Hypervolemia	Iatrogenic. Underlying disease, ie, CHF, renal failure.	Monitor intake and output, daily weights, CVP, breath sounds, peripheral edema. Consider administering more concentrated TNA solution.*
Hyperosmolar diuresis	High osmolarity of TNA.	Monitor intake and output, daily weights, CVP. Consider decreasing concentration or amount of fluid administered.*
Hepatic dysfunction	High concentration of carbohydrates and/or fats relative to protein in TNA.	Monitor liver function tests, triglyceride levels, presence of jaundice. Consider alteration in formula content.*
Hypercapnea	High carbohydrate content of fluid.	Consider changing formula to increase the proportion of fat relative to carbohydrate.
Lipid intolerance	Low birth weight or premature infant.	Monitor for bleeding (check stools for occult blood, coagulation studies, platelet levels). Monitor O_2 levels for impaired oxygenation.
	History of liver disease. History of elevated triglycerides.	Monitor for fat overload syndrome: monitor triglyceride levels and liver function tests, hepatosplenomegaly, decreased coagulation, cyanosis, dyspnea. Monitor allergic reaction: nausea, vomiting, headache, chest pain, back pain, fever. Administer lipid-containing solutions slowly, initially, while observing for symptoms.
Lipid particulate aggregation	Unstable mixture of dextrose solution with lipid emulsion.	Observe for cracking or creaming of fluid, and avoid use of fluid with these characteristics.

WBC: white blood cell; CHF: congestive heart failure; CVP: central venous pressure.
* Obtain orders from health care provider.

PROCEDURE GUIDELINES 18-2 ◆ Administration of Total Nutrient Admixture (TNA) (Similar procedure for total parenteral nutrition [TPN] and other components)

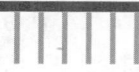

EQUIPMENT

Volume control infuser
Bag of TNA
Administration tubing with luer-lock connections
1.2-micron filter
Hypoallergenic tape, 1 in.
Face mask (optional)

Clean gloves
Sterile dressing kit to include:
 Alcohol swab sticks (3)
 Povidone-iodine sticks (3)
 Sterile gloves
 Transparent dressing

PROCEDURE

NURSING ACTION	RATIONALE
To change bag and bottle:	
PREPARATORY PHASE	
1. Remove TNA from refrigerator at least 1 hour before hanging.	1. Decreases incidence of hypothermia, pain, and venospasm.
2. Inspect fluid for presence of cracking or creaming.	2. Indicates fluid separation, do not use. If infusing TPN, solution should be clear without clouding.
3. Wash hands.	3. Prevents bacterial contamination.
PERFORMANCE PHASE	
1. Using strict sterile technique, attach tubing (with filter) to TNA bag and purge of air.	1. Prevent air embolus. * Tubing should be changed on a regular basis (every 2–3 days). Filter will be different for TPN, because lipids are not included.
2. Close all clamps on new tubing. Insert tubing into volume control infuser.	
3. If venous access device (VAD) has a clamp at proximal end, clamp tubing.	3. Prevents air embolus if VAD is inserted in a central vein.
4. If no clamp is available on central VAD, instruct patient to Valsalva maneuver (bear down and hold breath) while new tubing is connected.	4. Valsalva's maneuver creates positive pressure, preventing air from getting sucked into tubing.
5. Sterilely connect tubing to hub of VAD, making certain the connection is securely fastened using leur-lock connections.	5. Prevents disconnection of tubing.
6. Open all clamps and regulate flow through volume control infuser.	
FOLLOW-UP PHASE	
1. Monitor administration hourly, assessing for integrity of fluid and administration system and patient tolerance and complications.	1. See Table 18-3 for complications of TNA.
2. Document tubing change and fluid administration, observations, presence of complications, and any treatment given.	
PATIENT EDUCATION	
1. Teach patient signs and symptoms of complications, including sepsis, phlebitis, extravasation, and to report any changes to nursing personnel.	1. Patient can assist nursing personnel in monitoring therapy and detecting complications.
2. If patient is to be discharged to home with TNA, begin instruction regarding proper storage, handling, and administration of TNA. Include family members as appropriate.	2. Long-term therapy may be indicated in burns, emaciation due to cancer treatment, and other conditions. Home care nurses will reinforce your teaching.
To change central venous catheter dressing:	
PREPARATORY PHASE	
1. Obtain equipment.	
2. Explain procedure to patient.	

(continued)

PROCEDURE (cont'd)	NURSING ACTION	RATIONALE
	3. Place patient in a comfortable supine position and turn head away from site. 4. Wash hands. 5. Don mask (optional).	3. Turning patient's head away from site will decrease possible microbial contamination of site. 4. All precautions are taken to prevent bacterial contamination.

PERFORMANCE PHASE

1. Don clean gloves and carefully remove old dressing.
2. Inspect insertion site for complications.
3. Clean insertion site with each alcohol swab beginning at insertion site and moving outward in a circular pattern.
4. Repeat using each povidone-iodine swab.
5. Allow to dry.
6. Remove adhesive backing of transparent dressing. Center dressing over site.
7. Loop and tape tubing to skin using 1-in. tape. Do not tape over dressing.

2. Observe for edema, erythema, tenderness, and leakage of fluid.
3. Moves potential contaminants away from insertion site.
4. Provides for removal of bacteria from insertion site.
5. Drying allows adhesive dressing to adhere securely.
6. Application of transparent dressing provides a bacterial barrier while allowing full visualization of insertion site.
7. Prevent dislodgement of tubing.

FOLLOW-UP PHASE

1. Document dressing change and observation of insertion site.
2. Observe insertion site frequently for signs of complications.

2. Observe for edema, erythema, tenderness, and leakage of fluid.

PATIENT EDUCATION

1. Teach patient signs and symptoms of infection, phlebitis, and fluid extravasation and to report any changes to nursing personnel.
2. If patient is to be discharged to home with TNA, begin instruction regarding sterile dressing change. Include family members as appropriate.

1. Patient may be first to notice complications.
2. Because risk of sepsis is so great, sterile technique is still required for home dressing changes.

Nutritional Disorders

◆ OBESITY

Obesity is an overabundance of body fat resulting in body weight 20% over the average weight for the person's age, height, sex, and body frame.

Pathophysiology/Etiology

1. There is increasing evidence that heredity plays a part in the development of obesity. Identical twins raised apart are more likely to have similar amounts of body fat than fraternal twins raised separately.
2. Environment plays a role.
   a. Some evidence shows that children reared by obese parents have an increased tendency toward obesity as well.
   b. In addition, social class may influence weight, that is, higher social class may be associated with more weight-conscious behavior.
3. A variety of psychologic factors may contribute to weight gain, including depression and anxiety.
4. Physiologic factors
   a. Endocrine abnormalities (rare causes of obesity)—Cushing's syndrome, hypothyroidism, hypogonadism, or hypothalamic lesions.
   b. Age—advancing age may be associated with obesity often due to changes in activity level or in women, due to hormonal changes; early childhood and the start of puberty may also be associated with obesity.
      (1) Overeating after puberty may increase the total number of fat cells.
      (2) Despite dieting, these extra fat cells can never be eliminated, only decreased in size.

Clinical Manifestations

1. Body weight greater than 20% of normal
2. Increased weight is correlated with increased incidence of:
   a. Cardiovascular disease
   b. Diabetes mellitus

Diagnostic Evaluation

1. Nutritional assessment—to evaluate dietary habits.
2. Anthropometric and physical assessment—to evaluate increased body fat and effects of obesity on body.
3. Selected hormonal studies (thyroid, adrenal)—to look for underlying cause.

Management

A. *Conservative Measures*
1. Diet therapy
   a. One thousand calories per day must be eliminated from a diet to lose 1 kg (2.2 lb) of body weight per week.
   b. A 1,200 calorie diet for women and a 1,500 calorie diet for men with variations depending on patient size and activity level are basic to diet management. Fats should compose no more than 30% of all calories, proteins approximately 20% to 25%, and carbohydrates constituting the remaining portion.
   c. A balance of food groups is essential to maintain vitamin and nutrient balance. Nutrient supplements may be necessary (iron, B_6, zinc, and folate).
   d. Food preparation should include seasoning with herbs, onion, garlic, and pepper, and foods should be baked, broiled, steamed, or sautéed using minimal polyunsaturated oil.
   e. Food attractively arranged on smaller plates using whole rather than processed foods and eaten slowly will assist the overall process.
2. Exercise—A daily exercise program may include walking or other aerobic activity for approximately one-half hour per day.
3. Behavior modification is a cornerstone of any successful diet.
   a. Identify and eliminate situations or cues leading to overeating or high-calorie foods with use of a food diary.
   b. Provide for positive reinforcement of proper dietary habits.
   c. Should a lapse in diet habits occur, focus on a prompt and positive return to appropriate dietary habits.
   d. Stress reduction techniques, such as visual imagery or progressive relaxation; peer support may be helpful.

B. *Pharmacotherapy* Anorectic medications such as amphetamines and serotonin reuptake inhibitors reduce appetite and stimulate weight loss initially. However, tolerance develops within 2 to 4 weeks and weight is rapidly regained when the drugs are discontinued. Numerous long-term studies have failed to show success with these agents.

C. *Surgical Interventions* Numerous surgical procedures have been used, however, gastroplasty is the current

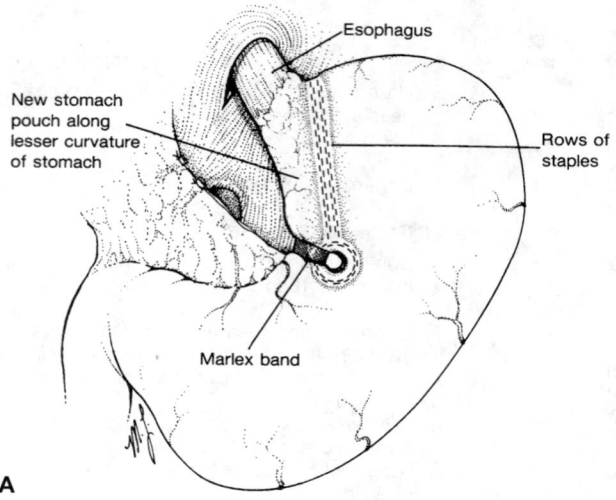

A

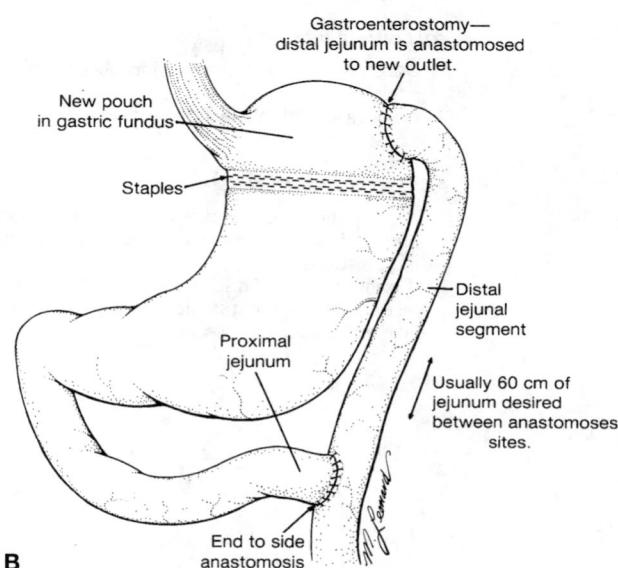

B

FIGURE 18-3 **(A)** *Gastroplasty with vertical banding.* **(B)** *Gastric bypass with Roux-en-y anastomosis.*

procedure of choice. These therapies are generally reserved for morbidly obese patients unable to lose weight through the above therapies (Fig. 18-3).

1. Gastroplasty—most common procedure is vertical banding involving creation of a 30-mL pouch along the lesser gastric curvature with a small outlet created with the use of a ring of plastic at the distal end to prevent dilation.
2. Gastric bypass—a Roux-en-Y gastroenterostomy is constructed by first creating a 50-mL pouch in the proximal stomach by stapling horizontally and completely separating the smaller proximal stomach pouch from the larger distal stomach pouch. To this proximal pouch, the distal jejunum is attached, thus bypassing the distal stomach pouch. The transected proximal portion of the jejunum is anastomosed to the distal jejunum.

Complications

1. Obesity is a risk factor for diabetes, gallbladder disease, osteoarthritis, high blood pressure, and coronary artery disease.
2. Vitamin and mineral deficiencies as a result of surgical intervention and/or severely restricted diet
   a. A moderate, well-balance weight reduction diet will generally not cause deficiencies, although a general vitamin/mineral supplement may be used.
   b. A very-low-calorie diet (fewer than 800 to 1,000 calories/day) will require careful monitoring and vitamin/mineral supplements.

Nursing Assessment

1. Obtain a complete nutritional assessment (may be in collaboration with a nutritionist).
2. Assess behavioral/emotional components of eating, coping mechanisms, and past successes/failures with dieting.

Nursing Diagnoses

A. Altered Nutrition: More Than Body Requirements related to high-calorie, high-fat diet and limited exercise
B. Fluid Volume Deficit related to gastroplasty or gastric bypass surgery

Nursing Interventions

A. Modifying Nutritional Intake
1. Assist patient in assessing current dietary habits and identifying poor dietary habits.
2. Assist patient in developing appropriate diet plan based on likes and dislikes, activity level, and lifestyle.
3. Suggest behavior modification strategies, such as shortening lunch break, preventing access to quick snacks, eating only at mealtimes at the table.
4. Provide emotional support to patient during weight-reduction efforts through positive reinforcement and creative problem solving.
5. Provide patient with alternative coping mechanisms, including stress reduction techniques, such as progressive relaxation and guided imagery.
6. Assess patient's ability to tolerate exercise through measurement of vital signs before, during, and after exercise and asking about symptoms of shortness of breath and chest pain.

B. Preventing Complications Postoperatively
1. Provide initial postoperative care as for gastric resection (see p.).
2. When bowel sounds return, give oral fluids to prevent dehydration.
3. If fluids are tolerated, begin six small feedings for a total of 600 to 800 calories.
4. Observe for and report increased pain and distention, which may indicate leakage at staple sites or obstruction.
5. Monitor vital signs and wound for signs of wound infection and dehiscence.

6. Watch for and report signs of dehydration (thirst, oliguria, dry mucous membranes) and hypokalemia (muscle weakness, anorexia, nausea, decreased bowel sounds, and dysrhythmias).
7. Warn patient that overeating will cause vomiting and painful esophageal distention.
8. Stress the importance of good dietary habits and behavior modification to lose weight, because gastroplasty is only an adjunct to treatment.
9. Encourage close long-term follow-up for monitoring of weight loss and nutritional status. Additional long-term complications include esophagitis and malnutrition.

Patient Education

1. Discuss fat, carbohydrate, and protein; their inclusion in common foods; and their calories per gram.
2. Describe the five basic food groups and their placement on the food pyramid.
3. Explain the purpose of a balanced diet and the need for vitamins and minerals.
4. Review the health hazards of obesity and recent evidence that repeated losing and regaining of weight carries a greater risk of heart disease.
5. Advise patient of plateau period that may occur without weight loss for some time, but not to get discouraged.
6. Tell patient to keep a food diary to show to nutritionist and to weigh self no more than once a week.
7. Refer to agencies such as: American Dietetic Association; 216 West Jackson Boulevard; Chicago, IL 60606-6995; 800-366-1655; and TOPS (Take Pounds Off Sensibly); P.O. Box 07360; 4575 South Fifth Street; Milwaukee, WI 53207; 414-482-4620.

Evaluation

A. Five-pound weight loss over first month
B. No abdominal distention, nausea or vomiting, or wound infection

◆ ANOREXIA NERVOSA

Anorexia nervosa is an eating disorder characterized by self-induced weight loss greater than 15% of minimally normal weight for age and height and associated with psychological and endocrine abnormalities. Periods of starvation may be mixed with gorging and purging.

Pathophysiology/Etiology

1. A semistarvation state with glucose and protein sparing, fat utilization, endocrine changes, and fluid and electrolyte disturbances is induced.
   a. Loss of fat stores
   b. Decreased protein synthesis
   c. Hypothalamic/pituitary dysfunction—decrease in follicle stimulating hormone (FSH), luteinizing hormone (LH), and estrogen
   d. Decrease in thyroid hormone
   e. Decrease in catecholamines
2. The biopsychosocial etiologic components of this disease interact differently in each patient.

a. Biologic/genetic predisposition remains unclear.
b. Psychologic components include
   (1) Distorted body image.
   (2) Fear of gaining weight.
   (3) Self-esteem very dependent on body image.
   (4) Ability to achieve weight loss viewed as a sign of self-control.
   (5) Denial of problem.
c. Social influences
   (1) Most patients are between the age of 14 and 24, and 90% are female.
   (2) Seen most often in the middle and upper class social strata.
   (3) Patients may relate high family expectations.
   (4) Frequent peer/social pressure to strive toward an aesthetic of thinness.

Clinical Manifestations

1. Symptoms vary widely and often are dependent on the severity of illness.
2. Physical signs and symptoms include loss of adipose tissue and weight loss of greater than 15% of ideal body weight, bradycardia, hypotension, cold intolerance, hypothermia, dry skin, thinning scalp hair, lanugo, amenorrhea for 3 consecutive months, decreased libido, constipation, and abdominal pain.
3. Psychological manifestations include perfectionistic and/or obsessive-compulsive behavior with high performance expectations, anxiety, increased exercise activity, inhibited or destructive social interactions, sleep disturbance, depression, and diminished sexual interest.

Diagnostic Evaluation

1. Serum chemistry may show electrolyte imbalance that may be life threatening (decreased chloride, potassium, phosphate, magnesium, zinc levels); increased blood urea nitrogen (BUN), creatinine, liver function tests, bicarbonate, amylase; and decreased albumin levels.
2. Hormone studies may show decreased LH, FSH, estrogen, testosterone (in men), and thyroid hormone and decreased response to luteinizing hormone–releasing hormone.
3. Complete blood count may show decreased white blood cells and hematocrit, indicating starvation's effect on immunity and anemia.
4. Electrocardiogram to detect dysrhythmias or signs of electrolyte imbalance.
5. Urinalysis may show ketonuria.

Management

1. Dietary modification to achieve gradual weight gain and normal eating habits.
2. Enteral/parenteral feeding may be necessary if prescribed diet cannot be maintained by patient and physical status warrants.
3. Individual counseling—focuses on patient's need to control weight, alteration in body image, and associated diagnoses, including depression and suicidal ideation.

4. Antidepressants may be tried as well as other pharmacologic agents for associated psychiatric problems.

Complications

1. Severe electrolyte disturbances, especially hypokalemia; dehydration; and anemia
2. Cardiac dysrhythmias, hypotension, cardiac arrest
3. Amenorrhea and other endocrine dysfunctions

Nursing Assessment

1. Obtain detailed dietary history as well as complete review of systems, including psychological, gynecologic, endocrine, GI systems, activities of daily living, and exercise history.
2. Perform physical examination, including vital signs, height and weight, heart rate and rhythm, bowel sounds, and observation for hematemesis and dental caries (which may indicate self-induced vomiting).

Nursing Diagnoses

A. Altered Nutrition: Less Than Body Requirements related to self-restricted intake
B. Body Image Disturbance related to weight

Nursing Interventions

A. *Promoting Weight Gain*
1. Monitor daily intake and output and weight (before breakfast).
2. Assess bowel function. Promote fluids and activity to prevent constipation if the patient cannot tolerate food high in fiber.
3. Encourage small, frequent meals or snacks of high-calorie foods and beverages. Liquid nutritional supplements may be best tolerated.
4. Provide positive reinforcement for improved intake and weight gain.

B. *Fostering a Healthy Body Image*
1. Establish a trusting relationship and provide for patient's safety and security needs.
2. Be alert for lying and manipulation that the patient may display to preserve control.
3. Involve patient in the treatment plan, offering choices to increase patient's sense of control.
4. Encourage patient to verbalize feelings about body image, self-concept, fears, and frustrations.
5. Emphasize the importance of counseling, stress management, assertiveness training, and other therapies.

Patient Education/ Health Maintenance

1. Teach principles of nutrition and healthful diet and eating habits. Discuss food matter-of-factly to avoid reinforcing the patient's preoccupation with food.

2. Teach the effect of starvation on both physiologic and psychological functioning.
3. Involve the patient's family and significant others in the treatment plan, as appropriate.
4. Describe the dangers of using laxatives and diuretics in weight control, such as electrolyte imbalances, dehydration, and bowel atony.
5. Refer to agencies such as: Anorexia Nervosa and Associated Disorders, 703-831-3438; and the Eating Addiction Disorder Access Helpline, 1-800-362-2644.

Evaluation

A. One-pound weight gain over 1 week
B. Verbalizes satisfaction with body image and weight

◆ BULIMIA NERVOSA

Bulimia is recurrent episodes of binge eating and a feeling of lack of control over eating behavior during these episodes, with associated inappropriate methods to prevent weight gain, including self-induced vomiting, excessive use of laxatives, diuretics, fasting, or excessive exercise. These episodes occur at least twice a week for 3 months. Self-image is significantly influenced by body weight and shape.

Pathophysiology/Etiology

1. Onset of illness often occurs in late adolescence or early 20s and is approximately 10 times more common in young women than in young men.
2. There is some association of bulimia with a personal or family history of obesity, substance abuse, depression, anxiety, or mood disorders.
3. Self-induced vomiting may result in electrolyte imbalance (hypokalemia, hyponatremia, hypochloremia, elevated bicarbonate) or esophageal tears or gastric rupture.
4. Starvation and its physiologic effects may or may not be evident as they are in anorexia nervosa.

Clinical Manifestations

1. The course of the disease may be chronic or intermittent over many years.
2. Weight is often maintained within normal range or may be significantly elevated or decreased.
3. Binge eating may be followed by inappropriate compensatory mechanisms, including self-induced vomiting, self-induced diarrhea through the use of laxatives or cathartics, the use of diuretics, excessive fasting, and excessive exercise.
4. Physical signs may include callouses or skin changes on hands and fingers, loss of dental enamel, swollen lymph nodes, and bad breath or mouthwash smell on breath due to self-induced vomiting.
5. Endocrine changes, such as amenorrhea, may be present.

Diagnostic Evaluation

1. Serum chemistry for electrolytes, blood urea nitrogen, and creatinine, and bicarbonate—may be abnormal, indicating fluid and electrolyte imbalances.
2. Additional tests may include thyroid function tests, luteinizing hormone, follicle stimulating hormone, estrogen, and electrocardiogram to determine effects of bulimia on body.

Management

1. Nutritional plan to accomplish weight goal (gain or loss).
   a. Balanced diet with incremental inclusion of foods previously perceived by patient as "fattening."
   b. Exercise.
2. Psychological counseling and support.
   a. Assist patient to develop insight into behavior and a more realistic body image.
   b. Assist patient to develop effective coping strategies and problem-solving mechanisms.

Complications

1. Fluid and electrolyte disturbances, particularly hypokalemia, metabolic alkalosis, and associated cardiac dysrhythmias
2. Obesity or anorexia nervosa
3. Dental erosion
4. Esophageal tear or gastric rupture

Nursing Assessment

1. Perform complete nutritional assessment.
2. Evaluate fluid and electrolyte status and manifestations of associated problems.
3. Assess for signs and symptoms of depression, anxiety, personality disorder, and associated eating behaviors and history of family dysfunction.

Nursing Diagnoses

A. Altered Nutrition: More/Less than Body Requirements related to binge/purge behavior
B. Ineffective Individual Coping related to lack of control over eating habits

Nursing Interventions

A. *Attaining Appropriate Weight*
1. Assist patient to select well-balanced diet and maintain appropriate eating habits.
   a. Educate patient to choose low-fat foods in small portions to gain control of caloric intake.
   b. Encourage patient to keep a food log and to eat only at mealtime.
2. Provide positive reinforcement for appropriate eating behaviors.

3. Teach patient the risks associated with abnormal eating behavior and benefits of maintaining healthful nutritional and exercise habits.
4. Assess daily weight, intake and output, urine for ketones, and serum electrolytes to determine physical response to nutritional interventions.

B. *Improving Coping*
1. Encourage patient to set realistic goals for weight and appearance.
2. Assist patient to identify and implement alternative coping strategies in times of stress, including expression and exploration of feelings, problem solving, appropriate use of exercise, and relaxation techniques.
3. Include family in counseling and teaching sessions, as appropriate.
4. Set limits so patient will feel in control of self.

Patient Education/Health Maintenance

1. Stress the importance of maintaining follow-up and counseling.
2. Refer to agencies such as: American Anorexia/Bulimia Association; 293 Central Park West #1R, New York, NY 10024, 212-501-8351; and Eating Disorder Information Center, 200 Elizabeth Street, CW1-328, Toronto, Ontario, Canada M5G 2C4, 416-340-4156.

Evaluation

A. Well-balanced dietary intake without evidence of vomiting
B. Verbalizing correct problem-solving approach

◆ MALABSORPTION SYNDROME

Malabsorption syndrome is a group of symptoms and physical signs occurring as a result of poor nutrient absorption in the small intestine, particularly fat absorption, with a resultant decrease in absorption of fat-soluble vitamins A, D, E, and K. Poor absorption of other nutrients including carbohydrates, minerals, and proteins may also occur.

Pathophysiology/Etiology

Malabsorption has multiple etiologies, including gallbladder or pancreatic disease, lymphatic obstruction, vascular impairment, or bowel resection. Outlined below are two common causes.

1. Celiac sprue—malabsorption of fat resulting from atrophy of villi and microvilli of the small intestine due to an intolerance to gluten found in common grains, such as wheat, rye, oats, and barley.
2. Lactase deficiency—often of genetic origin, this digestive enzyme deficiency prevents the digestion of lactose found in milk, causing osmosis of water into the lumen of the intestine.

Clinical Manifestations

1. Steatorrhea
2. Abdominal distention and pain
3. Flatulence
4. Anorexia, fatigue, weight loss, edema
5. Vitamin deficiency—fat soluble (A, D, E, K)
6. Protein deficiency and negative nitrogen balance

Diagnostic Evaluation

1. Fecal fat analysis—72-hour stool collection—may be increased.
2. Serum measurement of vitamin levels, total protein, and albumin may be decreased.
3. Prothrombin time may be prolonged due to vitamin K deficiency.

Management

1. Treatment of the underlying cause if possible by eliminating causative agents, such as grains or milk.
2. Promotion of adequate nutritional intake through a carefully designed diet substituting alternatives to the offending agent and ensuring replacement of deficient nutrients through oral, enteral, or parenteral therapy.

Complications

1. Dehydration
2. Electrolyte imbalance with possible cardiac dysrhythmias
3. Protein deficiency with muscle atrophy and edema
4. Vitamin deficiency with tetany, bleeding, and anemia
5. Skin breakdown

Nursing Assessment

1. Assess fluid and electrolyte status through careful monitoring of intake and output, daily weight, serum electrolytes, vital signs, and other signs and symptoms of dehydration and electrolyte imbalance.
2. Assess GI function through observation of frequency and characteristics of stool, bowel sounds, and presence of distention, pain, and other associated symptoms.
3. Assess nutritional status.

Nursing Diagnoses

A. Altered Nutrition: Less Than Body Requirements related to malabsorption of nutrients
B. Fluid Volume Deficit related to loss of fluid through stool
C. Pain related to abdominal distention and cramps
D. Risk for Impaired Skin Integrity related to irritation of anal area by stool

Nursing Interventions

A. *Improving Nutritional Status*
1. Ensure that diet is free of causative agent(s), such as milk or wheat products.
2. Provide diet high in missing nutrients, including proteins, carbohydrates, fats, vitamins, and minerals.
3. Teach patient to use substitute products for causative agents, such as gluten-free flour, corn, soybean, milk substitutes.
4. Monitor weight and characteristics of stool closely.

B. *Restoring Fluid Balance*
1. Monitor intake and output and urine-specific gravity.
   a. Include watery stool in output.
   b. Be aware that edema is due to low serum proteins, not to fluid overload.
2. Monitor vital signs frequently, based on condition.
3. Be alert for dehydration—orthostatic hypotension, tachycardia, decreased skin turgor, dry mucous membranes, thirst, oliguria.
4. Observe for signs and symptoms of potential electrolyte disturbances—nausea, vomiting, dysrhythmias, tremors, seizures, anorexia, weakness—and report abnormal results of serum electrolytes.
4. Administer IV fluids or parenteral or enteral nutrition as ordered.

C. *Relieving Pain*
1. Assess timing, frequency, and character of pain and its relationship to food.
2. Encourage Fowler's position and frequent change in position for comfort.
3. Administer analgesics, antidiarrheals, and antiflatulents as ordered.

D. *Maintaining Tissue Integrity*
1. Provide meticulous perineal care after each stool with application of hydrophobic ointments if necessary to prevent skin breakdown.
2. Give careful attention to general skin condition, assessing for redness, breakdown, and poor turgor, and maintain general skin integrity through cleanliness, lubrication, padding of bony prominences, frequent turning, and adequate hydration and nutrition.

Patient Education/ Health Maintenance

1. Provide nutritional counseling for patient and/or family, particularly if symptoms are secondary to food intolerance, stressing foods to avoid and carefully reading all food labels, appropriate food substitutions, and necessary nutritional supplements.
2. Advise regarding signs and symptoms indicating worsening of disease—increased frequency of stool, diarrhea or steatorrhea, increased pain.

Evaluation

A. Weight maintained
B. Vital signs stable, urinary output adequate
C. Verbalizes decreased pain after meals
D. No skin breakdown noted

◆ VITAMIN AND MINERAL DEFICIENCIES

Vitamins are organic compounds found in natural foods and are needed for growth, reproduction, good health, and resistance to infection. Minerals are inorganic compounds found in nature and serve a variety of physiologic functions. Specific requirements depend on age, activity, metabolic rate (increased fever), and special processes, such as pregnancy, lactation, and disease processes.

See Table 18-4 for management of vitamin and mineral imbalances.

TABLE 18-4   Vitamin and Mineral Requirements and Imbalances

Vitamin, RDA Requirements	Function	Clinical Manifestations of Imbalance	Diagnostic Evaluation	Management
Vitamin A (Retinol) RDA: 4,000–5,000 I.U. Fat soluble	Tissue maintenance via antioxidant ability. Skeletal and soft tissue growth and development. Visual adaptation to light and dark. Supports reproductive function.	Deficiency: Night blindness, xerophthalmia, keratinization, generalized mucosa dryness/damage, vomiting, diarrhea, weight loss, urinary and vaginal infections, tooth decay, follicular hyperkeratosis. Toxicity: Yellow-orange skin coloring, hair loss, joint pain, dry skin, mouth soreness, anorexia, vomiting, cirrhosis.	Deficiency: History and physical findings are helpful in diagnosis of most vitamin imbalances. Serum level less than 35 mg/dl suggests vitamin deficiency.	Deficiency: Replacement therapy of 30,000 I.U. to treat night blindness Good dietary sources of Vitamin A are green and yellow fruits and vegetables and liver. In patients with malabsorption of fat soluble vitamins and patients with low dietary intake of Vitamin A, i.v. supplements are required.

(continued)

TABLE 18-4 Vitamin and Mineral Requirements and Imbalances
(continued)

Vitamin, RDA Requirements	Function	Clinical Manifestations of Imbalance	Diagnostic Evaluation	Management
Vitamin B$_1$ (Thiamine) RDA: 1.0–1.5 mg Water soluble	Carbohydrate metabolism. Necessary for neurologic, gastric, cardiac, and musculoskeletal function.	Deficiency: Appetite loss, constipation, dyspnea, fatigue, irritability, nervousness, memory loss, paresthesias, muscle pain. Toxicity: Very large doses may be given generally without difficulty, although anaphylaxis has been reported.	Deficiency: Erythrocyte transketolase activity less than 15–20%.	Deficiency: Treat underlying cause. High protein diet with supplemental B complex vitamins. Food sources rich in thiamine are brewer's yeast, meat, wheat germ, and enriched grains and beans. Parenteral therapy with 50–100 mg/day followed by 5–10 mg/day p.o.
B$_2$ (Riboflavin) RDA: 0.6 mg/1,000 kcal Water soluble	Carbohydrate metabolism. Promotes growth, red blood cell formation, and healthy eyes and skin.	Deficiency: Sore throat, cheilosis, dermatitis, burning and itching of eyes, tearing and vascularization of corneas; late-stage symptoms include neuropathy and growth retardation. Toxicity: Flushing, gastric irritation, liver enzyme elevation.	Deficiency: Erythrocyte glutathione activity greater than 1.2–1.3. Decreased urinary riboflavin levels.	Deficiency: Good dietary sources of B$_2$ are dairy products, vegetables, enriched grains, eggs, nuts, and liver. Oral supplements of 5–15 mg/day. Toxicity: Supportive measures.
B$_6$ (Pyridoxine) RDA: 1.6–2 mg Water soluble	Promotes protein metabolism. Maintains neurologic function and RBC production.	Deficiency: Anemia, weakness, glossitis, cheilosis, irritability, seizures. Toxicity: Neuromuscular damage.	Deficiency: Pyridoxal phosphate levels less than 50 ng/ml	Deficiency: Oral supplementation—10–20 mg. Good dietary sources of B$_6$ are bananas, brewer's yeast, fish, meat, whole grains, and liver. Individuals taking oral contraceptives or isoniazid may need to supplement their diets with pyridoxine. Pregnancy also increases need.
B$_{12}$ (Cobalamin) RDA: 2 mcg Water soluble	Maintains neurologic function and RBC development via hemoglobin synthesis.	Deficiency: Megaloblastic anemia, memory impairment, confusion, depression, fatigue, nervousness, decreased reflex response, balance impairment, speech difficulties, demyelination of the large fibers of the spinal cord, anorexia, vomiting, weight loss, yellowing of skin, abdominal pain, dyspnea, diarrhea, glossitis.	Deficiency: Serum levels of less than 100 pg/ml. Decreased hematocrit with elevation of MCV. Schilling test also measures absorption of radioactive B$_{12}$.	Deficiency: B$_{12}$ 200 mcg/day i.m. for 1 wk, then every month for life if deficiency is due to pernicious anemia. Oral vitamin B$_{12}$ may be necessary for strict vegetarians. Good dietary sources of B$_{12}$ are eggs, fish, organ meats, lean meat, dairy products.
Biotin RDA: 30–100 mcg Water soluble	Metabolism of proteins, fats, and carbohydrates.	Deficiency: Dry skin, fatigue, grayish skin discoloration, muscle pain, depression, insomnia and anorexia.		Deficiency: Good sources of biotin are egg yolks, vegetables, yeast, milk, grains.

(continued)

TABLE 18-4 Vitamin and Mineral Requirements and Imbalances
(continued)

Vitamin, RDA Requirements	Function	Clinical Manifestations of Imbalance	Diagnostic Evaluation	Management
Folate (folic acid) RDA: 180–200 mcg Water soluble	RBC formation. DNA and RNA synthesis and support of cell growth and reproduction. Prevention of birth defects.	Deficiency: Glossitis, diarrhea, megaloblastic anemia, digestive problems.	Deficiency: Serum level less than 3 ng.	Deficiency: Nutritional supplementation— 1 mg/day p.o. Avoid alcohol. Good sources of folate are citrus fuits, eggs, milk, green leafy vegetables, dairy products, organ meats, seafood, whole grains, and yeast.
Niacin RDA: 13–19 mg Water soluble	Metabolism of carbohydrates, fats and proteins. Works with thiamine and riboflavin for the production of cellular energy. Promotes skin, neurologic, and gastrointestinal function.	Deficiency: Apathy, fatigue, appetite loss, headaches, indigestion, muscle weakness, nausea, insomnia, dermatitis, diarrhea, confusion, disorientation, memory impairment, glossitis, and stomatitis.	Deficiency: Serum levels less than 30 mcg/100 ml. Diminished or absent metabolites in urine.	Deficiency: Good sources of niacin are eggs, lean meats, organ meats, poultry, seafood, fish, dairy products, nuts, whole and enriched grains, brewer's yeast. Nutritional supplementation: 10–150 mg. Supplemental niacin may also be necessary when taking oral contraceptives.
Pantothenic acid RDA: 4–7 mg Water soluble	Vital for overall metabolism. Aids in formation of carbohydrates, proteins, and fats. Aids in cortisone production, ATP production, stress tolerance, vitamin utilization, hemoglobin synthesis.	Deficiency: Diarrhea, hair loss, respiratory infections, nervousness, muscle cramps, premature aging, intestinal disorders, eczema, kidney disorders.		Deficiency: This vitamin is widely available in foods, especially organ meats, legumes, vegetables, and fruits.
Vitamin C RDA: 50–60 mg Water soluble	Antioxidant action decreases cellular dysfunction. Promotes wound healing. Aids in connective tissue, bone, tooth, and cartilage formation. Promotes capillary integrity. Promotes non-heme iron absorption.	Deficiency: Bleeding gums, tooth decay, nosebleeds, low infection resistance, bruising, anemia, delayed wound healing, anorexia, joint pain, lethargy. Toxicity: Gastrointestinal distress	Deficiency: Serum levels less than 0.1 mg/100 dl.	Deficiency: Nutritional supplementation: 100–1,000 mg/day of vitamin C. Good sources of vitamin C are citrus fruits, green leafy vegetables, broccoli, tomatoes, peppers, potatoes, strawberries. Avoid smoking.
Vitamin D RDA: 200–400 I.U. Fat soluble	Regulates calcium and phosphate absorption and metabolism and bone formation. Aids in renal phosphate clearance, myocardial function, nervous system maintenance and normal blood clotting.	Deficiency: Rickets, osteomalacia Toxicity: Hypercalcemia, bone pain, weakness	Deficiency: Low levels of vitamin D and calcium (calcium less than 8.5 mg/100 ml). Radiographic bone deformities. Abnormal bone densitometry.	Deficiency: Nutritional supplementation: Ergocalciferol, 25 mcg/day p.o. Good sources of vitamin D are egg yolks, yeast, enriched milk, fish liver oils. Exposure to sunlight.

(continued)

TABLE 18-4 Vitamin and Mineral Requirements and Imbalances
(continued)

Vitamin, RDA Requirements	Function	Clinical Manifestations of Imbalance	Diagnostic Evaluation	Management
Vitamin E (Tocopherol) RDA: 8–10 mg Fat soluble	Antioxidant action decreases cellular dysfunction. Aids in RBC formation.	Deficiency: Neuromuscular disturbances, including decreased reflexes, vibratory and position sense, and ataxia.	Deficiency: Serum levels less than 0.5 mg/dl.	Deficiency: Nutritional supplementation: 100–400 I.U./day p.o. Parenteral therapy may be necessary to treat neurologic symptoms. Good sources of vitamin E are vegetable oils, milk, eggs, meat, fish, green leafy vegetables.
Vitamin K RDA: 65–80 mcg Fat soluble	Promotes coagulation through the formation of prothrombin and other clotting factors.	Deficiency: Abnormal bleeding times, hemorrhage, epistaxis, hemetemesis and bleeding at any orifice or puncture site is possible.	Deficiency: Prothrombin time extended longer than PTT.	Deficiency: Administration of vitamin K 15 mg subcutaneously. Good sources of Vitamin K are: green leafy vegetables, liver, wheat germ, cheese, egg yolk, soy bean oil.
Minerals Calcium RDA: 800–1,200 mg	Aids in: Bone and tooth formation. Muscle contraction. Blood coagulation. Nerve impulse transmission. Cardiac function. Cell membrane permeability. Enzyme activation.	Deficiency: Tooth decay, muscle cramps, tetany, nervousness and delusion, cardiac palpitations, congestive heart failure, and paresthesias. Toxicity: Muscle weakness, diminished deep tendon reflexes, anorexia, nausea, vomiting, personality changes, decreased memory, renal disturbances.	Deficiency: Serum level less than 8.5 mg/dl. Toxicity: Serum level greater than 10.5 mg/dl.	Deficiency: Oral supplements of 1–2 g/day of elemental calcium. In severe hypocalcemia, 10 ml of 10% calcium gluconate i.v. administered no faster than 2 ml/min. Good sources of calcium are milk products, green leafy vegetables, whole grains, and egg yolks. Toxicity: Force fluids, diuretics, and limit dietary intake. Administration of phosphate salts and glucocorticoids may also be necessary.
Chromium RDA: 0.29 mg.	Maintains serum glucose levels. Maintains fat metabolism.	Deficiency: Glucose intolerance, vertigo, abdominal pain, shock, convulsions, anuria, dermatitis.	Deficiency: Serum levels less than 0.3 mg/ml.	Deficiency: Nutritional supplements: 50–200 mg/day. Good sources of chromium are brewer's yeast, whole grains, cereals.
Copper RDA: 1.5–3 mg	Hemoglobin synthesis. Maintenance of hemostasis. Energy production.	Deficiency: Hypochromic anemia, bone disease, weakness, skin lesions, altered respiratory status. Toxicity: Nausea, vomiting, diarrhea, abdominal pain, malaise.	Deficiency: In addition to diminished serum levels, 24-hour urine samples showing levels of urinary excretion of copper below 15–60 mcg/24 hr	Deficiency: Nutritional supplementation: 0.1 mg/kg/day p.o. I.V. supplementation—1–2 mg/day. Good sources of copper are nuts, seeds, organ meats and seafood.
Iodine RDA: 150 mcg	Thyroid hormone synthesis.	Deficiency: Hypothyroidism/goiter, nervousness, irritability, obesity, cold hands and feet, chills, brittle hair, fatigue, bradycardia, decreased cardiac output, thick tongue, hoarseness, poor memory, hearing loss, anorexia.	Deficiency: Low T_3 and T_4 levels. Thyroid scan.	Deficiency: Nutritional supplementation: 50–100 mg daily p.o. Good sources of iodine are iodized salt, seafood.

(continued)

TABLE 18-4 Vitamin and Mineral Requirements and Imbalances
(continued)

Vitamin, RDA Requirements	Function	Clinical Manifestations of Imbalance	Diagnostic Evaluation	Management
Iron RDA: 10–15 mg	Hemoglobin synthesis. Cellular oxidation. Transportation of oxygen.	Deficiency: Iron deficiency anemia, fatigue, tachycardia, palpitations, dyspnea, susceptibility to infection, brittle nails, cheilosis, glossitis.	Deficiency: Decreased hemoglobin, hematocrit, iron, and ferritin levels and increased total iron binding capacity.	Deficiency: Nutritional supplementation: 325 mg p.o. t.i.d.; Imferon 250 mg/day IM for each gram of hemoglobin below normal. IV supplementation: 1.5–2 g over 4–6 hr. Good sources of iron are: eggs, fish, organ meats, wheat germ, beans, lentils, beef, potatoes, and peas.
Magnesium RDA: 280–350 mg	Parathyroid hormone regulation. Acid–base balance. Enzyme activation. Smooth muscle regulation. Metabolism of carbohydrates and protein. Cell growth and reproduction.	Deficiency: Tetany, tremors, confusion, depression, tachycardia, dysrhythmias, seizures. Toxicity: Nausea, vomiting, drowsiness, muscle weakness, decreased deep tendon reflexes, hypotension, respiratory depression.	Deficiency: Serum levels less than 1.3 mEq/l. Toxicity: Serum levels greater than 2.1 mEq/l.	Deficiency: Nutritional supplementation: 1–2 g i.v. over 15 min. Good sources of magnesium are nuts, meat, grain, green vegetables, seafood, dairy products. Toxicity: Supportive measures.
Phosphorus RDA: 800–1200 mg	Nerve and muscle activity. Vitamin utilization. Kidney function. Metabolism of carbohydrates, proteins and fats. Cell growth and repair. Myocardial contraction. Energy production. Bone and tooth formation. Acid–base balance. Red blood cell function.	Deficiency: Anorexia, weakness, tremor, paresthesias, anemia, mental status change, hypoxia, osteomalacia. Toxicity: Tetany, soft tissue calcification, seizures, renal damage.	Deficiency: Serum levels less than 2.5 mg/dl Toxicity: Serum levels greater than 4.5 mg/dl	Deficiency: Nutritional supplementation: p.o. or i.v. phosphate. Good sources of phosphate are dairy products, eggs, fish, grains, meat, poultry, yellow cheeses, almonds, beans, cocoa, chocolate, liver, milk, peas, peanuts, walnuts, whole wheat, and rye. Toxicity: Administration of phosphate-binding agents (Amphojel). Hemodialysis or peritoneal dialysis.
Potassium RDA: 2,000–3,500 mg	Muscle contraction. Cardiac function. Protein synthesis. Nerve impulse transmission. Carbohydrate metabolism. Acid–base balance. Major intracellular cation.	Deficiency: Muscle weakness, fatigue, malaise, flaccidity, mental confusion, irritability, depression, dysrhythmias, hypotension, nausea, vomiting, anorexia, decreased GI motility, muscle cramps, paresthesias, hyperglycemia, polyuria, metabolic alkalosis. Toxicity: Muscle weakness, paralysis, paresthesias, nausea, vomiting, diarrhea, metabolic acidosis, prolonged cardiac conduction, ventricular dysrhythmias.	Deficiency: Serum levels less than 3.5 mEq/l. Toxicity: Serum levels greater than 5 mEq/l.	Deficiency: Nutritional supplementation: p.o. or i.v., i.v. replacement generally at a rate of 10 mEq/hr with careful cardiac monitoring and frequent measurements of serum potassium levels. Good sources of potassium are bananas, oranges, beef, prunes, beans, seafood, raisins. Toxicity: Infuse calcium gluconate 10% (10 ml). Sodium bicarbonate infusion. Insulin and glucose infusion. Oral or rectal exchange resins. Hemodialysis or peritoneal dialysis.

(continued)

TABLE 18-4 Vitamin and Mineral Requirements and Imbalances
(continued)

Vitamin, RDA Requirements	Function	Clinical Manifestations of Imbalance	Diagnostic Evaluation	Management
Sodium RDA: 500 mg	Maintains fluid balance. Cell membrane permeability and absorption of glucose. Bioelectric potential of tissues. Cardiac function. Acid–base balance. Regulation of neuromuscular function.	Deficiency: Muscle weakness, irritability, headache, seizures, nausea, vomiting, malaise, abdominal cramping, hypotension, tachycardia. Toxicity: Flushed skin, oliguria, agitation, thirst, dry mucous membranes, seizures.	Deficiency: Serum levels less than 135 mEq/l. Toxicity: Serum levels greater than 145 mEq/l.	Deficiency: Restrict free water intake. Infuse 0.9% saline solution if patient is hypovolemic. Infuse 3% saline and administer diuretic if sodium levels significantly low. Demeclocycline may be used to block ADH in the renal tubules to promote water excretion. Toxicity: Administer salt-free solutions such as D_5W followed by 0.45% saline solution. Low sodium diet. Administer vasopressin if diminished ADH is the cause.
Zinc RDA: 12–15 mg	Cellular metabolism. Maintenance of taste and smell. Burn and wound healing. Gonadal function. Maintenance of serum vitamin A concentration. Acid–base balance. Protein digestion. Promotion of growth.	Deficiency: Fatigue, hair loss, poor wound healing, impaired growth, bone deformities, loss of taste, anorexia, iron deficiency anemia, hypogonadism, hyperpigmentation. Toxicity: Diminished deep tendon reflexes, malaise, decreased level of consciousness, diarrhea, leukopenia.	Deficiency: Serum levels less than 75 mcg/dl	Deficiency: Nutritional supplementation: zinc sulfate 200 mg t.i.d. p.o. Good sources of zinc are liver, seafood, beans, lentils, oatmeal, wheat bran, eggs, peas, pasta, chicken, and milk. Toxicity: Supportive measures.

i.v.: intravenous; p.o.: by mouth; RBC: red blood cell; MCV: mean corpuscular volume; i.m.: intramuscular; ATP; adenosine triphosphate; PTT: partial thromboplastin time; t.i.d.: three times a day; GI: gastrointestinal; ADH: antidiuretic hormone.

Selected References

American Psychological Association. (1994). *Diagnostic and statistical manual of mental disorders*. Washington, DC: American Psychological Association.

Butler, T., & Yanowitz, F. (1994, June). Obesity I. *Cardiovascular Reviews and Reports*, 31-32, 39-44, 49-54.

Irwin, E. G. (1993). A focused overview of anorexia nervosa and bulimia: Etiological issues. Part 1. *Archives of Psychiatric Nursing*, 7(6), 342-346.

Irwin, E. G. (1993). A focused overview of anorexia nervosa and bulimia: Challenges to the practice of psychiatric nursing. Part 2. *Archives of Psychiatric Nursing*, 7(6), 347-352.

Metheny, N., et al. (1993). Effectiveness of pH measurements in predicting feeding tube placement: An update. *Nursing Research*, 42(6), 324-330.

Miller, D. & Miller, H. (1995). Giving meds through the tube. *RN*, 58(1), 44–47.

Riccardi, E. & Brown, D. (1994). Managing PEG tubes. *AJN*, 94(10), 29–31.

Rombeau, J., & Caldwell, M. (1993). *Clinical nutrition: parenteral nutrition*. Philadelphia: Saunders.

Shils, M., Olson, J., & Shike, M. (1994). *Modern nutrition in health and disease*. Philadelphia: Lea & Febiger.

Williams, S. R. (1993). *Nutrition and diet therapy*. St. Louis: Mosby-Year Book.

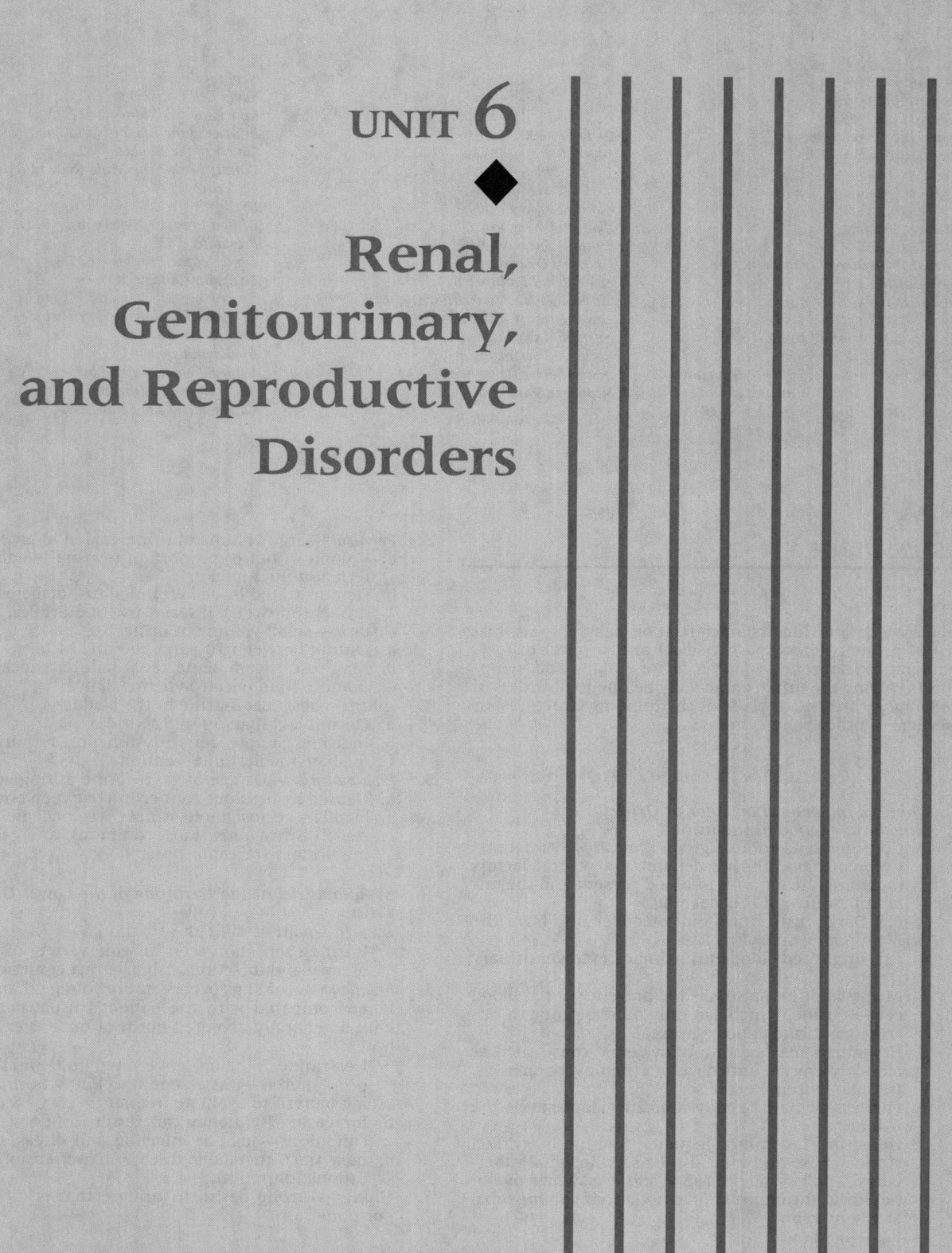

UNIT 6

◆

Renal,
Genitourinary,
and Reproductive
Disorders

CHAPTER 19 ◆

Renal and Urinary Disorders

Assessment

◆ SUBJECTIVE DATA

Subjective data include characterization of symptoms, history of present illness, past medical and surgical history, demographic data, and lifestyle factors. Signs and symptoms involving the urinary tract may be due to disorders of the kidneys, ureters, or bladder, surrounding structures, or disorders of other body systems.

Changes in Micturition (Voiding)

A. Changes in Amount or Color of Urine

1. *Hematuria*—blood in the urine
   a. Considered a serious sign and requires evaluation.
   b. Color of bloody urine depends on several factors including the amount of blood present and the anatomic source of the bleeding.
      (1) Dark, rusty urine indicates bleeding from the upper urinary tract.
      (2) Bright red bloody urine indicates lower urinary tract bleeding.
   c. Microscopic hematuria is the presence of red blood cells in urine, which can only be seen under a microscope; urine appears normal.
   d. Hematuria may be due to systemic cause such as blood dyscrasias, anticoagulant therapy, neoplasms, trauma, extreme exercise.
   e. Painless hematuria may indicate neoplasm in the urinary tract.
   f. Hematuria is common in patients with urinary tract stone disease and may also be seen in renal tuberculosis, polycystic disease of kidneys, acute pyelonephritis, thrombosis and embolism involving renal artery or vein.

2. *Polyuria*—large volume of urine voided in given time
   a. Volume is out of proportion to usual voiding pattern and fluid intake.
   b. Demonstrated in diabetes mellitus, diabetes insipidus, chronic renal disease, use of diuretics.

3. *Oliguria*—small volume of urine
   a. Output between 100 and 500 mL/24 h
   b. May result from acute renal failure, shock, dehydration, fluid–electrolyte imbalance.

4. *Anuria*—absence of urine in the bladder
   a. Output less than 50 mL/24 h
   b. Indicates serious renal dysfunction requiring immediate medical intervention.

5. *Pneumaturia*—passage of gas in urine during voiding
   a. Caused by fistulous connection between bowel and bladder, rectosigmoid cancer, regional ileitis, sigmoid diverticulitis (most common), and gas-forming urinary tract infections.

B. Symptoms Related to Irritation of the Lower Urinary Tract

1. *Dysuria*—pain or difficult urination
   a. Burning sensation seen in wide variety of inflammatory and infectious urinary tract conditions

2. *Frequency*—voiding occurs more often than usual when compared with the patient's usual pattern or with a generally accepted norm of once every 3 to 6 hours.
   a. Determine if habits governing fluid intake have been altered—it is essential to know normal voiding pattern to evaluate frequency.
   b. Increasing frequency can result from a variety of conditions—such as infection and diseases of urinary tract, metabolic disease, hypertension, medications (diuretics).

3. *Urgency*—strong desire to urinate that is difficult to postpone

a. Due to inflammatory conditions of the bladder, prostate, or urethra, acute bacterial infections, neurologic voiding dysfunctions, chronic prostatitis in men, and chronic posterior urethrotrigonitis in women.

4. *Nocturia*—excessive urination at night, which interrupts sleep
a. Causes include decreased renal concentrating ability or heart failure, diabetes mellitus, poor bladder emptying.

5. *Strangury*—slow and painful urination; only small amounts of urine voided
a. Blood staining may be noted.
b. Seen in severe cystitis.

C. ***Symptoms Related to Obstruction of the Lower Urinary Tract***
1. *Weak stream*—decreased force of stream when compared to usual stream of urine when voiding
2. *Hesitancy*—undue delay and difficulty in initiating voiding
a. May indicate compression of urethra, outlet obstruction, neurogenic bladder.
3. *Terminal dribbling*—prolonged dribbling or urine from the meatus after urination is complete
a. May be caused by urethral obstruction.
4. *Incomplete emptying*—feeling that the bladder is still full even after urination
a. Indicates either urinary retention or a condition that prevents the bladder from emptying well, leads to infection.

D. ***Types of Urinary Incontinence***
Urinary incontinence is the involuntary loss of urine; may be due to pathologic, anatomic, or physiologic factors affecting the urinary tract.

1. *Stress incontinence*—intermittent leakage of urine due to increased abdominal pressure, such as coughing, sneezing, or straining
a. Indicates weakness of sphincteric mechanism.
2. *Urge incontinence*—sensation of the need to urinate followed by sudden, involuntary loss of urine
a. Usually related to neurologic disease affecting the bladder or chronic irritation of the bladder wall.
3. *Overflow incontinence*—loss of urine caused by overdistention of the bladder
a. Associated with complete urinary retention.
4. *Total incontinence*—continuous leakage of urine from the bladder
a. Occurs with injury to the sphincteric mechanisms, bladder neck, and urethra.
5. *Enuresis*—involuntary voiding during sleep
a. May be physiologic to age of 3 years; thereafter, may be functional or symptomatic of obstructive disease (usually of lower urinary tract).

E. ***Urinary Tract Pain***
1. Genitourinary pain is not always present in renal disease, but is generally seen in the more acute conditions of the urinary tract.
2. Kidney pain—may be felt as a dull ache in costovertebral angle; or may be a sharp, colicky pain felt in the flank area that radiates to the groin or testicle.
a. Due to distention of the renal capsule; severity related to how quickly it develops.
3. Ureteral pain—felt in the back and radiates to the groin or scrotum if the upper ureter is the source, to the suprapubic area, penis, and urethra if the lower ureter is the source.

4. Bladder pain (lower abdominal pain or pain over suprapubic area)—may be due to bladder infection or overdistended bladder.
5. Urethral pain from irritation of bladder neck, from foreign body in canal, or from urethritis due to infection or trauma.
6. Pain in scrotal area due to inflammatory swelling of epididymis or testicle, or torsion of the testicle.
7. Testicular pain due to injury, mumps orchitis, torsion of spermatic cord.
8. Perineal or rectal discomfort due to acute prostatitis, prostatic abscess.
9. Back and leg pain due to cancer of prostate with metastases to pelvic bones.
10. Pain in glans penis is usually from prostatitis; penile shaft pain is from urethral problems.

F. ***Related Symptoms***
1. Gastrointestinal symptoms related to urologic conditions include nausea, vomiting, diarrhea, abdominal discomfort, paralytic ileus, and gastrointestinal hemorrhage with uremia.
2. Occur with urologic conditions because the gastrointestinal and urinary tracts have common autonomic and sensory innervation and because of renointestinal reflexes.
3. Fever and chills may also occur with infectious processes.

History

Seek the following historical data related to urinary and renal function:

1. What is (are) the patient's present and past occupation(s)? Look for occupational hazards related to the urinary tract—contact with chemicals, plastics, tar, rubber.
2. What is the patient's smoking history?
3. What is the past medical and surgical history, especially in relation to urinary problems?
4. Is there any family history of renal disease?
5. What childhood diseases did the patient have?
6. Is there a history of urinary tract infections? Did any occur before the age of 12?
7. Did enuresis continue beyond the usual age (past 3 years of age)?
8. Any history of genital lesions or sexually transmitted diseases (STDs)?
9. For the female patient: Number of children? Their ages? Any forceps deliveries? Catheterizations? When? Why? Any signs of vaginal discharge? Vaginal/vulvar itch or irritation?
10. Does the patient have diabetes mellitus? Hypertension? Allergies? Neurologic disease or dysfunction?
11. Has the patient ever been hospitalized for a urinary tract infection?
a. What diagnostic tests were performed? Cystoscopy? Urodynamics? Kidney x-ray procedures?
b. Was the patient catheterized? Were antibiotics given, either intravenously (IV) or orally?
12. Is the patient receiving any prescription or over-the-counter drugs that may affect renal or urinary function? Have any drugs been prescribed for renal or urinary problems?
13. Is the patient at risk for urinary tract infection?

◆ OBJECTIVE DATA

Objective data should focus on physical examination of the abdomen and the genitalia. Complete body system assessment may be indicated in some conditions, such as renal failure.

Examination of the Abdomen

1. Inspect the abdomen for any visible masses or bulges; auscultate for the presence of bowel sounds.
2. Percussion may reveal a distended bladder when dullness is found above the symphysis pubis.
3. Light palpation may detect tenderness or resistance; deep palpation can be used to assess the kidneys although this is difficult in most patients.
4. With the patient in a sitting position, tenderness of the costovertebral angle can be detected by placing the palm of your right hand over the costovertebral angle and striking your right hand with the fist of your left hand. Tenderness here indicates infection.

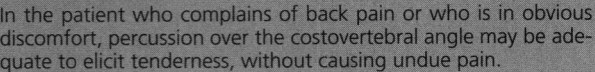

NURSING ALERT:
In the patient who complains of back pain or who is in obvious discomfort, percussion over the costovertebral angle may be adequate to elicit tenderness, without causing undue pain.

Examination of the Female Genitalia

1. Inspection of the female external genitalia may reveal inflammation, ulcerations, nodules, or lesions. Insert a finger into the vagina and milk the urethra by pressing upward from the inside outward—discharge from the meatus indicates urethral infection.
2. With the labia spread, ask the patient to bear down; a cystocele or urethrocele may be visible.
3. With two fingers in the vagina, ask the patient to contract her muscles around your fingers as long as possible; this allows for assessment of pelvic floor muscle strength.
4. Inspect the vaginal tissue for vascularity and evidence of atrophic vaginitis in which the tissue is smooth, pale, and dry.

Examination of the Male Genitalia

1. Inspect the urethral meatus for discharge.
2. Retract the foreskin and assess for hygiene and the presence of smegma.
3. Inspect the shaft of the penis, the glans, and prepuce for lesions or indurated areas.
4. Palpate the testis and the epididymis for evidence of inflammation, tenderness, or masses; palpate the scrotal contents for hydrocele or varicocele.
5. Inspect the inguinal and femoral areas for bulges or hernias; ask the patient to bear down or cough during this portion of the examination.

6. Perform a rectal examination in men over age 40; assess for size and consistency of the prostate as well as anal sphincter tone.

General Examination

1. Assess the patient's cardiac and respiratory status, including presence of adventitious lung sounds, cardiac arrhythmias, or evidence of congestive heart failure.
   a. Examination for jugular venous pressure, bulging neck vessels, and peripheral edema is important in patients suspected of having renal disease.
   b. Measure blood pressure, which may be elevated in renal disease.
2. Palpate inguinal lymph nodes for enlargement—important in patients suspected of having genitourinary cancer or STD.
3. Assess skin color and changes that may occur in chronic renal failure.

Diagnostic Tests

◆ LABORATORY STUDIES

Common laboratory studies pertaining to renal and urologic disorders include blood and urinary excretion tests for renal function, prostate-specific antigen (PSA), and urinalysis.

Tests of Renal Function

A. Description
1. Renal function tests are used to determine effectiveness of the kidneys' excretory functioning, to evaluate the severity of kidney disease, and to follow the patient's progress.
2. Renal function may be within normal limits until about 50% of renal function has been lost.
3. Best results are obtained by combining a number of clinical tests.

B. Nursing/Patient Care Considerations
See Table 19-1.

Prostate-Specific Antigen

A. Description
1. This amino acid glycoprotein is measured in the serum by a simple blood test.
2. PSA is specific to prostate disease, but not exclusive to prostate cancer.
3. Level rises continuously in the presence of prostate cancer.
4. Normal serum PSA level is less than 4.0 ng/mL.
   a. Levels of less than 10.0 ng/mL may be indicative of only benign prostatic hyperplasia (BPH) and not necessarily prostate cancer.
5. Patients who have undergone treatment for prostate cancer are monitored by PSA levels for recurrence.

TABLE 19-1 Tests of Renal Function

1. There is no single test of renal function; renal function is variable from time to time.
2. The rate of change of renal function is more important than the result of a single test.

Test	Purpose/Rationale	Test Protocol
Renal concentration test Specific gravity Osmolality of urine	Tests the ability to concentrate solutes in the urine. Concentration ability is lost early in kidney disease; hence, this test detects early defects in renal function.	Fluids may be withheld 12–24 h to evaluate the concentrating ability of the tubules under controlled conditions. Specific gravity measurements of urine are taken at specific times to determine urine concentration.
Creatinine clearance	Provides a reasonable approximation of rate of glomerular filtration. Measures volume of blood cleared of creatinine in 1 min. Most sensitive indication of early renal disease. Useful to follow progress of the patient's renal status.	Collect all urine over 24-h period. Draw one sample of blood within the period.
Serum creatinine	A test of renal function reflecting the balance between production and filtration by renal glomerulus. Most sensitive test of renal function.	Do test on blood serum.
Serum urea nitrogen (blood urea nitrogen [BUN])	Serves as index of renal excretory capacity. Serum urea nitrogen depends on the body's urea production and on urine flow. (Urea is the nitrogenous end-product of protein metabolism.) Affected by protein intake, tissue breakdown.	Do test on blood serum.
Protein	Random specimen may be affected by dietary protein intake. Proteinuria >150 mg/24 h may indicate renal disease.	Collect all urine over 24-h period.
Urine casts	Mucoproteins and other substances present in renal inflammation; help to identify type of renal disease (eg, red cell casts present in glomerulonephritis, fatty casts in nephrotic syndrome, white cell casts in pyelonephritis)	Collect random urine specimen.

B. Nursing/Patient Care Considerations
1. No patient preparation is necessary.
2. Some clinicians prefer not to perform digital rectal examinations of the prostate at the same time that a PSA is drawn, to prevent artificial elevation of PSA level, although this association has not been proven.

Urinalysis

A. Description
Involves examination of the urine for overall characteristics, such as appearance, pH, specific gravity, and osmolality, as well as microscopic evaluation for the presence of normal and abnormal cells.

1. *Appearance*—normal urine is clear.
   a. Cloudy urine (phosphaturia) is not always pathologic, related only to the precipitation of phosphates in alkaline urine. Normal urine may also develop cloudiness on refrigeration or from standing at room temperature.
   b. Abnormally cloudy urine (pyuria or chyluria)—due to pus, blood, epithelial cells, bacteria, fat, colloidal particles, phosphate, or lymph fluid.
2. *Odor*—normal urine has a faint aromatic odor.
   a. Characteristic odors produced by ingestion of asparagus, thymol.
   b. Cloudy urine with ammonia odor—urea-splitting bacteria such as *Proteus*, causing urinary tract infections.
   c. Offensive odor—may be due to bacterial action in presence of pus.
3. *Color* shows degree of concentration and depends on amount voided.
   a. Normal urine is clear yellow or amber because of the pigment urochrome.
   b. Dilute urine is straw-colored.
   c. Concentrated urine is highly colored; a sign of insufficient fluid intake.
   d. Cloudy or smoky colored—may be from hematuria, spermatozoa, prostatic fluid, fat droplets, chyle.
   e. Red or red-brown—due to blood pigments, porphyria, transfusion reaction, bleeding lesions in urogenital tract, some drugs.

f. Yellow-brown or green-brown—may reveal obstructive lesion of bile duct system or obstructive jaundice.

g. Dark brown or black—due to malignant melanoma, leukemia.

4. pH of urine reflects the ability of kidney to maintain normal hydrogen ion concentration in plasma and extracellular fluid; indicates *acidity* or *alkalinity* of urine.

   a. pH should be measured in fresh urine because the breakdown of urine to ammonia causes urine to become alkaline.

   b. Normal pH is around 6 (acid); may normally vary from 4.6 to 7.5.

   c. Urine acidity or alkalinity has relatively little clinical significance unless the patient is on special diet or therapeutic program or is being treated for renal calculous disease.

5. *Specific gravity* reflects the kidney's ability to concentrate or dilute urine; may reflect degree of hydration or dehydration.

   a. Normal specific gravity ranges from 1.005 to 1.025.

   b. Specific gravity is fixed at 1.010 in chronic renal failure.

c. In a person eating a normal diet, inability to concentrate or dilute urine indicates disease.

6. *Osmolality* is an indication of the amount of osmotically active particles in urine (specifically, it is the number of particles per unit volume of *water*). It is similar to specific gravity, but is considered a more precise test; it is also easy to do—only 1 to 2 mL urine is required.

   a. Average value is 300 to 1,090 mOsm/kg for female patients; 390 to 1090 mOsm/kg for male patients.

B. Nursing/Patient Care Considerations

1. Freshly voided urine provides the best results for routine urinalysis; some tests may require first morning specimen.

2. Obtain sample of about 30 mL.

3. Urine culture and sensitivities are often performed using the same specimen obtained for urinalysis; therefore, use clean-catch (Procedure Guidelines 19-1) or catheterization techniques.

4. Patients with urinary diversions, especially ileal conduit diversions, require special techniques to obtain urine that is not contaminated with bacteria from the intestinal diversion.

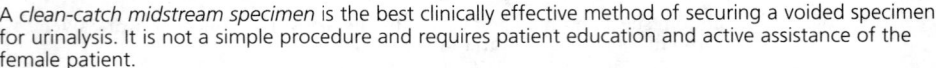

PROCEDURE GUIDELINES 19-1 ◆ Technique for Obtaining Clean-Catch Midstream Voided Specimen

A *clean-catch midstream specimen* is the best clinically effective method of securing a voided specimen for urinalysis. It is not a simple procedure and requires patient education and active assistance of the female patient.

EQUIPMENT
Antiseptic solution or liquid soap solution
Sterile water
4 × 4-inch sponges
Disposable gloves for nurse assisting female patient
Sterile specimen container

PROCEDURE

NURSING ACTION	RATIONALE
MALE PATIENT	
1. Instruct the patient to expose glans and cleanse area around meatus. Wash area with mild antiseptic solution or liquid soap. *Rinse thoroughly.*	1. The urethral orifice is colonized by bacteria. Urine readily becomes contaminated during voiding. Rinse antiseptic solution or soap solution thoroughly because these agents can inhibit bacterial growth in a urine culture.
2. Allow the initial urinary flow to escape.	2. The first portion of urine washes out the urethra and contains debris.
3. Collect the midstream urine specimen in a sterile container.	3. The midstream sample reflects the status of the bladder.
4. Avoid collecting the last few drops of urine.	4. Prostatic secretions may be introduced into urine at the end of the urinary stream.
5. Send specimen to laboratory immediately.	5. A culture should be performed as soon as possible to avoid multiplication of urinary bacteria and lysis of cells.
FEMALE PATIENT	
1. Ask the patient to separate her labia to expose the urethral orifice. If no one is available to assist the patient, she may sit backwards on the toilet seat facing the water tank or sit on (straddle) the wide part of the bedpan.	1. Keeping the labia separated prevents labial or vaginal contamination of the urine specimen. By straddling the toilet seat/bedpan, the patient's labia are spread apart for cleansing.
2. Cleanse the area around the urinary meatus with sponges soaked with antiseptic/soap solution. Rinse thoroughly. a. Wipe the perineum from the front to the back. b. Do not use sponges more than once.	2. The urethral orifice is colonized by bacteria. Urine readily becomes contaminated during voiding.

PROCEDURE (cont'd)	NURSING ACTION	RATIONALE

3. While the patient keeps the labia separated (see accompanying figure), instruct her to void forcibly.

3. This helps wash away urethral contaminants.

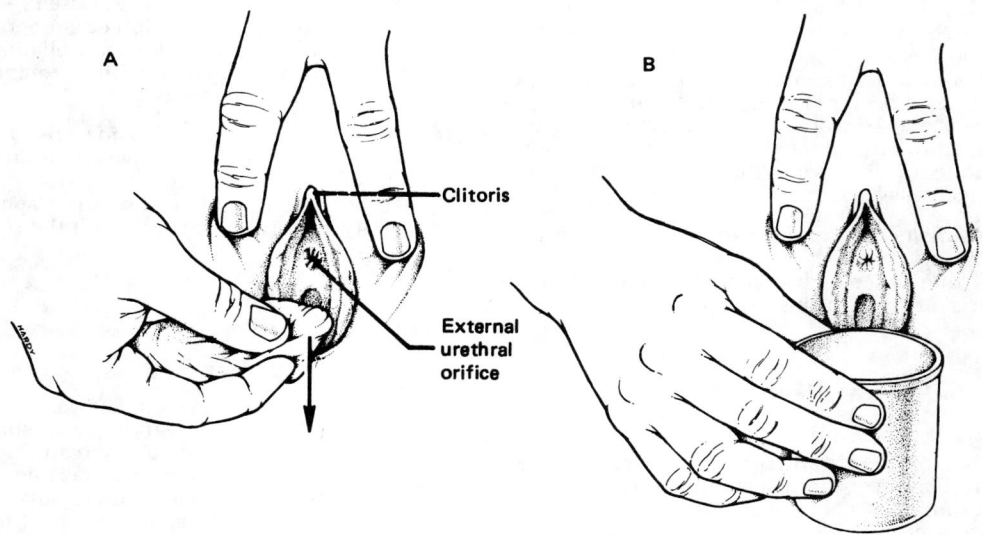

Obtaining a clean-catch midstream urine specimen in the female patient. (**A**) Instruct the patient to hold the labia apart and wash from high up front toward the back with gauze soaked in soap. (**B**) The collection cup is held so that it does not touch the body, and the sample is obtained only while the patient is voiding with the labia held apart.

4. Allow initial urinary flow to drain into bedpan (toilet) and then catch the midstream specimen in a sterile container, making sure that the container does not come in contact with the genitalia.

5. Send the specimen to the laboratory immediately.

4. The first portion of urine washes out the urethra. Have the patient remove the container from the stream while she is still voiding.

5. Too long an interval between collection and analysis cause contaminants to multiply in the urine and cells to lyse.

◆ RADIOLOGY/IMAGING

These tests include simple x-rays, x-rays with the use of contrast media, ultrasound, nuclear scans, and imaging through computed tomography (CT) and magnetic resonance imaging (MRI).

X-ray of Kidneys, Ureters, and Bladder (KUB)

A. Description
1. Consists of plain film of the abdomen.
2. Delineates size, shape, and position of kidneys.
3. Reveals any deviations, such as calcifications (stones), hydronephrosis, cysts, tumors, or kidney displacement.

B. Nursing/Patient Care Considerations No preparation is needed

Intravenous Pyelogram (IVP; Intravenous Urogram, IVU)

A. Description
1. IV introduction of a radiopaque contrast medium, which concentrates in the urine and thus facilitates visualization of the kidneys, ureter, and bladder.
2. The contrast medium is cleared from the bloodstream by renal excretion.

B. Nursing/Patient Care Considerations
1. Contraindicated in patients with renal failure, uncontrolled diabetes, or multiple myeloma.
2. Patients with known iodine/contrast material allergy must have steroid/antihistamine preparation; in some cases an anesthesiologist must be available.
3. Bowel preparation is necessary:
   a. Clear liquids only the day before the examination
   b. Cathartics/laxatives are given the evening before the examination.

    c. NPO after midnight the day of the examination (if scheduled for afternoon, clear liquids only in the morning).

Retrograde Pyelography

A. *Description*
1. Injection of opaque material through ureteral catheters, which have been passed up ureters into renal pelvis by means of cystoscopic manipulation. The opaque solution is introduced by gravity or syringe injection.
2. May be done if IVP provides inadequate visualization of the collecting system.

B. *Nursing/Patient Care Considerations* Contraindicated in patients with urinary tract infection, or with suspected perforation of the ureter or bladder; allergic reactions to contrast material are rare in this exam.

Cystourethrogram

A. *Description*
1. Visualization of urethra and bladder by x-ray after retrograde instillation of contrast material through a catheter. An examination of only the bladder is a *cystogram*; of only the urethra is a *urethrogram*.
2. Used to identify injuries, tumors, or structural abnormalities of the urethra or bladder; or evaluate emptying problems or incontinence (voiding cystourethrogram).

B. *Nursing/Patient Care Considerations*
1. Carries risk of infection due to instrumentation.
2. Allergy to contrast material is not a contraindication.
3. Additional x-rays may be taken after catheter is removed and patient voids (voiding cystourethrogram). Provide reassurance to allay patient's embarrassment.

Renal Angiography

A. *Description*
1. IV catheter is threaded through the femoral and iliac arteries into the aorta or renal artery.
2. Contrast material is injected to visualize the renal arterial supply.
3. Evaluates blood flow dynamics, demonstrates abnormal vasculature, and differentiates renal cysts from renal tumors.
4. May be done to embolize a kidney before nephrectomy for renal tumor.

B. *Nursing/Patient Care Considerations*
1. Clear liquids only after midnight before the examination; adequate hydration is essential. Continue oral medications (special orders needed for diabetic patients).
2. IV required.
3. May not be done on the same day as other studies requiring barium or contrast material.
4. Maintain bed rest for 8 hours after the examination, with the leg kept straight on the side used for groin access.
5. Observe frequently for hematoma or bleeding at access site. Keep sandbag at bedside for use if bleeding occurs.

Renal Scans

A. *Description*
1. Radiopharmaceuticals (also called radiotracers or isotopes) are injected IV.
    a. Tc-DTPA and Tc-MAG are used for anatomic visualization and evaluation of glomerular filtration.
2. Studies are obtained with a scintillation camera placed posterior to the kidney with the patient in a supine, prone, or sitting position.

B. *Nursing/Patient Care Considerations*
1. The patient should be well hydrated. Give several glasses of water before scan.
2. Furosemide (Lasix) or captopril (Capoten) may be administered in conjunction with the scan to determine their effects.

Ultrasound

A. *Description*
1. Uses high-frequency sound waves passed into the body and reflected back in varying frequencies based on the composition of soft tissues. Organs in the urinary system create characteristic ultrasonic images that are electronically processed and displayed as an image.
2. Abnormalities such as masses, malformations, or obstructions can be identified; useful in differentiating between solid and fluid-filled masses.
3. A noninvasive technique

B. *Nursing/Patient Care Considerations*
1. Ultrasound examination of the prostate is performed using a rectal probe. A Fleet's enema may be ordered just within hours of the examination.
2. Patient should not have had any studies using barium for 2 days before ultrasound of the kidney or bladder.

Computed Tomography/Magnetic Resonance Imaging

See descriptions, page 150.

◆ OTHER TESTS

Other tests that may be done to evaluate disorders of the renal and urologic systems include cystoscopy, urodynamic testing, and needle biopsy of the kidney.

Cystoscopy

A. *Description*
1. Cystoscopy is a method of direct visualization of the urethra and bladder by means of a cystoscope that is inserted through the urethra into the bladder. It has a self-contained optical lens system that provides a magnified, illuminated view of the bladder.
2. Uses include:
    a. To inspect bladder wall directly for tumor, stone, or ulcer and to inspect urethra for abnormalities or to assess degree of prostatic obstruction.

b. To allow insertion of ureteral catheters for radiographic studies, or before abdominal or genitourinary surgery.

c. To see configuration and position of ureteral orifices.

d. To remove calculi from urethra, bladder, and ureter.

e. To diagnose and treat lesions of bladder, urethra, and prostate.

B. *Nursing/Patient Care Considerations*
1. Simple cystoscopy is often performed in an office setting. More complicated cystoscopy involving resections or ureteral catheter insertions are done in the operating room cystoscopy suite.
2. The patient's genitalia are cleaned with an antiseptic solution just before the examination. A local topical anesthetic (Xylocaine gel) is instilled into the urethra before insertion of cystoscope.
3. Because fluid flows continuously through the cystoscope, the patient may feel an urge to urinate during the examination.
4. Contraindicated in patients with known urinary tract infection.
5. Nursing interventions after cystoscopic examination
   a. Monitor for complications: urinary retention, urinary tract hemorrhage, infection within prostate or bladder.
   b. Expect the patient to have some burning on voiding, blood-tinged urine, and urinary frequency from trauma to mucous membrane of the urethra.
   c. Administer or teach self-administration of antibiotics prophylactically as ordered to prevent urinary tract infection.
   d. Advise warm sitz baths or analgesics such as ibuprofen or acetaminophen to relieve discomfort after cystoscopy.
   e. Provide routine catheter care if urinary retention persists and an indwelling catheter is ordered.

Urodynamics

A. *Description*
Urodynamics is a term that refers to any of the following tests that provide physiologic and functional information about the lower urinary tract. They measure the ability of the bladder to store and empty urine.

1. Uroflowmetry (flow rate)—a record of the volume of urine passing through the urethra per unit of time (mL/s). It is shown on graph paper and gives information about the rate and flow pattern of urination.
2. Cystometrogram—graphic recording of the pressures exerted at varying phases of filling and emptying of the urinary bladder to assess its function. Pressures are also recorded on graph paper. Data about the ability of the bladder to store urine at low pressure and the ability of the bladder to contract appropriately to empty urine are obtained.
   a. One or more catheters are placed through urethra (or suprapubic area) and into bladder. The residual volume is measured if the patient recently voided, and the catheters are left in place.
   b. The catheters are connected to urodynamic equipment designed to measure pressure at the distal end of the catheter.

c. Water, saline, or contrast material is infused at a slow rate into the bladder.

d. When the bladder feels full, the patient is asked to "void." A normal detrusor contraction of the bladder appears as a sharp rise in bladder pressure on the graph. If the patient is unable to void (with catheters in place), the test is usually considered normal because it is difficult to void normally under these conditions.

3. Sphincter electromyelography (EMG) measures the activity of the pelvic floor muscles during bladder filling and emptying. EMG activity may be collected using surface (patch) electrodes placed around the anus or with percutaneous wire or needle electrodes.
4. Pressure–flow studies involve all of the above components, along with the simultaneous measurement of intra-abdominal pressure via a small tube with a fluid-filled balloon that is placed in the rectum. This permits better interpretation of actual bladder pressures without the influence of intra-abdominal pressure.
5. Video urodynamics use all of the above components. The fluid used to fill the bladder is contrast material, and the entire study is performed under fluoroscopy, providing radiographic pictures in combination with the data recorded on graph paper. Video urodynamics are reserved for patients with complicated voiding dysfunction.

B. *Nursing/Patient Care Considerations*
1. Contraindicated in patients with urinary tract infection.
2. Frequently performed by nurses; essential to provide information and support throughout the test to ensure clinically significant results.
3. Patients will have burning on urination afterward (due to instrumentation), encourage the patient to force fluids.
4. Short-term antibiotics are often given to prevent infection.

Needle Biopsy of Kidney

A. *Description* Performed by percutaneous needle biopsy through renal tissue or by open biopsy through a small flank incision; useful in securing specimens for electron and immunofluorescent microscopy to determine the diagnosis, treatment, and prognosis of renal disease

B. *Nursing/Patient Care Considerations*
1. Prebiopsy nursing management
   a. Ensure that coagulation studies are carried out to identify the patient at risk for postbiopsy bleeding and that serum creatinine and urinalysis are done.
   b. Ensure that patient fasts for several hours before the procedure, as ordered.
   c. Establish an IV line, as ordered.
   d. Describe the procedure to the patient, including holding breath (to stop movement of the kidney) during insertion of the biopsy needle.
2. Postbiopsy nursing management
   a. Place the patient in a prone position immediately after biopsy and on bed rest for 24 hours to minimize bleeding.
   b. Take vital signs every 5 to 15 minutes for first hour and then with decreasing frequency if stable to assess for hemorrhage, which is a major complication.
   c. Watch for rise or fall in blood pressure, anorexia, vomiting, or development of a dull, aching discomfort in abdomen.

d. Assess for flank pain (usually represents bleeding into the muscle) or colicky pain (clot in the ureter).

e. Assess for backache, shoulder pain, or dysuria.

f. Persistent bleeding may be suspected when an enlarging hematoma is palpable through the abdomen.

g. If perirenal bleeding develops, avoid palpating or manipulating the abdomen after the first examination has determined that a hematoma exists.

h. Collect serial urine specimens to evaluate for hematuria.

i. Assess for any patient complaints, especially frequency and urgency on urination.

j. Keep fluid intake at 3,000 mL daily if tolerated, unless the patient has renal insufficiency.

k. Check results of hematocrit and hemoglobin (done the following morning) to assess for anemia, unless the vital signs change before then.

l. Prepare for transfusion and surgical intervention for control of hemorrhage, which may necessitate surgical drainage or nephrectomy.

3. Instruct the patient on the following after biopsy:

a. Avoid strenuous activity, strenuous sports, and heavy lifting for at least 2 weeks.

b. Notify health care provider if any of the following occur: flank pain, hematuria, light-headedness and fainting, rapid pulse, or any other signs and symptoms of bleeding.

c. Report for follow-up 1 to 2 months after biopsy; will be checked for hypertension, and the biopsy area is auscultated for a bruit.

General Procedures/Treatment Modalities

◆ CATHETERIZATION

Catheterization may be done to relieve acute or chronic urinary retention, to drain urine preoperatively and postoperatively, to determine the amount of residual urine after voiding, or to determine accurate measurement of urinary drainage in critically ill patients. See Procedure Guidelines 19-2 and 19-3.

Suprapubic bladder drainage establishes drainage from the bladder by introducing a catheter percutaneously or by an incision through the anterior abdominal wall into the bladder. It may be done for acute urinary retention when urethral catheterization is not possible; for urethral trauma, stricture, or fistula to divert flow of urine from the urethra; or for obtaining an uncontaminated urine specimen for culture. See Procedure Guidelines 19-4.

PROCEDURE GUIDELINES 19-2 ◆ Catheterization of the Urinary Bladder

EQUIPMENT
Sterile gloves
Disposable sterile catheter set with single-use packet of lubricant
Antiseptic solution for periurethral cleansing (sterile)

Gloves, drape, sponges
Sterile container for culture
Bath blanket/sheet for draping
Standing lamp (preferred) or flashlight

SELECTION OF CATHETER SIZE
Use the smallest catheter capable of providing adequate drainage.

PROCEDURE	NURSING ACTION	RATIONALE
	FEMALE PATIENT	
	PREPARATORY PHASE	
	1. Put the patient at ease.	1. The patient will feel reassured if the procedure is explained and if she is handled gently and considerately.
	2. Open catheter tray using aseptic technique. Place waste receptacle in accessible place.	2. Catheterization requires the same aseptic precautions as a surgical procedure. The principal danger of catheterization is urinary tract infection, which is associated with increased morbidity and longer, more costly hospitalization.
	3. Direct light for visualization of genital area.	
	4. Place the patient in a supine position with knees bent, hips flexed, and feet resting on bed about 0.6 m (2 feet) apart. Drape the patient.	
	5. Position moisture-proof pad under the patient's buttocks.	
	6. Wash hands. Put on sterile gloves.	
	PERFORMANCE PHASE	
	1. Separate labia minora so that urethral meatus is visualized; one hand is to maintain separation of the labia until catheterization is finished.	1. This maneuver helps prevent labial contamination of the catheter (see accompany figure).

PROCEDURE (cont'd)

NURSING ACTION | RATIONALE

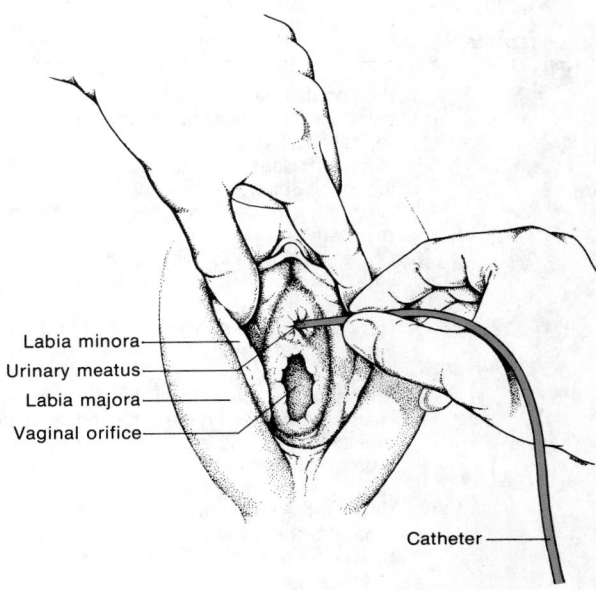

Labia minora—
Urinary meatus—
Labia majora—
Vaginal orifice—

Catheter—

Catheterization of urinary bladder in the female patient.

2. Cleanse around the urethral meatus with a povidone-iodine solution.

   a. Manipulate cleansing sponges with forceps, cleansing with downward strokes from anterior to posterior.
   b. Dispose of cotton sponge after each use.
   c. If the patient is sensitive to iodine, benzalkonium chloride or other cleansing agent is used.

3. Introduce well-lubricated catheter 5–7 cm (2–3 inches) into urethral meatus using strict aspectic technique.

   a. Avoid contaminating surface of catheter.
   b. Ensure that catheter is not too large or too tight at urethral meatus.

4. Allow some bladder urine to flow through catheter before collecting a specimen.

5. Pinch off catheter and remove gently when urine ceases to flow.

FOLLOW-UP PHASE

1. Dry area; make patient comfortable.
2. Measure urine and dispose of equipment.
3. Send specimen to laboratory as indicated.
4. Record time, procedure, amount, and appearance of urine.

MALE PATIENT

1. Carry out all of "preparatory phase" as for female patient except:
2. Place the patient in supine position with legs extended. Place the moisture-proof pad across upper thighs.

2. Bacteria that normally colonize the distal urethra may be introduced into the bladder during or immediately after catheter insertion. Inadequate preparation of the urethral meatus is a major cause of infection.

3. A well-lubricated catheter reduces friction and trauma to the meatus. The female urethra is a relatively short canal, measuring 3–4 cm in length.

   b. Too large a catheter may cause painful distention of the meatus and cause damage to the uroepithelium.

4. This is a representative bladder aliquot.

5. Pinching off the catheter prevents air from entering the bladder as the catheter is removed.

(continued)

PROCEDURE GUIDELINES 19-2 ◆ Catheterization of the Urinary Bladder
(continued)

PROCEDURE (cont'd)	

NURSING ACTION	RATIONALE
3. Position the perineal drape.	
4. Lubricate the catheter well with lubricant or prescribed topical anesthetic.	4. A well-lubricated catheter prevents urethral trauma (decreasing the opportunity for bacterial invasion).
5. Wash off glans penis around urinary meatus with an iodophor solution (Betadine) using forceps to hold cleansing sponges. Keep the foreskin retraction. Maintain sterility of dominant hand.	5. Cleanse urethral meatus from tip to foreskin with downward stroke on one side. Discard sponge. Repeat as required.
6. Grasp shaft of penis (with nondominant hand) and elevate it. Apply gentle traction to penis while catheter is passed.	6. This maneuver straightens the penile urethra and facilitates catheterization. Maintaining a grasp of the penis prevents contamination and retraction of penis.
7. Using sterile gloves, insert catheter into the urethra; advance catheter 15–25 cm (6–10 inches) until urine flows.	7. The male urethra is a canal extending from the bladder to the end of the glans penis. The length varies within wide limits; the average length is about 21 cm.
8. If resistance is felt at the external sphincter, slightly increase the traction on the penis and apply steady, gentle pressure on the catheter. Ask patient to strain gently (as if passing urine) to help relax sphincter.	8. Some resistance may be due to spasm of external sphincter. Inability to pass the catheter may mean that a urethral stricture or other forms of urethral pathology exist. The urethra may have to be dilated with sounds by a urologist.
9. When urine begins to flow, advance the catheter another 2.5 cm (1 inch).	9. Advancing the catheter ensures its position in the bladder.
10. Reduce (or reposition) the foreskin.	10. Paraphimosis (retraction and constriction of the foreskin behind the glans penis), secondary to catheterization, may occur if the foreskin is not reduced.

FOLLOW-UP PHASE
Same as for female patient.

PROCEDURE GUIDELINES 19-3 ◆ Management of the Patient With an Indwelling (Self-Retaining) Catheter and Closed Drainage System

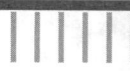

EQUIPMENT
Catheter tray with closed system of urinary drainage
Antibacterial solution for cleansing
Gauze squares
Single-use packet of lubricant

PROCEDURE	

NURSING ACTION	RATIONALE
GENERAL CONSIDERATIONS	
1. Catheterize the patient (p. 594), using a catheter that is preconnected to a closed drainage system.	1. A closed drainage system is one that is closed to outside air.
a. Advance catheter almost to its bifurcation (for male patient).	a. This prevents the balloon from becoming trapped in the urethra.
b. Inflate the balloon according to manufacturer's directions. Be sure catheter is draining properly before inflating balloon, then withdraw catheter slightly.	b. Inadvertent inflation of the balloon within the urethra is painful and causes urethral trauma.
2. Secure the indwelling catheter.	2. Properly securing the catheter prevents catheter movement and traction on the urethra.
a. Female: Tape the catheter and drainage tubing to the thigh. Male: Tape the catheter to the patient's thigh.	
b. Allow some slack of the tubing to accommodate the patient's movements.	
c. Keep the tubing over the patient's leg.	c. This tubing position helps prevent kinking or forming loops of stagnant urine.

PROCEDURE (cont'd)	NURSING ACTION	RATIONALE

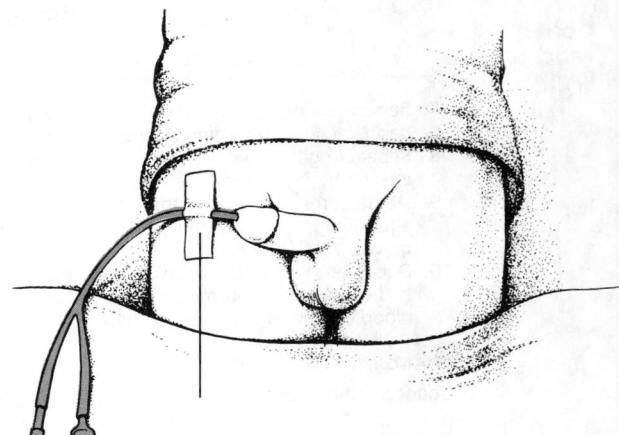

In the male patient, the indwelling catheter is taped to the thigh to straighten the angulation of the penoscrotal junction, thus reducing pressure on the urethra exerted by the catheter.

CARE OF THE INDWELLING CATHETER

NURSING ACTION

1. Cleanse around the area where catheter enters urethral meatus (meatal–catheter junction) with soap and water during the daily bath to remove debris.

2. Avoid using powders and sprays on the perineal area.
3. Avoid pulling on the catheter during cleansing.

RATIONALE

1. Suppurative drainage and encrustation occur at the exit of any tube. Infectious organisms can migrate to the bladder along the outside of any indwelling catheter; however, excessive manipulation of the catheter may promote migration of bacteria.
2. Powder can encrust and cause soreness and infection.
3. Pulling on the catheter may be painful. Backward and forward displacement of the catheter introduces contaminants into the urinary tract.

TO OBTAIN URINE FOR CULTURE

NURSING ACTION

1. Clamp the drainage tubing below the aspiration (sampling) port for a *few minutes* to allow urine to collect.

2. Cleanse the aspiration port with povidone-iodine or 70% alcohol.
3. Insert a sterile No. 21 gauge needle (attached to a sterile syringe) into the aspiration port of the catheter tubing.
4. Aspirate a small volume of urine for culture.
5. Remove needle from syringe and release urine carefully into sterile specimen container.
6. *Unclamp the drainage tube.*
7. Send specimen to laboratory immediately.

RATIONALE

1. Avoid separating catheter and connecting tube. Disconnection of the catheter and tubing is a major cause of urinary tract infection.

3. Avoid inserting needle into the shaft of the catheter because this may cause balloon deflation.

7. The specimen should be marked as a ''catheterized specimen'' because the presence of any number of colonies of an organism indicates a urinary tract infection.

TO IRRIGATE THE CATHETER

Note: This is not done unless obstruction is anticipated (bleeding following bladder/prostate surgery).

NURSING ACTION

1. Wash hands. Don gloves.
2. Using aseptic technique, pour sterile irrigating solution into sterile container.
3. Cleanse around catheter/drainage tubing connection with sterile gauze pads soaked in povidone-iodine solution.
4. Disconnect catheter from drainage tubing. Cover tubing with a sterile cap.
5. Place a sterile drainage basin under the catheter.
6. Connect a large volume syringe to the catheter and irrigate catheter using prescribed amount of sterile irrigant.

RATIONALE

3. If frequent irrigations are necessary to keep the catheter open, change the catheter as the catheter itself is probably contributing to the problem.

6. Instill about 30 mL irrigating solution at a time. Avoid instilling the solution forcibly to prevent bladder irritation and spasms.

(continued)

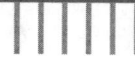

PROCEDURE GUIDELINES 19-3 ◆ Management of the Patient With an Indwelling (Self-Retaining) Catheter and Closed Drainage System *(continued)*

PROCEDURE (cont'd)	NURSING ACTION	RATIONALE

7. Remove syringe and place end of catheter over drainage basin, allowing returning fluid to drain into basin.

    7. This provides gravitational flow.

8. Repeat irrigation procedure until fluid is clear or according to physician's directives.

9. Disinfect the distal end of the catheter and end of drainage tubing; reconnect the catheter and tubing. Remove gloves. Wash hands.

10. Document type and amount of irrigating solution, color and character of returning fluid, presence of sediment/blood clots, and patient's reaction.

    10. Use irrigating equipment one time and then discard.

CHANGING THE CATHETER

Change catheter according to the needs of the patient.

An indwelling catheter should *not* be changed at arbitrarily fixed intervals.

PRINCIPLES OF CARE WHEN MANAGING A CLOSED DRAINAGE SYSTEM

1. Wash hands immediately before and after handling any part of the system. Wear clean disposable gloves when handling the drainage system.

    1. Hands are the major route of transmission of gram-negative bacteria.

2. Maintain unobstructed urine flow.

    a. Keep the drainage bag in a dependent position, below the level of the bladder.

    b. Urine should not be allowed to collect in the tubing, since a free flow of urine must be maintained to prevent infection.

    c. Keep the bag off the floor.

    2. Urine flow must be downhill.

    a. Raising the bag will cause reflux of contaminated urine from the bag into the patient's bladder.

    b. Improper drainage occurs when the tubing is kinked or twisted, allowing pools of drainage to collect in the loops of tubing.

    c. To prevent bacterial contamination.

3. To empty the drainage bag.

    a. Wash hands; don gloves.

    a. Empty the bag at regular intervals, taking care to see that the drainage valve/spout is not contaminated.

    b. Disinfect spigot. Empty the bag in a separate collecting receptacle for each patient. Disinfect spigot again.

    b. Each patient should have his own collecting receptacle that is labeled with his name and kept in his bathroom, not on the floor—to prevent cross-contamination.

    c. Avoid letting the drainage bag touch the floor.

    d. Change the drainage bag if contamination occurs, if the urine flow becomes obstructed, or if the connecting junctions start to leak.

MEASURES TO PREVENT CROSS-CONTAMINATION

1. Wash hands before and after handling the catheter/drainage system and between patients.

    1. Many urinary tract infections are due to extrinsically acquired organisms transmitted by cross-contamination.

2. Assign only one patient with an indwelling catheter to a room. If this is not possible, separate the infected patient with an indwelling catheter from an uninfected patient.

    2. There appears to be a greater risk of microbial transmission between catheterized patients.

3. Know the patients at risk.

    3. Female, elderly, debilitated, and critically ill patients, those in the postpartum state, and patients with obstructed or neurologically impaired bladders are at risk for infection.

COMMUNITY-BASED CARE TIP:
For care of catheter at home, instruct patient to:
1. Wash hands before and after handling the catheter.
2. Wash around urinary opening daily, taking care to avoid pulling on the catheter during cleansing.
3. Drink 8–12 glasses of fluids daily; increase fluid intake if urine becomes dark and concentrated.
4. Wipe all connecting junctions with alcohol before changing from leg-bag drainage to overnight bottle drainage.
5. Keep the drainage bag at a lower level than the bladder; do not place the bag on your chair.
6. Avoid letting the bag lay on its side as urine may flow back into the drainage tube.
7. Usually the catheter is not changed except when obstruction or malfunction occurs.
8. Inspect the catheter upon removal for evidence of encrustation; if there are no signs of encrustation and blocking of lumen, the interval between catheter changes may be increased.
9. Call healthcare provider if fever and/or cloudy, bloody, or odoriferous urine develops.

PROCEDURE GUIDELINES 19-4 ◆ Assisting the Patient Undergoing Suprapubic Bladder Drainage (Cystostomy)

Suprapubic bladder drainage is a method of establishing drainage from the bladder by introducing a catheter percutaneously or by an incision through the anterior abdominal wall into the bladder.

EQUIPMENT   Sterile suprapubic drainage system package (disposable)
Skin germicide for suprapubic skin preparation; sterile gloves
Local anesthetic agent if needed

PROCEDURE

NURSING ACTION	*RATIONALE*
PREPARATORY PHASE	
1. Place the patient in a supine position with one pillow under head.	
2. Expose the abdomen.	
PERFORMANCE PHASE (BY PHYSICIAN)	
1. The bladder is distended with 300–500 mL sterile saline via a urethral catheter, which is removed, or the patient is given fluids (PO or IV) before the procedure.	1. Distention of the bladder makes the bladder easier to locate by the suprapubic route.
2. The suprapubic area is surgically prepared. After the skin is dried, the needle entry point is located.	2. The needle entry point is in the midline, 2–3 cm above the symphysis pubis and directly over the palpable bladder.
3. The skin and subcutaneous tissues are infiltrated with local anesthesia.	3. An adequate level of local anesthesia is achieved to facilitate catheter introduction.
4. A small stab wound (incision) may be made.	
5. The catheter* is introduced via a guidewire, needle, or cannula through the incision and advanced in a slightly caudal direction.	5. Entrance into the bladder is usually felt and can be verified by free flow of urine.
6. The catheter is advanced until the flange is against the skin where it is secured with tape, a body seal system, or sutures.	6. Another method is to advance a long needle into the bladder until urine flow verifies the needle is in the bladder.
7. The catheter is connected to a sterile drainage system.	7. Aseptic technique is used in the area around the cystostomy tube.
8. Secure drainage tubing to lateral abdomen with tape.	8. Prevents undue tension on the catheter.
9. If the catheter is not draining properly, withdraw the catheter 2.5 cm (1 inch) at a time until urine begins to flow. Do not dislodge catheter from bladder.	
10. The drainage is maintained continuously for several days.	
11. If a "trial of voiding" is requested, the catheter is clamped for 4 h.	11. Usually, patients will void earlier after surgery with suprapubic drainage than with indwelling catheters.
a. Have the patient attempt to void while the catheter is clamped.	
b. After the patient voids, unclamp the catheter and measure residual urine.	
c. Usually, if the amount of residual urine is less than 100 ml on two separate occasions (AM and PM), the catheter may be removed.	
d. If the patient complains of pain or discomfort, or if the residual urine is over the prescribed amount, the catheter is usually left open.	
12. The catheter is removed upon request, and a sterile dressing is placed over the site. Usually the tract will close within 48 h.	12. Suprapubic drainage is considered more comfortable than an indwelling urethral catheter, it allows greater patient mobility, and there is less risk of bladder infection.
13. Monitor for complications.	13. Complications of this procedure: inadvertent peritoneal and bowel damage, leakage around catheter, kinking of catheter, hematuria, abdominal wall abscess.

* It is necessary to become familiar with the manufacturer's directions of the system being used.

◆ DIALYSIS

Dialysis refers to the diffusion of solute molecules through a semipermeable membrane, passing from the side of higher concentration to that of lower concentration. The purpose of dialysis is to maintain the life and well-being of the patient. It is a substitute for some kidney excretory functions but does not replace the kidneys' endocrine and metabolic functions.

Methods of dialysis include:

1. Peritoneal dialysis
    a. Intermittent peritoneal dialysis (acute or chronic)—see Procedure Guidelines 19-5
    b. Continuous ambulatory peritoneal dialysis
    c. Continuous cycling peritoneal dialysis—uses automated peritoneal dialysis machine overnight with prolonged dwell time during day.
2. Hemodialysis (see p. 601)

3. Continuous renal replacement therapy—special procedures such as continuous arteriovenous hemofiltration (CAV-H), continuous arteriovenous hemodialysis (CVA-HD), and continuous arteriovenous ultrafiltration. These use extracorporeal blood circulation through a small-volume, low-resistance filter to provide continuous removal of solutes and fluid in the intensive care setting.

Continuous Ambulatory Peritoneal Dialysis (Fig. 19-1)

Continuous ambulatory peritoneal dialysis (CAPD) is a form of intracorporeal dialysis that uses the peritoneum for the semipermeable membrane.

A. Procedure
1. A permanent indwelling catheter is implanted into the peritoneum; the internal cuff of the catheter becomes

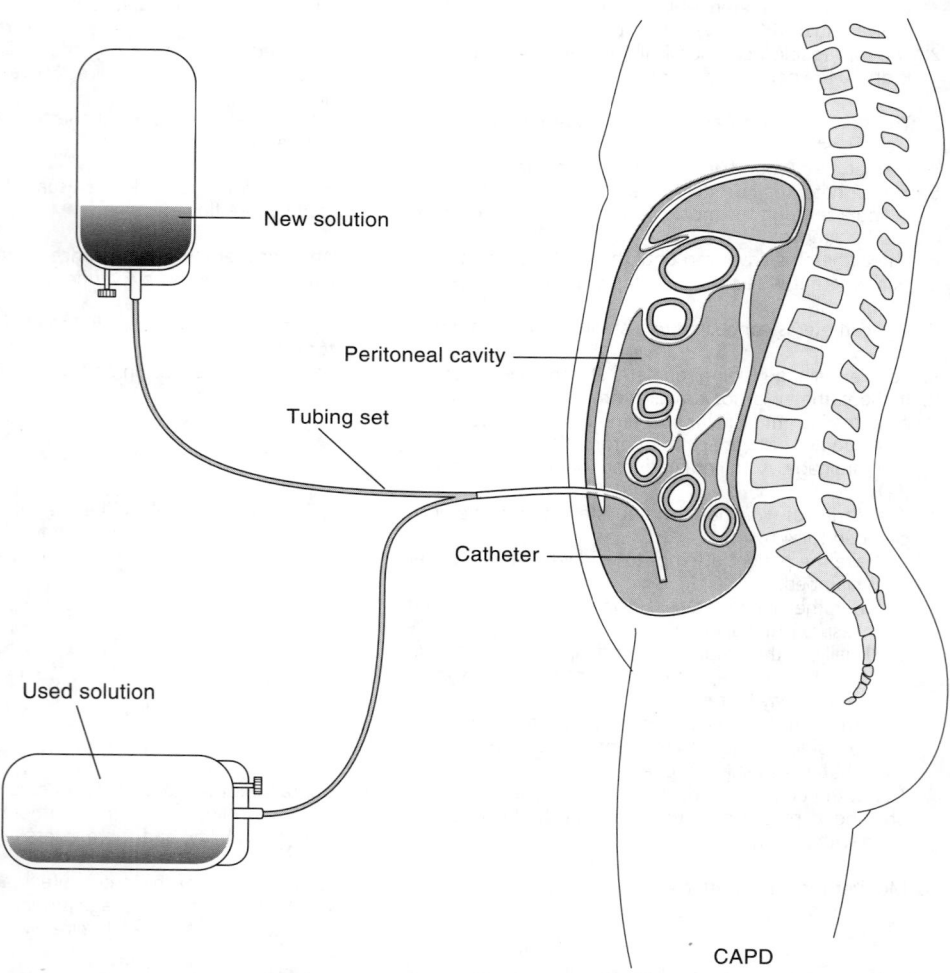

FIGURE 19-1 *Continuous ambulatory peritoneal dialysis. The peritoneal catheter is implanted through the abdominal wall. Fluid infuses into the peritoneal cavity and drains after prescribed time.*

embedded by fibrous ingrowth, which stabilizes it and minimizes leakage.

2. A connecting tube is attached to the external end of the peritoneal catheter, and the distal end of the tube is inserted into a sterile plastic bag of dialysate solution.

3. The dialysate bag is raised to shoulder level and infused by gravity into the peritoneal cavity (approximately 10 minutes for a 2-liter volume).

4. The typical dwell time is 4 to 6 hours.

5. At the end of the dwell time the dialysate fluid is drained from the peritoneal cavity by gravity. Drainage of 2 liters plus ultrafiltration takes about 10 to 20 minutes if the catheter is functioning optimally.

6. After the dialysate is drained, a fresh bag of dialysate solution is infused using aseptic technique, and the procedure is repeated.

7. The patient performs four to five exchanges daily, 7 days a week with an overnight dwell time allowing uninterrupted sleep; most patients become unaware of fluid in the peritoneal cavity.

B. Advantages Over Hemodialysis
1. Physical and psychological freedom and independence
2. More liberal diet and fluid intake
3. Relatively simple and easy to use
4. Satisfactory biochemical control of uremia

C. Complications
1. Infectious peritonitis, exit-site and tunnel infections.
2. Noninfectious catheter malfunction, obstruction, dialysate leak
3. Peritoneal–pleural communication, hernia formation
4. Gastrointestinal bloating, distention, nausea
5. Hypervolemia, hypovolemia
6. Bleeding

D. Patient Education
1. The use of CAPD as a long-term treatment depends on prevention of recurring peritonitis.
   a. Use strict aseptic technique when performing bag exchanges.
   b. Perform bag exchanges in clean, closed-off area without pets and other activities.
   c. Wash hands before touching bag.
   d. Inspect bag, tubing for defects and leaks.
2. Do not omit bag changes—this will cause inadequate control of renal failure.
3. Some weight gain may accompany CAPD—the dialysate fluid contains a significant amount of dextrose, which adds calories to daily intake.
4. Report signs and symptoms of peritonitis—cloudy peritoneal fluid, abdominal pain or tenderness, malaise, fever.

Hemodialysis

Hemodialysis is a process of cleansing the blood of accumulated waste products. It is used for patients with end-stage renal failure or for acutely ill patients who require short-term dialysis.

A. Procedure
1. The patient's access is prepared and cannulated.
2. Heparin is administered (unless contraindicated).
3. Heparinized blood flows through a semipermeable dialyzer in one direction and dialysis solution surrounds the membranes and flows in the opposite direction.

4. Dialysis solution consists of highly purified water to which sodium, potassium, calcium, magnesium, chloride, and dextrose have been added. Bicarbonate or acetate is also added to achieve the proper pH balance.

5. Through the process of diffusion, solute in the form of electrolytes, metabolic waste products, and acid–base components can be removed or added to the blood.

6. Excess water is removed from the blood (ultrafiltration).

7. The blood is then returned to the body through the patient's access.

B. Requirements for Hemodialysis
1. Access to the patient's circulation
2. Dialysis machine and dialyzer with semipermeable membrane
3. Appropriate dialysate bath
4. Time—approximately 4 hours, three times weekly
5. Place—dialysis center or home (if feasible)

C. Methods of Circulatory Access
1. Arteriovenous fistula (AVF)—creation of a vascular communication by suturing a vein directly to an artery
   a. Usually, radial artery and cephalic vein are anastomosed in nondominant arm; vessels in the upper arm may also be used.
   b. After the procedure, the superficial venous system of the arm dilates.
   c. By means of two large-bore needles inserted into the dilated venous system, blood may be obtained and passed through the dialyzer. The arterial end is used for arterial flow and the distal end for reinfusion of dialyzed blood.
   d. Healing of AVF requires several weeks; a central vein catheter is used in the interim.
2. Arteriovenous graft—arteriovenous connection consisting of a tube graft made from autologous saphenous vein or from polytetrafluoroethylene (PTFE).
3. Central vein catheters (CVC)—direct cannulation of veins (subclavian, internal jugular, or femoral)

C. Complications of Vascular Access
1. Infection
2. Catheter clotting
3. Central vein thrombosis or stricture
4. Stenosis or thrombosis
5. Ischemia of the hand
6. Aneurysm or pseudoaneurysm

D. Monitoring During Hemodialysis
1. Involves constant monitoring of hemodynamic status, electrolyte, and acid–base balance, as well as maintenance of sterility and a closed system.
2. Usually performed by a specially trained nurse who is well familiar with the protocol and equipment being used.

E. Lifestyle Management for Chronic Hemodialysis
1. Dietary management involves restriction or adjustment of protein, sodium, potassium, or fluid intake.
2. Ongoing health care monitoring includes careful adjustment of medications that are normally excreted by the kidney or are dialyzable.
3. Surveillance for complications
   a. Arteriosclerotic cardiovascular disease, congestive heart failure, disturbance of lipid metabolism (hypertriglyceridemia), coronary heart disease, stroke
   b. Intercurrent infection
   c. Anemia and fatigue
   d. Gastric ulcers and other problems
   e. Bone problems (renal osteodystrophy, aseptic necrosis of hip)—from disturbed calcium metabolism

f. Hypertension
g. Psychosocial problems: depression, suicide, sexual dysfunction
4. Supportive agencies: American Association of Kidney Patients; 1 David Blvd., Suite LL 1; Tampa, FL 33606; 1-800-749-AAKP; National Kidney Foundation; 2 Park Avenue; New York, NY 10016; 212-889-2210; American Kidney Fund; 6110 Executive Blvd.,Suite 1010; Rockville, MD 20852; and National Kidney and Urologic Diseases Information Clearing House; P. O. Box NKUDIC; Bethesda, MD 20862; 301-468-6345.

PROCEDURE GUIDELINES 19-5 ◆ Assisting the Patient Undergoing (Acute) Peritoneal Dialysis*

Peritoneal dialysis is a substitute for kidney function during renal failure. The peritoneum acts as a dialyzing membrane, and dialysate is delivered into the peritoneal cavity.

EQUIPMENT

Dialysis administration set (disposable, closed system)
Peritoneal dialysis solution as requested
Supplemental drugs as requested
Local anesthesia
Central venous pressure monitoring equipment

ECG
Suture set
Sterile gloves
Skin antiseptic

PROCEDURE

NURSING ACTION	RATIONALE
1. Prepare the patient emotionally and physically for the procedure.	1. Nursing support is offered by explaining procedure mechanics, providing opportunities for the patient to ask questions, allowing him to verbalize his feelings, and giving expert physical care.
2. See that the consent form has been signed.	
3. Weigh the patient before dialysis and every 24 h thereafter, preferably on an in-bed scale.	3. The weight at the beginning of the procedure serves as a baseline of information. Daily weight confirms ultrafiltration results and evaluates volume status.
4. Take temperature, pulse, respiration, and blood pressure readings before dialysis.	4. Measurement of vital signs at the beginning of dialysis is necessary for comparing subsequent changes in vital signs.
5. Have the patient empty bladder.	5. If the bladder is empty, there is less likelihood of perforating it when the trocar is introduced into the peritoneum.
6. Flush the tubing with dialysis solution.	6. The tubing is flushed to prevent air from entering the peritoneal cavity. Air causes abdominal discomfort and drainage difficulties.
7. Make the patient comfortable in a supine position. Have the patient and health care personnel wear masks.	7. This helps protect the patient from airborne contamination.

PERFORMANCE PHASE (BY THE PHYSICIAN)

The following is a brief summary of the method of insertion of a temporary peritoneal catheter (*done under strict asepsis*).

1. The abdomen is prepared surgically, and the skin and subcutaneous tissues are infiltrated with a local anesthetic.	1. Surgical preparation of the skin minimizes or eliminates surface bacteria and decreases the possibility of wound contamination and infection.
2. A small midline stab wound is made 3–5 cm below the umbilicus.	
3. The trocar is inserted through the incision with the stylet in place, or a thin stylet cannula may be inserted percutaneously.	
4. The patient is requested to raise head from the pillow after the trocar is introduced.	4. This maneuver tightens the abdominal muscles and permits easier penetration of the trocar without danger of injury to the intra-abdominal organs.
5. When the peritoneum is punctured, the trocar is directed toward the left side of the pelvis. The stylet is removed, and the catheter is inserted through the trocar and maneuvered into position.	
a. Dialysis fluid is allowed to run through the catheter while it is being positioned.	a. This prevents the omentum from adhering to the catheter, impeding its advancement or occluding its opening.
6. After the trocar is removed, the skin may be closed with a purse-string suture. (This is not always done.) A sterile dressing is placed around the catheter.	6. The catheter is attached to the skin to prevent loss of the catheter in the abdomen.

PROCEDURE (cont'd)	NURSING ACTION	RATIONALE

NURSING ACTION

7. Attach the catheter connector to the administration set, which has been previously connected to the container of dialysis solution (warmed to body temperature, 37°C.)

8. Drugs (heparin, potassium, antibiotic) are added in advance.

9. Permit the dialyzing solution to flow unrestricted into the peritoneal cavity (usually takes 5–10 min for completion). If the patient experiences pain, slow down the infusion.

10. Allow the fluid to remain in the peritoneal cavity for the prescribed time period (20–30 min). Prepare the next exchange while the fluid is in the peritoneal cavity.

11. Unclamp the outflow tube. Drainage should take approximately 20–30 min, although the time varies with each patient.

12. Check outflow for cloudy appearance, blood, and/or fibrin.

13. If the fluid is not draining properly, move the patient from side to side to facilitate the removal of peritoneal drainage. The head of the bed may also be elevated.

14. Ascertain if the catheter is patent. Check for closed clamp, kinked tubing, or air lock. *Never push the catheter in.*

15. When the outflow drainage ceases to run, clamp off the drainage tube and infuse the next exchange, using strict aseptic technique.

16. Take blood pressure and pulse q15min during the first exchange and every hour thereafter. Monitor the heart rate for signs of dysrhythmia.

17. Take the patient's temperature q4h (especially after catheter removal).

18. The procedure is repeated until the blood chemistry levels improve. The usual duration for short-term dialysis is 48–72 h. Depending on the patient's condition, he will receive 48–72 exchanges.

19. Keep an exact record of the patient's fluid balance during the treatment.

   a. Know the status of the patient's loss or gain of fluid at the end of each exchange. Check dressing for leakage and weight on gram scale if significant.
   b. The fluid balance should be about even or should show slight fluid loss or gain, depending on the patient's fluid status.

20. Promote patient comfort during dialysis.

   a. Provide frequent back care and massage pressure areas.
   b. Have the patient turn from side to side.
   c. Elevate head of bed at intervals.
   d. Allow the patient to sit in chair for brief periods if condition permits (only with surgically implanted catheter; with trocar, patient is usually on bedrest).

RATIONALE

7. The solution is warmed to body temperature for patient comfort and to prevent abdominal pain. Heating also causes dilatation of the peritoneal vessels and increases urea clearance.

8. The addition of heparin prevents fibrin clots from occluding the catheter. Potassium chloride may be added on request unless patient has hyperkalemia. Antibiotics are added for the treatment of peritonitis.

9. The inflow solution should flow in a steady stream. If the fluid flows in too slowly, the catheter may need to be repositioned, since its tip may be buried in the omentum, or it may be occluded by a blood clot. Flushing may help.

10. For potassium, urea, and other waste materials to be removed, the solution must remain in the peritoneal cavity for the prescribed time (dwell or equilibration time). The maximum concentration gradient takes place in the first 5–10 min for small molecules, such as urea and creatinine.

11. The abdomen is drained by a siphon effect through the closed system. Gravity drainage should occur fairly rapidly, and steady streams of fluid should be observed entering the drainage container. The drainage is usually straw-colored.

12. May be an early sign of peritonitis.

13. If the drainage stops, or starts to drip before the dialyzing fluid has run out, the catheter tip may be buried in the omentum. Rotating the patient may be helpful (or it may be necessary for the physician to reposition the catheter).

14. Pushing in the catheter introduces bacteria into the peritoneal cavity.

16. A drop in blood pressure may indicate excessive fluid loss from glucose concentrations of the dialyzing solutions. Changes in the vital signs may indicate impending shock or overhydration.

17. An infection is more apt to become evident after dialysis has been discontinued.

18. The duration of dialysis depends on the severity of the condition and on the size and weight of the patient.

19. Complications (circulatory collapse, hypotension, shock, and death) may occur if the patient loses too much fluid through peritoneal drainage. Large fluid losses around the catheter may not be noted unless the dressings are checked carefully.

20. The dialysis period is lengthy, and the patient becomes fatigued.

(continued)

PROCEDURE GUIDELINES 19-5 ◆ Assisting the Patient Undergoing (Acute) Peritoneal Dialysis* *(continued)*

PROCEDURE (cont'd) NURSING ACTION	RATIONALE
21. Observe for the following: a. Abdominal pain—note the time of discomfort during exchange cycle and duration of symptoms.	a. Pain may be caused by the dialyzing solution's not being at body temperature, incomplete drainage of the solution, chemical irritation, pressure by the catheter, peritonitis, or air pressing on the diaphragm, causing referred shoulder pain.
b. Dialysate leakage—change the dressings frequently, being careful not to dislodge the catheter; use sterile plastic drapes to prevent contamination.	b. Leakage around the catheter predisposes the patient to infection at the exit site and peritonitis. Dialysis may need to be terminated if leakage persists.
c. Place the patient in a more upright position and use smaller fluid volumes. 22. Keep accurate records. a. Exact time of beginning and end of each exchange: starting and finishing time of drainage b. Amount of solution infused and recovered c. Fluid balance d. Number of exchanges e. Medications added to dialyzing solution f. Pre- and postdialysis weight, plus daily weight g. Level of responsiveness at beginning, throughout, and at end of treatment h. Assessment of vital signs and patient's condition	

COMPLICATIONS

1. Peritonitis a. Watch for nausea and vomiting, anorexia, abdominal pain, tenderness, rigidity, and cloudy dialysate drainage. b. Send specimen of dialysate for white cell count and full set of cultures.	1. Peritonitis is the most common complication. Antibiotics may be added to dialysate and also given systemically.
2. Bleeding	2. A small amount of bleeding around the catheter is not significant if it does not persist. During the first few exchanges, blood-tinged fluid from subcutaneous bleeding is not uncommon. Small amounts of heparin may be added to inflow solution to prevent the catheter from becoming clogged.
a. A hematocrit of the drainage fluid may be taken to determine the amount of bleeding.	

* Automated closed-system peritoneal cycling machines are available.

◆ KIDNEY SURGERY

Kidney surgery may include nephrectomy (removal of the kidney), kidney transplantation for chronic renal failure, procedures to remove obstruction such as stones or tumors, and procedures to insert drainage tubes (nephrostomy). Incisional approaches vary, but may involve the flank, thoracic, and abdominal regions. Nephrectomy is most often performed for malignant tumors of the kidney but may also be indicated for trauma and kidneys that no longer function due to obstructive disorders and other renal disease. The absence of one kidney does not result in impaired renal function when the remaining kidney is normal.

Preoperative Management/ Nursing Care

1. Prepare patient for surgery with information about operating room routine, and administer preoperative antibiotics and bowel cleansing regimen.
2. Assess for risk factors for thromboembolism (smoking, oral contraceptive use, varicosities of lower extremities) and apply antiembolism stockings if ordered. Review leg exercises with patient and provide information about pneumatic/sequential compression stockings that will be used postoperatively.

3. Assess pulmonary status (presence of dyspnea, productive cough, other related cardiac symptoms) and teach deep-breathing exercises, effective coughing, and use of incentive spirometer.
4. If embolization of the renal artery is being done preoperatively for patients with renal cell carcinoma, monitor for and treat the following symptoms of postinfarction syndrome, which may last for up to 3 days:
   a. Flank pain
   b. Fever
   c. Leukocytosis
   d. Hypertension

Postoperative Management/ Nursing Care

1. Monitor vital signs and incisional area for evidence of bleeding or hemorrhage.

NURSING ALERT:
Use frequent and close observation of blood pressure, pulse, and respiration to recognize hemorrhage (and shock)—chief danger after renal surgery. Watch for pain, sanguinous drainage from drain site(s) or expanding flank mass. Prepare for rapid blood and fluid replacement and reoperation.

2. Assess for pulmonary complications of atelectasis, pneumonia, pneumothorax. Maintain good pulmonary toilet and chest tube drainage, if used (the proximity of the thoracic cavity to the operative area may result in the need for chest tube drainage postoperatively).
3. Maintain patency of urinary drainage tubes (nephrostomy, suprapubic, or urethral catheter) and ureteral stents as indicated.
4. Monitor lower extremities and respiratory status for thromboembolic complications.
5. Assess bowel sounds, abdominal distention, and pain that may indicate paralytic ileus and need for nasogastric decompression.
6. For kidney transplant patients, administer immunosuppressant drugs (corticosteroids in combination with azathioprine [Imuran] or similar agent) as ordered and monitor for early signs of rejection—temperature greater than 100.4°F (38.5°C), decreased urine output, weight gain of 3 lb or more overnight, pain or tenderness over the graft site, hypertension, increased serum creatinine.

Nursing Diagnoses

A. Pain related to surgical incision
B. Altered Urinary Elimination related to urinary drainage tubes or catheter(s)
C. Risk for Infection related to incision, potential pulmonary complications, and possibly immunosuppression
D. Risk for Fluid Volume Deficit or Excess related to fluid replacement needs and transplanted/remaining kidney function

Nursing Interventions

A. *Relieving Pain*
1. Assess pain location, level, and characteristics.
   a. Transient renal coliclike pain may be caused by passage of blood clots down the ureter; however, report any persistent increasing or unrelievable pain that may indicate obstruction of urinary drainage or hemorrhage.
2. Administer pain medications; evaluate effectiveness of patient-controlled analgesia (PCA).
3. Encourage patient to ambulate, splint incision to move or cough.

B. *Promoting Urinary Elimination*
1. Maintain patency of urinary drainage tubes and catheter(s) while in place. Prevent kinking or pulling.
2. Use handwashing and asepsis when providing care and handling urinary drainage system (especially important for the patient taking immunosuppressants).
3. Make sure indwelling catheter is dependent and draining.
   a. Report any decrease in output or excessive clots.
   b. Be alert for signs of urinary infection such as cloudy urine, fever, or bladder or flank ache.
4. Intervene to encourage removal of catheter when patient becomes ambulatory.
5. Maintain adequate fluid intake, IV or oral when allowed.

C. *Preventing Infection*
1. Monitor for fever, elevated leukocyte count, abnormal breath sounds.
2. Administer antibiotics as prescribed.
3. Assist patient with use of incentive spirometer, coughing and deep breathing, and ambulation to decrease risk of pulmonary infection. Provide meticulous care to chest tube sites.
4. Change dressings promptly if drainage is present—drainage is an excellent culture medium for bacteria.
5. Obtain specimens for bacteriologic testing of urine, wounds, sputum, and discontinued catheters, drains, and IV lines as indicated.
   a. Before removing catheters or urinary drains, disinfect skin around entry site, then remove. Using aseptic technique, cut off tip of catheter or drain and place in sterile container for laboratory culture.
6. Monitor vascular access to hemodialysis to ensure patency and watch for evidence of infection.
7. For kidney transplant patients, give oral antifungal—to prevent mucosal candidiasis, which often occurs due to immunosuppression.
8. Provide regular skin care and assist with hygiene.

D. *Maintaining Fluid Balance*
1. Closely monitor intake and output, especially after kidney transplantation.
   a. Expect normal urine output to be 30 to 100 mL/h.
   b. Report oliguria with less than 30 mL/h or polyuria of 100 to 500 mL/h.
2. Monitor serum electrolyte results and electrocardiogram (ECG) for changes associated with electrolyte imbalance.
   a. Report arrhythmias or other cardiac symptoms immediately.
3. Monitor blood pressure and heart rate, central venous pressure, and pulmonary artery pressure (if indicated) to anticipate adjustment of fluid replacement.
4. Avoid using dialysis access extremity for IV lines, intra-arterial monitoring, or restraints.
5. Prepare for hemodialysis in postoperative period until transplanted kidney is functioning well.

Patient Education/Health Maintenance

A. *After Nephrectomy*

1. Provide information about continued recovery from surgery; regular exercise, refraining from heavy lifting or strenuous activities, resumption of normal dietary intake.
2. Advise wearing a Medic Alert bracelet and inform all health care providers of solitary kidney status.
3. Encourage close follow-up and need to seek medical attention for any signs of urinary infection or urinary tract disease if only one kidney present to prevent damage to that kidney.

B. *After Kidney Transplantation*

1. Explain and reinforce symptoms of rejection—fever, chills, sweating, lassitude, hypertension, weight gain, peripheral edema, decrease in urine output. Acute rejection is common and usually reversible; often occurs in first 2 months after transplant.
2. Prepare patient for possible need for maintenance dialysis when rejection occurs. If the transplanted kidney is rejected, it may be removed in the initial postoperative period. For chronic rejection, the kidney is not commonly removed.
3. Explain continued protection of vascular access graft, which may still be enlarged, tender to palpation, associated with edema of overlying tissues.
4. Encourage compliance with laboratory tests (serum and urine chemistry, hematology, bacteriology) to monitor recipient's immune status and detect early signs of rejection.
5. Instruct patient and family about prescribed immunosuppressants and complications of therapy—infection or incomplete control of rejection.
   a. Review immunosuppressive medications in detail, including color identification of pills, dose schedules, side effects, and the necessity for taking the medication.
   b. Review other medications such as antacids to prevent stress ulcers, vitamins, and iron replacement.
6. Review in detail postoperative self-care regimen (may be inpatient or outpatient), including adequate fluid intake, daily weight, measurement of urine, stool test for occult blood, prevention of infection, exercise.
7. Instruct to report immediately:
   a. Decrease in urinary output
   b. Weight gain, edema
   c. Malaise, fever
   d. Graft swelling and tenderness (visible and palpable below the skin)
   e. Changes in blood pressure readings
   f. Respiratory distress
   g. Anxiety, depression, change in appetite or sleep
8. Advise avoidance of contact sports for life to prevent trauma to the transplanted kidney.
9. Stress that follow-up care after transplantation is a lifelong necessity.
10. For additional support and information refer to: American Association of Kidney Patients; 1 Davis Blvd., Suite LL 1; Tampa, FL 33606; 1-800-749-AAKP.

Evaluation

A. Verbalizes relief of pain
B. Urinary drainage clear without clots
C. Absence of fever or signs of infection
D. Vital signs stable; urine output 50 mL/h

◆ URINARY DIVERSION

Urinary diversion refers to diverting the urinary stream from the bladder so that it exits via a new avenue. A number of operative procedures may be performed to achieve this (Fig. 19-2). Methods of urinary diversion include:

1. *Ileal conduit* (or "Bricker's loop")—most common; transplants the ureters into an isolated section of the terminal ileum, bringing one end through the abdominal wall to create a stoma. Urine flows from the kidney into the ureters, then through the ileal conduit, and exits through urinary stoma. The ureters may also be transplanted into a segment of the transverse colon (colon conduit).

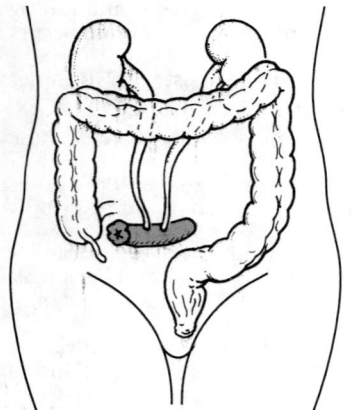
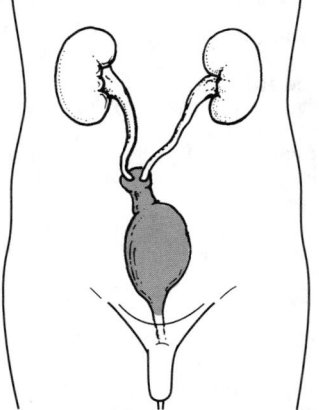
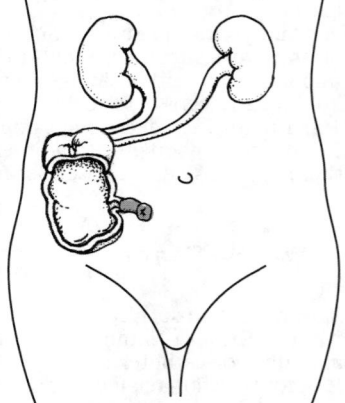

Ileal conduit   Orthotopic bladder replacement   Continent urinary reservoir

FIGURE 19-2 *Methods of urinary diversion.*

2. *Nephrostomy*—insertion of a catheter into the renal pelvis via an incision into the flank or by percutaneous catheter placement into the kidney. They are rarely placed for long periods of time; they are a short-term method of diverting urine away from an obstruction or lesion below the level of the renal pelvis.

3. Continent urinary diversion procedures—create a urinary reservoir from an intestinal segment that is either brought to the skin using a valve mechanism that permits catheterization, or is anastomosed directly to the proximal urethra (an option for men only).

   a. *Continent urinary reservoir* (Kock pouch, Indiana pouch, Mainz Pouch, and others)—transplants the ureters into a pouch created from small bowel or large and small bowel. Mechanisms to discourage ureteral reflux are used to implant the ureters into the pouch, including an intussuscepted nipple valve or tunneling the ureters through the taeniae of the bowel. The existing ileocecal valve, or a surgically created intussuscepted nipple valve, provides the continence mechanism. Patient does not have to wear an external appliance, but the procedure does require intermittent self-catheterization of the pouch.

   b. *Orthotopic bladder replacement* (Hemi-Kock pouch, Mainz pouch, "Le Bag," and others)—pouch created from small or large and small bowel is anastomosed to urethral stump in men; voiding is through the urethra. Patient usually has nocturnal incontinence; not all patients are candidates for this procedure.

Preoperative Management/ Nursing Care

1. Perform functional assessment including degree of manual dexterity and visual acuity—essential for stoma care or self-catheterization postoperatively.

2. Find out about patient's psychosocial resources including available support persons, education, occupation, and economic resources (including insurance coverage of ostomy supplies if needed), coping strengths, attitudes toward urinary diversion.

3. Prepare the bowel to prevent fecal contamination during surgery and the potential complication of infection.

   a. Clear liquids only and prescribed laxatives for mechanical cleansing of the bowel.

   b. Antibiotics as prescribed (nonabsorbable; active against enteric organisms) to reduce bacterial count in the bowel lumen.

4. Provide adequate hydration, including IV infusions, to ensure urine flow during surgery and to prevent hypovolemia.

5. Reinforce explanation of the procedure; ensure contact with enterostomal therapist before surgery. Advise patient that:

   a. For ileal or colon conduit the stoma site is planned preoperatively with the patient standing, sitting, and lying—to place the stoma away from bony prominences, skin creases, and scars, and where the patient can see it.

   b. Stoma site may also be marked even though continent urinary diversion procedure is planned, in case findings during surgery prevent continent procedure and standard ileal or colon conduit is necessary.

Postoperative Management/ Nursing Care

1. Monitor patient for immediate postoperative complications; wound infection, urinary or fecal anastomotic leakage, peritonitis, paralytic ileus, pelvic thrombophlebitis, pulmonary embolism, and necrosis of stoma.

2. Carefully monitor intake and output; assess urinary output for amount, patency of drainage catheter(s), and degree of hematuria.

3. Monitor pelvic gravity or suction drains—sudden increase in drainage suggests a urine leak; send specimen of drainage for blood urea nitrogen (BUN) and creatinine, if ordered. (Presence of measurable BUN and creatinine in the drainage indicates urine in drainage, confirming a urine leak.)

4. Ureteral stents are used to protect ureterointestinal anastomoses; stents will emerge from stoma or through separate wound (stents are not visible in orthotopic bladder replacement patients)—they are removed in 3 weeks.

Nursing Diagnoses

A. Altered Urinary Elimination related to urinary diversion
B. Pain related to surgery
C. Body Image Disturbance related to urinary diversion
D. Sexual Dysfunction related to reconstructive surgery and impotence (in men)

Nursing Interventions

A. *Achieving Urinary Elimination*
For ileal or colon conduit patients:

1. Maintain a transparent urostomy pouch over the stoma postoperatively to allow for easy assessment.

2. Inspect the stoma for color and size; whether it is flush, nippled, or retracted; and the condition of the skin around the stoma. Document baseline information for subsequent comparison.

   a. Stoma should be red, wet with mucus, soft, and slightly rubbery to the touch (stoma lacks nerve ending, so feeling in stoma is absent).

   b. Cyanotic stoma indicates poor circulation.

   c. Necrotic stoma is blue black or tan brown.

3. Report any bleeding, necrosis, sloughing, suture separation.

4. Check patency of ureteral stents.

5. Keep the pouch on at all times and observe normal urine (but not fecal) drainage at all times.

   a. Connect pouches to drainage bag when patient is in bed and record urine volume hourly.

   b. Initial urostomy pouch remains in place for several days postoperatively; it is changed every 3 to 5 days when patient teaching begins.

   For continent urinary diversion patients:

1. Maintain patency of drainage catheters placed into internal urinary pouch during surgery; irrigate with 30 mL saline every 2 to 4 hours to prevent obstruction from mucous accumulation.

2. Assess stoma—should be very small and flush.

3. Record urine output and character of urine.

4. Monitor output of pelvic drain (on gentle suction or gravity drainage) every 8 hours.
5. Advise patient that approximately 3 weeks after surgery the drainage catheter is removed from the pouch after a radiographic study ("pouch-o-gram") confirms healing of all anastomoses.

B. Controlling Pain
1. Administer analgesic medications or teach use of and monitor PCA (IV or epidural).
2. Assess response to pain control.
3. Provide positioning for comfort, alternating with ambulation, as able.

C. Resolving Body Image Issues
1. Assess patient's reaction to looking at new urinary stoma if applicable, provide reassurance and support.
2. Accept the patient's depression, which may be manifested in irritability or lack of motivation to learn.
   a. Give extra support until the patient can cope.
   b. Reinforce the concept that the stoma will be manageable.
   c. Acknowledge feelings of fear and anxiety as normal.
3. Encourage patient to gradually participate in care of stoma or catheters.
4. Encourage verbalization of feelings and concerns related to urinary diversion.
5. If possible, arrange for patient to speak with another patient who has undergone the same surgery; this provides realistic expectations and support for a positive outcome.
6. Help patient/family to gain independence through learning to manage the ostomy. Provide for demonstrations, supervised practice, written instructions, and return demonstrations until patient is independent in self-care.

D. Coping with Sexual Dysfunction
1. Be aware that most men experience impotence as a result of surgery; provide information or referrals about options including pharmacologic erection programs and penile prostheses.
2. Allow patient to express feelings related to loss of sexual function and encourage discussion with partner.
3. Tell women that they may usually resume sexual activity after healing is complete.

Patient Education/Health Maintenance

A. For Ileal or Colon Conduit Patients
1. Obtain and familiarize the patient with the appropriate equipment. Most urostomy pouching systems are disposable. The choice of pouch is determined by location of stoma, patient activity, body build, and economic status.
   a. Two-piece pouches consist of a skin barrier (or wafer) that fits around the stoma and adheres to the skin and a pouch that snaps onto the skin barrier.
   b. One-piece pouches are usually precut for the correct stoma size and include the adhesive; the pouch is applied directly to the peristomal skin.
2. Assist the patient to determine stoma size (for ordering correct appliance). The stoma will shrink considerably as edema subsides, and the opening is recalibrated every 3 to 6 weeks postoperatively.
   a. Measuring guides are included with most urostomy pouches.

b. The inside diameter of the skin barrier should not be more than $1/16$ to $1/8$ inch larger than the diameter of the stoma.
3. Teach how to change the pouch.
   a. Change pouch early in morning before taking fluids or before evening meal—urine output is lower at these times.
   b. Prepare the new pouching system according to manufacturer's directions.
   c. Wash the peristomal skin with noncream-based soap and water. Rinse and pat dry. *The skin must be dry or appliance will not adhere.*
   d. A gauze or tissue wick may be applied over the stoma to absorb urine while the appliance is being changed. Keep the skin free from direct contact with urine.

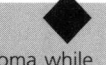

COMMUNITY-BASED CARE TIP:
Suggest the use of tampons to soak up urine from stoma while changing pouch.

   e. Center the skin barrier directly over the stoma and apply it carefully. Apply gentle pressure around appliance for secure adherence.
   f. Apply a belt to keep pouch in place if desired; it is especially useful in patients with soft abdomens.
4. Advise that additional adhesives, such as pastes or cements, are not usually necessary with a well fitting pouch.
5. Tell patient that frequency of pouch changes depends on the type of pouch used—generally pouches should be changed every 3 days (for one-piece pouches) to every 4 to 7 days (for two-piece pouches).
6. Advise emptying the pouch when it is a third to half full to prevent weight of urine from loosening adhesive seal—open drain valve (spigot) for periodic emptying.
7. Teach how to attach outlet on pouch to a bedside urinary drainage container with plastic tubing (at least 5 feet to allow turning) and how to secure tubing to leg to prevent twisting or kinking.
   a. Position the drainage bottle lower than the level of the bed—to enhance flow by gravity.
   b. Clean nighttime drainage equipment with vinegar and water. Rinse well.
8. Advise to drink liberal amounts of fluids to flush the conduit free of mucus and reduce possibility of urinary infection.
9. Teach that the stoma may bleed if it is bumped or rubbed; report bleeding that continues for several hours.
10. Advise carrying spare pouches in handbag or pocket and bringing an extra pouch to every visit with health care provider.
11. Advise wearing cotton (rather than nylon) underwear or the use of specially made underwear for ostomy patients that prevents contact between plastic pouch and skin. Heavy girdles are not allowed because they may cause chafing of the stoma and prevent free flow of urine.
12. Advise reporting problems with peristomal skin or with leakage from the pouch, or the development of fever, chills, pain, change in color of urine (cloudy, bloody), diminishing urine output.
13. For additional information and support refer to: United Ostomy Association, Inc.; 36 Executive Park, Suite 120; Irvine, CA 92714; 714-660-8624.

B. For Continent Ileal Urinary Reservoir Patients
1. Teach irrigation of catheter; this must be done every 4 to 6 hours at home.
2. Teach how to change stoma dressing or small urostomy pouch over pelvic drain that will stay in place for 3 weeks after surgery.
3. Instruct in use of leg bag or bedside urinary drainage bag while catheter remains in place.
4. Teach how to catheterize continent urinary diversion when healing is verified:
   a. Red rubber or plastic, straight or coudé catheters are used.
   b. Apply a small amount of water-soluble lubricant to the tip of the catheter.
   c. Use clean technique, wash hands before each catheterization.
   d. Maintain schedule of catheterizations during initial "training" period; to gradually allow the pouch to adapt to holding larger amounts of urine (every 2 hours during day/every 3 hours at night, increase by 1 hour each week for 5 weeks).
   e. After training period, catheterize four to five times a day, pouch should not hold more than 400 to 500 mL.
   f. Irrigate pouch with saline through catheter once a day to clear it of accumulated mucus.
5. Teach patient to report problems such as leakage of urine from stoma between catheterizations.
6. Tell patient to shower or bathe normally, wear normal clothing; only a small dressing or Band-aid need be worn over the stoma.
7. Advise drinking 8 to 10 glasses of water daily.

C. For Orthotopic Bladder Replacement
1. Teach patient to irrigate Foley catheter that will stay in place for 3 weeks after surgery; irrigate with 30 mL saline every 4 to 6 hours.
2. Instruct in use of leg bag or bedside drainage bag while catheter remains in place.
3. Instruct on how to change dressing or small urostomy pouch over pelvic drain while in place.
4. After healing of pouch is confirmed and catheter is removed, teach patient to "void."
   a. Voiding is accomplished by abdominal straining; mucus is expected in voided urine.
   b. Voiding schedule must be maintained for first 5 to 6 weeks; every 2 hours during day/every 3 hours at night, increase by 1 hour each week.
   c. Incontinence is anticipated after catheter is removed; usually more pronounced when patient is supine,
5. Teach patient to perform pelvic floor exercises, which must be done faithfully for the rest of life; as pelvic floor sphincter muscles strengthen, incontinence subsides. Most patients continue to have small amounts of nocturnal incontinence.
   a. Contract pelvic floor muscles (as if stopping stream of urine or flatus) for 5 to 10 seconds, then relax for 5 to 10 seconds.
   b. Repeat approximately 15 times for one set, and do 15 to 20 sets a day.
6. Provide information about absorbent products that may be used temporarily; also preventive skin care.
7. Instruct in clean self-catheterization, which may be needed if urethra becomes obstructed with mucus; pouch should be irrigated with saline if catheterization is necessary.

8. Reassure patient that time, patience, and continued adherence to voiding and exercise schedule will result in continence.

Evaluation

A. Urine draining via urinary diversion
B. Verbalizes good pain control
C. Discusses feelings about change in body image; seeks support through family
D. Verbalizes reasonable expectations about sexual function

◆ PROSTATIC SURGERY

Prostatic surgery may be done for BPH or prostate cancer. Surgical approach depends on size of the gland, severity of obstruction, age, underlying health, and prostatic disease.

Surgical Procedures

1. Transurethral resection of the prostate (TUR or TURP)—most common and done without an incision by means of endoscopic instrument
2. Open prostatectomy
   a. Suprapubic—incision into suprapubic area and through bladder wall; frequently done for BPH
   b. Perineal—incision between scrotum and rectal area; may be done for poor surgical risk patients but causes highest incidence of urinary incontinence and impotence
   c. Retropubic—incision at level of symphysis pubis; preserves nerves responsible for sexual function in 50% of patients

Preoperative Management/Nursing Care

Besides the routine preparation for surgery (see p. 76), provide the following nursing care.

1. Explain the nature of the procedure and the expected postoperative care, including catheter drainage, irrigation, and monitoring of hematuria.
2. Discuss complications of surgery and how patient will cope.
   a. Incontinence or dribbling of urine for up to 1 year following surgery; perineal (Kegel) exercises help regain urinary control.
   b. Retrograde ejaculation—seminal fluid released into bladder and eliminated in the urine rather than through the uretha during intercourse; impotence is usually not a complication of TUR but often a complication of open prostatectomy
3. Administer bowel preparation as prescribed, or instruct the patient in home administration and fasting after midnight.
4. Ensure that optimal cardiac, respiratory, and circulatory status have been achieved to decrease risk of complications.
5. Administer prophylactic antibiotics as ordered.

Postoperative Management/ Nursing Care

1. Maintain urinary drainage and monitor for hemorrhage.
2. Provide wound care and prevent infection.
3. Relieve pain and promote early ambulation.
4. Monitor for and prevent complications.
   a. Wound infection and dehiscence
   b. Urinary obstruction or infection
   c. Hemorrhage
   d. Thrombophlebitis, pulmonary embolism
   e. Urinary incontinence, sexual dysfunction

Nursing Diagnoses

A. Altered Urinary Elimination related to surgical procedure and urinary catheter
B. Risk for Infection related to surgical incision, immobility, and urinary catheter
C. Pain related to surgical procedure
D. Anxiety related to urinary incontinence, difficulty voiding, and sexual dysfunction

Nursing Interventions

A. *Facilitating Urinary Drainage*
1. Maintain patency of urethral catheter placed after surgery.
   a. Monitor flow of three-way closed irrigation and drainage system if used. (Continuous irrigation helps prevent clot formation, which can obstruct catheter, cause painful bladder spasms, and lead to infection.)
   b. Perform manual irrigation with 50 mL irrigating fluid using aseptic technique.
   c. Avoid overdistention of bladder, which could lead to hemorrhage.
   d. Administer anticholinergic medications to reduce bladder spasms, as ordered.
2. Assess degree of hematuria and any clot formation; drainage should become light pink within 24 hours.
   a. Report any bright red bleeding with increased viscosity (arterial)—may require surgical intervention.
   b. Report any increase in dark red bleeding (venous)—may require traction of the catheter so the inflated balloon applies pressure to prostatic fossa.
   c. Prepare for blood transfusion if bleeding persists.
3. Administer IV fluids as ordered and encourage oral fluids when tolerated to ensure hydration and urine output.

B. *Preventing Infection*
1. Maintain bed rest for the first 24 hours with frequent monitoring of vital signs, intake and output, and observation of incisional dressing, if present.
2. After 24 hours, encourage ambulation to prevent venous thrombosis, pulmonary embolism, and hypostatic pneumonia.
3. Observe urine for cloudiness or odor and obtain urine for evaluation of infection as ordered.
4. Administer antibiotics as prescribed.
5. Report any testicular pain, swelling, and tenderness that could indicate epididymitis from spreading infection.

6. Assist with perineal care if perineal incision is present to prevent contamination by feces.

C. *Relieving Pain*
1. Administer pain medication or monitor PCA as directed.
2. Position for comfort and tell the patient to avoid straining, which will increase pelvic venous congestion and may cause hemorrhage.
3. Administer stool softeners to prevent discomfort from constipation.
4. Make sure catheter is secured to patient's thigh and tubing is not creating traction on catheter, which will cause pain and potential hemorrhage.

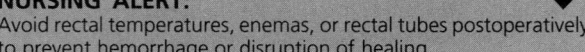

NURSING ALERT:
Avoid rectal temperatures, enemas, or rectal tubes postoperatively to prevent hemorrhage or disruption of healing.

D. *Reducing Anxiety*
1. Provide realistic expectations about postoperative discomfort and overall progress.
   a. Tell patient to avoid sexual intercourse, straining at stool, heavy lifting, and long periods of sitting for 6 to 8 weeks after surgery, until prostatic fossa is healed.
   b. Advise follow-up visits after treatment because urethral stricture may occur and regrowth of prostate is possible after TURP.
2. Reassure patient that urinary incontinence and frequency, urgency, and dysuria are expected after removal of catheter and should gradually subside.
   a. If sent home with catheter, will be removed in about 3 weeks when cystogram confirms healing.
   b. Discuss the use of absorbent products to contain urine leakage.
   c. Advise that incontinence is more pronounced when abdominal pressure is increased, such as coughing, laughing, straining.
3. Teach measures to regain urinary control.
   a. Have patient imagine there is an egg in his rectum, then squeeze the muscles to try to "break" it; hold the position, then relax. Caution on using abdominal muscles, which increases incontinence.
   b. Tell patient to stop urinary stream while voiding, hold for few seconds, then continue. Practice this 10 to 20 times an hour while not voiding.
3. Reinforce the risks for impotence as told by the surgeon. Remind patient that erectile function may not return for as long as 6 months.
4. Encourage patient to express fears and anxieties related to potential loss of sexual function, and to discuss concerns with partner.
5. Advise that options such as penile implant are available to restore sexual function if impotence persists.

Evaluation

A. Clear yellow drainage via catheter
B. Incision without drainage; afebrile
C. Verbalizes good pain relief
D. Verbalizes realistic expectations for urinary and sexual functioning

Urinary Disorders

◆ ACUTE RENAL FAILURE

Acute renal failure is a syndrome of varying causation that results in a sudden decline in renal function. It is frequently associated with an increase in the serum concentrations of urea (azotemia) and creatinine, oliguria (less than 500 mL urine/24 h), hyperkalemia and sodium retention.

Pathophysiology/Etiology

A. Causes
1. Prerenal causes—result from conditions that decrease renal blood flow (hypovolemia, shock, hemorrhage, burns, impaired cardiac output, diuretic therapy).
2. Postrenal causes—arise from obstruction or disruption to urine flow anywhere along the urinary tract.
3. Intrarenal causes—result from injury to renal tissue and is usually associated with intrarenal ischemia, toxins, immunologic processes, systemic and vascular disorders.

B. Clinical Course
1. Onset
   a. Begins when the kidney is injured and lasts from hours to days.
2. Oliguric–anuric phase (urine volume less than 400–500 mL/24 h)
   a. Accompanied by rise in serum concentration of elements usually excreted by kidney (urea, creatinine, uric acid, organic acids, and the intracellular cations—potassium and magnesium).
   b. There can be a decrease in renal function with increasing nitrogen retention even when the patient is excreting more than 2 to 3 liters of urine daily—called nonoliguric or high-output renal failure.
3. Diuretic phase
   a. Begins when the 24-hour urine volume exceeds 500 mL and ends when the BUN and serum creatinine levels stop rising.
4. Recovery phase
   a. Usually lasts several months to 1 year.
   b. Probably some scar tissue remains, but the functional loss is not always clinically significant.

Clinical Manifestations

1. *Prerenal*—decreased tissue turgor, dryness of mucous membranes, weight loss, hypotension, oliguria or anuria
2. *Postrenal*—difficulty in voiding; changes in urine flow
3. *Intrarenal*—fever, skin rash, edema
4. Changes in urine volume and serum concentrations of BUN, creatinine, uric acid, potassium, etc as described above.

Diagnostic Evaluation

1. Urinalysis—reveals proteinuria, hematuria, casts.
2. Rising serum creatinine and BUN levels

3. Urine chemistry examinations to distinguish various forms of acute renal failure
4. Renal ultrasonography—for estimate of renal size and to exclude a treatable obstructive uropathy

Management

A. Preventive Measures
1. Identify patients with preexisting renal disease.
2. Initiate adequate hydration before, during, and after operative procedures.
3. Avoid exposure to various nephrotoxins. Be aware that the majority of drugs or their metabolites are excreted by the kidneys.
4. Avoid chronic analgesic abuse—causes interstitial nephritis and papillary necrosis.
5. Prevent and treat shock with blood and fluid replacement. Prevent prolonged periods of hypotension.
6. Monitor urinary output and central venous pressure hourly in critically ill patients to detect onset of renal failure at the earliest moment.
7. Schedule diagnostic studies requiring dehydration so that there are "rest days," especially in aged who may not have adequate renal reserve.
8. Pay special attention to draining wounds, burns, etc, which can lead to dehydration and sepsis and progressive renal damage.
9. Avoid infection; give meticulous care to patients with indwelling catheters and IV lines.
10. Take every precaution to ensure that the right person receives the right blood—to avoid severe transfusion reactions, which can precipitate renal complications.

B. Corrective/Supportive Measures
1. Correct any reversible cause of acute renal failure (eg, improve renal perfusion; maximize cardiac output; surgical relief of obstruction).
2. Be alert for and correct underlying fluid excesses or deficits.
3. Correct and control biochemical imbalances—treatment of hyperkalemia.
4. Restore/maintain blood pressure.
5. Maintain nutrition.
6. Initiate hemodialysis, peritoneal dialysis, or continuous renal replacement therapy for patients with progressive azotemia and other life-threatening complications.

Complications

1. Infection
2. Arrhythmias due to hyperkalemia
3. Electrolyte (sodium, potassium, uric acid, calcium, phosphorus) abnormalities
4. Gastrointestinal bleeding due to stress ulcers
5. Multiple organ systems failure

Nursing Assessment

1. Determine if there is a history of cardiac disease, malignancy, sepsis, or intercurrent illness.

2. Determine if patient has been exposed to potentially nephrotoxic drugs (antibiotics, nonsteroidal anti-inflammatory drugs [NSAIDs], contrast agents, solvents).
3. Conduct an ongoing physical examination for tissue turgor, pallor, alteration in mucous membranes, blood pressure, heart rate changes, and edema.
4. Monitor urine volume.

Nursing Diagnoses

A. Fluid Volume Excess related to decreased glomerular filtration rate and sodium retention
B. Risk for Infection related to alterations in the immune system and host defenses
C. Altered Nutrition (Less than Body Requirements) related to catabolic state, anorexia, and malnutrition associated with acute renal failure
D. Risk for Injury related to gastrointestinal bleeding
E. Altered Thought Processes related to the effects of uremic toxins on the central nervous system (CNS)

Nursing Interventions

A. *Achieving Fluid and Electrolyte Balance*
1. Monitor for signs and symptoms of hypovolemia or hypervolemia (Table 19-2) because regulating capacity of kidneys is inadequate.
2. Monitor urinary output and urine specific gravity; measure and record intake and output including urine, gastric suction, stools, wound drainage, perspiration (estimate).
3. Monitor serum and urine electrolyte concentrations.
4. Weigh the patient daily to provide an index of fluid balance; expected weight loss is 0.25 to 0.5 kg ($1/2$–1 lb daily).
5. Adjust fluid intake to avoid volume overload and dehydration.
   a. Fluid restriction is not usually initiated until renal function is quite low.
   b. Give only enough fluids to replace losses during oliguric–anuric phase (usually 400–500 mL/24 h plus measured fluid losses).
   c. Fluid allowance should be distributed throughout the day.
   d. Avoid restricting fluids for prolonged periods for laboratory and radiologic examinations because dehydrating procedures are hazardous to patients who cannot produce concentrated urine.
   e. Restrict salt and water intake if there is evidence of extracellular excess (see Table 19-2).
6. Measure blood pressure at various times of the day with patients in supine, sitting, and standing positions.
7. Auscultate lung fields for rales.
8. Inspect neck veins for engorgement and extremities, abdomen, sacrum, and eyelids for edema.
9. Evaluate for signs and symptoms of hyperkalemia (see Table 19-2) and monitor serum potassium levels.
   a. Notify health care provider of value above 5.5 mg/L.
   b. Watch for ECG changes—tall, tented T waves; depressed ST segment; wide QRS complex.
10. Administer sodium bicarbonate or glucose and insulin to shift potassium into the cells.
11. Administer cation exchange resin (sodium polystyrene sulfonate [Kayexelate]) to provide more prolonged correction of elevated potassium.
12. Watch for cardiac arrhythmia and congestive heart failure from hyperkalemia, electrolyte imbalance, or fluid overload. Have resuscitation equipment on hand in case of cardiac arrest.
13. Instruct patient about the importance of following prescribed diet, avoiding foods high in potassium.
14. Prepare for dialysis when rapid lowering of potassium is needed.
15. Administer blood transfusions during dialysis to remove excess potassium.
16. Monitor normal acid–base balance
    a. Monitor arterial blood gases as necessary.
    b. Prepare for ventilator therapy if severe acidosis is present and/or respiratory problems develop.
    c. Administer sodium bicarbonate for symptomatic acidosis (bicarbonate deficit), see Table 19-2.

TABLE 19-2   Signs and Symptoms of Fluid and Electrolyte Imbalances

	Deficit	Excess
Volume	Acute weight loss (>5%), drop in body temperature, dry skin and mucous membranes, postural hypotension, longitudinal wrinkles or furrows of tongue, oliguria or anuria	Acute weight gain (>5%), edema, hypertension, distended neck veins, dyspnea, rales
Sodium	Abdominal cramps, apprehension, convulsions, fingerprinting on sternum, oliguria or anuria	Dry sticky mucous membranes, flushed skin, oliguria or anuria, thirst, rough and dry tongue
Potassium	Anorexia, abdominal distention, intestinal ileus, muscle weakness, tenderness, and cramps	Diarrhea, intestinal colic, irritability, nausea, parasthesias, flaccid paralysis, cardiac arrhythmias and arrest
Calcium	Abdominal cramps, positive Chovstek and Trousseau signs, tingling of extremities, tetany	Anorexia, nausea, vomiting, abdominal pain and distention, mental confusion
Bicarbonate	Deep, rapid breathing (Kussmaul), shortness of breath on exertion, stupor, weakness (metabolic acidosis)	Depressed respirations, muscle hypertonicity, tetany (metabolic alkalosis)
Magnesium	Positive Chovstek's sign, seizures, disorientation, hyperactive deep tendon reflexes, tremor	Hypotension, flushing, lethargy, dysarthria, hypoactive deep tendon reflexes, respiratory depression

d. Be prepared to implement dialysis for uncontrolled acidosis.

B. Preventing Infection
1. Monitor for all signs of infection. Be aware that renal failure patients do not always demonstrate fever and leukocytosis.
2. Remove bladder catheter as soon as possible; monitor for urinary tract infection.
3. Use intensive pulmonary hygiene—high incidence of lung edema and infection.
4. Carry out meticulous wound care.
5. If antibiotics are administered, care must be taken to adjust the dosage for the degree of renal impairment.

C. Maintaining Adequate Nutrition
1. Work collaboratively with dietitian to regulate protein intake according to impaired renal function because metabolites that accumulate in blood derive almost entirely from protein catabolism.
   a. Protein should be of high biologic value, rich in essential amino acids (dairy products, eggs, meat), so that the patient does not rely on tissue catabolism for essential amino acids.
   b. Low-protein diet may be supplemented with essential amino acids and vitamins.
   c. As renal function declines, protein intake may be restricted proportionately.
   d. Protein will be increased if the patient is on a dialysis program to allow for the loss of amino acids occurring during dialysis.
2. Offer high-carbohydrate feedings because carbohydrates have a greater protein-sparing power and provide additional calories.
3. Weigh daily.
4. Monitor BUN, creatinine, electrolytes, serum albumin, total protein, and transferrin.
5. Be aware that food and fluids containing large amounts of sodium, potassium, and phosphorus may need to be restricted.
6. Prepare for hyperalimentation when adequate nutrition cannot be maintained through the gastrointestinal tract.

D. Preventing Gastrointestinal Bleeding
1. Examine all stools and emesis for gross and occult blood.
2. Administer H_2-receptor antagonist such as cimetidine (Tagamet) or ranitidine (Zantac) or antacids as prophylaxis for gastric stress ulcers. If H_2-receptor antagonist is used, care must be taken to adjust the dose for the degree of renal impairment.
3. Prepare for endoscopy when gastrointestinal bleeding occurs.

E. Preserving Neurologic Function
1. Speak to the patient in simple orienting statements, using repetition when necessary.
2. Maintain predictable routine and keep change to a minimum.
3. Watch for and report mental status changes—somnolence, lassitude, lethargy, and fatigue progressing to irritability, disorientation, twitching, seizures.
4. Correct cognitive distortions.
5. Use seizure precautions—padded side rails, airway and suction equipment at bedside.
6. Encourage and assist patient to turn and move because drowsiness and lethargy may prevent activity.
7. Use music tapes to promote relaxation.

8. Prepare for dialysis, which may help prevent neurologic complications.

Patient Education/Health Maintenance

1. Explain that the patient may experience residual defects in kidney function for long period of time after acute illness.
2. Encourage reporting for routine urinalysis and follow-up examinations.
3. Advise avoidance of *any* medications unless specifically prescribed.
4. Recommend resuming activity gradually because muscle weakness will be present from excessive catabolism.

Evaluation

A. Blood pressure stable, no edema or shortness of breath
B. No signs of infection
C. Food intake adequate, maintaining weight
D. Stools heme negative
E. Appears more alert; sleeps less during the day

◆ CHRONIC RENAL FAILURE (CRF, END-STAGE RENAL DISEASE, ESRD)

Chronic renal failure is a progressive deterioration of renal function, which ends fatally in uremia (an excess of urea and other nitrogenous wastes in the blood) and its complications unless dialysis or a kidney transplant is performed.

Pathophysiology/Etiology

A. Causes
1. Hypertension; prolonged and severe
2. Diabetes mellitus
3. Glomerulopathies
4. Interstitial nephritis
5. Hereditary renal disease; polycystic disease
6. Obstructive uropathy
7. Developmental/congenital disorder

B. Consequences of Decreasing Renal Function
1. Rate of progression varies based on underlying cause and severity of that condition.
2. Stages: decreased renal reserve → renal insufficiency → renal failure → uremia
3. Retention of sodium and water causes edema, congestive heart failure, hypertension, ascites.
4. Decreased glomerular filtration rate (GFR) causes stimulation of renin–angiotensin axis and increased aldosterone secretion, which raises blood pressure.
5. Metabolic acidosis results from kidney's inability to excrete hydrogen ions, produce ammonia, and conserve bicarbonate.
6. Decreased GFR causes increase in serum phosphate, with reciprocal decrease in serum calcium and subsequent bone resorption of calcium.

7. Erythropoietin production by the kidney decreases, causing profound anemia.
8. Uremia affects the CNS, causing altered mental function, personality changes, seizures, and coma.

Clinical Manifestations

1. Gastrointestinal—anorexia, nausea, vomiting, hiccoughs, ulceration of gastrointestinal tract, and hemorrhage
2. Cardiovascular—hyperkalemic ECG changes, hypertension, pericarditis, pericardial effusion, pericardial tamponade
3. Respiratory—pulmonary edema, pleural effusions, pleural rub
4. Neuromuscular—fatigue, sleep disorders, headache, lethargy, muscular irritability, peripheral neuropathy, seizures, coma
5. Metabolic and endocrine—glucose intolerance, hyperlipidemia, sex hormone disturbances causing decreased libido, impotence, amenorrhea
6. Fluid, electrolyte, acid–base disturbances—usually salt and water retention but may be sodium loss with dehydration, acidosis, hyperkalemia, hypermagnesemia, hypocalcemia (see Table 19-2).
7. Dermatologic—pallor, hyperpigmentation, pruritus, ecchymoses, uremic frost
8. Skeletal abnormalities—renal osteodystrophy resulting in osteomalacia
9. Hematologic—anemia, defect in quality of platelets, increased bleeding tendencies
10. Psychosocial functions—personality and behavior changes, alteration in cognitive processes

Diagnostic Evaluation

1. Complete blood count (CBC)—anemia (a characteristic sign)
2. Elevated serum creatinine, BUN, phosphorus
3. Decreased serum calcium, bicarbonate, and proteins, especially albumin
4. Arterial blood gases—low blood pH, low CO_2, low bicarbonate (HCO_3)

Management

Goal: Conservation of renal function as long as possible.
1. Detection and treatment of reversible causes of renal failure (eg, bring diabetes under control; treat hypertension)
2. Dietary regulation—low-protein diet supplemented with essential amino acids or their keto analogues to minimize uremic toxicity and to prevent wasting and malnutrition
3. Treatment of associated conditions to improve renal dynamics
   a. Anemia—recombinant human erythropoietin (Epigen), a synthetic kidney hormone
   b. Acidosis—replacement of bicarbonate stores by infusion or oral administration of sodium bicarbonate
   c. Hyperkalemia—restriction of dietary potassium; administration of cation exchange resin

d. Phosphate retention—decrease dietary phosphorus (chicken, milk, legumes, carbonated beverages); administer phosphate-binding agents because they bind phosphorus in the intestinal tract.
4. Maintenance dialysis or kidney transplantation when symptoms can no longer be controlled with conservative management

Complications

1. Death

Nursing Assessment

1. Obtain history of chronic disorders and underlying health status.
2. Assess degree of renal impairment and involvement of other body systems by obtaining a review of systems and reviewing laboratory results.
3. Perform thorough physical examination including vital signs, cardiovascular, pulmonary, gastrointestinal, neurologic, dermatologic, and musculoskeletal systems.
4. Assess psychosocial response to disease process including availability of resources and support network.

Nursing Diagnoses

A. Fluid Volume Excess related to disease process
B. Altered Nutrition (Less than Body Requirements) related to anorexia, nausea, vomiting, and restricted diet
C. Impaired Skin Integrity related to uremic frost and changes in oil and sweat glands
D. Constipation related to fluid restriction and ingestion of phosphate-binding agents
E. Risk for Injury While Ambulating related to potential fractures and muscle cramps due to calcium deficiency
F. Noncompliance With the Therapeutic Regimen related to restrictions imposed by CRF and its treatment

Nursing Interventions

A. *Maintaining Fluid and Electrolyte Balance*
See interventions under acute renal failure, page 612.

B. *Maintaining Adequate Nutritional Status*
See interventions under acute renal failure, page 613.

C. *Maintaining Skin Integrity*
1. Keep skin clean while relieving itching and dryness.
   a. "Basis" soap
   b. Sodium bicarbonate added to bath water
   c. Oatmeal baths
   d. Bath oil to bath water
2. Apply ointments or creams for comfort and to relieve itching.
3. Keep nails short and trimmed to prevent excoriation.
4. Keep hair clean and moisturized.
5. Administer drugs for relief of itching if indicated.

D. *Preventing Constipation*
1. Be aware that phosphate binders cause constipation that cannot be managed with usual interventions.

2. Encourage high-fiber diet, bearing in mind the potassium content of some fruits and vegetables.
   a. Commercial fiber supplements (Fiberall; Fiber-Med) may be prescribed.
   b. Use stool softeners as prescribed.
   c. Avoid laxatives and cathartics that cause electrolyte toxicities (compounds containing magnesium or phosphorus).
   d. Increase activity as tolerated.

E. *Ensuring a Safe Level of Activity*
1. Monitor serum calcium and phosphate levels; watch for signs of hypocalcemia or hypercalcemia (see Table 19-2).
2. Inspect patient's gait, range of motion, and muscle strength.
3. Administer analgesics as ordered and provide massage for severe muscle cramps.
4. Monitor x-rays and bone scan results for fractures, bone demineralization, and joint deposits.
5. Increase activity as tolerated—avoid immobilization because it increases bone demineralization.
6. Administer medications as ordered:
   a. Phosphate-binding medications such as aluminum hydroxide (Amphojel) or calcium carbonate (Oscal) with meals and snacks to lower serum phosphorous
   b. Calcium supplements—between meals to increase serum calcium
   c. Vitamin D—increases absorption and utilization of calcium

F. *Increasing Understanding of and Compliance With Treatment Regimen*
1. Prepare patient for dialysis or kidney transplantation.
2. Offer hope tempered by reality.
3. Assess patient's understanding of treatment regimen as well as concerns and fears.
4. Explore alternatives that may reduce or eliminate side effects of treatment.
   a. Adjust schedule so rest can be achieved following dialysis.
   b. Offer smaller, more frequent meals to reduce nausea and facilitate taking medication.
5. Encourage strengthening of social support system and coping mechanisms to lessen the impact of the stress of chronic kidney disease.
6. Provide social work referral.
7. Contract with patient for behavioral changes if noncompliant with therapy or control of underlying condition.
8. Discuss option of supportive psychotherapy for depression.
9. Promote decision-making by the patient.
10. Refer patients and family members to renal support agencies (see p. 602).

Patient Education/Health Maintenance

To promote adherence to the therapeutic program, teach the following:

1. Weigh self every morning to avoid fluid overload.
2. Drink limited amounts *only* when thirsty.
3. Measure allotted fluids and save some for ice cubes; sucking on ice is thirst quenching.
4. Eat food before drinking fluids to alleviate dry mouth.
5. Use hard candy, chewing gum to moisten mouth.

Evaluation

A. Blood pressure stable, no excessive weight gain
B. Tolerating small feedings of low-protein, high-carbohydrate diet
C. No skin excoriation; reports some relief of itching
D. Passing small, firm stool daily
E. Ambulating without falls
F. Asking questions and reading education materials about dialysis

◆ LOWER URINARY TRACT INFECTIONS

A *urinary tract infection* is caused by the presence of pathogenic microorganisms in the urinary tract with or without signs and symptoms. Lower urinary tract infections may predominate at the bladder (cystitis) or urethra (urethritis). *Bacteriuria* refers to the presence of bacteria in the urine (10^5 bacteria/mL urine or greater generally indicates infection).

In *asymptomatic bacteriuria*, organisms are found in urine, but the patient has no symptoms.

Recurrent urinary tract infections may indicate the following:

Relapse—recurrent infection with an organism that has been isolated during a prior infection
Reinfection—recurrent infection with an organism distinct form previous infecting organism

Pathophysiology/Etiology

1. Ascending infection after entry via the urinary meatus
   a. Women are more susceptible to developing acute cystitis because of shorter length of urethra, anatomic proximity to vagina, periurethral glands, and rectum (fecal contamination), and the mechanical effect of coitus.
   b. Women with recurrent urinary tract infections often have gram-negative organisms at the vaginal introitus; there may be some defect of the mucosa of the urethra, vagina, or external genitalia of these patients that allows enteric organisms to invade the bladder.
   c. Poor voiding habits may cause increase in intravesical pressure, which tends to decrease blood flow to bladder mucosa.
   d. Acute infection in women most often arises from organisms of the patient's own intestinal flora (*Escherichia coli*).
2. In men, obstructive abnormalities (strictures, prostatic hyperplasia) are the most frequent cause.
3. Upper urinary tract disease may occasionally cause recurrent bladder infection.

Clinical Manifestations

1. Dysuria, frequency, urgency, nocturia
2. Suprapubic pain and discomfort
3. Microscopic or gross hematuria

Diagnostic Evaluation

1. Urine dipstick may react positively for blood, white blood cells, and nitrates indicating infection.
2. Urine microscopy shows red blood cells and many white blood cells per field without epithelial cells.

> **NURSING ALERT:**
> Urinalysis showing many epithelial cells is likely contaminated by vaginal secretions in women and is therefore inaccurate in indicating infection. Urine culture may be reported as contaminated, as well. Obtaining a clean-catch, midstream specimen is essential for accurate results.

3. Urine culture is used to detect presence of bacteria and for antimicrobial sensitivity testing.

Management

1. Antibiotic therapy according to sensitivity results
   a. A wide variety of antimicrobial drugs are available.
   b. Urinary infections usually respond to drugs that are excreted in urine in high concentrations; a potentially effective drug should rapidly sterilize the urine and thus relieve the patient's symptoms.
2. For uncomplicated infection
   a. Women with uncomplicated cystitis are usually treated with a 2- to 3-day course of antibiotics (trimethoprim-sulfamethoxazole [Bactrim], ofloxacin [Floxin], or nitrofurantoin [Macrodantin]).
   b. Men are treated with 7 to 10 days of antibiotic therapy.
   c. Follow-up culture to prove treatment effectiveness
   d. Side effects are nausea, diarrhea, drug-related rash, and vaginal candidiasis.
3. For complicated infection, see treatment of pyelonephritis (p. 618).

Complications

1. Pyelonephritis
2. Hematogenous spread resulting in sepsis

Nursing Assessment

1. Determine if patient had a history of urinary tract infections in childhood, during pregnancy, or has had recurring infections.
2. Question about voiding habits, personal hygiene practices, and methods of contraception (use of diaphragm or spermicides is associated with development of cystitis).

3. Ask if patient has any associated symptoms of vaginal discharge, itching, or irritation—dysuria may be prominent symptom of vaginitis or infection from sexually transmitted pathogens, rather than urinary tract infection.

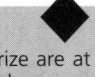

> **COMMUNITY-BASED CARE TIP:**
> Patients with indwelling catheters or who self-catheterize are at increased risk; review methods of handling catheters at home.

4. Examine for suprapubic tenderness, as well as abdominal tenderness, guarding, rebound, or masses that may indicate more serious process.

Nursing Diagnoses

A. Pain related to inflammation of the bladder mucosa
B. Knowledge Deficit related to prevention of recurrent urinary tract infection

Nursing Interventions

A. *Relieving Pain*
1. Administer or teach self-administration of antibiotic—eradication of infection is usually accompanied by rapid resolution of symptoms.
2. Encourage patient to take prescribed analgesics and antispasmodics if ordered.
3. Apply heat to the abdomen to relieve bladder spasms.
4. Encourage rest during the acute phase if symptoms are severe.
5. Encourage plenty of fluids to promote urinary output and to flush out bacteria from urinary tract.

B. *Increasing Understanding and Practice of Preventive Measures*
For women with recurrent urinary tract infections, give the following instructions:

1. Reduce vaginal introital concentration of pathogens by hygienic measures.
   a. Wash genitalia in shower or while standing in bathtub—bacteria in bath water may gain entrance into urethra.
   b. Cleanse around the perineum and urethral meatus after each bowel movement, with front to back cleansing to minimize fecal contamination of periurethral area.
2. Drink liberal amounts of water to lower bacterial concentrations in the urine.
3. Avoid irritants—coffee, tea, alcohol, cola drinks.
4. Decrease the entry of microorganisms into the bladder during intercourse.
   a. Void immediately after sexual intercourse.
   b. A single dose of an oral antimicrobial agent may be prescribed after sexual intercourse.
5. Avoid external irritants such as bubble baths and perfumed vaginal cleansers or deodorants.
6. Patients with persistent bacteria may require long-term antimicrobial therapy to prevent colonization of periurethral area and recurrence of urinary tract infection.

a. Take antibiotic at bedtime after emptying bladder to ensure adequate concentration of drug during overnight period because low rates of urine flow and infrequent bladder emptying predispose to multiplication of bacteria.

b. Use self-monitoring tests (dipsticks) at home to monitor for urinary tract infection.

Patient Education/Health Maintenance

1. Advise women with simple, uncomplicated cystitis that they do not require follow-up as long as symptoms are completely resolved with antibiotic therapy. Men usually need follow-up cultures and possibly additional testing if more than one episode of infection.
2. Instruct patient to void frequently (every 2–3 hours) and to empty bladder completely because this enhances bacterial clearance, reduces urine stasis, and prevents reinfection. Infrequent voiding distends the bladder wall, leading to hypoxia of bladder mucosa, which is then more susceptible to bacterial invasion.
3. Instruct patients who have had urinary tract infections during pregnancy to have follow-up studies.
4. Female patients with uncomplicated but recurrent cystitis may self-administer a 2- or 3-day course of antibiotics when symptoms begin if so prescribed.

Evaluation

A. Verbalizes relief of symptoms
B. Verbalizes self-care measures to prevent recurrence

◆ INTERSTITIAL CYSTITIS

Interstitial cystitis is a syndrome of chronic, cystitis-like symptoms in the absence of bacterial infection.

Pathophysiology/Etiology

1. The etiology of interstitial cystitis in unknown. Theories include an inflammatory or autoimmune process due to penetration of irritants into bladder tissue.
2. The bladder wall is chronically inflamed with no evidence of bacterial infection.
3. Occurs far more frequently in women than in men (10:1).

Clinical Manifestations

1. Extreme urinary frequency
2. Urgency and dysuria
3. Nocturia (more than twice)
4. Continuous bladder pain, may increase during voiding, may be diffuse perineal or suprapubic pain.
5. The duration of symptoms is often longer than 9 to 12 months when finally diagnosed.

Diagnostic Evaluation

1. Urine culture to rule out bacterial cystitis
2. Cystoscopy with biopsies and bladder distention; presence of bleeding or ulcerations on bladder distention is characteristic of many cases of interstitial cystitis.
3. Urodynamic tests often reveal a small bladder capacity with urgency and in some cases, small involuntary bladder contractions.
4. Diagnosis is often made by ruling out other potential causes of symptoms, including radiation or chemical cystitis, gynecologic or urologic malignancies, STD, urolithiasis, etc.

Management

1. Bladder distention during cystoscopy under general anesthesia relieves symptoms in 30% of patients.
2. Intravesical therapy with various substances including silver nitrate and dimethyl sulfoxide (DMSO) may be mixed with heparin, sodium bicarbonate, or prostaglandins.
3. Oral administration of tricyclic antidepressants (for their analgesic and anticholinergic effects); other drugs including pentosan polysulfate and nalmefene
4. Surgical intervention in extreme cases; bladder augmentation or cystectomy with urinary diversion

Complications

1. Psychosocial problems related to pain and urge incontinence
2. Secondary bacteriuria

Nursing Assessment

1. Assess voiding patterns including frequency, nocturia, urgency (a voiding diary is helpful). Determine if symptoms increase in relation to menstrual cycle or sexual intercourse.
2. Assess level of pain using a scale of 1 to 10; determine if pain increases during or after voiding and if bladder spasms occur.
3. Perform abdominal and pelvic examination if indicated to rule out gynecologic causes and to identify location of pain on palpation.
4. Assess significance of lifestyle alterations.

Nursing Diagnosis

A. Chronic Pain related to disease process
B. Altered Urinary Elimination related to frequency, urgency, dysuria, and nocturia
C. Ineffective Individual Coping related to interruption of lifestyle and chronic, unrelenting symptoms

Nursing Interventions

A. *Controlling Pain*
1. Administer pharmacologic agents as ordered to relieve pain; may be given orally or intravesically.

2. Instruct patient in comfort and preventive measures, application of heating pad, avoidance of bladder irritants (caffeine, alcohol, artificial sweeteners), electrostimulation therapy.
3. If prescribed, teach patient self-catheterization and the self-administration of intravesical medications.

B. Improving Urinary Elimination
1. Encourage patient to use a voiding diary as well as a dietary record to make associations between intake of certain foods or fluids and increase in symptoms.
2. Advise patient to restrict fluids only when necessary due to impending limited access to toilet facilities; normal fluid intake should be encouraged otherwise.
3. Assess patient's response to pharmacologic therapy.

C. Strengthening Coping
1. Refer for additional information to agencies such as: Interstitial Cystitis Association (ICA); (East Coast) P. O. Box 1553; Madison Square Station; New York, NY 10159; (West Coast) P. O. Box 151323 San Diego, CA 92115.

Patient Education/Health Maintenance

1. Teach patient mechanism of action and side effects of pharmacologic therapies.
2. Teach self-catheterization using clean technique if needed to self-administer medications.
3. Provide information about food and fluids known to be bladder irritants.
4. Teach patient nonpharmacologic methods to relieve pain.
5. Explore with patient positive coping strategies for self and family in dealing with chronic illness.

Evaluation

A. Verbalizes some relief of pain
B. Verbalizes less urgency, frequency, and nocturia
C. Seeks additional information and support

◆ BACTERIAL PYELONEPHRITIS

Bacterial pyelonephritis is an acute infection and inflammatory disease of the renal pelvis, tubules, and interstitial tissue of one or both kidneys.

Pathophysiology/Etiology

1. Pyelonephritis can result from any of the following sources of bacterial invasion or urinary obstruction:
   a. Enteric bacteria (*E. coli* most common organism)
   b. Secondary to vesicoureteral reflux (incompetence of ureterovesical valve, which allows urine to regurgitate into ureters, usually at time of voiding)
   c. Urinary obstruction/infection
   d. Trauma
   e. Blood-borne infection
   f. Renal disease
   g. Pregnancy

h. Metabolic disorders
2. Low-grade inflammation with interstitial infiltrations of inflammatory cells may lead to tubular destruction and abscess formation.
3. Chronic pyelonephritis may result in scarred, contracted, and nonfunctioning kidney(s).

Clinical Manifestations

1. Fever, chills
2. Costovertebral angle tenderness, flank pain (with or without radiation to groin)
3. Nausea, vomiting

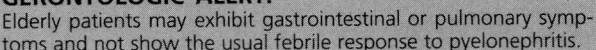

GERONTOLOGIC ALERT:
Elderly patients may exhibit gastrointestinal or pulmonary symptoms and not show the usual febrile response to pyelonephritis.

Diagnostic Evaluation

1. Urinalysis to identify leukocytes, bacteria, or pus in urine; gross or microscopic hematuria
2. Urine culture to identify antibody-coated bacteria in urine; bacteria invading kidney induce an antibody response that coats the bacteria—differentiates renal infection from bladder infection.
3. IVP to evaluate for urinary tract obstruction; other radiologic/urinary tests as necessary.

Management

1. Monitoring and supportive therapy for complications: bacteremia and gram-negative sepsis; papillary necrosis, leading to renal failure; renal abscess/perinephric abscess
2. Organism-specific antimicrobial therapy
   a. Usually immediate treatment is started to cover the prevalent gram-negative pathogens; subsequently adjusted according to culture results.
   b. Acute pyelonephritis usually caused by *E. coli*, which is sensitive to many antimicrobial drugs.
   c. A 2-week or more treatment regimen is needed for bacteriuria of renal origin.
3. Parenteral antimicrobial therapy may be necessary if patient cannot tolerate oral intake and is dehydrated; usually admitted to hospital if patient is acutely ill.
4. Maintenance therapy for chronic or recurring infections to preserve of renal function
   a. Continuous treatment with urine-sterilizing agents after initial antibiotic treatment has been used
   b. Continue for months to years until there is no evidence of inflammation, causative factors have been treated or controlled, and there is evidence of stability of renal function.
   c. Serial urine cultures and evaluation studies must be done for an indefinite period of time.
   d. Blood counts and serum creatinine determinations are required during long-term therapy.

Complications

1. Renal insufficiency possibly leading to CRF
2. Hypertension with chronic pyelonephritis
3. Renal abscess requiring treatment by percutaneous drainage or prolonged antibiotic therapy
4. Perinephric abscess

Nursing Assessment

1. Assess patient for fever, chills, flank pain, nausea, and vomiting.
2. Obtain vital signs; monitor for impending sepsis.
3. Obtain urologic history that could suggest recurrent infections or urinary tract obstruction.

Nursing Diagnoses

A. Hyperthermia due to infection
B. Pain related to renal swelling and edema

Nursing Interventions

A. *Reducing Body Temperature*
1. Administer or teach self-administration of antibiotics as prescribed and monitor for effectiveness and side effects.
2. Assess vital signs frequently and monitor intake and output; administer antiemetic medications to control nausea and vomiting.
3. Administer antipyretic medications as prescribed and according to temperature.
4. Use measures to decrease body temperature if indicated; cooling blanket, application of ice to armpits and groins, etc.
5. Correct dehydration by replacing fluids, orally if possible, or IV.
6. Collect serial urine specimens; monitor urine culture results for resolving infection.

B. *Relieving Pain*
1. Administer or teach self-administration of analgesic medications and monitor their effectiveness.
2. Use comfort measures such as positioning to locally relieve flank pain.
3. Assess patient's response to pain control measures.

Patient Education/Health Maintenance

1. Explain to patient possible causes of pyelonephritis and its signs and symptoms; review also signs and symptoms of lower urinary tract infection.
2. Review antibiotic therapy and importance of completing prescribed course of treatment and having follow-up urine cultures.
3. Explain preventive measures including good fluid intake, personal hygiene measures, and healthy voiding habits.

Evaluation

A. Afebrile
B. Verbalizes reduced pain

◆ ACUTE GLOMERULONEPHRITIS

Acute glomerulonephritis refers to a group of kidney diseases in which there is an inflammatory reaction in the glomeruli. It is not an infection of the kidney, per se, but rather the result of the immune mechanisms of the body.

Pathophysiology/Etiology

1. Occurs after an infection elsewhere in the body or may develop secondary to systemic disorders.
2. An antigen–antibody reaction produces immune complexes that lodge in the glomeruli, producing thickening of glomerular basement membrane.
3. Eventual scarring and loss of filtering surface may lead to renal failure.

Clinical Manifestations

1. Mild disease is frequently discovered accidentally through a routine urinalysis.
2. History of infection: pharyngitis from group A streptococcus, hepatitis B virus, endocarditis
3. Proteinuria, hematuria, oliguria
4. Puffiness of face, edema of extremities
5. Fatigue and anorexia
6. Hypertension (mild, moderate, or severe), headache
7. Anemia from loss of red blood cells into the urine
8. The clinical course of acute glomerulonephritis proceeds as follows from onset of symptoms to recovery—over 90% of patients regain normal renal function within 60 days:
   a. Diuresis usually starts 1 to 2 weeks after onset of symptoms.
   b. Renal clearances and blood urea concentration return to normal.
   c. Edema decreases and hypertension lessens.
   d. Microscopic proteinuria or hematuria may persist many months.

Diagnostic Evaluation

1. *Urinalysis*—hematuria (microscopic or gross), proteinuria, red cell casts, white blood cells, renal epithelial cells, and various casts in the sediment.
2. *Blood*—elevated BUN and creatinine levels, low albumin level, high lipid level, increased antistreptolysin titer (from reaction to streptococcal organism).
3. *Needle biopsy* of the kidney reveals obstruction of glomerular capillaries from proliferation of endothelial cells.

Management

1. Management is symptomatic and includes antihypertensives, diuretics, drugs for management of hyper-

kalemia (due to renal insufficiency), H_2 blockers (to prevent stress ulcers), and phosphate-binding agents (to reduce phosphate and elevate calcium).

2. Antibiotic therapy is initiated to eliminate infection (if still present).
3. Fluid intake is restricted.
4. Dietary protein is restricted moderately if there is oliguria and the BUN is elevated. It is restricted more drastically if acute renal failure develops.
5. Carbohydrates are increased liberally to provide energy and reduce catabolism of protein.
6. Potassium and sodium intake are restricted in presence of hyperkalemia, edema, or signs of congestive heart failure.
7. Therapy for rapidly progressive glomerulonephritis may include:
   a. Plasma exchange
   b. Immunosuppressants (corticosteroids; cyclophosphamide [Cytoxan])
   c. Dialysis—may be considered if fluid retention and uremia cannot be controlled

Complications

1. Hypertension, congestive heart failure, endocarditis
2. Fluid and electrolyte imbalances in the acute phase, hyperkalemia, hyperphosphatemia, hypervolemia
3. Malnutrition
4. Hypertensive encephalopathy, seizures
5. ESRD

Nursing Assessment

1. Obtain medical history; focus on recent infections or symptoms of chronic immunologic disorders (systemic lupus erythematosus, scleroderma).
2. Assess urine specimen for blood, protein, color, and amount.
3. Perform physical examination specifically looking for signs of edema, hypertension, and hypervolemia (engorged neck veins, elevated jugular venous pressure, adventitious lung sounds, cardiac arrhythmia).
4. Evaluate cardiac status and serum laboratory values for electrolyte imbalance.

Nursing Diagnoses

A. Altered Renal Tissue Perfusion related to damage to glomerular function
B. Fluid Volume Excess related to compromised renal function

Nursing Interventions

A. *Promoting Renal Function*
1. Monitor vital signs, intake and output and maintain dietary restrictions during acute phase.
2. Encourage bed rest during the acute phase until the urine clears and BUN, creatinine, and blood pressure normalize. (Rest also facilitates diuresis.)

3. Administer medications as ordered and evaluate patient's response to antihypertensives, diuretics, H_2 blockers, phosphate-binding agents and antibiotics (if indicated).

B. *Improving Fluid Balance*
1. Carefully monitor fluid balance; replace fluids according to the patient's fluid losses (urine, respiration, feces) and daily body weight as prescribed.
2. Monitor pulmonary artery pressure and central venous pressure, if indicated.
3. Monitor for signs and symptoms of congestive heart failure: distended neck veins, tachycardia, gallop rhythm, enlarged and tender liver, crackles at bases of lungs.
4. Observe for hypertensive encephalopathy, any evidence of seizure activity.

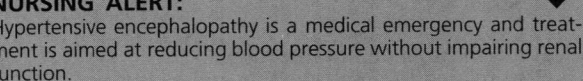

NURSING ALERT:
Hypertensive encephalopathy is a medical emergency and treatment is aimed at reducing blood pressure without impairing renal function.

Patient Education/Health Maintenance

1. Explain that the patient must have follow-up evaluations of blood pressure, urinary protein, and BUN concentrations to determine if there is exacerbation of disease activity.
2. Encourage patient to treat any infection promptly.
3. Tell patient to report any signs of decreasing renal function to obtain treatment immediately.

Evaluation

A. Urine output adequate; vital signs stable
B. No edema, shortness of breath, or adventitious heart or lung sounds

◆ NEPHROTIC SYNDROME

Nephrotic syndrome is a clinical disorder characterized by marked increase of protein in the urine (proteinuria), decrease in albumin in the blood (hypoalbuminemia), edema, and excess lipids in the blood (hyperlipidemia). These occur as a consequence of excessive leakage of plasma proteins into the urine because of increased permeability of the glomerular capillary membrane.

Pathophysiology/Etiology

1. Seen in any condition that seriously damages the glomerular capillary membrane
   a. Chronic glomerulonephritis
   b. Diabetes mellitus with intercapillary glomerulosclerosis
   c. Amyloidosis of kidney

d. Systemic lupus erythematosus
e. Renal vein thrombosis
f. Secondary to malignancy (older adults)
2. Hypoalbuminemia results in decreased oncotic pressure, causing generalized edema as fluid moves out of the vascular space.
3. Decreased circulating volume then activates the renin–angiotensin system causing retention of sodium and further edema.
4. Mechanism for increased lipids is unknown.

Clinical Manifestations

1. Insidious onset of pitting edema; weight gain
2. Marked proteinuria—leading to depletion of body proteins
3. Hyperlipidemia—may lead to accelerated atherosclerosis

Diagnostic Evaluation

1. Urinalysis—marked proteinuria, microscopic hematuria, urinary casts, appears "foamy."
2. 24-hour urine for protein (increased) and creatinine clearance (decreased)
3. Needle biopsy of kidney—for histologic examination of renal tissue to confirm diagnosis
4. Serum chemistry—decreased total protein and albumin, normal or increased creatinine, increased triglycerides, and altered lipid profile

Management

1. Treatment of causative glomerular disease
2. Corticosteroids or immunosuppressant agents to decrease proteinuria
3. General management of edema
   a. Sodium and fluid restriction
   b. Diuretics if renal insufficiency is not severe
   c. Infusion of salt-poor albumin
   d. Dietary protein supplements

Complications

1. Hypovolemia
2. Thromboembolic complications—renal vein thrombosis, venous and arterial thrombosis in extremities, pulmonary embolism, coronary artery thrombosis, cerebral artery thrombosis
3. Altered drug metabolism due to decrease in plasma proteins
4. Progression to end-stage renal failure

Nursing Assessment

1. Obtain history of onset of symptoms including changes in characteristics of urine and onset of edema.
2. Perform physical examination looking for evidence of edema and hypovolemia.
3. Assess vital signs, daily weights, intake and output, and laboratory values.

Nursing Diagnoses

A. Risk for Fluid Volume Deficit related to disease process
B. Risk for Infection related to treatment with immunosuppressants

Nursing Interventions

A. *Increasing Circulating Volume and Decreasing Edema*
1. Monitor daily weight, intake and output, and urine specific gravity.
2. Monitor central venous pressure (if indicated), vital signs, orthostatic blood pressure, and heart rate to detect hypovolemia.
3. Monitor serum BUN and creatinine to assess renal function.
4. Administer diuretics or immunosuppressants as prescribed and evaluate patient's response.
5. Infuse IV albumin as ordered.
6. Encourage bed rest for a few days to help mobilize edema; however, some ambulation is necessary to reduce risk of thromboembolic complications.
7. Enforce mild to moderate sodium and fluid restriction if edema is severe; provide a high protein diet.

B. *Preventing Infection*
1. Monitor for signs and symptoms of infection.
2. Monitor temperature and laboratory values for neutropenia.
3. Use aseptic technique for all invasive procedures and strict handwashing by patient and all contacts; prevent contact by patient with persons who may transmit infection.

Patient Education/Health Maintenance

1. Teach patient signs and symptoms of nephrotic syndrome; also review causes, purpose of prescribed treatments, and importance of long-term therapy to prevent ESRD.
2. Instruct patient in side effects of prescribed medications and methods of preventing infection if taking immunosuppressants.
3. Carefully review with patient and family dietary and fluid restrictions; consult dietitian for assistance in meal planning.
4. Discuss the importance of maintaining exercise, decreasing cholesterol and fat intake, and changing other risk factors such as smoking, obesity, and stress to reduce risk of severe thromboembolic complications.
5. In patients with severe disease, prepare for dialysis and possible transplantation.

Evaluation

A. Vital signs remain stable; edema decreased
B. No signs of infection

◆ NEPHROLITHIASIS/ UROLITHIASIS

Nephrolithiasis refers to renal stone disease; *urolithiasis* refers to the presence of stones in the urinary system. Stones, or calculi, are formed in the urinary tract from the kidney to bladder by the crystallization of substances excreted in the urine. The majority of stones (60%) are composed mainly of calcium oxalate crystals; the rest are composed of calcium phosphate salts, uric acid, struvite (magnesium, ammonium, and phosphate), or the amino acid cystine.

Pathophysiology/Etiology

1. Causes and predisposing factors
   a. Hypercalcemia and hypercalciuria caused by hyperparathyroidism, renal tubular acidosis, multiple myeloma, and excessive intake of vitamin D, milk, and alkali
   b. Chronic dehydration, poor fluid intake, and immobility
   c. Diet high in purines and abnormal purine metabolism (hyperuricemia and gout)
   d. Genetic disorders (cystinuria)
   e. Chronic infection with urea-splitting bacteria (*Proteus vulgaris*)
   f. Chronic obstruction with stasis of urine, foreign bodies within the urinary tract
   g. Excessive oxalate absorption in inflammatory bowel disease and bowel resection or ileostomy
   h. Living in warm, humid climate
2. Stones may be found anywhere in the urinary system and vary in size from mere granular deposits (called sand or gravel) to bladder stones the size of an orange.
3. Three of four patients with stones are men; in both sexes the peak age of onset is between 20 and 30 years.
4. Most stones migrate downward (causing severe colicky pain) and are discovered in the lower ureter. Spontaneous stone passage can be anticipated in 80% of patients with urolithiasis.
5. Some stones may lodge in the renal pelvis, ureters, or bladder neck causing obstruction, edema, secondary infection, and in some cases, nephron damage.
6. People who have had two stones tend to have recurrences.

Clinical Manifestations

1. Pain—pattern depends on site of obstruction (Fig. 19-3)
   a. Renal stones produce an increase in hydrostatic pressure and distention of the renal pelvis and proximal ureter causing renal colic. Pain relief is immediate following stone passage.
   b. Large ureteral stones produce symptoms or obstruction as they pass down the ureter (ureteral colic).
   c. Bladder stones produce symptoms similar to cystitis.

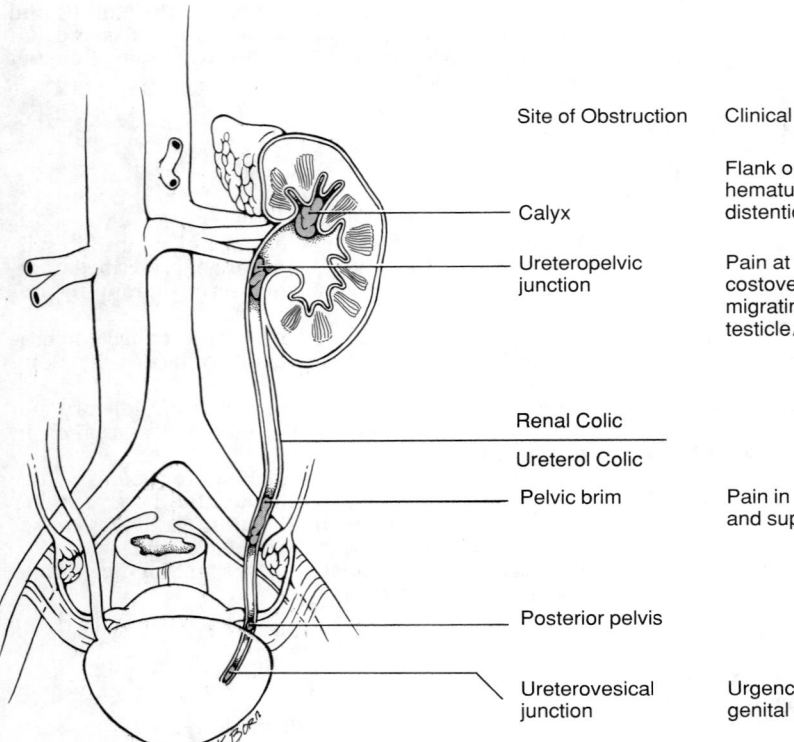

Site of Obstruction	Clinical Manifestations
Calyx	Flank or CVA pain, hematuria, abdominal distention
Ureteropelvic junction	Pain at flank or costovertebral angle, migrating to groin and testicle/labia minora
Renal Colic	
Ureterol Colic	
Pelvic brim	Pain in lateral flank and suprapubic area
Posterior pelvis	
Ureterovesical junction	Urgency, frequency, genital pain

FIGURE 19-3 *Areas where calculi may obstruct the urinary system. The ensuing clinical manifestations depend on the site of obstruction. Stones that have broken loose may obstruct the flow of urine, cause severe pain, and injure the kidney.*

2. Obstruction—stones blocking the flow of urine will produce symptoms of urinary tract infection; chills and fever.
3. Gastrointestinal symptoms—include nausea, vomiting, diarrhea, abdominal discomfort—due to renointestinal reflexes and shared nerve supply (celiac ganglion) between both the ureters and intestine.

Diagnostic Evaluation

1. IVP—to determine site and evaluate degree of obstruction
   a. Other uroradiologic studies are necessary when stones are radiolucent; retrograde or antegrade pyelography.
2. Analysis of available stone material—crystals can be identified by polarization microscopy, x-ray diffraction, and infrared spectroscopy.
3. Urinalysis—hematuria and pyuria; urine culture and drug sensitivity studies

Management

A. *Extracorporeal Shock Wave Lithotripsy (ESWL)*
Noninvasive technique and treatment of choice for stones less than 2 cm ($^3/_4$ inch) in diameter (80% of stones fall into this category).

1. High-energy shock waves are directed at the kidney stone, disintegrating it into minute particles that pass in the urine. (A *shock wave* is a large condensed wave of energy produced by high-speed motion.)
2. Patient is placed on specially designed table and immersed in a water bath or placed on an adjustable stretcher positioned over a cushion of water.
   a. In water bath model, shock waves travel through water surrounding the patient.
   b. In cushion model, a layer of gel lies between the stretcher and water; shock waves move through the cushion and gel.
3. Position of the kidney stone is located by x-rays and the shock waves are targeted directly at the stone. The shock waves do not affect soft tissue.

4. Eliminates need for surgery in majority of patients and can be repeated for recurrent stones with no apparent risk to kidney structure or function.
5. Complications include pain, urinary infection, and temporary bleeding around kidney.

B. *Percutaneous Nephrolithotomy (PCNL)*
For stones larger than 2.5 cm in diameter (Fig. 19-4).

1. Under fluoroscopic/ultrasound guidance, a needle is advanced into collecting system; guidewire is advanced into renal pelvis or ureter.
2. Tract is dilated with mechanical dilators or high-pressure balloon dilator until nephroscope can be inserted up against stone.
3. Stones can be broken apart with hydraulic shock waves or a laser beam administered via nephroscope; fragments are removed using forceps, graspers, or basket.
4. May be combined with ESWL.
5. Complications include hemorrhage, infection, and extravasation of urine.

C. *Percutaneous Stone Dissolution (Chemolysis)*
A multiholed nephrostomy tube (catheter) is placed in kidney; offers a pathway for introduction of solvent (depending on chemical composition of stone) to be infused into stone. A second catheter may be used for drainage.

1. Used for struvite, uric acid, and cystine stones.
2. May be used to shrink large stones before other retrieval methods or to irrigate debris after lithotripsy procedures.
3. Irrigating solution introduced at a continuous rate that patient can tolerate without flank pain or elevation of intrarenal pressure above 25 cm H_2O (most IV infusion pumps can be adapted for use and set to alarm should pressure exceed this level).
4. The patient receives antimicrobial agents before, during, and after procedure to maintain sterile urine.
5. Complications include infection (renal and perirenal abscesses, pyelonephritis, septic shock) and thrombophlebitis and pulmonary embolism (associated with immobilization).

D. *Ureteroscopy*
1. Used for distal ureteral calculi; may be used for mid-ureteral calculi

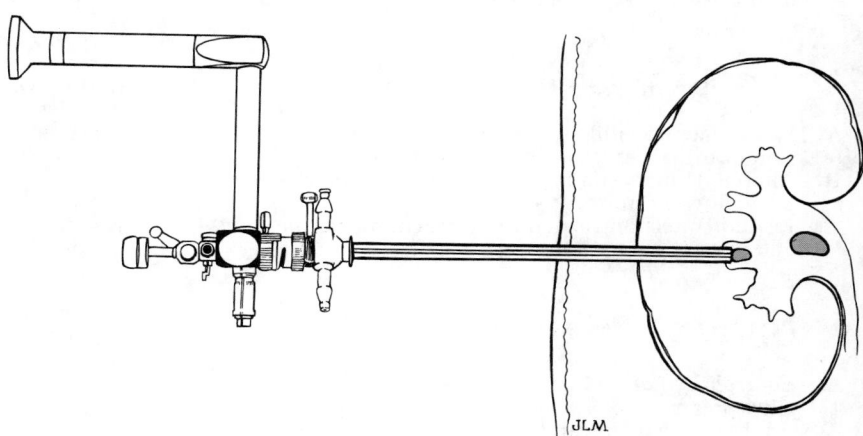

FIGURE **19-4** *A percutaneous nephrostomy tract permits access to the collecting system of the kidney for removal of kidney stones under direct vision via a nephroscope.*

2. Flexible or rigid ureteroscopes are used in conjunction with baskets or graspers.
3. Electrohydraulic, ultrasonic, or laser equipment may also be used to fragment stone.
4. A stent may be inserted and left in place after surgery to maintain patency of ureter.

E. Open Surgical Procedures
Indicated for only 1% to 2% of all stones.

1. *Pyelolithotomy*—removal of stones from kidney pelvis
   a. *Coagulum pyelolithotomy*—intraoperative injection of certain coagulation factors into the renal pelvis, producing a coagulum that entraps the stones and expedites their removal
2. *Nephrolithotomy*—incision into kidney for removal of stone
3. *Nephrectomy*—removal of kidney; indicated when kidney is extensively and irreparably damaged and is no longer a functioning organ; partial nephrectomy sometimes done.
4. *Ureterolithotomy*—removal of stone in ureter
5. *Cystolithotomy*—removal of stone from bladder

Complications

1. Obstruction—from remaining stone fragments
2. Infection—from dissemination of infected stone particles or bacteria resulting from obstruction
3. Impaired renal function—from prolonged obstruction before treatment and removal

Nursing Assessment

1. Obtain history focusing on family history of stones, episodes of dehydration, prolonged immobility, urinary tract infection, dietary and medication history.
2. Assess pain location and radiation; assess level of pain using a scale of 1 to 10. Observe for presence of associated symptoms: nausea, vomiting, diarrhea, abdominal distention.
3. Monitor for signs and symptoms of urinary tract infection: chills, fever, dysuria, frequency. Examine urine for hematuria.
4. Observe for signs and symptoms of obstruction: frequent urination of small amounts, oliguria, anuria.

Nursing Diagnoses

A. Pain related to inflammation, obstruction, and abrasion of urinary tract by migration of stones
B. Altered Urinary Elimination related to blockage of urine flow by stones
C. Risk for Infection related to obstruction of urine flow and instrumentation during treatment

Nursing Interventions

A. Controlling Pain
1. Give prescribed narcotic analgesic (usually IV or IM) until cause of pain can be removed.

a. Monitor patient closely for *increasing* pain, may indicate inadequate analgesia.
b. Very large doses of narcotics are often required to relieve pain, so monitor for respiratory depression and drop in blood pressure.
2. Encourage patient to assume position that brings some relief.
3. Reassess pain frequently using pain scale.
4. Administer antiemetics (IM or rectal suppository) as indicated for nausea.

B. Maintaining Urine Flow
1. Administer fluids orally or IV (if vomiting) to reduce concentration of urinary crystalloids and ensure inadequate urine output.

NURSING ALERT:
Avoid overhydration that may result in increased distention at stone location causing an increase in pain and associated symptoms.

2. Monitor total urine output and patterns of voiding. Report oliguria or anuria.
3. Strain all urine through strainer or gauze to harvest the stone; uric acid stones may crumble. Crush clots and inspect sides of urinal/bedpan for clinging stones or fragments.

COMMUNITY-BASED CARE TIP:
Advise patients at home to strain urine through a coffee filter.

4. Assist patient to walk, if possible, because ambulation may help move the stone through the urinary tract.

C. Controlling Infection
1. Administer parenteral or oral antibiotics as prescribed during treatment and monitor for side effects.
2. Assess urine for color, cloudiness, and odor.
3. Obtain vital signs and monitor for fever and symptoms of impending sepsis (tachycardia, hypotension).

Patient Education/Heath Maintenance

A. Recovery From Surgical Interventions for Stone Disease
1. Encourage fluids to accelerate passing of stone particles.
2. Teach about analgesics that still may be necessary for colicky pain, which may accompany passage of stone debris.
3. Warn that some blood may appear in urine for several weeks.
4. Encourage frequent walking to assist in passage of stone fragments.

B. Prevention of Recurrent Stone Formation
1. For patients with calcium oxalate stones
   a. Instruct on diet—avoid excesses of calcium and phosphorus; maintain a low-sodium diet (sodium restriction decreases amount of calcium absorbed in intestine).

b. Teach purpose of drug therapy—thiazide diuretics to reduce urine calcium excretion, allopurinol therapy to reduce uric acid formation.
2. For patients with uric acid stones
   a. Teach methods to alkalinize urine to enhance urate solubility.
   b. Instruct on testing urine pH.
   c. Teach purpose of taking allopurinol—to lower uric acid formation.
   d. Provide information about reduction of dietary purine intake (low protein—red meat, fish, fowl).
3. For patients with infection (struvite) stone
   a. Teach signs and symptoms of urinary infection (in patients with neurologic or spinal cord disease, teach use of dipsticks to evaluate urine for nitrites and leukocytes), encourage to report infection immediately; must be treated vigorously.
   b. Try to avoid prolonged periods of recumbency—slows renal drainage and alters calcium metabolism.
4. For patients with cystine stones—occur in *cystinuria*, a hereditary disorder of amino acid transport.
   a. Teach patient to alkalinize urine by taking sodium bicarbonate tablets (Soda Mint) to increase cystine solubility; instruct patient how to test urine pH with a pH indicator
   b. Teach patient about drug therapy with *d*-penicillamine (Depen)—to lower cystine concentration, or dissolution by direct irrigation with thiol derivatives.
   c. Explain importance of maintaining drug therapy consistently.
5. For all patients with stone disease
   a. Explain need for consistently increased fluid intake (24-hour urinary output greater than 2 liters)—lowers the concentration of substances involved in stone formation.
      (1) Drink enough fluids to achieve a urinary volume of 2,000 to 3,000 mL or more every 24 hours.
      (2) Drink larger amounts during periods of strenuous exercise, if you perspire freely.
      (3) Take fluids in evening to guarantee a high urine flow during the night.
   b. Encourage a diet low in sugar and animal proteins—refined carbohydrates appear to lead to hypercalciuria and urolithiasis; animal proteins increase urine excretion of calcium, uric acid, and oxalate.
   c. Increase consumption of fiber—inhibits calcium and oxalate absorption.
   d. Save any stone passed for analysis. (Only patients with more than one episode of urolithiasis are advised to have a metabolic evaluation).

Evaluation

A. Verbalizes reduced pain level
B. Urine output adequate with low specific gravity
C. Afebrile, urine clear

◆ RENAL CELL CARCINOMA

Renal cell carcinoma is the most common malignant renal tumor, occurring twice more frequently in men than in women. Most renal cell tumors are found in the renal parenchyma and develop with few (if any) symptoms.

Pathophysiology/Etiology

1. Unknown etiology; weak association with cigarette smoking
2. Most frequently occurs in persons between 50 and 60 years of age.
3. Aggressive cancer in which metastases occurs rapidly, often before diagnosis

Clinical Manifestations

1. Many renal tumors produce no symptoms and are discovered on routine physical examination as a palpable abdominal mass.
2. Fatigue, anemia, weight loss, and fever—from systemic effects of renal cancer
3. Classic triad (late symptoms)
   a. Hematuria—intermittent or continuous, microscopic or gross
   b. Flank pain—from distention of renal capsule, invasion of surrounding structures
   c. Palpable mass in flank

Diagnostic Evaluation

1. IVP—usually initial screening procedure
2. Ultrasonography—helpful in differentiating renal cyst from renal tumor; used as a complement to IVP.
3. CT or MRI—for patients with urographic findings suggesting tumor; useful for detecting, categorizing, and staging a renal mass.

Management

Goal: To eradicate the tumor and prevent metastasis

A. *Radical Nephrectomy*
Removal of kidney and associated tumor, adrenal gland, surrounding perirenal fat, Gerota's fascia, and possibly regional lymph nodes—provides maximum opportunity for disease control.

1. Performed through a vertical midline, subcostal, thoracoabdominal, or flank incision.
2. See page 604 for care of patient following renal surgery.

B. *Renal Artery Embolization*
Preoperative occlusion of renal artery followed by nephrectomy—for patient with large vascular tumor.

1. Catheter is advanced into renal artery.
2. Embolizing material (Gelfoam, steel coils, blood clot) is injected into artery and carried with arterial blood flow to occlude the tumor vessels.
3. Procedure decreases tumor vascularity and minimizes blood loss, relieves pain, and devitalizes the tumor preoperatively, thereby decreasing the chance for tumor cell dissemination at time of surgery.
4. Monitor for postinfarction syndrome (lasts 2–3 days)—severe abdominal pain, nausea, vomiting, diarrhea, fever.

5. Complications—arterial obstruction, bleeding, diminution of renal function

C. Chemotherapy/Immunotherapy

Renal cell carcinomas are generally refractory to chemotherapeutic agents, radiation, and hormonal manipulation.

1. Interleukin-2 (a lymphokine that stimulates growth of T lymphocytes) may offer some benefit to patients with metastatic renal cancer although toxicity is severe.

2. Interferon is also being investigated for possible beneficial effects in metastatic renal cell cancer.

Complications

1. Wide variety of metastatic sites (Fig. 19-5)

Nursing Assessment

1. Assess for clinical manifestations of systemic disease—fatigue, anorexia, weight loss, pallor, fever—as well as evidence of metastasis.

2. Monitor for side effects and complications of diagnostic tests and treatment.

3. Assess pain control and coping ability.

Nursing Diagnoses

A. Anxiety related to diagnosis of cancer and possibility of metastatic disease

B. Pain and Hyperthermia related to postinfarction syndrome

Also see page 605 for nursing diagnoses and interventions related to renal surgery.

Nursing Interventions

A. Reducing Anxiety

1. Explain each diagnostic test, its purpose, and possible adverse reactions. Ensure that informed consent has been obtained as indicated.

2. Assess patient's understanding about diagnosis and treatment options. Answer questions and encourage more thorough discussion with health care provider as needed.

3. Encourage patient to discuss fears and feelings; involve family and significant others in teaching.

B. Controlling Symptoms of Postinfarction Syndrome

1. Administer analgesics as prescribed to control flank and abdominal pain.

2. Encourage rest and assist with positioning for 2 to 3 days until syndrome subsides.

3. Obtain temperature every 4 hours and administer antipyretics as indicated.

4. Restrict oral intake and provide IV fluids while patient is nauseated.

5. Administer antiemetics as ordered.

Patient Education/Health Maintenance

1. Ensure that patient understands where and when to go for follow-up (surgeon, primary care provider, oncologist, and radiologist for metastatic work-up and treatment).

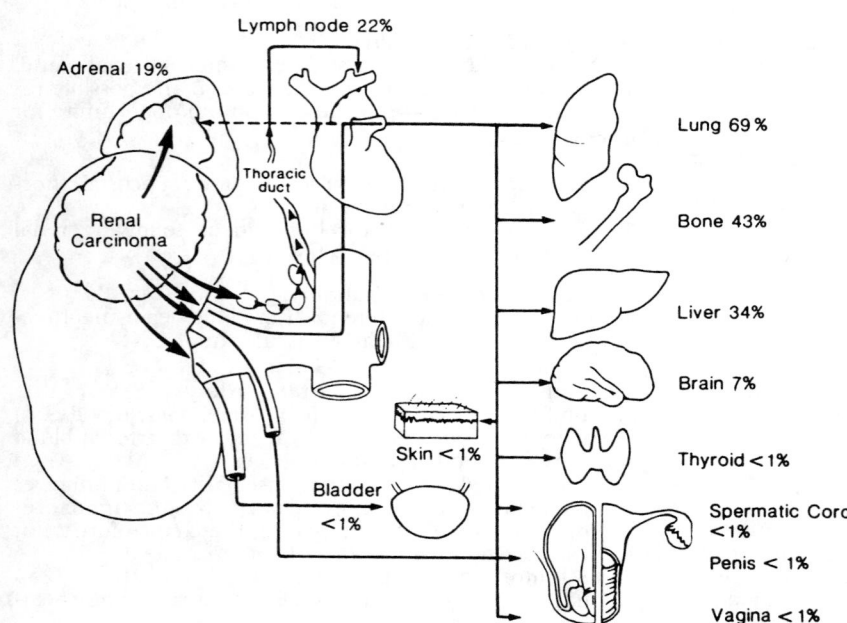

FIGURE 19-5 *Routes of common metastases from renal carcinoma. (From Semin Roentgenol 1987 Oct; 22[4]. Reproduced with permission.)*

2. Explain the importance of follow-up for hypertension and renal function, even if patient feels well.
3. Advise patient with one kidney to wear a Medic Alert bracelet and notify all health care providers because potentially nephrotoxic medications and procedures must be avoided.

Evaluation

A. Asks questions and verbalizes fears
B. Afebrile; states reduced pain

◆ INJURIES TO THE KIDNEY

Trauma to abdomen, flank, or back may produce renal injury. Suspicion is high in a patient with multiple injuries.

Pathophysiology/Etiology

1. *Blunt* trauma (falls, sporting accidents, motor vehicle accidents) can suddenly move the kidney out of position and in contact with a rib or lumbar vertebral transverse process, resulting in injury.
2. *Penetrating* trauma (gunshot and stab wounds) can injure the kidney if it lies in the path of the wound.
3. Renal trauma is classified according to severity of injury:
   a. Minor injuries—contusion, minor lacerations, hematomas
   b. Major injuries—major lacerations and rupture of kidney capsule (by expanding hematoma)
   c. Critical injuries—multiple and severe lacerations and renal pedicle injury (renal artery and vein are torn away from the kidney)
4. 80% of patients with renal trauma will have injuries to other organ systems also necessitating treatment.

Clinical Manifestations

1. Hematuria is common but not indicative of severity of injury.
2. Flank pain; perirenal hematoma
3. Nausea, vomiting, abdominal rigidity—from ileus (seen when there is retroperitoneal bleeding)
4. Shock—from severe/multiple injuries

Diagnostic Evaluation

1. History of injury—determine if injury was caused by blunt or penetrating trauma
2. Serial urine studies for hematuria
3. CT or MRI—defines lacerations, hematomas; detects extravasation of urine
4. IVP—to define extent of injury to involved kidney and the function of contralateral kidney

Management

1. Contusions and minor lacerations are managed conservatively with bed rest, IV fluids, and monitoring of serial urines for clearing of hematuria.

2. Major lacerations are surgically repaired.
3. Ruptures are surgically repaired, usually by partial nephrectomy.
4. Renal pedicle injury—this hemorrhagic emergency requires immediate surgical repair and possible nephrectomy.

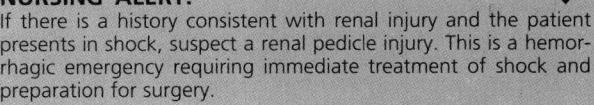

NURSING ALERT:
If there is a history consistent with renal injury and the patient presents in shock, suspect a renal pedicle injury. This is a hemorrhagic emergency requiring immediate treatment of shock and preparation for surgery.

Complications

1. Shock with cardiovascular collapse
2. Hematoma or urinoma formation, abscess formation
3. Hypertension
4. Pyelonephritis
5. Nephrolithiasis

Nursing Assessment

1. Obtain history of traumatic event and any history of renal disease.
2. Inspect for any abrasions, lacerations, or entrance and exit wounds to upper abdomen or lower thorax.
3. Monitor blood pressure and pulse—to assess for bleeding and impending shock; perirenal hemorrhage may cause rapid exsanguination.
4. Assess for presence and degree of hematuria.

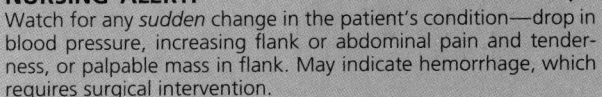

NURSING ALERT:
Watch for any *sudden* change in the patient's condition—drop in blood pressure, increasing flank or abdominal pain and tenderness, or palpable mass in flank. May indicate hemorrhage, which requires surgical intervention.

Nursing Diagnoses

A. Altered Renal Tissue Perfusion related to injury
B. Altered Urinary Elimination related to injury
C. Pain related to injury

Nursing Interventions

A. *Restoring and Maintaining Renal Perfusion*
1. Assess vital signs frequently, including blood pressure, heart rate, central venous pressure to monitor for hemorrhage and impending shock.
2. Assess abdomen and back for local tenderness and palpable mass, swelling, and ecchymosis, indicating hemorrhage or urine extravasation.

3. Outline original mass with marking pen for future comparison of size.
4. Establish IV access for support of blood pressure with fluids or vasopressors, replacement of blood, and perfusion of kidneys.
5. Monitor serial hematocrit determinations to be certain that continued bleeding is not occurring.

B. *Preserving Urinary Elimination*
1. Save, inspect, and compare each urine specimen—to follow the course and degree of hematuria.
   a. Label each specimen with date and time.
   b. If specimen is not grossly bloody, dipstick for blood or send to laboratory for microscopic examination.
2. Monitor intake and output carefully.
3. Give antibiotics as directed to discourage infection from perirenal hematoma or urinoma, or severely contaminated wounds.
4. Monitor for paralytic ileus (lack of bowel sounds) caused by retroperitoneal bleeding.
   a. Keep patient NPO until bowel sounds return.
   b. Administer IV fluids to maintain urine output.

C. *Controlling Pain*
1. Administer analgesic medication as prescribed; exercise caution with drugs that may aggravate hypotension or mask complications of hemorrhage.
2. Encourage bed rest and positioning of comfort until hematuria clears to facilitate healing of minor injuries.
3. Expect a low-grade fever with retroperitoneal hematomas as absorption of the clot occurs; administer antipyretics as ordered for comfort.

Patient Education/Health Maintenance

1. Instruct patient not to engage in strenuous activity for at least 1 month after blunt trauma to minimize incidence of delayed or secondary bleeding.
2. Teach patient signs and symptoms of late complications—infection and nephrolithiasis.
3. Advise patient to have blood pressure measured frequently and consistently to monitor self for hypertension.

Evaluation

A. Vital signs stable
B. Serial urines clearing
C. Reports decreased pain

◆ INJURIES TO THE BLADDER AND URETHRA

Injuries to the bladder and urethra commonly occur along with other trauma or may be due to surgical interventions.

Pathophysiology/Etiology

1. Bladder injuries are classified as follows:
   a. Contusion of bladder
   b. Intraperitoneal rupture
   c. Extraperitoneal rupture

   d. Combination intraperitoneal and extraperitoneal bladder rupture
2. Urethral injuries (occurring almost exclusively in men) are classified as follows:
   a. Partial or complete rupture
   b. Anterior or posterior urethral rupture
3. Injuries to the bladder and urethra are commonly associated with pelvic fractures and multiple trauma.
4. Certain surgical procedures (endoscopic urologic procedures, gynecologic surgery, surgery of the lower colon and rectum) also carry a risk of trauma to the bladder and urethra.
5. Intraperitoneal bladder rupture occurs when the bladder is full of urine and blunt trauma is sustained by the lower abdomen. The bladder ruptures at its weakest point, the dome. Urine and blood extravasate into the peritoneal cavity.
6. Extraperitoneal bladder rupture occurs when the lower bladder is perforated by a bony fragment during pelvic fracture or with a sharp instrument during surgery. Urine and blood extravasate into the pelvic cavity.
7. Urethral rupture occurs during pelvic fracture (posterior) or when the urethra or penis is manipulated accidentally during surgery or injury (anterior).

Clinical Manifestations

1. Inability to void
2. Hematuria; presence of blood at urinary meatus
3. Shock and hemorrhage—pallor, rapid and increasing pulse rate
4. Suprapubic pain and tenderness
5. Rigid abdomen—indicates intraperitoneal rupture
6. Absence of prostate on rectal examination in posterior urethral rupture
7. Swelling/discoloration of penis, scrotum, and anterior perineum in anterior urethral rupture

Diagnostic Evaluation

1. Retrograde urethrogram—to detect any rupture of urethra

NURSING ALERT:
If ruptured urethra is suspected, do not catheterize because catheterization may complete a partial urethral rupture. Urethrogram must be done first to determine patency of urethra.

2. Cystogram—to detect and localize perforation/rupture of bladder.
3. Plain film of abdomen—may show associated pelvic fracture.
4. Excretory urogram—to survey the kidneys for injury.

Management

A. *Bladder Injury*
1. Treatment instituted for shock and hemorrhage.
2. Surgical intervention carried out for intraperitoneal bladder rupture.

a. Extravasated blood and urine will first be drained and urine diverted with suprapubic cystostomy or indwelling catheter.
3. Small extraperitoneal bladder ruptures will heal spontaneously with indwelling suprapubic or Foley catheter drainage.
4. Large extraperitoneal bladder ruptures are repaired surgically.

B. **Urethral Injury**   Management is controversial

1. *Immediate repair*—urethra is manipulated into its correct anatomic position with reanastomosis after evacuation of hematoma.
2. *Delayed repair*—suprapubic cystostomy drainage for 6 to 12 weeks allows the urethra to realign itself while hematoma and edema resolve; then surgical reanastomosis.
3. *Two-stage urethroplasty*—reconstruction of the urethra occurs in two separate surgeries with urinary elimination diverted until final procedure.

Complications

1. Shock, hemorrhage, peritonitis
2. Urinary tract infection
3. Urethral stricture disease

Nursing Assessment

1. Obtain vital signs; assess for evidence of shock.
2. Obtain detailed history of injury if possible.
3. Inspect urinary meatus for evidence of bleeding.
4. Perform physical examination for symptoms of bladder rupture; dullness to palpation, rebound tenderness or rigidity.

Nursing Diagnoses

A. Risk for Fluid Volume Deficit related to trauma and resulting hemorrhage
B. Altered Urinary Elimination related to disruption of intact lower urinary tract
C. Pain related to traumatic injury
D. Fear related to traumatic injury and uncertain prognosis

Nursing Interventions

A. **Stablizing Circulatory Volume**
1. Monitor vital signs and central venous pressure frequently as indicated by condition.
2. Establish IV access and replace blood and fluids as ordered.

B. **Facilitating Urinary Elimination**
1. Inspect urethral meatus for blood, and if present, do not catheterize, but prepare for diagnostic evaluation and suprapubic cystostomy.
2. Obtain urine specimen, if possible, and assess for degree of hematuria and presence of infection.

3. Prepare patient for surgical repair by assisting with pre-operative work-up and describing postoperative experiences.
4. Postoperatively, maintain patency and flow of indwelling urinary catheter(s).
5. Inspect suprapubic incision and Penrose drains from perivesical areas for bleeding, extravasation of urine, or signs of infection.

C. **Controlling Pain**
1. Administer analgesics as ordered (once the patient's vital signs are stable).
2. Assess patient's response to pain control medications.
3. Position for comfort (usually semi-Fowler's position) if not contraindicated by other injuries, and prevent pulling of catheter tubing.

D. **Relieving Fears**
1. Provide information to the conscious patient throughout the stabilization and evaluation phase, prepare for surgery if impending.
2. Keep patient's family or significant others informed of condition and progress.
3. Provide information on long-term outcome of treatment.

Patient Education/Health Maintenance

1. Teach patient to care for indwelling catheters that will remain in place during healing or after surgery.
   a. Empty frequently.
   b. Cleanse catheter and insertion area with soap and water.
   c. Inspect urine for blood, cloudiness, or concentration.
   d. Drink plenty of fluids to keep urine flowing.
2. Teach patient to report signs and symptoms of urinary tract infection.
3. Instruct patient (after surgical repair of bladder rupture) that bladder capacity may be temporarily decreased—causing frequency and nocturia; this resolves over time.
4. Explain possibility of recurrent urethral stricture disease to patients with urethral injury; instruct in daily self-catheterization to dilate urethra if prescribed.
5. Inform patient (after severe urethral injury) of chance of impotence or incontinence.

Evaluation

A. Vital signs stable
B. Adequate urine output via catheter
C. Verbalizes relief of pain
D. Verbalizes reduction in fear

◆ CANCER OF THE BLADDER

Cancer of the bladder is the second most common urologic malignancy. Approximately 90% of all bladder cancers are transitional cell carcinomas, which arise from the epithelial lining of the urinary tract; transitional cell tumors can also occur in the ureters, renal pelvis and urethra. The remaining 10% of bladder cancers are adenocarcinoma, squamous cell carcinoma, or sarcoma.

Pathophysiology/Etiology

1. Many bladder tumors are diagnosed when the lesions are superficial, papillary tumors that are easily resected.
2. One-fourth of patients with bladder cancer present with nonpapillary, muscle invasive disease.
3. Bladder tumors tend to be heterogeneous (dissimilar) cancers; it is often difficult to predict the course they will take.
4. Metastases occur in the bladder wall and pelvis, para-aortic or supraclavicular nodes; in liver, lungs, and bone.
5. Although the specific etiology is unknown, it appears that multiple agents are linked to the development of cancer of the bladder, including:
   a. Cigarette smoking—the risk of developing bladder cancer is two to three times higher in smokers.
   b. Prolonged exposure to aromatic amines or their metabolites—generally dyes manufactured by the chemical industry and used by other industries
   c. Exposure to cyclophosphamide (Cytoxan), radiation therapy to the pelvis, chronic irritation of the bladder (as in long-term indwelling catheterization) and excessive use of the analgesic drug phenacetin, which has been taken off the market
6. Bladder cancer is the fourth most common cancer in men; it occurs three times more frequently in men; peak incidence occurs in the sixth to eighth decades.

Clinical Manifestations

1. Painless hematuria, either gross or microscopic—most characteristic sign
2. Dysuria, frequency, urgency—symptoms of bladder irritability
3. Pelvic or back pain—from distant metastases
4. Leg edema—from invasion of pelvic lymph nodes

Diagnostic Evaluation

1. Cystoscopy for visualization of number, location, and appearance of tumors; for biopsy
2. Urine and bladder washing for cytologic study
3. Urine for flow cytometry—uses a computer-controlled fluorescence microscope to scan and image the nucleus of each cell on a slide; based on the fact that cancer cells contain abnormally large amounts of DNA
4. IVP—may reveal filling defect indicative of bladder tumor, also to determine status of upper tracts
5. To evaluate for metastatic disease:
   a. Endoscopic examination with biopsies under anesthesia
   b. Bimanual examination of pelvis under anesthesia to determine degree of mobility, fixation of tumor, degree of extravesical extension
   c. CT or MRI—to evaluate extent of disease and tumor responsiveness
   d. Bone scan—to evaluate for bony metastases

Management

A. Surgery
1. Transurethral resection and fulguration—endoscopic resection for superficial tumors
   a. Usually combined with intravesical chemotherapy to prevent tumor recurrence.
   b. Complications include hemorrhage, infection, bladder perforation, and temporary irritative voiding.
   c. Laser irradiation of bladder tumors is also used to destroy tumors; however, it does not allow for tumor specimen collection for pathologic analysis.
2. Partial cystectomy when lesions are located only in the dome of the bladder, away from the ureteral orifices.
3. Radical cystectomy (removal of bladder) for invasive or poorly differentiated tumors
   a. Requires diversion of the urinary stream (see p. 606)
   b. In men, includes removal of bladder, prostate and seminal vesicles, proximal vas deferens, and part of proximal urethra.
   c. In women, consists of anterior exenteration with removal of bladder, urethra, uterus, fallopian tubes, ovaries, and segment of anterior wall of the vagina.
   d. May be combined with chemotherapy and radiation

B. Intravesical (Within the Bladder) Chemotherapy
1. Instillation of antineoplastic agent such as thiotepa, mitomycin C (Mutamycin), doxorubicin (Adriamycin); allows a high concentration of drug to come in contact with the tumor and urothelium with minimal systemic toxicity.
2. Instillation of immunotherapeutic agent bacillus Calmette-Guerin (BCG) stimulates immune response to prevent recurrence of transitional cell bladder tumors.
3. Patient is instructed as follows:
   a. Minimize fluid intake and avoid taking diuretic medications for several hours before the instillation period to maximize concentration of drug during treatment period.
   b. Change position as directed during instillation in an effort to have drug contact as much of urothelial surface as possible.
   c. Wash hands and perineal area after voiding the medication to prevent contact dermatitis.
   d. Do not void for 1 to 2 hours after instillation; then increase fluid intake and void frequently.
4. Course of treatment is weekly instillations for 6 to 8 weeks.
5. Complications from intravesical chemotherapy include urinary tract infection, irritative voiding symptoms, allergic reaction, bone marrow suppression, or systemic BCG reaction.
   a. A systemic BCG reaction occurs when fever higher than 100°F (37.7°C) persists for more than 24 hours; treated with antituberculosis agents.

C. Systemic Chemotherapy
1. Metastatic bladder cancer is a chemotherapeutically responsive disease; MVAC combination is widely used (methotrexate [Mexate], vinblastine [Velban], doxorubicin [Adriamycin] and cis-platin [Platinol]).

D. Radiation Therapy
1. May be internal or external

Complications

1. Metastasis

Nursing Assessment

1. Assess for hematuria, irritative voiding symptoms, risk factors (especially smoking history), weight loss, fatigue, and signs of metastasis.
2. Assess coping ability and knowledge of the disease.

Nursing Diagnoses

A. Altered Urinary Elimination related to hematuria and transurethral surgery
B. Pain related to irritative voiding symptoms and catheter-related discomfort
C. Anxiety related to diagnosis of cancer

Nursing Interventions

A. *Maintaining Urinary Elimination After Transurethral Surgery*
1. Maintain patency of indwelling urinary drainage catheter; manual irrigation is not recommended due to dangers of bladder perforation; continuous bladder irrigation may be used if necessary.
2. Ensure adequate hydration either orally or IV.
3. Monitor intake and output, including irrigation solution.
4. Monitor urine output for clearing of hematuria.

B. *Controlling Pain*
1. Administer analgesic medication for pelvic discomfort.
2. Administer anticholinergic medications or belladonna and opium suppositories to relieve bladder spasms.
3. Ensure patency of catheter drainage; do not irrigate unless specifically ordered.
4. Remove indwelling catheter as soon as possible after procedure.

C. *Relieving Anxiety*
1. Allow patient to verbalize fears and concerns.
2. Provide realistic information about diagnostic studies, surgery, and treatments.

Patient Education/Health Maintenance

1. Advise patient that irritative voiding symptoms and intermittent hematuria are possible for several weeks after transurethral resection of bladder tumor(s).
2. Teach patient importance of vigilant adherence to follow-up schedule; cystoscopy every 3 months for 1 year, then every 6 months to 1 year thereafter for the rest of patient's life (70% of superficial tumors will recur).
3. Review purpose and side effects of intravesical chemotherapy treatments (often not given until after recurrence).

Evaluation

A. Urine output adequate and clear

B. Verbalizes relief of pain and bladder spasms
C. Verbalizes lessened anxiety

Conditions of the Male Reproductive Tract

◆ URETHRITIS

Urethritis is inflammation of the urethra. It is usually an ascending infection in men. In women it is usually associated with cystitis (p. 615) or vaginitis (p. 664).

Pathophysiology/Etiology

1. Nongonococcal urethritis—urethritis not caused by gonococcus; however, a large number of cases are sexually transmitted by:
   a. *Chlamydia trachomatis* and *Ureaplasma urealyticum*—cause approximately 80% of nongonococcal urethritis.
   b. Other sexually transmitted organisms causing acute urethritis include herpes simplex virus, human papillomavirus or *Trichomonas vaginalis*.
   c. Incubation period 1 to 5 weeks
2. Gonococcal urethritis—caused by *N. gonorrhoeae*, sexually transmitted; usually most virulent and destructive
   a. Incubation period usually 2 to 5 days
3. Gonococcal and nongonococcal urethritis can both be present.
4. Nonsexually transmitted
   a. Bacterial urethritis—may be associated with urinary tract infection.
   b. From trauma—secondary to passage of urethral sounds, repeated cystoscopy, indwelling catheter
5. Postgonococcal urethritis—occurs after treatment for gonococcal urethritis; another pathogen, which was not treated, proliferates.

Clinical Manifestations

1. Often asymptomatic (except gonococcal)
2. Itching and burning around area of urethra
3. Urethral discharge: may be scant or profuse; thin, clear, or mucoid; or thick and purulent (gonococcal).
4. Dysuria and frequency
5. Penile discomfort

Diagnostic Evaluation

1. Gram stain—*N. gonorrhoeae* is detected as gram-positive diplococci on microscopic examination of urethral discharge or urine.
2. Culture of urethral discharge on selective medium
3. Fluorescent antibody stain—of urethral discharge—to detect *C. trachomatis* and *N. gonorrhoeae*
4. Wet mount microscopic examination of fresh urethral discharge—trichomonads may be visible and motile.

Management

1. Antimicrobial therapy with tetracycline class, some quinolones, or erythromycin class antibiotics—effective for most cases of nongonococcal urethritis; metronidazole (Flagyl) is used for *Trichomonas*.
2. Penicillinase-resistant penicillins, some cephalosporins, and quinolones may be used to treat gonococcal urethritis; one large-dose treatment is effective.

Complications

Depends on cause, but may include

1. Prostatitis, epididymitis, urethral stricture, sterility due to vasoepididymal duct obstruction
2. Rectal infection, pharyngitis, conjunctivitis, skin lesions, arthritis with gonococcal infection

Nursing Assessment

1. Obtain history of unprotected sexual contact.
2. Assess for signs and symptoms involving urinary and reproductive tracts.
3. Perform genital and abdominal examination to assess for extent of infection.

Nursing Diagnoses

A. Risk for Infection related to ascending or systemic spread of pathogens
B. Risk for Infection Transmission to sexual contacts

Nursing Interventions

A. *Resolving Infection and Preventing Complications*
1. Collect urethral swab of discharge, urine, and blood as ordered for laboratory examination.
2. Use universal precautions when handling specimens.
3. Administer antibiotics as prescribed.
   a. Usually ordered based on presumptive diagnosis before test results are back.
   b. Monitor for and advise patient of side effects or allergic reactions.

B. *Preventing Spread of Infection*
1. Encourage compliance with antimicrobial regimen for the prescribed time period.
2. Advise abstinence from sexual activity until treatment is complete and cure is established (usually 7–10 days).
3. Instruct the patient to avoid sexual activity with previous sexual partner until that person(s) has been tested and treated for infection as well.
4. The use of condoms may prevent transmission, but depends on technique.

Patient Education/Health Maintenance

1. Advise that barrier methods of contraception (condom; diaphragm) will reduce transmission of sexually transmitted organisms.

2. Emphasize that the patient must return in 4 to 7 days to assess results and determine if there is need for further treatment and tests.

Evaluation

A. Single dose therapy taken as ordered
B. Reports sexual contacts have been treated

◆ BENIGN PROSTATIC HYPERPLASIA (BPH)

Benign prostatic hyperplasia is enlargement of the prostate that constricts the urethra, causing urinary symptoms. One of four men who reach the age of 80 will require treatment for BPH.

Pathophysiology/Etiology

1. The process of aging and the presence of circulating androgens are required for the development of BPH.
2. The prostatic tissue forms nodules as enlargement occurs.
3. The normally thin and fibrous outer capsule of the prostate becomes spongy and thick as enlargement progresses.
4. The prostatic urethra becomes compressed and narrowed, requiring the bladder musculature to work harder to empty urine.
5. Effects of prolonged obstruction cause trabeculation (formation of cords) of the bladder wall, decreasing its elasticity.

Clinical Manifestations

1. In early or gradual prostatic enlargement, there may be no symptoms, because the detrusor musculature can initially compensate for increased urethral resistance.
2. Obstructive symptoms—hesitancy, diminution in size and force of urinary stream, terminal dribbling, sensation of incomplete emptying of the bladder, urinary retention
3. Irritative voiding symptoms—urgency, frequency, nocturia

Diagnostic Evaluation

1. Rectal examination—smooth, firm, symmetric enlargement of the prostate
2. Urinalysis to rule out hematuria and infection
3. Serum creatinine and BUN—to evaluate renal function
4. Serum PSA—to rule out cancer, but may also be elevated in BPH
5. Optional diagnostic studies for further evaluation:
   a. Urodynamics—measures peak urine flow rate, voiding time and volume, and status of the bladder's ability to effectively contract

b. Measurement of postvoid residual urine; by ultrasound or catheterization
c. Cystourethroscopy—to inspect urethra and bladder and evaluate prostatic size

Management

1. Patients with mild symptoms (in the absence of significant bladder or renal impairment) are followed annually; BPH does not necessarily worsen in all men.
2. Pharmacologic management
   a. α-Adrenergic blockers such as doxazosin (Cardura), prazosin (Minipress), terazosin (Hytrin)—relax smooth muscle of bladder base and prostate to facilitate voiding.
   b. Finasteride (Proscar)—antiandrogen effect on prostatic cells, reverses or prevents hyperplasia.
3. Balloon dilation of the prostatic urethra provides temporary relief of symptoms.
4. Surgery—TURP, transurethral incision of the prostate (TUIP), or open prostatectomy for very large prostates, usually by suprapubic approach
5. Newer approaches—laser surgery, insertion of prostatic stents or coils, microwave hyperthermia treatments

Complications

1. Acute urinary retention, involuntary bladder contractions, bladder diverticula and cystolithiasis
2. Vesicoureteral reflux, hydroureter, hydronephrosis
3. Gross hematuria, urinary tract infection

Nursing Assessment

1. Obtain history of voiding symptoms, including onset, frequency of day and nighttime urination, presence of urgency, dysuria, sensation of incomplete bladder emptying and decreased force of stream.
   a. Use symptom index to determine severity of symptoms and impact on patient's lifestyle. (Symptoms index is published in *Quick Reference Guide for Clinicians, #8: Benign Prostatic Hyperplasia: Diagnosis and Treatment* and can be obtained from the Agency for Health Policy and Research by calling 1-800-358-9295.)
2. Perform rectal (palpate size, shape, and consistency) and abdominal examination to detect distended bladder, degree of prostatic enlargement.
3. Perform simple urodynamic measures—uroflowmetry and measurement of postvoid residual, if indicated.

Nursing Diagnosis

A. Altered Urinary Elimination related to obstruction of urethra

Also see page 609 for care of the patient undergoing prostatic surgery.

Nursing Interventions

A. *Facilitating Urinary Elimination*
1. Provide privacy and time for patient to void.
2. Assist with catheter introduction with guidewire or via suprapubic cystotomy as indicated.
   a. Monitor intake and output.
   b. Maintain patency of catheter.
3. Administer medications as ordered and monitor for and teach patient about side effects.
   a. α-Adrenergic blockers—hypotension, orthostatic hypotension, syncope (especially after first dose); impotence; blurred vision; rebound hypertension if discontinued abruptly
   b. Finasteride (Proscar)—hepatic dysfunction; impotence; interference with PSA testing
4. Assess for and teach patient to report hematuria, signs of infection.

Patient Education/Health Maintenance

1. Explain to patient not undergoing treatment the symptoms of complications of BPH—urinary retention, cystitis, increase in irritative voiding symptoms. Encourage reporting these problems.
2. Teach patient to do perineal (Kegel) exercises after surgery to help gain control of voiding.
   a. Contract the perineal muscle as if to stop stream of urine or flatus, hold for 10 to 15 seconds, then relax.
   b. Repeat approximately 15 times (one set); do 15 sets per day.
3. Advise patient that irritative voiding symptoms do not immediately resolve after relief of obstruction; symptoms diminish over time.
4. Tell patient to avoid sexual intercourse, straining at stool, heavy lifting, and long periods of sitting for 6 to 8 weeks after surgery, until prostatic fossa is healed.
5. Advise follow-up visits after treatment because urethral stricture may occur and regrowth of prostate is possible after TURP.

Evaluation

A. Voiding adequate without residual urine
B. Describes surgical procedure and complications
C. No evidence of infection or abnormal bleeding

◆ PROSTATITIS

Prostatitis is an inflammation of the prostate gland. It is classified as bacterial prostatitis (acute or chronic), nonbacterial prostatitis, or prostatodynia.

Pathophysiology/Etiology

1. Acute bacterial invasion of prostate
   a. From reflux of infected urine into ejaculatory and prostatic ducts

b. From hematogenous (bloodstream) origin or lymphogenous spread
c. Secondary to urethritis—from ascent of bacteria from urethra
d. May be stimulated by urethral instrumentation or rectal examination of the prostate when bacteria are present.
2. Chronic bacterial prostatitis
  a. From bacteria ascending from urethra (urethritis)
  b. From hematogenous spread
3. Nonbacterial prostatitis
  a. Complication of urethritis (*Chlamydia* common cause)
4. Prostatodynia
  a. Symptoms of prostatitis in the absence of positive cultures or known etiologic cause; difficult to diagnose and manage.

Clinical Manifestations

1. Sudden chills and fever (moderate to high fever)
2. Bladder irritability—frequency, dysuria, nocturia, urgency, hematuria
3. Pain in perineum, rectum, lower back, lower abdomen, and penile head
4. Pain after ejaculation, symptoms of urethral obstruction

Diagnostic Evaluation

1. Culture and sensitivity tests of divided urine specimens.
  a. First 10 to 15 mL voided after cleansing is sent as urethral specimen.
  b. Next 50 to 75 mL of urine is collected as bladder specimen.
  c. Prostate is massaged and either prostatic fluid drips out by gravity and collected, or patient voids urine mixed with prostatic fluid.
2. Rectal examination frequently reveals exquisitely tender, painful, swollen prostate, warm to the touch.
3. Serum white blood cell count is elevated in bacterial prostatitis.

Management

1. Acute bacterial prostatitis—antimicrobial therapy (10–14 days) based on drug sensitivity; IV therapy may be required.
  a. Urinary retention is managed with suprapubic cystostomy; urethral catheterization should be avoided.
  b. Antipyretic medications to manage fever.
2. Chronic bacterial prostatitis—oral antibiotic therapy with ability to diffuse into prostate (quinolones such as lomefloxacin [Maxaquin] or ofloxacin [Floxin]; sulfonamide such as trimethoprim-sulfamethoxazole [Bactrim])
  a. Prolonged therapy may be necessary to control symptoms and prevent bacteriuria (12 weeks or more).
  b. Oral antispasmodic agents may provide relief from urinary frequency and urgency.
3. Nonbacterial prostatitis—1 to 2 weeks of oral antibiotics including tetracycline (Tetracyn), doxycycline (Vibramycin), or erythromycin (P.S.E.)

a. Therapy is directed toward control of symptoms—prostatic massage, anticholinergic or anti-inflammatory drugs, hot sitz baths.
4. Prostatodynia—α-adrenergic blockers and skeletal muscle relaxants may provide some relief of symptoms.
  a. Aggressive diagnostic intervention to rule out other conditions such as cancer of the prostate or interstitial cystitis

Complications

1. Bacteriuria, urethritis, epididymitis, prostatic abscess, bacteremia, septicemia
2. Acute urinary retention
3. Constipation

Nursing Assessment

1. Obtain history of previous lower urinary tract infections or STD, recent voiding patterns.
2. Perform examination of genitalia for urethral discharge; rectal examination (except in acute bacterial prostatitis due to tenderness and possibility of disseminating infection) to assess tenderness of prostate.
3. Collect specimens; urine for culture and expressed prostatic secretions.

Nursing Diagnoses

A. Hyperthermia related to infectious process
B. Pain related to prostatic inflammation
C. Chronic Pain related to chronic prostatitis, prostatodynia

Nursing Interventions

A. *Reducing Fever*
1. Start antibiotic therapy as soon as specimens obtained for culture.
2. Administer antipyretic medications; use cooling measures if necessary.
3. Keep the patient well hydrated, IV or orally, due to fluid loss through fever; however, avoid overhydration, which increases urine volume and reduces antibiotic concentration in urine.

B. *Relieving Pain*
1. Administer analgesic or anti-inflammatory medication as ordered.
2. Maintain bed rest in acute prostatitis to relieve perineal and suprapubic pain.
3. Maintain high-fiber diet and give stool softeners as needed to prevent constipation, which increases pain.

C. *Controlling Chronic Pain*
1. Administer or teach self-administration of analgesics, anti-inflammatory agents, α-adrenergic blockers, or skeletal muscle relaxants as ordered.
2. Advise warm sitz baths to relieve pain and promote muscular relaxation of pelvic floor and reduce potential for urinary retention.
3. Perform gentle prostatic massage if indicated (nonbacterial prostatitis only).

4. Assess patient's response to supportive measures and coping with chronic pain.

Patient Education/Health Maintenance

1. Instruct patient to take antibiotic as prescribed; emphasize importance of completing long course of therapy to prevent recurrence and resistance of organisms.
2. Teach patient symptoms of recurrence and of disseminated spread of infection.
3. Instruct patient in comfort measures; sitz baths (10–20 minutes) several times daily, continued use of stool softeners, avoid sitting for long periods of time.
4. Advise patient to avoid sexual arousal/intercourse during period of *acute* inflammation; sexual intercourse may be beneficial in the treatment of *chronic* prostatitis; chronic prostatic infection is *not* sexually transmissible.
6. Encourage prescribed follow-up because recurrence is possible.

Evaluation

A. Afebrile
B. Verbalizes relief of pain following analgesic
C. Verbalizes reduction of chronic pain

◆ CANCER OF THE PROSTATE

Cancer of the prostate is the second leading cause of cancer death among American men and is the most common carcinoma in men over 65 years of age.

Pathophysiology/Etiology

1. The incidence of prostate cancer is 40% higher in African American men.
2. The majority of prostate cancers arise from the peripheral zone of the gland; therefore, most prostatic cancers are palpable on rectal examination.

> **NURSING ALERT:**
> Annual rectal examination is recommended by the American Cancer Society for all men over 40 years of age. Annual rectal examination and PSA blood testing is recommended for all men over 50.

3. Prostate cancer can spread by local extension, by lymphatics, or via the bloodstream.
4. The etiology of prostate cancer is unknown; there is an increased risk for persons with a family history of the disease.
   a. The influences of infectious agents, including STDs, dietary fat intake, and industrial exposure to carcinogens remain unproven.

Clinical Manifestations

1. Most early stage prostate cancers are asymptomatic.
2. Symptoms due to obstruction of urinary flow
   a. Hesitancy and straining on voiding, frequency, nocturia
   b. Diminution in size and force of urinary stream
3. Symptoms due to metastases
   a. Pain in lumbosacral area radiating to hips and down legs (from bone metastases)
   b. Perineal and rectal discomfort
   c. Anemia, weight loss, weakness, nausea, oliguria (from uremia)
   d. Hematuria (from urethral or bladder invasion, or both)
   e. Lower extremity edema—occurs when pelvic node metastases compromise venous return.

Diagnostic Evaluation

1. Digital rectal examination—prostate can be felt through the wall of the rectum; hard nodule may be felt (Fig. 19-6).
2. Needle biopsy (through anterior rectal wall or through perineum) for histologic study of biopsied tissue or aspiration for cytologic study
3. Transrectal ultrasonography—a sonar probe placed in rectum
4. Serologic markers of prostate cancer
   a. PSA—usually greater than 10 ng/mL
   b. Prostatic acid phosphatase—elevated in advanced prostatic cancer
5. Excretory urogram—to demonstrate changes from ureteral obstruction
6. Metastatic work-up—chest x-ray, IVP, CT, or MRI (recently developed method of performing prostatic MRI with endorectal coil provides detailed images) and bone scan

Management

A. **Conservative Measures**
1. No treatment may be indicated in older men, over age 70 because prostate cancer may be slow growing and it is expected that many men will die from other causes. It is often recommended that these patients be followed closely with periodic PSA determinations and examination for evidence of metastases.
2. Symptom control for advanced prostatic cancer in which treatment is not effective
   a. Analgesics and narcotics to relieve pain
   b. Short course of radiotherapy for specific sites of bone pain
   c. IV administration of β-emitter agent (strontium chloride 89) delivers radiotherapy directly to sites of metastasis.
   d. TURP to remove obstructing tissue if bladder outlet obstruction occurs
   e. Suprapubic catheter placement

B. **Surgical Interventions (Curative)**
1. Radical prostatectomy—removal of entire prostate gland, prostatic capsule, and seminal vesicles; may include pelvic lymphadenectomy.

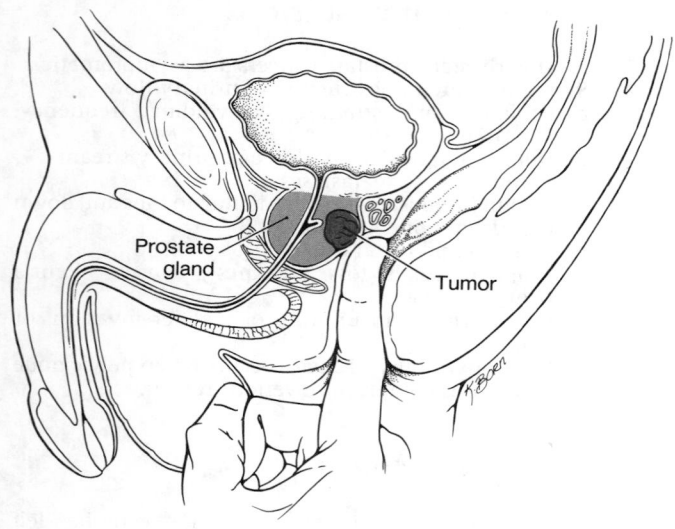

FIGURE 19-6 *The prostate gland can be felt through the wall of the rectum. The size of the gland, overall consistency, and the presence of any firm areas and nodules are noted.*

a. Complications include urinary incontinence, impotence, and rectal injury; however, better surgical dissection techniques may preserve sexual potency (see p. 609 for care of the patient undergoing prostatectomy).

3. Laparoscopic pelvic lymph node dissection may be performed before prostatectomy to accurately stage disease; positive lymph nodes would preclude radical prostatectomy.

4. Cryosurgery of the prostate freezes prostate tissue, killing tumor cells without removing the gland.

C. Radiation (Curative)

1. External beam radiation (using linear accelerator) focused on the prostate—to deliver maximum radiation dose to tumor and minimal dose to surrounding tissues.

2. Interstitial radiation—interstitial implantation of radioactive substances (brachytherapy) into prostate, which delivers doses of radiation directly to tumor while sparing uninvolved tissue.

3. Complications include radiation cystitis (urinary frequency, urgency, nocturia), urethral injury (stricture), radiation enteritis (diarrhea, anorexia, nausea), radiation proctitis (diarrhea, rectal bleeding), impotence.

D. Hormone Manipulation (Palliative)

1. Prostate cancer is a hormone-sensitive cancer. The aim of hormonal treatment is to deprive tumor cells of androgens or their by-products and thereby alleviate symptoms and retard progress of disease.

2. Bilateral orchiectomy (removal of testes) results in reduction of the major circulating androgen, testosterone. A small amount of androgen is still produced by adrenal gland.

3. Estrogen therapy (diethylstilbestrol [Stilphostrol])—suppresses release of luteinizing hormone, thereby indirectly decreasing testosterone levels.
   a. Therapy with estrogens leads to water retention, cardiovascular side effects, and gynecomastia (soreness and enlargement of breasts).

4. Other methods of achieving androgen deprivation

a. Luteinizing hormone-releasing hormone (LHRH) analogues (leuprolide [Lupron], goserelin acetate [Zoladex])—reduce testosterone levels as effectively as orchiectomy or estrogen.

b. Antiandrogen drugs (megestrol [Megace], flutamide)—block androgen action directly at the target tissues (testes and adrenals) and block androgen synthesis within the prostate gland.

c. Combination therapy with LHRH analogues and flutamide blocks the action of all circulating androgen.

5. Complications of hormonal manipulation include hot flashes, nausea and vomiting, gynecomastia, sexual dysfunction.

Complications

1. Bone metastasis—vertebral collapse and spinal cord compression, pathologic fractures

2. Complications of treatment

Nursing Assessment

1. Obtain history of current symptoms; assess for family history of prostate cancer.

2. Perform rectal and pelvic/abdominal examination to detect nodules on prostate, palpate lymph nodes, especially in supraclavicular and inguinal regions (may be first sign of metastatic spread), assess for flank pain, and distended bladder.

Nursing Diagnoses

A. Anxiety related to fear of disease progression and treatment options

B. Sexual Dysfunction related to effects of therapy

C. Pain related to bone metastases

Also see page 609 for care of the patient following prostatectomy.

Nursing Interventions

A. Reducing Anxiety
1. Help patient assess the impact of the disease and treatment options on quality of life.
2. Give repeated explanations of diagnostic tests and treatment options; help patient gain some feeling of control over disease and decisions.
3. Help patient/family set reachable goals.
4. Convey a sense of caring and reassurance in your physical care.

B. Achieving Optimal Sexual Function
1. Even though the patient may be ill while experiencing the effects of therapy, he may wonder about sexual function. Give him the opportunity to communicate his concerns and sexual needs.
2. Let patient know that decreased libido is expected after hormonal manipulation therapy and impotence may result from some surgical procedures and radiation.
3. Expect patient's behavior to reflect depression, anxiety, anger, and regression. Encourage ventilation of feelings and communication with partner.
4. Suggest options such as sexual counseling, learning other methods of sexual expression, and consideration of options for treatment of erectile dysfunction.

C. Controlling Pain
1. Administer and teach self-administration of narcotic analgesics as ordered; oral sustained-release narcotics, sustained-release transdermal patches, and subcutaneous or epidural patient-controlled infusion pumps are among the many options.
2. Encourage patient to take prescribed aspirin (Ecotrin), acetaminophen (Tylenol), or NSAIDs for reduction of mild pain or to supplement narcotic pain control regimen.
3. Be sure that patient is not undermedicated; help family and patient understand that addiction is not a concern.
4. Teach relaxation techniques such as imagery, music therapy, progressive muscle relaxation.
5. Use safety measures to prevent pathologic fractures from falls.
6. Encourage follow-up and palliative treatment such as radiation therapy to bony lesions for pain improvement.

Patient Education/Health Maintenance

1. Teach patient importance of follow-up for check of PSA levels and evaluation for disease progression.
2. Teach IM or subcutaneous administration of hormonal agents as indicated.
3. If bone metastasis has occurred encourage safety measures around the home to prevent pathologic fractures such as removal of throw rugs, using hand rail on stairs, using nightlights.
4. Advise reporting of symptoms of worsening urethral obstruction such as increased frequency, urgency, hesitancy, and urinary retention.

5. For additional information and support, refer to agencies such as: US TOO International Inc. (network of prostate cancer survivor support groups); One Heritage Plaza Building; 7501 Lemont Rd., Suite 215; Woodridge, IL 60517; 1-800-82USTOO; and American Foundation for Urologic Disease; 300 West Pratt St., Suite 401; Baltimore, MD 21201-2463; 1-800-242-2383.

Evaluation

A. Verbalizes understanding of sexual dysfunction and interest in seeking sexual counseling
B. Discusses treatment options, asks questions
C. Reports pain relief after narcotic administration

◆ TESTICULAR CANCER

Testicular cancer is a disease that occurs in younger men, between 25 and 35 years of age. It is relatively uncommon—6,600 cases are reported annually. It is the most treatable form of urologic cancer.

Pathophysiology/Etiology

1. The majority of testicular cancers are of germ cell origin; the most common germinal tumors in adults are seminoma, embryonal carcinoma, teratoma, and choriocarcinoma (the latter three are also called nonseminomas).
2. The etiology of testicular tumors is unknown, but there is a relationship between cryptorchidism (failure of the testes to descend into the scrotum) and tumor occurrence.
3. Testicular tumors metastasize to the retroperitoneal lymph nodes with subsequent involvement of the mediastinal lymph nodes, lungs, and liver.
4. Testicular germ cell tumors are considered potentially curable; seminomas are extremely responsive to radiation therapy, nonseminomas are sensitive to platinum-based chemotherapy.

Clinical Manifestations

1. Painless swelling or enlargement of the testis; accompanied by sensation of heaviness in scrotum
2. Pain in the testis (if patient has epididymitis or bleeding into tumor)
3. Symptoms of metastatic disease: cough, lymphadenopathy, back pain, abdominal mass

Diagnostic Evaluation

1. Elevated serum markers of human chorionic gonadotropin (HCG) and α-fetoprotein (AFP); assay of tumor markers also used for diagnosis, detection of early recurrence, staging, and monitoring response to therapy.
2. Scrotal ultrasonography—identifies location of lesion and differentiates between solid and cystic lesion.
3. Chest film—to seek pulmonary or mediastinal metastases.

4. CT scanning of chest, abdomen, and pelvis—to evaluate retroperitoneal lymph nodes and to follow progress of therapy.

Management

Choice of treatment depends on tumor histology and stage of disease.

A. Surgery
1. Inguinal orchiectomy—removal of testis and its tunica and spermatic cord
2. Retroperitoneal lymph node dissection (RPLND) is usually performed after orchiectomy in nonseminomas for staging and therapeutic purposes.
3. Complications of surgery
   a. RPLND causes infertility due to ejaculatory dysfunction.
   b. Modified nerve-sparing unilateral lymphadenectomy can be done on selected patients, thus preserving ejaculation.
   c. Unilateral orchiectomy eliminates half of germinal cells, thus reducing sperm count.
   d. Libido and ability to attain an erection are preserved.

B. Radiation Therapy
1. Radiation therapy to lymphatic drainage pathways (after orchiectomy in seminomas); cure rate is close to 99%.
2. Other testicle is shielded, usually preserving fertility.

C. Chemotherapy
1. Cisplatin combination therapy is used in treatment of nonseminomatous primary tumor and regional lymphatic metastases and in managing distant metastatic disease.
2. Discomforts of chemotherapy include significant nausea and vomiting, alopecia, myalgia, gastrointestinal cramping, and mucositis.

Complications

1. Infertility; loss of testicle
2. Retrograde ejaculation after retroperitoneal lymphadenectomy
3. Death from metastatic disease

Nursing Assessment

1. Examine testicular mass; ascertain when it was discovered and if it has changed or enlarged since initial discovery.
2. Examine supraclavicular and inguinal lymph nodes for enlargement.
3. Assess for symptoms of metastatic disease.

Nursing Diagnoses

A. Anxiety related to diagnosis of cancer and impending treatments

B. Body Image Disturbance related to loss of testicle and fertility
C. Risk for Injury related to complications of treatment

Nursing Interventions

A. Reducing Anxiety
1. Encourage the younger patient to investigate depositing sperm in sperm bank before surgery.
2. Provide realistic information about impending surgery or treatment; dispel myths associated with testicular disease, emphasize positive cure rates.

B. Preserving Body Image
1. Reassure patient that orchiectomy will not diminish virility, and retroperitoneal lymph node dissection will alter fertility and ejaculation but not libido, erection, and sensation.
2. Advise patient that gel-filled testicular prosthesis can be implanted that will preserve scrotal appearance and feel.
3. Refer the patient to a social worker or counselor as needed for problems and concerns with relationships, peers, or work life.

C. Preventing Complications of Treatment
1. Provide routine postoperative care, including early ambulation, respiratory care, and administration of pain medication.
2. Following RPLND monitor for paralytic ileus, which is common following extensive resection.
   a. Auscultate bowel sounds frequently and observe for abdominal distention.
   b. Withhold oral fluids until bowel sounds have returned.
   c. Report complaints of nausea and any vomiting.
   d. Begin nasogastric decompression, if indicated.
3. For nursing care involving radiation and chemotherapy see pages 102-113.

Patient Education/Health Maintenance

1. Teach all young men to perform monthly testicular self-examination; after orchiectomy patient should examine remaining testicle monthly. See Procedure Guidelines 19-6.
2. Review schedule for radiation treatments or chemotherapy; teach patient and family possible side effects; discuss expectations for treatment period.
3. Provide information about retrograde ejaculation after retroperitoneal lymph node dissection and alternatives for fertility.

Evaluation

A. Verbalizes understanding of treatment and complications
B. No abdominal distention noted
C. Discusses concerns about sexual function with staff and partner

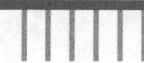

PROCEDURE GUIDELINES 19-6 ◆ Self-Examination for Testicular Tumor

1. The testis is easily accessible for self-examination. Most tumors are palpable and can be detected by self-examination.
2. The hormonally active years (15–35) are the tumor-prone years.

PROCEDURE	ACTION (BY PATIENT)	RATIONALE

1. Examine for testicular tumor periodically, preferably while showering/bathing.

2. Use both hands to palpate (feel). Carefully examine all scrotal contents.

3. Locate the epididymis; this is the irregular cordlike structure on the top and at the back of the testicle that stores and transports sperm. The spermatic cord (and vas) extends upward from the epididymis.
4. Feel each testis between the thumb and first two fingers of each hand.

5. Note size, shape, abnormal tenderness.

6. Stand in front of mirror and look for changes in size/shape of scrotum.

1. Detection of abnormalities is more readily accomplished after or during a warm shower or bath, when the scrotum wall is relaxed.
2. A small lump (nodule) can slip away from one hand. You can feel differences in weight between the testicles by using both hands.
3. It is important to know what the epididymis feels like so you will not confuse it with an abnormality.

4. The testes lie freely in the scrotum, are oval shaped, and measure 4–5 cm in length, 3 cm in width, and about 2 cm in thickness.
5. An abnormality may be felt as a firm area on the front or side of the testicle.
6. It is normal to find one testis larger than the other.

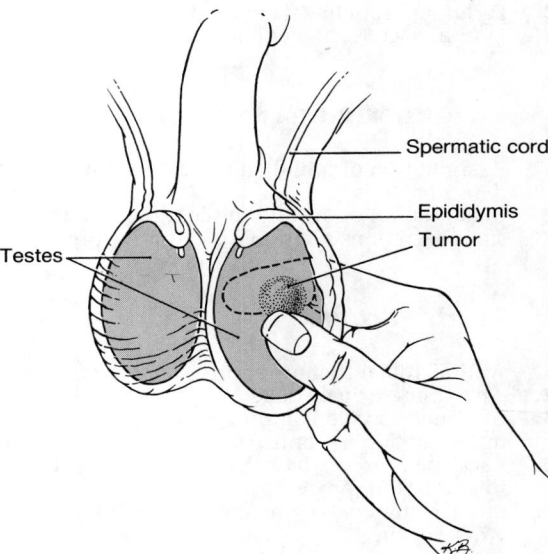

Palpation for testicular tumor. Using the fingertips and thumb, the epididymis, testes, and spermatic cord are located bilaterally.

7. Report any evidence of a small, pea-size lump or other abnormality.

◆ EPIDIDYMITIS

Epididymitis is an infection of the epididymis that usually spreads from the prostate or urinary tract to the epididymis via the ejaculatory duct and vas deferens.

Pathophysiology/Etiology

1. Occurs as a complication of urinary tract infection, urethral stricture disease, bacterial prostatitis, gonococcal or nongonococcal bacterial urethritis.
2. In men under 35, sexually transmitted organisms are the main etiologic agents, usually *C. trachomatis*, and *N. gonorrhoeae*.
3. In homosexual men, *E. coli* is a common cause.
4. In older men, the main causes are bladder outlet obstruction and urinary bacteria (*E. coli, Pseudomonas aeruginosa*)

Clinical Manifestations

1. Localized scrotal pain and tenderness
2. Edema, redness, and tenderness of scrotum
3. Dysuria, frequency, fever, nausea, vomiting
4. Pyuria, bacteriuria, leukocytosis

Diagnostic Evaluation

1. Examination of initial and midstream urine sample to detect bacteria
2. Examination of urethral discharge and expressed prostatic secretions to establish causative organism

Management

1. Antimicrobial therapy after collection of specimens
2. Analgesics for pain relief
3. Intermittent cold compresses to scrotum during acute inflammation to control swelling and for pain relief
4. Local heat or sitz bath later—to hasten resolution of inflammatory process
5. Stool softeners to prevent constipation, which may worsen pain

Complications

1. Spread of infection to testicle—epididymo-orchitis
2. Infertility; risk is greater when bilateral infection

Nursing Assessment

1. Obtain history of STD (or symptoms); urinary tract infection or prostatitis; recent urologic instrumentation or surgery.
2. Perform physical examination of genitals, assess for elevated temperature.

Nursing Diagnosis

A. Pain related to scrotal inflammation

Nursing Interventions

A. *Relieving Pain*
1. Administer or teach self-administration of analgesics as ordered—often NSAIDs or acetaminophen (Tylenol)—assess patient's response.
2. Encourage bed rest during the acute phase.
3. Apply scrotal support to relieve edema and discomfort, to improve venous drainage, and to take tension off the spermatic cord.
   a. Used rolled towel under scrotum or scrotal bridge.
   b. Suggest a cotton-lined athletic supporter for ambulation.
4. Apply ice bags or cool compresses until fever and acute swelling are relieved; then teach patient how to take warm sitz baths and apply heating pad or warm compresses.

Patient Education/Health Maintenance

Instruct the patient as follows:

1. Avoid straining (lifting, defecation, and sexual activity) until infection is under control.
2. Sex partners of patients with chlamydia or gonorrheal urethritis or epididymitis should be examined and treated.
3. It may take 2 to 4 weeks or longer for epididymis to return to normal.
4. Report signs of infection in the reproductive tract immediately to obtain treatment and prevent spread.
5. Obtain follow-up care to ensure complete resolution of infection; uncontrolled infection may impair fertility.
6. Use of condoms prevents further infection associated with sexual activity.

Evaluation

A. Verbalizes relief of pain

◆ GENITAL LESIONS CAUSED BY SEXUALLY TRANSMITTED DISEASES

Genital lesions are ulcerations or other skin or mucous membrane lesions that indicate infection with an STD and may actively shed the infecting organism.

Pathophysiology/Etiology

Causes include:

1. Syphilis—*Treponema pallidum*
2. Chancroid—*Haemophilus ducreyi*
3. Lymphogranuloma venereum (LGV)—specific subtypes of *C. trachomatis*

4. Genital herpes—herpes simplex virus (HSV-2)
5. Condylomata acuminata (genital warts)—specific sub-types of human papillomavirus (HPV)

Clinical Manifestations

See Table 19-3 for clinical manifestations, diagnosis, and treatment of genital lesions.

Patient Education/Health Maintenance

1. Explain transmission of STDs and preventive measures such as male or female condoms, abstinence, and mutual monogomy.
2. Encourage compliance with treatment regimen and follow-up to ensure cure before resuming sexual activity.
3. Explain that some shedding of herpes virus may occur even while asymptomatic, so patient must discuss this with partner; consider use of condoms at all times; and reduce risk of transmission by abstaining at the first sign of an outbreak (tingling sensation) until 1 to 2 weeks following resolution of symptoms.
4. For additional information and support refer to: STD National Hotline 1-800-227-8922 or 8923; (In California 1-800-982-5883).

◆ CARCINOMA OF THE PENIS

Carcinoma of the penis occurs primarily on the glans of the penis; it is frequently associated with poor personal hygiene and the accumulation of smegma under the skin of an uncircumcised penis. It primarily occurs in men over 60 and represents 0.5% of malignancies in men in the United States.

Pathophysiology/Etiology

1. Several types of penile lesions are potentially premalignant.
   a. Condylomata acuminata

TABLE 19-3 Characteristics and Management of Genital Lesions Caused by STDs

Disorder and Incubation	Clinical Manifestations	Diagnosis and Treatment
Herpes Genitalis—5–20 d	Clustered vesicles on erythematous, edematous base that rupture leaving shallow, painful ulcer that eventually crusts; mild regional lymphadenopathy; recurrent and may be brought on by stress, infection, pregnancy, sunburn.	Diagnostic tests include Tzank smear, viral culture, or antigen test of tissue or exudate from lesion. No cure, but symptomatic period is diminished by acyclovir (Zovirax) started with each recurrence; or recurrences greatly reduced or prevented by continuous treatment. Analgesics and sitz baths promote comfort.
Syphilis—10–90 d for primary; up to 6 mo following lesion (chancre) for secondary	Primary: nontender, shallow, indurated, clean ulcer; mild regional lymphadenopathy. Secondary: maculopapular rash including palms and soles, mucous patches, and condalomatous lesions; fever, generalized lymphadenopathy.	VDRL or rapid plasma reagin (RPR) blood test with confirmation by specific treponemal antibody tests. Preferred treatment is benzathine penicillin G (Bicillin LA) 2.4 million units IM in a single dose; Doxycycline (Vibramycin), tetracycline (Tetracyn), and possibly erythromycin (Eryc) may be used.
Chancroid—2–10 d	Vesiculopustule that erodes, leaving a tender, shallow or deep, well circumscribed ulcer with ragged, undermined borders and a friable base covered by purulent exudate; unilateral or bilateral large, tender inguinal lymph nodes (buboes) in 50% of patients.	May be identified on Gram, Giemsa, or Wright stain; must be cultured on special media. Treated with azithromycin (Zithromax), erythromycin (Eryc), or ceftriaxone (Rocephin) IM; Single dose regimens are available. Apply warm soaks to buboes.
LGV—3–21 d	Small, transient, nontender papule or superficial ulcer precedes firm, adherent unilateral inguinal and femoral lymph nodes (buboes) with characteristic groove in between (groove sign); may suppurate.	Microimmunofluorescence testing of bubo aspirate. Treatment of choice is doxycycline (Vibramycin), but erythromycin (Eryc) may be effective. Incision and excision of buboes should be avoided; aspiration may be helpful.
Condyloma acuminatum—3 wk to 3 mo, possibly years before grossly visible	Single or multiple, soft, fleshy, flat or vegetating growth(s) may occur on penis, anal area, urethra; no lymphadenopathy.	Diagnosed by Pap smear or biopsy. Topical therapy with podofilox 0.5% (Condylox) for external warts, podophyllin 10–25% solution, or trichloroacetic acid 80–90% (TCA)—may require multiple applications. Cryotherapy, electrodissection, electrocautery, carbon dioxide laser, and surgical excision may also be done. Recurrence is common.

b. Giant condylomata acuminata (Buschke-Lowenstein's tumor)
c. Erythroplasia of the glans (Queyrat's erythroplasia)
d. Leukoplakia
2. Lesions that ulcerate metastasize quickly to the regional inguinal and iliac lymph nodes.
3. Distant metastases occurs in the abdominal lymph nodes, liver, and lungs.

Clinical Manifestations

1. Disease process begins with a painless, wartlike growth or ulcer on the glans or coronal sulcus under the prepuce.
2. Phimosis (constriction of foreskin with inability to retract over glans) is present in approximately 50% of patients.
3. Lymphadenopathy; secondary infection of lesions

Diagnostic Evaluation

1. Biopsy of penile lesion and inguinal lymph nodes
2. Chest x-ray, bone scan, and CT scan (or MRI) to assess for metastases

Management

1. Localized lesions are surgically removed by partial penectomy, laser therapy or Moh's microresection; total penectomy with perineal urethroplasty is necessary for more involved tumors.
2. After other causes of lymphadenopathy are ruled out, bilateral inguinal lymphadenectomy may be performed.
3. Radiation therapy to primary lesion and lymph nodes may control the disease.

Complications

1. Disfigurement due to ulceration or treatment
2. Complications of lymphadenectomy—necrosis and infection of skin flap, chronic edema of lower extremities

Nursing Assessment

1. Obtain history of current lesion, history of STDs, and hygiene.
2. Perform genital examination for characteristics of lesion, phimosis, inguinal lymph node enlargement.

Nursing Diagnoses

A. Fear related to diagnosis of cancer
B. Body Image Disturbance related to partial or total penectomy

Nursing Interventions

A. *Resolving Fears*
1. Provide patient with opportunity to acquire information about causes and prognosis of disease.
2. Interpret diagnostic and staging results to patient.
3. Encourage realistic expectations regarding outcome of treatment.

B. *Enhancing Coping With Body Image Changes*
1. Maintain a nonjudgmental approach; allow patient to ventilate feelings about loss of part or all of penis.
2. Provide routine postoperative care confidently, watching for bleeding, monitoring urination, and anticipating pain.
3. Provide opportunity for patient to discuss alternate methods of sexual expression with knowledgeable professional.
   a. About 40% of patients are able to participate in sexual activity and stand to void after partial penectomy.
4. Monitor patient for symptoms of depression requiring intervention.

Patient Education/Health Maintenance

1. Instruct the uncircumcised patient about proper hygiene—importance of daily removal of all retained smegma.
2. Explain expected postoperative function of the penis in patient undergoing partial penectomy.
3. Describe how voiding will occur to the patient undergoing perineal urethroplasty.
4. Provide information about follow-up and monitoring for recurrences; or radiation and chemotherapy as appropriate.

Evaluation

A. Verbalizes understanding and acceptance of diagnosis and treatment plan
B. Discusses feelings and interest in seeking counseling

Selected References

American Cancer Society. (1993). *Cancer facts and figures 1993*. Atlanta: Author.
Boyd, S. D., Lieskovsky, G., & Skinner, D. G. (1991). Kock pouch bladder replacement. *Urologic Clinics of North America, 18,* 641-648.
Cavas, M., & Makay, S. (1991). The Indiana pouch: A continent urinary diversion system. *AORN Journal, 54*(3), 494-519.
Doughty, D. B. (Ed.). (1991). *Urinary and fecal incontinence: Nursing management.* St. Louis: Mosby-Year Book. 1991.
Gillenwater, J. Y., et al. (1990). *Adult and pediatric urology* (2nd ed., Vols. 1 & 2). Chicago: Year Book Medical Publishers.
Graham-Macaluso, M. (1991). Complications of peritoneal dialysis: Nursing care plans to document teaching. *ANNA Journal, 18,* 479-483.
Gray, M. L. (1992). *Genitourinary disorders.* St. Louis: Mosby-Year Book.

Hampton, B. G., & Bryant, R. A. (Eds.). (1992). *Ostomies and continent diversions: Nursing management.* St. Louis: Mosby-Year Book.

Hanno, P. M., & Wein, A. J. (1994). *A clinical manual of urology.* New York: McGraw-Hill.

Lassen, P. M., & Thompson, I. M. (1994). Treatment options for prostate cancer. *Urologic Nursing, 14*(1), 12-17.

McConnell, J. D., Barry, M. J., Bruskewitz, R. C., et al. (1994). *Benign prostatic hyperplasia: Diagnosis and treatment.* Clinical Practice Guideline, Number 8. AHCPR Publication No. 94-0582. Rockville, MD: Agency for Health Care Policy and Research, Public Health Service, US Department of Health and Human Services.

Mellinger, B. C. (1994). Human papillomavirus in the male: An overview. *AUA Update Series, 13*(13), 102-107.

Moore, S., Kuhrik, M., Shea, L., & Kuhrik, N. (1992). Nerve-sparing prostatectomy. *American Journal of Nursing, 92,* 59-64.

Rauscher, J., Farber, R. D., & Parra, R. O. (1992). Kock pouch: An internal ileal reservoir for continent urinary diversion. *AORN Journal, 56*(4), 666-678.

Reilly, N. J. (1994). Advances in quality of life after cystectomy: Urinary diversions. *Innovations in Urology Nursing, 5*(2), 17-22, 31-35.

Reilly, N. J. (1992). Urinary incontinence: New attitudes and treatment options. *Innovations in Urology Nursing, 3*(2), 1-4, 6, 15.

Rowland, R. G. (1990, Jan/Feb). A straightforward approach to urinary diversion. *Contemporary Urology,* 13-19.

Russell, K. J., & Blasko, J. C. (1993). Recent advances in interstitial brachytherapy for localized prostate cancer. *Problems in Urology, 7*(2), 260-278.

Sueppel, C. A. (1993). Postoperative pain in the adult urologic patient. *Innovations in Urology Nursing, 4*(1), 1, 15.

Switters, D. M., Soares, S. E., & de Vere White, R. W. (1992). Nursing care of the patient receiving intravesical chemotherapy. *Urologic Nursing, 12*(4), 136-139.

Thompson, J. M., McFarland, G. K., Hirsch, J. E., & Tucker, S. M. (Eds.). (1993). *Mosby's clinical nursing.* St. Louis: Mosby-Year Book.

Urinary Incontinence Guideline Panel. (1992). *Urinary incontinence in adults: Clinical practice guideline.* AHCPR Publication No. 92-0038. Rockville, MD: Agency for Health Care Policy and Research, Public Health Service, US Department of Health and Human Services.

Walsh, P. C., et al. (1992). *Campbell's urology* (6th ed., Vols. 1-3). Philadelphia: W. B. Saunders.

Winfield, H. N. (1993). Laparoscopic pelvic lymph node dissection for urologic pelvic malignancies. *Atlas of the Urologic Clinics of North America, 1*(2), 33-47.

Wozniak-Petrofsky, J. (1991). BPH: Treating older men's most common problem. *RN Magazine, 54*(7), 32-37.

CHAPTER 20 ◆

Gynecologic Disorders

General Overview

◆ THE MENSTRUAL CYCLE

The menstrual cycle is the the cyclical pattern of ovarian hormone secretion (estrogen and progesterone) under the control of pituitary hormones (luteinizing hormone [LH] and follicle-stimulating hormone [FSH]) that results in thickening of the uterine endometrium, ovulation, and menstruation. Cycle length varies among individuals.

Phases of the Menstrual Cycle

1. Menstrual or bleeding phase—day 1 of cycle; endometrial sloughing and discharge
2. Postmenstrual phase—4 to 5 days after period ends; thin endometrium
3. Proliferative phase—approximately 14 days before onset of next menstrual period, estrogen increases thickness of endometrium; includes ovulation, the expulsion of ovum from ovary.
4. Secretory phase—approximately days 16 to 23; corpus luteum forms and then regresses unless pregnancy occurs; thick endometrium due to increased progesterone.
5. Premenstrual phase—days 24 to 28; levels of LH and FSH fall due to increased levels of estrogen and progesterone.

Characteristics of Menstruation

Characteristics of Menstruation

Characteristic	Range	Average
Menarche (onset)	9–17 years of age	12.5 years
Cycle length	24–32 days	29 days
Flow—duration	1–8 days	3–5 days
Flow—amount	10–75 mL	35 mL
Menopause—onset	45–55 years of age	47–50

Assessment

◆ SUBJECTIVE DATA

Explore the patient's symptoms and perform a complete history to elicit important data such as the following.

Irregular Bleeding

1. Characteristics—What is the frequency, duration, and amount of flow? What is the color and consistency of blood? What are the size of clots? Any bleeding or spotting between periods, postmenopausal bleeding, or pain with bleeding? What was age at menarche? menopause?
2. Associated factors—What is the pregnancy and childbirth history? Is the patient sexually active? What method of contraception is used? Is the patient taking hormone replacement or oral contraceptives? Is the patient obese?
3. History—Any history of tumors or malignancy? Any family history of breast or ovarian cancer?
4. Significance—May indicate infection of the vagina or cervix; malignancy of the vulva, vagina, cervix or uterus; benign tumor of the uterus or ovarian cyst; pregnancy; endometriosis.

Vaginal Discharge

1. Characteristics—What is the color, amount, duration of the discharge? Any odor, itching, urinary symptoms, pain, fever, dyspareunia?
2. Associated factors—What is the sexual history, such as how many partners, what type of sexual activity, any symptoms in partner? Is barrier method of contraception used? Is patient menopausal or postmenopausal? On estrogen replacement? Any recent use of antibiotics?

3. History—Any history of sexually transmitted diseases (STDs)? Diabetes?
4. Significance—May indicate vaginitis, human papillomavirus (HPV), herpes simplex virus (HSV), pelvic inflammatory disease (PID), or genital malignancy.

Pelvic Pain

1. Characteristics—What is frequency, duration, severity, location of pain? What aggravates and what relieves it? Does it feel like heaviness in the pelvis?
2. Associated factors—Any fever, nausea, abnormal bleeding along with it? Has there been weight loss? Using any estrogen preparations? Is patient infertile?
3. History—Any history of STDs? Obstetric trauma or abdominal surgery?
4. Significance—May indicate condition arising from relaxed pelvic muscles, PID, endometriosis, cervical or uterine cancer.

◆ PHYSICAL EXAMINATION

Physical examination for a patient with a gynecologic disorder should focus on the abdomen and genitalia. Palpate the lower abdomen for any masses or tenderness. Inspect the external genitalia for any lesions, discharge, or tissue bulging from the vagina.

The nurse in a gynecologic or obstetric setting may perform a vaginal examination to obtain specimens for diagnostic studies as well as assess the patient's condition. See Procedure Guidelines 20-1.

Diagnostic Tests

Diagnostic tests for gynecologic disorders include a variety of laboratory tests, radiology or imaging studies, and office or ambulatory surgery procedures. Women with some gynecologic disorders such as endometriosis may undergo multiple invasive and surgical procedures to fully evaluate the problem.

PROCEDURE GUIDELINES 20-1 ◆ Vaginal Examination by the Nurse

EQUIPMENT

Perineal drape
Vaginal specula
Water-soluble lubricant
Sterile gloves

Long swab sticks
Pap smear equipment
Adequate lighting

PROCEDURE

PREPARATORY PHASE

1. Have the patient void before assistant positions her on examining table.
2. Position the patient on examining table (slip may be kept on, but other clothing from wait to knees is removed).
   a. Have buttocks at edge of table.
   b. Position feet in stirrups to assume dorsal lithotomy position.
   c. Make the patient as comfortable as possible with a small pillow under her head.
   d. Drape the patient to permit minimal exposure (but adequate for examiner).
3. Encourage the patient to relax; tell her what you are doing and what she may feel.
4. Adjust light for maximum focus.
5. Offer the patient a mirror to watch the examination in order to teach vulvar self-examination and about contraceptives as appropriate.

NURSING ACTION	*RATIONALE*
PERFORMANCE PHASE	
1. Be gentle and take your time; wash hands; don sterile gloves; lubricate fingers.	1. This promotes relaxation of the patient, making the procedure easier for both.
2. Observe external genitalia for apparent abnormalities, gently separate labia and continue visual inspection.	2. Note any evidence of irritation, infection, or abnormalities such as swelling, bleeding, erythema, discharge (other than clear and odorless).
3. To encourage relaxation in the patient, gently place the tip of one or two fingers into introitus.	3. Say to the patient, ''Tighten your muscles and squeeze my fingers—try hard—then relax.''
4. Identify cervix manually and depress the perneum downward with your fingers.	4. Downward pressure is away from the more sensitive anterior structures.
5. Lubricate speculum with warm water.	5. Any lubricant other than water may interfere with cytology results.
6. Gently insert warm speculum horizontally, passing it over your fingers and aiming it toward the cervix.	6. If it is preferred not to initially insert gloved fingers, the speculum is introduced vertically using a downward pressure; after entering the vestibule, the speculum is slowly rotated to the horizontal position.

(continued)

PROCEDURE GUIDELINES 20-1 ◆ Vaginal Examination by the Nurse
(continued)

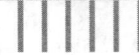

PROCEDURE (cont'd)	NURSING ACTION	RATIONALE

NURSING ACTION

7. Slowly open the speculum and lock into position. With slow manipulation, the speculum can be turned to permit visualization of the vaginal walls.
8. Inspect the cervix, which should be pink. Normally, the os is a dent, unless the woman has had children, in which case a slit is noted.

9. If Pap test is to be done, following procedure in accompanying figure.

RATIONALE

7. Walls normally are pink and moist. A pale white secretion may be noted.

8. If woman is taking an oral contraceptive, the cervix may be deep pink to red. A thread coming out of the cervix would suggest presence of an intrauterine device (IUD). Abnormal cervical signs include erosion, lacerations, and polyps.

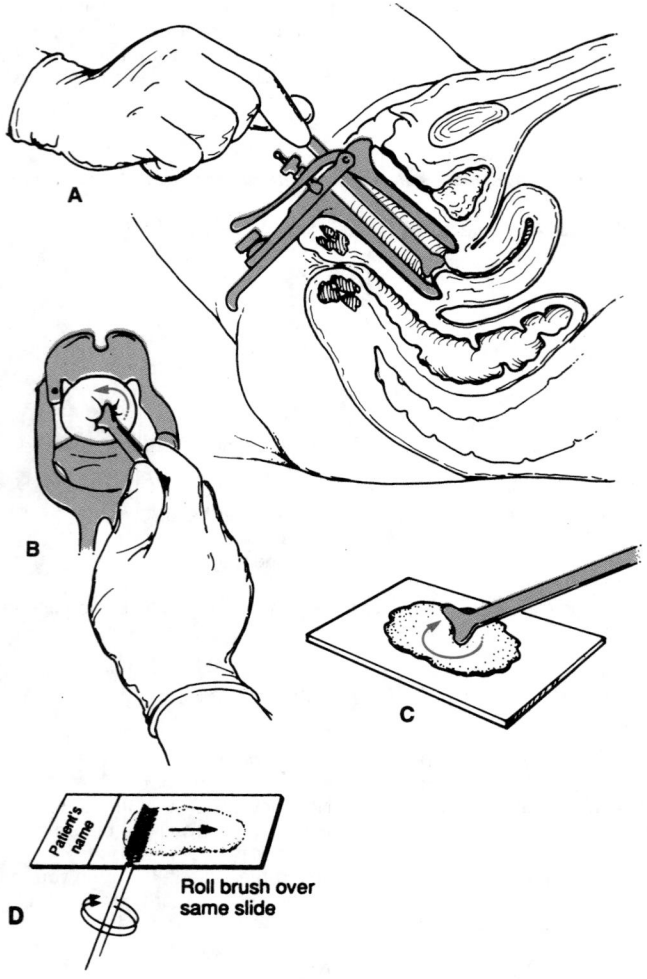

A cervical scrape of secretions for cytology is obtained by using a wooden Ayre spatula. (**A**) Shows the speculum in place: the Ayre spatula is inserted so that the longer end is placed snugly in the os. (**B**) A representative sample of secretions is obtained by rotating the spatula. (**C**) Cervical secretions are gently smeared on a glass slide in a single circular motion. (**D**) A cytobrush is rotated within the cervical os and smeared onto a glass slide. The slide is placed in the appropriate fixative immediately.

10. If indicated, swab cervix with Schiller's iodine solution to detect epithelial change. Or, swab vagina and cervix with acetic acid solution to detect lesions caused by human papilloma virus.

10. Cancer epithelium contains no glycogen and will not absorb iodine as normal epithelium will. Human papillomavirus lesions will be differentiated from normal epithelium by aceto-whitening.

PROCEDURE   *NURSING ACTION*   *RATIONALE*
(cont'd)

11. When removing speculum, hold it open until cervix is cleared, then withdraw speculum downward, applying pressure to posterior vaginal wall and allowing speculum to close as it is withdrawn.

11. By the time speculum is completely withdrawn, it will be closed.

12. For palpation (bimanual examination), see accompanying figure.

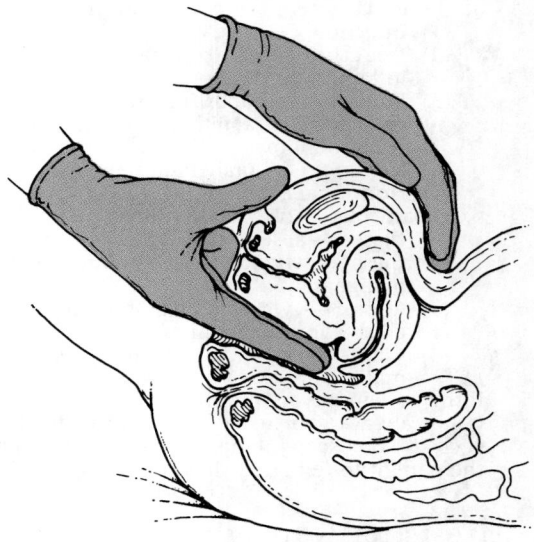

Bimanual examination of the pelvic organs.

FOLLOW-UP PHASE

1. Gently wipe the perineal area with soft tissue or gauze, using firm strokes from the pubic area back to beyond the rectum.

2. Instruct assistant in carefully helping the patient to remove feet from stirrups.

3. Elevate the lower third of the examining table to receive legs. Keep the patient covered with a sheet.

4. Assist the patient in sliding toward head end of table; provide a wide-based stool for her to step on as she gets off table.

5. Assist the patient in dressing if necessary. Answer any queries she may have.

1. This will remove secretions and liquid lubricant.

2. Both feet must be removed at the same time to reduce strain.

3. This permits the patient to assume dorsal recumbent position.

4. Do not rush the patient as she is getting off the table, as sudden shifting from recumbent to sitting position may cause a feeling of dizziness.

◆ LABORATORY TESTS

CA125

A. Description Tumor antigen used as a marker for ovarian cancer

B. Nursing/Patient Care Considerations
1. Tell patient that a blood test will be taken and the results will be ready in 1 to 3 days.
2. This is not a screening test for ovarian cancer; it is better measure of response to treatment.
3. Level may be elevated in benign gynecologic disease, hepatic cirrhosis, and in healthy women.

Cervical Cytology

A. Description A Papanicolaou smear of the cervix is obtained during pelvic examination to screen for cervical dysplasia or cancer. May also detect endometrial cancer, infections, and endocrine status

B. Nursing/Patient Care Considerations
1. Should not be performed during menses.
2. Instruct the patient to avoid douching for 24 hours before the examination—cellular deposits might wash away.

3. Recommend regular screening based on established guidelines.
   a. American College of Obstetrics and Gynecology and Planned Parenthood—annually; after hysterectomy, every 3 to 5 years if hysterectomy was not for cancer.
   b. American Cancer Society—every 3 years after two negative smears, may stop at age 65 if not high risk.
4. Classification by Bethesda system (preferred) or Papanicolaou number system
   a. Bethesda system (descriptive diagnosis)
      (1) Infection
      (2) Reactive and reparative changes (ie, inflammation)
      (3) Epithelial cell abnormalities (including atypia, squamous intraepithelial lesion, and squamous cell carcinoma)
      (4) Nonepithelial malignant neoplasm
      (5) Hormonal evaluation
   b. Papanicolaou (original classification system)
      (1) Class 1—absence of atypical or abnormal cells
      (2) Class 2—atypical cytology but no evidence of malignancy
      (3) Class 3—cytology suggestive of, but not conclusive for, malignancy
      (4) Class 4—cytology strongly suggestive of malignancy
5. If the patient has an abnormal smear, explain that this is not always conclusive but requires further testing such as colposcopy, biopsy, or conization. Encourage the patient to return for further testing.

Tests for Gonorrhea and Chlamydia

A. Description
1. Commonly known as DNA probe or antigen detection tests, a single specimen can detect both STD-causing organisms. Will detect even subclinical infection; can be used as screening test.
2. Can also be done by culture method, but takes longer and requires special processing of the specimen.

B. Nursing/Patient Care Considerations
1. Explain the procedure to the patient before taking the specimen.
2. Specimens should be taken from the woman without douching for 24 hours, from the man before urinating.
3. Obtain specimen with Dacron-tipped swab from cervical discharge in woman, urethral meatus in man. Small-tipped swabs are available for the urethra.
4. Send swab to laboratory in provided container with preservative.

◆ RADIOLOGY/IMAGING
Hysterosalpingogram

A. Description
1. This fluoroscopic x-ray study of the uterus and fallopian tubes is used to determine tubal patency, detect pathology in the uterine cavity, and identify peritoneal adhesions.
2. A bivalve speculum is introduced while the patient is in the lithotomy position and contrast medium is injected into the uterine cavity; contrast medium will enter the peritoneum in 10 to 15 minutes if tubes are patent.

B. Nursing/Patient Care Considerations
1. Determine date of last menstrual period—test is done a few days after menses ends, before ovulation.
2. Administer enema before procedure to decrease intestinal gas.
3. Administer prescribed medication to reduce anxiety.
4. After procedure, apply perineal pad for drainage of excess contrast medium or blood and instruct patient to notify health care provider if bloody drainage continues after 3 days or if any signs of infection are present.
5. Inform the patient that pain medication may be necessary for shoulder discomfort due to dye irritation of the phrenic nerve.

Pelvic Ultrasonography

A. Description A noninvasive test that uses high-frequency sound waves to form images of the interior pelvic cavity; used to detect uterine, tubal, ovarian, and pelvic cavity pathology, measure organ size, and evaluate pregnancy

B. Nursing/Patient Care Considerations
1. Inform patient that a full bladder is necessary to discriminate the bladder from the uterus, so not to void for several hours before the procedure.
2. Following the procedure, help the patient wipe off ultrasound gel from abdomen and allow her to empty her bladder.
3. Abnormalities are represented as different densities that differentiate solid from cystic masses and can help make a diagnosis; however, explain to the patient that further testing may be necessary.

◆ OTHER DIAGNOSTIC TESTS
Colposcopy

A. Description Examination of the cervix with a bright light and magnification of 10 to 40 times; done to determine distribution of abnormal squamous epithelium and to pinpoint areas from which biopsy tissue can be taken

B. Nursing/Patient Care Considerations
1. Procedure is preferably done when cervix is least vascular (usually a week after the end of the menstrual flow).
2. Explain nature of procedure to patient and tell her that no anesthesia will be needed because the cervix lacks pain receptors.
3. Help patient into lithotomy position, drape her appropriately, and provide emotional support throughout the procedure. Provide distraction techniques such as music and posters (hung on the ceiling) as appropriate.
4. Biopsy tissue is preserved in 10% formalin, labeled, and sent to the laboratory. Suturing and packing may be necessary if bleeding occurs.
5. After procedure, assist patient in rising slowly and give the following discharge instructions:
   a. Avoid heavy lifting for 24 hours.
   b. Packing will remain in place for 12 to 24 hours.
   c. There may be some bleeding; however, more than that of a normal period must be reported to health care provider.
   d. Obtain health care provider's instructions regarding douching and sexual relations.

Conization

A. Description Excision of a cone-shaped piece of tissue from the cervix for diagnostic and therapeutic purposes, including the area where the squamous and columnar epithelial tissue meet (transformation zone). The transformation zone is the area of most cervical cancers

B. Nursing/Patient Care Considerations
1. Explain to the patient that this test is a minor surgical procedure requiring local anesthesia.
2. Following excision, bleeding is controlled by cauterization or suturing and packing.
3. The patient may be observed for several hours after the procedure.
4. Advise the patient to avoid tampons, douching, and intercourse for 2 weeks.

Culdoscopy

A. Description Operative procedure in which an incision is made through the perineum into the posterior vaginal cul-de-sac so that a culdoscope can be inserted to visualize the uterus, tubes, broad ligaments, uterosacral ligaments, rectal wall, sigmoid, and even the small intestine

B. Nursing/Patient Care Considerations
1. Prepare patient as for any vagnial surgery.
2. Explain to patient that she will receive either local, general, or regional anesthesia and that she will be helped into the knee–chest position.
3. Following the procedure, the scope is withdrawn and sutures are placed.
4. The patient will be observed for several hours; make sure follow-up instructions have been given by the health care provider.

Hysteroscopy

A. Description Endoscopic visualization of the uterine cavity used to stage endometrial cancer, check tubal patency, determine the cause of uterine bleeding, remove polyps or fibroids, and observe the placement/appearance of interuterine devices (IUDs)

B. Nursing/Patient Care Considerations
1. Administer prescribed sedative before the procedure and explain that a local anesthetic will also be injected into the cervix in the operating room.
2. The patient will be assisted into lithotomy position and the perineum and vagina will be cleansed immediately before sterile draping.
3. Explain that sounds are inserted into the cervical canal for dilation before insertion of the hysteroscope. With the scope in place, a concentrated solution of dextran is slowly infused into the endometrial cavity to distend it and allow for viewing.
4. Observe patient for several hours and give discharge instructions.
   a. Over-the-counter analgesics may be needed for minor discomfort if analgesic has not been prescribed.
   b. Notify the health care provider of severe cramping or bleeding.

Endometrial Biopsy

A. Description
1. Procedure is done with local anesthetic to obtain cells from the uterine lining to assist in the diagnosis of endometrial cancer, menstrual disorders, and infertility.
2. During speculum examination, a uterine sound is placed, followed by a curet or suction device to withdraw specimen.

B. Nursing/Patient Care Considerations
1. Assist patient into dorsal lithotomy position and explain procedure.
2. Administer prostaglandin inhibitor to decrease uterine cramping postoperatively.
3. Label specimen, place in formalin, and send to laboratory.
4. Inform patient that she may experience light bleeding and occasional cramping for a few days.
5. Instruct patient to report fever, chills, and increased bleeding.

Dilation and Curettage

A. Description
1. This common gynecologic surgery for diagnostic and therapeutic purposes consists of widening of the cervical canal with a dilator and scraping the uterine cavity with a curet.
2. Performed to control uterine bleeding, secure endometrial and endocervical tissue for cytologic examination, and treat incomplete abortion.

B. Nursing/Patient Care Considerations
1. Prepare the patient for the procedure by answering questions, requesting that she void, administering an enema if ordered, and administering a sedative as directed.
2. Immediately postoperatively, monitor vital signs at frequent intervals—potential for hemorrhage exists.
3. Monitor perineal pads/bed for amount of bleeding; report excessive bleeding.
4. Offer prescribed analgesics for low back and pelvic pain; cramping may occur for 2 to 3 days due to dilation of the cervix.
5. Instruct patient to maintain bed rest for remainder of day to decrease cramping and bleeding.
6. Instruct patient to use perineal pads at home and to report fever, heavy bleeding, and severe cramping.
7. Instruct patient to avoid strenuous activity until bleeding stops.
8. Discuss with patient that the procedure does not affect sexual functioning, but that she should refrain from sexual intercourse, douching, and tampons for at least 2 weeks, according to preference of health care provider.

Laparoscopy

A. Description Endoscopic visualization of the pelvic and abdominal cavities through a small incision below the umbilicus; used to evaluate pelvic pain and infertility, treat endometriosis adhesions, and perform tubal sterilizations (the most common use)

B. *Nursing/Patient Care Considerations*
1. Prepare patient by ensuring that she has remained NPO, answering questions about the procedure, and administering a sedative and enema if ordered.
2. Inform patient that she may experience shoulder or abdominal discomfort after the procedure from the injection of carbon dioxide given to separate the intestines from pelvic organs.
3. Patient will receive local, general, or regional anesthesia, and be placed in Trendelenberg position to displace the intestines for better visualization.
4. Following procedure, monitor bleeding and vital signs, administer analgesics.
5. Inform patient that passing gas and bowel movements may be difficult initially due to the manipulation of the intestines; ambulation and fluids will be helpful.
6. Advise patient not to have intercourse or perform strenuous activity for 2 to 3 days and to report bleeding, cramping, or fever.

General Procedures/Treatment Modalities

◆ FERTILITY CONTROL

Nurses working with women in the gynecologic setting or in any setting may be involved in contraceptive counseling.

Basic Principles

1. *Contraception* is the prevention of fertility on a temporary basis.
2. *Sterilization* is the permanent prevention of fertility. Both female and male sterilization procedures can be performed. Some procedures can be reversed but with possible complications and variable success rates.
3. Contraception effectiveness depends on motivation, which is a result of education, culture, religion, and personal situation. It is best to include both partners in any contraception decision.
4. Nurses should be familiar with contraceptive methods and educate patients without moral judgment.
5. Failure rate (pregnancy) is determined by experience of 100 women for 1 year and is expressed as pregnancies per 100 woman-years.

Contraceptive Methods

See Table 20-1.

Sterilization Procedures

A. *General Considerations*
1. Tubal sterilization is frequently performed for birth control. Hysterectomy or oophorectomy, performed for other reasons, also results in sterility.
2. Male sterilization by vasectomy has also become increasingly common.

3. Informed consent is needed. The couple should be thoroughly counseled about the permanence of the procedure.

B. *Tubal Sterilization*
1. Approaches
   a. Abdominal—most frequently used: may be postpartum laparotomy, minilaparotomy, or laparoscopy. Laparoscopy with electrocoagulation is frequently performed. It is a safe and effective procedure.
   b. Vaginal—incision in posterior vagina (colpotomy) with the uterine tube pulled through it; higher rate of complications—infection.
2. Techniques—vary by surgeon preference
   a. Electrocoagulation—most common; burn section of tube with or without excision; low reversal rate
   b. Pomeroy—tube tied in midsection and section removed; may be reversed
   c. Fimbriectomy—fimbriated end removed and end tied; irreversible
   d. Cornual resection—remove section of tube nearest uterus and suture cornual opening closed
   e. Silastic bands—plastic or metal clips to occlude tube; may be reversed
3. Complications
   a. Failure to successfully block the tubes—pregnancy or tubal pregnancy
   b. Hemorrhage, infection, uterine perforation, damage to bowel or bladder
4. Nursing interventions
   a. Assess motivation for sterilization and level of knowledge about the procedure. Counsel as necessary.
   b. Teach patient that there is no effect on hormones and menstruation will continue.
   c. Teach patient that there should not be any adverse effect on sexual response.
   d. Other birth control methods are discontinued immediately before the procedure.
   e. Prepare the patient to expect some abdominal soreness for several days but to report any bleeding, increasing pain, or fever.
   f. Sexual intercourse and strenuous activity should be avoided for 2 weeks.

Contraceptive Research

1. Vaginal rings that release progestin may be available. Placed around the cervix, vaginal rings may be effective for 3 months, are removed during coitus, and require careful vaginal hygiene. Other implantable hormones in various delivery systems to provide contraception for several months to several years are being developed to rival Norplant.
2. RU-486 (Mifepristone) is a progesterone antagonist that prevents implantation and leads to menses. Administered by mouth within 10 days of an expected period, it produces a medical abortion in most patients. If combined with a prostaglandin suppository, it causes an abortion in up to 95% of patients up to 5 weeks after conception.
3. Birth control vaccines are being developed to interfere with hormones and sperm antigens to prevent pregnancy. A male vaccine to interfere with spermatogenesis is a possibility.

TABLE 20-1 Contraceptive Methods

Methods	Definition	Procedure	Advantages	Disadvantages
Natural Methods				
1. Periodic abstinence	Abstain from intercourse during fertile period of each cycle.	Determine fertile period by: 1. Calendar method—ovulation occurs 14 d before next menstrual period. 2. Cervical mucus method—increase in mucus at time of ovulation; clear and stringy. 3. Basal body temperature—drops immediately before ovulation and rises 24–72 h after ovulation 4. Symptothermal method—combines 2 & 3.	1. No health hazards 2. Inexpensive 3. Religiously acceptable 4. Increased knowledge of cycles	1. 20% failure rate 2. Requires consistent record-keeping
2. Coitus interruptus	Withdrawal of penis from vagina when ejaculation is imminent.	Must withdraw before ejaculation so that ejaculation occurs away from female genitalia.	1. No cost 2. No health hazards 3. Always available	1. Failure rate of 19%; preejaculatory fluid may contain sperm. 2. Interruption of sexual act
3. Lactation	Breast-feeding has a contraceptive effect due to prolactin's inhibition of luteinizing hormone, which maintains menstruation.	Breast-feed on demand, around the clock, without formula supplementation.	1. No health hazards 2. No cost	1. Unreliable 2. Need to use other method such as spermicide or barrier, which have no effect on breast milk.
Barrier Methods				
1. Condom	Rubber or processed collagenous tissue sheaths, placed over erect penis to prevent semen from entering vagina Note: female condom is also available.	1. Place condom over erect penis. 2. Leave dead space at tip of condom (from which air has been expelled) to allow room for ejaculate. 3. Use spermicide on exterior for added protection. 4. Grasp ring around condom at withdrawal to avoid leaving condom in vagina.	1. Failure rate is low with proper use (3%) 2. Prevention of STD 3. Inexpensive 4. No health hazard 5. May help premature ejaculation by decreasing sensitivity 6. Increases male involvement in contraception	1. Decreased sensitivity 2. Interruption of sexual act 3. Sensitivity to rubber may be a problem. 4. Failure rate with typical use is 12%
2. Diaphragm	Rubber cap shaped like a dome with a flexible rim	1. Check for holes. 2. Place spermicide inside dome. 3. Place diaphragm against and covering cervical opening, behind lower edge of pubic bone. 4. Leave in place for at least 6 h after intercourse.	1. Failure rate with perfect use is 6%; 18% with typical use. 2. Protection against STDs and possibly cervical neoplasia	1. Occasional toxic shock or allergic reactions 2. May experience pelvic discomfort
3. Cervical cap	Rubber cap, shaped like a cup with a tall dome and flexible rim.	Place spermicide inside cap and place cap over cervical opening prior to intercourse.	1. Failure rate similar to diaphragm 2. May decrease risk of STDs	1. Risk of TSS, cervicitis, and PID 2. Requires frequent followup.

(continued)

TABLE 20-1 Contraceptive Methods *(continued)*

Methods	Definition	Procedure	Advantages	Disadvantages
Spermicides	Nonoxynol-9 or octoxynol-9 available in a variety of forms: foam, jelly, cream, suppository, tablet	Place next to cervix before intercourse; better if used with a barrier method.	May kill STD agents	1. Less effective if not used with barrier method; generally 21% failure rate 2. Some patients are allergic. 3. May cause birth defects if pregnancy results
Intrauterine Devices	Small device made of plastic with exposed copper or progesterone-release system; acts to inhibit uterine wall implantation.	1. Physician inserts device; slowly and usually at time of menses. 2. Check IUD string regularly—at least once a month—or after each intercourse when it is first inserted.	1. Failure rate low, 2% or less 2. Convenient; permits spontaneous intercourse 3. Replaced every 1–6 y	1. Risk of PID and resultant tubal damage and infertility 2. May cause spotting, bleeding, or pain 3. Risk of spontaneous abortion 4. Risk of uterine rupture
Hormones 1. Combination oral contraceptives	Tablets containing estrogen to inhibit ovulation and progestin to make cervical mucus impenetrable to sperm—lowest effective doses are used.	Take for 21 d with 7 d off or 28 d (if 7 d of placebos are included).	1. As low as 0.1% failure rate 2. Decreased risk of endometriosis, ovarian and endometrial cancer, benign breast disease 3. Possible decreased risk of PID 4. Aid in menstrual disorders 5. Improves acne	1. Increased risk of cardiovascular disease (higher in women who smoke) 2. Questionable risk of breast, cervical cancer 3. May experience nausea, vomiting, headache, weight gain 4. Must remember to take at same time daily.
2. Progestin-only oral contraceptive (Mini-pill)	Smaller doses of progestins than in combined oral contraceptives	Take every day.	1. As low as 0.5% failure rate. 2. Avoids estrogen-related side effects and possibly cardiovascular risks 3. May offer protection against PID	1. May cause irregular menses, spotting, amenorrhea
3. Postcoital contraception (Morning-after pill)	May be combined estrogen and progestin, high-dose estrogen, or progestin	Must be started within 24–72 h after intercourse.	1. Very effective	1. May be religiously opposed 2. Not FDA-approved for postcoital method 3. May cause birth defects
4. Progesterone implant (Nor-plant).	Progesterone release system made up of five silastic rods.	Implanted in subcutaneous fat of upper arm.	1. Long-term (up to 5 y) 2. Convenient 3. Only 0.9% failure rate	1. May cause irregular bleeding, spotting, amenorrhea, acne, headaches 2. May be difficult to remove 3. High initial expense
5. Progesterone injection (Depo-Provera).	Intramuscular injection of long acting progesterone	Initial injection within first 5 d of menses, then every 3 months	1. Convenient 2. Only 0.3% failure rate	1. Requires every 3-month follow-up 2. May cause irregular bleeding, spotting, amenorrhea

PROCEDURE GUIDELINES 20-2 ◆ Vaginal Irrigation

EQUIPMENT Sterile reservoir for irrigating fluid—can or bag.
Sterile irrigating fluid as prescribed (1,000–4,000 mL) at
40.5°–43.3°C (105°–110°F)
Tubing, connecting tubes, and clamp (sterile)
Irrigating vaginal nozzle (sterile)

Bedpan or douche pan
Waterproof pad
Sterile cotton balls, cleansing solution
Gloves

PROCEDURE

NURSING ACTION	RATIONALE
PREPARATORY PHASE	
1. Check physician's directives for amount and temperature of irrigating fluid. Prepare equipment.	
2. Identify patient and explain the procedure. Place patient in dorsal recumbent position with waterproof pad under her.	2. To permit gravity to assist in allowing fluid to reach distal areas of vagina.

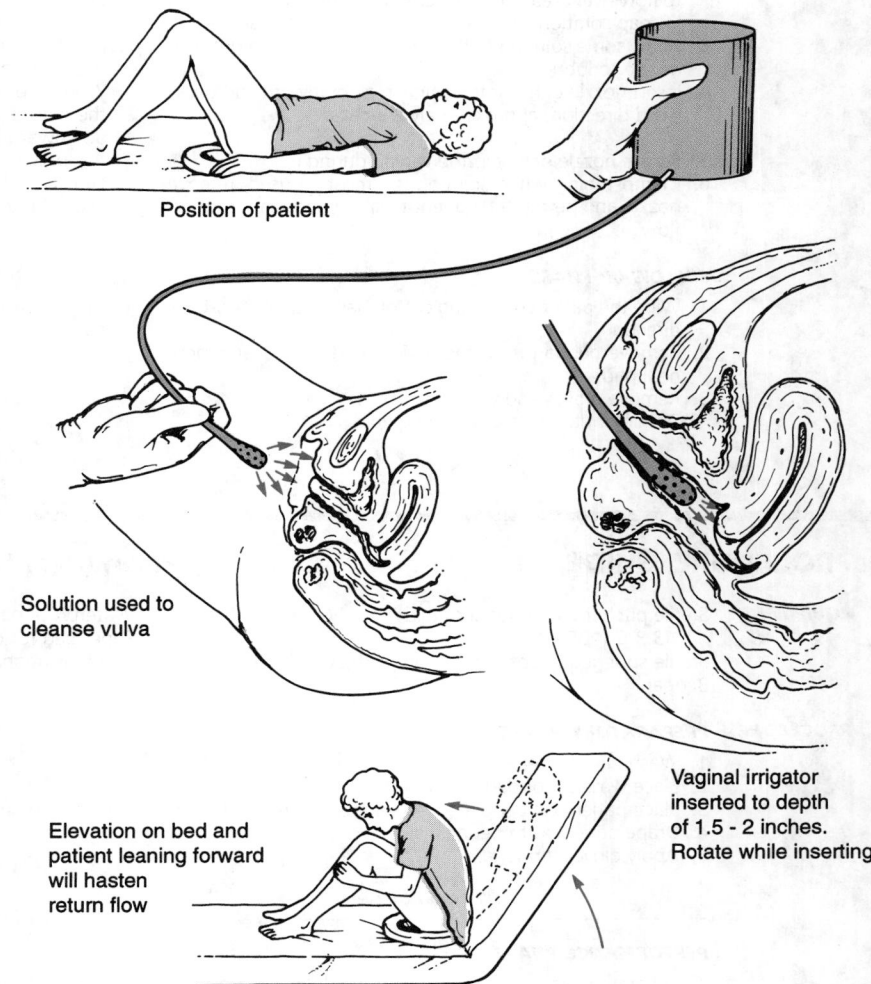

Position of patient

Solution used to
cleanse vulva

Vaginal irrigator
inserted to depth
of 1.5 - 2 inches.
Rotate while inserting.

Elevation on bed and
patient leaning forward
will hasten
return flow

Vaginal irrigation. The nurse wears gloves while doing this procedure.

(continued)

PROCEDURE GUIDELINES 20-2 ◆ Vaginal Irrigation *(continued)*

PROCEDURE *(cont'd)*

NURSING ACTION	RATIONALE
3. Wash hands.	
4. Have the patient void before beginning irrigation.	4. A full bladder would prevent adequate distention of vagina by solution.
5. Drape the patient	5. To prevent chilling and undue exposure.
6. Arrange irrigating receptacle at a level just above the patient's hips (not more than ½ meter, ie, 18 inches above hips) so that fluid flows easily but gently.	6. The higher the fluid source, the greater the pressure.

PERFORMANCE PHASE

NURSING ACTION	RATIONALE
1. Put on gloves.	1. Clean gloves may be used, but sterile gloves should be used if there is an open wound.
2. Cleanse vulva by separating labia and allowing solution to flow over area; if insufficient, use cotton balls saturated in soap solution, cleanse from front toward anal area.	2. Materials found around vaginal meatus may be introduced into vagina and cervix. This is to be avoided.
3. Allow some solution to flow through tubing and out over nozzle to lubricate it.	3. Moisture provides lubrication and less resistance when one surface is moved against another.
4. Insert nozzle gently into vagina in a downward and backward direction, approximately 2 inches.	4. When the patient is in a dorsal recumbent position, the natural anatomic position of the vagina is in the downward-backward direction.
5. Rotate nozzle gently in the vagina during inflow.	5. All surfaces are irrigated when nozzle is rotated.
6. Clamp tubing when solution is almost all used, remove nozzle and permit the patient to sit on bedpan for return flow.	6. Gravity will assist in allowing return flow to drain from vaginal tract.

FOLLOW-UP PHASE

NURSING ACTION	RATIONALE
1. Wipe the patient dry, using cotton balls in a front-to-back direction.	1. Drying the area prevents skin excoriation and promotes comfort.
2. Remove bedpan from the patient and apply sterile perineal pad.	
3. Remove gloves and wash hands.	
4. Document amount of returned fluid.	

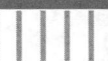

PROCEDURE GUIDELINES 20-3 ◆ Vulvar Irrigation (Perineal Care)

EQUIPMENT

Sterile pitcher with irrigating fluid (300–500 mL) 40.5°–43.3°C (105°–110°F)
Sterile sponge forceps and cotton pledgets
Bedpan

Waterproof pad
Paper bag for cotton pledget disposal
Gloves (optional)

PROCEDURE

PREPARATORY PHASE

1. Wash hands. Prepare equipment.
2. Place waterproof pad under patient.
3. Place patient on bedpan in dorsal recumbent position with knees flexed and separated.
4. Drape patient with perineal area exposed.
5. Apply gloves (optional).

PERFORMANCE PHASE

NURSING ACTION	RATIONALE
1. Separate labia with nondominant hand. Pour warmed irrigating solution gently over vulva from a sterile pitcher.	1. Materials will be flushed from perineal area into bedpan.
2. Cleanse perineal area with cotton pledget held in a sponge holder, use a front-to-back direction and discard each sponge in a plastic or paper bag after one use.	2. Friction facilitates cleansing process and the removal of soil. Follow aseptic technique, cleanse urethral and vaginal areas first, then external labia, then anus.
3. Dry perineal area using dry cotton pledgets in same fashion as for cleansing.	3. Cleansing from front to back assists in preventing intestinal organisms from entering vaginal area.

PROCEDURE (cont'd)	NURSING ACTION	RATIONALE

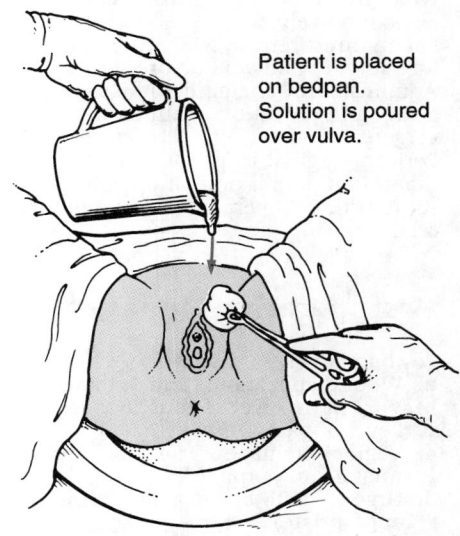

Patient is placed on bedpan. Solution is poured over vulva.

Sterile pledgets are used to cleanse; then area is dried.

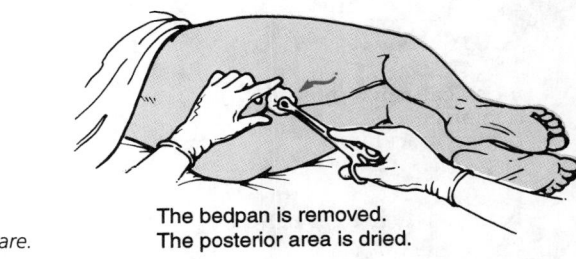

Perineal care.

The bedpan is removed. The posterior area is dried.

FOLLOW-UP PHASE
1. Apply sterile perineal pad.
2. Wash hands.

1. To maintain cleanliness and provide comfort for patient.

◆ VULVAR AND VAGINAL IRRIGATION

Vulvar irrigation is done to cleanse the perineal area after urination or a bowel movement to minimize infection after surgery. Vaginal irrigation is done to cleanse or disinfect the vagina and adjacent tissues before surgery or to soothe inflamed tissue after surgery. See Procedure Guidelines 20-2 and 20-3.

◆ HYSTERECTOMY

Hysterectomy is the surgical removal of the uterus. Sixty-five percent of these procedures occur during reproductive years.

Types of Hysterectomy

A. Abdominal
1. Subtotal hysterectomy—corpus of uterus is removed, but cervical stump remains.
2. Total hysterectomy—entire uterus is removed, including cervix; tubes and ovaries remain.
3. Total hysterectomy with bilateral salpingo-oophorectomy—entire uterus, tubes, and ovaries are removed.

B. Vaginal Removal of uterus through the cervix and vagina; cervical stump may remain

Preoperative Management

1. Determine if patient knows reason for hysterectomy, what the procedure involves, and what to expect postoperatively.
2. Patient must remain NPO from midnight the night before surgery and void before surgery.
3. Administer an enema before surgery to evacuate the bowel and prevent contamination and trauma during surgery.
4. Perform vaginal irrigation before surgery and ensure that a skin prep is done if ordered.
5. Administer preoperative medication to help the patient relax.

Postoperative Management

1. Postoperatively, assess for:
   a. Wound appearance and drainage
   b. Vital signs, level of consciousness
   c. Level of pain
   d. Vaginal drainage (serous, bloody)
   e. Intake and output
   f. Urge to void, bladder distention, residual urine (if appropriate)
   g. Clarity, color, and sediment of urine
   h. Homan's sign or impaired circulation
2. Promote exercise and ambulation to prevent thromboembolus, facilitate voiding, and stimulate peristalsis.

Complications

1. Incisional/pelvic infection
2. Hemorrhage
3. Urinary tract injury

Nursing Diagnoses

A. Pain related to surgical procedure
B. Altered Pattern of Urinary Elimination related to decreased bladder sensation
C. Risk for Infection related to surgical procedure
D. Self-Esteem Disturbance related to alteration in female organs
E. Sexual Dysfunction related to alteration in reproductive organs and function

Nursing Interventions

A. **Relieving Pain**
1. Assess pain location, level, and characteristics.
2. Administer prescribed pain medications.
3. Encourage patient to splint incision when moving.
4. Encourage patient to ambulate as soon as possible to decrease flatus and abdominal distention.
5. Institute sitz baths or ice packs as prescribed to alleviate perineal discomfort.

B. **Promoting Urinary Elimination**
1. Monitor intake and output, bladder distention, signs and symptoms of bladder infection.
2. Maintain patency of indwelling catheter if one is in place.
3. Catheterize patient intermittently if uncomfortable or has not voided in 8 hours.
4. Check for residual urine after patient voids; should be less than 100 mL. Continue to check if more than 100 mL or bladder infection may develop.
5. Encourage patient to empty bladder around the clock, not only when feeling the urge, due to loss of sensation of bladder fullness.
6. Encourage fluid intake to decrease risk of urinary infection.

C. **Preventing Infection**
1. Assess vaginal drainage for amount, color, and odor, assess incision site and temperature.
2. Administer antibiotics as prescribed.
3. Assist use of incentive spirometer, coughing and deep breathing, and ambulation to decrease risk of pulmonary infection.

D. **Strengthening Self-Esteem**
1. Allow patient to discuss her feelings about herself as a woman.
2. Reassure patient she is still feminine.
3. Encourage patient to discuss her feelings with her spouse or significant other.
4. Reassure patient that she will not go through premature menopause if her ovaries were not removed.

E. **Regaining Sexual Function**
1. Discuss changes regarding sexual functioning such as shortened vagina and possible dyspareunia due to dryness.
2. Offer suggestions to improve sexual functioning.
   a. Use of water-soluble lubricants
   b. Change position—female dominant offers more control of depth of penetration.

Patient Education/Health Maintenance

1. Advise patient that a total hysterectomy with bilateral salpingo-oophorectomy produces a surgical menopause. Patient may experience hot flashes, vaginal dryness, and mood swings unless hormonal replacement therapy is instituted.
2. Advise her against sitting too long at one time, as in driving long distances, because of the possibility of pooling of blood in the pelvis and causing thromboembolism.
3. Suggest that the patient delay driving a car until the third postoperative week because even pressing the brake pedal puts stress on the lower abdomen.
4. Tell the patient to expect a tired feeling for the first few days at home and, therefore, not to plan too many activities for the first week. She will be able to perform most of her usual daily activities within a month, and feel herself again within 2 months.
5. Tell the patient not to feel discouraged if at times during convalescence she experiences depression, feels like crying, and seems unusually nervous. This is common but will not last.
6. Remind the patient to ask her surgeon about any strenuous or lifting activities, which are usually delayed for 4 to 6 weeks.

7. Reinforce instructions given by the surgeon on intercourse, douching, and use of tampons, which are usually discouraged for 4 to 6 weeks. Sexual intercourse should be resumed cautiously to prevent injury and discomfort. Showers are permitted, but tub baths are deferred until healing is sufficient.
8. Instruct the patient to report fever over 37.8°C (100°F), heavy vaginal bleeding, drainage, and foul odor of discharge.
9. Emphasize the importance of follow-up and routine physical and gynecologic examinations.

Evaluation

A. Verbalizes decreased pain
B. Voids every 8 hours of sufficient quantity
C. Absence of fever and signs of infection
D. Verbalizes positive statements about self and positive outlook on recovery
E. Verbalizes understanding of possible changes in sexual functioning and what to do about it

Menstrual Conditions

◆ DYSMENORRHEA

Dysmenorrhea is painful menstruation; most common of gynecologic dysfunctions.

Pathophysiology/Etiology

A. *Primary*
1. Absence of pelvic lesion; usually intrinsic to uterus.
2. Current research supports increased prostaglandin production by the endometrium as the chief cause.
3. May also be due to hormonal, obstructive, and psychological factors.

B. *Secondary* Due to lesion such as endometriosis, pelvic infection, congenital abnormality, uterine fibroids

Clinical Manifestations

1. Pain may be due to increased uterine contractility and decreased endometrial flow.
2. Characteristics of pain—colicky or dull, usually in lower mid-abdominal region, spasmodic or constant.
3. May also experience nausea, vomiting, diarrhea, headache, chills, tiredness, nervousness, and low backache.

Diagnostic Evaluation

Tests to rule out underlying lesion:

1. Chlamydia and gonorrhea tests—may show infection.
2. Pelvic ultrasound—may detect tumor, endometriosis.
3. Possibly, hysteroscopy and laparoscopy—primarily to detect endometriosis.

Management

(Of primary dysmenorrhea; treatment of secondary dysmenorrhea is aimed at underlying pathology)

1. Local heat; such as heating pad to increase blood flow and decrease spasms
2. Exercise to increase endorphin release, which decreases pain perception, and to suppress prostaglandin release
3. Nonnarcotic analgesics, especially nonsteroidal anti-inflammatory agents (ibuprofen, naproxen) for their antiprostaglandin action
4. Oral contraceptives to decrease flow and contractility of the uterus
5. In some cases, dilation and curettage may be helpful.
6. Usually self-limiting without complications

Nursing Assessment

1. Obtain menstrual and gynecologic history that could suggest underlying pathology.
2. Assess level of pain using scale of 1 to 10; assess patient's emotional response to pain.
3. Obtain vital signs, including temperature, to rule out infection.
4. Perform abdominal and pelvic examination (if indicated) to assess for underlying lesions.

Nursing Diagnosis

A. Pain related to menstrual flow

Nursing Interventions

A. *Controlling Pain*
1. Administer pharmacologic agents as ordered to control pain and menstrual flow.
2. Apply heating pad to lower back or abdomen as desired by patient.
3. Assess patient's response to pain control measures.

Patient Education/Health Maintenance

1. Explain to patient possible causes of dysmenorrhea.
2. Teach patient nonpharmacologic methods to reduce pain.
   a. Apply heating pad to lower mid-abdomen or back or take warm tub baths.
   b. Exercise regularly (30 minutes, 3 times a week).
3. Teach patient to use prescribed medications effectively by taking medication at beginning of discomfort and repeating as necessary, especially on first day of menses.
4. Teach patient side effects of medications.
5. Encourage patient to reduce stress through adequate sleep, good nutrition, exercise, and coping with stressors.
6. Discuss patient's feelings toward menstruation (hygienic issues, inconvenience, female identity).

Evaluation

A. Describes methods to reduce pain and verbalizes reduced pain level

◆ PREMENSTRUAL SYNDROME

Premenstrual syndrome is a group of symptoms such as headache, irritability, depression, breast tenderness, and bloating that is clearly related to onset of menstruation.

Pathophysiology/Etiology

1. Linked to hormonal imbalances, prostaglandins, endorphins, psychological factors such as attitudes and beliefs related to menstruation and environmental factors such as nutrition and pollution.
2. Most common in women in their thirties.
3. May occur in 25% to 50% of menstruating women.

Clinical Manifestations

1. Symptoms may begin 7 to 14 days before onset of menstrual flow; diminish 1 to 2 days after menses begins.
2. Physical—edema of extremities, abdominal fullness, breast swelling and tenderness, headache, vertigo, palpitations, acne, backache, constipation, thirst, weight gain.
3. Behavioral—irritability, fatigue, lethargy, depression, anxiety, crying spells.
4. Diagnosis based on clinical manifestations; usually no diagnostic evaluation is necessary.

Management

1. Restrict sodium, caffeine, tobacco, alcohol, and refined sweets.
2. Aerobic exercise
3. Vitamin B_6 supplements
4. Progesterone replacement therapy
5. Prostaglandin inhibitors
6. Diuretics to decrease fluid retention and weight gain
7. Anxiolytic agents
8. Counseling
9. Oophorectomy (removal of ovaries) for severe cases in women who do not desire children
10. Usually self-limiting without complications

Nursing Assessment

1. Ask patient to describe symptoms and their onset and means of relief.
2. Assess patient's diet, activity, and rest habits.
3. Assess patient's emotional response to symptoms and methods of coping.

Nursing Diagnosis

A. Anxiety related to symptoms and lack of control over condition

Nursing Interventions

A. *Reducing Anxiety*
1. Administer medications as ordered; warn patient that diuretics will cause increased urination and anxiolytics may cause drowsiness or cognitive impairment.
2. Provide emotional support for patient and significant others.

Patient Education/Health Maintenance

1. Encourage patient to keep a diary for several consecutive months including dates, cycle days, stressors, symptoms and their severity to determine if therapy is effective.
2. Instruct patient in the use and side effects of prescribed medications.
3. Teach patient possible causes of syndrome and nonpharmacologic methods to alleviate distress, such as dietary modifications, exercise, and rest.
4. Teach stress reduction techniques such as imagery and deep breathing.
5. Refer for further resources and support to groups such as: PMS Access; P. O. Box 9326; Madison, WI 53715; 1-800-222-4767.

Evaluation

A. Verbalizes reduced anxiety, increased control over condition

◆ AMENORRHEA

Amenorrhea is absence of menstrual flow.

Pathophysiology/Etiology

A. *Primary*
1. Menarche does not occur by age 16.
2. Due to chromosomal, hormonal, nutritional, psychogenic disorders, or pregnancy

B. *Secondary*
1. Menstruation stops for three cycle intervals, or 6 months of amenorrhea in a woman who previously menstruated.
2. May be due to normal pregnancy or lactation, menopause, psychogenic, hormonal, nutritional, or exercise-related disorders.
   a. Excessive exercise or inadequate nutrition with decreased body fat stores is a significant cause of amenorrhea in young women.
3. Some medications, such as phenothiazines and oral contraceptives, may also induce amenorrhea.

Diagnostic Evaluation

1. Pregnancy test
2. Progesterone challenge test
   a. Positive—bleeding occurs—chronic anovulation is most likely.
   b. Negative—no bleeding occurs—may indicate organ failure—other tests are needed.
3. Hormonal levels—LH and FSH—to detect ovarian failure
4. Prolactin level to rule out pituitary tumor
5. Genetic karyotyping to detect chromosome abnormalities

Management

1. Discontinue causative medications.
2. Nutritional, exercise, or psychological counseling as indicated
   a. Recommend decreased exercise in athletes to increase body fat stores and decrease stress.
3. Hormonal replacement therapy

Complications

1. It has been theorized that prolonged amenorrhea may lead to atypia of the endometrium.

Nursing Assessment

1. Assess for signs of chromosomal disorders such as abnormal genitalia, masculinization, short stature, and characteristic facies.
2. Assess for signs of pituitary tumor such as headache, visual disturbances, dizziness.
3. Assess weight and body build along with change in weight and nutritional and exercise habits that may indicate anorexia or loss of body fat due to exercise.
4. Assess emotional status, areas of stress, and coping ability.

Nursing Diagnoses

A. Altered Nutrition (Less than Body Requirements) related to poor dietary habits and/or rigorous exercise
B. Ineffective Individual Coping related to school, job, relationships, etc

Nursing Interventions

A. **Meeting Nutritional Requirements**
1. Explore patient's body image, knowledge on the five food groups, behavior regarding meals, and exercise routine and point out misconceptions, dangerous behavior, and ideas for improvement.
2. Monitor weight gain, increase in body fat, and return of menstrual cycles.

B. **Strengthening Coping**
1. Provide emotional support for patient and family.

2. Point out ineffective coping mechanisms and teach relaxation techniques and more positive coping mechanisms such as confrontation.

Patient Teaching/Health Maintenance

1. Teach patient the physiology of the normal menstrual cycle and possible causes for amenorrhea.
2. Teach proper use and side effects of medications prescribed.
3. Teach the patient to chart menstrual periods on a calendar and maintain regular gynecologic and medical follow-up.

Evaluation

A. Verbalizes adequate dietary intake, decreased exercise
B. Weight increased and menses resumed

◆ DYSFUNCTIONAL UTERINE BLEEDING

Dysfunctional uterine bleeding (DUB) is abnormal uterine bleeding that has no organic cause, such as tumor, infection, or pregnancy.

Pathophysiology/Etiology

1. DUB is frequently caused by immature hypothalamic stimulation in adolescents.
2. DUB is caused by anovulation in any age group, especially in teens and perimenopausal women, due to impaired follicular formation or rupture, or corpus luteum dysfunction.
3. Ovarian failure in perimenopausal women frequently causes DUB.
4. Temporary estrogen withdrawal at ovulation may cause midcycle ovulatory bleeding.
5. Emotional lability, malnutrition, and changes in exercise may cause changes in gonadotropin release at the hypothalamic level, causing altered menstrual pattern.

Clinical Manifestations

1. Abnormal bleeding may occur in any of the following patterns:
   a. *Oligomenorrhea*—markedly diminished menstrual flow; may also be irregular, but consistent periods with long intervals.
   b. *Menorrhagia*—excessive bleeding during regular menstruation; can be increased in duration or amount.
   c. *Metorrhagia*—bleeding from uterus between regular menstrual periods; significant because it is usually a symptom of disease.
   d. *Polymenorrhea*—frequent menstruation occurring at intervals of less than 3 weeks.

Diagnostic Evaluation

Tests are done to rule out pathologic causes of abnormal bleeding.

1. Pregnancy test
2. Complete blood count (CBC) to detect anemia and platelet count and coagulation screen to rule out blood dyscrasia
3. Pap smear to rule out malignancy
4. Thorough examination to rule out trauma or foreign body
5. Chlamydia and gonorrhea tests to rule out PID
6. Pelvic ultrasound to rule out ovarian cysts and tumors and uterine fibroids and tumors
7. Hysteroscopy to detect uterine fibroids, polyps, and other lesions
8. Endometrial biopsy to determine hormonal effect on uterus and rule out malignancy
9. Laparoscopy to evaluate for endometriosis

Management

1. Treat underlying anemia with iron, possible transfusions (only significant complication).
2. Progesterone therapy to stop acute bleeding
3. Oral contraceptives to control chronic bleeding
4. Androgen therapy with danazol (Danocrine) to reduce menstrual blood loss
5. Dilation and curettage

Nursing Assessment

1. Ask the patient for menstrual and gynecologic history, sexual activity, and possibility of pregnancy.
2. Assess frequency, duration, and amount of menstrual flow.
3. Assess for other symptoms of underlying pathology such as pelvic pain, fever, and abdominal masses or tenderness.
4. Assess for signs and symptoms of anemia—fatigue, shortness of breath, pallor, tachycardia.

Nursing Diagnoses

A. Fatigue related to excessive blood loss
B. Fear of Bleeding Through Clothing related to excessive or unpredictable bleeding

Nursing Interventions

A. *Increasing Energy Level*
1. Encourage good dietary intake with increased sources of iron—fortified cereals and breads, meat (especially red meat), and green leafy vegetables.
2. Administer oral iron preparations with meals to prevent nausea. Treat constipation as necessary.
3. Monitor hemoglobin and infuse packed red blood cells as ordered.
4. Help limit patient's exertion and administer oxygen by nasal cannula if ordered.

B. *Relieving Fear*
1. Review pattern of menstrual flow with patient and help her plan for excessive bleeding.
2. Suggest wearing double tampons (if able) and double sanitary pads.
3. Tell patient to expect heavy gush of blood on arising from lying or reclining position.
4. Prepare patient to carry an adequate supply of sanitary products and a change of clothing until bleeding is under control.

Patient Education/Health Maintenance

1. Teach the patient the cause of dysfunctional uterine bleeding and the about the diagnostic process to rule out pathologic causes of abnormal bleeding.
2. Teach the patient to prevent anemia by eating a diet high in iron, along with vitamin C or citrus fruit to enhance absorption of iron.
3. Teach about hormonal therapy and what side effects to expect, as well as what to expect of bleeding—bleeding should stop within 2 to 7 days following short-term progesterone therapy, and should stop within first week of oral contraceptives but start again in fourth week as regular menstrual period.
4. Advise patient to keep a calendar or log of menses.

Evaluation

A. Verbalizes adequate energy to perform activities
B. Verbalizes more confidence in ability to conceal bleeding

◆ MENOPAUSE

Menopause is described as the physiologic cessation of menses.

Pathophysiology/Etiology

1. Menopause is caused by failing ovarian function and decreased estrogen production by the ovary.
2. Climacteric is the transition period (perimenopausal) during which the woman's reproductive function gradually diminishes and disappears. It usually occurs at about age 50.
3. Artificial or surgical menopause may occur secondary to surgery or radiation involving the ovaries.

Clinical Manifestations

1. Genitalia—atrophy of vulva, vagina, urethra results in dryness, bleeding, itching, burning, dysuria, thinning of pubic hair, loss of labia minora, decreased lubrication.
2. Sexual function—dyspareunia, decreased intensity and duration of sexual response, but can still have active function.

3. Vasomotor—60% to 70% of women experience "hot flashes," which may be preceded by an anxious feeling and accompanied by sweating.
4. Osteoporosis—decreased bone mass results in increased hip fractures, spinal compression fractures.
5. Cardiovascular—increased coronary artery disease, cholesterol level, and palpitations may occur.
6. Psychological—insomnia, irritability, anxiety, memory loss, fear, and depression may be experienced.

Diagnostic Evaluation

1. Hormonal levels of LH and FSH (increased), and estradiol (decreased) may be done to confirm menopause.

Management

1. Estrogen replacement therapy
   a. Indicated to reduce symptoms and to prevent osteoporosis and coronary artery disease.
   b. Topical preparations may be used for atrophic vaginitis.
   c. Progesterone preparation also given if uterus is intact to prevent endometrial hyperplasia and possible cancer.
2. Vaginal lubricants such as Replens to decrease vaginal dryness and dyspareunia.
3. Vitamin E and B supplements—to decrease hot flashes.
4. Calcium supplements to prevent bone loss.

Complications

1. Osteoporosis has been clearly linked to estrogen depletion in menopause.
2. Coronary artery disease rarely develops in women before menopause and has been associated with the effects of estrogen depletion on blood vessels.
3. Vulvovaginitis or trauma related to a dry, estrogen-depleted epithelium.

Nursing Assessment

1. Obtain history of patient's symptoms, menstrual cycle.
2. Obtain history for other risk factors for coronary artery disease and osteoporosis.
3. Assess genitalia for atrophy, dryness, and elasticity.
4. Assess patient's emotional response to menopause.

Nursing Diagnosis

A. Altered Sexual Patterns related to symptoms and psychological impact of menopause

Nursing Interventions

A. *Maintaining Sexual Patterns*
1. Provide patient with information related to estrogen replacement therapy, including dosage schedule, route, side effects, and what to expect of menstrual bleeding. Women who still have a uterus can expect a period at the end of every month if they are taking hormones cyclically. A newer method of hormone replacement, giving estrogen and lower dose progesterone daily, may cause some irregular spotting for 3 months to up to 1 year, then most women experience no bleeding.
2. Explore with patient her feelings about menopause, clear up misconceptions about sexual functioning, and encourage her to discuss her feelings with her partner.
3. Instruct patient how to use water-based lubricant for intercourse to decrease dryness.

Patient Teaching/Health Maintenance

1. Teach patient that sexual functioning does not decrease during menopause but may even increase due to loss of fear of pregnancy and increased time if children are grown.
2. Teach patient about foods that are high in calcium—dairy products, broccoli, and some fortified cereals—and to maintain weight-bearing activites to prevent osteoporosis.
3. Counsel patient on reducing risk factors for coronary artery disease.
4. Encourage patient to keep regular medical and gynecologic follow-up visits.
5. Advise patient that vulvovaginal infection and trauma are possible due to the dryness of the tissue, and to seek prompt evaluation if pain and discharge occur.

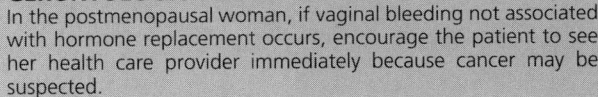

GERONTOLOGIC ALERT:
In the postmenopausal woman, if vaginal bleeding not associated with hormone replacement occurs, encourage the patient to see her health care provider immediately because cancer may be suspected.

Evaluation

A. Verbalizes confidence in sexual function and identity, decreased symptoms

Infections/Inflammation of the Vulva, Vagina, and Cervix

◆ VULVITIS

Vulvitis is inflammation of the vulva.

Pathophysiology/Etiology

A. *Causative Factors*
1. Infections—*Trichomonas*, molluscum contagiosum, bacteria, fungi
2. Irritants
   a. Urine, feces, vaginal discharge

b. Close-fitting, synthetic fabrics
c. Chemicals such as laundry detergents, vaginal sprays, deodorants, perfumes

3. Carcinoma

B. *Predisposing Factors*
1. Illnesses such as diabetes mellitus and dermatologic disorders
2. Atrophy due to menopause

Clinical Manifestations

1. Pruritus—more acute at night, aggravated by warmth
2. Reddened, edematous tissue, possible ulceration
3. Pain, burning, dyspareunia
4. Exudate—possibly profuse and purulent
5. Lesions of molluscum contagiosum are multiple, from 1 mm to 1 cm in size, and filled with white caseous material.

Diagnostic Evaluation

1. Vulvar smears and cultures—may show infectious organism.
2. Biopsy of vulvar tissue—may be necessary to rule out malignancy.

Management

1. Anti-infectives to treat infectious agents
2. Topical steroids to treat inflammation
3. Topical or systemic estrogen to treat atrophy
4. Treatment of underlying disorder
5. Molluscum contagiosum may be treated by scalpel excision or silver nitrate or electrical cautery.

Complications

1. Scarring and chronic discomfort

Nursing Assessment

1. Question the patient regarding medical history, symptoms, sexual activity.
2. Determine use of any chemical-containing products on undergarments or directly on vulva.
3. Examine the genitalia and lymph nodes.

Nursing Diagnosis

A. Pain related to vulvar inflammation

Nursing Interventions

A. *Relieving Pain*
1. Administer prescribed medications and instruct patient on their use, method of application, and side effects.
2. Provide sitz baths or cool compresses to soothe and cleanse vulva.

Patient Education/Health Maintenance

1. Teach patient hygienic principles.
   a. Wipe from front to back after voiding.
   b. Use cotton with warm water and bland soap for cleansing, pat dry.
   c. Apply nonirritating powder such as cornstarch.
2. Teach patient to avoid chemical irritants such as sprays, perfumed soaps, new laundry detergents, static-control dryer sheets.
3. Teach patient to avoid mechanical irritants such as tight clothing, synthetic fabrics and undergarments; replace these with loose-fitting cotton undergarments.
4. Teach patient how to use sitz bath and cool compresses at home and to avoid scratching.
5. Teach patient that some infections such as *Trichomonas* and molluscum contagiosum are sexually transmitted, so partner needs to seek treatment before intercourse is resumed.

Evaluation

A. Verbalizes increased comfort level

◆ BARTHOLIN CYST/ABSCESS

Bartholin cyst or abscess, also called bartholinitis, is an infection of the greater vestibular gland, causing cyst or abscess formation.

Pathophysiology/Etiology

1. These glands lie on both sides of the vagina at the base of the labia minora; lubricate the vagina.
2. If they become obstructed secondary to infection, abscess or cyst formation may occur (Fig. 20-1).
3. Abscess or cyst may spontaneously rupture or enlarge and become painful.
4. Most commonly caused by sexual transmission of infection.

Clinical Manifestations

1. Asymptomatic cyst
2. Pain, erythema, tenderness, swelling
3. If abscess is present: pain, edema, cellulitis

Diagnostic Evaluation

1. Culture to identify infectious organisms

Management

1. May be treated conservatively with warm soaks or sitz baths; antibiotics if cellulitis is present.
2. May need incision and drainage; provides immediate relief, but may recur.

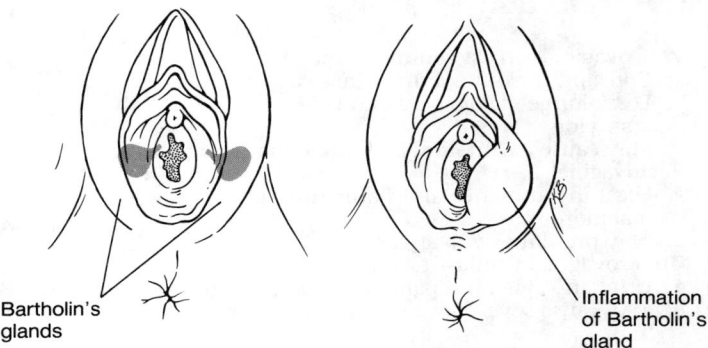

Bartholin's glands

Inflammation of Bartholin's gland

FIGURE 20-1 *Site and infection of vestibular gland.*

3. Marsupialization, for recurrent abscesses
 a. Contents are opened and drained, then edges of abscess are sutured to edges of external incision to keep cavity open.
 b. Healing occurs from within the area of the abscess.

Complications

Scarring from recurrent infection and rupture

Nursing Assessment

1. Obtain history of sexual activity including new partners, history of STDs.
2. Inspect labia minora for warmth, erythema, swelling.
3. Assess for signs of other STDs—rash, genital ulcers, vaginal discharge.

Nursing Diagnoses

A. Pain related to infection, enlargement of gland
B. Risk for Infection Transmission related to STD

Nursing Interventions

A. *Relieving Pain*
1. Administer pain medications and antibiotics as ordered; explain side effects to patient.
2. Instruct patient to apply warm soaks or sitz bath 3 to 4 times a day for 15 to 20 minutes to promote comfort and drainage.
3. Encourage patient to remain in bed as much as possible because pain is exacerbated by activity.
4. Prepare patient for incision and drainage if indicated.
5. For marsupialization: apply ice packs intermittently for 24 hours to reduce edema and provide comfort; thereafter, warm sitz baths or a perineal heat pack or lamp provide comfort.

B. *Preventing Infection Transmission*
1. Explain to patient that infection may have been caused by sexually transmitted infection.
2. Tell patient to instruct her partner to be tested for STDs.

3. Advise the patient to abstain from intercourse until cyst or abscess has completely resolved and she has completed all her antibiotics.

Patient Education/Health Maintenance

1. Review principles of perineal hygiene with patient.
2. Discuss STDs and methods of prevention.
3. Encourage patient to follow up for recurrent abscess because surgical treatment is often necessary.

Evaluation

A. Verbalizes relief of pain
B. At follow-up, verbalizes abstinence from intercourse and shows good signs of healing with no recurrence of infection

◆ VAGINAL FISTULA

A *vaginal fistula* is an abnormal, tortuous opening between the vagina and another hollow organ.

Pathophysiology/Etiology

A. *Causes*
1. Obstetric injury, especially in long labors and in countries with inadequate obstetric care
2. Pelvic surgery—hysterectomy or vaginal reconstructive procedures
3. Carcinoma—extensive disease or complication of treatment such as radiation therapy

B. *Types*
1. *Vesicovaginal fistula* is an opening between the bladder and vagina.
2. *Rectovaginal fistula* is an opening between the rectum and vagina.
3. *Ureterovaginal fistula* is an opening between the ureter and vagina.

Clinical Manifestations

1. Vesicovaginal—most common type of fistula
   a. Constant trickling of urine into vagina
   b. Loss of urge to void because bladder is continuously emptying
   c. May cause excoriation and inflammation of vulva
2. Rectovaginal
   a. Fecal incontinence and flatus through the vagina; malodorous
   b. May present as vulvar cancer
3. Ureterovaginal fistula—rare
   a. Urine in vagina but patient still voids regularly
   b. May cause severe urinary tract infections

Diagnostic Evaluation

1. Methylene blue test—following instillation of this dye in bladder
   a. Methylene blue appears in vagina in vesicovaginal fistula.
   b. Methylene blue does not appear in vagina in ureterovaginal fistula.
2. Indigo carmine test—following a negative methylene blue test, indigo carmine is injected intravenously. If dye appears in vagina, this indicates ureterovaginal fistula.
3. Intravenous pyelogram helps detect presence and location of fistula and presence of hydroureter and hydronephrosis.
4. Cystoscopy—performed to determine number and location of fistulas

Management

1. Fistulas recognized at time of delivery should be corrected immediately.
2. Treatment of postoperative fistulas may be delayed for 2 to 3 months to allow treatment of infection.
3. Surgical closure of opening via vaginal or abdomianl route (when patient's tissues are healthy)
4. Fecal or urinary diversion procedure may be required for large fistulas.
5. Rarely, a fistula may heal without surgical intervention.
6. Medical approach
   a. Prosthesis to prevent incontinence and allow tissue to heal; done for patients who are not surgical candidates.
   b. Prosthesis is inserted into vagina; it is connected to drainage tubing leading to a leg bag.

Complications

Hydronephrosis, pyelonephritis, and possible renal failure with ureterovaginal fistula.

Nursing Assessment

1. Obtain obstetric, gynecologic, and surgical history.
2. Monitor intake and output and voiding pattern.
3. Assess drainage on perineal pads.
4. Watch for signs of infection such as fever, chills, flank pain.

Nursing Diagnoses

A. Risk for Infection related to contamination of urinary tract by vaginal flora or contamination of the vagina by rectal organisms
B. Altered Urinary Elimination related to fistula

Nursing Interventions

A. *Preventing Infection*
1. Encourage frequent sitz baths.
2. Perform vaginal irrigation as ordered, and teach the patient the procedure.
3. Before repair surgery, administer prescribed antibiotics to reduce pathogenic flora in the intestinal tract.
4. After rectovaginal repair
   a. Maintain patient on clear liquids as prescribed to limit bowel activity for several days.
   b. Encourage rest because of debilitation.
   c. Administer warm perineal irrigations to decrease healing time and increase comfort.

B. *Maintaining Urinary Drainage*
1. Suggest the use of perineal pads or incontinence products preoperatively.
2. After versicovaginal repair
   a. Maintain proper drainage from indwelling catheter to prevent pressure on newly sutured tissue.
   b. Administer vaginal or bladder irrigations gently because of tenderness at operative site.
   c. Maintain strict intake and output records.
3. If medical management is indicated, teach patient the use of prosthetic device.
4. Encourage patient to express feelings about her altered route of elimination, and share them with significant other.

Patient Education/Health Maintenance

1. Teach patient to report signs of infection early.
2. Teach patient to cleanse perineum gently and follow surgeon's instructions on when to resume intercourse and strenuous activity.
3. Advise patient to keep regular follow-up appointments.

Evaluation

A. No signs of infection—afebrile, no complaints of flank pain or difficulty voiding.
B. Clear urine flows from catheter postoperatively. Patient voids without difficulty after catheter removal.

◆ VAGINITIS

Vaginitis is inflammation of the vagina due to infectious pathogens.

Pathophysiology/Etiology

1. May be due to sexually transmitted organisms or overgrowth of other common organisms.
2. Normal vaginal secretions due to estrogen secretion and acidity inhibit the growth of pathogens.
3. Conditions such as diabetes, pregnancy, stress, and menopause alter normal vaginal environment.
4. Types of vaginitis (Table 20-2)
   a. Simple (contact)
   b. *Gardnerella*
   c. *Trichomonas*
   d. *Candida albicans*
   e. Atrophic

Clinical Manifestations

1. Vaginal itching, irritation, burning
2. Odor, increased or unusual vaginal discharge
3. Dyspareunia, pelvic pain, dysuria
4. May be asymptomatic

Diagnostic Evaluation

1. Wet smear for microscopic examination
   a. Saline slide—discharge mixed with saline; useful in detecting *Gardnerella* and *Trichomonas* organisms.
   b. Potassium hydroxide (KOH); useful in detecting *C. albicans*. If fishy odor is noted, suspect *Gardnerella* organisms.
2. Vaginal pH—use Nitrazie paper.
   a. Normal pH—4.0 to 4.5
   b. *Gardnerella*—5.0 to 5.5
   c. *Trichomonas*—5.5+
3. Pap smear—may detect any type of vaginitis.
4. Chlamydia and gonorrhea cultures or DNA probe—to rule out chlamydia or gonorrhea cervicitis

Management

1. Anti-infectives (oral or vaginal preparations)
2. Estrogen replacement (oral or vaginal preparation)

Nursing Assessment

1. Obtain a health history including questions specific to the condition.
   a. Nature of discharge. Cheeselike, frothy, puslike, thick or thin, scant? When was it first noticed? Character, color, odor? Other symptoms: dysuria, itching, dyspareunia?
   b. Menstrual history. Age at menache, menopause; length of cycles, duration and amount of flow, dysmenorrhea, amenorrhea, dysfunctional bleeding?
   c. Disease history. Presence of diabetes mellitus in patient or family? Other debilitating diseases? Control of these? Previous vaginal infections? STDs?
   d. Pregnancy history
   e. Sexual history. Partner(s), how active sexually? Its nature? Urogenital infections in partner? Nature of contraceptives?
   f. Medications being taken. Purpose?
   g. Vaginal hygiene. Use of douches, deodorants, sprays, ointments; types of tampons, bubble bath, shower/bath, nature of clothing (tight fitting)?
2. Perform a physical examination including vaginal examination and obtain vaginal discharge specimens as indicated.

Nursing Diagnoses

A. Pain related to vaginal irritation
B. Impaired Tissue Integrity related to vaginal infection
C. Sexual Dysfunction related to abstinence secondary to treatment.

Nursing Interventions

A. *Relieving Pain*
1. Instruct patient to discontinue use of irritating agents, such as bubble baths, vaginal douches.
2. Suggest patient take cool baths or sitz baths and pat dry or dry with hair dryer on low setting.
3. Encourage patient to wear loose cotton undergarments.
4. Encourage patient to take prescribed steroids and analgesics.
5. Provide emotional support.

B. *Restoring Tissue Integrity*
1. Teach patient to cleanse perineum before applying medication.
2. Demonstrate application of prescribed medication.
3. Emphasize importance of taking prescribed medication for full length of therapy and as directed; teach patient side effects.
4. Instruct patient on the proper technique for douching.
5. Stress importance of follow-up visits.

C. *Restoring Sexual Function*
1. Emphasize importance of abstinence until therapy is complete and sexual partner has been treated, if indicated.
2. Tell patient that use of condoms may be protective but may produce irritation during treatment.
3. Instruct patient in the use of water-soluble lubricant if vagina is dry and atrophic.

Patient Education/Health Maintenance

1. Teach causes of vaginitis and their symptoms so patient can seek treatment promptly.
2. Teach patient about all STDs and means of prevention.
3. Teach measures to prevent vaginitis.
   a. Wipe from front to back after toilet use.
   b. Keep area clean and dry.
   c. Wear loose cotton clothing—to absorb moisture and provide good circulation.
   d. Change sanitary pads, tampons frequently so they do not become saturated.
   e. Avoid bubble baths, vaginal deodorants, sprays, and douches.

TABLE 20-2   Types of Vaginitis

Description	Manifestations	Management
Simple Vaginitis (Contact Vaginitis) An inflammation of the vagina, with discharge; this may be due to invading organisms, irritation, poor hygiene. *Urethritis* often accompanies vaginitis because of the proximity of the urethra to the vagina. Predisposing factors: Contact allergens, excessive perspiration, synthetic underclothing, poor hygiene, foreign bodies (tampons, condoms, diaphragms that have been left in too long)	1. Increased vaginal discharge with itching, redness, burning, and edema. 2. Voiding and defecation aggravate the above symptoms.	1. Enhance the natural vaginal flora by administering a weak acid douche, 15 mL of vinegar to 1,000 mL water, (1 T white vinegar to 1 qt water). 2. Stimulate the growth of lactobacilli (Döderlein's bacilli) by administering beta-lactose vaginal suppository; this dissolves with body heat, and the sugar then acts. 3. Foster cleanliness by meticulous care after voiding and defecation. 4. Discontinue use of causative agent.
***Gardnerella* Vaginitis (Nonspecific or Bacterial)** An inflammation of the vagina heretofore referred to as "nonspecific vaginitis," because it is not caused by *Trichomonas*, *Candida*, or gonorrhea. It is considered an STD.	1. Vaginal discharge with odor. 2. Itching and burning may suggest concomitant organisms present. 3. It is benign in that when the discharge is wiped away, underlying tissue is healthy and pink. 4. Vaginal pH is between 5.0 and 5.5. 5. May be asymptomatic.	1. Metronidazole (Flagyl) taken orally for 7 d or topical clindamycin (Cleocin) or metronidazole. 2. Alcohol intake should be avoided during Flagyl treatment to avoid nausea and vertigo. Flagyl has been associated with teratogenic effects and should not be used in pregnant women during first trimester. 3. Treating partners is contoversial unless the condition is recurrent; if so, Flagyl is usually prescribed.
***Trichomonas* Vaginalis** A condition produced by a protozoan, (pear-shaped and mobile), that thrives in an alkaline environment. Remissions may occur, but organism remains resistant to treatment in the urinary tract.	1. Copious malodorous discharge; may be frothy and yellow-green in color. 2. May have pruritus, dyspareunia, and spotting. 3. Red, speckled (strawberry) punctate hemorrhages on the cervix. 4. May also have vulvar edema, dysuria, and hyperemia secondary to irritation of discharge.	1. Destroy infective protozoa by taking metronidazole (Flagyl) (orally), usually single dose of 2 g. NOTE: Flagyl is contraindicated in the first trimester of pregnancy. 2. Prevent reinfection by treating male concurrently with Flagyl. 3. Avoid alcohol during treatment.
Candida albicans A fungal infection caused by *Candida albicans* Incidence— several factors have been found to be significantly associated with the incidence of *C. albicans:* 1. Steroid therapy 2. Obesity 3. Pregnancy 4. Antibiotic therapy 5. Diabetes mellitus 6. Oral contraceptives 7. Frequent douching 8. Chronic debilitative diseases Characteristics 1. *C. albicans* is a normal inhabitant of the intestinal tract and therefore a frequent contaminant of the vagina. 2. Because this fungus thrives in an environment rich in carbohydrates, it is seen commonly in patients with poorly controlled diabetes. 3. This infection is observed in patients who have been on antibiotic or steroid therapy for a while (reduces natural protective organisms in vagina).	1. Vaginal discharge is thick and irritating; white or yellow patchy, cheese-like particles adhere to vaginal walls. 2. Itching is the most common complaint. 3. May also experience burning, soreness, dyspareunia, frequency, and dysuria.	1. Eradicate the fungus by applying antifungal vaginal cream, or vaginal suppository for 3 or 4 nights as ordered. 2. Treat the symptomatic or uncircumcised partner by applying antifungal cream under the foreskin nightly for 7 nights. 3. For severe or recurrent cases can use systemic antifungal.

TABLE 20-2 **Types of Vaginitis** (continued)

Description	Manifestations	Management
Atrophic Vaginitis This is a common postmenopausal occurrence due to atrophy of the vaginal mucosa secondary to decreased estrogen levels; more susceptible to infection.	1. Vaginal itching, dryness, burning, dyspareunia, and vulvar irritation. 2. May also have vaginal bleeding. **NURSING ALERT:** ❖❖ In the postmenopausal woman, if vaginal bleeding occurs, encourage the patient to see her health care provider immediately because cancer may be suspected.	Because this is a manifestation of general body estrogenic depletion, the patient should be treated with oral, water-soluble, natural, conjugated estrogen (Premarin). The condition reverses itself under treatment, which must be maintained. If infection is also present, this is treated. Estrogenic or cortisone vaginal cream or transdermal patch may be prescribed.

    f. If patient insists on using douches, use a mild vinegar solution (2 tsp white vinegar to 1 qt water).

3. For recurrent *Candida* infections, encourage good control if diabetic, or encourage patient to be tested for diabetes. Teach all patients to eliminate concentrated carbohydrates from diet to prevent recurrence.

Evaluation

A. Verbalizes relief of pain
B. Vaginal mucosa pink, with normal amount and color of secretions
C. Reports safe, satisfying sexual activity

◆ CONDYLOMA ACUMINATUM

Condyloma acuminatum is venereal warts caused by infection with HPV.

Pathophysiology/Etiology

1. Sexually transmitted; highly contagious
2. Caused by HPV types 6 and 11
3. Incubation period of up to 8 months

Clinical Manifestations

1. Single or multiple soft, fleshy painless growths of the vulva, vagina, cervix , or anal area
2. May be subclinical infection and still contagious
3. Occasional vaginal bleeding, discharge, odor and dyspareunia

Diagnostic Evaluation

1. Pap smear—shows characteristic cellular changes (koilocytosis).

2. Acetic acid swabbing on vaginal examination will whiten lesions and make them more identifiable.
3. Anoscopy may be necessary to identify anal lesions.

Management

1. External lesions may be treated by patient with multiple applications of podofilox (Condylox).
2. Noncervical lesions may be treated by health care provider with topical preparations such as podophyllin, trichloroacetic acid, or 5-fluorouracil.
3. Cryotherapy, electrocautery, laser treatment, or local excision of large or cervical lesions
4. Highly recurrent—may require retreatment

Complications

1. Implicated in cervical intraepithelial neoplasia.
2. May cause neonatal laryngeal papillomatosis if infant born through infected birth canal.
3. Obstruction of anal canal, vagina by enlarging lesions

Nursing Assessment

1. Obtain history of STDs, Pap smears, sexual partners.
2. Inspect external genitalia for lesions, perform vaginal examination.

Nursing Diagnosis

A. Risk for Infection Transmission related to HPV

Nursing Interventions

A. *Preventing HPV Transmission*
1. Encourage sexual abstinence during therapy; condoms may not prevent infection, depending on location of lesions.

2. Advise patient of possibility of recurrence or reinfection if partner is not treated.

3. Advise patient of risk to neonate during delivery; patient should receive close prenatal care if pregnant.

Evaluation

A. Patient and partner exhibit no signs of recurrence at follow-up visits.

◆ HERPES GENITALIS

Herpes genitalis is a viral infection that causes lesions of the cervix, vagina, and external genitalia.

Pathophysiology/Etiology

1. Caused by HSV, usually type 2
2. Sexually transmitted
3. An estimated 40 million people are infected in the United States.
4. Recurrent infection; virus lies dormant in dorsal root ganglia of spinal nerves between outbreaks.

Clinical Manifestations

1. Lesions occur 2 to 10 days after initial exposure, along with fever, malaise, lymphadenopathy and headache for primary infection.
2. Lesions are preceded by sensation of tingling; proceed from vesicles on erythematous, edematous base to painful ulcers that crust and heal without scars.
3. Internal lesions may cause watery discharge, dyspareunia.
4. Recurrent lesions may be stimulated by fever, stress, illness, menses, sunburn.
5. Occasionally infection may be asymptomatic.

Diagnostic Evaluation

1. Viral culture—identifies HSV.
2. Pap smear—may show characteristic cellular changes.
3. Tzanck smear—fluid from vesicle or scraping from base of ulcer is stained to show characteristic changes.
4. Antibody tests for screening and diagnosis

Management

1. Acyclovir (Zovirax)—suppresses virus and decreases length, severity, and shedding of infection.
 a. May be given topically (least effective), orally, or intravenously (for severe infections or in immunocompromised patients).
 b. Given intermittently as soon as occurrence is identified; or continuously in the oral form to suppress recurrences in severe and frequent infections.
2. Pain medication
3. Local comfort measures such as lidocaine jelly, sitz baths, and compresses

4. Immunization is under investigation for high-risk individuals (multiple partners or partner with herpes genitalis).

Complications

1. Meningitis
2. Neonatal infection if infant born through infected canal

Nursing Assessment

1. Question patient abut frequency and type of sexual activity; discomfort noted.
2. Question patient about pruritus, burning, tenderness, urinary symptoms, unusual discharge.
3. Assess patient's view of herpes; stigmas, misconceptions, fears.
4. Inspect genitalia for lesions, erythema, edema. Use speculum to examine vagina and cervix.

Nursing Diagnoses

A. Pain related to HSV outbreak
B. Impaired Skin Integrity related to herpetic lesions
C. Self-Esteem Disturbance related to stigma attached to herpes
D. Sexual Dysfunction related to potential transmission of herpes

Nursing Interventions

A. *Relieving Pain*
1. Demonstrate and encourage the use of warm sitz baths to increase blood supply to the areas and facilitate healing.
2. Instruct patient to keep the area clean and dry. Pat dry with a clean towel or use blow dryer. Wear loose cotton undergarments and loose clothing.
3. Encourage bed rest if case is severe.
4. Administer pain medications as prescribed.
5. Encourage patient to void in a warm sitz bath if urination is painful.
6. Insert indwelling catheter if urination is extremely painful or retention occurs.
7. Encourage fluid intake.

B. *Restoring Skin Integrity*
1. Administer acyclovir and teach patient its proper use, side effects.
2. Keep lesions clean and dry.
3. Teach patient not to rub or scratch lesions.
4. Apply moist tea bags to lesions while lying down. Tannic acid facilitates healing.

C. *Improving Self-Esteem*
1. Explore with patient her feelings about herpes and its effects on relationships.
2. Reiterate that when patient is feeling better physically, her feelings about herself will improve.

3. Discuss effects of stress on future outbreaks. Assist patient to identify stressors in her life and cope with stress. Review stress reduction methods such as relaxation breathing and imagery.
4. Encourage patient to discuss her feelings with family and significant others.

D. *Restoring Satisfying Sexual Function*
1. Teach patient to avoid intercourse from first sign of active outbreak to complete resolution of lesions, at least 2 weeks with primary infection, about 1 week with recurrent infections.
2. Teach patient that shedding of virus through genital secretions is possible even during asymptomatic period, so partner must be notified.
3. Inform patient that partner should use condoms for intercourse, but they may not be fully protective.
4. Explore possibility of noncoital aspects of sexual relationship.

Patient Education/Health Maintenance

1. Inform patient that initial outbreak is more painful than recurrent outbreaks, and that outbreaks vary from monthly to only several per year.
2. Teach patient to recognize precipitating factors.
3. Encourage regular follow-up for Pap smears to detect cervical changes early.
4. Remind patient of the effects on a neonate and the importance of notifying her health care provider if she becomes pregnant.
5. Tell patient that oral lesions can occur with HSV-2 due to transmission by oral intercourse, but that most oral cold sores are due to HSV-1 infection.
6. Refer patient to herpes support groups such as: Help; (local listings in telephone directory or call 301-369-1323)

Evaluation

A. Verbalizes decreased pain
B. Skin intact, without signs of secondary infection, scarring
C. Verbalizes improved self-esteem
D. Reports satisfying sexual activity

◆ CERVICITIS

Cervicitis is inflammation of the cervix.

Pathophysiology/Etiology

1. Cervicitis is usually caused by the sexually transmitted bacteria *Neisseria gonorrhoeae* or *C. trachomatis* but may be caused by other nonsexually transmitted organisms.
2. *C. trachomatis* is the most common sexually transmitted pathogen in both men and women in the United States, with an incidence of 197.5 cases per 100,000 people.

Clinical Manifestations

1. May be asymptomatic or have vaginal discharge.
   a. Gonorrhea—may be profuse, purulent discharge.
   b. Chlamydia—may be clear mucoid to creamy discharge.
2. May have dysuria and mild pelvic discomfort.
3. Cervix may be covered by thick mucopurulent discharge and be tender, erythematous, edematous, and friable.

Diagnostic Evaluation

1. Antigen detection tests for gonorrhea and chlamydia
2. Possible Gram stain and cervical culture for offending organisms

Management

1. Appropriate antibiotic agents—may be one dose regimen or a week of therapy, oral or parenteral.
2. Treatment may be given despite isolation of offending organism based on presumed pathogens.

Complications

1. PID
2. Disseminated gonococcal infection—arthritis and skin manifestations
3. Infertility

Nursing Assessment

1. Obtain history of sexual activity, any symptoms or infections in partner.
2. Perform abdominal and vaginal examination for tenderness caused by possible spread to pelvic organs.

Nursing Diagnoses

A. Pain related to inflammation of cervix
B. Risk for Infection Transmission related to STD

Nursing Interventions

A. *Relieving Pain*
1. Advise patient to use analgesic, such as over-the-counter products as directed.
2. Encourage rest and light activity until infection has been treated.
3. If discharge is profuse, suggest sitz baths to cleanse vulva.

B. *Preventing Infection Transmission*
1. Advise abstinence from sexual intercourse until treatment has been completed and follow-up culture is negative, if indicated.
2. Ensure that partner is treated at the same time if there is a high probability of gonorrhea or chlamydia.

Patient Education/Health Maintenance

1. Teach about all STDs and their symptoms.
2. Explain the treatment regimen to patient and advise her of side effects.
3. Encourage abstinence, monogamy, or safer sex methods such as male and female condom use.
4. Stress the importance of follow-up examination and testing to ensure eradication of infection. Recurrence rates are highest in younger patients.
5. For further information on STDs refer patients to agencies such as: American Foundation for the Prevention of Venereal Disease; 799 Broadway, Suite 638; New York, NY 10003; 212-759-2069.

Evaluation

A. Verbalizes relief of pain
B. At follow-up, states compliance with abstinence and treatment of partner

Problems Resulting From Relaxed Pelvic Muscles

◆ CYSTOCELE AND URETHROCELE

Cystocele is a downward displacement (protrusion) of the bladder into the vagina. *Urethrocele* is a downward displacement of the urethra into the vagina.

Pathophysiology/Etiology

1. Associated with obstetric trauma to fascia, muscle, and ligaments during childbirth (results in poor support).
2. Often becomes apparent years later, when genital atrophy associated with aging occurs.
3. May also be due to congenital defect or appear after hysterectomy.

Clinical Manifestations

1. May be asymptomatic in early stages.
2. Pelvic pressure or heaviness, backache, nervousness, fatigue
3. Urinary symptoms—urgency, frequency, incontinence, incomplete emptying
4. Aggravated by coughing, sneezing, standing for long periods, and obesity, which increase intra-abdominal pressure.
5. Relieved by resting or lying down.

Diagnostic Evaluation

1. Pelvic examination identifies condition.
2. Urinalysis and culture are done to rule out infection.

Management

1. Vaginal pessary—plastic device inserted into vagina as temporary treatment to support pelvic organs.
   a. Prolonged use may lead to necrosis and ulceration.
   b. Should be removed and cleaned every 1 to 2 months.
2. Estrogen therapy after menopause to decrease genital atrophy.
3. Surgery—if cystocele is large and interferes with bladder functioning
   a. May do anterior vaginal colporrhaphy (repair of anterior vaginal wall).
   b. Complications of surgery include urinary retention, bleeding (requires vaginal packing).

Complications

1. Urinary incontinence and infection

Nursing Assessment

1. Obtain history of obstetric trauma, abdominal surgery, menopause, use of estrogen.
2. Ask about urinary symptoms, pain.
3. Observe perineum while patient bears down or is in upright position for bulge from vagina.

Nursing Diagnoses

A. Pain related to pelvic pressure
B. Stress Incontinence related to relaxed pelvic muscles, displaced organs
C. Urinary Retention related to displaced organs

Nursing Interventions

A. *Relieving Pain*
1. Encourage periods of rest with legs elevated to relieve strain on pelvis.
2. Advise use of mild analgesics as necessary.
3. Provide postoperative care.
   a. Encourage voiding every 4 to 8 hours to reduce pressure so that no more than 150 mL will accumulate in bladder—catheterization or use of an indwelling catheter may be required.
   b. Administer perineal care to the patient after each voiding and defecation.
   c. Use a heat lamp to help dry the incision line and enhance the healing process.
   d. Use available sprays for anesthetic and antiseptic effects.
   e. Apply an ice pack locally to relieve congestion and discomfort.
   f. Administer analgesics as prescribed for relief of pain.

B. *Controlling Incontinence*
1. Teach patient Kegel pelvic floor exercises to regain muscle tone.
   a. Practice while voiding by stopping the flow of urine for 3 to 5 seconds, then releasing for 5 seconds.

b. Patient can then tighten pelvic floor muscle at any time, repeat 10 times, three times a day, increase as able.

2. Encourage patient to void frequently, respond to the urge to void promptly.
3. Warn patient to avoid straining to prevent incontinence.

C. *Preventing Urinary Retention*
1. Encourage fluids to decrease bacterial flora in the bladder.
2. Catheterize patient if retention is suspected.
3. Obtain urine specimen for culture and sensitivity if infection is suspected.

Patient Education/Health Maintenance

1. Teach women to avoid straining, remain active, avoid obesity, and perform Kegel exercises to minimize pelvic relaxation in their older years.
2. Encourage prompt attention to symptoms of urinary tract infection—dysuria, frequency, foul-smelling urine.

Evaluation

A. Patient verbalizes reduced pain.
B. Patient reports decreased frequency of incontinence.
C. Patient voids regularly without symptoms of infection.

◆ RECTOCELE/ENTEROCELE

Rectocele is displacement (protrusion) of the rectum into the vagina. *Enterocele* is displacement of intestine into the vagina.

Pathophysiology/Etiology

1. Posterior vaginal wall becomes weakened, allowing displacement.
2. Weakening caused by obstetric trauma, childbirth, pelvic surgery, aging.

Clinical Manifestations

1. Pelvic pressure or heaviness, backache, perineal burning
2. Constipation—may have difficulty in fecal evacuation; patient may use fingers into vagina to push feces up so defecation may occur.
3. Incontinence of feces and flatus—if tear between rectum and vagina
4. Visible protrusion into vagina
5. Symptoms are aggravated by standing for long periods.

Diagnostic Evaluation

1. Vaginal examination reveals condition.

2. May use Sims speculum to uplift cervix and fully evaluate condition.

Management

1. Pessary—plastic device inserted into vagina to aid pelvic support
2. Estrogen replacement to prevent atrophy
3. Surgery—if rectocele is large enough to interfere with bowel functioning—posterior colpoplasty (perineorrhaphy)—repair of posterior vaginal wall.

Complications

1. Total fecal incontinence

Nursing Assessment

1. Obtain history of childbirth, pelvic surgery, symptoms of bowel function.
2. Observe for bulge into vagina while patient bears down or is in upright position.
3. Monitor bowel movements.

Nursing Diagnoses

A. Pain related to pelvic pressure
B. Constipation related to displaced rectum/bowel

Nursing Interventions

A. *Relieving Pain*
1. Encourage periods of rest with legs elevated to relieve pelvic strain.
2. Encourage use of mild analgesics as needed.
3. Postoperative care
   a. Suggest low Fowler's position to decrease edema and discomfort.
   b. Administer perineal care to the patient after each voiding and defecation.
   c. Use a heat lamp to help dry the incision line and enhance the healing process.
   d. Use ice packs locally to relieve congestion and discomfort.
   e. Administer analgesics and stool softeners as ordered.

B. *Relieving Constipation*
1. Teach patient to increase fluid and fiber in diet.
2. Encourage use of stool softeners or bulk laxatives to make passage of stool easier.
3. Use of enema may be necessary to prevent straining.

Patient Education/Health Maintenance

1. Advise patient to avoid straining and obesity, which may cause return of rectocele or enterocele.

Evaluation

A. Verbalizes reduced pain
B. Soft stool passed daily

◆ UTERINE PROLAPSE

Uterine prolapse is an abnormal position of the uterus in which the uterus protrudes downward.

Pathophysiology/Etiology

1. Uterus herniates through pelvic floor and protrudes into vagina (prolapse) and possibly beyond the introitus (procidentia).
2. Usually due to obstetric trauma and overstretching of musculofascial supports.
3. Degrees
   a. First degree—cervix, without straining or traction, is at the introitus.
   b. Second degree—cervix extends over the perineum.
   c. Third degree—the entire uterus (or most of it) protrudes.

Clinical Manifestations

1. Backache or abdominal pain
2. Pressure and heaviness in vaginal region
3. Bloody discharge due to cervix rubbing against clothing or inner thighs
4. Ulceration of cervix
5. Symptoms are aggravated by obesity, standing, straining, coughing, or lifting a heavy object, due to increased intra-abdominal pressure.

Diagnostic Evaluation

1. Pelvic examination identifies condition.

Management

1. Surgical correction is recommended treatment with an anterior and posterior repair; effective and permanent.
2. Vaginal pessary—plastic device inserted into vagina as temporary or palliative measure if surgery cannot be done.
3. Abdominal sarcopexy—to anchor vagina
4. Estrogen cream—to decrease genital atrophy

Complications

1. Necrosis of cervix, uterus

Nursing Assessment

1. Obtain history of childbirth and surgery.
2. Ask about symptoms and aggravating factors.
3. Examine patient in lying or standing position; if cervix not readily visible, spread labia gently, do not attempt to insert speculum.

Nursing Diagnoses

A. Pain related to downward pressure and exposed tissue
B. Impaired Tissue Integrity related to exposed cervix and uterus
C. Sexual Dysfunction related to loss of vaginal cavity

Nursing Interventions

A. *Relieving Pain*
1. Administer sitz baths and explain procedure to patient.
2. Provide heating pad for low back or lower abdomen.
3. Administer pain medications as ordered.
4. Check for proper placement of pessary.
5. Increase fluid intake and encourage patient to void frequently to prevent bladder infection.

B. *Maintaining Cervical and Uterine Mucosal Integrity*
1. For second and third degree prolapse, apply saline compresses frequently.
2. Provide postoperative care.
   a. Administer perineal care to patient after each voiding and defecation.
   b. Use a heat lamp to help dry the incision line and enhance healing process.
   c. If urinary retention occurs, catheterize or use indwelling catheter until bladder tone is regained.
   d. Apply an ice pack locally to relieve congestion.
   e. Promote ambulation but prevent straining to reduce pelvic pressure.

C. *Restoring Sexual Function*
1. Discuss with patient noncoital sexual activity before treatment is instituted.
2. Explain to patient that sexual intercourse is possible with pessary; however, vaginal canal may be shortened.
3. Reinforce surgeon's instructions postoperatively about waiting to have vaginal penetration.
4. Encourage patient to explore with partner ways to engage in sexual activity without strain and with greatest comfort.

Evaluation

A. Verbalizes reduced pain
B. Cervix and uterus without ulceration
C. Verbalizes satisfying sexual activity

Gynecologic Tumors

◆ CANCER OF THE VULVA

Cancer of the vulva is most commonly carcinoma of the labia majora or clitoris; it may also originate as urethral tumor.

Pathophysiology/Etiology

1. Most common in women over 60 years of age; number of new cases has increased due to increase in elderly population.
2. Represents 3% to 4% of gynecologic cancers.
3. The cause is unknown, but associated with history of infections such as HPV or HSV.
4. Spread primarily through lymphatic system; rare distant metastasis.

Clinical Manifestations

1. Lesion present for several months—reddened, pigmented, white, or slightly elevated or ulcerated.
2. Vulvar pruritus, pain
3. Discharge or bleeding; may be foul smelling due to secondary infection.
4. Dysuria due to invasion of urethra with bacteria.
5. Edema of tissues
6. Lymphadenopathy

Diagnostic Evaluation

Biopsy of lesion and lymph nodes. If lesion is small may be excised at time of biopsy. Most lesions are squamous cell carcinoma.

Management

1. Carcinoma in situ (noninvasive) is usually treated by simple vulvectomy. Laser therapy may also be used.
2. Invasive carcinoma—radical or modified radical vulvectomy with bilateral groin lymph node resection.
    a. Pelvic nodes also may be removed if involvement is suspected.
    b. If cancer is confined to the vulva, there is a 90% 5-year survival rate after surgery.
3. Advanced carcinoma—pelvic exenteration or surgery and radiation as a palliative measure.
    a. Radiation has a limited role due to tumor insensitivity and complications such as severe vulvitis.
    b. Chemotherapy is primarily investigational. May shrink lesion so surgery can be less extensive.

Complications

1. Lymphatic spread
2. Complications after vulvectomy are common—wound breakdown, lymphedema, leg cellulitis, and vaginal stenosis.

Nursing Assessment

1. Obtain history of lesion, including when the patient first noticed it and any change in appearance.
2. Obtain gynecologic history, especially past infections.
3. Palpate lymph nodes and perform pelvic examination.

Nursing Diagnoses

A. Fear related to cancer and radical surgery
B. Impaired Tissue Integrity related to surgery
C. Sexual Dysfunction related to vulvectomy

Nursing Interventions

Preoperative

A. ***Relieving Fear***
1. Have the patient describe what her understanding is regarding the problem; answer questions and clear up misconceptions.
2. Emphasize the positive outcomes of the prescribed treatment plan; reinforce what the surgeon has already described to her.
3. Prepare patient for surgery and describe to her the postoperative appearance of the wound, use of drains, urinary catheter, etc. (Fig. 20-2).
    a. Shave a wide area to include perineal, pubic, and inguinal areas.
    b. Cleanse the vulva the night before with hexachlorophene or povidone–iodine shower or scrub.
    c. Administer an enema to evacuate intestinal tract before surgery; there will be no bowel movement for 2 to 3 days postoperatively.

Postoperative

B. ***Promoting Tissue Healing***
1. Maintain drainage and compression of tissues to remove fluid that could cause edema and prevent wound healing. Empty drains as needed (at least every 8 hours).
2. Keep wound clean and dry.
    a. Sterile dressing changes as prescribed.
    b. Apply heat lamp if prescribed to increase circulation and healing.
    c. Perform perineal care or sitz baths after each bowel movement or voiding (after catheter removed).
    d. Maintain patency of urinary catheter (about 10 days) to prevent wound contamination with urine.

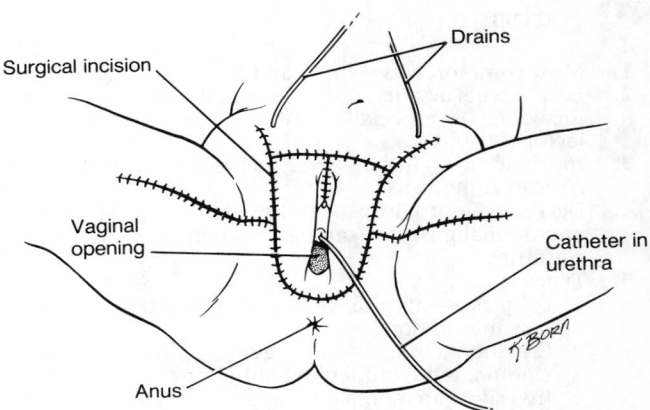

FIGURE 20-2 *Postoperative appearance after radical vulvectomy.*

e. Encourage low Fowler's position to promote comfort and reduce tension on sutures.
f. Prevent straining with defecation by providing a low- residue diet initially, stool softeners, later as ordered.
g. While patient is on bed rest, administer anticoagulants as prescribed and encourage leg exercises to prevent thrombus/embolus formation. Encourage careful ambulation the day after surgery while preventing perineal tension.

C. *Restoring Sexual Function*
1. Encourage patient to ventilate feelings about sexual mutilation, altered functioning.
2. Tell patient that if vagina is still intact, vaginal intercourse is still possible.
3. Inform patient of changes that may occur due to surgery—loss of sexual arousal if clitoris is removed, shortening of vagina, decreased lubrication.
4. Help patient explore alternate methods of sexual intimacy and encourage her to discuss feelings with her partner.

Patient Education/Health Maintenance

1. Encourage follow-up visits for additional therapy if required.
2. Encourage regular health check ups and screening for cancer and other age-related illness.
3. Encourage early evaluation of any suspicious lesions, bleeding, or discharge.

Evaluation

A. Verbalizes reduced fear
B. Perineum healed without complications
C. Verbalizes satisfying sexual function

◆ CANCER OF THE CERVIX

Cancer of the cervix is a common gynecologic malignancy.

Pathophysiology/Etiology

1. Most common between 35 and 55 years of age.
2. Early sexual activity, multiple sexual partners, and history of STDs, especially HPV and HSV, are major risk factors.
3. Incidence is higher in lower socioeconomic status and African Americans.
4. Decreased mortality rate in United States, but most frequent malignancy among women in developing countries.
5. Types
   a. Dysplasia—atypical cells with some degree of surface maturation
   b. Carcinoma in situ—cytology similar to invasive carcinoma, but confined to epithelium
   c. Invasive carcinoma—stroma is involved; 90% are of the squamous cell type. Spreads by local invasion and lymphatics to vagina and beyond.

Clinical Manifestations

1. Early disease is usually asymptomatic.
2. Initial symptoms are postcoital bleeding, irregular vaginal bleeding or spotting between periods or after menopause, and malodorous discharge.
3. As disease progresses, bleeding becomes more constant and is accompanied by pain that radiates to buttocks and legs.
4. Weight loss, anemia, and fever signal advanced disease.

Diagnostic Evaluation

1. Pap smear—routine screening measure; abnormal results warrant further diagnostic tests such as colposcopy and biopsy or conization.
2. Staging laparotomy—to evaluate metastasis outside the pelvis
3. Metastatic work-up—intravenous pyelogram, cystoscopy, sigmoidoscopy

Management

A. *Radiotherapy* Usual treatment for all stages

1. Intracavitary—radium via applicator
2. External—via linear accelerator or cobalt

B. *Surgery*
1. Hysterectomy
   a. Performed if childbearing no longer desired.
   b. Usually combined with radiation therapy for carcinoma in situ and invasive carcinoma.
   c. May cause impaired bladder function.
2. Pelvic exenteration
   a. Is the surgical removal of the vagina, uterus, uterine tubes, ovaries, bladder, rectum, and supporting structures and the creation of an ileal conduit and fecal stoma.
   b. Performed for very advanced disease if radiation therapy cannot be used; also for recurrent cancer.
   c. Vaginal reconstruction may be done.
3. Conization—if childbearing is desired, depending on stage of cancer.

C. *Other Procedures*
1. Laser therapy—tissue destruction for dysplasia
2. Cryosurgery—freezing destruction
3. Loop electrosurgical excision procedure (LEEP)—removes abnormal tissue with thin wire loop.

D. *Chemotherapy* Adjuvant with surgery or radiation

Complications

1. Spread to bladder and rectum; metastasis to lungs, mediastinum, bones, and liver.
2. Complications of intracavitary radiotherapy are cystitis, proctitis, vaginal stenosis, uterine perforation.
3. Complications of external radiation are bone marrow depression, bowel obstruction, fistula.

Nursing Assessment

1. Obtain history of Pap smears, sexual activity, past STDs.
2. Obtain history of any symptoms.
3. Assess understanding of disease and responses such as guilt, fear, denial, anxiety.

Nursing Diagnoses

A. Anxiety related to cancer, treatment
B. Body Image Disturbance related to surgical treatment

Nursing Interventions

A. Relieving Anxiety
1. Assist patient to seek information on stage of cancer, treatment options.
2. Prepare patient for hysterectomy or other surgery (see p. 655 for nursing interventions for hysterectomy).
3. Prepare patient for radiation therapy to the uterus (see p. 676 for nursing interventions for radiation therapy).

B. Enhancing Body Image
1. Provide emotional support during treatment.
2. Encourage patient to take pride in appearance by dressing, putting on makeup, etc. as able.
3. Encourage activity and socialization as patient feels able.

Patient Education/Health Maintenance

1. Explain the importance of life long follow-up regardless of treatments, to determine the response to treatment and detect spread of cancer.
2. Refer to cancer support group in community.

Evaluation

A. Reports decreased anxiety, increased ability to make decisions
B. Reports continued interest in appearance and femininity

◆ CANCER OF THE CORPUS UTERI

Cancer of the corpus uteri is usually adenocarcinoma of the endometrium of the fundus or body of the uterus.

Pathophysiology/Etiology

1. Most common gynecologic cancer and fourth leading cancer in women.
2. Most patients are over 55 years of age.

3. Cause is unknown but associated with increased estrogen stimulation, as in obesity, late menopause, nulliparity, and unopposed estrogen replacement.

Clinical Manifestations

1. Irregular bleeding before menopause or postmenopausal bleeding
2. Vaginal discharge—watery, usually malodorous
3. Pain, fever, and bowel and bladder dysfunctions are late signs.
4. Anemia secondary to bleeding

Diagnostic Evaluation

1. Pelvic examination—enlarged uterus may be palpated.
2. Endocervical aspirate—shows abnormal cells.
3. Endometrial biopsy—may be false negative.
4. Dilation and curettage—most accurate diagnostic tool.
5. Metastatic work-up—includes x-ray studies and cystoscopy.

Management

1. Hysterectomy with bilateral salpingo-oophorectomy (see p. 655)—primary therapy.
2. Radiation therapy (intracavitary or external)—preoperative and postoperative; complications include hemorrhagic cystitis, renal ulceration, or proctitis.
3. Hormonal therapy—progestational agents may alter receptor sites in endometrium for estrogen and thus decrease growth (for metastatic disease).
4. Chemotherapy—for metastatic and recurrent disease; low response rate of short duration.

Complications

1. Spread throughout the pelvis; metastasis to lungs, liver, bone, and brain

Nursing Assessment

1. Obtain history of menses, pregnancy, estrogen replacement.
2. Ask about irregular or postmenopausal bleeding, other symptoms.
3. Assess patient's response to possible diagnosis of cancer—fear, guilt, denial.

Nursing Diagnoses

A. Pain related to disease process
B. Fear related to cancer, treatment options

Nursing Interventions

A. Relieving Pain
1. Administer pain medications as prescribed and monitor patient's response.
2. Encourage use of relaxation techniques such as deep breathing, imagery, and distraction to help promote comfort.

B. Relieving Fear
1. Support patient through the diagnostic process and reinforce information given by health care provider about treatment options.
2. Prepare patient for radiation therapy, if indicated (see below).
3. Prepare patient for hysterectomy, if indicated (see p. 655).
4. Provide complete and concise explanations for all care you provide; emphasize the positive aspects of patient's recovery.

Patient Education/Health Maintenance

1. Explain the importance of reporting any postmenopausal bleeding.
2. Encourage keeping follow-up visits.
3. Explain that surgery or radiation treatment does not prevent satisfying sexual activity.
4. Refer to local cancer support group.

Evaluation

A. Verbalizes decreased pain
B. Verbalizes decreased fear

◆ NURSING CARE OF THE PATIENT RECEIVING RADIATION THERAPY TO THE UTERUS

Procedural Considerations

1. Applicators (tamdems and ovoids) are positioned in the endocervical canal and vagina in the operating room with the patient under anesthesia.
2. On recovery from anesthesia, x-rays are taken to check correct placement.
3. Radiologist then inserts radioactive material (radium or cesium) into applicator, which remains in place 24 to 72 hours. Therapy is individualized according to the stage of disease and the patient's response to and tolerance of radiation.
4. External radiation over pelvis may be supplemented to eliminate cancer spread via lymphatic system.

Nursing Interventions

A. Patient Preparation
1. Advise the patient that you will be administering an enema and vaginal douche and inserting an indwelling catheter before placement of applicator in the operating room.
2. Encourage patient to bring diversional activities because she will remain on bed rest during radiation treatment.
3. Instruct patient on radiation safety measures:
   a. Neither patient or secretions are radioactive.
   b. Do not touch source of radiation.
   c. Notify someone immediately if source is dislodged.
   d. When applicators are removed, there is no radioactivity remaining.
   e. Radioactivity is monitored by specially trained personnel.
   f. No pregnant visitors or children under 18 years old are allowed.
   g. Lead shields may be used to decrease radiation emanating from the patient.
4. Reinforce that help is readily available.

B. During Radiation Treatment
1. Maintain patient on strict bed rest on her back with head of bed elevated 20° to 30°. Patient may be log rolled three or four times per day. Use egg-crate mattress.
2. Have patient bathe upper body. Perineal care and linen changes are done only when absolutely necessary.
3. Maintain patient on a low-residue diet to prevent bowel movements, which could dislodge the apparatus. Encourage the patient to eat a variety of small rather than large servings.
4. Inspect indwelling catheter frequently to ensure proper drainage. A distended bladder may cause severe radiation burns.
5. Encourage fluids to prevent bladder infection.
6. Observe for signs and symptoms of radiation sickness—nausea, vomiting, fever, diarrhea, abdominal cramping.
7. Check applicator position every 8 hours, and monitor amount of bleeding and drainage (a small amount is normal).
8. Check patient frequently to minimize anxiety, but minimize time spent at bedside to reduce radiation exposure.

C. During Radiation Removal
1. Make sure that sterile gloves, long forceps, and lead container are available.
2. Check number of tubes removed against number applied; should be noted in chart.
3. Practice radiation precautions in handling and returning source to radiation department.
4. Administer a cleansing enema and douche before the patient gets out of bed.
5. Provide assistance during ambulation because of postural hypotension from prolonged bed rest.

◆ MYOMAS OF THE UTERUS

Myomas (fibroids, leiomyomas, fibromyomas) are benign tumors of the uterine myometrium (smooth muscle).

Pathophysiology/Etiology

1. Develop in women 25 to 40 years old.
2. May shrink after menopause.

3. Unknown cause but occur frequently in all women, most commonly in African American women.

Clinical Manifestations

1. Small myomas do not cause symptoms.
2. First indication may be palpable mass.
3. Irregular bleeding—usually menorrhagia.
4. Pain comes form pressure on adjacent organs—possibly heavy feeling in pelvis.
5. Secondary symptoms include fatigue due to anemia, urinary disturbances, and constipation.

Diagnostic Evaluation

1. Ultrasound—to identify size and location of myomas.
2. Cytology, dilation and curettage, etc to rule out cancer.

Management

1. Myomectomy may be done for small tumor.
2. Hysterectomy for large or numerous tumors.
3. Gonadotropin-releasing hormone antagonist (Lupron) therapy to create hypoestrogenic environment and try to shrink tumors

Complications

Infertility, habitual abortion

Nursing Assessment

1. Ask about pain, menstrual irregularity, and possible urinary symptoms, constipation.
2. Perform abdominal and bimanual examination to palpate masses.
3. Assess patient's understanding of condition as benign.

Nursing Diagnosis

A. Pain related to tumor growth

Nursing Interventions

A. *Relieving Pain*
1. Teach patient the proper use, side effects of analgesics.
2. Encourage patient to avoid long periods of standing; rest with pelvis in dependent position periodically to achieve comfort.
3. Encourage patient to void frequently to avoid increased pressure from distended bladder.
4. Advise use of high-fiber diet to prevent constipation.
5. Prepare patient for surgery, if indicated.

Patient Education/Health Maintenance

1. Tell patient to report increased symptoms, worsening bleeding because myomas may be enlarging and treatment may be indicated.
2. Reassure patient that myomas do not become malignant, but she should keep regular follow-up visits for cancer screening.

Evaluation

A. Verbalizes control of pain

◆ OVARIAN CYSTS

Ovarian cysts are benign growths arising from ovarian components.

Pathophysiology/Etiology

1. Often arise from functional changes in the ovary—from graafian follicle or from persistent corpus luteum.
2. May develop from abnormal embryonic epithelium—dermoid cysts.
3. Frequently found during childbearing years; masses found in women over age 50 have greater chance of being malignant.

Clinical Manifestations

1. May be asymptomatic or cause minor pelvic pain.
2. Menstrual irregularity
3. Tender, palpable mass
4. Rupture causes acute pain and tenderness, may mimic appendicitis or ectopic pregnancy.

Diagnostic Evaluation

1. Pelvic sonogram to determine size and characteristics
2. Pregnancy test to rule out ectopic pregnancy
3. Biopsy (at time of surgery) is done for suspicious cysts.

Management

1. Functional cysts less than 5 cm in diameter may be treated with oral contraceptives for 1 to 3 months in attempt to suppress them.
2. Surgery for large or leaking cyst by laparoscopy or laparotomy

Complications

1. Rupture may cause peritoneal inflammation.

Nursing Assessment

1. Obtain history of recent menses—irregular bleeding and spotting often signal follicular cyst, delayed menses followed by prolonged bleeding signals corpus luteal cyst.
2. Perform abdominal examination for tenderness, guarding, and rebound, which may indicate rupture.

Nursing Diagnoses

A. Pain related to abnormal growth
B. Risk for Fluid Volume Deficit Postoperatively related to change in intra-abdominal pressure following tumor removal

Nursing Interventions

A. Relieving Pain
1. Encourage the use of analgesics as prescribed.
2. Teach the patient the proper use of oral contraceptives if prescribed, along with side effects; encourage follow-up monthly to determine if cyst is resolving.
3. Tell the patient that heavy lifting, strenuous exercise, and sexual intercourse may increase pain.

B. Maintaining Fluid Volume
1. Prepare the patient for surgery as indicated.
2. Postoperatively monitor vital signs frequently and maintain intravenous (IV) infusion while NPO.
3. Assess frequently for abdominal distention due to fluid and gas pooling in abdominal cavity.
4. Apply abdominal binder to help prevent distention.
5. Place the patient in semi-Fowler's position for greatest comfort and encourage early ambulation to reduce distention (help patient arise slowly to prevent orthostatic hypotension).
6. Administer antiemetics and insert a nasogastric tube as ordered to prevent vomiting.
7. As distention resolves, assess bowel sounds and advance oral intake slowly.

Patient Education/Health Maintenance

1. Reassure patient that in most cases, ovarian function remains, and she remains fertile.
2. Reassure patient about low malignancy rate of cysts.
3. Encourage patient to report recurrent symptoms or worsening of pain if cyst is being treated medically.

Evaluation

A. Verbalizes reduced pain
B. Vital signs stable, no orthostasis

◆ OVARIAN CANCER

Ovarian cancer is a common gynecologic malignancy, with high mortality due to advanced disease by time of diagnosis.

Pathophysiology/Etiology

1. Peak incidence is in fifth decade.
2. Cause is unknown but associated with high-fat diet; smoking; alcohol; use of talcum powder perineally; history of breast, colon, or endometrial cancer; and family history of breast or ovarian cancer.
3. Epithelial cell tumors constitute 90%; germ and stromal cell tumors 10%.

Clinical Manifestations

1. No early manifestations
2. First manifestations—(vague) abdominal discomfort, indigestion, flatulence, anorexia, pelvic pressure, weight gain or loss, ovarian enlargement
3. Late manifestations—include abdominal pain, ascites, pleural effusion, intestinal obstruction

Diagnostic Evaluation

1. Pelvic examination—to detect enlargement, nodularity, immobility of the ovaries
2. Pelvic sonography and computed tomography (CT) scan—not helpful for early detection
3. Laparoscopy—to visualize mass
4. Paracentesis or thoracentesis—if ascites or pleural effusion is present
5. Laparotomy—to stage the disease and determine effectiveness of treatment
6. CA125—increase signifies progression

Management

1. Total abdominal hysterectomy with bilateral salpingo-oophorectomy and omentectomy is usual treatment due to delayed diagnosis.
2. Chemotherapy—more effective if tumor is optimally debulked; usually follows surgery due to frequency of advanced disease; may be given IV or intraperitoneal.
3. Radiation therapy usually added—intraperitoneal or external.
4. Immunotherapy with interferon or hormonal therapy with tamoxifen (Tamofen), an antiestrogen agent, may be used.
5. Second-look laparotomy may be done after adjunct therapies to take multiple biopsies and determine effectiveness of therapy.

Complications

1. Direct intra-abdominal or lymphatic spread

Nursing Assessment

1. Obtain history of irregular menses, pain, postmenopausal bleeding.
2. Ask about vague gastrointestinal-related complaints.
3. Ask about history of other malignancy and family history of breast or ovarian cancer.
4. Perform bimanual examination for palpable mass.

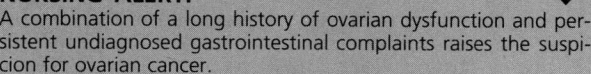

NURSING ALERT:
A combination of a long history of ovarian dysfunction and persistent undiagnosed gastrointestinal complaints raises the suspicion for ovarian cancer.
    A palpable ovary in a postmenopausal woman is abnormal and should be evaluated as soon as possible.

Nursing Diagnoses

A. Ineffective Coping related to advanced stage of cancer
B. Altered Nutrition (Less than Body Requirements) related to nausea and vomiting from chemotherapy
C. Body Image Disturbance related to hair loss from chemotherapy
D. Pain related to surgery

Nursing Interventions

A. Strengthening Coping
1. Provide emotional support through diagnostic process, allow patient to ventilate feelings, and encourage positive coping mechanisms.
2. Administer anxiolytic and analgesic medications as prescribed and teach patient and caregivers the potential side effects.
3. Refer patient to cancer support group.

B. Maintaining Adequate Nutrition
1. Administer or teach patient or caregiver to administer antiemetics as needed for nausea and vomiting.
2. Encourage small, frequent, bland meals or liquid nutritional supplements as able.
3. Assess the need for IV fluids if patient is vomiting.

C. Maintaining Body Image
1. Prepare patient for body image changes with chemotherapy (ie, hair loss).
2. Encourage patient to prepare ahead of time with turbans, wig, hats, etc.
3. Encourage patient to enhance appearance with makeup, clothing, jewelry, etc., as she is used to.
4. Stress the positive effects of patient's treatment plan.

D. Relieving Pain
1. Prepare patient for surgery as indicated; explain the extent of incision, presence of IVs, catheter, packing and drain tubes expected (see Hysterectomy, p. 655).
2. Postoperatively, administer analgesics as needed and explain to patient she may be drowsy.
3. Reposition frequently and encourage early ambulation to promote comfort and prevent side effects.

Patient Education/Health Maintenance

1. Explain to patient the onset of menopausal symptoms with ovary removal.
2. Tell patient that disease progression will be monitored closely by laboratory tests, and second look laparoscopy may be necessary.

3. Female relatives of patient should notify their doctors; biannual pelvic examinations may be necessary.
4. For women who have not had breast or ovarian cancer, oral contraceptives may decrease the risk of ovarian and endometrial cancer.

Evaluation

A. Openly discusses prognosis, asks appropriate questions, makes plans for short-term future
B. Weight maintained
C. Verbalizes satisfaction in appearance with wig
D. Verbalizes good control over pain

Other Gynecologic Conditions

◆ PELVIC INFLAMMATORY DISEASE

Pelvic inflammatory disease is an infection that may involve the fallopian tubes, ovaries, uterus, or peritoneum.

Pathophysiology/Etiology

1. Incidence has been increasing; high recurrence rate due to reinfections.
2. Causative agents include *N. gonorrhoeae*, *C. trachomatis*, and *Mycoplasma hominis*.
3. Predisposing factors include multiple sexual partners, early onset of sexual activity, use of IUDs (wick promotes ascension of bacteria), and procedures such as therapeutic abortion, cesarean sections, and hysterosalpingograms.

Clinical Manifestations

1. Pelvic pain—most common presenting symptom; usually dull and bilateral

NURSING ALERT:
Localized right or left lower quadrant tenderness with guarding, rebound, or palpable mass signifies tubo-ovarian abscess with peritoneal inflammation. Immediate evaluation and surgical intervention are necessary to prevent rupture and widespread peritonitis.

2. Fever—especially with gonococcal infections
3. Cervical discharge—mucopurulent
4. Cervical motion tenderness—especially with gonococcal infections
5. Irregular bleeding
6. Gastrointestinal symptoms—nausea, vomiting, acute abdomen usually signify abscess.
7. Urinary symptoms—dysuria, frequency
8. Presentation with *Chlamydia* may be mild.

Diagnostic Evaluation

1. Endocervical culture—to identify organisms
2. CBC—shows elevated leukocytes.
3. Laparoscopy—provides direct visualization of the fallopian tubes.

Management

1. Antibiotics—combinations of tetracyclines, penicillins, quinolones, and cephalosporins, orally or parenterally

COMMUNITY-BASED CARE TIP:
If patient with PID is to be treated at home, stress the importance of follow-up, usually in 48 hours to determine if oral antibiotic treatment is effective. Advise the patient to report any worsening of symptoms immediately.

2. Inpatient treatment required if uncertain diagnosis, abscess, pregnancy, severe infection, unable to take oral fluids, prepubertal, or more aggressive antibiotics required to preserve fertility.
3. Surgical treatment may be necessary to drain abscess or later to treat adhesions or tubal damage.

Complications

1. Abscess rupture and sepsis
2. Infertility—due to adhesions of fallopian tubes and ovaries
3. Ectopic pregnancy—due to inability of fertilized egg to pass stricture

Nursing Assessment

1. Obtain history of menstruation, contraception, sexual activity, including number of partners, STD history, symptoms in sexual partner.
2. Assess level of pain, fever, and vital signs for hypotension and increased pulse indicating hypovolemia.
3. Perform abdominal and pelvic examinations, if indicated—be alert for abdominal tenderness, rebound, guarding, or presence of a mass.
4. Assess patient's feelings about having an STD.

Nursing Diagnoses

A. Pain related to pelvic inflammation and infection
B. Fluid Volume Deficit related to fever and decreased oral intake

Nursing Interventions

Also see Nursing Care Plan 20-1.

A. Relieving Pain
1. Administer or teach self-administration of analgesics as prescribed.

2. Advise patient to rest in bed for first 1 to 3 days and apply heating pad to pelvis for comfort.
3. Administer or teach self-administration of antibiotics as prescribed. Keep strict dosage schedule and notify health care provider if dose lost through vomiting.

B. Restoring Fluid Balance
1. Monitor vital signs and intake and output closely.
2. Administer antiemetics as indicated.
3. Maintain IV infusion of fluids until oral intake adequate.
4. Provide clear fluids, followed by soft bland diet as tolerated.

Patient Education/Health Maintenance

1. Encourage compliance with antibiotic therapy for full length of prescription.
2. Stress the need for sexual abstinence until follow-up visit and testing ensure cure.
3. Advise testing and possible treatment for all sexual partners.
4. Educate about safer sexual practice.

Evaluation

A. Verbalizes relief of pain
B. Vital signs stable; urine output adequate

◆ ENDOMETRIOSIS

Endometriosis is the abnormal proliferation of uterine endometrial tissue outside the uterus.

Pathophysiology/Etiology

1. May also be found outside the pelvic cavity; an intact uterus is not needed to have endometriosis.
2. Peaks in women aged 25 to 45; may occur at any age. Increased risk in siblings, women with shorter menstrual cycles and longer duration of flow. More common in whites than African Americans, and in women who do not exercise and are obese.
3. Responds to ovarian hormonal stimulation—estrogen increases it, progestins decrease it.
   a. Bleeds during uterine menstruation, resulting in accumulated blood and inflammation and subsequent adhesions and pain.
   b. Regresses during amenorrhea (ie, pregnancy and menopause) and oral contraceptive and androgen use.
4. Theories of origin
   a. May be embryonic tissue remnants that differentiate as a result of hormonal stimulation and spread via lymphatic or venous channels.
   b. May be transferred via surgical instruments.
   c. May be due to retrograde menstruation through uterine tubes into peritoneal cavity.

NURSING CARE PLAN 20-1 ◆ *Care of the Patient With Pelvic Inflammatory Disease*

You are assigned Janice Smith, a 17-year-old with acute PID. From your assessment and your knowledge of PID, you develop your plane of care.

Subjective data: Janice tells you she has severe lower abdominal pain, vaginal discharge, fever, and nausea and vomiting that has made her unable to eat or drink for 2 days. She feels weak and dizzy. She admits to being sexually active with a new partner without condoms. She is on oral contraceptives and her last menstrual period was 1 week ago.

Objective data: Vital signs are—temperature 39°C (102.2°F), pulse 98, BP 94/60, respirations 24. On examination you note lower abdominal tenderness and mild guarding without rebound. On speculum examination, Janice has purulent cervical discharge. On bimanual examination, she has cervical motion tenderness and bilateral adnexal tenderness without masses.

NURSING DIAGNOSIS: Pain, related to pelvic infection

GOAL: Pain will be reduced.

NURSING INTERVENTIONS	RATIONALE	EVALUATION
1. Administer analgesics as prescribed. Alert patient to side effect of drowsiness.	1. Analgesics provide pain relief. Knowledge of side effects enhances patient compliance.	1. Verbalizes reduced severity of pain after medication.
2. Assist patient to position of pelvic dependence, with head and feet elevated slightly.	2. Promotes drainage of infection without strain on pelvic structures.	2. Resting in pelvic dependent position.
3. Encourage patient to apply heating pad to lower abdomen or low back.	3. Promotes circulation and relief of inflammation, promotes comfort.	3. Uses heating pad properly.

NURSING DIAGNOSIS: Fluid Volume Defecit related to fever and decreased oral intake

GOAL: Fluid balance will be restored.

NURSING INTERVENTIONS	RATIONALE	EVALUATION
1. Maintain IV fluids as ordered.	1. IV fluids replace circulating fluid volume.	1. Denies dizziness. BP 106/64, pulse 88.
2. Administer antiemetics as prescribed.	2. Antiemetics prevent vomiting.	2. No vomiting.
3. Monitor intake and output.	3. Provides feedback on fluid replacement.	3. Intake equals output.
4. Restart oral intake with ice chips and sips of water when vomiting has ceased for 2 h.	4. Will not distend stomach and produce vomiting.	4. Ice chips and sips of water tolerated without vomiting.

NURSING DIAGNOSIS: Risk for Infection Transmission related to sexual activity

GOAL: Infection will not be transmitted or recur.

NURSING INTERVENTIONS	RATIONALE	EVALUATION
1. Advise abstinence until repeat cultures prove cure at follow-up, about 2 weeks following treatment.	1. Abstinence is the only sure method of preventing transmission of organisms.	1. Reports understanding of abstinence, need for follow-up.
2. Tell patient to advise partner(s) to seek treatment.	2. All partners must receive treatment to break the chain of transmission.	2. Partner has been advised by patient.
3. Teach patient methods of preventing infection with STDs—abstinence, monogomy, proper use of condoms.	3. Safe sexual behavior reduces risk of STDs.	3. Describes proper use of condoms.

Clinical Manifestations

1. Depends on sites of implantation; may be asymptomatic.
2. Pelvic pain—especially during or before menstruation.
3. Dyspareunia
4. Painful defecation—if implants are on sigmoid colon or rectum.
5. Abnormal uterine bleeding
6. Persistent infertility
7. Hematuria, dysuria, flank pain—if bladder involved

Diagnostic Evaluation

1. Pelvic and rectal examinations—tender, fixed nodules or ovarian mass or uterine retrodisplacement; nodules may not be palpable.
2. Laparoscopy—for definitive diagnosis to view implants and determine extent of disease.
3. Other studies include ultrasound, CT, and barium enema to determine extent of organ involvement.

Management

A. *Medical*
1. Danazol (Danocrine)—most commonly used drug; synthetic androgen suppresses endometrial growth. Contraindicated in pregnancy.
2. Progestins—create a hypoestrogenic environment.
3. Gonadotropin-releasing hormone antagonist (Lupron) injections over a 6-month period—create hypoestrogenic environment.
4. Oral contraceptives—use small amount of estrogen, maximum amount of progestin and androgen effect to decrease implant size.

B. *Surgical*
1. Laparoscopic surgery—preferred procedure to remove implants and lyse adhesions; not curative; high recurrence rate.
2. CO_2 laser laparoscopy—for minimal to moderate disease; vaporizes tissue; may be done at same time as diagnosis; good pregnancy rate.
3. Laparotomy—for severe endometriosis or persistent symptoms.
4. Presacral neurectomy—to decrease central pelvic pain; preserves fertility.
5. Hysterectomy—if fertility is not desired and symptoms are severe; ovaries are preserved if not affected.

Complications

1. Infertility
2. Rupture of cyst—mimics ruptured appendix.

Nursing Assessment

1. Obtain history of symptoms to determine spread and severity of disease.
2. Assess pain—level, location, characteristics.

3. Perform abdominal, pelvic, rectal examinations to assess for areas of tenderness, nodules.
4. Assess for impact of endometriosis, infertility on patient, relationship with significant other.

Nursing Diagnoses

A. Pain related to hormonal stimulation, adhesions
B. Self-Esteem Disturbance related to difficult management of disease, infertility

Nursing Interventions

A. *Reducing Pain*
1. Teach use of analgesics, as prescribed, along with side effects.
2. Encourage use of heating pad to painful areas, as needed.
3. Teach patient relaxation techniques to control pain, such as deep breathing, imagery, and progressive muscle relaxation.
4. Encourage patient to try position changes for sexual intercourse if experiencing dyspareunia.

B. *Increasing Self-Esteem*
1. Include patient in treatment planning; answer questions about drug and surgical treatment so she can make informed choices.
2. Encourage adequate rest and nutrition.
3. Provide emotional support and encourage patient to discuss treatment of infertility with her physician.
4. Prepare patient for surgery as indicated.

Patient Education/Health Maintenance

1. Instruct patient in the side effects of prescribed medication; for example, danazol (Danocrine) may cause voice changes, increased facial hair, acne, weight gain, decreased breast size, and vasomotor reactions.
2. Refer patient to support groups such as: Endometriosis Association; 8585 North 76th Place; Milwaukee, WI 53223; 1-800-992-3636.

Evaluation

A. Verbalizes reduced pain
B. Verbalizes increased self-esteem

◆ TOXIC SHOCK SYNDROME

Toxic shock syndrome (TSS) is a condition caused by a bacterial toxin (*Staphylococcus aureus*) in the bloodstream; it can be life-threatening.

Pathophysiology/Etiology

1. Cause is uncertain, but 70% of cases are associated with menstruation and tampon use.

2. Research studies suggest that magnesium-absorbing fibers in tampons may account for lower levels of magnesium in the body; this contributes to providing an ideal condition for toxin production by the bacteria.
3. TSS has been observed in nonmenstruating individuals with conditions such as cellulitis, surgical wound infection, vaginal infections, subcutaneous abscesses, and with the use of contraceptive sponge, diaphragm, and tubal ligation.
4. Oral contraceptives may be protective against TSS by increasing lactobacilli in vaginal flora.

Clinical Manifestations

1. Sudden onset of fever greater than 39°C (102°F)
2. Vomiting and profuse watery diarrhea
3. Rapid progression to hypotension and shock within 72 hours of onset
4. Mucous membrane hyperemia
5. Sometimes, sore throat, headache, and myalgia
6. Rash (similar to sunburn) that develops 1 to 2 weeks after onset of illness and is followed by desquamation, particularly of the palms and soles

Diagnostic Evaluation

1. Blood, urine, throat, and vaginal/cervical cultures; possibly cerebrospinal fluid culture—to detect/rule out infectious organism.
2. Tests to rule out other febrile illnesses—Rocky Mountain spotted fever, Lyme disease, meningitis, Epstein-Barr or coxsackie virus.

Management

1. Fluid and electrolyte replacement to increase blood pressure and prevent renal failure
2. Vasopressor medications (ie, dopamine) as needed
3. Antibiotics (ie, penicillins or cephalosporins) may decrease the rate of relapse.
4. The use of steroids and immunoglobulins is controversial.

Complications

1. Cardiovascular collapse and renal failure due to shock

Nursing Assessment

1. Determine menstrual history, use of tampons, or whether there has been recent skin infection, childbirth, or surgery.
2. Determine vital signs and assess temperature and blood pressure as indicated; hemodynamic monitoring may be needed.

Nursing Diagnoses

A. Hyperthermia related to infectious process

B. Fluid Volume Deficit related to toxin effects
C. Impaired Skin Integrity related to latent desquamation

Nursing Interventions

A. **Reducing Body Temperature**
1. Administer antipyretics as ordered.
2. Use cooling measures such as sponge baths and hypothermia blanket, if indicated.
3. Monitor core body temperature frequently.

B. **Restoring Fluid Volume**
1. Perform hemodynamic monitoring as indicated (ie, arterial line, central venous pressure, or pulmonary artery pressure).
2. Maintain strict intake and output measurement.
3. Insert indwelling catheter to monitor urine output.
4. Administer IV fluids and vasopressors as ordered to control hypotension.
5. Monitor respiratory status for pulmonary edema and respiratory distress syndrome due to fluid overload from increased fluid replacement.
6. Administer diuretics as ordered if edema results.

C. **Restoring Skin Integrity**
1. Tell patient to expect desquamation of skin, as in peeling sunburn.
2. Protect skin and avoid use of harsh soaps and alcohol that cause drying.
3. Tell patient to apply mild moisturizer and avoid direct sunlight until healed.
4. Advise patient that reversible hair loss may occur 1 to 2 months after TSS.

Patient Education/Health Maintenance

1. Tell patient to expect fatigue for weeks to months after TSS.
2. Tell patient not to use tampons in future to reduce risk of recurrence.
3. Encourage follow-up examination and cultures.
4. Teach prevention of TSS.
   a. Alternate use of pads with tampons, avoid super absorbency tampons.
   b. Change tampons frequently and do not wear one longer than 8 hours; 4 hours maximum in heavy discharge time.
   c. Be careful of vaginal abrasions that can be caused by some applicators.
   d. Be alert to symptoms of TSS.

Evaluation

A. Afebrile
B. Normotensive, good urine output
C. Skin heals without scarring.

Selected References

Bernubi, G. (Ed.). (1994). *Obstetric and gynecologic emergencies.* Philadelphia: J. B. Lippincott.

Brucks, J. A., et al. (1992). Practical tips for assessment and management of vulvar and vaginal human papillomavirus. *Nurse Practitioner Forum, 3*(3), 169-176.

Chuong, C. J., Pearsall-Otey, L. R., & Rosenfeld, B. L. (1995). A practical guide to relieving PMS. *Contemporary Nurse Practitioner, 1*(3), 31-37.

Dunnihoo, D. R. (1992). *Fundamentals of gynecology and obstetrics* (2nd ed.). Philadelphia: J. B. Lippincott.

Farro, S. (1994). *Sexually transmitted diseases in obstetrics and gynecology.* Philadelphia: J. B. Lippincott.

Gerchufsky, M. (1995). Updating family planning options. *Advance for Nurse Practitioners, 3*(5), 18-23.

Glass, R. H. (Ed.). (1992). *Office gynecology* (4th ed.). Baltimore: Williams & Wilkins.

Hatcher, R. A., Stewart, F., & Trussell, J. (1994). *Contraceptive technology* (16th ed.). New York: Irvington Publishers.

Hillis, S. D., Nakashima, A., Marchbanks, P. A., et al. (1994). Risk factors for recurrent *Chlamydia trachomatis* infection in women. *American Journal of Obstetrics and Gynecology, 170*(3), 801-806.

Screening for gynecologic malignancies in primary care. (1993). *Emergency Medicine, 25*(4), 109-116.

1993 Sexually Transmitted Diseases Treatment Guidelines. (1993, Sept. 24). *MMWR, 42*(RR-14), 1-102.

Tamlyn-Leaman, K., et al.(1992). Cervical intraepithelial neoplasia: Clinical update and implications for nursing practice. *Canadian Oncology Nursing Journal, 2*(4), 137-139.

CHAPTER 21 ◆

Breast Conditions

Assessment of the Breast

◆ SUBJECTIVE DATA

Obtain a nursing history about specific breast complaints as well as general health information from the patient to plan care and appropriate patient teaching.

Breast Manifestations

1. Palpable lumps—date noted; affected by menstruation; changes noted since detection
2. Nipple discharge—date of onset, color, unilateral or bilateral, spontaneous or provoked
3. Pain or tenderness—localized or diffuse, cyclic or constant, unilateral or bilateral
4. Date of last mammogram and result
5. Patient's practice of breast self-examination (BSE)

History

A. General Information
1. Age
2. Past medical/surgical history; injuries; bleeding tendencies
3. Medications including current or prior use of oral contraceptives/hormones

B. Gynecologic and Obstetric History
1. Menarche
2. Date of last menstrual period
3. Pregnancies, miscarriages, abortions, deliveries
4. Lactational history
5. Prior breast history
6. Family history of breast cancer

◆ PHYSICAL EXAMINATION

Perform a breast examination, as outlined in Procedure Guidelines 21-1. Remind all women of the importance of routine checkups with breast examination. BSE is an essential first step in prevention of breast cancer.

Guidelines for Early Detection

The American Cancer Society recommends the following for early detection of breast cancer:

1. BSE—once a month; age 20 and over.
2. Clinical examination—see a doctor or nurse for a physical breast examination.
   a. Age 20 to 40, every 3 years.
   b. Over 40, every year.
3. Mammography—have first mammogram by age 40.
   a. Age 40 to 49, have a mammogram every 1 to 2 years.
   b. Age 50 and over, have a mammogram every year.

GERONTOLOGIC ALERT:
Normal breast changes in the elderly include drooping, flaccid breasts due to decreased subcutaneous tissue from decreased estrogen levels. Nipple size and erection are also reduced.

PROCEDURE GUIDELINES 21-1 ◆ Examination of the Breast by the Nurse

PURPOSE
1. To detect abnormalities in the breasts
2. To teach a woman how to perform breast self-examination

EQUIPMENT Good lighting and a private, warm setting

PROCEDURE

NURSING ACTION	RATIONALE
SITTING POSITION	
1. Wash your hands under warm water and dry them. Apply powder if they feel "sticky."	1. The breast is sensitive to cold. Powder reduces friction.
2. Have the woman strip to her waist and sit comfortably facing the examiner. Observe breast for abnormalities.	2. This provides an opportunity to observe breasts for lack of symmetry and for gross signs such as redness, irritated nipple, dimpling, orange peel skin.
3. Have patient raise arms overhead.	3. Changes in lower half of breast are more visible.
4. Palpate cervical and supraclavicular area.	4. Note whether lymph nodes are enlarged, fixed, moveable, or difficult to locate.
5. Palpate axillary nodes; hold the woman's forearm in your left palm while you check nodes with your right fingertips. Repeat on other side.	5. Same as 4 above.
6. Have patient place hands on hips and press.	6. Flexes pectoral muscles, accentuates skin dimpling or masses.
LYING POSITION	
1. Instruct the patient to lie down with her right arm under her head. Place a small pillow under the right shoulder.	1. This will spread breast tissue evenly over chest wall.
2. With the finger pads of two or three fingers, gently palpate breast tissue beginning at the upper outer quadrant. a. Proceed in an orderly pattern around the breast and repeat the first quarter examined. b. Repeat procedure for other breast.	2. The sensitive fingers, proceeding in a kneading fashion, can detect thickened, lumpy or "buckshot" tissue between the patient's skin and chest wall. Because the majority of breast lesions are in the upper outer quadrant, this segment is double checked.
3. Recognize that there is a prolongation of the axillary extension of normal breast tissue that may extend high into axilla.	3. This is normal if symmetrical and may be abnormal if asymmetrical.
4. Check areolar area for crustiness, nipple discharge, signs of infection. If nipple discharge is observed, note if from single or multiple ducts. May hemoccult to check for hidden blood.	4. A nipple discharge may be benign or may be related to cancer.
5. Record findings and report abnormalities to the health care provider.	5. Diagram may be useful for future reference.
6. Instruct the patient in performing self-examination on her own. Encourage her to ask any questions; provide her with appropriate literature.	6. Ninety percent of women discover their own abnormalities.

Diagnostic Tests

◆ LABORATORY TESTS

Nipple Discharge Cytology

A. *Description* Secretions are smeared on a slide, fixed and submitted for cytologic examination. This is not considered a reliable test because of its high false-negative rate

B. *Nursing/Patient Care Considerations*
1. Wash nipple area with water and pat dry before obtaining specimen if crusting of drainage is present.
2. Gently milk breast and express fluid to obtain a large drop on nipple.
3. Carefully touch slide to drop and draw slide across nipple to obtain smear.
4. Spray with fixative or drop into container with fixative.
5. Inform patient of results promptly because of anxiety and explain that other tests may be needed.

Estrogen and Progesterone Receptors

A. *Description*
1. Evaluates cancer cells from tissue biopsy to determine presence of receptor sites.
2. If such sites are present, the patient is more likely to respond to endocrine manipulation as adjuvant therapy.
3. About 60% are estrogen-receptor positive. (Positive results—more than 10 fmol/mg protein).

B. Nursing/Patient Care Consideration Tell patient that the test may help select appropriate chemotherapy, especially estrogen-blocking agents

Additional Laboratory Tests

A. Tumor Aggressiveness Tests To evaluate the aggressiveness of a tumor and its potential to regrow

1. Proliferation/S phase—cell kinetic study that shows percent of cells in S phase in a tumor and gives an indication of proliferative capacity.
2. DNA ploidy—measurement of DNA content of a tumor; interpreted as favorable or unfavorable.
3. Cathepsin D—studies suggest that high cathepsin D levels may be correlated with greater recurrence, lower survival, and poor prognosis, particularly in patients with negative nodes.

B. Tests to Detect Metastasis
1. Increased values on liver function tests may indicate possible liver metastasis.
2. Increased calcium and alkaline phosphatase levels may indicate possible bony metastasis.

◆ RADIOLOGY/IMAGING

Mammography

A. Description
1. Low-dose x-ray of breast used to screen for breast abnormalities or may be used when a lump is found on physical examination. Most sensitive method of early detection of breast cancer; can detect patients with clustered microcalcifications, early in breast cancer.
2. Compression of the breast is used to reduce the amount of radiation absorbed by the breast tissue and separate overlapping tissue.
3. Two views are taken routinely, craniocaudal and mediolateral; other views are done as necessary.
4. Best performed at a facility that is accredited by the American College of Radiology. The machines and staff at these facilities have met specific quality criteria.
5. Mammography is not routinely done if a woman is pregnant.
6. The breasts of young women tend to be extremely dense and are poorly suited to mammography.
7. False-negative results occur even in the best facilities; figure may reach 10%.

B. Nursing/Patient Care Considerations
1. Recommend regular screening based on established guidelines (see p. 685). Tell women that routine screening mammography has been shown to reduce mortality from breast cancer. Procedure takes about 15 minutes.
2. Remind woman not to apply deodorant, cream, or powder to breast, nipple, or underarm areas on examination day.
3. Advise that some discomfort may be felt from compressing the breast.
4. Alert patient that extra views do not imply that the patient has breast cancer.

NURSING ALERT:
Fewer than 50% of women obtain regular screening mammograms based on the established guidelines. Because health teaching is an important nursing role, nurses should be educating women about the importance of routine screening.

Ultrasonography

A. Description
1. Uses high-frequency sound waves to get an image of the breast.
2. Most useful test after mammography; helps determine if a lump is a cyst or a solid mass.
3. May be used if patient is pregnant or is less than 35 years old.

B. Nursing/Patient Care Considerations Advise that this test is painless and noninvasive.

Additional Imaging Studies

A. Galactography
1. A contrast mammogram is obtained by injection of water-soluble contrast medium into a duct for patient with persistent bloody nipple discharge. It is a time-consuming procedure that is not routinely used.
2. It may outline an intraductal papilloma.
3. Its ability to differentiate benign from malignant lesions is limited.

B. Magnetic Resonance Imaging (MRI)
1. May be used to rule out malignancy in nonpalpable breast lesions; useful in women with dense breasts.
2. It is expensive and not useful for generalized screening.
3. See page 151 for description of MRI.

C. Metastatic Work-up
1. May include x-rays (ie, chest x-ray), bone scan, or computed tomography (CT) scan to detect presence of metastasis.

◆ OTHER TESTS

Besides laboratory tests and imaging studies, biopsy methods are commonly used to evaluate breast conditions. A biopsy is the only certain way to learn whether a breast lump or suspicious area seen on a mammogram is cancerous.

Fine Needle Aspiration

A. Description
1. Uses a thin needle and syringe to collect tissue or drain lump after using a local anesthetic. If it is a cyst, removing the fluid will collapse it; no other treatment may be needed.
2. Normal cyst fluid appears straw-colored or greenish. Fluid should be sent for cytology if it appears suspicious—clear or bloody; otherwise it is discarded.
3. This office procedure uses local anesthetic with results usually within 24 hours.

4. It has limited sensitivity possibly due to insufficient acquisition of cytologic material.

B. *Nursing/Patient Care Considerations*
1. Inform the patient of small risk of hematoma and infection.
2. Band-aid applied after procedure; usually no discomfort.
3. Solid lesions may warrant an excisional biopsy.

Needle Biopsy

A. *Description*
1. Office procedure using local anesthetic that removes a small piece of breast tissue using a needle with a special cutting edge.
2. For palpable lesions with a high suspicion of malignancy. May provide a tissue diagnosis quickly—usually about 24 hours, without doing an excisional biopsy to plan definitive surgery.

B. *Nursing/Patient Care Considerations*
1. Inform the patient of small risk of hematoma and infection.
2. Tell patient that several passes may be necessary to obtain specimen, with minor discomfort.
3. Pressure dressing applied after procedure.
4. Recommend use of acetaminophen (Tylenol) or ibuprofen (Advil) for any postprocedure discomfort—usually minimal if any.

Stereotactic Core Needle Biopsy

A. *Description*
1. An x-ray-guided method for localizing and sampling nonpalpable lesions detected on mammography with 90% to 95% sensitivity in detecting breast cancer.
2. Performed as an outpatient procedure with the patient lying prone on a special table using an automated biopsy gun.
3. Following local anesthetic, a needle is placed in the lesion with confirmation of its position on stereotactic x-ray views. Multiple samples are taken from different portions of the lesion.
4. The procedure is quicker and less expensive than mammographically guided needle localization followed by surgical excisional biopsy and is an alternative to surgical excisional biopsy.

B. *Nursing/Patient Care Considerations*
1. Inform patient that it is a 1-hour outpatient procedure that requires no special preparation.
2. Complications may include minor bleeding, hematoma, and infection.
3. Explain that nonspecific, suspicious, or atypical findings may result in proceeding to excisional biopsy.
4. Remind patient that area in question will not be removed, only sampled.

Excisional Biopsy

A. *Description*
1. Surgical removal of a palpable or nonpalpable lesion. A frozen section may be done for immediate tissue diagnosis.

2. Excisional biopsy or lumpectomy is entire removal of a mass; incisional biopsy is partial removal of a mass.
3. In the past 10 years the number of screening mammograms has increased, which has led to an increase in the number of breast biopsies done for nonpalpable abnormalities.
4. This outpatient procedure may be performed under local or general anesthesia.
5. Curvilinear incision is usually made directly over the mass, which is excised en bloc including a 1-cm grossly free margin of tissue.

B. *Nursing/Patient Care Considerations*
1. Pressure dressing is placed, which can be removed in 24 to 48 hours.
2. Inform patient to watch for bleeding, hematoma, and signs of infection.
3. Recommend analgesics for discomfort and wearing a support bra for comfort.

Needle Localization With Biopsy

A. *Description*
1. Performed when there is a nonpalpable mammographic finding.
2. Mammogram is used as a guide for placing a needle at the site of the breast change after injecting some local anesthetic.
3. A wire may be left in place for the surgeon or dye may be injected to mark the site.
4. Excisional biopsy is then done (see above).

B. *Nursing/Patient Considerations* Inform patient that this may be a tedious procedure because of having to remain fairly immobile while the breast is compressed in the mammogram machine and different views are obtained

General Procedures/Treatment Modalities

◆ BREAST SELF-EXAMINATION

Breast self-examination is an inexpensive, risk-free method to detect cancer. When lumps are discovered at an early stage, they have a better chance for long-term survival. Figure 21-1 presents guidelines for teaching patients.

Patient Education

A. *General Points to Emphasize*
1. Examine breasts once a month, just after the menstrual period, because breasts are less engorged and a tumor is easier to detect, and at regular monthly intervals after the cessation of menses.
2. Compare findings with the opposite breast.
3. Remind patient that 90% of breast lumps are not cancer.
4. Do not neglect men when teaching BSE—1% of breast cancers are in men.

• LOOK FOR CHANGES • FEEL FOR CHANGES •

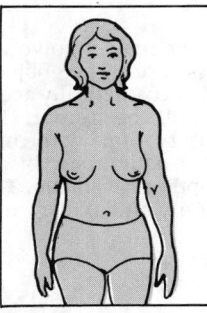

Hands at side.

Compare for symmetry.
Look for changes in:
• shape
• color

Check for:
• puckering
• dimpling
• skin changes
• nipple changes

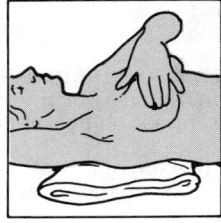

Lie down with a towel under right shoulder; raise right arm above the head.

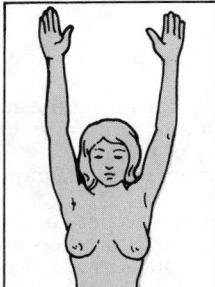

Hands over head.

Check front and side view for:
• symmetry
• puckering
• dimpling

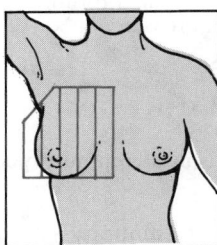

Examine area from:
• underarm to lower bra line
• across to breast bone
• up to collar bone
• back to armpit

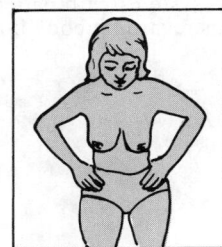

Hands on hips, press down, bend forward.

Check for:
• symmetry
• nipple direction
• general appearance

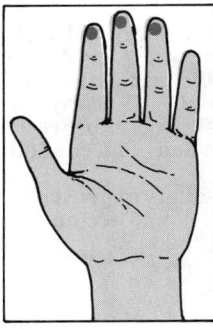

Use the pads of the three middle fingers of the left hand.

Hold hand in bowed position.

Move fingers in dime-size circles.

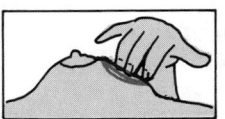

Use three levels of pressure:
• light
• medium
• firm

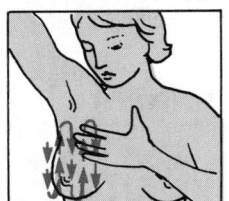

Examine entire area using vertical strip pattern.

Now check your left breast with your right hand in the same way. If there are any lumps, knots, or changes, tell your doctor right away.

FIGURE 21-1 Breast self-exam.

NURSING ALERT:
Nurses play an important role in promoting BSE. Women report increased frequency of BSE when taught by a nurse.

B. Suggestions for Patients Who Find BSE Difficult
1. Tenderness—gentle self-examination may be more effective and less painful than examination by someone else.
2. Cystic breasts—recommend professional examination annually, and instruct patient to compare changes in breasts from one month to the next.
3. Large, pendulous breasts—encourage woman to support her breast with her hand to palpate thoroughly; lying down may help to flatten breasts.

Community Health Education

Implement patient teaching of BSE on a community level by:

1. Teaching BSE to women in the community—schools, churches, women's groups.
2. Reinforcing that early detection is associated with decreased mortality.
3. Helping patients and families establish and maintain support networks.
4. Knowing the resources available and making people aware of them.
   a. National Cancer Institute—staff can answer questions and send booklets about cancer. Toll-free number is 1-800-4-CANCER.
   b. American Cancer Society—offers many services to patients and their families. Call toll-free number for local information: 1-800-ACS-2345.

◆ SURGERY FOR BREAST CANCER

Surgery for breast cancer may involve mastectomy or a breast-preserving procedure. The objective of breast-preserving procedures is a cosmetically acceptable breast after complete excision of the tumor. Research studies comparing breast conservation with mastectomy have demonstrated equivalent patient survival. See Table 21-1 for surgical approach options available. The following discussion covers mastectomy and axillary node dissection.

Preoperative Management/Nursing Care

See page 76 for routine preoperative care. In addition:

1. Explain the nature of the procedure and expected postoperative care including drain care, location of the incision, and mobility of the arm.
2. Reinforce information about diagnosis and possibility of further therapy.
3. Recognize the extreme anxiety and fear that the patient, family, and significant others are experiencing.
   a. Discuss patient's concerns and usual coping mechanisms.
   b. Explore support systems with patient.
   c. Discuss concerns regarding body image changes.

GERONTOLOGIC ALERT:
Assessment of preoperative mental status of the older patient will help determine if a cognitive change occurs postoperatively.

TABLE 21-1 Types of Surgery for Breast Cancer

Procedure	Description	Indications
Lumpectomy (excisional biopsy)	Removal of tumor and surrounding tissue	For diagnosis of an abnormal mammographic finding or palpable breast lump
Quadrantectomy (partial mastectomy)	Removal of a breast quadrant that includes the tumor area and overlying skin	Normal to large-sized breasts
Axillary dissection	Surgical removal of the axillary lymph nodes	Performed as part of breast-preserving procedure, mainly for prognosis, staging, and local/regional disease control
Simple mastectomy*	Surgical removal of the breast and a few of the axillary lymph nodes close to the breast	Prophylactic: Performed in carefully selected patients who are high risk for developing breast cancer
Modified radical mastectomy*	Surgical removal of the entire breast and the axillary lymph nodes	Advanced disease, large or multifocal tumors; women with very small breasts in whom local excision of tumor will be cosmetically unacceptable; ineligibility for radiation therapy
Radical mastectomy*	Removal of entire breast, pectoral muscles, axillary nodes	Rarely done today—may be performed for advanced disease

* Mastectomy may be followed by immediate or delayed reconstruction.

Potential Complications

1. Infection
2. Hematoma, seroma
3. Lymphedema
4. Paresthesia, pain of axilla and arm
5. Impaired mobility of arm

Postoperative Management/ Nursing Care

See page 80 for routine postoperative care. In addition:

1. Assess dressing and wound after dressing is removed for erythema, edema, tenderness, odor, and drainage.
   a. Initial dressing may consist of gauze held in place by elastic, tape, or clear occlusive dressing wrap.
   b. Usually removed in within 24 hours.
   c. Incision may remain open to air or Ace wrap may be replaced if patient prefers.
2. Assess drainage via suction drain for amount, color, and odor and record.
   a. May have 100 to 200 mL serous to serosanguineous drainage in the first 24 hours.
   b. Report if grossly bloody or excessive in amount.
3. Assess arm for edema, erythema, and pain.
4. Teach patient drain care, exercises.
5. Assess knowledge of surgical outcome and BSE.
6. Inquire about female relatives, especially sisters, daughters, and mother who may need closer breast cancer surveillance.

NURSING ALERT:
Mastectomy patients may have an elastic wrap bandage that should fit snugly but not so tightly that it hinders respiration. It should fit comfortably and support unaffected breast.

GERONTOLOGIC ALERT:
Signs and symptoms of infection may not be obvious in older patients. Assess patients for mental status changes or urinary incontinence.

Nursing Diagnoses

A. Impaired Physical Mobility related to impaired movement of arm on operative side
B. Knowledge Deficit of care of incision, arm, and performance of BSE
C. Altered Tissue Perfusion of affected arm related to lymphedema
D. Body Image Disturbance related to loss of breast (for mastectomy patient)
E. Anxiety related to diagnosis of cancer
F. Altered Sexuality Patterns related to loss of breast and diagnosis of breast cancer
G. Compromised Family Coping related to diagnosis of cancer

Nursing Interventions

In addition to routine postoperative interventions, provide the following care.

A. **Mobilizing Affected Arm**
1. Assess patient's ability to perform self-care and factors impeding performance.
2. Initially encourage wrist and elbow flexion and extension. Encourage use of arm for washing face, combing hair, applying lipstick, and brushing teeth. Encourage patient to gradually increase use of arm.
3. Encourage patient to avoid abduction initially to help prevent seroma formation.
4. Support arm in sling if prescribed to prevent abduction of the arm.
5. Instruct and provide patient with exercises to do when permitted (Table 21-2).

B. **Increasing Knowledge**
1. Explain how wound will gradually change and that the newly healed wound may have less sensation because of severed nerves.
2. Instruct patient on signs of infection, hematoma, or seroma formation to be reported.
3. Teach patient to bathe incision gently and blot carefully to dry, and later, with approval, massage the healed incision gently with cocoa butter to encourage circulation and increase skin elasticity.
4. Teach care of drains, if appropriate—empty contents, measure and record.
5. Teach care of affected arm (Table 21-3).
6. Teach importance of BSE, mammograms, and regular follow-up visits.
7. Encourage discussion with health care provider about pregnancy after breast cancer, if indicated.

C. **Promoting Lymphatic Drainage**
1. Instruct patient in potential problem of lymphedema—at particular risk are patients who undergo axillary node dissection in combination with radiation therapy to axilla.
2. Do not take blood pressure, draw blood, inject medications or start intravenous lines in affected arm. Post sign over bed.
3. Elevate affected arm on pillows, above level of heart, and hand above elbow to promote gravity drainage of fluid.
4. Teach patient to massage affected arm if prescribed to increase circulation and decrease edema.
5. Provide patient with information on arm and hand care (see Table 21-3).

D. **Enhancing Body Image**
1. Assess mastectomy patient's knowledge of prosthesis and reconstruction options, and provide information as needed.
2. Discuss patient's views on how her body image has been altered.
3. Suggest clothing adjustments to camouflage loss of breast.
4. Assist patient to obtain a temporary prosthesis (may be provided by Reach to Recovery). First prosthesis should be light and soft to allow incision to heal. She may wear heavier type usually 4 to 8 weeks after surgeon's approval has been secured. Provide information regarding where to obtain permanent prosthesis and bras.

TABLE 21-2 Exercises for the Rehabilitation of the Patient Following Mastectomy

Exercise	Equivalent Daily Activities
1. Stand erect. Lean forward from waist. Allow arms to hang. Swing arms from side to side together; then in opposite direction. Next: swing arms from front to back together; then in opposite direction.	Broom sweeping Vacuum cleaning Mopping floor Pulling out and pushing in drawers Weaving Playing golf
2. Stand erect facing wall with palms of hand flat against wall; arms extended. Relax arms and shoulders and allow upper part of body to lean forward against hands. Push away to original position; repeat.	Pushing self out of bath tub Kneading bread Breast stroke—swimming Sawing or cutting types of crafts
3. Stand erect facing wall with palms of hands flat against wall. Climb the wall with the fingers; descend, repeat.	Raising windows Washing windows Hanging clothes on line Reaching to an upper shelf
4. Stand erect and clasp hands at small of back; raise hands; lower; repeat. Clasp hands back of neck; reach downward; upward; repeat.	Fastening brassiere Buttoning blouse or dress Pulling up a dress zipper Fastening beads Washing the back
5. Toss a rope over the shower curtain rod. Hold the ends of the rope (knotted) in each hand and alternately pull on each end. Using a see-saw motion and with arms outstretched, slide the rope up and down over the rod.	Drying the back with a bath towel Raising and lowering a window blind Closing and opening window drapes
6. Flex and extend each finger in turn.	Sewing, knitting, crocheting Typing, painting, playing piano or other musical instrument

5. Encourage patient to discuss feelings with partner.
6. Encourage patient to allow herself to experience the grief process over the loss of her breast and to learn to cope with these feelings.

E. *Reducing Anxiety*
1. Familiarize patient with Reach to Recovery (an American Cancer Society program consisting of volunteers who have had mastectomies or breast-preserving procedures, who visit postoperatively in the hospital to provide support and information) after clearing with patient's health care provider.
2. Discuss patient's usual coping mechanisms.
3. Encourage and assist family to support patient.

4. Assist patient to maintain control by planning care with her and incorporating her usual routines.
5. Refer for postmastectomy support group as needed and desired.
6. Offer list of community resources.
7. Remind patient that stress related to breast cancer and mastectomy may persist for a year or more and to seek help.
8. Include family in supportive interventions and measures to increase coping skills.

F. *Maintaining Sexual Activity*
1. Discuss effect of diagnosis and surgery on view of self as a woman.
2. Explore alternative means of sexual activity such as changing position during intercourse to decrease pressure on incision.
3. Encourage patient to discuss concerns with partner.
4. Assist patient and partner to look at incision when ready.

Evaluation

A. Moves affected arm within prescribed limits
B. States care of incision, drains, follow-up guidelines
C. Absence of infection or swelling in affected arm
D. Expresses positive body image
E. Exhibits minimal anxiety
F. Reports satisfactory sexual activity and sexuality

◆ BREAST RECONSTRUCTION AFTER MASTECTOMY

Breast reconstruction (mammoplasty) may be performed immediately or as long after surgery as desired. Benefits include improved psychological coping due to improved

TABLE 21-3 Hand and Arm Care to Help Prevent Lymphedema and Infection

After a mastectomy or axillary dissection, the arm may swell because of the excision of lymph nodes and their connecting vessels. Circulation of lymph fluid is slowed making it more difficult for the body to combat infection. Special precautions should be taken to prevent lymphedema and infection.
Avoid burns while cooking or smoking.
Avoid sunburns.
Have all injections, vaccinations, blood samples, and blood pressure tests done on the other arm whenever possible.
Use an electric razor with a narrow head for underarm shaving to reduce the risk of nicks and scratches.
Carry heavy packages or handbags on the other arm.
Never cut cuticles; use hand cream or lotion instead.
Wear watches or jewelry loosely, if at all, on the operated arm.
Wear protective gloves when gardening and when using strong detergents, etc.
Use a thimble when sewing.
Avoid harsh chemicals and abrasive compounds.
Use insect repellent to avoid bites and stings.
Avoid elastic cuffs on blouses and nightgowns.

From *Mastectomy: A treatment for breast cancer.* NIH Publication No. 91-658

body image and self-esteem. Demand for postmastectomy reconstruction has been increasing. Cost is usually covered by insurance.

Implants

Indicated for patients with inadequate breast tissue and skin of good quality.

A. Description
1. Uses prosthetic implants placed in pocket under skin or pectoralis muscle.
2. If opposite breast is ptotic (protruding downward), mastopexy may be necessary for symmetry.
3. Silicone implants are available only to mastectomy patients for reconstruction.
4. Complications include capsular contracture resulting in firmness; may be painful, cause infection.
5. Tissue expanders may be necessary before implants are inserted.
   a. Inflatable envelope is placed under muscle or skin and is filled with saline once incision is healed (about 4 weeks).
   b. Saline is instilled every 1 to 3 weeks until the expander is beyond desired size.
   c. Later, expander is removed and a permanent implant is placed.
   d. Some types of expanders may be left in permanently.
6. Advantages of implant reconstruction over other methods—only one incision; less fibrosis.
7. Disadvantage—may take months.

B. Nursing Care/Patient Considerations
1. Teach signs and symptoms of infection, hematoma, migration, and deflation.
2. Teach patient to massage breast to decrease capsule formation around implant.
3. Teach patient she may feel discomfort with the expansions, if used.

Flap Grafts

A. Description
1. Transfer of skin, muscle, and subcutaneous tissue from another part of the body to the mastectomy site.
2. Two types
   a. Latissimus dorsi—skin, fat, and muscles of back between shoulder blades are tunneled under skin to front chest.
   b. Transverse rectus abdominis myocutaneous (TRAM) flap—muscle, fat, skin, and blood supply are tunneled to breast area.
3. Disadvantages include cost, several hospitalizations required, slow process (done in stages), increased morbidity.
4. Complications include flap loss, hematoma, infection, seroma, and abdominal hernia.

B. Nursing Care/Patient Considerations
1. Assess flap and donor site for color, temperature, and wound drainage.
2. Control pain.
3. Provide support with bra or abdominal binder to maintain position of prosthesis.

4. Teach patient to perform BSE monthly and that she may have some asymmetry.

Nipple–Areolar Reconstruction

1. Usually done at a separate time from breast reconstruction.
2. Uses skin and fat from reconstructed breast for nipple, and upper thigh for areola; tanning or tattoo done to obtain appropriate color.

◆ OTHER SURGERIES OF THE BREAST

Reduction mammoplasty may be done for cosmetic purposes or to relieve uncomfortable symptoms. Augmentation mammoplasty is considered a cosmetic procedure.

Reduction Mammoplasty

A. Description
1. Removal of excess breast tissue, which also involves a reduction in skin and possible transposition of nipple–areolar complex.
2. Used for alleviation of symptoms that may include back and neck pain, muscle spasm, and grooving at the shoulders secondary to bra straps.
3. Complications include hematoma, infection, necrosis of skin flap, and nipple inversion.

B. Nursing/Patient Care Considerations
1. Explore reasons patient may desire surgery.
2. Discuss postoperative expectations with patient.
3. Nursing interventions are similar to those in the patient undergoing reconstruction.

Augmentation Mammoplasty

A. Description
1. Enlarging of the breasts with the use of implants.
2. Implants may be made of silicone or saline—currently the FDA has limited use to saline implants only.
3. Complications include hematoma, wound infection, diminished sensation of the nipple, and capsular contracture resulting in firmness of the breast.

B. Nursing/Patient Care Considerations
1. Discuss patient's expectations preoperatively.
2. Nursing interventions are similar to those in the patient undergoing reconstruction with implants.

Disorders of the Breast

◆ FISSURE OF THE NIPPLE

A *fissure* is a type of ulcer that develops in the nipple(s) of a nursing mother.

Etiology/Clinical Manifestations

1. May be caused by lack of preparation of nipples in the prenatal period.
2. Condition aggravated by sucking infant.
3. Nipple appears sore and irritated.
4. Nipple bleeds.
5. Infection may result.

Management/Nursing Interventions

1. Wash nipples with sterile saline solution.
2. Use artificial nipple for nursing.
3. If above does not initiate healing process, stop nursing and use breast pump.
4. Teach proper breast-feeding techniques to prevent fissures.
   a. Wash, dry, and lubricate nipples in prenatal period in preparation for nursing.
   b. Make sure infant's mouth covers areola.
   c. Keep nipple clean by washing and drying after each nursing period.
   d. Use lanolin cream to prevent cracking; must remove before breast-feeding.

◆ NIPPLE DISCHARGE

Nipple discharge may be serous, serosanguineous, bloody, purulent, or multicolored. It is commonly associated with benign conditions; occasionally malignancy is responsible.

Etiology/Clinical Manifestations

1. Galactorrhea—bilateral, nonspontaneous, multiple duct, milky gray or green discharge usually seen in patients in childbearing years.
   a. Commonly seen after pregnancy and can last for 1 to 2 years.
   b. Also may be secondary to excessive breast manipulation, increased production of prolactin, medication, an endocrine anovulatory syndrome, or pituitary adenoma.
2. Mastitis—usually unilateral, purulent (see below).
3. Discharge containing blood—usually due to intraductal papilloma (wart) or other benign lesion.

Management

Nursing interventions are aimed at alleviating anxiety and providing support to patient undergoing diagnostic testing.

A. Nonsurgical/Medical Management
1. Evaluate with clinical examination, test for occult blood, mammogram if over the age of 35.
2. May want to evaluate galactorrhea with a prolactin level.
3. Nonspontaneous milky gray or green discharge generally is not of pathologic significance.
4. Bromocriptine mesylate (Parlodel) may be given to suppress galactorrhea.
5. Treat for mastitis if purulent (see below).

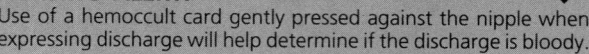

NURSING ALERT:
Use of a hemoccult card gently pressed against the nipple when expressing discharge will help determine if the discharge is bloody.

B. Surgical Management
1. Watery, serous, or bloody nipple discharges may require surgery.
2. Most commonly due to wartlike intraductal papilloma in one of larger collecting ducts at edge of areola. May be secondary to fibrocystic changes or duct ectasia.
3. Excisional biopsy and histologic examination must be done to rule out cancer.

◆ ACUTE MASTITIS

Acute mastitis is inflammation of the breast due to infection.

Pathophysiology/Etiology

1. Usually occurs at beginning of lactation in first-time breast-feeding mothers. May also occur later in chronic lactation mastitis and central duct abscesses.
2. Milk stasis may lead to obstruction, followed by non-infectious inflammation, then infectious mastitis.
3. Source of infection may be from hands of patient, personnel caring for patient, baby's nose or throat, or blood borne.
4. Most common pathogens—*Staphylococcus aureus, Escherichia coli, Streptococcus.*

Clinical Manifestations

1. Redness, warmth, edema, breast may feel doughy and tough.
2. Patient may complain of dull pain in affected area and may have nipple discharge.
3. Complication is mammary abscess (see below).

Management/Nursing Interventions

1. Diagnosis is usually made by characteristic manifestations.
2. Antibiotics are given.
3. May or may not have patient stop breast-feeding (controversial).
4. Apply heat to resolve tissue reaction; may cause increased milk production and worsen symptoms.
5. May apply cold to decrease tissue metabolism and milk production.
6. Have the patient wear firm breast support.
7. Encourage the breast-feeding patient to practice meticulous personal hygiene to prevent mastitis.

◆ MAMMARY ABSCESS

Mammary abscess is a localized collection of pus in a cavity of breast tissue.

Etiology/Clinical Manifestations

1. May follow acute mastitis if untreated.
2. Patient may have fever, chills, and malaise.
3. Affected area is sensitive and erythematous; may have palpable mass.
4. Pus may be expressed from nipple.

Management/Nursing Interventions

1. May perform needle aspiration if superficial mass.
2. Incision and drainage if deep.
3. A biopsy of the cavity wall may be done at time of incision and drainage to rule out breast carcinoma associated with abscess.
4. Administer antibiotics and analgesics, if ordered.
5. Apply hot, wet dressings to increase drainage and hasten resolution.

◆ FIBROCYSTIC CHANGES

Fibrocystic change is a general term that includes a variety of changes in the breast, namely, fibrosis and cystic dilatation of the ducts. May be present in 50% of women.

Pathophysiology/Etiology

1. Pathogenesis is not precisely known but is related to the cyclic stimulation of the breast by estrogen and represents a change from the normal stimulation and regression pattern of this process.
2. Occurs usually in women between 35 and 50 and is a source of considerable discomfort in a sizeable percentage of women.
3. Hormone replacement therapy may be associated with fibrocystic changes in a woman who had never experienced this previously.

Clinical Manifestations

1. Increased generalized breast lumpiness or excessive nodularity with tenderness, pain, and breast swelling. Symptoms may decrease after a menstrual period.
2. Lumps or cysts—soft or firm, single or multiple, smooth, round, and movable. Cysts may enlarge and become tender and painful. There may be many cysts of different sizes—some may be palpable.
3. Nipple discharge—may be present; milky, yellow or greenish.

Diagnostic Evaluation

1. Physical examination detects changes.
2. Mammography used to rule out calcification associated with malignancy.
3. Aspiration—if there is a palpable mass.
4. Cytology of cyst fluid is not cost effective and rarely of clinical value in fibrocystic breast changes.

Management

Usually geared toward relief of symptoms

A. **Surgical Management**
1. Needle aspiration and conservative medical follow-up if:
   a. The aspirate appears like normal cyst fluid and is not blood-stained.
   b. There is complete resolution of the cyst following aspiration.
   c. There are no signs to indicate an underlying neoplasm.
2. Surgical excision—indicated if a cyst keeps recurring after several aspirations, or a single solid discrete lump is present.

B. **Medical Management**
1. Sporadic discomfort may be relieved by over-the-counter analgesics.
2. Evening primrose oil—composed of essential fatty acids.
   a. Used in England as initial attempt to control cyclic breast pain. May be obtained over-the-counter in health food stores.
   b. Side effects include bloating and nausea.
3. Bromocriptine (Parlodel)—a dopamine agonist.
   a. May help with mastalgia by decreasing serum prolactin levels.
   b. Side effects include nausea, vomiting, headache, dizziness, and fatigue.
4. Contraceptives or supplemental progestins during the secretory phase of the menstrual cycle may help with pain control.
   a. Mastalgia that begins after initiating birth control pills may resolve after a few cycles.
   b. Switching to a lower estrogen/higher progesterone ratio may help.
5. Danazol (Danocrine)—a synthetic androgen used for severe fibrocystic changes to decrease hormonal stimulation of the breast by suppressing gonadotropins.
   a. Side effects include menstrual irregularity, weight gain, depression, bloating, and acne.
6. Tamoxifen (Tamofen)—blocks estrogen stimulation; side effects are minimal, may have hot flashes.

C. **Other Measures**
1. Diet modifications.
   a. Eliminating caffeine from the diet may help reduce symptoms in some women—coffee, tea, cola drinks, and chocolate.
   b. Adding vitamin E may be helpful with pain.
   c. Decreasing fat intake may improve swelling, tenderness, and nodularity.
2. Stopping tobacco has been suggested to relieve symptoms.
3. Prophylactic simple mastectomy—rarely indicated for intractable pain not relieved with medical therapy in women with multiple previous biopsies or biopsy evidence of a precancerous lesion.

Nursing Interventions/Patient Teaching

1. Emphasize the importance of monthly BSE—cysts may mask underlying cancer.

2. Reinforce patient's confidence in BSE by rechecking her findings.
3. Offer suggestions for alternative methods if BSE is difficult to do (ie, tender breasts).
4. Encourage patient to see health care provider regularly for examinations.
5. Recommend that the patient wear a good support bra.
6. Offer emotional support for her anxiety and fear of cancer.
7. Reassure that pain is common to many women and is rarely the only presenting sign of cancer.

◆ BENIGN TUMORS OF THE BREAST

Benign tumors of the breast are characterized clinically as benign lesions that are distinct and persistent over time. Approximately 90% are found by women themselves; 90% of breast lumps are benign.

Pathophysiology/Etiology

1. Fibrocystic changes—solid lumps may be fatty or fibrous tissue or fluid filled cysts (see above).
2. Galactocele—a milk-filled cyst.
3. Fibroadenoma—a benign breast tumor composed of epithelial and stromal components.
   a. Common in young women.
   b. There is a slight increase in the risk of breast cancer among women with fibroadenomas.
4. Other benign tumors include adenosis, intraductal papillomas, lipomas, and neurofibromatosis that may produce a papable mass.

Clinical Manifestations

1. Gross cysts—may be tender or nontender. Consistency depends on pressure of fluid within cyst and breast tissue around them; may be soft and fluctuant or may feel like a solid tumor if tense.
2. Galactocele—firm, nontender mass.
3. Fibroadenoma—may be a firm, smooth movable lump that is usually painless. Size does not usually fluctuate with menstrual cycle changes but tends to enlarge over time.

Diagnostic Evaluation

1. Physical examination, mammography, and ultrasound identify and characterize lesion.
2. Cyst aspiration—diagnostic aspiration is often curative in a galactocele or breast cyst.
3. If a lump does not respond to cyst aspiration, excisional biopsy remains the "gold standard" to rule out cancer.

Management/Nursing Interventions

1. Nonsuspicious or indeterminate masses in young women may be observed through one or two menstrual cycles for resolution of the mass.

2. In general, any distinct and persistent solid lump should have biopsy and possibly excision.
3. Nursing care is directed toward support as woman goes through diagnostic process.

◆ DISORDERS OF THE MALE BREAST

Disorders of the male breast may be benign or malignant.

Clinical Features

A. *Gynecomastia* Overdevelopment of breast tissue
1. Incidence greatest in adolescents and men over the age of 50.
2. Usually results from hormonal alterations—idiopathic, systemic disorders, drugs, neoplasms.
3. Pubertal gynecomastia usually disappears within 4 to 6 months.

B. *Breast Cancer* Resembles cancer of the breast in women
1. 1% of all breast cancers—incidence greatest in men in their sixties.
2. Poor prognosis because men may delay seeking treatment until disease is advanced.

◆ CANCER OF THE BREAST

Breast cancer or carcinoma is the leading cause of cancer in American women. One in 8 women will develop breast cancer.

Pathophysiology/Etiology

1. Most breast cancer begins in the lining of the milk ducts, sometimes in the lobule. Eventually it grows through the wall of the duct and into the fatty tissue. (See Table 21-4 for types of breast cancer.)
2. Family history accounts for approximately 7% of all breast cancers.
   a. Current genetic models attribute a significant portion of familial breast cancer to one or more dominantly inherited breast cancer susceptibility genes.
   b. BRCA1—susceptibility gene under study; high probability that carriers will develop breast cancer. Predictive testing not possible yet.
3. Present knowledge does not indicate that carcinogens play an important role in the development of breast cancer.
4. Hormones such as estrogen are not thought to produce cancer; however, they may influence the growth of breast cancer.

Epidemiology of Breast Cancer

A. *Incidence*
1. Approximately 183,400 new cases yearly (1,400 male)

TABLE 21-4   Types of Breast Cancer

Cell Type	Description	Incidence*	Comments
In situ			
Ductal (DCIS)	Well circumscribed in duct	28% Frequently found in combination with invasive cancer	Considered to be a precancerous condition—majority found by mammogram
Lobular (LCIS)	Solid proliferation of small cells within breast lobules	3–5% More frequent in premenopausal women	Nonpalpable mammographic finding. Precancerous. Tends to be bilateral, multicentric
Invasive			
Ductal	Classified on basis of microscopic appearance as ductal or lobular	75%	Characterized by stony hardness on palpation
Lobular	As above	5–10%	Relatively uncommon
Others			
Tubular Medullary Mucinous Papillary Sarcoma	Types frequently associated with above. Cell type must dominate to be assigned.	<10% of all breast cancers	Axillary metastasis uncommon in tubular; medullary associated with fast growth rate and favorable prognosis
Inflammatory	Applies to distinctive inflamed appearance of skin. No consistent histologic type	1–4%	Presents with erythema, warmth, tenderness, and edema. May be treated with chemotherapy or radiation therapy first
Paget disease of nipple	Usually associated with underlying intraductal or invasive carcinoma	2%	Presents as scaly, erythematous, periareolar eruption

* Percent greater than 100—Infiltrating carcinoma frequently includes small areas containing other special types or a combination of in situ and infilrating carcinoma is seen.

2. Second highest cause of deaths from cancer in American women (after lung cancer)—estimate for 1995 is 46,240 (240 men).

B.   Survival Rates
1. Lymph node status is the most important prognostic indicator of disease free survival.
   a. Five-year survival if localized to breast is 94% in white women, 84% in African American women.
   b. Five-year survival if spread to nodes is 74% in white women, 57% in African American women.
2. Age, staging, (tumor size, lymph node status, and presence of distant metastasis), nuclear grade, histologic differentiation, and treatment are important prognostic factors for survival (Tables 21-5 through 21-8).

C.   Risk Factors
1. Major—sex, increased age, prior history of breast cancer, and family history (especially mother, sisters). Approximate twofold risk in women with affected sister or mother, and this increases if more relatives were affected or if affected close relatives developed breast cancer before menopause.
2. Probable—nulliparity, first child after age 30, late menopause, early menarche, benign breast disease.
3. Controversial—oral contraceptive use (estrogen and progestin may stimulate tumor growth with long-term use), estrogen replacement therapy, alcohol use, obesity and increased dietary fat intake.

> **GERONTOLOGIC ALERT:**
> Age is the greatest single risk factor for the development of cancer. Cancer warning signals may be unheeded in older women.

Clinical Manifestations (Fig. 21-2)

1. A firm lump or thickening in breast, usually painless; 50% located in upper outer quadrant of breast. Enlargement of axillary or supraclavicular lymph nodes may indicate metastasis.
2. Nipple discharge—spontaneous, may be bloody, clear or serous.
3. Breast asymmetry—a change in the size or shape of the breast or abnormal contours as woman changes positions—compare one breast to other.
4. Nipple retraction or scaliness—especially in Paget's disease.
5. Late signs—pain, ulceration, edema, orange peel skin (peau d'orange) from interference of lymphatic drainage.

> **NURSING ALERT:**
> Pain is not usually an early warning sign of breast cancer.

TABLE 21-5 Staging of Primary Tumor (T) in Breast Cancer, American Joint Committee on Cancer and International Union Against Cancer

TX	Primary tumor cannot be assessed.
T0	No evidence of primary tumor
Tis*	Carcinoma in situ: intraductal carcinoma, lobular carcinoma in situ, or Paget's disease of the nipple with no tumor
T1	Tumor 2 cm or less in greatest dimension
	T1a 0.5 cm or less in greatest dimenstion
	T1b More than 0.5 but not more than 1 cm in greatest dimention
	T1c More than 1 cm but not more than 2 cm in greatest dimension
T2	Tumor more than 2 cm but not more than 5 cm in greatest dimension
T3	Tumor more than 5 cm in greatest dimension
T4†	Tumor of any size with direct extension to chest wall or skin
	T4a Extension to chest wall
	T4b Edema (including peau d'orange) or ulceration of the skin of the breast or satellite skin nodules confined to the same breast
	T4c Both (T4a and T4b)
	T4d Inflammatory carcinoma

* Note: Paget's disease associated with a tumor is classified according to the size of the tumor.
† Note: Chest wall includes ribs, intercostal muscles, and serratus anterior muscle but not pectoral muscle.

Diagnostic Evaluation

1. Mammography—most accurate method to detect nonpalpable lesion; cancer changes include microcalcifications to visible lesion.
2. Biopsy or aspiration—conclusive for cancer diagnosis and to determine type of breast cancer.
3. Estrogen/progesterone-receptor status, proliferation/S phase study, and other tests of tumor cells used to determine appropriate treatment and prognosis.
4. Laboratory tests to detect metastasis
   a. Increased values on liver function tests indicate possible liver metastasis.

TABLE 21-6 Staging of Regional Lymph Nodes (N) in Breast Cancer, American Joint Committee on Cancer and International Union Against Cancer

NX	Regional lymph nodes cannot be assessed (eg, previously removed)
N0	No regional lymph node metastasis
N1	Metatasis to movable ipsilateral axillary lymph node(s)
N2	Metastasis to ipsilateral axillary lymph node(s) fixed to one another or to other structures
N3	Metastasis to ipsilateral internal mammary lymph node(s)

TABLE 21-7 Staging of Distant Metastases (M) in Breast Cancer, American Joint Committee on Cancer and International Union Against Cancer

MX	Presence of distant metastasis cannot be assessed.
M0	No distant metastasis
M1	Distant metastasis (includes metastasis to ipsilateral supraclavicular lymph node[s])

   b. Increased calcium and alkaline phosphatase levels indicate possible bony metastasis.
5. Additional metastatic work-up includes chest x-ray, bone scan, possible brain and chest CT.

Management

Based on type and stage of breast cancer, receptors, and menopausal status. For women with localized breast cancer, information from clinical trials indicates that treatment with a breast-preserving procedure has similar survival rates as modified radical mastectomy.

A. Surgery
See page 690.

B. Radiation Therapy
1. In conjunction with breast-preserving procedure as adjuvant (additional) therapy to decrease incidence of local recurrence. Radiation directed to breast, chest wall, and remaining lymph nodes. Usually five treatments a week for 6 or 7 weeks. A "booster" or second phase of treatment may be given. May include implants of radioactive material after external treatment completed.
2. As primary therapy to shrink a large tumor to operable size.

TABLE 21-8 Stage Grouping for Breast Cancer, American Joint Committee On Cancer and International Union Against Cancer

Stage 0	Tis	N0	M0
Stage I	T1	N0	M0
Stage IIA	T0	N1	M0
	T1	N1	M0
	T2	N0	M0
Stage IIB	T2	N1	M0
	T3	N0	M0
Stage IIIA	T0	N2	M0
	T1	N2	M0
	T2	N2	M0
	T3	N1, N2	M0
Stage IIIB	T4	Any N	M0
	Any T	N3	M0
Stage IV	Any T	Any N	M1

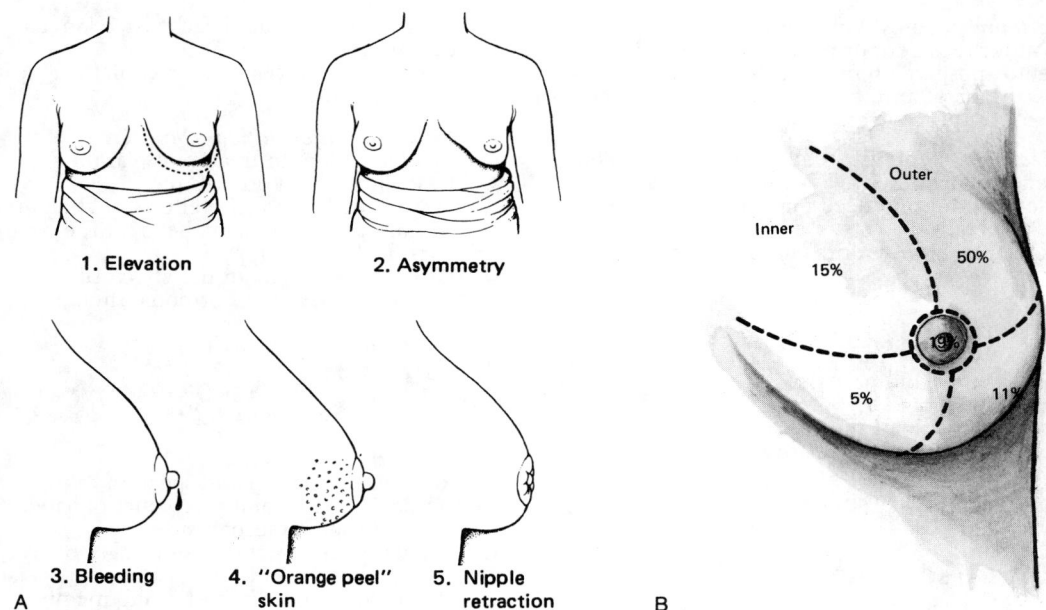

1. Elevation 2. Asymmetry

3. Bleeding 4. "Orange peel" skin 5. Nipple retraction

A

B

Outer

Inner

15%

50%

19%

5%

11%

FIGURE 21-2 *(A)* *Signs of cancer of the breast.* *(B)* *Distribution of carcinomas in different areas of breast.*

3. To alleviate pain caused by metastasis.
4. Side effects—mild fatigue, sore throat, dry cough, nausea, anorexia; later, skin will look and feel sunburned and eventually the breast becomes more firm. Complications include increased arm edema, decreased arm mobility, pneumonitis, and brachial nerve damage. See page for care of patient undergoing radiation therapy.

C. *Chemotherapy*
1. Major use is in adjuvant treatment postoperatively; usually begins 4 weeks after surgery (stressful for patient who just finished major surgery).
2. Treatments are given every 3 to 4 weeks for 6 to 9 months. Because the drugs differ in their mechanisms of action, combinations of agents are used to treat cancer.
3. Main drugs used for breast cancer include cyclophosphamide (Cytoxan), methotrexate (Mexate), 5-fluorouracil (5-FU), doxorubicin (Adriamycin). Paclitaxel (Taxol), an antimitotic cytotoxic agent, is being used now for advanced cancer.
4. Indications for chemotherapy include:
   a. Premenopausal women with positive lymph nodes, regardless of hormone-receptor status.
   b. Premenopausal women with negative lymph nodes, and poor prognostic factors, chemotherapy may be recommended.
   c. Postmenopausal women with positive lymph nodes and negative hormone-receptor status, chemotherapy may be considered.
5. Side effects include bone marrow suppression, nausea and vomiting, alopecia, weight gain/loss, fatigue, stomatitis, anxiety, depression, and premature menopause. (See p. 182 for nursing care of patient undergoing chemotherapy.)
6. Chemotherapy also used as primary treatment in inflammatory breast cancer and palliative treatment in metastatic disease or recurrence.

D. *Endocrine Therapy*
1. Antiestrogens, such as tamoxifen (Tamofen), bind estrogen receptors, thereby blocking effects of estrogen.
   a. Adjuvant systemic therapy after surgery. Greatest benefit in estrogen or progesterone receptor-positive patients, may also be used for metastases or recurrence.
   b. For postmenopausal women with positive nodes and positive hormone-receptor status, tamoxifen is the treatment of choice.
   c. Given for at least 2 years; oral administration twice a day.
   d. Side effects include hot flashes, irregular periods, vaginal irritation, nausea and vomiting, headaches.
2. Hormones may be used in advanced disease. Remissions may last months to several years. Agents commonly used include:
   a. Estrogens, such as diethylstilbestrol (DES) or ethinyl estradiol (Estinyl), in high doses to suppress follicle-stimulating hormone (FSH) and luteinizing hormone (LH) and may decrease endogenous estrogen production.
   b. Progestins may decrease estrogen receptors.
   c. Androgens may suppress FSH and estrogen production.
   d. Aminoglutethimide suppresses estrogen production by blocking adrenal steroids; "medical adrenalectomy," especially useful for women with bone and soft tissue metastases.
   e. Corticosteroids suppress estrogen/progesterone secretion from the adrenals.

E. *Bone Marrow Transplant*
1. Autologous method after high-dose chemotherapy; may be curative because it allows for high doses of drugs.
2. Especially indicated for stage 3 disease.

F. *Oophorectomy* Removal of ovaries
1. Treatment for recurrent or metastatic disease in estrogen receptor-positive premenopausal women.
2. Deprives tumor of primary estrogen source—remissions of 3 months to several years.

G. *Adrenalectomy* Removal of adrenal glands to eliminate androgen production (which converts to estrogen)
1. Rarely done because of need for long-term steroid replacement therapy.
2. Remissions may last 6 months to several years.

Complications

1. Metastasis—most common sites: lymph nodes, lung, bone, liver, and brain.
2. Signs and symptoms of metastasis may include bone pain, neurologic changes, weight loss, anemia, cough, shortness of breath, pleuritic pain, and vague chest discomfort.

Nursing Assessment

1. Assess general health status and presence of underlying chronic illnesses that may have an impact on patient's response to treatment.
2. Identify what the patient and family need to know regarding breast cancer and its treatment, and measures to decrease their impact. Base education on patient and family needs.
3. Determine level of anxiety, fears, and concerns.
4. Identify coping ability and availability of support systems.

Nursing Diagnoses

Also see page 690 for breast surgery care and Chapter 6, Cancer Nursing, page 99.
A. Anxiety related to diagnosis of cancer
B. Knowledge Deficit related to disease process and treatment options
C. Ineffective Individual and/or Family Coping related to diagnosis, prognosis, financial stress, and/or inadequate support

Nursing Interventions

A. *Reducing Anxiety*
1. Realize that a diagnosis of breast cancer is a devastating emotional shock to the woman. Support patient through the diagnostic process.

2. Interpret the results of each test in language the patient can understand.
3. Stress the advances made in earlier diagnosis and treatment options.

B. *Providing Information About Treatment*
1. Involve patient in treatment planning.
2. Describe surgical procedures.
3. Prepare patient for the effects of chemotherapy—encourage patient to plan ahead for the common side effects of chemotherapy.
4. Educate patient about the effects of radiation therapy.
5. Teach patient about hormonal therapy.

NURSING ALERT:
Document all components of patient care and teaching.

C. *Strengthening Coping*
1. Repeat information and speak in calm, clear manner.
2. Display empathy and acceptance of patient's emotions.
3. Explore coping mechanisms.
4. Evaluate where patient is in stages of acceptance.
5. Help patient identify and use support persons.
6. Obtain visit from support group member.
7. Refer for counseling, financial aid, etc.
8. Resources include American Cancer Society, National Institutes of Health.

Patient Education/Health Maintenance

1. Encourage patient to continue in close follow-up and report any new symptoms. Most women will be scheduled to be seen every 3 months for the first 2 years, every 6 months for the next 3 years, and once a year after 5 years.
2. Stress importance of continued yearly mammogram.
3. Inform patient that yearly laboratory work, bone scan, and chest x-ray may be appropriate.
4. Suggest to patient that psychological intervention may be necessary for anxiety, depression, or sexual problems.

Evaluation

A. Verbalizes less anxiety
B. Verbalizes understanding of all treatment options and their side effects
C. Identifies appropriate coping mechanisms and support systems

Selected References

Boyle, N., Bertin-Matson, K., & Bratschi A. (1994). A patient's guide to Taxol. *Oncology Nursing Forum, 21*(9), 1569-1572.

Champion, V. (1994). Beliefs about breast cancer and mammography by behavioral stage. *Oncology Nursing Forum, 21*(6), 1009-1014.

Donegan, W. L. (1992, Sept. 24). Evaluation of a palpable breast mass. *The New England Journal of Medicine, 327*(13), 937-942.

Dupont, W., Page, D., Parl, F., et al. (1994, July 7). Long-term risk of breast cancer in women with fibroadenoma. *The New England Journal of Medicine, 331*(1), 10-15.

Entrekin, N. (1992). Breast cancer. In J. C. Clark & R. F. McGee (Eds.). *Core curriculum for oncology nursing* (2nd ed.). Philadelphia: W. B. Saunders.

Fiorica, J. V. (1994). Fibrocystic changes. *Obstetrics and Gynecology Clinics of North America, 21*(3), 445-452.

Fiorica, J. V. (1994). Nipple discharge. *Obstetrics and Gynecology Clinics of North America, 21*(3), 453-460.

Fischera, S., & Frank, D. (1994). Attitudes, practices, and role of nurses in the use of mammography. *Cancer Nursing, 17*(3), 223-228.

Ganz, P. A. (1995). Advocating for the woman with breast cancer. *CA-A Cancer Journal, 45*(2), 114-125.

Goodman, M., & Harte, N. Breast cancer. In S. L. Groenwald, M. H. Frogge, M. Goodman, & C. H. Yarbro (Eds.). (1992). *Cancer nursing: Principles and practice* (2nd ed.). Boston: Jones and Bartlett.

Granda, C. (1994). Nursing management of patients with lymphedema associated with breast cancer therapy. *Cancer Nursing, 17*(3), 229-235.

Harden, J. T., & Girard, N. (1994). Breast reconstruction using an innovative flap procedure. *AORN Journal, 60*(2), 184-192.

Henderson, C. I. (1994, July 1). Adjuvant systemic therapy for early breast cancer. *Cancer Supplement, 74*(1), 401-409.

Kinne, D. W. (1991). The surgical management of primary breast cancer. *CA-A Cancer Journal for Clinicians, 41*(2), 71-84.

Lierman, L. M., Powell-Cope, G., Benoliel, J. Q., Georgiadou, F., &

Young, H. M. (1994). Using social support to promote breast self-examination performance. *Oncology Nursing Forum, 21*(6), 1051-1056.

Mansour, E., Ravdin, P., & Dressler, L. (1994, July 1). Prognostic factors in early breast carcinoma. *Cancer Supplement, 74*(1), 381-386.

Oberle, K., & Allen, M. (1994). Breast augmentation surgery: A women's health issue. *Journal of Advanced Nursing, 20,* 844-852.

Osteen, R. T. (1994, July 1). Selection of patients for breast conserving surgery. *Cancer Supplement, 74*(1), 366-370.

Schmidt, R. A. (1994). Stereotactic breast biopsy. *CA-A Cancer Journal for Clinicians, 44*(3), 172-191.

Wingo, P. A., Pong, T., & Bolden, S. (1995). Cancer statistics 1995. *CA-A Cancer Journal for Clinicians, 45*(1), 8-30.

UNIT 7

◆

Metabolic and
Endocrine Disorders

General Overview

◆ THE FUNCTION OF HORMONES

The endocrine system, along with the nervous system, maintains homeostasis. The endocrine glands produce hormones, chemical substances that are secreted into the bloodstream and exert a stimulatory or inhibitory effect on target tissues or glands. Hormones achieve their effect through binding with specific receptors located on the membrane on the target cell (eg, catecholamines) or by actually penetrating the cell membrane and forming a complex that influences cellular metabolism (eg, steroids). The target cell response may be reflected through the production and secretion of a second hormone or through a change in cell metabolism that alters the concentration of electrolytes or other substances in the bloodstream.

General Effects of Hormone Action

1. Regulate the overall metabolic rate as well as the storage, conversion, and release of energy
2. Regulate fluid and electrolyte balance
3. Initiate coping responses to stressors
4. Regulate growth and development
5. Regulate reproduction processes

Regulation of Hormones

1. Hormone secretion is typically controlled through a negative feedback system.
   a. Fall in blood concentration of hormone leads to activation of the regulator endocrine gland and release of its stimulator hormones.
   b. Elevations in blood concentration of target cell hormones or changes in blood composition resulting from target cell activity can cause inhibition of hormone secretion.

2. Endocrine disorders are manifested as states of hormone deficiency or hormone excess. The underlying pathophysiology may be expressed as:
   a. *Primary*—the secreting gland is releasing inappropriate hormone due to disease of the gland itself.
   b. *Secondary*—the secreting gland is releasing abnormal amounts of hormone due to disease in a regulator gland (eg, pituitary).
   c. *Tertiary*—the secreting gland is releasing inappropriate hormone due to hypothalamic dysfunction resulting in abnormal stimulation by the pituitary.
3. Abnormal hormone concentrations may also be caused by hormone-producing tumors (adenomas) located at a remote site.

Assessment

◆ HISTORY

Patients with diseases of the endocrine system commonly report nonspecific complaints. Often symptoms may reflect changes in general well-being such as fatigue, weakness, weight change, appetite, sleep patterns, or psychiatric status. A thorough review of systems is necessary to detect changes in a wide variety of body systems caused by an endocrine disorder (Table 22-1).

◆ PHYSICAL EXAMINATION

Objective findings may be obvious and related to the patient's complaints or may be "silent signs" of which the patient is completely unaware. Thorough physical examination of all body systems, particularly the skin and cardiovascular and neurologic systems may reveal key findings for endocrine dysfunction.

TABLE 22-1 Physical Assessment of Clinical Manifestations of Endocrine Dysfunction

Body System	Signs of Symptoms	Possible Causes
Cardiovascular	Tachycardia or tachyarrhythmia	Hyperthyroidism, Pheochromocytoma Adrenal insufficiency
	Bradycardia	Hypothyroidism
	Orthostatic hypotension	Adrenal insufficiency Hyperaldosteronism Pheochromocytoma
	Hypertension	Pheochromocytoma Hyperaldosteronism Cushing's syndrome Hyperparathyroidism Hypothyroidism Hyperthyroidism
	Congestive heart failure	Hypothyroidism Cushing's syndrome
Neurologic	Fatigue	Adrenal insufficiency Hypothyroidism Hyperparathyroidism
	Nervousness, tremor	Pheochromocytoma Hyperthyroidism
	Confusion, lethargy, or coma	Diabetic ketoacidosis Hypothyroidism Syndrome of inappropriate antidiuretic hormone
	Paresthesia	Hypothyroidism Hypoparathyroidism Diabetes mellitus
	Headache	Acromegaly Pituitary tumor Pheochromocytoma Hyperaldosteronism
	Psychosis	Hypothyroidism Hyperthyroidism Cushing's syndrome Adrenal insufficiency Hyperparathyroidism Syndrome of inappropriate antidiuretic hormone
	Chvostek's sign, Trousseau's sign	Hypoparathyroidism
	Increased reflexes	Hyperthyroidism
	Decreased reflexes	Hypothyroidism
Gastrointestinal	Anorexia	Addison's disease Hypothyroidism Hyperparathyroidism
	Peptic ulcer	Cushing's syndrome
	Diarrhea	Adrenal insufficiency
	Constipation	Hypothyroidism Hyperparathyroidism Pheochromocytoma
	Weight loss	Hyperthyroidism Hyperparathyroidism Pheochromocytoma Diabetes insipidus
	Hyperdefecation	Hyperthyroidism
	Abdominal pain	Addison's crisis Hyperparathyroidism Thyroid storm Myxedema

(continued)

TABLE 22-1 Physical Assessment of Clinical Manifestations of Endocrine Dysfunction *(continued)*

Body System	Signs of Symptoms	Possible Causes
Musculoskeletal	Weakness	Hyperthyroidism Hypothyroidism Cushing's syndrome Adrenal insufficiency Hyperparathyroidism Hypoparathyroidism Hyperaldosteronism
	Pathologic fractures	Hyperparathyroidism
	Joint pain	Hypothyroidism Acromegaly
	Bone pain	Hyperparathyroidism
	Bone thickening	Acromegaly
Urologic	Polyuria	Hyperparathyroidism Diabetes insipidus Diabetes mellitus Hyperaldosteronism
	Kidney stones	Hyperparathyroidism Acromegaly Cushing's syndrome
Integumentary	Hirsutism	Adrenal hyperfunction Acromegaly
	Hair loss	Hypoparathyroidism Hypothyroidism Cushing's syndrome
	Sparse body hair	Pituitary insufficiency Adrenal insufficiency Hypogonadism
	Hyperpigmentation	Addison's disease Hyperthyroidism Ectopic corticotropin production
	Profuse diaphoresis	Hyperthyroidism Pheochromocytoma
	Fine skin	Cushing's syndrome
	Coarse hair	Hypothyroidism
	Fine hair	Hyperthyroidism
	Edema	Cushing's syndrome
Reproductive	Amenorrhea	Hyperthyroidism Hypogonadism Cushing's syndrome Acromegaly Pituitary tumor
	Gynecomastia	Hypogonadism Pituitary tumor
	Loss of libido, impotence	Hypogonadism Hypothyroidism Adrenal insufficiency Diabetes mellitus
Ophthalmic/Visual	Exopthalamos	Graves' disease
	Diplopia	Graves' disease Pituitary tumor
	Visual field deficit	Pituitary tumor
	Periorbital swelling	Hypothyroidism Graves' disease
Body habitus	Round face, "buffalo hump"	Cushing's syndrome
	Abormally tall stature	Prepubertal growth Hormone excess

Diagnostic Tests

A variety of blood tests are available to evaluate endocrine function. These tests may measure the amount of hormone secreted by a specific endocrine gland, determine functioning of the hypothalamic–pituitary–thyroid axis, measure rate of functioning of an endocrine gland, or determine the presence of pathologic substances (eg, autoantibodies). Radiologic and imaging studies also evaluate endocrine disorders by measuring function and structure of the glands.

◆ TESTS OF THYROID FUNCTION

Serum Thyroxine (T_4)

A. Description
1. This is a direct measurement of the concentration of total T_4 in the blood using a radioimmunoassay technique.
2. It is an accurate index of thyroid function when T_4-binding globulin (TBG) is normal
3. Low plasma-binding protein states (malnutrition, liver disease) may give low values.
4. High plasma-binding protein values (pregnancy, estrogen therapy) may give high values.
5. It is used to diagnose hypo- and hyperfunction of the thyroid and to guide and evaluate thyroid hormone replacement therapy.

B. Nursing/Patient Care Considerations
1. When using test to monitor thyroid hormone therapy, should be performed at least 4 weeks after dosage adjustment due to long half-life of T_4.
2. Interpretation
   a. Hypothyroidism—below normal
   b. Hyperthyroidism—above normal
3. Iodides can elevate the results of thyroid tests; therefore, it is important to determine if the patient has had any recent tests using iodine as a contrast media.

Thyroid-Binding Globulin (TBG)

A. Description
1. This measures the concentration of the carrier protein for T_4 in the blood.
2. Because most T_4 is protein bound, changes in TBG will influence values of T_4.
3. Helpful in distinguishing between true thyroid disease and T_4 test abnormalities due to TBG excess or deficit.

B. Nursing/Patient Care Considerations Determine if the patient is taking estrogen or is pregnant, which can elevate TBG; results may be depressed by malnutrition, liver disease

Serum Triiodothyronine (T_3)

A. Description
1. Directly measures concentration of T_3 in the blood using a radioimmunoassay technique.
2. T_3 is less influenced by alterations in thyroid-binding proteins.

3. T_3 has a shorter half-life than T_4 and occurs in minute quantities in the active form.
4. Useful to rule out T_3 thyrotoxicosis, hyperthyroidism when T_4 is normal, and to evaluate effects of thyroid replacement therapy.

B. Nursing/Patient Care Considerations
1. T_3 can be transiently depressed in the acutely ill patient.
2. Interpretation
   a. Hypothyroidism—below normal
   b. Hyperthyroidism—above normal

T_3 Resin Uptake

A. Description
1. This is an indirect measure of thyroid function based on the available protein-binding sites in a serum sample that can bind to radioactive T_3.
2. The radioactive T_3 is added to the serum sample in the test tube.
3. Estrogen and pregnancy produce an increase in binding sites, causing a lowered percentage of binding by the available thyroid hormones.

B. Nursing/Patient Care Considerations
1. Results may be altered if patient has been taking estrogens, androgens, salicylates, or phenytoin.
2. Interpretation
   a. Hypothyroidism—below normal
   b. Hyperthyroidism—above normal

Free Thyroid Index (FTI)

A. Description Laboratory estimate of T_4 concentration with calculated adjustment for variations in patient's TBG concentration

B. Nursing/Patient Care Considerations Below normal in hypothyroidism; above normal in hyperthyroidism

Thyrotropin, Thyroid-Stimulating Hormone (TSH)

A. Description
1. Direct measure of TSH, the hormone secreted by the pituitary gland that regulates the production and secretion of T_4 by the thyroid gland.
2. Blood sample is analyzed by radioimmunoassay.
3. Useful in differentiating between thyroid disorders caused by disease of the thyroid gland itself and disorders caused by disease of the pituitary or hypothalamus. Also useful in detecting early stages of hypothyroidism and monitoring hormone replacement therapy.

B. Nursing/Patient Care Considerations
1. Interpretation
   a. In primary hypothyroidism, TSH levels are elevated.
   b. In secondary hypothyroidism (failure of the pituitary gland), TSH levels are low.
   c. In hyperthyroidism, TSH levels are low.

Thyrotropin-Releasing Hormone (TRH) Stimulation Test

A. Description
1. A baseline sample is drawn, then TRH is injected and blood samples are drawn to determine TSH levels at 30, 90, and 120 minutes.
2. Test determines patency of hypothalamic–pituitary axis.

B. Nursing/Patient Care Considerations
1. Interpretation
   a. Increased TSH should be seen.
   b. No rise in secondary hypothyroidism and no rise in hyperthyroidism
2. A subnormal response can occur in patients taking L-dopa or cortisol.

Thyroid Autoantibodies

A. Description
1. Used to detect the presence and titers of selected autoantibodies associated with some thyroid diseases.
   a. Thyroid-stimulating antibody (TSAb)—autoantibodies that stimulate the TSH receptor on the thyroid gland causing hyperfunction of the thyroid. Helpful in the diagnosis of Graves' disease.
   b. Thyroid microsomal antibodies (TMAb)—associated with Hashimoto's thyroiditis and Graves' disease.
   c. Thyroglobulin antibodies (TgAb)—elevated in the presence of Hashimoto's thyroiditis and Graves' disease.

◆ TESTS OF PARATHYROID FUNCTION

Parathyroid Hormone (PTH)

A. Description
1. Test is a direct measurement of PTH concentration in the blood using radioimmunoassay technique.
2. Results are usually compared with results of total serum calcium to determine likely cause of parathyroid dysfunction.
3. Range of normal values may vary by laboratory and method.

B. Nursing/Patient Care Considerations Elevated PTH in hyperparathyroidism; decreased PTH in hypoparathyroidism

Serum Calcium, Total

A. Description
1. This is a direct measurement of protein bound and "free" ionized calcium.
2. Ionized calcium fraction is best indicator of changes in calcium metabolism.
3. Results can be affected by changes in serum albumin, the primary protein carrier.
4. Useful in detecting alterations in calcium metabolism due to parathyroid disease or malignancy.

B. Nursing/Patient Care Considerations
1. Sample should be obtained from fasting patient and collected in tube with heparin as anticoagulant.
2. Test should be repeated on three different occasions to confirm parathyroid disease.
3. Elevations in serum calcium can be caused by dehydration, vitamin D intoxication, thiazide diuretics, immobilization, hyperthyroidism, or lithium therapy.
4. Low values may be seen in renal failure, chronic disease states, malabsorption syndrome, and vitamin D deficiency.
5. Interpretation
   a. Hyperparathyroidism, malignancy—elevated
   b. Hypoparathyroidism—below normal

Serum Calcium, Ionized

A. Description
1. About 45% to 50% of total serum calcium is in biologically active ionized form.
2. This is preferred method of testing changes in calcium metabolism due to parathyroid disease, malignancy, or neck surgery.

B. Nursing/Patient Care Considerations
1. Sample should be obtained from fasting patient and collected in tube with heparin as anticoagulant.
2. Test should be repeated on three different occasions to confirm parathyroid disease.
3. Interpretation
   a. Hyperparathyroidism, malignancy—elevated
   b. Hypoparathyroidism—below normal

> **NURSING ALERT:**
> Tourniquet use during blood sample collection for calcium studies should be kept to a minimum. Prolonged constriction will cause migration of plasma proteins into the bloodstream locally and results in spuriously high serum calcium values, pseudohypercalcemia.

Serum Phosphate

A. Description
1. Test measures the level of inorganic phosphorus in the blood.
2. Alteration in parathyroid function tends to have opposite effects on calcium and phosphorus metabolism.
3. Useful in confirming metabolic abnormalities affecting calcium metabolism.

B. Nursing/Patient Care Considerations Elevated in hypoparathyroidism; low values in hyperparathyroidism

◆ TESTS OF ADRENAL FUNCTION

Plasma Cortisol

A. Description
1. This is direct measure of the primary secretory product of the adrenal cortex by radioimmunoassay technique.
2. Serum concentration varies with circadian cycle so normal values vary with time of day and stress level of patient (8 AM levels typically double that of 8 PM levels).

3. Useful as an initial step in assessing adrenal dysfunction, but further work-up is usually necessary.

B. Nursing/Patient Care Considerations
1. A fasting sample is preferred.
2. Blood specimens should coincide with circadian rhythm with draw time indicated on laboratory slip.
3. Interpretation
   a. Cushing's syndrome—elevated
   b. Addison's disease—low values

24-Hour Urinary Free Cortisol Test

A. Description
1. Test measures cortisol production over a 24-hour period.
2. Useful in establishing diagnosis of hypercortisolism.
3. Less influenced by diurnal variations in cortisol.

B. Nursing/Patient Care Considerations
1. Instruct patient in appropriate collection technique.
2. Collection jug should be kept on ice and sent to laboratory promptly when collection completed.
3. Interfering factors
   a. Elevated values—pregnancy, oral contraceptives, spironolactone, stress
   b. Recent radioisotope scans can interfere with test results.

Dexamethasone Suppression Test (DST)

A. Description
1. This valuable test is used to evaluate adrenal hyperfunction.
2. Adrenal production and secretion of cortisol is stimulated by corticotropin (ACTH) from the pituitary gland.
3. Dexamethasone is a synthetic steroid effective in suppressing ACTH secretion.
4. In a normal individual, the administration of dexamethasone will inhibit ACTH secretion and cause cortisol levels to fall below normal.

B. Nursing/Patient Care Considerations
1. Explain the procedure to the patient.
   a. Overnight 1 mg DST (used primarily to identify those *without* Cushing's syndrome)
      (1) Give patient dexamethasone 1 mg orally at 11:00 PM.
      (2) Draw cortisol level at 8:00 AM before patient rises.
      (3) Expect suppressed cortisol levels (less than 5 μg/dL).
   b. High-dose overnight DST (helpful in distinguishing Cushing's *disease* from other forms of Cushing's syndrome)
      (1) Give patient dexamethasone 8 mg orally at 11:00 PM.
      (2) Draw cortisol level at 8:00 AM before patient rises.
      (3) Suppressed cortisol levels (less than 50% of baseline value) indicative of patient with ACTH-secreting pituitary adenoma (Cushing's *disease*).
      (4) Unsuppressed cortisol levels are associated with ectopic ACTH secretion (malignancy) or adrenal tumors.
2. Encourage patient to take dexamethasone with milk because it may cause gastric irritation.

Adrenocorticotropic (ACTH) Stimulation Test

A. Description
1. ACTH stimulates the production and secretion of cortisol by the adrenal cortex.
2. Demonstrates the ability of the adrenal cortex to respond appropriately to ACTH.
3. This is an important test in the evaluation of adrenal insufficiency but may not be able to distinguish primary insufficiency from secondary insufficiency.
4. Useful in determining if hypercortisolism is ACTH dependent (bilateral hyperplasia) or ACTH independent (adrenal tumor).

B. Nursing/Patient Care Considerations
1. Obtain baseline cortisol level.
2. Administer 0.25 mg ACTH (corsyntropin) intravenously (IV) or intramuscularly (IM).
3. Collect cortisol levels at times ordered (usually at 30 and 60 minutes).
4. Interpretation
   a. Range of normal responses may vary; however, typically a rise in cortisol of double baseline value is considered normal.
   b. Diminished response—adrenal insufficiency with low cortisol values, adrenal tumor with high cortisol values, prolonged glucocorticoid therapy
   c. Exaggerated response—adrenal hyperplasia with high cortisol values

Corticotropin Stimulation Test

A. Description
1. Test measures responsiveness of pituitary gland to corticotropin-releasing factor, a hypothalamic hormone that regulates pituitary secretion of ACTH.
2. Useful in differentiating the cause of excess cortisol secretion when ectopic source of ACTH is suspected.
3. In general, corticotropin will stimulate ACTH secretion in the pituitary but not in nonpituitary ACTH-secreting tissues.

B. Nursing/Patient Care Considerations
1. Describe procedure to patient.
   a. Patient is given corticotropin (1 μg/kg or 100 μg) IV.
   b. Blood samples for ACTH test are collected at −15, 0, 15, 30 60, 90, and 120 minutes.
2. Normal response is a rise in ACTH to at least double the baseline value.
3. Interpretation
   a. Brisk rise in ACTH double baseline value—Cushing's disease
   b. No response in ACTH—ACTH-independent Cushing's syndrome (adrenal tumor) or ectopic source of ACTH secretion (ectopic tumor)
   c. Test can produce false-negative response.

NURSING ALERT:
Infusion of corticotropin can cause flushing or slight reduction in blood pressure. Warn patients about these effects, monitor blood pressure, and ensure safety.

Urine Vanillylmandelic Acid (VMA) and Metanephrine

A. *Description*
1. Direct measure of metabolites of catecholamines secreted by the adrenal medulla
2. Metanephrine is a more reliable measure of catecholamine secretion.
3. Preferred method of diagnosing pheochromocytoma

B. *Nursing/Patient Care Considerations*
1. Obtain proper urine collection jug with HCl preservative and explain 24-hour urine collection to patient.
2. A wide range of medications and foods may alter test performed by some laboratories. Verify with the laboratory and health care provider the need to hold some medications such as sympathomimetics and methyldopa, and foods such as coffee, tea, vanilla extract, and bananas before and during urine collection.
3. Interpretation—pheochromocytoma: VMA greater than 10 μg/mg creatinine or greater than 10 mg/24 hours; metanephrine greater than 0.7 μg/mg creatinine or greater than 0.7 mg/24 hours

Plasma Catecholamines

A. *Description* Direct measure of circulating catecholamines using radioimmunoassay technique; more sensitive test than urine test but more prone to false-positive results

B. *Nursing/Patient Care Considerations*
1. Collect sample 20 to 30 minutes after venipuncture if possible to reduce the rise in catecholamine levels from pain and anxiety.
2. Collect the sample collected in a heparinized tube.
3. Interpretation—levels greater than 2,000 ng/L diagnostic for pheochromocytoma

Clonidine Suppression Test

A. *Description*
1. Based on the principle that catecholamine production by pheochromocytomas are autonomous as opposed to other causes of excess catecholamines, which are regulated by the sympathetic nervous system.
2. Clonidine (atapres) as a central α-adrenergic agonist suppresses production of catecholamines.
3. Useful in differentiating pheochromocytoma from essential hypertension when test results are inconclusive.

B. *Nursing/Patient Care Considerations*
1. Collect baseline catecholamine sample 20 to 30 minutes after venipuncture if possible to reduce the rise in catecholamine levels from pain and anxiety.
2. Give clonidine 0.3 mg orally.
3. After 3 hours, collect second catecholamine sample.
4. Interpretation—In patients without pheochromocytoma, a significant drop in catecholamines should be seen at 3 hours (less than 700 pg/mL), whereas in patients with pheochromocytoma, no drop in catecholamines will be evident.

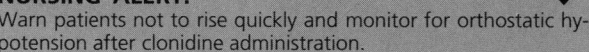

NURSING ALERT:
Warn patients not to rise quickly and monitor for orthostatic hypotension after clonidine administration.

Aldosterone (Urine or Blood)

A. *Description*
1. Direct measure of aldosterone, a hormone secreted by the adrenal cortex that regulates renal control of sodium and potassium, using radioimmunoassay technique
2. May be measured in the blood or in 24-hour urine collection sample.
3. Urine test is more reliable because it is less influenced by short-term fluctuations in the bloodstream.
4. Useful in the diagnosis of primary aldosteronism.

B. *Nursing/Patient Care Considerations*
1. Test results can be elevated by stress, strenuous exercise, upright posture, and medications such as diazoxide (Hyperstat), hydralazine (Apresoline), and nitroprusside (Nipride).
2. Test results may be decreased by excessive licorice ingestion and medications fludrocortisone (Florinef) and propranolol (Inderal).

◆ TESTS OF PITUITARY FUNCTION
Serum Growth Hormone (GH)

A. *Description* Direct radioimmunoassay measurement of human GH, secreted by the anterior pituitary gland; useful in the diagnosis of acromegaly, gigantism, pituitary tumors, or pituitary-related growth failure in children

B. *Nursing/Patient Care Considerations*
1. Blood sample is taken after an overnight fast.
2. Patient should be in restful and calm state before blood sample collection.
3. Normal range: men less than 5 ng/mL, women less than 8 ng/mL
4. Values less than 1 ng/mL suggest hypopituitarism.
5. May be elevated by the following medications: alcohol, L-dopa, oral contraceptives, α-antagonists, and β-adrenergic blocking agents.

Serum Prolactin

A. *Description* Direct radioimmunoassay measurement of prolactin, secreted by the anterior pituitary gland; useful in the diagnosis of pituitary tumors

B. *Nursing/Patient Care Considerations*
1. Blood sample is taken after an overnight fast.
2. Normal values: men 1 to 20 ng/mL, women 1 to 25 ng/mL
3. Values above 300 ng/mL highly suggestive of pituitary tumor
4. Elevated values may be caused by exercise or breast stimulation.
5. Medications that will elevate test results include phenothiazines, reserpine (Serpasil), estrogens, and tricyclic antidepressants.

Adrenocorticotrophic Hormone (ACTH)

A. Description
1. Direct measurement of ACTH concentration in the bloodstream by radioimmunoassay technique
2. One measure of pituitary gland function useful in providing important information regarding adrenal gland dysfunction
3. Useful in identifying cause of adrenal abnormalities when compared with serum cortisol levels.

B. Nursing/Patient Care Considerations
1. Blood sample should be collected in heparinized tube and put on ice immediately.
2. High stress levels in patient can invalidate results.
3. Interpretation
   a. Elevated levels with elevated cortisol—Cushing's disease or ectopic production of ACTH
   b. Elevated levels with low cortisol—Addison's disease
   c. Low levels with elevated cortisol—adrenal tumor
   d. Low levels with low cortisol–hypopituitarism

Insulin Tolerance Test

A. Description
1. Dynamic test measures pituitary response to induced hypoglycemia, particularly GH secretion and ACTH-stimulated cortisol production by the adrenal gland.
2. Useful in the diagnosis of functional hypopituitarism due to pituitary disease or after pituitary surgery.

B. Nursing/Patient Care Considerations
1. After overnight fast, insulin 0.1 unit/kg body weight is given IV.
2. Blood samples are collected usually at baseline, 30, 60, and 90 minutes after insulin dose.
3. The test is considered valid if blood glucose falls to half of baseline or less than 40 mg/dL.
4. Peak response is seen at 60 to 100 minutes.
5. For GH study, normal response should show a threefold rise in GH above baseline.
6. For adrenal response, a rise in cortisol by a factor of at least 1.5 is necessary to show normal response.
7. This test is contraindicated in individuals with epilepsy or heart failure. In persons with suspected adrenal insufficiency, ACTH stimulation test should be done first.

NURSING ALERT:
Test should be performed with health care provider present. Dextrose 50% solution should be available at bedside to treat hypoglycemia, if needed.

Water Deprivation Test

A. Description
1. Functional test of the adequacy of posterior pituitary secretion of antidiuretic hormone (ADH) and its ability to concentrate urine and maintain serum osmolality in the face of water deprivation.
2. Useful in determining the diagnosis and etiology of diabetes insipidus (DI).

B. Nursing/Patient Care Considerations
1. Test is begun by obtaining the patient's weight, serum and urine osmolality at time 0.
2. Patient weight, urine output volume, and osmolality are determined hourly.
3. Deprivation is continued until urine osmolality "plateaus" as evidenced by a change of less than 30 mOsm/kg over a 3-hour period, if the patient's weight decreases by 3%, or if cardiovascular instability occurs. At this point, serum osmolality is obtained.
4. If urine osmolality remains below that of serum (usually 300 mOsm/kg), the diagnosis of DI is confirmed and the second stage of the test, which distinguishes central and nephrogenic DI, is begun.
5. Artificial ADH (vasopressin 5 IU or DDAVP 1 μg) is given subcutaneously at this point to determine changes in urine osmolality at 30, 60, and 120 minutes in response to the injected hormone.
6. If the highest urine osmolality value obtained after injection is more than 50% over the preinjection value, DI is due to pituitary failure. If the osmolality value is less than 50% of preinjection value, then DI is due to renal disease.

NURSING ALERT:
Patients with suspected DI undergoing water deprivation test must be monitored closely because dehydration may occur rapidly in the individual with severe disease.

◆ RADIOLOGY/IMAGING

Radioactive ^{131}I Uptake

A. Description Measures thyroid uptake patterns of iodine as a whole, or within specified areas of the gland

B. Nursing/Patient Care Considerations
1. A solution of sodium iodide 131 is administered orally to the fasting patient.
2. After a prescribed interval, usually 24 hours, measurements of radioactive counts per minute are taken with a scintillator.
3. Normal thyroid will remove 15% to 50% of the iodine from the bloodstream.
4. Hyperthyroidism may result in the removal of as much as 90% of the iodine from the bloodstream (eg, Graves' disease) or, in the case of some forms of thyroiditis, a low uptake.
5. Hypothyroidism—reflected in low uptake

Thyroid Scan

A. Description
1. Rapid imaging of thyroid tissue, particularly suspicious nodules as contrast imaging agent is rapidly taken up by functioning tissue
2. Useful in the diagnosis of thyroid carcinoma.
3. Contrast media is usually administered IV.
   a. Technetium (^{99m}Tc) pertechnetate or ^{123}I is used for best images.
4. Images can be obtained from gamma counter within 20 to 60 minutes.

B. Nursing/Patient Care Considerations
1. May interfere with serum radioimmunoassay tests; contact laboratory to determine when blood test can be done.

2. Benign adenomas may be visualized as "hot" nodules, indicating increased uptake of iodine, or as "cold" nodules, indicating decreased uptake.

3. Malignant nodules usually take the form of "cold" nodules.

General Procedures/Treatment Modalities

◆ STEROID THERAPY

Steroid therapy is a treatment used in some endocrine disorders and a wide variety of other conditions. Steroids are hormones that affect metabolism and a number of body processes.

Classification of Steroids

(By major metabolic effects on body)

A. *Mineralocorticoids*
1. Concerned with sodium and water retention and potassium excretion
2. Example—aldosterone and 11-desoxycorticosterone

B. *Glucocorticoids (Corticosteroids, Steroids)*
1. Concerned with metabolic effects, including carbohydrate metabolism
2. Example—cortisol

C. *Sex Hormones*
1. Important when secreted in large amounts or when the growth of hormone-sensitive cancers are stimulated
2. Examples
   a. Androgens—testosterone
   b. Estrogens—estradiol
   c. Progestins—progesterone

Effects of Glucocorticoids

1. Antagonize action of insulin—promote gluconeogenesis, which provides glucose.
2. Increase breakdown of protein (inhibit protein synthesis).
3. Increase breakdown of fatty acids.
4. Suppress inflammation, inhibit scar formation, block allergic responses.
5. Decrease number of circulating eosinophils and leukocytes; decrease size of lymphatic tissue.
6. Exert a permissive action (allow the full effects) on catecholamines.
7. Exert a permissive action on functioning of central nervous system (CNS).
8. Inhibit release of adrenocorticotropin.
9. In summary, glucocorticoids are necessary to resist noxious stimuli and environmental change.

Uses of Steroids

1. Physiologically—to correct deficiencies or malfunction of a particular endocrine organ or system (eg, Addison's disease)

2. Diagnostically—to determine proper functioning of the endocrine system
3. Pharmacologically—to treat the following:
   a. Asthma and obstructive lung disease
   b. Acute rheumatic fever
   c. Blood conditions such as idiopathic thrombocytopenic purpura, leukemia, hemolytic anemia
   d. Allergic conditions—allergic rhinitis, anaphylaxis (following epinephrine)
   e. Dermatologic problems—drug rashes, contact dermatitis, atopic dermatitis
   f. Ocular diseases—conjunctivitis, uveitis
   g. Connective tissue disorders—systemic lupus erythematosus, rheumatoid arthritis
   h. Gastrointestinal problems—ulcerative colitis
   i. Organ transplant recipients—as an immunosuppressive agent
   j. Neurologic conditions—cerebral edema, multiple sclerosis

Preparing the Patient to Receive Steroid Therapy

1. Determine contraindications/precautions for such therapy.
   a. Peptic ulcer
   b. Diabetes mellitus
   c. Viral infections
2. Administer a tuberculin test, if indicated, before therapy, because steroids may suppress response to the test.
3. Assess the patient's own level of steroid secretion, if possible.
4. Explain the nature of the therapy, what is required of the patient, how long therapy will last, what adverse signs to watch for, and answer any questions.

Choice of Steroid and Method of Administration

1. May be given by a wide variety of methods—orally, parenterally, sublingually, rectally, by inhalation, or by direct application to skin or mucous membrane.
2. Combinations of steroids with other drugs should be avoided.
3. To help avoid steroid side effects, alternate-day therapy may be used.
4. May be given in initial high doses, then reduced; if the patient has been taking steroids for several weeks, doses must be tapered gradually to prevent Addisonian crisis.

Nursing Interventions

A. *Preventing Infection*
1. Encourage the patient to avoid crowds and the possibility of exposure to infection.
   a. Steroids may affect the circulating blood—resulting in decreased eosinophils and lymphocytes, increased red cells, and increased incidence of thrombophlebitis and infection.
2. Encourage exercise to prevent venous stasis.
3. Be aware that signs of infection/inflammation may be masked—fever, redness, swelling.
4. Practice and encourage good handwashing technique and asepsis.

B. *Preventing Nutritional and Metabolism Complications*
1. Determine whether the patient needs assistance in dietary control.
   a. Steroids may cause weight gain and an increase in appetite.
2. Encourage a high-protein, high-carbohydrate diet.
   a. Steroids affect protein metabolism; there may be negative nitrogen balance.
3. Encourage the patient to take steroids with milk or food.
   a. Steroids cause an increase in secretion of gastric HCl and have an inhibiting effect on secretion of mucus in the stomach; they may cause peptic ulcer.
4. Be on guard for early evidence of gastric hemorrhage such as melena, blood in vomitus.
5. Check urine for evidence of glucose.
   a. Steroids precipitate gluconeogenesis and insulin antagonism, which results in hyperglycemia, glucosuria, decreased carbohydrate tolerance.

C. *Observing for Bone Complications*
1. Be on the alert for the possibility of pathologic fractures. Stress safety measures to prevent injury.
   a. Steroids affect the musculoskeletal system, causing potassium depletion and muscular weakness.
   b. Steroids cause increased output of calcium and phosphorus, which may lead to osteoporosis.
2. Administer a diet high in calcium and protein.
3. Recommend a program of activities of daily living and weight-bearing; normal range of motion for the bedridden.

D. *Avoiding Electrolyte Disturbance*
1. Restrict sodium intake and increase potassium intake.
   a. Mineralocorticoid differs from other steroids, resulting in sodium retention and potassium depletion: edema, weight gain.
   b. Lemon juice is high in potassium and low in sodium.
   c. Avoid saline as a diluent in preparing injectable medications.
2. Check blood pressure frequently and weigh the patient daily.
3. Observe for evidence of edema.

E. *Monitoring for Behavioral Reactions*
1. Watch for convulsive seizures (especially in children).
   a. Steroids may alter behavior patterns, increase excitability, and affect the CNS.
2. Avoid overstimulating situations.
3. Recognize and report any mood deviating from the usual behavior patterns.
4. Report unusual behavior, haunting dreams, withdrawal, or suicidal tendencies.

F. *Preventing Stress Reactions*
1. Recommend that the patient carry an identification card indicating steroid therapy and name of health care provider.
   a. Steroids affect the hypothalamic–pituitary–adrenal system; this in turn affects the individual's ability to respond to stress.
2. Advise the patient to avoid extremes of temperature, as well as infections and upsetting situations.

G. *Preventing Injury and Promoting Healing*
1. Instruct the patient to avoid injury; stress safety precautions.
   a. Steroids interfere with fibroblasts and granulation tissue; there is altered response to injury, resulting in impaired growth and delayed healing.

2. Observe daily the healing process of wounds, particularly surgical wounds, to recognize the potential for wound dehiscence.

Patient Education/ Health Maintenance

1. Teach patient that steroids are valuable and useful medications, but if taken for longer than 2 weeks, they may produce certain side effects.
   a. "Acceptable" side effects may include weight gain (perhaps due to water retention), acne, headaches, fatigue, and increased urinary frequency.
   b. "Unacceptable" side effects that are to be reported to the health care provider are dizziness when rising from chair or bed (postural hypotension indicative of adrenal insufficiency), nausea, vomiting, thirst, abdominal pain, or pain of any type.
   c. Additional reportable side effects include convulsive seizures, feelings of depression or nervousness, or development of an infection.
2. Advise patient that a fall or automobile accident may precipitate adrenal failure—requires an immediate injection of hydrocortisone phosphate (Solu-Cortef).
3. Tell patients on long-term therapy that they should wear a Medic Alert tag and carry a kit with hydrocortisone as prescribed.
4. Instruct patient to inform any physician, dentist, or nurse in future contacts about steroid therapy.
5. Tell patient that regular follow-up visits to health care provider are required.

◆ CARE OF THE PATIENT UNDERGOING THYROIDECTOMY

Thyroidectomy involves the partial or complete removal of the thyroid gland to treat thyroid tumors, hyperthyroidism, or hyperparathyroidism.

Preoperative Management/ Nursing Care

1. The patient must be euthyroid at time of surgery, so thionamides are administered to control hyperthyroidism.
2. Iodide is given to increase firmness of thyroid gland and reduce its vascularity subsequent to blood loss.
3. An attempt is made to counteract the effects of hypermetabolism by maintaining a restful and therapeutic environment and providing a nutritious diet.
4. Prepare the patient for surgery physically and emotionally in the following ways.
   a. Make a special effort to ensure that patient has a good night's rest preceding surgery.
   b. Explain to the patient that speaking is to be minimized immediately postoperatively and that oxygen may be administered to facilitate breathing.
   c. Explain that postoperatively, fluids may be given IV to maintain fluid, electrolyte, and nutritional needs; IV glucose may also be given in the hours before the administration of anesthesic agents.

Complications

1. Hemorrhage, edema of the glottis, damage to laryngeal nerve
2. Hypothyroidism occurs in 5% of patients in first postoperative year; increases at rate of 2% to 3%/year.
3. Hypoparathyroidism occurs in about 4%; usually is mild and transient; requires calcium supplements IV and orally when more severe.

Postoperative Management/ Nursing Care

A. Observing for Hemorrhage and Airway Edema
1. Administer humidified oxygen as prescribed to reduce irritation of airway and prevent edema.
2. Move the patient carefully; provide adequate support to the head so that no tension is placed on the sutures.
3. Place the patient in semi-Fowler's position with the head elevated and supported by pillows; avoid flexion of neck.
4. Monitor vital signs frequently, watching for tachycardia and hypotension indicating hemorrhage (most likely between 12 and 24 hours postoperatively).
5. Observe for bleeding at sides and back of the neck, as well as anteriorly, when the patient is in dorsal position.
6. Watch for repeated clearing of the throat or complaint of smothering or difficulty swallowing, which may be early signs of hemorrhage.
7. Watch for irregular breathing, swelling of the neck, and choking—other signs pointing to the possibility of hemorrhage and tracheal compression.
8. Reinforce dressing if indicated.
9. Be alert for voice changes, which may indicate damage to laryngeal nerve.
10. Keep a tracheostomy set in the patient's room for 48 hours for emergency use.

B. Preventing Tetany
1. Watch for the development of tetany due to removal or disturbance of parathyroid glands through a progression of signs:
   a. Tingling of toes and fingers and around the mouth; apprehension
   b. Positive *Chvostek's sign*—tapping the cheek over the facial nerve causes a twitch of the lip or facial muscles (Fig. 22-1A).
   c. Positive *Trousseau's sign*—carpopedal spasm induced by occluding circulation in the arm with a blood pressure cuff (see Figure 22-1B).
2. Be prepared to treat hypocalcemic tetany.
   a. Position the patient for optimal ventilation; pillow removed to prevent head from bending forward and compressing trachea.
   b. Keep side rails padded and elevated and position the patient to prevent injury if a seizure occurs; do not use restraints because they only aggravate the patient and may result in muscle strain or fractures.
   c. Have equipment available to treat respiratory difficulties including airway, suction equipment, tracheostomy and cardiac arrest equipment.
   d. Monitor calcium levels. If in 48 hours, level falls below 7 mg/100 mL (3 mEq), IV calcium (gluconate, lactate) replacement is given.
   e. Use caution in IV administration of calcium to the patient who has renal disease or who is receiving digitalis preparations.

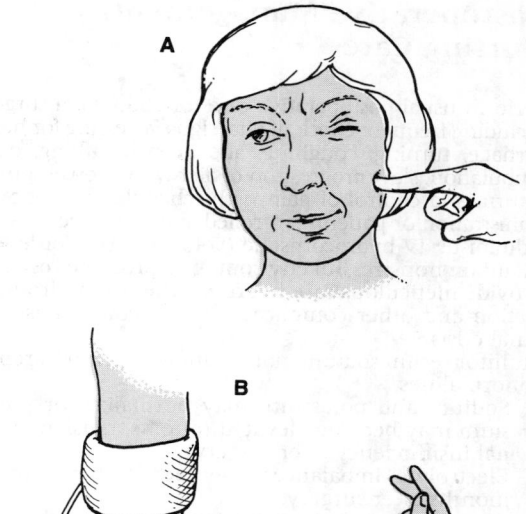

FIGURE 22-1 **(A)** *Chvostek's sign.* **(B)** *Trousseau's sign.*

◆ CARE OF THE PATIENT UNDERGOING ADRENALECTOMY

Adrenalectomy may be unilateral or bilateral to treat adrenal tumors, Cushing's syndrome, or hyperaldosteronism.

Preoperative Management/ Nursing Care

1. Reinforce explanation of surgery given by health care provider and give thorough description of nursing care. Point out where adrenal glands lie on top of kidneys and explain that incision may be on abdomen or loin area.
2. Stress the need for frequent blood pressure checks and glucocorticoid infusions before and after surgery to cover period of stress (surgery) because adrenal gland will be removed.
3. Prepare patient as you would for major abdominal surgery (see p. 494).

Complications

Hemorrhage, adrenal crisis

Postoperative Management/ Nursing Care

1. Perform usual postoperative care for abdominal surgery including frequent check of vital signs, assessing for hemorrhage, turning, coughing, and deep breathing, early ambulation, slow progression of diet when bowel sounds return, and control of pain with scheduled narcotic administration or patient-controlled analgesia (see p. 84).
2. Administer IV hydrocortisone (Solu-Cortef) as ordered.
3. Maintain nonstressful environment, promote rest, and provide meticulous care to protect the patient from infection and other complications that could cause adrenal crisis.
4. Monitor serum sodium, potassium, and glucose; report abnormalities.
   a. Sodium and potassium may normalize, or potassium may become elevated (due to transient adrenal insufficiency after surgery).
   b. Electrolyte imbalances may persist for 4 to 18 months after surgery.
   c. Hypertension may persist for 3 to 6 months after surgery.
   d. Hydrocortisone treatment causes glucose to rise and worsens control in diabetics; may require additional treatment.

◆ CARE OF THE PATIENT UNDERGOING TRANSPHENOIDAL HYPOPHYSECTOMY

1. Transphenoidal approach to pituitary removal is carried out through the nasal cavity, sphenoid sinus, and into the sella turcica (Fig. 22-2).
2. Advantages over intracranial approach to hypophysectomy include:

a. No need to shave head
b. No visible scar
c. Low blood loss, less need for transfusions
d. Lower infection rate
e. Well tolerated by frail and elderly patients
f. Good visualization of tumor field
3. Disadvantages include:
   a. Field of surgery restricted
   b. Potential cerebrospinal fluid (CSF) leak

Preoperative Management/ Nursing Care

1. Sinus infection is assessed for and treated, if necessary.
2. Hydrocortisone (Cortef) may be given preoperatively because the source of ACTH is being removed.
3. Prepare the patient physically and emotionally for surgery.
   a. Teach deep-breathing exercises.
   b. Caution the patient to avoid coughing and sneezing postoperatively to prevent CSF leak.

Complications

1. CSF leak, meningitis
2. Transient DI
3. Syndrome of inappropriate ADH secretion (SIADH)

Postoperative Management/ Nursing Care

1. Monitor vital signs, visual acuity, and neurologic status frequently.
2. Monitor fluid intake and output, urine specific gravity until DI has been ruled out.

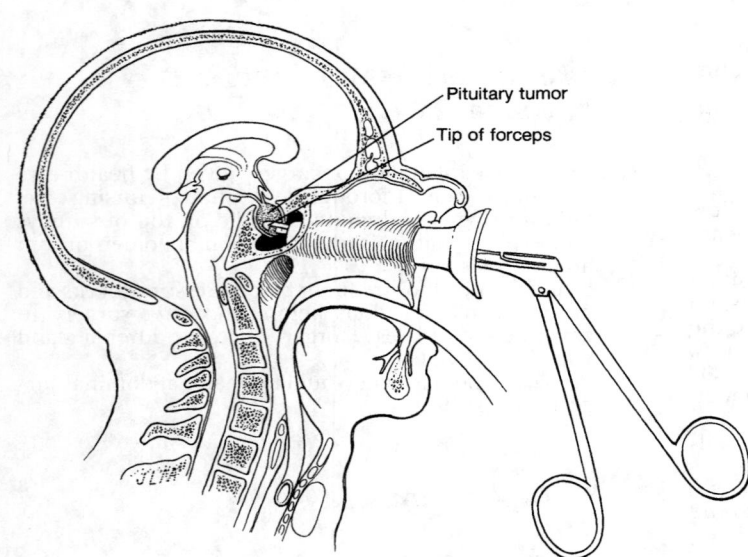

Pituitary tumor

Tip of forceps

FIGURE 22-2 Transsphenoidal approach to the pituitary. A special nasal speculum is used to view the sinus cavity. After the dura is opened, the tumor is removed using microcurettes or other specially designed instruments.

3. Monitor serum electrolyte and osmolality values to monitor for DI and SIADH.
4. Observe for signs of infection. Check incision within inner aspect of upper lip for drainage or bleeding.
5. Assess level of pain and administer analgesic or supervise patient-controlled analgesia.
6. Note frequency of nasal dressing changes and character of drainage. Prepare patient for packing removal one to several days postoperatively.
7. Encourage the use of a humidifier to prevent drying from mouth breathing.
8. Report persistent clear fluid from nose and increasing headache; could signal CSF leak.

Disorders of the Thyroid Gland

The thyroid gland affects the metabolic rate of all tissues, including the speed of chemical reactions, volume of oxygen consumed, and amount of heat produced. The stimulating effect is through the production and distribution of two hormones:

1. Levothyroxine (T_4)—contains four iodine atoms; maintains body's metabolism in a steady state; T_4 serves as a precursor of T_3.
2. Triiodothyronine (T_3)—contains three iodine atoms; is approximately five times as potent as T_4; has a more rapid metabolic action and utilization than T_4.

Most conversion of T_4 to T_3 occurs at the cellular level in the periphery. Some T_3 is produced in the thyroid gland.

◆ HYPOTHYROIDISM

This is a condition arising from inadequate amounts of thyroid hormone in the bloodstream.

Pathophysiology/Etiology

1. Primary hypothyroidism is the most common form of this condition and is generally due to (in order of frequency):
   a. Autoimmune disease (Hashimoto's thyroiditis)
   b. Use of radioactive iodine
   c. Destruction, suppression, or removal of all or some of the thyroid tissue by thyroidectomy
   d. Dietary iodide deficiency
   e. Subacute thyroiditis
   f. Lithium therapy
   g. Overtreatment with antithyroid drugs
2. Secondary hypothyroidism is due to inadequate secretion of TSH caused by disease of the pituitary gland (ie, tumor, necrosis).
3. Inadequate secretion of thyroid hormone leads to a general slowing of all physical and mental processes.
4. There is a general depression of most cellular enzyme systems and oxidative processes.
5. The metabolic activity of all cells of the body decreases, reducing oxygen consumption, decreasing oxidation of nutrients for energy, and producing less body heat.

6. The signs and symptoms of the disorder range from vague, nonspecific complaints that make diagnosis difficult, to severe symptoms that may be life-threatening if unrecognized and untreated.

Clinical Manifestations

1. Fatigue and lethargy
2. Weight gain
3. Complaints of cold hands and feet
4. Temperature and pulse become subnormal; unable to tolerate cold and desires increased room temperature
5. Reduced attention span; impaired short-term memory
6. Severe constipation; decreased peristalsis
7. Generalized appearance of thick, puffy skin; subcutaneous swelling in hands, feet, and eyelids
8. Hair thins; loss of the lateral one-third of eyebrow
9. Menorrhagia or amenorrhea; may have difficulty conceiving or experiences spontaneous abortion; decreased libido
10. Neurologic signs—polyneuropathy, cerebellar ataxia, muscle aches or weakness, clumsiness, prolonged deep tendon reflexes (especially ankle jerk)
11. Hyperlipoproteinemia and hypercholesterolemia
12. Enlarged heart on chest x-ray
13. Increased susceptibility to all hypnotic and sedative drugs and anesthetic agents
14. In severe hypothyroidism—hypotension, unresponsiveness, bradycardia, hypoventilation, hyponatremia, (possibly) convulsions, hypothermia, cerebral hypoxia, and myxedema
15. High mortality rate in the case of severe hypothyroidism (myxedema coma)

Diagnostic Evaluation

1. Low T_3 and T_4 levels
2. Elevated TSH levels in primary hypothyroidism
3. Elevation of serum cholesterol
4. Electrocardiogram (ECG)—sinus bradycardia, low voltage of QRS complexes, and flat or inverted T waves

Management

A. **Approach**
1. Depends on severity of symptoms—may necessitate replacement therapy in mild cases or lifesaving support and treatment in severe hypothyroidism and myxedema coma.
2. As thyroid hormone levels gradually return to normal, the patient is monitored closely to prevent complications resulting from sudden increases in metabolic rate and oxygen requirements.

B. **Restoration of Normal Metabolic State (Euthyroid)**
1. Thyroid hormone: T_4—levothyroxine (Synthroid, Levothroid); T_3—liothyronine (Cytomel); T_3 and T_4—thyroglobulin (Proloid) and liotrix (Euthroid, Thyrolar)
   a. Because T_3 acts more quickly than T_4, it is given via nasogastric tube if patient is unconscious.
   b. Sodium levothyroxine (Synthroid) is administered parenterally (until consciousness is restored) to restore T_4 level.

c. Later, the patient is continued on oral thyroid hormone therapy.

d. With rapid administration of thyroid hormone, plasma T_4 levels may initiate adrenal insufficiency; hence, steroid therapy may be started.

e. Mild symptoms in the alert patient or asymptomatic cases (with abnormal laboratory results only) require only initiation of low-dose thyroid hormone given orally.

2. Monitoring to anticipate treatment effects:
   a. Diuresis, decreased puffiness
   b. Improved reflexes and muscle tone
   c. Accelerated pulse rate
   d. A slightly higher level of total serum T_4
   e. All signs of hypothyroidism should disappear over a 3- to 12-week period.
   f. Decreasing TSH level

GERONTOLOGIC ALERT:
Care must be taken with elderly patients and those with coronary artery disease when starting thyroid hormone replacement to avoid coronary ischemia due to increased oxygen demands of heart. It is preferable to start with much lower doses and increase very gradually, taking 1 to 2 months to reach full replacement doses.

Nursing Assessment

1. Obtain history of symptoms, medication program, and past history of thyroid disease, surgery, or treatment.
2. Perform multisystem assessment, including cardiac, respiratory, neurologic, and gastrointestinal systems.

Nursing Diagnosis

(Also see Nursing Care Plan 22-1.)
A. Decreased Cardiac Output related to decreased metabolic rate and decreased cardiac conduction

Nursing Interventions

A. *Increasing Cardiac Output*
1. Monitor vital signs frequently to detect changes in cardiovascular status and ability to respond to stress.

2. Monitor ECG tracings to detect arrhythmias and deterioration of cardiovascular status.

3. Prevent chilling to avoid increasing metabolic rate, which, in turn, places strain on the heart. Provide bed socks, bed jacket, warm environment.

4. Avoid rapid rewarming techniques (warmed IV fluids, hypothermia blanket) because the resulting increased oxygen requirements and peripheral vasodilation may worsen cardiac failure.

5. Administer fluids cautiously, even though hyponatremia is present.

6. Administer all prescribed drugs with caution before and after thyroid replacement begins.
   a. Monitor the effects of sedatives, narcotics, and anesthetics closely because patient is more sensitive to these agents.
   b. After thyroid replacement is initiated, the thyroid hormones may increase the effects of digitalis (monitor pulse) and anticoagulants (watch for signs of bleeding).

7. Report occurrence of angina, and be alert for signs and symptoms of myocardial infarction and cardiac failure.

8. Monitor arterial blood gases to assess cardiopulmonary function.

Patient Education/ Health Maintenance

Instruct the patient about the following:

1. Thyroid hormone replacement therapy is a life-long treatment.
2. How and when to take medications
3. Signs and symptoms of insufficient and excessive medication; reinforce teaching by providing written instructions as well.
4. The necessity of having blood evaluations periodically to determine thyroid levels
5. Energy conservation techniques and need to increase activity gradually
6. Fluid intake and use of fiber to prevent constipation
7. Control of dietary intake to limit calories and reduce weight

Evaluation

A. Blood pressure and pulse rate stable

NURSING CARE PLAN 22-1 ◆ *Care of the Patient With Hypothyroidism*

You see Mrs. White in the clinic. She is a 45-year-old woman with a history of hypothyroidism, which has been treated with L-thyroxine .015 mg qd.
From your assessment and knowledge of hypothyroidism, you develop your teaching plan.

Subjective data: Mrs. White tells you that she has been feeling very tired lately and finds it hard to manage even the simplest of chores around the house. She complains of constipation, giving her a feeling of fullness and affecting her appetite. When asked about her medication, she states "Oh I ran out of those a few months ago and I never refilled the prescription. I was feeling fine so I didn't see any need to keep taking medicine."

(continued)

NURSING CARE PLAN 22-1 ◆ *Care of the Patient With Hypothyroidism* (continued)

Objective data: Vitals signs are—temperature 36.7°C (98.2°F), pulse 58, BP 100/60, respirations 12. On examination, you notice her skin is cool and dry to touch. She is wearing a sweater although it is a warm day outside. Bowel sounds are hypoactive. Knee jerk reflexes are sluggish.

Laboratory results: T_4—3.4 μg/dL (normal range 5–12 μg/dL)
TSH (thyroid-stimulating hormone) 25 μU/mL (normal range <7 μU/mL)

NURSING DIAGNOSIS: Constipation related to decreased bowel motility due to hypofunction of the thyroid gland

GOAL: The patient will resume normal bowel function.

NURSING INTERVENTIONS	RATIONALE	EVALUATION
1. Encourage increased intake of fluids.	1. Promotes passage of soft stools.	1. Drinks recommended amount of fluid each day.
2. Recommend foods high in fiber.	2. Increases bulk of stools and more frequent bowel movements.	2. Identifies and consumes foods high in fiber
3. Recommend patient monitor bowel function by recording frequency and consistency of stool.	3. Documents patient response to nursing interventions.	3. Patient reports bowel pattern has returned to normal.
4. Encourage increased mobility within patient's exercise tolerance.	4. Promotes evacuation of the bowel.	4. Participates in gradually increasing exercises.

NURSING DIAGNOSIS: Activity Intolerance related to reduced metabolic rate

GOAL: Exercise tolerance and participation in activities will increase.

NURSING INTERVENTIONS	RATIONALE	EVALUATION
1. Teach patient to space activities to promote rest and exercise as tolerated.	1. Promotes activity without overly stressing the patient.	1. Patient reports increased participation in activities of daily living.
2. Teach patient to keep a record of physical activity, noting duration, intensity and level of fatigue.	2. Promotes patient participation in care and promotes independence.	2. Patient provides reports of exercise tolerance and performance in daily activities.
3. Gradually increase level of activity as tolerated.	3. Demonstrates changes in patient activity tolerance.	3. Patient reports successful increases in activity tolerance.

NURSING DIAGNOSIS: Knowledge Deficit related to self-care needs for thyroid hormone replacement therapy

GOAL: Patient will demonstrate knowledge appropriate for self-care in thyroid replacement therapy.

NURSING INTERVENTIONS	RATIONALE	EVALUATION
1. Teach patient about the nature of chronic hypothyroidism and the purpose of thyroid hormone replacement therapy.	1. Provides rationale for adherence to prescribed hormone replacement.	1. Patient describes reason for thyroid hormone replacement therapy and describes regimen correctly.
2. Describe effects of thyroid hormone medication to patient.	2. Allows patient to appreciate benefits of therapy from the standpoint of her current physical complaints.	2. Patient states positive outcomes of thyroid hormone replacement therapy.

3. Describe signs and symptoms of underdose and overdose of medication.
  a. Underdosage—fatigue, slow pulse, constipation
  b. Overdosage—increased pulse or palpatations, sweating, difficulty sleeping, feeling jittery
	3. Allows patient to be an active participant in monitoring her therapy.	3. Patient identifies signs and symptoms indicative of overdose and underdose that should be reported to her health care provider promptly.

◆ HYPERTHYROIDISM

This hypermetabolic condition is characterized by excessive amounts of thyroid hormone in the bloodstream.

Pathophysiology/Etiology

1. More common in women than in men; occurs in about 2% of the female population.
2. Graves' disease (most prevalent)—diffuse hyperfunction of the thyroid gland with autoimmune etiology and associated with ophthalmopathy; most common in younger women; may subside spontaneously.
   a. Thyroid-stimulating antibody (TSA$_b$), an immunoglobulin found in the blood of patients with Graves' disease, is capable of reacting with the receptor for TSH on the thyroid plasma membrane and stimulating thyroid hormone production and secretion.
   b. May appear after an emotional shock, infection, or emotional stress.
3. Toxic nodular goiter (single or multiple)—more common in older women with preexisting goiter; will continue to be overactive unless eradicated or kept under suppressive therapy.
4. Hyperthyroidism is characterized by hypertrophy and hyperplasia of the thyroid gland, which is accompanied by increased vascularity and blood flow and enlargement of the gland.
5. Most of the clinical manifestations result from increased metabolic rate, excessive heat production, increased neuromuscular and cardiovascular activity, and hyperactivity of the sympathetic nervous system.
6. Hyperthyroidism ranges from a mild increase in metabolic rate to the severe hyperactivity known as thyrotoxicosis, thyroid storm, or thyroid crisis.
7. Hyperthyroidism can also be the result of ingestion of excessive amounts of thyroid hormone medication (factitious hyperthyroidism).

Clinical Manifestations

1. Nervousness, emotional lability, irritability, apprehension
2. Difficulty in sitting quietly
3. Rapid pulse at rest as well as on exertion (ranges between 90 and 160); palpitations
4. Heat intolerance; profuse perspiration; flushed skin (eg, hands may be warm, soft, moist)
5. Fine tremor of hands; change in bowel habits—constipation or diarrhea
6. Increased appetite and progressive weight loss; frequent stools
7. Muscle fatigability and weakness; amenorrhea
8. Atrial fibrillation possible (cardiac decompensation common in elderly patients)
9. Bulging eyes (exophthalmos)—produces a startled expression
10. Thyroid gland may be palpable and a bruit may be auscultated over gland.
11. Course may be mild, characterized by remissions and exacerbations.
12. It may progress to emaciation, extreme nervousness, delirium, disorientation, thyroid storm or crisis, and death.
13. Thyroid storm or crisis, an extreme form of hyperthyroidism, is characterized by hyperpyrexia, diarrhea, dehydration, tachycardia, arrhythmias, extreme irritation, delirium, coma, shock, and death if not adequately treated.
14. Thyroid storm may be precipitated by stress (surgery, infection) or inadequate preparation for surgery in a patient with known hyperthyroidism.

Diagnostic Evaluation

1. Elevated T_3 and T_4
2. Elevated serum T_3 resin uptake
3. Radioactive iodine uptake scan may be elevated or below normal depending on the underlying cause of the hyperthyroidism.

Management

A. Approach to Management

1. Treatment depends on causes, age of patient, severity of disease, and complications.
2. Remission of hyperthyroidism (Graves' disease) occurs spontaneously within 1 to 2 years; however, relapse can be expected in half the patients. Antithyroid drugs, radiation, or surgery may be used for treatment.
3. Nodular toxic goiter—surgery or use of radioiodine is preferred.
4. Thyroid carcinoma—surgery or radiation is used.
5. Goal of therapy: To bring the metabolic rate to normal as soon as possible and maintain it at this level.

B. Pharmacotherapy

1. Drugs that inhibit hormone formation
   a. Thionamides—propylthiouracil (PTU), methimazole (Tapazole)
   b. Act by depressing the synthesis of thyroid hormone by inhibiting peroxidase
   c. Given in divided daily doses (every 8 hours)
   d. Duration of treatment is determined by clinical criteria.
      (1) Thyroid gland becomes smaller.
      (2) Uptakes of T_4 and T_3 are measured to determine adequacy of dose.
      (3) Treatment continued until patient becomes clinically euthyroid; this varies from 3 months to 1 to 2 years; if euthyroidism cannot be maintained without therapy, then radiation or surgery is recommended.
      (4) Therapy is withdrawn gradually to prevent exacerbation.
2. Drugs to control peripheral manifestations of hyperthyroidism
   a. Propranolol (Inderal)
      (1) Acts as a β-adrenergic blocking agent
      (2) Abolishes tachycardia, tremor, excess sweating, nervousness
      (3) Controls hyperthyroid symptoms until antithyroid drugs or radioiodine can take effect
   b. Glucocorticoids—decrease the peripheral conversion of T_4 to T_3, a more potent thyroid hormone

C. Radioactive Iodine

1. Action—limits secretion of thyroid hormone by destroying thyroid tissue

2. Dosage is controlled so that hypothyroidism does not occur.

3. Chief advantage over thionamides is that a lasting remission can be achieved.

4. Chief disadvantage is that permanent hypothyroidism can be produced.

D. *Surgery*

1. Used for those with very large goiters, or those for whom the use of radioiodine or thionamides is contraindicated.

2. Subtotal thyroidectomy involves removal of most of the thyroid gland (see p. 712)

> **NURSING ALERT:** ❖
> Observe the patient for evidence of iodine toxicity: swelling of buccal mucosa, excessive salivation, coryza, skin eruptions. If these occur, iodides are discontinued.

E. *Emergency Management of Thyroid Storm*

1. Inhibition of new hormone synthesis with thionamides (PTU)

2. Inhibition of thyroid hormone release using iodine (Lugol's solution)

3. Inhibition of peripheral effects of thyroid hormones with propranolol (Inderal), corticosteroids, and thionamides (PTU)

4. Treatment aimed at systemic effects of thyroid hormones and prevention of decompensation
  a. Hyperthermia—cooling blanket, acetaminophen (Tylenol)
  b. Dehydration—administration of IV fluids and electrolytes

5. Treatment of precipitating event

Complications

1. Thionamide toxicity—agranulocytosis may occur suddenly.

2. Hypothyroidism if overtreated with antithyroid medication or radiation treatment is used.

3. Radiation thyroiditis (a transient exacerbation of hyperthyroidism) may occur as a result of leakage of thyroid hormone into the circulation from damaged follicles.

4. Infiltrative ophthalmopathy
  a. Occurs in 50% of patients with Graves' disease
  b. Features include exophthalmos, weakness of extraocular muscles, lid edema, lid lag.

Nursing Assessment

1. Obtain history of symptoms, family history of thyroid disease, medications, any recent physical stress, particularly infection.

2. Perform multisystem assessment, including cardiac, respiratory, neurologic, and gastrointestinal systems.

3. Closely monitor the patient's temperature for thyroid storm.

Nursing Diagnoses

A. Altered Nutrition (Less than Body Requirements) related to hypermetabolic state and fluid loss through diaphoresis

B. Risk for Impaired Skin Integrity related to diaphoresis, hyperpyrexia, restlessness, and rapid weight loss

C. Altered Thought Processes related to insomnia, decreased attention span, and irritability

D. Anxiety related to condition and concern about upcoming surgery/radioiodine treatment

Nursing Interventions

A. *Providing Adequate Nutrition*

1. Determine the patient's food and fluid preferences.

2. Provide high-calorie foods and fluids consistent with the patient's requirements.

3. Provide a quiet, calm environment at meals.

4. Restrict stimulants (tea, coffee, alcohol); explain rationale of requirements and restrictions to patient.

5. Encourage/permit the patient to eat alone if embarrassed or otherwise disturbed by voracious appetite.

6. Monitor IV infusion when prescribed to maintain fluid and electrolyte balance.

7. Monitor fluid and nutritional status by weighing the patient daily and keeping accurate intake and output records.

8. Monitor vital signs to detect changes in fluid volume status.

9. Assess skin turgor, mucous membranes, and neck veins for signs of increased or decreased fluid volume.

B. *Maintaining Skin Integrity*

1. Assess skin frequently to detect diaphoresis.

2. Bathe frequently with cool water; change linens when damp.

3. Avoid soap to prevent drying and use lubricant skin lotions to pressure points.

4. Protect and relieve pressure from bony prominences while immobilized or while hypothermia blanket is used.

C. *Promoting Normal Thought Processes*

1. Explain procedures to patient in an unhurried, calm manner.

2. Limit visitors; avoid stimulating conversations or television programs.

3. Reduce stressors in the environment; reduce noise and lights.

4. Promote sleep and relaxation through use of prescribed medications, massage, and relaxation exercises.

5. Minimize disruption of the patient's sleep or rest by clustering nursing activities.

6. Use safety measures to reduce risk of trauma or falls (padded side rails, bed in low position).

D. *Relieving Anxiety*

1. Encourage the patient to verbalize concerns and fears about illness and treatment.

2. Support the patient undergoing various diagnostic tests.
  a. Explain the purpose and requirements of each prescribed test.
  b. Explain results of tests if unclear to the patient or questions arise.

3. Clear up misconceptions about treatment options.

Patient Education/ Health Maintenance

1. Instruct the patient as follows:
  a. When to take medications

b. Signs and symptoms of insufficient and excessive medication
c. Necessity of having blood evaluations periodically to determine thyroid levels
d. Signs of agranulocytosis (fever, sore throat, upper respiratory infection) or rash, fever, urticaria, or enlarged salivary glands caused by thionamide toxicity
e. Signs and symptoms of thyroid storm (ie, tachycardia, hyperpyrexia, extreme irritation) and predisposing factors to thyroid storm (ie, infection, surgery, stress, abrupt withdrawal of antithyroid medications and adrenergic blocking agents)

2. Reinforce teaching by providing written instructions as well.

Evaluation

A. Food and fluid intake adequate, gaining weight
B. Skin cool, dry, and intact
C. Maintains concentration, follows conversation, and responds appropriately
D. Verbalizes concerns and questions about illness, treatment, and surgery

◆ SUBACUTE THYROIDITIS

A self-limiting, painful inflammation of the thyroid gland usually associated with viral infections.

Pathophysiology/Etiology

1. Affects younger women predominantly.
2. Acute inflammation results in sudden release of preformed T_3 and T_4 often causing symptoms of hyperthyroidism initially.
3. A clinical variant of this disorder, "silent thyroiditis" has been described that is similar to subacute thyroiditis; however, the symptoms may be milder and the thyroid gland is not painful. This disorder has been associated with onset within 6 months of the postpartum period in women.

Clinical Manifestations

1. Pain, swelling, thyroid tenderness, which lasts several weeks or months, then disappears
2. Temperature elevation, sore throat
3. Pain referred to the ear, making swallowing difficult and uncomfortable
4. Fever, malaise, chills
5. May develop clinical manifestations of hyperthyroidism (irritability, nervousness, insomnia, and weight loss) or hypothyroidism depending on the point of time in the natural course of the disease when the patient presents.

Diagnostic Evaluation

1. TSH level is low.
2. Radioactive iodine uptake is low.
3. Serum T_3 and T_4 levels are elevated.
4. Erythrocyte sedimentation rate is increased.

Management

1. Analgesics and mild sedatives
2. The patient may be placed on β-adrenergic blocking medications to reduce the symptoms of thyrotoxicosis.
3. Steroids may be administered for pain, fever, and malaise.
4. Aspirin or nonsteroidal anti-inflammatory agents may be used in mild cases to treat the symptoms of inflammation.

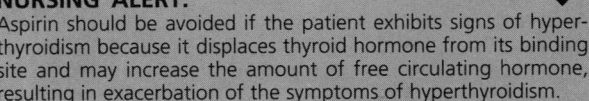

NURSING ALERT:
Aspirin should be avoided if the patient exhibits signs of hyperthyroidism because it displaces thyroid hormone from its binding site and may increase the amount of free circulating hormone, resulting in exacerbation of the symptoms of hyperthyroidism.

Complications

1. In about 10% of patients, permanent hypothyroidism occurs and long-term T_4 therapy is needed.

Nursing Assessment

1. Assess for signs and symptoms of hyperthyroidism (see p. 715).
2. Assess for level of discomfort.
3. Evaluate patient's coping skills with regard to pain.

Nursing Diagnosis

A. Pain related to inflammation of thyroid gland

Nursing Interventions

A. *Reducing Pain*
1. Explain all tests and procedures to patient/family.
2. Administer or teach self-administration of pain relief medication as prescribed.
3. Provide a restful environment.
4. Assess for degree of pain relief.
5. Notify health care provider if pain relief medications are inadequate for acceptable pain control.

Patient Education/ Health Maintenance

1. Explain all medications the patient is to continue at home.
2. Reassure patient that subacute thyroiditis usually resolves spontaneously over weeks to months.
3. Teach patient signs and symptoms of hypothyroidism (ie, fatigue and lethargy, weight gain, cold intolerance) that may be experienced and should be reported as inflammation of the gland subsides.

Evaluation

A. Verbalizes acceptable pain relief

◆ HASHIMOTO'S THYROIDITIS (LYMPHOCYTIC THYROIDITIS)

Hashimoto's thyroiditis is a chronic progressive disease of the thyroid gland caused by infiltration of lymphocytes and resulting in progressive destruction of the parenchyma and hypothyroidism if untreated.

Pathophysiology/Etiology

1. Cause is unknown; believed to be an autoimmune disease, genetically transmitted and perhaps related to Graves' disease.
2. Ninety-five percent of the cases affect women in their forties or fifties.
3. Possibly the most common cause of adult hypothyroidism
4. Appears to be increasing in incidence

Clinical Manifestations

1. Marked by a slowly developing, firm enlargement of the thyroid gland
2. Usually no gross nodules
3. Basal metabolic rate is usually low.
4. Periods of hyperthyroidism due to large amounts of T_3 and T_4 being released into bloodstream

Diagnostic Evaluation

1. T_3 and T_4 may be normal but usually become subnormal as the disease progresses.
2. TSH level is usually elevated.
3. Antithyroglobulin antibodies and antimicrosomal antibodies are virtually always present.
4. Normal or high concentration of thyroglobulin-binding protein

Management

1. Thyroid medications to maintain a normal level of circulating thyroid hormone; this is done to suppress production of TSH, to prevent enlargement of the thyroid, and to maintain a euthyroid state.
2. Surgical resection of goiter if tracheal compression, cough, or hoarseness occur
3. Careful follow-up to detect and treat hypothyroidism

Complications

1. Progressive hypothyroidism
2. Without treatment, Hashimoto's thyroiditis may progress from goiter and hypothyroidism to myxedema.

Nursing Assessment

1. Assess for signs and symptoms of hyperthyroidism and hypothyroidism.
2. Assess size of thyroid gland and symptoms of compression—neck tightness, cough, hoarseness.

Nursing Diagnosis

A. Anxiety related to enlargement of neck/thyroid gland

Nursing Interventions

A. *Reducing Anxiety*
1. Explain physiology of the disorder and reason for enlarging gland. Show anatomic pictures of thyroid gland, if possible.
2. Administer or teach self-administration of thyroid hormone to suppress stimulation on gland and possibly reduce size.
3. Reassure regarding slow progression of gland enlargement (over months) and the option of surgical resection if necessary.
4. Suggest wearing loose-necked clothing, avoiding jewelry or scarves around neck, and avoiding excessive neck flexion or hyperextension, which may aggravate feeling of compression.

Patient Education/ Health Maintenance

1. Teach signs of tracheal compression that should be reported to health care provider as soon as possible—difficulty breathing, cough, hoarseness.
2. Explain outcome of hypothyroidism and necessity of taking thyroid hormones every day for life.
3. Explain the need for regular medical follow-up to monitor thyroid hormone and TSH levels.

GERONTOLOGIC ALERT:
Careful and regular follow-up of elderly patients with Hashimoto's thyroiditis is especially important because the progression to hypothyroidism is usually subtle in the elderly and unlikely to be recognized promptly.

Evaluation

A. Verbalizes reduced anxiety, more relaxed, sleeping better

◆ CANCER OF THE THYROID

Carcinoma (cancer) of the thyroid is a malignant neoplasm of the gland.

Pathophysiology/Etiology

1. Incidence increases with age. The average age at time of diagnosis is 45.
2. There appears to be an association between external radiation to the head and neck in infancy and childhood and subsequent development of thyroid carcinoma. (Between 1949 and 1960, radiation therapy was often given to shrink enlarged tonsil and adenoid tissue, to treat acne, or to reduce an enlarged thymus.)
3. Papillary and well-differentiated adenocarcinoma (most common)
   a. Growth is slow, and spread is confined to lymph nodes that surround thyroid area.
   b. Cure rate is excellent after removal of involved areas.
4. Follicular (rapidly growing, widely metastasizing type)
   a. Occurs predominantly in middle-aged and elderly persons.
   b. Brief encouraging response may occur with irradiation.
   c. Progression of disease is rapid; high mortality rate.
5. Parafollicular—medullary thyroid carcinoma (MTC)
   a. Rare, inheritable type of thyroid malignancy, which can be detected early by a radioimmunoassay for calcitonin.

Clinical Manifestations

1. On palpation of the thyroid, there may be a firm, irregular, fixed, painless mass or nodule.
2. The occurrence of signs and symptoms of hyperthyroidism is rare.

Diagnostic Evaluation

1. A thyroid scan with ^{99m}Tc will detect a "cold" nodule with little uptake.
2. Fine needle aspiration biopsy
3. Surgical exploration

Management

1. Surgical removal is extensive, as required.
   a. Postsurgical radiation therapy is often done to reduce chances of recurrence.
   b. Follow-up includes periodic ^{131}I uptake scan to detect evidence of recurrence.
2. Thyroid replacement
   a. Thyroid hormone is administered to suppress secretion of TSH.
   b. Such treatment is continued indefinitely and requires annual checkups.
3. For unresectable cancer, patient is referred for treatment with ^{131}I, chemotherapy, or radiation therapy.

Complications

1. Untreated thyroid carcinoma can be fatal.

Nursing Assessment

1. Explore with patient feelings and concerns regarding the diagnosis, treatment, and prognosis.

Nursing Diagnosis

A. Anxiety related to concern about cancer, upcoming surgery

Nursing Interventions

Also see Care of the Patient Undergoing Thyroidectomy, p. 712.

A. *Allaying Anxiety*
1. Provide all explanations in a simple, concise manner and repeat important information as necessary because anxiety may interfere with patient's processing of information.
2. Stress the positive aspects of treatment, high cure rate as outlined by health care provider.
3. Encourage support by significant other, clergy, social worker, nursing staff, as available.

Patient Education/ Health Maintenance

1. Instruct the patient on thyroid hormone replacement and follow-up blood tests.
2. Stress the need for periodic evaluation for recurrence of malignancy.
3. Supply additional information or suggest community resources dealing with cancer prevention and treatment.

Evaluation

A. Discusses concerns with family, hospital clergy

Disorders of the Parathyroid Glands

The parathyroid glands are small, bean-sized structures embedded in the posterior section of the thyroid gland. Functions include the production, storage, and release of PTH (parathormone) in response to the serum level of ionized calcium. PTH increases serum calcium by decreasing elimination of calcium ions in the urine by the kidney, increasing absorption of calcium ions from the gut, and increasing bone contribution of calcium ions to the plasma.

◆ HYPERPARATHYROIDISM

Hyperparathyroidism is hypersecretion of PTH.

Pathophysiology/Etiology

1. Disorder is most common among women over the age of 50.
2. Primary hyperparathyroidism
   a. Single parathyroid adenoma is the most common cause (about 80% of cases).
   b. Parathyroid hyperplasia accounts for about 20% of cases.
   c. Parathyroid carcinoma accounts for less than 1% of cases.
3. Secondary hyperparathyroidism
   a. Primarily the result of renal failure

Clinical Manifestations

1. Decalcification of bones
   a. Skeletal pain, backache, pain on weight-bearing, pathologic fractures, deformities, formation of bony cysts
   b. Formation of bone tumors—overgrowth of osteoclasts
   c. Formation of calcium-containing kidney stones
2. Depression of neuromuscular function
   a. The patient may trip, drop objects, show general fatigue, loss of memory for recent events, emotional instability, changes in level of consciousness with stupor and coma.
   b. Cardiac arrhythmias, hypertension, cardiac standstill

Diagnostic Evaluation

1. Persistently elevated serum calcium (11 mg/100 mL); test is performed on at least two occasions to determine consistency of results.
2. Exclusion of other causes of hypercalcemia—malignancy (usually bone or breast), vitamin D excess, multiple myeloma, sarcoidosis, milk–alkali syndrome, drugs such as thiazides, Cushing's disease, hyperthyroidism
3. PTH levels are increased.
4. Serum calcium and alkaline phosphatase levels are elevated and serum phosphorus levels are decreased.
5. Skeletal changes are revealed by x-ray.
6. Early diagnosis often is difficult. (Complications may occur before this condition is diagnosed.)
7. Cine computed tomography (CT) will disclose parathyroid tumors more readily than x-ray.

Management

A. Treatment of Hypercalcemia
1. Hydration (IV saline) and diuretics—furosemide (Lasix) and ethacrynic acid (Edecrin)—to increase urinary excretion of calcium in patients *not* in renal failure
2. Oral phosphate may be used as an antihypercalcemic agent.
3. Plicamycin (Mithramycin), calcitonin (Cibacalcin), or etidronate disodium (Didronel) are effective in treating hypercalcemia by inhibiting bone resorption.
4. Dietary calcium is restricted, and all drugs that might cause hypercalcemia (thiazides, vitamin D) are discontinued.
5. Dialysis may be necessary in patients with resistant hypercalcemia or those with renal failure.
6. Digitalis is reduced because patient with hypercalcemia is more sensitive to toxic effects of this drug.
7. Monitoring of daily serum calcium, blood urea nitrogen (BUN), potassium, and magnesium levels
8. Removal of underlying cause

B. Treatment of Primary Hyperparathyroidism Surgery for removal of abnormal parathyroid tissue

Complications

1. Formation of renal stones, calcification of kidney parenchyma, renal shutdown
2. Ulceration of upper gastrointestinal tract leading to hemorrhage and perforation
3. Demineralization of bones, cysts and fibrosis of marrow—leading to fractures, especially of vertebral bodies and ribs
4. Hypoparathyroidism after surgery

Nursing Assessment

1. Obtain review of systems and perform multisystem examination to detect signs and symptoms of hyperparathyroidism.
2. Closely monitor patient's input and output and serum electrolytes, especially calcium level.

Nursing Diagnoses

A. Fluid Volume Deficit related to effects of elevated serum calcium levels
B. Altered Urinary Elimination related to renal calculi and calcium deposits in the kidneys
C. Impaired Physical Mobility related to weakness, bone pain, and pathologic fractures
D. Anxiety related to surgery
E. Risk for Injury related to hypocalcemia

Nursing Interventions

A. Achieving Fluid and Electrolyte Balance
1. Monitor fluid intake and output.
2. Provide adequate hydration—administer water, glucose, and electrolytes orally or IV as prescribed.
3. Prevent or promptly treat dehydration by reporting vomiting or other sources of fluid loss promptly.
4. Assist patient in understanding why and how to avoid dietary sources of calcium—dairy products, broccoli, calcium-containing antacids.

B. Promoting Urinary Elimination
1. Strain all urine to observe for stones.
2. Increase fluid intake to 3,000 mL/day to maintain hydration and prevent precipitation of calcium and formation of stones.

3. Instruct the patient about dietary recommendations for restriction of calcium.
4. Observe for signs of urinary tract infection, hematuria, and renal colic.
5. Assess renal function through serum creatinine and BUN levels.

C. *Increasing Physical Mobility*
1. Assist the patient in hygiene and activities if bone pain is severe or if the patient experiences musculoskeletal weakness.
2. Protect the patient from falls or injury.
3. Turn the patient cautiously and handle extremities gently to avoid fractures.
4. Administer analgesia as prescribed.
5. Assess level of pain and the patient's response to analgesia.
6. Encourage the patient to participate in mild exercise gradually as symptoms subside.
7. Instruct and demonstrate correct body mechanics to reduce strain, backache, and injury.

D. *Relieving Anxiety*
1. Encourage patient to verbalize fears and feelings about upcoming surgery.
2. Explain tests and procedures to the patient.
3. Reassure the patient about skeletal recovery.
   a. Bone pain diminishes fairly quickly.
   b. Fractures are treated by orthopedic procedures.
4. Prepare patient for surgery as for thyroidectomy (see p. 712).

E. *Monitoring for Hypocalcemia Postoperatively*
1. Monitor ECG to detect changes secondary to hypercalcemia. (During moderate elevations of serum calcium, QT interval is shortened; with extreme hypercalcemia, widening of the T wave is seen.)
2. Monitor serum calcium level and evaluate for signs and symptoms of hypocalcemia and onset of tetany (see p. 713).
   a. Observe calcium levels—if well below normal and if decline continues into the second week, the skeletal system is absorbing calcium and calcium administration may not be necessary.
   b. If some significant bone involvement was noted before surgery, as evidenced by elevated alkaline phosphatase level, elemental calcium may be ordered.

Patient Education/ Health Promotion

1. Instruct the patient about calcium-reducing medications.
   a. Calcitonin (Cibacalcin) is given subcutaneously— teach proper technique.
   b. Etidronate disodium (Didronel)—calcium-rich foods should be avoided within 2 hours of dose; therapeutic response may take 1 to 3 months.
   c. Plicamycin (Mithramycin)—antineoplastic drug that may cause nausea and vomiting, stomatitis; inspect oral mucosa regularly.
2. Teach signs and symptoms of tetany that the patient may experience postoperatively and should report to health care provider (numbness and tingling in extremities or around mouth).

Evaluation

A. Output equals intake, normal skin turgor, moist mucous membranes
B. No signs and symptoms of kidney stones or urinary tract infection; serum creatinine and BUN levels normal
C. Reports less bone and joint pain; using correct body mechanics
D. Verbalizes concerns and fears about surgery; appears less anxious
E. ECG without QT, T wave changes; no numbness or tingling reported

◆ HYPOPARATHYROIDISM

Hypoparathyroidism results from a deficiency of PTH and is characterized by hypocalcemia and neuromuscular hyperexcitability.

Pathophysiology/Etiology

1. The most common cause is accidental removal or destruction of parathyroid tissue or its blood supply during thyroidectomy or radical neck dissection for malignancy.
2. Decrease in gland function (idiopathic hypoparathyroidism); may be autoimmune or familial in origin
3. Malignancy or metastasis from a cancer to the parathyroid glands
4. Resistance to PTH action
5. With inadequate PTH secretion, there is decreased resorption of calcium from the renal tubules, decreased absorption of calcium in the gastrointestinal tract, and decreased resorption of calcium from bone.
6. Blood calcium falls to a low level, causing symptoms of muscular hyperirritability, uncontrolled spasms, and hypocalcemic tetany.
7. In response to decreased serum calcium levels and in the absence of PTH, the serum phosphate level rises and phosphate excretion by the kidneys decreases.

Clinical Manifestations

1. Tetany—general muscular hypertonia; attempts at voluntary movement result in tremors and spasmodic or uncoordinated movements; fingers assume classic tetanic position.
   a. Chvostek's sign—a spasm of facial muscles that occurs when muscles or branches of facial nerve are tapped
   b. Trousseau's sign—carpopedal spasm within 3 minutes after a blood pressure cuff is inflated 20 mm Hg above the patient's systolic pressure
   c. Laryngeal spasm
2. Severe anxiety and apprehension
3. Renal colic is often present if the patient has history of stones; preexisting stones loosen and migrate into the ureter.

Diagnostic Evaluation

1. Phosphorus level in blood is elevated.
2. Decrease in serum calcium level to a low level (7.5 mg/100 mL or less)
3. PTH levels are low in most cases; may be normal or elevated in pseudohypoparathyroidism.

Management

A. IV Calcium Administration
1. A syringe and an ampule of a calcium solution (calcium chloride, calcium gluceptate, calcium gluconate) are to be kept at the bedside at all times.
2. Most rapidly effective calcium solution is ionized calcium chloride (10%).
3. For rapid use to relieve severe tetany, infusion carried out every 10 minutes.
   a. All IV calcium preparations are administered slowly. It is highly irritating, stings, and causes thrombosis; patient experiences unpleasant burning flush of skin and tongue.

NURSING ALERT:
Too rapid calcium administration may cause cardiac arrest.
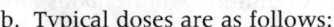

   b. Typical doses are as follows:
      (1) Calcium chloride—500 mg to 1 g (5–10 mL) as indicated by serum calcium; administer at rate of less than 1 mL/min of 10% solution.
      (2) Calcium gluconate—500 mg to 2 g (10–20 mL) at a rate of less than 0.5 mL/min of a 10% solution
      (3) Calcium gluceptate—1 to 2 g (5–10 mL) at a rate of less than 1 mL/min
4. A slow drip of IV saline containing calcium gluconate is given until control of tetany is ensured; then intramuscular or oral administration of calcium is prescribed.
5. Later, vitamin D is added to calcium intake—increases absorption of calcium and also induces a high level of calcium in the bloodstream.
   a. Thiazide diuretics may also be added due to their calcium-retaining effect on the kidney; doses of calcium and vitamin D may be lowered.
6. Administration of IV calcium seems to cause rapid relief of anxiety.

C. Other Measures
1. Treat kidney stones.
2. Monitor patient for hypercalciuria. Periodic 24-hour urinary calcium determinations are recommended.
3. Monitor blood calcium level periodically; variations in vitamin D may affect calcium levels.

Complications

1. Acute complications related to hypocalcemia include seizures, tetany, and mental disorders, all of which can be reversed with calcium therapy.
2. If onset of hypocalcemia is acute, the major concerns are laryngeal spasm, acute airway obstruction, and cardiovascular failure.

3. Long-term complications include subcapsular cataracts, calcification of the basal ganglia, and papilledema, (due to precipitation of calcium out of serum and deposition in tissue); shortening of the fingers and toes, and bowing of the long bones (due to inadequate PTH and additional genetic abnormalities). Of these complications, only papilledema is reversible.

Nursing Assessment

1. Perform multisystem assessment, focusing on neuromuscular system.
2. Closely monitor patient's input and output and serum electrolytes, especially calcium level.
3. Assess anxiety.

Nursing Diagnoses

A. Altered Nutrition (Less than Body Requirements) for calcium

Nursing Interventions

A. Maintaining Normal Serum Calcium Levels
1. Assess neuromuscular status frequently in patients with hypoparathyroidism and those at risk for hypocalcemia (patients in the immediate postoperative period after thyroidectomy, parathyroidectomy, radical neck dissection).
2. Check for Trousseau's and Chvostek's signs and notify health care provider if positive.
3. Assess respiratory status frequently in acute hypocalcemia and postoperatively.
4. Monitor serum calcium and phosphorus levels.
5. Promote high-calcium diet if prescribed—dairy products, green, leafy vegetables.
6. Instruct the patient about signs and symptoms of hypo- and hypercalcemia that should be reported.
7. Use caution in administering other drugs to the patient with hypocalcemia.
   a. The hypocalcemic patient is sensitive to digoxin (Lanoxin); as hypocalcemia is reversed, the patient may rapidly develop digitalis toxicity.
   b. Cimetidine (Tagamet) interferes with normal parathyroid function, especially in the patient with renal failure, which increases the risk of hypocalcemia.

Patient Education/Health Maintenance

1. Explain to the patient and family the function of PTH and the role of vitamin D and calcium in maintaining good health.
2. Discuss the importance of each medication prescribed for the control of hypocalcemia including vitamin D, calcium, and thiazide diuretic.
   a. Take medications as prescribed.
   b. Do not substitute with over-the-counter preparations without the advice and supervision of the health care provider.

3. Provide the patient with a written list of hypercalcemia and hypocalcemia and advise the patient to contact the health care provider immediately should signs of either condition develop.
4. Advise the patient to wear a Medic Alert tag.
5. Explain the need for periodic medical follow-up for life.

Evaluation

A. Verbalizes understanding of diet and medications; calcium level within normal limits

Disorders of the Adrenal Glands

The adrenal medulla, or inner portion of the gland, is not necessary to maintain life, but enables a person to cope with stress. It secretes two hormones:

1. *Epinephrine* (adrenalin) acts on α and β receptors to increase contractility and excitability of heart muscle, leading to increased cardiac output; facilitates blood flow to muscles, brain, and viscera; enhances blood sugar by stimulating conversion of glycogen to glucose in liver; and inhibits smooth muscle contraction.
2. *Norepinephrine* (noradrenaline) acts primarily on α receptors to increase peripheral vascular resistance, leading to increases in diastolic and systolic blood pressure.

The adrenal cortex, or outer portion of the gland, is essential to life. It secretes adrenocortical hormones—synthesized from cholesterol.

1. *Glucocorticoids* (cortisone and hydrocortisone) enhance protein catabolism and inhibit protein synthesis; antagonize action of insulin and increase blood sugar; increase synthesis of glucose by liver; influence defense mechanism of body and its reaction to stress; and influence emotional reaction.
2. *Mineralocorticoids* (aldosterone and desoxycorticosterone) regulate reabsorption of sodium; regulate excretion of potassium by renal tubules.
3. *Adrenosterones* (adrenal androgens) exert minimal effect on sex characteristics and function.

◆ PRIMARY ALDOSTERONISM

Primary aldosteronism refers to excessive secretion of aldosterone by the adrenal cortex.

Pathophysiology/Etiology

1. Excessive secretion of aldosterone results in the conservation of sodium and excretion of potassium primarily in the renal tubules, but also in he sweat glands, salivary glands, and in the gastrointestinal tract.
2. Usually caused by a cortical adenoma; also bilateral adrenal hyperplasia
3. Secondary aldosteronism occurs in conjunction with heart failure, renal dysfunction, or cirrhosis of the liver.

4. Women account for 70% of patients with aldosterone-secreting adenomas and the incidence of primary aldosteronism is four times higher among African Americans than among the general population.

Clinical Manifestations

1. Hypertension. (One to 2% of cases of hypertension are a result of primary aldosteronism, which usually can be treated successfully by surgical removal of the adenoma.)
2. A profound decline in blood levels of potassium (hypokalemia) and hydrogen ions (alkalosis) results in muscle weakness and inability of kidneys to acidify or concentrate urine, leading to excess volume of urine (polyuria).
3. A decline in hydrogen ions (alkalosis) results in tetany, paresthesia.
4. An elevation in blood sodium (hypernatremia) results in excessive thirst (polydipsia) and arterial hypertension.

Diagnostic Evaluation

1. Suspected in all hypertensive patients with spontaneous hypokalemia; also if hypokalemia develops concurrently with start of diuretics and remains after diuretics are discontinued.
2. Salt loading used as screening test—ingestion of at least 200 mEq/d (approximately 12 g salt) for 4 days does not influence the serum potassium level in the absence of aldosteronism, but will cause a decrease of serum potassium to less than 3.5 mEq/L in a patient with aldosteronism.
3. CT scanning to determine and localize cortical adenoma

Management

1. Removal of adrenal tumor—unilateral adrenalectomy
2. Management of underlying cause of secondary aldosteronism
3. Spironolactone (Aldactone) to treat both hypertension and potassium-depleted stages; therapy is needed 4 to 6 weeks before the full effect on blood pressure is seen.
   a. Side effects include reduced testosterone in men (decreased libido, impotence, gynecomastia) and gastrointestinal discomfort
   b. Amiloride (Midamor) may be used instead in sexually active men or in cases of gastrointestinal intolerance.
   c. Sodium restriction is necessary—no saline infusions, low-sodium diet.
   d. Potassium supplementation is usually necessary based on severity of deficit.
4. Addition of antihypertensive agent—thiazide diuretic such as triamterene (Dyrenium)

Complications

1. Long-term effects of untreated hypertension—stroke, renal failure, congestive heart failure

Nursing Assessment

1. Obtain history of symptoms such as muscle weakness, paresthesia, thirst, and polyuria.
2. Perform multisystem physical examination.
3. Evaluate blood pressure.

Nursing Diagnosis

A. Fluid Volume Excess related to sodium retention

Nursing Interventions

Also see Care of the Patient Undergoing Adrenalectomy, p. 713.

A. *Maintaining Normal Fluid and Sodium Balance*
1. Monitor fluid intake and output, daily weights, ECG changes for hypokalemia.
2. Teach low-sodium diet, administration of potassium supplements, as ordered; evaluate serum sodium and potassium results.
3. Monitor blood pressure; administer or teach self-administration of antihypertensives as ordered.
4. Assess for dependent edema; encourage activity, frequent repositioning, and elevation of feet periodically.

Patient Education/ Health Maintenance

1. Instruct patient regarding the nature of illness, the necessary treatment, and the need for continued medical care after discharge.
2. Instruct patient on the importance of following prescribed medical treatments.
   a. For medical management patient must remain on spironolactone (Aldactone) for life.
   b. Patient should report significant side effects if they interfere with sexual performance and quality of life.
   c. Glucocorticoid administration may be temporary after subtotal or unilateral adrenalectomy, chronic for bilateral adrenalectomy; dose may need to be increased during times of illness or stress.
3. Teach patient and family members how to take blood pressure readings, if indicated.

Evaluation

A. Intake equals urine output, daily weight stable

◆ CUSHING'S SYNDROME

Cushing's syndrome is a condition in which the plasma cortisol levels are elevated, causing signs and symptoms of hypercortisolism.

Pathophysiology/Etiology

1. Occurs 10 times more frequently in women than men.
2. The normal feedback mechanisms that control adrenocortical function are ineffective, resulting in secretion of adrenal cortical hormones despite adequate amounts of these hormones in the circulation.
3. The manifestations of Cushing's syndrome are the result of excess hormones (glucocorticoids, mineralocorticoids, and adrenal androgens).
4. Excess of one hormone or all the hormones can occur; the predominant hormone secreted in excess (usually glucocorticoids) determines the predominant symptoms.
5. Pituitary Cushing's syndrome (Cushing's disease)—hyperplasia of both adrenal glands due to overstimulation of the adrenal cortex by ACTH, usually from a pituitary adenoma or hyperplasia
   a. Most common cause of Cushing's syndrome
   b. Affects mostly women between 20 and 40 years of age
6. Adrenal Cushing's syndrome
   a. Associated with tumors of the adrenal cortex—adenoma or carcinoma
7. Ectopic
   a. Results from autonomous ACTH secretion by extrapituitary neoplasms
   b. Tumors elsewhere in body (such as lung) producing excess ACTH
8. Iatrogenic Cushing's syndrome caused by exogenous glucocorticoid administration

Clinical Manifestations

A. *Manifestations Due to Excess Glucocorticoids*
1. Weight gain/obesity
2. Heavy trunk; thin extremities
3. "Buffalo hump" (fat pad) in neck and supraclavicular area
4. Rounded face (moon face); plethoric, oily
5. Skin—fragile and thin; striae and ecchymosis, acne
6. Muscles—wasted due to excessive catabolism
7. Osteoporosis—characteristic kyphosis, backache
8. Mental disturbances—mood changes, psychosis
9. Increased susceptibility to infections

B. *Manifestations Due to Excess Mineralocorticoids*
1. Hypertension
2. Hypernatremia, hypokalemia
3. Weight gain
4. Expanded blood volume
5. Edema

C. *Manifestations Due to Excess Androgens*
1. Women experience virilism (masculinization)
   a. Hirsutism—excessive growth of hair on the face and midline of trunk
   b. Breasts—atrophy
   c. Clitoris—enlarges
   d. Voice—masculine
   e. Loss of libido
2. If exposed in utero—possible hermaphrodite
3. Males—loss of libido

Diagnostic Evaluation

1. Excessive plasma cortisol levels
2. An increase in blood glucose levels and glucose intolerance
3. Decreased serum potassium level
4. Reduced eosinophils
5. Elevated urinary 17-hydroxycorticoids and 17-ketogenic steroids
6. Elevation of plasma ACTH in patients with pituitary tumors
7. Very low plasma ACTH levels with adrenal tumor
8. Loss of diurnal variation of cortisol secretion
9. X-rays of the skull to detect erosion of the sella turcica by a pituitary tumor
10. Overnight DST, possibly with cortisol urinary excretion measurement
    a. Unsuppressed cortisol level in Cushing's syndrome caused by adrenal tumors
    b. Suppressed cortisol level in Cushing's disease caused by pituitary tumor
11. CT scan and ultrasonography to detect location of tumor

Management

A. Surgical/Radiation Tumor (adrenal or pituitary) is removed or treated with irradiation

1. The most recent development in the management of pituitary Cushing's syndrome in adults is transsphenoidal adenomectomy or hypophysectomy (pituitary removal), see p. 714.
2. Transfrontal craniotomy may be necessary when pituitary tumor has enlarged beyond sella turcica, see p. 373.
3. Hyperplasia of adrenals—bilateral adrenalectomy

B. Replacement Therapy Postoperatively
1. Adrenalectomy patients require a lifelong replacement therapy with the following:
    a. A glucocorticoid—cortisone (Cortef)
    b. A mineralocorticoid—fludrocortisone (Florinef)
2. After pituitary irradiation or hypophysectomy, patient may require adrenal replacement plus thyroid, posterior pituitary, and gonadal replacement therapy.
3. After transsphenoidal adenomectomy, patient requires hydrocortisone replacement therapy for periods of 12 to 18 months and additional hormones if excessive loss of pituitary function has occurred.
4. Protein anabolic steroids maybe given to facilitate protein replacement; potassium replacement is usually required.

C. Medical Treatment In patients unable to undergo surgery, cortisol synthesis-inhibiting medications may be used

1. Mitotane, an agent toxic to the adrenal cortex (DDT derivative)—known as medical adrenalectomy
    a. Nausea, vomiting, diarrhea, somnolence, and depression may occur with use of this drug.
2. Metyrapone (Metopirone) to control steroid hypersecretion in patients who do not respond to mitotane therapy

3. Aminoglutethimide blocks cholesterol conversion to pregnenolone, effectively blocking cortisol production.
    a. Side effects include gastrointestinal disturbances, somnolence, and skin rashes.

Complications

1. Possibility of recurrence in patients with adrenal carcinoma

Nursing Assessment

1. Observe patient for signs and symptoms of Cushing's disease.
2. Perform multisystem physical examination.
3. Monitor input and output, daily weights, and serum electrolytes.

Nursing Diagnoses

A. Impaired Skin Integrity related to altered healing, thin and fragile skin, and edema
B. Self-Care Deficit related to muscle wasting, osteoporosis, weakness, and fatigue
C. Disturbance in Self-Esteem related to altered physical appearance and emotional instability
D. Anxiety related to surgery

Nursing Interventions

A. Maintaining Skin Integrity
1. Assess skin frequently to detect reddened areas, breakdown or tearing of skin, excoriation, infection, or edema.
2. Handle skin and extremities gently to prevent trauma; protect from falls by use of side rails.
3. Avoid use of adhesive tape to reduce risk of trauma to skin on its removal.
4. Encourage the patient to turn in bed frequently or ambulate to reduce pressure on bony prominences and areas of edema.
5. Use meticulous skin care to reduce injury and breakdown.
6. Provide foods low in sodium to minimize edema formation.
7. Assess intake and output and daily weights to evaluate fluid retention.

B. Encouraging Active Participation in Self-Care
1. Assist the patient with ambulation and hygiene when weak and fatigued.
2. Assist the patient in planning schedule to permit exercise and rest.
3. Encourage the patient to rest when fatigued.
4. Encourage gradual resumption of activities as the patient gains strength.
5. Identify for the patient signs and symptoms indicating excessive exertion.
6. Instruct the patient in correct body mechanics to avoid pain or injury during activities.
7. Use assistive devices during ambulation to prevent falls and fractures.

8. Encourage foods high in potassium (bananas, orange juice, tomatoes), and administer potassium supplement as prescribed to counteract weakness related to hypokalemia.

C. *Increasing Self-Esteem*
1. Encourage the patient to verbalize concerns about illness, changes in appearance, and altered role functions.
2. Identify situations disturbing to the patient and explore with patient ways to avoid or modify those situations.
3. Be alert for evidence of depression; in some instances this has progressed to suicide; alert health care provider of mood changes, sleep disturbance, change in activity level, change in appetite, or loss of interest in visitors or other experiences.
4. Refer for counseling, if indicated.
5. Explain to the patient who has benign adenoma or hyperplasia that, with proper treatment, evidence of masculinization can be reversed.

D. *Reducing Anxiety*
1. Answer questions about surgery and encourage more thorough discussion with health care provider if patient not well informed.
2. Describe nursing care to expect in postoperative period.
3. Prepare the patient for abdominal surgery (see p. 494) or hypophysectomy (see p. 714) as indicated.

E. *Providing Postoperative Care*
1. Provide routine postoperative care for patient with abdominal surgery (see p. 495) or hypophysectomy (see p. 714).
2. Monitor closely for infection because glucocorticoid administration interferes with immune function; maintain aseptic technique, clean environment, and good handwashing.
3. Monitor thyroid function tests and provide hormone replacement therapy as ordered after hypophysectomy.
4. Monitor fluid intake and output and urine specific gravity to detect DI due to ADH deficiency after hypophysectomy.

Patient Education/ Health Promotion

1. Instruct patient on lifetime hormone replacement therapy and the need to follow up at regular intervals to determine if dosage is appropriate or detect side effects.
2. Instruct patient in proper skin care and in the prompt reporting of trauma or infection for medical treatment.
3. Teach patient to monitor urine or blood glucose or report for blood glucose tests as directed to detect hyperglycemia.
4. Help the patient prevent hyperglycemia and obesity by teaching a low-calorie, low-concentrated carbohydrate and fat diet and to increase activity as tolerated.
5. Encourage diet high in calcium (dairy products, broccoli) and weight-bearing activity to prevent osteoporosis due to glucocorticoid replacement.

Evaluation

A. Skin intact without evidence of breakdown, excoriation, infection, or trauma

B. Participates safely in activities of daily living
C. Verbalizes concerns about appearance, interacts well with visitors
D. Verbalizes understanding of surgery
E. Vital signs stable, pain controlled, no signs of infection

◆ ADRENOCORTICAL INSUFFICIENCY

Adrenocortical insufficiency occurs when there is inadequate secretion of the hormones of the adrenal cortex, primarily the glucocorticoids and mineralocorticoids.

Pathophysiology/Etiology

1. Primary adrenocortical insufficiency (Addison's disease)—destruction and subsequent hypofunction of the adrenal cortex, usually due to autoimmune process
2. Secondary adrenocortical insufficiency—ACTH deficiency from pituitary disease or suppression of hypothalamic–pituitary axis by corticosteroid treatment for nonendocrine disorders causes atrophy of adrenal cortex.
3. Inadequate aldosterone produces disturbances of sodium, potassium, and water metabolism.
4. Cortisol deficiency produces abnormal fat, protein, and carbohydrate metabolism; absence of cortisol during a period of stress can precipitate Addisonian crisis, an exaggerated state of adrenal cortical insufficiency, and lead to death.

Clinical Manifestations

1. Hyponatremia and hyperkalemia
2. Water loss, dehydration, and hypovolemia
3. Muscular weakness, fatigue, weight loss
4. Gastrointestinal problems—anorexia, nausea, vomiting, diarrhea, constipation, abdominal pain
5. Hypotension, hypoglycemia, low basal metabolic rate (BMR), increased insulin sensitivity
6. Mental changes—depression, irritability, anxiety, apprehension due to hypoglycemia and hypovolemia
7. Normal responses to stress lacking
8. Hyperpigmentation

Diagnostic Evaluation

1. Blood chemistry—decreased glucose, decreased sodium, increased potassium
2. Increased lymphocytes on complete blood count
3. Low fasting plasma cortisol levels; low aldosterone levels
4. 24-hour urine studies—decreased 17-ketosteroids, 17-hydroxycorticoids, and 17-ketogenic steroids; may be decreased
5. ACTH stimulation test—no rise in plasma cortisol and urinary 17-ketosteroids

Management

1. Restoration of normal fluid and electrolyte balance
   a. High-sodium, low-potassium diet and fluids

2. Treatment of glucocorticoid deficiency with agent such as hydrocortisone (Cortef) or prednisone (Orasone).
  a. Patients with chronic obstructive pulmonary disease and congestive heart failure may require preparations with low mineralocorticoid activity, such as methylprednisolone (Solu-Medrol), to prevent fluid retention.
3. Mineralocorticoid deficiency is treated with fludrocortisone (Florinef).

> **NURSING ALERT:**
> Overtreatment may be manifested by hypertension, edema from sodium and water retention, and weakness due to potassium loss.

4. Cardiovascular support if indicated
5. Immediate treatment if Addisonian crisis or circulatory collapse is imminent:
  a. IV sodium chloride solution to replace sodium ions
  b. Hydrocortisone (Cortef)
  c. Injection of circulatory stimulants such as atropine sulfate (Atropine), calcium chloride (Calcium), epinephrine (Adrenalin)
6. Diagnosis and treatment of underlying cause of adrenocortical insufficiency or addisonian crisis (eg, antibiotic therapy to treat infection if this is a factor in crisis)

Nursing Assessment

1. Obtain recent or past history of corticosteroid therapy, including length of treatment, dosage, and compliance.
2. Review history for sources of stress such as surgical procedures, infection, or development of other illness.
3. Perform thorough physical examination for manifestations of adrenocortical insufficiency or contributing factors.

Nursing Diagnoses

A. Fluid Volume Deficit related to renal losses of sodium and water
B. Risk for Injury related to ineffective stress response
C. Activity Intolerance related to decreased cortisol production and fatigue

Nursing Interventions

A. *Achieving Normal Fluid and Electrolyte Balance*
1. Assess fluid intake and output and serial daily weights.
2. Monitor vital signs frequently; a drop in blood pressure may suggest an impending crisis.
3. Monitor results of serum sodium and potassium.
4. Assess skin turgor and mucous membranes for dehydration.
5. Encourage diet high in sodium and fluid content; administer or teach self-administration of potassium supplements if prescribed.
6. Administer or teach self-administration of prescribed glucocorticoids and mineralocorticoids; document response.
7. Administer IV infusions of sodium, water, and glucose as indicated.

B. *Protecting Well-being*
1. Minimize stressful situations.
2. Protect the patient from infection.
  a. Control the patient's contacts so that infectious organisms are not transmitted.
  b. Protect the patient from drafts, dampness, exposure to cold.
  c. Prevent overexertion.
  d. Use meticulous handwashing and asepsis.
3. Assess comfort and emotional status of the patient.
  a. Control the temperature of the room to avoid sharp deviations in the patient's temperature.
  b. Maintain a quiet, peaceful environment; avoid loud talking and noisy radios.
4. Observe and report early signs of Addisonian crisis (sudden drop in blood pressure, nausea and vomiting, high temperature).

C. *Increasing Activity Tolerance*
1. Assist the patient with activities of daily living.
2. Provide for periods of rest and activity to avoid overexertion.
3. Provide for high-calorie, high-protein diet.

Patient Education/ Health Maintenance

1. Instruct the patient about the necessity for long-term therapy for adrenocortical insufficiency and medical follow-up.
  a. Inform the patient that therapy must be continued throughout life.
  b. Emphasize the importance of taking more hormones when under stress.
  c. Suggest that the patient carry an identification card indicating the type of medication being taken and health care provider's telephone number.
2. Instruct the patient about manifestations of excessive use of medications and reportable symptoms.
3. Identify actions to take to avoid factors that may precipitate addisonian crisis (infection, extremes of temperature, trauma).

Evaluation

A. Normal skin turgor, moist mucous membranes, stable vital signs
B. No signs of infection or stress
C. Carries out daily activities with minimal assistance

◆ PHEOCHROMOCYTOMA

Pheochromocytoma is a catecholamine-secreting neoplasm associated with hyperfunction of the adrenal medulla. It may appear wherever chromaffin cells are located; however, most are found in the adrenal medulla.

Pathophysiology/Etiology

1. Pheochromocytoma can occur at any age, but is most common between the ages of 30 and 60; it is uncommon in individuals over the age of 65.

2. Most pheochromocytoma tumors are benign; 10% are malignant with metastasis.
3. Tumors located in the adrenal medulla produce both increased epinephrine and norepinephrine; those located outside the adrenal gland tend to produce epinephrine only.
4. May occur as component of multiple endocrine neoplasia (MEN) II, an autosomal dominant syndrome characterized by pheochromocytoma, thyroid carcinoma, hyperparathyroidism, and Cushing's syndrome with excess ACTH.

Clinical Manifestations

1. Variation in signs and symptoms depends on the predominance of norepinephrine or epinephrine secretion and on whether secretion is continuous or intermittent.
2. Excess secretion of norepinephrine and epinephrine produces hypertension, hypermetabolism, and hyperglycemia.
3. Hypertension may be paroxysmal (intermittent) or persistent (chronic).
   a. Chronic form mimics essential hypertension; however, antihypertensives are not effective.
   b. Headaches and visual disturbances are common.
4. The hypermetabolic and hyperglycemic effects produce excessive perspiration, tremor, pallor or face flushing, nervousness, elevated blood glucose levels, polyuria, nausea, vomiting, diarrhea, abdominal pain, and paresthesia.
5. Emotional changes, including psychotic behavior, may occur.
6. Symptoms may be triggered by allergic reactions, physical exertion, emotional upset, or occur without identifiable stimulus.

Diagnostic Evaluation

1. VMA and metanephrine (metabolites of epinephrine and norepinephrine) are elevated in 24-hour urine sample.
2. Epinephrine and norepinephrine in urine and blood are elevated while patient is symptomatic.
3. CT scan and magnetic resonance imaging (MRI) of the adrenal glands or entire abdomen are done to identify tumor.
4. Clonidine suppression test is used to distinguish essential hypertension from pheochromocytoma.

Management

A. *Medical* Control of blood pressure and preparation for surgery

1. α-Adrenergic blocking agents such as phentolamine (Regitine) or phenoxybenzamine HCl (Dibenzyline) inhibit the effects of catecholamines on blood pressure.
   a. Effective control of blood pressure and blood volume may take 1 or 2 weeks.
   b. Surgery is delayed until blood pressure is controlled and blood volume has been expanded.

2. Catecholamine synthesis inhibitors such as metyrosine (Demser) may be used preoperatively or for long-term management of inoperable tumors.
   a. Side effects include sedation and crystalluria.

B. *Surgery* Unilateral or bilateral adrenalectomy or other tumor removal

Complications

1. Metastasis of tumor

Nursing Assessment

1. Obtain history of signs and symptoms patient has been experiencing.
2. Assess for predisposing factors that may be triggering signs and symptoms (ie, physical exertion, emotional upset, allergies).
3. Perform thorough physical examination to determine effects of hypertension.

Nursing Diagnoses

A. Anxiety related to the systemic effects of epinephrine and norepinephrine
B. Altered Tissue Perfusion related to hypotension during the postoperative period

Nursing Interventions

A. *Reducing Anxiety*
1. Remain with the patient during acute episodes of hypertension.
2. Ensure bed rest and elevate the head of bed 45° during severe hypertension.
3. Carry out tasks and procedures in calm, unhurried manner when with the patient.
4. Instruct the patient about use of relaxation exercises.
5. Reduce environmental stressors by providing calm, quiet environment. Restrict visitors.
6. Eliminate stimulants (coffee, tea, cola) from the diet.
7. Reduce events that precipitate episodes of severe hypertension—palpation of the tumor, physical exertion, emotional upset.
8. Administer sedatives as prescribed to promote relaxation and rest.
9. Monitor for orthostatic hypotension after administration of phentolamine (Regitine).
10. Encourage oral fluids and maintain IV infusion preoperatively to ensure adequate volume expansion going into surgery.

B. *Maintaining Tissue Perfusion Postoperatively*
1. Monitor vital signs, ECG, arterial blood pressure, neurologic status, and urine output closely postoperatively.
2. Assess for and report complications of hypertension, hypotension, and hyperglycemia.

3. Maintain adequate hydration with IV infusion to prevent hypotension. (Because reduction of catecholamines immediately postoperatively causes vasodilation and enlargement of vascular space, hypotension may occur.)
4. Monitor intake and output and laboratory results for BUN, creatinine, and glucose.

Patient Education/ Health Maintenance

1. Instruct the patient how and when to take medications.
   a. Warn patients taking metyrosine (Demser) of sedation and need to avoid taking other CNS depressants and participating in activities that require alertness; need to increase fluid intake to at least 2,000 mL/day to prevent kidney stones.
2. Inform patient regarding the need for continued follow-up for:
   a. Recurrence of pheochromocytoma
   b. Assessment of any residual renal or cardiovascular injury related to preoperative hypertension
   c. Documentation that catecholamines levels are normal 1 to 3 months postoperatively (by 24-hour urine)

Evaluation

A. Reports less anxiety during hypertensive episodes
B. Blood pressure stable, adequate urine output

Disorders of the Pituitary Gland

The pituitary gland (hypophysis) exerts prime control over the body's hormonal functions. It is located in the sella turcica at the base of the brain. Its function is regulated by the hypothalamus. The pituitary consists of two parts that are structurally and functionally separate, the anterior pituitary and the posterior pituitary. Hypothalamic control of the anterior pituitary is mediated by releasing factors secreted by the hypothalamus, whereas the posterior pituitary is regulated through direct neural stimulation. Hormones of the pituitary gland include:

Hormones	Target Tissue
Anterior Pituitary	
Growth hormone (GH)	Multiple sites
Thyroid stimulating hormone (TSH)	Thyroid gland
Adrenocorticotropic hormone (ACTH)	Adrenal glands
Prolactin	Breasts
Luteinizing hormone (LH)	Ovaries, testes
Folicle stimulating hormone (FSH)	Ovaries, testes
Melanocyte stimulating hormone (MSH)	Melanocytes (skin)
Posterior Pituitary	
Oxytocin	Uterus, breasts
Antidiuretic hormone (ADH)	Kidneys

◆ DIABETES INSIPIDUS

Diabetes insipidus (DI) is a disorder of water metabolism caused by deficiency of ADH, also called vasopressin, secreted by the posterior pituitary or by inability of the kidneys to respond to ADH (nephrogenic DI).

Pathophysiology/Etiology

1. Primary: idiopathic
2. Secondary: head trauma, neurosurgery, tumors (intracranial or metastatic), vascular disease (aneurysms, infarct), infection (meningitis, encephalitis)
3. Nephrogenic DI: long-standing renal disease, hypokalemia, some medications
4. Deficiency of ADH may be partial or complete.
5. DI may be transient or permanent.

Clinical Manifestations

1. Marked polyuria—daily output of 5 to 20 liters of very dilute urine; appearance of urine like that of water, with a specific gravity of 1.000 to 1.005, corresponding to a urine osmolality of 50 to 200 mOsm/kg.
2. Polydipsia (intense thirst)—drinks 4 to 40 liters of fluid daily; has craving for cold water.
3. High serum osmolality (above 295 mOsm) and high serum sodium level (greater than 145 mEq/L)

Diagnostic Evaluation

1. Serum osmolality—high; urine osmolality—low
2. Water deprivation test determines central and nephrogenic DI.
3. Measurements of serum and urine ADH—decreased to absent

Management

1. Administration of ADH or its derivative
   a. Vasopressin (Pitressin)—administered IM
      (1) Effective for 24 to 72 hours
      (2) Vial should be warmed and shaken vigorously before administering, to ensure uniform dispersion, because active component settles at bottom of vial.
   b. Lypressin (Diapid nasal spray)—absorbed through nasal mucosa
      (1) Duration of action 4 to 6 hours
      (2) May cause chronic nasal irritation
   c. Desmopressin acetate (DDAVP)—vasopressin derivative administered into the nose through a soft, flexible nasal tube
      (1) Duration of action 12 to 24 hours
2. For patients who have some residual hypothalamic ADH (determined by low levels of circulating ADH)
   a. Chlorpropamide (Diabinese)—potentiates action of vasopressin on renal-concentrating mechanism
   b. Clofibrate (Atromid-S)—probably acts by augmenting ADH secretion from posterior pituitary

c. Carbamazepine (Tegretol)—potentiates action of endogenous vasopressin

3. For patients with nephrogenic DI— chlorpropamide (Diabenese) or thiazide diuretics may be of value. Reversible by discontinuing causative medication if cause is drug related.

Complications

1. If untreated may result in death
2. Overtreatment of desmopressin (DDAVP) may cause hyponatremia and water intoxication.

> **GERONTOLOGIC ALERT:**
> Elderly patients are more sensitive to the effects of desmopressin (DDAVP), so ensure that overdosage does not occur and watch for early signs of hyponatremia and water intoxication—drowsiness, confusion, headache, anuria, weight gain—to prevent seizures, coma, and death.

Nursing Assessment

1. Obtain complete health history to determine possible cause of DI.
2. Assess hydration status.

Nursing Diagnosis

A. Risk for Fluid Volume Deficit related to disease process

Nursing Interventions

A. *Maintaining Adequate Fluid Volume*
1. Accurately measure fluid intake and output.
2. Obtain daily weights.
3. Monitor hemodynamic status, as indicated, via frequent blood pressure, heart rate, central venous pressure, and other measurements.
4. Provide patient with ample water to drink and administer IV fluids as indicated.
5. Monitor results of serum and urine osmolality and serum sodium tests.
6. Administer or teach self-administration of medication as prescribed and document patient response.

Patient Education/ Health Maintenance

1. Inform the patient that metabolic status must be monitored on a long-term basis because the severity of DI changes from time to time.
2. Advise patient to avoid limiting fluids to decrease urinary output; thirst is a protective function.
3. Advise patient to wear a Medic Alert tag stating that the wearer has DI.

4. Teach patient to be alert for signs of dehydration—decreased weight, decreased urine output, increased thirst, dry skin and mucous membranes; and overhydration—increased weight and edema and report these to the health care provider.
5. Tell the patient to consider eliminating coffee and tea from diet—may have an exaggerated diuretic effect.
6. Give written instruction on vasopressin administration. Have the patient demonstrate intranasal and injection technique.

Evaluation

A. Fluid intake equals output, weight stable

◆ PITUITARY TUMORS

Pituitary tumors represent a wide variety of cell types. Symptoms reflect tumor effects on target tissues or on local structures surrounding the pituitary gland.

Pathophysiology/Etiology

1. The cause of pituitary tumors is unknown.
2. Typically, pituitary tumors are characterized by size and by what hormones, if any, are secreted.
   a. Size
      (1) Microadenoma—less than 10 mm diameter
      (2) Macroadenoma—greater that 10 mm diameter
   b. Functional status
      (1) Hormone secreting—exaggerated hormone activity; may secrete multiple hormones
      (2) Nonsecreting—usually diminished hormone activity
3. Malignancy in pituitary tumors is rare.

◆ CLINICAL MANIFESTATIONS

1. "Mass effects"—effects of tumor on surrounding structures
   a. Headache
   b. Nausea and vomiting (in some cases)
   c. Impairment of cranial nerves II, III, IV, and VI on testing due to bilateral hemianopsia that results from pressure on the optic chiasm
   d. Visual disturbances such as visual field defects and diplopia
2. Endocrine effects—effects of hormone imbalances caused by tumor (Table 22-2)

Diagnostic Evaluation

1. Skull films (usually normal)
2. CT scan usually enhanced with contrast media, MRI shows mass.
3. Serum hormone levels to identify abnormalities suspected based on clinical evaluation
4. Provocative testing to detect hormone secretion abnormalities of the pituitary such as glucose tolerance test and DST

TABLE 22-2 Clinical Manifestations Associated With Hormone Effects of Pituitary Tumors

Hormone	Hyperpituitarism (increased secretion)	Hypopituitarism (diminished secretion)
Growth hormone (GH)	Gigantism (child)	Shortness of stature (child)
	Acromegaly (adult)	Silent (adult)
Prolactin	Infertility and galactorrhea (female)	Postpartum lactation failure
Adrenocorticotropic hormone (ACTH)	Cushing's disease	Adrenocortical insufficiency
Thyroid-stimulating hormone (TSH)	Hyperthyroidism	Hypothyroidism
Luteinizing hormone (LH)	Gonadal dysfunction	Hypogonadism
Follicle-stimulating hormone (FSH)		

Management

A. *Hypophysectomy* Removal of pituitary

1. Frontal craniotomy—uncommon approach except where tumor occupies broad area (see p. 373)
2. Transphenoidal hypophysectomy—direct approach through the sinus and nasal cavity to sella turcica (see p. 714)

B. *Other Methods of Pituitary Ablation*
1. Cryogenic destruction or stereotaxic radiofrequency coagulation
2. Radiation therapy
3. Drug therapy
   a. Bromocriptine (Parlodel) for prolactinomas and, in some instances, GH-secreting tumors
   b. Hormone replacement therapy for hypopituitarism

Complications

1. Hypothyroidism and adrenocortical insufficiency after ablation, requiring hormone replacement
2. Menstruation ceases and infertility occurs almost always after total or nearly total ablation.
3. Transient or permanent DI after surgery
4. Without treatment—death or severe disability due to stroke, blindness, or imbalances of ACTH, TSH, or ADH

Nursing Assessment

1. Obtain history of signs and symptoms.
2. Perform thorough neurologic examination as well as general physical examination to identify signs of hormone deficiency or excess.

Nursing Diagnoses

A. Anxiety related to ablation treatment
B. Ineffective Management of Therapeutic Regimen Postoperatively

Nursing Interventions

Also see Care of the Patient Undergoing Transphenoidal Hypophysectomy, p. 714.

A. *Reducing Anxiety*
1. Provide emotional support through the diagnostic process and answer questions about treatment options.
2. Prepare patient for surgery or other treatment by describing nursing care thoroughly.
3. Stress likelihood of positive outcome with ablation therapy.

B. *Promoting Management of the Therapeutic Regimen*
1. Teach patient the nature of hormonal deficiencies after treatment and the purpose of replacement therapy.
2. Instruct the patient in the early signs and symptoms of cortisol or thyroid hormone deficiency or excess and the need to report them.
3. Describe and demonstrate the correct method of administering prescribed medications.
4. Encourage patient in assuming active role in self-care through seeking information and problem-solving.

Patient Education/ Health Maintenance

1. Advise patient on temporary limitations in activities.
2. Teach patient the need for frequent initial follow-up and lifelong medical management when on hormonal therapy.
3. If applicable, advise patient on the need for postsurgery radiation therapy and periodic follow-up MRI and visual field testing.
4. Teach patient to notify health care provider if signs of thyroid or cortisol imbalance become evident.
5. Advise patient to wear Medic Alert tag.

Evaluation

A. States rationale for treatment, asks appropriate questions
B. Demonstrates correct medication administration

Selected References

Fitzgerald, P. (1992). *Handbook of clinical endocrinology* (2nd ed.). East Norwalk, CT: Appleton & Lange.

Graves, L. (1990). Disorders of calcium, phosphorus, and magnesium. *Critical Care Nursing Quarterly, 13*(3), 3-9.

Halloran, T. H. (1990). Nursing responsibilities in endocrine emergencies. *Critical Care Nursing Quarterly, 13*(3), 74-81.

Burrell, L. O. (Ed.). (1992). *Adult nursing in hospital and community settings*. East Norwalk, CT: Appleton & Lange.

Isley, W. (1990). Thyroid disorders. *Critical Care Nursing Quarterly, 13*(3), 39-49.

Johnson, J. L., & Felicetta, J. V. (1992). Hypothyroidism: A comprehensive review. *Journal of the American Academy of Nurse Practitioners, 4*(4), 131-138.

Johnson, J. L., & Felicetta, J. V. (1992). Hyperthyroidism: A comprehensive review. *Journal of the American Academy of Nurse Practitioners, 4*(1), 131-138.

Orth, D. N. (1995). Cushing's syndrome. *New England Journal of Medicine, 332*(12), 791-803.

Pagana, K. D., & Pagana, T. J. (1992). *Mosby's diagnostic and laboratory desk reference*. St. Louis: C. V. Mosby.

Reasoner, C. A. (1990). Adrenal disorders. *Critical Care Nursing Quarterly, 13*(3), 67-73.

Singer, P. A., Cooper, D. S., Levy, E. G., et al. (1995). Treatment guidelines for patients with hyperthyroidism and hypothyroidism. *JAMA, 273*(10), 808-812.

Winer, N. (1990). Pheochromocytoma. *Critical Care Nursing Quarterly, 13*(3), 14-22.

Yeomans, A. C. (1990). Assessment and management of hypothyroidism. *Nurse Practitioner, 15*(11), 8-16.

Diabetes Mellitus

General Considerations

Insulin Secretion and Function

1. Insulin is a hormone secreted by the beta cells of the islet of Langerhans in the pancreas.
2. Small amounts of insulin are released into the bloodstream in response to changes in blood glucose levels throughout the day.
3. Increased secretion or a bolus of insulin, released after a meal, helps maintain euglycemia.
4. Through an internal feedback mechanism that involves the pancreas and the liver, circulating blood glucose levels are maintained at a normal range of 60 to 120 mg/dL.
5. Insulin is essential for the utilization of glucose for cellular metabolism as well as for the proper metabolism of protein and fat.
   a. Carbohydrate metabolism—insulin affects the conversion of glucose into glycogen for storage in the liver and skeletal muscles, and allows for the immediate release and utilization of glucose by the cells.
   b. Protein metabolism—amino acid conversion occurs in the presence of insulin to replace muscle tissue or to provide needed glucose (gluconeogenesis).
   c. Fat metabolism—storage of fat, in adipose tissue and conversion of fatty acids from excess glucose, occurs only in the presence of insulin.
6. Glucose can be used in the endothelial and nerve cells without the aid of insulin.
7. Without insulin, plasma glucose concentration rises and glycosuria results.
   a. Absolute deficits in insulin result from decreased production of endogenous insulin by the beta cell of the pancreas.
   b. Relative deficits in insulin are caused by inadequate utilization of insulin at the cell receptor site.

Classification of Diabetes

A. *Insulin-Dependent Diabetes Mellitus (IDDM, Type I)*
1. Little or no endogenous insulin, requiring injections of insulin to control diabetes and prevent ketoacidosis
2. Five to 10% of all diabetic patients have IDDM.

3. Etiology: autoimmunity, viral, and certain histocompatibility (HLA) antigens, as well as a genetic component
4. Usual presentation is rapid with classic symptoms of polydipsia, polyphagia, polyuria, and weight loss.
5. Most commonly seen in patients under age 30, but can be seen in older adults.

B. *Non–Insulin-Dependent Diabetes Mellitus (NIDDM, Type 2)*
1. Caused by defect in insulin manufacture and release from the beta cell or insulin resistance in the peripheral tissues.
2. Approximately 90% of diabetic patients have NIDDM.
3. Etiology: strong heredity component, often associated with obesity
4. Usual presentation is slow and often insidious with symptoms of fatigue, weight gain, poor wound healing, and recurrent infection.
5. Found primarily in adults over 30 years of age.
6. Patients with this type of diabetes, but who eventually may be treated with insulin, are still referred to as having NIDDM or type II diabetes.

C. *Impaired Glucose Tolerance (IGT)*
1. Abnormality in glucose levels intermediate between normal and overt diabetes (formerly called latent or prediabetes)
2. Asymptomatic; it can progress to overt diabetes or remain unchanged.
3. May be a risk factor for the development of hypertension, coronary heart disease, and hyperlipidemias.

D. *Gestational Diabetes Mellitus (GDM)*
1. Defined as carbohydrate intolerance occurring during pregnancy.
2. Occurs in approximately 3% of pregnancies, and usually disappears after delivery.
3. Women with GDM are at higher risk for diabetes at a later date.
4. GDM is associated with increased risk of fetal morbidity.
5. Screening for GDM for *all* pregnant women should occur between the 24th and 28th weeks of gestation.

E. *Diabetes Associated With Other Conditions*
1. Certain drugs, chemicals, hormones, and genetic syndromes can decrease insulin activity resulting in hyperglycemia.
   a. Corticosteroids
   b. Cushing's disease or syndrome

2. Disease states affecting the pancreas affect insulin production.
   a. Pancreatitis, cancer of the pancreas

Diagnostic Evaluation

◆ LABORATORY TESTS

Laboratory tests include those tests used to make the diagnosis as well as measures to monitor short- and long-term glucose control.

Blood Glucose

A. Description Fasting blood sugar (FBS), drawn after a 12- to 14-hour overnight fast, evaluates circulating amounts of glucose; postprandial test drawn usually 2 hours after a well balanced meal to evaluate glucose metabolism; or random glucose, drawn at any time, nonfasting.

B. Nursing/Patient Care Considerations
1. For fasting glucose, ensure that patient has maintained 12-to 14-hour fast overnight; sips of water are allowed.
2. Advise patient to refrain from smoking before the glucose sampling because this affects the test results.
3. For postprandial test, advise patient that no food should be eaten during the 2-hour interval.
4. For random blood glucose, note the time and content of the last meal.
5. Interpret blood values as diagnostic for diabetes mellitus as follows:
   a. FBS greater than 140 mg/dL on two occasions
   b. Random blood sugar greater than 200 mg/dL and presence of classic symptoms of diabetes (polyuria, polydipsia, polyphagia, and weight loss)

> **NURSING ALERT:** ◆◆
> Capillary blood glucose values obtained by finger stick samples tend to be higher than values in venous samples.

Glucose Tolerance Test (GTT)

A. Description Evaluates insulin response to glucose loading. FBS is obtained before the ingestion of a 50- to 200-g glucose load (usual amount, 75 g) and blood samples are drawn at $1/2$, 1, 2, and 3 hours (may be 4- or 5-hour sampling).

B. Nursing/Patient Care Considerations
1. Advise patient that for accuracy in results, certain instructions must be followed:
   a. Usual diet and exercise pattern must be followed for 3 days before GTT.
   b. During GTT, the patient must refrain from smoking and remain seated.
   c. Oral contraceptives, salicylates, diuretics, phenytoin, and nicotinic acid can impair results and may be withheld before testing based on the advice of the health care provider.

2. Blood values diagnostic for diabetes mellitus are as follows: FBS less than 140 mg/dL and two GTTs with the 2-hour result greater than 200 mg/dL and one other value greater than 200 mg/dL after a 75-g glucose load.

Glycated Hemoglobin (Glycohemoglobin, Glycosylated Hemoglobin, HbA1$_c$)

A. Description Measures glycemic control over a 60- to 120-day period by evaluating the attachment of glucose to freely permeable erythrocytes during their 120-day life cycle.

B. Nursing/Patient Care Considerations
1. No prior preparation, such as fasting or withholding insulin, is necessary.
2. Test results can be affected by red blood cell disorders (eg, thalassemia, sickle cell anemia), room temperature, ionic charges, and ambient blood glucose values.
3. Many methods exist for performing the test, making it necessary to consult the laboratory for normal values.

C-Peptide Assay (Connecting Peptide Assay)

A. Description Cleaved from the proinsulin molecule during its conversion to insulin, C-peptide acts as a marker for endogenous insulin production.
Useful when the presence of insulin antibodies (from use of pork or beef insulin) interferes with direct insulin assay.

B. Nursing/Patient Care Considerations
1. Test can be performed after an overnight fast or after stimulation with Sustacal, intravenous (IV) glucose, or 1 mg glucagon subcutaneously.
2. Absence of C-peptide indicates no beta cell function, reflecting possible IDDM.

Fructosamine Assay

A. Description Glycosylated protein with a much shorter half-life than glycosylated hemoglobin, reflecting control over a shorter period of time, approximately 20 days. May be advantageous in patients with hemoglobin variants that interfere with the accuracy of glycosylated hemoglobin tests.

B. Nursing/Patient Care Considerations
1. Note if patient has hypoalbuminemia or elevated globulins because test may not be reliable.
2. Should not be used as a diagnostic test for diabetes mellitus.
3. No special preparation or fasting is necessary.

General Procedures/ Treatment Modalities

◆ BLOOD GLUCOSE MONITORING

Accurate determination of capillary blood glucose assists patients in the control and daily management of diabetes mellitus. Blood glucose monitoring helps evaluate effectiveness of insulin dosage; reflects glucose excursion after meals; assesses glucose response to exercise regimen; assists in the evaluation of episodes of hypoglycemia and hyperglycemia to determine appropriate treatment.

COMMUNITY-BASED CARE TIP:
Blood glucose meters are easily used in the home setting, giving the patient a sense of partnership in the control of diabetes, thus enhancing compliance and treatment effectiveness.

Procedure

1. Guidelines for glucose monitoring are included in Procedure Guidelines 23-1.
2. The most appropriate schedule for glucose monitoring is determined by the patient and health care provider.
   a. Medication regimens and meal timing are considered to set the most effective monitoring schedule.
   b. Scheduling of glucose tests should reflect cost effectiveness for the patient.
   c. Glucose monitoring is intensified during times of stress or illness or when changes in therapy are prescribed.
   d. Patients with NIDDM controlled with oral hypoglycemic agents or a single injection of intermediate-acting insulin may test glucose levels before breakfast and before supper or at bedtime (twice-a-day monitoring).
   e. Patients with IDDM using a multiple dose insulin regimen may test before meals and at bedtime, occasionally adding a 2 to 3 AM test (four to six times daily monitoring).

PROCEDURE GUIDELINES 23-1 ◆ Blood Glucose Monitoring Technique

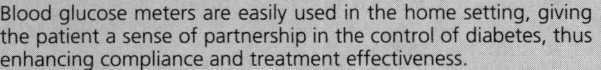

EQUIPMENT	Blood glucose meter	Alcohol wipe
	Test strip	2 × 2 gauze or clean tissue
	Disposable gloves	*Cotton ball
	Lancet/lancing device	

NURSING ACTION	RATIONALE
1. Prepare the finger to be lanced by having the patient wash hands in warm water and soap. Dry thoroughly. a. For convenience, an alcohol wipe may be used to cleanse the finger.	1. Washing in warm water will increase the blood flow to the finger.
2. Don disposable gloves.	2. Complies with CDC standards for blood-borne pathogens.
3. Turn on the glucose meter. a. Prepare the meter by validating the proper calibration with the strips to be used. (This usually involves matching a code number on the strip bottle to the code registered on the meter.)	a. Errors in glucose readings can result from miscalibrated or improperly coded meters.
4. The meter will indicate its readiness for testing blood glucose by message or symbol.	
5. Prick the patient's finger lateral to the fingertip using lancet/lancing device obtaining a large hanging drop of blood.	5. Capillary blood flow to the finger is best accessed along the lateral edges adjacent to the fingertip. a. Most inaccurate readings of blood glucose result from insufficient blood samples.
6. Apply the blood carefully to the strip test area.	6. The test area must be covered completely for accurate results.
7. Completing the test a. No-wipe system—the blood remains on the strip as the meter times and processes the result. b. Meters with a "wipe" system require that the nurse time the blood contact with the strip, wiping off the blood with a firm stroke with a cotton ball at the appropriate end time. The strip is inserted into the meter for the final result/reading.	b. Blood contact time with the test strip can vary with each glucose meter. Precise timing is crucial for accurate results. Consult the glucose meter instruction guide for the timing sequence necessary for your specific product.
8. The lanced finger is covered with a gauze or tissue until bleeding subsides. If necessary, a Band-aid is then applied.	

* Note: Universal precautions should be used throughout the procedure. All blood-contaminated items should be disposed of properly.

◆ URINE GLUCOSE AND KETONE MONITORING

Urine testing does not give an accurate reflection of current blood glucose values, but may be indicated as a general screening test or for home use by those who cannot perform blood glucose testing. Glycosuria is not present until the renal threshold for glucose is surpassed. An average adult renal threshold is 180 to 200 mg/dL indicating that blood glucose levels below the threshold yield negative urine test results.

Urine ketone testing evaluates the presence and amount of ketone bodies produced by the release of free fatty acids in times of poor glucose control. Insulin deficiency, with subsequent inability of the cells to use glucose, results in the breakdown of fat seen in the urine as ketones. Ketone testing is recommended whenever glucose levels are greater than 240 mg/dL or when illness is suspected.

Procedure

If urine tests are the method of choice, careful adherence to the proper procedure increases reliability.

1. Urine specimens tested must be second-voided samples (fresh urine collected 30 minutes after the initial voiding).
2. The urine testing product must be used as directed with special consideration to the timing of the urine application and reading of the final result.
3. Urine testing materials must be stored away from moisture in a cool, dry place and used within the specified time to maintain product performance.

> **NURSING ALERT:** ◆◆
> Urine test results evaluated as percentages cannot be accurately correlated with blood glucose levels.

4. Two methods are available for ketone testing.
   a. Ketostix—dip testing strip into urine sample, wait 30 seconds, and then compare to color chart on product bottle.
   b. Acetest tablets—with tablet on clean, white background, place one drop of urine onto the tablet; observe and compare to color chart.

◆ INSULIN THERAPY

Insulin therapy involves the subcutaneous injection of short-, intermediate-, or long-acting insulin at various times to achieve the desired effect. Short-acting regular insulin can also be given IV.

Self-Injection of Insulin

1. Teaching of self-injection of insulin should begin as soon as the need for insulin has been established.
2. Teach both the patient and another family member or significant other.
3. Use written and verbal instructions and demonstration techniques.

4. Teach injection first because this is the patient's primary concern; then teach loading the syringe.
5. See Procedure Guidelines 23-2 for technique.

Insulin Regimens

A. NPH Only
1. Used only in patients (NIDDM) who are capable of producing some exogenous insulin as a supplement for better glucose control.
2. Traditionally given as a morning dosage to assist with normalization of glucose during the afternoon and evening.
3. Evening or bedtime dosage can be helpful in controlling early morning hyperglycemia.
4. NPH can also be given twice daily (morning and bedtime) to eliminate afternoon hypoglycemia yet provide nighttime coverage (Fig. 23-1). Typically $2/3$ to $3/4$ of the daily dosage is given before breakfast and $1/3$ to $1/4$ is given at bedtime.

B. NPH/Regular
1. Short-acting regular insulin is added to NPH to promote postprandial glucose control.
2. Regular insulin added to morning NPH controls glucose elevations after breakfast.
3. Increased blood glucose levels after supper can be controlled by the addition of regular insulin before supper.
4. NPH and regular insulin given before breakfast and before supper is termed a "split-mix" regimen, providing 24-hour insulin coverage for IDDM (Fig. 23-2).

C. Intensive Insulin Therapy (ITT)
1. Designed to mimic the body's normal insulin responses to glucose
2. Uses multiple daily injections of insulin
3. NPH or ultralente insulin is used for basal insulin control.
4. Regular insulin acts as a premeal bolus given 30 minutes before each meal (Fig. 23-3).
5. 24-hour insulin coverage designed in this way can be flexible to meal times and physical activity.

D. Sliding Scale Versus Algorithm Therapy
1. Sliding scale therapy uses regular insulin to retrospectively correct hyperglycemia.
2. Algorithm therapy prospectively determines regular insulin dosages taking into account meal content and physical activity.

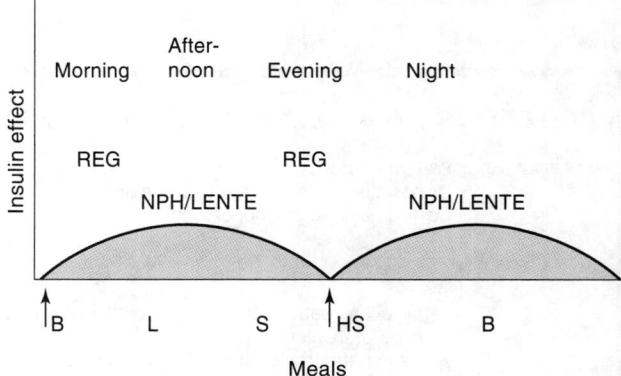

FIGURE 23-1 Insulin curve 1.

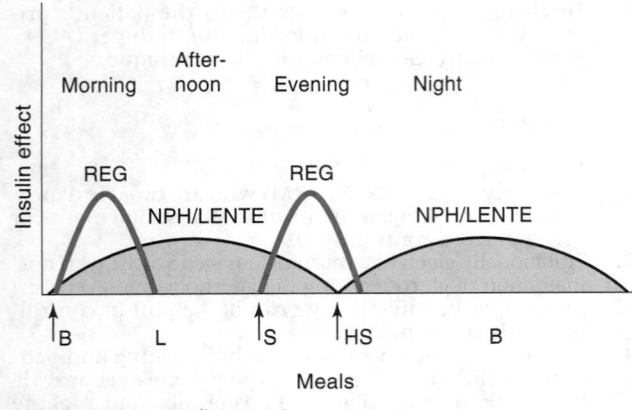

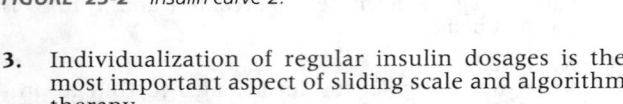

FIGURE 23-2 *Insulin curve 2.*

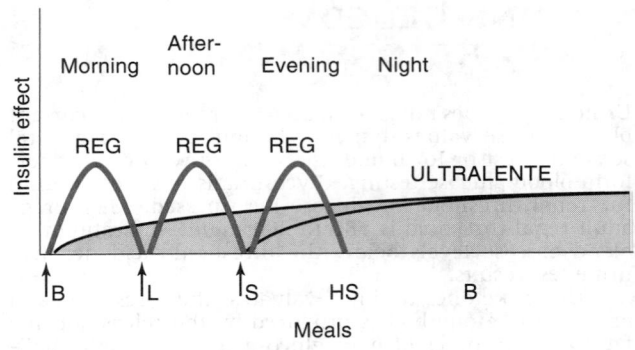

FIGURE 23-3 *Insulin curve 3.*

3. Individualization of regular insulin dosages is the most important aspect of sliding scale and algorithm therapy.
   a. The patient is encouraged to test blood glucoses to analyze insulin dose response.
   b. A pattern of increased blood glucose associated with certain foods (eg, pasta, pizza) can help determine the appropriate regimen of insulin dosage.
   c. Physical activity, which enhances insulin activity and decreases serum glucose, may indicate the need to reduce the dosage of premeal regular insulin.

E. *Continuous Subcutaneous Insulin Infusion (CSII)/Insulin Pump Therapy*
1. Provides continuous infusion of regular insulin via subcutaneous needle inserted in the abdomen.
2. The needle should be replaced every 48 hours or sooner if the site becomes painful or inflamed.
   a. Frequently, the insulin pump is removed for bathing, and tubing and needle are changed at that time.
   b. To reduce tubing and needle blockage, *buffered* regular insulin is used.
3. Intensive insulin management by pump therapy requires patient motivation.
   a. Blood glucose monitoring must be done at least four to six times each day.
   b. Frequent contact with health care team is necessary to adjust insulin dosage.
   c. Careful recordings of diet, insulin, and activity are required to evaluate adjustments.

d. Increased cost of insulin pump and infusion set compared to usual syringe method
e. Heightened risk of hypoglycemia with tighter glucose control
f. Danger of hyperglycemia exists should insulin pump fail to deliver correct insulin dosage.
g. Increased visibility of diabetes by use of an external device
4. Advantages of CSII in improving blood glucose control
   a. Insulin pump can deliver basal insulin at individualized programmed rates throughout a 24-hour period.
   b. Boluses of regular insulin given 30 minutes before eating allow for flexibility in meal content and timing.
   c. Supplements of regular insulin to rapidly correct blood glucoses can be easily given.

F. *Combination Oral Agent and Insulin Therapy*
1. Appropriate only in NIDDM; intermediate-acting insulin (NPH) is given in the evening and an oral hypoglycemic agent in the morning.
   a. No oral hypoglycemic agent is given in the evening.
   b. Lowering the FBS with evening insulin helps to achieve better glucose control during the day.
   c. Some patients may require Regular/NPH insulin injected before supper to assist with elevated postprandial evening glucoses.
   d. Diet and exercise continue to be of great therapeutic value.
   e. Use of this therapy remains controversial.

PROCEDURE GUIDELINES 23-2 ◆ Teaching Self-Injection of Insulin

EQUIPMENT   Prescribed bottle of insulin
Disposable insulin syringe and needle
Cotton ball and alcohol or alcohol wipe

TEACHING ACTION	*RATIONALE*
1. Give the patient the syringe containing the prescribed dose of insulin.	
2. Have patient wipe the skin with alcohol.	
3. Instruct the patient to hold the syringe as he would a pencil.	

PROCEDURE (cont'd)

NURSING ACTION	RATIONALE
4. Show the patient how to spread the skin taut on the anterior thigh, or form a skin fold by picking up subcutaneous tissue between the thumb and forefinger if the patient is thin.	4. Either of the techniques ensures that the needle tip is inserted into subcutaneous tissue and outside the muscle. Avoid pressing the skin tightly between the fingers because this is a common cause of local induration and infection.
5. Select areas of upper arms, abdomen, and upper buttocks for injection after patient becomes proficient with needle insertion (see accompanying figure).	5. The skin is loose and there is more subcutaneous fat in these areas. Systematic rotation of sites will keep the skin supple and favor uniform absorption of insulin

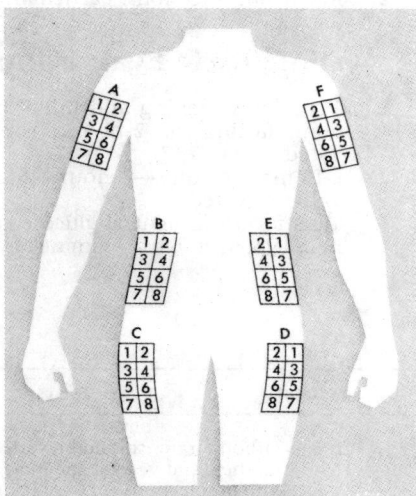

Rotate within each site and keep in mind the various rates of absorption in different sites. Exercising an injected site will also hasten insulin absorption. (From ADA Forecast—the Diabetics' Own Magazine. Vol 4[1]. Courtesy of Becton, Dickinson.)

6. Assist the patient to insert the needle with a quick thrust to the hub at a right angle to the skin surface.	6. The insulin is injected into deep subcutaneous tissue
7. Inject the insulin with slow, consistent pressure without aspiration.	
8. Instruct the patient to release the skin fold.	
9. Hold the alcohol sponge against the needle and gently withdraw the needle. Wipe area with alcohol sponge.	9. This maneuver prevents painful pulling of the skin as the needle is withdrawn.

TO LOAD THE SYRINGE

1. Roll the bottle of insulin (NPH and Lente) between the palms of the hands.	1. The rolling action mixes the insulin.
2. Wipe off the top of the insulin vial with an alcohol sponge.	
3. Inject approximately the same volume of air into the insulin vial as the volume of insulin to be withdrawn.	3. Air is injected into the vial to keep its contents under slight positive pressure and to make it easier to withdraw the insulin.

TO FILL A SYRINGE WITH LONG- AND SHORT-ACTING INSULIN MIXTURE

1. Wipe off the vial tops with an alcohol swab.
2. Inject air equal to the number of units to be injected into long-acting insulin first; withdraw needle.
3. Inject air into short-acting insulin bottle and withdraw prescribed amount of insulin
4. Then withdraw prescribed amount of insulin from long-acting insulin bottle.

Diabetes and Related Disorders

◆ DIABETES MELLITUS

Diabetes mellitus is a metabolic disorder characterized by hyperglycemia and results from defective insulin production, secretion, or utilization.

Pathophysiology/Etiology

1. Absolute or relative lack of insulin produced by the beta cell resulting in hyperglycemia
2. Defects at the cell receptor site, impaired secretory response of insulin to rises in glucose, and increased nocturnal hepatic glucose production (gluconeogenesis) as seen in NIDDM
3. Etiology of IDDM—viral, autoimmune, and environmental theories are under review.
4. Etiology of NIDDM—heredity/genetics and obesity play a major role.

Clinical Manifestations

Onset is abrupt with IDDM; insidious with NIDDM.

A. *Hyperglycemia*
1. Weight loss, fatigue
2. Polyuria, polydipsia, polyphagia
3. Blurred vision

B. *Altered Tissue Response*
1. Poor wound healing
2. Recurrent infections, particularly of the skin

Diagnostic Evaluation

1. Tests for screening and initial diagnosis include random, fasting, or 2-hour postprandial glucose—elevated (see p. 737)
2. GTT may be done—2-hour value and at least one other value elevated
3. Tests for assessment of glucose control are glycosylated hemoglobin and fructosamine assay—normal to elevated

TABLE 23-1 Meal Planning Guidelines

Principle	Action
1. Each meal should consist of a balance of carbohydrates, proteins, and fats.	1. a. Carbohydrates should be varied to include fruits, starches, and vegetables. b. Protein selections that are lean will help reduce fat and cholesterol intake. c. Fats should be used sparingly with < 10% of total calories derived from saturated fats. High in calories, fats contribute to weight gain in NIDDM.
2. Consistency in timing of meals and amounts of food eaten on a day-to-day basis help regulate blood glucose levels.	2. a. Avoid skipping or delaying meals. b. Measure portion sizes using a scale or measuring cups. c. Know the equivalent amounts of commonly used foods within a food group, eg, 1 slice of bread = $1/2$ cup cooked pasta.
3. Increase the intake of soluble and insoluble fiber.	3. a. Substitute foods high in fiber for processed foods when possible, eg, whole grain bread in place of white bread. b. Eat fresh fruit and vegetables in place of juices.
4. Avoid salt whenever possible.	4. a. Do not season foods with salt or salt-containing spices. b. Limit use of foods with "hidden" sodium content (eg, crackers, pickled foods, cheese, processed meats). c. Use salt-containing condiments sparingly (ketchup, soy sauce, gravies, bouillon).
5. Prepare foods to retain vitamins and minerals and reduce fats.	5. a. Do not fry foods. b. Bake, broil, or boil foods and discard fat. c. Steam vegetables to retain fiber. d. Avoid adding calories with butter sauces, fat back, and bacon. e. Trim all visible fat from meat; skim off fat from stews or other prepared dishes.
6. Distribute snacks in the meal plan depending on insulin/medication regimens, physical activity, and lifestyle.	6. a. Smaller, more frequent meals may enhance glucose control in NIDDM. b. Unplanned activity calls for an additional snack to avoid hypoglycemia.
7. Use alcohol only in moderation.	7. a. Always consume alcohol with food to avoid hypoglycemia. b. Do not omit food from meal plan in exchange for alcohol. c. Limit intake to 1–2 drinks per week. (4 oz dry wine, 12 oz beer, or 1.5 oz distilled liquor = 1 alcohol serving)
8. Use alternative nonnutritive, noncaloric sweeteners in moderation.	8. a. Limit "diet" soda intake to 2 L/d. b. Avoid frequent use of foods/beverages with concentrated sucrose.

TABLE 23-2 Oral Hypoglycemic Agents

Agent	Duration of Action	How Given
First Generation Sulfonyureas		
Tolbutamide (Orinase)	6–10 h	Divided doses
Chorpropamide (Diabinese)	36–60 h	Single dose
Acetohexamide (Dymelor)	10–20 h	Single or divided doses
Tolazamide (Tolinase)	12–24 h	Single or divided doses
Second Generation Sulfonyureas		
Glyburide (Micronase, Diabeta, Glynase)	12–24 h	Single or divided doses
Glipizide (Glibenese, Glucatrol)	10–18 h	Single or divided doses
(Glucatrol XL)	24 h	Single daily dose
Biguanides		
Metformin (Glucophage)	12-24h	Divided doses

Management

A. Diet
1. Dietary control with caloric restriction of carbohydrates and saturated fats to maintain ideal body weight
2. The goal of meal planning is to control blood glucose and lipid levels (Table 23-1).
3. Weight reduction is the primary treatment for NIDDM.

B. Exercise Regularly scheduled exercises to promote the utilization of carbohydrates, assist with weight control, enhance the action of insulin, and improve cardiovascular fitness

C. Medication
1. Oral hypoglycemic agents for patients with NIDDM who do not achieve glucose control with diet and exercise only (Table 23-2)
   a. Act by stimulating insulin secretion from functioning beta cells, possibly reducing hepatic glucose production, and by enhancing peripheral sensitivity to insulin.
   b. May cause hypoglycemic reactions.
2. Insulin therapy for patients with IDDM who require replacement (Table 23-3)
   a. May also be used for NIDDM when unresponsive to diet, exercise, and oral hypoglycemic agent therapy.
   b. Hypoglycemia may result, as well as rebound hyperglycemia (Somogyi effect).

Complications

A. Acute
1. Hypoglycemia occurs as a result of an imbalance in food, activity, and insulin/oral hypoglycemic agent.
2. Diabetic ketoacidosis (DKA) occurs primarily in IDDM during times of severe insulin deficiency or illness producing severe hyperglycemia, ketonuria, dehydration, and acidosis.
3. Hyperglycemic hyperosmolar nonketotic syndrome (HHNKS) affects patients with NIDDM, causing severe dehydration, hyperglycemia, hyperosmolarity, and stupor.

B. Chronic (Table 23-4)
1. In IDDM, chronic complications usually appear about 10 years after the initial diagnosis.

2. The prevalence of microvascular complications (retinopathy, nephropathy) and neuropathy is higher in IDDM.
3. Because of its insidious onset, chronic complications can appear at any point in NIDDM.
4. Macrovascular complications, in particular cardiovascular disease, occurring both in NIDDM and IDDM, is the leading cause of morbidity and mortality among persons with diabetes.

Nursing Assessment

1. Obtain a history of current problems, family history, and general health history.
   a. Has the patient experienced polyuria, polydipsia, polyphagia, and any other symptoms?
   b. Number of years since diagnosis of diabetes
   c. Family members diagnosed with diabetes, their subsequent treatment and complications
2. Perform a review of systems and physical examination to assess for signs and symptoms of diabetes, general health of patient, and presence of complications.
   a. General—recent weight loss or gain, increased fatigue, tiredness, anxiety
   b. Skin—skin lesions, infections, dehydration, evidence of poor wound healing
   c. Eyes—changes in vision—floaters, halos, blurred vision, dry or burning eyes, cataracts, glaucoma
   d. Mouth—gingivitis, periodontal disease
   e. Cardiovascular—orthostatic hypotension, cold extremities, weak pedal pulses, leg claudication
   f. Gastrointestinal—diarrhea, constipation, early satiety, bloating, or increased flatulence, hunger/thirst
   g. Genitourinary—increased urination, nocturia, impotence, vaginal discharge
   h. Neurologic—numbness and tingling of the extremities, decreased pain and temperature perception, changes in gait/balance

Nursing Diagnoses

A. Altered Nutrition (More than Body Requirements) related to intake in excess of activity expenditures

TABLE 23-3 Insulins Available in the United States

Type	Product*
Short-Acting Onset 0.25–1 h Peak 2–4 h Duration 5–7 h	Regular (L, NN)† Velosulin (NN) Humulin R (L) Novolin R (NN) Iletin II regular (L) Semilente (NN) Purified pork regular (NN) Iletin I regular (L) Iletin I semilente (L) Humulin BR (L) Velosulin Human R (NN)
Intermediate-Acting Onset 1–4 h Peak 2–15 h Duration 12–24 h	Semilente (L, NN) Semitard (NN) Protphane NPH (NN) NPH (L, NN) Monotard (NN) Insulatard (NN) Lente (L, NN) Lentard (NN) Humulin (L) Novulin N (NN) Iletin II lente (L) Iletin II NPH (L) Purified pork regular (NN) Purified pork NPH (NN) Insulatard NPH (NN) Iletin I NPH (L) Iletin I lente (L) Humulin L (lente) (L) Humulin N (NPH) (L) Novulin N (NPH) (NN) Insulatard NPH human (NN)
Long-Acting Onset 4–6 h Peak 10–30 h Duration 24–36 h	Ultralente (NN) Iletin II PZI (L) Iletin I PZI (L) Iletin I ultralente (L) Humulin U (ultralente) (L) Mixtard (NN) Humulin 70/30 (L) Novolin 70/30 (NN) Mixtard human 70/30 (NN)

> **NURSING ALERT** ◆◆
> Regular insulin is the *only* insulin that may be administered IV because all other insulin formulations are suspensions.

---

* Note: All insulins listed are U-100.
† Manufacturers: L, Lilly; NN, NovoNordisk.

B. Fear related to insulin injection
C. Risk for Injury (Hypoglycemia) related to effects of insulin, inability to eat
D. Activity Intolerance related to poor glucose control
E. Knowledge Deficit related to use of oral hypoglycemic agents
F. Risk for Impaired Skin Integrity related to decreased sensation and circulation to lower extremities
G. Ineffective Coping related to chronic disease and complex self-care regimen

Nursing Interventions

A. *Improving Nutrition*
1. Assess current timing and content of meals.
2. Advise patient on the importance of an individualized meal plan in meeting weight loss goals.
3. Discuss the goals of dietary therapy for the patient (see Table 23-1).
4. Assist the patient to identify problems that may have an impact on dietary adherence and possible solutions to these problems.
5. Explain the importance of exercise in maintaining/reducing body weight.
   a. Caloric expenditure for energy in exercise
   b. Carryover of enhanced metabolic rate and efficient food utilization
6. Assist patient to establish goals for weekly weight loss and incentives to assist in achieving them.
7. Strategize with the patient to address the potential social pitfalls of weight reduction.

B. *Teaching About Insulin*
1. Assist patient to reduce fear of injection by encouraging verbalization of fears regarding insulin injection, conveying a sense of empathy, and identifying supportive coping techniques.
2. Demonstrate and explain thoroughly the procedure for insulin self-injection (see p. 740).
3. Help patient to master technique by taking a step-by-step approach.
   a. Allow patient time to handle insulin and syringe to become familiar with the equipment.
   b. Teach self-injection first to alleviate fear of pain from injection.
   c. Instruct patient in filling syringe when he or she expresses confidence in self-injection procedure.

> **GERONTOLOGIC ALERT:** ◆
> Assess elderly patients for sensory deficits such as impaired vision, hearing, and fine touch, and tremors that may have an impact on learning and ability to self-administer insulin. Suggest use of an insulin pen or magnifying glass to assist with drawing up insulin.

4. Review dosage and time of injections in relation to meals, activity, and bedtime based on patient's individualized insulin regimen.

C. *Preventing Injury Secondary to Hypoglycemia*
1. Closely monitor blood glucose levels to detect hypoglycemia.
2. Instruct patient in the importance of accuracy in insulin preparation and meal timing to avoid hypoglycemia.
3. Assess patient for the signs and symptoms of hypoglycemia.
   a. Adrenergic—sweating, tremor, pallor, tachycardia, palpitations, nervousness from the release of adrenalin when blood glucose falls rapidly
   b. Neurologic—headache, light-headedness, confusion, irritability, slurred speech, lack of coordination, staggering gait from depression of central nervous system as glucose level progressively falls
4. Treat hypoglycemia promptly with 10 to 15 g of fast-acting carbohydrates.

(text continues on page 749)

TABLE 23-4 Chronic Complications of Diabetes Mellitus

Condition	Assessment	Intervention	Prevention/Teaching
MACROANGIOPATHY			
Cerebrovascular Disease Incidence: Twice as frequent in diabetes Hypertension, increased lipids, smoking, and uncontrolled blood glucose, increase risk of stroke and transient ischemic attack.	Increased blood pressure Change in mental status Hemiparesis Aphasia Clinical presentation mimics that of nondiabetic patient	Check blood glucose level to differentiate s/s of stroke vs. hypoglycemia. If stroke is suspected, do *not* give fast-acting carbohydrate as increased levels contribute to recurrence and ↑ mortality rates of strokes in patients with diabetes.	Maintain target goals of blood glucose avoiding severe hypoglycemia and hyperglycemia, which predispose the patient to cerebrovascular accident. In hypoglycemia, increased levels of adrenalin and catecholamines can produce cardiac arrhythmias. Hyperglycemia can lead to dehydration, which affects platelet aggregation.
Coronary Artery Disease Incidence: Increased vessel disease with more vessels affected in diabetes. Higher incidence of "silent" myocardial infarctions. Hyperglycemia contributes to atherosclerosis and vessel deterioration.	Severe coronary artery disease is often asymptomatic, seen only in ECG changes. ECG changes may indicate silent myocardial infarction. Symptoms can also present as pain in the jaw, neck, or epigastric area.	Usual medical treatment for angina prevails—sublingual nitroglycerin, oral nitrates. β-Adrenergic blockers and calcium channel blockers can also be used.	Emphasis must be placed on reducing cardiac risk factors, eg, cigarette smoking, hypertension, hyperlipidemias. Avoid wide fluctuations in blood glucose. Patients with autonomic neuropathy, which can cause orthostatic hypotension, should be carefully monitored when cardiac drug therapies are introduced. β-Adrenergic blockers can blunt or eliminate the clinical signs and symptoms of hypoglycemia.
Peripheral Vascular Disease Incidence: 50% of nontraumatic amputations are related to diabetes. Intermittent claudication, absent pedal pulses, and ischemic gangrene are increased in diabetes.	Physical examination of the lower extremities may reveal changes in skin integrity associated with diminished circulation. Decreased lower leg hair, absent or decreased anterior tibial or dorsal pedis pulses, poor capillary refill of toenails may occur. The extremity may appear pale/cool. Further examination for neurologic changes is indicated.	Any lesion, decrease in peripheral pulses, or change in skin color, temperature or sensation should be evaluated within 24–48 h. To ensure proper healing and prevent infection, treatment should begin as soon as possible and be carefully monitored. Mild antiseptics/antibiotic preparations are used to avoid further damage to the surrounding skin. Avoid the use of surgical tape to skin. Elevate affected leg to promote circulation and wound healing.	Foot care guidelines and smoking cessation must be stressed. Safe exercise guidelines and weight reduction as appropriate will further reduce risk of foot injury.

(continued)

TABLE 23-4 Chronic Complications of Diabetes Mellitus *(continued)*

Condition	Assessment	Intervention	Prevention/Teaching
MICROANGIOPATHY			
Retinopathy Incidence: Type I—10 y postdiagnosis 60% have some degree of retinopathy. Type II—approximately 20% present with retinopathy at diagnosis, which increases to 60–85% after 15 y. Appearance of hard exudates, blot hemorrhages, and microaneurysms on the retina in background retinopathy. Progresses to neurovascularization in proliferative diabetic retinopathy.	Usually asymptomatic in the early stages. Symptoms occurring with acute visual problems—"floaters," flashing lights, blurred vision may indicate hemorrhage or retinal detachment. Fundoscopic examination should be done by an ophthalmologist for full retinal visualization.	Laser therapy (photocoagulation) can be helpful in macular edema (focal laser) and proliferative retinopathy (panretinal laser). Reduction of active neovascularization by laser therapy reduces the risk of vitreous hemorrhage. Vitrectomy may be needed to treat retinal detachment or remove vitreous hemorrhage. During the acute phase, before laser therapy, patients must avoid activities that increase the chances of vitreous hemorrhage. (eg, weight lifting, high-impact aerobics)	Stress importance of annual eye examination with an ophthalmologist (preferably retina specialist). Optimal glucose control can prevent or slow the progression of retionopathy. Maintaining normal blood pressure also reduces the risk of retinopathy.
Nephropathy Incidence: Type I—with >20 y history of diabetes, approximately 40% will have renal disease. Type II—5–10 y after diagnosis 5–10% of patients develop nephropathy, with higher incidence in Native Americans, Hispanics, and African Americans. Thickening of the glomerular basement membrane, mesangial expansion, and renal vessel sclerosis are caused by diabetes. Subsequently, diffuse and nodular intercapillary glomerulosclerosis diminishes renal function.	Evidence of ↑ glomerular filtration rate. Microalbuminuria is the first clinical sign of renal disease. Elevation in BUN and creatinine indicate advanced renal disease. Gross proteinuria is further indication of renal deterioration.	Hypertension control, blood glucose control, and reduction of protein and sodium are essential. Angiotensin-converting enzyme inhibitors and calcium channel blockers are the drugs of choice to control blood pressure. In end-stage renal disease dialysis or transplantation may be necessary.	Frequent hypertension screening, noting any deviation from patient's normal reading. Early initiation of blood pressure control to prevent kidney damage. Excellent glucose control with insulin/oral agent adjustment to compensate for reduced kidney function, which predisposes the patient to hypoglycemia. Avoidance of nephrotoxic drugs, dyes, or renal procedures that may cause infection. Immediate treatment for any urinary tract infections.

(continued)

TABLE 23-4 Chronic Complications of Diabetes Mellitus *(continued)*

Condition	Assessment	Intervention	Prevention/Teaching
PERIPHERAL NEUROPATHY			
In general, neuropathy affects 60% of persons with diabetes, with nearly 100% showing signs and symptoms of slowing nerve conduction velocity. It can affect almost every organ system with varying specific symptoms. Distal symmetrical polyneuropathy involving the lower extremities is most commonly seen. In conjunction with peripheral vascular disease, neuropathy to the feet increases susceptibility to trauma and infection. Three clinical syndromes of distal symmetrical polyneuropathy can be seen: acute painful neuropathy, small fiber neuropathy, large fiber neuropathy.	Decreased light touch, vibratory, temperature sensation. Loss of foot proprioception, followed by ataxia, gait disturbances. Diminished ankle jerk response. Formation of "hammer toes," Charcot joint disease, which predispose patient to new pressure point areas. Hypersensitivity or other dysesthetic symptoms are experienced, followed by hypoestheis or anesthesia, which is not reversible.	All foot wounds or injuries are immediately evaluated. Culture and sensitivities ordered for any drainage present. Affected foot is elevated—avoid weight-bearing. Wet to dry dressings applied as ordered. Avoid use of caustic chemicals, dressing tapes. Use of systemic antibiotics as needed. Medication for painful neuropathy may include use of the tricyclic antidepressant drugs (eg, amitriptylline—Elavil) or topical application of capsaicin (Zostrix) ointment.	In general, blood glucose control is recommended, avoiding wide fluctuations. In patients who are poorly controlled, care must be taken to correct glucoses slowly to avoid increasing symptoms of neuropathy. Foot care guidelines. Smoking cessation. Frequent evaluation by podiatrist for modified foot wear, eg, orthotics, extra depth shoes. Safe exercise guidelines Weight reduction as necessary
AUTONOMIC NEUROPATHY			
Gastroparesis Incidence: Occurs in 25% of people with diabetes Characteristics: Delayed gastric emptying, prolonged pylorospasms and loss of the powerful contractions of the distal stomach to grind and mix foods.	Typical symptoms may include: Nausea/vomiting, early satiety, abdominal bloating, epigastric pain, change in appetite. Wide fluctuations in blood glucoses and postmeal hypoglycemia caused by poor glucose absorption. Visualization of the gut by upper gastrointestinal barium series may show retained food after an 8–12-h fast	Excellent glucose control to avoid hyperglycemia, which interferes with gut contractility. Avoidance of severe postmeal hypoglycemia by small frequent meals, low fat and low fiber. This diet is also helpful in bloating/early satiety. Medications to improve gut motility include: metoclopramide (Reglan) and cisapride (Pepcid).	Maintenance of excellent glucose control. Regular exercise improves/maintaines gut motility. Avoid use of laxatives.

(continued)

TABLE 23-4 Chronic Complications of Diabetes Mellitus (*continued*)

Condition	Assessment	Intervention	Prevention/Teaching
Diarrhea Incidence: Approximately 5% of diabetic patients Characteristics: Frequent, watery movements Mild steatorrhea Can be intermittent, persistent, or alternate with constipation.	Diarrhea occurs without warning, frequently at night or after meals. Fecal incontinence may be caused by loss of internal sphincter control and anorectal sensation. Other causes such as celiac sprue, pancreatic insufficiency, lactose intolerance must be investigated. Bacterial overgrowth in the bowel is also suspected.	Dietary changes may include: increased fiber, elimination of milk products. Sphincter-strengthening exercises may help. Medications: For diarrhea hydrophilic fiber supplement (Metamucil), cholestyramine (Questran), or synthetic opiates are used. Tetracycline, ampicillin are used for bacterial overgrowth.	Routine bowel elimination habits Maintenance of adequate hydration Excellent blood glucose control reduces dehydration. Inclusion of dietary fiber in the daily diet Daily exercise program that includes walking or swimming has been effective in encouraging bowel regularity.
Impotence/Sexual Dysfunction Incidence is not well documented due to inhibitions about reporting this problem to health care providers. Sexual dysfunction can involve changes in erectile ability, ejaculation, or libido.	Men: History of poor erectile function despite stimulation. Absence of early morning erection in response to increased hormonal levels. Women: May experience decreased vaginal lubrication and dyspareunia. Screening for use of ethanol or other medications associated with impotence (eg, antidepressants, antihypertensives).	Men: Referral to urologist for full examination is indicated. Treatment options may include papaverine (Povased) injections, noninvasive devices for promoting and maintaining erections or semirigid, or inflatable penile prosthesis. Women: Increase lubrication with use of water-based lubricant (K-Y jelly) or estrogen creams, which also may help thicken the vaginal mucosa, affecting dyspareunia.	Reduce consumption of alcohol, which may hasten or contribute to neuropathy. Maintain target ranges of blood glucose control to reduce likelihood of vaginal infections. Discuss alternative ways of maintaining intimacy.
Orthostatic Hypotension One of three syndromes associated with cardiovascular autonomic neuropathy, orthostatic hypotension occurs when the "postural reflex," which increases heart rate and peripheral vascular resistance is dysfunctional.	Patients may report episodes of syncope, weakness, or visual impairment particularly with positional changes. Evaluate blood pressure and pulse in both lying and standing position at each visit. Blood pressure changes that indicate neuropathic involvement: fall in systolic pressure of >30 mm Hg or fall in diastolic pressure of >10 mm Hg with change from lying to standing position.	Improvement in blood glucose control to prevent fluid loss from glycosuria. Moderate amounts of sodium may be used in the diet to encourage fluid retention during hot weather or strenuous exercise. Mechanical devices such as support stockings (full hose to waist) may decrease venous pooling. Drugs to enhance volume expansion may be used. (eg, fludrocortisone—Florine)	Encourage increased fluid intake to maintain hydration. Caution should be used in changing position from lying to standing. "Dangling" is recommended until blood pressure stabilizes. Avoid standing in one position, which may increase venous pooling.

a. Half cup (4 oz) juice, 3 glucose tablets, 4 sugar cubes, 5 to 6 pieces of hard candy may be taken orally.
b. Glucagon 1 mg (subcutaneously or intramuscularly) is given if the patient cannot ingest a sugar treatment. Family member or staff must administer injection.
c. IV bolus of 50 mL of 50% dextrose solution can be given if the patient fails to respond to glucagon within 15 minutes.

5. Encourage patient to carry a portable treatment for hypoglycemia at all times.

COMMUNITY-BASED CARE TIP:
A small tube of Cake Mate glossy decorating gel can be easily carried in a pocket or purse, contains about 15 g glucose, and can be easily squirted in the mouth for fast absorption during a hypoglycemic attack.

6. Assess patient for cognitive or physical impairments that may interfere with ability to accurately administer insulin.
7. Between-meal snacks as well as extra food taken before exercise should be encouraged to prevent hypoglycemia.
8. Encourage patients to wear an identification bracelet or card that may assist in prompt treatment in a hypoglycemic emergency.
   a. Identification bracelet may be obtained from Medic Alert Foundation International; 2323 Colorado; Tarlock, CA 95381
   b. Identification card may be requested from the American Diabetes Association; 1660 Duke St.; Alexandria, VA 22314

D. *Improving Activity Tolerance*
1. Advise patient to assess blood glucose level before strenuous exercise.
2. Instruct patient to plan exercises on a regular basis each day.
3. Encourage patient to eat a carbohydrate snack before exercising to avoid hypoglycemia.
4. Advise patient that prolonged strenuous exercise may require increased food at bedtime to avoid nocturnal hypoglycemia.
5. Instruct patient to avoid exercise whenever blood glucose levels exceed 250 mg/d and urine ketones are present.
6. Counsel patient to inject insulin into the abdominal site on days when arms or legs are exercised.

E. *Providing Information About Oral Hypoglycemic Agents*
1. Identify any barriers to learning, such as visual, hearing, low literacy, distractive environment.
2. Encourage active participation of the patient and family in the educational process.
3. Teach the action, use, and side effects of oral hypoglycemic agents.
   a. Sulfonylurea compounds promote the increased secretion of insulin by the pancreas and partially normalize both receptor and postreceptor defects.
   b. Metformin (Glucophage), a biguanide compound, appears to diminish insulin resistance. It decreases hepatic glucose production and intestinal reabsorption of glucose.
   c. Indicated only in NIDDM when glucose control has not been achieved through diet and exercise.

d. Contraindicated in patients with severe infections, surgery, gestational diabetes, or ketosis.
e. Most common side effect is hypoglycemia, particularly in the longer-acting agents. Small percentage of patients experience gastrointestinal disturbances, rash, pruritus, and facial flushing.

F. *Maintaining Skin Integrity*
1. Assess feet and legs for skin temperature, sensation, soft tissue injuries, corns, calluses, dryness, hammer toe or bunion deformation, hair distribution, pulses, deep tendon reflexes.
2. Maintain skin integrity by protecting feet from breakdown.
   a. Use heel protectors, special mattresses, foot cradles for patients on bed rest.
   b. Avoid drying agents to skin (eg, alcohol).
   c. Apply skin moisturizers to maintain suppleness and prevent cracking, fissures.
3. Instruct patient in foot care guidelines (Procedure Guidelines 23-3).
4. Advise the patient who smokes to stop smoking or reduce if possible, to reduce vasoconstriction and enhance peripheral blood flow.
   a. Help patient to establish behavior modification techniques to reduce smoking in hospital.

G. *Improving Coping Strategies*
1. Discuss with the patient the perceived effect of diabetes on lifestyle, finances, family life, occupation.
2. Explore previous coping strategies and skills that have had positive effects.
3. Encourage patient and family participation in diabetes self-care regimen to foster confidence.
4. Identify available support groups to assist in lifestyle adaptation.
5. Assist family in providing emotional support.

Patient Education/ Health Maintenance

A. *Survival Skills*
1. Targeted to the newly diagnosed or those undergoing stressful circumstances that preclude more in-depth education
2. Education focus—skills management, to include—insulin/oral agents, hypoglycemia treatment, blood glucose monitoring, and basic dietary information

B. *Lifestyle Management Skills*
1. Ongoing education of patient to include advanced skills and rationales for treatment, management
2. Educational focus—lifestyle management issues, to include sick day management (Table 23-5), exercise adjustments, travel preparations, foot care guidelines, intensive insulin management, and dietary considerations for dining out.
3. For additional information and support, refer to agencies such as: American Diabetes Association, Inc.; 1660 Duke St.; Alexandria, VA 22314; 703-549-1500; and American Dietetic Association; 216 West Jackson Blvd.; Chicago, IL 60606-6995; 1-800-366-1655.

Evaluation

A. Maintains ideal body weight
B. Demonstrates self-injection of insulin with minimal fear

C. Hypoglycemia identified and treated appropriately
D. Tolerates activity without compromise in glycemic control
E. Verbalizes appropriate use and action of oral hypoglycemic agents
F. No skin breakdown
G. Verbalizes initial strategies for coping with diabetes

◆ DIABETIC KETOACIDOSIS

Diabetic ketoacidosis (DKA) is an acute complication of diabetes mellitus (usually IDDM) characterized by hyperglycemia, ketonuria, acidosis, and dehydration.

PROCEDURE GUIDELINES 23-3 ◆ Foot Care Guidelines

Perform foot care and teach the patient the following guidelines

EQUIPMENT
Mirror (optional)
Magnifying glass (optional)
Moisturizing lotion
Lamb's wool
Scissors and nail file

TEACHING ACTION	RATIONALE
1. Inspect the feet carefully and daily for calluses, corns blisters, abrasions, redness, and nail abnormalities.	1. a. Use a small mirror to check bottom of each foot. b. Use a magnifying glass under good light if eyesight is poor, or have someone else check feet.
2. Bathe the feet daily in warm (never hot) water.	2. a. Do not soak the feet for prolonged periods (soaking is drying). b. Dry feet carefully, especially between the toes.
3. Massage the feet with an absorbable agent.	3. a. Use lanolin, nivea cream, or other cream moisturizers. b. Include between the toes of an autonomically denervated foot; loses its ability to sweat, and dries and cracks easily.
4. Prevent moisture between the toes to prevent maceration of the skin.	4. a. Insert lamb's wool between overlapping toes. b. Use foot powder, especially if feet perspire.
5. Wear well-fitting, noncompressive shoes and socks—long enough, wide enough, soft, supple, and low-heeled.	5. a. Buy shoes in the afternoon—feet are larger in the afternoon than in the morning. b. Have each foot measured before buying shoes—feet enlarge with age. c. Have the measurement taken while standing because foot is larger in the standing position. d. Do not "break in" shoes all at one time. e. Avoid rubber- or plastic-soled shoes, or vinyl shoes, which cause the feet to perspire and aggravate fungal infections. f. Avoid working in soft-soled bedroom slippers or other casual footwear.
6. Go to a podiatrist on a regular basis if corns, calluses, and ingrown toenails are present.	6. a. Cut toenails straight across to prevent ingrown toenails. b. File any rough corners with an emery board.
7. Avoid heat, chemicals, and injuries to the feet.	7. a. Do not go barefoot or expose feet to hot-water bottles, heating pads, caustic solutions, etc. b. Check bath temperature with thermometer or elbow before bathing. c. Switch off electric blanket before going to bed; wear socks at night to keep feet warm if necessary. d. Avoid sitting to close to a fire.
8. Inspect inside of shoes for foreign objects or areas of roughness.	8. a. Inspect seams and lining of shoes for possible areas of pressure or abrasion. b. Avoid the use of constricting sandals, high heels, or boots.
9. In an injury occurs to the foot:	9. a. Wash the area with mild soap and water. b. Cover with a dry sterile dressing without adhesive. c. Wear white cotton socks; dye in colored socks and wool may serve as irritants when skin is already irritated. d. Call health care provider.

TABLE 23-5 Sick Day Guidelines

1. Never omit insulin dosage.	1. a. Take, at least, the usual dosage of insulin. b. Keep regular insulin on hand for supplemental doses as prescribed by health care provider.
2. Monitor blood glucose and urine ketones q 2–4h	2. a. Whenever blood glucose is > 240 mg/dL, test urine ketones. b. Record all test results.
3. Drink plenty of fluids.	3. a. 6–8 oz of fluid every hour is recommended. b. If unable to eat, drink fluids that contain carbohydrates (eg, fruit juices, regular soda).
4. Contact health care provider if illness becomes severe or unmanageable.	4. a. Fever, nausea, vomiting, diarrhea increase dehydration. b. Signs and symptoms of infection—redness, swelling, drainage—need immediate attention. c. Large amount of urine ketones or other signs and symptoms of diabetic ketoacidosis, call health care provider immediately.

Pathophysiology/Etiology

1. Insulin deficiency prevents glucose from being used for energy, forcing the body to metabolize fat for fuel.
2. Free fatty acids, released from the metabolism of fat, are converted to ketone bodies in the liver.
3. Ketone bodies are organic acids that cause metabolic acidosis.
4. Increase in the secretion of glucagon, catecholamines, growth hormone, and cortisol, in response to the hyperglycemia caused by insulin deficiency, accelerates the development of DKA.
5. Osmotic diuresis caused by hyperglycemia creates a shift in electrolytes with losses in potassium, sodium, phosphate, and water.
6. Caused by inadequate amounts of endogenous or exogenous insulin.
   a. Frequently occurs due to failure to increase the dose of insulin during periods of stress (eg, infection, surgery, pregnancy).
   b. May occur in previously undiagnosed or untreated diabetics.

Clinical Manifestations

A. Early
1. Polydipsia, polyuria
2. Fatigue, malaise, drowsiness
3. Anorexia, nausea, vomiting
4. Abdominal pains, muscle cramps

B. Later
1. Kussmaul respiration (deep respirations)
2. Fruity sweet breath
3. Hypotension, weak pulse
4. Stupor and coma

Diagnostic Evaluation

1. Serum glucose level is usually elevated over 300 mg/dL, may be as high as 1,000 mg/dL.
2. Serum and urine ketone bodies are present.
3. Serum bicarbonate and pH are decreased due to metabolic acidosis, and P_{CO_2} is decreased as a respiratory compensation mechanism.
4. Serum sodium and potassium levels may be low, normal, or high due to fluid shifts and dehydration, despite total body depletion.
5. Blood urea nitrogen (BUN), creatinine, hemoglobin, and hematocrit are elevated due to dehydration.

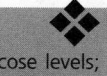

NURSING ALERT:
Severity of DKA cannot be determined by serum glucose levels; acidosis may be prominent with glucose level of 200 mg/dL or less.

6. Urine glucose is present in high concentration and specific gravity is increased reflecting osmotic diuresis and dehydration.

Management

1. IV fluids to replace losses from osmotic diuresis, vomiting
2. IV insulin drip—regular insulin only infused to increase glucose utilization and decrease lipolysis
3. Electrolyte replacement—sodium chloride and phosphate as required, potassium chloride and bicarbonate based on laboratory results.

Complications

1. Premature discontinuation of IV insulin can result in prolongation of DKA.
2. Too rapid infusion of IV fluids in cases of severe dehydration can cause cerebral edema and death.
3. Failure to institute subcutaneous insulin injections before discontinuation of IV insulin can result in extended hyperglycemia.

Nursing Assessment

1. Assess skin for dehydration—poor turgor, flushing, dry mucous membranes
2. Observe for cardiac changes reflecting dehydration, metabolic acidosis and electrolyte imbalance—hypotension, tachycardia, weak pulse, electrocardiographic changes: elevated P wave, flattened T wave or inverted, prolonged QT interval
3. Assess respiratory status—Kussmaul breathing, acetone breath characteristic of metabolic acidosis

4. Perform gastrointestinal assessment—nausea, vomiting, extreme thirst, abdominal bloating and cramping, diarrhea
5. Determine genitourinary symptoms—nocturia, polyuria
6. Observe for neurologic signs—crying, restless, twitching, tremors, drowsiness, lethargy, headache, decreased reflexes
7. Interview family or significant other regarding precipitating events to episode of DKA.
   a. Patient self-care management before hospitalization
   b. Unusual events that may have precipitated episode (eg, chest pain, trauma, illness)

Nursing Diagnoses

A. Fluid Volume Deficit related to hyperglycemia
B. Ineffective Management of Therapeutic Regimen related to failure to increase insulin during illness

Nursing Interventions

A. *Restoring Fluid and Electrolyte Balance*
1. Assess blood pressure and heart rate frequently depending on patient's condition; assess skin turgor and temperature.
2. Monitor intake and output every hour.
3. Replace fluids as ordered through peripheral IV line.
4. Monitor urine specific gravity to assess fluid changes.
5. Monitor capillary blood glucoses frequently.
6. Assess for symptoms of hypokalemia—fatigue, anorexia, nausea, vomiting, muscle weakness, decreased bowel sounds, paresthesia, arrhythmias, flat T waves, ST segment depression

NURSING ALERT:
Electrolyte levels may not reflect the total body deficit of potassium (primarily) and sodium (to a lesser extent) due to compartment shifts and fluid volume loss. Replacement is necessary despite normal to high values.

7. Administer replacement electrolytes and insulin as ordered.

NURSING ALERT:
Any interruption in insulin administration may result in reaccumulation of ketone bodies and worsening acidosis. Glucose will normalize before acidosis resolves so IV insulin is continued until bicarbonate levels normalize and subcutaneous insulin takes effect and the patient starts eating.

NURSING ALERT:
Flush the entire IV infusion set with solution containing insulin and discard the first 50 mL because plastic bags and tubing may absorb some insulin and the initial solution may contain decreased concentration of insulin.

8. Monitor serum glucose, bicarbonate, and pH levels periodically.
9. Provide reassurance about improvement of condition and that correction of fluid imbalance will help reduce discomfort.

B. *Preventing Further Episodes of DKA*
1. Review with patients precipitating events and causes of DKA.
2. Assist patient in identifying warning signs and symptoms of DKA.
3. Instruct patient in sick day guidelines (see p. 751).

Evaluation

A. Blood pressure and heart rate stable; glucose and bicarbonate levels improving
B. Verbalizes sick day guidelines correctly

◆ HYPERGLYCEMIC HYPEROSMOLAR NONKETOTIC SYNDROME

This is an acute complication of diabetes mellitus (particularly NIDDM) characterized by hyperglycemia, dehydration, and hyperosmolarity, but little or no ketosis.

Pathophysiology/Etiology

1. Prolonged hyperglycemia with glucosuria produces osmatic diuresis.
2. Loss of water, sodium, and potassium results in severe dehydration causing hypovolemia and hemoconcentration.
3. Hyperosmolarity is a result of excessive blood sugar and increasing sodium concentration in dehydration.
4. Insulin continues to be produced at a level that prevents ketosis.
5. Increased blood viscosity decreases blood flow to the organs creating tissue hypoxia.
6. Intracellular fluid and electrolyte shifts produce neurologic signs and symptoms.
7. Caused by inadequate amounts of endogenous/exogenous insulin to control hyperglycemia.
   a. Precipitating event may occur such as cardiac failure, burn, or chronic illness that increases need for insulin.
   b. Use of therapeutic agents that increase blood glucose levels (eg, glucocorticoids, immunosuppressive agents)
   c. Use of therapeutic procedures that cause stress or increase blood glucose levels (eg, hyperosmolar hyperalimenation, peritoneal dialysis).

Clinical Manifestations

A. *Early*
1. Polyuria, dehydration
2. Fatigue, malaise
3. Nausea, vomiting

B. Later
1. Hypothermia
2. Seizures, stupor, coma
3. Muscle weakness

Diagnostic Evaluation

1. Serum glucose and osmolality are greatly elevated.
2. Serum and urine ketone bodies are minimal to absent.
3. Serum sodium and potassium levels may be elevated, depending on degree of dehydration, despite total body losses.
4. BUN and creatinine may be elevated due to dehydration.
5. Urine specific gravity is elevated due to dehydration.

Management

1. Correct fluid and electrolyte imbalances with IV fluids.
2. Provide insulin via IV drip to lower plasma glucose.
3. Evaluate complications, such as stupor, seizures, shock, and treat appropriately.
4. Identify and treat underlying illnesses or events that precipitated HHNKS.

Complications

1. Too rapid infusion of IV fluids can cause cerebral edema and death.
2. HHNKS is a medical emergency, which if not treated properly, can cause death.
3. Patients who become comatose will need nasogastric tubes to prevent aspiration.

Nursing Assessment

1. Assess level of consciousness.
2. Assess for dehydration—poor turgor, flushing, dry mucous membranes.
3. Assess cardiovascular status for shock—rapid, thready pulse, cool extremities, hypotension, ECG changes.
4. Interview family or significant other regarding precipitating events to episode of HHNKS.
   a. Evaluate patient's self-care regimen before hospitalization.
   b. Determine precipitating events, treatments, or drugs that may have caused the event.

Nursing Diagnoses

A. Fluid Volume Deficit related to severe dehydration
B. Risk for Aspiration related to reduced level of consciousness and vomiting

Nursing Interventions

A. Restoring Fluid Balance
1. Assess patient for increasing signs and symptoms of dehydration, hyperglycemia, electrolyte imbalance.
2. Institute fluid replacement therapy as ordered (usually normal or half strength saline initially), maintaining patent IV line.
3. Assess patient for signs and symptoms of fluid overload, cerebral edema, as IV therapy progresses.
4. Administer regular insulin IV as ordered, and add dextrose to IV infusion as blood glucose falls below 300 mg/dL, to prevent hypoglycemia.
5. Monitor hydration status by monitoring hourly intake and output and urine specific gravity.

B. Preventing Aspiration
1. Assess patient's level of consciousness and ability to handle oral secretions.
   a. Cough and gag reflex
   b. Ability to swallow
2. Properly position patient to reduce possibility of aspiration.
   a. Elevate head of bed unless contraindicated.
   b. If nausea present use side-lying position.
3. Suction as often as needed to maintain patent airway.
4. Withhold oral intake until patient is no longer in danger of aspiration.
5. Insert nasogastric tube as indicated for gastric decompression.
6. Monitor respiratory rate and breath sounds for signs of aspiration pneumonia.
7. Provide mouth care to maintain adequate mucosal hydration.

Patient Education/ Health Maintenance

1. Advise the patient and family that it may take 3 to 5 days for symptoms to resolve.
2. Instruct patient and family in signs and symptoms of hyperglycemia and use of sick day guidelines (see p. 751).
3. Explain possible causes of HHNKS.
4. Review any changes in medication, activity, meal plan, or glucose monitoring for home care. It may not be necessary to continue insulin therapy following HHNKS; many patients can be treated with diet and oral agents.

Evaluation

A. Blood pressure stable, dehydration resolved
B. No evidence of aspiration

Selected References

American Diabetes Association (1991). *Physician's guide to non-insulin dependent (type II) diabetes: Diagnosis and treatment.* Alexandria, VA: Author.

Anderson, S. (1994). Seven tips for managing patients with diabetes. *AJN, 94*(9), 36-38.

Clore, J. (1995). New standards of care for diabetes mellitus. *Hospital Medicine, 31*(4), 26–33.

Davidson, J. K. (1991). *Clinical diabetes mellitus: A problem oriented approach* (2nd ed.). New York: Thieme Medical Publishers.

Fain, J. (1993). Diabetes. *Nursing Clinics of North America, 28*(10), 1-113.

Friesen, J., Pi-Sunyer, X., Thom, S. & Wishner, K. (1995). Questions and answers on diets for diabetes. *Contemporary Nurse Practitioner, 1*(2), 44–50.

Haire-Joshu, D. (1992). *Management of diabetes mellitus: Perspectives of care across the life span.* St. Louis: Mosby-Year Book.

Lebovitz, H. (1991). *Therapy for diabetes mellitus and related disorders.* Alexandria, VA: American Diabetes Association.

Peragallo-Dittko, V. (1995). Acute complications. *RN, 58*(8), 36–40.

Powers, M. A. (Ed.). (1988). *Nutrition guide for professionals: Diabetic education and meal planning.* American Diabetes Association and American Dietetic Association.

Tomky, D. (1995). Advances in monitoring. *RN, 58*(3), 38-44.

Disorders of the Blood

General Overview

Blood, the body fluid circulating through the heart, arteries, capillaries and veins, consists of plasma and cellular components. Plasma, the fluid portion, accounts for 55% of the blood volume. It is 92% water, 7% protein, and 1% inorganic salts, nonprotein organic substances such as urea, dissolved gases, hormones, and enzymes. Plasma proteins include albumin, fibrinogen, and globulins. Cellular components include erythrocytes (red blood cells), leukocytes and lymphocytes (white blood cells), and platelets. These cells are derived from pluripotent stem cells in the bone marrow, a process known as hematopoiesis (Fig. 24-1). The cellular components of blood account for 45% of the blood volume.

◆ CHARACTERISTICS OF CELLULAR COMPONENTS

Blood has multiple functions that are carried out by plasma or the cellular components (Table 24-1).

Erythrocytes (Red Blood Cells)

1. Enucleated, biconcave disc
2. Approximately 5 million erythrocytes per cubic millimeter of blood
3. Cell contents consist primarily of hemoglobin, essential for oxygen transport. Whole blood contains 14 to 15 g of hemoglobin per 100 mL of blood.
4. Circulate about 115 to 130 days before elimination by reticuloendothelial system, primarily in spleen and liver

Leukocytes (White Blood Cells) (Table 24-2)

1. Approximately 5,000 to 10,000 leukocytes per cubic millimeter of blood
2. Classified as granulocytes or mononuclear leukocytes
   a. Granulocytes account for about 70% of all white blood cells; have abundant granulocytes in cytoplasm; include neutrophils, basophils, and eosinophils.
   b. Mononuclear leukocytes have single-lobed nucleus and granule-free cytoplasm; include monocytes and lymphocytes.

Platelets (Thrombocytes)

1. Approximately 150,000 to 450,000 platelets per cubic millimeter of blood
2. Small particles without nuclei arise as a result of budding from giant cells (megakaryocytes) in bone marrow.
3. Primary function is to control bleeding through hemostasis.

Assessment

◆ SUBJECTIVE DATA

The patient presenting with a hematologic disorder may have a disruption of the hematologic, immune, and or coagulation system, producing a diverse array of symptoms. Patients often present with vague complaints of fatigue, frequent infections, swollen glands, and bleeding tendencies. Characterize these complaints and obtain a review of systems, concentrating on the neurologic, respiratory, cardiovascular, gastrointestinal, genitourinary, and integumen-

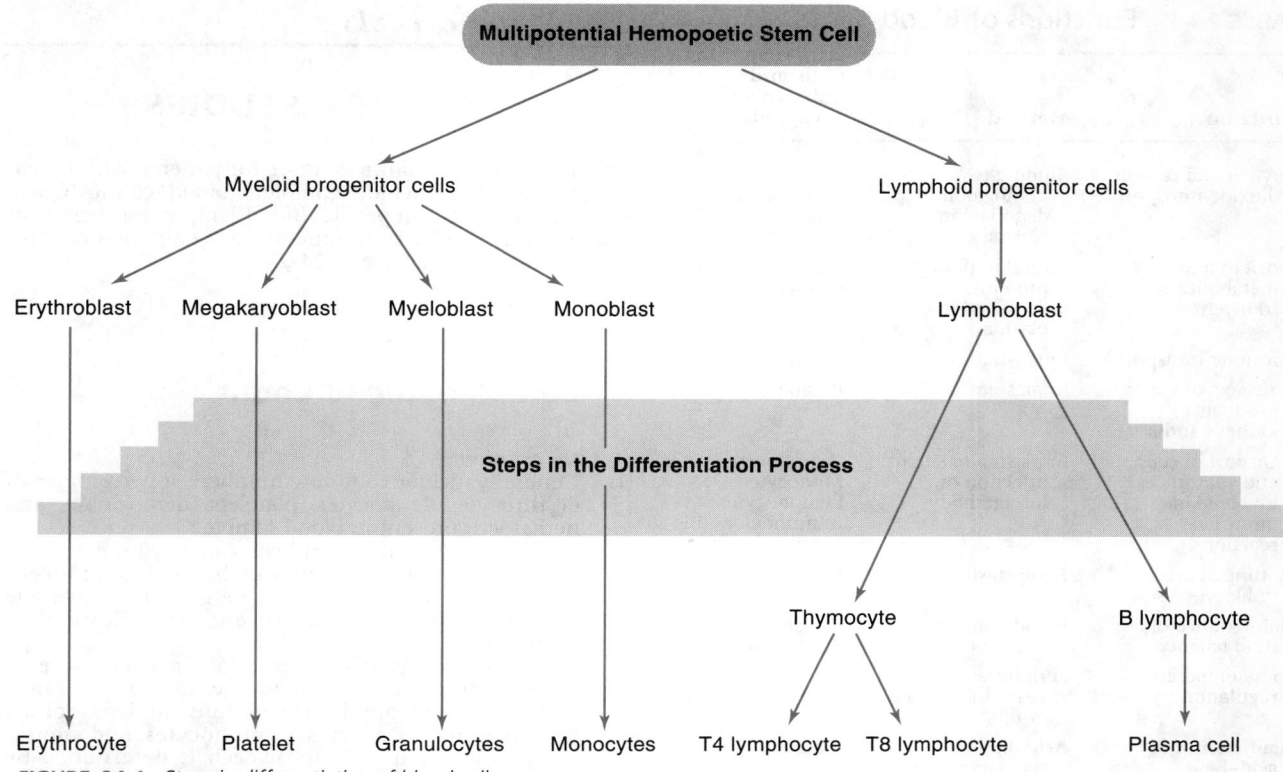

FIGURE 24-1 *Steps in differentiation of blood cells.*

tary systems to look for more clues of hematologic dysfunction.

Review of Systems

1. Skin and mucous membranes—Do you have any bruises, infections, drainage, or bleeding from wound sites?
2. Neurologic—Any dizziness, paresthesia, headache, confusion, disturbance in gait, fatigue, weakness?
3. Respiratory—Have you been experiencing shortness of breath, especially on exertion?
4. Cardiovascular—Do you have chest pain or palpitations?
5. Gastrointestinal—Have you noticed any bleeding from gums, abdominal pain, black stools, or blood-streaked emesis? How about any oral lesions, rectal pain, or diarrhea?
6. Genitourinary—Describe your menstrual flow. How often do you change pads? For how many days? Any blood in your urine or discomfort on urination?

Key History Questions

1. What are your present medications, any over-the-counter medications? What else have you taken in the past several months?

2. What medical problems have you had in the past? Any surgery? Ask specifically about partial or total gastrectomy, splenic injury or splenectomy, tendency to bleed (eg, with dental procedures), infectious diseases, human immunodeficiency virus (HIV) infection, cancer.
3. What is your occupation? Ask about exposure to substances such as benzene, pesticides, and ionizing radiation.
4. Any family history of hematologic or malignant disorder?
5. Determine the social history and lifestyle. Any use of recreational drugs or alcohol? What is the pattern of sexual activity?

◆ PHYSICAL EXAMINATION

Physical examination may produce abnormal assessment findings in a variety of body systems caused by anemia, uncontrolled bleeding or clotting, or altered immune function leading to infection in patients with hematologic disorders. Perform a systematic physical examination, paying careful attention to the cardiovascular, respiratory, and integumentary systems.

Key Examination Findings

1. Tachycardia; dyspnea; shiny smooth tongue; ataxia; pallor of conjunctivae, nail beds, lips, and oral mucosa—suggest anemia

TABLE 24-1   Functions of Blood

Function	Method	Cells and Substances Involved
Oxygen and carbon dioxide transport	Binding to hemoglobin; dissolved in plasma	Erythrocyte Hemoglobin Plasma
Nutrient and metabolite transport	Bound to plasma proteins; dissolved in plasma	Plasma proteins Plasma
Hormone transport	In plasma	Plasma
Transport of waste products to kidneys and liver	In plasma	Plasma
Transport of cells and substances involved in immune reactions	In plasma to site of infection or foreign body	Granulocytes Monocytes Lymphocytes Immunoglobulins Other substances
Clotting at breaks in blood vessels	Hemostasis	Platelets Clotting factors
Maintenance of fluid balance	Blood volume regulation	Water Electrolytes
Body temperature regulation	Peripheral vasoconstriction or dilation	
Maintenance of acid–base balance	Acid–base regulation	Electrolytes

2. Decreased blood pressure, altered level of consciousness, hematuria, tarry stools, petechiae, bleeding sites—suggest altered clotting
3. Fever; tachycardia; abnormal breath sounds; delirium; oral lesions; erythema, swelling, tenderness, and drainage of the skin—suggest infection

Diagnostic Tests

◆ LABORATORY STUDIES

Laboratory studies routinely done for patients with hematologic disorders include complete blood count (CBC), blood smear, and iron profile. Blood samples for these tests may be obtained by skin puncture or venipuncture (Procedure Guidelines 24-1 and 24-2).

Complete Blood Count

A. Description
1. Generally includes absolute numbers or percentages of erythrocytes, leukocytes, platelets, hemoglobin, and hematocrit present in blood sample.
   a. Erythrocyte (RBC) indices can be done to provide information on the size, hemoglobin concentration, and hemoglobin weight of an average RBC; aids in diagnosis and classification of anemias.
   b. Leukocyte (WBC) differential—can be done to determine the percentage of each type of granulocyte (neutrophils, eosinophils, and basophils) and nongranulocytes (lymphocytes and monocytes); absolute value of each is determined by multiplying the percentage by the total number of WBC; used to evaluate infection or potential for infection and identify various types of leukemia.

B. Nursing/Patient Care Considerations Blood sample can be drawn at any time without fasting or patient preparation; can be obtained by either venipuncture or skin puncture (if only small amount of blood is needed, but values may be lower in capillary blood).

TABLE 24-2   Characteristics of White Blood Cells

Cell	Major Function	Physical Characteristics
Neutrophil	Ingest and destroy microorganisms (phagocytosis)	Small cell, multilobed nucleus, most plentiful leukocyte
Eosinophil	Host resistance to helminthic infections; also allergic response	Bilobed nucleus; red-staining granules
Basophil	Allergic response	Bilobed nucleus; granules containing heparin and histamine
Monocyte	Phagocytosis	Large cell, kidney-shaped nucleus
B lymphocyte	Produce antibodies (immunoglobulins); humoral immunity	Small, agranular
T lymphocyte	Regulation of immune response; cellular immunity	Small, agranular; include cytotoxic, helper (T4), and suppressor (T8) T cells; identified by surface markers

Blood Smear

A. *Description* Blood specimen prepared for microscopic viewing using appropriate stains, allowing visual analysis of numbers and characteristics of cells present; can identify abnormal cells of certain anemias, leukemias, and other disorders that affect the blood stream.

B. *Nursing/Patient Care Considerations* Can be done from blood sample drawn for CBC; no additional sample is necessary.

Iron Profile

A. *Description*
Test completed on blood sample that generally includes levels of serum ferritin, iron, total iron-binding capacity, folate, vitamin B_{12} and is used to determine type and severity of anemia.

B. *Nursing/Patient Care Considerations* Recent administration of chloramphenicol, oral contraceptives, iron supplements, and corticotropin (ACTH) may affect results of serum iron and iron-binding capacity.

PROCEDURE GUIDELINES 24-1 ♦ Obtaining Blood by Skin Puncture

EQUIPMENT

Disposable lancet
Pipette and tubing
Slides

Alcohol sponges and dry sterile gauze pads
or
Prepared alcohol prep pads
Disposable gloves

PROCEDURE	NURSING ACTION	RATIONALE

PERFORMANCE PHASE

NURSING ACTION	RATIONALE
1. Wash hands and put on gloves.	1. Protects health care worker from possible exposure to blood.
2. Cleanse site (preferably ball of finger) with alcohol and dry with sterile gauze square.	2. If any alcohol remains, it will alter red cell morphology; also, blood will not collect into a compact drop but will run down the patient's finger.
3. Create stasis by pressing on the distal joint of the finger to produce redness at the end of the finger.	
4. Use a sterile disposable lancet, or an automated lancet.	4. This avoids the possibility of the transference of blood-borne viral diseases.
5. Prick the skin sharply and quickly with the lancet.	5. Pricking the skin sharply and quickly minimizes pain and produces a free-flowing sample.
6. Release pressure on the finger. Wipe off the first drop of blood.	6. Epithelial or endothelial cells may be found in the first drop of blood and render the count inaccurate. Also, platelets will begin to clump immediately in the blood at the puncture site.
7. Allow the blood to flow freely with an adequate puncture.	7. Pressing out the blood dilutes it with tissue fluid.
8. Obtain the blood sample: a. Fill the pipette or microhematocrit tube. b. Make blood slides according to the study required.	b. Gently touch the drop of blood to glass slides or cover slip.
9. Apply pressure over the wound with a dry gauze sponge until bleeding stops.	
10. Remove gloves, wash hands. Dispose of equipment and supplies in approved containers.	10. Protects health care workers from possible exposure to blood.

PROCEDURE GUIDELINES 24-2 ♦ Obtaining Blood by Venipuncture

EQUIPMENT

70% alcohol
Dry sterile sponges
5- and 10-mL syringe

No. 20-gauge needle(s)
or
Vacutainer assembly
Disposable gloves

PROCEDURE	NURSING ACTION	RATIONALE

PERFORMANCE PHASE

NURSING ACTION	RATIONALE
1. Reassure the patient. Explain that relatively little blood will be taken.	1. The patient is reassured when the nurse displays self-assurance and competence in relating to people and when performing technical skills.

(continued)

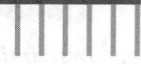

PROCEDURE GUIDELINES 24-2 ◆ Obtaining Blood by Venipuncture
(continued)

PROCEDURE (cont'd)	NURSING ACTION	RATIONALE
	2. Wash hands and put on gloves.	2. Protects health care worker from possible exposure to blood.
	3. Instruct the patient to extend his arm; the arm should be held straight at the elbow.	
	4. Apply the tourniquet directly above the elbow with just sufficient pressure to prevent venous return.	4. A tourniquet increases venous pressure and makes the vein more prominent and easier to enter.
	5. Inspect the area to visualize the vein, including the antecubital area, wrist, dorsum (back) of hand, and top of foot (if necessary). Palpate the vein.	5. Select a vein that is visible, palpable, and well fixed to surrounding tissue so that it does not roll away. (Not all veins are visible; some may be deep and can only be palpated.)
	6. Cleanse the skin with iodine and alcohol. Dry.	6. Cleansing the skin reduces pathogens.
	7. Fix chosen vein with the thumb and draw the skin taut immediately below the site before inserting needle to stabilize the vein.	7. The vein may roll beneath the skin when the needle approaches its outer surface (especially in elderly and extremely thin patients).
	8. Hold the syringe between the thumb and last 3 fingers with the bevel up and directly in line with the course of the vein. Insert the needle quickly and smoothly under the skin and into the vein.	
	9. Obtain blood sample by *gently* pulling back on the plunger.	9. Use minimal suction to prevent hemolysis of blood and collapse of the vein.
	10. Release the tourniquet as soon as specimen is obtained.	
	11. Withdraw the needle slowly.	11. Slow withdrawal of the needle is less painful.
	12. Apply a sterile dry gauze to puncture site and request patient to apply gentle but firm pressure to site for 2–4 min.	12. Firm pressure over the puncture site prevents leakage of blood into surrounding tissues with subsequent hematoma development. Merely flexing the arm may not prevent a hematoma, as the vein can slip to the side of the area where pressure is applied.
	13. Make the blood smear from the needle as desired.	
	14. Remove the needle from the syringe. As soon as possible after drawing the blood, gently eject the blood sample into a test tube containing an anticoagulant.	14. Slowly transfer the blood into the test tube *without* forming bubbles.
	15. Invert the tube gently several times to mix blood with anticoagulant.	15. For some tests, the blood is allowed to coagulate in the test tube.
	16. Label specimens correctly and send to laboratory immediately.	16. Specimens should go to the laboratory with a minimum of delay for optimum reliability.
	17. Dispose needle and syringe in appropriate containers to avoid possible spread of blood-borne viral diseases. Clean all spills with 10% bleach solution. Remove gloves and wash hands.	

◆ OTHER DIAGNOSTIC PROCEDURES

Bone Marrow Aspiration

A. Description
1. Aspiration of bone marrow from the iliac crest or sternum to obtain specimen to examine microscopically and biopsy. See Procedure Guidelines 24-3.
2. Purposes include diagnosis of hematologic disorders; monitoring of course of illness and response to treatment; diagnose other disorders such as primary and metastatic tumors, infectious diseases, and certain granulomas; and isolation of bacteria and other pathogens by culture.

B. Nursing/Patient Care Considerations
1. Give medication for pain and anxiety before or after the procedure as ordered.
2. Watch for bleeding and hematoma formation after procedure.

Lymph Node Biopsy

A. Description
1. Surgical excision or needle aspiration usually of a superficial lymph node in the cervical, supraclavicular, axillary, or inguinal region.
2. Performed to determine the cause of lymph node enlargement, distinguish between benign and malignant lymph node tumors, and stage metastatic carcinoma.

B. Nursing/Patient Care Considerations
1. Local anesthetic is usually given.
2. Specimen is placed in normal saline or 10% formaldehyde solution for transportation to the laboratory for cytologic and histologic evaluation.

┌───

PROCEDURE GUIDELINES 24-3 ◆ **Bone Marrow Aspiration and Biopsy**

EQUIPMENT Bone marrow aspiration tray
  Marrow aspiration needles with stylets
  Towels
  No. 25- and 22-gauge needles
  Two 20-mL syringes
  Three 5-mL syringes
  Local anesthetic (1% procaine or xylocaine)
  Sterile gauze squares
  Sterile gloves, drape

Skin antiseptic
Masks and protective eyewear for physician and nurse
  (check institutions policy)
Laboratory equipment
  Coverslips
  Microscopic slides
  Test tubes (plain and heparinized)
Scalpel blade and handle

PROCEDURE	*NURSING ACTION*	*RATIONALE*

PREPARATORY PHASE

1. Explain the procedure to the patient. Tell patient when the skin will be marked, antiseptic applied, and the needle puncture performed.
2. Give analgesic and/or tranquilizer as requested, 30 min before procedure. May not be necessary for aspiration.
3. Place the patient in prone or supine position.
4. The following sites are most frequently used:
   a. Posterior superior iliac crest
   b. Anterior iliac crest (if patient is very obese)
ILIAC CREST ASPIRATION/BIOPSY

PERFORMANCE PHASE (BY PHYSICIAN)

1. Position the patient on his abdomen (prone) or on his side with top knee flexed.
   a. The posterior iliac crest is located and marked.

   b. The skin area is prepared and draped. The marked area is infiltrated with local anesthetic through the skin and subcutaneous tissue to the periosteum of the bone.
   c. A small incision may be made.

   d. The bone marrow needle, with stylet in place, is introduced through the incision.

   e. The needle is advanced and rotated by using firm and steady pressure. When the needle is felt to enter the outer cortex of the bone marrow cavity, the stylet is removed and the syringe attached. Negative pressure is applied, and a small volume of blood and marrow is aspirated.
   f. A biopsy is taken by using a special needle equipped with a sharp cutting edge and a hollow core.
   g. After removal of needle, apply pressure to site, and dressing.

1. An explanation helps the patient to cope with anticipated stress. Tactile sensations (pressure, cold) can be misinterpreted as pain unless the patient is forewarned.
2. Analgesic and/or sedative may minimize pain, discomfort, and anxiety during procedure.

a. The iliac crest provides a large marrow cavity at the posterior superior iliac spine away from nearby abdominal organs.
b. Tell the patient he will experience a needle prick followed by a burning sensation. The periosteum is the region of greatest sensitivity.
c. The biopsy needle is large, and a small incision facilitates insertion.
d. The needle is pointed toward the anterior superior iliac spine and brought into contact with the posterior iliac spine.
e. There is usually decreased resistance when the bone marrow cavity is entered. The actual aspiration may cause brief pain, and the patient should be forewarned. Bone marrow appears rusty-red and normally has a thick, fluid-like consistency.

g. Prevents bleeding from puncture site. Dressing keeps site clean and dry until healed.

General Procedures/ Treatment Modalities

◆ SPLENECTOMY

The spleen is a fist-sized organ located in the upper left quadrant of the abdomen. It includes a central "white pulp" where storage and some proliferation of lymphocytes and other leukocytes occurs, and a peripheral "red pulp" involved in fetal erythropoiesis, and later in erythrocyte destruction and the conversion of hemoglobin to bilirubin. It may be surgically removed due to trauma or to treat certain hemolytic or malignant disorders with accompanying splenomegaly.

Preoperative Management/ Nursing Care

1. For general aspects of preoperative nursing management, see page 76.

2. Stabilization of preexisting condition:

    a. For trauma: volume replacement with intravenous (IV) fluids, evacuation of stomach via nasogastric tube to prevent aspiration, urinary catheterization to monitor urinary output, assessment for pneumothorax or hemothorax and possible chest tube placement

    b. For hemolytic or malignant disorder with accompanying thrombocytopenia: coagulation studies, administration of coagulation factors (eg, vitamin K, fresh frozen plasma, cryoprecipitate), platelet and red cell transfusions

3. Assist with preoperative pulmonary physical therapy and teaching.

Postoperative Management/ Nursing Care

1. For general aspects of postoperative nursing management, see page 80.

2. Prevent respiratory complications: hypoventilation and limited diaphragmatic movement, atelectasis of left lower lobe, pneumonia, left pleural effusion

3. Monitor for hemorrhage.

4. Administer narcotics for pain and watch for side effects.

5. Monitor fever.

    a. Postsplenectomy fever—mild, transient fever is expected.

    b. Persistent fever may indicate subphrenic abscess or hematoma; instruct patient to report.

6. Monitor daily platelet count: thrombocytosis (elevation of platelet count) may follow a few days after splenectomy and persist during first 2 weeks.

Potential Complications

1. Pancreatitis and fistula formation: tail of pancreas is anatomically close to splenic hilum.

2. Hemorrhage

3. Atelectasis and pneumonia

4. Overwhelming postsplenectomy infection (OPSI)—increased risk of developing a life-threatening bacterial infection with encapsulated organisms such as *Streptococcus pneumoniae, Neisseria meningitides,* or *Haemophilus influenzae.*

> **NURSING ALERT:** ❖
> The risk of OPSI is highest soon after splenectomy and in patients whose splenectomy occurred during childhood or for a malignant disease. Early symptoms include fever and malaise; the infection may progress within hours to sepsis and death, with a mortality rate as high as 50% to 70%. Patient education after splenectomy should include the risks of OPSI, recognition of early symptoms and promptly seeking medical attention, and the use of vaccinations against these bacteria, and in some cases, prophylactic antibiotics.

Nursing Diagnoses

A. Ineffective Breathing Pattern related to pain and guarding of surgical incision

B. Risk for Fluid Volume Deficit related to hemorrhage due to surgery of highly vascular organ

C. Risk for Injury (Thromboembolism) related to thrombocytosis

D. Risk for Infection related to surgical incision and removal of the spleen

E. Pain related to surgical incision

Nursing Interventions

A. *Maintaining Effective Breathing*

1. Assess breath sounds and report absent, diminished, or adventitious sounds.

2. Assist with aggressive chest physiotherapy and incentive spirometry.

3. Encourage early and progressive mobilization.

B. *Monitoring for Hemorrhage*

1. Monitor vital signs frequently and as condition warrants.

2. Measure abdominal girth and report abdominal distention.

3. Assess for pain and report increasing pain.

4. Prepare patient for surgical reexploration if bleeding is suspected.

C. *Avoiding Thromboembolic Complications*

1. Monitor platelet count daily.

2. If elevated, assess for possible thromboembolism.

    a. Assess skin color and temperature and pulses.

    b. Advise patient to report chest pain, shortness of breath, pain, or weakness.

D. *Preventing Infection*

1. Assess surgical incision daily or if increased pain, fever, or foul smell.

2. Maintain meticulous handwashing and change dressings using sterile technique.

3. Teach patient to report signs of infection (fever, malaise) immediately.

E. *Relieving Pain*

1. Administer narcotics or teach self-administration, as prescribed and as necessary to maintain level of comfort.

2. Warn patient of side effects such as nausea and drowsiness; watch for hypotension and decreased respirations.

3. Document dosage and response to medication.

Evaluation

A. Respirations unlabored, breath sounds clear

B. Vital signs stable, abdominal girth unchanged

C. Pulses strong, extremities warm and without pallor or cyanosis

D. Afebrile, no purulent drainage from incision

E. Verbalizes decreased pain

The Anemias

Anemia is the lack of sufficient circulating hemoglobin to deliver oxygen to tissues. Iron deficiency anemia, pernicious anemia, folic acid deficiency, and aplastic anemia are the anemias most often seen in adults.

◆ IRON DEFICIENCY ANEMIA (MICROCYTIC, HYPOCHROMIC)

Iron deficiency anemia is a condition in which the total body iron content is decreased below a normal level, affecting hemoglobin synthesis.

Pathophysiology/Etiology

1. May be due to chronic blood loss (gastrointestinal bleeding, excessive menstrual bleeding, hookworm infestation), iron malabsorption (small bowel disease, gastroenterostomy), increased requirements (during pregnancy, periods of rapid growth), insufficient intake (weight loss, inadequate diet).
2. Decreased hemoglobin may result in insufficient oxygen delivery to body tissues.
3. Most common type of anemia; major health problem in developing countries

Clinical Manifestations

1. Physical—headache, dizziness, tinnitus, palpitations, dyspnea on exertion, pallor of skin and mucous membranes, smooth, sore tongue, cheilosis (lesions at corners of mouth), koilonychia (spoon-shaped fingernails)
2. Behavioral—fatigue, pica (craving to eat unusual substances)

Diagnostic Evaluation

1. CBC and iron profile—decreased hemoglobin, hematocrit, serum iron, and ferritin; elevated red cell distribution width (RDW) and normal or elevated total iron-binding capacity (TIBC)
2. Determination of source of chronic blood loss may include sigmoidoscopy, colonoscopy, upper and lower gastrointestinal studies, stool and urine for occult blood examination.

Management

1. Correction of chronic blood loss
2. Oral or parenteral iron therapy
   a. Oral ferrous sulfate preferred and least expensive; treatment continues until hemoglobin level is normalized and iron stores replaced (up to 6 months).
   b. Parenteral therapy may rarely be used when patient unable to tolerate or noncompliant with oral therapy. May use iron dextran (Imferon) or iron sorbitex (Jectofer).

Complications

1. Severe compromise of the oxygen-carrying capacity of the blood may predispose to ischemic organ damage such as myocardial infarction or cerebrovascular accident.
2. Anaphylaxis to parenteral iron therapy

Nursing Assessment

1. Obtain history of symptoms, dietary intake, past history of anemia, possible sources of blood loss.
2. Examine for tachycardia, pallor, dyspnea, as well as signs of gastrointestinal or other bleeding.

Nursing Diagnoses

A. Altered Nutrition (Less than Body Requirements) related to inadequate intake of iron
B. Activity Intolerance related to decreased oxygen-carrying capacity of the blood
C. Altered Tissue Perfusion related to decreased oxygen-carrying capacity of the blood

Nursing Interventions

A. *Promoting Iron Intake*
1. Assess diet for inclusion of foods rich in iron. Arrange nutritionist referral as appropriate.
2. Administer iron replacement as ordered. Technique of parenteral iron administration:
   a. Allow small amount of air in syringe and use new 5-cm (2-inch) needle for injection to avoid tracking medication through subcutaneous tissue and resulting painful induration.
   b. Retract skin over muscle of upper outer quadrant of buttock laterally before inserting needle (Z-track technique) to prevent leakage along track and staining of skin.
   c. Inject deeply and slowly into upper outer quadrant of buttock. Wait a few seconds before withdrawing needle.

NURSING ALERT:
Anaphylactic reactions may occur after parenteral iron administration. Monitor patient closely for hypotension, angioedema, and stridor after injection. Do not administer along with oral iron.

B. *Increasing Activity Tolerance*
1. Assess level of fatigue and normal sleep pattern, determine activities that cause fatigue.
2. Assist in developing a schedule of activity, rest periods, and sleep.
3. Encourage conditioning exercises to increase strength and endurance.

C. *Maximizing Tissue Perfusion*
1. Assess patient for palpitations, chest pain, dizziness, and shortness of breath; minimize any activities that cause these symptoms.
2. Elevate head of bed and provide supplemental oxygen as ordered.
3. Monitor vital signs and fluid balance.

Patient Education/ Health Maintenance

1. Educate patient on proper nutrition and good sources of iron: select well balanced diet including animal pro-

teins, iron-fortified cereals and bread, green leafy vegetables, dried fruits, legumes, nuts.

2. Teach patient about iron supplementation. Take iron on empty stomach with full glass of water or fruit juice. Liquid forms may stain teeth; mix well with water/fruit juice and use straw. Anticipate some epigastric discomfort, change in color of stool to green or black, and in some cases nausea, constipation, or diarrhea. Keep iron medications away from children: overdose may be fatal.

3. Encourage follow-up laboratory studies and visits to health care provider.

Evaluation

A. Incorporates several foods high in iron into diet; takes prescribed iron supplementation as ordered
B. Tolerates increased activity; obtains sufficient rest
C. Vital signs stable without complaints of chest pain, palpitations, or shortness of breath

◆ MEGALOBLASTIC ANEMIA: PERNICIOUS

A megaloblast is a large, nucleated erythrocyte with delayed and abnormal nuclear maturation. Pernicious anemia is a type of megaloblastic anemia associated with vitamin B_{12} deficiency.

Pathophysiology/Etiology

1. Vitamin B_{12} is necessary for normal DNA synthesis in maturing RBCs.
2. Normal gastric mucosa secretes a substance called intrinsic factor, necessary for absorption of vitamin B_{12} in ileum. If a defect exists in gastric mucosa, or after gastrectomy or small bowel disease, intrinsic factor may not be secreted and orally ingested B_{12} not absorbed.
3. Primarily a disorder of elderly persons

Clinical Manifestations

1. Of anemia—pallor, fatigue, dyspnea on exertion, palpitations, angina pectoris, congestive heart failure
2. Of underlying gastrointestinal dysfunction—sore mouth, glossitis, anorexia, nausea, vomiting, loss of weight, indigestion, epigastric discomfort, recurring diarrhea or constipation
3. Of neuropathy (occurs in high percentage of untreated patients)—paresthesia involving hands and feet, gait disturbance, bladder and bowel dysfunction, psychiatric symptoms due to cerebral dysfunction

Diagnostic Evaluation

1. CBC and blood smear—decreased hemoglobin and hematocrit; marked variation in size and shape of RBCs with a variable number of unusually large cells
2. Folic acid (normal) and B_{12} levels (decreased)

3. Gastric analysis—volume and acidity of gastric juice diminished
4. Schilling test for absorption of vitamin B_{12} uses small amount of radioactive B_{12} orally and 24-hour urine collection to measure uptake—decreased

Management

1. Parenteral replacement with hydroxocobalamin or cyanocobalamin (B_{12}) is necessary.

Complications

1. Neurologic: paresthesia, gait disturbances, bowel and bladder dysfunction, and cerebral dysfunction may be persistent.

Nursing Assessment

1. Assess for pallor, tachycardia, dyspnea on exertion, exercise intolerance to determine patient's response to anemia.
2. Assess for paresthesia, gait disturbances, changes in bladder or bowel function, altered thought processes indicating neurologic involvement.
3. Obtain history of gastric surgery or gastrointestinal disease.

Nursing Diagnoses

A. Altered Thought Processes related to neurologic dysfunction in absence of vitamin B_{12}
B. Sensual/Perceptual Alterations (Kinesthetic) related to neurologic dysfunction in absence of vitamin B_{12}

Nursing Interventions

A. *Improving Thought Processes*
1. Administer parenteral vitamin B_{12} as prescribed.
2. Provide patient with quiet, supportive environment; reorient to time, place, and person if needed; give instructions and information in short, simple sentences and reinforce frequently.

B. *Minimizing the Effects of Paresthesia*
1. Assess extent and severity of any sensory or perceptual alterations.
2. Refer for physical therapy/occupational therapy as appropriate.
3. Provide safe, uncluttered environment; ensure personal belongings are within reach; provide assistance with activities as needed.

Patient Education/ Health Maintenance

1. Encourage monthly follow-up for vitamin B_{12} administration, should be continued for life.

2. Instruct patient to see health care provider approximately every 6 months for hematologic studies and gastrointestinal evaluation; may develop hematologic or neurologic relapse if therapy inadequate. Patients with pernicious anemia have higher incidence of gastric cancer and thyroid dysfunction; periodic stool examinations for occult blood, gastric cytology, and thyroid function tests are done.

Evaluation

A. Oriented, cooperative, and following instructions
B. Carrying out activities without injury

◆ MEGALOBLASTIC ANEMIA: FOLIC ACID DEFICIENCY

Chronic megaloblastic anemia due to folic acid (folate) deficiency

Pathophysiology/Etiology

1. Dietary deficiency, malnutrition, marginal diets; commonly associated with alcoholism
2. Impaired absorption in jejunum (eg, with small bowel disease)
3. Increased requirements (eg, with chronic hemolytic anemia, pregnancy)
4. Impaired utilization from folic acid antagonists (methotrexate) and other drugs (phenytoin, sulfamethoxazole, alcohol, oral contraceptives)

Clinical Manifestations

1. Of anemia: fatigue, weakness, pallor
2. Of folic acid deficiency: sore tongue, cracked lips

Diagnostic Evaluation

1. Vitamin B_{12} and folic acid level—folic acid will be decreased.

Management

1. Oral folic acid replacement

Complications

1. Folic acid deficiency has been implicated in the etiology of congenitally acquired neural tube defects.

Nursing Assessment

1. Obtain nutritional history.

2. Monitor level of dyspnea, tachycardia, and development of chest pain or shortness of breath for worsening of condition.

Nursing Diagnosis

A. Altered Nutrition (Less than Body Requirements) related to inadequate intake of folic acid

Nursing Interventions

A. *Improving Folic Acid Intake*
1. Assess diet for inclusion of foods rich in folic acid.
2. Arrange nutritionist referral as appropriate.
3. Assist alcoholic patient to obtain counseling and additional medical care as needed.

Patient Education/Health Maintenance

1. Teach patient to select balanced diet including green vegetables (asparagus, broccoli, spinach), yeast, liver and other organ meats, some fresh fruits; avoid overcooking vegetables.
2. Encourage pregnant patient to maintain prenatal care.

Evaluation

A. Eats appropriate and nutritious diet

◆ APLASTIC ANEMIA

Aplastic anemia is a disorder characterized by bone marrow hypoplasia or aplasia resulting in pancytopenia (insufficient numbers of RBCs, WBCs, and platelets).

Pathophysiology/Etiology

1. May be idiopathic or caused by exposure to chemical toxins; ionizing radiation; viral infections, particularly hepatitis; certain drugs (eg, chloramphenicol).
2. May be congenital (Fanconi's anemia)
3. Clinical course is variable and dependent on degree of bone marrow failure; severe aplastic anemia is generally fatal if untreated.

Clinical Manifestations

1. From anemia: pallor, weakness, fatigue, exertional dyspnea, palpitations
2. From infections associated with neutropenia: fever, headache, malaise; adventitious breath sounds; abdominal pain, diarrhea; erythema, pain, exudate at wounds or sites of invasive procedures
3. From thrombocytopenia: bleeding from gums, nose, gastrointestinal or genitourinary tracts; purpura, petechiae, ecchymoses

Diagnostic Evaluation

1. CBC and peripheral blood smear show decreased RBC, WBC, platelets (pancytopenia)
2. Bone marrow aspiration and biopsy: bone marrow is hypocellular or empty with greatly reduced or absent hematopoiesis.

Management

1. Removal of causative agent or toxin
2. Allogeneic bone marrow transplantation (BMT)—treatment of choice for patient with severe aplastic anemia (see p. 791)
3. Immunosuppressive treatment with corticosteroids, cyclophosphamide, (Cytoxan) antithymocyte globulin (ATG) or antilymphocyte globulin (ALG)
4. Androgens (oxymetholone or testosterone enanthate) may stimulate bone marrow regeneration; significant toxicity encountered.
5. Supportive treatment includes platelet and RBC transfusions, antibiotics, and antifungals.

Complications

1. Untreated severe aplastic anemia may be fatal, generally due to overwhelming infection. Even with treatment, morbidity and mortality due to infections and bleeding is high.

Nursing Assessment

1. Obtain thorough history including medications, past medical history, occupation, hobbies.
2. Monitor for signs of bleeding and infection.

Nursing Diagnoses

A. Risk for Infection related to granulocytopenia secondary to bone marrow aplasia
B. Risk for Injury related to bleeding

Nursing Interventions

A. *Minimizing Risk of Infection*
1. Care for patient in protective environment while hospitalized—private room with strict handwashing and avoidance of any contaminants.
2. Encourage good personal hygiene including daily shower or bath with mild soap, mouth care, and perirectal care after toileting.
3. Monitor vital signs including temperature frequently; notify health care provider of oral temperature of 38.3°C (101°F) or higher.
4. Minimize invasive procedures or possible trauma to skin or mucous membranes.
5. Obtain cultures of suspected infected sites or body fluids.

B. *Minimizing Risk of Bleeding*
1. Use only soft toothbrush or toothette for mouth care and electric razor for shaving; keep nails short by filing.
2. Avoid intramuscular injections and other invasive procedures.
3. Prevent constipation by use of stool softeners as prescribed.
4. Restrict activity based on platelet count and presence of active bleeding.
5. Monitor pad count for menstruating patient; avoid use of vaginal tampons.
6. Control bleeding by applying pressure to site, using ice packs and prescribed topical hemostatic agents.
7. Administer blood product replacement as ordered; monitor for allergic reaction, anaphylaxis, and volume overload.

Patient Education/ Health Maintenance

1. Teach patient how to minimize risk of bleeding: avoid falls or other injury; use electric razor rather than plain razor; use nail clippers or file rather than scissors; avoid blowing nose; use soft toothbrush or toothette for mouth care; use water-soluble lubricants as needed during sexual activity.
2. Teach patient how to minimize risk of infection: wash hands after contact with possible source of infection; immediately cleanse any abrasion or wound of mucous membranes or skin; monitor temperature and report any fever or other sign of infection immediately; avoid crowds and individuals with illnesses; avoid raw or undercooked foods; use condoms and other safe sex practices.
3. Advise patient to avoid exposure to potential bone marrow toxins: solvents, sprays, paints, pesticides.
4. Teach patient to take only prescribed medications; avoid aspirin and nonsteroidal anti-inflammatory drugs (NSAIDs), which may interfere with platelet function.
5. Resources include: Aplastic Anemia Foundation of America; P.O. Box 22689; Baltimore, MD 21203; 410-955-2803.

Evaluation

A. Remains afebrile with no signs/symptoms of infection
B. Episodes of bleeding are rapidly controlled

Myeloproliferative Disorders

Myeloproliferative disorders are disorders of the bone marrow resulting from abnormal proliferation of cells from the myeloid line of the hematopoietic system. They include polycythemia vera, acute lymphocytic and acute myelogenous leukemia, and chronic myelogenous leukemia.

◆ POLYCYTHEMIA VERA

This chronic myeloproliferative disorder involves all bone marrow elements, resulting in an increase in RBC mass and hemoglobin.

Pathophysiology/Etiology

1. Hyperplasia of all bone marrow elements results in:
   a. Increased RBC mass
   b. Increased blood volume and viscosity
   c. Decreased marrow iron reserve
   d. Splenomegaly
2. Underlying cause is unknown.
3. Usually occurs in middle and later years.

Clinical Manifestations

Result from increased blood volume and viscosity

1. Reddish purple hue of skin and mucosa, pruritus
2. Splenomegaly, hepatomegaly
3. Epigastric discomfort
4. Painful fingers and toes from arterial and venous insufficiency
5. Headache, fullness in head, dizziness, visual abnormalities, altered mentation from disturbed cerebral circulation
6. Weakness, fatigue, bleeding tendency
7. Hyperuricemia from increased formation and destruction of erythrocytes and leukocytes and increased metabolism of nucleic acids

Diagnostic Evaluation

1. CBC—elevated RBC and hemoglobin and hematocrit
2. Bone marrow aspirate and biopsy—hyperplasia

Management

1. Of hyperviscosity: phlebotomy (withdrawal of blood) at intervals determined by CBC results to reduce RBC mass; generally 250 to 500 mL removed at a time
2. Of marrow hyperplasia: myelosuppressive therapy, generally using IV radioactive phosphorus (^{32}P) or alkylating agent such as hydroxyurea
3. Of hyperuricemia: allopurinol

Complications

1. Thromboembolic events due to hyperviscosity including deep vein thrombophlebitis, myocardial and cerebral infarction, pulmonary embolism, and thrombotic occlusion of the splenic, hepatic, portal and mesenteric veins
2. Spontaneous hemorrhage due to venous and capillary distention and abnormal platelet function
3. Gout due to hyperuricemia
4. Congestive heart failure due to increased blood volume and hypertension
5. Myelofibrosis or acute leukemia may be terminal complications.

Nursing Assessment

1. Obtain history of symptoms including changes in skin, epigastric discomfort, bleeding tendencies, circulatory problems, or painful, swollen joints.

2. Monitor for signs of bleeding or thromboembolism.
3. Monitor for hypertension and signs and symptoms of congestive heart failure including shortness of breath, distended neck veins.

Nursing Diagnosis

A. Altered Tissue Perfusion (Multiple Organs) related to hyperviscosity of blood

Nursing Interventions

A. *Preventing Thromboembolic Complications*
1. Encourage or assist with ambulation.
2. Assess for early signs of thromboembolic complications—swelling of limb, increased warmth, pain.
3. Monitor CBC and assist with phlebotomy as ordered.

Patient Education/ Health Maintenance

1. Educate patient about risk of thrombosis; encourage patient to maintain normal activity patterns and avoid long periods of bed rest.
2. Advise patient to avoid taking hot showers or baths because rapid skin cooling worsens pruritus; use skin emollients; take antihistamines as prescribed.
3. Instruct patient to take only prescribed medications.
4. Encourage patient to report at prescribed intervals for follow-up blood (hematocrit) studies.

Evaluation

A. No signs or symptoms of thromboembolism

◆ ACUTE LYMPHOCYTIC AND ACUTE MYELOGENOUS LEUKEMIA

(See Nursing Care Plan 24-1.)

Leukemias are malignant disorders of the blood and bone marrow resulting in an accumulation of dysfunctional, immature cells, due to loss of regulation of cell division. They are classified as acute or chronic based on the development rate of symptoms, and further classified by the predominant cell type. Acute leukemias affect immature cells and are characterized by rapid progression of symptoms. When lymphocytes are the predominant malignant cell, the disorder is acute lymphocytic leukemia (ALL); when monocytes or granulocytes are predominant, it is acute myelogenous leukemia (AML), sometimes called acute nonlymphocytic leukemia (ANLL).

Pathophysiology/Etiology

1. The development of leukemia has been associated with:
   a. Exposure to ionizing radiation

b. Exposure to certain chemicals and toxins (eg, benzene, alkylating agents)
c. Human T-cell leukemia–lymphoma virus (HTLV-1) in certain areas of the world, including the Caribbean and southern Japan
d. Familial susceptibility
e. Genetic disorders (eg, Down syndrome, Fanconi's anemia)

2. About half of new leukemias are acute. About 85% of acute leukemias in adults are AML. ALL is most common cancer in children, with peak incidence between ages 2 and 9.

Clinical Manifestations

1. Common symptoms include pallor, fatigue, weakness, fever, weight loss, abnormal bleeding and bruising, lymphadenopathy (in ALL) and recurrent infections (in ALL)
2. Other presenting symptoms may include bone and joint pain, headache, splenomegaly, hepatomegaly, neurologic dysfunction.

Diagnostic Evaluation

1. CBC and blood smear—peripheral WBC count varies widely from 1,000 to 100,000/mm³; anemia may be profound; platelet count may be abnormal and coagulopathies may exist.
2. Bone marrow aspiration and biopsy—cells also studied for chromosomal abnormalities (cytogenetics) and immunologic markers to classify type of leukemia further.
3. Lymph node biopsy—to detect spread
4. Lumbar puncture and examination of cerebrospinal fluid (CSF) for leukemic cells (especially in ALL)

Management

1. To eradicate leukemic cells and allow restoration of normal hematopoiesis
   a. High-dose chemotherapy given as an induction course to obtain a remission (disappearance of abnormal cells in bone marrow and blood) and then in cycles as consolidation or maintenance therapy to prevent recurrence of disease (Table 24-3)
   b. Radiation, particularly of central nervous system (CNS) in ALL
   c. Autologous or allogeneic bone marrow transplant
2. Supportive care and symptom management

Complications

1. Leukostasis: in setting of high numbers (greater than 50,000/mm³) of circulating leukemic cells (blasts), blood vessel walls infiltrated and weakened, with high risk for rupture and bleeding, including intracranial hemorrhage
2. Disseminated intravascular coagulation (DIC)
3. Infection, bleeding, organ damage

Nursing Assessment

1. Take nursing history, focusing on weight loss, fever, incidence of frequent infections, progressively increasing fatigability, shortness of breath, palpitations, visual changes (retinal bleeding).
2. Ask about difficulty in swallowing, coughing, rectal pain.
3. Examine patient for enlarged lymph nodes, hepatosplenomegaly, evidence of bleeding, abnormal breath sounds, skin lesions.
4. Look for evidence of infection: mouth, tongue, and throat for reddened areas/white patches. Examine skin for breakdown, which is a potential source of infection.

Nursing Diagnoses

A. Risk for Infection related to granulocytopenia of disease and treatment
B. Risk for Injury related to bleeding secondary to bone marrow failure and thrombocytopenia

Nursing Interventions

A. *Preventing Infection*
1. Especially monitor for pneumonia, pharyngitis, esophagitis, perianal cellulitis, urinary tract infection, and cellulitis, which are common in leukemia and carry significant morbidity and mortality.
2. Monitor for fever, flushed appearance, chills, tachycardia; appearance of white patches in mouth; redness, swelling, heat or pain of eyes, ears, throat, skin, joints, abdomen, rectal and perineal areas; cough, changes in sputum; skin rash.
3. Check results of granulocyte counts. Concentrations under 500 mm³ make the patient at serious risk for infection.
4. Avoid invasive procedures and trauma to skin or mucous membrane to prevent entry of microorganisms.
5. Use the following rectal precautions to prevent infection.
   a. Avoid diarrhea and constipation, which can irritate the rectal mucosa.
   b. Avoid rectal thermometers.
   c. Avoid foods that increase bacterial colonization of the gastrointestinal tract such as fresh fruits, vegetables, raw meat, buttermilk.
   d. Keep perianal area clean.
6. Care for patient in protected environment with strict handwashing practice.
7. Encourage and assist patient with personal hygiene, bathing, and oral care.
8. Obtain cultures and administer antimicrobials promptly as directed.

B. *Preventing and Managing Bleeding*
1. Watch for signs of minor bleeding such as petechiae, ecchymosis, conjunctival hemorrhage, epistaxis, bleeding gums, bleeding at puncture sites, vaginal spotting, heavy menses.
2. Be alert for signs of serious bleeding such as headache with change in responsiveness, blurred vision, hemoptysis, hematemesis, melena, hypotension, tachycardia, dizziness.

3. Test all urine, stool, emesis for gross and occult blood.
4. Monitor platelet counts daily.
5. Administer blood components as directed.
6. Keep patient on bed rest during bleeding episodes.

Patient Education/ Health Maintenance

1. Teach patient infection precautions (see pp. 768).
2. Teach signs and symptoms of infection and who to notify.
3. Encourage adequate nutrition to prevent emaciation from chemotherapy.

4. Encourage regular dental visits to detect and treat dental infections and disease.
5. Teach avoidance of constipation with increased fluid and fiber, and good perianal care.
6. Teach good hygiene.
7. Teach bleeding precautions such as use of electric razor, avoidance of aspirin or NSAIDs, avoidance of sharp objects, avoidance of straining at stool or forceful nose-blowing.

Evaluation

A. Afebrile, without signs of infection
B. No signs of bleeding

NURSING CARE PLAN 24-1 ◆ *Care of the Patient With Acute Leukemia*

You are assigned Charles Wintry, a 48-year-old with acute myelogenous leukemia (AML) who has been admitted with neutropenia and thrombocytopenia following chemotherapy. From your assessment and your knowledge of AML, you develop your plan of care.

Subjective data: Charles tells you he has felt very tired over the past week and stopped working at his part-time store manager job. Since yesterday evening he has had a low-grade fever and pain in his chest with inspiration. He has also noticed new bruises on his lower legs and abdomen. This morning he had a nosebleed.

Objective data: Vital signs are temperature 38.3°C (101°F), pulse 104, BP 145/90, respirations 32. On examination you notice extensive petechiae; dried blood around the nares and gingival bleeding; warm, dry skin; and crackles heard in the bases of both lungs. CBC reveals 30,000 platelets, 1,200 WBCs with 450 neutrophils, and hematocrit of 32%.

NURSING DIAGNOSIS: Risk for Infection related to granulocytopenia secondary to leukemia or its treatment with chemotherapy and/or radiation

GOAL: Risk of infection will be minimized.

NURSING INTERVENTIONS	RATIONALE	EVALUATION
1. Place patient in protected environment (private room) with handwashing precautions strictly enforced.	1. Meticulous handwashing is the single most important method of preventing transmission of endogenous and exogenous nosocomial infections.	1. Staff and visitors comply with handwashing precautions.
2. Avoid exposure to all sources of stagnant water (eg, flower vases, denture cups, water pitchers, humidifiers) and plants.	2. Stagnant water and soil are good media for anaerobic bacterial growth.	2. Sources of possible bacterial growth are eliminated.
3. Encourage or assist with personal hygiene—mouth care, perirectal care, daily shower or bath with mild soap. Inspect skin and mucous membranes daily for possible signs of infection.	3. Skin care and good oral hygiene may help prevent skin, oral, respiratory, and gastrointestinal infections. Signs of infection may be minimal in neutropenic patient.	3. Skin remains clean and lubricated. Oropharynx has no lesions, plaques, or erythema.
4. Monitor vital signs q4h.	4. Infections may progress rapidly in immunocompromised patient.	4. Vital signs monitored and changes reported to health care provider.
5. Assess respiratory function q4h while symptoms present, otherwise q8h. Encourage ambulation, deep breathing, and coughing.	5. Neutropenic patient may have significant bacterial or fungal pneumonia with minimal changes on chest x-ray or physical examination.	5. Ambulates and uses incentive spirometer.

(continued)

NURSING CARE PLAN 24-1 ◆ Care of the Patient With Acute Leukemia (continued)

NURSING INTERVENTIONS	RATIONALE	EVALUATION
6. Assess for changes in mental status at least q8h including restlessness, irritability, confusion, headache, or changes in level of consciousness.	6. Mental status changes are often first subtle signs of sepsis.	6. Mental status remains normal.
7. Avoid invasive procedures if possible, eg, urinary catheterization. Use strict aseptic technique if procedure unavoidable.	7. Risk of infection from invasive procedure is high.	7. Invasive procedures minimized. Injections given IV.
8. Prevent rectal trauma by avoiding rectal temperatures, enemas, or suppositories. Use sitz bath and barrier cream for patient with diarrhea and hemorrhoids. Use stool softeners as needed to prevent constipation.	8. Perianal area is high risk site for infection, including rectal abscesses.	8. Perianal area remains clean and intact.
9. Obtain cultures of suspected infected sites or body fluids.	9. Pus may not be present with neutropenia. Cultures may reveal bacterial, fungal or viral pathogens.	9. Sputum sent for culture.
10. Report: 1) fever ≥ 101°F or 38.3°C; 2) significant change in vital signs, particularly hypotension, tachycardia, and/or tachypnea; 3) chills or rigors; 4) mental status changes.	10. Fever may be only response to infection in neutropenic patient. Patient is at risk for sepsis due to lack of normal immunologic response.	10. Fever reported.
11. Teach patient measures to prevent infection: avoid crowds; avoid raw or undercooked food; use condoms.	11. Potential for infection remains after discharge.	11. Patient states preventative measures.

NURSING DIAGNOSIS: Risk for injury related to bleeding secondary to thrombocytopenia, disseminated intravascular coagulation or leukostasis associated with leukemia

GOAL: Risk of bleeding will be minimized.

NURSING INTERVENTIONS	RATIONALE	EVALUATION
1. Assess for signs of bleeding at least q8h.	1. Overt and covert spontaneous bleeding is possible at platelet counts < 50,000/mm³.	1. No further bleeding noted.
2. Provide soft toothbrush or toothettes and mild mouthwash for mouth care.	2. Minimize damage to mucous membranes.	2. Uses soft toothbrush after meals for gentle cleansing.
3. Use only an electric razor for shaving. Keep fingernails and toenails short and smooth. Lubricate skin with mild lotion.	3. Minimize skin excoriation.	3. Wife brings electric razor from home.
4. Avoid IM injections, invasive procedures, rectal procedures. Use stool softeners to prevent constipation.	4. Minimize risk of bleeding.	4. Invasive procedures minimized. Injections given IV.
5. Restrict activity based on assessment of platelet count and presence of active bleeding.	5. Injury to muscles or spontaneous bleeding may be minimized by restricting activity at lower platelet counts.	5. Ambulates within room with assistance until bleeding controlled and platelet count stabilized.
6. Menstrual suppression may be necessary for females. Monitor pad count/amount. Avoid use of vaginal tampons.	6. Menorrhagia may be severe in thrombocytopenic patient.	6. N/A

(continued)

NURSING CARE PLAN 24-1 ◆ *Care of the Patient With Acute Leukemia* (continued)

NURSING INTERVENTIONS	RATIONALE	EVALUATION
7. Control bleeding by applying pressure to site, ice packs, and prescribed topical hemostatic agents such as microfibrillar collagen hemostat (Avitene) or thrombin (Fibrindex, Thrombinar).	7. Topical interventions generally adequate to control most bleeding episodes.	7. No further bleeding episodes.
8. Administer blood product replacement as ordered. Monitor for signs and symptoms of allergic reactions, anaphylaxis, and volume overload.	8. Platelet transfusions may be necessary when platelet count < 30,000/mm³ or with active bleeding. Other blood products (RBCs, fresh frozen plasma, cryoprecipitate) may also be required.	8. Platelet products given q2–3d until thrombocytopenia resolved.
9. Teach patient to avoid activities likely to cause injury (eg, contact sports) and other methods to prevent bleeding.	9. Risk for bleeding remains after discharge.	9. Patient states preventative measures.

NURSING DIAGNOSIS: Pain related to tumor growth, infection, or side effects of chemotherapy

GOAL: Pain will be controlled.

NURSING INTERVENTIONS	RATIONALE	EVALUATION
1. Assess at least q4h for presence, location, intensity, and characteristics of pain.	1. Pain is potentially distressing symptom. Pain may be symptom of infection.	1. Patient rates pain between 1 and 3 on scale 0–10 after first day.
2. Administer analgesics as ordered to control pain. Administer on regular schedule rather than PRN. Avoid aspirin and nonsteroidal anti-inflammatory medications in thrombocytopenic patients. If oral analgesics in optimal doses are not effective or not tolerated, consider IV route.	2. Analgesics on regular schedule at appropriate doses should be used to control pain. Aspirin and non-steroidal anti-inflammatory medications interfere with platelet function. IM and SC injections should be avoided in thrombocytopenia.	2. Oral analgesia (codeine 30 mg q4h) well tolerated.
3. Teach and use nonpharmacologic measures as appropriate (eg, application of heat and cold, relaxation exercises, distraction, imagery).	3. Nonpharmacologic measures may be useful adjunctive treatments for patients with pain.	3. Heat packs to right chest area provide additional relief.

NURSING DIAGNOSIS: Powerlessness related to diagnosis and perceived lack of support/resources

GOAL: Patient and family will be empowered to seek appropriate help.

NURSING INTERVENTIONS	RATIONALE	EVALUATION
1. Encourage verbalization of feelings regarding diagnosis, treatment plan, and anticipated course of illness.	1. Nurse–patient relationship allows appropriate discussion of concerns.	1. Verbalizes feelings appropriately.
2. Refer as needed to social worker, psychiatric liaison nurse, psychologist.	2. Further assistance and support may be needed.	2. Referred to social worker for assistance with financial concerns.
3. Share information regarding national and local resources.	3. National and local organizations may be significant sources of support for patients and families.	3. Attends American Cancer Society support group after discharge.

TABLE 24-3 Common Chemotherapeutic Drugs
Used in Acute Leukemias

Drug	Major Side Effects	Classification	Primary Use
Cytarabine (ARA-C, Cytosar-U)	Bone marrow suppression, nausea and vomiting, pulmonary toxicity, mucositis, lethargy, cerebellar toxicity, dermatitis, keratoconjunctivitis	Antimetabolite	Induction and consolidation therapy for AML
Daunorubicin (Cerubidine)	Bone marrow suppression, nausea and vomiting, alopecia, cardiotoxicity, vesicant	Antibiotic	Induction and consolidation therapy for AML
Doxorubicin (Adriamycin PFS)	Leukopenia, nausea and vomiting, alopecia, cardiotoxicity, photosensitivity, vesicant	Antibiotic	Induction and consolidation therapy for AML
L-asparaginase (Elspar)	Liver dysfunction, nausea and vomiting, hypersensitivity reaction, depression, lethargy	Miscellaneous: enzyme	Induction therapy for ALL
6-Mercaptopurine (6-MP, Purinethol)	Mild bone marrow suppression, gastrointestinal disturbances, hepatotoxicity	Antimetabolite	Maintenance therapy for ALL
Methotrexate (MTX, Folex)	Bone marrow suppression, stomatitis, nausea, diarrhea, hepatotoxicity, neurotoxicity with intrathecal doses	Antimetabolite	Intrathecal central nervous system treatment and prophylaxis for ALL; maintenance therapy for ALL
Prednisone (Orasone)	Appetite stimulation, mood alteration, Cushing's syndrome, hypertension, diabetes, peptic ulcer	Corticosteroid	Induction therapy for ALL
Vincristine (Oncovin, Vincasar)	Neurotoxicity, alopecia, vesicant	Plant alkaloid	Induction therapy for ALL

ALL, acute lymphocytic leukemia; AML, acute myelogenous leukemia.

◆ CHRONIC MYELOGENOUS LEUKEMIA (CML)

This chronic leukemia (ie, involving more mature cells than acute leukemia), also known as chronic granulocytic or chronic myelocytic leukemia, is characterized by proliferation of myeloid cell lines, including granulocytes, monocytes, platelets, and occasionally RBCs.

Pathophysiology/Etiology

1. Specific etiology unknown. Results from malignant transformation of pluripotent hematopoietic stem cell.

2. First cancer associated with chromosomal abnormality (the Philadelphia (Ph) chromosome), present in more than 90% of patients.
3. Accounts for 25% of adult leukemias and less than 5% of childhood leukemias. Generally ages 25 to 60 with peak incidence mid-forties.
4. With progression of illness, enters terminal phase resembling an acute leukemia consisting of accelerated phase or blast crisis.

Clinical Manifestations

1. Insidious onset, may be discovered during routine physical examination.

2. Common symptoms include fatigue, pallor, activity intolerance, fever, weight loss, night sweats, abdominal fullness (splenomegaly).

Diagnostic Evaluation

1. CBC and blood smear—large numbers of granulocytes (often more than 100,000/mm³), platelets—may be decreased
2. Bone marrow aspiration and biopsy—hypercellular, usually demonstrates presence of Ph chromosome

Management

A. *Chronic Phase*
1. Potentially curative treatment is offered by allogeneic (related or unrelated donor) BMT.
2. Palliative treatment, controlling symptoms, includes chemotherapy with agents such as busulfan (Myleran) or hydroxyurea (Hydrea); irradiation; splenectomy; or biotherapy (interferon).

B. *Accelerated Phase or Blast Crisis*
1. Attempts to restore chronic phase through use of high-dose chemotherapy, leukophoresis
2. Supportive care—generally terminal

Complications

1. Leukostasis
2. Infection, bleeding, organ damage
3. With exception of possible cures using BMT, CML is a terminal disease with unpredictable survival, on average 3 years.

Nursing Assessment

1. Obtain health history, focusing on fatigue, weight loss, night sweats, activity intolerance.
2. Assess for signs of bleeding and infection.
3. Evaluate splenomegaly, hepatomegaly.

Nursing Diagnosis

A. Fear of disease progression and death

For patient with CML in blast crisis, see Nursing Care Plan 24-1.

Nursing Interventions

A. *Allaying Fear*
1. Encourage appropriate verbalization of feelings and concerns.
2. Provide comprehensive patient teaching about disease, using methods and content appropriate to patient's needs.

3. Assist patient in identifying resources and support (eg, family and friends, spiritual support, community or national organizations, support groups).
4. Facilitate use of effective coping mechanisms.

Patient Education/ Health Maintenance

1. Teach patient to take medications as prescribed and monitor for side effects.
2. For information and support, refer to agencies such as: Leukemia Society of America; 600 Third Ave.; New York, NY 10016; 212-573-8484. (For additional agencies, see Table 24-4.)

Evaluation

A. Demonstrates effective coping skills and manages fear

Lymphoproliferative Disorders

Lymphoproliferative disorders result from proliferation of cells from the lymphoid line of the hematopoietic system. They include chronic lymphocytic leukemia, Hodgkin's disease, non-Hodgkin's lymphomas, and multiple myeloma.

◆ CHRONIC LYMPHOCYTIC LEUKEMIA (CLL)

This chronic leukemia (ie, involving more mature cells than acute leukemia) is characterized by proliferation of lymphocytes. Classified according to cell origin, it includes B cell (accounts for 95% of cases), T cell, lymphosarcoma, prolymphocytic leukemia, and hairy cell leukemia.

Pathophysiology/Etiology

1. Specific etiology unknown. Tends to cluster in families, much more common in western hemisphere. Male hormones may play role.
2. Most common leukemia in United States and Europe. Disease of later years (90% over age 50 years). Twice as common in men.
3. May be indolent for years, with gradual transformation to more malignant disease.

Clinical Manifestations

1. Insidious onset, may be discovered during routine physical examination.
2. Early symptoms may include history of frequent skin or respiratory infections, symmetrical lymphadenopathy, mild splenomegaly.
3. Symptoms of more advanced disease include pallor, fatigue, activity intolerance, easy bruising, skin lesions, bone tenderness, abdominal discomfort.

TABLE 24-4 Resources for Patients With Hematologic Malignancies

National and Local Organizations

American Cancer Society 1599 Clifton Rd., NE Atlanta, GA 30329 404-320-3333 or 1-800-ACS-2345	Patient education materials, CanSurmount and I Can Cope educational and support programs, durable medical equipment loans
Corporate Angel Network, Inc. Westchester County Airport, Bldg 1 White Plains, NY 10604 914-328-1313	Use of corporate aircraft to provide free travel to cancer patients going to check-ups, treatments or consultations
Leukemia Society of America 600 Third Ave. New York, NY 10016 212-573-8484 or 1-800-955-4572	Patient education materials, support groups, financial assistance (patient aid) program for patients with leukemia, Hodgkin's and non-Hodgkin's lymphoma
National Cancer Care Foundation 1180 Avenue of the Americas, 2nd floor New York, NY 10036 212-221-3300	Information related to nonmedical resources, support, financial aid
National Coalition for Cancer Survivorship 1010 Wayne Ave., 5th floor Silver Spring, MD 20910 301-650-8868	Network related to survivorship issues, sponsors National Cancer Survivors' Day, publishes Cancer Survivors Almanac of Resources
National Leukemia Association, Inc. 585 Stewart Ave., Suite 536 Garden City, NY 11530 516-222-1944	Information and financial aid
National Marrow Donor Program 3433 Broadway St., NE Minneapolis, MN 55413 612-627-5800	Information for patients and volunteer donors regarding unrelated bone marrow transplant
Office of Cancer Communications National Cancer Institute, Bldg 31, Rm 10A24 Bethesda, MD 20892 1-800-4-CANCER	National telephone hotline for information, patient education materials, research reports
Wellness Centers/Groups (name and address of nearest available from Office of Cancer Communications at 1-800-4-CANCER)	Psychosocial support including groups, hotlines, patient education materials, social activities

Newsletters and Magazines

BMT Newsletter c/o Susan Stewart 1985 Spruce Ave. Highland Park, IL 60035 708-831-1913	**NCCS Networker** National Coalition for Cancer Survivorship 1010 Wayne Ave Silver Spring, MD 20910 301-650-8868

Diagnostic Evaluation

1. CBC and blood smear—large numbers of lymphocytes (10,000 to 150,000/mm³), may also be anemia, thrombocytopenia, hypogammaglobulinemia
2. Bone marrow aspirate and biopsy—lymphocytic infiltration of bone marrow
3. Lymph node biopsy—to detect spread

Management

A. Symptom Control
1. Chemotherapy with chlorambucil (Leukeran), cyclophosphamide (Cytoxan), and prednisone (Orasone) to decrease lymphadenopathy and splenomegaly
2. Splenic irradiation or splenectomy for painful splenomegaly or platelet sequestration, hemolytic anemia
3. Irradiation of painful enlarged lymph nodes

B. Supportive Care
1. Transfusion therapy to replace platelets and RBCs
2. IV immunoglobulins or gamma globulin to treat hypogammaglobulinemia

Complications

1. Thrombophlebitis from venous or lymphatic obstruction due to enlarged lymph nodes
2. Infection, bleeding
3. Median survival depends on severity of disease, varies from 2 to 7 years.

Nursing Assessment

1. Obtain health history, focusing on history of infections, fatigue, bruising and bleeding, swollen lymph nodes.
2. Assess for signs of anemia, bleeding, or infection.
3. Evaluate splenomegaly, hepatomegaly, lymphadenopathy.

Nursing Diagnoses

A. Pain related to tumor growth, infection, or side effects of chemotherapy.
B. Activity Intolerance related to anemia and side effects of chemotherapy

Nursing Interventions

A. *Reducing Pain*
1. Assess frequently for pain and administer or teach patient to administer analgesics on regular schedule, as prescribed; monitor for side effects.
2. Teach the use of relaxation techniques such as relaxation breathing, progressive muscle relaxation, distraction and imagery to manage pain.

B. *Improving Activity Tolerance*
1. Encourage frequent rest periods alternating with ambulation and light activity as tolerated.
2. Assist with hygiene and physical care as necessary.
3. Encourage balanced diet or nutritional supplements as tolerated.
4. Teach patient to use energy conservation techniques while performing activities of daily living, such as sitting while bathing, minimizing trips up and down stairs, using shoulder bag or push cart to carry articles.

Patient Education/ Health Maintenance

1. Teach patient to minimize risk of infection (see p. 768).
2. Teach use of medications as ordered, and possible side effects and their management; also to avoid aspirin and NSAIDs, which may interfere with platelet function.
3. Refer for information and support (see Table 24-4).

Evaluation

A. States free of pain
B. Performs activities without complaints of fatigue

◆ HODGKIN'S DISEASE

Hodgkin's disease is a lymphoma. Lymphomas are malignant disorders of the reticuloendothelial system resulting in an accumulation of dysfunctional, immature lymphoid-derived cells. They are classified according to the predominant cell type and by the degree of malignant cell maturity (eg, well differentiated, poorly differentiated, or undifferentiated). Hodgkin's disease originates in the lymphoid system and involves predominantly lymph nodes.

Pathophysiology/Etiology

1. Etiology is unknown.
2. Characterized by appearance of "Reed-Sternberg" multinucleated giant cell in tumor. Generally spreads via lymphatic channels, involving lymph nodes, spleen, and ultimately extralymphatic sites.
3. May also spread via bloodstream to sites such as gastrointestinal tract, bone marrow, skin, upper air passages, and other organs.
4. Incidence demonstrates two peaks, at ages 20 to 40 and after age 60.

Clinical Manifestations

1. Common symptoms include painless enlargement of lymph nodes (generally unilateral), fever, chills, night sweats, weight loss, pruritus.
2. Wide variety of symptoms may occur if there is pulmonary involvement, superior vena cava obstruction, hepatic or bone involvement, etc.

Diagnostic Evaluation

Tests are used to determine extent of disease involvement before treatment and followed at regular intervals to assess response to treatment.

1. Lymph node biopsy—determines type of lymphoma.
2. CBC, bone marrow aspirate and biopsy—determine whether bone marrow is involved.
3. Radiographic tests (eg, x-rays, computed tomography [CT], magnetic resonance imaging [MRI])—detect deep nodal involvement.
4. Liver function tests, scan—determine hepatic involvement; liver biopsy may be indicated if results abnormal.
5. Lymphangiogram—detects size and location of deep nodes involved, including abdominal nodes, which may not be readily seen via computed tomography (CT).
6. Surgical staging (laparotomy with splenectomy, liver biopsy, multiple lymph node biopsies)—in selected patients

Management

Choice of treatment depends on extent of disease, histopathologic findings, and prognostic indicators. Hodgkin's disease is more readily cured than other lymphomas. More than one treatment strategy is available, and combinations of radiation and chemotherapy are commonly used.

A. *Radiation Therapy*
1. Treatment of choice for localized disease
2. Areas of body where lymph node chains are located can generally tolerate high radiation doses.
3. Vital organs are protected with lead shielding during radiation treatments.

B. *Chemotherapy*
1. Initial treatment often with MOPP regimen of nitrogen mustard (Mustargen), vincristine (Oncovin), procarbazine, and prednisone or ABVD regimen of doxorubicin (Adriamycin), bleomycin (Blenoxane), vinblastine (Valban), and DTIC (dacarbazine)

2. Three or four drugs may be given in intermittent or cyclical courses with periods off treatment to allow recovery from toxicities.

C. *Autologous or Allogeneic Bone Marrow Transplantation (see p. 791)*

Complications

1. Side effects of radiation or chemotherapy (see p. 102)
2. Dependent on location and extent of malignancy, but may include splenomegaly, hepatomegaly, thromboembolic complications, spinal cord compression

Nursing Assessment

1. Obtain health history, focusing on fatigue, fever, chills, night sweats, swollen lymph nodes.
2. Evaluate splenomegaly, hepatomegaly, lymphadenopathy.

Nursing Diagnoses

A. Impaired Tissue Integrity related to high-dose radiation therapy
B. Altered Oral Mucous Membranes related to high-dose radiation therapy

Nursing Interventions

A. *Maintaining Tissue Integrity*
1. Avoid rubbing, powders, deodorants, lotions, or ointments (unless prescribed) or application of heat/cold to treated area.
2. Encourage patient to keep treated area clean and dry, bathing area gently with tepid water and mild soap.
3. Encourage wearing loose-fitting clothes.
4. Advise patient to protect skin from exposure to sun, chlorine, temperature extremes.

B. *Preserving Oral and Gastrointestinal Tract Mucous Membranes*
1. Encourage frequent small meals, using bland and soft diet at mild temperatures.
2. Teach patient to avoid irritants such as alcohol, tobacco, spices, extreme food temperatures.
3. Administer or teach self-administration of pain medication or antiemetic before eating or drinking, if needed.
4. Encourage mouth care at least twice a day and after meals using soft toothbrush or toothette and mild mouth rinse.
5. Assess for ulcers, plaques, or discharge that may be indicative of superimposed infection.
6. For diarrhea switch to low-residue diet and administer antidiarrheals as ordered.

Patient Education/ Health Maintenance

1. Teach patient about risk of infection (see p. 768).

2. Teach patient how to take medications as ordered, their possible side effects and management.
3. Explain to patients that radiation therapy may cause sterility; men should be given opportunity for sperm banking before treatment; women may develop ovarian failure and require hormone replacement therapy.
4. Refer for information and support (see Table 24-4).
5. Reassure patient that fatigue will decrease after treatment is completed; encourage frequent naps and rest periods.

Evaluation

A. Skin intact without erythema or swelling
B. Oral mucosa intact, patient eating

◆ NON-HODGKIN'S LYMPHOMA

Non-Hodgkin's lymphomas are a group of malignancies of lymphoid tissue arising from T or B lymphocytes or their precursors.

Pathophysiology/Etiology

1. Association with defective or altered immune system; higher incidence in patients receiving immunosuppression for organ transplant, in HIV-positive individuals, and in presence of some viruses
2. Arise from malignant transformation of lymphocyte at some stage during development; level of differentiation and type of lymphocyte influences course of illness and prognosis.
3. Incidence rises steadily from about age 40.

Clinical Manifestations

1. Common symptoms include painless enlargement of lymph nodes (generally unilateral), fever, chills, night sweats, weight loss. Unlike Hodgkin's disease, is more likely to be advanced disease at presentation.
2. Wide variety of symptoms may occur if there is pulmonary involvement, superior vena cava obstruction, hepatic or bone involvement, etc.

Diagnostic Evaluation

1. Lymph node biopsy—to detect type
2. CBC, bone marrow aspirate and biopsy—to detect bone marrow involvement
3. X-rays, CT, and MRI to detect deep nodal involvement
4. Liver function tests, liver scan to detect liver involvement
5. Lymphangiogram—to evaluate lymph system involvement
6. Surgical staging (laparotomy with splenectomy, liver biopsy, multiple lymph node biopsies)

Management

1. Radiation therapy generally palliative, not curative

2. Chemotherapy: variety of regimens available including CHOP regimen of cyclophosphamide (Cytoxan), doxorubicin (Adriamycin), vincristine (Oncovin), and prednisone (Orasone) or BACOP regimen of bleomycin (Blenoxane), doxorubicin (Adriamycin), cyclophosphamide (Cytoxan), vincristine (Oncovin), and prednisone
3. Autologous or allogeneic BMT (see p. 791).

Complications

1. Complications of radiation therapy and chemotherapy (see p. 102)
2. Of disease: depends on location and extent of malignancy, but may include splenomegaly, hepatomegaly, thromboembolic complications, spinal cord compression

Nursing Assessment

1. Obtain health history, focusing on fatigue, fever, chills, night sweats, swollen lymph nodes, and history of illness or therapy causing immunosuppression.
2. Evaluate splenomegaly, hepatomegaly, lymphadenopathy.

Nursing Diagnosis

A. Risk for Infection related to altered immune response due to lymphoma and leukopenia caused by chemotherapy or radiation therapy

Nursing Interventions

A. *Minimizing Risk of Infection*
1. Care for patient in protected environment with strict handwashing observed.
2. Avoid invasive procedures, such as urinary catheterization, if possible.
3. Assess temperature and vital signs, breath sounds, level of consciousness, and skin and mucous membranes frequently for signs of infection.
4. Notify health care provider of fever greater than 38.3°C (101°F) or change in condition.
5. Obtain cultures of suspected infected sites or body fluids.

Patient Education/ Health Maintenance

1. Teach patient infection precautions (see p. 768).
2. Encourage frequent follow-up for monitoring of CBC and condition.

Evaluation

A. Remains afebrile with no signs or symptoms of infection

◆ MULTIPLE MYELOMA

Multiple myeloma is a malignant disorder of plasma cells.

Pathophysiology/Etiology

1. Etiology unknown; genetic and environmental factors, such as chronic exposure to low levels of ionizing radiation, may play a part.
2. Characterized by proliferation of neoplastic plasma cells derived from one B lymphocyte (clone) and producing a homogeneous immunoglobulin (M protein or Bence Jones protein) without any apparent antigenic stimulation.
3. Plasma cells produce osteoclast-activating factor (OAF) leading to extensive bone loss, severe pain, and pathologic fractures.
4. Abnormal immunoglobulin affects renal function, platelet function, resistance to infection, and may cause hyperviscosity of blood.
5. Generally affects the elderly (median age at diagnosis is 68 years) and is more common among African American men and women.

Clinical Manifestations

1. Constant, often severe bone pain due to bone lesions and pathologic fractures; sites commonly affected include thoracic and lumbar vertebrae, ribs, skull, pelvis, and proximal long bones.
2. Fatigue and weakness related to anemia due to crowding of marrow by plasma cells.
3. Proteinuria and renal insufficiency
4. Electrolyte disturbances including hypercalcemia (bone destruction), hyperuricemia (cell death, renal insufficiency)

Diagnostic Evaluation

1. Bone marrow aspiration and biopsy—demonstrate increased number and abnormal form of plasma cells.
2. CBC and blood smear—changes reflect anemia.
3. Urine and serum analysis for presence and quantity of abnormal immunoglobulin
4. Skeletal x-rays—osteolytic bone lesions

Management

1. Chemotherapy
   a. Oral melphalan (Alkeran) or cyclophosphamide (Cytoxan)
   b. Corticosteroids alone or in combination with chemotherapy
2. Plasmapheresis to treat hyperviscosity or bleeding
3. Radiation therapy for bone lesions
4. Other supportive care options
   a. Allopurinol (Zyloprim) and fluids to treat hyperuricemia
   b. Hemodialysis to manage renal failure
   c. Surgical stabilization and fixation of fractures
5. BMT in selected cases.

Complications

1. Pathologic fractures, spinal cord compression
2. Infections, particularly bacterial
3. Renal failure, pyelonephritis
4. Bleeding
5. Thromboembolic complications due to hyperviscosity
6. Patients with multiple myeloma have a median survival of 3 to 4 years.

Nursing Assessment

1. Obtain health history, focusing on pain, fatigue.
2. Evaluate for evidence of bone deformities and bone tenderness or pain.

Nursing Diagnoses

A. Pain (Bone) related to destruction of bone and possible pathologic fractures
B. Impaired Physical Mobility related to pain and possible fracture
C. Fear related to poor prognosis

Nursing Interventions

A. *Controlling Pain*
1. Assess for presence, location, intensity, and characteristics of pain.
2. Administer pharmacologic agents as ordered to control pain. Use adequate doses of regularly scheduled, around-the-clock analgesics.
3. Assess effectiveness of analgesics and adjust dosage or drug used as necessary to control pain.

B. *Promoting Mobility*
1. Encourage patient to wear back brace for lumbar lesion.
2. Recommend physical/occupational therapy consultation.
3. Discourage bed rest to prevent hypercalcemia but ensure safety of environment to prevent fractures.
4. Assist patient with measures to prevent injury and decrease risk of fractures. Advise avoidance of lifting and straining; use walker and other assistive devices as appropriate.

C. *Relieving Fear*
1. Develop trusting, supportive relationship with patient and significant others.
2. Encourage patient to discuss medical condition and prognosis with health care provider when patient is ready.
3. Ensure patient that you are available for support, to provide comfort measures, and answer questions.
4. Encourage use of patient's own support network, religious and community services, and national agencies (see Table 24-4).

D. *Monitoring for Complications*
1. Report any sudden, severe pain, especially of back which could indicate pathologic fracture.
2. Watch for nausea, drowsiness, confusion, polyuria, which could indicate hypercalcemia due to bony destruction or immobilization. Monitor serum calcium levels.
3. Check results of blood urea nitrogen and creatinine and urine protein tests to detect renal insufficiency, caused by nephrotoxicity of abnormal proteins in multiple myeloma.
4. Increase fluid intake, monitor intake and output, and weigh patient daily.

Patient Education/ Health Maintenance

1. Teach patient about risk of infection due to impaired antibody production (see p. 768).
2. Teach patient to take medications as prescribed and monitor for possible side effects; avoid aspirin and NSAIDs unless prescribed by physician because these drugs may interfere with platelet function.
3. Teach patient to minimize risk of fractures. Use proper body mechanics and assistive devices as appropriate; avoid bed rest, remain ambulatory.
4. Advise patient to report new onset of pain, new location, or sudden increase in pain intensity immediately. Report new onset or worsening of neurologic symptoms (eg, changes in sensation) immediately.
5. Encourage the patient to maintain high fluid intake (2–3 L/d) to avoid dehydration and prevent renal insufficiency; also not to fast before diagnostic tests.

Evaluation

A. States decreased pain
B. Ambulating without injury
C. Asking questions about disease, contacted support group

Bleeding Disorders

Bleeding disorders may be congenital or acquired and be caused by dysfunction in any phase of hemostasis (clot formation and dissolution). Bleeding disorders commonly seen in adults include thrombocytopenia, idiopathic thrombocytopenic purpura (ITP), disseminated intravascular coagulation (DIC), and von Willebrand's disease.

◆ THROMBOCYTOPENIA

Thrombocytopenia is a decrease in circulating platelet count (less than 100,000/mm³), and is the most common cause of bleeding disorders.

Pathophysiology/Etiology

A. *Classification by Etiology*
1. Decreased platelet production—infiltrative diseases of bone marrow, leukemia, aplastic anemia, myelofibrosis, myelosuppressive therapy, radiation therapy;

may include inherited disorders such as Fanconi's anemia and Wiskott-Aldrich syndrome.
2. Increased platelet destruction—infection, drug-induced, ITP, DIC
3. Abnormal distribution or sequestration in spleen
4. Dilutional thrombocytopenia—following hemorrhage, RBC transfusions

Clinical Manifestations

1. Usually asymptomatic
2. When platelet count drops below 20,000/mm^3:
   a. Petechiae occur spontaneously.
   b. Ecchymoses occur at sites of minor trauma (venipuncture, pressure).
   c. Bleeding may occur from mucosal surfaces, nose, gastrointestinal and genitourinary tracts, respiratory system, and within CNS.
   d. Menorrhagia is common.
   e. Excessive bleeding may occur after procedures (dental extractions, minor surgery, biopsies).

Diagnostic Evaluation

1. CBC with platelet count—decreased hemoglobin, hematocrit, platelets
2. Bleeding time, prothrombin time (PT), partial thromboplastin time (PTT)—prolonged

Management

1. Treat underlying cause.
2. Platelet transfusions
3. Steroids or IV immunoglobulins may be helpful in selected patients.

Complications

1. Severe blood loss or bleeding into vital organs may be life-threatening.

Nursing Assessment

1. Obtain health history, focusing on prior illnesses and episodes of bleeding, past surgical experiences, exposure to toxins or ionizing radiation, family history of bleeding.
2. Obtain complete list of current and recent medications (including over-the-counter preparations).
3. Perform complete physical examination for signs of bleeding.

Nursing Diagnosis

A. Risk for injury related to bleeding due to thrombocytopenia

Nursing Interventions

A. *Minimizing Bleeding*
1. Institute bleeding precautions—avoid use of plain razor, hard toothbrush or floss, intramuscular injections, tourniquets, rectal procedures or suppositories; administer stool softeners as necessary to prevent constipation; restrict activity and exercise when platelet count is less than 20,000/mm^3 or when there is active bleeding.
2. Monitor pad count/amount of saturation during menses; administer or teach self-administration of hormones to suppress menstruation as prescribed.
3. Administer blood products as ordered. Monitor for signs and symptoms of allergic reactions, anaphylaxis, and volume overload.
4. Evaluate all urine and stool for gross and occult blood.

Patient Education/ Health Maintenance

1. Teach patient bleeding precautions; also advise to avoid blowing nose, take only prescribed medications, avoid use of aspirin and NSAIDs, which may interfere with platelet function.
2. Demonstrate the use of direct, steady pressure at bleeding site if bleeding does develop.
3. Encourage routine follow-up for platelet counts.

Evaluation

A. Episodes of bleeding rapidly controlled

◆ IDIOPATHIC (IMMUNE) THROMBOCYTOPENIC PURPURA

Idiopathic thrombocytopenic purpura, or immune thrombocytopenic purpura, is an acute or chronic bleeding disorder resulting from immune destruction of platelets by antiplatelet antibodies.

Pathophysiology/Etiology

1. Autoantibodies of both IgG and IgM subclasses, directed against a platelet-associated antigen, lead to destruction of platelets in spleen, liver.
2. Acute disorder more common in childhood, typically following viral illness; has good prognosis with 80% to 90% recovering uneventfully.
3. Chronic disorder (more than 6-month course) most common at ages 20 to 40, more common in women.

Clinical Manifestations

1. Bruising, petechiae, bleeding from nares and gums, menorrhagia

Diagnostic Evaluation

1. Platelet count less than 20,000/mm³ (acute ITP); 30,000 to 70,000/mm³ (chronic ITP)
2. Assay for platelet autoantibodies sometimes helpful

Management

1. Supportive care: judicious use of platelet transfusions, control of bleeding
2. Corticosteroids, IV immunoglobulins (IVIG), danazol (Danocrine), azathioprine (Imuran), vincristine (Oncovin), vinblastine (Velban)
3. Splenectomy (see p. 761)

Complications

1. Severe blood loss or bleeding into vital organs may be life-threatening.

Nursing Assessment

1. Obtain history of bleeding episodes including bruising and petechiae, bleeding of gums, and heavy menses.
2. Perform physical examination for signs of bleeding.

Nursing Diagnosis

A. Risk for Injury related to bleeding due to thrombocytopenia

Nursing Interventions

A. *Minimizing Bleeding*
1. Institute bleeding precautions (see p. 766).
2. Monitor pad count/amount of saturation during menses; administer or teach self-administration of hormones to suppress menstruation as prescribed.
3. Administer blood products as ordered. Monitor for signs and symptoms of allergic reactions, anaphylaxis, and volume overload.
4. Evaluate all urine and stools for gross and occult blood.

Patient Education/ Health Maintenance

1. Teach patient bleeding precautions; also advise to avoid blowing nose, take only prescribed medications, avoid use of aspirin and NSAIDs, which may interfere with platelet function.
2. Demonstrate the use of direct, steady pressure at bleeding site if bleeding does develop.
3. Encourage routine follow-up for platelet counts.

Evaluation

A. Episodes of bleeding rapidly controlled

◆ DISSEMINATED INTRAVASCULAR COAGULATION

Disseminated intravascular coagulation is an acquired thrombotic and hemorrhagic syndrome in which there is abnormal activation of the clotting cascade and accelerated fibrinolysis. This results in widespread clotting in small vessels of the body with consumption of clotting factors and platelets, so that bleeding and thrombosis occur simultaneously.

Pathophysiology/Etiology

1. A syndrome arising in the presence of an underlying disorder or event:
   a. Overwhelming infections, particularly bacterial sepsis
   b. Obstetric complications—abruptio placentae, eclampsia, amniotic fluid embolism, retention of dead fetus
   c. Massive tissue injury—burns, trauma, fractures, major surgery, fat embolism
   d. Vascular and circulatory collapse, shock
   e. Hemolytic transfusion reaction
   f. Malignancy—particularly of lung, colon, stomach, pancreas

Clinical Manifestations

1. Signs of abnormal clotting: coolness and mottling of extremities; acrocyanosis (cold, mottled extremities with clear demarcation from normal tissue); dyspnea, adventitious breath sounds; altered mental status; acute renal failure; pain (eg, related to bowel infarction)
2. Signs of abnormal bleeding: oozing, bleeding from sites of procedures, IV catheter insertion sites, suture lines, mucous membranes, orifices; internal bleeding leading to changes in vital organ function, altered vital signs

Diagnostic Evaluation

1. Platelet count—diminished
2. PT and PTT—prolonged
3. Fibrinogen—decreased level
4. Fibrin split (degradation) products—increased level

Management

1. Treat underlying disorder.
2. Replacement therapy for serious hemorrhagic manifestations:
   a. Fresh frozen plasma—replaces clotting factors
   b. Platelet transfusions

c. Cryoprecipitate—replaces clotting factors
3. Supportive measures including fluid replacement, oxygenation, maintenance of blood pressure and renal perfusion
4. Heparin therapy (controversial)—inhibits clotting component of DIC

Complications

1. Thromboembolic—pulmonary embolism, cerebral, myocardial, splenic or bowel infarction, acute renal failure, tissue necrosis or gangrene
2. Hemorrhagic—cerebral hemorrhage is most common cause of death in DIC.

Nursing Assessment

1. Be aware that all seriously ill patients are at risk—monitor condition closely.
2. Assess for signs of bleeding and thrombosis, including chest pain, shortness of breath, hematuria, abdominal pain, headache, numbness and coolness of an extremity.

Nursing Diagnoses

A. Risk for Injury related to bleeding due to thrombocytopenia
B. Altered Tissue Perfusion (All Tissues) related to ischemia due to microthrombi formation

Nursing Interventions

A. *Minimizing Bleeding*
1. Institute bleeding precautions (see p. 766).
2. Monitor pad count/amount of saturation during menses; administer or teach self-administration of hormones to suppress menstruation as prescribed.
3. Administer blood products as ordered. Monitor for signs and symptoms of allergic reactions, anaphylaxis, and volume overload.
4. Avoid dislodging clots. Apply pressure to sites of bleeding for at least 20 minutes, use topical hemostatic agents. Use tape cautiously.
5. Maintain bed rest during bleeding episode.
6. If internal bleeding is suspected, assess bowel sounds and abdominal girth.
7. Evaluate fluid status and bleeding by frequent measurement of vital signs, central venous pressure, intake and output.

B. *Promoting Tissue Perfusion*
1. Keep patient warm.
2. Avoid vasoconstrictive agents (systemic or topical).
3. Change patient's position frequently and perform range of motion exercises.
4. Monitor electrocardiogram and laboratory tests for dysfunction of vital organs caused by ischemia—arrhythmias, abnormal arterial blood gases, increased blood urea nitrogen and creatinine, etc.

5. Monitor for vascular occlusion of brain (decreased level of consciousness, sensory and motor deficits, seizures, coma); eyes (visual deficits); bone (bone pain); pulmonary vasculature (chest pain, shortness of breath, tachycardia); extremity (cold, mottling, numbness); coronary arteries (chest pain, arrhythmias); bowel (pain, tenderness, decreased bowel sounds). Report immediately.

Patient Education/ Health Maintenance

1. Explanation of syndrome and its management is needed by patient and family members as part of reassurance and support during this critical illness.

Evaluation

A. Episodes of bleeding rapidly controlled
B. Alert, vital signs stable, urine output adequate, no complaints of chest pain or shortness of breath

◆ VON WILLEBRAND'S DISEASE

Inherited (autosomal dominant) or acquired bleeding disorder characterized by decreased level of von Willebrand factor and prolonged bleeding time.

Pathophysiology/Etiology

1. von Willebrand factor synthesized in vascular endothelium, megakaryocytes and platelets; enhances platelet adhesion as first step in clot formation, also acts as carrier of factor VIII in blood.
2. von Willebrand's is most common inherited bleeding disorder; includes multiple subtypes with varying severity
3. Acquired form is rare, generally appears late in life, often in association with lymphoma, leukemia, multiple myeloma, or autoimmune disorder.

Clinical Manifestations

1. Mucosal and cutaneous bleeding (eg, bruising, gingival bleeding, epistaxis, menorrhagia)
2. Prolonged bleeding from cuts or after dental and surgical procedures

Diagnostic Evaluation

1. Bleeding time—prolonged
2. von Willebrand's factor—decreased
3. Factor VIII—generally decreased

Management

1. Replacement of factor VIII via infusions of cryoprecipitate
2. Antifibrinolytic medication (Amicar) to stabilize clot formation before dental procedures and minor surgery
3. Desmopressin (DDAVP), a synthetic analogue of vasopressin, may be used to manage mild to moderate bleeding

Complications

1. Severe blood loss or bleeding into vital organs may be life-threatening.

Nursing Assessment

1. Obtain history of bleeding episodes such as menstrual flow.
2. Perform physical examination for signs of bleeding.

Nursing Diagnosis

A. Risk for Injury related to bleeding due to decreased level of factor VIII

Nursing Interventions

A. *Minimizing Bleeding*
1. Institute bleeding precautions—avoid use of plain razor, hard toothbrush or floss, intramuscular injections, tourniquets, rectal procedures or suppositories; administer stool softeners as necessary to prevent constipation; restrict activity and exercise when platelet count less than $20,000/mm^3$ or when there is active bleeding.
2. Monitor pad count/amount of saturation during menses; administer or teach self-administration of hormones to suppress menstruation as prescribed.
3. Administer blood products as ordered. Monitor for signs and symptoms of allergic reactions, anaphylaxis, and volume overload.

Patient Education/ Health Maintenance

1. Teach patient bleeding precautions; also advise to avoid blowing nose, take only prescribed medications, avoid use of aspirin and NSAIDs, which may interfere with platelet function.
2. Demonstrate the use of direct, steady pressure at bleeding site if bleeding does develop.
3. Encourage routine follow-up for platelet counts.

Evaluation

A. Episodes of bleeding rapidly controlled

Selected References

Acevedo, M. (1992). Blood dyscrasias: Polycythemia, idiopathic thrombocytopenic purpura, and thrombotic thrombocytopenic purpura. *Journal of Intravenous Nursing,* 15(1), 52-57.

Alkire, K., & Collingwood, J. (1990). Physiology of blood and bone marrow. *Seminars in Oncology Nursing,* 6(2), 99-108.

Bick, R. L. (1992). *Disorders of thrombosis and hemostasis: Clinical and laboratory practice.* Chicago: ASCP Press.

Bick, R. L. (1992). Disseminated intravascular coagulation. *Hematology/ Oncology Clinics of North America,* 6(6), 1259-1280.

Cardisco, M. E. (1994). Fighting DIC. *RN,* 57 (8), 36-40.

Collins, P. M. (1990). Diagnosis and treatment of chronic leukemia. *Seminars in Oncology Nursing,* 6(1), 31-43.

Groenwald, S. L., Frogge, M. H., Goodman, M., & Yarbro, C. H. (Eds.). (1993). *Cancer nursing: Principles and practice* (3rd ed.). Boston: Jones and Bartlett.

Holmberg, L. & Nilsson, I. M. (1992). von Willebrand's disease. *European Journal of Haematology,* 48, 127-141.

Huston, C. J. (1994). Disseminated intravascular coagulation. *AJN,* 94(8), 51.

Kirchner, J. T. (1992). Acute and chronic immune thrombocytopenic purpura: Disorders that differ in more than duration. *Postgraduate Medicine,* 92(6), 112-126.

Rostad, M. E. (1991). Current strategies for managing myelosuppression in patients with cancer. *Oncology Nursing Forum* (Suppl.) 18(2), 7-15.

Rubin, R. N., & Colman, R. W. (1992). Disseminated intravascular coagulation: Approach to treatment. *Drugs,* 44(6), 963-971.

Shivnan, J. C., Ohly, K. V., & Hanson, J. (1995). Bone marrow transplantation. Nolan, M, & Augustine, S. (eds.) Transplantation nursing. Norwalk, CT: Appleton-Lange, 239-289.

Sitton, E. (1992). Early and late radiation-induced skin alterations. Part I: Mechanisms of skin changes. *Oncology Nursing Forum,* 19(5), 801-807.

Sitton, E. (1992). Early and late radiation-induced skin alterations. Part II: Nursing care of irradiated skin. *Oncology Nursing Forum,* 19(6), 907-912.

Timmerman, P. R. (1993). Intravenous immunoglobulin in oncology nursing practice. *Oncology Nursing Forum,* 20(1), 69-75.

Whedon, M. B. (Ed.). (1991). *Bone marrow transplantation: Principles, practice, and nursing insights.* Boston: Jones and Bartlett.

Wright, J. E., & Shelton, B. K. (Eds.). (1993). *Desk reference for critical care nursing.* Boston: Jones and Bartlett.

Yeager, K. A., & Miaskowski, C. (1994). Advances in understanding the mechanisms and management of acute myelogenous leukemia. *Oncology Nursing Forum,* 21(3), 541-548.

CHAPTER 25

Transfusion Therapy and Bone Marrow Transplantation

Transfusion Therapy

◆ PRINCIPLES OF TRANSFUSION THERAPY

Because of the potentially life-threatening consequences of ABO incompatibility and the recent safety concerns about disease transmission through blood products, transfusion therapy has been limited to occasions when it is absolutely necessary. In addition, various transfusion options and stringent screening techniques before transfusion have been instituted. Blood product procurement, storage, preparation, and testing are regulated by the Food and Drug Administration, the American Association of Blood Banks, and the Joint Commission on Accreditation of Healthcare Organizations.

Blood Compatibility

A. **Antigens**
1. The surface membrane of the red blood cell (RBC) is characterized by the presence or absence of glycoproteins known as antigens.
2. More than 400 different antigens have been identified on the RBC membrane.
3. The clinically significant antigens number less than a dozen, and of these, only two antigenic systems (ABO and Rh) require routine prospective matching before the transfusion.
4. The ABO blood group system is clinically the most significant because A and B antigens elicit the strongest immune response.
5. The presence or absence of A and B antigens on the RBC membrane determines the individual's ABO group (Table 25-1). The ability to make A or B antigens is inherited.
6. Antibody formation in the absence of specific exposure to antigen is unique to the ABO system. Antibody directed against the missing antigen(s) will be produced by the age of 3 months in neonates.

B. **Antibodies**
1. Antibodies (or immunoglobulins) are proteins produced by B lymphocytes and consisting of two light and two heavy chains, forming a Y shape.

2. Antibodies generally have a high degree of specificity, interacting only with the antigen that stimulated their production.
3. The five classes of immunoglobulins are determined by differences in their heavy chains: IgG, IgA, IgM, IgD, IgE.
4. The interaction of antibodies and antigens triggers an immune response, the humoral immune response.
5. Antibodies against the A and B antigens are large IgM molecules. When they interact with and coat the A and B antigens on the RBC surface, the antibody/cell complexes clump together (agglutinate).
6. Antibody/cell complexes also activate the complement cascade, resulting in the release of numerous active substances and RBC lysis. The large antibody/cell complexes also become trapped in capillaries, where they may cause thrombotic complications to vital organs, and in the reticuloendothelial system, where they are removed from circulation by the spleen.
7. The extent of the humoral response elicited by anti-A and anti-B interaction with A and B antigens depends on the quantity of antibody and antigen.

C. **Other Red Blood Cell Antigens**
1. Non-ABO RBC antigen–antibody reactions usually do not produce powerful immediate hemolytic reactions, but several do have clinical significance.
2. After A and B, D is the most immunogenic antigen. It is part of the Rhesus system, which includes C, D, and E antigens.
   a. D (Rh)-negative individuals do not develop anti-D in the absence of specific exposure, but there is a high incidence of antibody development (alloimmunization) after exposure to D.
   b. Two common methods of sensitization to these RBC antigens are by transfusion or fetomaternal hemorrhage during pregnancy and delivery.
   c. Anti-D can complicate future transfusions and pregnancies. For the D (Rh)-negative individual, exposure to D should be avoided by the use of Rh-negative blood products. In the case of Rh-negative mother and Rh-positive fetus, exposure to D can be treated using Rh immunoglobulin, which will prevent anti-D formation.
   d. Exposure to RBC antigens from other antigenic systems (such as Lewis, Kidd, or Duffy) may also cause alloimmunization, which may become clinically significant in individuals receiving multiple blood products over long periods of time.

TABLE 25-1   Blood Group Antigens and Antibodies of ABO System

Blood Group	Antigen on RBC	Antibody in Plasma	Approximate Frequency of Occurrence in Population
A	A	anti-B	45%
B	B	anti-A	8%
AB	A and B	none	3%
O	none	anti-A and anti-B	44%

Blood Transfusion Options

A. Autologous Transfusion
1. Before elective procedures, the patient may donate blood to be set aside for later transfusion.
2. Autologous RBCs can also be salvaged during some surgical procedures or after trauma-induced hemorrhage by use of automated "cell-saver" devices or manual suction equipment.
3. Autologous blood products must be clearly labeled and identified.
4. Autologous transfusion eliminates the risks of alloimmunization, immune-mediated transfusion reactions, and transmission of disease, making it the safest transfusion choice.

NURSING ALERT: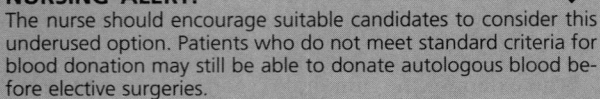
The nurse should encourage suitable candidates to consider this underused option. Patients who do not meet standard criteria for blood donation may still be able to donate autologous blood before elective surgeries.

B. Homologous Transfusion
1. By far the most common option, volunteer donors' blood products are assigned randomly to patients.
2. Before donation, volunteer donors receive information about the process, potential adverse reactions, tests that will be performed on donated blood, postdonation instructions, and education regarding risk for human immunodeficiency virus (HIV) infection and signs and symptoms.
3. Donors are screened against eligibility criteria designed to protect both donor and recipient (Table 25-2).

C. Directed Transfusion
1. In directed transfusion, blood products are donated by an individual for transfusion to a specified recipient.
2. This option may be used in certain circumstances (eg, a parent providing sole transfusion support for a child), but in general there is no evidence that directed donation reduces transfusion risks.

Blood Product Screening

A. Serologic Testing
1. Routine laboratory testing is performed to assess the compatibility of a particular blood product with the re-

cipient before release of the blood product from the blood bank.
   a. ABO group and Rh type: determines the presence of A, B, and D antigens on the surface of the patient's RBCs.
   b. Direct Coombs' test: determines the presence of antibody attached to the patient's RBCs.
   c. Crossmatch (compatibility test): detects agglutination of donor RBCs caused by antibodies in the patient's serum.
   d. Indirect Coombs' test: identifies the presence of lower molecular weight antibodies (IgG) directed against blood group antigens.

B. Screening for Infectious Diseases
1. Routine laboratory testing is performed to identify antigens or antibodies in donor blood that may indicate prior exposure to specific blood-borne diseases.
2. Such testing supplements other principles of donation designed to decrease the risk of disease transmission via blood products, including the use of volunteer donors, the exclusion of high-risk populations, and the screening of donors via health and social history.
3. Specific conditions screened for include:
   a. Hepatitis: tests for the presence of hepatitis B surface antigen and most recently, hepatitis C, the most common non-A, non-B hepatitis.
   b. HIV: tests for the presence of antibody against HIV, which indicates prior exposure to the virus.
      (1) All blood products in the United States have been screened since the test first became available in 1985.
      (2) Because antibody to the virus is not produced until at least 6 weeks after exposure, donor screening and exclusion of high-risk groups (eg, homosexual men, intravenous [IV] drug abusers, prostitutes, and sexual partners of

TABLE 25-2   General Blood Donor Eligibility Criteria

Age	Generally 17–66 y
Weight	Minimum 110 lb
Vital Signs	Afebrile, normotensive, pulse 50–100
Hemoglobin	Lower limit for females 12.5 g/dL, for males 13.5 g/dL.
History	Exposure to AIDS evaluated; high-risk groups deferred. International travel to malarial areas is cause for deferral. Pregnancy, recent (<6 wk) delivery, or blood transfusion during prior 6 mo is cause for temporary deferral. History of any hepatitis is cause for deferral.
Immunizations	Attenuated viral vaccines: 2-wk deferral. Rubella vaccine: 1 mo deferral. Rabies vaccine: 1-y deferral. Killed vaccines or toxoids: acceptable if symptom free.
Illnesses	Positive HIV test, diseases of heart, lungs, or liver, abnormal bleeding or history of cancer are causes for deferral.

high-risk individuals) remain important parts of preventing transmission of HIV via blood products.

   (3) A low risk of HIV transmission (estimated to be 1/100,000 units of blood) remains.

c. Cytomegalovirus (CMV): tests for the presence of antibody against CMV

   (1) Approximately 50% of blood donors have been exposed to CMV and 10% carry CMV virus in white blood cells (WBCs).

   (2) Patients with impaired immune function (eg, bone marrow and organ transplant recipients, premature babies) are at risk for CMV infection from transfused blood.

d. Syphilis: tests for the presence of antibody against the spirochete

e. Bacteria: Contamination of blood products with bacteria may occur during and after collection of blood. This risk is managed by maintenance of sterile technique during phlebotomy and blood processing procedures, correct storage techniques, visual inspection of blood products, and limitation on shelf life.

◆ ADMINISTRATION OF WHOLE BLOOD AND BLOOD COMPONENTS

Whole blood and blood components are administered to increase the amount of oxygen being delivered to the tissues and organs, to prevent or stop bleeding due to platelet defects or deficiencies or coagulation abnormalities, and to combat infection due to decreased or defective WBCs or antibodies (see Procedure Guidelines 25-1).

General Considerations

1. A unit of whole blood is usually separated into its various component parts shortly after collection.
2. Less than 3% of the blood collected nationwide is transfused as whole blood.
3. The use of blood components conserves the limited supply of blood, provides optimal therapeutic benefit, and reduces the risk of circulatory overload.

Whole Blood

A. Description
1. Consists of RBCs, plasma, plasma proteins, and about 60 mL anticoagulant/preservative solution in a total volume of about 500 mL.
2. Indications include acute, massive blood loss of greater than 1,000 mL, requiring the oxygen-carrying properties of RBCs as well as the volume expansion provided by plasma. In general, even acute loss of as much as one-third of a patient's total blood volume (1,000–1,200 mL) can be safely and rapidly replaced with crystalline or colloidal solutions.

B. Nursing/Patient Care Considerations
1. For rapid infusions of large volumes of whole blood, additional steps may be taken to deliver product rapidly and safely.

a. A small-pore (20–40 μm) filter may be used to remove microaggregates (platelets, WBCs) that have been identified in the lungs of massively transfused patients.

b. An approved blood warmer may be indicated to prevent hypothermia and cardiac arrhythmias associated with the rapid infusion of refrigerated solutions.

c. Electromechanical infusion devices to deliver blood at high flow rates can hemolyze RBCs and should be used with caution.

2. Observe closely for the most common acute complication associated with whole blood transfusion—circulatory overload (rise in venous pressure, distended neck veins, dyspnea, cough, crackles at bases of lungs).

3. Reduce the risk of hemolytic reactions by meticulously confirming ABO and Rh compatibility and patient identification before infusion (Table 25-3).

TABLE 25-3   ABO & Rh Compatibility Chart

WHOLE BLOOD

Recipient	A	B	O	AB	Rh Positive	Rh Negative
A	●					
B		●				
O			●			
AB				●		
Rh Positive					●	●
Rh Negative						●

RED BLOOD CELLS

Recipient	A	B	O	AB	Rh Positive	Rh Negative
A	●		●			
B		●	●			
O			●			
AB	●	●	●	●		
Rh Positive					●	●
Rh Negative						●

PLASMA

Recipient	A	B	O	AB	Rh Positive	Rh Negative
A	●			●		
B		●		●		
O	●	●	●	●		
AB				●		
Rh Positive					●	●
Rh Negative					●	●

The chart above identifies ABO and Rh compatibility when transfusing whole blood, red blood cells, and plasma. Components suspended in plasma, such as platelets and cryoprecipitate, usually follow plasma compatibility rules if the total volume exceeds 120 mL for an adult patient.

Packed Red Blood Cells

A. Description
1. Consist primarily of RBCs, a small amount of plasma, and about 100 mL anticoagulant/preservative solution in a total volume of about 250 to 300 mL/unit.
2. Packed RBCs are typically contaminated with WBCs that may increase the risk of minor transfusion reactions and alloimmunization. For patients receiving multiple blood products (eg, patients with leukemia, aplastic anemia), packed RBCs may be further manipulated to remove WBCs by washing or freezing the product in the blood bank or by the use of small-pore (20–40 μm) filters during administration.
3. Indications include restoration or maintenance of adequate organ oxygenation with minimal expansion of blood volume.
4. Dosage: average adult dose administered is 2 units; pediatric doses are generally calculated as 5 to 15 mL/kg.

B. Nursing/Patient Care Considerations
1. Infuse at the prescribed rate. Generally, a unit can be given to an adult in 90 to 120 minutes. Pediatric patients are usually transfused at a rate of 2 to 5 mL/kg per hour.
2. To reduce the risk of bacterial contamination and sepsis, RBCs must be transfused within 4 hours of leaving the blood bank.
3. Observe closely (particularly during first 15–30 minutes) for the most common acute complications associated with packed RBCs, allergic and febrile transfusion reactions. Signs and symptoms of the more serious, but rare, hemolytic transfusion reaction are usually manifested during infusion of the first 50 mL.

Platelet Concentrates

A. Description
1. Consist of platelets suspended in plasma. Products vary according to the number of units (each unit is a minimum of 5.5×10^{10} platelets) and the volume of plasma (50–400 mL).
2. Platelets may be obtained by centrifuging multiple units of whole blood and expressing off the platelet-rich plasma (multiple-donor platelets) or from a single volunteer platelet donor using automated cell separation techniques (apheresis). The use of single donor products decreases the number of donor exposures, thus decreasing the risk of alloimmunization and transfusion-transmitted disease.
3. Patients may become alloimmunized to human leukocyte antigens (HLA) through exposure to multiple platelet products. Apheresis products from HLA-matched platelet donors may be necessary. However, HLA-matched transfusions are often difficult to obtain due to the tremendous number of possible HLA combinations in the population.
4. Indications include prevention or resolution of hemorrhage in patients with thrombocytopenia or platelet dysfunction.
5. Dosage: Average dose is generally 1 unit of platelets for each 10 kg of body weight; however, patients who are actively bleeding or undergoing surgical procedures may require more.

B. Nursing/Patient Care Considerations
1. Infuse at the rate prescribed. Generally, the infusion can be completed within 20 to 60 minutes, depending on total volume.
2. Observe closely for the most common acute complications associated with platelet transfusions, allergic and febrile transfusion reactions.

Plasma (Fresh or Fresh Frozen)

A. Description
1. Consists of water (91%), plasma proteins including essential clotting factors (7%), and carbohydrates (2%). Each unit is the volume removed from a unit of whole blood (200–250 mL).
2. May be stored in a liquid state or frozen within 6 hours of collection.
3. Indications include treatment of blood loss or blood clotting disorders related to liver disease and failure, disseminated intravascular coagulation (DIC), over-anticoagulation with warfarin (Coumadin), all congenital or acquired clotting factor deficiencies, and dilutional coagulopathy resulting from massive blood replacement. Storage in liquid state results in the loss of labile clotting factors V and VIII, so that only plasma that has been fresh frozen can be used to treat factor V and VIII deficiencies.
4. Dosage: depends on clinical situation and assessment of prothrombin time (PT), partial thromboplastin time (PTT), or specific factor assays.

B. Nursing/Patient Care Considerations
1. Infuse at the rate prescribed. Generally, the infusion can be completed within 15 to 30 minutes, depending on total volume.
2. Observe closely for the most common acute complication associated with plasma infusion, volume overload.

Cryoprecipitate

A. Description
1. Consists of certain clotting factors suspended in 10 to 20 mL plasma. Each unit contains approximately 80 to 120 units of factor VIII (antihemophilic and von Willebrand factors), 250 mg fibrinogen, and 20% to 30% of the factor XIII present in a unit of whole blood.
2. Indications include correction of deficiencies of factor VIII (ie, hemophilia A and von Willebrand's disease), factor XIII, and fibrinogen (ie, DIC)
3. Dosage: Adult dosage is generally 10 units, which may be repeated every 8 to 12 hours until the deficiency is corrected or until hemostasis is achieved.

B. Nursing/Patient Care Considerations
1. Infuse at the rate prescribed. Generally, the infusion can be completed within 3 to 15 minutes.

Fractionated Plasma Products

A. Description
1. A variety of highly concentrated plasma protein products are commercially prepared by pooling thousands of single plasma units and extracting the desired protein. Most techniques involve heat or

chemical treatments, which eliminate the risk of transmitting blood-borne viruses such as hepatitis B and HIV.

2. Colloid solutions provide volume expansion in situations where crystalloid solutions are not adequate, such as therapeutic plasma exchange, shock, and massive hemorrhage. They may also be used in the treatment of acute liver failure, burns, and hemolytic disease of the newborn.
   a. Albumin is available as a 5% solution, which is oncotically equivalent to plasma, and a concentrated 25% solution.
   b. Plasma protein fraction (PPF) is available as a 5% solution. Rapid infusion of PPF has been associated with hypotension.
   c. Albumin and PPF are pasteurized and carry no risk of viral disease. They do not contain preservatives and should be used immediately after opening.
3. Immune serum globulins (ISGs) are concentrated aqueous solutions of gamma globulin containing high titers of antibody.
   a. Must be administered by deep intramuscular injection.
   b. Nonspecific ISG is prepared from random donor plasma and is used to increase gamma globulin levels and enhance general immune response in mild inherited or acquired immune disorders such as hypogammaglobulinemia.
   c. Specific ISG is prepared from donors who have high antibody titers to known antigens and is used to treat specific disorders or conditions. Hepatitis B immunoglobulin, varicella zoster immunoglobulin, and Rh immunoglobulin are examples of specific ISGs.
   d. ISGs carry no risk of hepatitis B, HIV, or other blood-borne infections.
   e. Problems associated with use include pain at the injection site, limitations on volume administered, loss of IgG into extravascular tissue, or by degradation at the injection site.
4. Intravenous immunoglobulins (IVIGs) are aqueous solutions of immunoglobulins at a higher concentration and given in larger volumes than ISGs.
   a. Like ISGs, they may be nonspecific or specific.
   b. Indications include chronic replacement therapy in patients with congenital or acquired immunodeficiency syndromes, acute autoimmune disorders such as immune thrombocytopenic purpura (ITP), and the treatment of chronic lymphocytic leukemia (CLL). There are also numerous investigational uses, such as Guillain-Barre syndrome, myasthenia gravis, rheumatoid arthritis, and viral infections such as CMV, adenovirus, and influenza.
   c. IVIGs do not appear to transmit HIV, but have been reported to transmit non-A, non-B hepatitis.
   d. Administration of IVIG should be closely monitored due to the possibility of anaphylactic reactions. Dosage and rate of infusion depend on the manufacturer's formulation.
5. Factor VIII concentrate is a lyophilized concentrate used to treat moderate to severe hemophilia A and severe von Willebrand's disease.
6. Factor IX concentrate is a lyophilized concentrate used to treat factor IX deficiency (Christmas disease).

B. *Nursing/Patient Care Considerations*
1. Product may be distributed by the pharmacy rather than the blood bank.
2. Check order and product insert to ensure proper dosage and administration route.

Granulocyte Concentrates

A. *Description*
1. Consist of a minimum of 1×10^{10} granulocytes, variable amounts of lymphocytes (usually less than 10% of the total number of WBCs), 6 to 10 units of platelets, 30 to 50 mL RBCs, and 200 to 400 mL plasma.
2. Obtained via apheresis, generally of multiple donors.
3. Indications include treatment of life-threatening bacterial or fungal infection unresponsive to other therapy in patient with severe neutropenia.
4. Dosage: generally 1 unit daily for approximately 5 to 10 days, discontinuing if no therapeutic response

B. *Nursing/Patient Care Considerations*
1. Transfuse granulocytes as soon as they are available. WBCs have a short survival time, and therapeutic benefit is directly related to dose and viability.
2. Premedicate per order to prevent adverse reactions, generally with antihistamine and acetaminophen. Steroids or meperidine may also be required.
3. Begin the transfusion slowly and increase to the rate prescribed and as tolerated. The recommended length of infusion is 1 to 2 hours.
4. Observe the patient closely throughout the transfusion for signs and symptoms of febrile, allergic, and anaphylactic reactions, which may be severe. Have emergency medications and equipment readily available.
5. Do not administer amphotericin B (Fungizone) immediately before or after granulocyte transfusion because pulmonary insufficiency has been reported with concurrent administration of amphotericin B and granulocytes. Many institutions recommend a 4-hour gap to avoid this risk.

Modified Blood Products

A. *Purpose*
1. To reduce the risk of specific transfusion-related complications, blood products may receive further processing or treatment
   a. Leukocytes are removed from blood products through filtration, washing, and freezing to reduce the risk of febrile, nonhemolytic transfusion reactions and alloimmunization to HLA antigens.
   b. Function and proliferation of donor lymphocytes are inhibited by irradiation, to decrease the risk of posttransfusion graft-versus-host disease (GVHD) in immunocompromised patients.

B. *Methods*
1. Filtration
   a. Standard filters (170 μm) effectively remove gross fibrin clots.

b. Microaggregate filters (approximately 40 μm) remove microscopic aggregates of fibrin, platelets, and leukocytes that accumulate in RBC products during storage. Their use is recommended during rapid, massive transfusion of whole blood or packed RBCs to prevent pulmonary complications. They may also decrease the incidence of febrile transfusion reactions by removing many of the leukocytes present.

c. Special leukocyte-depletion filters have been developed for use with platelet products that remove 80% to 95% of leukocytes and retain 80% of the platelets.

d. A product may be filtered before release from the blood bank, but more commonly is released with the appropriate filter that must be attached to the standard infusion set at the bedside per manufacturer's or blood bank's instructions.

2. Washing
   a. Washing RBCs or platelets with a normal saline solution removes 80% to 95% of the WBCs and virtually all of the plasma to reduce the incidence of febrile, nonhemolytic transfusion reactions.
   b. Washing requires an additional hour of processing time, and the shelf life of the product is reduced to 24 hours after this additional manipulation.

3. Freezing
   a. RBCs can be frozen within 7 days of blood collection, and then remain viable for 7 to 10 years.
   b. Removal of the hypertonic freezing preservative (glycerol) before transfusion eliminates all of the plasma and 99% of WBCs.
   c. Thawing and deglycerolization of RBCs requires an additional 90 minutes of preparation time and reduces shelf life to 24 hours after this additional manipulation.
   d. Freezing is also an effective method of storing rare blood types and autologous RBCs.

4. Irradiation
   a. Exposure of blood products to a measured amount of gamma irradiation inhibits lymphocyte function and proliferation without damaging RBCs, platelets, or granulocytes. This eliminates the ability of transfused lymphocytes to engraft in the immunocompromised transfusion recipient and the accompanying risk of posttransfusion GVHD.
   b. Patients at risk for posttransfusion GVHD include bone marrow and peripheral stem cell transplant recipients, premature neonates, and patients with congenital immunodeficiency disorders, Hodgkin's disease, and non-Hodgkin's lymphoma.

PROCEDURE GUIDELINES 25-1 ◆ Administering Blood/Blood Components

EQUIPMENT

Tourniquet
Iodine-containing skin antiseptic
Needle or venous catheter
Y-type blood infusion set

170-micron filter
Normal saline
Blood product as described

PROCEDURE	NURSING ACTION	RATIONALE

PREPARATORY PHASE

NURSING ACTION	RATIONALE
1. Inform the patient of the procedure, blood product to be given, approximate length of time, and desired outcome of transfusion.	1. Instruct the patient to report unusual symptoms immediately.
2. Obtain and record baseline vital signs.	2. If the patient's clinical status permits, delay transfusion if baseline temperature is greater than 38.5°C (101.7°).
3. Prepare infusion site. Select a large vein that allows patient some degree of mobility. Start the prescribed intravenous infusion.	3. Antecubital veins are not recommended for lengthy infusions. Prolonged restriction of arm movement is uncomfortable and inconvenient for the patient. In the event of an acute reaction, the intravenous catheter should be maintained with normal saline.

NURSING ALERT:
Crystalloid solutions other than 0.9% saline and all medications are incompatible with blood products. They may cause agglutination and/or hemolysis.

NURSING ACTION	RATIONALE
4. Obtain blood product from blood bank. Inspect for abnormal color, cloudiness, clots, and excess air. Read instructions on the product label regarding storage and infusion. Check expiration date.	4. Platelets are normally cloudy. If the transfusion cannot begin immediately, return product to blood bank. Blood out of proper storage for more than 30 min (above 10°C [50°F]) cannot be reissued. Never store blood in unauthorized refrigerators, such as those on the nursing unit.

PROCEDURE (cont'd)	NURSING ACTION	RATIONALE

NURSING ACTION

5. Verify patient identification
   a. Ask the patient to state his full name and compare with name on the wrist band. If the patient is unable to state his name, verify identity with an individual familiar with the patient.
   b. Compare the name and ID number on the wristband with the bag tag, transfusion form, and medical order.
   c. Confirm ABO and Rh compatibility by comparing the bag label, bag tag, medical record, and/or transfusion form.
   d. Check bag labels for expiration date and satisfactory serologic testing.

PERFORMANCE PHASE

1. Start infusion slowly (ie, 2 mL/min). Remain at bedside 15–30 min. If there are no signs of an adverse reaction, increase flow to the prescribed rate.

2. Observe the patient closely and check vital signs at least hourly until 1 h after transfusion. Report signs and symptoms of adverse reaction to physician immediately.
3. Record the following information on the patient's chart:
   a. Time and names of persons starting and ending the transfusion
   b. Names of individuals verifying patient ID
   c. Unique product identification number

   d. Product and volume infused
   e. Immediate response—for example, ''no apparent reaction''

RATIONALE

5. The majority of acute fatal transfusion reactions are caused by clerical errors. Patient and product verification is the single most important function of the nurse. It is strongly recommended that two qualified individuals perform this task. Do not proceed with the transfusion if there is any discrepancy. Contact the blood bank immediately.

1. Institutional policy may vary regarding flow rates and patient monitoring.
   Signs of a severe transfusion reaction (ie, acute hemolytic, anaphylactic) are usually manifested during infusion of the initial 50–100 mL.
2. Acute reactions may occur at any time during the transfusion.

3. Facts relating to the transfusion should be charted exactly.

   c. It must be possible to trace each transfusion product to the original blood donor.

◆ TRANSFUSION REACTIONS

Every transfusion of blood or blood components can result in an adverse reaction. Reactions can be placed into two general categories: acute and delayed.

Acute Reactions

1. Acute reactions may occur during the infusion or within minutes to hours after the blood product has been infused.
2. Acute reactions include allergic, febrile, septic, and hemolytic reactions and circulatory overload.
3. Because reactions may exhibit similar clinical manifestations, every symptom should be considered potentially serious and the transfusion discontinued until the cause is determined.
4. When a reaction is suspected, the health care provider should be notified immediately and blood bags with tubing from all products recently transfused should be returned to the blood bank for evaluation.
5. The following samples should also be obtained if an acute reaction is suspected.
   a. A clotted blood sample to examine serum for hemoglobin and confirm RBC group and type
   b. An anticoagulated blood sample for a direct Coombs' test to determine the presence of antibody on the RBCs
   c. The first voided urine sample to test for hemoglobinuria

6. Precautions must be taken to avoid the hemolysis of RBCs during venipuncture and sample collection because this could lead to invalid test results. Whenever possible, blood samples should be drawn from a fresh venipuncture and not from existing needles or catheters.
7. If the only symptoms are those resulting from a mild allergic reaction (eg, urticaria), extensive evaluation may not be necessary. In the event of a severe reaction (eg, hypotension, tachypnea), more tests may be required to determine the cause of the reaction.
8. Causes, clinical manifestations, management, and prevention of acute reactions are summarized in Table 25-4.

Delayed Reactions

1. Delayed reactions occur days to years after the transfusion.
2. Delayed reactions include delayed hemolytic reactions, iron overload (hemosiderosis), GVHD, infectious diseases (eg, hepatitis B, hepatitis C, CMV, Epstein-Barr virus, malaria, HIV).
3. Symptoms of a delayed reaction can vary from mild to very severe. Diagnosis may be complicated by the long incubation period between transfusion and reaction and the complexity of diagnostic tests.
4. Causes, clinical manifestations, management, and prevention of delayed reactions are summarized in Table 25-5.

TABLE 25-4 Acute Reactions to Blood Transfusion

Acute Reaction	Cause	Clinical Manifestations	Management	Prevention
Allergic	Sensitivity to plasma protein or donor antibody, which reacts with recipient antigen	1. Flushing 2. Itching, rash 3. Urticaria, hives 4. Asthmatic wheezing 5. Laryngeal edema 6. Anaphylaxis	1. Stop transfusion immediately. Keep vein open (KVO) with normal saline. Notify health care provider and blood bank. 2. Give antihistamine as directed (diphenhydramine). 3. Observe for anaphylaxis—prepare epinephrine if respiratory distress is severe. 4. If hives are the only clinical manifestation, the transfusion can sometimes continue at a slower rate. 5. Send blood samples and blood bags to blood bank. Collect urine samples for testing.	Before transfusion, ask patient about past reactions. If patient has history of anaphylaxis, alert physician, have emergency drugs available, and remain at bedside for the first 30 min.
Febrile, nonhemolytic	Hypersensitivity to donor WBCs, platelets, or plasma proteins	1. Sudden chills and fever 2. Headache 3. Flushing 4. Anxiety	1. Stop transfusion immediately and KVO with normal saline. Notify physician and blood bank. 2. Send blood samples and blood bags to blood bank. Collect urine samples for testing. 3. Check temperature $1/2$ h after chill and as indicated thereafter. 4. Give antipyretics as prescribed—treat symptomatically.	Given antipyretic (acetaminophen or aspirin) before transfusion as directed. Leukocyte-poor blood products may be recommended for future transfusions.
Septic reactions	Transfusion of blood or components contaminated with bacteria	1. Rapid onset of chills 2. High fever 3. Vomiting; diarrhea 4. Marked hypotension	1. Stop transfusion immediately and KVO with normal saline. Notify physician and blood bank. 2. Obtain cultures of patient's blood and return blood bags with administration set to blood bank for culture. 3. Treat septicemia as directed—antibiotics, IV fluids, vasopressors, steroids.	Do not permit blood to stand at room temperature longer than necessary. Warm temperatures promote bacterial growth. Inspect blood for gas bubbles, clotting, or abnormal color before transfusion Complete infusions within 4 h. Change administration set after 4 h of use.
Circulatory overload	Fluid administered at a rate or volume greater than the circulatory system can accommodate. Increased blood in pulmonary vessels and decreased lung compliance.	1. Rise in venous pressure 2. Distended neck veins 3. Dyspnea 4. Cough 5. Crackles at base of lungs	1. Stop transfusion and KVO with normal saline. Notify physician. 2. Place patient upright with feet in dependent position. 3. Administer prescribed diuretics, oxygen, morphine, and aminophylline.	Concentrated blood products should be given whenever positive. Transfuse at a rate within the circulatory reserve of the patient. Monitor central venous pressure of patient with heart disease.

(continued)

TABLE 25-4 Acute Reactions to Blood Transfusion *(continued)*

Acute Reaction	Cause	Clinical Manifestations	Management	Prevention
Hemolytic reaction	Infusion of incompatible blood products: 1. Antibodies in recipient's plasma attach to transfused RBCs, hemolyzing the cells either in circulation or in the reticuloendothelial system. 2. Antibodies in donor plasma attach to recipient RBCs, causing hemolysis (may result from infusion of incompatible plasma—less severe than incompatible RBCs).	1. Chills; fever 2. Low back pain 3. Feeling of head fullness; flushing 4. Oppressive feeling 5. Tachycardia, tachypnea 6. Hypotension, vascular collapse 7. Hemoglobinuria, hemoglobinemia 8. Bleeding 9. Acute renal failure	1. Stop transfusion immediately—KVO with 0.9% saline. 2. Notify physician and blood bank. 3. Treat shock, if present 4. Draw testing samples, collect urine sample. 5. Maintain blood pressure with IV colloid solutions. Give diuretics as prescribed to maintain urine flow, glomerular filtration, and renal blood flow. 6. Insert indwelling catheter to monitor hourly urine output. Patient may require dialysis if renal failure occurs.	Meticulously verify patient identification—from sample collection to product infusion. Begin infusion slowly and observe closely for 30 min—consequences are in proportion to the amount of incompatible blood transfused.

Bone Marrow and Peripheral Stem Cell Transplantation

Bone marrow transplantation (BMT) is a lifesaving treatment with application in a number of malignant and nonmalignant disorders. Several decades of research have advanced this technology from an experimental treatment of last resort to the preferred method of intervention for selected diseases. Although the basic procedures are now well established, this field continues to grow rapidly through ongoing research in areas such as the use of peripheral stem cells and the application of biologic response modifiers.

◆ PRINCIPLES OF TRANSPLANTATION

Types of Transplant

The type of transplant selected is contingent on factors such as the underlying disorder, the availability of a histocompatible (HLA-matched) donor, and the clinical condition of the patient.

A. Autologous Bone Marrow Transplantation
1. Bone marrow is removed from the patient during an operative harvesting procedure, frozen, and reinfused after the patient has undergone high-dose chemotherapy and possibly radiotherapy.
2. Advantages: readily available and generally lower morbidity and mortality
3. Disadvantages: marrow must be disease free, sufficient quantity of cellular marrow must be aspirable, and generally higher rate of relapse

B. Syngeneic Bone Marrow Transplantation
1. Bone marrow is removed from an identical twin during an operative harvesting procedure and infused into the patient, who has undergone high-dose chemotherapy and possibly radiotherapy.

2. Advantages: patient's marrow does not need to be harvestable (as in early relapse, aplastic anemia, CML), generally lower morbidity and mortality
3. Disadvantages: higher relapse rate than in allogeneic

C. Allogeneic Bone Marrow Transplantation
1. Bone marrow is removed from a donor who is generally a complete HLA match, is most often a sibling or other close relative (related) but may be a volunteer donor (unrelated). As with other types of BMT, this is done during an operative harvesting procedure and infused into the patient, who has undergone high-dose chemotherapy and possibly radiotherapy.
2. Advantages: patient's marrow does not need to be harvestable (as in early relapse, aplastic anemia, CML, genetic disorders), lowest rate of relapse (presumed due to a graft-versus-leukemia effect)
3. Disadvantages: risk for GVHD, generally higher morbidity and early mortality than other types of BMT

D. Peripheral Stem Cell Transplantation
1. Although hematopoietic stem cells are primarily found in the bone marrow, they can also be found in the peripheral circulation in smaller numbers. This finding has led to the development of methods to harvest peripheral stem cells (also called peripheral blood progenitor cells).
2. Peripheral stem cells are collected using multiple apheresis procedures, usually after the patient has been treated to increase the number of circulating stem cells by methods such as timed administration of chemotherapy or growth factors. This technology is generally applied in the autologous setting but has also been used for allogeneic donors. The cells are stored and later reinfused into the patient, following high-dose chemotherapy and possibly radiotherapy.
3. Advantages: Patient's marrow does not need to be harvestable (as in hypocellular or tumor-contaminated bone marrow); no operative risk, particularly with adjuvant use of growth factors; has a low risk of morbidity and mortality and eliminates lengthy hospital stays; may be used alone or in conjunction with autologous bone marrow.
4. Disadvantages: New method, long-term benefits not yet known

TABLE 25-5 Delayed Reactions to Transfusion Therapy

Delayed Reaction	Cause	Clinical Manifestations	Management	Prevention
Delayed hemolytic reaction	The destruction of transfused RBCs by antibody not detectable during crossmatch, but formed rapidly after transfusion. Rapid production may occur because of antigen exposure during previous transfusions or pregnancy.	1. Fever 2. Mild jaundice 3. Decreased hematocrit	Generally, no acute treatment is required, but hemolysis may be severe enough to cause shock and renal failure. If this occurs, manage as outlined under acute hemolytic reactions.	The crossmatch blood sample should be drawn within 3 d of blood transfusion. Antibody formation may occur within 90 d of transfusion and/or pregnancy.
Iron overload (hemosiderosis)	Deposition of iron in the heart, endocrine organs, liver, spleen, skin, and other major organs as a result of multiple, long-term transfusions (aplastic anemia, thalassemia)	1. Diabetes 2. Decreased thyroid function 3. Arrhythmias 4. CHF and other symptoms related to major organ failure	1. Treat symptomatically. 2. Deferoxamine (Desferal), which chelates, and removes accumulated iron through the kidneys; administered IV, IM, or SC.	
Graft-versus-host disease	Engraftment of lymphocytes in the bone marrow of immunosuppressed patients setting up an immune response of the graft against the host.	1. Erythematous skin rash 2. Liver function test abnormalities 3. Profuse, watery diarrhea	1. Immunosupression with corticosteroids, cyclosporine A. 2. Symptomatic management of pruritius, pain 3. Fluid and electrolyte replacement for diarrhea	Transfuse with irradiated blood products.
Infectious disease 1. Hepatitis B	Hepatitis B virus transmitted from blood donor to recipient via infected blood products.	1. Elevated liver enzymes (SGPT and SGOT) 2. Anorexia, malaise 3. Nausea and vomiting 4. Fever 5. Dark urine 6. Jaundice	Usually resolves spontaneously within 4–6 wk. Can result in permanent liver damage. Treat symptomatically.	Screen blood donors, temporarily rejecting those who may have had contact with the virus. Those with a history of hepatitis after age 11 are permanently deferred; pretest all blood products (EIA).
2. Hepatitis C (formerly non-A, non-B hepatitis)	Hepatitis C virus transmitted from blood donor to recipient via infected blood products.	Similar to serum B hepatitis, but symptoms are usually less severe. Chronic liver disease and cirrhosis may develop.	Symptoms usually mild and require no treatment.	Pretest all blood donors (ALT, anti-HBc antibody, anti-hepatits C antibody).
3. Epstein-Barr virus, cytomegalovirus, malaria	Transmitted through infected blood products.			Question prospective blood donors, regarding colds, flu, foreign travel.
4. Acquired immunodeficiency syndrome	HIV virus transmitted from blood donor to recipient via infected blood products.	1. Night sweats 2. Unexplained weight loss 3. Lymphadenopathy 4. Pneumocystis pneumonia 5. Kaposi's sarcoma 6. Diarrhea	AZT may delay onset of AIDS symptoms. Active disease is treated symptomatically.	Test each donor for HIV antibody. Reject prospective high-risk donors: males who have had sex with another male since 1977; users of self-injected IV drugs; male or female partners of prostitutes; hemophiliacs or their sexual partners; sexual partners of those with AIDS or high risk for AIDS; immigrants from Haiti or sub-Saharan Africa

(continued)

TABLE 25-5 Delayed Reactions to Transfusion Therapy *(continued)*

Delayed Reaction	Cause	Clinical Manifestations	Management	Prevention
5. HTLV-1 associated myelopathy and tropical spastic paraparesis (HAM/TSP) Adult T-cell leukemia	Human T-lymphotropic virus type 1 (HTLV-1) transmitted from blood donor to recipient via blood products.	Signs of neuromuscular disease Signs of T-cell leukemia	HTLV-I-infected individuals have a low risk of developing disease (3–5%). Incubation period 10–20 y. Should disease occur, treat symptomatically	Screen all prospective blood donors for anti-HTLV-I antibody.
6. Syphilis	Spirochetemia caused by *Treponema pallidum*. Incubation 4–18 wk	1. Presence of chancre 2. Regional lymphadenopathy 3. Generalized rash	Penicillin therapy	Test blood prior to transfusion (rapid plasma reagin—RPF). Organism will not remain viable in blood stored 24–48 h at 4°C.

The Human Leukocyte Antigen System and Transplantation

1. The immune-mediated recognition of the differences in HLA antigens is the first step in the rejection of a transplanted organ or graft or in GVHD.
2. The HLA antigens are complex proteins expressed on the surface of all nucleated cells (A, B, C antigens) or cells of the immune system (D antigens).
   a. More than a hundred different antigens have been identified.
   b. Antigens are classified according to the locations on chromosome 6, which encodes them.
   c. The genetically inherited mixture of antigens of an individual expressed on cell surfaces is the phenotype or tissue type of that individual.
3. Although considerably more complex, determination of HLA type is similar to ABO testing.
   a. Lymphocytes are mixed with antibody directed against known HLA antigens. Lymphocytes will survive if the antigen is absent and will be inactivated if it is present. This method identifies HLA-A, -B, and -C antigens.
   b. Donor and recipient lymphocytes are mixed and cultured together. This test, the mixed lymphocyte culture (MLC), identifies HLA-D antigens. Survival of both sources of cells indicates compatibility.
   c. New techniques for determining the genetic HLA code in an individual use DNA probes. These tests are highly accurate, but their use remains limited due to the specialized techniques and high cost.
4. Siblings have a 1 in 4 chance of having identical sets of HLA antigens. With a decreasing national birthrate, however, only 35% of patients in the United States can anticipate having an HLA-identical sibling.
5. Due to the complexity of the HLA system, unrelated individuals have less than a 1 in 5,000 chance of having identical HLA types. The establishment of the National Bone Marrow Donor Registry in 1987 maintains a computerized list of potential HLA-typed bone marrow donors and provides assistance to patients seeking an unrelated donor. Information on becoming a volunteer bone marrow donor or initiating a computerized search for a donor can be obtained by calling the National Marrow Donor Program at 1-800-654-1247.

Indications

1. If an HLA-matched related donor is available, allogeneic BMT is generally considered the treatment of choice in certain disorders, including:
   a. Severe aplastic anemia
   b. Inherited immunodeficiency disorders such as severe combined immunodeficiency disease and Wiskott-Aldrich syndrome
   c. Chronic myelogenous leukemia (CML)
2. Allogeneic BMT has also been used with varying success in the treatment of other genetic disorders (eg, thalassemia).
3. Allogeneic and autologous BMT and more recently, peripheral stem cell transplant, are also widely applied in other malignancies, where success rates depend largely on factors such as the age of the patient, current disease status, the extent of prior treatment, and coexisting morbidity.
4. Diseases and disorders treated with this technology are summarized in Table 25-6.

◆ HARVESTING OF BONE MARROW AND PERIPHERAL STEM CELLS

Evaluation of Recipient

1. Eligibility criteria include age (generally under 55 for allogeneic and under 65 for autologous BMT) and availability of suitable bone marrow or peripheral stem cell source.
2. Before undergoing BMT an extensive work-up ensures that the patient's disease is treatable with BMT and that the patient has no limitations increasing the risk of mortality. Specific criteria may vary among transplant centers and treatment protocols, but generally include:
   a. Disease-specific evaluation of severity and extent of current disease manifestations
   b. Adequate cardiac function: generally left ventricular ejection fraction greater than 45%
   c. Adequate pulmonary function: generally forced expiratory capacity and forced vital capacity greater than 50%

TABLE 25-6 Indications for Bone Marrow Transplanation

Allogeneic	Autologous
Nonmalignant	
Aplastic anemia	Acute myeloid leukemia
	Acute lymphocytic leukemia
Myelofibrosis	Hodgkin's disease
Wiskott-Aldrich syndrome	Non-Hodgkin's lymphoma
Thalassemia	Multiple myeloma
Severe combined immunodeficiency diseases	Selected solid tumors
Mucopolysaccharidoses	Breast
Osteopetrosis	Lung
Lipid storage diseases	Neuroblastoma
	Testicular/germ cell
Malignant	Ovarian
Acute myeloid leukemia	Colon
Acute lymphocytic leukemia	Melanoma
Chronic myelogenous leukemia	Sarcomas
Hodgkin's disease	Gliomas
Non-Hodgkin's lymphoma	Renal cell
Preleukemia	Pancreatic
Burkitt's lymphoma	Gastric
Multiple myeloma	
Selected solid tumors	

   d. Adequate renal function: generally creatinine less than 2 mg/dL

   e. Adequate hepatic function: generally bilirubin less 2 mg/dL

   f. No active infections (including HIV)

   g. No coexisting severe or uncontrolled medical conditions

Evaluation of Donor

1. Because bone marrow donation for allogeneic or syngeneic BMT is an elective procedure with no benefit to the donor, great care is taken to ensure that the potential donor is fit for surgery and understands the potential risks. Evaluation generally includes:
   a. Thorough medical history and physical examination
   b. Chest x-ray
   c. Electrocardiogram
   d. Laboratory evaluation (complete blood count, chemistry profile, testing for CMV, hepatitis B and C, HIV and syphilis, ABO and Rh determination, coagulation studies)
2. Informed consent including potential donor complications must be obtained.
   Relatively common complications include:
   a. Bruising
   b. Pain at aspiration sites
   c. Mild bleeding
      Rare complications include:
   d. Adverse effects of anesthesia (general, spinal, or epidural)

   e. Infection of aspiration sites

   f. Persistent pain

   g. Transient neuropathies

3. Because of the significant loss of blood volume and RBCs during the harvest procedure, donors are advised to give 1 or 2 units of autologous blood 1 to 3 weeks before surgery, which may be reinfused during marrow collection if needed.

Harvesting Procedure

A. **Bone Marrow (Autologous or Allogeneic)**
1. Performed under epidural, spinal, or general anesthesia under sterile conditions in operating room.
2. An aspiration needle is used to puncture the skin and then puncture the iliac crest multiple times without exiting the skin, removing marrow in 2- to 5-mL aliquots (samples).
3. Marrow is drawn up into heparinized syringes and filtered to remove fibrin clots and other debris.
4. Marrow may be infused immediately, treated and infused, or frozen in a preservative solution containing dimethylsulfoxide (DMSO) until needed.
5. Bone marrow donation is a relatively safe operative procedure with few serious complications. A review of 3,000 cases reported to the International Bone Marrow Transplant Registry found only two donor deaths, neither of which was a result of the harvest procedure itself.

B. **Postharvest Care of the Donor**
1. Procedure is generally done as same-day care, with discharge after recovery from anesthesia.
2. Observe for potential complications (bleeding, hypotension due to fluid loss).
3. Instruct patient to resume normal activities gradually over the week following donation.
4. Instruct patient to keep aspiration sites clean and dry and observe for signs of infection (redness, swelling, warmth or discharge at sites, fever, malaise).
5. Provide adequate analgesia (frequently acetaminophen with codeine) and instruct patient related to pain management.
6. Arrange follow-up appointment with primary care provider in 2 to 3 weeks for complete blood count.

C. **Harvesting of Peripheral Stem Cells**
1. Involves donor preparation by "priming" hematopoietic system by using timed sequential growth factors or chemotherapy before collection to increase number of circulating stem cells.
2. Large-bore central catheter suitable for apheresis procedures is inserted.
3. Approximately 5 to 10 apheresis procedures are performed to collect sufficient numbers of suitable cells.
4. Cells are frozen in a preservative solution containing DMSO until needed.

◆ PREPARATION AND PERFORMANCE OF THE TRANSPLANT

Preparation of Recipient

1. Long-term central catheter is inserted for multiple IV treatments, total parenteral nutrition, and phlebotomies.

2. High-dose chemotherapy or radiotherapy is administered to:
   a. Destroy residual tumor cells
   b. Suppress immune response against new marrow
   c. Create space within marrow for new cells
3. Symptoms immediately associated with high-dose chemotherapy or radiotherapy regimens used in BMT may include:
   a. Severe nausea and vomiting (with most regimens)
   b. Cardiomyopathy, hemorrhagic cystitis (with cyclophosphamide [Cytoxan])
   c. Seizures (with busulfan [Myleran])
   d. Fever, generalized erythema, parotitis (with total body irradiation)

Reinfusion of Bone Marrow or Peripheral Stem Cells

NURSING ALERT:
Unlike all other blood products administered to BMT recipients, bone marrow and peripheral stem cells should never be irradiated. In addition, infusion pumps and filters should be avoided because they may remove or damage stem cells.

A. ABO Compatible Untreated Allogeneic Bone Marrow
1. Administered over 2 to 4 hours from large blood infusion bag, generally via large lumen of central catheter.
2. Volume depends on size of recipient and cellularity of bone marrow; generally 500 to 2,000 mL.
3. Potential immediate adverse reactions are generally related to volume overload, allergic reactions (urticaria, chills, fever), or pulmonary compromise (related to fat emboli or clumped aggregates of cells).
4. Emergency medications should be available and the recipient closely monitored throughout the infusion.

B. ABO Incompatible Allogeneic Bone Marrow
1. ABO incompatible bone marrow is processed after harvesting to remove incompatible RBCs and plasma.
   a. Although this processing is highly effective, the recipient should be considered at risk for intravascular RBC hemolysis.
   b. The recipient should be well hydrated with fluids containing sodium bicarbonate before and after the infusion to ensure adequate renal perfusion and urine alkalinization.
2. Administered over 2 to 4 hours from blood infusion bag, generally via large lumen of central catheter.
3. Volume after removal of RBCs is usually 200 to 600 mL.
4. Potential immediate adverse reactions are generally related to allergic reactions (urticaria, chills, fever) or intravascular hemolysis (hemoglobinuria, potential anaphylactic reaction).
5. Emergency medications should be available and the recipient closely monitored throughout the infusion.

C. Treated Allogeneic Bone Marrow (eg, T-cell Depleted)
1. Allogeneic bone marrow may be treated before infusion with a variety of methods to remove T cells as a method of preventing GVHD. Methods include:
   a. Monoclonal antibodies
   b. Counterflow centrifugation (elutriation)
   c. Positive selection of CD34+ cells

2. These manipulations may alter total volume and result in RBC and plasma removal. Management of reinfusion incorporates the principles described under allogeneic ABO compatible and incompatible bone marrow reinfusion.

D. Autologous Bone Marrow
1. Autologous bone marrow is thawed by immersion in a warm water bath immediately before infusion.
2. Administered via slow IV push (if in syringes) or from small infusion bags, generally through large lumen of central catheter.
3. Volume depends on size of recipient and amount of bone marrow harvested; usually 100 to 500 mL.
4. Potential immediate adverse reactions are generally related to use of DMSO as preservative solution and include:
   a. Histamine-release reaction (flushing, feeling of chest tightness, abdominal cramping, nausea)
   b. Cardiac arrhythmias, especially bradycardia
   c. Anaphylaxis
5. Emergency medications should be available and the recipient closely monitored throughout the infusion; cardiac monitoring is recommended.

E. Peripheral Stem Cells
1. Peripheral stem cells are thawed by immersion in a warm water bath immediately before infusion.
2. Administered via slow IV push (if in syringes) or from small infusion bags, generally through large lumen of central catheter.
   a. Volume depends on size of recipient and amount of peripheral stem cells harvested; often a large volume.
   b. May be administered over many hours or even several days due to large volume and high DMSO content.
   c. Recipient may require premedication with antihistamine and antiemetic.
3. Potential immediate adverse reactions are generally related to use of DMSO as preservative solution and include:
   a. Histamine-release reaction (flushing, feeling of chest tightness, abdominal cramping, nausea)
   b. Cardiac arrhythmias, especially bradycardia
   c. Anaphylaxis
4. Emergency medications should be available and the recipient closely monitored throughout the infusion; cardiac monitoring is recommended.

Posttransplant Care

A. General Considerations
1. Significant complications requiring specialized medical and nursing care may occur during the first few weeks and months after BMT.
2. Nursing care is aimed at early identification and treatment of problems, and includes:
   a. Comprehensive physical and psychosocial assessment
   b. Immediate notification of health care provider of any abnormal assessment parameters found
   c. Expert management of problems that may occur after BMT such as nausea, vomiting, pain, fatigue, anxiety, delirium
   d. Prevention of infection
   e. Prevention of bleeding

B. *Hematopoietic Complications*
1. BMT patients are at risk for life-threatening bacterial, viral, and fungal infections due to their profound immunosuppression.
    a. BMT patients are generally cared for in a protective environment, ranging from single hepafiltered rooms to strict laminar airflow and isolation in sterile environment.
    b. Additional preventive interventions vary widely and include elaborate disinfection procedures; modified or sterile diets; prophylactic antibiotics, antivirals, and antifungals; surveillance cultures.
2. The megakaryocyte is generally the last cell produced by new bone marrow, and platelet counts may take months to return to normal.
    a. BMT patients require frequent assessment for signs and symptoms of overt or covert bleeding, protection from injury, and support with platelet products.
3. Anemia is a frequent complication due to loss of RBCs through aging, destruction, bleeding, and routine phlebotomy.
    a. BMT patients require frequent RBC transfusions.

C. *Gastrointestinal Complications*
1. Mucositis may develop due to high-dose chemotherapy and radiation therapy that destroy rapidly dividing cells, including cells lining the mouth and esophagus.
    a. Management includes meticulous oral hygiene, local and systemic analgesia, and antimicrobial therapy.
2. Nausea and vomiting may arise from multiple causes, including high-dose chemotherapy, infection, gastrointestinal bleeding, acute GVHD, and medications.
    a. Management includes pharmacologic and nonpharmacologic interventions, replacement of fluids and electrolytes, and support of nutritional requirements.
3. Diarrhea may be due to multiple causes, including high-dose chemotherapy, infection, gastrointestinal bleeding, GVHD, and medications.
    a. Management includes cautious use of antidiarrheals, replacement of fluids and electrolytes, support of nutritional requirements, protection of perirectal skin from excoriation.

D. *Renal and Genitourinary Complications*
1. Renal failure may arise from multiple causes, including drug toxicity, infection, and ischemia.
    a. Management includes maintenance of fluid and electrolyte balance, monitoring of drug levels, and hemodialysis.
2. Hemorrhagic cystitis may occur as a result of high-dose cyclophosphamide (Cytoxan) or with certain viral infections.
    a. Management includes hydration, blood product support, continuous bladder irrigation, and invasive procedures such as instillation of alum or formalin.

E. *Hepatic Complications*
1. Veno-occlusive disease may occur as a result of damage to the liver from high-dose chemotherapy and radiation therapy; incidence approximately 20%.
    a. Signs and symptoms include hepatomegaly (generally painful), bilirubinemia, weight gain.
    b. May progress to hepatic encephalopathy, coagulopathies, coma and death in up to 50% of patients with veno-occlusive disease.
    c. Management is generally aimed at preventing further damage and treating symptoms.

F. *Pulmonary Complications*
1. Life-threatening pulmonary infections in BMT patients include bacterial pneumonias, fungal infections including aspergillosis, CMV pneumonitis, and less commonly, *Pneumocystis carinii* pneumonia (PCP), legionnaire's disease, toxoplasmosis, and tuberculosis.
    a. Preventive measures include encouragement of exercise, deep breathing and coughing; administration of CMV-screened blood products, high-dose acyclovir (Zovirax) or ganciclovir (Cytovene), and IVIG for allogeneic BMT patients at high risk for CMV; prophylactic sulfamethoxazole-trimethoprim (Bactrim) for patients at risk for PCP.
    b. Supportive care for symptomatic disease includes oxygen therapy, mechanical ventilation, and pulmonary hygiene.
2. Noninfectious pulmonary disease includes idiopathic pneumonitis, pulmonary fibrosis, and bronchiolitis obliterans.

G. *Graft-Versus-Host Disease*
1. Acute GVHD occurs in 40% to 60% of allogeneic BMT recipients even with HLA matching, generally within first 3 months after BMT as a manifestation of the immune response of activated donor T lymphocytes against the recipient's cells and organs.
    a. Affects the skin, liver, and gastrointestinal tract.
    b. Severity ranges from mild and self-limited erythematous rash to widespread blistering of skin, profuse watery diarrhea, and liver failure.
    c. Prophylaxis generally includes immunosuppression with medications such as cyclosporin A (Sandimmune) and methotrexate (Mexate); may also include T-cell depletion of bone marrow.
    d. Treatment generally includes increased doses of immunosuppressive medications and additional drugs such as corticosteroids, antithymocyte globulin, and monoclonal antibodies.
2. Chronic GVHD occurs in about 20% of long-term survivors, usually appears within first year after BMT.
    a. It has many similarities to autoimmune disorders such as scleroderma.
    b. It affects the skin, mouth, salivary glands, eyes, musculoskeletal system, liver, esophagus, gastrointestinal tract, vagina.
    c. Treatment generally consists of corticosteroids; may include other immunosuppressive medications.
    d. Immune system frequently suppressed beyond the effects of medications; patient is at risk for infections, particularly from encapsulated bacteria, and should receive prophylaxis with suitable antibiotic such as penicillin.

Long-term Sequelae and Survivorship Issues

1. Long-term disease-free survival varies from 10% for patients with resistant, aggressive leukemias or lymphomas to 75% to 80% for aplastic anemia.
2. Long-term complications of BMT include:
    a. Relapse of original disease
    b. Secondary malignancy
    c. Sterility
    d. Endocrine dysfunction
    e. Cataracts
    f. Chronic GVHD
    g. Aseptic necrosis

3. Survivorship issues after this intensive and potentially life-threatening treatment include:
   a. Feelings of isolation, guilt, and loss
   b. Altered family dynamics
   c. Readjustment to school or work setting
   d. Financial burden of BMT
   e. Chronic health problems and fatigue
   f. Difficulty obtaining adequate health insurance

4. Despite the complex issues BMT survivors face as they return to the task of living, several quality of life studies have demonstrated that the majority rate their quality of life highly, would choose to undergo BMT again, and frequently state that their experiences have added new dimensions of meaning and purpose to their lives.

Selected References

Antman, K. (1992). Hematopoietic stem cells: Clinical implications. *Marrow Transplantation Review, 2*(2), 27-29.

Baranowski, C. (1992). Current trends in blood component therapy: The evolution of a safer, more effective product. *Journal of Intravenous Nursing, 15*(3), 136-151.

Bodensteiner, D. C., et al. (1992). Use of blood components in cancer patients with bleeding. *Hematology/Oncology Clinics of North America, 6*(6), 1375-1391.

Bortin, M. M., et al. (1992). Increasing utilization of allogeneic bone marrow transplantation. *Annals of Internal Medicine, 116*(6), 505-512.

Coffland, F. I., & Sheleton, D. M. (1993). Blood component replacement therapy. *Critical Care Nursing Clinics of North America, 5*(3), 543-546.

Gerber, L. (1994). Autologous blood transfusion: Why and how. *Journal of Intravenous Nursing, 17*(2), 65-69.

Groenwald, S. L., Frogge, M. H., Goodman, M., & Yarbro, C. H. (Eds.). (1993). *Cancer nursing: Principles and practice* (3rd ed.). Boston: Jones and Bartlett.

Jarsak, P. F. & Riley, M. B. (1994). Autologous stem cell transplant: An overview. *Cancer Practice, 2*(2), 141-145.

Lowry, P. A., & Tabbara, I. A. (1992). Peripheral hematopoietic stem cell transplantation: Current concepts. *Experimental Hematology, 20*(8), 937-942.

Poe, S. S., et al. (1994). A national survey of infection prevention practices on bone marrow transplant units. *Oncology Nursing Forum, 21*(10), 1687-1694.

Shivnan, J. C., Ohly, K. V., & Hanson, J. (1995). Bone marrow transplantation. *In* Nolan, M. & Augustine, S. (eds.). *Transplantation nursing.* Norwalk, CT: Appleton-Lange, 239–289.

Whedon, M. B. (Ed). (1991). *Bone marrow transplantation: Principles, practice, and nursing insights.* Boston: Jones and Bartlett.

Wujcik, D., & Downs, S. (1992). Bone marrow transplantation. *Critical Care Nursing Clinics of North America, 4*(1), 149-166.

UNIT 9

◆

Immune and Autoimmune Related Disorders

CHAPTER 26 ◆

Allergy Problems

Underlying Principles

◆ THE ALLERGIC REACTION

An allergic reaction results from antigen–antibody reaction on a sensitized mast cell causing the release of chemical mediators. The reaction may be characterized by inflammation, increased secretions, and bronchoconstriction.

Definitions

1. *Antigen*—a substance that stimulates an immune reaction causing the production of antibodies
2. *Antibody*—a globulin (protein) produced by B cells as a defense mechanism against foreign materials
3. *Atopy*—a term referring to a genetic predisposition to develop allergic disease
4. *Immunity*
   a. *Humoral*—the process by which B lymphocytes produce circulating antibodies to act against antigens
   b. *Cell-mediated*—that portion of the immune system in which the participation of T lymphocytes and macrophages is predominant
5. *Mast cell*—a tissue cell that resembles a peripheral blood basophil and contains granules with chemical mediators
6. *Hypersensitivity*—reaction to an antigen following reexposure; there are four types; type I (immediate) and type IV (delayed) are considered allergic reactions.

Immunoglobulins

Antibodies that are formed by lymphocytes and plasma cells in response to an immunogenic stimulus comprise a group of serum proteins called immunoglobulins.

1. The abbreviation for immunoglobulin is Ig.
2. Antibodies combine with antigens in special ways (lock-and-key style).
3. There are five major classes of immunoglobulins.
   a. IgM—comprises 10% of immunoglobulin pool; found mostly in intravascular fluid and is primarily engaged in initial defense.
   b. IgG—major immunoglobulin accounting for 70% to 75% of secondary immune responses and in combating tissue infection.
   c. IgA—15% to 20% of immunoglobulins; predominantly found in seromucous secretions (such as saliva, tears) where it provides a primary defense mechanism.
   d. IgD—less than 1% of immunoglobulin pool; found on many circulating B lymphocytes, but function is unknown.
   e. IgE—only a trace found in serum; attaches to surface membrane of basophils and mast cells; responsible for immediate types of allergic reactions.

Immunologic Reactions (Fig. 26-1)

A. **Immediate Hypersensitivity (Type 1)**
1. Characterized by:
   a. Allergic reaction
   b. Occurs immediately after contact with the antigen.
   c. Causes release of chemical mediators.
2. Examples—anaphylaxis, allergic rhinitis, urticaria

B. **Products of Immediate Hypersensitivity (Chemical Mediators)**
1. Histamine—a bioactive amine stored in granules of mast cells and basophils
2. Serotonin—an amine released at the same time as histamine
3. Bradykinin—acts chiefly by increasing capillary permeability and contractility of smooth muscle
4. Platelet-activating factor (PAF)—has many properties; causes the aggregation of platelets
5. SRS-A—slow-reacting substance of anaphylaxis
6. Prostaglandins—potent vasodilators as well as potent bronchoconstrictors
7. ECF-A—causes an influx of eosinophils into the area of allergic inflammation

C. **Effects of Chemical Mediators and Their Manifestations**
1. Generalized vasodilation, hypotension, flushing
2. Increased permeability
   a. Capillaries of the skin—edema
   b. Mucous membranes—edema
3. Smooth muscle contraction
   a. Bronchioles—bronchospasm
   b. Intestines—abdominal cramps, diarrhea

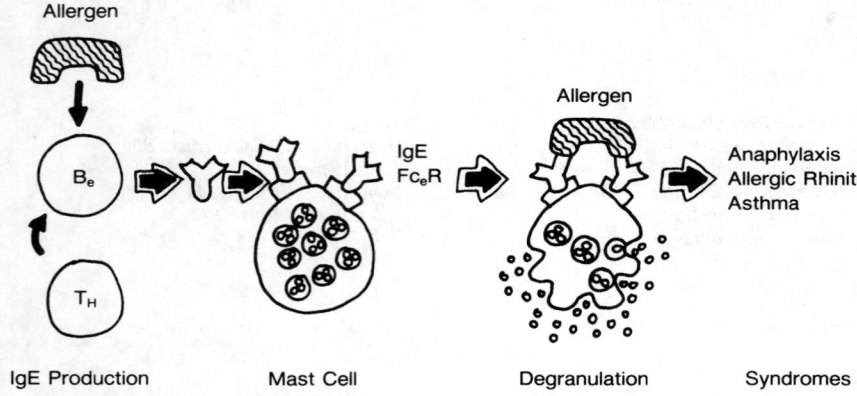

FIGURE 26-1 *Type I immediate hypersensitivity. Specific IgE is produced by B cells with T cell help as a result of allergen stimulation. The next step in sensitization is the attachment of the IgE antibody to the mast cell by the F_c receptor. When specific allergen reaches the sensitized mast cell and combines with the two adjacent antibody molecules on the surface of the cell, degranulation occurs, releasing chemical mediators that cause the symptoms associated with type I hypersensitivity.*

4. Increased secretions
   a. Nasal mucous glands—rhinorrhea
   b. Bronchioles—increased mucus in airways
   c. Gastrointestinal—increased gastric secretions
   d. Lacrimal—tearing
   e. Salivary—salivation
5. Pruritus (itching)
   a. Skin
   b. Mucous membrane

D. Delayed Hypersensitivity (Type IV)
1. Characterized by a cell-mediated reaction between antigens and antigen-responsive T lymphocytes.
2. Maximal intensity occurs between 24 to 48 hours.
3. Usually consists of erythema and induration.
4. Examples—tuberculin skin test; contact dermatitis such as poison ivy

Assessment and Diagnostic Tests

◆ EVALUATION OF THE PATIENT FOR ALLERGY

Evaluation includes:

1. The allergy history (Fig. 26-2)
2. Physical examination based on patient presentation and specific allergy condition
3. Skin testing (Procedure Guidelines 26-1 and 26-2)
4. Other tests as indicated for specific allergic conditions

Skin Testing

The purpose of skin testing is to identify antigens responsible for immediate hypersensitivity and to determine the level of sensitivity in an individual. The types of skin tests used in clinical allergy are epicutaneous (prick, puncture, or scratch) and intradermal methods. The skin test remains unequaled as a sensitive and effective test for the diagnosis of allergies.

A. Epicutaneous (Prick) Method
1. Advantages
   a. Safe—less chance for anaphylaxis due to minimal systemic absorption
   b. Efficient—results within 15 minutes
   c. Little discomfort to the patient
2. Disadvantages
   a. Less sensitive than the intradermal method
   b. Old or thick, leathery skin decreases reactivity.
   c. Drops have a tendency to run together, which would affect the accuracy of the test.

B. Intradermal Method
1. Advantages
   a. More sensitive than prick testing
2. Disadvantages
   a. Increased possibility for anaphylactic reactions
   b. Requires more time and skill to perform
   c. Increased discomfort to the patient
   d. Less specific than prick testing

Radioallergosorbent Test (RAST)

A. Description Measurement of allergen—specific IgE antibodies in serum samples after panel of allergens have been added to samples

B. Nursing/Patient Care Considerations
1. Allergy testing without the risk of causing severe allergic reaction
2. Obtain 4 to 10 mL venous blood for each panel of six allergens to be tested.
3. A positive RAST is greater than four times the control— diagnostic for allergy to a particular allergen.

(text continues on page 805)

ALLERGY SURVEY

Name _____ Age _____ Sex _____ Date _____

1. Reason for visit:
2. Do you have any of the following problems?

_____ Hay Fever   _____ Sinus problems   _____ Eczema
_____ Asthma   _____ Drug allergy   Other: (please specify)
_____ Hives   _____ Insect allergy   _____
_____ Food allergy _____ Skin rash   _____

3. Does anyone in your family have allergies? _____
4. Have you ever been tested for allergies? _____
   When? _____ Results _____
5. Do you smoke? _____ How much? _____ No. of years _____
6. Exercise habits: _____
7. Other significant past medical history _____
   _____

8. Current symptoms: (Circle one(s) that applies)

Nasal stuffiness/congestion   Mouth breathing   Shortness of breath
Sneezing   Snoring   Diminished sense of
Runny nose   Itching/irritation/redness/   smell
Itching   tearing of eyes
Postnasal drip   Cough
Sinus headaches   Chest tightness
Sinus infections   Wheezing

9. Do symptoms occur year 'round? _____
10. If not, during what seasons do your symptoms occur?

Summer   Fall   Winter   Spring

11. Where do symptoms occur? _____

Home   Office   School   Outdoors   Basement   Bedroom

12. Are symptoms made worse by:

Smoke   Heat   Humidity   Cold   Pollen   Pollution
Dust   Exposure to strong odors—ammonia, paint, perfume
Pets   Exercise   Eating   Drinking   Emotional stress

13. Have you had symptoms after eating? If so, list the foods _____
14. Do you have pets? _____ Dog _____ Cat   Other: _____
15. List any medications that you are currently taking, including over-the-counter drugs:

Do you know what they are for?

Are you aware of possible side effects?

16. Can you take aspirin without any adverse reactions?

17. In what way(s) has your health problem affected your lifestyle?

FIGURE 26-2 Allergy survey.

PROCEDURE GUIDELINES 26-1 ◆ Epicutaneous Skin Testing

EQUIPMENT

Antigens for testing
Controls
    Positive—histamine 1 mg/mL
    Negative—glycerol saline
Pricking device (sterile needle or lancet)
Alcohol swabs

Paper tissues
Skin marking pencil
Millimeter ruler
Tourniquet
Epinephrine 1:1000 aqueous solution for injection for
    emergency use

PROCEDURE

NURSING ACTION	RATIONALE
PREPARATORY PHASE	
1. Explain the procedure to the patient. Ask patient if he or she has taken antihistamines in the past 48–72 h.	1. Oral antihistamines taken 48–72 h before skin testing are likely to prevent a reaction from occurring.
2. Prepare the site (volar surface of forearm or back) by cleansing with alcohol.	2. The forearm is usually preferable because in the event of a significant local or systemic reaction, a tourniquet may be placed proximal to the skin test to slow the diffusion of the antigen into the circulation.
3. Mark the test sites with a skin marking pencil approximately 3–4 cm apart.	3. Sites need to be spaced appropriately so that reactions will remain distinct from one another, thus allowing an accurate reading.
IMPLEMENTATION PHASE	
1. Apply positive (histamine) and negative (glycerol saline) controls next to the appropriate markings. Introduce the tip of the pricking device at a 15–20° angle through each drop, lifting up and tenting the skin until the point pops loose without causing any bleeding. The pricking device must be wiped thoroughly with a paper tissue after each puncture.	1. Because of interpatient variability in cutaneous reactivity, it is necessary to include positive and negative controls whenever skin testing is performed. A response to the positive control confirms an immunologic ability to react. A response to the negative control indicates reactivity to the diluting solution and/or mechanical trauma. Care must be taken to prevent cross-contamination between antigens.
2. Apply small drops of antigens next to the skin markings and prick the drops as described above. Blot (do not rub) skin surface with paper tissue	2. Rubbing may cause redness and cross-contamination of antigens.
3. Instruct the patient not to scratch the test area during the 15-min waiting interval before the reactions are graded.	3. It is normal for sensitive individuals to have a pruritic sensation at the testing site because of the histamine released by the mast cells.
4. Observe the patient closely for signs of impending anaphylaxis (such as itching, flushing, lump in throat).	4. General systemic or anaphylactic reactions are rare, but do occur. If suspected, apply tourniquet above test site and administer 0.3 mL epinephrine 1:1000 subcutaneously.
FOLLOW-UP PHASE	
1. Fifteen minutes after pricking the antigens, measure the extent of induration (wheal) and erythema (flare) in two perpendicular axes through the center of the reaction; record in millimeters (see accompanying figure).	

PROCEDURE (cont'd)	NURSING ACTION	RATIONALE

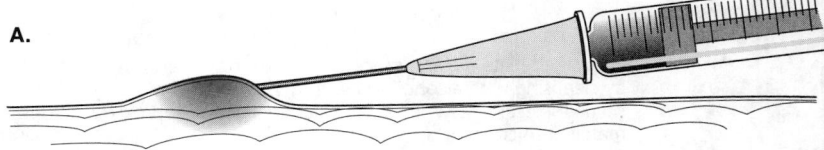

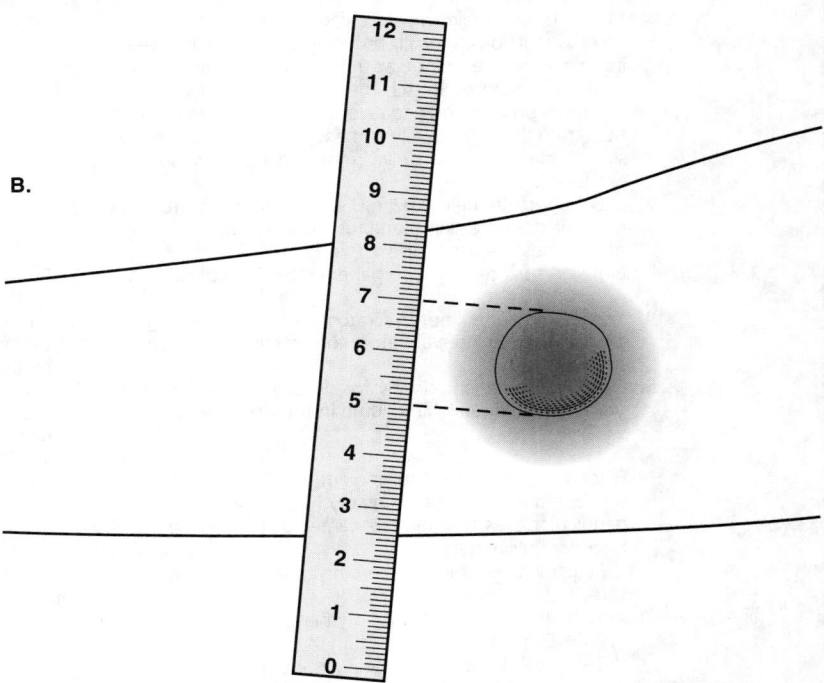

(A) Intradermal injection producing a wheal. *(B)* Measuring area of induration.

2. Document the procedure, test results, patient tolerance, and any other pertinent observations.

PROCEDURE GUIDELINES 26-2 ◆ Intradermal Skin Testing

EQUIPMENT
Antigens for testing
Controls
    Positive—histamine 0.1 mg/mL
    Negative—human serum albumin
1-mm tuberculin syringes with 26- or 27-gauge intradermal needle
Alcohol swabs

Paper tissues
Skin marking pencil
Millimeter ruler
Tourniquet
Gloves
Epinephrine for emergency use

PREPARATORY PHASE

1. Explain the procedure to the patient. Ask the patient if he or she has taken antihistamines in past 48–72 h.

1. Oral antihistamines taken 48–72 h before skin testing are likely to prevent a reaction from occurring.

(continued)

PROCEDURE GUIDELINES 26-2 ◆ Intradermal Skin Testing *(continued)*

PROCEDURE (cont'd)	NURSING ACTION	RATIONALE

2. Prepare the site (volar surface of forearm or upper arm) by cleansing with alcohol. Allow to dry.
3. Mark the test sites with a skin marking pencil approximately 3–4 cm apart.

3. Sites need to be spaced appropriately so that reactions will remain distinct from one another, thus allowing an accurate reading.

IMPLEMENTATION PHASE

1. Using sterile technique, draw up 0.05 mL of each testing material. All bubbles must be carefully expelled to avoid "splash reactions," which reduce precision. While wearing gloves, place syringe at a 10°–15° angle to the skin with the bevel up. Stretch the skin taut and insert 0.02 mL of the positive and negative controls. The bevel should penetrate the skin entirely and end between the layers of skin. A bleb approximately 2 mm in diameter should be produced.

1. Gloves should be worn when there is any possibility of exposure to blood or body fluids. Only small amount needs to be deposited into skin—enough to raise a bleb.

2. Inject approximately 0.02 mL of test antigens intradermally next to the skin markings. A different syringe and needle must be used for each antigen.

2. To avoid antigen and microbial contamination.

3. Blot skin surfaces dry with paper tissue. Do not rub.

3. Rubbing may cause redness and cross-contamination of antigens.

4. Instruct the patient not to scratch the test area during the 15-min waiting interval before the reaction is graded.

4. It is normal for sensitive individuals to have a pruritic sensation at the testing site because of the histamine released by the mast cells.

5. Observe the patient closely for signs of impending anaphylaxis (itching, flushing, lump in throat).

5. There is an increased possibility of anaphylactic reactions with intradermal skin testing. If suspected, apply tourniquet above test site, and administer 0.3 mL epinephrine 1: 1000 subcutaneously.

6. Fifteen minutes after applying antigens, measure the extent of induration (wheal) and erythema (flare) in two perpendicular axes through the center of the reaction and record in millimeters.
   Reactions are graded according to the following:
0	2 mm or less
1+	3–5 mm wheal with erythema
2+	6–10 mm wheal with erythema
3+	over 11–15 mm wheal without pseudopods*
4+	wheal over 15 mm with pseudopods

* Pseudopods—asymmetric extensions of wheal that indicate increased sensitivity.

FOLLOW-UP PHASE

1. Document the procedure, test results, patient tolerance, and any other pertinent observations.
2. Monitor for the following complications during and following testing.

2. Any significant reaction may be anxiety provoking for the patient, but anaphylaxis occurs suddenly and may be life-threatening.

Local Reactions—unusually large 4+ reactions
a. Apply prescribed steroid cream to affected area.
b. If no relief, administer prescribed oral antihistamine.
Vasovagal Reactions—fainting episode
a. Monitor vital signs.
b. Reassure the patient.
c. Finish skin testing if possible.
Systemic Anaphylaxis
a. Stop testing and apply tourniquet above skin testing site.
b. Administer epinephrine subcutaneously.

General Procedures/ Treatment Modalities

◆ IMMUNOTHERAPY

Immunotherapy is the desensitization of the immune system to a known allergen(s) that causes IgE, type I (immediate) hypersensitivity. It is indicated for significant symptoms of allergic rhinitis and asthma that cannot be controlled by avoidance of the allergen.

Although immunotherapy is not a cure, it does give relief for most people. Considerable compliance and time commitment are essential for successful therapy. See Procedure Guidelines 26-3.

Features of Immunotherapy

1. Specific allergen(s) are identified by skin testing (usually intradermal).
2. Serial injections are begun containing extracts from identified allergens (allergy serum).
3. Initially, small amount of very dilute allergy serum is given, usually at weekly intervals.

4. Amount and concentration are very slowly increased to maximum tolerable dose.
5. Then maintenance dose is injected every 2 to 4 weeks for a period of one to several years to achieve maximal benefit.

Precautions and Considerations

1. The danger of anaphylactic reaction exists after injection.
   a. Should only be given in health care facility with epinephrine (Adrenalin), trained personnel, and emergency equipment available.
   b. Patient should remain in office for 30 minutes after injection, after which the risk of anaphylaxis is greatly reduced.
   c. If large, local reaction (erythema, induration) occurs after an injection, the next dose should not be increased because a systemic reaction may occur.
2. If several weeks are missed, dosage may need to be decreased to prevent a reaction.
3. Medication such as antihistamines and decongestants should be continued until significant symptom relief occurs (may take 12–24 months).
4. Environmental controls should be maintained to enhance effectiveness of therapy.

PROCEDURE GUIDELINES 26-3 ◆ Giving an Allergy Injection

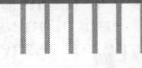

EQUIPMENT
Patient's individualized allergy serum
1 mL syringe

25- to 27-gauge ½ to ⅝-inch needle
Alcohol sponges

NURSING ALERT:
Because of the risk of anaphylaxis, have epinephrine (Adrenalin) 1:1000 readily available for injection.

PROCEDURE

NURSING ACTION	RATIONALE
PREPARATORY PHASE	
1. Check record and ask patient about reaction to last injection. Note how many weeks since last shot.	1. Local erythema and induration may have occurred during observation period or later.
2. Check order for prescribed dosage and any special instructions based on reaction history.	2. Significant reaction (greater than 2–3 cm and lasting 24 h) may require injection at same or lower dose. Missed weeks may require dosage adjustment.
3. Draw up dose, checking both strength of allergy serum and amount (usually 0.1–0.5 mL).	3. Serum will periodically be replaced with a stronger preparation.
PERFORMANCE PHASE	
1. Select the appropriate site for subcutaneous injection, usually the lateral upper arms. If two injections are necessary, give in opposite arms.	1. Because injections usually only given once a week, no need to use abdomen or thighs. Using different arms for two injections allows for determining which serum may have caused reaction if one occurs.
2. Cleanse site with alcohol and allow to dry.	2. Disinfects skin.
3. Grasp upper arm with nondominant hand so that tissue is elevated slightly.	3. Secures arm and subcutaneous tissue beneath outer skin.
4. Insert needle at 45°–90°, depending on thickness of subcutaneous tissue at the site.	4. Thickness of subcutaneous tissue varies among individuals.
5. Aspirate for blood return, and if none occurs, inject serum.	5. If blood enters syringe, dispose of it and begin again rather than injecting into a blood vessel.

(continued)

PROCEDURE GUIDELINES 26-3 ◆ Giving an Allergy Injection *(continued)*

PROCEDURE (cont'd)	NURSING ACTION	RATIONALE
	6. Withdraw syringe, cover site with alcohol sponge, and dispose of needle and syringe. Check site for bleeding or bruising.	6. Follow institution policy; do not resheath needle.

FOLLOW-UP PHASE

1. Have patient wait 30 min before leaving. Check for local reaction periodically and tell patient to report any sudden swelling, itching, or respiratory difficulty.
2. Record amount and concentration of serum; site given; and appearance of site after 30 min.
3. Dismiss patient with instructions on who to call if reaction occurs and when to return for next injection.

1. Significant local or systemic reaction may occur; most likely with increased dose.
2. Flow sheet serves as official documentation of medication given and may be reviewed by allergist when evaluating therapy.
3. May call allergist or primary care provider, or go to emergency room if systemic reaction occurs.

Allergic Disorders
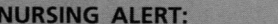

◆ ANAPHYLAXIS

Anaphylaxis is an immediate, life-threatening systemic reaction that can occur on exposure to a particular substance. It is a result of a type I hypersensitivity reaction in which chemical mediators released from mast cells affect many types of tissue and organ systems.

NURSING ALERT:
With immunotherapy (allergy shots), the risk of systemic reaction is always present. Skin testing can also result in systemic reactions. Have epinephrine 1:1,000 available during these procedures (with syringe and tourniquet) and have patient remain in office or clinic for at least 30 minutes after administration.

Pathophysiology/Etiology

1. May be caused by:
   a. Immunotherapy
   b. Stinging insects
   c. Skin testing
   d. Medications
   e. Contrast media infusion
   f. Foods
   g. Exercise
2. Release of chemical mediators results in massive vasodilation; increased capillary permeability, bronchoconstriction, and decreased peristalsis.

Clinical Manifestations

1. Respiratory—laryngeal edema, bronchospasm, cough, wheezing, lump in throat
2. Cardiovascular—hypotension, tachycardia, palpitations, syncope
3. Cutaneous—urticaria (hives), angioedema, pruritus, erythema (flushing)
4. Gastrointestinal—nausea, vomiting, diarrhea, abdominal pain, bloating

NURSING ALERT:
Before you administer any potentially harmful drug or other agent, ask patients if they have ever had a reaction to it. Do not rely on the chart alone.

Management

Prompt identification of signs and symptoms and immediate intervention are essential; the more quickly a reaction occurs, the more severe it tends to be.

A. Immediate Treatment
1. A tourniquet is applied above site of antigen injection (allergy injection, insect sting, etc) or skin test site—to slow the absorption of antigen into the system.
2. Epinephrine (Adrenalin) 1:1,000, 0.1 to 0.5 mL is injected subcutaneously or intramuscularly (IM) into opposite arm; may be repeated every 15 to 20 minutes if necessary—causes vasoconstriction, decreases capillary permeability, relaxes airway smooth muscle, and inhibits mast cell mediator release.

B. Subsequent Treatment
1. An adequate airway is established and epinephrine is administered by inhalation.
2. Hypotension and shock are treated with fluids and vasopressors.
3. Additional bronchodilators are given to relax bronchial smooth muscle.
4. H_1 antihistamines such as diphenhydramine (Benadryl) and possibly H_2 antihistamines such as ranitidine (Zantac) are given to block the effects of histamine.
5. Corticosteroids are given to decrease vascular permeability and diminish the migration of inflammatory cells; may be helpful in preventing late phase responses.

Complications

1. Cardiovascular collapse
2. Respiratory failure

Nursing Assessment

1. Emergently assess airway, breathing, and circulation (ABCs) if severe presentation and intervene with cardiopulmonary resuscitation as appropriate (see p. 942).
2. If less severe presentation, assess vital signs, degree of respiratory distress, and presence of angioedema.
3. Obtain a history of onset of symptoms and exposure to allergen.

Nursing Diagnoses

A. Impaired Breathing Pattern related to bronchospasm and laryngeal edema
B. Decreased Cardiac Output related to vasodilation
C. Anxiety related to respiratory distress and life-threatening situation

Nursing Interventions

A. *Restoring Effective Breathing*
1. Establish and maintain an adequate airway.
   a. If epinephrine has not stabilized bronchospasm, assist with endotracheal intubation, emergency tracheostomy, or cricothyroidotomy as indicated.
   b. Continually monitor respiratory rate, depth, and breath sounds for decreased work of breathing and effective ventilation.
2. Administer nebulized epinephrine or other bronchodilators, as ordered. Monitor heart rate (increased with bronchodilators).
3. Provide oxygen via nasal cannula at 2 to 5 L/min or by alternate means, as ordered.
4. Administer aminophylline and corticosteroids intravenously (IV), as ordered.

B. *Increasing Cardiac Output*
1. Monitor blood pressure by continuous automatic cuff, if available.
2. Administer rapid infusion of IV fluids to fill vasodilated circulatory system and raise blood pressure.
3. Monitor central venous pressure (CVP) to ensure adequate fluid volume and prevent fluid overload.
4. Insert indwelling catheter and monitor urine output hourly to ensure kidney perfusion.
5. Initiate and titrate vasopressor, as ordered, and based on blood pressure response.

C. *Reducing Anxiety*
1. Provide care in a quick, confident manner.
2. Remain responsive to the patient, who may remain alert, but not completely coherent due to hypotension, hypoxemia, and effects of medication.
3. Keep family/significant others informed of patient's condition and the treatment being given.
4. When patient is stable and alert, give simple, honest explanation of anaphylaxis and the treatment that was given.

Patient Education/ Health Maintenance

Instruct patients as follows:

1. Read labels and be familiar with the generic name of the drug thought to cause a reaction.
2. Discard all unused drugs. Make sure any drug kept in the medicine cabinet is clearly labeled.
3. Familiarize yourself with drugs that may cross-react with a drug to which you are allergic.
4. Always know the names of every drug that you take.
5. Be extremely careful about everything you eat if you have a known sensitivity to a food product—allergic compounds are often hidden in a preparation (such as monosodium glutamate).
6. Teach the patient at risk for anaphylaxis about the potential seriousness of these reactions.
7. Educate patients to recognize the early signs and symptoms of anaphylaxis.
8. Persons allergic to bee stings should avoid wearing brightly colored or black clothes, perfumes, and hair spray. Shoes should be worn at all times.
9. For exercise-induced anaphylaxis, patients should exercise in moderation, preferably with another person, and in a controlled setting where assistance is readily available.
10. If food is associated with exercise-induced anaphylaxis, wait at least 2 hours after eating to exercise.
11. Instruct the patient in the self-injection technique for the administration of epinephrine and to carry it at all times.
12. Provide the patient with information on epinephrine (Epi-Pen; Ana-Kit), including the action of the drug, possible side effects, and the importance of prompt administration at the first sign of a systemic reaction.
13. Instruct patients to wear a Medic Alert bracelet or tag at all times.

Evaluation

A. Respirations 28/min and deep with moderate wheezing and aeration throughout lung fields
B. Blood pressure and CVP within normal range; urine output adequate
C. Patient responsive and cooperative

◆ ALLERGIC RHINITIS

Allergic rhinitis is an inflammation of the nasal mucosa caused by an allergen that affects 8% to 10% of the population.

Pathophysiology/Etiology

1. Type I hypersensitivity causing local vasodilation and increased capillary permeability
2. Brought about by airborne allergens
   a. Seasonal—offending allergen is a pollen or mold; symptoms are episodic.
   b. Perennial—offending allergen is dust, dust mites, mold, or animal dander; symptoms occur year round.

Clinical Manifestations

1. Nasal—mucous membrane congestion, edema, itching, rhinorrhea with clear secretions, sneezing
2. Eyes—edema, itching, burning, tearing, redness, dark circles under eyes (allergic) shiners
3. Ears—itching, fullness
4. Other—palatal itching, throat itching, nonproductive cough

Diagnostic Evaluation

1. Nasal smear—the presence of an increased number of eosinophils suggests allergic disease.
2. Skin testing—confirms a hypersensitivity to certain allergens.
3. RAST—positive for offending allergen(s)
4. Rhinoscopy—allows better visualization of the nasopharynx; useful to rule out physical obstruction (septal deviation, nasal polyps).

Management

A. *Avoidance*
1. Patients should minimize contact with offending allergens, regardless of other treatment.
2. Dust mites can be removed from carpeting through treatment with 3% tannic acid or benzyl benzoate (Ascarosan).

B. *Medications: Acute Phase*
1. H_1 antihistamines—block the effects of histamine on smooth muscle and blood vessels by blocking histamine receptor sites, thereby relieving the symptoms of allergic rhinitis.
2. Decongestants—shrink nasal mucous membrane by vasoconstriction.
3. Anticholinergic agents—inhibit mucous secretions.

C. *Medications: Preventive Therapy*
1. Intranasal cromolyn sodium (Nasalcrom)—mast cell stabilizer; hinders the release of chemical mediators. Mast cell stabilizers now are also available as oral preparation cromolyn (Gastrocrom) and ophthalmic solution cromolyn (Crolom) and lodoxamide (Alomide).
2. Corticosteroids (oral and intranasal)
   a. Reduce inflammation of nasal mucosa
   b. Prevent mediator release
   c. Only given systemically for a short course during a disabling attack

D. *Immunotherapy*
1. Regimen consists of administering subcutaneous injections of increasing amounts of an allergen to which the patient is sensitive in an attempt to decrease sensitivity and reduce the severity of symptoms.
2. Immunotherapy produces the following immunologic changes:
   a. Increases IgG-blocking antibody that combines with antigen before it reacts with IgE antibodies.
   b. May decrease IgE antibodies against specific antigens.
   c. Decreases mast cell sensitivity.
3. Possible adverse reactions of immunotherapy
   a. Systemic reactions—anaphylaxis is rare, but potentially fatal.
   b. Local reactions—consist of erythema and induration at the site of injection.

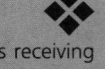

NURSING ALERT:
Note: Immunotherapy should not be given to patients receiving β-adrenergic blocking agents. It would be difficult to reverse a systemic reaction, should one occur.

Complications

1. Allergic asthma
2. Chronic otitis media, hearing loss
3. Chronic nasal obstruction, sinusitis

Nursing Assessment

1. Obtain history of severity and seasonality of symptoms.
2. Inspect for characteristic tearing, conjunctival erythema, pale nasal mucous membranes with clear discharge, allergic shiners, and mouth breathing.

Nursing Diagnosis

A. Breathing Pattern Ineffective related to nasal obstruction

Nursing Interventions

A. *Facilitating Normal Breathing Pattern*
1. Reassure patient that suffocation will not occur due to nasal obstruction; mouth breathing will occur.
2. Use a bedside humidifier and increase oral fluid intake to prevent drying of mucous membranes and increased insensible loss through mouth breathing.
3. Administer and teach self-administration of antihistamines, decongestants, and other medications as directed.
   a. Instruct patients on proper use of nasal inhalers—clear mucus from nose first, exhale, then inhale while releasing medication.
   b. Warn patient to avoid driving or other situations that require alertness if sedating antihistamines such as diphenhydramine (Benadryl) or chlorpheniramine (Chlor-Trimeton) have been prescribed.
   c. Do not use over-the-counter nasal decongestants for more than 2 to 3 days because their effect is short lived and a "rebound" effect causing nasal mucosal edema often occurs.

Patient Education/ Health Maintenance

A. *Immunotherapy*
1. Provide information on the purpose, method of administration, time frame of expected results, and the possible risks involved (local reactions, anaphylaxis).
2. Inform the patient that close observation for 30 minutes is essential after each injection.
3. Alert patient to the possibility of a delayed reaction that needs to be reported to the nurse or health care provider.

B. *Environmental Control* Advise patients on the following environmental modifications to reduce symptoms

1. Use nonallergic materials for bedding (pillows, blankets).
2. Keep clothing in a closet with door shut.
3. Avoid venetian blinds—use washable curtains.
4. Avoid stuffed animals and other dust collectors.
5. Encase mattress and boxsprings in zippered plastic covers.
6. Use synthetic pillows that can be washed and replaced frequently; bed linens should be washed in hot water (more than 130°F).
7. Damp-dust daily and wear a mask while doing it.
8. Eliminate upholstered furniture, shag carpets, and draperies.
9. Use air conditioning to reduce antigen load indoors.
10. Change furnace filters frequently.
11. Using a high-efficiency air filtering system may help.
12. Avoid smoking and smoke-filled areas.
13. Avoid rapid changes in temperature.
14. Patients allergic to animal danders should not have household pets—or should at least keep them out of the bedroom.
15. Avoid mold growth by using a fungicide in bathrooms, damp basements, food storage areas, and garbage containers.
16. Keep windows closed during high pollen season.
17. Avoid outdoor activities when high pollen/pollutants are in the air.

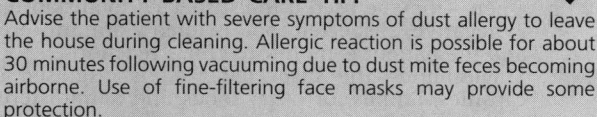

COMMUNITY-BASED CARE TIP:
Advise the patient with severe symptoms of dust allergy to leave the house during cleaning. Allergic reaction is possible for about 30 minutes following vacuuming due to dust mite feces becoming airborne. Use of fine-filtering face masks may provide some protection.

C. *Additional Resources*
American Academy of Allergy and Immunology
611 E. Wells St.
Milwaukee, WI 53202
800-822-2762

Asthma and Allergy Foundation of America
1125 15th St., NW
Suite 502
Washington, DC 20005
800-727-8462

Evaluation

A. Mouth breathing reduced; no complaints of dry mouth

◆ URTICARIA AND ANGIOEDEMA

Urticaria (hives) may affect 10% of the population at some time during their lives. Angioedema is a similar lesion but involves deep dermis and subcutaneous tissues. Urticaria and angioedema can occur individually or in combination.

Pathophysiology/Etiology

1. Acute urticaria
   a. Hives lasting less than 6 weeks
   b. A detectable cause is usually determined.
2. Chronic urticaria
   a. Hives lasting 6 weeks or longer
   b. The cause is undetermined in 75% to 90% of patients.
3. Causes include:
   a. Ingested substances—food, food additives, drugs
   b. Infections—viral, bacterial, parasitic
   c. Physical factors—heat, sun, cold, pressure, emotional stress

Clinical Manifestations

1. Raised, dime- to saucer-sized red edematous wheals
2. May affect any body region
3. Intense pruritus
4. Diffuse swelling with angioedema, especially of the lips, eyelids, cheeks, hands, and feet
5. Symptoms may develop within seconds or over 1 to 2 hours and may last up to 24 to 36 hours.

Diagnostic Evaluation

1. Laboratory—erythrocyte sedimentation rate (ESR) is often elevated.
2. Skin biopsy to rule out urticaria pigmentosa
3. Challenge testing to determine physical cause
   a. Exercise challenge
   b. Ice cube challenge
   c. Heat challenge
   d. Pressure challenge

Management

A. *Acute Urticaria*
1. Identification and elimination of causative factors
2. Medications
   a. H_1 antihistamine such as terfenadine (Seldane)
   b. Epinephrine (Adrenalin) 1:1,000 (0.3–0.5 mL subcutaneously) for extensive urticaria, angioedema
   c. Corticosteroids—limited to severe cases unresponsive to antihistamines

B. *Chronic Urticaria*
1. Elimination diet
2. Medications
   a. H_1 antihistamines
   b. H_2 antihistamines such as ranitidine (Zantac) may be of some value.
   c. Tricyclic antidepressants—doxepin (Adapin)—given for antihistaminic effect
   d. Topical agents to relieve itching (Lubriderm or oatmeal baths)

Complications

1. Neurovascular impairment due to swelling
2. Occasionally edema of the larynx or bronchi may occur

Nursing Assessment

1. Assess for time course over which lesions appear and disappear.
2. Assess for triggering factors.
3. Assess for family history of angioedema; may indicate hereditary angioedema rather than allergic reaction.

Nursing Diagnosis

A. Sensory/Perceptual Alteration related to pruritus

Nursing Interventions

A. *Relieving Pruritus*
1. Administer or teach self-administration of antihistamines, corticosteroids, and additional medications as prescribed.
2. Encourage the proper use of topical and over-the-counter agents, as directed.
3. Advise patient to avoid exposure to heat, exercise, sunburn, fever, anxiety, and alcohol—factors that may aggravate reactions due to vasodilation.
4. Warn patient to avoid triggers of exacerbation if identified.
5. Teach relaxation techniques and methods of distraction to enhance coping.
6. Assess effectiveness of therapy.

Patient Education/ Health Maintenance

1. Warn the patient to monitor for symptoms of laryngeal edema and seek medical intervention immediately if respiratory distress occurs.
2. Instruct patients in self-administration of epinephrine if there is a history of laryngeal edema.

Evaluation

A. Reports relief of pruritus with antihistamines and distraction methods

◆ FOOD ALLERGIES

Food allergies result when the body's immune system overreacts to certain otherwise harmless substances. Food allergies occur in 4% to 6% of children and less than 1% of adults although the perceived prevalence is much higher due to other existing adverse food reactions that cause similar symptoms.

Pathophysiology/Etiology

1. Food hypersensitivity—a true food allergy is an IgE-mediated response to a food allergen (protein).
2. Food intolerance—an abnormal physical response to a food or additive and is not immunologic.
   a. Toxicity (poisoning)—caused by toxins contained in foods, microorganisms, or parasites.
   b. Pharmacologic (chemical)—such as caffeine
   c. Idiosyncratic—etiology unknown
3. Common food allergens include cow's milk, eggs, shellfish, peanuts, soybean, and wheat.

Clinical Manifestations

1. Respiratory—rhinoconjunctivitis, sneezing, laryngeal edema, wheezing
2. Cutaneous—urticaria, angioedema, atopic dermatitis
3. Gastroenteritis—lip swelling, palatal itching, nausea, abdominal cramping, diarrhea
4. Neurologic—migraine headaches in some patients

Diagnostic Tests

1. Skin testing
   a. Limit to those foods suspected of provoking symptoms based on history.
   b. Only epicutaneous testing is done.
   c. Intradermal testing has not been demonstrated to have a high degree of clinical correlation.
2. RAST—positive
3. Oral challenge
   a. The suspected food is given to the patient in an attempt to identify the allergen by reproducing the symptoms caused by the initial reaction.
   b. Open—may be used if the suspected food skin test is negative; suspected food is openly administered and the patient is monitored for a reaction.
   c. Single-blind—the suspected food is disguised in capsules, liquids, or other foods and administered to the patient in increasing doses at intervals determined by history and may be interspersed with placebo. Some bias exists.
   d. Double-blind placebo-controlled—the most definitive technique to confirm or refute histories of food allergies. The suspected food is administerd in capsules or other vehicle that masks its identity and is interspersed with placebo so neither the health care provider/nurse nor patient knows whether the suspected food or placebo is being ingested.
5. Elimination diet
   a. To determine if the patient's symptoms will stop when certain foods are avoided
   b. Restrict one or two foods at a time if certain foods are suspected.
   c. If no particular food is suspected, a highly restricted diet for 7 to 14 days is preferable.

Management

1. Avoidance of specific foods is the only way of effectively preventing food allergy reactions.
2. Medications:
   a. Antihistamines—may modify IgE symptoms but will not eliminate them.
   b. Corticosteroids—only used in the treatment of food allergy if associated with eosinophilic gastroenteritis or gastroenteropathy.

c. Epinephrine (Adrenalin)—if history of anaphylaxis, patient should carry it at all times (Epi-Pen; Ana-Kit)

Complications

1. Anaphylaxis

Nursing Assessment

1. Assist with assessment for offending foods; encourage the patient to keep a food/symptom diary.
2. Assess compliance with prescribed diet and relief of symptoms.

Nursing Diagnosis

A. Altered Nutrition (Less than Body Requirements) related to restrictive diet

Nursing Interventions

A. *Promoting Adequate Nutrition*
1. Consult with dietitian to ensure a balanced diet that excludes identified allergens and incorporates patient's food preferences.
2. Administer dietary supplements as needed.
3. Explain hidden sources of foods to decrease the risk of unexpected exposure to an offending allergen. Encourage label reading.
4. Discuss alternative food preparation techniques and methods of substitution (such as using extra baking powder in place of eggs).
5. Administer and teach self-administration of medications, if necessary, to reduce abdominal cramping and diarrhea, which may deter food intake.
6. Monitor weight.

Patient Teaching/Health Education

1. Instruct the patient in self-injection technique for the administration of epinephrine if history of anaphylactic reaction.
2. Caution highly allergic patients about restaurant food; when eating out, patients should request ingredient information—such brochures are now available in many restaurants, including fast food establishments.
3. Advise patient that most young children and about one-third of older children and adults lose their food sensitivity after 1 to 2 years of avoidance. Compliance with elimination is the key. Sensitivity to fish and nuts is rarely lost, however.

Evaluation

A. Verbalizes acceptance of diet; weight stable

◆ BRONCHIAL ASTHMA

Bronchial asthma is characterized by variable, recurrent, reversible airway obstruction clinically manifested by intermittent episodes of wheezing and dyspnea. It is associated with hyperresponsiveness of the bronchi to various stimuli that may be antigen mediated (allergic).

Pathophysiology/Etiology

The basic defect appears to be an abnormality in the host, which intermittently leads to an increased constriction of smooth muscle, hypersecretion of mucus in the bronchial tree, and mucosal edema.

A. *Neuromechanisms (Autonomic Nervous System)*
1. Stimulation of the vagus nerve (which is responsible for bronchomotor tone) by viral respiratory infections, air pollutants, and other stimuli causes bronchoconstriction, increased secretion of mucus, and dilation of the pulmonary vessels.
2. β-Adrenergic receptor cells that line the airways are also responsible for bronchomotor tone. Abnormal functioning of these cells predisposes patients to bronchoconstriction.

B. *Antigen–Antibody Reaction*
1. Susceptible individuals form abnormally large amounts of IgE when exposed to certain allergens.
2. This immunoglobulin (IgE) fixes itself to the mast cells of the bronchial mucosa.
3. When the individual is exposed to certain allergens, the resulting antigen combines with the cell-bound IgE molecules, causing the mast cell to degranulate and release chemical mediators.
4. These chemical mediators act on bronchial smooth muscle to cause bronchoconstriction, on dilated epithelium to reduce mucociliary clearance, on bronchial glands to cause mucus secretion, on blood vessels to cause vasodilation and increased permeability, and on leukocytes to cause a cellular infiltration and inflammation.
5. Late-phase reactions (occurring 4–8 hours after the initial response) include the influx of neutrophils, eosinophils, lymphocytes, and monocytes.

C. *Bronchial Inflammation*
1. Occurs in both the immediate- and late-phase reactions caused by antigen–antibody response.
2. Factors other than allergens (such as noxious environmental stimuli) cause bronchial inflammation and hyperreactivity by mast cell activation.

Classification

A. *Extrinsic Asthma*
1. Hypersensitivity reaction to inhalant allergens (dust, dust mites, mold, pollens, feathers, and animal dander are the major ones)
2. Mediated by immunoglobin E (IgE mediated).

B. *Intrinsic Asthma*
1. No inciting allergen
2. Infection, often viral
3. Environmental stimuli (such as air pollution)

C. *Mixed Asthma*
Immediate type I reactivity appears to be combined with intrinsic factors.

D. *Aspirin-Induced Asthma*
1. Induced by ingestion of aspirin and related compounds.
2. "Triad" has been described as a combination of aspirin-induced asthma, nasal polyps, and sinusitis.

E. *Exercise-Induced Asthma*
Symptoms vary from slight chest tightness and cough to severe wheezing/cough and shortness of breath that usually occur within 5 to 20 minutes after exercise.

F. *Occupational Asthma*
1. Caused by inhalation of industrial fumes, dust, and gases.
2. Cough without associated wheezing is a more common symptom than in other forms of asthma.

Clinical Manifestations

1. Episodes of coughing
2. Wheezing
3. Dyspnea
4. Feeling of chest tightness

NURSING ALERT:
Do not be fooled by lack of wheezing on auscultation when the patient complains of severe shortness of breath. Airflow may be so restricted that wheezing ceases.

Diagnostic Evaluation

1. Laboratory—increased levels of IgE are usually seen in atopic asthma.
2. Pulmonary function testing—decreased—forced expiratory volume
3. Bronchial methacholine challenge—demonstrates airway hyperreactivity by the inhalation of a cholinergic agent in serial concentrations delivered by nebulization; a positive response is indicated by a 20% greater decrease in the forced expiratory volume in 1 second from the control value.
4. Skin testing to identify causative allergens
5. Sputum and nasal cytology (increased eosinophilia)
6. Chest x-ray to exclude other lung diseases

Management

The goal is to allow the person with asthma to live a normal life. It is important that the approach to management is structured and that the treatment is unique to the patient and his or her condition.

A. *Medications*
1. Include bronchodilators, corticosteroids, cromolyn sodium (Intal), antihistamines, and anticholinergics.
2. Aerosol therapy with β-adrenoceptor agonists, cromolyn sodium, and inhaled steroids form the basis of asthma treatment.

3. The most convenient and inexpensive method of aerosol delivery to patients is the metered-dose inhaler.

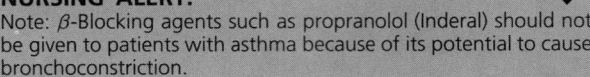

NURSING ALERT:
Note: β-Blocking agents such as propranolol (Inderal) should not be given to patients with asthma because of its potential to cause bronchoconstriction.

B. *Other Measures*
1. Environmental control (see allergic rhinitis, p. 809)
2. Immunotherapy (see allergic rhinitis, p. 808)
3. Dietary control. Foods that contain tartrazine (yellow dye no. 5) may cause asthma in aspirin-sensitive patients and should be avoided.
4. Exercise
   a. Regular aerobic exercise should be encouraged.
   b. Use of an inhaled β agonist or cromolyn taken 15 to 20 minutes before exercise will decrease postexercise bronchospasm.

Nursing Assessment

1. Review patient's record: ask about coughing, dyspnea, exertional changes, and increased mucous production.
2. Observe the patient and assess the rate, depth, and character of respirations, especially on expiration; observe for hyperinflation.
3. Auscultate the chest for breath sounds/wheezing.
4. Assess for triggers of asthma including
   a. Allergens
   b. Respiratory infections
   c. Inhalation of irritating substances (dust, fumes, gases)
   d. Environmental factors (weather, air pollution, and humidity)
   e. Exercise, particularly in cold weather
   f. Aspirin and its derivatives
   g. Sulfite-containing agents used as food preservatives
   h. Emotional factors
5. After acute episode subsides, attempt to determine patient's degree of compliance with medications/management regimen.

Nursing Diagnoses

A. Ineffective Breathing Pattern related to bronchospasm
B. Anxiety related to fear of suffocating, difficulty in breathing, death

Nursing Interventions

A. *Attaining Relief of Dyspneic Breathing*
1. Monitor vital signs, skin color, and degree of restlessness, which may indicate hypoxia.
2. Provide nebulization and oxygen therapy as prescribed.
3. Monitor airway functioning through peak flow meter or pulmonary function testing to assess effectiveness of treatment.
4. Encourage intake of fluids to liquefy secretions.
5. Instruct patient on positioning to facilitate breathing—sitting upright (leaning forward on a table).

6. Use chest physiotherapy/postural drainage to mobilize secretions.
7. Encourage patient to use adaptive breathing techniques (eg, pursed-lip breathing) to decrease the work of breathing.

B. Relieving Anxiety
1. Explain rationale for interventions to gain patient's co-operation. Provide care in prompt confident manner.
2. Help patient clarify source(s) of anxiety; suggest measures to reduce anxiety and control breathing.
3. Encourage and support efforts to comply with management plan.

Patient Education

1. Provide information on the nature of asthma methods of treatment.
2. Provide information regarding medications, including proper use of inhaler devices; stress avoiding overuse of inhalers and nebulizers.
3. Demonstrate the use of peak flow meters and recording of peak flow measurements.
4. Help patient to identify what triggers asthma, warning signs of an impending attack, and strategies for preventing an attack.
5. Teach adaptive breathing techniques and breathing exercises, such as pursed-lip breathing.
6. Discuss environmental control.
   a. Avoid persons with respiratory infections.
   b. Avoid substances and situations known to precipitate bronchospasm, such as irritants, gases, fumes and smoke.
   c. Wear a mask if cold weather precipitates bronchospasm.
   d. Stay inside when air pollution is high.
   e. See Patient Education, Allergic Rhinitis, page 809.
7. Promote optimal health practices, including nutrition, rest, and exercise.
   a. Encourage regular exercise to improve cardiorespiratory and musculoskeletal conditioning.
   b. Drink liberal amounts of fluids to keep secretions thin.
   c. Avoid taking sleeping pills after an asthma attack because these medications slow respirations and make breathing more difficult.
   d. Try to avoid upsetting situations.
   e. Use relaxation techniques, biofeedback management.
   f. Use community resources for smoking cessation classes, stress management, exercises for relaxation, etc.
8. For additional information and support, refer to: National Asthma Education Program, ROW Sciences, Inc.; P.O. Box 30105; Bethesda, MD 20824; 301-251-1222.

Evaluation

A. Wheezing reduced; peak flow improved
B. Verbalizes relief of anxiety

◆ STATUS ASTHMATICUS

Status asthmaticus is a severe form of asthma in which the airway obstruction is unresponsive to conventional drug therapy and lasts longer than 24 hours.

Contributing Factors

1. Infection
2. Overuse of tranquilizers
3. Nebulizer abuse
4. Dehydration
5. Inhalation of air pollutants
6. Noncompliance in taking medications
7. Sudden reduction in corticosteroids
8. Ingestion of aspirin or related drugs in aspirin-sensitive patient

Clinical Manifestations

1. Labored respirations, with increased effort on exhalation
2. Distended neck and face veins
3. Fatigue, headache, irritability, dizziness, impaired mental functioning—from hypoxia
4. Muscle twitching, somnolence, diaphoresis—from continued carbon dioxide retention
5. Tachycardia, elevated blood pressure
6. Heart failure and death from suffocation

Management and Nursing Interventions

1. Continuously or frequently monitor arterial blood gases, blood pressure, electrocardiogram, and respiratory rate.

NURSING ALERT:
In status asthmaticus, the return to a normal or increasing P_{CO_2} does not necessarily mean that the asthmatic patient is improving—it may indicate a fatigue state that develops just before the patient slips into respiratory failure.

2. Administer repeated aerosol treatments with bronchodilators such as albuterol (Ventolin) as prescribed—may perpetuate intractability—administer with caution until the metabolic and respiratory acidosis and hypoxemia have been corrected.
3. Monitor IV therapy.
   a. When IV fluids are administered, aminophylline (Aminophyllin) may be prescribed and administered slowly by constant infusion; the clinician must be constantly alert for signs of theophylline toxicity (tachycarida, nausea, vomiting, restlessness, dizziness).
   b. Corticosteroids are given to treat inflammation of airways; because these act slowly, their beneficial effects may not be apparent for several hours.

c. Fluids are given to treat dehydration and loosen secretions.

4. Provide continuous humidified oxygen via nasal cannula as prescribed. (Patients with associated chronic obstructive pulmonary disease or emphysema are at risk for depressed hypoxemic ventilatory drive, thus compounding respiratory insufficiency, so use oxygen cautiously.)

5. Initiate mechanical ventilation, if necessary.

6. Assist with mobilization of obstructing bronchial mucus.

a. Perform chest physiotherapy (chest wall percussion and vibration).

b. Administer expectorant and mucolytic drugs as prescribed.

c. Remove secretions by suctioning, or prepare for bronchoscopy if needed.

d. Provide adequate hydration.

7. Alleviate the patient's anxiety and fear by acting calmly and reassuring the patient during an attack. Stay with the patient until the attack subsides.

Selected References

Beltrani, V. S. (1993). Managing the patient with hives. *Dermatology Nursing, 5*(4), 281-288.

Borkgren, M. W. & Gronkiewicz, C. A. (1995). Update your asthma care from hospital to home. *AJN, 94*(1), 26-34.

Creticos, P. S. (1992). Immunotherapy with allergans. *The Journal of the American Medical Association, 268*(20), 2834-2839.

Kaliner, M., & Lemanske, R. (1992). Rhinitis and asthma. *The Journal of the American Medical Association, 268*(20), 2807-2829.

Mygrind, N. & Naclerio, R. (eds.) (1993). *Allergic and nonallergic rhinitis: Clinical aspects.* Philadelphia: W.B. Saunders.

Patterson, R., Zeiss, C. R., Grammar, L. C. & Greenberger, P. A. (1993). *Allergic diseases: Diagnosis and Management.* Philadelphia: J.B. Lippincott.

Salerno, M., Huss, K., & Huss, R. W. Allergen avoidance in the treatment of dust-mite allergy and asthma. (1992). *The Nurse Practitioner, 17*(10), 53-65.

Valentine, M. D. (1992). Anaphylaxis and stinging insect hypersensitivity. *The Journal of the American Medical Association, 268*(20), 2830-2833.

Winbourn, M. (1994). Food allergy, the hidden culprit. *Journal of the American Academy of Nurse Practitioners, 6*(11), 515-522.

HIV Disease and AIDS

◆ DEVELOPMENT AND TRANSMISSION OF HIV DISEASE AND AIDS

Acquired immunodeficiency syndrome (AIDS) is defined as the most severe form of a continuum of illnesses associated with human immunodeficiency virus (HIV) infection. It causes a slow degeneration of the immune system with the development of opportunistic infections and malignancies. HIV disease implies the entire course of HIV infection from asymptomatic infection and early symptoms to AIDS.

Pathophysiology/Etiology

1. The causative agent is a retrovirus that infects and depletes the "protector" cells of the immune system called lymphocytes. B lymphocytes secrete antibodies into the body fluids or humors and this is known as *humoral immunity*. T lymphocytes can penetrate living cells, a process called *cell-mediated immunity*.
2. Monocytes and macrophages, whose role is to present antigen to T cells thereby initiating the body's immune response, are also infected by HIV.
3. Once HIV has entered the body, it attaches most efficiently to CD4 molecules, which are predominantly located on the cell membrane of T4 helper lymphocytes. HIV destroys the CD4 molecule as it enters to infect the T4 lymphocyte.
4. With progressive invasion of HIV, cellular and humoral immunity decline and opportunistic infections that characterize this disease begin to emerge.
5. Body fluids known to transmit HIV are blood, vaginal secretions, semen, and breast milk.
6. HIV is transmitted by injection of blood or blood components, sexual contact (vaginal/anal intercourse, oral sex), and perinatally from an infected mother to the child.

High-Risk Groups for HIV Transmission

1. Homosexual or bisexual men
2. Intravenous (IV) drug users
3. Transfusion and blood product recipients (before 1985)
4. Heterosexual contacts of HIV-positive individuals
5. Newborn babies of mothers who are HIV positive

Natural History of HIV Disease

A. **After Exposure to HIV Infection**
1. Most persons infected with HIV show no immediate symptoms or signs of illness. However, some people experience a brief flulike illness referred to as acute retroviral syndrome. It is not known what significance, if any, the occurrence of this syndrome has on the prognosis of the disease. However, it is known that the immune system is compromised by a sudden decrease in T4 helper cells for a brief period.
2. Seroconversion occurs when the person has developed enough antibody to HIV that the serologic test is positive. It takes 3 to 6 months for seroconversion to occur.
3. Staging of HIV disease is based on the medical findings and the CD4 count. A normal CD4 count is 800 to 1,000/cu mm. Because HIV destroys a CD4 molecule as it enters the T4 lymphocyte, CD4 count diminishes over time. Therefore, measurement of CD4 is used to evaluate the stage of HIV infection (Fig. 27-1).

B. **Development of AIDS-Related Diseases**
1. Appears years after exposure to HIV
2. Due to declining immunity, frequent infections, severe opportunistic infections, and malignancies develop.

Clinical Manifestations

1. Pulmonary manifestations
   a. Persistent cough with and without sputum production, shortness of breath, chest pain, fever
   b. From *Pneumocystis carinii* pneumonia (most common), bacterial pneumonia, *Mycobacterium tuberculosis*, disseminated *Mycobacterium avium* complex, cytomegalovirus (CMV), *Histoplasma*, Kaposi's sarcoma, *Cryptococcus*, *Legionella*, and other pathogens
2. Gastrointestinal manifestations
   a. Diarrhea, weight loss, anorexia, abdominal cramping, rectal urgency (tenesmus)
   b. From enteric pathogens including *Salmonella*, *Shigella*, *Campylobacter*, *Entamoeba histolytica*, CMV, *M. avium* complex, herpes simplex, *Strongyloides*, *Giardia*, *Cryptosporidium*, *Isospora belli*, *Chlamydia*, and others

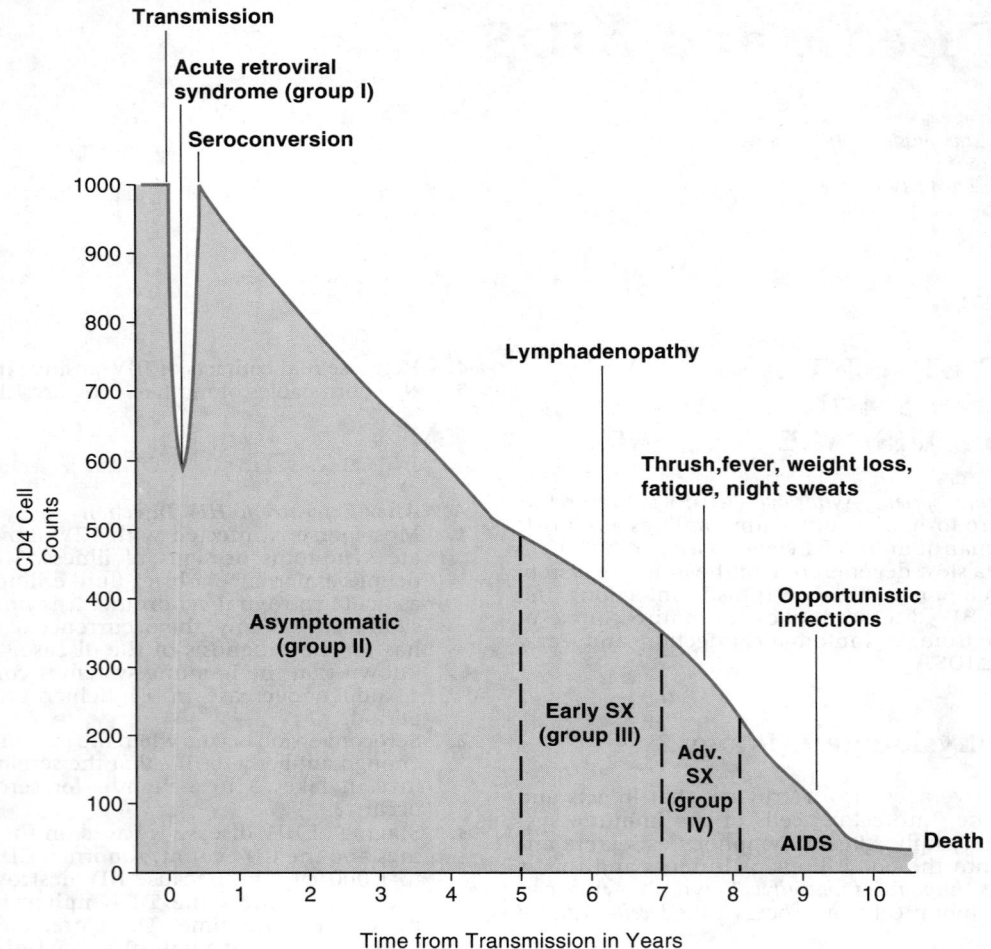

FIGURE 27-1 *Natural history of HIV disease.*

3. Oral manifestations
   a. Appearance of oral lesions, white plaques on oral mucosa, and angular cheilitis from *Candida albicans* of mouth and esophagus
   b. Vesicles with ulceration from herpes simplex virus
   c. White thickened lesions on lateral margins of tongue from hairy leukoplakia
   d. Oral warts due to human papillomavirus (HPV) and associated gingivitis
   e. Periodontitis progressing to gingival necrosis
4. Central nervous system (CNS) manifestations
   a. Cognitive, motor, and behavioral symptoms (AIDS dementia complex/HIV encephalopathy)
   b. Demonstrated by mental slowing, impaired memory and concentration, loss of balance, lower extremity weakness, ataxia, apathy, and social withdrawal
   c. From CNS toxoplasmosis, cryptococcal meningitis, herpes virus infections, CMV (causing retinopathy and blindness), and CNS lymphoma
6. Malignancies
   a. Kaposi's sarcoma (aggressive tumor involving skin, lymph nodes, gastrointestinal tract, and lungs)

   b. Non-Hodgkin's lymphoma (p. 766) and lymphomas (p. 775)
   c. Cervical carcinoma (p. 674)

Diagnostic Evaluation

1. History of risk factors/high-risk behaviors
2. Positive blood test for HIV
   a. Enzyme-linked immunosorbent assay (ELISA)—serologic test for detecting antibody to HIV
   b. Western blot test—used to confirm a positive result on ELISA test
   c. Once infected with HIV, it can take the body 3 to 6 months to develop enough antibody to HIV for the test result to be positive, resulting in a false-negative test if evaluated early.
   d. Occasionally, a sample that tests reactivity by ELISA may give an indeterminate result by Western blot. The cause of an indeterminate result may be early HIV seroconversion or error during interpretation of the test. The test should be repeated every 2 to 3 months until Western blot becomes positive or there is no longer suspicion of HIV disease.

3. Lymphocyte panel shows decreased CD4 count.
4. A complete blood count (CBC) may show anemia and a low white blood cell count.
5. Presence of indicator disease (eg, *P. carinii* pneumonia, candidiasis of esophagus, Kaposi's sarcoma, etc.)
6. Diagnostic procedures (biopsies, imaging procedures, etc.) of the organ system involved to confirm opportunistic infection, malignancy, or other causes

7. Neuropsychological testing—to identify cognitive deficits associated with AIDS dementia complex

Complications

1. Repeated overwhelming opportunistic infections (Table 27-1)
2. Respiratory failure
3. Wasting

TABLE 27-1 Opportunistic Infections and Drug Therapies

Name	Clinical Manifestations	Diagnostic Tests	Medications
Pneumocystis carinii pneumonia (PCP)	Cough; dry or scant white sputum production Shortness of breath Low grade fever	Chest x-ray Sputum culture for silver stain Bronchoscopy	Trimethoprim/ sulfamethoxazole (Bactrim) Pentamidine (Pentam) (IV only) Dapsone (Dapsone)
Candida esophagitis/ oral	White coating in mouth White coating down throat Sensation of food getting caught in throat while swallowing	Gross observation Microscopy for hyphae Endoscopy	Nystatin (Mycostatin) Clotrimazole (Mycelex) Ketoconazole (Nizoral) Fluconazole (Diflucan) Amphotericin B (Fungizone)
Mycobacterium avium complex (MAC)	Weakness Weight Loss Diarrhea Fever, chills	Blood culture for acid-fast bacteria	Micobutin (Rifabutin) Rifampin (Rifadin) Ethambutol (Myambutol) Isoniazid (INH) Clarithromycin (Biaxin)
Kaposi's sarcoma	Pink, purple, or brown spots Pain, edema of affected area	Gross observation Biopsy	Alpha-interferon (Alferon) Vincristine (Oncovin) Bleomycin (Blenoxane)
Toxoplasmosis	Fever Headache Change in mental status Confusion Lethargy Frank psychosis	Computed tomography Magnetic resonance imaging Serum *Toxoplasma* antibodies	Pyrimethamine (Daraprim) Sulfadiazine (Microsulfon) Clindamycin (Cleocin)
Tuberculosis	Cough; dry or scant frothy white/pink sputum Shortness of breath Fever Lymphadenopathy	Positive purified protein derivative (≥5 mm induration) Chest x-ray Sputum culture for acid-fast bacteria	Isoniazid (INH) Rifampin (Rifadin) Pyrazinamide (Daraprim) Ethambutol (Myambutol)
Cryptosporidium	Severe diarrhea Severe abdominal cramping	Stool culture for *Cryptosporidium*	Octreotide (Somatostatin)
Cryptococcal meningitis	Headache Confusion, memory loss Nausea Seizures Change in mental status Fever Photophobia	Cerebral spinal fluid culture for cryptococcosis	Amphotericin B (Fungizone) Flucytosine (Ancobon) Fluconazole (Diflucan)
Cytomegalovirus (CMV)	Visual changes; floaters/ blindness Difficulty swallowing Nausea, vomiting Abdominal cramping	Ophthalmologic examination Blood, urine, tissue culture for CMV	Gancyclovir (Cytorene) Foscarnet (Foscavir)

HIV encephalopathy/ AIDS dementia complex	Early: Inattention
	    Reduced concentration
	    Forgetfulness
	    Slowed movements
	    Clumsiness
	    Ataxia
	    Apathy
	    Agitation
	Late: Paraplegia
	    Mutism
	    Vegetative state
		Computed tomography
		Magnetic resonance imaging
		Cerebral spinal fluid evaluation
			Zidovudine (Retrovir, AZT)—high doses

Management

A. Underlying Considerations
1. Treatments are available at this time for the underlying immunodeficiency.
2. HIV vaccine studies are showing initial promise as a treatment to prolong life in those already infected with HIV.
3. Treatment is available for some opportunistic infections and other diseases associated with AIDS. Although individual response to treatment is highly variable, treatment of opportunistic infections may last months or even for the rest of the patient's life.
4. Management requires the expertise of many specialties: infectious disease, pulmonary medicine, gastroenterology, neurology, obstetrics and gynecology, dentistry, surgery, and psychiatry; nursing; nutrition; and social work.

B. Specific Treatment
1. Antiviral therapy; zidovudine (AZT), dideoxyinosine (ddi), zalcitabine (ddc) (Table 27-2)
   a. Therapy is started at CD4 count of 500/cu mm or less.
   b. Decreases viral replication.
   c. Prolongs quality of life; some studies show an extension of life by 1 to 2 years.
   d. May not be tolerated well due to side effects.

> **NURSING ALERT:**
> If a patient taking ddi develops abdominal pain or vomiting, discontinue the medication immediately and notify the health care provider. There has been mortality associated with DDI and acute pancreatitis.

2. *P. carinii* pneumonia prophylaxis: trimethoprim-sulfamethoxazole (Bactrim), dapsone, aerosolized pentamidine

   a. Therapy is started at a CD4 cell count of 200/cu mm or less.
   b. Decreases frequency, morbidity, and mortality of *P. carinii* pneumonia infection.

C. Supportive Care
1. Treatment of reversible illnesses
2. Nutritional support
3. Palliation of pain
4. Dental management
5. Evaluation and management of psychological and social aspects of AIDS
6. Treatment to relieve symptoms (cough, diarrhea)
7. Antidepressant drugs; psychiatric interventions

◆ NURSING MANAGEMENT OF HIV DISEASE AND AIDS

Nursing Assessment

1. Obtain history of risk factors, constitutional signs and symptoms, recent infections, positive blood test for HIV antibodies.
2. Review patient's present complaint(s) such as cough, shortness of breath, diarrhea.
3. Evaluate nutritional status by assessing for weight loss, body mass depletion, decreased skin-fold thickness and mid-arm muscle circumference, hypoalbuminemia, decreased iron-binding capacity, selenium deficiency, anemia.
4. Assess respiratory rate, depth, and auscultate lungs for breath sounds; assess for skin color and temperature, palpable lymph nodes, and evidence of fever, night sweats.
5. Inspect mouth for lesions; examine skin for rash, sores, Kaposi's sarcoma lesions. Record number, size, and locations.
6. Ask about bowel patterns, changes in habits, constipation, abdominal cramping, number and volume of stools, presence of perianal pain and ulceration.
7. Is patient oriented to time, place, and person? Affect? Any problem with memory and concentration? Headaches? Seizures?

TABLE 27-2 Antiviral Therapy

Drug/Dosage	Indications	Adverse Reactions	Monitoring
Zidovudine (AZT, Retrovir) 100 mg 5 times a day	CD4 count <500	Nausea, fatigue (initial month on drug) Anemia, myalgias, leukopenia, granulocytopenia	CBC every 2 wk
Dideoxyinosine (ddi, Videx) 200 mg twice a day (weight dependent)	Intolerance to AZT Failure on AZT (CD4 decline and/or development of opportunistic infection)	Pancreatitis Peripheral neuropathy	CBC, liver function tests, amylase monthly for 3 mo; then every other month if stable
Zalcitabine (ddc, HIVID) 0.75 mg three times a day	Intolerance to AZT and ddi (other than peripheral neuropathy) Failure on AZT and ddi (CD4 decline or development of opportunistic infection)	Peripheral neuropathy Headache Oral and esophageal ulcers	CBC, liver function tests, amylase monthly for 3 mo; then every other month if stable

8. How much does the patient know about AIDS? Etiology? Signs and symptoms? Mode of transmission? Methods for limiting exposure?
9. Find out as much as possible about patient's premorbid personality, experience and skills, social support system.

Nursing Diagnoses

A. Fear of disease progression, treatment effects, isolation, and death related to having AIDS
B. Risk for Infection related to immunodeficiency and neutropenia secondary to medications/treatment
C. Altered Nutrition (Less than Body Requirements) related to disease/treatment effects
D. Altered Oral Mucous Membranes related to opportunistic infection
E. Diarrhea related to disease/treatment effects
F. Altered Thought Processes (Impaired Cognition and Dementia) related to disease effects
G. Hyperthermia related to HIV infection, opportunistic infection, or visceral involvement by Kaposi's sarcoma
H. Altered Breathing Pattern related to opportunistic infections and noninfectious disorders (Kaposi's sarcoma of the lung)
I. Other nursing diagnoses could include:
   1. Fatigue related to underlying HIV infection and reactive depression
   2. Disturbances in Body Image related to rapid body changes from debilitating disease
   3. Helplessness related to inexperience with illness, sense of loss of control, depression, and vulnerability associated with AIDS
   4. Pain related to infection, peripheral neuropathies, nodules of Kaposi's sarcoma, diarrhea
   5. Anticipatory Grieving related to awareness of implications of AIDS, dying and death, unfinished business, multiple bereavements, and changes in lifestyle
   6. Ineffective Family Coping related to crisis created by AIDS, guilt, fear, overwhelming caretaking responsibilities

NURSING ALERT:
Never assume the family/loved ones know that the patient is HIV positive. Always ask the patient who knows of the HIV status. Confidentiality regarding the HIV infection must be maintained. However, encourage the patient to share the diagnosis to decrease isolation. Offer to be with the patient when the diagnosis is shared with the family; role playing before you meet with family/loved ones can be helpful.

Nursing Interventions

A. *Reducing Fear*
1. Maintain nonjudgmental attitude and nonprejudicial approach.
2. Anticipate that the patient may pass through series of stages: initial crisis, transitional stage, acceptance state, and preparation for death.
3. Allow patient to use denial as a protective mechanism—gives some control over when and how patient will control mortality.

   a. Expect some displaced anger; avoid being personally affronted by patient's anger.
   b. Allow patient to acknowledge reality of the situation without false reassurance.
4. Explain that symptoms of anxiety and depression are common initially but generally improve with time and support.
5. Anticipate that drug abusers may exhibit antisocial behaviors, feelings of alienation and isolation.
6. Provide careful discussion and clarification of treatment options.
7. Help patient set realistic goals and expectations.
8. Offer counseling services, especially when AIDS is initially diagnosed and as patient enters terminal phase of illness.
9. Obtain social service referral for available resources and services such as housekeeping, food shopping, community support services, cancer counseling agencies, Social Security Administration.
10. Help patient identify and strengthen personal resources such as positive coping skills, relaxation techniques, strong support network, and optimistic outlook.
11. Encourage patient to join a support group—helpful in defusing stressful issues and in developing strategies to cope with the disease.
12. Observe for emerging psychiatric problems, especially in persons who are socially isolated, those with guilt about sexuality and lifestyle, and those with poor accommodation.
13. Provide information on advance directives and encourage patient to arrange personal business because cognitive deterioration may make it impossible for patient to act on own behalf at a later date.

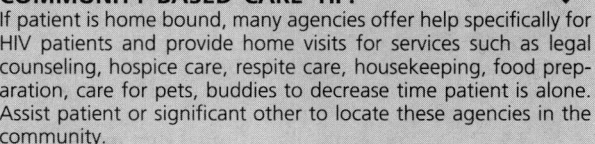

COMMUNITY-BASED CARE TIP:
If patient is home bound, many agencies offer help specifically for HIV patients and provide home visits for services such as legal counseling, hospice care, respite care, housekeeping, food preparation, care for pets, buddies to decrease time patient is alone. Assist patient or significant other to locate these agencies in the community.

14. Allow discussion of nature and management of death—minimizes negative impact of ever-present threat of death.
   a. Assure patient of palliative care, pain control, and help with anxiety and depression.
   b. Respect the right of the patient to participate in treatment decisions (ie, to limit therapy and life-prolonging interventions).

B. *Preventing Infection*
1. Have a high index of suspicion for infection even when clinical manifestations are subtle or absent—opportunistic infections may be reactivated at any time during the course of the disease.
2. Follow universal precautions for all patients.
3. Administer prescribed pharmacologic agents; some infections are not treatable with currently available regimens.
4. Administer and teach patient/family good skin care—a break in the skin is a source of secondary infection; use position changes, emollient lotions, special pads and beds, and attend to hydration and nutrition.
5. Maintain cleanliness of environment.

6. Use aseptic techniques when performing invasive procedures.
7. Teach patient to make the most of what remains of the immune system by minimizing the risk of disease.
   a. Avoid exposure to persons with infections—may activate HIV.
   b. Turn, cough, and do breathing exercises, especially when confined to bed.
   c. Avoid continuing injection drug use and unprotected sex with an HIV-positive partner to prevent repeated exposure to HIV.
   d. Instruct visitors about handwashing before entering and leaving the room.
   e. Advise patient/family to wash hands before preparing food and prepare foods on clean surfaces.
   f. Advise patient not to eat raw or undercooked foods.
   g. Tell the patient to have someone else clean a cat box or bird cage; if that is not possible, use rubber gloves.

C. *Improving Nutritional Status*
 1. Monitor nutritional status by weighing, recording dietary intake and calorie count, taking anthropometric measurements, and evaluating serum albumin, blood urea nitrogen, protein, and transferrin levels.
 2. Monitor for sore throat that progresses to dysphagia or odynophagia (pain on swallowing) or persistent heartburn—suggestive of esophageal candidiasis.
 3. Consult with dietitian to develop strategies for nutrition care including additional calories and nutritional supplements to maintain strength, comfort, and level of functioning.
 4. Include patient in decision-making regarding nutrition care.
 5. Alter timing of drug administration to improve intake with meals.
   a. Administer or teach patient to administer prescribed antiemetic 30 minutes before meals.
   b. Try to give drug infusions after meals.
 6. For patient with oral/esophageal pain from candida esophagitis, herpetic esophagitis, endotracheal Kaposi's sarcoma:
   a. Administer prescribed antifungal therapy.
   b. Avoid highly seasoned or acidic foods.
   c. Offer fluids and blenderized foods to minimize chewing and ease swallowing.
   d. Suggest nutrition-dense supplements such as instant breakfast drinks or protein-fortified juices for home care.
 7. Encourage patient to maximize intake during periods he or she is feeling better.
 8. Discourage excessive alcohol intake—has immunosuppressive effect.
 9. Make appropriate community referral if patient is unable to shop or prepare meals.
 10. Encourage small, frequent meals because these may make best use of limited absorptive capacity.
 11. Keep in mind that elemental diets/nutritional supplements may become intolerable to patient as anorexia progresses; prepare patient for enteral or parenteral feedings when necessary.

D. *Relieving Oral Discomfort*
 1. Ask about persistent sore throat, dysphagia, heartburn—all these symptoms are suggestive of oral/esophageal candidiasis.
 2. Examine mouth for oral candidiasis and other lesions.

3. Administer or teach patient to administer prescribed antifungal mouth rinses or lozenges for oral candidiasis or acyclovir (Zovirax) for herpes simplex.
4. Perform or encourage oral care two to three times a day.

E. *Minimizing the Effects of Diarrhea*
 1. Keep in mind that gastrointestinal infections and diarrhea decrease absorptive efficiency.
 2. Tell patient to monitor stools for blood and try to determine if bleeding is before, with, or after bowel movement to help determine source of bleeding.
 3. Monitor intake and output; assess skin and mucous membranes for poor turgor and dryness, indicating dehydration.
 4. Administer fluids and electrolytes as prescribed.
 5. Advise patient to rest to achieve bowel rest.
 6. Use enteric precautions.
 7. Plan regimen of skin care including cleansing/blotting/drying of the anal area, application of ointment or skin barrier cream.
 8. Advise patient to eliminate caffeine, alcohol, dairy products, food high in fats, fresh juices, and acidic juices if diarrhea persists. Drink liquids at room temperature.
 9. Advise patient to avoid foods that increase intestinal motility and distention such as gas-forming fruits and vegetables.
 10. Advise patient to report symptoms and signs of increased weakness, dizziness, and continuing weight loss.

F. *Managing Altered Thought Processes*
 1. Remember that the brain is a critical target organ for HIV infection.
 2. Provide daily assessment of mental status; monitor for changes in behavior, memory, concentration ability, and motor system dysfunction—patient may become vegetative and unable to ambulate.
   a. Onset of dementia is usually insidious but may be abrupt, precipitated by acute infection.
 3. Reorient patient frequently; use calendar, clock, family/friends' pictures, lists, structured plan of care.
 4. Provide for patient safety: bed rails up; call signal available; things within patient's reach.
 5. Give repeated reassurance.
 6. Assess for depressive or suicidal symptoms—AIDS represents a significant risk for suicide.
 7. Anticipate necessity of guardianship, durable power of attorney for health care, and informed consent if patient has AIDS dementia complex because patient may have poor insight and become indifferent to illness.

G. *Reducing Fever*
 1. Frequently assess for chills, fever, tachycardia, and tachypnea.
 2. Teach patient/caregiver to keep a temperature chart.
 3. Encourage high fluid intake to replace insensible water losses incurred by fever/diaphoresis.
 4. Administer or teach patient to administer antipyretics as prescribed.
 5. Teach patient or caregiver to report a change in fever pattern or significant change in condition.

H. *Improving Breathing Pattern*
 1. Provide supplemental oxygen as ordered.
 2. Watch for *sudden* change in respiratory function—patient may be developing a secondary infection.

3. Administer or teach patient to administer prescribed narcotic for postinfectious cough, a complication of *P. carinii* pneumonia and viral pneumonia.
4. Encourage smoking cessation to enhance pulmonary ciliary defense.
5. Administer saline nebulization to induce sputum collection for culture and sensitivity.
   a. Wear mask and gloves during sputum collection.
   b. Instruct patient to brush tongue, buccal surfaces, teeth, and palate with water before sputum induction—to remove superficial squamous epithelial cells and their adherent bacteria and foreign material.
   c. Instruct patient to gargle and rinse mouth with tap water.
6. Answer questions and support patient's decision for or against resuscitation and mechanical ventilation.

Patient Education/ Health Maintenance

1. Indicate that patient is a source of infection to others and should take actions to prevent transmission (no exchange of blood or body fluids).
2. Encourage patient to disclose HIV status to sex and needle-sharing partners.
3. Emphasize to HIV-positive woman that children should be tested for HIV.
4. Discuss family planning with HIV-positive woman; the rate of transmission from mother to newborn is approximately 30%. If she does not want more children, discuss birth control options.
5. Establish a primary care provider for the patient and encourage the need for regular follow-up care.
   a. Should include yearly Pap smears for women, routine dental, and eye examinations.
6. Teach patient to recognize and report important symptoms.
   a. Change in pattern/magnitude of temperature elevation.
   b. Development of a new focal complaint: skin spots, sore mouth, diarrhea.
7. Emphasize to injection drug users that continued use may expose them to additional infection and such infections may activate viral replication.
8. Encourage patient to modify sexual behaviors for safer sex.

a. Use latex male condoms supplemented by creams and jelly containing a viricidal agent.
   b. If a man will not use a condom, the woman should use a female condom.
   c. Refrain from oral and anal sex.
   d. Encourage patient to read literature from various AIDS action groups on "safe sex" techniques.
9. If a substance abuser:
   a. Enroll in a treatment program.
   b. Do not share needles ("works").
   c. If no access to unused needles, clean needles before using with a bleach/water solution.
10. Teach patient to optimize immune system function by sound dietary practices, exercise, and regular periods of sleep; promote changes in the direction of more healthful living.
11. Refer patient to resources such as:

National AIDS Hotline
Operates 24 hours a day, 7 days a week; offers information on transmission, prevention, testing, and local referrals.
1-800-342-AIDS
Spanish—1-800-344-7432
TDD Service for the deaf—1-800-243-7889

National AIDS Information Clearinghouse
P. O. Box 6003
Rockville, MD 20850
General information for health care providers

HIV Telephone Consultation Service—1-800-933-3413

On-line data bases
MEDLINE/AIDS Line
National Library of Medicine
8600 Rockville Pike
Bethesda, MD 20894

Evaluation

A. Speaks openly about HIV disease with health care providers, significant others
B. Neutrophil count greater than 1,000
C. Eating three to four meals a day
D. Oral mucosa without lesions
E. Reports formed stools one to three times a day
F. Appropriate responses to questions of self, time, and place; verbalizes accurate account of activities
G. Afebrile with a normal heart rate
H. Respirations unlabored, rate 20/min; no cough or sputum production

Selected References

Bartlett, J. G. (1994). *Medical management of HIV infection.* Glenview, IL: Physicians & Scientists Publishing Company.
Bartlett, J. G., & Finkbeiner, A. K. (1991). *The guide to living with HIV infection.* Baltimore: Johns Hopkins University Press.
Broder, S., Merigan, T., & Bolognesi, D. (Eds.). (1994). *AIDS medicine.* Baltimore: Williams & Wilkins.
Centers for Disease Control. (1989). Interpretation and use of the Western

blot assay for serodiagnosis of human immunodeficiency virus type 1 infections. *MMWR, 38*(S-7), 1-7.
Chan, M., & Cello, J. (1991). Management of AIDS related diarrhea. *AIDS Patient Care, 5*(4), 175-177.
Cohen, F., & Durham, J. (Eds.). (1993). *Women, children, and HIV/AIDS.* New York: Springer.
Cooper, D. A., Gatell, J. M., Kroon, S., et al. (1993). Zidovudine in persons with

asymptomatic HIV infection and CD4+ cell counts greater than 400 per cubic millimeter. *The New England Journal of Medicine, 329*(5), 297-352.
DeVita, V. T. J., Hellman, S., & Rosenberg, S. A. (Eds.). (1988). *AIDS: Etiology, diagnosis, and prevention* (2nd ed.). Philadelphia: J. B. Lippincott.
Flaskerud, J. H. (1992). *AIDS/HIV infection: A reference guide for nursing professionals.* Philadelphia: W. B. Saunders.

Fox, R. C., Aiken, L. H., & Messikomer, C. M. (1990). The culture of caring: AIDS and the nursing profession. *The Milbank Quarterly, 68*(2), 226-256.

Newshan, G., & Wainapel, S. (1993). Pain characteristics and their management in persons with AIDS. *Journal of the Association of Nurses in AIDS Care, 4*(2), 53-59.

Porcher, F. (1992). HIV-infected pregnant women and their infants: Primary health care implications. *Nurse Practitioner, 17*(11), 46-54.

Sande, M. A., Carpenter, C. C., Cobbs, C. G., Holmes, K. K., & Sanford, J. P. (1993). Antiviral therapy for adult HIV-infected patients. *The Journal of the American Medical Association, 270*(21), 2583-2589.

Sande, M. A., & Volberding, P. A. (Eds.). (1995). *The medical management of AIDS*, 4th ed. Philadelphia: W. B. Saunders.

Santangelo, J., & Schnack, J. (1991). Primary care intervention and management for adults with early HIV infection. *Nurse Practitioner, 16*(6), 9-15.

Schmidt, J. (1992). Case management problems and homecare. *Journal of the Association of Nurses in AIDS Care, 3*(3), 37-44.

Twiname, B. (1993). The relationship between HIV classification and depression and suicidal intent. *Journal of the Association of Nurses in AIDS Care, 4*(4), 28-35.

U.S. Department of Health and Human Services, Public Health Service. (1994). *Evaluation and management of early HIV infection*. AHCPR Publication No. 94-0572.

U.S. Department of Health and Human Services, Public Health Service, Centers for Disease Control and Prevention. (1992). 1993 revised classification system for HIV infection and expanded surveillance case definition for AIDS among adolescents and adults. MMWR, 41, No. RR-17.

U.S. Department of Health and Human Services, Public Health Service, Centers for Disease Control and Prevention. (1993). Update: Barrier protection against HIV infection and other sexually transmitted diseases. *MMWR, 42*, 30.

CHAPTER 28

Connective Tissue Disorders

General Overview

Connective tissue makes up a large portion of the interstitial tissue of the skin and musculoskeletal system. Structures include bone, cartilage, tendons, ligaments as well as the less compact connective tissue making up the structures supporting and surrounding organs and cells. These tissues are metabolically active, constantly turning over and replacing their large and molecular components. The interaction between the molecular components and the inflammatory cells (mostly white blood cells [WBCs]) produces chemicals that are important to initiating disease and determining which connective tissue is affected.

◆ MUSCULOSKELETAL AND RELATED ASSESSMENT

Assessment for connective tissue disorders focuses on the musculoskeletal system but also involves remote body systems. Clues to connective tissue disorders may be found in the skin, eyes, lungs, and neurologic system.

Presenting Symptoms

Obtain history of presenting symptoms including duration and intensity.

1. Musculoskeletal pain—characteristics
2. Joint swelling
3. Presence of morning stiffness
4. Constitutional symptoms
    a. Fever
    b. Weight loss
    c. Anorexia
    d. Fatigue
5. Involvement of other body symptoms
    a. Skin
    b. Ocular
    c. Pulmonary
    d. Neurologic
    e. Mucous membranes
6. Family history of rheumatic or autoimmune disorders.

Physical Examination Findings

1. Musculoskeletal examination
    a. Pain on palpation or range of motion
    b. Joint swelling, warmth, or erythema
    c. Joint motion restriction
    d. Pain, swelling, or warmth of soft tissues surrounding joints
2. Skin
    a. Skin rash or other abnormalities such as thickening
    b. Alopecia
3. Oral mucosa
    a. Ulcerations
    b. Dryness
4. Ocular
    a. Conjunctival inflammation
    b. Dryness
5. Pulmonary
    a. Adventitious sounds
    b. Friction rub
6. Neurologic
    a. Depression
    b. Psychosis
    c. Foot drop
    d. Muscle weakness
    e. Strokelike findings

Diagnostic Tests

◆ LABORATORY STUDIES
Antinuclear Antibody (ANA)

A. Description A test for the presence of antibodies to nucleoprotein (autoantibodies or a heterogeneous group of gamma globulins); highly sensitive for detecting systemic lupus erythematosus (SLE), but is nonspecific (high false-positive rate).

B. Nursing/Patient Considerations
1. Note drug therapy because many drugs may cause false-positive results.
2. Results will be reported in a staining pattern (speckled, homogeneous, peripheral, nucleolar), if positive, which correlates to various types of connective tissue disorders and various subsets of SLE (Table 28-1).
3. Titer will also be reported with positive ANA but does not reflect disease activity or prognosis.

Rheumatoid Factor (RF)

A. Description Test for the presence of macroglobulin found in the blood of patients with rheumatoid arthritis

TABLE 28-1   ANA Staining Patterns and Connective Tissue Disorders

ANA Pattern	Connective Tissue Disorder
Peripheral (rim, ring, membranous)	Active SLE, usually with renal disease
Homogenous (diffuse)	SLE, RA
Speckled	SLE, RA, scleroderma, Sjögren's syndrome, mixed connective tissue disorder
Nucleolar	Scleroderma

ANA, antinuclear antibody; RA, rheumatoid arthritis; SLE, systemic lupus erythematosus

(RA) and other disorders. RF has properties of an antibody and may be directed against immunoglobulin.

B.   Nursing/Patient Care Considerations
1.   It is not a highly sensitive or specific test.
2.   May be positive in 30% to 60% of patients with RA, SLE, and Sjögren's syndrome. May be false positive in endocarditis, tuberculosis, syphilis, sarcoidosis, cancer, viral infections, patients with skin or renal allographs, and in some liver, lung, or kidney disease.
3.   Negative RF does not exclude the diagnosis of RA.
4.   Certain disease manifestations such as severe joint involvement and extra-articular manifestations may be more frequent in those with high titer RF.

Erythrocyte Sedimentation Rate (ESR)

A.   Description
1.   Test determines the rate at which red blood cells (RBCs) fall out of unclotted blood in 1 hour.
2.   Based on premise that inflammatory and other disease processes create changes in blood proteins causing aggregation of RBCs that makes them heavier.

B.   Nursing/Patient Considerations
1.   ESR is generally but not always elevated in the majority of rheumatic illnesses.
2.   Result may be elevated by pregnancy, menstruation, medications such as heparin and oral contraceptives, and advanced age. Result may be reduced by elevated blood glucose or albumin, high phospholipids, or drugs such as corticosteroids or high-dose aspirin.
3.   Most beneficial in monitoring progress of an inflammatory disease.

Complement

A.   Description
1.   Complement is a complex cascade system that activates proteins as part of the body's defense against infection.
2.   Specific components include C1q, C2, C3, and C4 and measurement helps determine immune complex formation or presence of a gammaglobulinemia.

3.   Complement levels are decreased in certain autoimmune diseases due to complement consumption and due to activation of proteolytic enzymes and tissue damage.

B.   Nursing/Patient Care Considerations
1.   Obtain venous blood sample and send to laboratory promptly because complement deteriorates at room temperature.
2.   Serial measurements may be helpful in monitoring the activity of some rheumatic diseases; decreased levels indicate increased disease activity.

◆ OTHER TESTS
Synovial Fluid Analysis

A.   Description
1.   A sample of synovial (joint) fluid is analyzed for several components.
     a.   Color
     b.   Clarity/turbidity
     c.   Viscosity
     d.   WBC count with differential
     e.   Presence and identification of crystals
2.   Arthrocentesis is a sterile procedure requiring antiseptic cleaning agent, local anesthetic, and 18-gauge needle, and a 10- to 20-mL syringe.

B.   Nursing/Patient Care Considerations
1.   Patients are generally apprehensive about having a needle inserted into their joint. They generally require reassurance and explanation of the importance of information derived from test results.
2.   Results help to differentiate infection and inflammation due to connective tissue disorder or inflammatory arthritis (Table 28-2).

General Procedures/ Treatment Modalities

◆ PHARMACOLOGIC AGENTS

Connective tissue disorders may be treated with a variety of drugs to relieve pain and halt or minimize the disease process. Drug therapy may be long-term and require frequent evaluation for adverse reactions (Table 28-3).

◆ PHYSICAL/OCCUPATIONAL THERAPY

Physical and occupational therapy provide a multimodal program to help reduce pain and improve joint function. Many other measures can be taught to patients to practice at home. Components of the program may include:

*   Joint conservation
*   Splinting
*   Range-of-motion exercises
*   Application of heat and cold
*   Endurance/aerobic conditioning
*   Energy conservation
*   Modification of home/work environment

TABLE 28-2 Synovial Fluid Analysis

	Color	WBC Count	Viscosity	Crystals
Normal	Clear, yellow	200	Normal	None
Osteoarthritis	Clear, slightly turbid	200–600	Low	None
Gout	Turbid	2,000–75,000	Low	Monosodium urate
Inflammatory arthritis				
RA	Turbid, yellow	2,000–75,000	Low	None
SLE				
Sjögren's				
Psoratic				
Septic arthritis	Pus very turbid	Generally 80,000	Low	None

RA, rheumatoid arthritis; SLE, systemic lupus erythematosus; WBC, white blood cell

Joint Conservation

Teach or reinforce the following practices:

1. Perform activities using good body mechanics.
2. Maintain ideal body weight—extra weight places undue stress on weight-bearing joints.
3. Use large joints to perform activities—spread the load over as many joints as possible.
4. Perform activities in smooth movements to avoid trauma induced by abrupt movements.

Energy Conservation

Teach or reinforce the following practices:

1. Organize materials, utensils, and tools.
2. Perform lengthy activities in a seated position.
3. Work at an even pace—avoid rushing.
4. Delegate work to others when possible.

Splinting

1. Frequently used for wrists and hands.
2. Ensure proper application.
3. Periodically inspect for skin irritation, neurovascular compromise, or improper fit.
4. Usually worn during acute stage of inflammation to protect joint.

Exercise

Instruct/reinforce correct method of exercise:

1. Avoid exercising inflamed joints—putting these joints through range-of-motion one to two times per day when inflamed is sufficient.
2. Perform exercises daily as prescribed.
3. Aerobic conditioning exercises may be indicated when disease activity permits.
4. Walking, biking, swimming, and water walking for 30 minutes three times a week.

COMMUNITY-BASED CARE TIP:
Encourage patient to exercise regularly, choosing an activity that is inexpensive, convenient, enjoyable, and not dependent on the weather. Suggest dancing, mall walking, use of stationary bicycle in the home, or contacting the local YMCA about special programs for arthritis.

Other Measures

1. Reinforce correct use and application of heat and cold.
2. Obtain and teach correct use of assistive devices.
3. Reinforce use of behavior modification and relaxation techniques as adjuncts to therapy.
4. Advise patient to modify home and work environments as needed.
5. Advise patient to seek counseling regarding sexuality if joint pain and inflammation are barriers to performance.

The Disorders

◆ RHEUMATOID ARTHRITIS

Rheumatoid arthritis is a general term used to describe what may be a heterogeneous group of inflammatory diseases affecting both joints and other organ systems.

Pathophysiology/Etiology

1. Immunologic processes result in inflammation of synovium, producing antigens and inflammatory byproducts leading to destruction of articular cartilage, edema, and production of a granular tissue called pannus (Fig. 28-1).
2. Granulation tissue forms adhesions leading to decreased joint mobility.
3. Similar adhesions can occur in supporting structures, such as ligaments and tendons, causing contractures and ruptures further affecting joint structure and mobility.

TABLE 28-3 Drug Therapy for Connective Tissue Disorders

Drug	Action	Adverse Effects

Anti-inflammatory Agents
Salicylates
Aspirin (may be buffered or enteric coated
Nonsteroidal anti-inflammatory drugs (NSAIDs)
  Ibuprofen (Motrin)
  Fenoprofen (Nalfon)
  Naproxen (Naprosyn)
  Tolmetin (Tolectin)
  Sulindac (Clinoril)
  Meclofenamate (Meclomen)
  Ketroprofen (Orudis)
  Salsalate (Disalcid)
  Diclofenac (Voltaren)
  Nabumetone (Relafen)
  Ketorolac (Toradol)
  Oxaprozin (Day Pro)
  Flurbiprofen (Ansaid)
  Diflunisal (Dolobid)
  Piroxicam (Feldene)
  Etodolac (Lodine)
  Indomethacin (Indocin)
	Anti-inflammatory, antipyretic, and analgesic effects
	Anti-inflammatory and analgesic effects
	Mechanism of action may be related to inhibition of prostaglandin synthesis (prostaglandins have a role in inflammatory process, pain, and fever)
	Nonsteroidal antirheumatic agents for adjunctive treatment of rheumatoid arthritis
	Sometimes remarkably effective in control of articular symptoms
		Tinnitus, gastric intolerance or gastrointestinal bleeding and purpuric tendencies
		Gastrointestinal irritation: nausea, vomiting, epigastric distress, precipitation and reactivation of peptic ulcer, hepatitis
		Hematologic: bone marrow depression, anemia, leukopenia, thrombocytopenia purpura
		Decrease in renal function can precipitate renal failure
		CNS: Headache, dizziness, drowsiness, aseptic meningitis
		Cardiovascular: edema, dyspnea palpitations

Disease-Modifying Agents
Gold compounds (Chrysotherapy)
  Oral:
    Auranofin (Ridaura)
  Injectable:
    Gold sodium thiomalate (Myocrisine)
    Aurothioglucose (Solganal)
 	
Antimalarial agents
  Hydroxychloroquine sulfate (Placquenil)
  Chloroquine phosphate (Aralen)
 	
Chelating agents
  Penicillamine (Cuprimine; Depen)
	Mechanism of action unclear
	Anti-inflammatory, anti-arthritic, and immunomodulating effects
	
	Remission–induction agents for rheumatoid arthritis
	Used also in certain forms of lupus
	
	Mechanism of action poorly understood
	Used in active progressive rheumatoid arthritis
		Cutaneous reactions ranging from dermatitis to life-threatening exfoliative dermatitis
		Renal toxicity
		Thrombocytopenia and marrow aplasia
		Nitritoid reaction with IM gold
		Ocular toxicity (retinopathy that can result in permanent loss of vision; blurred vision, night blindness, scotoma
		Can cause severe toxic reactions: mucocutaneous, renal, gastrointestinal, hepatic, and hematologic toxicities

Immunosuppressives
Methotrexate (Mexate)
Azathioprine (Imuran)
 	
Cyclophosphamide (Cytoxan)
 	
Cyclosporine (Sandimmune)
 	
Corticosteroids
  Prednisone (Orasone)
  Prednisolone (Delta-Cortef)
  Triamcinalone (Kenalog)
  Betamethasome (Celestone)
  Hydrocortisone (Cortef)
  Dexamethasone (Decadron)
  Methylprednisolone (Medrol)
	Exert anti-inflammatory effect by inhibition of cellular replication
	Used in patients with inflammatory synovitis refractory to other therapy
	Alkylating agent that interferes with the growth of rapidly dividing cells
	
	Inhibition of immunocompetent lymphocytes also inhibits lymphokine production and release
	Potent anti-inflammatory drugs may also reduce immune response
	Usually used for short-term management of patients with severe limitations
		Bone marrow suppression, hepatic and pulmonary toxicity reduce resistance to infection
		
		Possibility of a malignancy occurring many years later after initiating therapy can cause sterility, urinary bladder, fibrosis, cystitis
		Renal dysfunction, tremor, hypertension, gum hyperplasia
		
		Osteoporosis, tractures, avascular necrosis
		Gastric ulcers, infection, susceptibility
		Hirsutism, acne, moon facies, abnormal fat deposition, edema, emotional disorders, menstrual disorders
		Hyperglycemia, hypokalemia
		Hypertension, cataracts

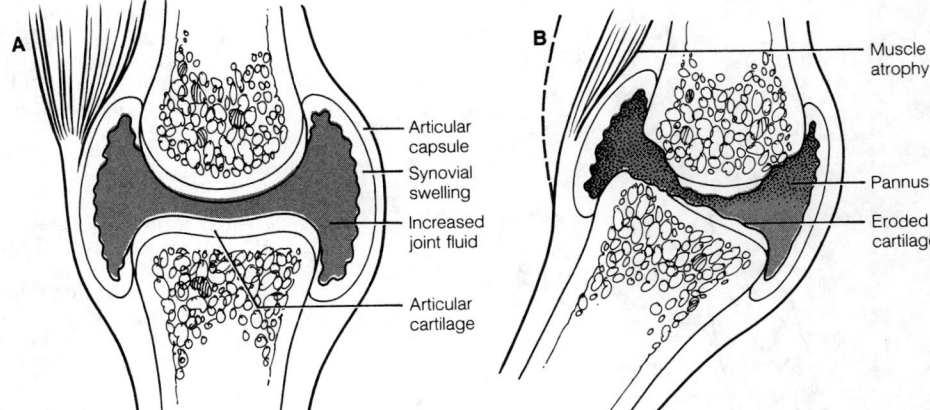

FIGURE 28-1 *Pathophysiology of rheumatoid arthritis. (A) Joint structure with synovial swelling and fluid accumulation in joint. (B) Pannus, eroded articular cartilage with joint space narrowing, muscle atrophy, and ankylosis.*

4. The etiology is unknown but is probably a combined effect of environmental, demographic, infectious, and genetic factors.
5. An infectious agent has not been identified but many infectious processes can produce a polyarthritis similar to RA.
6. Women are affected more frequently than men.

Clinical Manifestations

1. Arthritis
   a. Bilateral, symmetric arthritis affects any diarthrodial joint but most often involves the hands, wrists, knees, and feet (Fig. 28-2).
2. Skin manifestations
   a. Rheumatoid nodules—elbows, occiput, sacrum
   b. Vasculitic changes—brown, splinterlike lesions in fingers or nail folds
3. Cardiac manifestations
   a. Acute pericarditis
   b. Conduction defects
   c. Valvular insufficiency
   d. Coronary arteritis
   e. Cardiac tamponade—rare
4. Pulmonary manifestations
   a. Asymptomatic pulmonary disease
   b. Pleural effusion
   c. Interstitial fibrosis
   d. Laryngeal obstruction due to involvement of the cricoarytenoid joint—rare
5. Neurologic manifestations
   a. Mononeuritis multiplex
      (1) Wrist drop
      (2) Foot drop
   b. Carpal tunnel syndrome
   c. Compression of spinal nerve roots
6. Systemic manifestations
   a. Fever
   b. Fatigue
   c. Weight loss

Diagnostic Evaluation

1. Complete blood count (CBC)—normochromic anemia
2. RF—positive in a large percentage of patients

3. ESR—elevated
4. Synovial fluid analysis—see Table 28-2.
5. X-rays
   a. Hands/wrists—marginal erosions of the proximal interphalangeal (PIP), metacarpophalangeal (MCP), and carpal joints; generalized osteopenia
   b. Cervical spine—erosions producing atlantoaxial subluxation
6. Magnetic resonance imaging (MRI)—spinal cord compression resulting from C1—C2 subluxation and compression of surrounding vascular structures
7. Bone scan—"increased uptake" in the joints involved in RA
8. Synovial biopsy
   a. Presence of inflammatory cells associated with RA
   b. Excludes other causes of polyarthritis by noting the absence of other pathologic findings.

Management

1. Pharmacologic
   a. Nonsteroidal anti-inflammatory drugs (NSAIDs)—to relieve pain and inflammation
   b. Disease-modifying antirheumatic drugs (DMARDs)—to reduce disease activity
   c. Corticosteroids—to reduce inflammatory process
2. Local comfort measures
   a. Application of heat and cold
   b. Use of splints
   c. Use of transcutaneous electrical nerve stimulation (TENS) unit
   d. Iontophoresis—delivery of medication through the skin using direct electrical current
3. Nonpharmacologic modalities
   a. Behavior modification
   b. Relaxation techniques
4. Surgery
   a. Synovectomy
   b. Arthrodesis—joint fusion
   c. Total joint replacement

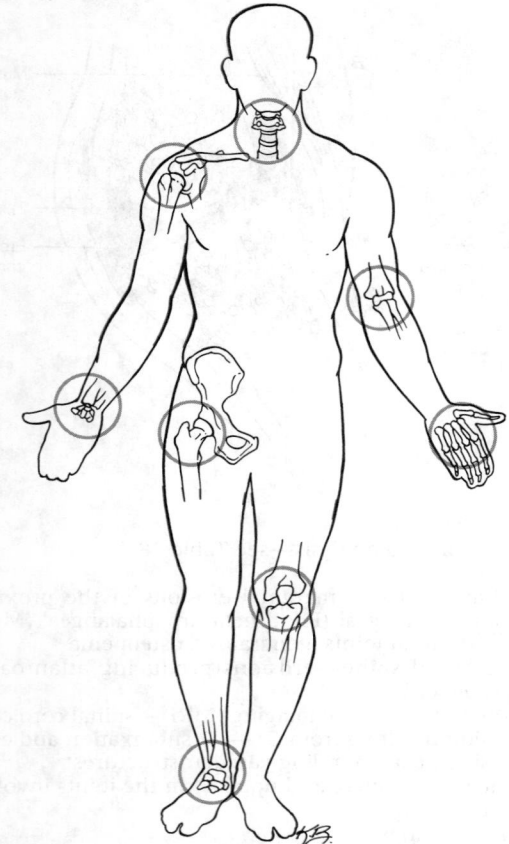

FIGURE 28-2 *Rheumatoid arthritis characteristically involves the joints of the hands, wrists, feet, ankles, knees, elbows, and the glenohumeral and acromioclavicular joints and the hips. The articulations of the cervical spine are also affected.*

Complications

1. Loss of joint function due to bony adhesions and damage of supporting structures
2. Anemia of chronic disease

Nursing Assessment

1. Perform joint examination if indicated.
   a. Determine range of motion.
   b. Presence or absence of joint effusions
2. Presence of deformities
   a. Swan neck—PIP joints hyperextend
   b. Boutonniere—PIP joints flex
   c. Ulnar deviation—fingers point toward ulna
3. Assess pain.
4. Assess functional status.
   a. Class I—no restriction of ability to perform normal activities
   b. Class II—moderate restriction, but adequate for normal activities
   c. Class III—marked restriction, inability to perform most duties of usual occupation or self-care
   d. Class IV—incapacitation or confinement to bed or wheelchair
5. Assess for signs and symptoms indicating adverse reaction to medications.

Nursing Diagnoses

A. Chronic Pain related to disease process
B. Impaired Physical Mobility related to pain and limited joint motion
C. Self-Care Deficit related to limitations secondary to disease process
D. Ineffective Individual Coping related to pain, physical limitations, and chronicity of RA

Nursing Interventions

Controlling Pain
1. Apply local heat or cold to affected joints for 15 to 20 minutes three to four times a day.
   a. Avoid temperatures likely to cause skin or tissue damage by checking temperature of warm soaks or covering cold packs with a towel.
2. Administer or teach self-administration of pharmacologic agents.
   a. Advise patient on when to expect pain relief based on mechanism of action of the drug.
3. Encourage use of adjunctive pain control measures.
   a. Progressive muscle relaxation
   b. TENS
   c. Biofeedback

B. Optimizing Mobility
1. Encourage warm bath or shower in the morning on arising to decrease morning stiffness.
2. Encourage measures to protect affected joints.
   a. Perform gentle range-of-motion exercises.
   b. Use splints.
   c. Assist with activities of daily living if necessary.
3. Encourage exercise consistent with degree of disease activity.
4. Refer to physical therapy and occupational therapy.

C. Promoting Self-Care
1. Provide pain relief before self-care activities.
2. Provide privacy and an environment conducive to performance of daily activities.
3. Schedule adequate rest periods.
4. Discuss importance of promoting the patient's self-care at an appropriate level with patient and family.
5. Help patient attain appropriate assistive devices such as raised toilet seats, special eating utensils, and zipper pulls.
   a. Contact occupational therapist, social worker, or Arthritis Foundation for information.

D. Strengthening Coping
1. Be aware of potential problems in job, child care, maintenance of home, and social and family functioning that may result from RA.
2. Encourage patient to ventilate problems and feelings.
3. Assist with problem-solving approach to explore options and gain control of problem areas.
4. Reinforce effective coping mechanisms.
5. Refer to social worker or mental health counselor as needed.

Patient Education/ Health Maintenance

1. Instruct patient and family in the nature of disease.
   a. Chronic nature of RA with characteristic exacerbations and remissions over time
   b. Disease can have systemic affects resulting in constitutional symptoms and involvement of other organ systems.
   c. Severity of RA is variable but most patients are *not* confined to bed or wheelchair.
   d. There is no cure for RA; avoid "miracle cures" and quackery.
2. Educate about pharmacologic agents.
   a. Medication must be taken consistently to achieve maximum benefit.
   b. Most medications used in the treatment of RA require periodic laboratory testing to monitor for potential adverse reactions.
   c. Advise patient of possible adverse reactions of medications and need to report adverse reactions to health care provider.
   d. Reinforce to patient the need for lifelong treatment.

Evaluation

A. Reports reduction in pain
B. Wears wrist splints correctly and performs range-of-motion exercises twice a day
C. Maintains independent toiletry, bathing, and feeding
D. Verbalizes concerns about cleaning/cooking; meets with occupational therapist

◆ SYSTEMIC LUPUS ERYTHEMATOSUS

Systemic lupus erythematosus (SLE) is a chronic, multisystem disease that is most likely a failure of immune regulation.

Pathophysiology/Etiology

1. The T lymphocyte system is affected for unknown reasons and the failure of its regulatory system may result in an inability to slow or halt the production of inappropriate autoantibodies.
2. B lymphocyte-stimulating factors are produced and this too may lead to production of autoantibodies.
3. Autoantibodies may combine with other elements of the immune system to activate immune complexes. These immune complexes and other immune system constituents combine to form complement, which is deposited in organs, causing inflammation and tissue necrosis.
4. More women are affected than men.

Clinical Manifestations

1. Skin
   a. "Butterfly" rash characterized by erythema and edema
   b. Ring-shaped lesions involving the shoulders, arms, and upper back
   c. Discoid lesions resulting in erythematous, scaly plaques on the face, scalp, external ear, and neck alopecia are common.
2. Arthritis
   a. Generally bilateral, symmetric involving the hands and wrists as well as other joints
   b. Can resemble RA and may be mistaken for it especially early in the course of the disease.
   c. Unlike RA, the arthritis is nonerosive, that is, no joint destruction is seen on x-ray.
   d. Tendon involvement is common and may lead to deformities or tendon rupture.
3. Cardiac
   a. Pericarditis
   b. Pleural effusion
   c. Myocarditis
   d. Endocarditis
   e. Coronary arteritis—less common
4. Pulmonary
   a. Pleuritis
   b. Pleural effusion
   c. Lupus pneumonitis
   d. Pulmonary hemorrhage
   e. Pulmonary embolism
5. Gastrointestinal
   a. Oral ulcers
   b. Acute or subacute abdominal pain
   c. Pancreatitis
   d. Spontaneous bacterial peritonitis
   e. Bowel infarction
6. Renal—occurs in 50% of patients with as many as 15% developing renal failure
   a. Nephritis
      (1) Mesangial nephritis—mild form, can be reversible, best prognosis
      (2) Focal segmental glomerulonephritis—active necrotic or sclerosing lesions
      (3) Proliferative—may be focal or diffuse. Diffuse carries good prognosis
      (4) Membranous nephritis—may persist for years without serious renal function decline. May present as nephrotic syndrome.
      (5) Sclerosing nephritis—increase in the amount of matrix material in the glomeruli.
   b. Renal thrombosis—rare
7. Central nervous system
   a. Neuropsychiatric disorders
      (1) Depression
      (2) Psychosis
   b. Transient ischemic attacks/stroke
   c. Epilepsy
   d. Migraine headache
   e. Myelopathy
   f. Guillain-Barré syndrome
   g. Chorea and other movement disorders
8. Hematologic
   a. Hemolytic anemia
   b. Leukopenia
   c. Thrombocytopenia
9. Constitutional
   a. Fever
   b. Weight loss
   c. Fatigue

Diagnostic Evaluation

1. CBC—leukopenia, anemia (may be hemolytic), thrombocytopenia
2. ANA—positive in more than 90% of patients with SLE; predominant pattern is homogeneous.
3. ESR—generally elevated
4. Complement levels—generally decreased when disease is active.
5. Urinalysis—hematuria, proteinuria, and "active sediment" (RBC casts).
6. 24-hour urine for protein and creatinine clearance
7. Chest x-ray may show changes.
8. X-ray of hands and wrists—nondestructive arthritis
9. Computed tomography (CT) scan or MRI
   a. Brain—to define any neurologic manifestations
   b. Abdomen—to rule out other abdominal processes in a patient with abdominal pain
10. Cerebral arteriogram—to look for evidence of cerebral vasculitis

Management

A. Pharmacologic
1. NSAIDs—to reduce pain and inflammation
2. Antimalarials—to decrease disease activity
3. Corticosteroids—to reduce inflammatory process
4. Immunosuppressives—to suppress immune process

B. Nonpharmacologic
1. Avoid direct exposure to sunlight to reduce the chance of exacerbation.
2. Behavior modification to prevent exacerbations and reduce symptoms
3. Joint protection and energy conservation

Complications

1. Renal failure
2. Permanent neurologic impairment
3. Infection
4. Death due to disease process

Nursing Assessment

1. Obtain clinical history, review of systems, and perform physical examination for characteristic findings.
2. Assess for signs and symptoms of infection and other adverse reactions to medications.
3. Assess patient's and family's ability to cope with impact of chronic disease.

Nursing Diagnoses

A. Chronic Pain related to inflammation of joints and juxta-articular structures
B. Powerlessness related to unpredictable course of disease
C. Risk for Impaired Skin/Oral Mucous Membrane Integrity related to skin/oral lesions
D. Fatigue related to chronic inflammatory process
E. Altered Urinary Elimination related to renal involvement

Nursing Interventions

A. Reducing Pain
1. Administer and teach self-administration of medications to reduce disease activity and additional analgesics as ordered.
2. Suggest the use of hot or cold applications, relaxation techniques, and nonstrenuous exercise to enhance pain relief.

B. Increasing Control Over Disease Process
1. Instruct patient in avoidance of factors that may exacerbate disease.
   a. Avoid exposure to sunlight and ultraviolet light.
      (1) Use sunscreen 15 SPF or greater.
      (2) Wear protective clothing, light weight, long sleeves, hats.
      (3) Avoid prolonged exposure to sun.
   b. Avoid exposure to drugs/chemicals.
      (1) Hairspray
      (2) Hair coloring agents
      (3) Medications—obtain provider advice before taking medications.
2. Teach self-administration of pharmacologic agents to reduce disease activity.
3. Encourage good nutrition, sleep habits, exercise, rest, and relaxation to improve general health and help prevent infection.
4. Encourage ventilation of feelings, counseling, or referrals to social work, occupational therapy, as needed.

C. Maintaining Skin and Mucous Membrane Integrity
1. Apply topical corticosteroids to skin lesions as ordered.
2. Suggest alternate hairstyles, wearing scarves, wigs to cover significant areas of alopecia.
3. Encourage good oral hygiene and inspect mouth for oral ulcers.
   a. Avoid hot or spicy foods that may irritate oral ulcers.
   b. Apply topical agents or analgesics to reduce pain and promote eating.

D. Reducing Fatigue
1. Advise patient that fatigue level will fluctuate with disease activity.
2. Encourage patient to modify schedule to include several rest periods during the day; pace activity and exercise according to body's tolerance; use energy conservation techniques in daily activities.
3. Teach relaxation techniques such as deep breathing, progressive muscle relaxation, and imagery to reduce emtional stress that causes fatigue.

E. Preserving Urinary Elimination
1. Assist with monitoring of urinary status as indicated by degree of renal involvement.
   a. Monitor intake and output and urine specific gravity.
   b. Measure urine protein, microalbumin, or obtain 24-hour creatinine clearance, as ordered.
   c. Check test results of serum blood urea nitrogen (BUN) and creatinine.
2. See page 600 for the care of patients on dialysis.

Patient Education/ Health Maintenance

1. Stress that close follow-up is mandatory, even in times of remission to detect early progression of organ involvement and alter drug therapy.
2. Advise on the use of special cosmetics to cover skin lesions.
3. Advise about reproduction.
   a. Avoid pregnancy during time of severe disease activity.
   b. Immunomodulators may have teratogenic effects.
   c. Use of some drugs for treatment of SLE can result in sterility.
4. For additional information and support, refer to agencies such as: Lupus Foundation Greater Atlanta Chapter; 340 Interstate North Parkway, Suite 455; Atlanta, GA 30339; 404-952-3891.

Evaluation

A. Reports pain reduction
B. Verbalizes appropriate use of medications, avoidance of sun and chemicals, and need for nutrition and sleep to minimize disease process
C. Reports oral ulcers healing without interference with appetite
D. Urine output adequate; specific gravity stable

◆ SYSTEMIC SCLEROSIS

Systemic sclerosis is a generalized disorder of connective tissue characterized by hardening and thickening of the skin (scleroderma), blood vessels, synovium, skeletal muscles, and internal organs. Fibrotic, degenerative, and inflammatory changes including vascular insufficiency result in changes in joints and several organ systems.

Pathophysiology/Etiology

1. The changes seen in the skin and internal organs in systemic sclerosis are most likely due to overproduction of collagen by fibroblasts.
2. The etiology of systemic sclerosis is unknown.
3. Systemic sclerosis affects three to four times as many women as men.

Clinical Manifestations

A. *Skin*
1. Bilateral symmetric swelling of the hands and sometimes the feet
2. After the edematous phase, the skin becomes hard and thick.
3. Digits, dorsum of hand, neck, face, and trunk are involved.
4. Normal landmarks in skin are absent—no skin folds.
5. Increased or decreased skin pigmentation
6. Skin changes may regress after several years.
7. Telangiectasia—on tongue, face, fingers, and lips
8. Areas of calcinosis—late in the course of disease
9. Raynaud's phenomenon

B. *Gastrointestinal*
1. Esophageal dysmotility—resulting in reflux and dysphagia
2. Distal esophageal dilation and esophagitis
3. Barrett's metaplasia—may predispose to adenocarcinoma of the esophagus.
4. Duodenal atrophy dilitation—may cause postprandial abdominal pain, malabsorption, diarrhea, and abdominal distention.
5. Colonic hypomotility—resulting in constipation

C. *Musculoskeletal*
1. Joint pain
2. Polyarthritis—large and small joints affected
3. Carpal tunnel syndrome
4. Flexion contractures
5. Inflammatory muscle atrophy

D. *Cardiac*
1. Left ventricular dysfunction
2. Myocardial involvement—congestive heart failure and atrial and ventricular arrhythmias
3. Right ventricular involvement—secondary to pulmonary disease

E. *Pulmonary*
1. Interstitial fibrosis
2. Restrictive lung disease
3. Pulmonary hypertension

F. *Renal*
1. Scleroderma renal crisis—rapid malignant hypertension with encephalopathy

G. *Localized Scleroderma*
1. CREST—*C*alcinosis, *R*aynaud's phenomenon, *E*sophageal dysmotility, *S*clerodactyly, *T*elangectasia
2. Morphea and linear scleroderma—scleroderma lesions appear as streaks or bands in linear scleroderma. Morphea lesions may be several centimeters in diameter and have a purple border. There is generally no visceral involvement in localized scleroderma.

Diagnostic Evaluation

1. CBC and ESR—generally normal
2. RF—positive in approximately 30% of patients
3. ANA—generally positive with speckled or nucleolar patterns
   a. Scl 70—positive in diffuse cutaneous disease
   b. Anticentromere antibody—highly specific for limited cutaneous disease
4. X-ray of hands and wrists—muscle atrophy, osteopenia, osteolysis
5. Barium swallow—esophageal dysmotility
6. Pulmonary function test—decreased diffusion capacity and vital capacity
7. Multiple gated image analysis—to determine left ventricular function
8. Endoscopy—to biopsy for Barrett's metaplasia
9. Esophageal manometry—to determine contractile capacity of esophageal muscles

Management

A. *Pharmacologic*
1. Penicillamine (Depen) to decrease disease activity
2. Calcium channel blockers—for Raynaud's phenomenon

3. NSAIDs—for arthralgias and polyarthritis
4. H₂ blockers and omeprazole (Prilosec)—for reflux
5. Antibiotics—for malabsorption due to bacterial over-growth
6. Antihypertensive agents
7. Metaclopromide (Reglan) and cisapride (Propulsid)—for intestinal dysmotility

B. *Nonpharmacologic*
1. Skin lubricants
2. Avoidance of factors associated with exacerbation of Raynaud's phenomenon
3. Biofeedback

Complications

1. Skin ulcers
2. Malabsorption
3. Esophageal adenocarcinoma
4. Pulmonary hypertension
5. Renal failure
6. Congestive heart failure
7. Death due to disease process

Nursing Assessment

1. Focus physical assessment on:
   a. Skin ulcers, thickening
   b. Joint examination—flexion contractures
   c. Heart and lung examination—for signs and symptoms of congestive heart failure, hypertension
   d. Gastrointestinal function
2. Determine nutritional status.

Nursing Diagnoses

A. Altered Peripheral Tissue Perfusion related to Raynaud's phenomenon
B. Risk for Impaired Skin Integrity related to effects of disease process
C. Altered Nutrition (Less than Body Requirements) related to impaired swallowing and gastrointestinal involvement
D. Body Image Disturbance related to effects of disease

Nursing Interventions

A. *Maintaining Tissue Perfusion*
1. Teach patient to identify Raynaud's phenomenon.
   a. Characteristic color change of the fingers–blue, white, red
   b. Coldness, pallor, numbness, pain
2. Teach patient to reduce factors associated with precipitation or exacerbation of Raynaud's phenomenon.
   a. Dress warmly—cover head and extremities, keep trunk warm.
   b. Discontinue tobacco usage.
   c. Avoid prolonged exposure to cold.
      (1) Weather
      (2) Artificially controlled environments (ie, air conditioning)
      (3) Limit contact with cold food items such as frozen foods, ice cube trays—use gloves or tongs.

3. Protect ulcerated digits and observe for signs of infection.

B. *Preserving Skin Integrity*
1. Use moisturizers on skin daily.
2. Advise patient to avoid use of drying soaps and detergents.
3. Use protective padding (eg, elbow pads) to protect the skin from friction or trauma.
4. Inspect skin daily for cracking, ulceration, and signs of infection.

C. *Achieving Optimal Nutritional Status*
1. Ensure patient is in proper position for meals to avoid aspiration (ie, in chair if possible).
2. Provide smaller, more frequent feedings of well balanced diet.
3. Encourage patient to remain upright after meals for 45 to 60 minutes and raise head of bed during sleep to avoid reflux.
4. Administer or teach self-administration of medications to prevent nausea and reflux as ordered.
5. Encourage good oral hygiene and frequent dental visits.
6. Advise to use lubricating agents, if necessary, to treat dry mouth and teach stretching exercises of mouth to maintain aperture.
7. Weigh weekly and ask patient to keep food diary.

D. *Strengthening Body Image*
1. Encourage patient to take an active role in treatment plan to feel in control of body changes.
2. Explain that changes may be gradual and slow, and that, although not noticeable, internal organ involvement is even more important than external changes.
3. Suggest continuance of activities that patient enjoys and fostering of strong support network.
4. Refer for counseling as needed.

Patient Education/ Health Maintenance

1. Explain all diagnostic tests and their purpose in detecting gastrointestinal, pulmonary, renal, or cardiac involvement.
2. Teach about drug treatment including adverse reactions.
3. Advise on fluid and sodium restriction if congestive heart failure has been identified.
4. Advise on modifying activity and using oxygen to prevent dyspnea due to restrictive lung disease.
5. Encourage regular follow-up and prompt attention to worsening symptoms.
6. Refer to agencies such as: Scleroderma Federation; One Newbury Street, Peabody Office Building; Peabody, MA 01960; 1-800-422-1113.

Evaluation

A. Relates factors precipitating Raynaud's phenomenon
B. Reports no skin cracking or ulceration
C. Reports no weight loss
D. Reports participating in community and church activities and groups

◆ GOUT

Gout is a disorder of purine metabolism characterized by elevated uric acid levels and deposition of urate (usually in the form of crystals) in joints and other tissues.

Pathophysiology/Etiology

Gout results from an overabundant accumulation and subsequent deposition of uric acid in the body. This can occur in one of two ways.

A. *Overproduction of Uric Acid* **(10% of cases)**

1. Inherited enzyme defects
2. Certain disease conditions
   a. Myleoproliferative disorders
   b. Lymphoproliferative disorders
   c. Ethanol abuse
   d. Cancer chemotherapy
   e. Hemolytic anemias
   f. Psoriasis

B. *Underexcretion of Uric Acid* **(90% of cases)**

1. Renal disease
2. Endocrine disorders
3. Medications and chemicals
   a. Diuretics
   b. Ethanol (alcohol)
   c. Low-dose aspirin
   d. Pyrazinamide—antituberculosis agent
   e. Lead
4. Volume depletion states—nephrogenic diabetes insipidus

Clinical Manifestations

A. *Acute Gouty Arthritis*
1. Generally affects one joint—often the first metatarsophalangeal joint called podagra
2. Other joints can be affected such as ankle, tarsals, knee; upper extremities less commonly involved.
3. Pain, warmth, erythema, and swelling of tissue surrounding the affected joint.
4. Fever may occur.
5. Onset of symptoms is sudden; intensity is severe.
6. Duration of symptoms is self-limiting; lasts approximately 3 to 10 days without treatment.

B. *Chronic Tophaceous Gout*
1. Occurs if acute gout is inadequately treated or goes untreated.
2. Characterized by development of tophi or deposits of uric acid in and around joints, cartilage, and soft tissues.
3. Arthritis is more chronic in nature with discrete attacks less common.
4. Arthritis can produce bone erosions and subsequent bony deformities that can resemble RA.

C. *Renal Disease*
1. Caused by hyperuricemia (persistent elevation of uric acid in the blood).
2. Kidney stones are composed of uric acid.
3. Deposition of uric acid in kidney tissue

Diagnostic Evaluation

1. Synovial fluid analysis
   a. Identification of monosodium urate crystals under polarized microscopy
   b. Synovial WBC count can range from 2,000 to 100,000/mm^3.
   c. Culture of synovial fluid to rule out infection
2. 24-hour urine for uric acid to determine overproduction of uric acid versus underexcretion.
3. ESR—elevated
4. X-rays of affected joints show changes consistent with diagnosis of gout.

Management

A. *Pharmacologic*
1. NSAIDs—for acute attacks to relieve pain and swelling
2. Colchicine—for prevention of acute attacks as well as their treatment
   a. Intravenous (IV) for acute attacks
   b. Oral at onset of an attack, taken hourly until first signs of toxicity (diarrhea)
3. Corticosteroids
   a. Intra-articular if attack confined to one joint
   b. Oral—in short tapering course if other treatments contraindicated or if attack involves many joints

B. *Urate-Lowering Agents*
1. Uricosuric drugs such as probenacid (Benamid) interfere with tubular reabsorption of uric acid.
2. Allopurinol (Zyloprim)—interferes with conversion of hypoxanthine and xanthine to uric acid.
   a. Side effects include skin rash (including exfoliative rashes), hypersensitivity syndrome (fever, eosinophilia, leukocytosis, worsening renal failure, hepatocellular injury, rash); bone marrow depression is rare.

C. *Nonpharmacologic*
1. Avoidance of obesity
2. Avoidance of alcohol
3. Low purine diet gives only a minor decrease in serum uric acid levels.

Complications

1. Uric acid kidney stone
2. Urate nephropathy
3. Erosive, deforming arthritis

Nursing Assessment

1. Obtain history for factors predisposing to gout.
2. Perform physical examination.
   a. Inspect involved joint.
   b. Seek presence of tophi.
      (1) Pinna of ear
      (2) Olecranon bursa
      (3) Achilles tendon
3. Assess pain and pain relief pattern if attack is acute.

Nursing Diagnoses

A. Pain related to acute arthritis
B. Impaired Physical Mobility related to arthritis

Nursing Intervention

A. Relieving Pain
1. Administer and teach self-administration of pain relieving medications as prescribed.
2. Encourage adequate fluid intake to assist with excretion of uric acid and decrease likelihood of stone formation.
3. Instruct patient in need to take prescribed medications consistently because interruptions in therapy can precipitate acute attacks.

B. Facilitating Mobility
1. Elevate and protect affected joint during acute attack.
2. Assist with activities of daily living.
3. Encourage exercise and maintenance of routine activity in chronic gout, except during acute attacks.
4. Protect draining tophi by covering and applying antibiotic ointment as needed.

Patient Education/ Health Maintenance

1. Instruct patient and family in nature of disease.
   a. Generally acute attacks are followed by periods of remission.
   b. Once need for chronic treatment has been determined it will generally be life long.
2. Encourage to avoid alcohol.
3. Avoid rapid weight loss by fasting or crash diets because rapid weight loss results in production of chemicals that compete with uric acid for excretion from the body, resulting in increased uric acid levels.
4. Avoid medications known to increase uric acid levels.
5. Advise prompt treatment of acute attack to reduce joint damage associated with repeated attacks.
6. Instruct in signs and symptoms of allopurinol hypersensitivity syndrome and need to report promptly.
7. Review foods containing purines (sardines, anchovies, shellfish, organ meats) if low-purine diet has been advised.

Evaluation

A. Reports relief of pain
B. Performs activities of daily living with minimal assistance

◆ SJÖGREN'S SYNDROME

Sjögren's syndrome is a chronic inflammatory autoimmune process affecting the lacrimal and salivary glands. The disease can be primary or secondary. Secondary Sjögren's syndrome is seen most commonly in RA but can be seen in SLE and some other connective tissue diseases.

Pathophysiology/Etiology

1. The etiology of the syndrome is unknown but is thought to include several factors: genetic predisposition, immunologic, infectious, and hormonal.
2. It is thought that antibodies directed at exocrine glands are produced, leading to disturbed function of the involved tissue.
3. Lymphocytes are found infiltrating affected tissues.
4. Sjögren's syndrome occurs primarily in middle-aged women.

Clinical Manifestations

1. Ocular—decreased tear formation leading to kertoconjunctivitis, photophobia
2. Oral—xerostomia (dry mouth) due to diminished production of saliva, mucosal ulcers, stomatitis
3. Salivary gland enlargement—unilateral or bilateral
4. Nasal dryness, epitaxsis, nasal ulcers
5. Dryness of bronchial tree, hoarseness, recurrent otitis media, pneumonia, and bronchitis
6. Gastrointestinal—dysphagia, pancreatitis, hypo- or achlorhydria, autoimmune liver disease
7. Renal—renal tubular acidosis, nephrogenic diabetes insipidus
8. Skin—xerodermia (dry skin), urticaria, purpura
9. Neuromuscular—cranial nerve dysfunction, polymyopathy, sensory and motor neuropathy, seizures, multiple sclerosis-like syndrome
10. Thyroid—autoimmune thyroiditis (Hashimoto's thyroiditis)
11. Cardiovascular—Raynaud's phenomenon, vasculitis, babies born to mothers with Sjögren's syndrome may be born with congenital heart block.
12. Sex organs—vaginal dryness, dyspareunia
13. Musculoskeletal—nonerosive polyarthritis

Diagnostic Evaluation

1. CBC—mild anemia, leukopenia present in 30% of patients
2. ESR—elevated in 90% of patients
3. RF—positive in 75% to 90% of patients
4. ANA—positive in 70% of patients; speckled and nucleolar patterns are most common.
5. Antibodies to SSA/SSB—test to detect antibodies to specific nuclear proteins
   a. SSA—positive in patients with Sjögren's syndrome and SLE
   b. SSB—positive in 60% of patients with Sjögren's syndrome; also in patients with SLE
6. Organ-specific antibodies—antibodies directed against specific organ tissues have been found.
   a. Gastric
   b. Thyroid
   c. Smooth muscle
   d. Salivary gland
   e. Lacrimal gland
7. Salivary scintigraphy—salivary gland function is measured by determining excretion of radioisotope dye.
8. X-rays of affected joints to rule out erosive arthritis
9. Salivary gland biopsy—to determine lymphocytic infiltration of tissue

Management

A. *Pharmacologic*
1. Corticosteroids—used in severe cases
2. Cyclophosphamide (Cytoxan)—used in severe cases
3. Antifungal agents—used for oral candidiasis

B. *Nonpharmacologic*
1. Symptomatic relief of dryness
   a. Artificial tears
   b. Saliva substitutes—commercial
   c. Frequent use of nonsugar liquids, gums, and candies
   d. Vaginal lubricants
   e. Use of occlusive goggles at bedtime to prevent drying
2. Dental care
   a. Frequent brushing and flossing
   b. Topical fluoride treatments
   c. Avoidance of high-sucrose foods

Complications

1. Ocular complications such as corneal ulceration, corneal opacification, vascularization of the cornea, infection, glaucoma, cataract formation
2. Tooth loss
3. Pulmonary fibrosis
4. Pulmonary hypertension
5. Obstructive airway disease
6. Chronic atrophic gastritis
7. Chronic pancreatitis
8. Abnormal liver function tests
9. Primary biliary cirrhosis
10. Renal tubular function abnormalities and membranous and membranoproliferative glomerulonephritis
11. Subcortical dementia

Nursing Assessment

1. Obtain history of signs and symptoms, emphasizing dryness.
2. Perform physical examination including oral cavity, eyes, skin, lungs, gastrointestinal, and neurologic systems.
3. Assess nutritional status because decreased saliva makes eating difficult.

Nursing Diagnoses

A. Altered Oral Mucous Membrane related to disease process
B. Risk for Impaired Skin Integrity related to dryness
C. Altered Nutrition (Less than Body Requirements) related to disturbances in saliva production, taste, and difficulty swallowing
D. Sexual Dysfunction related to discomfort of decreased vaginal secretions

Nursing Interventions

A. *Maintaining Mucous Membranes*
1. Inspect oral mucosa for oral candida, ulcers, saliva pools, and dental hygiene.

2. Instruct and assist patient in proper oral hygiene.
   a. At least twice daily brushing
   b. Frequent rinsing with antiseptic mouthwash
3. Encourage frequent intake of noncaffeinated, nonsugar liquids. Keep pitcher filled with cool water.
4. Promptly report any ulcers or signs of infections.

B. *Protecting Skin Integrity*
1. Instruct and assist patient with daily inspection of skin for areas of trauma or potential breakdown.
2. Apply lubricants to skin daily.
3. Avoid shearing forces and encourage or perform frequent position changes.

C. *Promoting Adequate Nutritional Intake*
1. Increase liquid intake with meals.
2. Assist and instruct patient to avoid choosing spicy or dry foods from menu choices.
3. Suggest small, more frequent meals.
4. Weigh weekly and review diet history for deficiency in basic nutrients.

D. *Promoting Optimal Sexual Functioning*
1. Encourage patient to discuss sexual difficulty and explain its relation to disease process.
2. Advise on proper use of water-soluble vaginal lubrication.
3. Suggest alternate positioning and practices to prevent discomfort.
4. Teach patient to report symptoms of vaginitis—discharge, irritation, itching—because infection may result from altered mucosal barrier.

Health Maintenance/ Patient Education

1. Advise patient of commercially available artificial saliva preparations, artificial tears, moisturizing nasal sprays, artificial vaginal moisturizers.
2. Encourage frequent dental visits. Dental cavities are more frequent in Sjögren's syndrome.
3. Advise patient to check with health care provider before using any medications because many, such as diuretics, tricyclic antidepressants, and antihistamines, have the side effect of mouth dryness.
4. Advise patient to wear protective eyewear while outdoors.

Evaluation

A. Demonstrates proper oral hygiene
B. Reports skin without cracking, scaling, or other lesions
C. Maintains weight
D. Describes correct use of water-soluble lubricant

◆ POLYARTERITIS NODOSA (PAN)

Polyarteritis nodosa is characterized by an inflammation of small to medium-sized blood vessels. Any organ can be affected; however, the kidney, gastrointestinal system, peripheral nerves, skin, and joints are most commonly involved.

Pathophysiology/Etiology

1. Inflammation due to deranged immunologic processes results in disruption of the blood vessel walls.
2. The affected vessels may narrow as a result of injury or develop aneurysms especially at vessel branching points.
3. Sometimes associated with hepatitis B or hepatitis C infection.
4. Men affected more than women.

Manifestations

1. Constitutional symptoms—fever, weight loss, fatigue, arthralgias, myalgias
2. Skin—palpable purpura, ulcers, changes in fingers and toes due to ischemia
3. Cardiac—coronary artery aneurysm, congestive heart failure
4. Gastrointestinal—abdominal pain, hematemesis, melena, thrombosis of mesenteric vessels
5. Kidneys—proteinuria, hematuria, presence of RBC casts, hypertension
6. Neurologic—peripheral neuropathy (sensory and motor), seizures (rare)
7. Sex organs—testicular pain

Diagnostic Evaluation

1. CBC—decreased hemoglobin and hematocrit (normochromic anemia)
2. ESR—generally elevated
3. Serum albumin—decreased
4. Complement levels—decreased
5. Hepatitis B and hepatitis C antigen—found in some patients
6. RF—sometimes positive
7. Arteriography—aneurysms
8. Biopsy—to elevate condition of blood vessels. Biopsy site may depend on patient's symptoms.

Management

1. Corticosteroids
2. Immunosuppressants such as cyclophosphamide (Cytoxan) and azathioprine (Imuran)

Complications

1. Hypertension
2. Coronary artery disease
3. Congestive heart failure
4. Cerebrovascular disease
5. Renal failure
6. Death

Nursing Assessment

1. Obtain history for constitutional symptoms, vascular changes, and manifestations of internal organ involvement.

2. Perform physical examination including the skin, neurologic system, heart and lungs, and measurement of blood pressure.

Nursing Diagnoses

A. Risk for Infection related to immunosuppressive therapy
B. Altered Peripheral Tissue Perfusion related to vasculitis

Nursing Interventions

A. Preventing Infection
1. Advise patient to avoid known sources of infection.
   a. Anyone with a contagious disease
   b. Crowds during cold and flu season
   c. Stagnant water
2. Practice and teach frequent handwashing.
3. Report any signs of infection such as cough, dysuria, sore throat, wound drainage; fever may be absent due to altered inflammatory response to medications.
4. Monitor CBC results for leukocyte and absolute neutrophil counts.

B. Promoting Tissue Perfusion
1. Inspect skin for rash, ulcers, ischemic digits, (cold, numb or painful, pale).
2. Protect extremities from trauma and keep warm to enhance blood flow.
3. Administer anti-inflammatory and immunosuppressive agents as ordered and based on patient's response. Stress compliance.

C. Monitoring for Complications
1. Be alert for signs of mesenteric ischemia—abdominal pain after meals, vomiting, diarrhea.
2. Provide small, high-caloric meals.
3. Medicate for pain as needed.

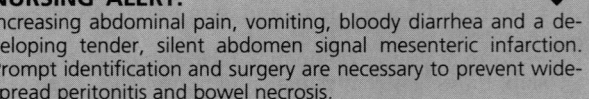

NURSING ALERT:
Increasing abdominal pain, vomiting, bloody diarrhea and a developing tender, silent abdomen signal mesenteric infarction. Prompt identification and surgery are necessary to prevent widespread peritonitis and bowel necrosis.

4. Periodically assess the lower extremities for foot drop and decreased sensation.
5. Teach protective measures to prevent injury from hot water, stepping on sharp objects, etc.
6. Monitor renal function through intake and output measurement, urine dipstick, urine specific gravity, and laboratory studies as ordered. Report abnormalities promptly.
7. Administer and teach self-administration of antihypertensive agents as ordered.

Patient Education/ Health Maintenance

1. Instruct patient and family in nature of disease.
   a. Course of disease is acute.
   b. Untreated disease has poor survival rate.
   c. Organ destruction and death are not uncommon.

Evaluation

A. Verbalizes sources of infection
B. Reports fingers without ulceration or signs of ischemia
C. Reports no abdominal pain after meals, no vomiting or diarrhea

◆ PSORIATIC ARTHRITIS

Psoriatic arthritis is an inflammatory arthritis that can be seen in patients with psoriatic skin disease or psoriatic nail disease.

Pathophysiology/Etiology

1. Disease manifestation is probably an interaction among immune, genetic, and environmental factors.
2. Psoriatic arthritis occurs in approximately 5% to 7% of patients with psoriasis.

Clinical Manifestations

A. *Inflammatory Arthritis*
1. Asymmetric arthritis involving a few joints (approximately 50% of patients)
   a. Small joints in the fingers and toes
   b. Hips, knees, ankles, and wrists
   c. Inflammation of tendon sheaths occurs, producing "sausage digits."
2. Distal interphalangeal joint—approximately 5% to 10% of patients
3. Arthritis mutilans— less than 5% of patients
   a. Severe, extensive joint destruction usually of the hands and feet
   b. Patients usually have extensive skin disease and inflammation of the sacroiliac joints.
4. Symmetric polyarthritis—approximately 25% of patients
   a. May have a clinical picture that is the same as RA, including having a positive RF.
5. Spinal arthritis—approximately 20% to 40% of patients.
   a. Arthritis affects the sacroiliac joints and may also involve all regions of the spine.

B. *Skin Involvement*
1. Psoriasis may be mild or severe.
2. Arthritis may precede the development of skin disease.
3. Nail disease is present in the large majority of patients with psoriatic arthritis.
   a. Nail pitting
   b. Nail thickening
   c. Separation of the nail from the underlying nail bed
   d. "Spoon-shaped" nails

C. *Extra-articular Manifestations*
1. Eye inflammation
   a. Conjunctivitis
   b. Iritis
2. Pulmonary fibrosis
3. Aortic insufficiency

Diagnostic Evaluation

1. CBC—may show anemia.
2. ESR—may be elevated.
3. Synovial fluid analysis—WBC count in synovial fluid between 1,000 and 15,000 cells/mm^3.
4. X-rays
   a. Hands and wrists—joint erosion in the small joints of the fingers; resorption of the distal bone tufts of the fingers
   b. Sacroiliac joints—involvement may be unilateral or bilateral.
   c. Spine—syndesmophytes on vertebrae may be present at any or all levels.
5. Skin biopsy shows characteristic hyperkeratosis and other changes.

Management

A. *Pharmacologic*
1. NSAIDs—to reduce pain and inflammation
2. Intra-articular or soft tissue injection of steroids
3. Gold—to modify disease
4. Methotrexate (Mexate)—to suppress immune response
5. Antimalarials—may exacerbate skin disease in some patients.
6. Topical steroids to treat skin disease
7. Treatments with psoralen plus ultraviolet A (PUVA) light to treat skin disease

B. *Nonpharmacologic*
1. Range of motion exercises
2. Application of heat or cold

C. *Surgical Reconstruction*

Complications

1. Anemia of chronic disease
2. Altantoaxial, lateral, and subaxial subluxations of the cervical spine have been seen.

Nursing Assessment

1. In addition to assessment of arthritis component, assess skin integrity, extent of lesions, itching, discomfort.

Nursing Diagnoses

Same as for RA; in addition:
A. Altered Skin Integrity related to psoriatic process

Nursing Interventions

A. *Promoting Skin Integrity*
1. Protect skin from excessive friction and trauma to prevent development of new lesions (Koebner phenomenon).
2. Apply topical agents after scales have been removed through soaking and gentle rubbing.

3. Encourage the use of warm clothes, good fluid intake, and good diet because extensive lesions may cause excessive fluid and plasma protein loss through skin.

Patient Education/ Health Maintenance

Same as for RA; in addition:

1. Encourage close follow-up for both arthritis and dermatologic components of the disorder.

2. Advise patient to check with health care provider before taking any additional drugs such as β-adrenergic blockers and other drugs that may exacerbate psoriasis.
3. For additional information refer to such agencies as: National Psoriasis Foundation; 6443 S.W. Beaverton Highway, Suite 210; Portland, OR 97221; 504-244-7404.

Evaluation

Same as for RA; in addition:
A. Describes appropriate procedure for removing scales and applying topical agent

Selected References

Carpenito, L. J. (Ed.). (1991). *Nursing care plans and documentation*. Philadelphia: J. B. Lippincott.

Cash, J. M. (1991). Drug therapy: Second-line drug therapy for rheumatoid arthritis. *New England Journal of Medicine, 19*, 1368-1375.

Kelley, W., Harris E., Ruddy, S., & Sledge, C. (Eds.). (1989). *Textbook of rheumatology*. (3rd ed.). Philadelphia: W. B. Saunders.

Pigg, J. S. (1995). Rheumatoid arthritis: How allied health professionals can help. *Journal of Musculoskeletal Medicine, 12*(2), 27–39.

Pinals, R. S. (1994). Current concepts: Polyarthritis and fever. *New England Journal of Medicine, 11*, 769-774.

Schumacher, H. R., Jr. (Ed.). (1993). *Primer on the rheumatic diseases*. (10th ed.). Atlanta, GA: The Arthritis Foundation.

Star, V. L. & Hochberg, M. C. (1994). Gout; steps to relieve acute symptoms, prevent further attacks. *Consultant, 34*(12), 1697–1706.

Varga, J. & Jimenez, S. A. (1995). Modulation of collagen gene expression: Its relation to fibrosis in systemic sclerosis and other disorders. *Annals of Internal Medicine, 122*(1), 60–62.

UNIT 10

◆

Musculoskeletal Disorders

Assessment

◆ SUBJECTIVE DATA

A great deal can be learned about musculoskeletal disorders from subjective data. History of injury, description of symptoms, and associated personal health and family history can give clues to the underlying problem and appropriate care for that problem.

Common Manifestations of Musculoskeletal Problems

A. Pain
1. Where is the pain located?
   a. Joint(s), as in osteoarthritis
   b. Muscles or soft tissue, as in contusions, sprains, or strains.
   c. Bone, as in fractures or tumors.
2. Is it sharp, as in a fracture or sprain, or dull, as in a bone tumor?
3. Does pain radiate?
   a. To buttocks or legs, as in low back pain
   b. To thigh or knee, as in hip fracture

B. Limited Range of Motion
1. Is stiffness present; how long does it last?
   a. Present in morning for less than 30 minutes with osteoarthritis
   b. May persist and is associated with acute pain when due to spasm of low back strain
2. Is swelling present and limiting mobility?
   a. May be due to fracture
   b. May be soft tissue injury, such as sprain, strain, or contusion
3. How does limited mobility affect activities of daily living?

C. Associated Symptoms
1. Any sensory or motor deficits, such as numbness, paresthesias, or weakness, indicating neurovascular compromise?

2. Any weight loss, fever, or malaise, as in bone tumors?
3. Any bony nodules or deformity, as in osteoarthritis?

History

A. Mechanism of Injury
1. How did the injury occur? Essential for all trauma, including fractures, contusions, sprains, and strains to help identify the extent of injury.
2. What was the progression of symptoms?
3. If not an acute injury, was there any repetitive movement or strain that may have contributed to problem, as in tendinitis?

B. Medical History
1. Any history of corticosteroid use that predisposes to osteoporosis?
2. Is the woman postmenopausal? On estrogen replacement? If estrogen deficient, may predispose to osteoporosis.
3. Any history of prostate, breast, or lung cancer, which may metastasize to the bone?
4. What are other chronic conditions that may affect immobility imposed by casting, traction, or surgery?

C. Social/History
1. What is the patient's occupation, which may contribute to low back strain or osteoarthritis?
2. What activities or sports does the patient participate in, such as running or tennis, that may cause tendinitis?
3. Are there risk factors for osteoporosis, such as smoking, inactivity, or lack of exposure to the sun?
4. Is there a family history of osteoporosis or arthritis?

◆ OBJECTIVE DATA

Data on current system condition and functional abilities are secured through inspection, palpation, and measurement. Always compare with contralateral side (one side of the body to the other).

Musculoskeletal System

A. *Skeletal Component*
1. Note deviation from structural normal—bony deformities, length discrepancies, alignment, amputations.
2. Identify abnormal motion and crepitus (grating sensation), as found with fractures.

B. *Joint Component*
1. Identify swelling that may be due to inflammation or effusion.
2. Note deformity associated with contractures or dislocations.
3. Evaluate stability, which may be altered.
4. Estimate range of motion, both actively and passively.

C. *Muscle Component*
1. Inspect for size and contour of muscles.
2. Assess coordination of movement.
3. Palpate for muscle tone.
4. Estimate strength through cursory evaluation (ie, handshake) or scaled criteria (ie, 0 = no palpable contraction; 5 = normal range of motion against gravity with full resistance).
5. Measure girth to note increases due to swelling or bleeding into muscle or decreases due to atrophy (difference of more than 1 cm is significant).
6. Identify abnormal clonus (rhythmic contraction and relaxation) or fasciculation (contraction of isolated muscle fibers).

Additional Assessment

A. *Neurovascular Component*
1. Assess circulatory status of involved extremities by noting skin color and temperature, peripheral pulses, capillary refill response, pain.
2. Assess neurologic status of involved extremities by the patient's ability to move distal muscles and description of sensation (eg, paresthesia).
3. Test reflexes of extremities.
4. Compare all to uninjured/unaffected extremity.

B. *Skin Component*
1. Inspect traumatic injuries (eg, cuts, bruises).
2. Assess chronic conditions (eg, dermatitis, stasis ulcers).
3. Note hair distribution and nail condition.
4. Inspect for Heberden's or Bouchard's nodes.

Diagnostic Tests

◆ RADIOLOGIC/IMAGING STUDIES

Many radiologic and imaging studies are helpful in evaluating musculoskeletal problems to rule out fracture or skeletal changes and to differentiate soft tissue injury.

X-rays

A. *Description*
1. Of bone—to determine bone density, texture, integrity, erosion, changes in bone relationships.
2. Of cortex—to detect any widening, narrowing, irregularity.
3. Of medullary cavity—to detect any alteration in density.
4. Of involved joint—to show fluid, irregularity, spur formation, narrowing, changes in joint contour.
5. Tomogram—special x-ray technique for detailed view of special plane of bone

B. *Nursing/Patient Care Considerations*
1. Tell the patient that proper positioning is important to obtain a good x-ray, so cooperation is essential.
2. Advise patient to remove all jewelry, clothing with zippers or snaps, change from pockets, or other items that may interfere with x-ray.

Bone Scan

A. *Description* Parenteral injection of bone-seeking radiopharmaceutical (such as gallium); concentration of isotope uptake revealed in primary skeletal disease (osteosarcoma), metastatic bone disease, inflammatory skeletal disease (osteomyelitis); fracture

B. *Nursing/Patient Care Considerations*
1. Advise patient that laxative may be needed before the procedure.
2. Injectable radionuclide may be given 24 to 72 hours before the scan.
3. Reassure patient that there is no pain and that scan will take 1 to 2 hours.
4. Breast-feeding should be discontinued for at least 4 weeks after test to prevent radionuclide exposure to infant.

Bone Densitometry

A. *Description* A noninvasive study that yields an actual measurement of bone density and is diagnostic for osteoporosis

B. *Nursing/Patient Care Considerations*
1. No special preparation or restrictions.
2. Have patient remove clothing and all jewelry or other metal objects.
3. Advise patient to lie still with hips flexed during test; technician will remain in room.
4. Reassure that radiation exposure is minimal.

Magnetic Resonance Imaging (MRI)

A. *Description* Uses magnetic fields to demonstrate differences in hydrogen density of various tissues. Demonstrates tumors and soft tissue (muscle, ligament, tendon) abnormalities

B. *Nursing/Patient Care Considerations*
1. Prepare patient for need to lie still for about 1 hour; repetitive clanging noise of machine will be heard; patients may feel closed in.
2. Practice relaxation techniques, such as relaxation breathing and imagery, ahead of time.
3. Some patients may need sedation; claustrophobic patients may be unable to undergo procedure or may need open MRI.

4. Contradicted for patients with metal implants, prosthetic valves, surgical clips, pacemakers, and orthopedic hardware.

NURSING ALERT:
Patients with metal implants, metal braces, or pacemakers are unable to undergo MRI.

Other Tests

1. Arthrogram—injection of radiopaque substance or air into joint cavity to outline soft tissue structures (e.g., meniscus) and contour of joint
2. Myelogram—injection of contrast medium into subarachnoid space at lumbar spine to determine level of disc herniation or site of tumor (see p. 363).
3. Diskogram—injection of small amount of contrast medium into lumbar disk abnormalities.
4. Arthrocentesis—insertion of needle into joint and aspiration of synovial fluid for purposes of examination.
5. Arthroscopy—endoscopic procedure that allows direct visualization of joint structures (synovium, articular surfaces, menisci, ligaments) through a large-bore needle. May be combined with arthrography.
6. Nerve studies—to differentiate nerve root compression, muscle disease (eg, dystrophy, myositis), peripheral neuropathies, central nervous system–anterior horn cell neuropathies, neuromuscular junction problems.
   a. Electromyography (EMG)—measures electrical potential generated by the muscle during relaxation and contraction.
   b. Nerve conduction velocities—measure the rate of potential generation along specific nerves (speed of impulse conduction).

General Procedures/ Treatment Modalities

◆ CRUTCH WALKING

Crutches are artificial supports that assist patients who need aid in walking because of disease, injury, or a birth defect.

Preparation for Crutch Walking

Goals: Develop power in the shoulder girdle and upper extremities that bear the patient's weight in crutch walking. Strengthen and condition the patient.

A. *Strengthening the Muscles Needed for Ambulation*
Instruct the patient as follows:

1. For quadriceps setting:
   a. Contract the quadriceps muscle while attempting to push the popliteal area against the mattress and raise the heel.
   b. Maintain the muscle contracture for the count of 5.
   c. Relax for the count of 5.

d. Repeat this exercise 10 to 15 times hourly.
2. For gluteal setting:
   a. Contract or pinch the buttocks together for a count of 5.
   b. Relax for the count of 5.
   c. Repeat 10 to 15 times hourly.

B. *Strengthening the Muscles of the Upper Extremities and Shoulder Girdle*
Instruct the patient as follows:

1. Flex and extend arms slowly while holding traction weights; gradually increase poundage of weight and number of repetitions to increase strength and endurance.
2. Do push-ups while lying in a prone position.
3. Squeeze rubber ball—increases grasping strength.
4. Raise head and shoulders from bed; stretch hands forward as far as possible.
5. Sit up on bed or chair.
   a. Raise body from chair by pushing hands against chair seat (or mattress).
   b. Raise body out of seat. Hold. Relax.

C. *Measuring for Crutches*
1. When the patient is lying down (an approximate measurement):
   a. Instruct the patient to wear shoes he or she will be using for walking.
   b. Measure from the anterior fold of the axilla to the sole of the foot. Then add 5 cm (2 in.).
   c. Alternatively, subtract 40 cm (16 in.) from the patient's height.
2. When the patient is standing erect:
   a. Stand the patient against the wall with feet slightly apart and away from the wall.
   b. The crutches should be fitted with large rubber suction tips.
   c. The elbow is flexed 30 degrees with the hand resting on the grip.
   d. There should be a two-finger-width insertion between the axillary fold and the hand grip. A foam-rubber pad on the underarm piece will relieve pressure on the upper arm and thoracic cage.
   e. The tip of the crutch is placed 15 to 20 cm (6–8 in.) lateral to the forefoot.

D. *Teaching the Crutch Stance*
1. Have the patient wear well-fitting shoes with firm soles.
2. Before using the crutches, have the patient stand by a chair on the unaffected leg to achieve balance.
3. Position the patient against a wall with head in a neutral position.
4. Tripod position—basic crutch stance for balance and support.
   a. Crutches rest approximately 20 to 25 cm (8–10 in.) in front of and to the side of the patient's toes (Fig. 29-1).
   b. Taller patient requires a wider base, whereas shorter patient needs a narrower base.
5. Teach the patient to support weight on hands; weight borne on the axillae can damage the brachial plexus nerves and produce "crutch paralysis."

Teaching the Crutch Gait

1. Crutch walking requires balance, coordination, and a high energy cost; these can be acquired with diligent and regular practice.

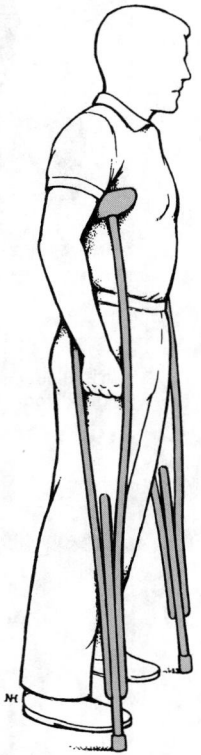

FIGURE 29-1 *The tripod position is the basic crutch stance for balance and support.*

2. Practice balancing with crutches while leaning against the wall.
3. Practice shifting body weight in different positions while standing with crutches.
4. The selection of the crutch gait depends on the type and severity of the disability and the patient's physical condition, arm and trunk strength, and/or body balance.

5. Teach the patient at least two gaits—a faster gait to be used for swiftness and a slower one to be used in crowded places.
6. Instruct the patient to change from one gait to another—relieves fatigue, because a different combination of muscles is used.

Crutch Gaits

A. *Four-Point Gait (Four-Point Alternate Crutch Gait)*
1. This is a slow but stable gait; the patient's weight is constantly being shifted.
2. Four-point gait can be used only by patients who can move each leg separately and bear a considerable amount of weight on each of them.
3. Crutch–foot sequence (Fig. 29-2):
  a. Right crutch
  b. Left foot
  c. Left crutch
  d. Right foot

B. *Three-Point Gait* This is used when one leg is involved
Crutch–foot sequence (Fig. 29-3):
1. Both crutches and the involved lower leg are moved forward simultaneously.
2. Then the stronger lower extremity is moved forward while most of the body weight is put on the crutches.

C. *Two-Point Gait* This is a progression from the four-point gait that allows faster ambulation
Crutch–foot sequence (Fig. 29-4):
1. Weight is borne on both lower extremities and both crutches.
2. Advance right foot and left crutch together.
3. Then advance left foot and right crutch together.

Crutch Maneuvering Techniques

A. *Standing Up*
1. Move forward to the edge of the chair with the strong leg slightly under the seat.
2. Place both crutches in the hand on the side of the affected extremity.

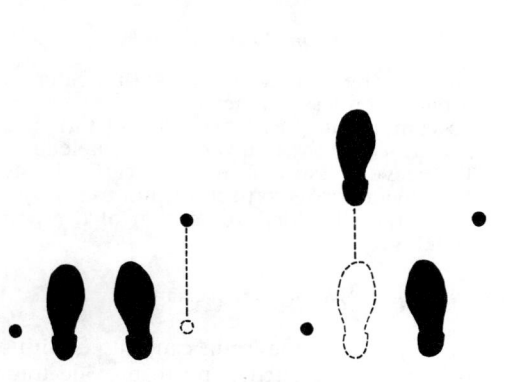

Right crutch forward   Advance left foot

FIGURE 29-2 *Four-point gait.*

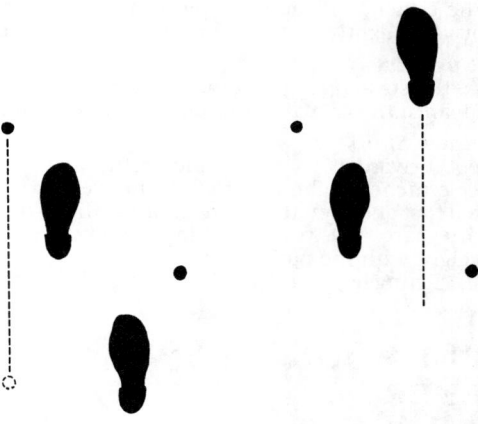

Left crutch forward   Advance right foot

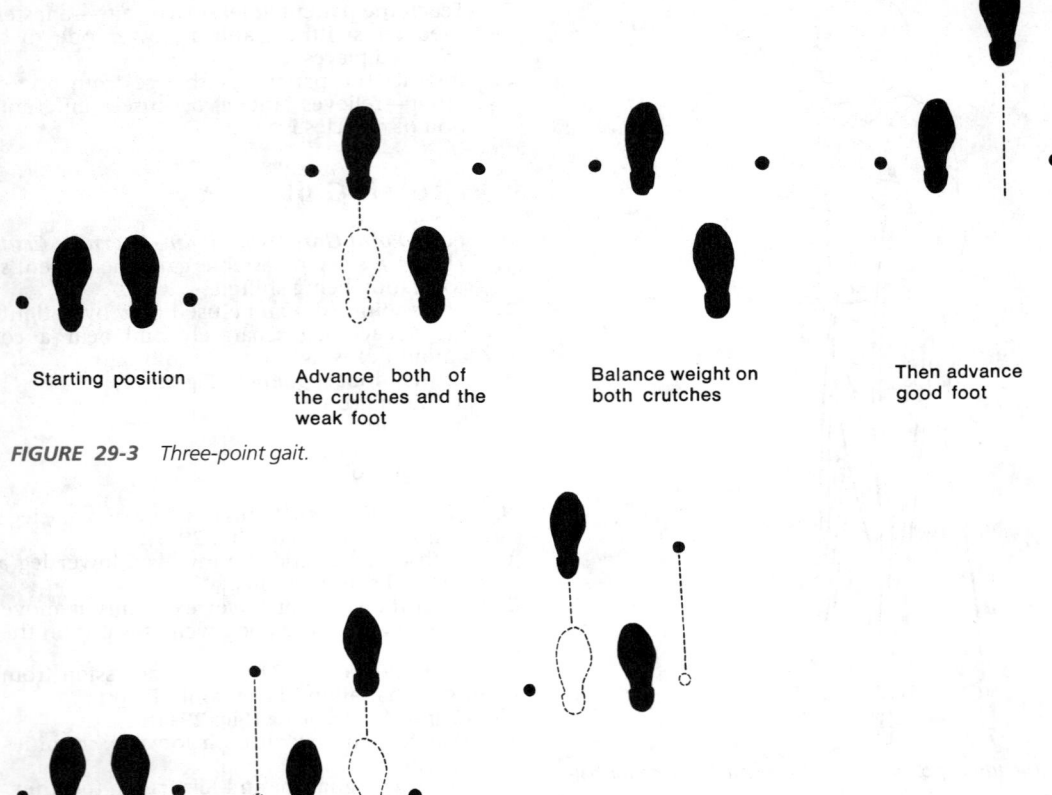

FIGURE 29-3 *Three-point gait.*

Starting position

Advance both of
the crutches and the
weak foot

Balance weight on
both crutches

Then advance
good foot

Starting position

Advance right foot and
left crutch

Then advance left foot
and right crutch simulta-
neously.

FIGURE 29-4 *Two-point gait.*

3. Push down on the hand pieces while raising the body to a standing position.

B. Sitting in a Chair
1. Grasp the crutches at the hand pieces for control and bend forward slightly while assuming a sitting position.

C. Going Up Stairs
1. Advance the stronger leg first up to the next step.
2. Then advance the crutches and the weaker extremity.

D. Going Down Stairs
1. Place feet forward as far as possible on the step.
2. Advance crutches to the lower step. The weaker leg is advanced first and then the stronger one—the stronger extremity shares the work of raising and lowering the body weight with the patient's arms.
   Note: Strong leg goes up stairs first and down stairs last.

◆ AMBULATION WITH A WALKER

A walker provides more support than crutches or a cane for the patient who has poor balance and cannot use crutches. It gives stability but does not permit a natural reciprocal walking pattern. Teach the following sequence:

1. Lift the walker, placing it in front of you while leaning your body slightly forward.
2. Take a step or two into the walker.
3. Lift the walker and place it in front of you again.

◆ AMBULATION WITH A CANE

A cane is used for balance and support:

1. To assist the patient to walk with greater balance and support and less fatigue.
2. To compensate for deficiencies of function normally performed by the neuromuscular skeletal system.
3. To relieve pressure on weight-bearing joints.
4. To provide forces to push or pull the body forward or to restrain the forward motion of the patient while walking.

Principles of Cane Use

1. An adjustable aluminum cane fitted with a 3.75 cm ($1\frac{1}{2}$ in.) rubber suction tip to provide traction while walking gives optimal stability to the patient.
2. With bilateral disease, using two canes give better balance and weight relief.

3. To fit for a cane:
   a. Have patient flex elbow at a 30-degree angle and hold the cane 15 cm (6 in.) lateral to the base of fifth toe.
   b. Adjust the cane so that the handle is approximately level with the greater trochanter.
4. Alternatively, while the patient is standing with arms at side, the handle of the cane should line up with the crease in wrist.

Technique for Walking With a Cane

1. Hold the cane in the hand opposite to the affected extremity (ie, the cane should be used on the good side)—allows partial weight-bearing relief as the cane is in contact with the floor at the same time as the affected extremity.
2. Advance the cane at the same time the affected leg is moved forward.
3. Keep the cane fairly close to the body to prevent leaning.
4. If the patient is unable to use the cane in the opposite hand, the cane may be carried on the same side and advanced when the affected leg is advanced.
5. To go up and down stairs:
   a. Step up on unaffected extremity.
   b. Then place cane and affected extremity on the step.
   c. Reverse this procedure for the descending steps.
   d. The strong leg goes up first and comes down last.

◆ CASTS

A cast is an immobilizing device made up of layers of plaster or fiberglass (water-activated polyurethane resin) bandages molded to the body part that it encases. See Procedure Guidelines 29-1 and 29-2 for application and removal of a cast.

Purposes

1. To immobilize and hold bone fragments in reduction.
2. To apply uniform compression of soft tissues.
3. To permit early mobilization.
4. To correct and prevent deformities.
5. To support and stabilize weak joints.

Types of Casts

A. Short-Arm Cast Extends from below the elbow to the proximal palmar crease

B. Gauntlet Cast Extends from below the elbow to the proximal palmar crease, including the thumb (thumb spica)

C. Long-Arm Cast Extends from upper level of axillary fold to proximal palmar crease; elbow usually immobilized at right angle

D. Short-Leg Cast Extends from below knee to base of toes

E. Long-Leg Cast Extends from upper thigh to the base of toes; foot is at right angle in a neutral position

F. Body Cast Encircles the trunk stabilizing the spine

G. Spica Cast Incorporates the trunk and extremity

1. Shoulder spica cast—a body jacket that encloses trunk, shoulder, and elbow.
2. Hip spica cast—encloses trunk and a lower extremity.
   a. Single hip spica—extends from nipple line to include pelvis and extends to include pelvis and one thigh.
   b. Double hip spica—extends from nipple line or upper abdomen to include pelvis and extends to include both thighs and lower legs.
   c. One-and-a-half hip spica—extends from upper abdomen, includes one entire leg, and extends to the knee of the other.

H. Cast-Brace External support about a fracture that is constructed with hinges to permit early motion of joints, early mobilization, and independence

1. Cast bracing is based on the concept that some weight-bearing is physiologic and will promote the formation of bone and contain fluid within a tight compartment that compresses soft tissues, providing a distribution of forces across the fracture site.
2. Cast-brace is applied after initial edema and pain have subsided and there is evidence of fracture stability.

I. Cylinder Cast Can be used for upper of lower extremity. Used for fracture or dislocation of knee (lower extremity) or elbow dislocation (upper extremity)

Complications of Casts

1. Compartment syndrome—Trauma or surgery affecting an extremity will produce swelling (result of hemorrhage from bone and surrounding tissue and of tissue edema). Vascular insufficiency and nerve and muscle compression due to unrelieved swelling can cause irreversible damage to an extremity.
2. Pressure of cast on neurovascular and bony structures causes necrosis, pressure sores, and nerve palsies.
3. Immobility and confinement in a cast, particularly a body cast, can result in multisystem problems.
   a. Nausea, vomiting, and abdominal distention associated with cast syndrome (superior mesenteric artery syndrome, resulting in diminished blood flow to the bowel), adynamic ileus, and possible intestinal obstruction.
   b. Acute anxiety reaction symptoms (ie, behavioral changes and autonomic responses—increased respiratory and heart rate, elevated blood pressure, diaphoresis) associated with confinement in a space.
   c. Thrombophlebitis and possible pulmonary emboli associated with immobility and ineffective circulation (eg, venous stasis).
   d. Respiratory atelectasis and pneumonia associated with ineffective respiratory effort.
   e. Urinary tract infection—Renal and bladder calculi associated with urinary stasis, low fluid intake, and calcium excretion associated with immobility.
   f. Anorexia and constipation associated with decreased activity.
   g. Psychological reaction (eg, depression) associated with immobility, dependence, and loss of control.

◆ NURSING PROCESS OVERVIEW: THE PATIENT WITH A CAST

Nursing Assessment

1. Assess neurovascular status of the extremity with a cast for signs of compromise.
   a. Pain
   b. Swelling
   c. Discoloration—pale or blue
   d. Cool skin distal to injury
   e. Tingling or numbness (paresthesia)
   f. Pain on passive extension (muscle stretch)
   g. Slow capillary refill; diminished or absent pulse
   h. Paralysis
2. Assess skin integrity of casted extremity. Be alert for:
   a. Severe initial pain over bony prominences; this is a warning symptom of an impending pressure sore. Pain increases when ulceration occurs.
   b. Odor
   c. Drainage on cast

NURSING ALERT:
Do not ignore the complaint of pain of the patient in a cast. Suspect circulatory complications or a pressure sore. Notify health care provider if symptoms persist. Cast may have to be split or removed.

3. Carefully assess for positioning and potential pressure sites of the casted extremity.
   a. Lower extremity—heel, malleoli, dorsum of foot, head of fibula, anterior surface of patella.
   b. Upper extremity—medial epicondyle of humerus, ulnar styloid.
   c. Plaster jackets or body spica casts—sacrum, anterior and superior iliac spines, vertebral borders of scapulae.
4. Assess cardiovascular, respiratory, and gastrointestinal systems for possible complications of immobility.
5. Assess psychological reaction to illness, cast, and immobility.

Nursing Diagnoses

A. Altered Peripheral Tissue Perfusion related to swelling and constrictive bandage/cast
B. Impaired Physical Mobility related to condition and casting

Nursing Interventions

A. *Maintaining Adequate Tissue Perfusion*
1. Elevate the extremity on cloth-covered pillow above the level of the heart. Keep the heel off the mattress.
2. Avoid resting cast on hard surfaces or sharp edges that can cause denting or flattening of the cast and consequent pressure sores.
3. Handle moist cast with palms of hands.
4. Turn patient every 2 hours while cast dries.

5. Assess neurovascular status hourly during the first 24 hours, then less frequently as condition warrants and swelling resolves.
6. If symptoms of neurovascular compromise occur:
   a. Notify health care provider immediately.
   b. Bivalve the cast—split cast on each side over its full length into two halves.
   c. Cut the underlying padding—blood soaked padding may shrink and cause constriction of circulation.
   d. Spread cast sufficiently to relieve constriction.
7. If symptoms of pressure area occur, cast may be "windowed" (hole cut in it) so that the skin at the pain point can be examined and treated. The window must be replaced so that the tissue does not swell and cause additional pressure problems at window edge (Fig. 29-5).

B. *Minimizing the Effects of Immobility*
1. Encourage the patient to move about as normally as possible.
2. Encourage compliance with prescribed exercises to avoid muscle atrophy and loss of strength.
   a. Active range of motion for every joint that is not immobilized at regular and frequent intervals.
   b. Isometric exercises for the muscles of the casted extremity. Instruct patient to alternately contract and relax muscles without moving affected part.
3. Reposition and turn patient frequently.
4. Avoid pressure behind knees, which reduces venous return and predisposes to thromboembolism.
5. Use antiembolism stockings as prescribed.
6. Administer prophylactic anticoagulants as prescribed.

NURSING ALERT:
Persons at high risk include older adults and persons with previous thromboembolism, obesity, congestive heart failure, or multiple trauma. They may require prophylaxis against thromboembolism.

7. Encourage deep-breathing exercises and coughing at regular intervals to prevent atelectasis and pneumonia.
8. Observe for symptoms of cast syndrome—nausea, vomiting, abdominal distention, abdominal pain, and decreased bowel sounds.

NURSING ALERT:
Cast syndrome (superior mesenteric artery syndrome) is a rare sequela of cast application, yet it is a potentially fatal complication. It is important to teach patients about this syndrome, because this can develop as late as several weeks after cast application.

9. Encourage the patient to drink liberal quantities of fluid—to avoid urinary infection and calculi secondary to immobility.

C. *Providing Additional Care*
1. Encourage balanced nutritional intake.
   a. Assess the patient's food preferences. Serve small meals.
   b. Provide natural bowel stimulants (eg, fiber).
   c. Monitor bowels and use a bowel program if necessary.
2. If symptoms of cast syndrome develop, report immediately.
   a. Place patient in a prone position, if tolerated, to relieve pressure symptoms.
   b. Use nasogastric suction as prescribed.

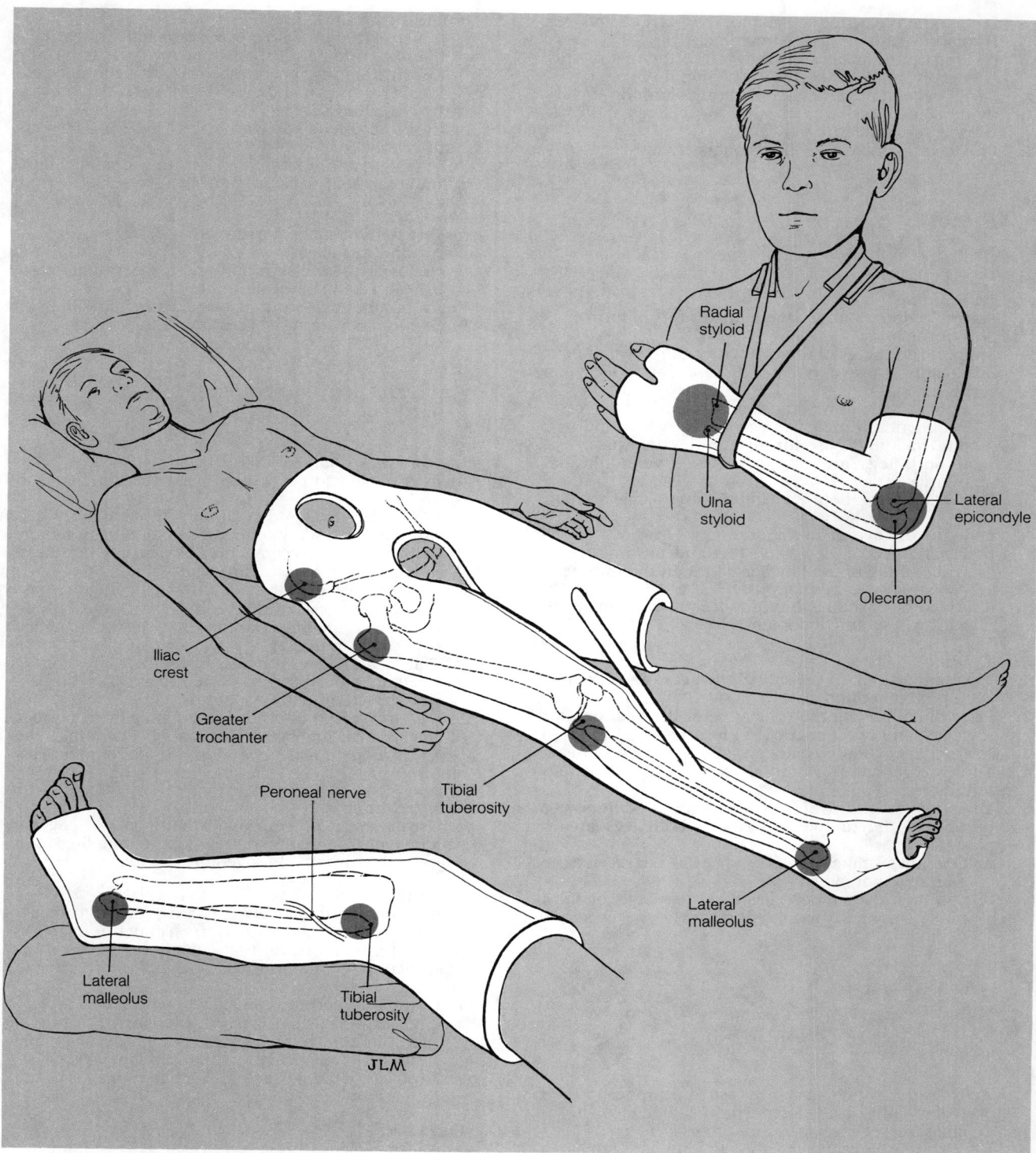

FIGURE 29-5 *Pressure areas in different types of casts.*

c. Maintain electrolyte balance by intravenous replacement of fluids as prescribed.
d. Prepare the patient for removal of the cast or surgical relief of duodenal obstruction if necessary.
3. Facilitate patient participation in care planning and activities. Encourage verbalization of feelings and concerns regarding casting.
4. Provide and encourage diversional activities.

Specific Care for Patient in Spica/ Body Cast

A. Positioning
1. Place a bedboard under the mattress for uniform support of the body.
2. Support the curves of the cast with cloth-covered flexible pillows—prevents cracking and flat spots while cast is drying.
   a. Place three pillows crosswise on bed for body cast.
   b. Place one pillow crosswise at the waist and two pillows lengthwise for affected leg for spica cast. If both legs are involved, use two additional pillows.
3. Encourage the patient to maintain physiologic position by:
   a. Using the overhead trapeze.
   b. Placing good foot flat on bed and pushing down while lifting himself or herself up on the trapeze.
   c. Avoiding twisting motions.
   d. Avoiding positions that produce pressure on groin, back, chest, and abdomen.

B. Turning
1. Move the patient to the side of the bed using a steady, even pulling motion.
2. Place pillows along the other side of the bed; one for the chest and two (lengthwise) for the legs.
3. Instruct the patient to place arms at side or above head.
4. Turn the patient as a unit. Avoid twisting the patient in the cast.
5. Turn the patient toward the leg not encased in plaster or toward the unoperated side if both legs are in plaster.
   a. One nurse stands at other side of bed to receive the patient's shoulders.
   b. Second nurse supports leg in plaster while the third nurse supports the patient's back as he or she is turned.

NURSING ALERT:
Do not grasp cross bar of spica cast to move the patient. The purpose of the bar is to strengthen the cast.

   c. Turn the patient in body cast to a prone position twice daily—provides postural drainage of bronchial tree; relieves pressure on back.
6. Keep the cast level by elevating the lumbar sacral area with a small pillow when the head of the bed is elevated.

C. Hygienic Care
1. Provide hygienic care of the patient.

2. Protect cast from soiling.
   a. Cover perineum with a towel and apply spray (lacquer-type) to perineal area of cast. Tuck 10-cm (4-in.) strips of thin polyethylene sheeting under perineal area of cast and tape to cast exterior. Replace when soiling occurs.
   b. Clean outside of cast with dry cleanser on almost-dry cloth.
3. Roll the patient onto fracture bedpan; use small pillow in lumbosacral area for support.

D. Skin Care
1. Inspect skin for signs of irritation:
   a. Around cast edge.
   b. Under cast—pull skin taut and inspect under cast, using a flashlight for illumination.
2. Reach up under cast and massage accessible skin.
3. Protect the toes from the pressure of the bedding.

Patient Education/Health Maintenance

A. Neurovascular Status
1. Instruct patient to check neurovascular status and to control swelling.
   a. Watch for signs and symptoms of circulatory disturbance, including blueness or paleness of fingernails or toenails accompanied by pain and tightness, numbness, cold or tingling sensation.
   b. Elevate affected extremity and wiggle fingers/toes.
   c. Apply ice bags as prescribed ($\frac{1}{3}-\frac{1}{2}$ full) to each side of the cast, making sure that they do not make indentations in plaster.
   d. Call health care provider promptly if excessive swelling, paresthesia, persistent pain, pain on passive stretch, or paralysis occurs.
2. Instruct patient to alternate ambulation with periods of elevation to the cast when seated. Encourage the patient to lie down several times daily with cast elevated.

B. Skin Irritation
1. Advise patient to prevent skin irritation at cast edge by padding edges of cast with moleskin or "petaling" cast edges with strips of adhesive tape.

C. Exercise
1. Instruct patient to actively exercise every joint that is not immobilized and to perform isometric exercises (contract muscles without moving joint) of those immobilized to maintain muscle strength and to prevent atrophy.
2. Tell patient to perform hourly when awake.
   a. Leg cast—"Push down on the popliteal (knee) space, hold it, relax, repeat." Move toes back and forth; bend toes down, then pull them back.
   b. Arm cast—"Make a fist, hold it, relax, repeat." Move shoulders.

D. Cast Care
1. Advise to avoid getting cast wet, especially padding under cast—causes skin breakdown as plaster cast becomes soft.
2. Warn against covering a leg cast with plastic or rubber boots, because this causes condensation and wetting of the cast.

3. Instruct to avoid weight bearing or stress on plaster cast for 24 hours.
4. Instruct to report to health care provider if the cast cracks or breaks; instruct the patient not to try to fix it.
5. Teach how to clean the cast:
   a. Remove surface soil with slightly damp cloth.
   b. Rub soiled areas with household scouring powder.
   c. Wipe off residual moisture.

E. *Teaching Safety Measures* Avoid walking on wet floors or sidewalks, to prevent falls; do not place objects under the cast, to prevent pressure and injury to the skin

F. *After Cast Is Removed*
1. Instruct to cleanse skin with mild soap and water, blot dry, and apply emollient lotion to dry skin.

2. Warn against scratching the skin.
3. Advise to continue prescribed exercises. Gradually resume activities, and elevate extremity to control swelling.

Evaluation

A. No pain, discoloration, or sensory or motor impairment of affected extremity; warm, with good capillary refill
B. Ambulating with assistance; performing active range of motion and isometric exercises every 1 to 2 hours
C. No signs of complications

PROCEDURE GUIDELINES 29-1 ◆ Application of a Cast

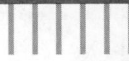

EQUIPMENT   Plaster or synthetic bandages in desired widths
*Stockinette (tubular knitted material)
*Cast padding (roll padding)
Splints (for reinforcement)

*Cotton, polyester, or polyurethane foam padding for bony prominences
Cast knives, scissors
Polyethylene sheeting or newspaper—to protect floor
Disposable gloves—to protect hands of operator

Material needs to be nonabsorbent if non-plaster cast is used.

Large, plastic-lined pail of water at room temperature—21°–24°C (70°–75°F)—or as recommended by cast material manufacturer
Cast finishing hand cream for synthetic cast as needed

UNDERLYING CONSIDERATIONS
1. The application of a cast requires 2–3 persons: one to apply the plaster (operator), one to dip and hand the plaster bandages to the operator, and a third person to hold the extremity in correct position. (Body spicas may require additional personnel.)
2. The time required for the cast to become rigid varies with the material used—generally 2–6 minutes.
3. There should be no movement of the extremity while the cast is being applied and set.
4. In general, the joints above and below the involved bone are immobilized.

PROCEDURE

NURSING ACTION	RATIONALE
PREPARATORY PHASE	
1. Spread polyethylene sheeting or newspaper on floor.	
2. Explain to the patient that there will be a feeling of warmth as the plaster is applied.	2. Heat is produced by crystallization as plaster sets. The reaction of water with plaster of paris liberates heat.
3. Apply stockinette and roll cast padding on the extremity or part to be immobilized. a. Apply roll padding as smoothly and snugly as possible so that each turn overlaps the preceding turn by ½ the width of the roll. b. Extra pieces of padding may be placed over bony prominences: olecranon process, malleoli, patella.	3. Padding is used to pad the sharp cast margins for patient comfort and to prevent pressure areas, minimize circulatory problems, and facilitate cast removal. It is applied from the distal to the proximal end of the extremity. When too much padding is used, it may shift and produce pressure areas under the cast.
4. While keeping the thumb under the forward edge of the bandage, submerge the plaster bandage vertically in water (room temperature) for a minute or so, or until bubbles cease to rise. Check directions on synthetic cast materials.	4. Water that is too warm will accelerate setting time, may cause a burn, and may result in excessive plaster loss by loosening the adhesive agents that bond the plaster to the fabric.
5. Expel excess water by squeezing (not wringing) toward the center of the bandage; hand bandage to operator with free end hanging loose.	5. The cast will dry more quickly (and thus will acquire maximum strength sooner) if a well-squeezed plaster bandage is used. Maximum strength is achieved by synthetic casts through chemical reaction in about ½ hour.

(continued)

PROCEDURE GUIDELINES 29-1 ♦ Application of a Cast *(continued)*

PROCEDURE *(cont'd)*	**NURSING ACTION**	**RATIONALE**

PERFORMANCE PHASE (BY OPERATOR)

NURSING ACTION	RATIONALE
1. Starting at the distal end, roll the bandage gently and evenly on the extremity overlapping the preceding turn by ½ the width of the roll.	1. Roll inward toward the patient's body for ease of control.
2. Keep the bandage moving and in constant contact with the surface of the extremity. Smooth and rub down successive layers or turns of each bandage into the layers below with the thumbs and thenar eminences (mound on the palm) in circumferential and longitudinal directions.	2. This keeps the cast uniformly thick. Rubbing the plaster as it is applied will form a smooth, solid, and well-fused cast. Avoid indenting the cast with the fingertips, as this may produce pressure sores on underlying skin. Handle fresh casts with palms.
3. Take tucks in the lower border of the bandage by lifting the bandage off the surface (without tension) and overlapping it in a V-shaped fashion.	3. Tucking the bandage helps to contour the cast to the changing circumference of the extremity. Do not twist or reverse the bandage to change its direction, as this produces sharp cutting edges.
4. Trim the cast to size with a sharp knife. Fold stockinette over edges of cast and anchor with cast material.	4. Stockinette produces smooth, comfortable edges on cast. Do not pull too vigorously on the stockinette, as this may cause pressure on bony prominences.
5. Finish synthetic cast with cast hand cream as indicated.	5. Smooths rough exterior surface.
6. Ask the patient if there is any discomfort or pain.	6. If a patient complains of pain, it may be due to manipulation of fracture during setting; pain should subside rapidly. If it persists, the cast and encircling dressings are split to avoid constriction, circulatory problems, and pressure sores.

FOLLOW-UP PHASE

NURSING ACTION	RATIONALE
1. Support the cast with the palm of the hand while moving the patient. Avoid indentations from tips of fingers.	1. Finger indentation on a fresh cast can produce pressure sores.
2. Expose the cast to warm, circulating, dry air. Or blow air over cast with a circulating fan to increase the evaporation of water.	2. Avoid covering the cast when it is drying, as this delays drying time. Usually the plaster cast will reach its maximum temperature 5–15 minutes after it is applied and will then cool rapidly. The ultimate plaster cast strength is obtained after the cast is dry (up to 48 hours, depending on outside temperature and humidity). The synthetic cast strength is maximum within 30 minutes of application and not dependent on being dry.
3. Clean equipment and store ready for use.	

PROCEDURE GUIDELINES 29-2 ♦ Removal of a Cast

EQUIPMENT
Cast cutter—an electric saw with circular blade that oscillates and is connected to a vacuum collector
Cast spreader
Plaster knife
Scissors
Felt-tip pen

PROCEDURE	**NURSING ACTION**	**RATIONALE**

PREPARATORY PHASE

NURSING ACTION	RATIONALE
1. Describe to the patient how and where the cast cutter will be used and the expected sensations.	1. Reassures the patient that the cutter produces vibrations but not pain.
2. Determine whether or not the cast is padded.	2. An electric plaster cast cutter should not be used on unpadded casts.
3. Determine where the cut will be made. Mark, with a felt pen, the area to be cut.	3. The line should be in front of the lateral malleolus and behind the medial malleolus on a lower extremity cast. An upper extremity cast is usually split along the ulnar or flexor surface.

PROCEDURE (cont'd)	NURSING ACTION	RATIONALE

PERFORMANCE PHASE

1. Inform the patient to shield eyes.
2. Grasp the electric cutter as illustrated.
3. Rest the thumb on the cast.

4. Turn on the electric cutter. Push the blade firmly and gently through the cast while holding the thumb against the cast to steady the blade while cutting through the cast.
5. As the blade cuts through the plaster, a sudden lack of resistance is felt; plaster will "give" (or "dip") when the cut is completed.
6. Lift the cutting blade up a degree (but not out of the cutting groove) and advance the blade at a slightly higher or lower level. The cast is cut by a series of alternating pressure and linear movements along the line of the cut (see accompanying figure).

1. Plaster dust may be irritating to the eyes.

3. The thumb serves as a depth gauge and acts as a guard in front of the blade.

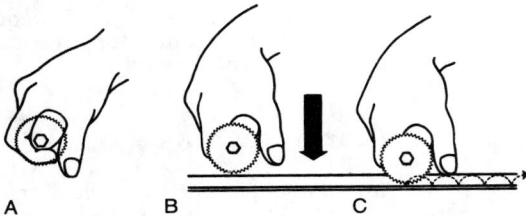

A   B   C

Operating a cast cutter. (Photo courtesy Stryker Corporation)

7. Avoid drawing the cutting blade along the extremity in a single motion.

8. Cut the cast on both sides. Then rock the anterior portion of the cast over the posterior portion.
9. Insert the blades of the cast spreader in the cut trough. Separate the 2 halves with the spreader at several sites along the cast split. Separate the cast with the hands.
10. Cut through the padding and stockinette with scissors, keeping the scissor blade that is closest to the skin parallel to the skin.
11. Lift the extremity carefully out of the posterior portion of the cast. Support the extremity so that it is maintained in the same position as when in the cast.

7. This will cut the skin. If saw blade is in contact with padding too long, the patient will feel burning sensation on skin from rapidly oscillating blade.
8. This maneuver allows the operator to determine if the cast is completely cut.

10. Use bandage scissors; place the flat blade closest to the skin.

11. When the support of the cast has been removed, stresses and strain are placed on parts that have been at rest.

AFTER REMOVAL OF CAST

1. Cleanse the skin gently with mild soap and water. Blot dry. Apply a skin cream.

2. Emphasize the importance of continuing the prescribed exercises, reporting for physical therapy, etc.

1. Explain to the patient that the skin will be scaly and the extremity will appear "thin" from disuse. Reassure him or her that it will take a few weeks to regain normal appearance and function.
2. Exercises are necessary to redevelop and increase strength and function. Pain and stiffness may be expected after cast removal.

◆ TRACTION

Traction is force applied in a specific direction. To apply the force needed to overcome the natural force or pull of muscle groups, a system of ropes, pulleys, and weights is used. See Procedure Guidelines 29-3: Application of Buck's Extension Traction.

Purposes of Traction

1. To reduce and immobilize fracture.
2. To regain normal length and alignment of an injured extremity
3. To lessen or eliminate muscle spasm.
4. To prevent deformity.
5. To give the patient freedom for "in-bed" activities.
6. To reduce pain.

Types of Traction

A. Running Traction
1. A form of traction in which the pull is exerted in one plane.
2. May use either skin or skeletal traction.
3. Buck's extension traction (Fig. 29-6) is an example of running skin traction.

B. Balanced Suspension Traction
1. Uses additional weights to counterbalance the traction force and floats the extremity in the traction apparatus.
2. The line of pull on the extremity remains fairly constant despite changes in the patient's position

Application of Traction

Traction may be applied to the skin or to the skeletal system.

A. Skin Traction
1. Accomplished by applying a light force that pulls on tape, sponge rubber, or special device (boot, cervical halter, pelvic belt) that is in contact with the skin.
2. The pulling force is transmitted to the musculoskeletal structures.
3. Skin traction is used as a temporary measure in adults to control muscle spasm and pain.
4. It is used before surgery in the treatment of hip fracture (Buck's extension), and femoral shaft fractures (Russell's traction).
5. Pelvic and cervical traction are used for treatment of back disorders or injuries. Skin traction may be used definitively to treat fractures in children.

B. Skeletal Traction (Figs. 29-7 and 29-8).
1. Traction applied by the orthopedic surgeon under aseptic conditions using wires, pins, or tongs placed through bones.
2. Skeletal traction is used most frequently in treating fractures of the femur, humerus (supracondylar fractures), tibia, and cervical spine.

Complications

1. Infection of pin tracts in skeletal traction
2. Skin breakdown and dermatitis under skin traction
3. Complications of immobility
   a. Stasis pneumonia
   b. Thrombophlebitis
   c. Pressure ulcers

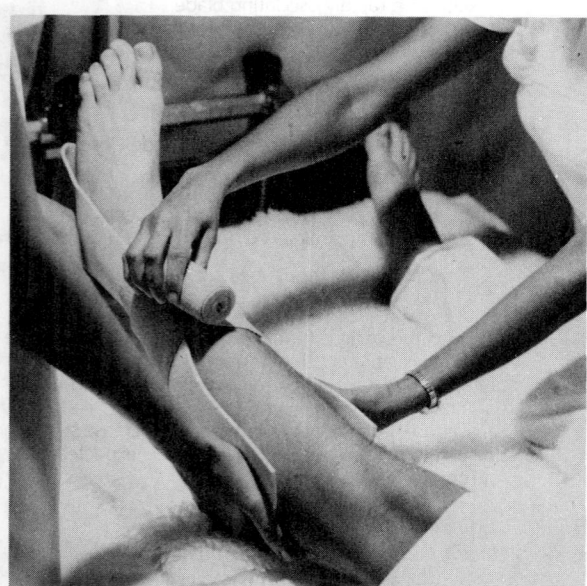
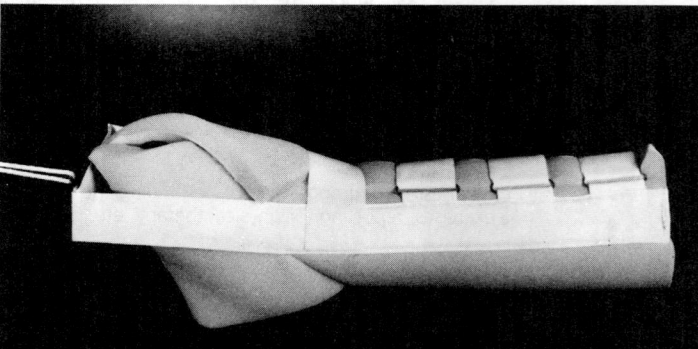

FIGURE 29-6 (Left) *Applying elastic bandage for Buck's extension traction.* (Right) *Prepadded boot that may be used in Buck's extension. (Photo of boot courtesy of All Orthopedic Appliances)*

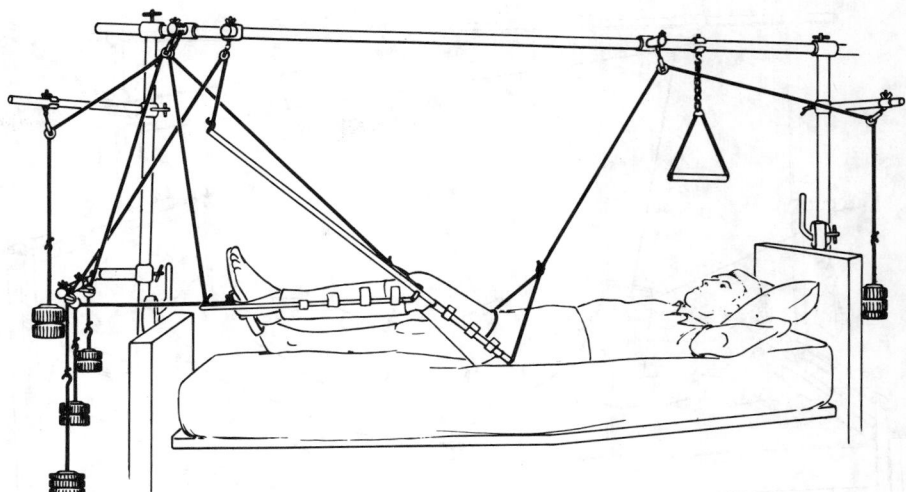

FIGURE 29-7 *Balanced skeletal traction using Thomas leg splint and Pearson attachment.*

d. Urinary infection and calculi
e. Constipation

◆ NURSING PROCESS OVERVIEW: THE PATIENT IN TRACTION

Nursing Assessment

1. Assess for pain, deformity, swelling, motor and sensory function, and circulatory status of the affected extremity.
2. Assess skin condition of the affected extremity, both under skin traction and around skeletal traction, as well as over body prominences throughout the body.
3. Assess for signs and symptoms of complications.
4. Assess traction equipment for safety and effectiveness
   a. The patient is placed on a firm mattress.
   b. The ropes and the pulleys should be in alignment.
   c. The pull should be in line with the long axis of the bone.
   d. Any factor that might reduce the pull or alter its direction must be eliminated.
      (1) Weights should hang freely.
      (2) Ropes should be unobstructed and not in contact with the bed or equipment.
      (3) Help the patient to pull himself or herself up in bed at frequent intervals.

> **NURSING ALERT:**
> Traction is *not* accomplished if the knot in the rope or the footplate is touching the pulley or the foot of the bed or if the weights are resting on the floor. Never remove the weights when repositioning the patient who is in skeletal traction, because this will interrupt the line of pull.

   e. The amount of weight applied in skin traction must not exceed the tolerance of the skin. The condition of the skin must be inspected frequently.

f. Cover exposed sharp ends of skeletal pins with cork or other pin covering to protect patient and caregivers from injury.
5. Assess emotional reaction to condition and traction as well as understanding of the treatment plan.

Nursing Diagnoses

A. Impaired Physical Mobility related to traction therapy and underlying pathology
B. Risk for Impaired Skin Integrity related to pressure on soft tissues
C. Risk for Infection related to bacterial invasion at skeletal traction site
D. Altered Peripheral Tissue Perfusion related to injury or traction therapy

Nursing Interventions

A. *Minimizing the Effects of Immobility*
1. Encourage active exercise of uninvolved muscles and joints to maintain strength and function. Dorsiflex feet hourly to avoid development of footdrop and aid in venous return.
2. Encourage deep breathing hourly to facilitate expansion of lungs and movement of respiratory secretions.
3. Auscultate lung fields twice a day.
4. Encourage fluid intake of 2,000 to 2,500 mL daily.
5. Provide balanced high-fiber diet rich in protein; avoid excessive calcium intake.
6. Establish bowel routine through use of diet and/or stool softeners, laxatives, and enemas, as prescribed.
7. Prevent pressure on the calf and evaluate periodically for the development of thrombophlebitis.
8. Check traction apparatus at repeated intervals—the traction must be continuous to be effective, unless prescribed as intermittent, as with pelvic traction.
   a. *With running traction,* the patient may not be turned without disrupting the line of pull.

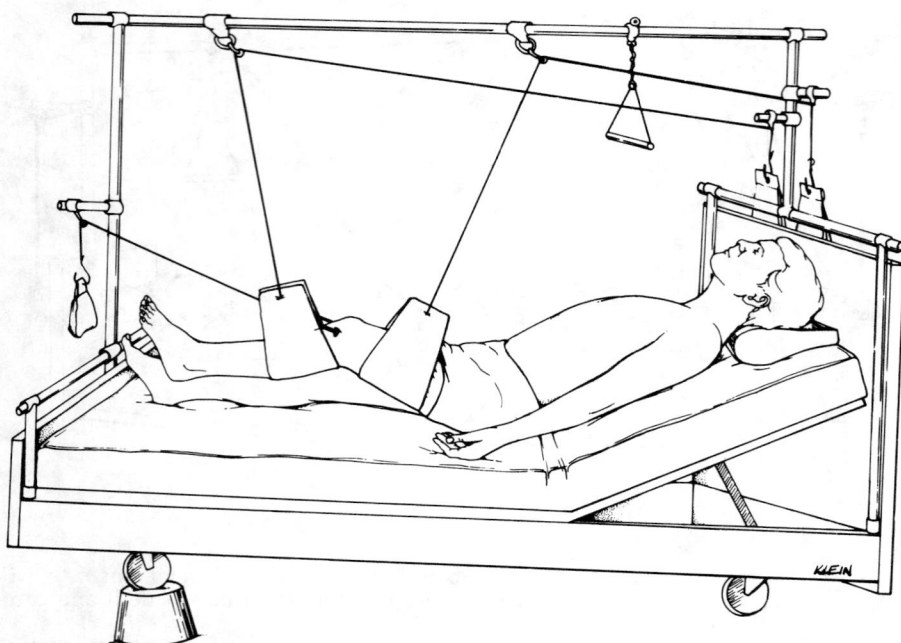

FIGURE 29-8 *Balanced skeletal traction using slings for support and suspension.*

b. *With balanced suspension traction,* the patient may be elevated, turned slightly, and moved as desired.

> **NURSING ALERT:** ❖
> Every complaint of the patient in traction should be investigated immediately.

B. *Maintaining Skin Integrity*
1. Examine bony prominences frequently for evidence of pressure or friction irritation.
2. Observe for skin irritation around the traction bandage.
3. Observe for pressure at traction–skin contact points.
4. Report complaint of burning sensation under traction.
5. Relieve pressure without disrupting traction effectiveness.
    a. Ensure that linens and clothing are wrinkle-free.
    b. Use lambs wool pads, heel/elbow protectors, and special mattresses as needed.
6. Special care must be given to the back at regular intervals, because the patient maintains a supine position.
    a. Have patient use trapeze to pull self up and relieve back pressure.
    b. Provide backrubs.

C. *Avoiding Infection at Pin Site*
1. Monitor vital signs for fever or tachycardia.
2. Watch for signs of infection, especially around the pin tract.
    a. The pin should be immobile in the bone and the skin wound should be dry. Small amount of serous oozing from pin site may occur.
    b. If infection is suspected, percuss gently over the tibia; this may elicit pain if infection is developing.

c. Assess for other signs of infection: heat, redness, fever.
3. If directed, clean the pin tract with sterile applicators and prescribed solution/ointment—to clear drainage at the entrance of tract and around the pin, because plugging at this site can predispose to bacterial invasion of the tract and bone.

D. *Promoting Tissue Perfusion*
1. Assess motor and sensory function of specific nerves that might be compromised.
    a. Peroneal nerve—Have patient point great toe toward nose; check sensation on dorsum of foot; presence of footdrop.
    b. Radial nerve—Have patient extend thumb; check sensation in web between thumb and index finger.
    c. Median nerve—Thumb–middle finger apposition; check sensation of index finger.
2. Determine adequacy of circulation (eg, color, temperature, motion, capillary refill of peripheral fingers or toes).
    a. With Buck's traction, inspect the foot for circulatory difficulties within a few minutes and then periodically after the elastic bandage has been applied.
3. Report promptly if change in neurovascular status is identified.

Patient Education/Health Maintenance

1. Teach the patient the purpose of traction therapy.
2. Delineate limitations of activity necessary to maintain effective traction.

3. Teach use of patient aids (eg, trapeze).
4. Instruct the patient not to adjust or modify traction apparatus.
5. Instruct the patient in activities designed to minimize effects of immobility on body systems.
6. Teach the patient necessity for reporting changes in sensations, pain, movement, etc.

Evaluation

A. Exercising as instructed; deep breathing hourly; fluid intake 1,800 mL/24 hours; Homans' sign negative
B. No signs of skin breakdown under traction bandage or over body prominences
C. No drainage, redness, or odor at pin site
D. No motor or sensory impairment; good capillary refill, color, and warmth of extremity

◆ EXTERNAL FIXATION

External fixation is a technique of fracture immobilization in which a series of transfixing pins is inserted through bone and attached to a rigid external metal frame (Fig. 29-9). The method is used mainly in the management of open fractures with severe soft tissue damage.

Advantages

1. Permits rigid support of severely comminuted open fractures, infected nonunions, and infected unstable joints.
2. Facilitates wound care (frequent debridements, irrigations, dressing changes) and soft tissue reconstruction (delayed wound closure, muscle flaps, skin grafts).
3. Allows early function of muscles and joints.
4. Allows early patient comfort.

Ilizarov External Fixator

A. ***Purpose*** May be used for limb lengthening, correction of angulation and rotation defects, and in treatment of nonunion

B. ***Components***
1. This fixator apparatus consists of through-the-bone tension wires placed above and below the treatment site.
2. The wires are attached to fixator rings surrounding the limb.
3. The rings are connected to one another by telescoping rods.

C. ***Management***
1. Adjustments are made daily at about 1 mm per day, stimulating callus and bone formation.
2. Patient compliance is essential.
3. Weight bearing is encouraged.
4. When the desired length or correction is achieved, the fixator is left in place without further adjustment until bone healing occurs.

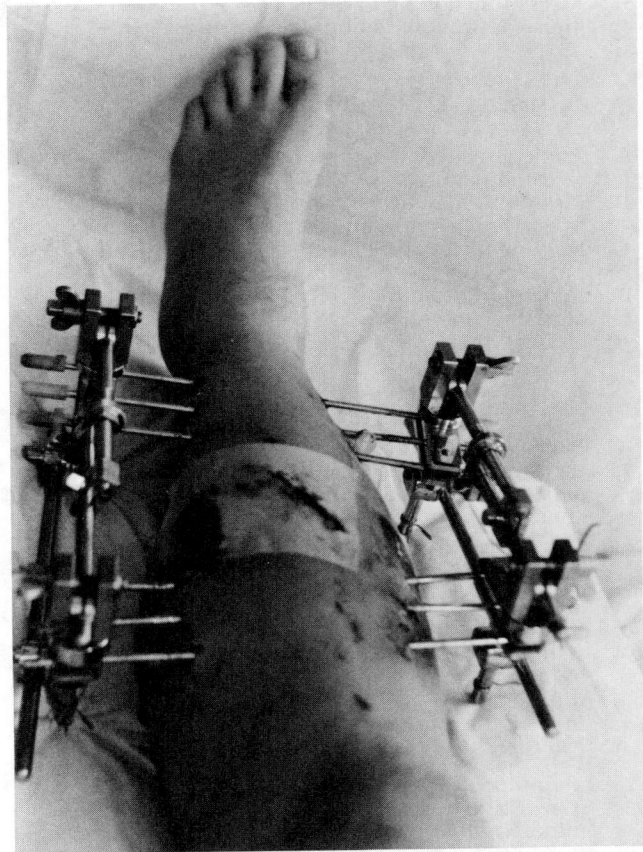

FIGURE 29-9 *External fixation device used for reduction and immobilization of open fracture, allowing treatment of soft tissue wounds. (From Smeltzer S and Bare B. Textbook of Medical-Surgical Nursing, 8th ed. Philadelphia: J. B. Lippincott, 1996.)*

Application of External Fixator

1. Under general anesthesia, the skin is cleansed and transfixing pins are inserted into the bone through small incisions above and below the fracture.
2. After reduction of the fracture, the appliance is stabilized by adjusting and tightening the bars connecting the sets of pins.
3. The sharp pin heads are covered with plastic, cork, or rubber covers to protect the other extremity and caregivers.

Nursing Assessment

1. Determine the patient's understanding of procedure and fixation device.
2. Evaluate neurovascular status of involved body part.
3. Inspect each pin site for redness, drainage, tenderness, pain, and loosening of the pin.
4. Inspect open wounds for healing, infection, or devitalized tissue.

5. Assess functioning of other body systems affected by injury or immobilization.

Nursing Diagnoses

A. Anxiety related to appearance of external fixation device and wound
B. Risk for Peripheral Neurovascular Dysfunction related to swelling, fixator, and underlying condition
C. Risk for Infection related to open injury and skeletal pin insertion
D. Impaired Physical Mobility related to presence of fixator and condition

Nursing Interventions

A. *Relieving Anxiety*
1. If possible, before placement of the device, reassure the patient that although the fixator appears clumsy and cumbersome, it should not hurt once it is in place.
2. Emphasize the positive aspects of this device in treating complex musculoskeletal problems.
3. Encourage the patient to verbalize reaction to the device.
4. Inform the patient that greater mobility can be achieved with an external fixation device, thereby minimizing the development of other system problems.
5. Involve the patient in care and in the management of external fixator.

B. *Maintaining Intact Neurovascular Status*
1. Assess neurovascular status frequently: every 15 to 60 minutes while swelling is significant and later every 2 to 8 hours.
2. Establish baseline of functioning for comparative monitoring. Complex musculoskeletal injuries frequently result in disruption of soft tissue functioning.

> **NURSING ALERT:**
> Assess neurovascular status frequently and *record findings.*

3. Elevate extremity to reduce swelling.
   a. Extremity can be suspended by hanging the fixator directly on the traction frame.
   b. Suspension is for control of edema and not for application of traction force.
4. Report any change in neurovascular status.

C. *Avoiding Infection*
1. Provide site and fixator care:
   a. Cleanse pin sites and remove crusts with sterile cotton applicator, using solution and/or ointment, as prescribed, or established standard of care.
      (1) Crusts formed by serous drainage can prevent fluid from draining and cause infection.
      (2) A small amount of serous drainage from the pin sites is normal.

   b. Note and report inflammation, swelling, tenderness, and purulent drainage at pin site.
   c. Note skin tension at pin site—tension can cause discomfort.
   d. Report loosened pins.
   e. Cleanse fixator with clean cloth and water as needed.
2. Wound care:
   a. The open wounds at the fracture site are usually treated by daily dressing changes.
   b. Use sterile technique.
   c. Note wound appearance. Monitor healing. Report signs of infection.
3. Monitor for local and systemic indicators of infection.

D. *Encourage Mobility*
1. Encourage the patient to participate in care activities.
2. Assure the patient that pain associated with injury will diminish as tissue reactions to injury and manipulation resolve and healing progresses.
3. Inform the patient that the external fixator maintains the fracture in a very stable position and that the extremity can be moved. Adjustment of the fixator is done by the health care provider. (Patient is taught how to adjust the Ilizarov fixator.)
4. To move the extremity, grasp the frame and assist the patient to move. Reassure the patient that the fixator can withstand normal movement.
5. Teach quadriceps exercises and range-of-motion exercises for joints: usually started on first postoperative day.
6. Teach crutch walking when soft tissue swelling has diminished; encourage weight bearing as prescribed.

Patient Education/Health Maintenance

1. Instruct to inspect around each pin site daily for signs of infection and loosening of pins. Watch for pain, soft tissue swelling, and drainage.
2. Teach how to cleanse around each pin daily, using aseptic technique. *Do not touch wound with hands.*
3. Advise to clean fixator regularly—to keep it free of dust and contamination.
4. Warn against *tampering with clamps or nuts*—can alter compression and misalign fracture.
5. Review weight bearing and other restrictions associated with injury and treatment regimen.
6. Encourage the patient to follow rehabilitation regimen.

Evaluation

A. Verbalizes understanding of and comfort with fixator device
B. Swelling relieved; neurovascular status intact
C. No drainage or signs of infection at pin sites
D. Ambulating with crutches as directed

PROCEDURE GUIDELINES 29-3 ◆ Application of Buck's Extension Traction

Buck's extension skin traction is used as a temporary measure to provide immobility, support, and comfort until definitive treatment is accomplished.

EQUIPMENT Foam Buck's traction boot or traction tape and 10-cm (4-in.) elastic bandage
Spreader block or metal spreader
Pulley, nylon rope, and weights (2.3–3.1 kg [5–7 lb] is usual (amount of weight is prescribed by physician)
Sheepskin pad
Shock blocks or adjustable bed for Trendelenburg's position

PROCEDURE

NURSING ACTION	RATIONALE
PREPARATORY PHASE	
1. Place bedboard under the mattress. Bed position is flat or in Trendelenburg's position. This depends on the size of the patient and the weight applied.	1. Elevating the foot of the bed (countertraction) helps prevent the patient from sliding down toward the foot of the bed.
2. Question the patient to determine previous skin conditions (contact dermatitis). Inspect skin for evidences of atrophy, abrasions, and circulatory disturbances.	2. The skin must be in healthy condition to tolerate skin traction.
3. Make sure that the skin of the extremity is clean and dry.	3. Clean, dry skin helps traction tape adherence.
4. Document the neurovascular status of the extremity, any evidence of skin problems or varicosities.	
PERFORMANCE PHASE	
1. Position the patient in center of bed in good alignment.	1. For effective line of pull.
IF TRACTION TAPE IS USED:	
2. Apply continuous traction tape to medial and lateral aspects of lower leg (below knee and loosely around foot to allow for attachment of spreader).	2. Avoid pressure over malleoli and head of fibula. Pressure sores develop rapidly over bony prominences. Pressure over the region of the fibular head and common peroneal nerve may produce peroneal palsy and footdrop.
3. Have a second person elevate and support the extremity under the ankle and knee while the elastic bandage is applied. Beginning at the ankle, wrap the elastic bandage snugly over the tape up to the tibial tubercle.	3. The elastic bandage holds tape to the skin and helps prevent slipping.
4. Attach a spreader block (or metal spreader) to the distal end of the tape. Attach a rope to the spreader block and pass it over a pulley fastened to the end of the bed and gently apply weights.	4. The spreader block prevents pressure along the side of the foot. The spreader should not be too narrow (causes pressure sores on ankle) or too wide (pulls traction tape away from the heel).
5. Place a sheepskin pad under the leg (or use a commercial heel protector).	5. Sheepskin is used to reduce friction of the heel against the bed.
IF FOAM BOOT IS USED:	
1. Apply antiembolitic stockings if prescribed.	1. Prophylactic measure in high-risk population.
2. Place leg in foam boot, adjusting it so that the heel is in the heel of the boot.	2. Preventing sore heels is a primary concern.
3. Secure Velcro bootstraps, avoiding excessive pressure on malleoli and fibular head.	3. Pressure over bony prominences causes skin breakdown, and pressure on peroneal nerve may result in footdrop.
4. Attach rope to built-in spreader plate, pass it over pulley, and apply weights gently.	4. The rope should move unobstructed and the weights should hang free of the bed and not touch the floor.

◆ ORTHOPEDIC SURGERY

Types of Surgery

1. Open reduction—reduction and alignment of the fracture through surgical incision.
2. Internal fixation—stabilization of the reduced fracture with use of metal screw, plates, nails, or pins.
3. Bone graft—placement of autologous or homologous bone tissue to replace, promote healing of, or stabilize diseased bone.
4. Arthroplasty—repair of a joint; may be done through arthoscope (arthoscopy) or open joint repair.
5. Joint replacement—type of arthroplasty that involves replacement of joint surface(s) with metal or plastic materials.
6. Total joint replacement—replacement of both articular surfaces within a joint.
7. Meniscectomy—excision of damaged meniscus (fibrocartilage) of the knee.
8. Tendon transfer—movement of tendon insertion point to improve function.

9. Fasciotomy—cutting muscle fascia to relieve constriction or contracture.
10. Amputation—removal of a body part.
    Note: Joint replacement and amputation will be covered separately.

Preoperative Management/ Nursing Care

1. Assess nutritional status: hydration, protein, and caloric intake. Maximize healing and reduce risk of complications by providing intravenous fluids, vitamins, and nutritional supplements as indicated.

GERONTOLOGIC ALERT:
Many elderly are at risk for poor healing due to undernutrition.

2. Determine if person has had previous corticosteroid therapy—could contribute to current orthopedic condition (aseptic necrosis of the femoral head, osteoporosis) as well as affect the patient's response to anesthesia and the stress of surgery. May need corticotropin postoperatively.
3. Determine if the person has an infection (cold, dental, skin, urinary tract infection)—could contribute to development of osteomyelitis after surgery. Administer preoperative antibiotics as ordered.
4. Prepare patient for postoperative routines: coughing and deep breathing, frequent vital sign and wound checks, repositioning.
5. Have the patient practice voiding in bedpan or urinal in recumbent position before surgery. This helps reduce the need for postoperative catheterization.
6. Acquaint the patient with traction apparatus and the need for splint or cast, as indicated by type of surgery.

Postoperative Management/ Nursing Care

1. Monitor neurovascular status and try to relieve swelling caused by edema and bleeding into tissues.
2. Immobilize the affected area and limit activity to protect the operative site and stabilize musculoskeletal structures.
3. Monitor for hemorrhage and shock, which may result from significant bleeding and poor hemostasis of muscles that occurs with orthopedic surgery.
4. Take measures to prevent complications of immobility through aggressive and vigilant postoperative care

Complications

1. Compartment syndrome
2. Shock
3. Atelectasis and pneumonia
4. Osteomyelitis, wound infections
5. Thromboembolism
6. Fat embolus

Nursing Diagnoses

A. Risk for Fluid Volume Deficit related to hemorrhage
B. Ineffective Breathing Pattern related to effects of anesthesia, analgesics, and immobility
C. Risk for Peripheral Neurovascular Dysfunction related to swelling
D. Pain related to surgical intervention
E. Risk for Infection related to surgical intervention
F. Impaired Physical Mobility related to immobilization therapy and pain

Nursing Interventions

A. *Monitoring for Shock and Hemorrhage*
1. Evaluate the blood pressure and pulse rates frequently—rising pulse rate or slowly falling blood pressure indicates persistent bleeding or development of a state of shock.
2. Monitor for hemorrhage—orthopedic wounds have a tendency to ooze more than other surgical wounds
   a. Measure suction drainage if used.
   b. Anticipate up to 500 mL of drainage in the first 24 hours, decreasing to less than 30 mL per 8 hours within 48 hours, depending on surgical procedure.
   c. Report increased wound drainage or steady increase in pain of operative area.
3. Administer intravenous fluids and/or blood products as ordered.

B. *Promoting Effective Breathing Pattern*
1. Avoid or give respiratory depressant drugs in minimal doses. Monitor respiration depth and rate frequently. Narcotic analgesic effects may be cumulative.
2. Change position every 2 hours—mobilizes secretions and helps prevent bronchial obstruction.
3. Encourage use of incentive spirometer and coughing and deep-breathing exercises every 2 hours.
4. Auscultate lungs for atelectasis and retention of secretions.

C. *Monitoring Peripheral Neurovascular Status*
1. Watch circulation distal to the part where cast, bandage, or splint has been applied.
2. Prevent constriction leading to interference with blood or nerve supply.
3. Elevate affected extremity and apply ice packs as directed to reduce swelling and bleeding into tissues.
4. Observe toes and fingers for healthy color and good capillary refill.
5. Check pulses of affected extremity; compare with unaffected extremity.
6. Note skin temperature.
7. Document observations.

NURSING ALERT:
If neurovascular problems are identified, notify surgeon and loosen cast or dressing at once.

D. *Relieving Pain*
1. Institute pain relief measures as prescribed.
2. Be aware that muscle spasms may contribute to pain experience.
3. Administer prescribed parenteral medications to control pain during the first few postoperative days.

a. Avoid injection sites near operative site.
b. Swelling and edema in operative area reduce absorption.
c. Rotate injection sites.
4. Use patient-controlled analgesia according to standards of care.

E. Preventing Infection
1. Monitor vital signs for fever, tachycardia, or increased respiratory rate, which may indicate infection.
2. Examine incision for redness, increased temperature, swelling, and induration.
3. Note character of drainage.
4. Evaluate complaints of recurrent or increasing pain.
5. Administer antibiotic therapy as prescribed.
6. Maintain aseptic technique for dressing changes and wound care.

F. Minimizing the Effects of Immobility
1. Encourage the patient to exercise by self with a planned program of exercise as soon as possible after surgery.
2. Have the patient flex knee, extend the knee with hip still flexed, and then lower the extremity to the bed.
3. Encourage the patient to move fingers and toes periodically.
4. Advise the patient to move joints that are not fixed by traction or appliance through their range of motion as fully as possible.
5. Suggest muscle-setting exercises (quadriceps setting) if active motion is contraindicated.
6. Apply antiembolism stockings as prescribed.
7. Give prophylactic anticoagulants as directed (eg, heparin, warfarin, aspirin).
8. Encourage early resumption of activity.

G. Providing Additional Nursing Care
1. Watch for signs and symptoms of anemia—especially after fracture of long bones:
a. Fatigue
b. Shortness of breath
c. Pallor
2. Monitor hemoglobin and hematocrit levels. Report below-normal results to health care provider.
3. Encourage high-iron diet and administer blood products and iron supplements as directed.
4. Provide a balanced diet and increase fluids and fiber to reduce incidence of constipation associated with immobility.
5. Avoid giving large amounts of milk to orthopedic patients on bed rest—adds to calcium pool in the body and demands more calcium excretion by the kidneys, predisposing to the formation of urinary calculi.
6. Maintain urinary output and prevent infection and calculi by increased fluid intake.
7. Watch for urinary retention—elderly men with some degree of prostatism may have difficulty in voiding.

Patient Education/Health Maintenance

1. Teach the patient activities that will minimize the development of complications (eg, turning, coughing, and deep breathing).
2. Instruct the patient in dietary considerations to facilitate healing and minimize development of constipation and renal calculi.

3. Inform the patient of techniques that facilitate moving while minimizing associated discomforts (eg, supporting injured area and practicing smooth, gentle position changes).
4. Encourage long-term follow-up and physical therapy exercises as prescribed to regain maximum functional potential.

Evaluation

A. Blood pressure stable; drainage from wound less than 30 mL
B. Respirations 22, deep; performing effective deep breathing and coughing every 2 hours
C. Extremity beyond operative site neurovascularly intact
D. Verbalizes decreased pain
E. Afebrile; incision without drainage
F. Ambulating as directed

◆ ARTHROPLASTY AND TOTAL JOINT REPLACEMENT

Arthroplasty is reconstructive surgery to restore joint motion and function and to relieve pain. It generally involves replacement of bony joint structure by a prosthesis.
Total joint arthroplasty is the replacement of both articular surfaces with metal or plastic components. The most common types of joint replacement (Fig. 29-10) include:
Total hip replacement (total joint arthroplasty)—the replacement of a severely damaged hip with an artificial joint. Although a large number of implants are available, most consist of a metal femoral component topped by a spherical ball fitted into a plastic acetabular socket.
A *total knee arthroplasty* is an implant procedure in which tibial, femoral, and patellar joint surfaces are replaced because of destroyed knee joint.

Clinical Indications

1. For patients with unremitting pain and irreversibly damaged joints:
a. Primary degenerative arthritis (osteoarthritis)
b. Rheumatoid arthritis
2. Selected fractures (eg, femoral neck fracture)
3. Failure of previous reconstructive surgery (osteotomy, cup arthroplasty, femoral neck fracture complications—nonunion, avascular necrosis)
4. Congenital hip disease
5. Pathologic fractures from metastatic cancer
6. Joint instability

Considerations

1. The prostheses are of various designs and may be fixed to the remaining bone by cement, press fit, or bone ingrowth.
2. Selection of the prosthesis and fixation technique depends on individual patient's bone structure, joint stability, and other individual characteristics, including age, weight, and activity level.

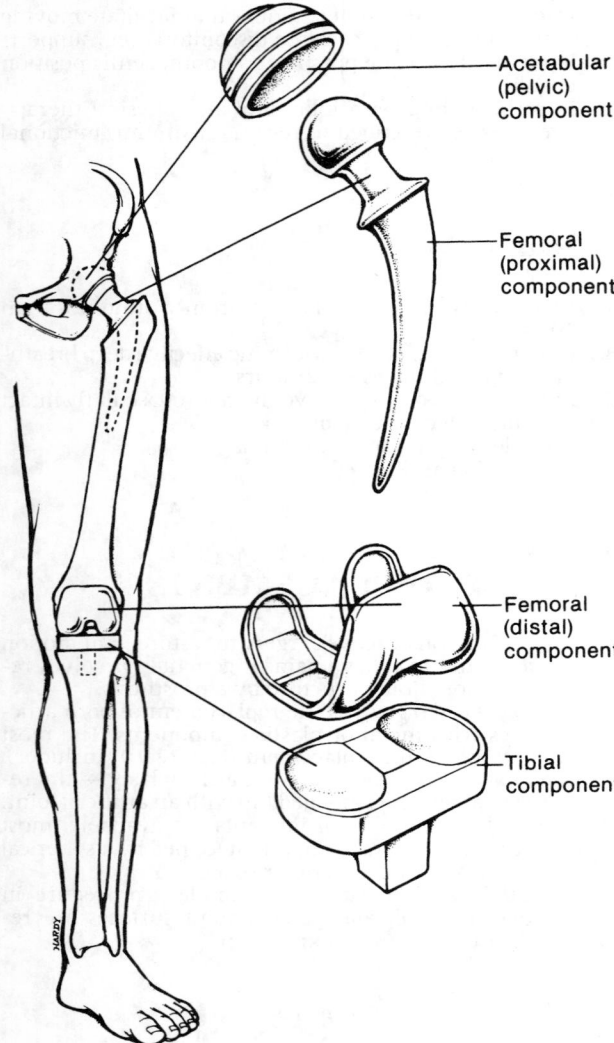

- Acetabular (pelvic) component
- Femoral (proximal) component
- Femoral (distal) component
- Tibial component

FIGURE 29-10 *Hip and knee replacement.*

3. Arthroplasty is an exacting and meticulous procedure. To reduce the risk of an infected prosthesis, special precautions are carried out in the operating room (impermeable operating room attire, clean air system) to reduce particulate matter and bacterial count of the air.

Preoperative Management/Nursing Care

1. Assess patient for infections (bladder, dental, skin)—potential foci of infection for seeding prosthesis infection.
2. Provide preoperative patient teaching.
   a. Educate the patient concerning postoperative regimen (eg, extended exercise program will be carried out after surgery—atrophied muscles must be reeducated and strengthened).
   b. Teach isometric exercises (muscle setting) of quadriceps and gluteal muscles; teach active ankle motion.
   c. Teach bed-to-wheelchair transfer without going beyond the hip flexion limits (usually 45 degrees).
   d. Practice nonweight- and partial weight-bearing ambulation with ambulatory aid (walker, crutches) to facilitate postoperative ambulation.
   e. Demonstrate abduction splint, knee immobilizer, or continuous passive motion if equipment will be used postoperatively.
3. Use antiembolism stockings to minimize development of thrombophlebitis.
4. Give meticulous skin preparation with antimicrobial solution to reduce skin microorganisms, a potential source of infection.
5. Administer antibiotics as prescribed to ensure therapeutic blood level during and immediately after surgery. Antimicrobials usually are given immediately preoperatively, intraoperatively, and postoperatively to reduce incidence of infection.
6. Thoroughly assess cardiovascular, respiratory, renal, and hepatic function and institute measures to maximize general health condition.

Postoperative Management/ Nursing Care

A. Use of Appropriate Positioning To prevent dislocation of prosthesis and facilitate healing
Note: Numerous modifications are required in positioning these patients postoperatively.
1. After hip arthroplasty:
   a. The patient is usually positioned supine in bed.
   b. The affected extremity is held in slight abduction by either an abduction splint or pillow or Buck's extension traction to prevent dislocation of the prosthesis.
   c. Avoid acute flexion of the hip.

> **NURSING ALERT:**
> The patient must not adduct or flex operated hip—may produce dislocation. Signs of joint dislocation include shortened extremity, increasing discomfort, inability to move joints.

   d. Two nurses turn the patient on unoperated side while supporting operated hip securely in an abducted position; the entire length of leg is supported by pillows.
      (1) Use pillows to keep the leg abducted; place pillow at back for comfort.
      (2) Use overhead trapeze to assist with position changes.
   e. The bed is usually not elevated more than 45 degrees; placing the patient in an upright sitting position puts a strain on the hip joint and may cause dislocation.
   f. A fracture bedpan is used. Instruct the patient to flex the unoperated hip and knee and pull up on the trapeze to lift buttocks onto pan. Instruct the patient *NOT* to bear down on the operated hip in flexion when getting off the pan.
2. After knee arthroplasty:
   a. The knee may be immobilized in extension with a firm compression dressing and an adjustable soft extension splint or long-leg plaster cast.

b. Leg is elevated on pillows to control swelling.
c. Alternatively, continuous passive motion may be started to facilitate joint healing and restoration of joint range of motion.

B. Deterring Complications
1. Provide aggressive care and continuous assessment
2. Prevent thromboembolism by continuous use of sequential compression devices while patient is in bed. Discontinue when patient is ambulatory.

C. Promoting Early Ambulation
1. Within 2 days after surgery, short periods of standing may be ordered.
   a. Monitor for orthostatic hypotension.
   b. Weight bearing may be limited with ingrowth prosthesis to prevent disruption of bone growth.
2. Transfers to the chair or ambulation with aids, such as walkers, are encouraged as tolerated and based on patient's condition and type of prosthesis.

Nursing Diagnosis

Also see Orthopedic Surgery, p. 858.

A. Impaired Physical Mobility related to prosthetic joint

Nursing Interventions

See also p. 858.

A. Promoting Mobility
After hip arthroplasty:
1. Use an abduction splint or pillows while assisting the patient to get out of bed.
   a. Keep the hip at maximum extension.
   b. Instruct the patient to pivot on unoperated extremity.
   c. Assess the patient for orthostatic hypotension.
2. When the patient is ready to ambulate, teach him or her to advance the walker and then advance the operated extremity to the walker, permitting weight bearing as prescribed.
3. With increased stability, assist patient to use crutches or cane as prescribed.
4. Encourage practice of physical therapy exercises to strengthen muscles and prevent contractures.
After knee arthroplasty:
1. Assist patient with transfer out of bed into wheelchair with extension splint in place.
2. Ensure that no weight bearing is permitted until prescribed by the orthopedic surgeon.
3. Apply continuous passive motion equipment or carry out passive range-of-motion exercises as prescribed.

Patient Education/Health Maintenance

Instruct the patient as follows:

1. Continue to wear elastic stockings after going home until full activities are resumed.
2. Avoid excessive hip adduction, flexion, and rotation after hip arthroplasty.
   a. Avoid sitting in low chair/toilet seat.
   b. Keep knees apart; do *not* cross legs.
   c. Limit sitting to 30 minutes at a time—to minimize hip flexion and the risk of prosthetic dislocation and to prevent hip stiffness and flexion contracture.
3. Continue quadriceps setting and range-of-motion exercises as directed.
   a. Have a *daily* program of stretching, exercise, and rest throughout lifetime.
   b. Do not participate in any activity placing undue or sudden stress on joint (jogging, jumping, lifting heavy loads, becoming obese, excessive bending and twisting).
   c. Use a cane when taking fairly long walks.
4. Use self-help and energy-saving devices:
   a. Handrails by toilet
   b. Raised toilet seat if there is some residual hip flexion problem
   c. Bar-type stool for shower and kitchen work
5. Lie prone twice daily for 30 minutes.
6. Report for follow-up evaluation and testing.
7. Monitor for late complications—deep infection, increased pain and/or decreased function associated with loosening of prosthetic components, implant wear, dislocation, fracture of components, avascular necrosis or dead bone caused by loss of blood supply, heterotrophic ossification (formation of bone in periprosthetic space).
8. Use supportive equipment (crutches, canes, raised toilet seat) as prescribed.
9. Take prophylactic antibiotic if undergoing any procedure known to cause bacteremia (tooth extraction, manipulation of genitourinary tract).
10. Avoid MRI studies because of implanted metal component.

Evaluation

A. Maintaining proper positioning without evidence of complications

◆ AMPUTATION

Amputation is the total or partial surgical removal of an extremity. Amputation is considered a surgical reconstructive procedure.

Indications

1. Inadequate tissue perfusion, such as results with diabetes mellitus or other peripheral vascular diseases
2. Severe trauma
3. Malignant tumor
4. Congenital deformity

Types of Amputation

A. Open (Guillotine)
1. Used with infection and patients who are poor surgical risks.
2. Wound heals by granulation or secondary closure in about a week.

B. *Closed (Myoplastic)*
1. Residual limb is covered by a flap of skin.
2. Flap of skin is sutured posteriorly.

Surgical Considerations

1. The surgeon considers possible limb salvage techniques.
   a. Revascularization
   b. Hyperbaric oxygenation
   c. Tumor resection with bone grafting
2. Determines level for amputation based on level of maximal viable tissue for wound healing.
3. Develops a functional, nontender, pressure-tolerant residual limb.

Types of Dressings

A. *Soft Dressing*
1. Secured with elastic bandage.
2. Permits wound inspection.
3. Used with patients who should avoid early weight bearing (eg, those with peripheral vascular disease).

B. *Closed, Rigid Plaster Dressing*
1. Applied immediately after surgery.
2. Controls edema.
3. Supports circulation, promoting healing.
4. Minimizes pain on movement.
5. Shapes residual limb.
6. Permits attachment of prosthetic extension (pylon) and early ambulation.

Preoperative Management/ Nursing Care

1. Hemodynamic evaluation is performed through testing, such as angiography, arterial blood flow, xenon[133]—to determine optimal amputation level.
2. Culture and sensitivity tests of draining wounds as done to assist in control of infection preoperatively.
3. Evaluation of sound (contralateral) extremity is performed to determine functional potential postoperatively.
4. Evaluation of cardiovascular, respiratory, renal, and other body systems is necessary to determine preoperative condition of patient and reduce the risks of surgery by optimizing function.

> **NURSING ALERT:**
> Amputation of the lower extremity can be a life-threatening procedure, especially in patients older than age 60 with peripheral vascular disease. Significant morbidity accompanies above-knee amputations because of associated poor health and disease as well as the complications of sepsis and malnutrition and the physiologic insult of amputation.

5. Evaluate and improve nutritional status with adequate protein to enhance wound healing.
6. Teach exercises to strengthen muscles for use of ambulatory aids (lower limb amputee).
   a. Flex and extend arms while holding traction weights.

b. Do push-ups from a prone position if feasible.
   c. Do sit-ups from a seated position if feasible.
7. Teach use of ambulatory aids.
   a. Instills confidence in ability.
   b. Maintains mobility.
   c. Prepares for postoperative mobility.
8. Explain to the patient that he or she will continue to "feel" (phantom sensations) the amputated body part for some time.
9. Support the patient emotionally.
   a. Support concept of amputation as a surgical reconstructive procedure.
   b. Explore patient's perception of procedure and effect on lifestyle.
   c. Avoid unrealistic and misleading reassurance—management of prosthesis can be slow and painful.

Postoperative Management/ Nursing Care

1. Monitor for complication—hemorrhage, infection, unrelieved phantom pain, nonhealing wound.
2. Initiate rehabilitation through physical therapy and prosthetic fitting (if indicated).
   a. Diabetes mellitus, heart disease, infection, stroke, chronic obstructive pulmonary disease, peripheral vascular disease, and increasing age are factors limiting rehabilitation.
   b. Wound breakdown, infection, and delay in healing of residual limb delay rehabilitation.
3. Promote psychological acceptance of body image change.

Nursing Diagnoses

A. Risk for Fluid Volume Deficit related to hemorrhage from disrupted surgical hemostasis
B. Altered Tissue Perfusion related to edema and tissue responses to surgery and prosthesis
C. Ineffective Coping related to change in body image and self-care
D. Pain related to surgical procedure and phantom sensations
E. Impaired Physical Mobility related to amputation, muscle weakness, change in body weight distribution

Nursing Interventions

> **NURSING ALERT:**
> Prevention of complications associated with a major operation and facilitation of early rehabilitation are essential to prevent prolonged disability. Frequent monitoring of the patient's physiologic responses to anesthesia, surgery, and immobility are required.

A. *Monitoring Fluid Balance*
1. Monitor patient for systemic symptoms of excessive blood loss—hypotension, tachycardia, diaphoresis, decreased alertness.

2. Watch for excessive wound drainage.
   a. Keep tourniquet (in view) attached to end of bed to apply to residual limb (stump) if excessive bleeding occurs.
   b. Reinforce dressing as required, using aseptic technique.
   c. Measure suction drainage.
   d. Maintain accurate record of bloody drainage on dressing and in drainage system.
3. Monitor intake and output for fluid balance.

B. *Maintaining Adequate Tissue Perfusion*
1. Control edema.
   a. Elevate residual limb to promote venous return.
   b. Use air splint if prescribed.
2. Maintain pressure dressing.
   a. Reapply if necessary, using sterile dressing secured with elastic bandage.
   b. Notify surgeon if rigid cast dressing comes off.

C. *Supporting Effective Coping*
1. Accept patient responses to loss of body part (ie, depression, withdrawal, denial, frustration).

2. Encourage expression of fears and concerns.
3. Recognize that modification of body image takes time.
4. Encourage participation in rehabilitation planning and self-care.
5. Assist patient to adapt to changes in self-care activities.
   a. Upper extremity amputation—encourage independence in one-handed self-care activities using one-handed aids (eg, one-handed knife), as needed.
   b. Lower extremity amputation—encourage mobility using transfer assistance and ambulatory aids as needed.

D. *Controlling Pain*
1. Surgical pain
   a. Assess the patient's pain experience.
   b. Administer prescribed medications as needed to control postoperative pain.
   c. Use nonpharmaceutical pain management techniques, such as progressive muscle relaxation and imagery.
   d. Recognize that increasing discomfort may indicate presence of hematoma, infection, or necrosis.

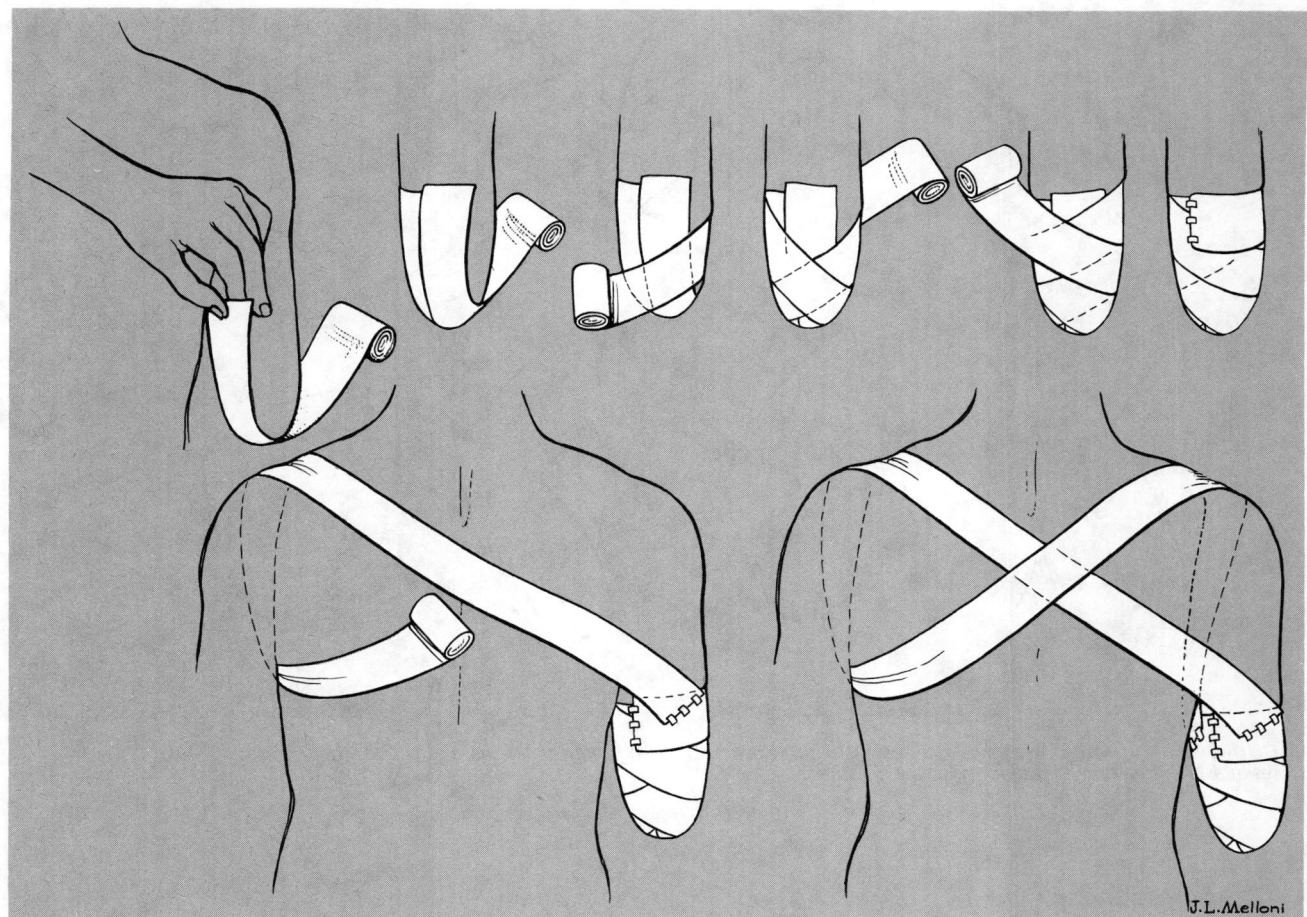

FIGURE 29-11 *Wrapping above-elbow residual limb. Elastic bandaging reduces edema and shapes the residual limb for the prosthesis. Bandage may need to be secured by wrapping across back and shoulders.*

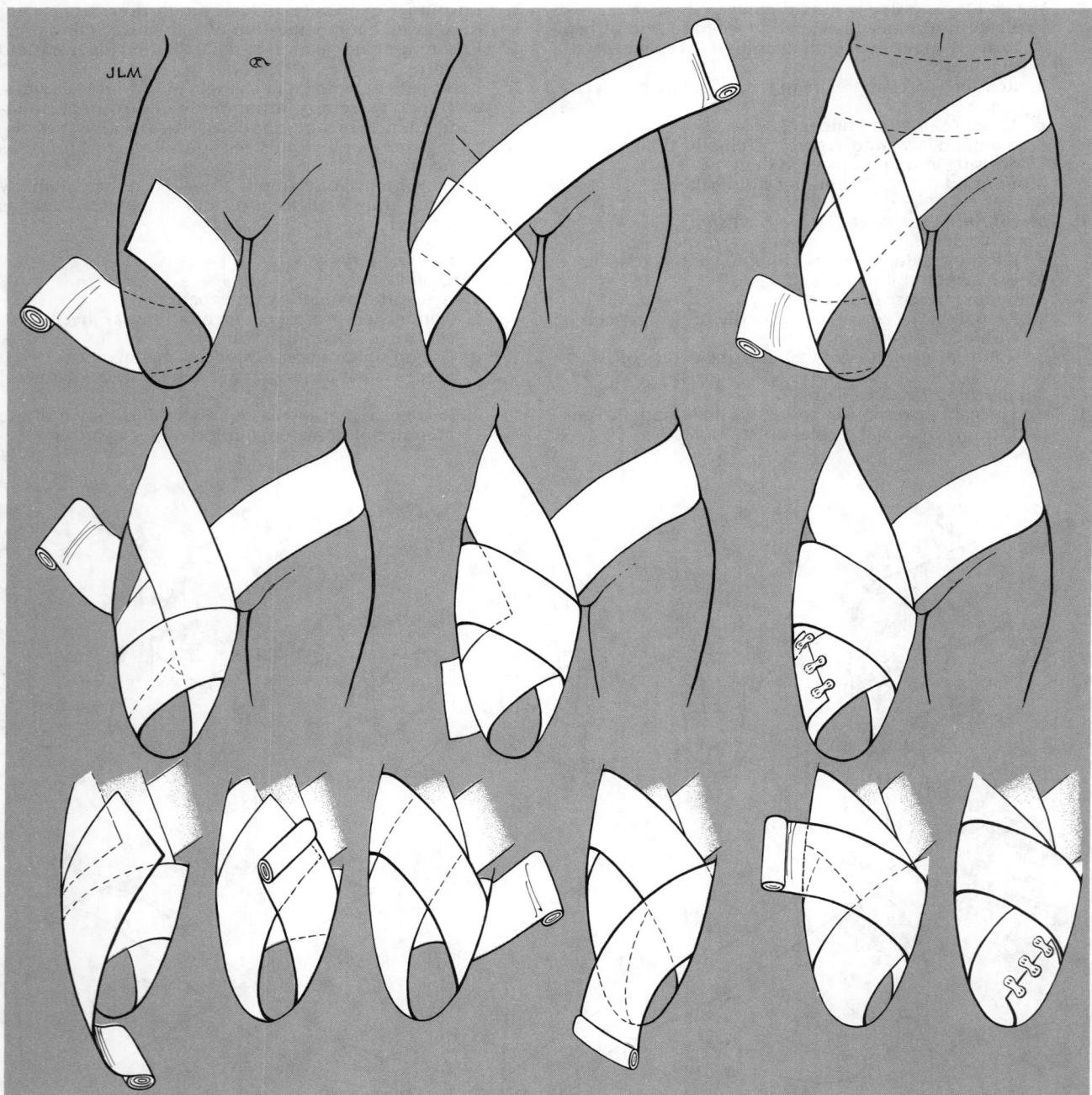

FIGURE 29-12 *Wrapping above-knee residual limb. Elastic bandaging reduces edema and shapes the residual limb in a firm conical form for the prosthesis.*

2. Phantom sensations (pain)
  a. Anticipate complaint of pain and sensation located in the missing limb ("phantom pain").
  b. Use physical modalities (eg, wrapping, temperature changes) and transcutaneous electrical nerve stimulation, if prescribed, in relieving discomfort.
  c. Encourage patient activity to decrease awareness of phantom limb pain.
  d. Reassure the patient that phantom limb pain will diminish over time.

E. *Promoting Physical Activity*
1. Encourage frequent repositioning in bed.
2. Teach patient to avoid long periods in one position.
  a. Avoids dependent edema.
  b. Avoids flexion deformity.
  c. Avoids skin pressure areas.
3. Prevent deformities.
  a. Lower extremity amputations—hip flexion contracture (avoid placing residual limb on pillow; encourage prone position twice a day) and abduction deformity (use trochanter roll; avoid pillow between legs).
  b. Upper extremity amputations—postural abnormalities (encourage good posture).
4. Encourage active range of motion and muscle-strengthening exercises when prescribed to:
  a. Minimize muscle atrophy.
  b. Increase muscle strength.
  c. Prepare residual limb for prosthesis.
5. Promote reestablishment of balance (amputation alters distribution of body weight).
  a. Transfer to chair within 48 hours after surgery.
  b. Instruct and guard lower limb amputee during balance exercises (ie, arise from chair; stand on toes holding onto chair; bend knee holding onto chair; balance on one leg without support; hop on one foot while holding onto chair).
6. Supervise ambulation, use of wheelchair, and self-care activities.

Patient Education/Health Maintenance

1. Teach patient and family how to wrap residual limb with elastic bandage to control edema and to form a firm conical shape for prosthesis fitting (Figs. 29-11 and 29-12).
  a. Wrapping generally begins 1 to 3 days after surgery or after hard plaster dressing is removed.
  b. Use diagonal figure-eight bandaging technique.
  c. Wrap distal to proximal to maintain pressure gradient and to control edema.
  d. Begin wrapping with minimal tension and increase as wound heals and sutures are removed.
  e. Flatten skin at ends of incision to ensure conical stump shape.
  f. Rewrap residual limb a couple of times a day and as necessary to achieve a smooth, graded tension dressing.
  g. Rewrap if patient complains of more pain—dressing is probably too tight.
  h. Keep residual limb wrapped at all times except when bathing.
2. Teach patient residual limb conditioning.
  a. Push the residual limb against a soft pillow.

  b. Gradually push residual limb against harder surfaces.
  c. Massage healed residual limb to soften scar, decrease tenderness, and improve vascularity.
3. Fitting of prosthesis
  a. Note residual limb contour.
  b. Assess for residual limb contraction.
  c. When maximum shrinkage occurs, the prosthetist measures and fits the prosthesis.
  d. Adjustments are made by the prosthetist to minimize skin problems.
4. Continuing care of residual limb and prosthesis.
  a. Instruct patient to wash and dry limb thoroughly at least twice a day, removing all soap residue, to prevent skin irritation and infection.
  b. Avoid soaking residual limb because it results in edema.
  c. Inspect residual limb and skin under prosthesis harness daily for pressure, irritation, and actual skin breakdown.
  d. Wear residual limb sock/cotton underwear—to absorb perspiration and to avoid direct contact between prosthetic socket/harness and skin.
  e. Avoid wrinkles in residual limb sock—potential pressure areas.
  f. Wipe the socket of prosthesis with a damp cloth when prosthesis is removed for evening.
  g. Have prosthesis checked periodically.
5. Teach patient to protect the remaining extremity from injury and to secure prompt treatment of problems.

Evaluation

A. Vital signs stable; dressing reinforced once in 4 hours
B. Pressure dressing intact; stump elevated without edema
C. Patient participating in plan of care; expressing concerns about independence
D. Verbalizes relief of incisional pain; dull phantom sensation tolerable
E. Performing range of motion actively; transferring to wheelchair with assistance

Musculoskeletal Trauma

◆ CONTUSIONS, STRAINS, AND SPRAINS

A *contusion* is an injury to the soft tissue produced by a blunt force (blow, kick, or fall). A *sprain* is an injury to ligamentous structures surrounding a joint; it is usually caused by a wrench or twist resulting in a decrease in joint stability. A *strain* is a microscopic tearing of the muscle caused by excessive force, stretching, or overuse.

Clinical Manifestations

A. *Contusion*
1. Hemorrhage into injured part (ecchymosis)—from rupture of small blood vessels; also associated with fractures
2. Pain, swelling, and discoloration

3. Hyperkalemia may be present with extensive contusions, resulting in destruction of body tissue and loss of blood

B. Strain
1. Hemorrhage into the muscle
2. Swelling
3. Tenderness
4. Pain with isometric contraction
5. May be associated spasm

C. Sprain
1. Rapid swelling—due to extravasation of blood within tissues
2. Pain on passive movement of joint
3. Increasing pain during first few hours due to continued swelling

Management

1. X-ray may be done to rule out fracture.
2. Immobilize in splint, elastic wrap, or compression dressing to support weakened structures and control swelling.
3. Apply ice for first 24 hours.
4. Analgesics usually include nonsteroidal anti-inflammatory drugs (NSAIDs).
5. Severe sprains may require surgical repair and/or cast immobilization.

Nursing Interventions/Patient Education

1. Elevate the affected part. Maintain splint or immobilization as prescribed.
2. Apply cold compresses for the first 24 hours (20 to 30 minutes at a time)—to produce vasoconstriction, decrease edema, and reduce discomfort.
3. Apply heat to affected area after 24 hours (20 to 30 minutes at a time) four times a day—to promote circulation and absorption.
4. Assess neurovascular status of contused extremity every hour to every 4 hours as the patient's condition indicates.
5. Instruct the patient on use of pain medication as prescribed.
6. Ensure correct use of crutches or other mobility aid with or without weight bearing, as prescribed.
7. Educate on need to rest injured part for about a month to allow for healing.
8. Teach the patient to resume activities gradually.
9. Teach the patient to avoid excessive exercise of injured part.
10. Teach the patient to avoid reinjury by "warming up" before exercise.

◆ TENDINITIS

Tendinitis is an inflammation of a tendon caused by a lack of sufficient lubrication of the tendon sheath. May be caused by acute strain on tendon structure or by chronic overuse.

Clinical Manifestations

1. Onset of pain may occur immediately after activity or delayed up to a day later. Range-of-motion and resistance testing is painful.
2. Sudden onset of sharp pain in calf and hearing/feeling a "snap" is associated with tendon rupture, as in Achilles tendinitis due to running injuries.
3. Mild swelling occurs and the tendon sheath is tender to the touch.

Management

1. X-rays not usually diagnostic.
2. Thompson's test helps with diagnosis of Achilles rupture. Patient kneels on chair or lies prone. Examiner squeezes calf of affected leg. Normal response: foot moves downward, denoting intact tendon. If foot does not move, tendon is assumed to be ruptured.
3. Initial treatment includes rest, ice, compression, elevation (RICE).
4. Splinting or casting for up to 6 weeks in functional position usually necessary.
5. Surgical intervention may be necessary.
6. Physical therapy to regain strength and function.

Nursing Interventions/Patient Education

1. Ensure understanding of need for proper immobilization for full time period even though fracture is not present.
2. Encourage the use of warm compresses after 24 hours to relieve pain and inflammation.
3. Advise patient not to return to full activity until strength is equal to unaffected extremity.
4. Teach proper warm-up before exercise/sports activities (stretching of all major tendons).

◆ TRAUMATIC JOINT DISLOCATION

A *dislocation of a joint* occurs when the surfaces of the bones forming the joint are no longer in anatomic contact—this is a medical emergency because of associated disruption of surrounding blood and nerve supplies.

1. Shoulder, fingers, elbow are most common joints to dislocate.
2. Mechanism of injury can be anterior, posterior, lateral, or medial force. Posterior dislocation is the most common.

Clinical Manifestations

1. Pain
2. Deformity
3. Change in the length of the extremity
4. Loss of normal movement

5. X-ray confirmation of dislocation without associated fracture

Management

1. Immobilize part while the patient is transported to emergency department, x-ray department, or clinical unit.
2. Secure reduction of dislocation (bring displaced parts into normal position) as soon as possible to prevent circulatory or nerve impairments; usually performed under anesthesia.
3. Stabilize reduction until joint structures are healed to prevent permanently unstable joint or aseptic necrosis of bone.

Nursing Interventions/Patient Education

1. Assess neurovascular status of extremity before and after reduction of dislocation.
2. Administer or teach self-administration of pain medications, such as NSAIDs.
3. Ensure proper use of immobilization device after reduction.
4. Review instructions for activity restrictions and need for physical therapy and follow-up.

◆ KNEE INJURIES

The knee ligaments provide stability to the knee joint. These ligaments promote rotational stability (anterior and posterior cruciate ligaments [ACL]) and prevent varus and valgus instability (medial and lateral collateral ligaments). Pieces of cartilage that stabilize the knee internally are known as the medial and lateral menisci. Anterior cruciate ligament injuries and medial meniscus tears are common due to sports injuries.

Clinical Manifestations

1. Severe stresses are applied to the knee during many sports activities (eg, soccer, skiing, running).
2. Injury to knee structures occurs during rapid position changes involving flexing and twisting of the joint.
3. Torn cartilage (meniscus) causes pain, tenderness, joint effusion, clicking sensations, and decreased range of motion.
4. Knee ligaments may be torn, resulting in pain on ambulation, swelling, and joint instability. The patellar tendon may rupture.

Management

1. Special assessment techniques are done to detect anterior cruciate ligament injury (Table 29-1).
2. Magnetic resonance imaging shows injury to soft tissue involved.
3. Some injuries may be immobilized (splint, brace, or cast) and treated with physical therapy.
4. ACL reconstruction frequently indicated.
   a. Arthroscopic surgery preferred synthetic ligaments selected where ligaments failed. Graft rejection is a complication.
   b. Postoperative continuous passive motion used.
   c. Postoperative ACL rehabilitation program includes progressive range of motion, bracing (not done with synthetic ligaments).
   d. Long-term bracing during sports controversial.
5. Meniscal injury—damaged cartilage removed.
   a. Arthroscopic or open meniscectomy.
   b. Rehabilitation includes progressive range of motion and quadriceps strengthening.

Nursing Interventions/Patient Education

1. After arthoscopic surgery, ensure proper use of crutches as indicated and encourage pain control through medications as prescribed and rest, ice, compression, and elevation.

TABLE 29-1 Assessment Techniques for Anterior Cruciate Ligament Injury

Test	Description	Positive Finding
Anterior drawer test	Place patient supine with knee in 90 degrees of flexion with foot flat on table. Proximal tibia is pulled forward by examiner using 2 hands.	Tibia subluxes (dislocates) forward on femur.
Lachman test	Place patient supine with knee in 15–20 degrees of flexion. Distal femur is grasped by examiner with one hand while the other hand grasps the proximal tibia and applies forward pressure.	Tibia subluxes forward on femur.
Pivot shift test (evaluates anterolateral rotational stability)	Place patient supine with knee slightly flexed. Examiner grasps patient's ankle in one hand and places palm of other hand over the lateral aspect of the knee distal to the joint. Lower leg is extended and internally rotated, applying a valgus (lateral) stress to knee.	Tibia subluxes and reduces itself ("pivots and shifts")

2. For open joint surgery, see care of the patient undergoing orthopedic surgery, p. 857.
3. Teach patient strengthening exercises for affected extremity.
4. Teach patient to prevent fatigue through rest periods, conservation of energy.
5. Advise on prevention of injuries using proper equipment and footwear for sports.

◆ FRACTURES

A *fracture* is a break in the continuity of bone. A fracture occurs when the stress placed on a bone is greater than the bone can absorb. Muscles, blood vessels, nerves, tendons, joints, and other organs may be injured when fracture occurs.

Types of Fractures

1. *Complete*—involves the entire cross section of the bone, usually displaced (not normal position).
2. *Incomplete*—involves a portion of the cross section of the bone or may be longitudinal.
3. *Closed (simple)*—skin (mucous membranes) not broken.
4. *Open (compound)*—skin broken, leading directly to fracture.
   a. Grade I—minimal soft tissue injury.
   b. Grade II—laceration greater than 1 cm without extensive soft tissue flaps.
   c. Grade III—extensive soft tissue injury, including skin, muscle, neurovascular structure, with crushing.
5. *Pathologic*—through an area of diseased bone (osteoporosis, bone cyst, bone tumor, bony metastasis).

Patterns of Fracture

(See Fig. 29-13.)

1. *Greenstick*—one side of the bone is broken and the other side is bent.
2. *Transverse*—straight across the bone.
3. *Oblique*—at an angle across the bone.
4. *Spiral*—twists around the shaft of the bone.
5. *Comminuted*—bone splintered into more than three fragments.
6. *Depressed*—fragment(s) indriven (seen in fractures of the skull and facial bones).
7. *Compression*—bone collapses in on itself (seen in vertebral fractures).
8. *Avulsion*—fragment of bone pulled off by ligament or tendon attachment.
9. *Impacted*—fragment of bone wedged into other bone fragment.

GERONTOLOGIC ALERT:
Osteoporosis is a major risk for fractures, particularly hip and vertebral compression fractures.

10. *Fracture–dislocation*—fracture complicated by the bone being out of the joint.
11. *Other*—described according to anatomic location: epiphyseal, supracondylar, midshaft, intraarticular, etc.

Clinical Manifestations

A. *Physical Findings*
1. Pain at site of injury
2. Swelling
3. Tenderness
4. False motion and crepitus (grating sensation)
5. Deformity
6. Loss of function
7. Ecchymosis
8. Paresthesia

B. *Altered Neurovascular Status*
1. Injured muscle, blood vessels, nerves
2. Compression of structures resulting in ischemia
3. Findings:
   a. Progressive uncontrollable pain
   b. Pain on passive movement
   c. Altered sensations (paresthesia)
   d. Loss of active motion
   e. Diminished capillary refill response
   f. Pallor

C. *Shock*
1. Bone is very vascular.
2. Overt hemorrhage through open wound.
3. Covert hemorrhage into soft tissues (especially with femoral fracture) or body cavity, as with pelvic fracture.
4. May be fatal if not detected.

Diagnostic Evaluation

1. X-ray and other imaging studies to determine integrity of bone.
2. Blood studies (complete blood count, electrolytes) with blood loss and extensive muscle damage—may show decreased hemoglobin and hematocrit.
3. Arthroscopy to detect joint involvement.
4. Angiography if associated with blood vessel injury.
5. Nerve conduction and electromyogram studies to detect nerve injury.

Management

(Emergency management—see p. 951.)

A. *Factors Influencing Choice of Fracture Management*
1. Type, location, and severity of fracture.
2. Soft tissue damage.
3. Age and health status of patient, including type and extent of other injuries.

B. *Goals*
1. To regain and maintain correct position and alignment.
2. To regain the function of the involved part.
3. To return the patient to usual activities in the shortest time and at the least expense.

C. *Process*
1. *Reduction*—setting the bone; refers to restoration of the fracture fragments into anatomic position and alignment.
2. *Immobilization*—maintains reduction until bone healing occurs (see Figs. 29-14 and 29-15).
3. *Rehabilitation*—regaining normal function of the affected part.

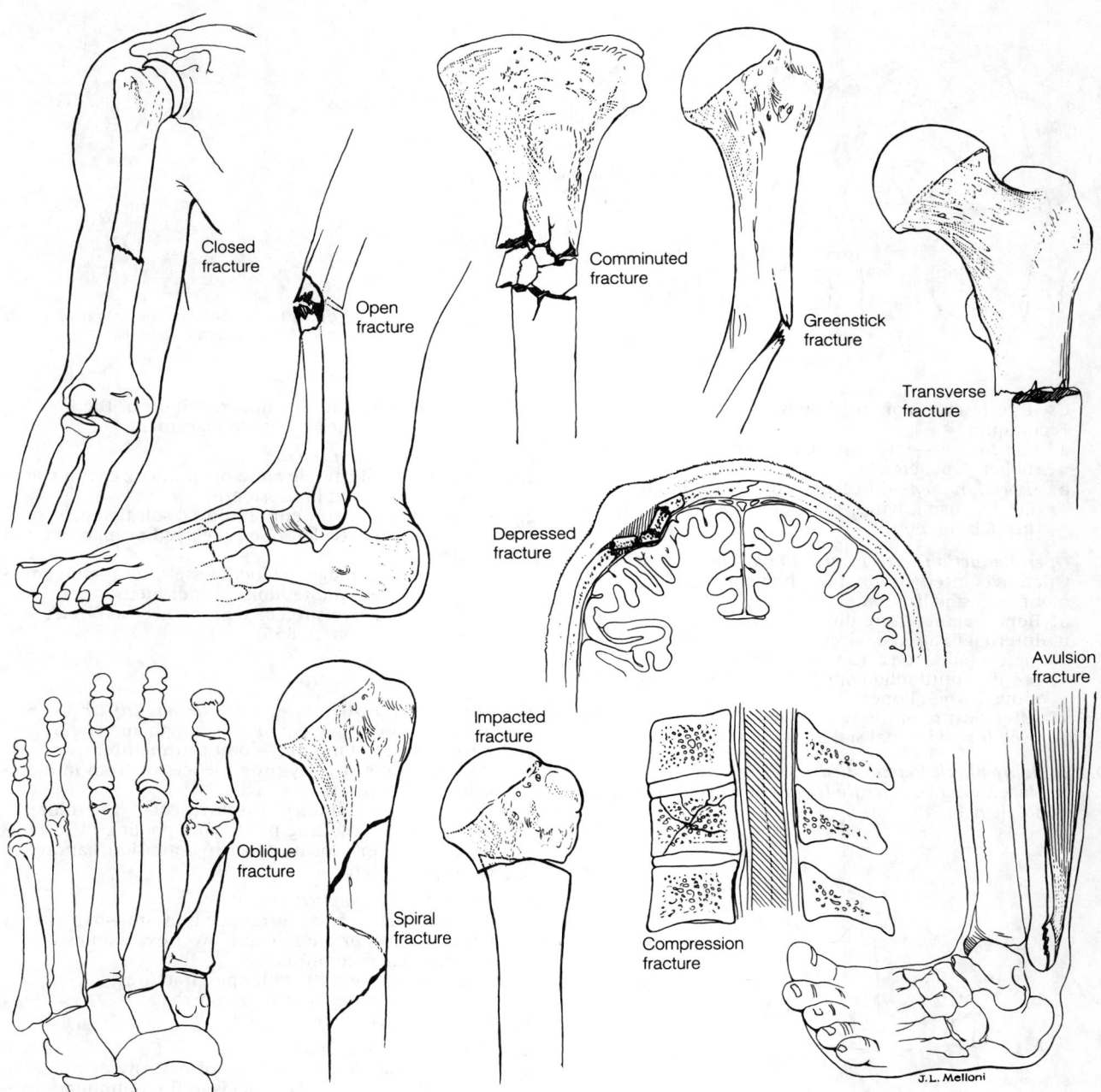

FIGURE 29-13 *Patterns of fractures.*

Approaches

Vary by specific site of fracture (Table 29-2).

A. *Closed Reduction*
1. Bony fragments are brought into *apposition* (ends in contact) by manipulation and manual traction—restores alignment.

2. May be done under anesthesia for pain relief and muscle relaxation.
3. Cast or splint applied to immobilize extremity and maintain reduction (see Casts, p. 845).

B. *Traction*
1. Pulling force applied to accomplish and maintain reduction and alignment (see Traction, p. 852).

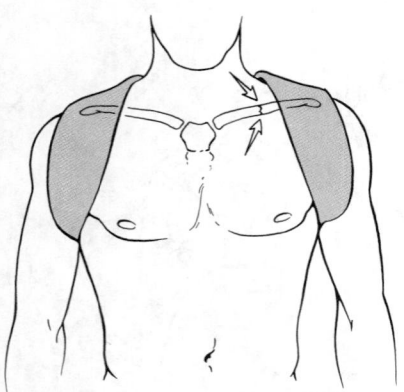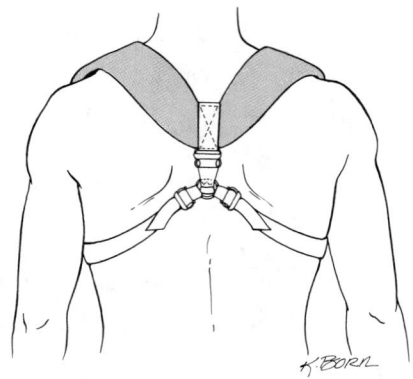

FIGURE 29-14 Method for immobilizing a clavicular fracture with a clavicular strap.

2. Used for fractures of long bones.
3. Techniques
   a. *Skin traction*—force applied to the skin using foam rubber, tape, etc.
   b. *Skeletal traction*—force applied to the bony skeleton directly, using wires, pins, or tongs placed into or through the bone.

C. **Open Reduction With Internal Fixation**
1. Operative intervention to achieve reduction, alignment, and stabilization.
   a. Bone fragments are directly visualized.
   b. Internal fixation devices (metal pins, wires, screws, plates, nails, rods) used to hold bone fragments in position until solid bone healing occurs (may be removed when bone is healed).
   c. After closure of the wound, splints or casts may be used for additional stabilization and support.

D. **Endoprosthetic Replacement**
1. Replacement of a fracture fragment with an implanted metal device.

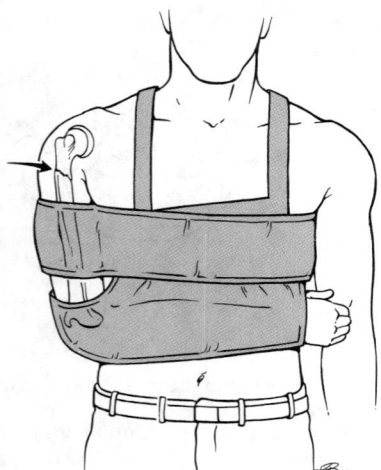

FIGURE 29-15 Immobilization of fracture of upper humerus can be achieved with conventional sling and swathe.

2. Used when fracture disrupts nutrition of the bone or treatment of choice is bony replacement.

E. **External Fixation Device**
1. Stabilization of complex and open fracture with use of a metal frame and pin system.
2. Permits active treatment of injured soft tissue.
   a. Wound may be left open (delayed primary wound closure).
   b. Repair of damage to blood vessels, soft tissue, muscles, nerves, and tendons as indicated.
   c. Reconstructive surgery may be necessary (see External Fixation, p. 855).

Complications

A. **Complications Associated With Immobility**
1. Muscle atrophy, loss of muscle strength and endurance.
2. Loss of range of motion—joint contracture.
3. Pressure sores at bony prominences or from immobilizing device pressing on skin.
4. Diminished respiratory, cardiovascular, gastrointestinal function, resulting in possible pooling of respiratory secretions, orthostatic hypotension, anorexia, constipation, etc.

B. **Other Acute Complications**
1. Venous stasis and thromboembolism—particularly with fractures of the hip and lower extremities
2. Neurovascular compromise
3. Infection—especially with open fractures
4. Shock—due to significant hemorrhage
5. Pulmonary emboli

C. **Fat Emboli Syndrome**
1. Associated with embolization of marrow or tissue fat or platelets and free fatty acids to the pulmonary capillaries, producing rapid onset of symptoms
2. Clinical manifestations
   a. Respiratory distress—tachypnea, hypoxemia, crackles, wheezes, acute pulmonary edema, interstitial pneumonitis
   b. Mental disturbances—irritability, restlessness, confusion, disorientation, stupor, coma due to systemic embolization, and severe hypoxia
   c. Fever
   d. Petechiae in buccal membranes, hard palate, conjunctival sacs, chest, anterior axillary folds, due to occlusion of capillaries

TABLE 29-2 Fractures of Specific Sites

Site and Mechanism	Management	Nursing/Patient Care Considerations
Clavicle—fall on shoulder	1. Closed reduction and immobilization with clavicular strap (Fig. 29-14), figure-8 bandage, or sling 2. ORIF for marked displacement, severely comminuted fracture, and extensive soft tissue injury	1. Pad axilla to prevent nerve damage from pressure of immobilizer 2. Assess neurovascular status of arm 3. Teach exercises of elbow, wrist, and fingers 4. Teach shoulder exercises through full range of motion as prescribed
Proximal humerus—fall on outstretched arm; osteoporosis is predisposing factor	1. Many remain in alignment and are supported by a sling and swathe or Belpeau bandage for comfort (Fig. 29-15) 2. If displaced, treated with reduction under x-ray control, open reduction, or replacement of humeral head with prosthesis	1. Place a soft pad under the axilla to prevent skin maceration 2. Encourage shoulder range-of-motion exercises after specified period of immobilization to prevent frozen shoulder 3. Instruct patient to lean forward and allow affected arm to abduct and rotate

Shaft of humerus—direct fall, blow to arm, or auto injury; damage to radial nerve may occur	1. Immobilize with sling and swathe, splint, or hanging cast
	2. A hanging cast is applied for its weight to correct displaced fractures with shortening of the humeral shaft
	3. ORIF for associated vascular injury or pathologic fracture, followed by support in sling
		1. Hanging cast must remain unsupported to maintain traction
		  a. Teach patient to avoid supporting elbow in lap or arm on pillow
		  b. Patient should sleep in upright position to maintain 24-hour traction.
		2. Encourage exercise of fingers immediately after application of cast
		3. Teach pendulum exercises of arm as prescribed to prevent frozen shoulder

Elbow and forearm—fall on elbow, outstretched hand, or direct blow (sideswipe injury)	1. Treatment depends on specific characteristics of fracture—ORIF, arthroplasty, external fixaton, casting 2. Closed drainage system may be used to decrease hematoma formation and swelling	1. Assess neurovascular status of forearm and hand 2. If radial pulse weakens or disappears, report immediately to prevent irreversible ischemia 3. Elevate arm to control edema 4. Encourage finger and shoulder exercises

Wrist—Colles' fracture is common (1.2–2.5 cm above the wrist with dorsal displacement of lower fragment); caused by fall on outstretched palm; often associated with osteoporosis	1. Closed reduction with splint or cast support
	2. Percutaneous pins and external fixator or plaster cast
		1. Elevate arm above level of heart for 48 hours after reduction to promote venous and lymphatic return and reduce swelling
		2. Watch for swelling of fingers and check for constricting bandages or cast
		3. Teach finger exercises to reduce swelling and stiffness
		  a. Hold hand above level of heart
		  b. Move fingers from full extension to flexion
		  c. Hold and release
		  d. Repeat at least 10 times every half hour when awake for as long as swelling occurs
		4. Encourage daily prescribed exercises to restore full extension and supination

Hand—caused by numerous injuries	1. Splinting for undisplaced fractures of fingers 2. Debridement, irrigation and Kirchner wire fixation for open fractures 3. Reconstructive surgery may be necessary for complex injuries	1. Provide aggressive care and encouragement with rehabilitation plan to regain maximal function of hand.

(continued)

TABLE 29-2 **Fractures of Specific Sites** *(continued)*

Site and Mechanism	Management	Nursing/Patient Care Considerations

Hip (proximal femur)—occur frequently in older adults, women with osteoporosis, and with falls
Types:
1. Intracapsular—femoral neck within joint capsule
2. Extracapsular—femoral neck between greater and lesser trochanter (intertrochanteric) or of femoral shaft
3. Subtrochanteric—of femur just below level of lesser trochanter
	1. Hip fracture identified by shortening and external rotation of affected leg; pain in hip or knee; inability to move leg
	2. Immobilization with Buck's extension traction until surgery
	3. Surgery as soon as medically stable; choice depends on location, character, and patient factors
	  a. Internal fixation with nail, nail-plate combination, multiple pins, screw, or sliding nails
	  b. Femoral prosthetic replacement
	  c. Total hip replacement
		1. Provide constant monitoring and nursing care to reduce the risk of complications, such as pneumonia, thrombophlebitis, fat emboli, dislocation of prosthesis, infection, and pressure sores
		2. Administer aspirin, warfarin (Coumadin), or low-dose subcutaneous heparin as ordered
		3. Use sequential compression devices as ordered
		4. Provide meticulous skin care to prevent breakdown
		  a. Use trapeze for patient to assist with position changes
		  b. Use special bed or mattress as indicated
		  c. Inspect heels daily and use heel protection measures
		5. Prevent urinary tract infection by increasing fluids and encouraging frequent voiding
		6. Keep affected leg in abduction and neutral rotation
		7. Teach quadriceps setting exercise to prevent muscle atrophy of affected leg

Femoral shift	1. Closed reduction and stabilization with skeletal traction—Thomas leg splint with Pearson attachment; followed by use of orthosis (cast-brace) to allow weight bearing 2. Open reduction with hardware or with bone grafting may be necessary 3. External fixator may be used	1. Marked concealed blood loss may occur; watch for signs of shock initially and anemia later 2. Examine skin under the ring of the Thomas splint for signs of pressure
Knee—direct blow to knee area; involve distal shaft of femur (supracondylar), articular surfaces, or patella	1. Closed reduction and/or immobilization through casting, traction, braces, splints 2. ORIF 3. Goal is to preserve knee mobility	1. Elevate extremity by raising foot gatch of bed 2. Evaluate for effusion—report and loosen pressure dressing if pain is severe; prepare for joint aspiration 3. Teach quadriceps setting exercises and limited weight bearing as prescribed
Tibia and fibula/ankle—distal tibia or fibula, malleoli, or talus fractures generally result from forceful twisting of ankle and often associated with ligament disruption; also high incidence of open fractures of tibial shaft, because tibia lies superficially beneath the skin	1. Closed reduction and toe to groin cast for closed fractures, later replaced by short leg cast or orthosis 2. ORIF may be necessary for some closed fractures 3. External fixator for open fracture	1. Elevate lower leg to control edema 2. Avoid dependent position of extremity for prolonged periods 3. Prepare patient for long immobilization period, as union is slow (12–16 weeks, longer for open and comminuted fractures) 3. Prepare patient for stiff ankle joint following immobilization
Foot—metatarsal fracture due to crush injuries of foot	1. Immobilization with cast, splint, or strapping	1. Encourage partial weight bearing as allowed 2. Elevate foot to control edema

(continued)

TABLE 29-2 Fractures of Specific Sites *(continued)*

Site and Mechanism	Management	Nursing/Patient Care Considerations
Thoracic and lumbar spine—trauma from falls, contact sports, or auto accidents, or excessive loading may cause fracture of vertebral body, lamina, spinous and transverse processes; usually stable compression fractures	1. Suspected with pain that is worsened by movement and coughing and radiates to extremities, abdomen, or intercostal muscles; and presence of sensory and motor deficits 2. Bed rest on firm mattress and pain relief followed by progressive ambulation and back strengthening to treat stable fractures; takes about 6 weeks to heal 3. ORIF with Harrington rod, body cast, or laminectomy with spinal fusion may be necessary for unstable or displaced fractures	1. Use log roll technique to change positions 2. Monitor bowel and bladder dysfunction, as paralytic ileus and bladder distention may occur with nerve root injury 3. Assist patient to ambulate when pain subsides, no neurologic deficit exists, and x-rays reveal no displacement 4. Teach proper body mechanics and back preservation techniques 5. Encourage weight reduction 6. Teach patient with osteoporosis the importance of safety measures to avoid falls

Pelvis—sacrum, ilium, pubic, ischium, and coccyx fractures may occur from auto accidents, crush injuries, and falls; most are stable fractures that do not involve the pelvic ring and have minimal displacement	1. Emergency management to treat multiple trauma, shock from intraperitoneal hemorrhage, and injury to internal organs is necessary (see p. 952)
	2. Bed rest for several days followed by progressive weight bearing for stable fracture
	3. Prolonged bed rest, external fixation, ORIF, skeletal traction, or pelvic sling are options for unstable fracture
		1. Monitor and support vital functions as indicated
		2. Observe urine output for blood indicating genitourinary injury
		3. Do not attempt to insert urethral catheter until patency of urethra is known; incidence of urethral injury in males is high with anterior fractures
		4. Assist the patient being treated in pelvic sling
		  a. Fold sling back over buttocks to enable the patient to use bedpan
		  b. Reach under sling to give skin care; line sling with sheepskin
		  c. Loosen sling only as directed

NURSING ALERT:
Restlessness, confusion, irritability, and disorientation may be the first signs of fat embolism syndrome. Confirm hypoxia with arterial blood gas analysis. Young adults (20 to 30 years old) and older adults (60 to 70 years old) with multiple fractures or fractures of long bones or pelvis are particularly susceptible to development of fat emboli.

D. Bone Union Problems
1. *Delayed union* (takes longer to heal than average for type of fracture)
2. *Nonunion* (fractured bone fails to unite)
3. *Malunion* (union occurs but is faulty—misaligned)

◆ NURSING PROCESS OVERVIEW: THE PATIENT WITH A FRACTURE

Nursing Assessment

1. Ask patient how the fracture occurred—mechanism of injury important in determining possible associated injuries.
2. Ask patient to describe location, character, and intensity of pain to help determine possible source of discomfort.

3. Ask patient to describe sensations in injured extremity—to aid in evaluation of neurovascular status.
4. Observe patient's ability to change position—to assess functional mobility.
5. Note patient's emotional status and behavior—indicators of ability to cope with stress of injury.

NURSING ALERT:
Change in behavior and/or cerebral functioning may be an early indicator of cerebral anoxia from shock or pulmonary or fat emboli.

6. Assess patient's support system; identify current and potential sources of assistance/caregiving.
7. Review findings on past and present health status—to aid in formulating plan of care.
8. Conduct physical examination.
   a. Examine skin for lacerations, abrasions, ecchymosis; note areas of swelling and edema.
   b. Auscultate lungs to establish baseline assessment of respiratory function.
   c. Assess pulses and blood pressure; assess peripheral tissue perfusion, especially in injured extremity, to establish circulatory status baseline.
   d. Determine neurologic status (sensations and movement) of extremity distal to injury.
   e. Note length, alignment, and immobilization of injured extremity.

f. Evaluate behavior and cognitive functioning of patient to determine ability to participate in care planning and patient education activities.

GERONTOLOGIC ALERT:
Assessment of patient's health and functional abilities before fracture and available support system facilitate development of realistic rehabilitation and discharge goals.

Nursing Diagnoses

A. Risk for Fluid Volume Deficit related to hemorrhage and shock
B. Impaired Gas Exchange related to immobility and potential pulmonary emboli or fat emboli
C. Risk for peripheral neurovascular dysfunction
D. Risk for injury related to thromboembolism
E. Pain related to injury
F. Risk for Infection related to open fracture or surgical intervention
G. Bathing/Hygiene Self Care Deficit related to immobility
H. Impaired Physical Mobility related to injury/treatment modality
I. Risk for Disuse Syndrome related to injury and immobilization
J. Post-Trauma Response

Nursing Interventions

A. *Evaluating for Hemorrhage and Shock*
1. Monitor vital signs as frequently as clinical condition indicates, observing for hypotension, elevated pulse, cold clammy skin, restlessness, pallor.
2. Watch for evidence of hemorrhage on dressings or in drainage containers.
3. Review laboratory data; report abnormal values.
4. Administer prescribed fluids/blood to maintain circulating volume.
5. Monitor intake and output.

B. *Monitoring for Impaired Gas Exchange*
1. Evaluate changes in mental status and restlessness that may indicate hypoxia.
2. Review diagnostic evaluation data—especially arterial blood gas values and chest x-ray.
3. Position to enhance respiratory effort.
4. Encourage coughing and deep breathing to promote lung expansion and diminish pooling of pulmonary secretions.
5. Administer oxygen as prescribed.
6. Report any sudden or progressive changes in respiratory status.

C. *Preventing Neurovascular Compromise*
1. Monitor neurovascular status for compression of nerve, diminished circulation, development of compartment syndrome.
   a. *Pain*—progressive, localized, deep throbbing, persistent, unrelieved by immobilization and medications
   b. *Pain*—on passive stretch
   c. *Weakness* progressing to paralysis
   d. *Altered sensation*, hypothesis, anesthesia
   e. *Poor capillary refill response*
   f. *Skin color*—pale, cyanotic

g. *Elevated compartment pressure*—palpable tightness of muscle compartment, elevated measured tissue pressure
h. *Pulselessness*

NURSING ALERT:
Monitoring the neurovascular integrity of the injured extremity is essential. Development of *compartment syndrome* (increased tissue pressure causing hypoxemia) leads to permanent loss of function in 6 to 8 hours. This situation must be identified and managed promptly.

2. Reduce swelling.
   a. Elevate injured extremity (unless compartment syndrome is suspected—may contribute to vascular compromise).
   b. Apply cold to injury if prescribed.
3. Relieve pressure caused by immobilizing device as prescribed (such as bivalving cast, rewrapping elastic bandage, or splinting device).
4. Relieve pressure on skin to prevent development of pressure sore.
   a. Frequent repositioning
   b. Skin care
   c. Special mattresses

D. *Preventing Development of Thromboembolism*

GERONTOLOGIC ALERT:
Older adults with fractures, trauma, immobility, obesity, or history of thrombophlebitis are at high risk for developing thromboembolism.

1. Encourage active and passive ankle exercises.
2. Use elastic stockings and sequential compression devices, as prescribed.
3. Elevate legs to prevent stasis, avoiding pressure on blood vessels.
4. Encourage mobility; change position frequently; encourage ambulation.
5. Administer anticoagulants as prescribed.
6. Monitor for development of thrombophlebitis.
   a. Note complaint of pain and tenderness in calf.
   b. Report calf pain
   c. Report increased size and temperature of calf.

E. *Relieving Pain*
1. Secure data concerning pain.
   a. Have the patient describe the pain, location, characteristics (dull, sharp, continuous, throbbing, boring, radiating, aching, etc.)
   b. Ask the patient what causes the pain, makes the pain worse, relieves the pain, etc.
   c. Evaluate the patient for proper body alignment, pressure from equipment (casts, traction, splints, appliances).
2. Initiate activities to prevent or modify pain.
   a. Assist the patient with pain-reduction techniques—cutaneous stimulation, distraction, guided imagery, transcutaneous electrical nerve stimulation, biofeedback, etc.
   b. Immobilize injured part.
   c. Position the patient in correct alignment.
   d. Support splinted fracture above and below fracture when repositioning or moving the patient.
   e. Reposition patient with slow and steady motion; use additional personnel as needed.

f. Elevate painful extremity to diminish venous congestion.

g. Apply heat or cold modalities as prescribed.

h. Modify environment to facilitate rest and relaxation.

3. Administer prescribed pharmaceuticals as indicated. Encourage use of less potent drugs as severity of discomfort decreases.

4. Establish a supportive relationship to assist patient to deal with discomfort.

5. Encourage the patient to become an active participant in rehabilitative plans.

F. Monitoring for Development of Infection

1. Cleanse, debride, and irrigate open fracture wound as prescribed as soon as possible to minimize chance of infection.

a. Open fractures are contaminated.

b. Begin prescribed antibiotic therapy promptly after wound culture obtained.

2. Use sterile technique during dressing changes to minimize infection of wound, soft tissues, and bone.

3. Evaluate patient for elevation of temperature at regular intervals.

4. Note elevated white blood cell counts.

5. Report areas of inflammation and swelling around incision or open wound.

6. Report purulent drainage.

7. Obtain specimens for culture and sensitivity to determine causative organism.

8. Administer antibiotic therapy as prescribed.

G. Promoting Self-Care Activities

1. Encourage participation in care.

2. Arrange patient area and personal items for patient convenience to promote independence.

3. Modify activities to facilitate maximum independence within prescribed limits.

4. Allow time for patient to accomplish task.

5. Teach safe use of mobility and other aids.

6. Assist with activities of daily living as needed.

7. Teach family how to assist patient while promoting independence in self-care.

H. Promoting Physical Mobility

1. Perform active and passive exercises to all nonimmobilized joints.

2. Encourage patient participation in frequent position changes, maintaining supports to fracture during position changes.

3. Minimize prolonged periods of physical inactivity, encouraging ambulation when prescribed.

4. Administer prescribed analgesics judiciously to decrease pain associated with movement.

I. Preventing Development of Disuse Syndrome

1. Teach and encourage isometric exercises to diminish muscle atrophy.

2. Encourage use of immobilized extremity within prescribed limits.

J. Promoting Positive Psychological Response to Trauma

1. Monitor patient for symptoms of post-trauma stress disorder.

a. Memory of event; anger, helplessness, vulnerability, mood swings, depression, cognitive impairment, sleep disturbance, increased dependency, social withdrawal

2. Assist patient to move through phases of post-traumatic stress (outcry, denial, intrusiveness, working through, completion).

3. Establish trusting therapeutic relationship with patient.

4. Encourage patient to express thoughts and feelings about traumatic event.

5. Encourage patient to participate in decision making to reestablish control and overcome feelings of helplessness.

6. Teach relaxation techniques to decrease anxiety.

7. Encourage development of adaptive responses and participation in support groups.

8. Refer patient to psychiatric liaison nurse or refer for psychotherapy, as needed.

Patient Education/Health Maintenance

1. Explain basis for fracture treatment and need for patient participation in therapeutic regimen.

2. Promote adjustment of usual lifestyle and responsibilities to accommodate limitations imposed by fracture.

3. Instruct the patient to actively exercise joints above and below the immobilized fracture at frequent intervals.

a. Isometric exercises of muscles covered by cast—start exercise as soon as possible after cast application.

b. Increase isometric exercises as fracture stabilizes.

4. After removal of immobilizing device (eg, cast, splint), have the patient start active exercises and continue with isometric exercises.

5. Instruct the patient on exercises to strengthen upper extremity muscles if crutch walking is planned.

6. Instruct the patient in methods of safe ambulation—walker, crutches, cane.

7. Emphasize instructions concerning amount of weight bearing that will be permitted on fractured extremity.

8. Discuss prevention of recurrent fractures—safety considerations, avoidance of fatigue, proper footwear.

9. Encourage follow-up medical supervision to monitor for union problems.

10. Teach symptoms needing attention, such as numbness, decreased function, increased pain, elevated temperature.

11. Encourage adequate balanced diet to promote bone and soft tissue healing.

Evaluation

A. Vital signs stable; urine output adequate

B. Respirations unlabored; alert and oriented

C. No signs of neurovascular compromise

D. No calf pain reported: Homan's sign negative

E. Reports decreased pain with elevation, ice, and analgesic

F. Afebrile; no wound drainage

G. Performing hygiene and dressing practices with minimal assistance

H. Performing active range of motion correctly

I. Using affected extremity for light activity as allowed

J. Denies acute symptoms of stress; reports working through feelings about trauma

Other Musculoskeletal Disorders

◆ LOW BACK PAIN

Low back pain is characterized by an uncomfortable or acute pain in the lumbosacral area associated with severe spasm of the paraspinal muscles, often with radiating pain.

Pathophysiology/Etiology

Multiple causes:

1. Mechanical (joint, muscular, or ligamentous sprain)
2. Degenerative disk disease; acute herniation of disk(s)
3. Lack of physical activity and exercise; weakness of musculature of back
4. Arthritic conditions
5. Diseases of bone (osteoporosis, vertebral fracture, Paget's disease, metastatic carcinoma)
6. Congenital disorders
7. Systemic diseases
8. Infections of disk spaces or vertebrae
9. Spinal cord tumors
10. Referred pain from other areas

Clinical Manifestations

1. Pain localized or radiating to buttocks or to one or both legs
2. Paresthesias, numbness, and/or weakness of lower extremities
3. Spasm in acute phase
4. Bowel/bladder dysfunction

Diagnostic Evaluation

1. X-rays of lumbar spine are usually negative
2. Computed tomography of spine to detect arthritic changes, degenerative disk disease, tumor, and other abnormalities.
3. Myelography—to confirm and localize disk herniation.
4. Magnetic resonance imaging—to detect any pathology: disherniation, soft tissue injury, etc.
5. Electromyography of lower extremities—to detect nerve changes related to back pathology.
6. Diskogram—detects herniated disk.

Management

For management of herniated disk, see p. 413. For management of spinal cord tumors, see p. 407.

1. Rest in bed in a supine to semi-Fowler's position with hips and knees flexed—to relieve painful muscle and ligament sprain, heal soft tissue injury, remove stress from lumbar sacral area, relieve tension on sciatic nerves, and open the posterior part of the intervertebral spaces.

a. Acute spasm and pain should subside in 3 to 7 days if there is no nerve involvement or other serious underlying disease.
b. Isometric exercises should be done hourly while on bed rest, if possible.
2. Heat or ice used to relax muscle spasm and relieve discomfort. Follow heat with massage.
3. Medications
a. Oral pain medication and muscle relaxants: NSAIDs frequently used.
b. Painful trigger points may be injected with hydrocortisone/xylocaine for pain relief (by physician).
c. Parenteral pain medication in acute severe pain syndromes.
4. Lumbosacral support may be used—provides abdominal compression and decreases load on lumbar intervertebral disks.
5. Transcutaneous electrical nerve stimulation may be helpful in relieving pain.
6. Psychiatric intervention may be needed for the patient with chronic depression, anxiety, and low back syndrome.
a. Psychotropic medication may be used for treatment of depression and anxiety, which potentiate pain.
b. Focus on getting back to functional state after long disability.

Complications

1. Spinal instability, infection, sensory and motor deficits
2. Chronic pain
3. Malingering and other psychosocial reactions

Nursing Assessment

1. Obtain history to determine when, where, and how the pain occurs, aggravating or relieving factors, relationship of pain to specific activities, presence of numbness or paresthesia.
2. Perform physical exam of neurologic system—spots localized weakness of extremities and reflex and sensory loss.
3. Perform musculoskeletal exam for changes in strength, tone, and range of motion.
4. If condition chronic, assess coping ability of patient and family/significant others.
5. Assess effect of illness on daily living—work, school, etc.

Nursing Diagnoses

A. Pain related to injury
B. Impaired Physical Mobility related to pain

Nursing Interventions

A. *Relieving Pain*
1. Advise the patient to rest in bed on firm mattress or with bedboards beneath mattress for support. (Bed rest may eliminate the need for pain medications.)
2. Keep pillow between flexed knees while in side-lying position—minimizes strain on back muscles.

3. Apply heat (moist towels; hydrocollator packs) or ice as prescribed.
4. Administer or teach self-administration of pain medications and muscle relaxants, as prescribed.
   a. Give NSAIDs with meals to prevent gastrointestinal upset and bleeding.
   b. Muscle relaxants may cause drowsiness.

B. *Promoting Mobility*

1. Encourage range of motion of all uninvolved muscle groups.
2. Suggest gradual increase of activities and alternating activities with rest in semi-Fowler's position.
3. Avoid prolonged periods of sitting.
4. Encourage the patient to discuss problems that may be contributing to backache.
5. Encourage the patient to do prescribed back exercises (Fig. 29-16). Exercise keeps postural muscles strong, helps recondition the back and abdominal musculature, and serves as an outlet for emotional tension.

Patient Education/Health Maintenance

Instruct the patient to avoid recurrences as follows:

1. Standing, sitting, lying, and lifting properly are necessary for a healthy back.
2. Alternate periods of activity with periods of rest.
   a. Avoid prolonged *sitting* (intradiskal pressure in lumbar spine is higher during sitting), standing, and driving.
   b. Change positions and rest at frequent intervals.
   c. Avoid assuming tense, cramped positions.
   d. Sit in a straight-back, fairly high-seated chair. Sit with the knees higher than the hips. Use a footstool.
   e. Flatten the hollow of the back by sitting with the buttocks "tucked under." Pelvic tilt (small of back is pressed against a flat surface)—decreases lordosis.
   f. Avoid knee and hip extension. When driving a car, have the seat pushed forward as necessary for comfort. Place a cushion in the small of the back for support.
3. When standing for any length of time, rest one foot on a small stool or wooden box to relieve lumbar lordosis.
4. Avoid fatigue, which contributes to spasm of back muscles.
   a. Sleep on a firm mattress.
   b. Avoid sleeping in a prone position.
   c. When lying on the side, place a pillow under the head and one between the flexed knees to reduce strain on the back muscles.
5. Pick up objects or loads correctly.
   a. Maintain a straight spine.
   b. Flex knees and hips while stooping.
   c. Keep load close to body.
   d. Lift with the legs.
   e. Avoid twisting trunk while lifting.
   f. Avoid lifting above waist level and reaching up for any length of time.
6. *Daily exercise is important in the prevention of back problems.*
   a. Do prescribed back exercises twice daily.
      (1) Strengthens back, leg, and abdominal muscles.
   b. Walking outdoors (progressively increasing distance and pace) is recommended.
   c. Reduce weight if necessary.
      (1) Decreases strain on back muscles.

Evaluation

A. Verbalizes relief of pain with rest and medication
B. Performs back exercises correctly

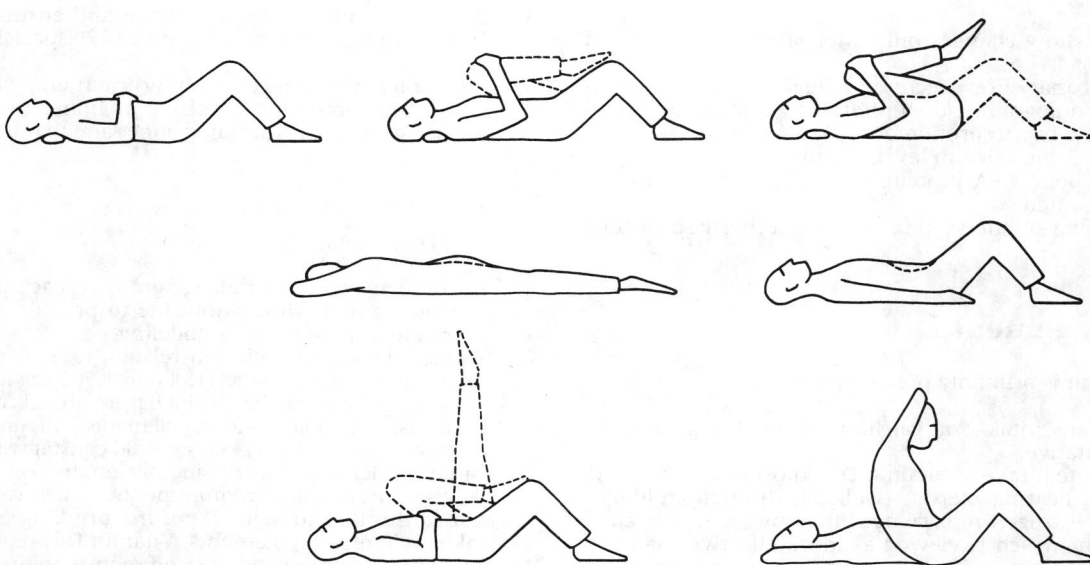

FIGURE 29-16 *Back exercises to strengthen abdominal and postural muscles, to stretch contracted back muscles, and to maintain flexibility.*

◆ OSTEOPOROSIS

Osteoporosis is a condition in which the bone matrix is lost, thereby weakening the bones and making them more susceptible to fracture.

Pathophysiology/Etiology

1. The rate of bone resorption increases over the rate of bone formation, causing loss of bone mass.
2. Calcium and phosphate salts are lost, creating porous, brittle bones.
3. Occurs most frequently in postmenopausal women.
4. Other factors include:
   a. Age
   b. Inactivity
   c. Chronic illness
   d. Medications, such as corticosteroids
   e. Calcium and vitamin D deficiency
   f. Family history
   g. Smoking
   h. Diet—Caffeine has been linked as a risk factor
   i. Race—Whites and Asians have higher risk incidence

Clinical Manifestations

1. Asymptomatic until later stages
2. Fracture after minor trauma may be first indication. Most frequent fractures associated with osteoporosis include fractures of the distal radius, vertebral bodies, proximal humerus, pelvis, and proximal femur (hip).
3. May have vague complaints related to aging process (stiffness, pain, weakness)
4. Estrogen deficiency may be noted

Diagnostic Evaluation

1. X-rays show changes only after 30% to 60% loss of bone.
2. Studies that show decreased density of bone—computed tomography, dual photon absorptiometry, dual energy x-ray absorptiometry (DEXA)
3. Serum/urine calcium levels normal
4. Serum bone GLA-protein—a marker for bone turnover; elevated.
5. Bone biopsy shows thin, porous, otherwise normal bone.

Management

Management is primarily preventative.

1. Adequate intake of calcium—1 to 1.5 g may be preventative.
2. Adequate intake of vitamin D (exposure to sunlight).
3. Weight-bearing exercise (walking) throughout life.
4. Use of estrogen replacement therapy for menopausal women, which is viewed as more effective than calcium supplements. Ideally, start within 5 years of menopause before osteoporosis is established, but may be of benefit in late stages as well.
5. Prevention of falls in the elderly to prevent fractures.

6. Other agents, such as 25-hydroxyvitamin D, calcitonin, etidronate disodium (Didronel), and thiazide diuretics may have some benefit but are not proven.

Complications

1. Fractures

Nursing Assessment

1. Obtain history of risk factors for osteoporosis, history of fractures, and other musculoskeletal disease.
2. Assess risk for falls and fractures—sensory or motor problems, improper footwear, lack of knowledge of safety precautions, etc.

Nursing Diagnosis

A. Chronic Pain related to vertebral compression fractures in late stages of osteoporosis

Nursing Interventions

A. Reducing Pain
1. Administer narcotic analgesics as ordered for acute exacerbations of pain.
2. Encourage replacement with nonnarcotic pain relievers as soon as possible to avoid addiction.

GERONTOLOGIC ALERT:
Prolonged use of narcotics in the elderly is especially dangerous due to impairment of mental status and may contribute to falls and other accidents.

3. Assist with putting on back brace and ensure proper fit. Encourage use as much as possible, especially while ambulatory.
4. Encourage compliance with physical therapy appointments and practicing exercises at home to increase muscle strength surrounding bones and to relieve pain.

Patient Education/Health Maintenance

1. Encourage exercise for all age groups. Teach the value of walking daily throughout life to provide stress required for strong bone remodeling.
2. Provide dietary education in relation to adequate daily intake of 800 mg or more (1,000 to 1,500 mg ideally) of calcium. Calcium can be obtained through milk and dairy products, vegetables, and supplements. Anyone with a history of urinary tract stones should consult with health care provider before increasing calcium intake.
3. Advise on vitamin D requirements, which can be obtained through sunlight exposure, drinking milk, and taking vitamin supplements. Vitamin D is required for calcium absorption and use and requirements increase with age.
4. Encourage young women at risk to maximize bone mass through nutrition and exercise.

5. Suggest that perimenopausal women confer with the physician concerning need for calcium supplements and estrogen therapy.
6. Teach strategies to prevent falls. Assess home for hazards (eg, scatter rugs, slippery floors, extension cords, adequate lighting). Encourage use of walking aids when balance is poor and muscle strength weakens.

COMMUNITY-BASED CARE TIP:
Identify women at high risk for osteoporotic fractures in the community—frail, elderly white or Asian women with poor dietary intake of dairy products and little exposure to sun—and provide education and safety measures to prevent falls and fracture.

Evaluation

A. Pain tolerable with nonnarcotic analgesics

◆ OSTEOARTHRITIS

Osteoarthritis, or degenerative joint disease, is a chronic, noninflammatory, slowly progressing disorder that causes deterioration of articular cartilage. It affects weight-bearing joints (hips and knees) as well as joints of the distal interphalangeal and proximal interphalangeal joints of the fingers.

Pathophysiology/Etiology

1. Changes in articular cartilage occur first; later, secondary soft tissue changes may occur.
2. Progressive wear and tear on cartilage leads to thinning of joint surface and ulceration into bone.
3. Leads to inflammation of the joint and increased blood flow and hypertrophy of subchondral bone.
4. New cartilage and bone formation at joint margins results in osteophytosis (bone spurs), altering the size and shape of bone.
5. Generally affects adults age 50 to 90; equal in males and females.
6. Cause is unknown, but aging and obesity are contributing factors. Previous trauma may cause secondary osteoarthritis.

Diagnostic Evaluation

1. No specific laboratory examination.
2. X-rays of affected joints show joint space narrowing, osteophytes, and sclerosis.
3. Radionuclide imaging (bone scan)—shows increased uptake in affected bones.
4. Analysis of synovial fluid differentiates osteoarthritis and rheumatoid arthritis.

Management

1. Conservative management includes physical therapy, analgesic therapy, and nonnarcotics education on joint conservation techniques to stop the progression of degeneration.

2. Surgical intervention is considered when the pain becomes intolerable to the patient and mobility is severely compromised. Options include osteotomy, debridement, joint fusion, arthroscopy, and arthroplasty.

Complications

1. Limited mobility
2. Neurologic deficits associated with spinal involvement

Nursing Assessment

1. Obtain history of pain, and its characteristics: which joint(s) involved.
2. Evaluate range of motion and strength.
3. Assess effect on activities of daily living and emotional status.

Nursing Diagnoses

A. Pain related to joint degeneration and muscle spasm
B. Impaired Physical Mobility related to pain and limited joint motion
C. Self Care Deficits (feeding, bathing/hygiene, dressing/grooming, toileting) related to pain limited joint movement

Nursing Interventions

A. *Relieving Pain*
1. Advise patient to take prescribed NSAIDs or over-the-counter analgesics as directed to relieve inflammation and/or pain. May alternate with narcotic analgesic, if prescribed.

GERONTOLOGIC ALERT:
Elderly patients are at greater risk for gastrointestinal bleeding associated with NSAID use. Encourage administration with meals and monitor stool for occult blood.

2. Provide rest for involved joints—excessive use aggravates the symptoms and accelerates degeneration.
   a. Use splints, braces, cervical collars, traction, lumbosacral corsets as necessary.
   b. Have prescribed rest periods in recumbent position.
3. Advise patient to avoid activities that precipitate pain.
4. Apply heat as prescribed—relieves muscle spasm and stiffness; avoid prolonged application of heat—may cause increased swelling and flare symptoms.
5. Teach correct posture and body mechanics—postural alterations lead to chronic muscle tension and pain.
6. Advise sleeping with a rolled terrycloth towel under the neck—for relief of cervical osteoarthritis.
7. Provide crutches, braces, or cane when indicated—to reduce weight-bearing stress on hips and knees.
8. Teach use of cane in hand on side opposite involved hip/knee.
9. Advise wearing corrective shoes and metatarsal supports for foot disorders—also help in the treatment of arthritis of the knee.

10. Encourage weight loss to decrease stress on weight-bearing joints.
11. Support the patient undergoing orthopedic surgery for unremitting pain and disabling arthritis of joints (see p. 857).

B. *Increasing Physical Mobility*
1. Encourage activity as much as possible without causing pain.
2. Teach range-of-motion exercises to maintain joint mobility and muscle tone for joint support, to prevent capsular and tendon tightening, and to prevent deformities. Avoid flexion and adduction deformities.
3. Teach isometric exercises and graded exercises to improve muscle strength around the involved joint.
4. Advise putting joints through range of motion after periods of inactivity (eg, automobile ride).

C. *Promoting Independence in Activities of Daily Living*
1. Suggest performing important activities in morning, after stiffness has been abated and before fatigue and pain become a problem.
2. Advise on modifications, such as wearing looser clothing without buttons, placing bench in tub or shower for bathing, sitting at table or counter in kitchen to prepare meals.
3. Help with obtaining assistive devices, such as padded handles for utensils and grooming aids, to promote independence.
4. Refer to occupational therapy for additional assistance.

Patient Education/Health Maintenance

1. Suggest swimming or water aerobics (offered by the YMCA) as a form of nonstressful exercise to preserve mobility.
2. Encourage adequate diet and sleep to enhance general health.
3. Refer for additional information and support to local chapter of the Arthritis Foundation.

Evaluation

A. Reports reduction in pain while ambulatory
B. Performs range-of-motion exercises
C. Dresses, bathes self, and grooms with assistive devices

◆ BONE TUMORS

Musculoskeletal neoplasms include primary sarcomas, metastatic bone disease, and benign tumors of the bone.

Pathophysiology/Etiology

A. *Benign Bone Tumors*   Osteoid osteoma, chondroma, and osteoclastoma (benign giant cell tumor) are examples of benign bone tumors. Malignant transformation occurs with some.

B. *Malignant Bone Tumors*
1. Chondrosarcoma and osteosarcoma are examples of primary malignant bone tumors. Hematogenous spread to the lung occurs.
2. Multiple myeloma is a malignant neoplasm arising from the bone marrow.

C. *Metastatic Bone Tumors*
1. Metastatic bone tumors are most frequently associated with cancers of the breast, prostate, and lung (primary malignancy site).
2. Bone metastasis most frequently occurs in the vertebrae and results in pathologic fracture.

Clinical Manifestations

1. Pain in the involved bone—from effects of tumor (destruction, erosion, and expansion of tumor)
   a. Generally mild to constant pain, which may be worse at night or with activity
   b. Pain will be acute with fracture
   c. Neurologic symptoms may present with nerve root compression
2. Swelling and limitation of motion and joint effusion
3. *Physical findings*
   a. Palpable, tender, fixed bony mass
   b. Increase in skin temperature over mass
   c. Superficial veins dilated and prominent

Diagnostic Evaluation

1. X-ray will usually reveal bone tumor; may show increased or decreased bone density.
2. Computed tomography (CT) and/or MRI demonstrate soft tissue involvement and location of tumor(s).
3. Bone scan—helpful in detecting initial extent of malignancy, planning therapy, defining level of amputation, and following course of radiation/chemotherapy
4. Serum alkaline phosphatase—usually increased
5. Bence Jones protein in urine with multiple myeloma
6. Biopsy of bone—to confirm suspected diagnosis
7. Chest x-ray and lung scan—to determine if metastases are present
8. Arteriography—to assess soft tissue involvement

Management

A multidisciplinary approach in a cancer center is often preferred. The basic objective is to halt the progression of the tumor by destroying or removing the lesion. Treatment depends on the type of tumor. Combinations of chemotherapy, surgery, and/or radiation may be indicated as most appropriate for specific type of tumor.

A. *Surgery*
1. Tumor curettage or resection with bone grafting may be used.
2. Limb-salvaging procedures involve resection of affected bone and surrounding normal muscle tissue and reconstruction using metallic prostheses or allografts for bone/joint replacement and skin grafting, as needed.
3. Amputation is necessary in some cases.

B. *Chemotherapy* May be used as preoperative, adjunctive, and palliative treatment

1. Chemotherapy may be administered before (to shrink the tumor) and after (to destroy metastases) surgery.
2. Chemotherapy used in combination to achieve a greater patient response at a lower toxicity rate and to minimize potential problems of drug resistance and may be given in varying courses separated by rest periods.

C. *Radiotherapy*
1. Tumor irradiation may be used.
2. Prophylactic lung irradiation may be performed—to suppress metastases.

D. *Other Therapies*
1. Immunotherapeutic approach may be selected.
2. Hormone therapy may be used with metastatic tumors of the breast and prostate.
3. If pathologic fracture occurs, the fracture is managed with open reduction and internal fixation or other fracture treatment method.

Complications

1. Lack of tumor control and metastases
2. Pathologic fracture
3. Hypercalcemia from bone destruction

Nursing Assessment

1. Obtain history of progression of disease; presence of pain, fever, weight loss, malaise.
2. Examine for painless mass.
3. Review records for evidence of pathologic fracture.
4. Assess knowledge of cancer, experiences with family or others, and present coping.

Nursing Diagnoses

A. Pain related to effects of tumor
B. Risk for trauma related to altered bone structure
C. Ineffective Individual Coping related to diagnosis and treatment options

Nursing Interventions

See also Orthopedic Surgery, p. 857, and Amputation, p. 861.

A. *Relieving Pain*
1. Use multiple approaches to reduce discomfort.
2. Administer pain medications $\frac{1}{2}$ hour before ambulation or other uncomfortable movement.
3. Support painful extremities on pillows.

B. *Preventing Pathologic Fractures*
1. Assist the patient in movement with gentleness and patience.
2. Avoid jarring the patient or bed.
3. Support joints when repositioning the patient.
4. Guard the patient to avoid falls.
5. Create a hazard-free environment.

C. *Strengthening Coping Abilities*
1. Create a supportive environment.
2. Use psychological support services as needed.
3. Answer questions and clear up misconceptions about treatment options.

Patient Education/Health Maintenance

1. Teach about particular treatment selected. See p. 102 for information on chemotherapy, and p. 111 for radiation therapy information.
2. Encourage appropriate follow-up and diagnostic testing for recurrence.
3. Refer for additional information and support to: American Cancer Society; 19 West 56th Street; New York, NY 10019; 212-586-8700.

Evaluation

A. Reports decreased pain with ambulation
B. No signs or symptoms of fractures
C. Verbalizes understanding of treatment options and strength to make decisions

Selected References

Cunningham, M.E. (1994). Bursitis and tendinitis. *Orthopaedic Nursing, 13*(5), 13-16.

Fecht-Gramley, M.E. (1994). Emergency! Recognizing compartment syndrome. *AJN, 94*(10), 41.

Maher, A., Salmond, S., & Pellino, T. (Eds.). (1993). *Orthopaedic nursing.* Philadelphia: Saunders.

Polan, M.L. (1995). Value of early screening for osteoporosis. *Contemporary Nurse Practioner, 1*(1), 19–25.

Rodts, M.F. (Ed.). (1991). Orthopaedic nursing, sports nursing. *Nursing Clinics of North America, 26*(1).

Salmond, S., Mooney, N.E., & Verdisco, L. (Eds.). (1991). *Core curriculum for orthopaedic nursing in edition.* 2nd Ed. Pitman, NJ: National Association of Orthopaedic Nurses.

Styreula, L. (1995). Traction basics: Part III, types of traction. *Orthopaedic Nursing, 13*(4), 34–44.

◆

Integumentary Disorders

Dermatologic Disorders

General Overview

◆ DESCRIPTION OF SKIN LESIONS

Dermatologic conditions are usually described by the type of lesion that appears on the skin as well as their shape and configuration. See Figure 30-1 for types of skin lesions.

Primary Lesions

1. Macula—flat, circumscribed discoloration of skin; may have any size or shape.
2. Papule—solid, elevated lesion less than 1 cm (0.4 in.) in diameter.
3. Nodule—raised, solid lesion larger than 1 cm (0.4 in.) in diameter.
4. Vesicle—circumscribed elevated lesion less than 1 cm (0.4 in.) that contains fluid.
5. Bulla—a vesicle or blister larger than 1 cm (0.4 in.) in diameter.
6. Pustule—circumscribed raised lesion that contains pus; may form as a result of purulent changes in a vesicle.
7. Wheal—elevation of the skin lasting less than 24 hours caused by edema of the dermis; may be surrounding erythema or blanching.
8. Plaque—solid, elevated lesion on the skin or mucous membrane, larger than 1 cm (0.4 in.) in its largest diameter; psoriasis is commonly manifested as plaques on the skin; leukoplakia is an example of plaques on mucous membranes.
9. Cyst—soft or firm mass in the skin filled with semisolid or liquid material contained in a sac.

Secondary Lesions

Secondary lesions involve changes that take place in primary lesions that modify them.

1. Scales—heaped-up, horny layers of dead epidermis; may develop as a result of inflammatory changes.
2. Crusts—covering formed by the drying of serum, blood, or pus on the skin.
3. Excoriations—linear scratch marks or traumatized area of skin.
4. Fissures—cracks in the skin, usually from marked drying and long-standing inflammation.
5. Ulcer—lesion formed by local destruction of the epidermis and part or all of the underlying dermis.
6. Lichenification—thickening of skin accompanied by accentuation of skin markings.
7. Scar—new formation of connective tissue that replaces the loss of substance in the dermis as a result of injury or disease.
8. Atrophy—diminution in size or loss of skin cells causing thinning of the skin.

Shape and Configuration

After the type of lesion is identified, the shape, configuration or arrangement (in relation to each other), and their pattern of distribution is noted (Fig. 30-2). The following are descriptions frequently used:

Annular—ring-shaped
Circinate—circular
Confluent—lesions run together or join
Discoid—disk-shaped
Discrete—lesions remain separate
Generalized—widespread eruption
Grouped—clustering of lesions
Guttate—droplike
Herpetiform—grouped vesicles
Iris—ring or a series of concentric circles
Linear—in lines
Multiform—more than one kind of skin lesion
Nummular—coin-shaped
Polymorphous—occurring in several or many forms
Reticulated—lacelike network
Serpiginous—snakelike or creeping eruption
Telangiectasia—tiny, superficial, dilated cutaneous vessel; can be seen as a red thread or line
Zosteriform or dermatomal—bandlike distribution limited to one or more dermatomes of skin

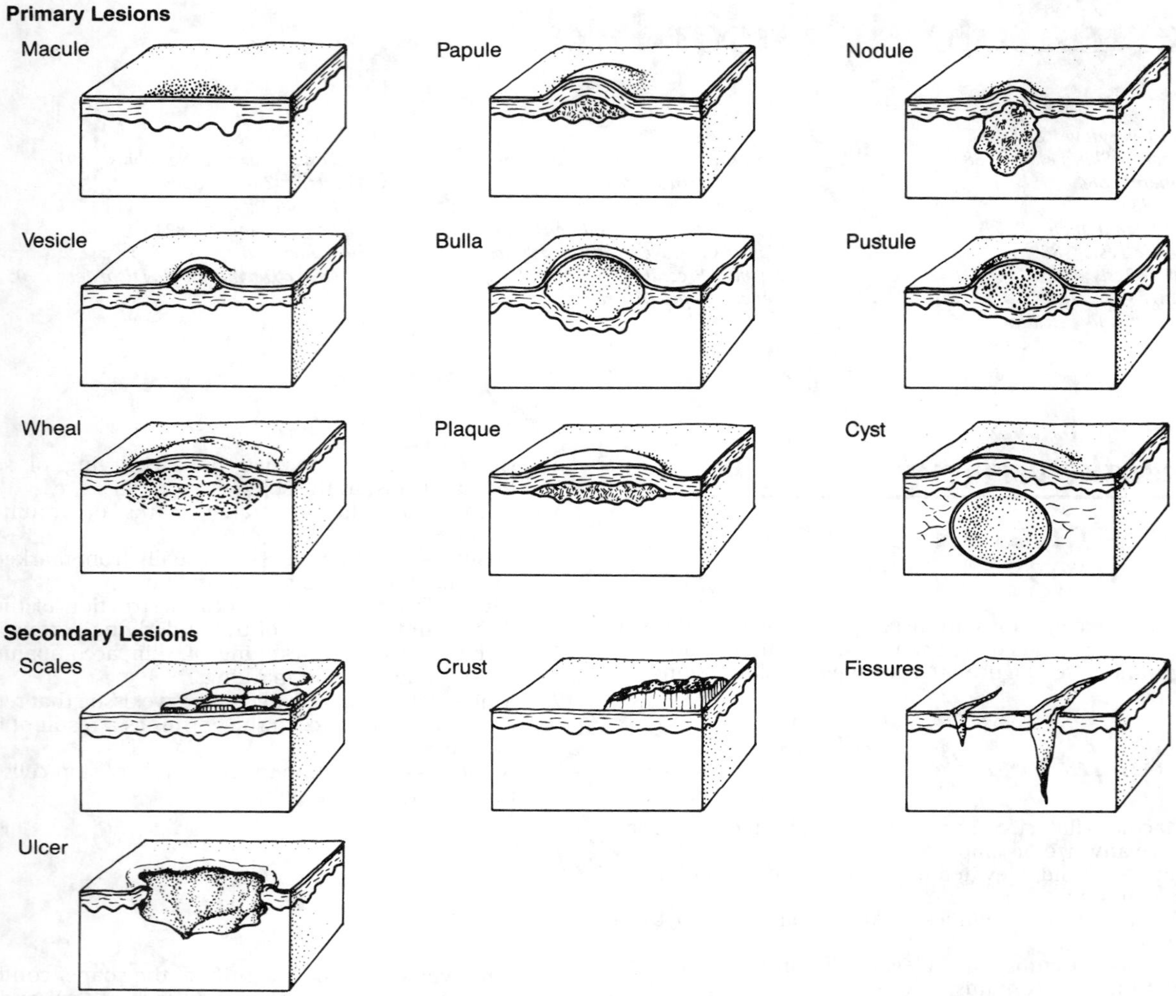

Primary Lesions

Macule

Papule

Nodule

Vesicle

Bulla

Pustule

Wheal

Plaque

Cyst

Secondary Lesions

Scales

Crust

Fissures

Ulcer

FIGURE 30-1 *Types of skin lesions. (From Smeltzer, S.C. and Bare, B.G. (1996). Textbook of medical-surgical nursing (8th ed). Philadelphia, JB Lippincott.)*

Assessment

◆ HISTORY

By obtaining a history of rash or other complaints related to dermatologic conditions, you will understand characteristics of the problem and their effect on the patient that will help in planning care.

Characteristics of Rash

1. When did the rash first occur? Was the onset sudden or gradual?
2. What site was first affected? Describe the spread and severity.
3. What was the color and configuration of the rash initially? Has it changed?
4. Is there associated itching, burning, tingling, pain, or numbness?
5. Has it been constant or intermittent?

Associated Factors

1. What makes the rash worse or better? Is it seasonal? Affected by stress?
2. What medications are being taken? What topical products have been used? What effect did they have?
3. What skin products are used? What chemicals have come into contact with the skin, such as laundry detergent, cleaning products, insecticides.
4. Has there been pet contact?
5. What is the patient's occupation? Any hobbies, such as gardening or hiking?
6. What is the sexual history and chance of sexually transmitted disease exposure?

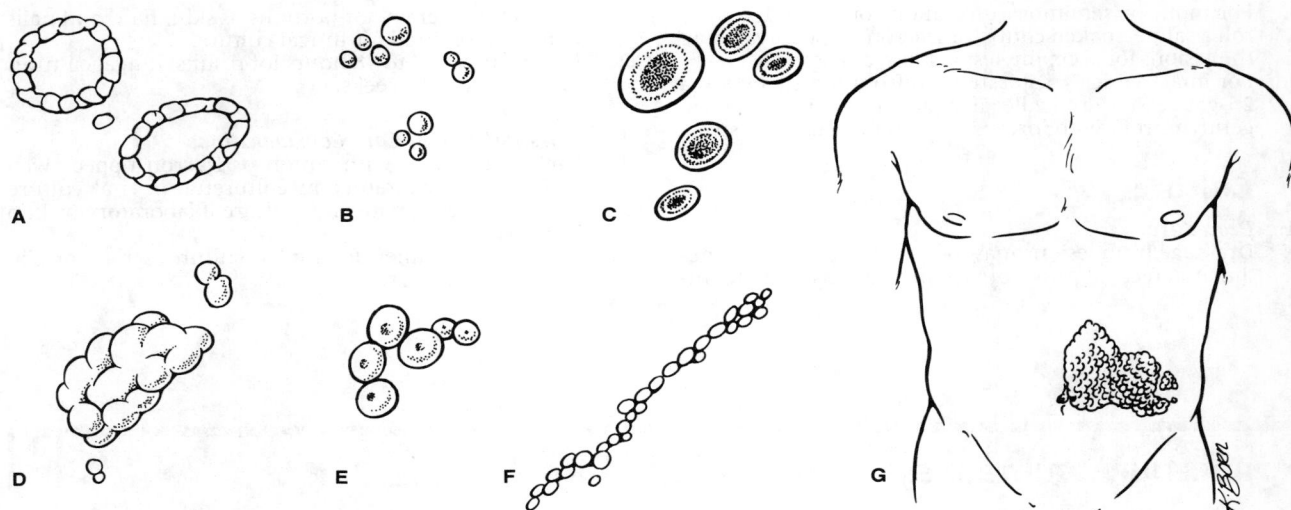

FIGURE 30-2 *Shape and arrangement of skin lesions:* **(A)** *annular;* **(B)** *grouped;* **(C)** *iris;* **(D)** *confluent;* **(E)** *herpetiform;* **(F)** *linear;* **(G)** *zosteriform.*

Medical History

1. Is there a history of hay fever, asthma, hives, eczema, or allergies?
2. Has the patient had this particular rash or other skin disorders in the past?
3. What is the family history of skin disorders?
4. Are there any chronic medical problems?

◆ PHYSICAL EXAMINATION

Focus your examination on the skin, hair, and nails. Some dermatologic conditions affect other body systems, however, so perform a general physical exam as indicated.

Examination of the Skin, Hair, and Nails

1. Ask the patient to show you the area of concern and examine the skin surface under good lighting conditions. You may have to examine the entire skin if the condition is generalized.
2. Note the distribution and configuration of skin lesions. Compare right and left sides of the body.
3. Note the shape, border, texture, and surface of the lesions.
4. Palpate the lesions for texture, warmth, and tenderness.
5. Use a metric ruler to determine size of lesions and to serve as a baseline for comparison with subsequent measurements.
6. Examine the scalp, nails, and oral mucosa.
7. Perform diascopy—gently press a glass slide or Lucite rule over a skin lesion to detect blanching (caused by dilated blood vessels).
8. Use a Wood's light to inspect for fluorescent changes with some fungal infections.
9. For dark-skinned individuals, look for black, purple, or gray lesions and palpate carefully to determine if rash is present.

Diagnostic Tests

◆ LABORATORY TESTS

Some dermatologic conditions can be evaluated by laboratory tests of microscopy and culture. See Procedure Guidelines 30-1: Skin Scrapings for Scabies, to obtain a skin scraping for scabies.

Microscopy

A. **Description**
1. A sample is taken by scraping, swabbing, or aspirating a skin lesion and transferred to a glass slide for direct observation or staining.
   a. Direct visualization of scrapings mixed with mineral oil for visualization of scabies mites or the nits of lice clinging to hair.
   b. A Tzanck smear is obtained from vesicular fluid or a moist ulcer and stained to detect characteristics of herpes simplex virus, herpes zoster, and varicella (chicken pox).
   c. Potassium hydroxide may be added to skin scrapings on a glass slide and heated to dissolve skin cells to detect hyphae and spores in fungal infections.
   d. Gram stain may be performed to tentatively identify bacteria in certain skin infections.

B. **Nursing/Patient Care Considerations**
1. Use the side of a glass slide or a scalpel held at a 45-degree angle to gently scrape the skin of a dry lesion or inflamed area; only mild discomfort and pinpoint bleeding should occur.

2. For moist or semimoist ulcerations or crusted lesions, roll a saline-soaked cotton or Dacron-tipped swab over the lesion; for weeping lesions, use a dry swab.

3. For intact vesicles, aspirate fluid from the edge with a 25-gauge sterile needle; if vesicle is partially broken, gently unroof with forceps and obtain fluid on a swab.

Culture

A. *Procedure*

1. Drainage from lesions may be cultured on specific media to detect causative organism and sensitivity to an-

timicrobial therapy, or portions of skin, hair, and nails may be submitted for fungal culture.

2. Usually takes 24 to 48 hours for results; fungal cultures may take 4 to 5 weeks.

B. *Nursing/Patient Care Considerations*

1. Obtain specimen with cotton or Dacron-tipped swab and send to laboratory in culturette or viral culture container; refrigerate viral culture if laboratory pickup is delayed.

2. To obtain specimen for fungal culture, scrape or clip the affected skin, hair, or nails.

PROCEDURE GUIDELINES 30-1 ◆ Skin Scrapings for Scabies

PURPOSE   To demonstrate the mite *Sarcoptes scabiei* (or its ova or feces) in skin scrapings removed from burrows or papules.

EQUIPMENT   Hand lens
Mineral oil in dropper bottle
Scalpel and scalpel blade, No. 15
Glass slide/coverslip
Microscope

PROCEDURE | *NURSING ACTION* | *RATIONALE*

PREPARATORY PHASE

1. Place a small drop of oil in the middle of a glass slide.

PERFORMANCE PHASE

1. Inspect for the burrows of Sarcoptes scabiei *on webs of fingers, lower abdomen, pubic and axillary areas, legs, arms (see accompanying figure).*

1. The female scabies mite, ova, and fecal deposits may be found in burrows on the skin.

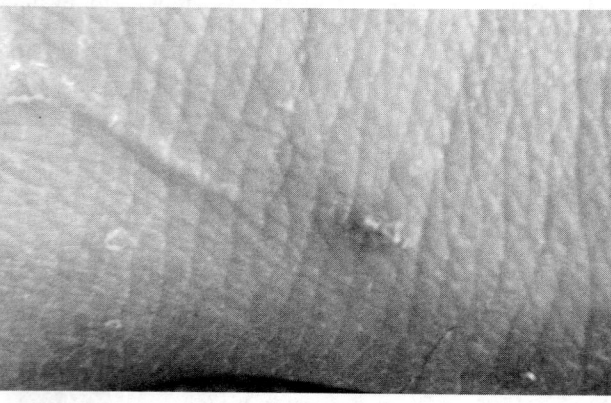

Burrow in the epidermis made by the mite Sarcoptes scabiei. (Photo courtesy Michael Rosenbaum, M.D.)

2. Apply a small amount of mineral oil on unexcoriated burrows or papule.

2. The mineral oil causes the mite to float and enhances visualization.

3. Scrape the involved skin with the scalpel blade.

4. Transfer the scrapings to the prepared glass slide and apply coverslip; or pick out the mite with a disposable needle and transfer it to a glass slide.

4. To avoid air bubble.

5. Examine the slide with a scanning lens of the microscope.

5. Look for the mites, eggs, egg casings, and fecal pellets (which outnumber living organisms).

◆ OTHER TESTS

Patch Testing

A. Description
1. A series of suspected allergens are applied to the skin on patches and inspected 48 hours later for reaction; documents the cause of contact dermatitis or allergy.

B. Nursing/Patient Care Considerations
1. Do not apply allergens to inflamed skin, because testing will exacerbate condition.
2. Apply patches to clean, dry, hairless skin on the back or ventral surface of the forearm that has been prepared by blotting with adhesive tape 10 to 12 times to remove the outer layers of epidermis.
3. Remove patches after 48 hours and note redness, inflammation, or induration; observe 48 hours later for delayed reaction.
4. Remove patches immediately if pain, pruritus, or irritation develops.

Skin Biopsy

A. Procedure
1. Removal of a piece of skin by shave, punch, or excision technique to detect malignancy or other characteristics of skin disorders.
   a. Shave biopsy—scalpel used to remove raised lesions, leaving lower layers of dermis intact.
   b. Punch biopsy—special instrument used to remove round core of lesion, containing all layers of skin. Core is usually closed with sutures.
   c. Excisional biopsy—scalpel and scissors used to remove entire lesion; suturing required.

B. Nursing/Patient Care Considerations
1. Position the patient comfortably with the site exposed, and explain that a local anesthetic will be given.
2. After the biopsy, apply pressure to the site to stop bleeding and apply a dressing.
3. Place the biopsy specimen in a container with 10% formaldehyde and transport it to the lab.

General Procedures/Treatment Modalities

◆ BATHS AND WET DRESSINGS

A therapeutic bath is used to apply medication to the entire skin surface and is useful in treating widespread eruptions and general pruritus. Baths soothe, soften, reduce inflammation, and relieve itching and dryness. See Table 30-1 for types and desired effects. Wet dressings and soaks are damp compresses containing water, normal saline solution, aluminum acetate solution, or magnesium sulfate solution.

TABLE 30-1 Therapeutic Baths

Bath Solution and Medication	Desired Effect
Water	To remove crusts and relieve inflammation
Saline	Used for widely disseminated lesions
Colloidal—oatmeal or Aveeno	Antipruritic and demulcent
Sodium bicarbonate	Cooling
Starch	Soothing
Tar baths (follow package directions) Alma-Tar, Balnetar, Lavatar, Polytar	Tar baths are used for psoriasis and chronic eczematous conditions
Bath oils Alpha-keri, Lubath, Nutraderm	Bath oils are used for antipruritic and emollient soothing properties
Bath Oil	Used for acute and subacute eczematous eruptions

They may be either sterile or unsterile, warm or cool, depending on the skin condition and area to which their applied.

Therapeutic Baths

A. Indications
1. Vesicular, bullous, and ulcerative disorders.
2. Acute inflammatory conditions.
3. Erosions and exudative, crusted surfaces.

B. Nursing/Patient Care Considerations
1. Prepare the bath or teach the patient to prepare a warm bath at 32°C to 38°C (90°F–100°F) and with the tub half full, to add the prescribed quantity of medication, and to mix thoroughly to prevent sensitivity reaction.
2. Rub the skin gently after 15 minutes to remove loosened scales, if indicated; do not rub inflamed skin.
3. Keep the room and water at comfortable temperatures and limit bathing to 20 to 30 minutes; the bath area should be well ventilated if tars are used, because they are volatile.

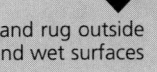

COMMUNITY-BASED CARE TIP:
Tell the patient to use a bath mat inside the tub and rug outside the tub, because medication may make the tub and wet surfaces slippery.

4. Blot skin dry with a towel and apply emollient or topical medication to moist skin, if prescribed.

Open Wet Dressings

A. Indications
1. Bacterial infections that require drainage.

2. Inflammatory and pruritic conditions.
3. Oozing and crusting conditions.

B. *Nursing/Patient Care Considerations*
1. Apply dressing to affected area or teach patient to apply and moisten to the point of slight dripping; remoisten as necessary.
2. Apply ice cubes to solution if cooling is desired; use warm tap water if warming is desired.
3. Rewarm or cool every 5 minutes, because compresses reach body temperature quickly.
4. Apply for 15 minutes three to four times a day unless otherwise indicated.
5. Keep the patient warm and do not treat more than one-third of body at a time, because open wet dressings can cause chilling and hypothermia.

COMMUNITY-BASED CARE TIP:
Prevent burns by measuring temperature of solution with a bath thermometer or testing tap water on wrist before applying compress. Do not use microwave ovens to warm dressings, because uneven heating can occur.

◆ DRESSINGS FOR SKIN CONDITIONS

Occlusive Dressing

An occlusive dressing is formed by an airtight plastic or vinyl film applied over medicated skin (usually corticosteroids) to enhance absorption of medication and promote moisture retention.

A. *Indications*
1. Skin conditions with thick scaling, such as psoriasis.

B. *Nursing/Patient Care Considerations*
1. Wash area and pat dry.
2. Apply medication while skin is still moist.
3. Cover with plastic wrap, vinyl gloves, plastic bag.
4. Seal with paper tape at edges or cover with other dressing to hold in place.

NURSING ALERT:
Excessive use of occlusive dressings containing corticosteroids may cause skin atrophy, striae, telangiectasia, folliculitis, non-healing ulceration, erythema, and systemic absorption of corticosteroids.
  Do not apply to ulcerated or abraded skin, remove within 12 to 24 hours, and do not apply with high-potency corticosteroids.

Other Dressings

Other dressing materials may be used as dry dressings to protect the skin, keep affected areas clean, and absorb drainage or to cover medication or hold occlusive dressings in place.

A. *Nursing/Patient Care Considerations*
1. Apply dry gauze dressing using clean technique (unless sterile technique is indicated by open wounds).
2. Wrap extremities with elastic or cotton-rolled bandages or apply tape.

COMMUNITY-BASED CARE TIP:
Advise patient to use alternative dressing materials, such as disposable gloves for the hands, cotton socks for the feet, sheets or towels for large areas, disposable diapers or towels folded in diaper fashion for the groin, washcloths for the axilla, cotton T-shirt or cotton pajamas for the trunk, turban or plastic shower cap for the scalp, or mask made from gauze for the face with holes cut for the eyes, mouth, and nose.

◆ WOUND COVERAGE: GRAFTS AND FLAPS

Wound coverage using grafts and flaps is a type of reconstructive (plastic) surgery performed to improve the skin's appearance and function.

Description

A. *Skin Graft*
1. A section of skin tissue is separated from its blood supply and transferred as free tissue to a distant (recipient) site; it must obtain nourishment from capillaries at the recipient site.
2. In dermatology, skin grafting is used to repair defects resulting from excision of skin tumors and to cover areas of denuded skin.
3. Definitions
   a. *Autografts*—grafts done with tissue transplanted from the patient's own skin.
   b. *Allografts*—involve the transplant of tissue from one individual of the same species; these grafts are also called *allogenic* or *homografts*.
   c. *Xenograft* or *heterograft*—involves the transfer of tissue from another species.
4. Classification by thickness
   a. *Split thickness* (thin, intermediate, or thick)—graft that is cut at varying thicknesses and is used to cover large wounds or defects for which a full-thickness graft or application is impractical.
   b. *Full thickness*—graft consists of epidermis and all of the dermis without the underlying fat; used to cover wounds that are too large to close primarily. They are used frequently to cover facial defects, because they neither contract nor develop unsightly pigmentation.

B. *Skin Flaps*
1. A *flap* is a segment of tissue that has been left attached at one end (called a *base* or *pedicle*), while the other end has been moved to a recipient area. It is dependent for its survival on functioning arterial and venous blood supplies and lymphatic drainage in its pedicle or base.
   a. *Free flap* or free-tissue transfer—one that is completely severed from the body and is transferred to another site; receives early vascular supply from mi-

crovascular anastomosis with vessels at recipient site.
2. Flaps may consist of skin, mucosa, muscle, adipose tissue, omentum, and bone.
3. Used for wound coverage and to provide bulk, especially when bone, tendon, blood vessels, or nerve tissue is exposed.
4. Flaps offer the best aesthetic solution, because a flap retains the color and texture of the donor area.
5. Flaps are classified according to the method of movement, composition, location, or function.

Preoperative Management/ Nursing Care

1. Explain the procedure to the patient.
   a. Graft obtained by razor blade, skin-grafting knife, electric or air-powered dermatome/drum dermatome.
   b. Skin is taken from the "donor" or "host" site and applied to the wound/defect site, called the "recipient site" or "graft bed."
   c. Process of revascularization and reattachment of the skin graft to the recipient bed is referred to as a "take."
   d. Series of operations may be required for some types of flaps.
2. Maintain clean and dry donor and recipient sites; cleanse as prescribed.

Postoperative Management/ Nursing Care

Educate the patient on the following care:

1. Keep the affected part immobilized as much as possible.
2. Keep the affected extremity elevated, as the new capillary connections are fragile and excess venous pressure may cause rupture. Wear an elastic stocking to counteract venous pressure.
3. Inspect the dressing daily. Report unusual drainage or signs of an inflammatory reaction.
4. After 2 to 3 weeks, mineral oil or a lanolin cream may be massaged around the wound to stimulate circulation.
5. Expect some loss of sensation in the grafted area for a time.

◆ AESTHETIC PROCEDURES (COSMETIC SURGERY)

Aesthetic procedures are a type of reconstructive (plastic) surgery performed to reconstruct or alter congenital or acquired defects or to restore or improve the body's appearance.

Description

Types of procedures include:

1. *Rhytidectomy*—(face lift) done through various techniques and incisions to alleviate skin folds and wrinkles to improve the appearance of the aging face.

2. *Blepharoplasty*—done by scalpel or carbon dioxide laser excision to remove excess skin or fat from the upper and lower eyelids.
3. *Dermabrasion*—(skin planing) uses a special instrument to abrade the skin and remove the epidermis and superficial dermis to improve the appearance.
4. *Body contouring*—(liposuction) reduces localized deposits of fat not amenable to weight loss, with a cannula aided by suction or fitted to a syringe; may be done on the face, neck, breasts, abdomen, flanks, hips, buttocks, and extremities.

Preoperative Management/ Nursing Care

Advise the patient of the following:

1. Local or general anesthetic will be administered.
2. Cleanse skin with antiseptic agent the night before surgery, if prescribed.
3. Make sure patient thoroughly understands procedure and has discussed the risks and benefits with the health care provider before surgery.

Postoperative Management/ Nursing Care

Provide the following patient education:

1. Expect the face or affected part to be swollen, bruised, and numb for several days to weeks.
2. Rest for 24 to 48 hours after the procedure.
3. Elevate the head at night for 2 weeks after the procedure.
4. Avoid bending and lifting following rhytidectomy, which may increase edema and provoke bleeding.
5. Apply iced gauze compresses to eyes to reduce edema after blepharoplasty.
6. After dermabrasion, do not pluck at crusts, because new epithelium will be injured; wash face and apply emollient as directed.
7. After liposuction, drink lots of fluids and avoid aspirin or ibuprofen for at least 1 week to prevent bleeding.
8. Notify the health care provider if sudden pain develops—suggests hematoma or abscess.
9. Cleanse face, apply emollient, perform massage, and avoid makeup as directed.
10. Avoid direct sunlight for 2 to 3 months and begin the practice of using sunscreen with sun protection factor of 15 or greater.

Complications

1. Hematoma formation
2. Necrosis, scarring, or irregularity of skin
3. Excessive bleeding
4. Partial facial paralysis with rhytidectomy
5. Abscess formation or wound infection

Dermatologic Disorders

◆ CELLULITIS

Cellulitis is an inflammation of the subcutaneous tissue of the skin.

Pathophysiology/Etiology

1. Caused by infection with group A beta-hemolytic streptococci, *Staphylococcus aureus, Haemophilus influenzae,* or other organisms.
2. Usually results from break in skin.
3. Infection can spread rapidly through lymphatic system.

Clinical Manifestations

1. Tender, warm, erythematous, and swollen area that is well demarcated.
2. Tender, warm, erythematous streak extending proximally from the area, indicating lymph vessel involvement.
3. Possible fluctuant abscess or purulent drainage.
4. Possible fever, chills, headache, malaise.

Diagnostic Evaluation

1. Gram stain and culture of drainage.
2. Blood cultures.

Management

1. Oral antibiotics (penicillinase-resistant penicillins, cephalosporins, or quinolones) may be adequate to treat small localized areas of cellulitis of legs or trunk.
2. Parenteral antibiotics may be needed for cellulitis of the hands, face, or lymphatic spread.
3. Surgical drainage and debridement for suppurative areas.

Complications

1. Tissue necrosis
2. Septicemia

Nursing Assessment

1. Obtain history of trauma to skin, needle stick, insect bite, or wound.

2. Observe for expanding borders and lymphatic streaking; palpate for fluctuance of abscess formation.
3. Watch for signs of antibiotic sensitivity—shortness of breath, urticaria, angioedema, measleslike skin rash, or severe skin reaction, such as erythema multiforme or toxic epidermal necrolysis.

Nursing Diagnoses

A. Risk for Impaired Skin Integrity related to infectious process
B. Pain related to inflammation of subcutaneous tissue

Nursing Interventions

A. *Protecting Skin Integrity*
1. Administer, or teach patient to administer, antibiotics as prescribed; teach dosage schedule and side effects.
2. Maintain intravenous infusion or venous access to administer intravenous antibiotics, if indicated.
3. Elevate affected extremity to promote drainage from area.
4. Administer warm soaks to relieve inflammation and promote drainage.
5. Prepare patient for surgical drainage and debridement, if necessary.

B. *Relieving Pain*
1. Encourage comfortable position and immobilization of affected area.
2. Administer, or teach patient to administer, analgesics as prescribed; monitor for side effects.
3. Use bed cradle to relieve pressure from bed covers.

Patient Education/Health Maintenance

1. Ensure that patient understands dosage schedule of antibiotics and the importance of complying with therapy to prevent complications.
2. Advise patient to notify health care provider immediately if condition worsens; hospitalization may be necessary.
3. Outpatient-treated cellulitis should be observed within 48 hours of starting antibiotics to determine adequacy of treatment.
4. Teach patients with impaired circulation or sensation proper skin care and inspection of skin for trauma.

Evaluation

A. Skin is normal color and temperature, nontender, nonswollen, and intact
B. Patient actively moving extremity; verbalizes no pain

◆ TOXIC EPIDERMAL NECROLYSIS

Toxic epidermal necrolysis is a severe, potentially fatal skin disease associated with erythema and epidermal sloughing.

Pathophysiology/Etiology

1. Exact mechanism is unknown but can be induced by a variety of drugs, including sulfonimides, anticonvulsants, nonsteroidal anti-inflammatory agents, and vaccines.
2. Resembles second-degree burns with sloughing of skin at epidermal/dermal junction.

Clinical Manifestations

1. Malaise, fatigue, vomiting, and diarrhea may be prodromal symptoms.
2. Sudden onset of urticaria and erythema, then large bullae appear.
3. Within hours coma may develop; fever.
4. Bullae become confluent and slough in large sheets, leaving moist, erythematous surface.
5. Positive Nikolsky's sign (desquamation of skin on light pressure).
6. Ulceration of lips and buccal mucosa; conjunctivitis.

Diagnostic Evaluation

1. Skin pathology to determine level of separation.
2. Possible cultures of blood and body fluids to differentiate infection.

Management

1. Treatment in intensive care unit or regional burn center, because toxic epidermal necrolysis has similar pathophysiologic characteristics to those of extensive burns.
2. Treatment of affected skin:
   a. Wounds are cleansed in operating room with anesthesia; loose skin and blisters removed, necrotic areas debrided to prevent infection.
   b. Temporary biologic dressings (porcine cutaneous xenographs, amnion, collagen-based skin substitute, or plastic semipermeable dressings) applied to prevent secondary skin infection while awaiting reepithelialization.
3. All nonessential drugs are stopped immediately.
4. Fluid replacement therapy, as necessary, and possible enteral nutrition if extensive oral involvement.
5. Topical antimicrobial dressings to enhance reepithelialization.
6. Ophthalmologic examination and removal of corneal adhesions as necessary.

Complications

1. Sepsis
2. Pneumonia
3. Blindness

Nursing Assessment

1. Obtain medication and immunization history.
2. Monitor vital signs and level of consciousness closely, because condition is rapidly progressive.
3. Monitor fluid and nutritional status through daily weight, vital signs, and laboratory test results (electrolytes, blood urea nitrogen and creatinine, albumin and total protein).

Nursing Diagnoses

A. Impaired Skin Integrity related to sloughing
B. Risk for Fluid Volume Deficit related to transudation of fluid into bullae
C. Pain related to exposed dermal nerve endings
D. Altered Oral Mucous Membranes related to oral lesions

Nursing Interventions

A. Restoring Skin Integrity
1. Place patient on warmed air-fluidized bed to distribute weight with minimal shearing forces.
2. Use extreme care in handling patient, because skin is very fragile; obtain assistance in moving patient.
3. Gently apply warm, wet compresses of prescribed antiseptic solution to reduce bacterial population of wound surface.
4. Inspect xenograft several times daily for dislodgement or purulence; these will require new xenograft.
5. Watch for new areas of toxic epidermal necrolysis; note and record progression of skin slough and chart progress.
6. Patient should be in private room on reverse isolation to prevent infection.
7. Provide nutritional supplements through enteral feeding to ensure healing.

B. Maintaining Fluid Balance
1. Monitor vital signs for falling blood pressure or rising pulse, indicating hypovolemia; use an indwelling arterial catheter to avoid cuff pressure on the skin.
2. Measure hourly urine output.
3. Weigh patient daily.
4. Give intravenous fluids as prescribed.
5. Assess bowel sounds and give oral fluids as tolerated.

C. Reducing Pain
1. If patient is unable to verbalize, watch for facial expressions, guarding, or increased pulse and respirations to indicate pain.

2. Administer analgesics as prescribed and as required, possibly around the clock; monitor for side effects and document effectiveness.
3. Provide distraction through music or other measures to promote relaxation.
4. Provide emotional support and encouragement.

D. *Protecting Mucous Membranes*
1. Use meticulous oral hygiene:
   a. Inspect oral cavity daily; note any changes.
   b. Rinse mouth with normal saline, diluted hydrogen peroxide, or other solution to remove debris and cleanse ulcerations.
   c. Apply petroleum jelly or other lubricant/protectant to cracked, swollen lips.
2. Assess urethral, vaginal, and anal regions for ulcerations or bleeding.
3. Inspect eyes and remove crusts from eyelid margins using damp compresses or saline-soaked swabs; apply eyedrops as prescribed.

Patient Education

1. Advise patient to use sunscreen of at least 15 sun protection factor and avoid direct sunlight during the healing phase, and continue to use sunscreen.
2. Advise patient to avoid suspected medication in the future.

Evaluation

A. New epithelium noted without scarring
B. Output equals input; weight and vital signs remain stable
C. Patient verbalizes reduced pain
D. Oral mucosa intact

◆ HERPES ZOSTER

Herpes zoster (shingles) is an inflammatory condition in which a virus produces a painful vesicular eruption along the distribution of the nerves from one or more dorsal root ganglia. The prevalence increases with age.

Pathophysiology/Etiology

1. Caused by a varicella-zoster virus, which is a member of a group of DNA viruses.
2. Virus is identical to the causative agent of varicella (chicken pox). After the primary infection, the varicella-zoster virus may persist in a dormant state in the dorsal nerve root ganglia. The virus may emerge from this site in later years, either spontaneously or in association with immunosuppression, to cause herpes zoster.

Clinical Manifestations

1. Eruption may be accompanied or preceded by fever, malaise, headache, and pain; pain may be burning, lancinating, stabbing, or aching.
2. Inflammation is usually unilateral, involving the cranial, cervical, thoracic, lumbar, or sacral nerves in a bandlike configuration.
3. Vesicles appear in 3 to 4 days.
   a. Characteristic patches of grouped vesicles appear on erythematous, edematous skin.
   b. Early vesicles contain serum; they later rupture and form crusts; scarring usually does not occur unless the vesicles are deep and involve the dermis.
   c. If ophthalmic branch of the facial nerve is involved, patient may have a painful eye.
   d. In normal host, lesions resolve in 2 to 3 weeks.
4. A susceptible person can acquire chicken pox if he or she comes in contact with the infective vesicular fluid of a zoster patient. A person with a history of chicken pox is immune and thus is not at risk from infection after exposure to zoster patients.

NURSING ALERT:
Varicella-zoster virus may be a life-threatening condition to the patient who is immunosuppressed, who is receiving cytotoxic chemotherapy, or who is a bone marrow transplant recipient.

Diagnostic Evaluation

1. Culture of varicella-zoster virus from lesions or detection by fluorescent antibody techniques, including viral detection using monoclonal antibodies (MicroTrak).

Management

1. Antiviral drugs, particularly acyclovir (Zovirax), interfere with viral replication; may be used in all cases but especially for treatment of immunosuppressed and/or debilitated patients.
2. Corticosteroids *early* in illness—given for severe herpes zoster if symptomatic measures fail; given for anti-inflammatory effect and relief of pain. Controversial.
3. Pain management; aspirin, acetaminophen, nonsteroidal anti-inflammatory drugs, narcotics—useful during the acute stage, but not generally effective for postherpetic neuralgia.

Complications

1. Chronic pain syndrome (post-herpetic neuralgia) characterized by constant aching and burning pain or intermittent lancinating pain or hyperesthesia of affected skin after it has healed.

2. Ophthalmic complications with involvement of ophthalmic branch of trigeminal nerve with keratitis, uveitis, corneal ulceration, and possibly blindness.
3. Facial and auditory nerve involvement resulting in hearing deficits, vertigo, and facial weakness.
4. Visceral dissemination—pneumonitis, esophagitis, enterocolitis, myocarditis, pancreatitis.

Nursing Diagnoses

A. Pain related to inflammation of cutaneous nerve endings
B. Impaired Skin Integrity related to rupture of vesicles

Nursing Interventions

A. *Controlling Pain*
1. Assess patient's level of discomfort and medicate as prescribed; monitor for side effects of pain medications.
2. Teach patient to apply wet dressings for soothing effect.
3. Encourage diversional activities.
4. Teach relaxation techniques, such as deep breathing, progressive muscle relaxation, and imagery to help control pain.

B. *Improving Skin Integrity*
1. Apply wet dressings to cool and dry inflamed areas by means of evaporation.
2. Apply lotions (calamine)—for cooling and soothing and drying effect of the powder that remains on skin after evaporation.
3. Apply antibacterial ointments (after acute stage) as prescribed to soften and separate adherent crusts and prevent secondary infection.

Patient Education/Health Maintenance

1. Teach patient to use proper hand-washing technique to avoid spreading herpes zoster virus.
2. Advise patient not to open the blisters to avoid secondary infection and scarring.
3. Reassure that shingles is a viral infection of the nerves; "nervousness" does not cause shingles.
4. A caregiver may be required to assist with dressings and meals. In older persons, the pain is more pronounced and incapacitating. Dysesthesia and skin hypersensitivity are distressing.

Evaluation

A. Patient verbalizes decreased pain
B. Reepithelialization of skin without scarring

◆ PEMPHIGUS

Pemphigus is a serious autoimmune disease of the skin and mucous membranes characterized by the appearance of blisters (bullae) of various sizes on apparently normal skin and mucous membranes (mouth, esophagus, conjunctiva, vagina) (Fig. 30-3). Familial benign chronic pemphigus (Hailey-Hailey disease) is a familial type of pemphigus appearing in adult life, affecting particularly the axillae and groin.

Pathophysiology/Etiology

1. The cause is unknown.
2. Certain drugs, other autoimmune diseases, and genetics may play a role in its development.
3. Many variants of pemphigus exist.

Clinical Manifestations

1. Initial lesions may appear in oral cavity; flaccid blisters (bullae) may arise on normal or erythematous skin.
   a. The bullae enlarge and rupture, forming painful raw and denuded areas that eventually become crusted.
   b. The eroded skin heals slowly; eventually, widespread areas of the body may become involved.
   c. In the mouth, the blisters are usually multiple, of varying size and irregular shape, painful, and persistent. Oral lesions may appear initially, along with lesions of the mucous membranes of the pharynx and esophagus; the conjunctivae, larynx, urethra, cervix, and rectum may be become affected as well.
2. An offensive odor may emanate from the bullae.

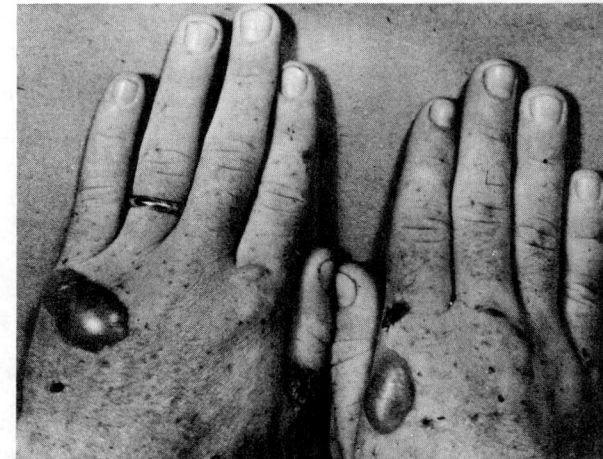

FIGURE 30-3 *Pemphigus—bullous dermatitis of hand (vesicles). (Photo courtesy Armed Forces Institute of Pathology)*

3. Positive Nikolsky's sign—separation of epidermis when minimal pressure is applied to the skin. Downward pressure on a bulla will cause it to expand laterally.

Diagnostic Evaluation

1. Skin biopsies of blisters and surrounding skin—demonstrates *acantholysis* (separation of epidermal cells from each other).
2. Immunofluorescent studies of serum—reveal circulating antibodies (pemphigus antibodies).

Management

1. Corticosteroids in large doses to control the disease and keep skin free of blisters.
2. Immunosuppressive agents such as cyclophosphamide (Cytoxan), azathioprine (Imuran) are used alone or in combination with steroids—for immunosuppressive and steroid-sparing effect.
3. Plasmapheresis—reinfusion of specially treated plasma cells; temporarily decreases serum level of antibodies.
4. Treatment of denuded skin.

Complications

1. Infections (skin, pneumonia, septicemia)
2. Psychosis
3. Side effects from corticosteroids; gastrointestinal bleeding; central nervous system toxicity; hyperglycemia

Nursing Diagnoses

A. Altered Oral Mucous Membrane related to ruptured bullae
B. Impaired Skin Integrity related to ruptured bullae
C. Risk for Fluid Volume Deficit related to transudation of fluid into bullae
D. Body Image Disturbance related to widespread or chronic skin lesions

Nursing Interventions

A. *Restoring Oral Mucous Membrane Integrity*
1. Inspect oral cavity daily; note and report any changes—oral lesions heal slowly.
2. Keep oral mucosa clean and allow regeneration of epithelium—secondary infection may be associated with offensive odor from oral lesions. *Candida albicans* infection of the mouth frequently seen in patients on high-dose steroid therapy; look for white patches.
3. Give topical oral therapy as directed.

4. Offer prescribed mouthwashes through a straw to rinse mouth of debris and to soothe ulcerative areas.
5. Teach patient to apply petrolatum to lips frequently.
6. Use cool-mist therapy to humidify environmental air.

B. *Restoring Skin Integrity*
1. Keep skin clean and eliminate debris and dead skin—the bullae will clear if epithelium at the base is clean and not infected.
2. Obtain swab of bullous fluid for cultures—most common organism is *Staphylococcus aureus*.
3. Administer cool, wet dressings and/or baths or teach patient to administer to soothe and cleanse skin—patients with large areas of blistering have a characteristic odor that is lessened when secondary infection is under control.
   a. After the bath, dry and cover with talcum powder as directed—enables the patient to move more freely in bed. Fairly large amounts are necessary to keep clothes and sheets from sticking.
4. The nursing management of patients with blistering or bullous skin conditions is similar to that of the patient with a burn (see p. 910).

C. *Achieving Fluid Balance*
1. Evaluate for fluid and electrolyte imbalance—extensive denudation of the skin leads to fluid and electrolyte imbalance.
   a. Monitor serum albumin and protein levels.
   b. Monitor vital signs for hypotension or tachycardia
   c. Weigh patient daily
2. Administer intravenous saline solutions as directed.
3. Encourage the patient to maintain hydration; suggest cool nonirritating fluids.
   a. Suggest soft, high-protein, high-calorie diet or liquid supplements (Ensure, Sustacal, eggnogs, milkshakes) that will not be irritating to oral mucosa but will replace lost protein.

D. *Promoting Positive Body Image*
1. Develop a trusting relationship with the patient.
2. Educate patient and family about the disease and its treatment—reduces uncertainty and clears up misconceptions.
3. Encourage expression of anxieties, embarrassment, discouragement.
4. Encourage patient to maintain social contacts and activities among support network.

Patient Education

Instruct the patient as follows:

1. The disease may be characterized by relapses that require continuing therapy to maintain control.
2. Long-term administration of immunosuppressive drugs is associated with numerous side effects and risks—hyperglycemia, osteoporosis, psychosis, adrenal suppression, and increased risk of cancer. Report for health care follow-up regularly.
3. Monitor skin/mouth for recurrence of pemphigus activity.

Evaluation

A. Oral mucous membranes pink with healing lesions and no signs of infection
B. Skin with intact bullae, healing lesions, and no signs of infection
C. Vital signs stable; urine output adequate
D. Patient expressing concerns and planning activities

◆ BENIGN TUMORS

Benign tumors are common skin growths. Most do not require any treatment but are important to recognize to differentiate malignant lesions.

Characteristics of Benign Tumors

A. Seborrheic Keratoses Tumors are benign wartlike lesions of varying size and color, ranging from light tan to black; most common skin tumors in middle-aged and elderly persons

B. Actinic (Solar) Keratoses Premalignant skin lesions appearing as rough, scaly patches with underlying erythema that develop as a consequence of prolonged exposure to ultraviolet rays
1. Develop in chronic sun-exposed areas of body; may gradually transform into squamous cell cancer.
2. Many available treatments, including liquid nitrogen cryosurgery and curettage.

C. Verrucae (Warts) Common, benign skin tumors caused by human papilloma virus

1. Warts often do not need treatment, because they tend to disappear spontaneously.
2. Treatment options:
  a. Freezing with liquid nitrogen—causes destruction of wart while sparing rest of skin.
  b. Area may be treated surgically with curettage or electrodesiccation.
  c. Application of salicylic acid, topical fluorouracil, topical vitamin A acid, or other irritants may be helpful, especially for flat warts.

D. Angiomas (Birthmarks) Benign vascular tumors involving the skin and subcutaneous tissue

1. May occur as flat, violet-red patches (port-wine angiomas) or as raised, bright-red nodular lesions (strawberry angiomas). Strawberry angiomas may involute spontaneously, whereas port-wine angiomas usually persist indefinitely.
2. Most patients use masking cosmetics (Covermark) to camouflage the defect.
3. Laser is being used with good success.

E. Pigmented Nevi (Moles) Common skin tumors of various sizes and shapes, ranging from yellowish to brown to black

1. May be flat, macular lesions or elevated papules or nodules that occasionally contain hair.
2. Majority of pigmented nevi are harmless; however, in rare cases, malignant changes supervene and a melanoma develops at the site of the nevus.
3. Treatment
  a. Nevi at sites subject to repeated irritation from clothing or jewelry can be removed for comfort.
  b. Nevi that show change in size or color or that become symptomatic (itch or bleed) or develop notched borders should be removed to determine if malignant changes have occurred. This is especially true for nevi with irregular borders or variations of red, blue, and/or blue-black colors.

F. Keloids Benign overgrowths of connective tissue at site of scar or trauma in predisposed individuals

1. More prevalent among black race.
2. Usually asymptomatic—may cause disfigurement and cosmetic concern.
3. Management—intralesional corticosteroid therapy, surgical removal, radiation.

◆ CANCER OF THE SKIN

Skin cancer is the most common malignancy; basal and squamous cell carcinomas are easily curable due to early diagnosis and slow progression. These cancers are locally invasive and tend not to metastasize. Conversely, malignant melanomas are less common and metastasize eventually.

Pathophysiology/Etiology

1. Most basal and squamous cell carcinomas are located on sun-exposed areas and are directly related to ultraviolet radiation. *Sun damage is cumulative.*
2. Risk factors for skin cancer include:
  a. Fair complexion, blue eyes, blond or red hair
  b. Working outdoors
  c. Elderly with sun-damaged skin
  d. History of x-ray treatment of skin conditions
  e. Exposure to certain chemical agents (arsenicals, nitrates, tar and pitch, oils, and paraffins)
  f. Burn scars, damaged skin in areas of chronic osteomyelitis, fistulae openings
  g. Long-term immunosuppressive therapy
  h. Genetic susceptibility
  i. Multiple dysplastic nevi—moles that are larger, irregular, more numerous, or variable colors—or family history of dysplastic nevi
  j. Congenital nevi.
3. Types of skin cancer:
  a. Basal cell carcinoma—arises from basal layers of the epidermis or hair follicle; most common type, rarely metastasizes.

b. Squamous cell carcinoma—arises from the epidermis; metastasis occurs more often than with basal cell carcinoma.

c. Malignant melanoma—arises from nevocytic cells in the upper dermis; can metastasize.

Clinical Manifestations

A. Basal Cell Carcinoma
1. Lesions often begin as small nodules with a rolled, pearly, translucent border with telangiectasia, crusting, and occasionally ulceration (Fig. 30-4).
2. Appear most frequently on sun-exposed skin, frequently on face between hairline and upper lip.
3. If neglected, may cause local destruction, hemorrhage, and infection of adjacent tissues, producing severe functional and cosmetic disabilities.

B. Squamous Cell Carcinoma
1. Appears as reddish rough, thickened, scaly lesion with bleeding and soreness or may be asymptomatic; border may be wider, more infiltrated, and more inflammatory than basal cell carcinoma (Fig. 30-5).
2. May be preceded by leukoplakia (premalignant lesion of mucous membrane) of the mouth or tongue, actinic keratoses, scarred or ulcerated lesions.
3. Seen most commonly on lower lip, rims of ears, head, neck, and backs of the hands.

C. Malignant Melanoma
See Figure 30-6.

1. Melanoma in situ
   a. Earliest phase, difficult to recognize because clinical changes are minimal.
2. Superficial spreading melanoma (most common).

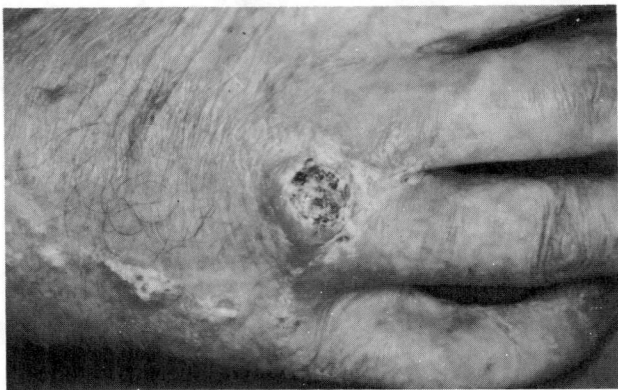

FIGURE 30-5 Squamous cell carcinoma. (Courtesy, Mervyn L. Elgart, M.D.)

a. Circular, with irregular outer portions; the margins may be flat or elevated and palpable.
b. Has combination of colors—hues of tan, brown, and black mixed with gray, bluish black, or white.
c. May be dull pink-rose color in a small area within the lesion.
d. Occurs anywhere on body; usually affects middle-aged persons.

3. Nodular melanoma
   a. Spherical blueberry-like nodule with relatively smooth surface and relatively uniform blue-black, blue-gray, or reddish blue color.
   b. May be polypoidal and elevated, with smooth surface of rose-gray or black color.
   c. Occurs commonly on torso and extremities.
   d. Invades directly into the subjacent dermis (vertical growth) and hence has a poorer prognosis.

4. Lentigo maligna melanoma
   a. First appears as tan, flat macula—malignant degeneration is manifested by changes in color, size, and topography
   b. Slowly evolving; occurs on exposed skin surfaces of persons in the 5th or 6th decade.

5. Acrolentiginous melanoma (uncommon)
   a. Irregular pigmented macules, which develop nodules; may become invasive early.
   b. Occurs commonly on palms, soles, nail beds, and rarely on mucous membranes.
   c. Most common type of melanoma in blacks.

Diagnostic Evaluation

1. Excisional biopsy (for histopathologic diagnosis) and microstaging determination of thickness and level of invasion; helps determine treatment and prognosis.

Management

Method of treatment depends on tumor location, cell type (location and depth), history of previous treat-

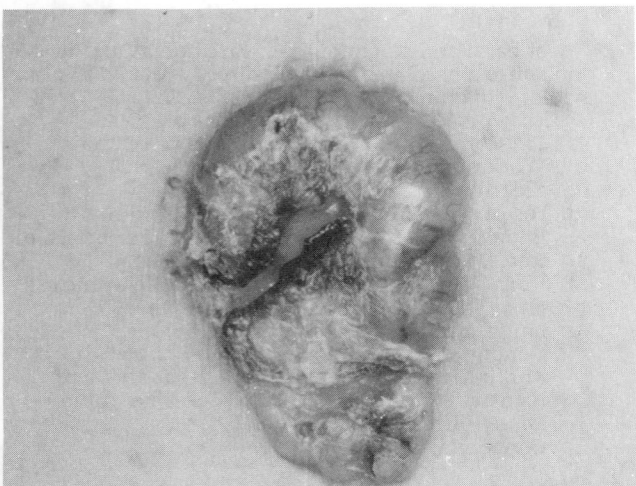

FIGURE 30-4 Basal cell carcinoma. (Courtesy, Mervyn L. Elgart, M.D.)

ment, and whether it is invasive or if metastasis has occurred.

1. Curettage followed by electrodessication—usually done on small tumors of basal or squamous cell type (less than 1 to 2 cm).
2. Surgical excision; may be followed by simple closure, flap or graft.
3. Microscopically controlled surgery—immediate microscopic examination is made of frozen or chemically fixed sections for evidence of cancer cells. Layers are removed until no more cancer cells are seen.
4. Radiation therapy—can be done for cancer of eyelid, tip of nose, in or near vital structures such as facial nerve or where tissue sparing is difficult with other forms of treatment; also used for extensive malignancies where goal is palliation or when other medical conditions contraindicate other forms of therapy.
5. Regional perfusion—chemotherapeutic agent may be perfused directly into area containing melanoma by mechanically controlling arterial and venous blood flow; allows higher concentration of cytotoxic drug to be delivered to site, with less systemic toxicity.
6. Systemic chemotherapy—generally used for recurrence of metastasis or palliation; may be combined with autologous bone marrow transplantation or several agents used in combination.
7. Other therapeutic regimens—topical fluorouracil, interferon, retinoids, photoradiation.

Complications

1. Regional or systemic metastasis (frequently central nervous system).

Nursing Assessment

1. Have a high index of suspicion for persons at risk.
2. Ask about sunbathing habits. Question patient about pruritus, tenderness, pain, or bleeding, which are not features of a benign nevus (mole).
3. Ask about changes in preexistingmoles or development of a new pigmented lesion.
4. Use a magnifying lens in a brightly lit room to look for variegated color and irregular border and surface in the mole. Use side lighting to assess for subtle elevation.
5. Examine entire skin surface, including scalp, genital area, gluteal folds, and soles of feet.
6. Examine diameter of mole; melanomas are often larger than 6 mm; look for lesions situated near the mole.

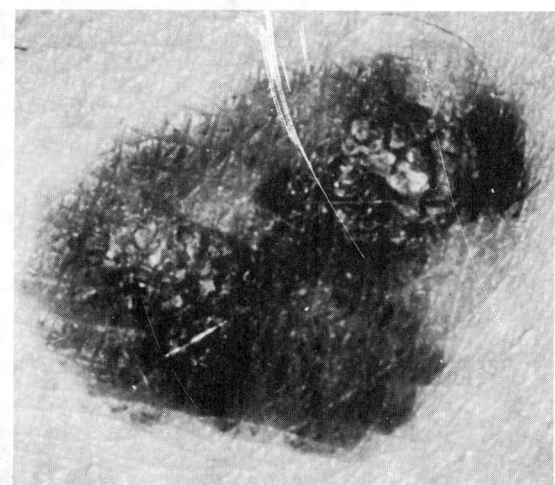

A

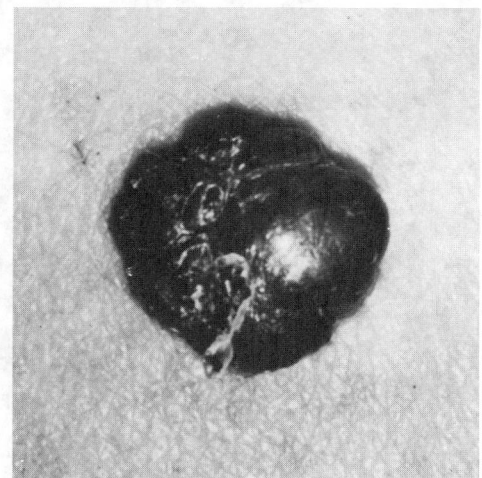

B

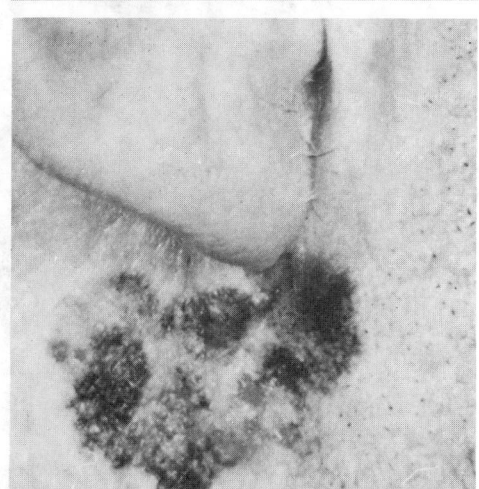

C

FIGURE 30-6 **(A)** *Superficial spreading melanoma; note irregular border.* **(B)** *Nodular melanoma.* **(C)** *Lentigo-maligna melanoma; note irregular pigment pattern. (Photos courtesy Arthur J. Sober, M.D.)*

NURSING ALERT:
Any skin lesion that changes in size or color, bleeds, ulcerates, or becomes infected may be skin cancer.

Nursing Diagnoses

A. Knowledge Deficit related to risk factors for skin cancer
B. Anxiety related to diagnosis of cancer

Nursing Interventions

1. Encourage follow-up skin examinations and instruct the patient to examine skin monthly as follows:
   a. Use a full-length mirror and a small hand mirror to aid in examination.
   b. Learn where moles/birthmarks are located.
   c. Inspect all moles and other pigmented lesions; report any change in color, size, elevation, thickness, or development of itching or bleeding.
2. Teach the patient to use a sunscreen with a sun protection factor of at least 15 routinely for the rest of life and *never become sunburned*.
   a. Sunlight permanently damages the skin and can be cumulative.
   b. Do not try to tan if skin burns easily, never tans, or tans poorly.
   c. Avoid unnecessary exposure to the sun, especially during times when ultraviolet radiation is most intense (10:00 AM to 3:00 PM).
   d. Wear protective clothing (long sleeves, broad-brimmed hat, high collar, long pants, etc.)—however, clothing does not provide complete protection, because up to 50% of sun's damaging rays can go through clothes.
   e. Do not use sunlamps for indoor tanning; avoid commercial tanning salons.
B. *Reducing Anxiety*
1. Allow patient to express feelings about the seriousness of diagnosis.
2. Answer questions; clarify information and correct misconceptions.
3. Emphasize use of positive coping skills and support system.

Patient Education/Health Maintenance

1. Encourage lifelong follow-up with dermatologist and/or primary care provider with every-6-month skin examinations.
2. Encourage all individuals to have moles removed that are accessible to repeated friction and irritation, congenital, or suspicious in any way.
3. Teach all individuals the importance of sun-avoidance measures; teach proper use of sunscreen:
   a. Sunscreens with a sun protection factor of 15 or greater offer good protection.
   b. Sunscreens should be used from infancy through old age.
   c. Sunscreens should be applied before going outdoors to all areas that may be exposed and preferably before dressing.
   d. Sunscreen should not come off easily, but periodically reapply, especially after swimming or bathing.
   e. Protect lips with a lip balm that contains a sunscreen with the highest sun protection factor.
3. For more information, refer patients to agencies such as: The Skin Cancer Foundation; 245 Fifth Avenue, Suite 2402; New York, NY 10016; 212-725-5176.

Evaluation

A. No signs of mole change or tumor recurrence
B. Patient verbalizes decreased anxiety

◆ OTHER DERMATOLOGIC DISORDERS

See Table 30-2 and Figure 30-7.

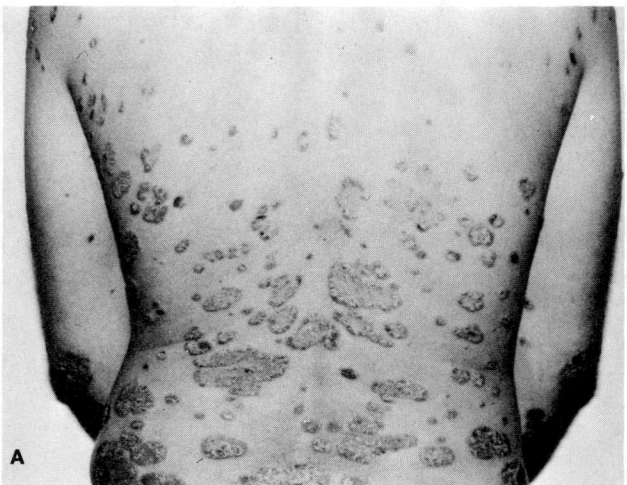

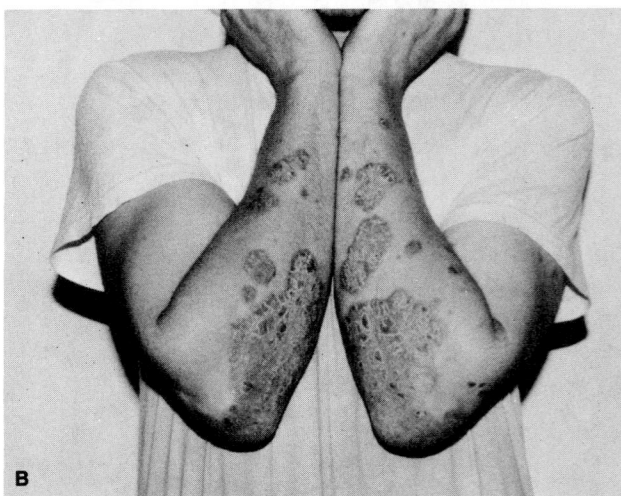

FIGURE 30-7 The lesions of psoriasis appear as red raised patches of skin covered with silvery scales that, in time, coalesce, forming irregularly shaped patches. (Photos courtesy the National Psoriasis Foundation)

TABLE 30-2 Other Dermatologic Disorders

Name/Description	Clinical Manifestations	Management	Nursing/Patient Care Considerations
Bacterial Infections			
Folliculitis—inflammation of the hair follicle	1. Single or multiple papules or pustules. 2. Commonly seen in the beard area of men and on women's legs from shaving.	1. Twice daily cleansing with antibacterial soap. 2. Topical antibiotic ointment. 3. Systemic antibiotics for recurrent or recalcitrant cases.	1. Advise warm compresses to relieve inflammation.
Furunculosis—perifollicular abcess (boil) caused by *Staphylococcus aureus;* Carbuncles are two or more confluent furuncles	1. Tender, circumscribed, erythematous area whose center may become fluctuant and suppurate. 2. Commonly occur on the back of neck, axillae, buttocks.	1. Warm compresses to reduce inflammation and promote drainage. 2. When area becomes fluctuant, incision and drainage can be performed, followed by packing. 3. Furuncles of the ear canal, nares, upper lip, and nose may require systemic antibiotic treatment, because these areas drain directly into cranial venous sinuses.	1. Encourage the use of warm compresses. 2. Warn patient not to squeeze or incise the lesion. 3. If severe or recurrent, look for underlying immunosuppression by disorders such as diabetes, AIDS, alcoholism, or malnutrition.
Paronychia—inflammation of skin folds surrounding the fingernail	1. Tender, purulent, erythematous swelling of nail border 2. Chronic and recurrent paronychia cause horizontal ridges at base of nail.	1. Incision and drainage for acutely inflamed paronychia. 2. Fungicidal or bactericidal ointment for chronic paronychia. 3. Systemic antibiotic treatment usually is necessary. 4. Prevention of trauma and maceration.	1. Encourage soaking in warm water for 10–15 minutes 3–4 times a day while acutely inflamed to relieve pain and promote drainage. 2. Identify persons with work-related chronic paronychia (bartenders, dishwashers, housekeepers) and recommend use of rubber gloves over thin cotton gloves when working around moisture.
Erysipelas—streptococcal infection involving the superficial dermal lymphatics, usually of the face	1. Prodromal—malaise, fever, chills, headache, vomiting, joint pain. 2. Local— redness, warmth, swelling, and characteristic raised indurated border. 3. Leukocytosis. 4. Advancing edge of the patch with extension. 5. May vessiculate.	1. Oral, I.M., or I.V. antibiotics, usually penicillin derivatives.	1. Ice or cold compresses may be soothing.
Intertrigo—superficial inflammation and secondary infection where two skin surfaces are in apposition	1. Erythematous and mascerated rash. 2. There may be erosions, fissures, and drainage. 3. Burning and itching.	1. Topical antibacterial and antifungal agents.	1. Teach patient to prevent skin maceration by separating opposing skin surfaces with gauze or cotton material. 2. Skin surfaces should be dried thoroughly after bathing with a hair dryer on low setting. 3. Talcum powder can be applied lightly to the area after drying. 4. Loose, airy clothing should be worn.

(continued)

TABLE 30-2 Other Dermatologic Disorders *(continued)*

Name/Description	Clinical Manifestations	Management	Nursing/Patient Care Considerations
Mycotic (fungal) Infections Tinea pedis—ringworm of the foot; Tinea corporis—ringworm of the body; Tinea cruris—ringworm of the groin; Tinea capitis—ringworm of the scalp	1. Caused by the dermatophyte *Trichophyton, Epidermophyton,* or *Microsporum.* 2. Erythematous, inflamed, and vesicular lesions of feet. 3. Scaling erythematous patches of body or head with central clearing. 4. Dull red or brownish rash of upper inner thighs and groin with scaling borders. 5. Itching and irritation.	1. Examination of rash under Wood's light shows characteristic fluorescence with certain fungi. 2. Skin scraping from leading edge shows characteristic spores and hyphae with KOH preparation under microscope. 3. Treat with topical antifungals or systemic antifungals for severe cases. 4. Reduction of moisture in groin, between toes.	1. Advise washing 1–2 times daily with water and mild soap, then applying talc powder or cornstarch to well dried area. 2. Use hair dryer set on low temperature to dry tender areas. 3. Encourage wearing cotton socks and underwear and light, airy clothing to promote evaporation. 4. Warn about contamination from feet to groin or other areas of the body by hands or clothing. 5. Encourage use of open shoes or canvas sneakers and avoidance of plastic or rubber soled shoes or boots and tight shoes with tinea pedis. 6. Wash contaminated clothing in hot water.
Tinea vesicolor—superficial fungal infection by *Malassezia furfur*	1. Patchy macular or mildly scaly rash of upper trunk and upper arms; yellowish or brownish in light skinned people, hypopigmented in dark skin. 2. Mild itching and scaling	1. Identified by fluorescence on Wood's light examination. 2. Microscopic examination with KOH preparation of skin scraping shows characteristic "spaghetti and meatballs" appearance of hyphae and spores. 3. Treat with topical antifungals or selenium sulfide. 4. Systemic antifungal may be used.	1. Common in high temperature, high humidity environments. 2. Advise patient that discoloration may persist after fungus has been eradicated; lost pigmentation will resolve with sun exposure. 3. Tell patient that recurrence is common after 2–12 weeks if prophylactic treatment is not given periodically.
Onychomycosis (tinea unguium)—infection of the nail by fungus	1. Discoloration (white, yellow, or darkened) of the nail. 2. Nail becomes brittle, cracked, irregular, loosened. 3. May be some inflammation and pain.	1. Identification of offending fungus by microscopic examination of shavings with KOH or by culture. 2. Treatment with appropriate antifungal, either topical or systemic, for prolonged period—3–6 months or longer. 3. Surgical removal of nail may be necessary.	1. Encourage patient to comply with lengthy treatment, as fungal infections of the nail are difficult to treat. 2. Examine patient for other areas of tinea infection (feet, groin), encourage treatment, and teach patient that infection may be spread from fingernails by scratching. 3. After nail removal, advise patient to keep hand or foot elevated for several hours, and change dressing daily by applying gauze and antibiotic ointment or other prescribed medication until nail bed is dry.
Parasitic Infections Pediculosis capitis—head lice; Pediculosis corporis—body lice; Pediculosis pubis—crab louse infestation of the genital region	1. Itching is primary complaint. 2. Lice and nits may be seen in seams of clothing (body lice) or clinging to hairs (pubic lice).	1. Treatment for pediculosis corporis involves washing with soap and water and washing all infested clothing and linens with hot water. Alternatively, clothes may be dry-cleaned or ironed, paying close attention to the seams.	1. Advise patient that pediculosis pubis is considered a sexually transmitted disease; partners must be examined and treated. 2. Teach patient the proper use of medication:

(continued)

TABLE 30-2 Other Dermatologic Disorders *(continued)*

Name/Description	Clinical Manifestations	Management	Nursing/Patient Care Considerations
	3. Skin excoriation in affected area. 4. Erythematous macules or wheals may appear at puncture sites. 5. Gray-blue macules may appear on trunk or inner thighs with pediculosis pubis.	2. Pediculosis capitis and pubis are treated with a topical antiparasitic preparation such as lindane (Kwell) or permethrin (Nix). 3. Manual removal of nits (eggs) may be performed, and retreatment in 3–7 days is rocommended. 4. Petroleum may be applied to eyelashes, then lice and nits removed with swab or tweezers or pilocarpine drops can be used to paralyze the lice.	a. Apply lotion or cream after bathing to affected hairy and adjacent areas, wash off after 8–12 hours. b. Alternatively, apply shampoo to affected hairy areas and lather for 4–5 minutes, rinse and let hair dry. c. Use fine-tooth comb to remove nits. 3. Urge patient to wash all clothing, towels, linens, combs, and hair accessories that may be contaminated. 4. Advise patient not to use antiparasitic preparations if pregnant or use more frequently than recommended.
Scabies—superficial infestation by itch mite; transmitted by close personal contact	1. Itching, more intense at night 2. Small erythmatous papules and short, wavy burrows are seen on skin surface. 3. Frequently seen between fingers or in groin area. 4. Spares head and scalp except in children under 1 year of age	1. Parasite identified by microscopic examination of skin scraping. 2. Treated with antiparasitic such as lindane (Kwell) or crotamiton (Eurax). 3. Machine wash and dry clothing and linens on hot cycle. 4. Topical or systemic steroids may be needed to treat symptoms of allergic reaction to mites. **GERONTOLOGIC ALERT:** Infestation with scabies may be a problem in nursing homes, particularly among debilitated patients who require extensive hands-on care.	1. Teach proper use of medication: a. Apply thin layer from neck downward, with particular atention to hands, feet, and intertriginous areas; every inch of skin must be treated because mites are migrating. Apply to dry skin. (Wet skin allows more penetration and the possibility of toxicity.) b. Leave medication on for 8–12 hours but no longer, as this will irritate the skin. Then wash thoroughly. 2. Advise patient to avoid close contact for 24 hours after treatment to prevent transmission. 3. Encourage treatment of sexual and close contacts simultaneously. 4. Tell patient that itching may persist for days to weeks following treatment due to an allergic reaction to mites; retreatment is not necessary.

(continued)

TABLE 30-2 Other Dermatologic Disorders *(continued)*

Name/Description	Clinical Manifestations	Management	Nursing/Patient Care Considerations
Viral Infections Herpes simplex—acute vesicular eruption caused by herpes simplex virus type 1 or 2	1. Prodromal pain, burning, or tingling, possible fever and malaise. 2. Tiny vesicles appear on erythematous, swollen base; they rupture, forming painful ulcers, crusting, and eventual healing. 3. Can occur anywhere, especially near mucocutaneous junctions.	1. Tzanck smear from scraping of ulcer or fluid from vesicle shows characteristic giant cells with intranuclear inclusions; also diagnosed by fluorescent antibody detection or viral culture. 2. Antiviral treatment with acyclovir (Zovirax) for acute infection or continuous suppressive therapy to prevent or lessen recurrence. 3. Analgesics may be needed for widespread and genital eruptions.	1. Teach patient that herpes simplex can be transmitted by close and sexual contact; good personal hygiene and hand washing are required for facial cases; sexual abstinence or condom use are required for genital cases. 2. Recurrence may be brought on by fever, illness, emotional stress, menses, pregnancy, sunlight, and other factors. 3. Advise patients with active herpes simplex infection to avoid contact with immunosuppressed individuals (diabetes, HIV disease, cancer or cancer treatment, alcoholism, malnutrition, etc.), because herpes simplex infection can be severe in these individuals. 4. Tell patients that lesions usually resolve in 1–2 weeks without scarring.
Other Conditions Contact dermatitis— inflammatory condition caused by exposure to irritating or allergenic substances, such as plants, cosmetics, cleaning products, soaps and detergents, hair dyes, metals and rubber.	1. Itching, burning, erythema, and vesiculation at point of contact. 2. Progresses to weeping, crusting, drying, fissuring, and peeling. 3. Lichenification (thickening of skin) and pigmentation changes may occur with chronicity.	1. Topical or oral steroids, depending on severity. a. Oral steroids usually given in tapered dose—start with high dose and gradually decrease to provide greatest anti-inflammatory effect without adrenal suppression. 2. Removal or avoidance of causative agent. 3. Antipruritics—systemic or topical antihistamines or topical calamine preparations. 3. Desensitization to poison ivy and other substances may be accomplished for those who have severe reactions and cannot avoid contact.	1. Take thorough history to determine causative agent or contributing factors; have patient keep log of activities and symptoms if unsure of irritant. 2. Teach patient to use allergen-free products, wear gloves and protective clothing, and wash and rinse skin thoroughly and wash clothing after contact. 3. Advise patient that rash is not contagious, not even oozing lesions of poison ivy; however, contaminated clothing may cause spread of poison ivy in those who are sensitive. 4. Advise patient to perform patch test by applying substance behind ear or on inside of wrist before trying new cosmetics, soaps, or hair products.
Psoriasis—chronic inflammatory disorder in which epidermal turnover occurs 6–9 times faster than normal (Fig. 30-7)	1. Erythematous, raised patches covered by silvery scales. 2. Symmetrically affects the knees, elbows, sacrum, scalp, external ears, genitalia, perianal area, nails, and dorsa of hands. 3. About 10% of cases include arthritis.	1. Coal tar preparations retard and inhibit the rapid production of epidermal cells. a. Preparation is applied for a period; may then by washed off; this is followed by carefully graded doses of ultraviolet radiation, which produces mild redness and desquamation. b. Daily tar shampoo followed by application of steroid lotion may be used for scalp lesions.	1. Instruct patient to take daily tub bath to soften scales; gentle rubbing with bath brush may be necessary to remove scales. 2. Apply topical preparations after removing scales. 3. Goggles should be worn during ultraviolet light therapy to prevent eye injury.

(continued)

TABLE 30-2   Other Dermatologic Disorders (*continued*)

Name/Description	Clinical Manifestations	Management	Nursing/Patient Care Considerations
		2. Anthralin preparations (a distillate of crude coal tar) are useful for especially thick and resistant psoriatic plaques. 3. Topical steroids with occlusive dressing to penetrate plaques and decrease inflammation. 4. Intralesional steroid injections. 5. Systemic therapy with methotrexate (Mexate), retinoids (Tegison), hydroxyurea (Hydrea), or cyclosporine (Sandimmune) for severe cases. 6. PUVA therapy—ingestion of psoralen, a photosensitizer, before ultraviolet light exposure	4. Encourage patient to comply with frequent laboratory monitoring of blood counts and liver function while on methotrexate, since this drug may be toxic. 5. Warn patient that PUVA therapy causes photosensitization for the rest of the day, so protective clothing, wraparound sunglasses, and sunscreen must be worn. 6. Encourage patients on PUVA therapy to comply wth periodic eye exams, because cataracts are an adverse effect. 7. For more information, contact: The National Psoriasis Foundation 6443 S. W. Beaverton Highway, Suite 210, Portland, OR 97221, 503-244-7404.
Exfoliative dermatitis—chronic extensive scaling and inflammation of the skin; may be idiopathic or related to preexisting skin conditions, drug reactions, or underlying malignancy	1. Starts as patchy erythema, with possible fever, chills, and malaise. 2. Rapid spread until whole integument is involved. 3. Skin color changes to scarlet, desquamates, and may ooze serous fluid. 4. Pruritus, hair loss, secondary infection.	1. Discontinuation of offending drug or treatment of underlying condition. 2. Systemic corticosteroids should control most cases. 3. Supportive treatment—bed rest, warm environment, fluid and electrolyte replacement. 4. Soothing baths and topical emollients for symptomatic relief. 5. Possible use of immunosuppressants—azathioprine (Imuran), methotrexate (Mexate), and cyclophosphamide (Cytoxan).	1. Monitor fluid balance and electrolyte values 2. Watch for signs of secondary infection and report so antimicrobial therapy can be started. 3. Watch for signs of heart failure caused by chronically increased cutaneous blood flow. 4. Teach patient how to relieve itching with oatmeal baths and emollient creams. 5. Tell patient to avoid environments with temperature fluctuations to avoid chilling. 6. Advise patient to avoid all irritants.
Alopecia—hair loss, may be idiopathic (alopecia areata), male-pattern, physiologic, or due to hair pulling (trichotillomania); also due to scarring from other skin or systemic disorders	1. Patterned, patchy, or diffuse hair loss. 2. Inflammation and scarring with some types. 3. Physiologic alopecia may be associated with hormonal changes (childbirth), nutritional factors, or toxin exposure.	1. Treatment of underlying cause. 2. Minoxidil (Rogaine) may cause fine hair regrowth in male-pattern baldness and alopecia areata. 3. Other methods of hair replacement—surgical grafting of hair follicles, hair weaving, hair pieces.	1. Explain that alopecia areata and physiologic loss are usually temporary and self-limiting. 2. Encourage women to change hairstyle or wear hairpieces or turbans until hair grows back after childbirth. 3. Counsel men on the slow, limited effects of minoxidil treatment and stress that effects reverse when treatment is stopped.
Seborrheic dermatitis—chronic, superficial inflammatory skin disorder	1. Crusted pinkish or yellow patches. 2. Loose scales that may be dry, moist, or greasy. 3. Mild itching. 4. Affects the scalp, eyebrows, eyelids, nasolabial creases, lips, ears, chest, axillae, umbilicus, groin.	1. Selenium sulfide (Selsun), tar (Pentrax), zinc, or resorcinol shampoo to scalp several times a week. 2. Corticosteroid lotions or creams. 3. For eyelid margin involvement (blepharitis), daily debridement with cotton-tipped applicator and baby shampoo, and ophthalmic steroid ointment or lotion.	1. Advise patient of chronic nature of seborrhea and that condition may be exacerbated by perspiration, neuroleptic drugs, and emotional stress; also seen more frequently in persons with Parkinson's disease, HIV disease, diabetes mellitus, malabsorption syndromes, and epilepsy.

(continued)

TABLE 30-2 Other Dermatologic Disorders *(continued)*

Name/Description	Clinical Manifestations	Management	Nursing/Patient Care Considerations
		4. For external ear canal involvement, corticosteroid cream.	2. Teach patient to apply topical preparations as prescribed. 3. Advise baby shampoo use only and gently rubbing with swab near eyes to prevent irritation of conjunctiva in seborrheic blepharitis.

Hidradenitis suppurative—chronic plugging and secondary infection of the apocrine glands of the groin and axilla	1. Development of tender red nodules that enlarge, rupture, and suppurate.
	2. Sinus tracts develop with recurrent lesions, leading to continuous inflammation and drainage.
		1. Initial treatment involves prolonged antibiotics and systemic or intralesional corticosteroids, however, progression of the conditon is likely.
		2. Surgical treatment necessary when chronic suppuration and fistulas develop:
		  a. Incision and drainage
		  b. Cauterization of sinus tracts
		  c. Excision with possible skin grafting.
		3. Isotretinon (Accutane), antiandrogens, and x-ray treatment may be helpful but not curative.
			1. Advise patient to use antibacterial soap and keep axilla and groin dry to reduce bacterial colonization of the skin.
			2. Advise patient to avoid shaving of hair in affected area to prevent trauma and possible infection.
			3. Advise patient to avoid use of deodorant or other chemicals on affected area.
			4. Teach patient the signs of bacterial infection—purulent drainage, odor, pain—that call for notification of health care provider and treatment with antibiotics.
			5. Encourage use of warm compresses to relieve inflammation.

Bullous pemphigoid— chronic bullous disease of the elderly of unknown etiology	1. Tense vesicles and bullae arise on normal or erythematous skin, rupture, and heal without scarring. 2. Occurs on flexor aspects of the body, axilla, inguinal areas, abdomen, and occasionally on mucous membranes.	1. Systemic corticosteroid treatment if widespread involvement. 2. Condition may remit within 2–4 years even without treatment.	1. Keep skin clean and dry to reduce chances of secondary infection. 2. If patient is immobilized, encourage positioning to prevent undue pressure on lesions; may cause premature rupture and secondary infection. 3. Be sure to differentiate from early pressure sore development and treat pressure sores appropriately. 4. Advise patient that lesions usually heal without scarring.
Acne vulgaris— obstruction and inflammation of sebaceous glands and follicles	1. Closed comedones (whiteheads). 2. Open comedones (blackheads). 3. Papules, pustules, nodules, cysts, or abcesses may develop. 4. Primary sites are face, chest, upper back, and shoulder.	1. Topical benzoyl peroxide— antibacterial and comedolytic. 2. Topcal retinoic acid (retin-A)— comedolytic. 3. Topical antibiotics—suppress growth of *Propionibacterium acnes* and produce decrease in comedones, papules, and pustules without sytemic side effects. 4. Systemic antibiotics—long-term, low-dose therapy for more inflammatory and extensive causes.	1. Advise patient to wash face gently with mild soap and water 1–2 times daily. 2. Teach proper application of topical preparation—use sparingly and decrease frequency if irritation and redness develop. 3. Teach side effects of systemic antibiotics. 4. Ensure that women of childbearing potential are using contraceptives and that a negative pregnancy test has been obtained before starting Accutane therapy.

(continued)

TABLE 30-2 Other Dermatologic Disorders *(continued)*

Name/Description	Clinical Manifestations	Management	Nursing/Patient Care Considerations
		5. Retinoid therapy—(Accutane) inhibits sebum production and secretion; for severe, disfiguring cystic acne. 6. Estrogen therapy—antiandrogenic effect decreases sebum production. 7. Intralesional steroid injection—for inflamed lesions. 8. Dermabrasion—surgical planing or chemical peels to smooth surface configuration of old scars.	5. Encourage follow-up and monitoring of laboratory tests while on Accutane for elevated liver enzymes, cholesterol and triglycerides, and decreased HDL. 6. Advise patient on Accutane to notify health care provider of persistent headache—could signal pseudotumor cerebri. 7. Tell patient that initiation of therapy may worsen symptoms for several weeks, but to continue treatment. 8. Advise not to squeeze pimples and avoid friction around face. 9. Advise use of water-based and hypoallergenic cosmetics. 10. Encourage balanced diet and avoidance of foods believed to aggravate acne.

HDL: high-density lipoprotein; AIDS: acquired immunodeficiency syndrome; I.M.: intramuscular; I.V.: intravenous; HIV: human immunodeficiency virus; PUVA: psoralen-ultraviolet-light (treatment); KOH: potassium hydroxide.

Selected References

Abel, E. A. (1992). Contact dermatitis: recognition and management. *Hospital Medicine, 28*(11), 101-108.

Agency for Toxic Substances and Disease Registry. (1993). Contact dermatitis and urticaria from environmental exposures. *American Family Physician, 48*(5), 773-780.

DeVilley, R. L., Jacobs, J. P., Szpumar, C. A., et al. (1994). Androgenital alopecia in the female: Treatment with 2% topical minoxidil solution. *Archives of Dermatology, 130*(3), 303-307.

Fitzpatrick, T. B., Eisen, A. Z., Wolff, K., et al. (1993). Dermatology in general medicine (4th ed.). New York: McGraw-Hill.

Goldstein, B. G., & Goldstein, A. O. (1992). *Practical dermatology.* St. Louis: Mosby-Yearbook.

Landis, B. J. Facial cosmetic surgery: A primary care perspective. *The Nurse Practitioner, 19*(11), 71-76.

Shegal, V. N., et al. Atopic dermatitis: Clinical criteria. (1993). *International Journal of Dermatology, 32*(9):628-637.

Sokoloff, F. (1994). Identification and management of pediculosis. *The Nurse Practitioner, 19*(8), 62-64.

Stiller, M. J., et al. (1993). Treatment of dermatophytoses II: New topical antifungal drugs. *International Journal of Dermatology, 32*(9):638-641.

Swartz, S. M., et al. (1993). The technique of patch testing: role of the office staff. *Dermatology Nursing, 5*(2), 133-137.

Burns

Etiology and Physiology of Burns

Burns are a form of traumatic injury caused by thermal, electrical, chemical, or radioactive agents.

Inhalation injury and associated pulmonary complications are a significant factor in mortality and morbidity from burn injury (50% to 60% of fire deaths are secondary to inhalation injury).

◆ ETIOLOGY AND INCIDENCE

1. More than 2 million injuries and 7,000 to 9,000 deaths occur as a result of fire and burns each year in the United States.
2. Most accidents occur at home. The second most frequent occurring place of injury is at work.
3. Flame injury is the leading cause of accidents for adults, and scalding is the leading cause of accidents for children.
4. Teenage boys have a high incidence of electrical injuries.
5. The very young and the elderly are at greatest risk for burn injuries.
6. Smoking, often combined with alcohol intake, is associated with at least half of major fire injuries and deaths.
7. Males are more commonly injured by burns than are females.

Pathophysiology

A. Burn Injury
1. A burn injury usually results from energy transfer from a heat source to the body. Type of burn injury may be flame/flash, contact, scald (water, grease, etc.), chemical, electrical, inhalation, or any thermal source. Many factors alter the response of body tissues to these sources of heat.
   a. Local tissue conductivity—bone is most resistant to the heat source accumulation. Lesser resistance is seen in nerves, blood vessels, and muscle tissue.
   b. Adequacy of peripheral circulation.
   c. Skin thickness, insulating material of clothing, or dampness of the skin.
2. Physiologic reaction to a burn is similar to inflammatory process.
   a. Adjacent intact vessels dilate, causing redness and blanching with pressure.
   b. Platelets and leukocytes begin to adhere to the vascular endothelium as an early event in the inflammatory process.

   c. Increased capillary permeability produces wound edema.
   d. An influx of polymorphonuclear leukocytes and monocytes occurs at the injury site.
   e. Eventually, new capillaries, immature fibroblasts, and newly formed collagen fibrils appear within the wound. This supports the regenerating epithelium or forms a granulating tissue bed to accept a skin graft.
3. Burns may be partial or full thickness (Fig. 31-1).
   a. *Partial-thickness* burn injuries involve the epidermis and upper portions of the dermis. Some of the dermal appendages remain, from which the wound can spontaneously re-epithelialize.
   b. In *full-thickness* injuries, all layers of the skin and sometimes underlying tissues are destroyed. Grafting usually is required to close the wound.
4. Burn depth is directly related to the temperature of the burning agent and the duration of contact with body tissue.
   a. Below 44°C (112°F), no local damage occurs unless exposure is for a protracted period.
   b. At 49°C (120°F), it takes 5 minutes' exposure to create a full-thickness burn.
   c. At 52° degrees C (125°F), the time requirement is 2 minutes, and at 60°C (140°F), only 6 seconds are required.
   d. At 70°C (159°F) it takes 1 second to create a full thickness burn in a healthy adult; less time or temperature in children or the elderly.

B. Inhalation Injury
1. May be upper airway (supraglottic) and incur injury in minutes to hours or may involve lower airway and cause adult respiratory distress syndrome (ARDS). This can occur in as little as 4 hours. Thermal injury can be seen in lower airway with steam or drug activity, such as free basing. Adult respiratory distress syndrome most simply as pulmonary edema of noncardiac origin may be seen in children.
2. Carbon monoxide (CO) is a colorless, odorless, tasteless, nonirritating gas produced from incomplete combustion of carbon-containing materials.
3. Affinity of hemoglobin for CO is 200 times greater than for oxygen.
4. Toxicity depends on concentration of CO in inspired air and the length of time of exposure.
   a. A carboxyhemoglobin of less than 10 ppm is not a cause for alarm.
   b. From 10 to 20 ppm bears watching and should be correlated with the spirometry results. (Smokers have been known to have carboxyhemoglobin levels of 15 to 18 ppm).
   c. Levels of 20 to 50 ppm can produce fatigue, irritability, cardiac dysrhythmias, ataxia, vomiting, syncope, possible coma, increased blood pressure, tin-

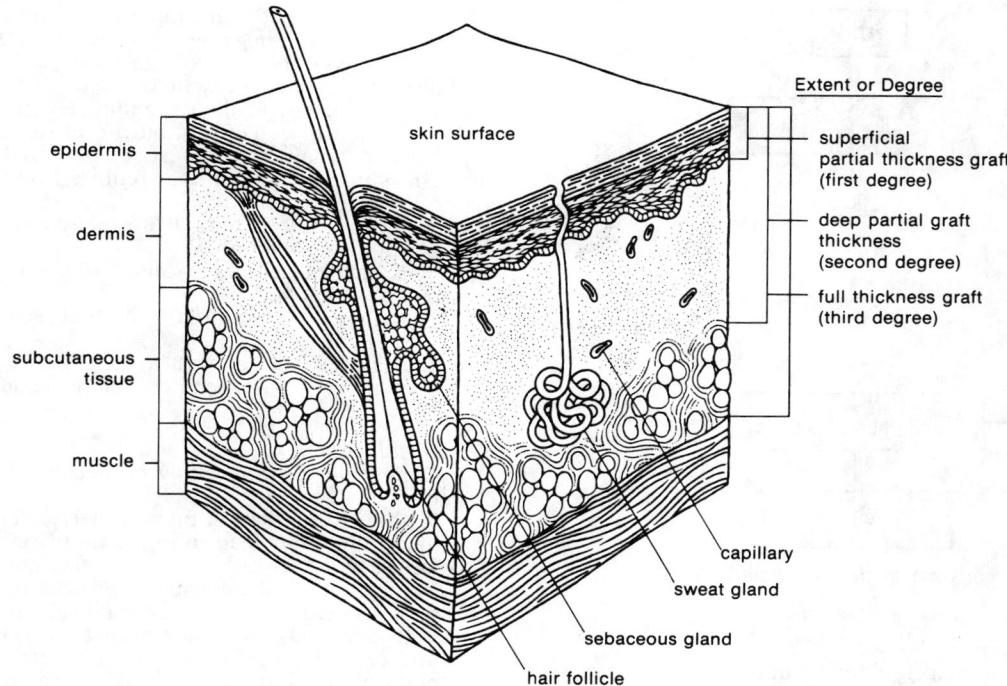

FIGURE 31-1 *Cross-section of skin depicting blood supply, depth of burn, and relative thickness of skin grafts. (From The Burn Patient, Ethicon)*

nitus, dystopia, ventricular dysrhythmias, severe alterations of consciousness, neurologic compromise, loss of consciousness, deep coma, hypertension, convulsions, paralysis, areflexia. This is considered a severe to lethal exposure.

5. Sulfur dioxide and nitrous oxide are toxic agents inhaled in soot. In the presence of water, they form corrosive acids and alkalies that are extremely toxic.
6. Toxic fumes from burning plastic are more dangerous than smoke.
   a. Noxious gases include hydrogen cyanide, hydrochloric acid, sulfuric acid, halogens, and perhaps phosgene.
7. Restrictive pulmonary complications can occur because of the tourniquet effect of edema seen with circumferential chest burns. Lung compliance and alveolar gas exchange can also be decreased because of noncardiogenic pulmonary edema (ARDS).

Systemic Changes in Major Burns

Major burns involve more than 25% of total body surface area (TBSA).

A. *Fluid Shifts*
1. In addition to changes in the local burned area, there are alterations and disruptions in the vascular and other systems of the body.
2. The water-vapor barrier for the body is the outermost layer of epidermis. When it is rendered nonfunctioning, severe systemic reactions from fluid losses can occur.
3. Fluid volume deficit is directly proportional to extent and depth of burn injury.
4. Capillary permeability increases, permitting fluid and protein to move from vascular to interstitial spaces (edema results) for the first 24 to 36 hours, peaking at 12 hours postburn. Protein-rich fluid is lost in blebs of the burned tissues as well as by weeping of second-degree wounds and surface of full-thickness wounds. With reduced vascular volume, the patient will go into shock if untreated.
5. Capillary permeability starts to change in about 48 hours, but protein lost in interstitial spaces may remain there for 5 days to 2 weeks before returning to the vascular system.
   a. When fluid mobilizes (moves from interstitial spaces back to vascular compartment), patients with good cardiac and renal function will diurese.
   b. Patients with impaired cardiac or renal function are in danger of fluid overload and pulmonary edema at this time.
6. Red blood cell mass is also diminished, because of thrombosis, sludging, and red blood cell death from thermal injury; as fluid escapes from capillary walls, however, blood concentrates and the hematocrit rises, causing sluggish flow (Fig. 31-2).
7. Capillary stasis may cause ischemia and even necrosis.
8. The body attempts to compensate for losses of plasma volume.
   a. Constriction of vessels.
   b. Withdrawal of fluid from undamaged extracellular space.
   c. The patient is thirsty. (Oral fluids are not given until bowel sounds are heard or until patient is no longer intubated).

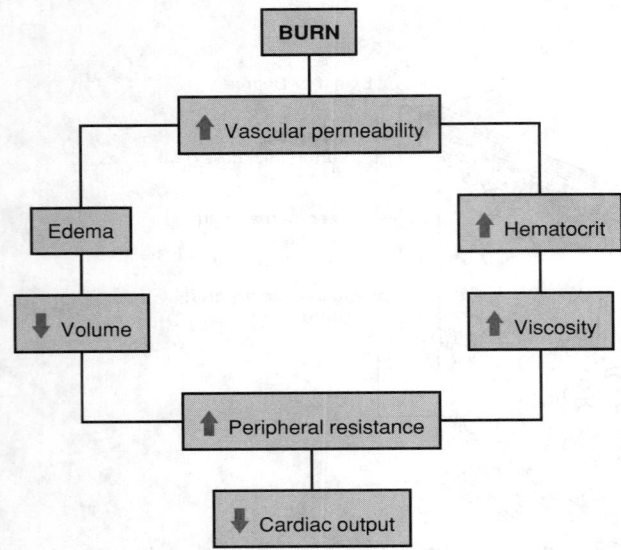

FIGURE 31-2 *Hemodynamic changes in burn injury.*

B. **Hemodynamics**
1. Lessened circulating blood volume results in decreased cardiac output initially and increased pulse rate.
2. There is a decreased stroke volume as well as a marked rise in peripheral resistance (due to constriction of arterioles and increased hemoviscosity).
3. This results in inadequate tissue perfusion, which may in turn cause acidosis, renal failure, and irreversible burn shock.
4. Electrolyte imbalance may also occur.
   a. Hyponatremia usually occurs during the 3rd to 10th day due to fluid shift.
   b. The burn injury also causes hyperkalemia initially due to cell destruction, followed by hypokalemia as fluid shifts occur and potassium is not replaced.

C. **Metabolic Demands**
1. Catecholamine release appears to be the major mediator of the hypermetabolic response to burn injury.
2. "Burn fever" is common and is dependent on depth of burn and percentage of TBSA involved. Temperatures of 102°F to 103°F (38.8°C–39.4°C) are common as "fever spikes."
3. Healing a large surface area requires much energy; glucose is the primary metabolic fuel.
4. Because total body glucose stores are limited and stored liver and muscle glycogen is exhausted within the first few days postburn, hepatic glucose synthesis (gluconeogenesis) increases.
5. Insulin levels decrease early postburn, and patients develop hyperglycemia. They continue to be hyperglycemic when insulin levels increase, probably due to increased gluconeogenesis.
6. Skeletal and visceral protein is mobilized to meet increased nutritional demands.
7. With adequate fluid resuscitations, the patient's weight will increase during the first few days. Fluid mobilization will result in weight loss, as will the catabolic response. Nutritional support in the form of enteral and/or total parenteral nutrition may be necessary. Weight loss from fluid resuscitation usually starts within 3 to 4 days postresuscitation.

8. Despite all nutritional support, it is almost impossible to counteract a negative nitrogen balance; the sooner a burn wound is closed, the more rapidly a positive nitrogen balance is reached.
9. The resting metabolic expenditure increases linearly with amount of TBSA; a burn of 40% to 50% TBSA has a metabolic rate almost twice normal.
10. The adult burn patient may require 3,000 to 5,000 calories or more per day.
    a. A burn of less than 10% usually requires minimal supplementation.
    b. A high-protein, high-calorie diet is necessary for a 10% to 20% burn.
    c. Between 20% and 30% enteral feedings are generally necessary.
    d. Between 30% and 40% TBSA burns generally require total parenteral nutrition to meet nutritional needs.

D. **Renal Needs**
1. Glomerular filtration may be decreased in extensive injury.
2. Without resuscitation or with delay, decreased renal blood flow may lead to high output or oliguric renal failure and decreased creatinine clearance.
3. Hemoglobin and myoglobin, present in the urine of patients with deep muscle damage often associated with electrical injury, may cause acute tubular necrosis and call for a greater amount of initial fluid therapy and osmotic diuresis.

E. **Pulmonary Changes**
1. Hyperventilation and increased oxygen consumption are associated with major burns.
2. The majority of deaths from fire are due to smoke inhalation.
3. Overzealous fluid resuscitation and the effects of burn shock on cell membrane potential may cause pulmonary edema, contributing to decreased alveolar exchange. Therefore, with an inhalation injury, it may be necessary to keep the patient slightly less hydrated.
4. Initial respiratory alkalosis resulting from hyperventilation may change to respiratory acidosis associated with pulmonary insufficiency as a result of major burn trauma.

F. **Hematologic Changes**
1. Thrombocytopenia, abnormal platelet function, depressed fibrinogen levels, inhibition of fibrinolysis, and a deficit in several plasma clotting factors occur postburn.
2. Anemia results from the direct effect of destruction of red blood cells due to burn injury, reduced life span of surviving red blood cells, overt or (more commonly) occult blood loss from duodenal or gastric ulcers, and blood loss during diagnostic and therapeutic procedures.

G. **Immunologic Activity**
1. The loss of the skin barrier and presence of eschar favor bacterial growth.
2. Granulation tissue, richly vascular, resists bacteria.
3. Abnormal inflammatory response after burn injury causes a decreased delivery of antibiotics, white blood cells, and oxygen to the injured area.
4. Hypoxia, acidosis, and thrombosis of vessels in the wound area impair host resistance to pathogenic bacteria.
5. Several major immunoglobulins, complement, and serum albumin are decreased soon after the burn occurs.

6. Depressed cellular immunity is reflected by lymphocytopenia, impaired delayed skin sensitivity, decreased allograft rejection potential, depletion of thymus-dependent lymphoid tissue, and increased susceptibility to fungi, viruses, and gram-negative organisms.
7. Burn wound sepsis
   a. After colonization of the burn wound surface by bacteria, subeschar and intrafollicular colonization develop. Intraeschar and subeschar colonization may progress to invasion of subadjacent, nonburned, previously viable tissue.
   b. A bacterial count of 10^5/g tissue as determined by burn wound biopsy indicates burn wound sepsis.
   c. The wound is fully colonized in 3 to 5 days.
8. Seeding of bacteria from the wound may give rise to systemic septicemia.

H. Gastrointestinal
1. As a result of sympathetic nervous system response to trauma, peristalsis decreases, and gastric distention, nausea, vomiting, and paralytic ileus may occur.
2. Ischemia of the gastric mucosa and other etiologic factors put the burn patient at risk for duodenal and gastric ulcer, manifested by occult bleeding and, in some cases, life-threatening hemorrhage.

◆ ASSESSMENT AND DIAGNOSTIC EVALUATION

As with all trauma victims, a primary and secondary trauma survey, including assessment of airway, breathing, and circulation as well as vital signs, is done. Other assessment parameters specific to the burn injury focus on extent and severity of burn injury and inhalation injury.

Severity of Burns

Severity of burns is determined by:

1. Depth—first, second, third degree
2. Extent—percentage of TBSA
3. Age—the very young and very old have a poor prognosis; the prognosis alters after age 45.
4. Area of the body burned—face, hands, feet, perineum, and circumferential burns require special care.
5. Medical history and concomitant injuries and illness.
6. Inhalation injury.

Assessment for Inhalation Injury

1. If victim was burned in closed area, there should be a high index of suspicion that smoke inhalation has occurred.
2. Evaluate all patients in closed-space fires for presence of symptoms of carbon monoxide poisoning: headache, visual changes, confusion, irritability, decreased judgment, nausea, ataxia, collapse.
3. Question the patient about types of things that burned in this room—type of carpet, vinyl articles, synthetics.
4. Observe for upper body burns, erythema or blistering of lips, buccal mucosa or pharynx, singed nasal hair, soot in oropharynx, dark gray or black sputum (Fig. 31-3).

5. Listen for hoarseness and crackles. Increasing hoarseness, stridor, and/or drooling are indicators for increasing immediacy for intubation.
6. Obtain arterial blood gases (ABGs), carboxyhemoglobin levels, and spirometry.
7. Direct visualization of the vocal cords may be necessary. Further visualization may be accomplished through bronchoscopy if necessary.
8. A chest x-ray should be obtained as a baseline.

Signs and Symptoms of Toxicity From Carbon Monoxide

CO Blood Level	Manifestations
0–10%	None
	Smokers may normally have 10% CO level
10%–20%	Headache, visual disturbance, angina in patients with cardiovascular disease, slowed mental function
20%–40%	Tight feeling in head, rapid fatigue from muscular effort, decreased muscular coordination, confusion, irritability, ataxia, nausea, vomiting, increased pulse rate, decreased blood pressure, dysrhythmias
40%–60%	Pulmonary and cardiac dysfunction, collapse, coma, convulsions
Over 60%	Often fatal

With the increasing use of synthetics, toxicity from aldehydes, cyanide, and other substances are increasing and must be considered.

Extent of Body Surface Burned

1. Anatomic location—burns affecting hands, feet, face, and perineum require specialized care. Circumferential burns also require special attention and may require escharotomy.
2. Determination is based on the use of tables for this purpose, such as the "rule of nines" (Fig. 31-4), the Lund and Browder chart (see p. 911), or the rule of the palm. The patient's palm is approximately 1% of the TBSA burned. Calculation of the percentage of TBSA burned serves as a guide for fluid therapy.
3. Repeat assessment may be performed on the 2nd or 3rd day to verify demarcation of burned areas.

Depth of Burn and Triage Criteria

1. It may be difficult to differentiate between second- and third-degree wounds initially. If the areas appear wet and are particularly sensate, then a second-degree (partial-thickness) injury is likely. If the area is less painful or insensate, the hairs are easily pulled out, and the area appears dry and is firm to touch, then it is most likely a third-degree (full-thickness) burn (Table 31-1).

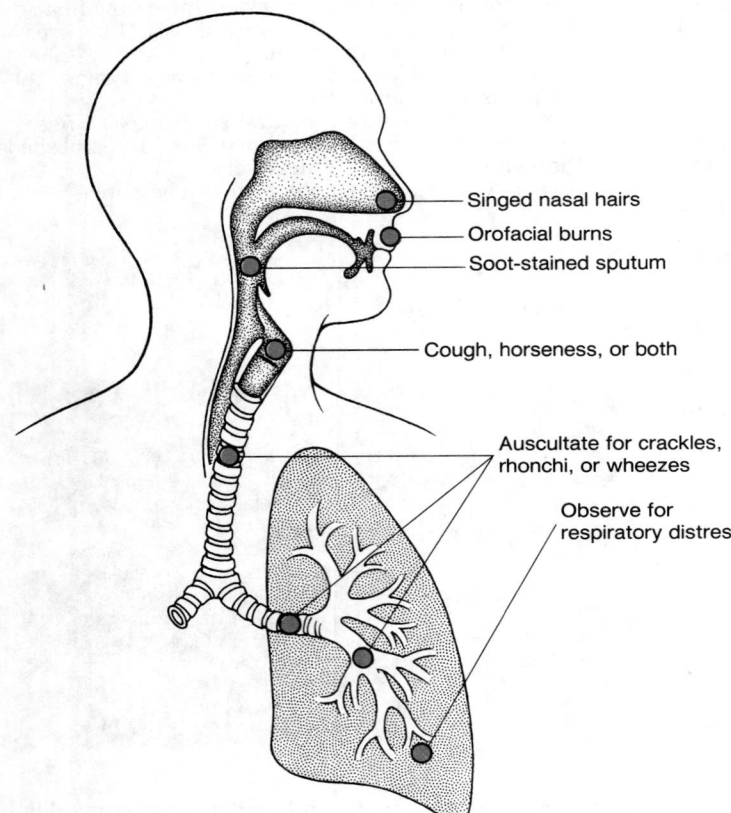

Singed nasal hairs
Orofacial burns
Soot-stained sputum

Cough, horseness, or both

Auscultate for crackles, rhonchi, or wheezes

Observe for respiratory distress

FIGURE 31-3 In the nursing history, determine whether the victim was in a closed area during the fire and whether he or she lost consciousness. If any of the above physical findings are noted in addition to the nursing history data, the victim should be taken to the hospital or burn center for further evaluation. Baseline arterial blood gas measurements (to detect hypoxemia) should be taken immediately on admission.

2. Reassess daily for first few days, because second-degree burn can convert to a third-degree injury.

3. Second- and third-degree burns of certain extent, chemical burns, electrical burns, burns of certain areas of the body, and any airway or inhalation injury should be triaged to a regional burn center (Table 31-2).

◆ TREATMENT OF BURNS

Management of the acute burn injury includes hemodynamic stabilization, metabolic support, wound debridement, use of topical antibacterial therapy, biologic dressings, and wound closure. Prevention and treatment of complications, including infection and pulmonary damage, and rehabilitation are also of major importance. The patient will also require physical therapy, occupational therapy, psychiatric and nutritional support.

Hemodynamic Stabilization

A. Intravenous Fluid Therapy
1. Immediate intravenous (IV) fluid resuscitation is indicated for:

a. Adults with burns involving more than 15% to 20% of body surface area.
b. Children with burns involving more than 10% to 15% of body surface area.
c. Patients with electrical injury, the elderly, or anyone with cardiac or pulmonary disease and compromised response to burn injury. Those patients will require meticulous monitoring and may require a modification of fluid requirements.

2. The goal is to give sufficient fluid to allow perfusion of vital organs without overhydrating the patient and risking later complications and circulatory overload.

3. Generally a crystalloid (Ringer's lactate) solution is used initially. Colloid is used during the 2nd day (5% albumin, plasmate, or hetastarch).

4. One of several formulas may be used to determine the amount of fluid to be given in the first 48 hours.
a. The Parkland formula is most commonly used.
b. The Brooks and Evans formulas may also be used.

5. Parkland formula:
a. First 24 hours—4 mL of Ringer's lactate × weight in kg × % TBSA burned.
b. One-half amount of fluid is given in the first 8 hours, calculated from the time of injury. If the starting of fluids is delayed, then the same amount of fluid is given over the remaining time. Remember to deduct any fluids given in the prehospital setting.

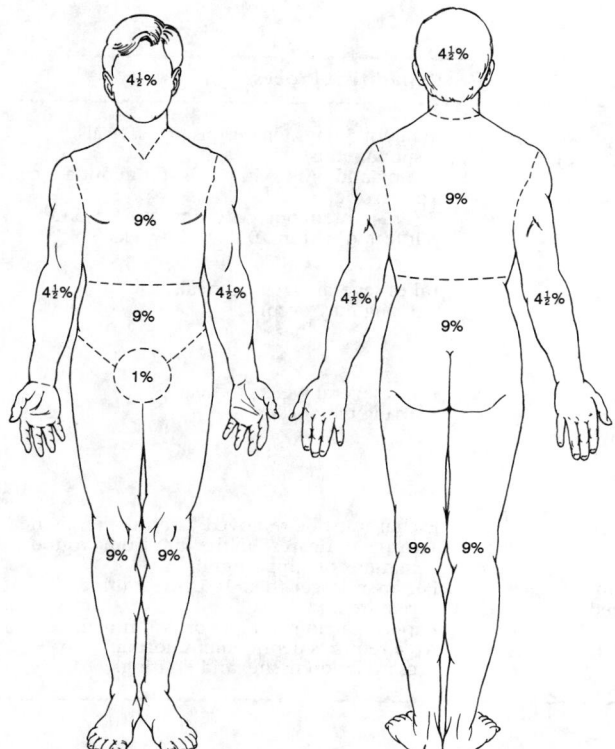

FIGURE 31-4 *Rule of nines for calculating total burn surface area (TBSA).*

c. The remaining half of the fluid is given over the next 16 hours. Example:

Patient's weight: 70 kg % TBSA burn: 80%
4 mL × 70 kg × 80% TBSA = 22,400 mL of Ringer's lactate
1st 8 hours = 11,200 mL or 1,400 mL/hour
2nd 16 hours = 11,200 mL or 700 mL/hour

d. Second 24 hours:
0.5 mL colloid × 70 kg × 80% TBSA/24 hours + 2,000 mL 5% dextrose in water run concurrently over the 24-hour period. Example:

0.5 mL × 70 kg × 80% = 2,800 mL colloid + 2,000 mL 5% D/W yields
117 mL colloid/hour
84 mL 5% D/W per hour

e. Boluses of crystalloid or colloid may be necessary to keep a urinary output of 0.5 to 1 mL/kg/hour.

B. Additional Interventions
1. Enzymatic agents applied to the burn wound may be used for more rapid debridement of eschar.
2. In surgical excision, primary or tangential, all nonviable tissue is removed down to a viable base, which is covered with biologic dressings: heterograft, homograft (both temporary), or autograft.

3. Fluids may be titrated to achieve a urinary output of 30 to 50 mL/hour (0.5 mL to 1.0 mL/kg/hour in an adult and approximately 1 mL/kg/hour in a child).
4. An indwelling urinary catheter is needed to monitor response to fluid therapy.
5. Weigh the patient on admission and then daily.
6. Elevate extremities.
7. Monitor peripheral pulses.
8. Administer humidified oxygen through a nasal cannula, mask, or ventilator support.

Metabolic Support

1. Initially, keep the patient on nothing-by-mouth status until bowel sounds return (1 to 2 days). However, small amounts (5 to 10 mL/hour) of isotonic enteral tube feedings are often started within 24 hours to help maintain a functioning gastrointestinal tract. Small amounts of erythromycin (Sumycin) may be used to encourage gastrointestinal motility.
2. Reduce metabolic stress by allaying pain, fear, and anxiety and maintaining a warm environment.
3. Nutritional management must be aggressive to combat acute nutritional deficiency and weight loss; a positive nitrogen balance should be the goal throughout the postburn care.
4. When bowel sounds return, administer oral fluids and advance diet as tolerated.
5. Offer more solid food after 2 to 3 days postburn as tolerance to food improves.
   a. Build up daily caloric intake to match daily caloric expenditure.
   b. Provide 3 g protein/kg body weight: 20% of needed calories in form of fats; remainder in carbohydrates.
6. When caloric requirements cannot be met by enteral feedings, it may be necessary to initiate total parenteral nutrition (amino acids, carbohydrates, and fat emulsions).
7. Provide potassium and vitamin and mineral supplements (zinc, iron, vitamin C).

Wound Cleansing and Debridement

Treatment of the burn wound includes daily or twice-daily wound cleansing with debridement, or hydrotherapy (tubbing) and dressing changes. Early excision of deep second- and third-degree burns is the goal.

1. Burn wounds must be cleansed initially and usually daily with a mild antibacterial cleansing agent and saline solution or water.
   a. This may be done in the hydrotherapy tub, in the bathtub, shower, or at the bedside.
   b. See Hydrotherapy, below.
2. Nonviable tissue (eschar) may be removed through natural, enzymatic, mechanical, and/or surgical debridement.
3. Burn eschar will begin to separate from the underlying viable tissue by a natural process of bacterial growth, which causes a lysis of protein at viable–nonviable tissue interface.
4. Eschar can be removed through daily or twice-daily dressing changes and use of forceps and scissors at time of wound cleansing.

TABLE 31-1 Assessment of Burn Injury

Extent or Degree	Assessment of Extent	Reparative Process
First degree	Pink to red: slight edema, which subsides quickly. Pain may last up to 48 hours; relieved by cooling. (Sunburn is a typical example.)	In about 5 days, epidermis peels, heals sponaneously. Itching and pink skin persist for about a week. No scarring. Heals spontaneously if it does not become infected within 10 days–2 weeks.
Second degree	*Superficial:* Pink or red; blisters form (vesicles); weeping, edematous, elastic. Superficial layers of skin are destroyed; wound moist and painful.	Takes several weeks to heal. Scarring may occur.
	Deep dermal: Mottled white and red: edematous reddened areas blanch on pressure. May be yellowish but soft and elastic—may or may not be sensitive to touch; sensitive to cold air. Hair does not pull out easily.	Takes several weeks to heal. Scarring may occur.
Third degree	Destruction of epithelial cells—epidermis and dermis destroyed. Reddened areas do not blanch with pressure. Not painful; inelastic; coloration varies from waxy white to brown; leathery devitalized tissue is called *eschar.* Destruction of epithelium, fat, muscles, and bone.	Eschar must be removed. Granulation tissue forms to nearest epithelium from wound margins or support graft. For areas larger than 3–5 cm, grafting is required. Expect scarring and loss of skin function. Area requires debridement, formation of granulation tissue, and grafting.

5. Enzymatic agents applied to the burn wound may be used for more rapid debridement of eschar.
6. In surgical excision, facial or tangential, all nonviable tissue is removed to a viable base or fascia and is then covered with a biologic dressing, that is, xenograft, allograft, or autograft. This may be a temporary or permanent covering procedure.

Hydrotherapy

Hydrotherapy ("tubbing," "tanking," or "showering") is the bathing of the burn patient in a tub of water or with a water shower to facilitate cleansing and debridement of the burned area.

A. *Advantages*
1. Topical medications, adherent dressings, and eschar are more easily removed.
2. Provides an opportunity for the patient to practice range-of-motion exercises.
3. Total assessment of the burn area is facilitated; total body cleansing can be achieved.

B. *Disadvantages*
1. Loss of body heat; sodium loss also occurs in tub water.
2. Uncomfortable to the patient and at times painful.
3. Maintenance of I.V. lines and ventilator care may be difficult during tubbing.
4. The patient's anxiety level often increases, and there is often a fear of drowning as well as the discomfort of the experience.

C. *Interventions*
1. Describe the procedure to the patient who is experiencing hydrotherapy for the first time.

2. Select the time for future tubbings in collaboration with the patient; administer a pain-control medication, if prescribed, before the treatment so that maximum benefit is realized. Use nursing activities to assist patient with the pain experience.
3. If the patient has an indwelling catheter, drain and plug it, or maintain a closed system to avoid contamination.
4. Aseptic technique is adhered to as closely as possible in preparing the patient for hydrotherapy, during hydrotherapy, and then in redressing wounds of the patient after therapy.
5. During hydrotherapy, after cleansing of the wounds, debride wound, shave adjacent areas at health care provider's direction, shampoo hair, and gently wash normal skin.
6. Limit hydrotherapy to as brief a time as possible to decrease the loss of body temperature and subsequent chilling.
7. Never leave the patient unattended in the tub.
8. Respect the patient's feelings and expressions of stress, pain, cold, and fatigue.
9. After treatment, the patient may be weighed before being carefully dressed and returned to the unit.
10. Document significant data, including status of the wound.

Topical Antimicrobials

Topical medications are used to cover burn areas and to reduce the number of organisms.

A. *Principles*
1. They are applied directly to the burn area as ointments, creams, or solutions, or they may be incorporated in single-layer dressings that do not stick to the wound but permit drainage.

TABLE 31-2 Triage Criteria for Determining When it is Advisable to Transfer a Patient to a Burn Center

Burned area second degree and third degree
  (age <10 or >50): 10%
Burned area second degree and third degree
  (age >10 or <50): 20%
Burned area third degree: >5% at any age
Chemical burn
Electrical injury
Burn of face, hands, feet, or perineum or circumferential burns
Burn accompanied by airway or inhalation injury

2. Dressings may take the form of commercial multilayered pads, standard 4 × 4 gauze pads, or several layers of stretch bandage (Kerlex type).
3. If gauze or pads are used, they may be held in place by stretch gauze or net tube dressings.
4. When wet dressings are used, that is, after a surgical procedure, then the same dressings are used. They are remoistened every 4 to 6 hours, as ordered. Heat loss may be prevented by limiting evaporative loss with a dry blanket and by warming the bed or using a heat cradle.
5. When wet dressings are used, 20-ply gauze will help retain solution at the proper concentration if rewet every 4 hours. A dry top layer of stockinette or a cotton bath blanket prevents evaporative heat loss.
6. Desired characteristics in a topical antimicrobial:
   a. Demonstrates action against a broad spectrum of bacteria.
   b. Has the ability to diffuse through the wound and penetrate the eschar.
   c. Nontoxic and noninjurious to body tissue.
   d. Inexpensive, pleasant to use, odorless or has pleasant odor; will not stain skin or clothing.
   e. Will not cause resistant strains of pathogenic organisms to develop.
7. Generally, all of the previously applied topical cream should be removed and the wound gently cleansed before applying new cream with each dressing change. Extremity dressings should be wrapped distally to proximally, taking care to avoid circulatory compromise when edema occurs or dressing is too tight.
8. There is no "ideal" topical antimicrobial.

B. **Types of Topical Antimicrobial Agents**
See Table 31-3.

Surgical Management

Early excision and grafting is the basic goal.

A. **Tangential Excision**
1. A special blade is used to slice off thin layers of damaged skin until live tissue is evidenced by capillary bleeding.
2. Commonly used with deep partial-thickness burns and is followed with immediate coverage with a biosynthetic or biologic dressing or an autograft.

B. **Fascial (Primary) Excision**
1. The skin, lymphatics, and subcutaneous tissue are removed, down to fascia, with either immediate auto-

grafting or temporary coverage with biologic or biosynthetic dressings.
2. This is repeated until all the deep burn areas are removed.

C. **General Consideration**
1. Early surgical intervention reduces the potential for wound infection and speeds the course of hospital care.
2. Operative excision is very stressful metabolically and incurs heavy blood loss; therefore, more conservative measures may be indicated for some patients.
3. As a general consideration, up to 190 mL of blood may be lost per 1% of burn excised in the adult patient.

Burn Wound Coverings

A. **Types of Burn Wound Coverings**
See Table 31-4.

B. **Biologic Dressings**
1. *Biologic dressings* are used to cover large surfaces of the body. Usually they are split-thickness grafts harvested either from human cadavers or other mammalian donors, such as pigs. Human amnion may also be used.
2. An *allograft* is a graft of skin taken from a person other than the burn victim and applied to a burn wound temporarily (a cadaver is the most common source).
3. A *xenograft* or *heterograft* is a segment of skin taken from an animal, such as a pig. It is useful in preparing debrided area for grafting and is really a biologic dressing.

C. **Donor Criteria**
1. Skin color unimportant, because it is only a temporary graft.
2. Donor should be an adult, free of infection.

D. **Purpose and Benefits**
1. Decreases heat, fluid, and protein losses.
2. Reduces bacterial proliferation.
3. Closes wound temporarily; enhances production and protection of granulation tissue.
4. Protects exposed neurovascular and muscle tissue as well as tendons.
5. Reduces pain and facilitates patient comfort.
6. Acts as a test graft to determine when granulating wounds will accept autograft successfully.
7. Provides an effective donor-site dressing.

E. **Clinical Procedures**
1. Allograft (cadaver) skin is the most popular temporary biologic dressing.
2. Devitalized tissue is first removed surgically or enzymatically.
3. Allograft is applied directly (shiny side down) to the denuded area. Before applying, it may be dipped in saline solution. It may be trimmed to fit the wound.
4. The grafts are usually secured with Steri-Strips. Staples or sutures may be used as well. The graft is covered with wet Adaptic (bibiotic solution or saline) and covered with stretch gauze, and this is again wet down with the appropriate solution.
5. The wound remains unchanged initially for 3 to 5 days, during which time it is wet down every 4 to 6 hours.
6. After the initial takedown, dressings are changed daily.
7. If allograft or xenograft is used, the wound bed may be prepared for permanent autografting.

F. **Biosynthetic Dressings**
1. Temporary biosynthetic dressings that help prevent bacterial contamination.

TABLE 31-3 Topical Antimicrobial Agents for Burns

Topical Agent	Description and Indications	Disadvantages	Nursing Implications
Silver sulfadizane 1% Silvadene (Marion Laboratories) SSD (Boots–Flint, Inc.)	A white, crystalline, highly insoluble compound in an opaque, odorless, water-miscible cream Exerts antimicrobial effect at level of cell membrane and cell wall Active against gram-negative and gram-positive bacteria and yeasts Penetration of silver sulfadiazine into wound is intermediate between silver nitrate and mefenide Systemic toxicity is rare Most widely used agent and least common incidence of side effects	May cause transient leukopenia that disappears after 2–3 days of treatment May increase possibility of kernicterus and should not be used in pregnant women in last trimester, premature infants, or neonates <2 months Impairment of hepatic and renal function that results in decreased excretion of drug constituents may preclude therapeutic benefits of continued silver sulfadiazine administration Exposure to sunlight produces gray discoloration Crystalluria and methemoglobinemia are rare toxic effects Protracted use may be associated with emergene of sulfadiazine resistance	Use with either open treatment, light or occlusive dressings Apply with sterile gloved hand directly to wound or applied to gauze dressing 0.16 cm ($^1/_{16}$ in.) thick, once or twice daily after thorough wound cleansing Silver sulfadiazene will be discontinued if WBC are less than 1,500 in an adult or less than 2,000 in a child. WBC count usually recovers in 2–4 days and application may be resumed.
Mafenide acetate 10% cream or 5% solution Sulfamylon	Usually supplied in water-miscible, hydroscopic cream base Active against most gram-positive ortanisms and particularly, *Clostrídia* sp. Active against common gram-negative burn wound pathogens but has little antifungal activity Not significantly bound by protein and wound exudate Good penetrating power and useful for control of established invasive burn wound infection	Painful during and for a while after application A potent carbonic anhydrase inhibitor resulting in metabolic acidosis therefore not used if > 20% TBSA Brisk alkaline diuresis and inappropriate polyuria may result when used on patients with a large burn surface area Compensatory hyperventilation and pulmonary failure may ensue if mafenide is not discontinued Hemolytic anemia is a rare complication	Cream is applied with or without dressing if possible. Must be reapplied every 12 hours to maintain therapeutic effectiveness Therapeutic solution concentration is maintained with bulky wet dressings, rewet every 2–4 hours Applicaton is associated with significant pain Hypersensitivity evidenced by maculopapular rash; is treated with antihistamines and/or discontinuing use Requires careful monitoring of pulmonary status and acid–base and fluid balance
Silver nitrate (0.5% solution)	Clear solution with low toxicity and significant antimicrobial effect against common burn wound pathogens Minimal absorption occurs because of the insolubility of its chloride and other salts Nonallergenic and not usually painful on application Best use is prophylaxis against infection	Can cause electrolyte abnormalities by depleting serum sodium, chloride, potassium, and magnesium Methemoglobinemia is a rare complication Stains everything (including normal skin) brown or black	Monitor electrolyte balance carefully; supplementation with sodium and potassium salts is routinely needed for patients with extensive burns Use bulky dressings, rewet every 2–4 hours, to maintain therapeutic concentration Maintain patient warmth and minimize transcutaneous evaporative water loss with dry top layer, such as stockinette or bath blanket
Other topical agents Cerium nitrate (1.74% solution) Cerium nitrate combined with silver sulfadiazine cream Povidone-iodine (1% cream; also in foam and solution forms) (Betadine) Gentamicin (0.1% ointment) (Garamycin) Nitrofurazone (0.2% ointment) (Furacin) Polymixin B-bacitracin ointment (Polysporin) Bibiotic solution (Bacitracin powder 5,000 units and polymixin powder 200,000 units to 1 liter of 0.9% saline solution)			

2. Used when permanent autograft is unavailable or unnecessary (as when partial-thickness wounds will heal spontaneously over time).
3. Biobrane (Woodruff Laboratories) consists of a custom-knit nylon fabric mechanically bonded to an ultrathin silicone rubber membrane, to which collagenous peptides of porcine skin are covalently bonded.
   a. Has a longer shelf life and lower cost than biologic dressings, such as pigskin.
   b. Is widely used for coverage of shallow wounds awaiting epithelialization, excised wounds awaiting autografts, widely meshed autografts until closure of interstices, and donor sites awaiting healing.

G. *Artificial Dermis*
1. Method being studied in selected burn centers to improve survival of patients with massive burns and little donor skin available.
2. Composed of a porous collagen-chondroitin 6-sulfate fibrillar mat covered with a thin Silastic sheet.
3. Used with an epidermal graft to provide a permanent cover that is at least as satisfactory as other available grafting techniques.
4. Used with donor sites that are thinner and that heal faster; seems to result in less hypertrophic scarring than the usual grafting methods.

H. *Wound Closure*
1. Skin grafting is usually required or preferred with full-thickness burns greater than 3 to 5 cm in diameter or in deep partial-thickness wounds or in areas of function.
2. After gradual eschar removal and development of a base of granulating tissue or in the presence of viable tissue after excision, grafts of the patient's own skin (autografts) are applied.
3. Sheet grafts or meshed grafts, providing wider expansion from donor sites, may be used.
4. Blood flow is established by the 3rd or 4th day, and by the 7th to 10th day postgrafting, vascular continuity, and wound closure have been established.
5. Cultured epithelial autografts may be used for patients with large burns and little available donor skin.
   a. Biopsies of unburned skin are cultured in a specialized laboratory to yield confluent sheets of epithelial cells suitable for grafting in about 3 weeks.
   b. Available donor sites can be used for coverage of the most functional or posterior surfaces, and the more delicate cultured epithelial autografts can be used to cover other large areas.
   c. Additional experience is needed to determine the long-term durability of cultured epithelial autografts, which may be lifesaving treatment for the severely burned.
6. Many partial-thickness burn wounds will heal spontaneously within a few weeks, provided they are protected from infection.
7. The donor site requires meticulous care and may be covered with a synthetic dressing (Biobrane, etc.), scarlet red, or an antimicrobial cream. If a cream is used, the wound must be dressed.

Prevention and Treatment of Complications

Primary causes of morbidity and mortality in burn victims are those related to infection and pulmonary problems.

1. Intravenous antibiotics may be given prophylactically to prevent gram-positive infection.
2. Topical antibacterial agents help to retard the proliferation of pathogenic organisms until wound closure occurs spontaneously or through surgical intervention.
3. Broad-spectrum antibiotics may be necessary to treat systemic gram-positive and gram-negative infections and sometimes fungal infection.
4. Critical diagnostic parameters include observing for signs of burn-wound sepsis, obtaining quantitative and qualitative wound biopsy, checking for signs of systemic septicemia, and taking blood for cultures.
5. Meticulous pulmonary care is essential, because pneumonia (especially if patient remains intubated) is common.
6. Severe inhalation injury, including ARDS, can contribute significantly to mortality, even though the burn wound size may be small.

◆ NURSING MANAGEMENT OF THE BURN PATIENT

Nursing Assessment

1. Obtain a thorough history, including:
   a. Causative agent—hot water, chemical, gasoline, flame, etc.
   b. Duration of exposure.
   c. Circumstances of injury, including whether in closed or open space, accidental or intentional, or self-inflicted.
   d. Age.
   e. Initial treatment, including first aid, prehospital emergency care (including fluids, intubation, etc.), or care rendered in another facility (emergency department, etc.).
   f. Preexisting medical problems—heart disease, diabetes, ulcers, alcoholism, chronic obstructive pulmonary disease, epilepsy, psychosis.
   g. Current medications.
   h. Concomitant injuries (eg, from fall, explosions, assaults).
   i. Evidence of inhalation injury.
   j. Allergies.
   k. Tetanus immunization status.
   l. Height and weight.
2. Take photograph of burned area (with patient permission) for medical record of extent of burn.
3. Perform ongoing assessment of hemodynamic and respiratory status, condition of wounds, and signs of infection.

Nursing Diagnoses

A. Impaired Gas Exchange related to inhalation injury
B. Ineffective Breathing Pattern related to circumferential chest burn, upper airway obstruction, or ARDS
C. Decreased Cardiac Output related to fluid shifts and hypovolemic shock
D. Altered Peripheral Tissue Perfusion related to edema and circumferential burns
E. Risk for Fluid Volume Excess related to fluid resuscitation and subsequent mobilization 3 to 5 days postburn

TABLE 31-4 Burn Wound Coverings

Description	Indications	Source or Form	Nursing Considerations
Amnion (rarely used) Amnionic and chorionic membranes collected from human placentas under sterile conditions	To protect partial-thickness burns To temporarily cover granulation tissue awaiting autograft	Obstetric department frees membranes from placenta and processes for short-term storage	Apply to clean wounds Change every 48 hours; wound may be left open to air or redressed immediately
Allograft/Homograft Human cadaver skin, about 0.015-in. thick Preferred biologic dressing	To debride untidy wounds To protect granulation tissue after escharotomy To cover excised wound immediately To serve as test graft before autograft	Fresh, cryopreserved homografts available from tissue banks throughout U.S.	Remember that length of time dressing is left in place varies greatly Observe for exudate; also, watch for local and systemic signs of infection and rejection
Xenograft Heterograft Pigskin similar to human skin, harvested after slaughter, then cryopreserved or lyophilized for long-term storage	Same as for homograft To cover meshed autografts To protect exposed tendons To cover partial-thickness burns that are eschar-free and clean or only slightly contaminated	Available in fresh, frozen, or lyophilized form, in rolls or sheets; also available meshed and impregnated with silver sulfadiazine	Change every 2–5 days; wound may be dressed or left open Observe for signs of infection
Biobrane Nylon fabric bonded to silicon rubber membrane, containing collagenous porcine peptides Elastic and durable; adheres to wound surface until removed or sloughed by spontaneous reepithelialization	To cover donor graft sites To protect clean, superficial, partial-thickness burns and excised wounds awaiting autografts To cover meshed autografts	Individually packaged sterile sheets of various sizes; also in glove-shaped form for hand burns	Remember that Biobrane is useful for wounds awaiting autograft because it can be left in place 3–14 days or longer and it is permeable to antimicrobials, which can be applied over it
Duo-Derm Hydroactive dressing that interacts with moisture on skin, creating bond that makes it adhere Interacts with wound exudate to produce soft, moist gel, facilitating removal	To cover small partial-thickness burns To prevent bacterial contamination	Individual, peelable, "blister" packages containing sheets of various sizes (from 3 × 3 to 8 × 12 in.)	Use size that allows dressing to extend beyond wound onto healthy skin Be careful to distinguish pus from liquefied material that normally remains in wound
Op-Site Thin, transparent elastic film that adheres to dry surfaces, conforms to body contours, and stretches with movement Occulsive and waterproof; permeable to moisture, vapor, and air	To cover clean partial-thickness burns and clean donor sites and to reduce pain from these wounds To provide moist environment for reepithelialization	Individual, sterile, peelable packages of sheets in various sizes	Maintain closed dressing; if exudate forms, drain aseptically with needle and syringe; seal hole with Op-Site patch Check for pooling of exudate in dependent areas
N-terface Surface material used between burn and outer dressing Translucent, nonabsorbent, and nonreactive; permeable to air and fluid	To cover partial-thickness burns and newly applied autografts To eliminate shearing of epithelium and protect healing tissue	Sterile, indvidually packaged strips, sheets, or rolls of various sizes	Remember that N-terface will shorten time it normally takes to change dressing, eliminating soaking and other steps required with conventional gauze dressing

(continued)

TABLE 31-4 Burn Wound Coverings *(continued)*

Description	Indications	Source or Form	Nursing Considerations
Vigilon Colloidal suspension on a polyethylene mesh support Permeable to gases and water vapor; provides moist environment Compatible with topical preparations	To clean small partial-thickness burns	Individual sterile or nonsterile sheets in various sizes	For occlusive use, remove one polyethylene film backing and place uncovered side on wound; for nonocclusive use, remove both backings and secure over wound with gauze or tape Change daily

Reprinted with permission. Bayley E and Smith G. The three degrees of burn care. Nursing 87 1987 Mar; 17(3): 34–41. Copyright @1987, Springhouse Corporation, Springhouse, PA. All rights reserved.

F. Impaired Skin Integrity related to burn injury and surgical interventions (donor sites)
G. Altered Urinary Elimination related to indwelling catheter
H. Ineffective Thermoregulation related to loss of skin microcirculatory regulation and hypothalamic response
I. Risk for Infection related to loss of skin barrier and altered immune response
J. Impaired Physical Mobility related to edema, pain, skin and joint contractures
K. Altered Nutrition: Less Than Body Requirements related to hypermetabolic response to burn injury
L. Risk for Injury related to decreased gastric motility and stress response
M. Pain related to injured nerves in burn wound and skin tightness
N. Ineffective Individual Coping related to fear and anxiety
O. Body Image Disturbance related to cosmetic and functional sequelae of burn wound

Nursing Interventions

A. *Achieving Adequate Oxygenation and Respiratory Function*
1. Provide humidified 100% oxygen until carbon monoxide level is known. (*CAUTION:* Adjust oxygen flow rate for patient with chronic obstructive pulmonary disease as prescribed.) If the patient is stable, try to get the initial ABG on room air.
2. Assess for signs of hypoxemia (anxiousness, tachypnea, tachycardia), and differentiate this from pain.
3. Suspect respiratory injury if burn occurred in an enclosed space.
4. Observe for and report erythema or blistering of buccal mucosa; singed nasal hairs; burns of lips, face, or neck; increasing hoarseness.
5. Monitor respiratory rate, depth, rhythm, cough.
6. Auscultate chest and note breath sounds.
7. Note character and amount of respiratory secretions. Report carbonaceous sputum, tracheal tissue.
8. Observe for signs of inadequate ventilation and begin serial monitoring of ABGs and oxygen saturation.
9. Provide mechanical ventilation, continuous positive airway pressure, or positive end-expiratory pressure if requested.

10. Keep intubation equipment nearby, and be alert for signs of respiratory obstruction.
11. In mild inhalation injury:
    a. Provide humidification of inspired air.
    b. Encourage coughing and deep breathing.
    c. Maintain pulmonary toilet.
12. In moderate to severe inhalation injury:
    a. Initiate more frequent bronchial suctioning.
    b. Closely monitor vital signs, urinary output, and ABGs.
    c. Administer bronchodilator treatments as ordered.
    d. For additional respiratory problems, it may be necessary to have patient intubated and placed on mechanical ventilation.

B. *Maintaining Adequate Tidal Volume and Unrestricted Chest Movement*
1. Observe rate and quality of breathing; report if progressively more rapid and shallow.
2. Assess tidal volume; report decreasing volume to health care provider.
3. Encourage deep breathing and incentive spirometry (may use sigh control on ventilator as needed).
4. Place patient in semi-Fowler's position to permit maximal chest excursions if there are no contraindications, such as hypotension or trauma.
5. Ensure that chest dressings are not constricting.
6. Prepare the patient for escharotomy and assist as indicated.

C. *Supporting Cardiac Output*
1. Position the patient to increase venous return.
2. Give fluids as prescribed.
3. Monitor vital signs, including apical pulse, respirations, central venous pressure, pulmonary artery pressures, and urine output at least hourly.
4. Determine cardiac output as requested.
5. Monitor sensorium.
6. Document all observations, and particularly note trends in vital sign changes.

D. *Promoting Peripheral Circulation*
1. Remove all jewelry and clothing.
2. Elevate extremities.
3. Monitor peripheral pulses hourly. Use Doppler as necessary.
4. Prepare the patient for escharotomy if circulation is impaired.
5. Monitor tissue pressure.

E. *Facilitating Fluid Balance*
1. Titrate fluid intake as tolerated. The initial resuscitation formula is only a base.

GERONTOLOGIC ALERT:
The elderly and those with impaired renal function, cardiovascular disease, and pulmonary disease are more likely to develop fluid overload. Proceed with caution.

2. Maintain accurate intake and output records.
3. Weigh the patient daily.
4. Monitor results of serum potassium and other electrolytes.
5. Be alert to signs of fluid overload and congestive heart failure, especially during initial fluid resuscitation and immediately afterward, when fluid mobilization is occurring.
6. Administer diuretics as ordered.

F. *Protecting and Reestablishing Skin Integrity*
1. Cleanse wounds and change dressings twice daily. Use an antimicrobial solution or mild soap and water. Dry gently. This may be done in the hydrotherapy tank, bathtub, shower, or at the bedside.
2. Perform debridement of dead tissue at this time. May use gauze, scissors, or pickups or forceps as appropriate. Try to limit time to 20 to 30 minutes depending on the patient's tolerance. Additional analgesia may be necessary.
3. Apply topical bacteriostatic agents as directed. Cream or ointment is applied $1/8$ inch thick.
4. Dress wounds as appropriate—using conventional burn pads, gauze rolls, or any combination. Dressings may be held in place as necessary with gauze rolls or netting.
5. For grafted areas, use extreme caution in removing dressings; observe for and report serous or sanguineous blebs or purulent drainage. Redress grafted areas according to protocol.
6. Observe all wounds daily and document wound status on the patient's record.
7. Promote healing of donor sites by:
   a. Preventing contamination of donor sites that are clean wounds.
   b. Opening to air for drying postoperatively if gauze or impregnated gauze dressing is used. If exudate occurs after the first 24 hours, swab the area for culture and apply an antimicrobial topical cream. If the culture is positive, treatment will be in accord with sensitivities.
   c. Following health care provider's or manufacturer's instructions for care of sites dressed with synthetic materials.
   d. Allowing dressing to peel off spontaneously.
   e. Cleansing healing donor site with mild soap and water once dressings are removed; lubricating site twice daily and as needed.

G. *Preventing Urinary Infection*
1. Maintain closed urinary drainage system and ensure patency.
2. Observe color, clarity, amount of urine frequently.
3. Empty drainage bag frequently.
4. Provide catheter care, such as washing with soap and water.

5. Encourage removal of catheter and use of urinal, bedpan, or commode as soon as frequent urine output determinations are not required.

H. *Promoting Stable Body Temperature*
1. Be efficient in care; do not expose wounds unnecessarily.
2. Maintain warm ambient temperatures.
3. Use radiant warmers, warming blankets, or adjustment of the bed temperature to keep the patient warm.
4. Obtain urine, sputum, and blood cultures for temperatures greater than 38.9°C (102°F) rectal or core temperature or if chills are present.
5. Provide a dry top layer for wet dressings to reduce evaporative heat loss.
6. Warm wound cleansing and dressing solutions to body temperature.
7. Use blankets in transporting patient to other areas of the hospital.
8. Administer antipyretics as prescribed.

I. *Avoiding Wound and Systemic Infection*
1. Wash hands with antibacterial cleansing agent before and after all patient contact.
2. Use barrier garments—isolation gown or plastic apron—for all care requiring contact with the patient or the patient's bed.
3. Cover hair and wear mask when wounds are exposed or when performing a sterile procedure.
4. Use sterile examination gloves for all dressing changes and all care involving patient contact.
5. Maintain proper concentration of topical antibacterial agents used in wound care.
6. Be alert for reservoirs of infection and sources of cross-contamination in equipment, assignment of personnel, etc.
7. Check history of tetanus immunization and provide passive and/or active tetanus prophylaxis as prescribed.
8. Change I.V. tubing and lines according to Centers for Disease Control and Prevention recommendations.
9. Administer antibiotics as prescribed and be alert for toxic effects and incompatibilities.
10. Assess wounds daily for local signs of infection—swelling and redness around wound edges, purulent drainage, discoloration, loss of grafts, etc.
11. Be alert for early signs of septicemia, including changes in mentation, tachypnea, and decreased peristalsis as well as later signs, such as increased pulse, decreased blood pressure, increased or decreased urine output, facial flushing, increased and later decreased temperatures, increasing hyperglycemia, and malaise. Report to health care provider promptly.
12. Promote optimal personal hygiene for the patient, including daily cleansing of unburned areas, meticulous care of teeth and mouth, shampooing of hair every other day, shaving of hair in or near burned areas, meticulous care of I.V. and urinary catheter sites.
13. Inspect skin carefully for signs of pressure and breakdown.
14. Observe for and report signs of thrombophlebitis or catheter-induced infections.
15. Prevent atelectasis and pneumonia through chest physical therapy, postural drainage, meticulous pulmonary technique, and, if indicated, tracheostomy care.

J. *Promoting Range of Motion and Ability to Perform Activities of Daily Living*
1. Ensure consultation with physical and occupational therapists, who will exercise the patient at least once or twice daily as necessary.

2. Encourage the patient to be as active as possible and to perform active range-of-motion exercises throughout the day.

3. Maintain splints in proper position as prescribed by occupational therapist; remove splints on regular schedule and observe for signs of skin irritation before reapplying.

4. Position the patient to decrease edema and avoid flexion of burned joints.

5. Coordinate pain management and other care to allow optimal effort during periods of physical exercise.

6. Initiate passive and active range-of-motion and breathing exercises during early postburn period.

7. Plan with therapists for a conditioning regimen that gradually increases energy expenditure and tolerance for activity.

8. Act as advocate for the patient's need for rest by coordinating the patient's therapeutic and social activities and prioritizing interventions and visits.

9. Help the patient achieve adequate relaxation and sleep through medication and environmental measures.

K. Ensuring That Nutritional Intake Will Meet Metabolic Demands

1. Weigh the patient daily with dressings removed.

2. Obtain consultation from dietitian for calculation of nutritional needs based on age, weight, height, and burn size. Two of the more popular formulas used to estimate nutritional needs are the Harrison-Benedict and Curreri formulas.

3. Administer vitamins and mineral supplements as prescribed.

4. Minimize metabolic stress by allaying fears, pain, and anxiety and by maintaining a warm environmental temperature.

5. Generally, for burns less than 10% TBSA, a well-balanced diet with emphasis on protein intake is necessary. For burns involving 10% to 20% TBSA, a high-protein, high-calorie diet is ordered. From 20% to 30% TBSA, supplementary enteral nutrition is necessary. Between 30% and 40%, total parenteral nutrition is usually implemented.

6. When the patient is ready for oral fluids, observe tolerance. If there are no problems, advance the diet as tolerated.

7. Provide nasogastric tube feedings as prescribed, using caution to prevent aspiration by checking tube placement before each feeding and checking amount of gastric aspirate.

8. Administer IV hyperalimentation and fat emulsions prescribed with usual nursing precautions.

9. Keep record of caloric intake.

10. Encourage the patient to feed self.

11. Supplement meals with between-meal high-protein, high-caloric snacks, such as milkshakes or foods brought from home according to patient's preference.

L. Preventing Paralytic Ileus and Stress Ulcer

1. Keep on nothing-by-mouth status until bowel sounds resume.

2. Assess bowel sounds every 2 to 4 hours while acutely ill. (Decreased peristalsis may be an early sign of septicemia.)

3. Decompress stomach with nasogastric tube on low intermittent suction until bowel sounds resume.

4. Recent practice now encourages small amounts of tube feedings, 5 to 10 mL/hour, immediately following the initial injury to help preserve the function of the gut and prevent paralytic ileus or stress ulcer.

5. Check amount and pH of gastric drainage or aspirate and report change.

6. Administer histamine-2 blockers and antacids as prescribed. This will help prevent or diminish the occurrence of stress (Curling's) ulcers.

7. Heed complaints of nausea while intubated by checking for abdominal distention, tube placement, residual aspirate.

8. Provide mouth care every 4 hours while intubated.

9. Test stools for occult bleeding.

M. Reducing Pain

1. Assess for pain periodically; do not wait for complaints of pain to intervene.

2. Determine previous experience with pain, the patient's response, and coping mechanisms.

3. Offer analgesics before wound care or before particularly painful treatments.

4. Change the patient's position when possible, supporting extremities with pillows.

5. Reduce anxiety by approaches such as sensory-oriented explanations of procedures.

6. Teach relaxation techniques, such as imagery, breathing exercises, and progressive muscle relaxation, to help the patient cope with pain.

7. Allow the patient to make choices regarding care whenever possible, thus allowing some measure of input and control in care.

N. Enhancing Effective Coping Strategies

1. Assess the patient's coping mechanisms from past history and current behavior.

2. Provide opportunities for the patient to express thoughts, feelings, fears, and anxieties regarding injury.

3. Explore with the patient alternative mechanisms for coping with the burn injury and its consequences.

4. Assure the patient of the normality of responses and the effect that time and healing will likely have on current concerns.

5. Interpret patient behavior to concerned family members and significant others.

6. Respect current coping mechanisms and discourage them only when an appropriate alternative can be provided.

7. Support family and friends' communications and visits if this is noted to help the patient.

8. Assess need for mental health consultation.

9. Offer antianxiety medications as prescribed.

O. Preserving Positive Body Image

1. Gather data on the patient's preburn self-image and life-style.

2. When ready, encourage the patient to express concerns regarding changes in self-image or life-style that may result from burn injury.

3. Be honest, but positive, in responding to the patient and family.

4. Positively reinforce appropriate, effective coping mechanisms.

5. Arrange for the patient to see face (if burned) with appropriate supportive personnel before being placed/transferred to a room with access to a mirror.

6. Arrange for the patient to talk with other patients who have had a similar injury and are progressing satisfactorily.

7. Encourage participation in a burn survivor's group, such as the Phoenix Society or other local support group.

8. Use and emphasize the concept of being a burn survivor. Survivors continue onward. Avoid the use of the term "burn victim," because it enhances the sick role.

Patient Education/Health Maintenance

Health education is closely related to rehabilitation as the burn patient prepares to return to a productive place in society. Functional and cosmetic reconstruction is accomplished, and the patient attempts to integrate a new self-concept into social realities. Broadly viewed, health education focuses on biologic, psychological, and social parameters.

1. Assist the patient in transition from dependence on the health team to independence by assisting the patient to communicate needs and functional abilities to others.
2. Guide the patient in thinking positively about self. Promote ability to redirect others' attention from the scarred body to the self within.
3. Demonstrate and explain wound care procedures to be continued after discharge:
   a. Wash hands.
   b. Cleanse small open wounds with mild soap in tub or shower.
   c. Rinse well with tap water.
   d. Pat dry with clean towel.
   e. Apply prescribed topical agent and/or dressing.
4. Teach patient to observe for local signs of wound infection:
   a. Increased redness of normal skin around burn area.
   b. Increased cloudy yellow pus or drainage.
   c. Increased pain, foul odor in burn area.
   d. Elevated body temperature.
5. Instruct the patient in measures to lubricate and enhance comfort of healing skin:
   a. After cleansing, use moisturizers such as cocoa butter, Nivea, Absorbase, Eucerin, or other nonperfumed hand lotion at least twice a day or more frequently as needed.
   b. Wear clean white underwear and clothing free of irritating dyes until wounds are well healed.
   c. Take antipruritics as prescribed.
   d. Stay in a cool environment if itching occurs.
   e. Protect skin from further trauma; use a sunscreen numbered 24 or higher.
   f. Discuss summer precautions to include a hat with a full wide brim if there were facial or neck burns. Also limit exposure to sun, because the affected areas will sunburn more easily and tan more deeply.
   g. Advise the patient that if wearing a pressure vest with or without sleeves or tights that the Occupational Safety and Health Administration standards for work in a hot environment as well as the need for oral fluid replacement should be used.
6. Advise patient to develop a schedule to incorporate exercise regimen as prescribed by physical therapist.

   a. Suggest scheduling exercises immediately after wound cleansing and application of topical agent, because skin may be more pliable and less sensitive to stretching then.
7. Instruct the patient in use and care of splints and pressure garments.
   a. Cleanse with mild soap and rinse well daily.
   b. Keep away from heat; dry garment by laying it flat on towels.
   c. Wear garment as prescribed. This is usually 23 out of 24 hours/day. The garment is usually worn for 1 to $1\frac{1}{2}$ years.
   d. Small open wounds should be covered with a light dressing under splints or pressure garments.
   e. Small superficial wounds smaller than 1.5 cm are usually treated with an antiseptic drying agent, such as merbromin 4% or 10%, twice a day.
   f. Observe for signs of skin breakdown. Reassure the patient that the small blister formation is normal and generally lessens after the first year.
   g. Wear/bring splints and pressure garments to follow-up visits to be checked for proper fit.
8. Review with the patient and family common emotional responses during convalescence (depression, withdrawal, grieving, dreaming, anxiety, guilt, excessive sensitivity, emotional lability, insomnia, fear of future), and discuss usual temporary nature of these as well as effective coping mechanisms. Make sure that the patient has a phone number or referral to the counselor should he or she want to make follow-up appointments.
9. Ensure that information has been given about follow-up evaluations and home health care services, as needed, in the interim.
10. For additional information and support, contact agencies such as: The American Burn Association, New York Hospital Burn Center; Room L 706; 525 E. 68th St., New York, NY 10021.

Evaluation

A. Carboxyhemoglobin below 10, ABGs within normal limits, respiratory rate 12 to 28
B. Tidal volume within normal limits
C. Pulse 110 or below, blood pressure stable
D. Peripheral pulses strong
E. Weight stable, no edema, lungs clear
F. Wounds clean and granulating
G. Catheter patent, urine clear and quantity sufficient
H. Temperature normal to low-grade fever, no chills
I. No signs of infection
J. Normal range of motion achieved and performing activities of daily living independently
K. Less than 5% weight loss from baseline
L. No gastric distention, aspirate and stool hemoccult negative
M. Reports minimal pain after analgesic administration
N. Using appropriate coping mechanisms
O. Verbalizing fears and concerns after viewing self in mirror

Selected References

Civetta, J. M., Taylor, R .W., & Kirby, R. R. (1992). *Critical care.* Philadelphia: J.B. Lippincott.

Davies, M. P., Evans, J., & McGonigle, R. (1994). The dialysis debate: Acute renal failure in burn patients. *Burns 20*(1), 71-73.

Faldmo, L., & Kravitz, M. (1993). The management of acute burn and burn shock resuscitation. *AACN Clinical Issues in Critical Care Nursing, 4*(2), 351-366.

Gilespie, R. (ed.) (1994). *Advanced Burn Life Support Instructors Manual.* Lincoln, NE: ABLS.

Haparick, E., & Munster, A. (1990). *Respiratory injury: Smoke inhalation and burns.* New York: McGraw-Hill.

Hudak, C. M., & Gallo, B. M. (1994). *Critical care nursing: A holistic approach.* Philadelphia: J.B. Lippincott.

Locke, G. Infection precautions in a burn unit. (1994). *Nursing Standard, 7*(48): 25-29.

Munster, A., & Parsons, L. (1991). Management of patient burns: Role of the laboratory in assessment and monitoring. *Critical Care Report, 2*(3), 360-364.

Munster, A. M., Smith-Meek, M., & Sharkey, P. (1994). The effect of early surgical intervention on mortality and cost effectiveness in burn care. *Burns, 20*(1), 61-64.

Rodeneaver, G., Baharestani, M. M., Brabec, M. E., Byrd, H. J., Salzberg, C. A., Spencer, P., & Vogelpohl, T. S. (1994). Wound healing and wound management: focus on debridement. *Advances in Wound Care, 7*(1), 22-24, 26-29, 32-36.

Saffle, J. R., Sullivan, J. J., Tuohig, G. M., & Larson, C. M. (1993). Multiple system organ failure in patients with thermal injury. *Critical Care Medicine, 21*(11), 1673-1683.

Smith, D. J., Thompson, P. D., Gardner, W. L., & Rodrigues, S. L. 1994. Burn wounds: Infection and healing. *American Journal of Surgery, 167*(1A), 465-485.

UNIT 12

◆

Infectious Diseases

CHAPTER 32 ◆

Infectious Diseases

General Considerations

◆ THE INFECTION PROCESS

The transmission of an infectious agent is accomplished by an infectious source, a vector of spread, and a susceptible host.

Causative Agent

Types: bacterium, virus, fungus, parasite, rickettsia, helminth, etc.

1. Pathogenicity—ability to cause disease.
2. Virulence (disease severity) and invasiveness (ability to enter and move through tissue).
3. Infective dose—number of organisms needed to initiate infection.
4. Organism specificity (host preference), antigenic variations.
5. Elaboration of toxins.

Reservoir

The environment in which the agent is found.

1. Human—humans are the reservoir of diseases that are more dangerous to humans than to other species.
2. Animal—responsible for infestations with trophozoites, worms, etc.
3. Nonanimal—street dust, garden soil, lint from bedding.

Mode of Escape from Reservoir

1. Respiratory tract (most common in humans).
2. Gastrointestinal tract.
3. Genitourinary tract.
4. Open lesions.
5. From bloodstream or tissues by insect bites, hypodermic needles, or surgical instruments.

Mode of Transmission

There are four main routes of transmission.

A. Contact Transmission
1. Direct contact—person to person.
2. Indirect contact—usually an inanimate object.
3. Droplet contact—from coughing, sneezing, or talking by an infected person.

B. Vehicle Route (Through Contaminated Items)
1. Food—salmonellosis.
2. Water—shigellosis, legionellosis.
3. Drugs—bacteremia resulting from infusion of a contaminated infusion product.
4. Blood—hepatitis B.

C. Airborne Transmission
1. Droplet nuclei—residue of evaporated droplets that remain suspended in air.
2. Dust particles in the air containing the infectious agent.
3. Organisms shed into environment from skin, hair, wounds, or perineal area.

D. Vectorborne Transmission
1. Via contaminated or infected arthropods, such as flies, mosquitoes, and ticks.

Mode of Entry of Organisms Into Human Body

1. Respiratory tract
2. Gastrointestinal tract
3. Genitourinary tract
4. Direct infection of mucous membranes/break in skin

Host Factors

Illness after entrance of infection into the body depends on:

1. Number of organisms to which host is exposed; duration of exposure.
2. Age, genetic constitution of host, and general physical, mental, and emotional health and nutritional status of host.
3. Status of hematopoietic system; efficacy of reticuloendothelial system.
4. Absent or abnormal immunoglobulins.
5. The number of T lymphocytes and their ability to function.

Diagnostic Tests

◆ COLLECTION OF SPECIMENS

Proper collection of specimens is important to maximize the outcome of laboratory tests for the diagnosis of infectious diseases. A variety of laboratory tests can be performed to make a presumptive or definitive diagnosis so that therapy can begin.

Principles

1. It is imperative that specimens be collected and handled very carefully if the causative agent for infection is to be identified correctly.
2. Specimens should be collected during the acute phase of infection and before the initiation of antibiotic therapy, if possible.
3. Obtain an adequate amount of the specimen necessary for tests.
4. Avoid potential contamination of the specimen by using proper collection instruments and containers.

5. Label the container properly with the name of the patient, source of the specimen, date, time collected, and test to be performed.

> **NURSING ALERT:** ◆
> Use universal precautions during the collection of specimens.

Types of Specimen Collection

A. **Blood**
1. Normally a sterile body fluid.
2. Specimens obtained by venipuncture are preferred over sampling from vascular catheters.
3. Blood cultures should be performed serially over 24 hours or drawn concurrently from more than one site.
4. Aseptic technique is essential to avoid contaminating the specimen with organisms colonizing the skin.
5. Cleanse the site of venipuncture with povidone–iodine and allow to dry. If the patient is allergic to iodine preparations, use 70% alcohol.
6. The diaphragm tops of the culture bottles are not sterile and must be wiped with povidone–iodine or alcohol before injection of blood.

TABLE 32-1 Guide for Adult Immunization

Category	Vaccine	Comments
Age (yr)		
18–24	Td* (0.5 mL IM)	Booster every 10 yr at mid-decades (age 25, 35, 45, etc.) for those who completed primary series
	Measles† (MMR, 0.5 mL SC × 1 or 2)	Post-high school institutions should require two doses of live measles vaccine (separated by 1 month), the first dose preferably given before entry
	Mumps‡ (MMR, 0.5 mL SC × 1)	Especially susceptible males
	Rubella‡ (MMR, 0.5 mL SC × 1)	Especially susceptible females; pregnancy now or within 3 months postvaccination is contraindication to vaccination
	Influenza	Advocated for young adults at increased risk of exposure (military recruits, students in dorms, etc.)
25–64	Td*	As above
	Mumps‡	As above
	Measles† (MMR, 0.5 mL SC × 1)	Persons vaccinated between 1963 and 1967 may have received inactivated vaccine and should be revaccinated
	Rubella‡ (MMR, 0.5 mL SC × 1)	Principally females ≤ 45 yr with childbearing potential; pregnancy now or within 3 months postvaccination is contraindication to vaccination
>65	Td*	As above
	Influenza (0.5 mL IM)	Annually, usually in November
	Pneumococcal (23 valent, 0.5 mL IM)	Single dose; efficacy for elderly not established, but case control and epidemiology studies suggest 60–70% effectiveness in preventing pneumococcal bacteremia (*NEJM* 325:1453, 1991)

IM: intramuscular; MMR: measles, mumps, and rubella; SC: subcutaneously.
* Td—Diphtheria and tetanus toxoids absorbed (for adult use). Primary series is 0.5 mL IM at 0, 4 wk and 6–12 months; booster doses at 10-year intervals are single doses of 0.5 mL IM. Adults who have not received at least 3 doses of Td should complete the primary series. Persons with unknown histories should receive the series.
† Persons are considered immune to measles if there is documentation of receipt of two doses of live measles vaccine after the first birthday, prior physician diagnosis of measles, laboratory evidence of measles immunity or birth before 1957.
‡ Persons are considered immune to mumps if they have a record of adequate vaccination, documented physician diagnosed disease, or laboratory evidence of immunity. Persons are considered immune to rubella if they have a record of vaccination after their first birthday or laboratory evidence of immunity. (A physician diagnosis of rubella is considered nonspecific.)
(From: Bartlett, John G. Pocketbook of Infectious Disease Therapy.)
(Adapted from: Guide for Adult Immunization, American College of Physicians, 2nd Ed., Philadelphia, PA 1-178, 1990; MMWR 40(RR12):1–94, 1991)

BOX 32-1 Universal Precautions

1. Gloves must be worn for touching blood and any body fluid visibly contaminated with blood, for touching mucous membranes and nonintact skin of all patients and for handling items or surfaces soiled with blood or body fluids. Gloves should be changed between procedures on the same patient and between each patient.
2. Gowns or aprons must be worn when contamination of clothing with blood or body fluids is anticipated.
3. Masks and protective eyewear must be worn when performing procedures likely to generate sprays or splashes of blood or body fluids into the eyes, nose or mouth.
4. Hands and other skin surfaces must be washed immediately if contaminated with blood or body fluids.
5. Needles and other sharps are *never* to be manipulated by hand (e.g. recapped, purposely bent or broken, removed from syringes or handles). All sharps are placed in puncture-resistant containers for disposal.
6. Blood spills are to be cleaned up promptly with an appropriate germicide such as a phenolic or hypochlorite solution.
7. All items soiled with blood or bloody body fluids are placed and transported in bags that prevent leakage.

7. DO NOT CHANGE NEEDLES ON THE SYRINGE BETWEEN INJECTIONS OF BLOOD INTO THE CULTURE BOTTLES. The risk of needlestick with a blood-contaminated sharp is too great.

B. **Urine**
1. Normally a sterile body fluid.
2. A clean-catch *midstream* urine collection provides the best method for obtaining a specimen to detect a urinary tract infection. The urinary meatus must be cleaned with povidone–iodine.
3. Patients who are catheterized should have the specimen withdrawn using a sterile needle and syringe from the catheter sampling port. Clamp the collection tube for about 30 minutes before taking the sample.
4. Urine specimens must be transported to the laboratory within 30 minutes or refrigerated for up to 5 hours.
5. Urine specimens that have greater than 100,000 colonies of bacteria per milliliter of urine are indicative of infection.

C. **Stool**
1. Obtained to culture organisms that are not part of the normal bowel flora (ie, salmonella, shigella, rotavirus).
2. Patient should defecate into a container. Stool specimens should not contain urine or water from the toilet bowl.
3. Fecal specimens can be obtained directly from the rectum using a sterile swab.

D. **Sputum**
1. Specimen needs to be from the lower respiratory tract, not oropharyngeal secretions. The laboratory will perform a Gram's stain on all sputum specimens to determine if they are representative of pulmonary secretions. A specimen containing a majority of cells from squamous epithelium will be rejected.

2. The most common method of collection is expectoration from a cooperative patient with a productive cough.
3. A sputum specimen can be collected in a sputum trap from patients who have artificial airways and require suctioning.
4. If a patient cannot produce sputum, sputum induction using an aerosol nebulizer may assist with loosening thickened secretions.
5. Bronchoscopy may be required to obtain sputum if induction fails.

E. **Wounds**
1. Specimens are cultured for aerobic and anaerobic organisms.
2. Using a sterile cotton-tipped swab, collect as much exudate as possible. Avoid swabbing surrounding skin.
3. Place the swab immediately in transport culture tube and take to the laboratory.

◆ LABORATORY TESTS
Microbiologic Evaluation

A. **Microscopy**
1. Microscopic examination distinguishes tissue cells from microorganisms.
2. Stains are added to highlight the structural characteristics of microorganisms (ie, Gram stain, acid-fast stains to isolate mycobacteria).
3. Classification is done according to their shape and size; gram-positive versus gram-negative, rods versus cocci, bacteria versus viruses.
4. Results of microscopy are usually available within minutes, which permits the initiation of treatment based on a presumptive diagnosis.

B. **Culture**
1. Allows for positive identification of the organism.
2. Different culture media are used for suspected pathogens. Liquid medium is used for blood specimens, because fewer microorganisms can be grown. Solid medium will grow polymicrobial cultures.
3. Recovery of the pathogen from cultures will vary based on the type of microorganism, the type of specimen, and the stage of illness. Many common pathogens, such as *Staphylococci*, *Streptococci*, and *Enterococcus*, will be identified in 48 hours.
   a. Fungal organisms may take up to 10 days to culture.
   b. Viruses may take weeks to grow in culture.

C. **Antibiotic Susceptibility Testing**
1. Antibiotics are added to a culture to determine whether the microorganism is inhibited from growing or is dead.
2. Agar diffusion method—a pure culture of the microorganism is exposed to a paper disk impregnated with a known amount of antibiotic, which diffuses from the disk into the culture.
   a. Minimum inhibitory concentration—amount of drug that will inhibit visible growth—is measured by the size of the zone around the disk in which growth is inhibited.
   b. The results of agar diffusion tests are reported as "resistant" if growth is not altered, "sensitive" if growth is inhibited, and "intermediate" if results are uncertain.

3. Tube dilution method—uses either broth or agar as the medium.
   a. Different concentrations of an antibiotic are added to a known number of organisms to determine the minimum inhibitory concentration.
   b. An organism is considered sensitive to a drug if the antibiotic blood levels can be attained at two to four times the minimum inhibitory concentration.

White Blood Cell Count

1. Nonspecific tests that provide important information about the inflammatory response of a patient as well as the response to therapy.
2. The total number of circulating leukocytes and the differential (given as a percent of the total white blood cell count) may change during a bacterial or viral infection.
3. During an acute bacterial infection, the white blood cell count increases (>11,000/mm^3), accompanied by increased neutrophils and increased bands (immature neutrophils) in the differential. The shift in differential reflects phagocytic activity.

Immunologic Tests

1. Pathogens that are antigenic stimulate antibodies that can be detected in the serum of patients.
2. Detection of antibodies is *not* diagnostic of current infection.
3. Antigen–antibody reactions must be evaluated over a period of time.
4. Immunoglobulin M antibody production peaks during active infection and decreases during convalescence.
5. Immunoglobulin G antibodies peak during convalescence and persist.
6. A fourfold rise in antibody titer during convalescence indicates concurrent infection.

General Procedures/Treatment Modalities

◆ IMMUNIZATION

Immunity is the resistance that an individual has against disease. Specific immunity to a particular organism implies that an individual has either generated the appropriate antibody in his or her own body or received ready-made antibodies from another source.

Immunity may be natural (not acquired through previous contact with the infectious agent) or acquired (resistance acquired by the host as a result of previous exposure to the disease). Acquired immunity may be *passive* or *active*. See Table 32-1 for recommended adult immunizations.

Active Immunity

Active immunity is immunization that has been produced by naturalor acquired stimulation so that the body produces its own antibodies.

1. It may result from clinical or subclinical infection (the person gets the disease), by vaccination with live or killed microorganisms or their antigens, or by inactivated vaccines and toxoids.
2. The organisms have been treated by heating or by chemical inactivation to destroy their harmful properties without destroying their ability to stimulate antibody protection.
3. Depending on age and health status, adults may be immunized against tetanus, diphtheria, measles, and rubella, and high-risk groups (those older than age 65 years and those with chronic heart, lung, and metabolic disease) may be immunized against influenza, pneumococcal pneumonia, and hepatitis B.

Passive Immunity

Passive immunity to a disease is a state of relatively short-lived immunity produced by the injection of serum containing antibodies that have been formed in another host.
Types of preparation for passive immunity:

1. Nonspecific immunoglobulin—used for immune maintenance of selected immunodeficient persons as well as for passive immunization against hepatitis A and possibly measles.
2. Specific immunoglobulins—contain high levels of antibody against specific pathogens that include hepatitis B, rabies, varicella zoster, and tetanus.
3. Animal serum or antitoxins—may cause an anaphylaxis-like reaction or serum sickness.

◆ PREVENTION OF TRANSMISSION OF INFECTION IN THE HEALTH CARE FACILITY

Fundamental Aspects

1. Hand washing is the single most important procedure for the prevention of disease transmission. The combination of soap and water and friction on the hands will remove the transient flora acquired through direct care of patients and the handling of environmental fomites. The use of an antimicrobial soap product with residual activity is recommended for staff working with high-risk patients, such as neonates, immunocompromised oncology or transplant patients, and intensive care patients. Gloves are not a substitute for hand washing.
2. Largely because of the human immunodeficiency virus epidemic, the Centers for Disease Control and Prevention recommended a strategy to minimize the risk of transmission of bloodborne pathogens in the workplace. *Universal Blood and Body Fluid Precautions* requires that all patients' blood and body fluids be considered potentially infected with a bloodborne pathogen (eg, hepatitis B, hepatitis C, human immunodeficiency virus; see Box 32-1).

> **NURSING ALERT:** ❖
> The use of universal precautions has been mandated by the Occupational Safety and Health Administration of the U.S. Department of Labor.

3. Ensure the maintenance of a clean environment. Routine cleaning of walls and curtains is not indicated unless they become visibly soiled.
4. Soiled linen should be handled as little as possible and with minimal agitation. The risk of disease transmission from linen is negligible.
5. Disinfect reusable equipment between patients with an appropriate germicide.
6. Private rooms may be indicated based on the epidemiology of the infectious disease. For example, private rooms with special ventilation are required for patients with pulmonary or laryngeal tuberculosis. The special ventilation criteria are:
   a. Minimum of six air changes per hour.
   b. Negative air pressure in relation to the corridor.
   c. Exhausting of air from the room directly to the outside or subjecting the air to high-efficiency filtration before recirculating to other areas.
      Private rooms are useful for spatial segregation of patients colonized/infected with an organism spread by direct contact, such as methicillin-resistant *Staphyloccocus aureus* (MRSA). Additionally, private rooms may be used for patients with poor hygienic habits or for patients who are immunocompromised and for whom consequences of infection are likely to be serious.

Isolation Techniques

1. Isolation precautions are required for certain infected patients to prevent the spread of disease to other patients, staff, and visitors.
   a. Isolation precautions are used to isolate the infection, *not* the patient.
   b. The Centers for Disease Control and Prevention recommends the use of either a disease-specific isolation system or a category-specific isolation system.
   c. A more generic approach to isolation is called *body substance isolation.*
2. Disease-specific isolation—diagnosis-based system that considers the epidemiology of each infectious disease individually. The barriers (private room, masks, gowns, gloves) required to interrupt transmission are specified, thereby eliminating "overisolation."
3. Category-specific isolation—includes six categories of isolation, which are determined by the mode of transmission of the diseases grouped together in a category. This system may lead to overisolation, because many different diseases are grouped into the categories, leading to unnecessary precautions being applied to some diseases. The categories are:
   a. Strict isolation—designed for highly contagious infections that are spread by both airborne droplet nuclei and contact transmission.
      (1) Examples include varicella, disseminated herpes zoster, and the viral hemorrhagic fevers.
      (2) Technique includes a private room with negative airflow and the use of masks, gowns, and gloves for all persons entering the room.
   b. Contact isolation—designed for highly transmissible infections that are not spread by airborne droplet nuclei but are transmitted primarily by close and direct contact.
      (1) Examples include viral respiratory infections in children, such as respiratory syncytial virus (RSV) or any colonization/infection with a multiple-drug resistant bacteria, such as vancomycin-resistant *Enterococcus.*
      (2) Patients with large draining wounds require contact precautions.
      (3) Technique includes a private room, masks for those personnel providing close direct care to the patient, gowns if soiling is likely, and gloves for touching infective material.
   c. Respiratory isolation—designed to prevent transmission of diseases spread over short distances through the air (droplet transmission).
      (1) Examples include children with *Haemophilus influenzae*, epiglottitis, meningitis, or pneumonia; patients with serious meningococcal disease; mumps and pertussis.
      (2) Technique includes a private room or cohorting patients with the same organism and masks for those personnel providing close direct care to the patient.
   d. Tuberculosis or acid-fast bacillus (AFB) isolation—designed for patients suspected or known to have pulmonary or laryngeal tuberculosis.
      (1) Technique includes a private room with negative airflow and the use of appropriate respiratory protection (see p. 224).
   e. Enteric precautions—designed to prevent infections that are transmitted by direct or indirect contact with fecal material, such as *Salmonella* gastroenteritis.
      (1) Technique includes a private room only if the patient has poor hygiene and is likely to contaminate the environment, gowns if soiling is likely, and gloves for touching infective material.
   f. Drainage/secretion precautions—designed to prevent infections transmitted by direct or indirect contact with purulent material or other drainage from an infected body site.
      (1) Technique includes gowns if soiling is likely and gloves for touching infective material.
4. Body substance isolation—an alternative to diagnosis-driven isolation systems. Focuses on the isolation of all moist body substances from all patients through the use of barriers, primarily gloves.
   a. The system is based on the premise that it is the unrecognized transmissible agent present in body substances that is the most problematic in hospital-acquired infection.
   b. The use of barriers is dictated not by the patients' diagnosis but by the type of interaction with the patient.
   c. A "Stop Sign Alert" is placed on the doors of patients with diseases spread via the airborne route.
   d. The system emphasizes the restriction for nonimmune personnel not entering the rooms of patients with measles, mumps, rubella, and varicella.

Infectious Disorders

See Table 32-2.

TABLE 32-2 Selected Infectious Diseases

Disease & Infectious Agent	Clinical Manifestations	Incubation Period	Diagnostic Tests
Vector-Transmitted Fevers			
Rocky Mountain Spotted Fever *Rickettsia rickettsii*	Systemic, febrile illness. Rash usually occurs by the 6th day with a progression from macular to maculopapular to petechial. Fever, headache, myalgia, nausea, and vomiting.	Related to the size of the inoculum. Usually 1 week with a range of 1–14 days.	Immunofluorescence of body tissue may identify rickettsiae during the 3rd or 4th day of illness. Serology—increase in antibody titer can usually be detected after 7–10 days of illness, but may be delayed for 4 or more weeks if antibiotic therapy is begun early. Titers wane rapidly in late convalescence. Complement fixation—titers rise later in illness (10–14th day) and persist longer.
Lyme Disease *Borrelia burgdorferi*	Erythema migrans is the best clinical marker—an annular skin lesion that appears at the site of the tick bite and expands over a period of days to weeks and develops central clearing. Lesion is warm to touch but not painful. Flulike symptoms—malaise, fever, headache, stiff neck, myalgia. Inflamed painful arthritis. Limb weakness. Bell's palsy.	3–32 days	IgM antibodies peak during the 3rd to 6th weeks after disease onset. IgG antibodies slowly rise and peak months later when arthritis is present. Early in the illness, high sedimentation rate, elevated serum IgM level, or an increased SGOT level.
Viral Infections			
Influenza Types A, B and C with many mutagenic strains	Acute, usually self-limited febrile illness associated with upper and lower respiratory infection. Characterized by a severe and protracted cough, myalgias coryza, and mild sore throat.	24–72 hours	Tissue culture of nasal or pharyngeal secretions. Fluorescent antibody staining of secretions.
Mononucleosis Epstein-Barr Virus (EBV)	Produces a generalized lymph node hyperplasia. Characterized by fever, exudative pharyngitis, splenomegaly, and lymphadenopathy.	4–6 weeks	Differential WBC—lymphocytes and monocytes >50%, with more than 10% being atypical lymphocytes. Serology—heterophil agglutination antibody present usually by the end of 1st week. Not useful diagnostic tool in children under 5 years of age. If negative, EBV IgM and IgG may be performed. EBV IgM elevated 1:80 to 1:160 drops rapidly after clinical disease. EBV IgG elevated 1:80 is suggestive, >1:5 suggests immunity.

Management	Complications	Nursing Considerations
Tetracycline (Sumycin) (25–50 mg/kg per day) or chloramphenicol (Chloromycetin) (50 mg/kg per day) administered orally in 4 divided doses. Appropriate doses of IV preparations may be substituted during the initial toxic state. Medication continued for 5–7 days. Supportive therapy including fluid replacement, control of fever and management of anemia with transfusion of packed red cells.	Shock. Disseminated intravascular coagulation (DIC). Thrombosis and gangrene. Cardiac arrhythmias. Neurologic sequelae. Renal failure. Coma & death.	1. Not communicable person to person. 2. Instruct the patient that relapse of illness may occur and that reoccurrence of symptoms should be reported immediately. 3. The best means of prevention is the avoidance of tick-infested areas. While working or playing in infested areas, inspection of the body and clothing should be performed every 3–4 hours. 4. Ticks should be removed from the skin with tweezers or forceps to avoid leaving mouth parts in the skin. 5. Use of insect repellents are useful for repelling ticks.
Tetracycline (Sumycin) 250 mg four times a day or phenoxymethyl penicillin (Betapen-VK) 500 mg four times a day or erythromycin (Eryc) 250 mg four times a day for at least 10 days or up to 20 days if symptoms persist. For meningitis/cranial or peripheral neuropathies—IV penicillin G (Duracillin) 20 million units a day or ceftriaxone (Rocephin) 2 g/d for 14–21 days. Lyme arthritis—IV penicillin G 20 million units a day for 10 days.	Meningeal irritation leading to meningitis, encephalitis. Chorea. Atrioventricular block.	1. Not communicable person to person. 2. The best means of prevention is the avoidance of tick-infested areas. While working or playing in infested areas, inspection of the body and clothing should be performed every 3–4 hours. 3. Ticks should be removed from the skin with tweezers or forceps to avoid leaving mouth parts in the skin. 4. Use of insect repellents are useful for repelling ticks.
Aspirin (A.S.A.) or acetaminophen (Tylenol) for control of fever. Amantadine (Symmetrel) 100 mg PO BID for duration of epidemic (5–6 weeks) as prophylaxis for high-risk persons. Amantadine is given as therapy within 24–48 hours of symptoms until 48 hours after symptoms resolve. Agent-specific antibiotics for bacterial complications. Vaccine must be repeated yearly in the fall for viral strain expected. Recommended for any person at risk for complications of influenza.	Secondary bacterial pneumonia. Primary viral pneumonia.	1. Maintain bed rest for at least 48 hours after fever subsides. 2. Force fluids. 3. Encourage high-risk persons to receive the influenza vaccine in the fall of each year. 4. Continue antibiotics prescribed for bacterial complications for defined time period (usually 7–10 days). 5. Report symptoms of secondary infection (purulent nasal drainage or sputum, ear pain, increase in fever) to health care provider.
Supportive therapy to include aspirin (A.S.A.) or acetaminophen (Tylenol) for sore throat and fever, bed rest. Surgical removal of the spleen for splenic rupture. Corticosteroids for severe neurologic complications, thrombocytopenic purpura, or hemolytic anemia.	Splenic rupture. Thrombocytopenic purpura. Hemolytic anemia. Pericarditis. Hepatitis. Encephalitis.	1. Convalescence may be as long as 3–4 weeks. 2. Patients with splenomegaly should avoid activity that may increase the risk of injury to the spleen, such as contact sports and heavy lifting. 3. Report any excess bruising or bleeding, jaundice, or abnormal CNS functioning.

(continued)

TABLE 32-2 Selected Infectious Diseases *(continued)*

Disease & Infectious Agent	Clinical Manifestations	Incubation Period	Diagnostic Tests
Cytomegalovirus (CMV)	Ordinarily asymptomatic. Clinical disease in the adult resembles mononucleosis. More extensive organ involvement in the immunosuppressed host—hepatitis, pneumonitis, arthralgias may occur. Congenital infections are serious and lead to irreversible CNS damage.	Unknown; 3–8 weeks following transfusion; in neonates 3–12 weeks following delivery-produced infection.	Differential WBC count—increase in lymphocytes, many atypical. Complement fixation—fourfold rise in titer in adult or child suggestive of current infection. Positive cell culture of urine, cervical secretions, or biopsy tissue. Differential diagnosis: heterophil agglutination negative.
Rabies Rabies virus	Initial symptoms nonspecific and consist of malaise, fatigue, headache, anorexia, and fever. May have pain or paresthesia at the site of exposure. Usually lasts 2–10 days. Followed by the acute neurologic period which includes hyperactivity, disorientation, hallucinations, seizures, nuchal stiffness, or paralysis. In 50% or more of cases, hydrophobia (fear of water) is present. Usually lasts 2–7 days and ends either with death or with onset of coma. Coma occurs 4–10 days after onset of symptoms and may last for hours or months. Respiratory arrest usually occurs, followed by death.	20–90 days. Shorter when the site of the bite is on the head (25–48 days) than when it is on an extremity (46–78 days).	Measurement of rabies neutralizing antibody by the rapid fluorescent focus inhibition test. Virus isolation from saliva, CSF, urine sediment, and tracheal secretions most successful in the first 2 weeks of clinical illness.
Protozoan Infections Malaria *Plasmodium vivax, P. falciparum, P. malariae,* and *P. ovale*	Malarial paroxysm characterized by high fever, chills, rigor is the hallmark of acute malaria. Prodromal period from 1 to several days before the onset of the paroxysms and may complain of malaise, headache, myalgia, and fatigue. Moderate splenomegaly and tender hepatomegaly. Coagulopathic.	Variable depending on the strain.	Diagnosis of malaria rests on the demonstration of parasites in stained peripheral blood smears. Twice-daily smears on several days required. If more than 5% of the RBCs are parasitized, *P. falciparum* should also be suspected. Leukopenia, hemolytic anemia (normocytic, normochromic), platelets decreased (less than 50,000/mm^3). Urine reveals small amounts of protein. Liver function tests reveal elevated transaminase level and increase in indirect serum bilirubin.
Amebiasis *Entamoeba histolytica*	*Nondysenteric colitis:* Recurring episodes of loose stools. Vague abdominal pain. Hemorrhoids with occasional rectal bleeding. *Dysenteric colitis:* Intense, intermittent, bloody, mucous diarrhea.	Variable—3 days to months; usually 2–4 weeks.	Microscopic examination of stool, rectal secretions; positive for trophozoites or cysts of protozoan.

Management	Complications	Nursing Considerations
Supportive therapy for control of fever and sore throat. Corticosteroids for neurologic and hematologic complications. Hyperimmune gamma globulin (Gammar) as a prophylactic agent for patients undergoing marrow transplantation.	Congenital infection leads to neurologic defects (severe mental retardation, microcephaly, psychomotor retardation). Immunocompromised host—progressive pneumonitis, hemolytic anemia, hepatitis, pericarditis, and GI ulceration.	1. Convalescence may be as long as 3–4 weeks. 2. Patients with splenomegaly should avoid activity that may increase the risk of injury to the spleen, such as contact sports and heavy lifting. 3. Report any excess bruising or bleeding, jaundice, or abnormal CNS functioning.
Rabies is a disease best controlled through prevention rather than treatment. Supportive therapy to manage neurologic, respiratory, and cardiac symptoms. Isolation of the patient using masks, gowns, and gloves. Use of high-dose passive rabies immunoglobulin (Imogam) or vaccine (Imovax) after the onset of illness has not been successful. Interferon of unproven value.	Most complications occur in the coma phase and include: Increases in intracranial pressure. Hypothalamic involvement producing inappropriate secretion of ADH (antidiuretic hormone) and/or diabetes insipidus. Autonomic dysfunction leading to hypertension, hypotension, cardiac dysrhythmias or hypothermia. Hypoxia.	1. No tests available to diagnose rabies before onset of clinical disease. 2. Preexposure prophylaxis should be offered to persons at high risk for exposure to rabies, such as veterinarians, veterinary students, and certain laboratory workers with human diploid cell rabies vaccine (HDCV). 3. Bites from animals, particularly dogs and cats, should be thoroughly cleaned with soap and water immediately. 4. Domestic dogs and cats should be quarantined for 10 days. 5. Wild animal carriers include skunk, bat, fox, coyote, racoon, bobcat, and other carnivores. 6. Postexposure prophylaxis must include the use of human rabies immunoglobulin followed by HDCV unless preexposure prophylaxis with HDCV had been administered. HDCV requires 5 doses IM.
Patients with *P. falciparum* infection should be hospitalized. If *P. falciparum* infection is ruled out, therapy with chloroquine (Aralen) can be instituted on an outpatient basis. General management should include: IV fluids and electrolytes—restrict fluids in cerebral edema. Assisted ventilation with pulmonary edema. Dialysis in renal failure. Transfusions in anemia. Heparin or fresh-frozen plasma in coagulopathy.	Splenic rupture. Renal failure. Hepatic failure. Pulmonary edema. Perivascular edema and hemorrhage in cerebral cortex. Disseminated intravascular coagulation (DIC).	1. Patients with *P. vivax* or *P. ovale* may have recurrence of symptoms and should report them immediately. 2. Patients should return for blood examination 4–5 days after completion of treatment. 3. Travelers to malaria-endemic countries should follow preventive measures: Proper use of mosquito netting at night. Clothing that minimizes contact with mosquitoes. Use of insect repellents. Chemoprophylaxis with chloroquine or hydroxychloroquine (Plaquenil).
Treatment regimens depend on the severity of the illness. Acute dysentery is best treated with metronidazole (Flagyl) followed by iodoquinol (Diodoquin) if cyst passage persists.	Perforated bowel. Hemorrhage. Systemic deterioration. Anemia. Hepatic abscess.	1. Instruct patient to wash hands thoroughly after defecating to prevent transmission to others. 2. Household and sexual contacts should seek medical examination and treatment. 3. Instruct patient on safe sexual practices. 4. Travelers to areas where the water supply is not chemically treated or protected from sewage should boil all water used for drinking and cooking. 5. Relapses after treatment are common. Follow-up should be scheduled at 6 weeks and 6 months after treatment.

(continued)

TABLE 32-2 Selected Infectious Diseases *(continued)*

Disease & Infectious Agent	Clinical Manifestations	Incubation Period	Diagnostic Tests
Giardiasis *Giardia lamblia*	*Acute:* Explosive, foul-smelling diarrheal stool. Abdominal cramping and flatulence. Nausea. *Chronic:* Intermittent loose stools. Increased flatulence and distention. Vague abdominal discomfort.	5–25 days; median 7–10 days.	Examination of stool; positive for cysts or trophozoites of the *G. lamblia* protozoan.
Hookworm *Ancylostoma duodenale,* *A. ceylonicum, Necator* *americanus*	Chronic debilitating disease leading to iron-deficiency anemia and hypoproteinemia that result from intestinal blood loss to the hookworm.	Symptoms may develop after a few weeks to many months, depending on intensity of infection.	Microscopic examination of cultured specimen positive for larva.
Trichinosis *Trichinella spiralis*	Clinical disease highly variable; can range from inapparent infection to a fulminating fatal disease. Sudden appearance of muscle soreness and pain accompanied by edema of upper eyelids. Ocular signs progress to subconjunctival, subungual, and retinal hemorrhages; pain; and photophobia. Remittent fever is usual, sometimes as high as 104°F. Gastrointestinal symptoms such as diarrhea.	5–45 days depending on the number of worms involved; usually 8–15 days after ingestion of infected meat.	Skeletal muscle biopsy not earlier than 10 days after exposure to infection demonstrates the *Trichinella* larvae. Serology; complement fixation, fluorescent antibody—fourfold increase in antibody titer 2 weeks after infection. Differential WBC count—increase in eosinophils.

Fungal Infections
Histoplasmosis
Histoplasma capsulatum
	May be asymptomatic with only hypersensitivity to histoplasmin.
	Four other clinical forms of disease:
	  1. Acute pulmonary histoplasmosis characterized by pleural and substernal chest pain, fever, weakness, dry or productive cough, erythema multiforme, and erythema nodosum.
	  2. Acute disseminated with hepatosplenomegaly, high fever, and prostration.
	  3. Chronic pulmonary histoplasmosis characterized by purulent sputum, hemoptysis, and chronic low-grade fever.
		5–18 days after exposure, commonly 10 days.	Complement fixation shows increase in antibodies within 3–4 weeks; fourfold increase suggests disease progression.
			Fungal culture positive for *H. capsulatum.*
			Chest x-ray—Acute findings: transient parenchymal pulmonary infiltrates resembling lobar pneumonia. Chronic: Progressively enlarging areas of necrosis with or without cavitation.

Management	Complications	Nursing Considerations
Metronidazole (Flagyl) is the drug of choice. Quinacrine (Atabrine) is an alternative.	Chronic diarrhea. Malabsorption.	1. Instruct patient to wash hands thoroughly after defecating to prevent transmission to others. 2. Household and sexual contacts should seek medical examination and treatment. 3. Instruct patient on safe sexual practices. 4. Travelers to areas where the water supply is not chemically treated or protected from sewage should boil all water used for drinking and cooking. 5. Relapses after treatment are common. Follow-up should be scheduled at 6 weeks and 6 months after treatment.
Mebendazole (Vermox) 100 mg BID for 3 days or pyrantel pamoate (Antiminth) single oral dose of 11 mg/kg up to total of 1 g/day. Iron therapy to correct anemia.	Immunosuppressed individuals—septicemia and death.	1. Follow-up examination of the stool 2 weeks after therapy is necessary. 2. Nutrition counseling and taking iron supplements is recommended until deficiencies are corrected. 3. Family members and close contacts should be examined and treated for parasites. 4. Thorough hand washing after defecation is critical.
Thiabendazole (Mintezol) within 24 hours of eating infected meat–25 mg/kg/day for 1 week. Supportive therapy for respiratory, neurologic, and cardiac sequelae.	Respiratory failure or pneumonia. Myocarditis. Encephalitis. Death.	1. Instruct patient to thoroughly wash hands after defecation. 2. Proper cooking of pork to 150°F is necessary. 3. Family members and close contacts of patients should be examined and treated for parasites.
Amphotericin B (Fungizone) 5–10 mg initial dose, increasing 10 mg/day until 50 mg is attained, then 50 mg 3 times/week until 2.5 g has been administered. Corticosteroids and diphenhydramine (Benadryl) to minimize the side effects of amphotericin.	Pneumonia. Progressive emphysema. Hepatosplenomegaly. Severe prostration. Death.	1. Medical follow-up is indicated for 1 year after treatment to prevent relapses.

(continued)

TABLE 32-2 Selected Infectious Diseases *(continued)*

Disease & Infectious Agent	Clinical Manifestations	Incubation Period	Diagnostic Tests
	4. Chronic disseminated histoplasmosis with variable symptoms, such as unexplained fever, anemia, patchy pneumonia, mucosal ulcers of the mouth, larynx, stomach, or bowel.		
Bacterial Infections Typhoid Fever *Salmonella typhi*	Acute enteric fever manifested by sustained bacteremia and microabscess formation and ulceration of the distal ileum. Gastrointestinal symptoms generally follow the systemic manifestations.	1–3 weeks.	Culture of urine and/or stool positive for *Salmonella typhi* during 2nd week. Culture of blood positive for *S. typhi* during 1st week. Leukopenia. Anemia.
Botulism *Clostridium botulinum*	Severe intoxication characterized by visual difficulty, dysphagia, and dry mouth. Followed by descending symmetrical flaccid paralysis. Vomiting and constipation or diarrhea may be present initially.	12–36 hours, sometimes several days after eating contaminated food.	Culture of *C. botulinum* from stool or stomach contents. Serum positive for botulinal toxins.
Tetanus *Clostridium tetani*	Acute disease induced by an exotoxin of the tetanus bacillus. Painful muscular contractions, primarily of the masseter and neck muscles. Abdominal rigidity. Generalized spasms frequently induced by sensory stimuli—opisthotonos (arching of the trunk) and risus sardonicus (distorted grin).	Usually 3–21 days; average 3–10 days.	Organism rarely recovered from the site of infection. No detectable antibody response.
Staphylococci *Staphylococcus aureus* Coagulase-negative staphylococci; *S. epidermidis, S. haemolyticus*	Skin and soft tissue infections—furuncles (boils), impetigo, carbuncles, cellulitis, abscesses, and infected lacerations. Seeding of the bloodstream may lead to pneumonia, osteomyelitis, septicemia, endocarditis, meningitis, hepatic abscess, splenic abscess, perinephritic abscess.	Variable; usually 4–10 days.	Confirmed by isolation of the organism from culture.

Management	Complications	Nursing Considerations
IV fluids and electrolytes. Bed rest. Avoid antispasmodics, laxatives, and salicylates. Chloramphenicol (Chloromycetin) or ampicillin (Omnipen) either IV or PO. Immunization is advised for travelers to areas of high endemicity. Ampicillin may terminate the chronic carrier state and is preferred in intravascular infection.	Endocarditis. Meningitis. Pneumonia. Pyelonephritis. Osteomyelitis. Intestinal perforation and hemorrhage. Septicemia.	1. Transmitted by contaminated food or water and via direct fecal–oral route. 2. Relapses occur in 5–10% of untreated cases and may be more common following antibiotic therapy. Report symptoms immediately. 3. Instruct patient to wash hands thoroughly after defecation and before preparing food. 4. Family and close contacts should be examined and treated. 5. Typhoid is communicable for as long as the infective organism is in the feces or urine, which may persist for up to 1 year.
IV and IM administration as soon as possible of trivalent botulinum antitoxin. IV fluids and electrolytes. Intensive care to anticipate and manage respiratory failure: mechanical ventilation. Report to health department immediately.	Death from respiratory failure.	1. All patient contacts known to have eaten the same food should have gastric lavage, high enemas, and cathartics and kept under close medical supervision. 2. Instruct patient/patient contacts to wash hands thoroughly after defecation and before handling food. 3. No questionable canned food should ever be tasted.
High case fatality rate 30–90%. Tetanus immune globulin. Wound care to include cleaning and irrigation. Sedatives and muscle relaxants. Neuromuscular blockade for treatment of severe uncontrolled spasms (pancurmonium [Pavulon]). Cardiac monitoring. Sympathetic blocking agents for management of hypertension and tachycardia (propranolol [Inderal]).	Cardiac arrest. Bacterial shock. Autonomic disturbances.	1. Refer persons with skin injuries for tetanus prophylaxis. 2. Remind adults to receive a tetanus booster every 10 years.
Penicillinase-resistant penicillins (nafcillin 'Unipen) and the cephalosporins (cephalothin 'Keflin). Vancomycin 'Vancocin is treatment of choice for methicillin-resistant *S. aureus.* Incision of abscesses to permit drainage of pus. In severe systemic infection, the selection of antibiotics should be governed by results of susceptibility tests on the isolates.	Septicemia. Embolic skin lesions. Death.	1. Monitor patient's response to prescribed therapy. 2. Emphasize meticulous hand washing among patients and visitors. 3. Contain purulent drainage with a dressing. 4. Place soiled dressings in a paper bag before disposal.

(continued)

TABLE 32-2 Selected Infectious Diseases *(continued)*

Disease & Infectious Agent	Clinical Manifestations	Incubation Period	Diagnostic Tests
Streptococci *Streptococcus pyogenes,* group A with approximately 80 serologically distinct types	Streptococcal pharyngitis. Wound and skin infections— impetigo, cellulitis, erysipelas. Scarlet fever (streptococcal sore throat with a rash that occurs if infectious agent produces erythrogenic toxin to which patient is not immune).	Short; usually 1–3 days.	Identification of group A streptococcal antigen in pharyngeal secretions (rapid strep test). Isolation of the organism by culture.
Syphilis (*Treponema pallidum,* a sexually transmitted infection)	Primary: indurated, painless, clean ulcer (chancre); may be bilateral inguinal adenopathy. Secondary: macular-papular rash including palms and soles; fever; generalized adenopathy, condyloma lata	Usually 3 weeks, but may be up to 3 months; signs of secondary syphilis develop about 6 weeks after healing of chancre.	Nonspecific serologic tests such as RPR and VDRL; confirmed by specific antitreponemal antibody tests such as FTA-ABS and MHA-TP; dark-field examination of lesion exudate for organism.

IV: intravenous; SGOT: serum glutamic oxaloacetic transaminase; PO: by mouth; BID: twice daily; WBC: white blood cell; ASA: acetylsalicylic acid; CNS: central nervous system; GI, gastrointestinal; CSF: cerebrospinal fluid; RBC: red blood cell.

Management	Complications	Nursing Considerations
Penicillin (Betapen-VK) is the drug of choice. Therapy should be continued for at least 10 days. Erythromycin 'Eryc for penicillin-allergic patients.	Septicemia. Acute glomerulonephritis. Rheumatic fever.	1. Repeated attacks of sore throat or other streptococcal disease due to different types of streptococci are relatively frequent. 2. Make sure the patient understands the importance of completing the course of antimicrobial therapy. 3. Emphasize the relationship of streptococcal infections to heart disease and glomerulonephritis.
Primary and Secondary: benzathine penicillin (Bicillin LA) G 2.4 million units IM in a single dose; in penicillin allergy, if not pregnant, doxycycline 100 mg, twice a day for 2 weeks; erythromycin is an inferior substitute in pregnant, penicillin-allergic patients	Tertiary syphilis with cardiac, dermatologic, neurologic, and other systemic manifestations	1. Warn patient of possible Jarisch-Herxheimer reaction—fever, myalgias, headache, hypotension—within 24 hours of treatment. 2. Ensure that sexual activity is not resumed until treatment is complete for both patient and partner. 3. Consider testing for HIV and other sexually transmitted diseases. 4. Encourage follow-up at 3 months for repeat serologic testing.

Selected References

Bartlett, J. (1993). *Pocket book of infectious disease therapy.* Baltimore: Williams & Wilkins.

Benenson, A. S. (1990). *Control of communicable diseases in man* (15th ed.). American Public Health Association.

Bennett, J., & Brachman, P. (1992). *Hospital infections.* (3rd ed.). Boston: Little, Brown.

Federal Register. (1991). *Occupational exposure to bloodborne pathogens: Final rule.* Occupational Safety and Health Administration Department of Labor.

Grimes, D. (1991). *Infectious diseases.* St. Louis: Mosby Year Book.

Hoeprich, P. D. (ed.) (1994). *Infectious Diseases.* Philadelphia: J. B. Lippincott.

Osguthorpe, N. C. and Morgan, E. P. (1995). An immunization update for primary health care providers. *Nurse Practitioner, 20*(6), 52, 54, 60–65.

Peter, G. (ed.) (1994). *1994 Red Book: Report of the Committee on Infectious Diseases (23rd ed.).* Elk Grove Village, IL: American Academy of Pediatrics.

Pugliese, G. (1991). *Universal precautions.* American Hospital Publishing.

Update on Adult Immunization. (1991). *MMWR, 40,* RR-12.

Wenzel, R. P. (1993). *Prevention and control of nosocomial infections* (2nd ed.). Baltimore: Williams & Wilkins.

UNIT 13

◆

Emergency Nursing

CHAPTER 33 ◆

Emergency Nursing

Basic Approach to Emergency Care

Emergency care can be defined as the episodic and crisis-oriented care provided to patients with serious or potentially life-threatening injuries or illnesses. The philosophy of emergency care includes the concept that an emergency is whatever the patient or family considers it to be.

◆ EMERGENCY ASSESSMENT

A systematic approach to the assessment of an emergency patient is essential. Often the most dramatic injury is not the most serious. The primary and secondary survey provide the emergency nurse with a methodical approach to help identify and prioritize patient needs.

Primary Assessment

1. The initial rapid assessment of the patient is meant to identify life-threatening problems (airway, breathing, and circulation). If conditions are identified that present an immediate threat to life, appropriate interventions are required before proceeding to the secondary assessment.

NURSING ALERT:
Conditions that present an immediate threat to life include obstructed or compromised airway, respiratory arrest, compromised respirations, cardiac arrest, and profuse bleeding. Intervene immediately.

2. The first step in the primary assessment is to determine if the patient is conscious. If the patient is conscious, the primary assessment can be performed at a glance.
   a. A patient who is alert and talking indicates that there is breathing and circulation.
   b. A conscious patient also indicates that circulation is adequate and enough blood is being circulated to the brain.
   c. If, however, the patient is not fully conscious, the primary assessment should proceed step by step.
3. In seriously injured or ill patients, it is recommended to add two more letters to the primary survey: D—disability, and E—expose.

NURSING ALERT:
If the patient is unconscious, assume there is a serious neck or spinal cord injury until proven otherwise.

4. Airway—Does the patient have an open airway?
5. Breathing—Is the patient breathing?
6. Circulation—Is circulation in immediate jeopardy?
   a. Is there a pulse?
   b. Is there profuse bleeding?
7. Disability—assess level of consciousness and pupils (a more complete neurologic survey will be completed in the secondary survey).
   a. Assess level of consciousness using the AVPU scale:
      (1) A—Is the patient alert?
      (2) V—Does the patient respond to voice?
      (3) P—Does the patient respond to painful stimulus?
      (4) U—The patient is unresponsive even to painful stimulus.
8. Expose—undress the patient to look for clues to injury or illness, such as wounds or skin lesions.

Secondary Assessment

The secondary survey is a systematic, brief (2–3 minutes) examination of the patient from head to toe. The purpose is to detect and prioritize additional injuries or to detect signs of underlying medical conditions.

A. History
1. If possible, a brief history of the chief complaint, accident, or illness is taken from the patient or an accompanying person—relative, prehospital provider.
   a. What is the mechanism of injury—the circumstances, forces, location, and time of injury?
   b. When did the symptoms appear?
   c. Was the patient unconscious after the accident?
   d. How did the patient reach the hospital?
   e. What was the health status of the patient before the accident or illness?
   f. Is there a history of illness?
   g. Is the patient currently taking any medications?
   h. Does the patient have any allergies?
   i. Is the patient under a health care provider's care (name of provider)?
   j. Was treatment attempted before arrival at the hospital—home remedies, over-the-counter medication, or prehospital emergency medical services care?

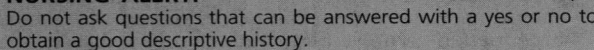

NURSING ALERT:
Do not ask questions that can be answered with a yes or no to obtain a good descriptive history.

B. Vital Signs
1. Routinely includes temperature, pulse rate, respiratory rate, and blood pressure.
2. When obtained early in the assessment, they help to establish complete baseline information.

C. Head-to-Toe Assessment
1. General appearance
   a. Position/posture/gait
   b. Level of consciousness—restlessness is a danger signal
   c. Behavior and degree of distress
   d. Cooperation
   e. Skin condition and color
2. Head/Scalp
   a. Bleeding
   b. Deformity and depressions
   c. Facial symmetry
3. Ears
   a. Blood
   b. Clear fluid (cerebrospinal fluid [CSF])
   c. Battle's sign (bluish discoloration of the mastoid area)
4. Eyes
   a. Pupil size and reaction to light
   b. Extraocular motions
   c. Orbital ecchymosis
   d. Gross vision
   e. Conjunctivae—examine for pallor or cyanosis
5. Nose
   a. Blood
   b. Clear fluid (CSF)

6. Mouth
   a. Missing teeth
   b. Cyanosis of the lips
   c. Foreign material/vomitus
7. Neck
   a. Tracheal deviation
   b. Jugular distention
   c. Tenderness
8. Chest
   a. Symmetry
   b. Tenderness/pain
   c. Ecchymosis
   d. Subcutaneous emphysema
   e. Soft tissue injuries
   f. Breath sounds
   g. Heart sounds
9. Abdomen
   a. Distention/rigidity
   b. Tenderness/pain
   c. Guarding
   d. Bowel sounds
   e. Soft tissue injuries
10. Pelvis
   a. Stability
   b. Tenderness
11. Genitalia
   a. Bleeding
   b. Wounds/trauma
   c. Priapism
   d. Rectal tone
   e. Pain
12. Extremities
   a. Pain
   b. Deformity and bruises
   c. Pulses
   d. Sensation and strength
   e. Soft tissue injury
   f. Capillary refill
   g. Edema
13. Posterior (observe cervical spine precautions in trauma patients)
   a. Soft tissue injury
   b. Spinal tenderness
   c. Pain or tenderness

Focused Assessment

1. A more detailed assessment of deviations from normal or problems identified in the secondary survey.
2. If more then one focused assessment is necessary, any problem identified with the pulmonary system, cardiovascular system, or neurologic system should be assessed first.

◆ TRIAGE

Triage is a French verb meaning "to sort." Most patients entering an emergency department are greeted by a triage nurse. The role of the triage nurse is to do a brief evaluation of the patient to determine a level of acuity or priority of care. Thus, the triage nurse acts as a gatekeeper, sorting patients into categories, ensuring that the more seriously ill are treated first.

Priorities of Care/Triage Categories

Standardized triage categories are usually developed within each emergency department. Most common triage systems consist of three levels of acuity.

A. Emergent I
1. Conditions requiring immediate medical interventions. Any delay in treatment is potentially life or limb threatening.
2. Includes conditions such as:
   a. Airway compromise
   b. Cardiac arrest
   c. Severe shock
   d. Cervical spine injury
   e. Multisystem trauma
   f. Altered level of consciousness
   g. Eclampsia

B. Urgent II
1. Patients who present as stable but whose condition requires medical intervention within a few hours. There is no immediate threat to life or limb for these patients.
2. Conditions include:
   a. Fever
   b. Minor burns
   c. Minor musculoskeletal injuries
   d. Dizziness
   e. Lacerations

C. Nonemergent III
1. Patients who present with chronic or minor injuries. There is no danger to life or limb by having these patients wait to be seen. These patients are in no obvious distress.
2. Conditions include:
   a. Chronic low back pain
   b. Routine medication refills
   c. Dental problems
   d. Missed menses

◆ PSYCHOLOGICAL CONSIDERATIONS

Body trauma is an insult to physiologic and psychological homeostasis; it requires both physiologic and psychological healing.

Approach to the Patient

1. Understand and accept the basic anxieties of the acutely traumatized patient. Be aware of the patient's fear of death, mutilation, and isolation.
   a. Personalize the situation as much as possible—speak, react, and respond in a warm manner.
   b. Give explanations on a level that the patient can grasp—an informed patient can cope with psychological/physiologic stress in a more positive manner.
   c. Accept the rights of the patient and family to have and display their own feelings.
   d. Maintain a calm and reassuring manner—helps the emotionally distressed patient or family to mobilize their psychological resources.

2. Understand and support the patient's feelings concerning loss of control (emotional, physical, and intellectual).
3. Treat the unconscious patient as if conscious—touch, call by name, and explain every procedure that is done. Avoid making negative comments about the patient's condition.
   a. Orient the patient to person, time, and place as soon as he or she is conscious; reinforce by repeating this information.
   b. Bring the patient back to reality in a calm and reassuring way.
   c. Encourage the family, when possible, to orient the patient to reality.
4. Be prepared to handle all aspects of acute trauma; know what to expect and what to do—alleviates the nurse's anxieties and increases the patient's confidence.

Approach to the Family

1. Inform the family where the patient is, and give as much information as possible about the treatment he or she is receiving.
2. Recognize the anxiety of the family and allow them to talk about their feelings—allow expressions of remorse, anger, guilt, and criticism.
3. Allow the family to relive the events, actions, and feelings preceding admission to the emergency department.
4. Deal with reality as gently and quickly as possible; avoid encouraging and supporting denial.
5. Assist the family to cope with sudden and unexpected death. Some helpful measures include the following:
   a. Take the family to a private place.
   b. Talk to all of the family together—so that they can mourn together.
   c. Assure the family that everything possible was done; inform them of the treatment rendered.
   d. Avoid using euphemisms, such as "passed on." Show the family that you care by touching, offering coffee, etc.
   e. Allow family to talk about the deceased—permits ventilation of feelings of loss. Encourage family to talk about events preceding admission to the emergency department.
   f. Encourage family to support each other and to express emotions freely: grief, loss, anger, helplessness, tears, disbelief.
   g. Avoid volunteering unnecessary information (patient was drinking, etc.).
   h. Avoid giving sedation to family members—may mask or delay the grieving process, which is necessary to achieve emotional equilibrium and prevent prolonged depression.
   i. Encourage family members to view the body if they wish to do so—helps to integrate the loss (cover mutilated areas).
      (1) Go with family to see the body.
      (2) Show acceptance of the body—by touching—to give family "permission" to touch and talk to the body.
      (3) Spend a few minutes with the family, listening to them.
6. Encourage the emergency department staff to discuss among themselves their reaction to the event—to share intense feelings for review and for group support.

Cardiopulmonary Resuscitation and Airway Management

Cardiopulmonary resuscitation (CPR) is a technique of basic life support for the purpose of oxygenating the brain and heart until appropriate, definitive medical treatment can restore normal heart and ventilatory action. Management of foreign-body airway obstruction or cricothyroidotomy may be necessary to open the airway before CPR can be performed.

◆ CARDIOPULMONARY RESUSCITATION

See Procedure Guidelines 33-1: Cardiopulmonary Resuscitation.

Indications

1. Cardiac arrest
   a. Ventricular fibrillation
   b. Ventricular tachycardia
   c. Asystole
   d. Pulseless electrical activity
2. Respiratory arrest
   a. Drowning
   b. Stroke
   c. Foreign-body airway obstruction
   d. Smoke inhalation
   e. Drug overdose
   f. Electrocution/injury by lightning
   g. Suffocation
   h. Accident/injury
   i. Coma
   j. Epiglottitis

Assessment

1. Immediate loss of consciousness.
2. Absence of breath sounds or air movement through nose or mouth.
3. Absence of palpable carotid or femoral pulse; pulselessness in large arteries.

Complications

1. Postresuscitation distress syndrome (secondary derangements in multiple organs).
2. Neurologic impairment, brain damage.

NURSING ALERT: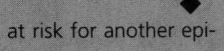
The patient who has been resuscitated is at risk for another episode of cardiac arrest.

PROCEDURE GUIDELINES 33-1 ◆ Cardiopulmonary Resuscitation

EQUIPMENT

Trained personnel
Arrest board
Oral airway
Bag and mask device

Intravenous (IV) setup
Defibrillator
Emergency cardiac drugs
Electrocardiograph machine

PROCEDURE	NURSING ACTION	RATIONALE

ASSESSMENT

1. Determine unresponsiveness: tap or gently shake patient while shouting, "Are you OK?"
2. Activate emergency medical service (EMS) (call local emergency telephone number or 911) if outside hospital.
3. Place patient supine on a firm, flat surface. Kneel at the level of the patient's shoulders. If the patient has suspected head or neck trauma, the rescuer should move the patient only if absolutely necessary.
4. Open the airway.
   a. *Head-tilt/Chin-lift Maneuver:*
      Place one hand on the patient's forehead and apply firm backward pressure with the palm to tilt the head back.
      Then, place the fingers of the other hand under the bony part of the lower jaw near the chin and lift up to bring the jaw forward and the teeth almost to occlusion.

1. This will prevent injury from attempted resuscitation on a person who is not unconscious.

3. This enables the rescuer to perform rescue breathing and chest compression without moving the knees.

   a. In the absence of sufficient muscle tone, the tongue and/or epiglottis will obstruct the pharynx and larynx.

      This supports the jaw and helps tilt the head back.

PROCEDURE (cont'd)	NURSING ACTION	RATIONALE

b. *Jaw-thrust Maneuver:*
Grasp the angles of the patient's lower jaw and lifting with both hands, one on each side, displace the mandible forward, while tilting the head backward.

c. The jaw-thrust technique without head tilt is the safest method for opening the airway in the presence of suspected neck injury.

BREATHING

ASSESSMENT
Determine presence or absence of spontaneous breathing.

1. Place ear over patient's mouth and nose while observing the chest, *look* for the chest to rise and fall, *listen* for air escaping during exhalation, and *feel* for the flow of air.

2. Perform rescue breathing—Mouth-to-mouth: While keeping the airway open, pinch the nostrils closed using the thumb and index finger of the hand that is on the forehead. Take a deep breath, open mouth wide, and place it outside of the patient's mouth, creating an airtight seal.
Ventilate the patient with two full breaths (1–1½ seconds each breath), taking a breath after each ventilation.
If the initial ventilation attempt is unsuccessful, reposition the patient's head and repeat rescue breathing.

Rationale:

1. Keep maintaining an open airway.

2. This prevents air from escaping from the patient's nose.

Adequate ventilation is indicated by seeing the chest rise and fall, feeling the air escape during ventilation and hearing the air escape during exhalation.

CIRCULATION

ASSESSMENT
Determine pulselessness.

1. While maintaining head-tilt with one hand on the forehead, palpate the carotid or femoral pulse. If pulse is not palpable, start external chest compressions.

Rationale:

1. Cardiac arrest is recognized by pulselessness in the large arteries of the unconscious, breathless patient. If there is a palpable pulse, but no breathing present, initiate rescue breathing at rate of 12 × per minute (once every 5 seconds) after initial two breaths.

EXTERNAL CHEST COMPRESSIONS
Consist of serial, rhythmic applications of pressure over the lower half of the sternum.

1. Kneel as close to side of patient's chest as possible. Place the heel of one hand on the lower half of the sternum, 3.8 cm. (1½ inches) from the tip of the xiphoid. The fingers may either be extended or interlaced but must be kept off the chest.

2. While keeping your arms straight, elbows locked, and shoulders positioned directly over your hands, quickly and forcefully depress the lower half of the patient's sternum straight down, 3.8–5 cm. (1½–2 inches).

3. Release the external chest compression completely and allow the chest to return to its normal position after each compression. The time allowed for release should equal the time required for compression. Do not lift the hands off the chest or change position.

4. Use 80 compressions per minute (100 if possible). For one rescuer, do 15 compressions at a rate of 80–100 per minute and then perform two ventilations; re-evaluate the patient.

Rationale:

1. The long axis of the heel of the rescuer's hand should be placed on the long axis of the sternum; thus the main force of the compression will be on the sternum and decrease the chance of rib fracture.

3. Release of the external chest compression allows blood flow into the heart.

4. Rescue breathing and external chest compressions must be combined. Check for return of carotid pulse. If absent, resume CPR with 2 ventilations followed by compressions. For CPR performed by health professionals, mouth-to-mask ventilation is an acceptable alternative for rescue breathing.

(continued)

PROCEDURE GUIDELINES 33-1 ◆ Cardiopulmonary Resuscitation
(continued)

PROCEDURE (cont'd)	NURSING ACTION	RATIONALE
	5. For CPR performed by two rescuers, the compression rate is 80–100 per minute. The compression–ventilation ratio is 15:1 with a pause for ventilation (1–1½ seconds) 6. While resuscitation proceeds, simultaneous efforts are made to obtain and use special resuscitation equipment to manage breathing and circulation and provide definitive care.	6. Definitive care includes defibrillation, pharmacotherapy for dysrhythmias and acid-base disturbances, and ongoing monitoring and skilled care in an intensive care unit.

* Adapted from: Guidelines for cardiopulmonary resuscitation and emergency cardiac care. JAMA 1992;268(16):2172–2198.

◆ FOREIGN-BODY AIRWAY OBSTRUCTION

Foreign-body obstruction of the airway may be either partial or complete.

The *Heimlich maneuver* (subdiaphragmatic–abdominal thrusts) is recommended for relieving foreign-body airway obstruction in the adult. See Procedure Guidelines 33-2: Management of Foreign-Body Airway Obstruction.

Assessment

1. Weak, ineffective cough
2. High-pitched noises on inspiration
3. Respiratory distress
4. Inability to speak or breathe
5. Cyanosis
6. Collapse

PROCEDURE GUIDELINES 33-2 ◆ Management of Foreign-Body Airway Obstruction

PROCEDURE	EMERGENCY ACTION	RATIONALE

	HEIMLICH MANEUVER WITH CONSCIOUS PATIENT SITTING OR STANDING
	 1. Stand behind the patient; wrap your arms around waist and proceed as follows:
	   a. Make a fist with one hand, placing the thumb side of the fist against the patient's abdomen in the midline, slightly above the navel and well below the xiphoid process. Grasp the fist with the other hand.
	   b. Press your fist into the patient's abdomen with a quick upward thrust. Each new thrust should be a separate and distinct maneuver.
		b. A subdiaphragmatic abdominal thrust, by elevating the diaphragm, can force air from the lungs to create an artificial cough intended to move and expel an obstructing foreign body in the airway.

	HEIMLICH MANEUVER WITH UNCONSCIOUS PATIENT LYING DOWN 1. Position patient supine with face up. 2. Kneel astride the patient's thighs, facing head. 3. Place the heel of one hand against the patient's abdomen in the midline slightly above the navel and well below the tip of the xiphoid; place the second hand directly on top of the first. 4. Press into the abdomen with a quick upward thrust. **FINGER SWEEP** 1. Open patient's mouth by grasping both the tongue and lower jaw between the thumb and fingers and lift the mandible (tongue–jaw lift).	1. This maneuver is to be used only in the unconscious patient. This action draws the tongue away from the foreign body that may be lodged there.

PROCEDURE (cont'd)	NURSING ACTION	RATIONALE
	2. Insert the index finger of the other hand down along the inside of the cheek and deeply into the throat to the base of the tongue.	
	3. Use a hooking action to dislodge the foreign body and maneuver it into the mouth for removal.	3. Take care not to force the object deeper into the throat.
	CHEST THRUST WITH CONSCIOUS PATIENT STANDING OR SITTING	
	1. Stand behind the patient with arms under axillae to encircle the patient's chest.	1. This technique is to be used only in advanced stages of pregnancy or in markedly obese person.
	2. Place thumb side of your fist on middle of patient's sternum, taking care to avoid xiphoid process and rib cage margins.	
	3. Grasp your fist with the other hand and perform backward thrusts until the foreign body is expelled or patient becomes unconscious.	3. Each thrust is administered with the intent of relieving the obstruction.
	CHEST THRUST WITH UNCONSCIOUS PATIENT LYING DOWN	
	1. Place the patient on back and kneel close to the side of body.	This maneuver is used only in the advanced stages of pregnancy or when the rescuer cannot apply the Heimlich maneuver effectively to the unconscious, markedly obese person.
	2. Place the heel of your hand on the lower half of the sternum.	
	3. Deliver each chest thrust slowly and distinctly with the intent of relieving the obstruction.	

Adapted from: Guidelines for cardiopulmonary resuscitation and emergency care. JAMA 1992;268(16):2172–2198.

◆ CRICOTHYROIDOTOMY

Cricothyroidotomy is the puncture or incision of the cricothyroid membrane to establish an emergency airway in certain emergency situations when endotracheal intubation or tracheostomy are not possible or are contraindicated. See Procedure Guidelines 33-3: Cricothyroidotomy.

Indications

1. Compromised airway and inability to intubate or perform tracheostomy:
   a. Foreign-body obstruction.
   b. Trauma to head and neck.
3. Allergic reaction causing laryngeal edema.

PROCEDURE GUIDELINES 33-3 ◆ Cricothyroidotomy

EQUIPMENT   No. 11 gauge needle or scalpel with No. 11 scalpel blade

PROCEDURE	NURSING ACTION	RATIONALE
	1. Extend the neck. Place a towel roll beneath the shoulders.	1. So that the cricothyroid membrane can be palpated readily.
	2. Identify the prominent thyroid cartilage (Adam's apple) and allow your finger to descend in the midline to the depression between the lower border of the thyroid cartilage and the upper border of the cricoid cartilage (see accompanying figure).	2. This depression represents the cricothyroid membrane.

(continued)

PROCEDURE GUIDELINES 33-3 ◆ Cricothyroidotomy (continued)

PROCEDURE (cont'd)	NURSING ACTION	RATIONALE

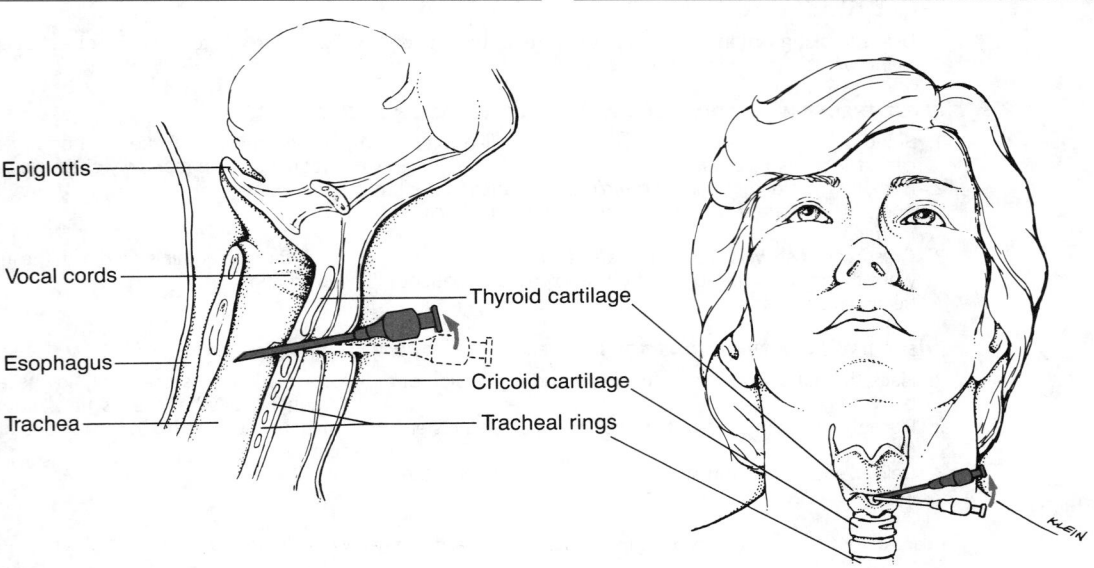

Cricothyroidotomy, or cricothyroid membrane puncture.

3. Insert a needle or any sharp instrument at a 10- to 30-degree caudal direction in the midline just above the upper part of the cricoid cartilage.
4. Listen for air passing back and forth through the needle synchronously with the patient's respirations.
5. Direct the needle downward and posteriorly.

6. Tape the needle with adhesive for stability.

7. An alternate method is to make a transverse incision overlying the cricothyroid membrane and a similar incision through the membrane itself.
   The membrane incision is spread and a tracheostomy tube is inserted and directed into the trachea.
8. Prepare for endotracheal intubation/tracheostomy.

9. Potential complications: bleeding, aspiration.

5. To avoid injury to the vocal cords (located cephalad to the cricothyroid membrane).
6. To prevent laceration or perforation of the posterior tracheal wall.

8. After the patient is stabilized, a more permanent means of ventilatory support is implemented.

Injuries to the Head, Spine, and Face

◆ HEAD INJURIES

Head injuries can include fractures to the skull and face, direct injuries to the brain (as from a bullet), and indirect injuries to the brain (such as a concussion, contusion, or intracranial hemorrhage). Any time the skull is fractured, the patient is said to have an open head injury. If the skull is intact, the term "closed head injury" is used. Head injuries commonly occur from motor vehicle accidents, assaults, or falls.

Concussion—a temporary loss of consciousness that results from a transient interruption of the brain's normal functioning.

Contusion—a bruising of the brain tissue. Actual small amounts of bleeding into the brain tissue.

Intracranial hemorrhage—significant bleeding into a space or a potential space between the skull and the brain. This is a serious complication of a head injury with a high mortality rate due a rising intracranial pressure and the potential for brain herniation. Intracranial hemorrhages can be classified as epidural hematomas, subdural hematomas, or subarachnoid hemorrhages, depending on the site of bleeding.

NURSING ALERT:
Assume a cervical spine fracture for any patient with a significant head injury, until proven otherwise.

Primary Assessment

1. Airway—assess for vomitus, bleeding, and foreign objects.
2. Breathing—assess for abnormally slow or shallow respirations. An elevated PCO_2 can worsen cerebral edema.
3. Circulation—assess pulses and bleeding.

Primary Interventions

1. Open the airway using the jaw-thrust technique without head tilt. Oral suction equipment (to handle heavy vomitus) should be at hand.
2. Administer high-flow O_2: the most common cause of death from head injury is cerebral anoxia.
3. Assist inadequate respirations with a bag-valve mask. In general, head-injured patients should be hyperventilated with a respiratory rate of 20 to 25 breaths per minute. Hyperventilation lowers the PaO_2, causing cerebral vasoconstriction and minimizing cerebral edema.
4. Control bleeding—do not apply pressure to the injury site. Apply a bulky loose dressing. Do not attempt to stop the flow of blood or CSF from the nose or ears; apply a loose dressing if needed.
5. Initiate an intravenous (IV) line to run at a keep-vein-open rate.

Subsequent Assessment

1. History
   a. Mechanism of injury.
   b. Duration of loss of consciousness.
   c. Memory of the event.
   d. Position found.
2. Level of consciousness
   a. Change in the level of consciousness is the most sensitive indicator of a change in the patient's condition.
   b. Glasgow Coma Score (see p. 368).
3. Vital signs
   a. Hypertension and bradycardia indicate an increasing intracranial pressure.
   b. Head-injured patients may have associated cardiac dysrhythmias, noted by an irregular pulse or a fast pulse.
   c. Changing patterns of respiration or apnea may indicate a head injury.
   d. Elevated temperature—high temperatures are associated with head injury.
4. Unequal or unresponsive pupils.
5. Confusion or personality changes.
6. Impaired vision.
7. One or both eyes appear sunken.
8. Seizure activity.
9. Battle's sign—a bluish discoloration behind the ears (indicates a possible basal skull fracture).
10. Rhinorrhea or otorrhea (indicative of leakage of CSF).
11. Periorbital ecchymosis (indicates anterior basilar fracture).

General Intervention

1. Keep the neck in a neutral position with the cervical spine immobilized.
2. Hyperventilation to reduce intracranial pressure.
3. Establish an IV line of normal saline or Ringer's lactate—fluid volume should be restricted.
4. Be prepared to manage seizures—if seizures occur they should be controlled immediately.
5. Maintain normothermia.
6. Pharmacologic interventions
   a. Diazepam (Valium)—to control seizures.
   b. Steroids—to reduce swelling and brain cell oxygen requirements.
   c. Mannitol (Osmitrol)—to reduce cerebral edema and decrease intracranial pressure.
   d. Barbiturate coma.
   e. Antibiotics.
7. Prepare for immediate surgical intervention if patient shows evidence of neurologic deterioration.

◆ CERVICAL SPINE INJURIES

Injuries to the cervical spine are serious, because the crushing, stretching, and rotational shear forces exerted on the cord at the time of trauma can produce severe neurologic deficits. Edema and cord swelling contribute further to the loss of spinal cord function.

Any person with a head, neck, or back injury or fractures to the upper leg bones or to the pelvis should be suspected of having a potential spinal cord injury until proven otherwise.

Primary Assessment

1. Provide immediate immobilization of the spine while performing assessment.
2. Airway.
3. Breathing.
   a. Intercostal paralysis with diaphragmatic breathing—indicates cervical spinal cord injury.
   b. In conscious patient, observe for increased respiratory rate and difficulty in speaking due to shortness of breath.
4. Circulation.

Primary Interventions

1. Immobilize the cervical spine.
2. Open the airway using the jaw-thrust technique without head tilt.
3. If the patient needs to be intubated, it may be done nasally.
4. If respirations are shallow, assist with a bag-valve mask.

Subsequent Assessment

1. Assess the position of the patient when found.
   a. Forearms flexed across their chest—C-6 injury.
   b. Arms stretched out above head—cervical injury.
2. Hypotension and bradycardia accompanied by warm dry skin—suggests "spinal shock."
3. Neck and/or back pain/extremity pain or burning sensation to the skin.
4. History of unconsciousness.
5. Total sensory loss and motor paralysis below level of injury.
6. Loss of bowel and bladder control; usually urinary retention and bladder distention.
7. Loss of sweating and vasomotor tone below level of cord lesion.
8. Priapism—persistent erection of penis.
9. Hypothermia—due to the inability to constrict peripheral blood vessels and conserve body heat.
10. Loss of rectal tone.

General Interventions

> **NURSING ALERT:**
> A spinal cord injury can be made worse during the acute phase of injury, resulting in permanent neurologic damage. Proper handling is an immediate priority.

1. Monitor blood gas values serially.
2. Prepare for nasotracheal intubation—to prevent regurgitation and aspiration from gastric dilation and ileus.
3. Initiate IV access.
4. Insert an indwelling urinary catheter to avoid bladder distention.
5. Monitor for hypotension, hypothermia, and bradycardia.
6. Continue with repeated neurologic examinations to determine if there is deterioration of the spinal cord injury.
7. Be prepared to manage seizures.
8. Pharmacologic interventions:
   a. High dose steroids.
   b. Diazepam (Valium)—for seizure control.

◆ MAXILLOFACIAL TRAUMA

Injuries to the head frequently result in facial lacerations and fractures to the facial bones, that is, nasal fractures, orbital fractures, maxillary fractures, and mandibular fractures.

Primary Assessment

1. Initiate immobilization of the spine while performing assessment.
2. Airway—obstruction can occur due to tongue swelling (fractured jaw), bleeding, or broken or missing teeth.
3. Breathing—may be impaired due to an obstructed airway.
4. Circulation—control bleeding.

Primary Interventions

1. Establish and maintain an airway. This includes having high-flow suction available, inserting an oral airway, or assisting with intubation. A nasopharyngeal airway should only be used if there is no evidence of nasal fractures or CSF leakage from the nose.
2. Control bleeding—do not apply pressure to the injury site. Apply a bulky loose dressing. Do not attempt to stop the flow of blood or CSF from the nose or ears; apply a loose dressing if needed.

Subsequent Assessment

1. Examine the mouth for broken or missing teeth.
2. Assess for a potential eye injury, vision loss, double vision, or pain in the eye.
3. Examine the eye for dysconjugate gaze—discoordination of eye movements.
4. Paralysis of the upward gaze is indicative of an inferior orbit fracture (blowout fracture).
5. Crepitus or a crackling feeling on palpation around the nose usually indicates a nasal fracture.
6. Malocclusion of the teeth is indicative of a maxilla or mandible fracture.
7. A palpable flattening of the cheek and a loss of sensation below the orbit may indicate a zygoma (cheekbone) fracture.
8. Spasms of the jaw (trismus) and mobility of the jaw indicate a maxilla fracture.
9. Rhinorrhea or otorrhea (indicative of leakage of CSF).

General Interventions

1. Gently apply ice to areas of swelling or ecchymosis—this may reduce further swelling and pain. However, if you suspect an injury to the eye itself, do not apply ice.
2. If other injuries permit, elevate the head of the bed.
3. Possible pharmacologic interventions:
   a. Morphine (Duramorph)—pain management.
   b. Diazepam (Valium)—sedation.
4. With the potential for a CSF leak, the patient should be instructed not to blow the nose, cough, or sneeze because of the potential for transmitting infection to the brain or eyes.

Injuries to Soft Tissue, Bones, and Joints

◆ SOFT TISSUE INJURIES

Soft tissue injuries involve the skin and underlying subcutaneous tissue and muscles. They can be classified as open or closed injuries. A **closed wound** is an injury to the soft tissue but without a break in the skin. Closed wounds include:

1. Contusion—bleeding beneath the skin into the soft tissue. The bleeding can be minor or extensive. Extensive bleeding can cause severe pain and swelling, leading to a compromise of vital structures.
2. Hematoma—a well-defined pocket of blood and fluid beneath the skin.

An **open wound** is an injury to soft tissue with a break in the skin. Generally, they are more serious than closed injuries due to the potential for blood loss and infection. Open wounds include:

1. Abrasion—a superficial loss of skin resulting from rubbing or scraping the skin over a rough or uneven surface.
2. Laceration—a tear in the skin. Can be a partial- or full-thickness cut. Can be defined as incisional or jagged.
3. Puncture—occurs when the skin is penetrated by a pointed object. Can be penetrating (entrance wound only) or perforating (entrance and exit wound). Generally, puncture wounds do not cause serious external bleeding, but there may be significant internal bleeding and damage to vital organs.
4. Avulsion—involves a tearing off or loss of a flap of skin.
5. Amputation—traumatic cutting or tearing off of a finger, toe, arm, or leg.

Primary Assessment

1. Always assure the adequacy of airway, breathing, and circulation before initiating treatment.
2. If the bleeding from the injury has been significant, be aware of the clinical symptoms and signs of shock.
   a. Skin pale, mottled, cold, and/or diaphoretic.
   b. Tachycardia (rapid, weak pulse).
   c. Tachypnea (rapid, shallow breathing).
   d. Hypotension (falling blood pressure is a late sign of shock).
   e. Restlessness, confusion, and anxiety.
3. Assess for arterial or venous bleeding. Arterial bleeding is bright red and usually spurts from the wound. Venous bleeding is darker red and will flow steadily from a wound.

Primary Interventions

The primary goal and nursing intervention are to control severe bleeding.

> ◆
> **NURSING ALERT:**
> Wounds that result in severe arterial bleeding should be considered life threatening and treatment is second only to CPR.

A. Direct Pressure
1. Most external bleeding can be controlled by direct pressure.
2. Cover the injury with sterile dressings.
3. Apply firm direct pressure to the site of injury.
4. Pressure should be maintained until the bleeding stops, a pressure dressing is applied, or definitive treatment is undertaken.

5. If the dressing becomes saturated, reinforce the dressing; do not remove the dressing.
6. After bleeding has stopped, apply a pressure dressing.
   a. A pressure bandage is made by securing several gauze pads over the injury with a rolled gauze bandage.
   b. A pressure dressing allows the nurse freedom to continue assessing the patient or attend to other injuries.
   c. After applying a pressure dressing, always ensure that the patient has a pulse distal to the dressing. If no pulse is present, the dressing may be too tight.

B. Elevation
1. Elevating the injured area while applying direct pressure helps to control bleeding. This measure uses gravity to slow the blood flow and to promote clotting.
2. If possible, the injured area should be elevated above the level of the heart.
3. Do not raise a limb if a fracture is suspected or if elevation causes the patient pain or discomfort.

C. Pressure Points
1. Pressure points are used when direct pressure and elevation cannot control bleeding alone or when direct pressure cannot be applied to a bleeding site due to a protruding bone or an embedded object.
2. Pressure points are located between the site of injury and the heart where a main artery passes over a bone or underlying muscle mass (Fig. 33-1).
3. Locate the pressure point and apply firm, steady pressure with the fingers or the heal of the hand.
4. If heavy bleeding still is not controlled and the patient may exsanguinate, a tourniquet may be used or a vascular clamp can be applied to the artery. Apply a tourniquet only as a last resort.

Subsequent Assessment

1. Expose the wound, cut away clothing if necessary. Do not remove any impaled objects.
2. Assess for the presence of concomitant injuries.
3. Assess vascular status distal to the injury and compare it to the uninjured extremity.
   a. Color of the injured extremity—pallor suggests poor arterial perfusion and cyanosis suggests venous congestion.
   b. Test capillary refill time by depressing the fingernail until it blanches and seeing how long until the nail bed returns to pink. A capillary refill time greater than 2 seconds suggests decreased arterial capillary perfusion.
   c. Test pulses distal to the injury—generally, they should be full and strong.
4. Perform a neurologic assessment of the injured extremity to determine peripheral nerve insult, possibly caused by direct injury, compression, or edema.
   a. Sensory function—while the patient's eyes are closed, lightly touch the area distal to the injury.
   b. Motor function—have patient move extremity distal to the injury.
5. Determine tetanus immunization status.
6. History of the injury, including when and how the wound occurred. Any wound that is more than 6 hours old is considered at high risk for infection, and primary closure by suturing may not be an option.
7. Allergies to local anesthesia, epinephrine, and antibiotics.

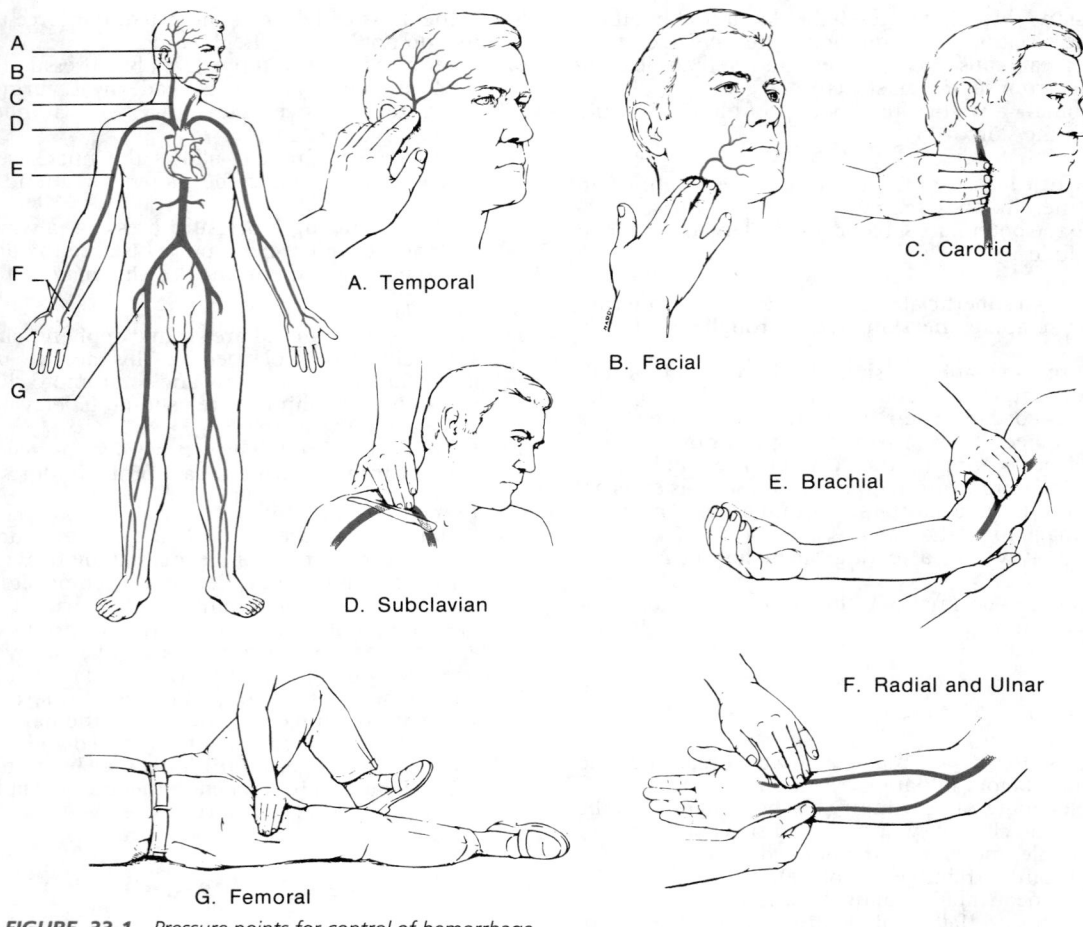

FIGURE 33-1 *Pressure points for control of hemorrhage.*

General Interventions

A. *Wound Preparation*
1. Shave the area surrounding area of the wound, but only shave what is necessary. Eyebrows are never shaved.
2. Irrigate gently and copiously with isotonic sterile saline solution or sterile water to remove dirt and debris.
   a. A catheter-tip syringe may be used to create a hydraulic action.
   b. General rule—irrigate with 50 mL per inch of wound per hour of age of wound. Use more irrigant for grossly contaminated wounds.
   c. If the wound is grossly contaminated, the wound may need to be cleaned with a surgical scrub sponge and then irrigated.
   d. The wound may be anesthetized first if the patient cannot tolerate the wound irrigation and cleaning.
3. The wound is infiltrated with local anesthetic intradermally through the wound margins or by regional nerve block.
4. Devitalized tissue and foreign matter are removed—devitalized tissue inhibits wound healing and enhances chance of bacterial infection.

B. *Wound closure*
1. Closure by *primary intent*
   a. Wound is repaired without delay following the injury; yields the fastest healing.
   b. Primary closure may be with sutures, skin tapes, staples, or tissue adhesives.
2. Closure by *secondary intent*
   a. Wound is allowed to granulate on its own without surgical closure.
   b. Wound is cleansed and covered with a sterile dressing.
3. Closure by *tertiary intent* or *delayed primary closure*
   a. Wound is cleansed and dressed.
   b. Patient returns in 3 to 4 days for definitive closure.

C. *Wound dressing*
1. Dressing should be applied in three layers.
   a. The first layer is the contact layer. This should consist of a nonabsorbent hydrophilic dressing that will allow exudate to pass through to the second layer without wetting the contact layer. Examples of contact layer dressings are: Adaptic, petroleum gauze, and Xeroform gauze.
   b. The second layer is the absorbent layer and is usually constructed of surgical dressing pad or 4 × 4 gauze dressings.

c. The third layer is the outer wrap that holds the dressing in place. The outer wrap may consist of rolled gauze and tape.

D. Pharmacologic Interventions
1. Give antimicrobial treatment as directed, depending on how the injury occurred, age of wound, presence of soil-infection potential.
2. Give tetanus prophylaxis as indicated, based on patient's immunization status and wound. For inadequate primary immunization, both tetanus toxoid and tetanus immune globulin are given.

Tetanus Prophylaxis in Routine Wound Management—United States

History of Adsorbed Tetanus Toxoid (Doses)	Clean, Minor Wounds		All Other Wounds*	
	Td†	TIG	Td†	TIG
Unknown or < three	Yes	No	Yes	Yes
≥ Three‡	No§	No	No‖	No

* Such as, but not limited to, wounds contaminated with dirt, feces, soil, saliva, etc.; puncture wounds; avulsions; and wounds resulting from missiles, crushing, burns, and frostbite.
† For children under 7 years old, DTP (DT, if pertussis vaccine is contraindicated) is preferred to tetanus toxoid alone. For persons 7 years old and older, Td is preferred to tetanus toxoid alone.
‡ If only three doses of *fluid* toxoid have been received, a fourth dose of toxoid, preferably an adsorbed toxoid, should be given.
§ Yes, if more than 10 years since last dose.
‖ Yes, if more than 5 years since last dose. (More frequent boosters are not needed and can accentuate side effects.)
(Source: MMWR Morbid Mortal Wkly Rep 34:405, 1986.)

E. Patient Education
1. Inform the patient that pain should subside in 24 hours.
2. Acetaminophen (Tylenol) or prescribed analgesic to be taken for the first 24 hours after a simple laceration.
3. If pain reappears, a wound infection may be suspected.
4. Recommend that the wound be elevated to limit accumulation of fluid in the wound's interstitial spaces.
   a. Elevate extremity for first 48 hours.
   b. Sleep with the head elevated if facial lacerations are present.
   c. Advise that health care provider be contacted if there is sudden or persistent onset of pain, fever/chills, bleeding, rapid swelling, foul odor, purulent fluid, or redness surrounding the wound.

◆ INJURIES TO BONES AND JOINTS

Injuries to bones and joints are common injuries. They are usually obvious injuries and may be dramatic in nature. However, rarely are these injuries life threatening. Fractures may be caused by direct trauma, that is, projectiles, crush injuries, or by indirect trauma, that is, bones being pulled apart or rotational forces. In addition, bones may be fractured due to pathologic reasons. A pathologic fracture is due to a weakness in the bone secondary to a disease process, such as metastatic cancer. For the classification of fractures, see p. 868.

Other injuries include:

1. **Dislocation**—complete displacement or separation of a bone from its normal place of articulation. It may be associated with a tearing of the ligaments. The shoulder, elbow, fingers, hips, and ankles are the joints most frequently affected.
2. **Subluxation**—a partial disruption of the articulating surfaces.
3. **Sprains**—injuries in which ligaments are partially torn or stretched. These types of injuries are usually caused by a twisting of a joint beyond its normal range of motion. The severity can range from mild to severe. The more seriously injured ligaments may resemble a fracture.
4. **Strains**—a stretching or tearing of muscle and tendon fibers. Usually caused by overexertion or overextension.

Primary Assessment

1. Always ensure the adequacy of airway, breathing, and circulation before initiating treatment.
2. Occult blood loss into a closed space from the fracture may be significant enough to produce hypovolemic shock. Death by exsanguination can occur from pelvic and femoral fractures. Estimated blood loss from closed fractures in liters:
   a. Tibia—1.5 L
   b. Femur—2 L
   c. Pelvis—6 L
   d. Humerus—2 L
3. A fractured cervical spine, pelvic fracture, or fractured femur may produce life-threatening injuries. Posterior dislocations of the hip are life- and limb-threatening emergencies due to the potential for blood loss and the disruption in blood supply to the head of the femur. Unless this dislocation is promptly reduced, the patient may develop avascular necrosis of the femoral head and subsequently may require a hip replacement.

Primary Interventions

1. Support airway, breathing, and circulation if compromised.
2. Initiate IV line and treat for shock if evident.
3. Protect injured part from movement or further trauma.

Subsequent Assessment

1. Seek information on the mechanism of injury.
   a. How did the injury occur?
   b. In what position was the limb after the injury?
   c. Did the person fall? How many feet did the person fall?
   d. What was the direction and amount of force? Certain musculoskeletal injuries commonly occur together.
2. Assess for the presence of concomitant injuries.
   a. A fractured calcaneus as the result of a fall from a great height may also include a compression fracture of the spine.

b. A fractured patella from an motor vehicle accident may also have a fractured or dislocated femur.
c. A fractured pelvis may occur with lumbosacral spine fractures and bladder injuries.
3. Perform a neurovascular assessment to include the area above and below the injury.
   a. Assess for ischemia to the extremity.
      (1) Pallor suggests poor arterial perfusion.
      (2) Cyanosis suggests venous congestion.
      (3) A capillary refill time greater than 2 seconds suggests decreased arterial capillary perfusion.
      (4) Palpate the pulse distal to the extremity—it should be full and strong.
      (5) Loss of a pulse or coldness of the extremity distal to the injury indicates pressure on an artery and may require immediate medical intervention.
   b. Assess neurologic supply of the injured extremity to determine peripheral nerve insult. Damage to a peripheral nerve can be the result of a direct injury, compression, or edema.
      (1) Test sensory function—with the patient's eyes closed lightly touch the area distal to the injury.
      (2) Test motor function—have patient move extremity distal to the injury.
      (3) Numbness or paralysis indicates pressure on the nerves and may require immediate medical interventions.
4. Examine the bones and joints adjacent to the injury. If there was enough force to produce one injury, there may be other injuries.
5. Signs and symptoms of fractures:
   a. Pain and tenderness over the fracture site.
   b. A grating or crepitus over the fracture site.
   c. Swelling, due to internal bleeding and edema.
   d. Deformity, unnatural position, or movement where there is no joint.
   e. Loss of use or guarding.
   f. Discoloration due to bleeding into the surrounding tissue.
   g. Shortening of an extremity or rotation of the extremity.
6. Signs and symptoms of dislocations:
   a. Loss of joint motion—the joint may appear "frozen."
   b. Obvious deformity—a lump, ridge, or excavation.
   c. Severe pain.
7. Signs and symptoms of sprains:
   a. Pain in the joint area.
   b. Swelling.
   c. Limited use or movement.
   d. Discoloration.
8. Signs and symptoms of strains:
   a. Pain located in a muscle or its tendon, not a bone or a joint.
   b. Swelling is usually minimal.
9. Closely monitor vital signs.

General Interventions

A. Severely Injured
1. Initiate an IV line and start volume replacement with Ringer's lactate.
2. Immobilize the injury—this will prevent further damage and will help to relieve the pain.

3. Prepare the patient for the operating room for open reduction, closed reduction, internal fixation, and/or wound care.
4. Antibiotics may be started.

B. Other Interventions
1. Elevate to prevent or limit swelling.
2. Apply ice packs or cold compresses; ice should not be placed directly on the skin.
3. Cover open fractures with a sterile dressing.
4. Splint the extremity in as good alignment as possible until definitive care is complete. Immobilize the joint above and below the fracture.
5. Handle the part gently and as little as possible.

C. Assess for Compartment Syndrome
1. Increased pressure within an extremity resulting from bleeding and swelling into a closed space, causing pressure on vital structures.
2. The six P's (signs and symptoms) of compartment syndrome are:
   a. Pain—development of a different type of pain or the return of pain after treatment/splinting had caused pain relief.
   b. Pallor—a deterioration in skin color and an increase in the capillary refill time.
   c. Pulselessness.
   d. Paresthesias.
   e. Paralysis—a late sign.
   f. Puffiness—a late sign.

Shock and Internal Injuries

◆ SHOCK

Shock is the common denominator in a wide variety of disease processes that presents as an immediate threat to life. Simply defined, shock is inadequate tissue perfusion. This inadequate tissue perfusion is the result of failure of one or more of the following: 1) the heart—pump failure; 2) blood volume; 3) arterial resistance vessels; and 4) the capacity of the venous beds. Any condition that significantly effects any of the above may precipitate a shock state.
Shock is classified as:

1. *Hypovolemic shock*—occurs when a significant amount of fluid is lost from the intravascular space. This fluid may be blood, plasma, or electrolyte solution. May result from hemorrhage, burns, or fluid shifts.
2. *Cardiogenic shock*—occurs when the heart fails as a pump. Primary causes of this failure are myocardial infarction, serious cardiac dysrhythmias, and myocardial depression. Secondary causes include mechanical restriction of cardiac function or venous obstruction, such as occurs with cardiac tamponade, vena cava obstruction, or tension pneumothorax.
3. *Septic shock*—occurs as the result of bacteria and their products circulating in the blood. The primary cause is the vasoactive mediators released by gram-negative bacteria affecting almost every physiologic system. Any septic focus has the potential to produce septic shock.
4. *Other types*—include spinal shock, neurogenic shock, anaphylactic shock, and hypoglycemic shock.

Primary Assessment and Interventions

1. Rapid recognition and prompt intervention are essential to increase the chance of survival, because a downward spiral of physiologic responses will occur if shock is not treated.
2. The initial priorities in the assessment are the same for all types of shock.
   a. Is the airway open?
   b. Is the patient breathing?
   c. Is there a circulation problem?
3. Initiate immediate interventions as indicated.
   a. Resuscitate as necessary.
   b. Administer oxygen to augment oxygen-carrying capacity of arterial blood.
   c. Start cardiac monitoring.
   d. Control hemorrhage.

Subsequent Assessment

1. Assess level of consciousness.
   a. Important indicator of shock because it reflects cerebral perfusion.
   b. Changes may include:
      (1) Confusion
      (2) Irritability
      (3) Anxiety
      (4) Agitation
      (5) Inability to concentrate
   c. Watch for increasing lethargy progressing to obtundation and coma, indicating progression of shock.
2. Monitor arterial blood pressure.
   a. If the patient can compensate for the shock state, the blood pressure may initially rise approximately 20%. A significant change in blood pressure may not occur until late.
   b. Narrowing pulse pressure—early in shock, the diastolic pressure may rise due to an initial vasoconstriction produced by release of catecholamines from the sympathetic nervous system.
   c. A fall in the systolic pressure—there is no absolute value in blood pressure that indicates a shock state. It is the deviation from normal that is important. However, it is generally accepted that a systolic pressure below 80 mm Hg or a mean arterial pressure below 60 mm Hg is indicative of shock.
3. Pulse quality and rate changes.
   a. The rate usually is increased.
   b. Weak thready pulse due to decreased cardiac output and increased peripheral vascular resistance.
4. Assess urinary output.
   a. A decrease in renal blood flow or pressure will result in decreased urinary output.
   b. Ideally in an adult, the urine output should be 50 mL/hour. An output of less than 25 mL/hour may indicate shock.
5. Assess capillary perfusion.
   a. Pale, ashen, mottled, cold, and sweaty skin indicates potent vasoconstriction.
   b. A capillary refill time greater than 2 seconds indicates vasoconstriction.
6. Also assess for:
   a. Subjective feeling of impending doom.
   b. Metabolic acidosis due to anaerobic metabolism within the cells.
   c. Excessive thirst.
   d. Hyperthermia if septic shock.

General Interventions

1. Administer O_2 to maintain the PaO_2 at 80 to 100 torr. This will augment oxygen-carrying capacity of arterial blood.
   a. One hundred percent oxygen by nonrebreather face mask.
   b. Intubation if the patient is unable to manage secretions or is ventilating poorly.
   c. If intubated, the patient may be hyperventilated to help control the acidosis.
2. Fluid resuscitation.
   a. Two large-bore IV lines should be established.
   b. Ringer's lactate is the initial fluid choice. Normal saline is the second choice, because hyperchloremic acidosis may develop if massive amount of normal saline is infused.
   c. Rate of infusion depends on severity of blood loss and clinical evidence of hypovolemia.
   d. Fresh whole blood is infused when there is massive blood loss.
   e. Additional platelets and coagulation factors are given when large amounts of blood are needed, because replacement blood is deficient in clotting factors.
   f. Warm the blood (commercial warmer or basin of warm water)—massive blood replacement has a cooling effect that can cause cardiac dysrhythmias, paradoxical hypotension, decreased oxyhemoglobin dissociation, or cardiac arrest.
3. Insert an indwelling urinary catheter.
   a. Record urinary output every 15 to 30 minutes.
   b. Urinary volume reveals adequacy of kidney and visceral perfusion.
4. Apply pneumatic antishock garment, also known as military antishock trousers (MAST), if available—to control internal bleeding and to facilitate blood flow to vital areas (Fig. 33-2). (Its primary use is for hypovolemic shock secondary to bleeding in the lower part of the body.)
5. Maintain patient in supine position with the legs elevated. *(This position is contraindicated in patients with head injuries.)*

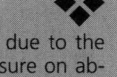

NURSING ALERT:
Trendelenburg's position is no longer recommended due to the potential for respiratory compromise due to the pressure on abdominal organs.

6. Electrocardiogram (ECG) monitoring—dysrhythmias may contribute to shock.
7. Maintain ongoing nursing surveillance of *total patient*—blood pressure, heart rate, respiratory rate, skin temperature, color, central venous pressure, arterial blood gases, urinary output, ECG, hematocrit, hemoglobin, coagulation profiles, and electrolytes—to assess patient response to treatment.
8. Immobilize fractures to minimize blood loss.
9. Maintain normothermia.
   a. Too much heat produces vasodilatation, which counteracts the body's compensatory mechanism of vasoconstriction and also increases fluid loss through perspiration.
   b. A patient who is in septic shock should be kept cool, because high fever will increase the cellular metabolic effects of shock.
10. Pharmacologic interventions:
    a. Inotropes are used in cardiogenic shock
       (1) Isoproterenol (Isuprel)
       (2) Digoxin (Lanoxin)
       (3) Dobutamine (Dobutrex)

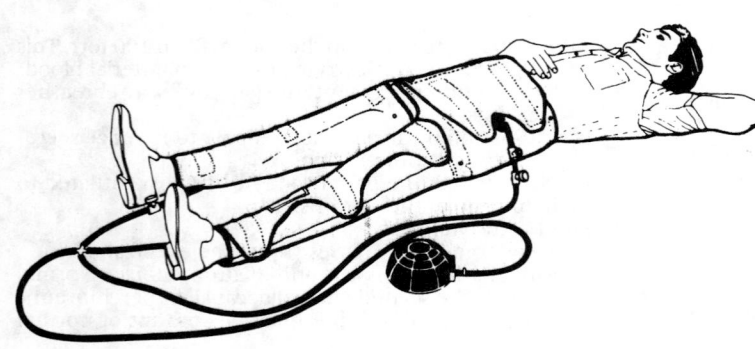

FIGURE 33-2 *The Military Anti-Shock Trouser (MAST) is a garment designed to correct internal bleeding and hypovolemia by the application of counter pressure around the legs and abdomen. This creates an artificial peripheral resistance and helps sustain coronary perfusion. It should be applied as soon as possible after injury, preferably before the patient is transferred to the emergency department. (Courtesy of David Clark Co., Inc., Worcester, MA 01604)*

   b. Vasopressors
     (1) Dopamine (Intropin)
     (2) Norepinephrine (Levophed)
     (3) Metaraminol (Aramine)
   c. Antibiotics—broad spectrum for septic shock.

◆ ABDOMINAL INJURIES

Abdominal injuries account for a large percentage of trauma-related injuries and deaths. The visceral organs contained within the abdomen can be classified as either hollow or solid. Damage to a hollow organ can result in acute peritonitis leading to shock within a few hours, and damage to a solid organ can result in lethal hemorrhage. Abdominal injuries may be classified as either penetrating or blunt.

Penetrating abdominal injury—usually the result of gunshot wounds or stab wounds. The mechanism that caused the penetrating abdominal trauma may cross the diaphragm and enter the chest. The opposite can also occur.

Blunt abdominal injury—usually caused by motor vehicle accidents or falls. Trauma to the abdomen is frequently associated with extraabdominal injuries, that is, chest, head, and extremity injuries and severe concomitant trauma to multiple intraperitoneal organs. Causes more delayed complications, especially if there is injury to liver, spleen, or blood vessels, which can lead to substantial blood loss into the peritoneal cavity.

Primary Assessment and Interventions

1. Assess airway, breathing, and circulation.
2. Initiate resuscitation as indicated.
3. Control bleeding and prepare to treat shock.
4. If there is an impaled object in the abdomen, leave it there. Stabilize the object in place with bulky dressings along the sides of the object.

Subsequent Assessment

1. Obtain a history of the mechanism of the injury, type of weapon, and estimated amount of blood loss.
   a. If the patient was stabbed, how long was the blade?
   b. Was the person who stabbed the patient a man or a woman?
     (1) Men usually hold a knife underhand and stab/thrust upward.
     (2) Women usually will stab/thrust downward with an overhand motion.
   c. Time of onset of symptoms.
   d. Passenger location (driver frequently sustains spleen/liver rupture).
2. Inspect the abdomen for obvious signs of injury (penetrating injury, bruises).
3. Evaluate for signs and symptoms of hemorrhage—frequently accompanies abdominal injury, especially if the liver and spleen have been traumatized.
4. Note tenderness, rebound tenderness, guarding, rigidity, and spasm.
   a. Press the area of maximal tenderness (let the patient point to the area).
   b. Remove the fingers quickly to check for rebound tenderness; pain at suspected point indicates peritoneal irritation.
5. Ask about referred pain: Kehr's sign—pain radiating to the left shoulder is a sign of blood beneath the left diaphragm; pain in right shoulder can result from laceration of liver.
6. Look for increasing abdominal distention. Measure abdominal girth at umbilical level early in assessment—serves as a baseline from which changes can be determined.
7. Auscultate for bowel sounds—a silent abdomen accompanies peritoneal irritation.
8. Auscultate for loss of dullness over solid organs (liver, spleen)—indicates presence of free air; dullness over regions normally containing gas may indicate presence of blood.
9. Look for chest injuries, which frequently accompany intraabdominal injuries.
10. Cullen's sign—a slight bluish discoloration around the naval is a sign of hemoperitoneum.
11. Pain is a poor indicator of the extent of the abdominal injury. Rebound tenderness and boardlike rigidity are indicative of a significant intraabdominal injury.
12. A rectal exam should be done on all patients and a pelvic exam on all female patients. The presence of blood on a gloved hand is indicative of trauma.
13. Continually assess vital signs, urinary output, central venous pressure readings, hematocrit values, and neurologic status. Tachypnea, tachycardia, and hypotension may be clues to intraabdominal bleeding.

General Interventions

1. Goals are to control bleeding and maintain blood volume and prevent infection.

2. Keep the patient quiet and on the stretcher, because movement may fragment or dislodge a clot in a large vessel and produce massive hemorrhage.
3. Cut the clothing away from the wound.
4. Count the number of wounds.
5. Look for entrance and exit wounds.
6. If the patient is comatose, immobilize the cervical spine until after cervical films are taken and cleared.
7. Apply compression to external bleeding wounds and occlusion of chest wounds.
8. Insert two large-bore IV lines and infuse Ringer's lactate. If possible, one of the lines should be in a central venous location.
9. Insert a nasogastric tube to decompress the abdomen. This will serve to empty the stomach, relieve gastric distention, and facilitate abdominal assessment. In addition, if blood is found, it may indicate stomach injury or esophageal injury.
10. Cover protruding abdominal viscera; do not attempt to replace the protruding organs into the abdomen. Use sterile saline dressings to protect viscera from drying.
11. Cover open wounds with dry dressings.
12. Withhold oral fluids to prevent increased peristalsis and vomiting.
13. Insert an indwelling urethral catheter to ascertain the presence of hematuria and to monitor urinary output. If a fracture of the pelvis is suspected, a catheter should not be placed until the integrity of the urethra is ensured.
14. Pharmacologic interventions
    a. Tetanus prophylaxis.
    b. Broad-spectrum antibiotics, because bacterial contamination is a frequent complication (depending on history and nature of wound).
15. Prepare for peritoneal lavage when there is uncertainty about intraperitoneal bleeding. See Procedure Guidelines 33-4: Peritoneal Lavage.
16. Prepare for surgery if the patient shows evidence of unexplained shock, unstable vital signs, peritoneal irritation, bowel protrusion or evisceration, significant penetrating injury, significant gastrointestinal bleeding, or peritoneal air.
17. Prepare the patient for diagnostic procedures.
    a. Urinalysis—as a guide to possible urinary tract injury and to monitor urine output.
    b. Serial hemoglobin and hematocrit levels—their trend reflects presence or absence of bleeding.
    c. Complete blood count—white blood cell count is generally elevated with trauma.
    d. Serum amylase—elevation usually indicates pancreatic injury or perforations of gastrointestinal tract.
    e. Computed tomography scans—permit detailed evaluation of abdominal and retroperitoneal injuries.
    f. Abdominal and chest x-rays—may reveal free air beneath diaphragm, indicating ruptured hollow viscus.

PROCEDURE GUIDELINES 33-4 ◆ Peritoneal Lavage

Peritoneal lavage is a technique of irrigation of the peritoneal cavity and examination of the irrigating fluid to evaluate the effects of trauma to the abdomen (see accompanying figure).

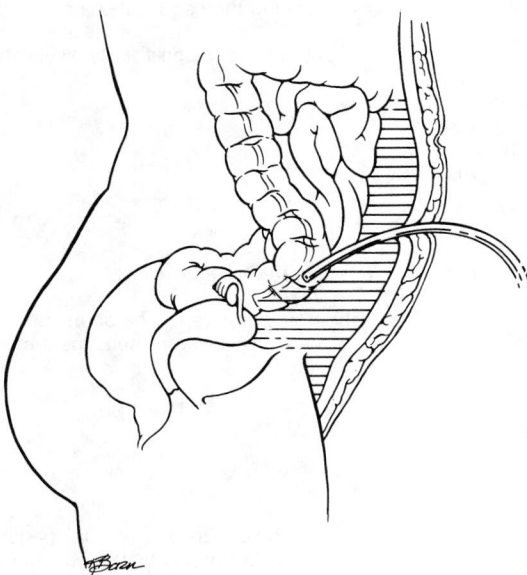

Peritoneal lavage.

(continued)

PROCEDURE GUIDELINES 33-4 ◆ Peritoneal Lavage *(continued)*

EQUIPMENT Peritoneal dialysis tray   Peritoneal dialysis catheter (multiple perforations)
Sterile solution (lactated Ringer's solution)   Local skin anesthetic; sterile gloves
IV tubing; IV pole

PROCEDURE

NURSING ACTION	RATIONALE

PREPARATORY PHASE

1. Explain the procedure to the patient; see that the consent form has been signed.
2. Insert indwelling catheter into the bladder.
3. Prepare the abdomen as for surgery.

4. Place the patient in a supine position.
5. Fill the IV tubing with solution using aseptic technique.

2. To prevent puncture of urinary bladder.
3. To minimize or eliminate surface bacteria and decrease the possibility of wound contamination and infection.

PERFORMANCE PHASE (BY THE PHYSICIAN)

1. The skin is infiltrated 2–3 cm (0.7–1.2 in.) below the umbilicus in the midline with local anesthetic.

2. A small vertical incision is made at the chosen site.
3. Bleeding vessels are carefully ligated.
4. The peritoneum is opened under direct vision and the peritoneal catheter is inserted into the peritoneal cavity, *OR*
5. A needle is passed intraabdominally, a flexible wire is passed through the needle, and a catheter is guided over the wire.
6. A syringe is attached to the catheter, and the peritoneal cavity is aspirated.

7. If no blood (or less than 10 mL) is present, the catheter is attached to the IV tubing; 500–1000 mL of solution is infused into the peritoneal cavity through the IV tubing attached to the dialysis catheter.
8. After the solution is infused, the empty IV bag is removed from the pole and lowered below the abdominal level (near the floor).
9. The peritoneal dialysis catheter is removed, and the wound is closed (unless laparotomy is necessary).
10. The fluid recovered from the peritoneal cavity is examined visually and is usually sent to the laboratory for cell counts and microscopic inspection of spun-down sediment.

1. The midline area is relatively avascular. Epinephrine may be injected with local anesthetic to produce capillary constriction and prevent a false-positive tap.

3. Ligation of vessels helps avoid a false-positive lavage.
4. There are various methods (open or percutaneous) of introducing the catheter into the peritoneal space.

6. If more than 10 mL of blood is obtained or the fluid contains bile, feces, or particulate matter, the test is considered positive and the patient is prepared for immediate laparotomy (incision into abdominal cavity).
7. If not contraindicated by the patient's condition, he or she may be turned from side to side to ensure that the solution reaches all parts of the abdominal cavity.

8. Lowering the bag creates a siphon effect to drain the excess fluid. As much of the fluid as possible is siphoned out of the peritoneal cavity by gravity.

INTERPRETATION OF LAVAGE FLUID

Clear fluid indicates a lack of significant intraperitoneal bleeding.
Criteria for positive results:
Aspiration of free blood from peritoneal cavity
Red blood cells > 100,000 per mm³
White blood cells > 500 per mm³
Amylase > 110 IU/dL
Presence of bile, bacteria, or fecal or food particles in lavage fluid

This indicates a negative test.

If the test is positive, a laparotomy is usually done. Indeterminate or equivocal results merit monitoring and investigation.

FOLLOW-UP PHASE

1. Assess the patient for complications.

2. Watch the patient closely for any type of deterioration.

1. Complications include visceral perforation, wound hematoma, perforated bowel, puncture of bladder, laceration of major vessels, infection.
2. Repeated physical examinations of the abdomen should be performed when intraabdominal injury is suspected.

◆ MULTIPLE INJURIES

The patient with multiple injuries requires rapid and definitive interventions during the 1st hour after the trauma to increase chance of survival; this 1st hour has been called the "golden hour." During this time, multiple assessments and interventions may be performed simultaneously by the health care team.

Primary Assessment and Interventions

A. Airway
1. Assume a cervical spine injury and open the airway using the jaw-thrust technique without head tilt.
2. Apply suction to clear the trachea and bronchial tree. Remove debris from mouth, that is, broken teeth, mucus.
3. Insert an oropharyngeal airway—to prevent occlusion by the tongue, avoid flexing the head.
4. Prepare for endotracheal intubation if adequate airway cannot be maintained.
5. If upper airway trauma or edema exists, a cricothyroidotomy may be indicated.

B. Breathing
1. Note the character and symmetry of chest wall motion and pattern of breathing. Assess for open wounds, deformity, and flail segments.
2. Auscultate the lungs and assess for tracheal deviation. If a tension pneumothorax is present, the trachea will shift from the midline.
3. Ask the conscious patient if experiencing difficulty in breathing or chest pain with breathing.
4. Administer oxygen by 100% nonrebreather mask or assist the patient's ventilations by bag-valve-mask system to alleviate hypoxia.
5. Suspect serious intrathoracic injuries if respiratory distress continues after adequate airway has been established.
6. Assess the overall effectiveness of ventilations.

C. Circulation
1. Assess cardiac function and treat cardiac arrest (hypoxia, metabolic acidosis, and chest trauma may precipitate cardiac arrest).
   a. For cardiac arrest, start closed chest compression and ventilation.
   b. If the chest wall is unstable (flail chest), emergency thoracotomy and manual compression may be necessary.
2. Control hemorrhage.
   a. Apply pressure over bleeding points if hemorrhage is overt.
   b. Expect significant blood loss in patients with fractures to the shaft of the femur, multiple fractures, or pelvic trauma.
   c. Use tourniquet(s) for massive arterial bleeding from extremities that cannot be halted with pressure.
   d. Prepare for immediate surgical intervention if patient is bleeding internally.
3. Palpate the carotid pulse and note its rate and quality. In addition, assess the femoral and radial pulses to determine an approximate systolic pressure.
   a. If the carotid pulse is present, the systolic pressure is at least 60 mm Hg.
   b. If the femoral pulse is present, the systolic pressure is at least 70 mm Hg.
   c. If the radial pulse is present, the systolic pressure is at least 80 mm Hg.
4. Prevent and treat hypovolemic shock.
   a. Insert at least two (sometimes four) IV lines, one above diaphragm and one below. Use venous cutdown if necessary.
   b. Initiate a central venous catheter to monitor the patient's response to fluid infusion—to prevent fluid overload and as a route for fluid infusion.
   c. Fluid resuscitation—Ringer's lactate or normal saline is given for volume replacement until blood is available.
   d. Administer blood—massive transfusions have a cooling effect that can cause cardiac irritability and arrest; blood should be warmed.
5. Note presence or absence of pulses in fractured extremities.

D. Neurologic
1. Assess level of responsiveness, pupil size and reactivity, motor power, and reflexes.
2. Determine a Glasgow Coma Score as a baseline (see p. 368).
3. If signs of increased intracranial pressure exist, intracranial pressure monitoring may be instituted.

Subsequent Assessment and Interventions

1. The goals are rapid determination of the extent of the injuries and treatment prioritization.
2. Monitor ECG—to detect life-threatening dysrhythmias.
3. Insert indwelling urethral catheter and monitor urinary output to aid in diagnosis of shock and monitor effectiveness of therapy. Do not force the catheter—the patient may have a ruptured urethra.
4. Perform an ongoing clinical evaluation to observe for improvement or deterioration, such as changes in vital signs, improvement in level of responsiveness, skin warmth, and speed of capillary filling.
5. Prepare for immediate surgical intervention if the patient does not respond to fluids or blood—inability to restore blood pressure and circulatory volume in the patient usually indicates major internal bleeding.
6. Splint fractures to prevent further trauma to soft tissues and blood vessels and to relieve pain.
7. Examine the patient for abdominal pain, muscular rigidity, tenderness, rebound tenderness, diminished bowel sounds, hypotension, and shock.
8. Prepare for peritoneal lavage to assess for intraperitoneal bleeding.
9. Draw blood for laboratory studies (type and cross-matching, hemoglobin, hematocrit, baseline complete blood count, electrolytes, blood urea nitrogen (BUN), glucose, prothrombin time).
10. Insert a nasogastric tube to prevent vomiting and aspiration.
11. Prepare for laparotomy if the patient shows continuing signs of hemorrhage and deterioration.
12. Continue to monitor urinary output every 30 minutes—reflects cardiac output and state of perfusion of visceral organs.
13. Assess for hematuria and oliguria.

14. Evaluate the patient for other injuries and institute appropriate treatment, including tetanus immunization.
15. Perform a more thorough physical examination after resuscitation and management of the aforementioned priorities.

Environmental Emergencies

◆ HEAT EXHAUSTION

Heat exhaustion is the inadequacy or the collapse of peripheral circulation due to volume and electrolyte depletion. Heat exhaustion is one condition in the spectrum of heat-related illnesses, including heat rash, heat edema, heat cramps, and heat syncope. Untreated heat exhaustion may progress to heatstroke.

Primary Assessment and Interventions

1. Expect the patient to be alert without significant cardiorespiratory or neurologic compromise.
2. If vital functions are significantly impaired, suspect secondary condition, such as myocardial infarction or stroke.

Subsequent Assessment

1. Obtain history of headache, fatigue, dizziness, muscle cramping, and nausea.
2. Inspect skin—usually pale, ashen, and moist.
3. The temperature may be normal, slightly elevated, or as high as 104°F (40°C).
4. Measure vital signs for hypotension, orthostatic changes, tachycardia, and tachypnea.
5. The patient will be awake but may give a history of syncope or confusion.
6. Laboratory analysis will show hemoconcentration and hyponatremia (if sodium depletion is the primary problem) or hypernatremia (if water depletion is the primary problem).
7. The ECG may show dysrhythmias without evidence of infarction.

General Interventions

1. Move the patient to a cool environment and remove all the clothing.
2. Position the patient supine with the feet slightly elevated.
3. If the patient complains of nausea or vomiting, do not give fluids by mouth.
4. Start an IV line with Ringer's lactate or normal saline until electrolyte results are confirmed.
5. Monitor the patient for changes in the cardiac rhythm and vital signs. Vital signs should be taken at least every 15 minutes until the patient is stable.
6. Provide fans and cool sponge baths as cooling methods.
7. Provide patient education.

a. Advise the patient to avoid immediate reexposure to high temperatures; the patient may remain hypersensitive to high temperatures for a considerable length of time.
b. Emphasize the importance of maintaining an adequate fluid intake, wearing loose clothing, and reducing activity in hot weather.
c. Athletes should monitor fluid losses, replace fluids, and use a gradual approach to physical conditioning, allowing sufficient time for acclimatization.

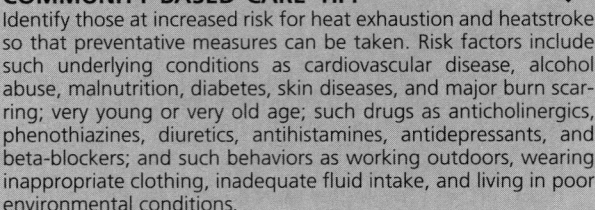

COMMUNITY-BASED CARE TIP:
Identify those at increased risk for heat exhaustion and heatstroke so that preventative measures can be taken. Risk factors include such underlying conditions as cardiovascular disease, alcohol abuse, malnutrition, diabetes, skin diseases, and major burn scarring; very young or very old age; such drugs as anticholinergics, phenothiazines, diuretics, antihistamines, antidepressants, and beta-blockers; and such behaviors as working outdoors, wearing inappropriate clothing, inadequate fluid intake, and living in poor environmental conditions.

◆ HEATSTROKE

Heatstroke is a medical emergency that can result in significant morbidity and mortality. It is defined as the combination of hyperpyrexia (105°F [40.6°C]) and neurologic symptoms. It is caused by a shutdown or failure of the heat-regulating mechanisms of the body.

Primary Assessment and Interventions

1. Assess airway, breathing, and circulation.
2. Level of consciousness may be altered.
3. Expect to intervene immediately if cardiovascular collapse occurs.

Subsequent Assessment

1. Obtain a history from accompanying person about environmental conditions, activity, underlying health, and medications that may have contributed to heatstroke.
2. Perform a neurologic assessment.
   a. Initially the patient may exhibit bizarre behavior or irritability. This may progress to confusion, combativeness, deliriousness, and coma.
   b. Other central nervous system disturbances include tremors, seizures, fixed and dilated pupils, and decerebrate or decorticate posturing.
3. Assess vital signs.
   a. Temperature greater than 105°F (40.6°C).
   b. Hypotension.
   c. Rapid pulse, may be bounding or weak.
   d. Rapid respirations.
4. The skin may appear flushed and hot; in early heatstroke, the skin may be moist, but as the heatstroke progresses, the skin will become dry as the body loses its ability to sweat.
5. Arterial blood gasses show metabolic acidosis.

General Interventions

NURSING ALERT:
Once the diagnosis of heatstroke is made or suspected, it is imperative to reduce patient's temperature.

1. Provide cooling measures.
   a. Reduce the core (internal) temperature to 39°C (102°F) as rapidly as possible.
   b. Evaporative cooling is the most efficient. Spray tepid water on the skin while electric fans are used to blow continuously over the patient to augment heat dissipation.
   c. Apply ice packs to neck, groin, axillae, and scalp (areas of maximal heat transfer).
   d. Soak sheets/towels in ice water and place on patient, using fans to accelerate evaporation/cooling rate.
   e. Immerse patient in cold water (controversial because it may result in peripheral vasoconstriction and may decrease the body's heat loss).
   f. If the temperature fails to decrease, initiate core cooling: iced saline lavage of stomach, cool-fluid peritoneal dialysis, cool-fluid bladder irrigation, or cool-fluid chest irrigations.
   g. Place the patient on a hypothermia blanket.
   h. Discontinue active cooling when the temperature reaches 39°C (102°F). In most cases, this will reduce the chance of overcooling, because the body temperature will continue to fall after cessation of cooling.
2. Oxygenate patient to supply tissue needs that are exaggerated by the hypermetabolic condition: 100% nonrebreather mask or intubate the patient if necessary to support a failing cardiorespiratory system.
3. Monitor condition.
   a. Monitor and record the core temperature continually during cooling process to avoid hypothermia; also, hyperthermia may recur spontaneously within 3 to 4 hours.
   b. Monitor the vital signs continuously, including ECG, central venous pressure, blood pressure, pulse, and respiratory rate.
   c. Perform frequent (every 30 minutes) neurologic assessments.
4. Replace fluids.
   a. Start IV infusion using Ringer's lactate to replace fluid losses, maintain adequate circulation, and facilitate cooling.
   b. At least one IV line should be a central line.
   c. Fluid replacement is based on the patient's response and laboratory results.

GERONTOLOGIC ALERT:
Vigorous fluid replacement in the elderly or those with underlying cardiovascular disease may cause pulmonary edema.

5. Other measures:
   a. Dialysis for renal failure.
   b. Diuretics such as mannitol (Osmitrol) to promote diuresis.
   c. Anticonvulsant agents to control seizures.
   d. Potassium for hypokalemia and sodium bicarbonate to correct metabolic acidosis, depending on laboratory results.
   e. Antipyretics are not useful in treating heatstroke. They may contribute to the complications of coagulopathy and hepatic damage.
   f. Intense shivering may be controlled by diazepam (Valium). Shivering will generate heat and increase the metabolic rate.
   g. Patients with depleted clotting factors may be treated with platelets or fresh-frozen plasma.
6. Insert a Foley catheter with a urimeter and measure urinary output at least hourly—acute tubular necrosis is a complication of heatstroke.
7. Perform continuous ECG monitoring and frequent cardiovascular assessments for possible ischemia, infarction, and dysrhythmias.
8. Perform serial laboratory testing (clotting parameters, electrolytes, glucose, and serum enzymes).
9. The patient should be admitted to an intensive care unit; complications can occur including heart failure, cardiovascular collapse, hepatic failure, renal failure, disseminated intravascular coagulation, and rhabdomyolysis.
10. Monitor the patient for the development of seizures and provide for a safe environment in case of seizures.

◆ FROSTBITE

Frostbite is trauma due to exposure to freezing temperatures that cause actual freezing of the tissue fluids in the cell and intracellular spaces, resulting in vascular damage. The areas of the body most likely to develop frostbite are the earlobes, cheeks, nose, hands, and feet. Frostbite may be classified as frostnip (initial response to cold, reversible), superficial, and deep.

Primary Assessment and Interventions

1. If not alert, assess airway, breathing, and circulation.
2. Deficits may indicate coexisting hypothermia or underlying condition.
3. Protect frostbitten tissue while performing other interventions.

Subsequent Assessment

A. **Frostnip**
1. History of gradual onset.
2. Skin appears white.
3. Numb, painfree.

B. **Superficial Frostbite**
1. Damage is limited to the skin and subcutaneous tissue.
2. The skin will appear white and waxy.
3. On palpation, the skin will feel stiff but the underlying tissue will be pliable, soft, and have its normal "bounce."
4. Sensation is absent.

C. **Deep Frostbite**
1. Skin will appear white, yellow-white, or mottled blue-white.

2. On palpation, the surface will feel frozen and the underlying tissue will feel frozen and hard.

3. The affected part is completely insensitive to touch.

General Interventions

1. Frostnip may be treated by placing a warm hand over the chilled area.

2. Leave the frostbitten area alone until definitive rewarming is undertaken. Pad the extremity to prevent damage from trauma.

COMMUNITY-BASED CARE TIP:
Once definitive rewarming of a frostbitten extremity has started, it must not be stopped. Refreezing of a partially thawed extremity reverses ice crystal formation in tissues and increases tissue damage and loss.

3. Handle the part gently to avoid further mechanical injury.

4. Remove all constricting clothing that can impair circulation, including watchbands and rings.

5. Rewarming:
  a. Rewarm the extremity by controlled and rapid rewarming. Rewarm with a temperature of 37°C to 40°C (98.6°F to 104°F) in a fairly large tepid water bath where the part can be fully immersed without touching the side or bottom. If clothing, socks, or gloves are frozen to the extremity, they should be left on and removed after rewarming.
  b. More warm water may be added to the container by removing some cooled water and adding warm water.
  c. Slow rewarming is less effective and may increase tissue damage.
  d. Dry heat is not recommended for rewarming.
  e. The rewarming procedure may take 20 to 30 minutes.
  f. Rewarming is complete when the area is warm to the touch and pink or flushed.
  g. Do not rub or massage a frostbitten extremity: the ice crystals in the tissue will lacerate delicate tissue.

5. Pharmacologic interventions:
  a. Narcotics for pain control.
  b. Antibiotics if there is an open wound.
  c. Tetanus prophylaxis.

6. Protect the thawed part from infection. Large blisters may develop in 1 hour to a few days after rewarming; these blisters should not be broken.

7. Place sterile gauze or cotton between affected fingers/toes to absorb moisture.

8. Use strict aseptic technique during dressing changes—frostbite injuries make the patient susceptible to infection. Make sure any dressings are loosely applied.

9. Elevate the part to help control swelling.

10. Use a foot cradle to prevent contact with bedding if the feet are involved—prevents further tissue injury.

11. Perform a physical assessment to look for concomitant injury (soft tissue injury, dehydration, alcohol coma, fat embolism due to fracture, immobility).

12. Restore electrolyte balance; dehydration and hypovolemia occur frequently in frostbite victims.

13. Whirlpool bath for the affected extremity—to aid circulation, debride dead tissue, and help prevent infection.

14. Escharotomy (incision through the eschar)—to prevent further tissue damage, allow for normal circulation, and permit joint motion.

15. Fasciotomy (incision in fascia to release pressure on the muscles, nerves, blood vessels)—to treat compartment syndrome.

16. Encourage hourly active motion of the affected digits to promote maximum restoration of function and to prevent contractures.

17. Advise patient not to use tobacco because of the vasoconstrictive effects of nicotine, which further reduce the already deficient blood supply to injured tissues.

18. Perform serial laboratory testing (urinalysis and serum enzymes) to monitor for the complications of rhabdomyolysis and subsequent renal failure.

◆ HYPOTHERMIA

Hypothermia is a condition in which the core (internal) temperature of the body is less than 35°C (95°F) as a result of exposure to cold. In response to a decreased core temperature, the body will attempt to produce or conserve more heat by 1) shivering, which produces heat through muscular activity; 2) peripheral vasoconstriction, to decrease heat loss; and 3) raising the basal metabolic rate. Hypothermia may be classified as mild, moderate, or severe.

GERONTOLOGIC ALERT:
The elderly are at greater risk for hypothermia due to altered compensatory mechanisms.

Primary Assessment and Interventions

NURSING ALERT:
Extreme caution should be used in moving or transporting patients, because the heart is near fibrillation threshold.

1. Assess airway and breathing
  a. Spontaneous respirations may be extremely slow and imperceptible.
  b. Assist breathing and oxygenation with supplemental O_2 at 100% or a bag-valve-mask device.
  c. If intubation is necessary, extreme caution should be used, because ventricular fibrillation may be precipitated.

2. Assess circulation.
  a. If the body temperature falls below 30°C (86°F), the heart sounds may not be audible even if the heart is still beating. Tissues conduct sound poorly at low temperatures.
  b. Blood pressure readings may be extremely difficult to hear, because cold tissue conducts sound waves poorly.
  c. Pupil reflexes may be blocked by a decrease in cerebral blood flow, so the pupils may appear fixed and dilated.
  d. A patient with a heartbeat may present like a patient in cardiac arrest with fixed dilated pupils, no pulse, and no blood pressure. Provide CPR until further evaluation through ECG and hemodynamic monitoring.

Subsequent Assessment

1. There is progressive deterioration marked by apathy, poor judgment, ataxia, dysarthria, drowsiness, and eventually coma.
2. Speech is slow and may be slurred.
3. Shivering may be suppressed below a temperature of 32.2°C (90°F).
4. Cardiac dysrhythmias—cold disrupts the conduction system of the heart, and a variety of dysrhythmias may be seen. A hypothermic heart is extremely susceptible to ventricular fibrillation. Very cold hearts do not respond to drugs or defibrillation.
5. The heartbeat and the blood pressure may be so weak that the peripheral pulsations become undetectable.
6. Urine output may increase in response to peripheral vasoconstriction, "cold diuresis."
7. Initial tachypnea followed by slow and shallow respirations, possibly 2 or 3 a minute in severe hypothermia.
8. Fruity or acetone odor to the breath, because the body may be metabolizing fat as a result of decreased insulin levels.

General Interventions

Goal: Rewarm without precipitating cardiac dysrhythmias.

A. *Supportive Measures*
1. Handle the patient *carefully and gently*—to avoid triggering ventricular fibrillation.
2. Continuously monitor core temperatures with a low reading rectal thermometer.
3. Continuously monitor ECG. Because you may be unable to obtain a pulse due to the hypothermia, rely on the cardiac monitor to determine the need for CPR.
4. Monitor the patient's condition through vital signs, central venous pressure, urinary output, arterial blood gas values, and blood chemistry determinations.
5. Maintain an arterial line for recording blood pressure and to facilitate blood sampling—allows rapid detection of acid–base disturbances and assessment of adequacy of ventilation and oxygenation.
6. Start IV therapy with normal saline. Ringer's lactate is not recommended, because the cold liver may not be able to metabolize the lactate.

B. *Rewarming Techniques*
The type of rewarming depends on the degree of hypothermia. Rewarming should continue until the core temperature is 34°C (93.2°F). If the patient is in cardiac arrest, rewarming should continue until a temperature of 32°C (89.6°F) has been reached. Death in hypothermia is defined as a failure to revive after rewarming.

1. Passive external rewarming (temperature above 28°C [82.4°F]).
   a. Remove all the wet or cold clothing and replace with warm clothing.
   b. Provide insulation by wrapping the patient in several blankets.
   c. Provide warmed fluids to drink.
   d. Disadvantage: slow process.
2. Active external rewarming (temperature above 28°C [82.4°F]).
   a. Provide external heat for the patient, warm hot water bottles to the armpits, neck, or groin. (Do not apply hot water bottles directly to the skin.)
   b. Warm water immersion.
   c. Disadvantages:
      (1) Causes peripheral vasodilation, returning cool blood to the core, causing an initial lowering of the core temperature.
      (2) Acidosis due to the "washing out" of lactic acid from the peripheral tissues.
      (3) An increase in the metabolic demands before the heart is warmed to meet these needs.
3. Active core rewarming (temperature below 28°C [82.4 F]).
   a. Inhalation of warmed, humidified oxygen by mask or ventilator.
   b. Warmed IV fluids.
   c. Warmed gastric lavage.
   d. Peritoneal dialysis with warmed standard dialysis solution.
   e. Mediastinal irrigation through open thoracotomy has been used successfully but has serious complications.
   f. Cardiopulmonary bypass.
   g. Disadvantage of active core rewarming is the invasiveness of the procedures.

Toxicologic Emergencies

Toxicology is the study of the harmful effect of various substances on the body. Poisons are substances that are harmful to the body no matter how much or in what manner they enter the body. Drugs become toxic when they are taken in excess quantities or manners that are not therapeutic. Alcohol is considered a drug. The treatment goals of toxicologic emergencies are first, supportive; second, prevent or minimize absorption; third, provide an antidote.

◆ INGESTED POISONS

Ingested poisons can produce immediate or delayed effects. Immediate injury is caused when the poison is caustic to the body tissues, that is, a strong acid or a strong alkali. Other ingested poisons must be absorbed into the bloodstream before they become harmful. Ingested poisoning may be accidental or intentional.

Primary Assessment and Interventions

1. Maintain an open airway—some ingested substances may cause soft tissue swelling of the airway.
2. Attain control of the airway, ventilation, and oxygenation; in the absence of cerebral or renal damage, the patient's prognosis depends largely on successful management and support of vital functions.

Subsequent Assessment

1. Identify the poison.
   a. Try to determine the product taken: where, when, why, how much, who witnessed the event, time since ingestion.
   b. Call the poison control center in the area if an unknown toxic agent has been taken or if it is necessary to identify an antidote for a known toxic agent.
2. Continue the focused assessment, observing any significant deviations from normal. Different poisons will affect the body in different ways.

3. Obtain blood and urine tests for toxicology screening. Gastric contents may also be sent for toxicology screening in serious ingestions.
4. Monitor neurologic status, including mentation; monitor the course of vital signs and neurologic status over time.
5. Monitor for fluid and electrolyte imbalance.

General Interventions

A. *Supportive Care*
1. Initiate large-bore IV access.
2. Administer oxygen for respiratory depression.
3. Monitor and treat shock.
4. Prevent aspiration of gastric contents by positioning (on side with head down), use of oropharyngeal airway, and suctioning.
5. Give supportive care to maintain vital organ systems.
6. Insert an indwelling urinary catheter to monitor renal function.
7. Support the patient having seizures; many poisons excite the central nervous system, or the patient may convulse from oxygen deprivation.
8. Monitor and treat for complications: hypotension, coma, cardiac dysrhythmias, and seizures.
9. Psychiatric evaluations may be done after the patient is stabilized.

B. *Minimizing Absorption*
1. The primary method for preventing or minimizing absorption is to administer activated charcoal with a cathartic to hasten excretion. Newer superactivated charcoals can reduce absorption of a toxic substance by as much as 50%. Administering activated charcoal plus a cathartic is just as effective or more effective than gastric lavage.
   a. Administration of oral-activated charcoal—adsorbs the poison on the surface of its particles and allows it to pass with the stool. Multiple doses may be administered.
   b. Activated charcoal is usually mixed in tap water to make a slurry.

2. The secondary method for preventing or minimizing absorption is induction of emesis with syrup of ipecac. This procedure should be done only if the patient is conscious and has a good gag reflex. It is most effective within 30 minutes of ingestion of poison.
   a. Syrup of ipecac, 30 mL by mouth followed by two glasses of water is the usual adult dose.
   b. For children between age 1 and 12, give 15 mL followed by 8 to 16 ounces of water.

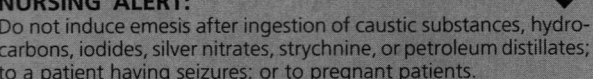

NURSING ALERT:
Do not induce emesis after ingestion of caustic substances, hydrocarbons, iodides, silver nitrates, strychnine, or petroleum distillates; to a patient having seizures; or to pregnant patients.

3. Gastric lavage for the obtunded patient (see Procedure Guidelines 33-5: Assisting With Gastric Lavage). Save gastric aspirate for toxicology screens.
4. Procedures to enhance the removal of the ingested substance if the patient is deteriorating.
   a. Forced diuresis with urine pH alteration—to enhance renal clearance.
   b. Hemoperfusion (process of passing blood through an extracorporeal circuit and a cartridge containing an adsorbent, such as charcoal, after which the detoxified blood is returned to patient).
   c. Hemodialysis—used in selected patients to purify blood and accelerate the elimination of circulating toxins.
   d. Repeated doses of charcoal—for binding nonabsorbed drugs/toxins.
   e. Gastric lavage may be used in conjunction with activated charcoal and a cathartic to maximize elimination of the substance.

C. *Providing an Antidote*
1. An antidote is a chemical or physiologic antagonist that will neutralize the poison.
2. Administer the specific antidote as early as possible to reverse or diminish effects of the toxin.

PROCEDURE GUIDELINES 33-5 ◆ Assisting With Gastric Lavage

Gastric lavage is the aspiration of the stomach contents and washing out of the stomach by means of a gastric tube (see accompanying figure).

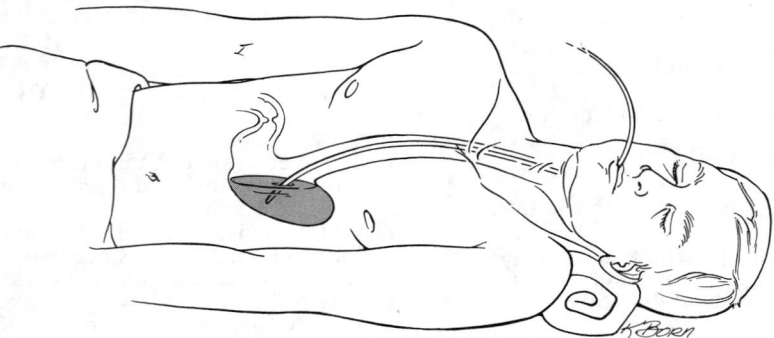

Gastric lavage.

PURPOSES
1. To remove unabsorbed poison after poison ingestion.
2. To diagnose gastric hemorrhage and for the arrest of hemorrhage.
3. To cleanse the stomach before endoscopic procedures.
4. To remove liquid or small particles of material from the stomach.

EQUIPMENT

Large-bore orogastric tubes or large-bore Ewald tube
Large irrigating syringe with adapter
Large plastic funnel with adapter to fit stomach tube
Water-soluble lubricant

Lavage fluid (warm saline or other prescribed solution)
Bucket for aspirate
Mouth gag; nasotracheal or endotracheal tubes with inflatable cuffs
Containers for specimens

PROCEDURE

EMERGENCY DEPARTMENT/TEAM ACTION	RATIONALE
1. Remove dental appliances and inspect oral cavity for loose teeth.	1. To prevent accidental aspiration.
2. Measure the distance on the lavage tube between the bridge of the nose and the xiphoid process. Mark with indelible pencil or tape.	2. This is a rule-of-thumb measurement of the distance the tube is passed to reach the stomach; avoids curling/kinking of excess tubing.
3. Lubricate the tube with water-soluble lubricant.	
4. If the patient is comatose, he or she is intubated with a cuffed nasotracheal or endotracheal tube.	4. A cuffed endotracheal tube prevents aspiration of gastric contents.
5. Place the unconscious patient in a left lateral position with the head (lowered approximately 15 degrees downward), neck, and trunk forming a straight line.	5. This position decreases passage of gastric contents into the duodenum during lavage and minimizes the possibility of aspiration into lungs.
6. Pass the tube via the oral (or nasal) route while keeping the head in a neutral position. Pass the tube to the adhesive marking or about 50 cm (20 in.). After the lavage tube is passed, the head of the table is lowered. Have standby suction available.	6. The depth of insertion of the tube will vary with the height of the patient. If the tube enters the larynx instead of the esophagus, the patient will experience coughing and dyspnea.
7. Submerge free end of tube below water level at the moment of the patient's exhalation or auscultate the stomach during injection of air with a syringe to confirm gastric location.	7. If tube is inadvertently in the lungs, the water will bubble with each exhalation.
8. Aspirate the stomach contents with syringe attached to the tube before instilling water or antidote. Save the specimen for analysis.	8. Aspiration is performed to remove the stomach contents. Initial gastric aspirates are saved for toxicologic analysis.
9. Remove syringe. Attach funnel to the stomach tube or use 50-mL syringe to put lavage solution in gastric tube. Volume of fluid placed in the stomach should be small.	9. Overfilling of the stomach may cause regurgitation and aspiration or force the stomach contents through the pylorus.
10. Elevate funnel above the patient's head and pour approximately 150–200 mL of solution into funnel.	10. The lavage fluid is left in place about 1 minute and then allowed to drain.
11. Lower the funnel and siphon the gastric contents into the bucket.	11. The fluid should flow in freely and drain by gravity.
12. Save samples of first two washings.	12. Keep track of fluid input/output to be sure that most of fluid is being removed.
13. Repeat lavage procedure until the returns are relatively clear and no particulate matter is seen.	13. This usually requires a total volume of at least 2 L, some clinicians advocate 5–20 L.
14. At the completion of lavage:	
a. Stomach may be left empty.	
b. An adsorbent (powder form of activated charcoal mixed with water to form a slurry, the consistency of thick soup) may be instilled in the tube and allowed to remain in the stomach.	b. Activated charcoal adsorbs a variety of drugs and toxic agents onto its surface and is used to prevent the gastrointestinal absorption of various substances. It renders the poison inaccessible to the circulation, thereby reducing its toxicity.
c. A saline cathartic may be instilled in the tube.	c. A cathartic facilitates the transit of the charcoal and remains of the ingested substance through the intestinal tract.
15. Pinch off tube during removal or maintain suction while tube is being withdrawn.	15. Pinching off the tube prevents aspiration and the initiation of the gag reflex. Keeping the patient's head lower than the body also gives this protection.
16. Give the patient a cathartic if prescribed. Warn the patient that stools will turn black from the charcoal.	16. A cathartic may be given if the poison has no corrosive action on the bowel. The cathartic will help remove unabsorbed material from the intestine.

◆ CARBON MONOXIDE POISONING

Carbon monoxide poisoning is an example of an inhaled poison and is the result of the inhalation of the products of incomplete hydrocarbon combustion. It may occur as an industrial or household accident or as an attempted suicide. Carbon monoxide exerts its toxic effect by binding to circulating hemoglobin to reduce the oxygen-carrying capacity of the blood. The affinity between carbon monoxide and hemoglobin is 200 to 300 times that between oxygen and hemoglobin. (Carbon monoxide combines with hemoglobin to form carboxyhemoglobin.) As a result, tissue anoxia occurs.

Primary Assessment

1. Assess airway and breathing.
   a. Respiratory depression may be present.
   b. If the carbon monoxide poisoning is due to smoke inhalation, stridor (indicative of laryngeal edema due to thermal injury) may be present.

Primary Interventions

1. Provide 100% oxygen by tight-fitting mask. (The elimination half-time of carboxyhemoglobin, in serum, for a person breathing room air is 5 hours 20 minutes. If the patient breathes 100% oxygen, the half-time is reduced to 80 minutes; 100% oxygen in a hyperbaric chamber will reduce the half-life in 23 minutes.)
2. Intubate if necessary to protect the airway.

Subsequent Assessment

1. A thorough history is important: determine the type and length of exposure as well as possible other fumes inhaled. An underlying anemia, cardiac disease, or pulmonary disease may place a person at higher risk.
2. Determine level of consciousness—the patient may appear intoxicated from cerebral hypoxia; confusion may progress rapidly to coma.
3. Assess complaints of headache, muscular weakness, palpitation, dizziness.
4. Inspect skin—may be pink, cherry red, or cyanotic and pale—*skin color is not a reliable sign.*
5. Monitor vital signs—increased respiratory and pulse rates are generally present. Be alert for for altered breathing patterns and respiratory failure.
6. Listen for rales or wheezes in the lungs (with smoke inhalation, indicates adult respiratory distress syndrome).
7. Obtain arterial blood samples for carboxyhemoglobin levels.
   a. Normal is less than 12%.
   b. Severe carbon monoxide poisoning is present when levels are greater than 30% to 40%.

General Interventions

1. History of exposure to carbon monoxide justifies immediate treatment.

2. Goals are to reverse cerebral and myocardial hypoxia and hasten carbon monoxide elimination.
3. Give 100% oxygen at atmospheric or hyperbaric pressures to reverse hypoxia and accelerate elimination of carbon monoxide. Patients should receive hyperbaric oxygen for central nervous system or cardiovascular system dysfunction.
4. Use continuous ECG monitoring, treat dysrhythmias, and correct acid–base and electrolyte abnormalities.
5. Observe the patient constantly—psychoses, spastic paralysis, visual disturbances, and deterioration of personality may persist after resuscitation and may be symptoms of permanent central nervous system damage.

◆ INSECT STINGS

Insect stings or bites are injected poisons that can produce either local or systemic reactions. Local reactions are characterized by pain, erythema, and edema at the site of injury. Systemic reactions usually begin within minutes and produce mild to severe and life-threatening reactions.

Primary Assessment and Interventions

1. Assess airway, breathing, and circulation.
2. Anaphylactic reactions may produce unconsciousness, laryngeal edema, and cardiovascular collapse.
3. Epinephrine is the drug of choice—the amount and route depends on the severity of the reaction.
4. Administer a bronchodilator to help relieve the bronchospasm.
5. Initiate an IV with Ringer's lactate.
6. Prepare for CPR.

Subsequent Assessment

1. Obtain history of insect sting, previous exposure, and allergies.
2. Inspect skin for local reaction—erythema, edema, pain at site of injury— as well as generalized pruritus, urticaria, and angioedema.
3. Continue to monitor blood pressure and respiratory status for dyspnea, wheezing, and stridor.

General Interventions

1. Apply ice packs to site to relieve pain.
2. Elevate extremity with large edematous local reaction.
3. Administer oral antihistamine for local reactions.
4. Clean the wound thoroughly with soap and water or an antiseptic solution.
5. Administer tetanus prophylaxis if not up to date.
6. Provide patient education.
   a. Always have epinephrine on hand (Epi-Pen).
   b. Wear medical emergency bracelets indicating hypersensitivity.
   c. Instructions when sting occurs:
      (1) Take epinephrine immediately if stung.
      (2) Remove stinger with one quick scrape of fingernail.

(3) Do not squeeze venom sac, because this may cause additional venom to be injected.
(4) Report to nearest health care facility for observation.
d. Avoid exposure.
(1) Avoid locales with stinging insects (camp and picnic sites).
(2) Stay away from insect feeding areas—flower beds, ripe fruit orchards, garbage, fields of clover.
(3) Avoid going barefoot outdoors—yellow jackets may nest on ground.
(4) Avoid perfumes, scented soaps, bright colors—attract bees.
(5) Keep car windows closed.
(6) Spray garbage cans with rapid-acting insecticide, and keep areas meticulously clean.

◆ SNAKEBITES

The majority of snakes in the United States are not poisonous. The poisonous varieties are pit vipers (rattlesnakes and copperheads) and coral snakes. Bites by these snakes may result in envenomation, an injected poisoning.

Primary Assessment and Interventions

1. Assess airway, breathing, and circulation if patient is not alert.
2. Severe envenomation may lead to neurotoxicity with respiratory paralysis, shock, coma, and death.
3. Be prepared to resuscitate and provide advanced life support.

Subsequent Assessment

1. Get a description of the snake, the time of the snakebite, and the location of the bite. Bites to the head and trunk may progress more rapidly and be more severe.
   a. Pit vipers have triangular shaped heads, vertical shaped pupils, indentations between the eyes and nostrils, and long fangs.
   b. Coral snakes are small, brightly colored, with short fangs and teeth behind them, and with a series of bands of yellow, red, yellow, and black (in that order).
2. Assess for local reactions—burning, pain, swelling, and numbness at the site. Local reactions to coral snakebites may be delayed several hours and be very mild.
3. A few hours after the bite, hemorrhagic blisters may occur at the site, and the entire extremity may become edematous.
4. Watch for signs of systemic reactions, including nausea, sweating, weakness, lightheadedness, initial euphoria followed by drowsiness, difficulty in swallowing, paralysis of various muscle groups, signs of shock, seizures, and coma.
5. Monitor vital signs closely, because tachycardia or bradycardia may develop.

General Interventions

1. Keep the patient calm and at rest in a recumbent position with the affected extremity immobilized.
2. Administer oxygen.

3. Start an IV line with normal saline or Ringer's lactate.
4. Administer antivenin and be alert to allergic reaction (antivenin is horse serum based).
5. Administer vasopressors in the treatment of shock.
6. Monitor for bleeding and administer blood products for coagulopathy.

◆ DRUG INTOXICATION

Substance abuse includes the use of specific substances that are intended to alter mood or behavior.

Drug abuse is the use of drugs for other than legitimate medical purposes. There is a growing tendency among drug users to take a variety of drugs simultaneously (polydrug abuse), including alcohol, sedatives, hypnotics, and marijuana, which may have additive effects. The clinical manifestations may vary with the drug used (Table 33-1), but the underlying principles of management are essentially the same.

Overdose refers to the toxic effects that occur when a drug is taken in a larger than normal dose.

Primary Assessment and Interventions

1. Assess the presence and adequacy of respirations.
2. Attain control of the airway, ventilation, and oxygenation.
3. Intubate and/or provide assisted ventilation in severe respiratory depressed patients or in patients lacking gag or cough reflexes. If possible, intubation should be held off until a trial dose of naloxone (Narcan) is given.
4. Begin external cardiac compression and ventilation in the absence of heartbeat.

Subsequent Assessment

1. Do a thorough physical examination to rule out insulin shock, meningitis, head injury, stroke, or trauma.
2. If the patient is unconscious, consider all possible causes of loss of consciousness.
3. Monitor level of consciousness continuously.
4. Monitor vital signs frequently—some drugs will cause depressed vital signs, others will elevate the vital signs.
5. Monitor the pupils—"extreme miosis" (pinpoint pupils) may indicate narcotic overdose.
6. Look for needle marks and external evidence of trauma.
7. Perform a rapid neurologic survey: level of responsiveness, pupil size and reactivity, reflexes, and focal neurologic findings.
8. Keep in mind that many drug abusers take multiple drugs simultaneously.
9. Be aware that there is a high incidence of human immunodeficiency virus and infectious hepatitis among drug users.
10. Examine the patient's breath for characteristic odor of alcohol, acetone, etc.
11. Try to obtain a history of the drug experiences (from the person accompanying the patient or from the patient).

TABLE 33-1 Specific Drug Overdose Presentations and Interventions

Type of Drug	Presentation	Interventions
CNS stimulants 　Amphetamines 　Designer drugs (MDA, Ecstasy, Ice, Eve) 　Cocaine (can be smoked in freebase or 　　crack form, snorted, or injected)	Palpitations, feeling of impending doom, tachycardia, hypertension, dysrhythmia, myocardial ischemia/infarction; euphoria, agitation, combativeness, confusion, hallucinations, paranoia, aggressive or violent behavior, suicide attempts, hyperpyrexia, seizures. When the drug wears off—depression, exhaustion, irritability, sleeplessness.	Secure airway, breathing, and circulation. Monitor ECG and provide oxygen for ishcemia. Sedate as necessary. Administer antiarrhythmics for ventricular dysrhythmia. Administer diazepam (Valium) for seizures. Closely monitor hemodynamic status and provide IV fluids as indicated.
Hallucinogens 　Lysergic acid 　　diethylamide (LSD) 　Phencyclidine HCl (PCP) 　Mescaline 　Psilocybin mushrooms 　Jimson weed seeds	Marked anxiety bordering on panic, confusion, incoherence, hyperactivity, hallucinations, hazardous behavior, convulsions, coma, circulatory collapse, death. Flashbacks may occur months to years after initial drug use.	Try to talk the patient down by understanding what patient is going through, reducing fears, and establishing contact with reality. Reduce sensory stimuli, encourage patient to keep eyes open, and stay with patient. Monitor for hypertensive crisis and evidence of trauma. Sedate if hyperactivity cannot be controlled, and place patient in a protected environment.
Narcotics 　Heroin (may be cut with other 　　ingredients in 20:1 to 200:1 ratio) 　Morphine and its derivatives 　Codeine and its derivatives	Hypotension, respiratory depression leading to apnea, miosis, drowsiness progressing to stupor and coma.	Administer naloxone (Narcan) 0.4 to 2 mg IV or by endotracheal tube (effective in 1–2 minutes). Maintain an open airway but defer intubation until naloxone given, if possible. Monitor for reappearance of symptoms and readminister naloxone or provide continuous infusion, as necessary. Protect the patient from harm (may be combative on awakening).
Sedatives 　Barbiturates such as amobarbital 　　(Amytal) and secobarbital (Seconal) 　Benzodiazepines such as diazepam 　　(Valium) and flurazepam (Dalmane) 　Other sedative/hypnotics such as 　　chloral hydrate (Noctec) and 　　glutethimide (Doriden)	Incoordinations, ataxia, impaired thinking and speech, lethargy to coma, early miosis; later, fixed and dilated pupils, hypoventilation, hypotension, hypothermia, decreased reflexes.	Administer flumazenil (Romazicon) to reverse or diminish effects of benzodiazepines. Administer activated charcoal. Protect the airway. For hypotension, infuse with Ringer's lactate and give vasopressors.
Alcohol 　Intoxication generally occurs with 　　blood levels greater than 100 mg/dL. 　　Levels over 400 mg/dL are due to 　　rapid consumption of alcohol and 　　represent a medical emergency.	Slurred speech, incoordination, ataxia, belligerent behavior ranging to stupor and coma; odor of alcohol on breath and clothing; respiratory depression.	Protect the airway. Closely monitor for CNS and respiratory depression. Draw blood for ethanol concentration, electrolytes, glucose, and drug screen using nonalcohol skin cleanser. Assess for head injury and other trauma and organic disease. Administer IV fluids, magnesium sulfate (to reduce risk of seizures), thiamine (to prevent Wernicke-Korsakoff syndrome), and glucose (to treat hypoglycemia).

CNS: central nervous system; ECG; electrocardiogram.

General Interventions

1. Goals:
   a. Support the respiratory and cardiovascular functions.
   b. Give definitive treatment for drug overdose.
   c. Prevent further absorption, enhance drug elimination, and reduce its toxicity.
2. Measure arterial blood gases for hypoxia due to hypoventilation or for acid–base derangements.
3. Continuously monitor ECG.
4. Draw blood samples for testing glucose, electrolytes, blood urea nitrogen, creatinine, and appropriate toxicologic screen.
5. Initiate IV fluids.
6. Administer oxygen.
7. Pharmacologic interventions:
   a. Give specific drug antagonist if drug is known.
   b. Naloxone hydrochloride (Narcan) for central nervous system depression.
   c. Dextrose 50% IV to rule out hypoglycemic coma.
8. If the drug was taken by mouth, the primary method for preventing or minimizing absorption is to administer activated charcoal with a cathartic to hasten excretion. Mix activated charcoal with water to make a slurry. Follow with a cathartic. Multiple doses may be administered.
9. Vomiting may be induced if the patient is seen *early* after ingestion; save vomitus for toxicologic study.
10. Use gastric lavage if the patient is unconscious or if there is no way to determine when the drug was ingested; save gastric aspirate. In patients lacking gag or cough reflexes, perform this procedure only after intubation with cuffed endotracheal tube to prevent aspiration of stomach contents.
11. Take rectal temperature—extremes of thermoregulation (hyperthermia/hypothermia) must be recognized and treated.
12. Treat seizures with diazepam (Valium).
13. Assist with hemodialysis/peritoneal dialysis for potentially lethal poisoning.
14. Catheterize the patient, because the drug or metabolites are excreted by the urine.
15. Do not leave the patient alone, because there is a potential for the patient to harm self or emergency department staff.
16. Anticipate complications—sudden death from cerebral hypoxia, dysrhythmias, seizures, respiratory arrest, myocardial infarction.
17. Always suspect mixtures of medications and alcohol.

◆ ALCOHOL WITHDRAWAL DELIRIUM

Alcohol withdrawal delirium (delirium tremens, or alcoholic hallucinosis) is an acute toxic state that follows a prolonged bout of steady drinking or sudden withdrawal from prolonged intake of alcohol. It may be precipitated by acute injury or infection. Symptoms can begin as early as 4 hours after a reduction of alcohol intake and usually peak at 24 to 48 hours, but may last up to 2 weeks.

NURSING ALERT: ❖
Alcohol withdrawal delirium is a serious complication and is life threatening.

Primary Assessment and Interventions

1. Patient will present alert, unless experiencing a seizure.
2. If the patient is having a seizure, ensure the airway.

Subsequent Assessment

1. Assess for major symptoms—may occur independently or in combination.
   a. "Shakes"
   b. Seizures
   c. Hallucinations
2. Obtain drinking history, including the severity of past withdrawal episodes and any recent drug intake. Be aware that alcoholics tend to underestimate drinking habits.
3. Assess complaints of nausea and vomiting, malaise, weakness, anxiety, or fear.
4. Perform thorough examination for signs of autonomic hyperreactivity—tachycardia, diaphoresis, elevated temperature, dilated but reactive pupils—as well as any coexisting illnesses or injuries (head injury, pneumonia, metabolic disturbances).
5. Observe behavior for talkativeness, restlessness, agitation, or preoccupation.

General Interventions

1. Protect the patient from injury. The hallucinations may be visual, tactile, or auditory and are frequently of a frightening nature.
2. Take a breath analyzer reading—indicates where patient is in the withdrawal process.
3. Using a nonalcohol swab, draw blood for measurement of ethanol concentration, toxicologic screen for other drugs of abuse, and other tests as directed.
4. Pharmacologic interventions:
   a. Diazepam (Valium) or chlordiazepoxide (Librium) for sedation. Sedate the patient with sufficient dosage of medication to produce adequate relaxation and to reduce agitation, prevent exhaustion, and promote sleep.
   b. Diazepam (Valium) or phenytoin (Dilantin) for seizure control.
5. Monitor vital signs every 30 minutes.
6. Place the patient in a private room where close observation can take place.
7. Maintain electrolyte balance and hydration through oral or IV route—fluid losses may be extreme because of profuse perspiration, vomiting, and agitation.
8. Assess respiratory, hepatic, and cardiovascular status of patient—pneumonia, liver disease, and cardiac failure are complications.
9. Observe for hypoglycemia and treat appropriately. Hypoglycemia may accompany alcoholic withdrawal because alcohol depletes liver glycogen stores and impairs gluconeogenesis; many patients also suffer from malnutrition.
   a. Administer thiamine followed by parenteral dextrose if liver glycogen is depleted.

b. Give orange juice, Gatorade, or other carbohydrates to stabilize blood sugar and to counteract tremulousness.

Behavioral Emergencies

A *behavioral emergency* is an urgent, serious disturbance of behavior, affect, or thought that makes the patient unable to cope with his or her life situation and interpersonal relationships.

A patient presenting with a psychiatric emergency may be overactive or violent, depressed, or suicidal.

◆ VIOLENT PATIENTS

Violent and aggressive behavior is usually episodic and is a means of expressing feelings of anger, fear, or hopelessness about a situation.

Assessment

1. Assess for overactivity, aggression, or anger out of proportion to the circumstances.
2. Determine risk factors for violence, including:
   a. Intoxicated with drugs/alcohol.
   b. Going through drug or alcohol withdrawal.
   c. Acute paranoid schizophrenic states, acute organic brain syndrome, acute psychosis, paranoia, or borderline personality.

General Interventions

1. Goals are to bring violence under control and protect patient and staff from harm.
2. Establish control.
   a. Keep the door of the room open, and be in clear view of the staff.
   b. Help the patient bring violence under control.
      (1) Give the patient space. Do not make any sudden movement.
      (2) Avoid touching an agitated patient or standing too close.
      (3) Ask if he or she has a weapon. Request that it be placed in a neutral area.
      (4) If the patient will not surrender weapon, leave the room and allow security personnel/police to handle the situation.
   c. Try not to leave the patient alone—this may be interpreted as rejection or the patient may try to harm self.
   d. Adopt a calm, nonconfrontational approach and remain in control of the situation—external calm and structure may help the patient gain control.
3. Provide emotional support.
   a. Talk and listen to the patient.
   b. Crisis intervention is best done with an attitude of interest in the patient's well-being and with an attempt to "tune in" to the patient while remaining firm.

c. Acknowledge the patient's state of agitation, for example, "I want to work with you to relieve your distress."
   d. Give the patient the opportunity to ventilate anger verbally; avoid challenging the delusional state.
   e. Try to hear what the patient is saying.
   f. Convey the expectation of appropriate behavior and make the patient aware that help is available for him or her to gain control.
   g. Administer prescribed tranquilizer to reduce anxiety and hyperactivity, if verbal management techniques fail to attenuate the patient's tension.
4. Secure assistance.
   a. Allow security personnel/police to intervene if patient does not become calm.
   b. Use restraints when absolutely necessary but with minimal force.
   c. Have a specific plan and enough well-trained personnel available when applying restraints; if patient is intoxicated, restrain in a left lateral position and monitor closely for aspiration.
   d. Talk reassuringly while applying restraints; use empathetic and supportive verbal interactions.
   e. Monitor patient continuously after restraints are applied; check circulation of restrained extremities.

◆ DEPRESSION

Depression may be seen as the presenting condition at the health care facility or may be masked by the presentation of anxiety and somatic complaints.

Assessment

1. Observe for sadness, apathy, feelings of worthlessness, self-blame, suicidal thoughts, desire to escape, worsening of mood in morning, anorexia, weight loss, sleeplessness, lessening interest in sex, reduction of activity or ceaseless activity.
2. The agitated, depressed individual may exhibit motor restlessness and severe anxiety.

General Interventions

1. Listen to the patient in a calm, unhurried manner.
2. The patient will benefit from ventilation of feelings.
3. Give the patient an opportunity to talk about problems.
4. Anticipate that the patient may be suicidal.
5. Attempt to find out if the patient has thought about or attempted suicide.
   a. "Have you ever thought about taking your own life?"
   b. The patient is generally relieved because of the opportunity to discuss feelings.
6. Find out if there is an illness, perceived or real.
7. Assess whether there has been sudden worsening of depression.
8. Notify relatives about a seriously depressed patient. Do not leave the patient alone, because suicide is usually an act committed in solitude.
9. Give antidepressant and antianxiety agents as prescribed.
10. Point out to the patient that depression is treatable.

11. Be aware of crisis and supportive services in the community: telephone counseling and referral, suicide prevention centers, group therapy, marital and family counseling, drug/alcohol counseling, adolescent counseling, or befriending programs.
12. Refer for psychiatric consultation or to psychiatric unit.

◆ SUICIDE IDEATION

Suicide is the eighth leading cause of death in the United States and the second lethal killer of young people.

Assessment

1. Assess for risk factors:
   a. Associated psychiatric illness (affective disorders and substance abuse in adults; conduct disorders and depression in young people).
   b. Personality traits such as aggression, impulsivity, depression, hopelessness, borderline personality disorder, or antisocial personality.
   c. Persons who have experienced early loss, decreased social support, chronic illness, or recent divorce.
   d. Genetic and familial factors: family history of suicide, certain psychiatric disorders or alcoholism; alcohol and substance abuse.
2. Determine whether patient has communicated *suicidal intent*, such as preoccupation with death or talking of someone else's suicide.
3. Determine whether patient has ever attempted suicide—the risk is much greater in these persons.
4. Determine if there is a specific plan for suicide and a means to carry out the plan.

General Interventions

1. Use crisis intervention (a form of brief psychotherapy) to determine suicide potential, discover areas of depression and conflict, find out about the patient's support system, and determine whether hospitalization, psychiatric referral, etc. is warranted.
2. Treat the consequences of the suicide attempt (eg, gunshot wound, drug overdose).
3. Prevent further self-injury—a patient who has made a suicide gesture may do so again.
4. Admit to intensive care unit (if condition warrants), arrange follow-up care, or admit to psychiatric unit, depending on assessment of suicide potential.

Alleged Sexual Assault

◆ RAPE

Rape is defined as unlawful carnal knowledge of a female forcibly and against her will. Carnal knowledge is defined as penetration of genitalia, no matter how slight, by the penis. Rape is also committed if intercourse occurs while the women is sleeping, unconscious, or under the influence of alcohol or drugs. A male who is sexually assaulted is sodomized. Sodomy is oral or anal penetration.

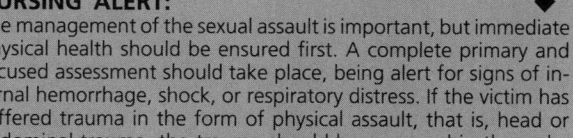

NURSING ALERT:
The management of the sexual assault is important, but immediate physical health should be ensured first. A complete primary and focused assessment should take place, being alert for signs of internal hemorrhage, shock, or respiratory distress. If the victim has suffered trauma in the form of physical assault, that is, head or abdominal trauma, the trauma should be managed in the order of established priorities.

Assessment

A. Initiating a Supportive Relationship
1. The manner in which the patient is received and treated in the emergency department is important to the future psychological well-being of the patient.
   a. Call the rape-crisis intervention counselor (if available), who will meet the patient/family in the emergency department.
   b. Do not leave patient alone. Accept the emotional reactions of the patient (hysteria, stoicism, overwhelmed feeling, etc.)
2. Emotional trauma may be present for weeks, months, or years. Patient's reaction to rape has been called the "rape trauma syndrome." Patients may go through phases of psychological reactions:
   a. Acute phase (disorganization)—shock, disbelief, fear, anxiety, guilt, humiliation, suppression of feelings—may last for months to years.
   b. Phase of denial and unwillingness to talk about incident, followed by phase of heightened anxiety, fear, flashbacks, sleep disturbances, hyperalertness, and psychosomatic reactions.
   c. Phase of reorganization—putting incident into perspective.

B. Interviewing the Patient
1. Consent should be obtained for the examination, the collecting of cultures/evidence, and for release of information to law enforcement agencies.

NURSING ALERT:
Most emergency departments have commercially prepared rape evidence collection kits as well as written protocols for treatment of injuries, legal documentation, and sexually transmitted disease and pregnancy prevention.

2. Record history of event in the patient's own words.
3. Ask if the patient has bathed, douched, gargled or brushed teeth, changed clothes, or urinated or defecated since attack—may alter interpretation of subsequent findings.
4. Record time of admission, time of examination, date and time of alleged sexual assault, and the general appearance of the patient.
   a. Document any evidence of trauma—discoloration, bruises, lacerations, secretions, torn and bloody clothing.
   b. Record emotional state.

Interventions

A. Preparing for Physical Examination
1. Assist the patient to undress over a sheet/large piece of paper to obtain debris.

2. Place each item of clothing in a separate paper bag (plastic bags promote moisture retention, which may lead to formation of mold and mildew, which can destroy evidence).
3. Label bags appropriately; give to appropriate law enforcement authority.
4. Advise the patient of the nature and necessity of each procedure; give the rationale for each question asked.

B. Physical Examination
1. Examine the patient (from head to toe) for injuries, especially to the head, neck, breasts, thighs, back, and buttocks.
2. Assess for external evidence of trauma (bruises, contusions, lacerations, stab wounds).
3. Assess for dried semen stains (appearing as crusted, flaking areas) on the patient's body.
4. Inspect fingers for broken nails and tissue and foreign materials under nails.
5. Assist in conducting oral examination to determine secretion status of patient compared with that of assailant.
   a. Obtain a saliva specimen.
   b. Take prescribed cultures of gum and tooth areas.
6. Document evidence of trauma with body diagrams or photographs.

C. Pelvic and Rectal Examinations
1. Examine perineum and thighs with an ultraviolet light (Wood's lamp); areas that are found to fluoresce may indicate semen stains. Urine and other stains may also fluoresce.
2. Note color and consistency of any discharge present.
3. Use water-moistened vaginal speculum for examination; do not use lubricant (contains chemicals that may interfere with later forensic testing of specimens and acid phosphatase determinations).

D. Obtaining Laboratory Specimens
1. Collect vaginal aspirate, which is examined for presence or absence of motile/nonmotile sperm.
2. Use sterile swab to draw from vaginal pool for acid phosphatase, blood group antigen of semen, and precipitin test against human sperm and blood.
3. Obtain separate smears from the oral, vaginal, and anal areas.
4. Obtain swabs of body orifices for gonorrhea and chlamydia testing (to determine preexisting infection or new infection if patient is not presenting immediately).
5. Trim areas of pubic hair suspected of containing semen; obtain several pubic hairs with follicles; place in separate containers and identify these as patient's pubic hairs.
6. Obtain blood serum for syphilis; a sample of serum may be frozen and saved for future testing.
7. Collect foreign material (leaves, grass, dirt) and place in appropriate container.
8. Examine rectum for signs of trauma, blood, and semen stains.
9. Conduct a pregnancy test if there is possibility that patient is pregnant.

10. Label all specimens with name of patient, date, time of collection, body area from which specimen was obtained, and names of personnel collecting specimens to preserve chain of evidence; give to designated person (crime laboratory, etc.) and obtain an itemized receipt.
11. Photographs are taken by designated person.

E. Other Interventions
1. Treat physical trauma as with any patient.
2. Protect patient against sexually transmitted diseases.
   a. Specimens obtained for sexually transmitted diseases, including gonorrhea, cannot be immediately obtained (positive cultures taken in the immediate postrape period will only reflect existing disease).
   b. In addition, follow-up visits cannot be ensured, so some health care providers may treat the patient as if they have been exposed to a known case of gonorrhea or chlamydia.
   c. Antibiotic choices include single-dose, 7-day injectable or oral treatment of the following:
      (1) Cephalosporins, such as ceftriaxone (Rocephin) or cefoxitin (Mefoxin).
      (2) Tetracyclines such as doxycycline (Vibramycin)
      (3) Quinolones such as ciprofloxacin (Cipro) or ofloxacin (Floxin)
      (4) Erythromycins or macrolides such as azithromycin (Zithromax).
3. Protect patient against pregnancy.
   a. It is important to determine whether pregnancy existed before the attack.
   b. Negative pregnancy test should be obtained before administering postcoital therapy.
   c. Hormonal treatment to prevent pregnancy—"morning after pill."
      (1) Oral norgestrel (Nordette) or estradiol (Ovral).
      (2) Oral diethylstilbestrol (Stilphostrol).
      (3) Conjugate estrogen (Premarin) oral or IV.
4. Allay fear of acquired immunodeficiency syndrome.
   a. It is important to determine the existence of the human immunodeficiency virus before initiating therapy. An informed consent is obtained and the patient is tested for human immunodeficiency virus (HIV) exposure.
   b. Prophylactic treatment with zidovudine (azidothymidine [AZT]) may be considered.
5. Possible prophylactic scabies treatment.
6. Provide the patient with cleansing facilities, including a cleansing douche, shower, and mouthwash.

F. Providing for Follow-up Services
1. Make an appointment for follow-up surveillance for pregnancy and sexually transmitted disease.
2. Inform the patient of counseling services to prevent long-term psychological effects; counseling services should be made available to the family.
3. Encourage the patient to return to previous level of functioning as soon as possible.
4. The patient should be accompanied by a family member or friend when leaving the health care facility.

Selected References

Alspach, J. G. (Ed.). (1991). *Core curriculum for critical care.* (4th ed.). Philadelphia: W.B. Saunders.

Caroline, N. L. (1991). *Emergency care in the streets.* Boston: Little, Brown.

Emergency Cardiac Care Committee and Subcommittees, American Heart Association. (1992). Guidelines for cardiopulmonary resuscitation and emergency cardiac care. *Journal of the American Medical Association, 268*(16), 2172-2198.

Emergency Nurses Association. (1992). *Emergency nursing core curriculum* (4th ed.). Philadelphia: W.B. Saunders.

Hopkins, A. G. (1994). The trauma nurse's role with families in crisis. *Critical Care Nurse, 14*(2), 35-43.

Kitt, S., & Kaiser, J. (Eds.). (1990). *Emergency nursing: A physiologic and clinical perspective.* Philadelphia: W.B. Saunders.

Malestic, S. L. (1995). Fight violence with forensic evidence. *RN, 58*(1), 30–32.

Molitor, L. (1992). *Emergency department triage handbook.* Gaithersburg, MD: Aspen.

Nettina, S. M., & Drake, D. K. (1994). Recognition and management of heat-related illness. *Nurse Practitioner, 19*(8): 43–47.

Parker, V. F. (1995). Battered. *RN, 58*(1), 26–29.

Rosen, P., & Barkin, R. M. (Eds.). (1992). *Emergency medicine concepts and clinical practice* (3rd ed.). Philadelphia: C.V. Mosby.

Weinman, S. A. (1993). Emergency management of drug overdose. *Critical Care Nurse, 13*(6), 45-51.

Wright, J. E., & Shelton, B. K. (Eds.). (1993). *Desk reference for critical care nursing.* Boston: Jones and Barlett.

PART III ◆

Maternity and Neonatal Nursing

CHAPTER 34 ◆

Maternal and Fetal Health

Introduction to Maternity Nursing

Providing care to childbearing families is aimed at the ideal of having every pregnancy result in a healthy mother, baby, and family unit. The nurse today faces many evolving and challenging issues in achieving this goal. Such advances as in vitro fertilization and embryo freezing have afforded individuals opportunities once never thought possible. There are an increasing number of high-risk pregnancies resulting from such factors as drug abuse, acquired immunodeficiency syndrome, late or no prenatal care, teenage pregnancies, and pregnancies to women older than 35 years. Technologic advances in high-risk obstetric units, fetal monitoring, sonography, and neonatal intensive care units are now providing the means to improve maternal health and save fetuses and infants who would not have survived years ago.

Regionalization of obstetric services is being implemented so that childbearing families have access to the technologic advances and skilled personnel capable of managing pregnancy or neonatal complications. Childbearing families are also being offered alternate types of care in birthing centers, birthing rooms in hospitals, home deliveries, alternate methods used during delivery, and changes in hospital policies, such as having children and others present during labor and delivery.

Economic changes in the health care climate are also affecting the practice of nursing as cost containment considerations have shortened the hospital length of stay. Some hospitals have adopted a practice of 24-hour discharge after delivery coordinated with home health care follow-up.

This combination of advancing technology, pregnancy risk factors, and changing economics challenges the nurse to be a highly skilled clinician and outstanding communicator.

◆ TERMINOLOGY USED IN MATERNITY NURSING

Gestation—pregnancy or maternal condition of having a developing fetus in the body.
Embryo—developing organism during first 8 weeks.
Fetus—human conceptus from 8 weeks until delivery.
Viability—capability of living, usually accepted as 24 weeks, although survival is rare.
Gravida—a woman who is or has been pregnant, regardless of pregnancy outcome.

Nulligravida—a woman who is not now and never has been pregnant.
Primigravida—a woman pregnant for the first time.
Multigravida—a woman who has been pregnant more than once.
Para—refers to past pregnancies that have reached viability.
Nullipara—a woman who has never completed a pregnancy to the period of viability. The woman may or may not have experienced an abortion.
Primipara—refers to a woman who had completed one pregnancy to the period of viability regardless of the number of infants delivered and regardless of the infant being live or stillborn.
Multipara—refers to a woman who has completed two or more pregnancies to the stage of viability.

A woman pregnant for the first time is a primigravida and is described as Gravida 1 Para 0. A woman who delivered one fetus to the period of viability and who is pregnant again is described as Gravida 2, Para 1. A woman with two abortions and no viable children is Gravida 2, Para 0.

◆ OBSTETRIC HISTORY

In some obstetric services, a woman's obstetric history is summarized by a series of four digits, such as 5-0-2-5. These digits correspond with the abbreviation F/TPAL.

F/T represents full-term deliveries, 38 or more weeks.
P represents preterm deliveries, 20 to 37 weeks.
A represents abortions, elective or spontaneous loss of a pregnancy before the period of viability.
L represents the number of children living. If a child has died, further explanation is needed for clarification.

If, for example, a particular woman's history is summarized as Gravida 7, Para 5, 5-0-2-5, then she has been pregnant seven times, delivered five times past the age of viability, had five term deliveries, zero preterm deliveries, two abortions, and five living children.

The Expectant Mother

◆ MANIFESTATIONS OF PREGNANCY

Pregnancy may be determined by cessation of menses, enlarged uterus, and a positive result on a pregnancy test. These and the many other manifestations of pregnancy are classified into three groups: presumptive, probable, and positive.

Presumptive Signs and Symptoms

1. Cessation of menses—pregnancy is suspected if more than 10 days have elapsed since the time of the expected onset. Suggestive of pregnancy in a woman with a previously spontaneous, cyclic, and predictable menses.
2. Breast changes.
   a. Breasts enlarge and become tender. Veins in breasts become increasingly visible.
   b. Nipples become larger and more pigmented.
   c. Colostrum, a thin, milky fluid, may be expressed in the second half of pregnancy.
   d. Montgomery's glands, small elevations on the areolae, may appear.
3. Abdominal striae (*striae gravidarum*)—sometimes appear on the breasts, abdomen, and thighs because of the stretching, rupture, and atrophy of the deep connective tissue of the skin.
4. Nausea and vomiting (morning sickness)—occurs mainly in the morning, but may occur at any time of the day, lasting a few hours. Usually disappears spontaneously near the end of the first trimester.
5. *Quickening* (sensations of fetal movement in the abdomen)—occurs between the 16th and 20th week after the onset of the last menses.
6. Frequency of urination.
   a. Caused by pressure of the expanding uterus on the bladder.
   b. Decreases when the uterus rises out of the pelvis.
   c. Reappears when the fetal head engages in the pelvis at the end of pregnancy.
7. Fatigue—characteristic of early pregnancy.

Probable Signs and Symptoms

1. Enlargement of abdomen—at about 12 weeks' gestation, the uterus can be felt through the abdominal wall, just above the symphysis.
2. Changes in shape, size, and consistency of the uterus.
   a. Uterus enlarges, elongates, and decreases in thickness as pregnancy progresses.
   b. *Hegar's sign*—lower uterine segment softens 6 to 8 weeks after the onset of the last menstrual period.
3. Changes in cervix.
   a. *Chadwick's sign*—bluish or purplish discoloration of cervix and vaginal wall.
   b. *Goodell's sign*—softening of the cervix, may occur as early as 4 weeks.
   c. With inflammation and carcinoma during pregnancy, the cervix may remain firm.
4. Intermittent contractions of the uterus (*Braxton Hicks contractions*)—painless, palpable contractions occurring at irregular intervals, more frequently felt after 28 weeks. They usually disappear with walking or exercise.
5. *Ballottement*—a sinking and rebounding of the fetus in its surrounding amniotic fluid in response to a sudden tap on the uterus (occurs near midpregnancy).
6. Changes in levels of human chorionic gonadotropin in maternal plasma and urine.
7. Leukorrhea—increase in vaginal discharge.

Positive Signs and Symptoms

1. Fetal heart tones (FHTs)—usually heard between 16th and 20th week of gestation with a fetoscope.
2. Fetal movements felt by the examiner (after about 20 weeks' gestation).
3. Outlining of the fetal body through the maternal abdomen in the second half of pregnancy.
4. Sonographic evidence (after 8 weeks' gestation).

◆ MATERNAL PHYSIOLOGY DURING PREGNANCY

Duration of Pregnancy

1. Averages 280 days or 40 weeks from the 1st day of the last normal menstrual period.
2. Duration may also be divided into three equal parts, or trimesters, of slightly more than 13 weeks or 3 calendar months each.
3. *Estimated date of confinement* is calculated by adding 7 days to the date of the 1st day of the last menstrual period and counting back 3 months (*Nägele's rule*).
   a. For example, if a woman's last menstrual period began on September 10, 1991, her estimated date of confinement would be September 10, 1991, plus 7 days = September 17, 1991, minus 3 months = June 17, 1991.

Changes in Reproductive Tract

A. **Uterus**
   1. Enlargement during pregnancy involves stretching and marked hypertrophy of existing muscle cells.
   2. In addition to an increase in the size of the uterine muscle cells, there is an increase in fibrous tissue, elastic tissue, blood vessels, and lymphatics.
   3. Enlargement and thickening of the uterine wall is most marked in the fundus.
   4. By the end of the 3rd month (12 weeks), the uterus is too large to be contained wholly within the pelvic cavity—it can now be palpated suprapubically.
   5. As the uterus rises out of the pelvis, it rotates somewhat to the right because of the presence of the rectosigmoid on the left side of the pelvis.
   6. By 20 weeks' gestation, the fundus has reached the level of the umbilicus.
   7. By 36 weeks, the fundus has reached the xiphoid.
   8. During the last 3 weeks, the uterus descends slightly—because of fetal descent into pelvis. Walls of uterus become thinner.
   9. Changes in contractility occur—from the first trimester, irregular painless contractions occur (Braxton Hicks contractions). In latter weeks of pregnancy, these contractions become stronger and more regular.
   10. There is a progressive increase in uteroplacental blood flow during pregnancy.

B. **Cervix**
   1. Pronounced softening and cyanosis—due to increased vascularity, edema, hypertrophy, and hyperplasia of the cervical glands.
   2. Clot of very thick mucus obstructs the cervical canal (cervical plug).

3. Erosions of cervix, common during pregnancy, represent an extension of proliferating endocervical glands and columnar endocervical epithelium.

C. Ovaries
1. Ovulation ceases during pregnancy; maturation of new follicles is suspended.
2. One corpus luteum functions during early pregnancy (first 8 weeks), producing mainly progesterone.

D. Vagina and Outlet
1. Increased vascularity, hyperemia, and softening of connective tissue in skin and muscles of perineum and vulva.
2. Chadwick's sign noted—characteristic violet color due to increased vascularity and hyperemia.
3. Vaginal walls prepare for labor: mucosa increases in thickness, connective tissue loosens, and small-muscle cells hypertrophy.
4. Vaginal secretions increase; pH is 3.5 to 6—because of increased production of lactic acid from glycogen in the vaginal epithelium by *Lactobacillus acidophilus*. (Acid pH probably aids in keeping vagina relatively free of pathogenic bacteria.)

Changes in the Abdominal Wall

1. Striae gravidarum (stretch marks) may develop—reddish, slightly depressed streaks in the skin of abdomen, breast, and thighs (become glistening silvery lines after pregnancy).
2. *Linea nigra* may form—a line of dark pigment extending from the umbilicus down the midline to the symphysis. Often during the first pregnancy, the *linea nigra* occurs at the height of the uterus. During subsequent pregnancies, the entire line may be present early in gestation.
3. *Diastasis recti* may occur as muscles (rectus) separate. If severe, a part of the anterior uterine wall may be covered only by a layer of skin, fascia, and peritoneum.

Breast Changes

1. Tenderness and tingling occur in early weeks of pregnancy.
2. Increase in size by 2nd month—hypertrophy of mammary alveoli.
3. Nipples become larger, more deeply pigmented, and more erectile early in pregnancy.
4. Colostrum may be expressed by second trimester.
5. Areolae become broader and more deeply pigmented. The depth of pigmentation varies with the individual's complexion.
6. Scattered through the areola are a number of small elevations (glands of Montgomery), which are hypertrophic sebaceous glands.

Metabolic Changes

Numerous and intensive changes occur in response to rapidly growing fetus and placenta.

A. Weight Gain Averages
11.5 to 16 kg (25 to 35 lb)

Area	Kg	Lb
Fetus	3.2–3.4	7.0–7.5
Placenta	0.5–0.7	1.0–1.5
Amniotic fluid	0.9	2.0
Uterus	1.1	2.5
Breast tissue	0.7–1.4	1.5–3.0
Blood volume	1.6–2.3	3.5–5.0
Maternal stores	1.8–4.3	4.0–9.5

B. Water Metabolism
1. The average woman retains 6 to 8 L of extra water during the pregnancy.
2. Approximately 4 to 6 L of fluid cross into the extracellular spaces. This creates a physiologic increase in blood volume.
3. Many pregnant women experience edema of the legs and ankles at the end of the day. This is most common in the third trimester.

C. Protein Metabolism
1. Fetus, uterus, and maternal blood are rich in protein rather than in fat or carbohydrates.
2. At term, fetus and placenta contain 500 g of protein or approximately half of the total protein increase of pregnancy.
3. Approximately 500 g more of protein are added to the uterus, breasts, and maternal blood in the form of hemoglobin and plasma proteins.

D. Carbohydrate Metabolism
1. Pregnancy can initiate diabetes.
2. Diabetes mellitus may be aggravated by pregnancy.
3. Clinical diabetes appears in some women only during pregnancy.
4. During pregnancy, there is a "sparing" of glucose used by maternal tissues and a shunting of glucose to the placenta for use by the fetus.
5. Human placental lactogen (placental hormone) promotes lipolysis, increases plasma free fatty acids, and thereby provides alternative fuel sources for the mother.
6. Human placental lactogen, estrogen, progesterone, and an insulinase produced by the placenta oppose the action of insulin during pregnancy.

E. Fat Metabolism
1. Total circulating red blood cells increase about 40% to 50% during pregnancy; therefore, iron requirements are increased to 20 to 40 mg daily. This often exceeds dietary intake.
2. Supplemental iron is valuable during pregnancy and for several weeks after pregnancy or lactation.
3. During the last half of pregnancy, iron is transferred to fetus and stored in the fetal liver. This store lasts 3 to 6 months.

Changes in Cardiovascular System

A. Heart
1. Diaphragm is progressively elevated during pregnancy; heart is displaced to the left and upward, with the apex moved laterally.

2. Heart sounds—an exaggerated splitting of the first heart sound, a loud, easily heard third sound.
3. Heart murmurs—systolic murmurs are common and usually disappear after delivery.

B. Circulation
1. Cardiac volume increases by 40% to 50% from the beginning to the end of pregnancy, causing slight hypertrophy of the heart and increased cardiac output.
2. In the supine position, the large uterus compresses the venous return from the lower half of the body to the heart. This may cause arterial hypotension, referred to as the *supine hypotensive syndrome*. Cardiac output increases when the woman turns from her back to her left side.
3. Femoral venous pressure increases—because of retardation of blood flow from lower extremities as a result of pressure of enlarged uterus on pelvic veins and inferior vena cava.
4. Pulse rate usually increases 10 to 15 beats/minute during pregnancy.
5. Blood pressure—during the first half of pregnancy there is a slight decrease in systolic and diastolic blood pressure. During the last half of pregnancy, the blood pressure gradually returns to prepregnancy levels.
6. Increased cutaneous blood flow dissipates excess heat caused by increased metabolism of pregnancy.

C. Hematologic Changes
1. Total volume of circulating red blood cells increases; hemoglobin concentration at term averages 12 g/dL.
2. Leukocyte count is elevated to 25,000 or more during labor—cause unknown; probably represents the reappearance in the circulation of leukocytes previously shunted out of active circulation.
3. Blood coagulation—fibrinogen levels increase 50%. Other clotting factors that increase include factor VII (proconvertin), factor VIII (antihemophilic globulin), factor IX (plasma thromboplastin component), and factor X (Stuart factor). Factor II (prothrombin) increases slightly, whereas factors XI (plasma thromboplastin antecedent) and XIII (fibrin-stabilizing factor) decrease during pregnancy. There is no significant change in the number, appearance, or function of platelets.

Changes in Respiratory Tract

1. Hyperventilation occurs—increase in respiratory rate, tidal volume (45%), and minute volume (40%).
2. Increased total volume lowers blood PCO_2, causing mild respiratory alkalosis that is compensated for by lowering of the bicarbonate concentration.
3. Increased respiratory rate and reduced PCO_2 are probably induced by progesterone and estrogen to a lesser degree on the respiratory center.
4. Diaphragm is elevated during pregnancy—chiefly by the enlarging uterus.
5. Thoracic cage expands by means of flaring of the ribs—result of increased mobility of rib attachments.

Changes in Urinary Tract

1. Ureters become dilated and elongated during pregnancy because of mechanical pressure and perhaps the effects of progesterone. When the uterus rises out of the uterine cavity, it rests on the ureters, compressing them at the pelvic brim. Dilation is greater on the right side—left side is cushioned by the sigmoid colon.
2. Glomerular filtration rate increases early in pregnancy, and the increase persists almost to term. Renal plasma flow increases early in pregnancy and decreases to nonpregnant levels in the third trimester. These changes may be due to placental lactogen.
3. Glucosuria may be evident—because of the increase in glomerular filtration without increase in tubular resorptive capacity for filtered glucose.
4. Proteinuria does not occur normally, except for slight amounts during or just after vigorous labor.
5. Toward the end of pregnancy, pressure of the presenting part impedes drainage of blood and lymph from the bladder base, often leaving the area edematous, easily traumatized, and more susceptible to infection.

Changes in Gastrointestinal Tract

1. Gums may become hyperemic and softened and may bleed easily.
2. A localized vascular swelling of the gums may appear—called *epulis of pregnancy*.
3. Stomach and intestines are displaced upward and laterally by the enlarging uterus. Heartburn is common, caused by reflux of acid secretions in the lower esophagus.
4. Tone and motility of gastrointestinal tract decrease, leading to prolongation of gastric emptying due to large amount of progesterone produced by the placenta.
5. Hemorrhoids are common because of elevated pressure in veins below the level of the large uterus and constipation.
6. Distention of the gallbladder is common along with a decrease in emptying time and thickening of bile.
7. Liver function tests yield significantly different results during pregnancy.

Changes in Endocrine System

1. *Pituitary gland* enlarges slightly.
2. *Thyroid* is moderately enlarged because of hyperplasia of glandular tissue and increased vascularity.
   a. Basal metabolic rate increases progressively during normal pregnancy (as much as 25%)—because of metabolic activity of fetus.
   b. Level of protein-bound iodine and thyroxine rises sharply and is maintained until after delivery—because of increased circulatory estrogen.
3. *Adrenal* secretions considerably increased—amounts of aldosterone increase as early as 15th week.
4. *Pancreas*—Because of the fetal glucose needs for growth, there are alterations in maternal insulin production and usage.
   a. Estrogen, progesterone, cortisol, and human placental lactogen decrease maternal utilization of glucose.
   b. Cortisol also increases maternal insulin production.
   c. Insulinase, an enzyme produced by the placenta, deactivates maternal insulin.
   d. These changes result in an increased need for insulin, and the islets of Langerhans increase their production of insulin.

Changes in Integumentary System

1. Pigmentary changes occur because of melanocyte-stimulating hormone, the level of which is elevated from the 2nd month of pregnancy until term.
2. Striae gravidarum appear in later months of pregnancy as reddish, slightly depressed streaks in the skin of the abdomen and occasionally over the breasts and thighs.
3. A brownish black line of pigment is often formed in the midline of the abdominal skin—known as *linea nigra.*
4. Brownish patches of pigment may form on the face—known as *chloasma,* or "mask of pregnancy."
5. Angiomas (vascular spiders), minute red elevations commonly on the skin of the face, neck, upper chest, and arms, may develop.
6. Reddening of the palms (*palmar erythema*) may also occur.

Changes in Musculoskeletal System

1. The increasing mobility of sacroiliac, sacrococcygeal, and pelvic joints during pregnancy is a result of hormonal changes.
2. This mobility contributes to alteration of maternal posture and to back pain.
3. Late in pregnancy, aching, numbness, and weakness in the upper extremities may occur because of lordosis, which ultimately produces traction on the ulnar and median nerves.
4. Separation of the rectus muscles due to pressure of the growing uterus creates a diastasis recti. If this is severe, a portion of the anterior uterine wall is covered by only a layer of skin, fascia, and peritoneum.

Pelvis

A. Bones of the Pelvis
The pelvis is composed of four bones:

1. Two innominate bones (hip bones) form sides and front.
2. Sacrum and coccyx form the back.
   Pelvic bones are held together by fibrocartilage of the symphysis pubis and several ligaments.

B. Divisions of the Pelvis
1. False pelvis—lies above an imaginary line called the *linea terminalis* (Fig. 34-1). Function of the false pelvis is to support the enlarged uterus.
2. True pelvis lies below the pelvic brim or linea terminalis; it is the bony canal through which the infant must pass. It is divided into three parts: the inlet, the midpelvis, and the outlet.
   a. Inlet
      (1) Upper boundary of true pelvis—bounded by upper margin of symphysis pubis in front, linea terminalis on sides, and sacral promontory (1st sacral vertebra) in back.
      (2) Largest diameter of inlet is transverse (Fig. 34-2).
      (3) Smallest diameter of inlet is anteroposterior.
      (4) Anteroposterior diameter is most important diameter of inlet: measured clinically by *diagonal conjugate*—distance from lower margin of symphysis to the sacral promontory (usually 12.5 cm) (Fig. 34-3).
      (5) *Obstetric conjugate*—distance between inner surface of symphysis and sacral promontory measured by subtracting 1.5 to 2 cm (thickness of symphysis) from the diagonal conjugate. It is usually 11 cm.
   b. Midpelvis
      (1) Bounded by inlet above and outlet below—the true bony cavity.
      (2) Diameters cannot be measured clinically.
      (3) Clinical evaluation of adequacy is made by noting the ischial spines. Prominent spines that protrude into the cavity indicate a contracted midpelvic space.
   c. Outlet
      (1) Lowest boundary of the true pelvis.
      (2) Bounded by lower margin of symphysis in front, ischial tuberosities on sides, tip of sacrum posteriorly.
      (3) Most important diameter clinically is distance between the tuberosities (usually 9 cm).

C. Shapes of the Pelvis
There are four main types of pelvic shapes (Fig. 34-4).

1. Gynecoid (normal female pelvis)
2. Android

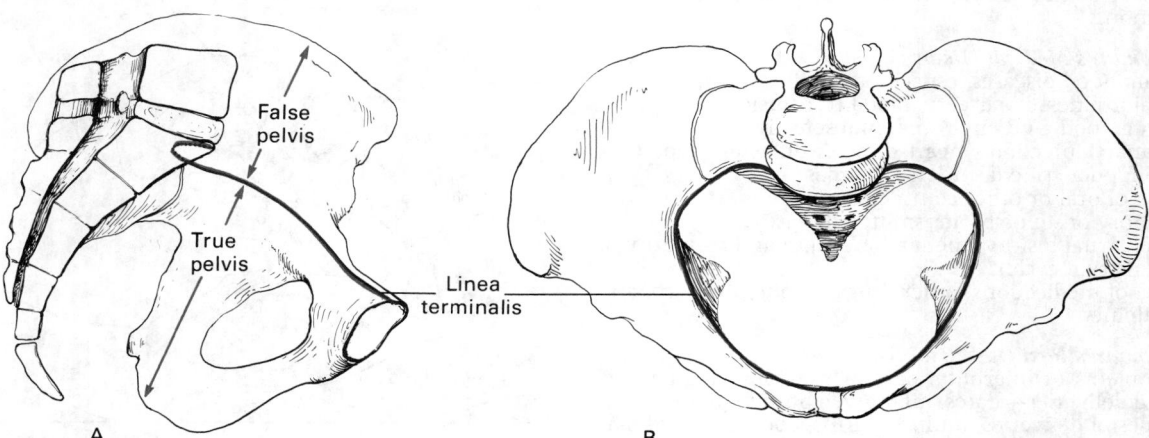

FIGURE 34-1 **(A)** Side view of the true and false pelvis. **(B)** Front view showing linea terminalis (pelvic brim).

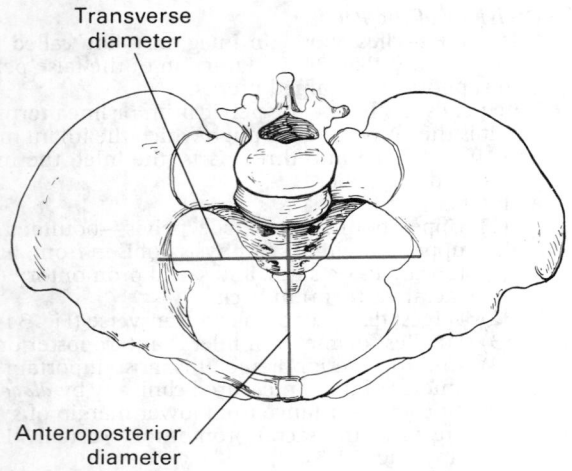

FIGURE 34-2 *Inlet of normal female pelvis showing transverse and anteroposterior diameters.*

3. Anthropoid
4. Platypelloid

◆ PRENATAL ASSESSMENT

Health History

A. Age
1. Adolescents have an increased incidence of anemia, pregnancy-induced hypertension, preterm labor, small-for-gestational-age infants, cephalopelvic disproportion, and dystocia.
2. Older women have an increased incidence of hypertension, pregnancies complicated by underlying medical problems, and infants with genetic abnormalities.

B. Family History
Congenital disorders, hereditary diseases, multiple pregnancies, diabetes, heart disease, hypertension, mental retardation.

C. Woman's Medical History
1. Childhood diseases, especially rubella.
2. Major illnesses, surgery, blood transfusions.
3. Drug, food, and environmental sensitivities.
4. Urinary infections, heart disease, diabetes, hypertension, endocrine disorders, anemias.
5. Use of oral or other contraceptives.
6. History of sexually transmitted diseases.
7. Menstrual history (menarche, length and regularity of menstrual cycle).
8. Use of medications, other drugs, alcohol, tobacco, and caffeine.

D. Woman's Past Obstetric History
1. Problems of infertility, date of previous pregnancies, and deliveries—dates, infant weights, length of labors, types of deliveries, multiple births, abortions, and maternal, fetal, and neonatal complications.
2. Woman's perception of past pregnancy, labor, and delivery for herself and effect on her family.

E. Woman's Present Obstetric History
1. Gravidity, parity.
2. Date of last menstrual period.
3. Estimated date of birth—expected date of confinement.
4. Signs and symptoms of pregnancy—amenorrhea, breast changes, nausea and vomiting, fetal movement, fatigue, urinary frequency, skin pigmentary changes. Expectations for her present pregnancy, labor, and delivery.
5. Rest and sleep patterns—length, quality, and regularity of rest and sleep.
6. Activity and employment—exercise patterns, type and hours of employment, plans for continued employment.
7. Sexual activity—sexual satisfaction, frequency and positions during intercourse, alternative practices used to achieve sexual satisfaction.
8. Diet history—weight gain, eating patterns (times and frequency of eating daily), social or cultural dietary habits, number of servings of food from five food groups (Table 34-1), and calories, protein, vitamins, and minerals consumed daily.
9. Psychosocial status—emotional changes she is experiencing, woman's and family's reactions to present pregnancy, support system—family's and friends' willingness to provide support, woman's present coping with lifestyle changes caused by the pregnancy.

Laboratory Data

A. Urinalysis
1. Urine is tested for glucose and protein.
2. Glucose may be present in small amounts because the glomerular filtration rate is increased without the same increase in kidney tubular reabsorption.
3. Protein in the urine should be reported because it may be a sign of a hypertensive disorder of pregnancy or renal problems.
4. If the urine is cloudy and bacteria or leukocytes are present, a urine culture is done.

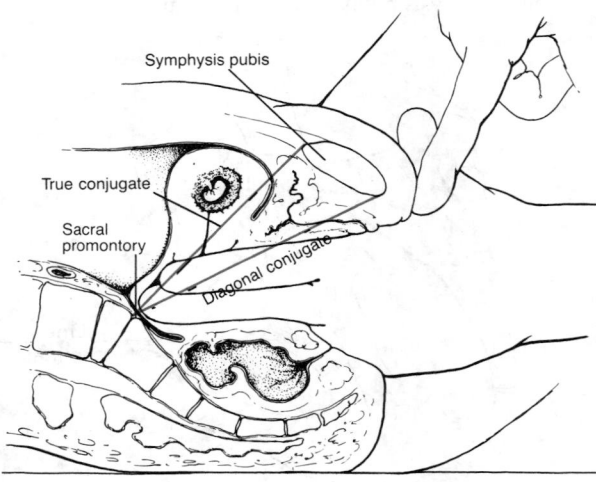

FIGURE 34-3 *Method of obtaining diagonal conjugate diameter.*

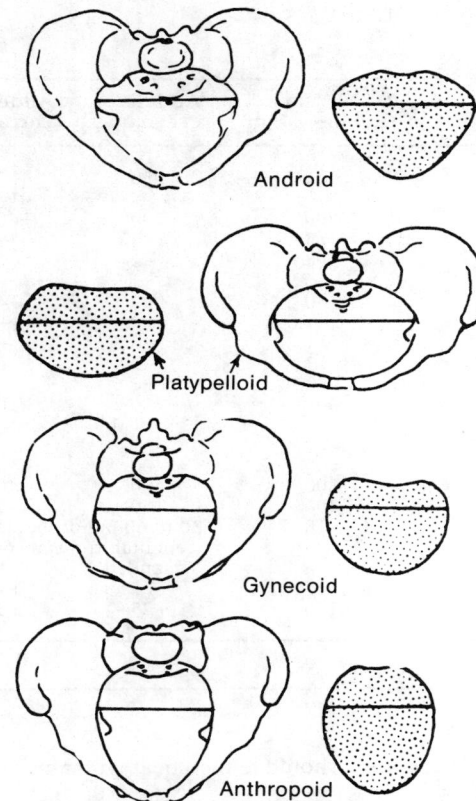

FIGURE 34-4 *The four types of female pelvis. Android—male-type pelvis. Platypelloid—broad pelvis with shortened anteroposterior diameter and flattened, oval, transverse shape. Gynecoid—typical female pelvis in which inlet is round instead of oval. Anthropoid—pelvis in which anteroposterior diameter is equal to or greater than the transverse diameter.*

B. Blood
1. Determination of hematocrit and hemoglobin levels and description of the morphology of the red blood cells are done to find evidence of anemias, such as sickle cell or Mediterranean anemia.
2. Hemoglobin levels average 12 g/dL.
3. Blood type, Rh factor, and antibody screen—if the woman is found to be Rh negative or to have a positive antibody screen, her partner is screened and a maternal antibody titer is drawn as indicated.
   a. Coombs, test—retested at 28 weeks in the Rh negative woman for detection of antibodies.
   b. Rh$_o$(D) immune globulin (RhoGAM) given at 28 weeks as indicated.
4. Glucose—diabetic screening done at 24 to 28 weeks.
   a. One hour 50-g glucose load test.
5. Alpha-fetoprotein—done at 15 to 18 weeks. High maternal levels after 18 weeks may indicate a neural tube defect in the fetus, however, this test has high false-positive results.

C. Infection
1. Venereal Disease Research Lab (VDRL) or Fluorescent Treponemal Antibody Absorption Test (FTA-ABS) tests for syphilis are done on the initial visit; repeat VDRL at 32 weeks as indicated.
2. Gonorrhea—cervical cultures are usually done at the initial visit and when symptoms are present.
3. Herpes—all possible lesions are cultured, and the cervix is cultured weekly beginning 4 to 8 weeks before delivery.
4. Chlamydia—done at the initial visit and when symptoms are present.
5. Rubella titer—if nonimmune, less than 1:8, immunize postpartum.
6. Hepatitis B surface antigen.
7. Human immunodeficiency virus (HIV)—screen is done on high-risk women.

D. Other Tests
1. Toxoplasmosis—done as indicated for women at risk.
2. Tuberculin skin tests—done as indicated.
3. Papanicolaou smear—done unless recent results available.

Physical Assessment

A. General Exam
1. The woman is asked to empty her bladder before the examination so that during vaginal examination her uterus and pelvic organs may be readily palpated.
2. Evaluation of the woman's weight and blood pressure.
3. Examination of eyes, ears, and nose—nasal congestion during pregnancy may occur as a result of peripheral vasodilation.
4. Examination of the mouth, teeth, throat, and thyroid—gums may be hyperemic and softened because of increased progesterone.
5. Inspection of breasts and nipples—breasts may be enlarged and tender; nipple and areolar pigment may be darkened.
6. Auscultation of heart.
7. Auscultation and percussion of the lungs.

B. Abdominal Examination
1. Examination for scars or striations, diastasis (separation of the rectus muscle), or umbilical hernia.
2. Palpation of the abdomen for height of the fundus (palpable after 13 weeks of pregnancy); measurement recorded and used as guideline for subsequent calculations.
3. Palpation of the abdomen for fetal outline and position—third trimester
4. Check of FHT—FHTs are audible with a doppler after 12 to 13 weeks and at 18 weeks with a fetoscope.
5. Record fetal position, presentation, and FHTs.

C. Pelvic Examination
1. The woman is placed in lithotomy position.
2. Inspection of external genitalia.
3. Vaginal examination—done to rule out abnormalities of the birth canal and to obtain cytologic smear (Papanicolaou and, if indicated, smears for gonorrhea, vaginal trichomoniasis, candidiasis, herpes, and chlamydia).
4. Examination of the cervix for position, size, mobility, and consistency. Cervix is softened and bluish (increased vascularity) during pregnancy.
5. Identification of the ovaries (size, shape, and position).
6. Rectovaginal exploration to identify hemorrhoids, fissures, herniation, or masses.
7. Evaluation of pelvic inlet—anteroposterior diameter by measuring the diagonal conjugate.

TABLE 34-1 Recommended Dietary Allowances of Selected Nutrients for Pregnancy and Lactation

Nutrient	11–14 Years (101 lb–62 in.)	15–18 Years (120 lb—64 in.)	19–22 Years (120 lb—64 in.)	23–50 Years (120 lb—64 in.)	Added for Pregnancy	Added for Lactation
Protein (g)	46	46	44	44	+30	+20
Fat-soluble vitamins						
Vitamin A (μg RE)	800	800	800	800	+200	+400
Vitamin D (μg)	10	10	7.5	5	+5	+5
Vitamin E (mg αTE)	8	8	8	8	+2	+3
Water-soluble vitamins						
Vitamin C (mg)	50	60	60	60	+20	+40
Thiamine (mg)	1.1	1.1	1.1	1.0	+0.4	+0.5
Riboflavin (mg)	1.3	1.3	1.3	1.2	+0.3	+0.5
Niacin mg NE	15	14	14	13	+2	+5
Vitamin B_6 (mg)	1.8	2.0	2.0	2.0	+0.6	+0.5
Folacin (μg)	400	400	400	400	+400	+100
Vitamin B_{12} (μg)	3.0	3.0	3.0	3.0	+1.0	+1.0
Minerals						
Calcium (mg)	1200	1200	800	800	+400	+400
Phosphorus (mg)	1200	1200	800	800	+400	+400
Magnesium (mg)	300	300	300	300	+150	+150
Iron (mg)	18	18	18	18	30 to 60 mg of supplemental iron is recommended	
Zinc (mg)	15	15	15	15	+5	+10
Iodine (μg)	150	150	150	150	+25	+50

(From Food and Nutrition Board, National Academy of Sciences—National Research Council.)

8. Evaluation of midpelvis—prominence of the ischial spines.
9. Evaluation of pelvic outlet—distance between ischial tuberosities and mobility of coccyx.

Subsequent Prenatal Assessments

1. Uterine growth and estimated fetal growth (Fig. 34-5).
   a. Fundus at symphysis pubis indicates 12 weeks' gestation.
   b. Fundus at umbilicus indicates 20 weeks' gestation.
   c. Fundus 28 cm from top of symphysis pubis indicates 28 weeks' gestation.
   d. Fundus at lower border of rib cage indicates 36 weeks' gestation.
   e. Uterus becomes globular and drops indicates 40 weeks' gestation.
2. A greater fundal height suggests:
   a. Multiple pregnancy.
   b. Miscalculated due date.
   c. Polyhydramnios (excessive amniotic fluid).
   d. Hydatidiform mole (degeneration of villi into grapelike clusters; fetus does not usually develop).
3. A lesser fundal height suggests:
   a. Intrauterine fetal growth retardation.
   b. Error in estimating gestation.
   c. Fetal or amniotic fluid abnormalities.
   d. Intrauterine fetal death.
4. Fetal heart tones—palpate abdomen for fetal position.
   a. Normal—120 to 160 beats/minute.
5. Weight—major increase in weight occurs during second half of pregnancy; usually between 0.22 kg (0.5 lb)/week and 0.44 kg (1 lb)/week. Greater weight gain may indicate fluid retention and hypertensive disorder.

6. Blood pressure—should remain near woman's normal baseline.
7. Hemoglobin; VDRL—rechecked at beginning of the third trimester and as indicated.
8. Culture smears for gonorrhea, chlamydia, and herpes, as indicated.
9. Urinalysis—for protein, glucose, blood, and nitrates.
10. Alpha-fetoprotein—done at 15 to 18 weeks.
11. Diabetic screening done at 24 to 28 weeks.
12. Administer RhoGAM as indicated at 28 weeks.
13. Edema—check the lower legs, face, and hands.
14. Evaluate discomforts of pregnancy—fatigue, heartburn, hemorrhoids, constipation, and backache.
15. Evaluate eating and sleeping patterns, general adjustment and coping with the pregnancy.
16. Evaluate concerns of the woman and her family.
17. Evaluate preparation for labor, delivery, and parenting. See Box 34-1 for a patient education list.

◆ HEALTH EDUCATION AND INTERVENTION

Nursing Diagnoses

A. Pain (backache, leg cramps, breast tenderness) related to physiologic changes of pregnancy
B. Altered Nutrition, Less Than Body Requirements related to morning sickness and heartburn and lack of knowledge of requirements in pregnancy
C. Altered Urinary Elimination, (frequency) related to increased pressure from the uterus
D. Constipation related to physiologic changes of pregnancy and pressure from the uterus

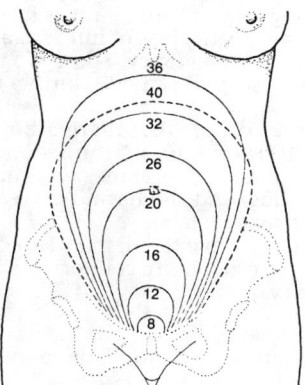

FIGURE 34-5 *Height of fundus. (From Danforth's Obstetrics and Gynecology. 7th ed. Philadelphia, JB Lippincott, 1994)*

E. Impaired Tissue Integrity related to pressure from the uterus and increased blood volume
F. Anxiety/Fear related to the birth process and infant care
G. Altered Role Performance related to the demands of pregnancy
H. Activity Intolerance related to physiologic changes of pregnancy and enlarging uterus

Nursing Interventions

A. ***Minimizing Pain***
1. Teach the woman to use good body mechanics—wear comfortable, low-heeled shoes with good arch support, try the use of a maternity girdle.
2. Instruct the woman in the technique for pelvic rocking exercises.
3. Encourage the woman to take rest periods with her legs elevated.
4. Inform the woman that adequate calcium intake may decrease leg cramps.
5. Instruct the woman to dorsiflex the foot while applying pressure to the knee to straighten the leg for immediate relief of leg cramps.
6. Instruct the woman to wear a fitted, supportive brassiere.
7. Instruct the woman to wash her breasts and nipples with water only.
8. Instruct the woman to apply vitamin E or lanolin cream to the breast and nipple area. Lanolin is contraindicated for women with allergies to lamb's wool.

B. ***Minimizing Morning Sickness and Heartburn and Maintaining Adequate Nutrition***
1. Encourage the woman to eat low-fat protein foods and dry carbohydrates, such as toast and crackers.
2. Encourage the woman to eat small, frequent meals.
3. Instruct the woman to avoid brushing her teeth soon after eating.
4. Instruct the woman to get out of bed slowly.
5. Encourage the woman to drink soups and liquids between meals to avoid stomach distention.

6. Instruct the woman in the use of antacids; caution against the use of sodium bicarbonate because it results in the absorption of excess sodium and fluid retention.
7. Teach the woman the importance of good nutrition for herself and her fetus. Review the basic food groups with appropriate daily servings.
   a. Seven servings of protein foods, including one serving of a vegetable protein.
   b. Three servings of milk or milk products.
   c. Seven servings of grain products.
   d. One serving of vitamin C–rich vegetable or fruit.
   e. Three servings of other fruits and vegetables.
   f. Three servings of unsaturated fats.
8. Inform the woman that average weight gain in pregnancy is 25 to 35 lb. About 2 to 5 lb are gained in the first trimester and about 1 lb per week for the remainder of the gestation.
   a. Average weight gain for overweight women is 15 to 25 lb.
   b. Adolescent weight gain should be about 5 lb more than for adult women if within 2 years of starting menses.
   c. Women with a multiple pregnancy should gain between 35 and 45 lb.
   d. Average weight gain for underweight women is 28 to 40 lb.
9. Advise the woman to limit the use of caffeine.
10. Inform the woman that alcohol should be limited or eliminated during pregnancy; no safe level of intake has been established.
11. Inform the woman that smoking should be eliminated or severely reduced during pregnancy; risk of spontaneous abortion, fetal death, low birth weight, and neonatal death increases with increased levels of maternal smoking.
12. Inform the woman that ingesting any drug during pregnancy may affect fetal growth and should be discussed with her physician.

BOX 34-1 *Patient Education Checklist*

1. Importance of keeping scheduled prenatal care appointments:
     Weeks 1–28, every month
     Weeks 28–36, every 2 weeks
     Weeks 36–delivery, every week
2. Discomforts of pregnancy and strategies for relief
3. Nutritional requirements and sample diet
4. Importance of exercise and proper body mechanics
5. Danger symptoms of pregnancy—require reporting to health care provider:
   Visual disturbances—blurring, spots, or double vision
   Vaginal bleeding, new or old blood
   Edema of the face, fingers, and sacrum
   Headaches—frequent, severe, or continuous
   Fluid discharge from vagina
   Unusual or severe abdominal pain
   Chills, fever, or burning on urination
   Epigastric pain (severe stomachache)
   Muscular irritability or convulsions
   Inability to tolerate food or liquids, leading to severe nausea and/or hyperemesis

C. ***Minimizing Urinary Frequency***
1. Instruct the woman to limit fluid intake in the evening.
2. Instruct the woman to void before going to bed.
3. Encourage the woman to void after meals.

D. ***Avoiding Constipation***
1. Instruct the woman to increase fluid intake to at least eight glasses of water a day. One to two quarts of fluid a day is desirable.
2. Teach the woman that foods high in fiber should be eaten daily.
3. Encourage the woman to establish regular patterns of elimination.
4. Encourage daily exercise, such as walking.
5. Inform the woman that over-the-counter laxatives should be avoided and that bulk-forming agents may be prescribed if indicated.

E. ***Maintaining Tissue Integrity***
1. Encourage the woman to take frequent rest periods with her legs elevated.
2. Instruct the woman to wear support stockings and wear loose fitting clothing for leg varicosities.
3. Instruct the woman to rest periodically with a small pillow under the buttocks to elevate the pelvis for vulvar varicosities.
4. Instruct the woman to avoid constipation, apply cold compresses, take sitz baths, and use topical anesthetics, such as Tucks, for the relief of anal varicosities (hemorrhoids).
5. Provide reassurance that varicosities will totally or greatly resolve after delivery.

F. ***Reducing Anxiety and Fear and Promoting Preparation for Labor, Delivery, and Parenthood***
1. Encourage the woman/couple to discuss their knowledge, perceptions, and expectations of the labor and delivery process.
2. Provide information on childbirth education classes and encourage them to attend.
3. Encourage a tour of the birth facility.
4. Discuss coping and pain control techniques for labor and birth.
5. Inform the woman/couple of common procedures during labor and birth.
6. Provide guidelines for coming to the birth facility.
7. Encourage the woman/couple to discuss their perceptions and expectations of parenthood and their "idealized child."
8. Discuss the infant's sleeping, eating, activity, and response patterns for the 1st month of life.
9. Discuss physical preparations for the infant, such as a sleeping space, clothing, feeding, changing, and bathing equipment.
10. Discuss plans for returning to work and child care arrangements.
11. Discuss the importance of planning time for themselves and each other apart from the newborn.
12. Provide information and encourage attendance at baby care, breast-feeding, and parenting classes.
13. Answer any questions the woman/couple may have.

G. ***Enhancing Role Changes***
1. Encourage discussion of feelings and concerns regarding the new role of mother and father.
2. Provide emotional support to the woman/couple regarding the altered family role.

3. Discuss physiologic causes for changes in sexual relationships, such as fatigue, loss of interest, and discomfort from advancing pregnancy. Some women experience heightened sexual activity during the second trimester.
4. Teach the woman/couple that there are no contraindications to intercourse or masturbation to orgasm provided the woman's membranes are intact, there is no vaginal bleeding, and she has no current problems or history or premature labor.
5. Teach the woman/couple that female superior or side-lying positions are often more comfortable in the latter half of pregnancy.

H. ***Minimizing Fatigue***
1. Teach the woman reasons for fatigue and have her plan a schedule for adequate rest.
   a. Fatigue in the first trimester is due to increased progesterone and its effects on the sleep center.
   b. Fatigue in the last trimester is due mainly to carrying increased weight of the pregnancy.
   c. About 8 hours of rest is needed at night.
   d. Inability to sleep may be due to excessive fatigue during the day.
   e. In the latter months of pregnancy, sleeping on the side with a small pillow under the abdomen may enhance comfort.
   f. Frequent 15- to 30-minute rest periods during the day are important to avoid overfatigue.
   g. Whenever possible, the woman should work while sitting with her legs elevated.
   h. The woman should avoid standing for prolonged periods of time, especially during the third trimester.
   i. To promote placental perfusion, the woman should not lie flat on her back—the left lateral position provides the best placental perfusion.
2. Help the woman plan for adequate exercise.
   a. In general, exercise during pregnancy should be in keeping with the woman's prepregnancy pattern and type of exercise.
   b. Activities or sports that have a risk of bodily harm (skiing, snowmobiling, horseback riding) should be avoided.
   c. During pregnancy, endurance during exercise may be decreased.
   d. Exercise classes for pregnant women that concentrate on toning and stretching have resulted in enhanced physical condition, increased self-esteem, and greater social support as a result of being in the exercise group.

Evaluation

A. Verbalizes understanding of proper body mechanics and wears low-heeled shoes
B. Identifies the basic food groups and describes meals to include needed servings for pregnancy
C. Reports limited fluid intake in the evening
D. Describes foods high in fiber
E. Wears support stockings and loose-fitting clothing
F. Discusses expectations for labor, delivery, and parenthood and attends educational classes
G. Verbalizes an understanding of the physiologic causes that may change the sexual relationship
H. Reports engaging in regular exercise

◆ PSYCHOSOCIAL ADAPTATION OF PREGNANCY

Rubin's Framework for Maternal Role Assumption

1. Attainment of motherhood role occurs with each pregnancy.
2. Involves a series of cognitive operations.
   a. Mimicry—The woman begins observing and modeling her behavior after other pregnant women.
   b. Role play—The woman begins acting out behaviors of a mother. For example, the woman will rock a baby to sleep.
   c. Searching for a role "fit"—The woman has perceptions of how the motherhood role will be. She observes others' behaviors to determine how well they fit with her expectations of the motherhood role.
   d. Grief work—The woman experiences a sense of loss of her "old" self as she prepares to begin her new role as a mother.
3. Maternal task
   a. Safe passage—the mother seeks to ensure a safe passage for her fetus and self throughout her pregnancy. During the first trimester the focus is on self-safety; in the third trimester the safety of the fetus is inseparable from self-safety.
   b. Acceptance by other—acceptance of this child by each family member.
   c. Binding-in to the child—maternal perception of the child as a real person.
   d. Giving of oneself—the most complex task, in which the mother is learning to give to the unborn child and placing the unborn child's need in relation to her own needs.

The Fetus

◆ GENERAL CONSIDERATIONS

Previously, methods used to determine how well the fetus was growing and maturing consisted of evaluating uterine growth and listening to fetal heart sounds. Advances in knowledge and technology have provided newer methods for assessing fetal well-being and maturity. Improved methods for assessment and diagnosis enable early intervention for improved outcome.

Fetal Growth and Development

See Figure 34-6.

A. *First Lunar Month*   Fertilization to 2 weeks of embryonic growth
1. Implantation is complete.
2. Primary chorionic villi forming.
3. Embryo develops into two cell layers (bilaminar embryonic disk)
4. Amniotic cavity appears.

B. *Second Lunar Month*   3 to 6 weeks of embryonic growth
1. At the end of 6 weeks of growth, the embryo is approximately 1.2 cm long.
2. Arm and leg buds are visible; arm buds are more developed with finger ridges beginning to appear.
3. Rudiments of the eyes, ears, and nose appear.
4. Lung buds are developing.
5. Primitive intestinal tract is developing.
6. Primitive cardiovascular system is functioning.
7. Neural tube, which forms the brain and spinal cord, closes by the 4th week.

C. *Third Lunar Month*   7 to 10 weeks of growth
1. The middle of this period (8 weeks) marks the end of the embryonic period and the beginning of the fetal period.
2. At the end of 10 weeks of growth, the fetus is 6.1 cm from crown to rump and weighs 14 g.
3. Appearance of external genitalia.
4. By the middle of this month, all major organ systems have formed.
5. The membrane over the anus has broken down.
6. The heart has formed four chambers (by 7th week).
7. The fetus assumes a human appearance.
8. Bone ossification begins.
9. Rudimentary kidney begins to secrete urine.

D. *Fourth Lunar Month*   11- to 14-week-old fetus
1. At the end of 14 weeks of growth, the fetus is 12 cm crown–rump length and 110 g.
2. Head erect; lower extremities well developed.
3. Hard palate and nasal septum have fused.
4. External genitalia of male and female can now be differentiated.
5. Eyelids are sealed.

E. *Fifth Lunar Month*   15- to 18-week-old fetus
1. At the end of 18 weeks of growth, the fetus is 16 cm crown–rump length and 320 g.
2. Ossification of fetal skeleton can be seen on x-ray.
3. Ears stand out from head.
4. Meconium is present in the intestinal tract.
5. Fetus makes sucking motions and swallows amniotic fluid.
6. Fetal movements may be felt by the mother (end of month).

F. *Sixth Lunar Month*   19–22-week-old fetus
1. At the end of 22 weeks of growth, the fetus is 21 cm crown–rump length and 630 g.
2. Vernix caseosa covers the skin.
3. Head and body (lanugo) hair visible.
4. Skin is wrinkled and red.
5. Brown fat, an important site of heat production, is present in neck and sternal area.
6. Nipples are apparent on the breasts.

G. *Seventh Lunar Month*   23–26-week-old fetus
1. At the end of 26 weeks of growth, the fetus is 25 cm crown–rump length and 1,000 g.
2. Fingernails present.
3. Lean body.
4. Eyes partially open; eyelashes present.
5. Bronchioles are present; primitive alveoli are forming.
6. Skin begins to thicken on hands and feet.
7. Startle reflex present; grasp reflex is strong.

H. *Eighth Lunar Month*   27–30-week-old fetus
1. At the end of 30 weeks of growth, the fetus is 28 cm crown–rump length and 1,700 g.
2. Eyes open.
3. Ample hair on head; lanugo begins to fade.
4. Skin slightly wrinkled.

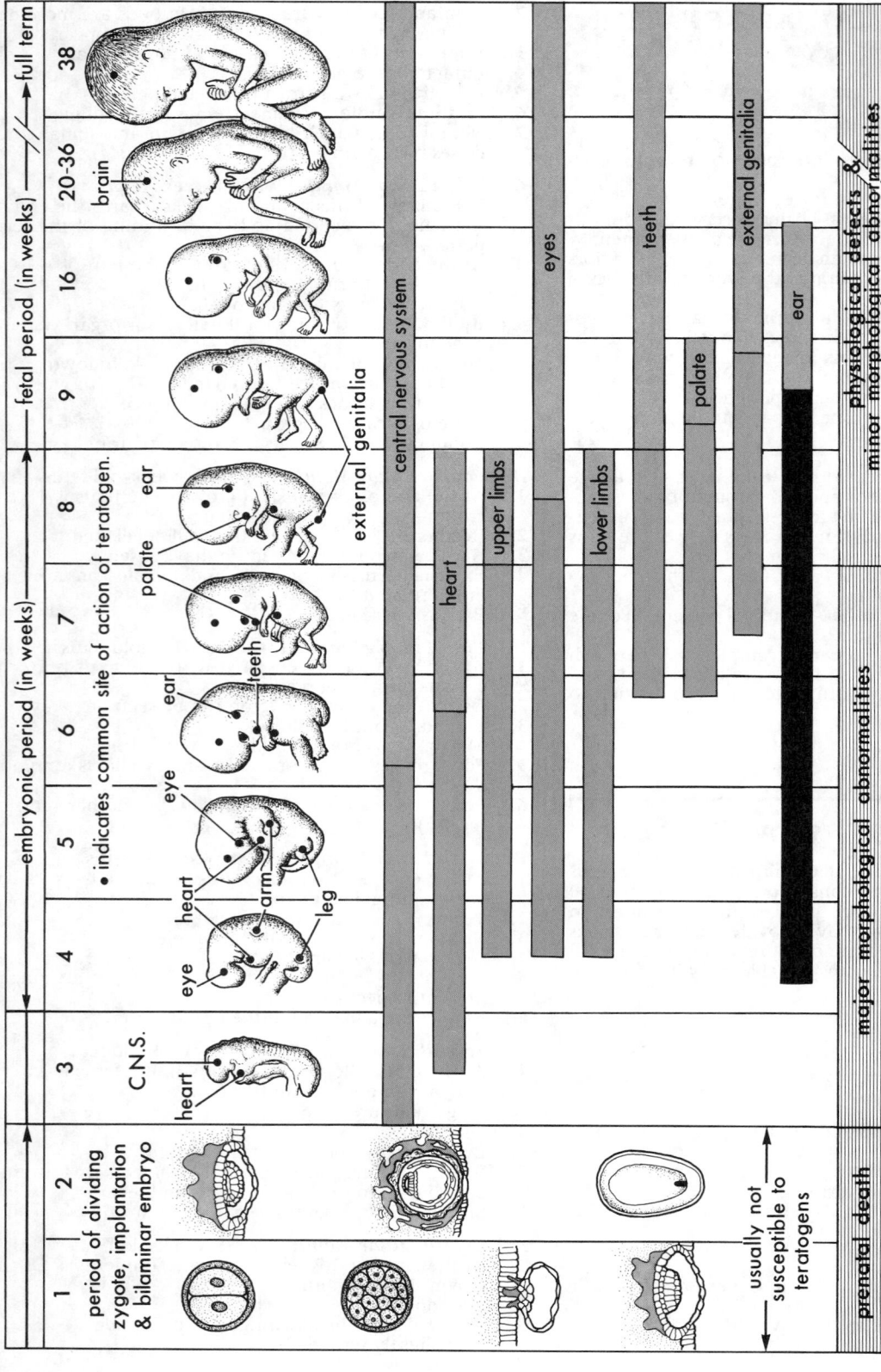

FIGURE 34-6 Schematic illustration of the sensitive or critical periods in human development. During the first 2 weeks of development, the embryo is usually not susceptible to teratogens. During these predifferentiation stages, a substance either damages all or most of the cells of the embryo, resulting in its death, or damages only a few cells, allowing the embryo to recover without developing defects. The left (shaded) sides of the bars denote highly sensitive periods; the right sides indicate stages that are less sensitive to teratogens. (From Moore KL. The Developing Human: Clinically Oriented Embryology. 4th ed. Philadelphia, WB Saunders, 1988.)

5. Toenails present.
6. Testes in inguinal canal, begin descent to scrotal sac.
7. Surfactant coats much of the alveolar epithelium.

I. **Ninth Lunar Month** 31–34-week-old fetus
1. At the end of 34 weeks of growth, the fetus is about 32 cm crown–rump length and 2,500 g.
2. Fingernails reach fingertips.
3. Skin pink and smooth.
4. Testes in scrotal sac.

J. **Tenth Lunar Month** 35- to 38-week-old fetus; end of this month is also 40 weeks from onset of last menstrual period
1. End of 38 weeks of growth, fetus is about 36 cm crown–rump length and 3,400 g.
2. Ample subcutaneous fat.
3. Lanugo almost absent.
4. Toenails reach toe tips.
5. Testes in scrotum.
6. Vernix caseosa mainly on the back.
7. Breasts are firm.

Fetal Circulation

See Figure 34-7.

◆ ASSESSMENT OF FETAL MATURITY AND WELL-BEING

Maternal History and Examination

A. **History**
1. The woman's general health.
2. History of current pregnancy and identified risk factors.
3. Health during previous pregnancies.
4. Outcome of previous pregnancies.
5. Estimation of fundal height.

Fetal Heart Tones

A. **Description** Fetal heart tones are representative of the fetal heart rate and are an indicator of oxygen perfusion to the fetal brain and heart. The evaluation of fetal heart tones is indicated in routine assessment of fetal well-being, in determining gestational age, and in cases of threatened abortion or other abnormalities. Fetal heart tones can be heard using techniques that amplify sound

1. Doppler at approximately 10 weeks' fetal gestation.
2. Fetoscope (fetal stethoscope) at approximately 20 weeks' fetal gestation.
3. Electronic fetal monitoring testing is usually done when the fetus is considered viable; around 24 weeks' gestation.
4. Rate—between 120 and 160 beats/minute.
5. In latter months of pregnancy, fetal heart sounds found.
   a. Near the woman's midline in fetal occipitoanterior positions.
   b. Lateral to midline in fetal occipitotransverse positions.
   c. In the woman's flank in fetal occipitoposterior positions.
   d. Below the woman's umbilicus in cephalic presentations.
   e. At or above the woman's umbilicus in breech presentations.
6. Failure to hear FHTs at the expected time may be due to maternal obesity, polyhydramnios, error in date calculation, or fetal death.

B. **Nursing/Patient Care Considerations**
1. Explain equipment, purpose, and procedure to the woman.
2. Assist the woman to a side-lying or semi-Fowler's position. Position may affect the ability to clearly hear the heart tones.
3. Document findings on the woman's chart and/or monitor strip along with date, time, activity level, medications, and other information per health care facility's guidelines.
4. Discontinue electronic fetal monitoring as indicated according to guidelines.
5. Communicate appropriate information to the woman and other personnel.

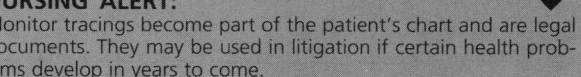

NURSING ALERT:
Monitor tracings become part of the patient's chart and are legal documents. They may be used in litigation if certain health problems develop in years to come.

Fetal Movement

A. **Description** Fetal movements or "kick counts" may be evaluated daily by the pregnant woman to provide reassurance of fetal well-being

1. It is an inexpensive and noninvasive method of evaluation.
2. Fetal movements are counted for 60 minutes three times a day, usually after meals.
3. The health care provider must be notified if:
   a. There are fewer than 10 movements in 12 hours.
   b. An increase of violent movements, followed by decreased movement.
   c. No movement for 8 hours.

B. **Nursing/Patient Care Considerations**
1. Instruct the woman to lie on her side and place her hands on the largest part of her abdomen and concentrate on fetal movement.
2. Instruct the woman to use a clock and record the movements felt.
3. Request the woman to explain the procedure so that her understanding is ensured.

Maternal Serum Alpha-Fetoprotein

A. **Description**
Maternal serum alpha-fetoprotein (AFP) levels are analyzed at 16 to 18 weeks' gestation to identify certain birth defects and chromosomal abnormalities during pregnancy

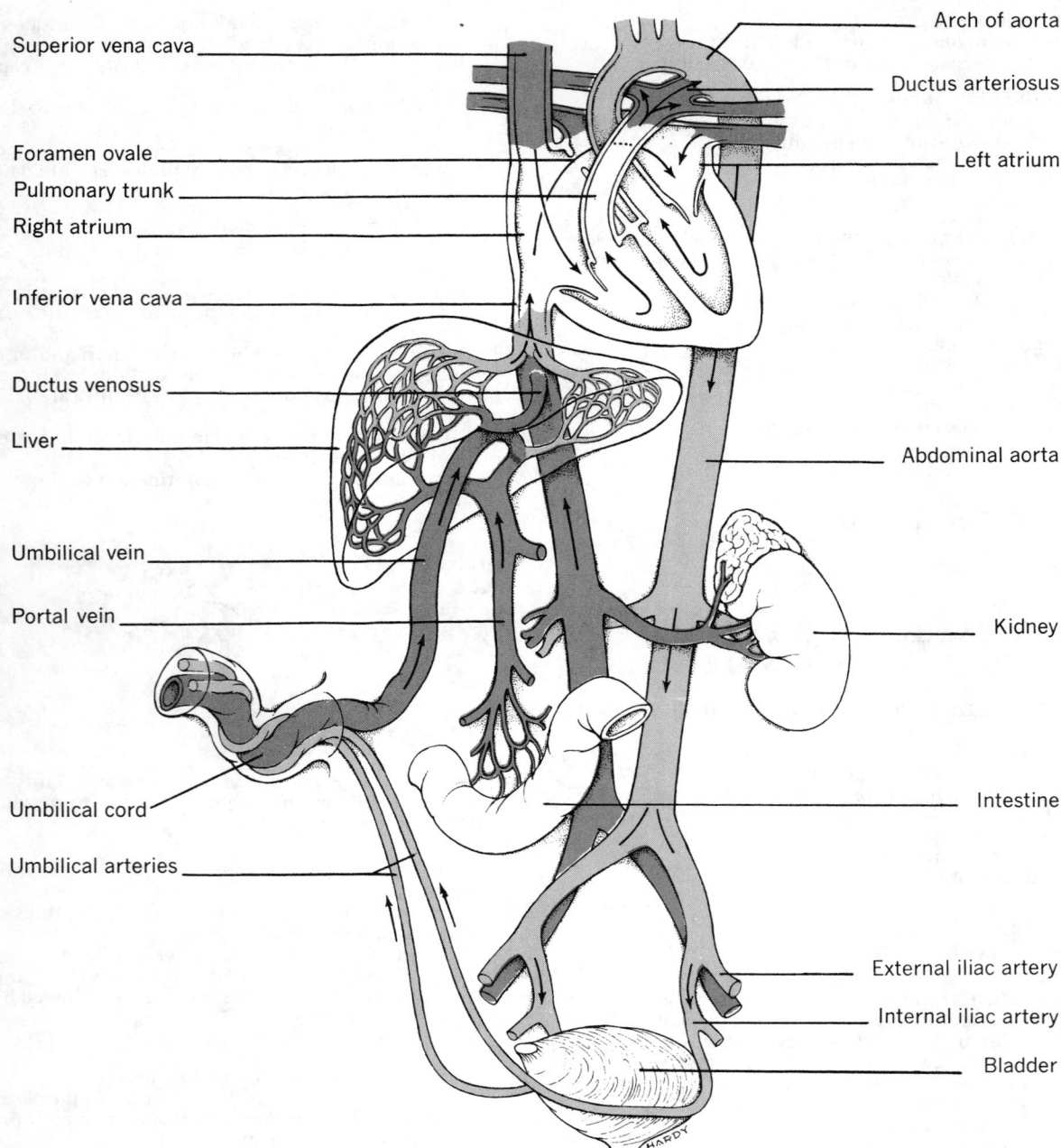

Superior vena cava

Foramen ovale

Pulmonary trunk

Right atrium

Inferior vena cava

Ductus venosus

Liver

Umbilical vein

Portal vein

Umbilical cord

Umbilical arteries

Arch of aorta

Ductus arteriosus

Left atrium

Abdominal aorta

Kidney

Intestine

External iliac artery

Internal iliac artery

Bladder

FIGURE 34-7 *Diagram of the fetal circulation shortly before birth. Arrows indicate course of blood.*

1. Elevated AFP levels are associated with neural tube defects, Rh isoimmunization, multiple gestation, maternal diabetes mellitus, and fetoplacental dysfunction.
2. Decreased levels are associated with Down's syndrome.

3. Follow-up for abnormal high or low levels includes ultrasound examination and amniocentesis.

B. *Nursing/Patient Care Considerations*
1. Obtain health and pregnancy history, including the date of the woman's last menstrual period and risk fac-

tors. Accurate dating of the pregnancy is crucial to interpret the results of the serum levels.
2. Explain the purpose and procedure for the test.
3. Discuss the woman's concerns.

Ultrasound

A. Description Ultrasound is a noninvasive, safe technique that uses reflected sound waves as they travel in tissue to produce a picture. A clear gel is applied to the woman's abdomen or transducer, and the transducer is moved along the abdomen by the examiner producing images on a screen

1. Uses in the first trimester of pregnancy include:
   a. Early confirmation of pregnancy and determination of the estimated date of confinement.
   b. Diagnosis of an ectopic pregnancy.
   c. Detection of an intrauterine device.
   d. Evaluation of placental location.
   e. Diagnosis of a multiple gestation.
2. Uses in the second trimester include:
   a. Evaluation of fetal growth, weight, and gestational age.
   b. Evaluation of the placenta for placenta previa or separation associated with vaginal bleeding.
   c. Evaluation of fetal presentation and position.
   d. Evaluation of fetal abnormalities.
   e. Evaluation of fetal viability.
   f. Determination of the Biophysical Profile Score.
   g. Evaluation of amniotic fluid volume.
   h. Guidance for amniocentesis.

B. Nursing/Patient Care Considerations
1. Explain the purpose and procedure to the woman, emphasizing the need to remain still.
2. Inform the woman of the need for a full bladder before the procedure.
3. Instruct the woman to drink 3 to 4 glasses of water if the bladder is not full.
4. Instruct the woman not to void until the procedure is over.
5. Remove the lubricant from the woman's abdomen after the procedure.

Amniocentesis

A. Description Amniocentesis is a procedure in which amniotic fluid is removed from the uterine cavity by insertion of a needle through the abdominal and uterine walls and into the amniotic sac. The procedure, usually performed between 16 and 18 weeks' gestation, is used in prenatal diagnosis of genetic or metabolic diseases, fetal lung maturity, and in the treatment of polyhydramnios. Risks associated with the procedure are very low

1. In determination of genetic or metabolic diseases, the procedure is useful for women 35 years of age or older, family history of metabolic disease, previous child with a chromosomal abnormality, family history of chromosomal abnormality, patient or husband with a chromosomal abnormality, or a possible female carrier of an X-linked disease.
2. In determination of lung maturity, the lecithin/sphingomyelin (L/S) ratio of the amniotic fluid is analyzed.
   a. When the ratio of lecithin to sphingomyelin is 2:1 or greater, the fetal lung is considered mature and the incidence of respiratory distress syndrome in the newborn is low.
   b. Results may be less reliable with maternal diabetes or if the fluid is contaminated with blood or meconium.
3. The presence of phosphatidylglycerol, one of the last lung surfactants to develop, is the most reliable indicator of fetal lung maturity.
4. A rapid foam test, mixing amniotic fluid, ethanol, and normal saline, is also used to determine the presence of mature L/S ratios. Adequate amounts of lecithin are present when a stable foam ring forms and remains on top of the solution after vigorous shaking (shake test).
5. In the treatment of polyhydramnios ($\geq$2,000 mL amniotic fluid), amniocentesis may be performed to drain excess fluid and relieve pressure. Polyhydramnios is associated with specific fetal abnormalities, such as trisomy 18, anencephaly, and spina bifida.

B. Nursing/Patient Care Considerations
1. Reduce anxiety related to the procedure.
   a. Reduce the parents' anxiety by determining their understanding of the procedure and the meaning it holds for them.
   b. Explain the procedure before it begins and answer any questions they have.
   c. Provide explanations during the procedure, correct misinformation they may have, and make sure they know when the results will be available and how they may obtain the results as soon as possible.
2. Reduce pain and discomfort related to the procedure.
   a. Reduce discomfort by having the mother lie comfortably on her back with her hands and a pillow under her head. Relaxation breathing may help.
   b. Ensure adequate time between infiltration of local anesthetic and introduction of needle into the amniotic sac.
3. Reduce potential for traumatic injury to fetus, placenta, or maternal structures.
   a. Have the woman empty her bladder if the fetus is more than 20 weeks' gestation to avoid injury to the woman's bladder. If the fetus is less than 20 weeks' gestation, the woman's full bladder will hold the uterus steady and out of the pelvis. The placenta is localized with the use of ultrasound.
   b. Obtain maternal vital signs and a 20-minute fetal heart rate tracing to serve as a baseline to evaluate possible complications.
   c. Monitor the woman during and after the procedure for signs of premature labor or bleeding.
   d. Tell the woman to report signs of bleeding, unusual fetal activity or abdominal pain, cramping, or fever while at home after the procedure.

Chorionic Villus Sampling (CVS)

A. Description
Chorionic villus sampling involves obtaining samples of chorionic villus (tissue of fetal origin) to test for genetic disorders of the fetus.

1. Using an ultrasound picture, a catheter is passed vaginally into the woman's uterus, where a sample of chorionic villus tissue is snipped off or obtained by suction.

2. Samples can be obtained earlier in pregnancy than can fetal cells obtained through amniocentesis. Biopsy is performed between 8 and 12 weeks of pregnancy.
3. Results from CVS are available in 1 to 2 weeks.
4. Complications include rupture of membranes, intrauterine infection, spontaneous abortion, hematoma, fetal trauma, or maternal tissue contamination.
5. Incidence of fetal loss is about 2% to 5%.

B. *Nursing/Patient Care Considerations*
1. Obtain maternal vital signs.
2. Instruct the woman to void.
3. Inform the woman that a small amount of spotting is normal, but heavy bleeding or passing clots or tissue should be reported.
4. Instruct the woman to rest at home for a few hours after the procedure.

Percutaneous Umbilical Blood Sampling

A. *Description*
Percutaneous umbilical blood sampling, or cordocentesis, involves a puncture of the umbilical cord for aspiration of fetal blood under ultrasound guidance.

1. It is used in the diagnosis of blood incompatibilities, anemias, and genetic studies.
2. Transfusion to the fetus may be done with this procedure.

B. *Nursing/Patient Care Considerations*
1. Explain the procedure to the woman.
2. Provide support to the woman during the procedure.
3. Monitor the woman after the procedure for uterine contractions and the fetal heart rate for distress.

Nonstress Test (NST)

A. *Description* The NST is used to evaluate fetal heart rate accelerations that normally occur in response to fetal activity in a fetus in good condition. Accelerations are indicative of an intact central and autonomic nervous system

1. Maternal indications include postdates, Rh sensitization, maternal age 35 or older, chronic renal disease, hypertension, collagen disease, sickle cell disease, diabetes, premature rupture of membranes, history of stillbirth, vaginal bleeding in the second and third trimesters.
2. Fetal indications include decreased fetal movement, intrauterine growth retardation, fetal evaluation after an amniocentesis, oligohydramnios or polyhydramnios.
   a. Criteria for a reactive NST include two accelerations within 20 minutes, each lasting at least 15 seconds with a fetal heart rate increased by 15 beats/minute above baseline in response to fetal activity. The test period should be a minimum of 40 minutes to allow for fetal rest cycle patterns.
   b. In a nonreactive NST, the above criteria are not met. The test period may be extended to allow for fetal rest cycles. Fruit juice may be given, or abdominal manipulation may stimulate the fetus.
   c. The test is unsatisfactory if the fetal heart rate tracing is not adequate for interpretation.

B. *Nursing/Patient Care Considerations*
1. Explain the procedure and equipment to the woman.
2. Assist the woman to a semi-Fowler's position in bed and apply the external fetal and uterine monitors.
3. Instruct the woman to make a mark on the monitor strip each time fetal movement is felt. The nurse will do this if the woman cannot.
4. Evaluate the response of the fetal heart rate immediately after fetal activity.
5. Monitor the woman's blood pressure and uterine activity for deviations during the procedure.

Acoustic Stimulation Test

A. *Description* Vibroacoustic stimulation, using an artificial larynx, is used to stimulate the fetus and assess its reaction to the sound

1. This test may be as good a screening tool as the NST, because the loud noise stimulates the fetus and notes ability to respond to the noise by increasing heart rate.
2. One method of evaluation indicates that a reactive acoustic stimulation test will have at least one acceleration of at least 15 beats/minute lasting 2 minutes or two accelerations with an increase of 15 beats/minute lasting 15 seconds within 5 minutes of stimulation.

B. *Nursing/Patient Care Considerations*
1. Explain procedure and equipment to the woman.
2. Assist woman to a semi-Fowler's position in bed.
3. Apply external fetal monitors to the woman.
4. Observe for reactivity.

Oxytocin Challenge Test, Stress Test, or Contraction Stress Test

A. *Description* This test is used to evaluate the ability of the fetus to withstand the stress of uterine contractions as would occur during labor. It is used with decreasing frequency, because it may stress an already stressed fetus

1. The test is usually used when a woman has a nonreactive NST.
2. The test is contraindicated in women with third trimester bleeding, multiple gestation, incompetent cervix, or premature rupture of membranes.

B. *Nursing/Patient Care Considerations*
1. Obtain maternal vital signs.
2. Instruct the woman to void.
3. Assist the woman to a semi-Fowler's or side-lying position in bed.
4. Obtain a 30-minute strip of the fetal heart rate and uterine activity for baseline data.
5. Administer diluted oxytocin through an intravenous line infusion pump as indicated until three contractions occur within 10 minutes. This may take 1 to 2 hours.
6. Discontinue the infusion when the test is complete.

Biophysical Profile

A. *Description* The biophysical profile uses ultrasonography and NST to assess five variables in determining fetal well-being

1. Nonstress test—looking for acceleration in relation to fetal movements.
2. Amniotic fluid volume—assessing for one or more pockets of amniotic fluid measuring 1 cm in two perpendicular planes.
3. Fetal breathing—one or more episodes lasting at least 30 seconds.
4. Gross body movements—three or more body or limb movements in 30 minutes.
5. Fetal tone—one or more episodes of active extension with return to flexion.

   For each variable, if the criteria are met, a score of 2 is given. For an abnormal observation, a score of 0

or 1 is given. A score of 8 to 10 is considered normal, 6 is equivocal, and 4 or less is abnormal.

B. Nursing/Patient Care Considerations
1. Explain the purpose and procedure to the woman.
2. Inform the woman that a full bladder may be necessary.
3. Instruct the woman to drink 3 to 4 glasses of water if the bladder is not full.
4. Remove the lubricant from the woman's abdomen after the procedure.
5. Instruct the woman to void after the procedure.

Selected References

Borrie, M. M., et al. (1994). *Foundations of maternal newborn nursing.* Philadelphia: W.B. Saunders.

Carpenito, L J. (1993). *Handbook of nursing diagnosis* (5th ed.). Philadelphia: J.B. Lippincott.

Carrington, B. W., et al. (1993). The need for family planning services for women delivering with little or no prenatal care [editorial]. *Woman and Health, 20*(1), 1-9.

Cogswell, M. E., et al. (1995). Gestational weight gain among average weight and overweight women—what is excessive. *American Journal of Obstetrics and Gynecology, 172*(2), 705–12.

Creasy, R. K., & Resnik, R. (1994). *Maternal-fetal medicine principles and practice* (3rd ed.). Philadelphia: W.B. Saunders.

Cunningham, F. G., et al. (1993). *Williams obstetrics* (19th ed.). Norwalk, CT: Appleton and Lange.

Dickason, E. J., et al. (1994). *Maternal-infant nursing care* (2nd ed.). St. Louis: Mosby-Year Book.

Di Iorio, C., et al. (1992).Patterns of nausea during first trimester of pregnancy. *Clinical Nursing Research, 1*(2), 127-140, discussion 141-143.

Fried, P. (1993). Prenatal exposure to tobacco and marijuana: Effects during pregnancy, infancy, and early childhood. *Clinical Obstetrics and Gynecology, 36*(2), 319-337.

Luke, B. (1994). Maternal-fetal nutrition. *Clinical Obstetrics and Gynecology, 37*(1), 93-109.

May, K. A., & Mahlmeister, L. R. (1994). *Maternal and neonatal nursing-family centered care* (3rd ed.). Philadelphia: J.B. Lippincott.

McFarland, G. K., & McFarlane, E. A. (1993). *Nursing diagnosis and intervention* (2nd ed.). St. Louis: Mosby-Year Book.

Newman, V., et al. (1993). Clinical advances in the management of severe nausea and vomiting during pregnancy. *Journal of Obstetric, Gynecologic, and Neonatal Nursing, 22,* 483-490.

Randall, B. P. (1993). Growth versus stability: older primiparous woman as a paradigmatic case for persistence. *Journal of Advanced Nursing, 18*(4), 518-525.

Worthington, R., et al. (1993). *Nutrition in pregnancy and lactation* (5th ed.). St. Louis: Mosby-Year Book.

CHAPTER 35

Nursing Management During Labor and Delivery

The Labor Process

From the initial prenatal visits, the nurse needs to emphasize that labor and delivery are normal physiologic processes. The pregnant woman often approaches the time of delivery with major concerns of her personal well-being, that of her unborn child, and fear of a difficult and painful labor. Addressing these concerns and minimizing her discomfort should be of paramount importance to all participants involved in the care of the mother and her fetus.

◆ GENERAL CONSIDERATIONS

Prepared Childbirth

Previously, the term *natural childbirth* was used to describe one approach to giving birth. To some, natural childbirth meant delivery without analgesic or anesthesia, whereas to those who had developed the approach it simply meant being prepared for childbirth through prenatal education and training. This preparation gave the woman a method of coping with the discomforts of labor and delivery. To avoid the suggestion that analgesia or anesthesia is unavailable to the woman during labor and delivery should she need it, the term *prepared childbirth* is now used instead of natural childbirth.

A. Method of Grantly Dick-Read
1. This method is based on the idea that fear and anticipation of pain arouse natural protective tensions in the body, both psychic and muscular.
2. Fear stimulates the sympathetic nervous system and causes the circular muscle of the cervix to contract.
3. The longitudinal muscles of the uterus then have to act against increased cervical resistance, causing tension and pain.
4. Tension and pain aggravate fear, which produces a vicious cycle of tension, pain, and fear.
5. A minor degree of pain, magnified by fear, becomes unbearable.
6. According to Dick-Read, prenatal courses and training reduce fear, overcome ignorance, and build a woman's self-confidence. Included in this method are:
   a. Explanations of fetal development and childbirth.
   b. Descriptions of methods available to relieve pain.
   c. Exercises that strengthen certain muscles and relax others.
   d. Breathing techniques that will enable the woman to relax in the first stage of labor and work effectively with muscles used during delivery.
   e. Explanations of the value of improved physical health and emotional stability for childbirth.
   f. The woman is not told that labor and delivery will be painless; analgesia and anesthesia are available if needed or desired.
   g. The woman is given empathic understanding and support during labor by her partner, the nurse, and the health care provider.

B. Psychoprophylactic or Lamaze Method
1. Psychoprophylactic childbirth has a rationale based on Pavlov's concept of pain perception and his theory of conditioned reflexes (the substitution of favorable conditioned reflexes for unfavorable ones). The Lamaze method is an example of this technique.
2. The woman is taught to replace responses of restlessness, fear, and the loss of control with more useful activity. A high level of activity can excite the cerebral cortex efficiently to inhibit other stimuli, such as pain in labor.
3. The mother-to-be is taught exercises that strengthen the abdominal muscles and relax the perineum.
4. Breathing techniques to help the process of labor are practiced.
5. The woman is conditioned to respond with respiratory activity and disassociation or relaxation of the uninvolved muscles, while controlling her perception of the stimuli associated with labor.
6. One method of control consists of breathing normally while silently mouthing the words to a song and simultaneously tapping the rhythm with the fingers.
7. Similarity between the Dick-Read and Lamaze methods:
   a. Fear, which enhances the perception of pain, may diminish or disappear when the woman understands the physiology of labor.
   b. Because psychic tension enhances perception of pain, relaxation is achieved more easily in a calm, agreeable atmosphere with supportive persons nearby.
   c. Muscular relaxation and a specific type of breathing diminish or abolish the pains of labor.

C. The Leboyer Method of Delivery
1. The *Leboyer method* is based on the premise that the infant suffers psychological shock at the time of deliv-

ery. An effort is made to reduce the contrast between the intrauterine environment and the outside world.

2. Gentle, controlled delivery—prenatal education, support from family and personnel to decrease anxiety, fear, and tension.

3. Emphasis on providing protection to the craniosacral axis by gently supporting the newborn infant's head, neck, and sacrum. The craniosacral axis is completely relaxed, and lost body heat is restored in a warm water bath.

4. Avoiding overstimulation of the newborn sensorium— the infant is allowed to breathe spontaneously; cutting the cord is delayed to permit placental blood transfusion for improved respiration.

5. Importance of maternal–infant bond—skin-to-skin contact with mother is provided, and infant is fondled and stroked.

D. Home Delivery

1. *Home delivery,* although controversial, has won increasing support in recent years.

2. Motivations for home delivery:
   a. Belief that home birth has significant advantages for the family and the newborn infant.
   b. Objection to the impersonal and authoritarian atmosphere of the hospital environment with enforced separation of woman and family.
   c. Desire to avoid such practices as routine cesarean delivery for breech presentation, episiotomy, forceps delivery, oxytocin stimulation, routine monitoring of the fetal heart tones, and other practices associated with hospitals.
   d. Risk of in-hospital infections; belief that infant is immune to own-home bacteria.
   e. Rising costs of hospitalization.

3. Contraindications
   a. High-risk indications for infant and mother.
   b. Patient with history of premature or postdate delivery in previous pregnancy.
   c. Woman with medical or emotional complications.
   d. Patient who cannot be quickly transported to a hospital.

4. Alternatives
   a. Alterations of hospital setting to a family-centered approach.
   b. Birthing centers for low-risk women with adequate facilities for emergency care.
   c. Properly educated and motivated support personnel.

Initiation of Labor

The exact mechanism that initiates labor is unknown. Theories include:

1. Uterine stretch theory—uterus becomes stretched and pressure increases, causing physiologic changes that initiate labor.

2. As pregnancy progresses, there is a gradual rise in the amount of circulating oxytocin.

3. As pregnancy advances, progesterone is less effective in controlling rhythmic uterine contractions that normally occur. In addition, there also may be an actual decrease in the amount of circulating progesterone.

4. There is increased production of prostaglandins by fetal membranes and uterine decidua as pregnancy advances.

5. In later pregnancy, the fetus produces increased levels of cortisol that inhibit progesterone production from the placenta.

Factors Affecting Labor

Successful labor and delivery depend on adequate pelvic dimensions, adequate fetal dimensions and presentation, and adequate uterine contractions.

A. Pelvic Dimensions

1. Adequate pelvic inlet (anteroposterior diameter; normal shape),

2. Adequate midpelvis (ischial spines do not protrude into bony canal).

3. Adequate outlet (adequate distance between tuberosities; mobile coccyx).

4. Adequacy of pelvic dimensions determined by pelvic examination during pregnancy and again with the onset of labor.

B. Fetal Dimensions
Important fetal dimensions influenced by fetal size, posture, lie, and presentation. Fetal position is also an important factor in successful labor.

1. *Fetal size*—with excessive size, fetal skull bones may not be able to override enough to be accommodated in the bony pelvic cavity.

2. *Fetal posture*—fetus assumes a characteristic posture in later pregnancy to accommodate to the uterine cavity. The fetal head is flexed, back is bent, and extremities are flexed. Flexed head allows smallest diameter of fetal head to present and pass through the birth canal (Fig. 35-1).

3. *Fetal lie*—fetus assumes a lie (comparison of the fetal long axis to the long axis of the woman) that is either transverse or longitudinal. In a longitudinal lie (99% of all births), the fetal head will present (cephalic presentation) or the buttocks or feet will present (breech presentation). In a transverse lie, the shoulder presents.

4. *Fetal presentation*—whichever portion of the infant is deepest in the birth canal and is felt on vaginal examination is referred to as the presenting part; this determines fetal presentation.

5. *Fetal position*—designation of landmark of fetal presenting part (occiput, mentum, sacrum, acronium) to right or left, and anterior, posterior, or transverse portion of the woman's pelvis. For example, a fetus presenting by the vertex with occiput on the left anterior part of the woman's pelvis would have presentation and position described as LOA, or left occiput anterior (see Fig. 35-2).

C. Fetal Head
In approximately 95% of all births, the fetal head presents first. The sutures and fontanelles provide important landmarks for determining fetal position during a vaginal exam (Fig. 35-3).

1. Bones of the fetal skull
   a. Occipital bone posteriorly.
   b. Two parietal bones on the sides.
   c. Two temporal bones anteriorly.
   d. Two frontal bones anteriorly.

2. Sutures of the fetal skull—membranous spaces between the bones of the fetal skull.
   a. Frontal suture—between the two frontal bones.
   b. Sagittal—between the two parietal bones.
   c. Coronal—between the frontal and parietal bones.
   d. Lambdoid—between the back of the parietal bones and the margin of the occipital bone.

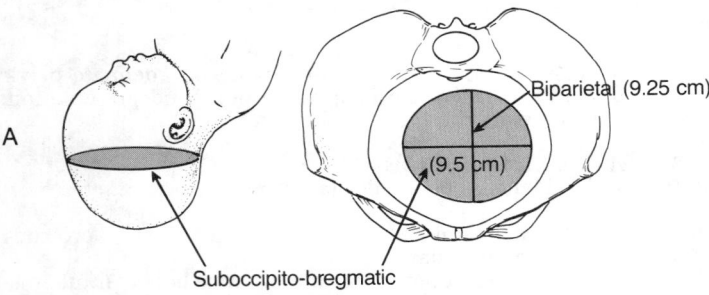

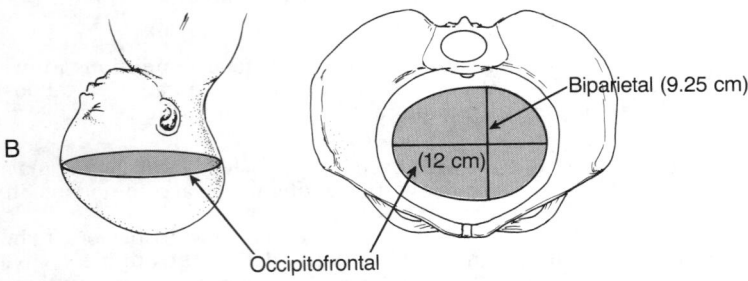

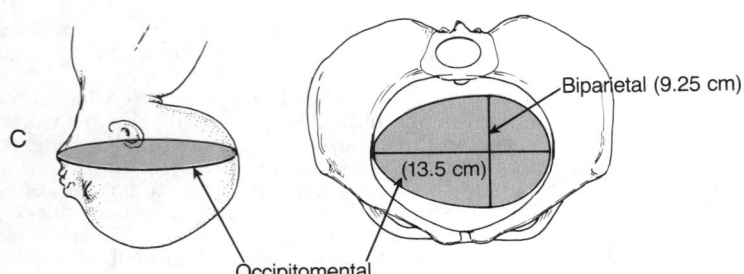

FIGURE 35-1 (A) *Complete flexion allows smallest diameter of head to enter pelvis.* **(B)** *Moderate extension causes larger diameter to enter pelvis.* **(C)** *Marked extension forces largest diameter against pelvic brim, but head is too large to enter pelvis.*

3. Fontanelles—irregular spaces formed where two or more sutures meet. Sutures and fontanelles allow fetal skull bones to overlap in order to pass through the maternal pelvis.
   a. Anterior fontanelle—junction of the sagittal, frontal, and coronal sutures—closes by 18 months of age.
   b. Posterior fontanelle—located where the sagittal suture meets the lambdoidal (smaller than anterior)—closes at 6 to 8 weeks of age.

D. Uterine Contractions
Successful labor also depends on uterine contractions occurring at regular intervals and having adequate intensity.

1. Uterine contractions are involuntary.
2. During uterine contractions, the active upper portion of the uterus becomes thicker, while the lower uterine segment stretches and becomes thinner.

3. At the completion of a contraction, the upper uterine segment retains its shortened, thickened cell size and with each succeeding contraction becomes thicker and shorter. Cells of the lower uterine segment become thinner and longer with each contraction. This mechanism is greatly responsible for the progress of the fetus through the birth canal.

Events Preliminary to Labor

1. *Lightening* (the settling of the fetus in the lower uterine segment) occurs 2 to 3 weeks before term in the primigravida and later, during labor, in the multigravida.
   a. Breathing becomes easier as the fetus falls away from the diaphragm.
   b. Lordosis of the spine is increased as the fetus enters the pelvis and falls forward. Walking may become more difficult; leg cramping may increase.

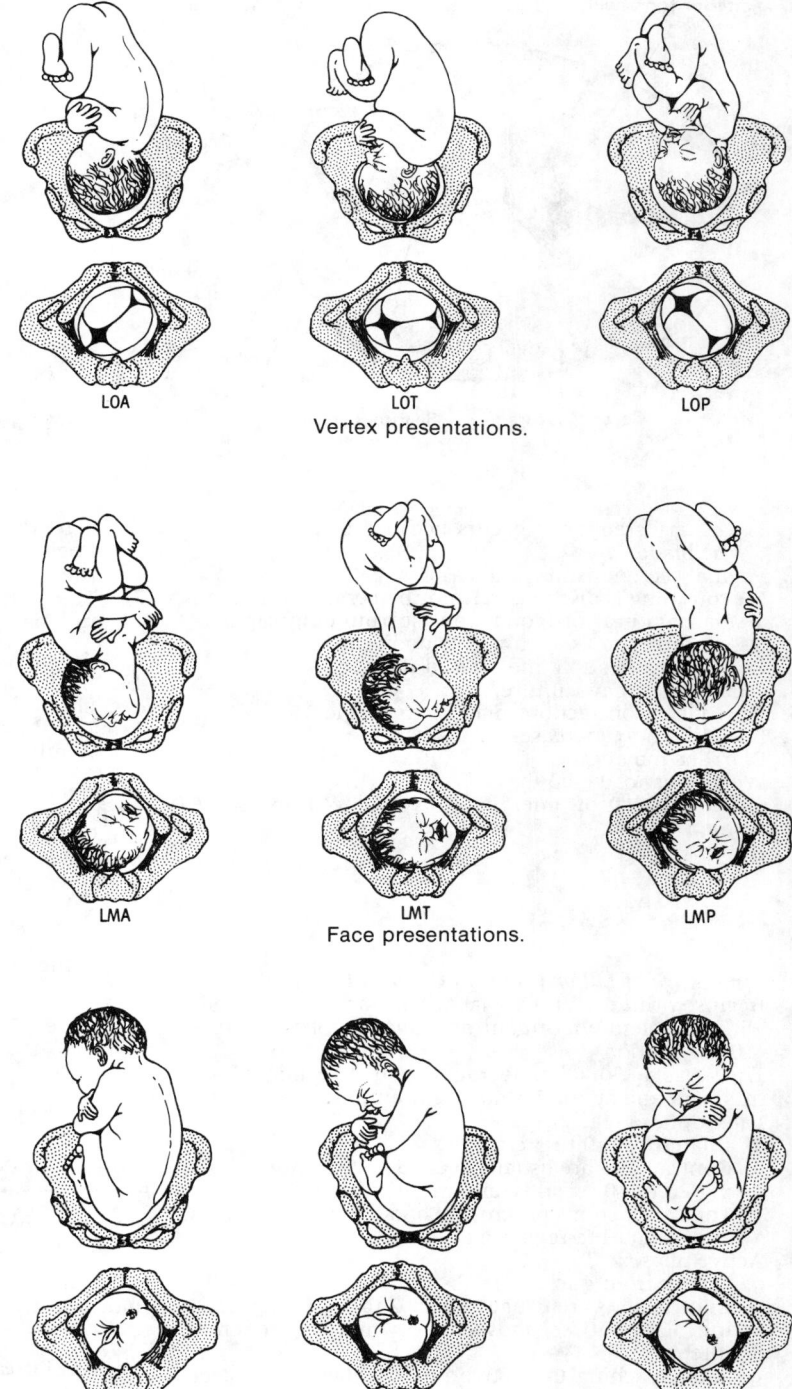

LOA   LOT   LOP

Vertex presentations.

LMA   LMT   LMP

Face presentations.

LSA   LST   LSP

Breech presentations.

FIGURE 35-2 *Fetal presentations. A three-letter abbreviation is used to describe the relationship of the presenting part to the maternal pelvis. Standard landmarks for the fetal presenting part are as follows: O, occiput (head); S, sacrum (buttocks); Sc, scapula (shoulders); M, mentum (chin). The maternal pelvis is divided into the following segments: R, right; L, left; A, anterior (front); P, posterior (back); T, transverse. First, identify which side the presenting part is facing in the pelvis: R or L. Next, identify the landmark that is presenting: O, S, Sc, M. Finally, identify the direction the presenting part is facing in the pelvis: A, P, or T. (From Benson, RC. Handbook of Obstetrics and Gynecology. Los Altos, CA: Lange Medical Publication.)*

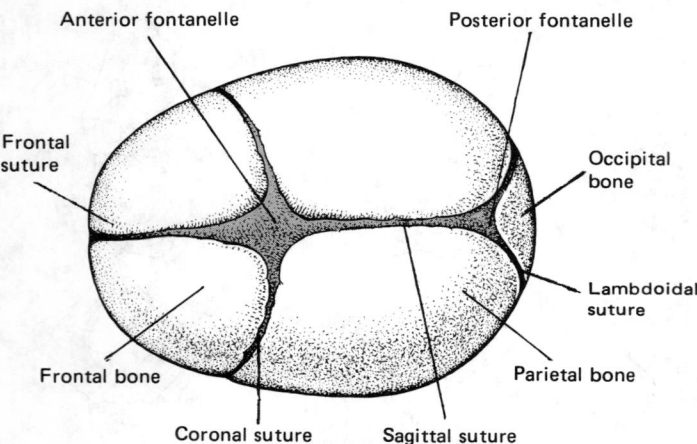

FIGURE 35-3 *Fetal head.*

c. Urinary frequency occurs because of pressure on the bladder.
2. Vaginal secretions may increase.
3. Mucous plug is discharged from the cervix along with a small amount of blood from surrounding capillaries—referred to as "show" ("bloody show").
4. Cervix becomes soft and effaced (thinned).
5. Membranes may rupture.
6. False labor contractions may occur (Table 35-1).
7. Backache may increase.
8. Diarrhea may occur.
9. Weight loss of 1 to 3 lb.
10. Sudden burst of energy is experienced by some women.

Stages of Labor

A. *First Stage of Labor (Stage of Cervical Dilation)*
1. Begins with the first true labor contractions and ends with complete effacement and dilation of the cervix (10 cm dilation).
2. The first stage of labor averages about 13.3 hours for a nullipara and about 7.5 hours for a multipara.
3. Latent phase (early):
   a. Dilates from 0 to 4 cm.
   b. Contractions are usually every 5 to 20 minutes, lasting 20 to 40 seconds, and of mild intensity.
   c. The contractions progress to about every 5 minutes and establish a regular pattern.
4. Active phase:
   a. Dilates from 4 to 7 cm.
   b. Contractions are usually every 2 to 5 minutes; lasting 30 to 50 seconds and of mild to moderate intensity.
   c. After reaching the active phase, dilation averages 1.2 cm per hour in the nullipara and 1.5 cm per hour in the multipara.
5. Transitional phase:
   a. Dilates from 8 to 10 cm.
   b. Contractions are every 2 to 3 minutes, lasting 50 to 60 seconds and of moderate to strong intensity. Some contractions may last up to 90 seconds.

B. *Second Stage of Labor, or Stage of Expulsion*
1. Begins with complete dilation and ends with birth of the baby.
2. The second stage may last from 1 to 1½ hours in the nullipara and from 20 to 45 minutes in the multipara.

C. *Third Stage of Labor, or Placental Stage*
1. Begins with delivery of the baby and ends with delivery of the placenta.
2. The third stage may last from a few minutes up to 30 minutes.

D. *Fourth Stage*
Lasts from delivery of the placenta until the postpartum condition of the woman has become stabilized (usually 1 hour after delivery).

Mechanisms of Labor

1. If the woman's pelvis is adequate, size and position of the fetus are adequate, and uterine contractions are

TABLE 35-1 True and False Labor Contractions

True Labor Contractions	False Labor Contractions
Result in progressive cervical dilation and effacement	Do not result in progressive cervical dilation and effacement
Occur at regular intervals	Occur at irregular intervals
Interval between contractions decreases	Interval between contractions remains the same or increases
Intensity increases	Intensity decreases or remains the same
Located mainly in back and abdomen	Located mainly in lower abdomen and groin
Generally intensified by walking	Generally unaffected by walking
Not affected by mild sedation	Generally relieved by mild sedation

regular and of adequate intensity, the fetus will move through the birth canal.

2. The position and rotational changes of the fetus as it moves down the birth canal will be affected by resistance offered by the woman's bony pelvis, cervix, and surrounding tissues.
3. The events of engagement, descent, flexion, internal rotation, extension, external rotation, and expulsion overlap in time (Fig. 35-4).

A. Engagement
When biparietal diameter of fetal head has passed through pelvic inlet:

1. Primigravidas—occurs up to 2 weeks before onset of labor.
2. Multigravidas—usually occurs with onset of labor.
3. Because biparietal diameter is narrowest diameter of fetal head and anteroposterior diameter is narrowest of pelvic inlet, the fetal head usually enters pelvis in a transverse position.

B. Descent
Occurs throughout labor and is essential for fetal rotations prior to birth.

1. Accomplished by force of uterine contractions on fetal portion in fundus; during second stage of labor, bearing down increases intra-abdominal pressure, thus augmenting effects of uterine contractions.
2. Station is the relationship of the level of the presenting part to the ischial spines. The degree of descent is described as:
   a. Floating—fetal presenting part is not engaged in pelvic inlet (Fig. 35-5).
   b. Fixed—fetal presenting part has entered pelvis.
   c. Engagement—fetal presenting part (usually biparietal diameter of fetal head) has passed through pelvic inlet.
   d. Stations that are −1, −2, −3, or −4 occur when the presenting part is 1, 2, 3, or 4 cm above the level of the ischial spines (Fig. 35-6).
   e. Station 0 occurs when the presenting part is at the level of the ischial spine.
   f. Station +1, +2, +3, or +4 is when the presenting part is 1, 2, 3, or 4 cm below the ischial spines. A station of +4 indicates that the presenting part is on the pelvic floor.

C. Flexion
Resistance to descent causes head to flex so that the chin is close to the chest; this causes the smallest fetal head diameter, the suboccipitobregmatic (9.5 cm), to present through the canal.

D. Internal Rotation
In accommodating the birth canal, the fetal occiput rotates anteriorly from its original position toward the symphysis. This movement results from the shape of the fetal head, space available in the midpelvis, and contour of the perineal muscles. The ischial spines project into the midpelvis, causing the fetal head to rotate anteriorly to accommodate to the available space.

E. Extension
As the fetal head descends further, it meets resistance from the perineal muscles and is forced to extend. The fetal head becomes visible at the vulvovaginal ring; its largest diameter is encircled (crowning), and the head then emerges from the vagina.

F. External Rotation
When the head emerges, the shoulders are undergoing internal rotation as they turn in the midpelvis to accommodate the projection of the ischial spines. The head, now born, rotates as the shoulders undergo this internal rotation.

G. Expulsion
After delivery of the infant's head and internal rotation of the shoulders, the anterior shoulder rests beneath the symphysis pubis. The posterior shoulder is born, followed by the anterior shoulder and the rest of the body.

Nursing Assessment and Interventions

◆ WHEN LABOR BEGINS

Nursing responsibilities when labor begins include history taking and performing a vaginal exam to determine presentation and position of the fetus and condition of the cervix and membranes.

History and Baseline Data

1. Introduce yourself; ask for name of woman's health care provider and if he or she has been notified that the woman was coming to the hospital or birth center.
2. Establish baseline information.
   a. Assess gravidity, parity, expected date of delivery of confinement.
   b. When did contractions begin? How far apart are they? How long do they last?
   c. Have the membranes ruptured? Color? Consistency? Amount of fluid?
   d. Is there any bloody show?
   e. How much discomfort is the woman experiencing?
   f. What, if any, problems has the woman had in this pregnancy? Problems in past pregnancies?
   g. Blood type and Rh?
3. Establish baseline maternal and fetal vital signs.
   a. Temperature—elevation suggests a possible infection or dehydration.
   b. Pulse—evaluate between contractions; may be slightly elevated over the resting rate.
   c. Respirations—evaluated between contractions.
   d. Blood pressure—evaluated between contractions.
      (1) A slight elevation over baseline may be attributed to anxiety.
      (2) A blood pressure with a systolic elevation of 30 mm Hg or greater than 140 mm Hg and a diastolic elevation of 15 mm Hg or greater than 90 mm Hg suggests hypertension and requires further evaluation.
   e. Assess the fetal heart rate (FHR); if a fetal monitor is to be used, run a 30-minute strip for baseline data.
4. Obtain a urine specimen—test the urine for glucose and protein. Protein results may be positive if the membranes have ruptured.

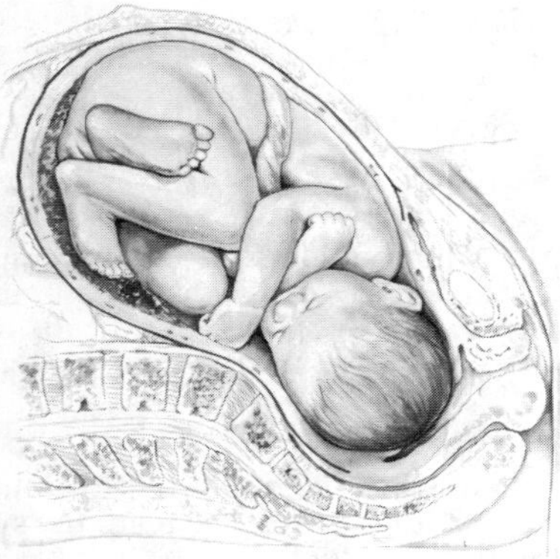

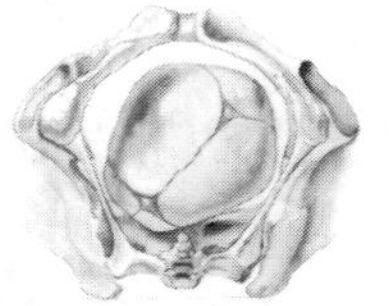

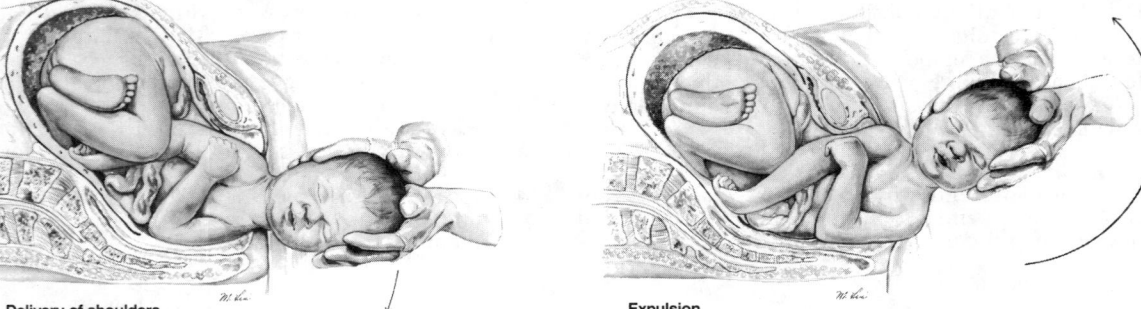

Engagement, descent flexion

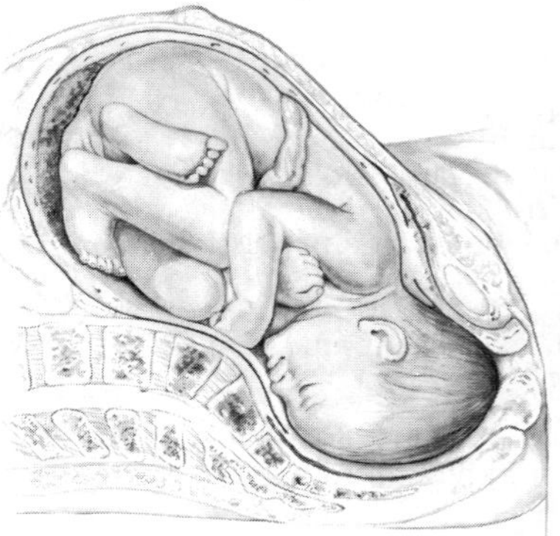

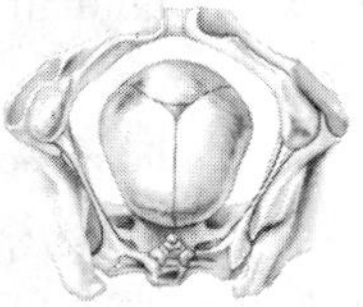

Internal rotation

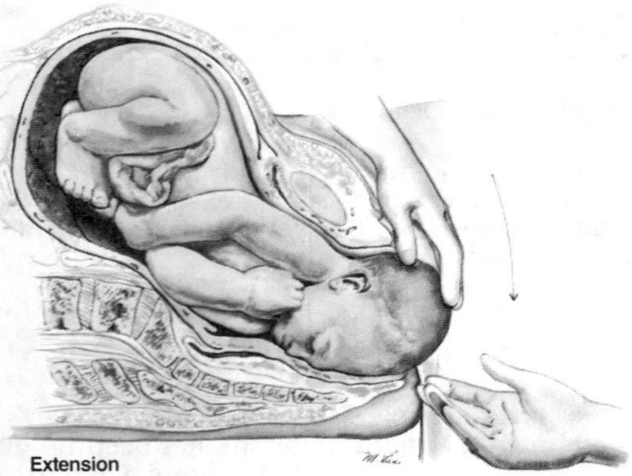

Extension

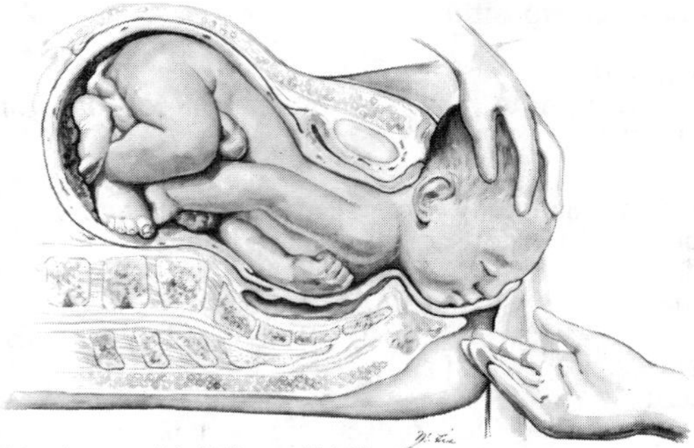

Extension complete (delivery of fetal head)

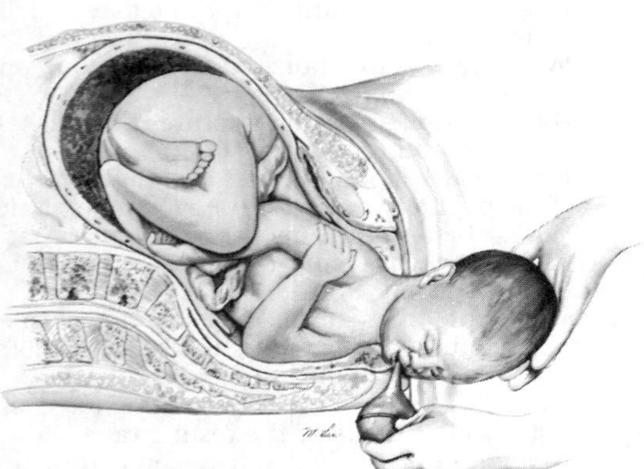

Aspiration of trachea

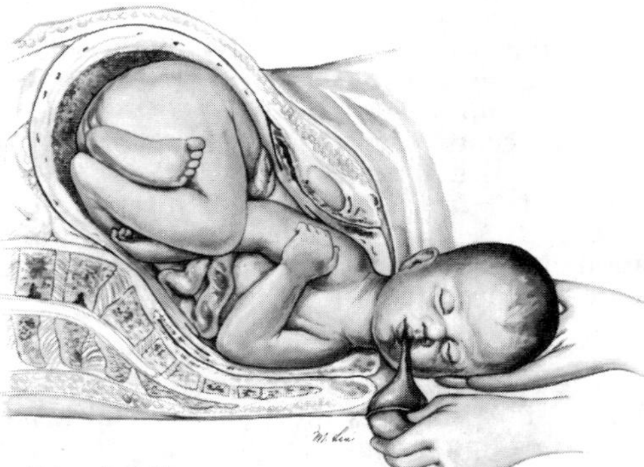

External rotation

Delivery of shoulders

Expulsion

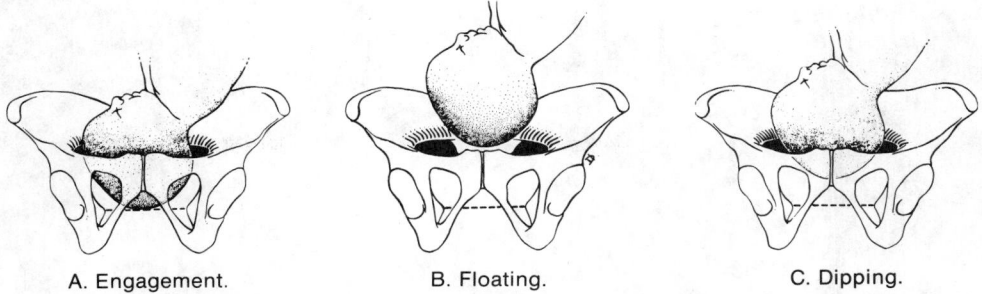

A. Engagement.   B. Floating.   C. Dipping.

FIGURE 35-5 *Engagement, floating, and dipping. (From Oxom H and Foote WR. Human Labor and Birth. New York, Appleton–Century–Crofts)*

Methods for Determining Fetal Presentation

A. Vaginal Examination and Determination of Fetal Landmarks Presenting

B. Leopold's Maneuvers
Determined by abdominal palpitation (Fig. 35-7).

1. First maneuver (Fig. 35-7A)—to determine if fetal head or breech is in uterine fundus. Palpate sides of uterus and fundus. Head feels hard and round, freely movable and ballotable; breech feels large, nodular, softer.
2. Second maneuver (Fig. 35-7B)—to determine the position of the fetal extremities, the fetal back, and the anterior shoulder. Place hands on the sides of the abdomen to identify the location of the back and small parts. Palpate down sides of uterus applying gentle but deep pressure. On side of fetal back, a long continuous structure will be felt; side with fetal extremities will feel nodular, reflecting portions of fetal extremities.
3. Third maneuver (Fig. 35-7C)—to determine the portion of the fetus that is presenting and if engagement has occurred. Grasp the lower uterine segment between the thumb and fingers of one hand to feel the presenting part. If presenting part is movable, engagement has not occurred; if engagement has occurred, fetal part feels fixed in the pelvis. The head is at inlet or in pelvis in 90% of women.
4. Fourth maneuver (Fig. 35-7D)—to confirm the findings of the third maneuver and to determine the flexion of the vertex. Turn and face the woman's feet. Gently move the fingers down the sides of the uterus. The cephalic prominence is felt on the side where there is greater resistance to the descent of the fingers into the pelvis.

C. Ultrasonography
See page 989.

Assessing Fetal Heart Tones

Fetal heart tones are auscultated with a DeLee Hillis fetoscope, or doppler.
1. Determine the position, presentation, and lie of the fetus by palpation. As internal rotation and descent occur, the location of the fetal heart tone changes, swinging gradually from the lateral to the medial area and dropping until immediately before birth, when it is above the pubic bone (Fig. 35-8).
2. Place the fetoscope or doppler on the abdomen over the back or chest of fetus. Avoid friction noises caused by fingers on the abdominal surface area.
3. Differentiate between fetal heart tone and other abdominal sounds.
   a. *Fetal heart tone*—a rapid crisp or ticking sound.
   b. *Uterine bruit*—a soft murmur, caused by the passage of blood through dilated uterine vessels; is synchronous with maternal pulse.
   c. *Funic souffle (uterine souffle)*—a hissing sound produced by passage of blood through the umbilical arteries; it is synchronous with the FHR.
4. Listen and count the rate for 1 full minute; note the location and character when counting.
5. Check the rate before, during, and after a contraction to detect any slowing or irregularities.
6. Check the fetal heart tone immediately after the rupture of membranes; a sudden release of fluid may cause a prolapse of the umbilical cord.

Assessing Uterine Contractions

Intensity, frequency, duration:

1. Place fingertips gently on the fundus.
2. As contraction begins, tension will be felt under the fingertips. Uterus will become harder, then slowly soften.
3. The intensity may be described as follows:
   a. Mild—the uterine muscle is somewhat tense.

FIGURE 35-4 *Mechanism of delivery for a vertex presentation. (From Whitley N. A manual of clinical obstetrics (1985). Philadelphia, JB Lippincott.)*

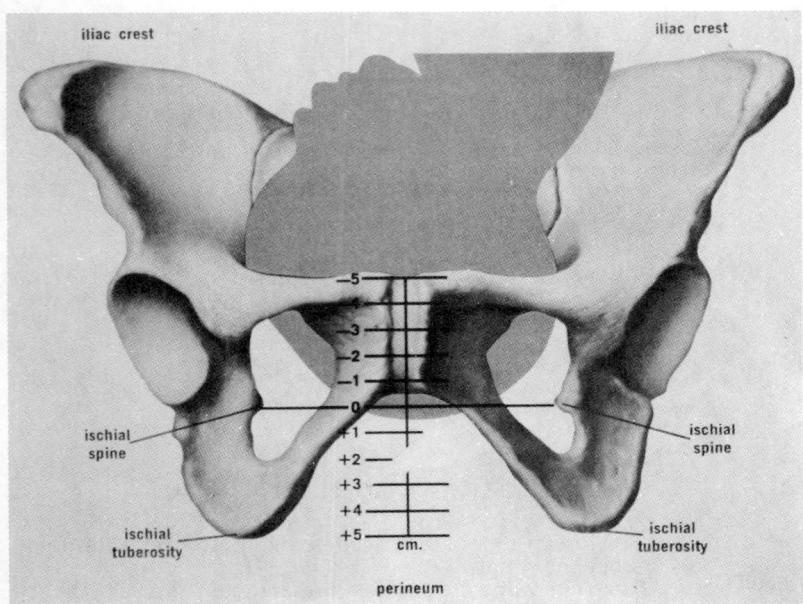

iliac crest   iliac crest

ischial spine

ischial spine

ischial tuberosity

ischial tuberosity

cm.

perineum

FIGURE 35-6 *Stations of presenting part. The location of the presenting part in relation to the level of the ischial spines is designated station and indicates the degree of advancement of the presenting part through the pelvis. Stations are expressed in centimeters above (minus) or below (plus) the level of the ischial spines (zero). (Courtesy of Ross Laboratories)*

b. Moderate—the uterine muscle is moderately firm.
c. Strong (hard)—the uterine muscle is so firm that it seems almost boardlike.
4. The frequency is measured in minutes—represents the time from the beginning of one contraction until the beginning of the next.
5. Duration of a contraction is timed from the moment the uterus first begins to tighten until it relaxes again.
6. As labor progresses, the character of the contractions changes and they last longer.
7. When the cervix becomes completely dilated (the transition stage), the contractions become very strong, last for 60 seconds, and occur at 2- to 3-minute intervals.

> **❖ NURSING ALERT:**
> If any contraction lasts longer than 90 seconds and is not followed by a period of uterine muscle relaxation, notify the health care provider immediately. Uterine rupture and fetal hypoxia may occur.

Vaginal Examination

See Figure 35-9.

1. Place the woman in lithotomy position.
2. Conduct examination gently, under aseptic conditions.
3. Evaluate the following:
   a. Condition of cervix.
      (1) Hard or soft (in labor, cervix is soft).
      (2) Effaced and thin or thick and long (in labor, cervix is thin and effaced.
      (3) Easily dilatable or resistant.
      (4) Closed or open (dilated); degree of dilation.
   b. Presentation
      (1) Breech, cephalic (head), or shoulder.
      (2) Caput succedaneum (edema occurring in and under fetal scalp) present (small or large).

(3) Station identified: engaged, floating.
c. Position
   (1) Cephalic presentation (identification of the sagittal suture and of its direction).
   (2) Location of posterior fontanelle
d. Membranes
   (1) Intact
   (2) Ruptured
      (a) Drainage of fluid
      (b) Passage of meconium
   (3) Usually increases frequency and intensity of uterine contractions.
   (4) Contraindicated in presence of vaginal bleeding, premature labor, or abnormal fetal presentation or position.

Assessing Woman's/Couple's Expectations and Concerns

1. What are their concerns?
2. How anxious are they?
3. What has been their preparation for labor (type, by whom, and when)?
4. What is their understanding of the labor process?
5. What are their expectations of the labor and delivery process (prepared childbirth, anesthesia, analgesics, use of birthing room, etc.)?
6. How well are they coping and how well are they communicating with each other?
7. Review written birth plan with the couple.

◆ FETAL MONITORING

The purposes of *continuous fetal monitoring* during labor are to monitor the progress of a woman's contraction pattern and to monitor the condition of the fetus in response to the stress of uterine contractions.

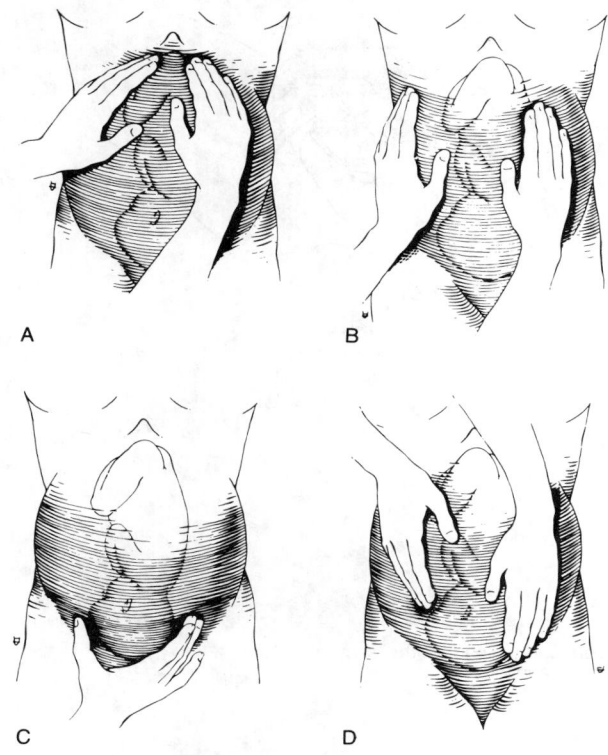

FIGURE 35-7 *Leopold's maneuvers.*

External Monitoring (Indirect Monitoring)

Separate transducers are secured to the woman's abdomen: a tokodynamometer (tocotransducer) measures abdominal tension, and an ultrasonic transducer transmits fetal heart sounds into electrical signals that record on a graph chart.

> **NURSING ALERT:**
> The external monitoring of uterine contractions is not accurate for intensity. External monitoring of FHR is not accurate for variability.

1. The ultrasonic transducer device should be applied over the area of the abdomen where the sharpest fetal heart sound is heard. Lubricate the face of the transducer with a thin layer of ultrasonic gel to aid in the transmission of sounds.
2. The transducer will need to be readjusted when the fetus changes positions.
3. The tokodynamometer recording uterine contractions will need to be reapplied over the fundus as the fetus and uterus descend during labor.

Internal Monitoring (Direct Monitoring)

A method of recording intrauterine pressure and FHR through internal measurements, this method is more accurate than external monitoring.

1. Fetal electrocardiograph—obtained by screwing a small spiral electrode into the presenting part (the membranes must be ruptured, the cervix dilated at least 2 to 3 cm, the presenting part must be accessible and identifiable).
2. Uterine contractions are recorded by means of a water-filled catheter placed in the uterine cavity behind the presenting part. The catheter is filled with sterile water and is connected to an external pressure transducer that converts the pressure values in millimeters of mercury (mm Hg) on the graph.
3. Monitor strips record the fetal heart and uterine contraction simultaneously.

Interpretation

A. *Baseline Rate*
1. Fetal heart rate is initially evaluated for the baseline rate.
2. Baseline rate is the FHR when the mother is not in labor, when the fetus is not moving, between contractions, and when the fetus is not being stimulated.
3. Fluctuations in the heart rate are either accelerations or decelerations.

B. *Tachycardia*
1. An FHR of 160 or more, or more than 30 beats/minute above the normal baseline rate for at least 10 minutes.
2. Etiology—early fetal hypoxia, fetal immaturity, maternal fever, maternal hyperthyroidism, maternal ingestion of parasympatholytic and beta-sympathomimetic drugs, amnionitis, fetal anemia, fetal cardiac dysrhythmias, and fetal heart failure.

C. *Bradycardia*
1. A baseline FHR below 120 for at least 10 minutes.
2. Fetal bradycardia above 90 beats/minute in the third stage of labor is not considered abnormal unless there is a loss of variability.
3. Etiology—late or profound fetal hypoxia, maternal hypotension, prolonged umbilical cord compression, hypothermia, maternal ingestion of beta-adrenergic blocking drugs, and anesthetics.

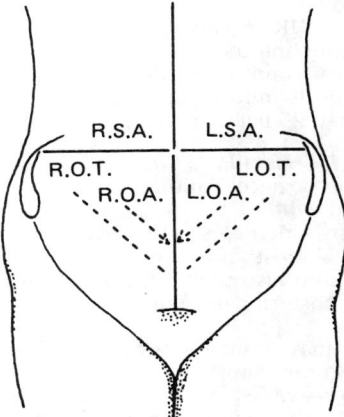

FIGURE 35-8 *Fetal heart tone locations on the abdominal wall indicating possible corresponding fetal positions and the effects of the internal rotation of the fetus.*

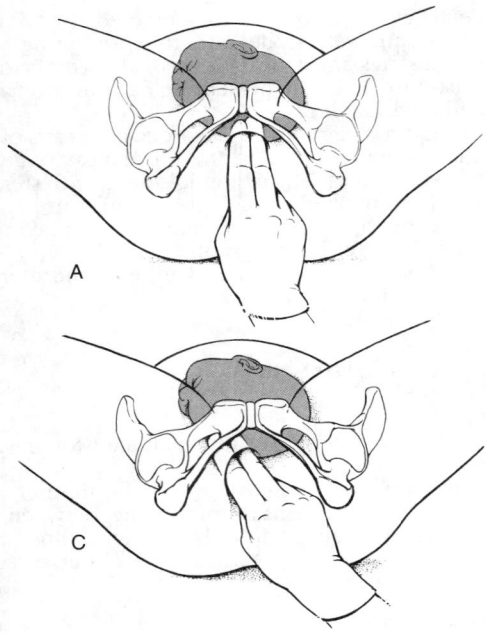
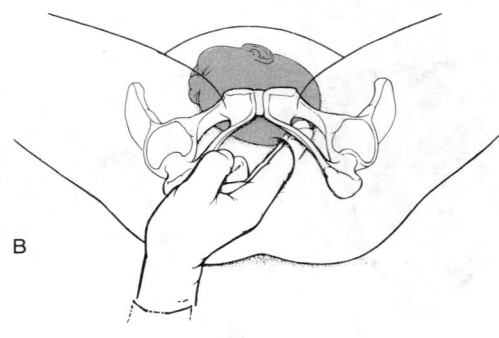

FIGURE 35-9 *Vaginal examination.* **(A)** *Determining the station and palpating the sagittal suture.* **(B)** *Identifying the posterior fontanelle.* **(C)** *Identifying the anterior fontanelle.*

D. Variability
1. Beat-to-beat changes in FHR that result from the interplay between the sympathetic and parasympathetic nervous systems.
2. Variability indicates normal neurologic function in relation to heart rate and also fetal reserve.
3. Short-term variability—the beat-to-beat change in FHR.
4. Long-term variability—the rhythmic changes in the heart rate, usually 3 to 5 cycles/minute.
5. Short- and long-term variability tend to increase and decrease together.
6. Normal variability is 6 to 25 beats/minute and is described below.
7. Overview of FHR variability:
   a. 0 to 2 beats/minute, no variability.
   b. 3 to 5 beats/minute, minimal variability.
   c. 6 to 25 beats/minute, moderate variability.
   d. More than 25 beats/minute, marked variability.

E. Periodic Fetal Heart Rate Changes
1. Acceleration or deceleration of FHR are due to stress experienced by the fetus.
2. Acceleration—increases in the FHR.
   a. Etiology—most often fetal movements or fetal stimulation; also seen with breech presentations, occiput posterior presentations, and uterine contractions.
   b. Shape—may or may not resemble the shape of the uterine contraction.
   c. Recovery—varies, and if accelerations occur with contractions, they may return to baseline as the uterine pressure decreases.
   d. Treatment—observe the tracing for late or variable decelerations later in labor.

3. Early decelerations
   a. Etiology—head compression from uterine contractions, vaginal examination, scalp stimulation; also frequently seen in women who are completely dilated.
   b. Shape—mirror image of the contraction, and all look the same.
   c. Onset—early in the contraction, with the peak being at the acme of the contraction.
   d. Recovery—returns to baseline by the end of the contraction.
   e. Treatment—none.
4. Late decelerations
   a. Etiology—uteroplacental insufficiency.
   b. Shape—uniform in shape with a reverse mirror image of the contraction phase.
   c. Onset—late in the contraction, usually after the acme of the contraction with the low point of the deceleration occurring well after the acme.
   d. Recovery—returns to baseline after the end of the contraction.
   e. Treatment—aimed at increasing uteroplacental perfusion.
      (1) Includes changing maternal position, with the left lateral being the position of choice, correcting any hypotension through increasing the maintenance intravenous fluids.
      (2) Oxytocin is stopped.
      (3) Oxygen is administered by face mask at 8 to 12 L/minute.
5. Variable decelerations
   a. Etiology—cord compression that can result from maternal position, prolapsed cord, cord around a fetal part, a short cord, and a true knot in the cord.
   b. Shape—variable, and does not follow the uterine contraction; frequently are shaped like a "U" or "W."

c. Onset—variable, frequently preceded by an acceleration.
d. Recovery—occurs rapidly, often followed by an acceleration.
e. Treatment—involves changing of maternal position, observing that the return occurs quickly and that there is no loss of variability.
6. Combined deceleration patterns do occur and make identification of the patterns difficult.

F. *Unusual Patterns*
1. The sinusoidal pattern is characterized by a waveform of rhythmic regular oscillations occurring evenly above and below the baseline.
   a. Short-term variability is decreased or absent.
   b. Fetal heart rate ranges between 120 and 160.
   c. Seen in the presence of fetal anemia and fetal hypoxia.
   d. Seen after narcotic analgesic administration for a temporary period, and in this instance is not associated with a compromised fetal outcome.

◆ FIRST STAGE OF LABOR— LATENT PHASE

Nursing Diagnoses

A. Altered Nutrition: Less Than Body Requirements related to food restriction during labor
B. Fluid Volume Deficit related to decreased oral intake
C. Anxiety related to concern for self and the fetus
D. Pain related to uterine contractions and/or position of the fetus

Nursing Interventions

A. *Maintaining Nutrition and Hydration*
1. Provide clear liquids and ice chips as allowed.
2. Evaluate urine for ketones and glucose.
3. Administer intravenous fluids as indicated.

B. *Relieving Anxiety*
1. Establish a relationship with the woman/couple.
2. Provide information on the health care facility's policies and procedures.
3. Inform the woman/couple of maternal status and fetal status and labor progress.
4. Explain all procedures and equipment used during labor.
5. Answer any questions the woman/couple have.
6. Review the birth plan and make appropriate revisions.
7. Monitor maternal vital signs
   a. Temperature every 4 hours, unless elevated or membranes ruptured, then every 2 hours.
   b. Pulse and respirations every hour unless receiving pain medication, then every 15 to 30 minutes or as indicated.
   c. Blood pressure every hour unless hypertension or hypotension exists or woman has received pain medication or anesthesia. Then evaluate more frequently based on findings or as indicated.
8. Monitor FHR.
   a. Evaluate once an hour for 15 to 20 minutes for intermittent monitoring

b. Evaluate the monitor strip at least hourly with continuous monitoring.
c. Evaluate immediately and after each of the next 5 contractions on rupture of the membranes.

C. *Controlling Pain*
1. Encourage ambulation as tolerated if membranes are not ruptured and the presenting part is engaged. (This may vary according to health care provider.)
2. Encourage diversional activities, such as reading, talking, watching TV, playing cards, listening to music.
3. Review, evaluate, and teach proper breathing techniques.
   a. Slow-paced breathing—Relax, take one deep breath and exhale slowly and completely. Breathe deeply, slowly, rhythmically throughout contraction. Follow with another deep, complete breath. Take about six to nine breaths a minute.
   b. Modified-paced breathing—Take one deep breath and exhale slowly and completely. Breathe regularly at more shallow level. When stronger contraction occurs, breathe more quickly with very light breaths. Then take deep breath and exhale slowly.
   c. Patterned-paced breathing—Concentrate on breathing in controlled manner. Take a deep breath and exhale slowly and completely. At beginning of contraction, take a fairly deep breath. Then engage in modified paced breathing. After a certain number of breaths the woman exhales with a more forceful puff or blow. The number of breaths before the more forceful exhalation can range between two and six or the ratio of breaths to blows may be constant. This breathing pattern is most often used during transition.
4. Encourage a warm shower.
5. Encourage relaxation techniques.
6. Provide comfort measures
   a. Give back rubs.
   b. Assist the woman to change position.
   c. Reposition external monitors as needed.

Evaluation

A. Tolerates fluids well and urine negative for ketones and glucose
B. Verbalizes positive statements about self and fetus
C. Reports pain decreased from comfort strategies

◆ FIRST STAGE OF LABOR— ACTIVE/TRANSITION PHASE

Nursing Diagnoses

A. Anxiety related to concern for self and fetus
B. Pain related to uterine contractions and/or nausea and vomiting
C. Altered Urinary Elimination related to epidural anesthesia or from pressure of the fetus
D. Ineffective Individual Coping related to discomfort
E. Risk for Infection related to rupture of the membranes
F. Impaired Physical Mobility related to medical interventions and/or discomfort

G. Ineffective Breathing Pattern related to pain and fatigue

Nursing Interventions

A. *Relieving Anxiety*
1. Monitor maternal vital signs and FHR and keep the woman/couple informed of the maternal and fetus status.
   a. Maternal temperature every 4 hours unless elevated or membranes ruptured, then every 2 hours.
   b. Blood pressure, pulse, respirations every 30 minutes unless receiving pain medication or epidural anesthesia; then at least every 15 minutes or more frequently as indicated until stable.
   c. Evaluate FHR every 30 minutes unless using continuous monitoring.
   d. Evaluate once an hour for 10 to 15 minutes with intermittent monitoring.
2. Provide encouragement and support.
3. Involve the support person in the woman's care.

B. *Minimizing Pain*
1. Encourage position changes for comfort.
2. Assist the woman with breathing and relaxation techniques as needed.
3. Provide back, leg, and shoulder massage as needed.
4. Administer prescribed analgesia as needed (Table 35-2).
   a. Confirm that the woman has no known allergies to the drug.
   b. Describe effects of the drug, such as making the woman feel sleepy, relaxed, and more comfortable.
   c. Evaluate vital signs after drug administration.
   d. Observe for signs and symptoms of a drug reaction.
   e. Evaluate FHR pattern. Decreased variability and a sinusoidal pattern are sometimes seen after narcotic administration to the mother.
   f. Maintain intravenous fluids as indicated.
5. Assist with regional anesthesia (epidural) if needed.
   a. Administer intravenous fluid bolus of Ringer's lactate as indicated.
   b. Assist with positioning the woman.
   c. Monitor the FHR during the procedure and assess for a nonreassuring pattern.
   d. Monitor the woman's blood pressure, pulse, and respirations every 2 to 3 minutes after the procedure, then every 15 minutes thereafter or as indicated.
   e. Observe for hypotension, nausea and vomiting, and light-headedness after the procedure. If these occur:
      (1) Increase the rate of the intravenous fluid
      (2) Flatten the head of the bed and put in Trendelenburg's if necessary.
      (3) Turn the woman to her side.
      (4) Administer oxygen face mask at 8 to 10 L/minute.
      (5) Have ephedrine available
   f. Provide safe environment.
   g. Document on the woman's record and monitor strip according to institutional policy.

TABLE 35-2 Obstetric Analgesia and Anesthesia

Drug	Comment
Narcotic Analgesics Meperidine (Demerol) Butorphanol (Stadol) Nalbuphine (Nubain) Fentanyl (Sublimaze)	Decreases fear and anxiety, promotes physical relaxation and rest between contractions; may cause nausea and vomiting; respiratory depression is the main side effect and is seen primarily in the newborn.
Ataractics Promethazine (Phenergan) Promazine (Sparine) Hydroxyzine (Vistaril)	May be used in combination with narcotics; potentiates narcotics; may be used as an antiemetic.
Barbiturates Sodium secobarbital (Seconal) Sodium pentobarbital (Nembutal) Sodium phenobarbital (Luminal)	Produces sedation and hypnosis.
Epidural narcotics	Used with a local anesthetic to provide pain relief with a decreased motor block in labor. Used postoperatively to promote long-acting analgesia.
Epidural Block	Used for labor to provide a sensory block up to the T-10–T-12 level. Medication is given through the epidural catheter. Used for cesarean section and postpartum tubal ligation by increasing the level of anesthesia up to T-4–T-6.
Subarachnoid Block (Spinal)	Used for such surgical procedures as a cesarean section and postpartum tubal ligation. The procedure is quicker and easier to perform. There is no catheter for the procedure. Medication lasts for a finite period of time.
Local Anesthesia	Used for pain control of the perineal area for an episiotomy or repair during a vaginal delivery.
Pudendal Block	Used during the second stage of labor just before delivery to numb the lower vaginal canal and the perineum for delivery. May also be used to provide pain relief for a forceps delivery if the woman doesn't have an epidural.
General Anesthesia	Used for emergency delivery involving cesarean section; if the woman refuses regional anesthesia; if regional anesthesia cannot be performed.

C. *Encouraging Bladder Emptying*
1. Encourage the woman to void every 2 hours at least 100 mL.
2. Palpate the lower abdomen and evaluate for a distended bladder.
3. Assist with enabling the woman to void by providing time and privacy, running the sink water gently, providing a perineal bottle of warm water for the woman to squirt against her perineum.
4. Catheterize (in and out) when necessary.
5. Monitor intake and output.

D. *Strengthening Coping with Active Labor and Transition*
1. Assist the woman with breathing and relaxation techniques.
2. Encourage a positive attitude.
3. Encourage the labor coach to assist with coping strategies.
4. Provide comfort measures, which may include:
   a. Back and leg rubs.
   b. A cool cloth to face, neck, abdomen, or back.
   c. Ice chips to moisten mouth.
   d. An emesis basin.
   e. Clean pads and linens as needed.
   f. A quiet environment.
   g. Repositioning, either side is preferable, with pillow and blanket. Supports as needed.
5. Encourage the woman to deal with one contraction at a time.
6. Provide reassurance and encouragement during each contraction.
7. Provide information on the contraction's ascent, peak, and descent.
8. Encourage resting between contractions.
9. Encourage the woman not to push with feelings of rectal pressure until complete cervical dilation has occurred. Assisting her with panting may be helpful.

E. *Preventing Intrauterine Infection*
1. Take the woman's temperature and record every 2 hours.
2. Change the pads and linens when wet or soiled.
3. Provide perineal care after voiding and as needed.
4. Discourage the use of perineal pads, because they create a warm, moist environment for bacteria.
5. Minimize vaginal exams.
6. Observe for fetal tachycardia.
7. Assess complete blood count as indicated.

F. *Maintaining Mobility*
1. Provide information regarding limitations and opportunities for movement with electronic fetal monitoring.
2. Encourage the woman to be out of bed ambulating and/or sitting in a chair while being monitored, if indicated.
3. Encourage position change in bed every hour or as indicated.
4. Assist with back rubs, leg massage, and leg exercises while in bed.

G. *Encouraging Effective Breathing Techniques*
1. Assist the woman with altering her breathing and relaxation techniques as needed to maintain control.
2. Inform the woman that the urge to push is common during transition and is usually due to rapid fetal descent, the dilating cervix, and uterine contractions. Pushing with feelings of rectal pressure before complete cervical dilatation should be avoided due to risks of increasing cervical edema and lacerations.

3. Assist the woman to avoid pushing prematurely by:
   a. Maintaining close eye contact during breathing.
   b. Breathing with the woman, having her blow out strong, short breaths.
4. Awaken the woman before the beginning of each contraction so that she can gain control of her breathing if she has partial amnesia between contractions.

Evaluation

A. Verbalizes positive statements about self and fetus
B. Reports pain decreased from comfort strategies and medical interventions
C. Bladder remains undistended and the woman voids or bladder is emptied for 100 mL or more
D. Directs strategies for decreasing discomfort
E. Absence of fever and signs of infection
F. Changes position during labor
G. Uses breathing techniques during contractions

◆ SECOND STAGE OF LABOR
Nursing Diagnoses

A. Fear/Anxiety related to impending delivery
B. Pain related to descent of the fetus
C. Risk for Infection related to episiotomy and/or tissue trauma.

Nursing Interventions

A. *Minimizing Fear and Anxiety*
1. Monitor maternal vital signs as follows:
   a. Blood pressure—every 5 to 30 minutes depending on the woman's status.
   b. Pulse and respirations—every 15 to 30 minutes.
   c. Temperature—every 2 hours once membranes have ruptured.
2. Monitor FHR and uterine contractions every 15 minutes in low-risk women and every 5 minutes in high-risk women.
   a. Early decelerations and some fetal bradycardia may occur due to head compression.
   b. There is normally no loss of variability during pushing.
   c. Contractions may become less frequent, but intensity does not decrease.
3. Explain procedures and equipment during pushing and delivery.
4. Keep the woman/couple informed of their status.
5. Provide frequent, positive encouragement.
   a. Use of a mirror often allows the woman to see her progress.
6. Assist and instruct the woman in the pushing technique.
   a. Take a full, cleansing breath, in through the nose and out through the mouth, at the beginning and end of each contraction.
   b. Push only during contractions.
   c. Push down toward the perineum with the abdominal muscles and try to keep the rest of the body relaxed.
   d. For each push, take a breath and push for 6 to 7 seconds while exhaling slightly.

B. *Promoting Comfort*
1. Assist the woman to a comfortable position.
   a. Left or right lateral, squatting, or semisitting positions may be used.
   b. Assist the woman with pulling her legs back so that her knees are flexed.
   c. Teach the woman to put her chin to her chest so that her body forms a "C" shape while pushing.
2. Evaluate bladder fullness and encourage voiding or catheterize as needed.
3. Evaluate effectiveness of anesthesia as indicated.

C. *Preventing Infection and Promoting Safety*
1. Prepare the birthing room or delivery room using aseptic technique, allowing ample time for setup before delivery.
2. Prepare the infant resuscitation area for delivery.
3. Prepare necessary items for newborn care.
4. Notify necessary personnel to prepare for delivery.
5. Transfer the primigravida to the delivery room when the fetal head is crowning. The multigravida is taken earlier depending on fetal size and speed of fetal descent.
6. Place all side rails up before moving. Instruct the woman to keep her hands off the rails, and move from the bed to the delivery table between contractions.
7. Position the woman for delivery using a large cushion for her head, back, and shoulders. Elevate the head of the bed. Stirrups or footrests may be used for leg or foot support. Pad the stirrups. Place both legs in the stirrups at the same time to avoid ligament strain, backache, or injury.
8. Cleanse the vulva and perineal areas once the woman is positioned for delivery.
   a. Cleanse from the mons to the lower abdomen.
   b. Then cleanse the groin to the inner thigh on each side.
   c. Then cleanse each labia.
   d. Finally, cleanse the introitus.
9. Guide the woman step-by-step during the delivery process.
   a. When the fetal head is encircled by the vulvovaginal ring, an episiotomy may be performed to prevent tearing.
   b. When the head is delivered, mucus is wiped from the face, and the mouth and nose are aspirated with a bulb syringe.
   c. If loops of umbilical cord are found around the infant's neck, they are loosened and slipped from around the neck. If the cord cannot be slipped over the head, it is clamped with two clamps and cut between the two clamps.
   d. After this step, the woman is asked to give a gentle push in order that the infant's body may be quickly delivered.
   e. After delivery of the infant's body and cutting of the cord, the infant is shown to the parents and then placed on the maternal abdomen or taken to the radiant warmer for inspection and identification procedures.
10. Practice universal precautions during labor and delivery.

Evaluation

A. Verbalizes positive statements about delivery outcome
B. Reports decreased pain from proper positioning
C. Absence of fever

◆ THIRD STAGE OF LABOR

Nursing Diagnosis
A. Impaired Tissue Integrity related to placental separation

Nursing Interventions

A. *Promoting Tissue Integrity*
1. Ask the woman to bear down gently, or fundal pressure may be applied to facilitate delivery of the placenta on signs of separation (Fig. 35-10). These include the following:
   a. The uterus rises upward in the abdomen.
   b. The umbilical cord lengthens.
   c. Trickle or spurt of blood appears.
   d. The uterus becomes globular in shape.
2. Evaluate the placenta for size, shape, and cord site implantation.
3. Check to see that the placenta and membranes are complete.
4. Evaluate and massage the uterine fundus until firm.
5. Evaluate vaginal bleeding.
6. Administer Pitocin as indicated to assist with maintaining uterine tone.
7. Inspection and repair of lacerations of the vagina and cervix are made by the birth attendant.

Evaluation

A. An intact placenta is delivered

◆ IMMEDIATE CARE OF THE NEWBORN

Nursing Diagnoses

A. Ineffective Airway Clearance related to nasal and oral secretions from delivery
B. Ineffective Thermoregulation related to environment and immature ability for adaptation
C. Risk for Injury related to immature defenses of the newborn

Nursing Interventions

A. *Promoting Airway Clearance and Transitioning of the Newborn*
1. Wipe mucus from the face and mouth and nose. Aspirate with a bulb syringe.
   a. If meconium is present before the delivery, mechanical suctioning of the nasopharynx with an 8 or 10 French catheter is done.
   b. Suctioning is done by the birth attendant when the head is delivered.
2. Clamp the umbilical cord approximately 2.5 cm (1 in.) from the abdominal wall with a cord clamp.
   a. Cord clamping is done by the birth attendant.
   b. Count the number of vessels in the cord—fewer than three vessels has been associated with renal and cardiac anomalies.

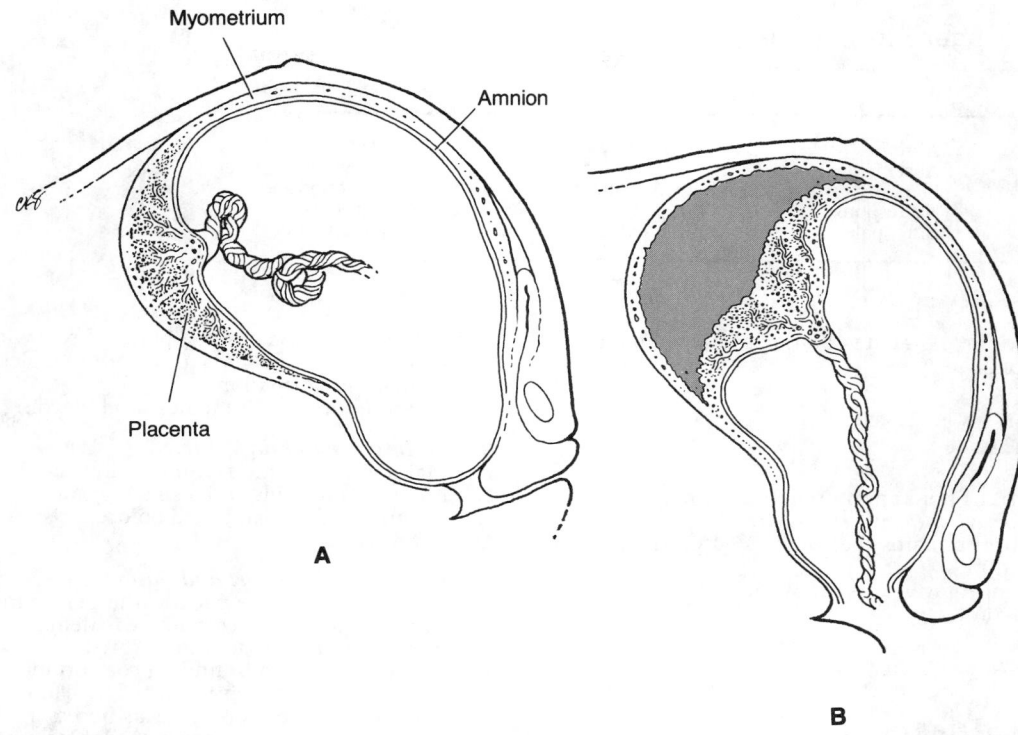

FIGURE 35-10 *Placental separation.* **(A)** *Placenta attached to uterine wall.* **(B)** *Placenta separated from uterine wall.*

3. Evaluate the newborn's condition by the Apgar scoring system (Table 35-3) at 1 and 5 minutes after birth.
   a. Newborns scoring 7 to 10 are free of immediate stress.
   b. Newborns scoring 4 to 6 are moderately depressed.
   c. Newborns scoring 0 to 3 are severely depressed.

B. *Promoting Thermoregulation*
1. Dry the newborn immediately after delivery.
   a. A wet, small newborn loses up to 200 calories per 1 kg/minute in the delivery room through evaporation, convection, and radiation. Drying the infant cuts this heat loss in half.
2. Cover the newborn's head with a cotton stocking cap to prevent heat loss.
3. Wrap the newborn in warm blankets.
4. Place the newborn under a radiant heat warmer, or place the newborn on the mother's abdomen with skin-to-skin contact.
5. Provide a warm, draft-free environment for the newborn.
6. Take the newborn's axillary temperature—a normal temperature is between 36.4°C and 37.2°C (97.5°F–99.0°F).

C. *Preventing Injury and Infection*
1. Administer prophylactic treatment against ophthalmia neonatorum (gonorrheal or chlamydial).
   a. Treatment may be with silver nitrate drops, erythromycin, or tetracycline antibiotic ophthalmic ointment or drops.

   b. If the mother has a positive gonococcal or chlamydial culture, the newborn will require further treatment.
   c. Treatment is mandatory in all states.
2. Administer a prophylactic injection of vitamin K.
   a. This is done to prevent a neonatal hemorrhage during the first few days of life before the infant begins to produce its own vitamin K.
3. Place matching identification bracelets on the mother and the newborn.
   a. Bracelets are placed on the newborn's arms or legs.
   b. A similar bracelet is placed on the mother. The father or significant other may also wear a bracelet matching the mother's.
   c. Information includes the mother's name, hospital number, newborn's sex, race, and date and time of birth.
   d. Fingerprints of the mother and footprints of the newborn may also be done for the family. If footprints are to be done, remove all vernix from the foot before inking to improve the quality of the footprint.
   e. Complete all identification procedures before the infant is taken from the delivery room.
4. Weigh and measure the infant.
   a. Normal newborn weight is 2,700 to 4,000 g (6–9 lb).
   b. Normal newborn length is 48 to 53 cm (19–21 inches).
5. Administer hepatitis B vaccine.
   a. Vaccination of all infants born in the United States is recommended within 12 hours after birth for the

TABLE 35-3 Apgar Scoring Chart

Sign	0	1	2
Heart rate	Absent	Slow (less than 100)	Over 100
Respiratory effort	Absent	Slow, irregular	Good, crying
Muscle tone	Flaccid	Some flexion of extremities	Active motion
Reflex irritability	No response	Cry	Vigorous cry
Color	Blue, pale	Body pink, extremities blue	Completely pink

prevention of acute and chronic hepatitis B infection.

Evaluation

A. Newborn transitions appropriately as evidenced by Apgar score between 7 and 10
B. Temperature remains between 36.4°C and 37.2°C (97.5°F–99.0°F)
C. Identification bracelets on newborn and initial newborn care complete

◆ FOURTH STAGE OF LABOR

Nursing Diagnoses

A. Risk for Injury related to uterine atony and hemorrhage
B. Fluid Volume Deficit related to decreased oral intake, bleeding, and diaphoresis
C. Pain/Fatigue related to tissue trauma and birth process
D. Altered Urinary Elimination related to epidural or spinal anesthesia and tissue trauma
E. Sensory/Perceptual Alterations (tactile) related to effects of regional anesthesia
F. Altered Parenting related to the newborn and/or inexperience

Nursing Interventions

A. *Promoting Uterine Contraction and Controlling Bleeding*
1. Monitor blood pressure, pulse, and respirations every 15 minutes for 1 hour, then every $\frac{1}{2}$ hour to 1 hour until stable or transferred to the postpartum unit.
2. Take temperature every 4 hours unless elevated, then every 2 hours.
3. Evaluate the following at the time vital signs are taken:
   a. Uterine fundal tone, height, and position. The uterus should be firm around the level of the umbilicus, at the midline.
   b. Amount of vaginal bleeding.
      (1) Scant—blood only on tissue when wiped or less then 1-in. stain on perineal pad within 1 hour.
      (2) Small/light—less than 4-in. stain on perineal pad within 1 hour.
      (3) Moderate—less than 6-in. stain on perineal pad within 1 hour.

      (4) Heavy—saturated perineal pad within 1 hour.
   c. Perineum for edema, discoloration, bleeding, or hematoma formation.
   d. Episiotomy for intactness and bleeding.

B. *Maintaining Fluid Volume*
1. Maintain intravenous fluids as indicated.
2. Provide oral fluids and a snack or meal as tolerated.
3. Encourage drink and food before assisting the woman out of bed.

C. *Relieving Discomfort and Fatigue*
1. Apply a covered ice pack to the perineum for an episiotomy, perineal laceration, or edema.
2. Administer analgesics as indicated.
3. Assist the woman in finding comfortable positions.
4. Assist the woman with a partial bath and perineal care, and change linens and pads as necessary.
5. Allow for privacy and rest periods between postpartum checks.
6. Provide warm blankets and reassure the woman that tremors are common during this period.

D. *Encouraging Bladder Emptying*
1. Evaluate the bladder for distention.
2. Encourage the woman to void.
   a. Provide adequate time and privacy.
   b. The sound from a running faucet may stimulate voiding.
   c. Gently squirting tepid water against the perineum in a perineal bottle may help.
3. Catheterize the woman (in and out) if the bladder is full and she is unable to void.
   a. Birth trauma, anesthesia, and pain from lacerations and episiotomy may reduce or alter the voiding reflex.
   b. Bladder distention may displace the uterus upward and to the side.

E. *Assessing Return of Sensation*
1. Evaluate mobility and sensation of the lower extremities.
2. Evaluate vital signs.
3. Remain with the woman and assist her out of bed for the first time. Evaluate her ability to support her weight and ambulate.
4. Do not provide hot fluids if sensation is decreased.

F. *Promoting Parenting*
1. Show the newborn to the mother and father or support person immediately after birth when possible.
2. Encourage the mother and/or father to hold the baby as soon as possible.
3. Teach the mother/parents to hold the newborn close to their faces, about 8 to 12 inches, when talking to the baby.

4. Have the mother/parents look at and inspect the baby's body to familiarize themselves with their child.
5. Assist the mother with breast-feeding during the first 2 hours after birth. This is often a period of quiet alert time for the newborn and he or she will often readily take to the breast.
6. Provide quiet alone time in a low-lighted room for the family to become acquainted.
7. Observe and record the reaction of the mother/parents to the newborn.

Evaluation

A. Vital signs remain stable, vaginal bleeding within normal limits of less than 500 mL since delivery, and uterus remains firm at the midline
B. Tolerates fluids well after delivery
C. Verbalizes decreased perineal pain and feeling more rested
D. Voids greater than 100 mL within 6 hours of delivery
E. Ambulates without problems
F. Interacts with the newborn

Special Considerations

◆ NEWBORN RESUSCITATION

This procedure is most effective when there is a simple, organized, and efficient system established in the birth area.

Causes

Asphyxia is the main reason for newborn resuscitation.

A. Primary Apnea
1. Intrauterine asphyxia may result in passage of meconium, fetal tachycardia, loss of variability, late decelerations, or prolonged bradycardia.
2. Infants born with primary apnea will need sensory stimuli (tactile or positive-pressure ventilation) to initiate respirations.

B. Secondary Apnea
1. Secondary apnea occurs when primary apnea is unresolved. The heart rate drops and spontaneous gasps occur.
2. May occur in utero or after birth.
3. At birth these infants are pale, flaccid, and bradycardiac. Spontaneous respirations will not occur with sensory stimuli because of the biochemical, neurologic, and circulatory changes that have occurred.

Steps in Newborn Resuscitation

1. Call for assistance if needed.
2. Place the infant in a warm radiant warmer in Trendelenburg's position.
3. Suction the mouth, then the nose with a bulb syringe or wall suction.
4. Dry off the trunk with warmed towels and attempt to keep the infant warm.

5. Assess respiratory and cardiac status.
6. Begin bag and mask ventilation.
   a. Use an inspiratory pressure of 20 to 30 cm water at a rate of 40 to 60 breaths/minute.
   b. Observe chest movement and auscultate for air movement in all lung fields.
7. Begin external cardiac massage at a rate of 100 to 120 compressions/minute if needed.
8. Assist with endotracheal intubation if needed.
9. Assist with insertion of an umbilical venous line for administration of medications and fluids if needed.
10. Transport when stable.

◆ EMERGENCY DELIVERY

In delivery under emergency conditions, consider the woman and infant as a unit; work to prevent infection, injury, and hemorrhage in woman and infant and to establish respirations in the newborn.

Interventions

1. Provide reassurance and instruct the woman in a calm, controlled manner.
2. Instruct the woman to assume a lithotomy position.
3. Wash hands and cleanse perineum. This should be done by the birth attendant if time permits.
4. Exert gentle pressure against the head of the fetus to control its progress and prevent too rapid a delivery.
   a. Use a clean or sterile towel.
   b. This prevents undue stretching of the perineum.
   c. This prevents sudden expulsion through the vulva with subsequent infant and maternal complications.
5. Encourage the woman to pant at this time to prevent bearing down.
6. Rupture the membranes by tearing them at the nape of the infant's neck. This is done if membranes have not ruptured by the time the head is delivered.
7. Wipe the infant's face and mouth with a clean towel. Suction the mouth and nose with a bulb syringe if available.
8. Check to see if the cord is wrapped around the infant's neck or other body part. If the cord is too tight to permit slipping it over the infant's head, it must be clamped in 2 places and cut between the clamps before the rest of the body is delivered.
9. Hold the infant's head in both hands and gently exert downward pressure toward the floor, thus slipping the anterior shoulder under the symphysis pubis.
10. Support the infant's body and head as it is born.
11. Hold the infant with the head down to help drain mucus; wipe away excess mucus from the mouth and nose; gentle rubbing of the back may stimulate breathing.
12. Place the infant on the mother's abdomen where she can see him or her after the infant cries.
13. Avoid touching the perineal area to prevent infection.
14. Avoid pulling on the cord, which might break and cause hemorrhage.
15. Watch for signs of placental separation.
16. Do the following when the placenta is delivered:
    a. Clamp the cord with a cord clamp when the cord stops pulsating. If a clamp is not available, tie off the cord with any suitable material several centimeters from the infant's abdomen.

b. Do not cut the cord; it can be cut later under more sterile conditions.

c. Wrap the infant and placenta in a blanket; keep the infant warm and close to the mother.

17. Check fundal contractions; massage if indicated. Putting the baby to breast may help the uterus to contract.

18. Place identification of some kind on the mother and infant.

19. Give the woman fluids.

20. Assist the woman to a suitable environment, if she is not in a bed or in a place where she can lie down.

21. Do not leave the woman alone.

22. Teach the woman to massage her fundus; explain why the cord has not been cut.

23. Record the time and date of birth.

Selected References

Aldrich, C. J., et al. (1995). Late fetal heart decelerations and changes in cerebral oxygenation during the first stage of labour. *British Journal of Obstetrics and Gynecology, 102*(1), 9–13.

Avery, G., et al. (1994). *Neonatology pathophysiology and management of the newborn* (4th ed.). Philadelphia: J.B. Lippincott.

Blackburn, S. T., & Loper, D. L. (1992). *Maternal, fetal and neonatal physiology: A clinical perspective.* Philadelphia: W.B. Saunders.

Cassidy, J. (1993). A picture-perfect birth. *RN, 56*(6), 45-46.

Creasy, R. K., & Resnik, R. (1994). *Maternal-fetal medicine principles and practice* (3rd ed.). Philadelphia: W.B. Saunders.

Dickason, E. J., et al. (1994). *Maternal-infant nursing care* (2nd ed.). St. Louis: Mosby-Year Book.

Gorrie, T. M., et al. (1994). *Foundations of maternal newborn nursing.* Philadelphia: W.B. Saunders.

Lucas, V. A. (1993). Birth: Nursing's role in today's choices. *RN, 56*(6), 38-44.

May, K. A., & Mahlmeister, L. R. (1994). *Maternal and neonatal nursing: Family centered care* (3rd ed.). Philadelphia: J.B. Lippincott.

Merenstein, G. B., & Gardner, S. L. (1993). *Handbook of neonatal intensive care* (3rd ed.). St. Louis: Mosby-Year Book.

Morrison, J. C., et al. (1993). Monitoring by auscultation or electronic means. *American Journal of Obstetrics and Gynecology, 168*(Pt 1), 63-66.

Rickford, F. (1993). Choice in childbirth. *Nursing Times, 89*(13), 19.

Sadler, C. (1993). Baby brainwave [news]. *Nursing Times, 89*(3), 18-19.

Spencer, J. A. (1992). Current methods of continuous fetal heart rate monitoring. *Professional Nurse, 8*(3), 173-175.

Thomson, A. M. (1993). Pushing techniques in the second state of labor. *Journal of Advanced Nursing, 18*(2), 171-177.

CHAPTER 36 ◆

Care of the Mother and Newborn During the Postpartum Period

Nursing Care of the Mother

◆ THE PUERPERIUM

The *puerperium* is the period beginning after delivery and ending when the woman's body has returned as closely as possible to its prepregnant state. The period lasts approximately 6 weeks.

Physiologic Changes of the Puerperium

1. Uterine changes
   a. The fundus is usually midline and about at the level of the woman's umbilicus after delivery. Within 12 hours of delivery, the fundus may be 1 cm above the umbilicus. After this, the level of the fundus descends about 1 finger breadth (or 1 cm) each day, until by the 10th day, it has descended into the pelvic cavity and can no longer be palpated.
   b. After delivery, *lochia*, a vaginal discharge consisting of fatty epithelial cells, shreds of membrane, decidua, and blood, is red (*lochia rubra*) for about 2 or 3 days. It then progresses to a paler or more brownish color (*lochia serosa*), followed by a whitish or yellowish color (*lochia alba*) in the 7th to 10th day. Lochia usually ceases by 3 weeks, and the placental site is completely healed by the 6th week.
2. The vaginal walls, uterine ligaments, and muscles of the pelvic floor and abdominal wall regain most of their tone during the puerperium.
3. Postpartum diuresis occurs between the 2nd and 5th postpartum days, as extracellular water accumulated during pregnancy begins to be excreted. Diuresis may also occur shortly after delivery if urinary output was obstructed because of the pressure of the presenting part or if intravenous fluids were given to the woman during labor.
4. Breasts
   a. With loss of the placenta, circulating levels of estrogen and progesterone decrease while levels of prolactin increase, thus initiating lactation in the postpartum woman.
   b. *Colostrum*, a yellowish fluid containing more minerals and protein but less sugar and fat than mature breast milk and having a laxative effect on the infant, is secreted for the first 2 days postpartum.
   c. Mature milk secretion is usually present by the third postpartum day but may be present earlier if a woman breast-feeds immediately after delivery.
   d. Breast engorgement with milk, venous and lymphatic stasis, and swollen, tense, and tender breast tissue may occur between days 3 and 5 postpartum.

Emotional and Behavioral Status

1. After delivery, the woman may progress through Rubin's stages of "taking in" and "taking hold."
   a. Taking in
      (1) May begin with a refreshing sleep after delivery.
      (2) Woman exhibits passive, dependent behavior.
      (3) Woman is concerned with sleep and the intake of food, both for herself and for the infant.
   b. Taking hold
      (1) Woman begins to initiate action and to function more independently.
      (2) Woman may require more explanation and reassurance that she is functioning well, especially in caring for her infant.
      (3) As the woman meets success in caring for the newborn, her concern extends to other family members and their activities.
2. Some women may experience a euphoria in the first few days after delivery and set unrealistic goals for activities after discharge from the birthing place.
3. Many women may experience temporary mood swings during this period because of the discomfort, fatigue, and exhaustion after labor and delivery and because of hormonal changes after delivery.
4. Some mothers may experience "postpartum blues" at about the third postpartum day and exhibit irritability, poor appetite, insomnia, tearfulness, or crying. This is a temporary situation. Severe or prolonged depression is usually a sign of a more serious condition.
5. Nursing research findings indicate that new mothers identified the postpartum needs listed below. Coping with:
   a. The physical changes and discomforts of the puerperium, including a need to regain their prepregnancy figure.
   b. Changing family relationships and meeting the needs of family members, including the infant.
   c. Fatigue, emotional stress, feelings of isolation, and being "tied down."
   d. A lack of time for personal needs and interests.

◆ NURSING ASSESSMENT

Immediate Postpartum Assessment

The first hour after delivery of the placenta (fourth stage of labor) is a critical period; postpartum hemorrhage is most likely to occur at this time (see p. 1049).

Subsequent Postpartum Assessment

1. Check firmness of the fundus at regular intervals.
2. Inspect the perineum regularly for frank bleeding.
   a. Note color, amount, and odor of the lochia.
   b. Count the number of perineal pads that are saturated in each 8-hour period.
3. Assess vital signs at least twice daily and more frequently if indicated.
4. Assess for bowel and bladder elimination.
5. Evaluate interaction and care skills of mother and family with infant.
6. Assess for breast engorgement and condition of nipples if breast-feeding.
7. Inspect legs for signs of thromboembolism, and assess Homans' sign.
8. Assess incisions for signs of infection and healing.
9. If a patient is Rh negative, evaluate the need for $Rh_o(D)$ immune globulin (RhoGAM). If indicated, administer the RhoGAM within 72 hours of delivery.
10. If the woman is not rubella immune, a rubella vaccination may be given, and pregnancy must be avoided for at least 3 months.

◆ NURSING MANAGEMENT

Nursing Diagnoses

A. Risk for Fluid Volume Deficit related to blood loss and effects from anesthesia
B. Altered Urinary Elimination related to birth trauma
C. Colonic Constipation related to physiologic changes from birth
D. Risk for Infection related to birth process
E. Fatigue related to labor
F. Pain related to perineal discomfort from birth trauma, hemorrhoids, and physiologic changes from birth
G. Altered Health Maintenance related to lack of knowledge of postpartum care
H. Altered Health Maintenance related to lack of knowledge of newborn care
I. Ineffective Breastfeeding related to lack of knowledge and inexperience

Nursing Interventions

A. *Monitoring for Hypotension and Bleeding*
1. Monitor vital signs every 4 hours during the first 24 hours, then every 8 to 12 hours. Observe for the following:
   a. Decreased respiratory rate below 14 to 16 breaths per minute may occur after receiving epidural narcotics or narcotic analgesics.
   b. Increased respiratory rate greater than 24 breaths per minute may be due to increased blood loss, pulmonary edema, or a pulmonary embolus.
   c. Increased pulse rate greater than 100 beats per minute may be present with increased blood loss, fever, or pain.
   d. Decrease in blood pressure 15 to 20 mm Hg below baseline pressures may indicate decreased fluid volume or increased blood loss.
2. Assess the woman for light-headedness and dizziness when sitting upright or before ambulating.
   a. Evaluate orthostatic blood pressures.
   b. Have the woman lie in bed if symptoms exist.
3. Assess vaginal discharge for amount and presence of clots (Fig. 36-1).
4. Evaluate lower extremity sensory and motor function before ambulation if the woman had regional anesthesia.
5. Encourage food and drink as tolerated.
6. Maintain intravenous line as indicated.
7. Monitor postpartum hemoglobin and hematocrit.

B. *Encouraging Bladder Emptying*
1. Observe for the woman's first void within 6 to 8 hours after delivery.
2. Palpate the abdomen for bladder distention if the woman is unable to void or complains of fullness after voiding.
   a. Uterine displacement from the midline suggests bladder distention
   b. Frequent voidings of small amounts of urine suggest urinary retention with overflow.
3. Catheterize the woman (in and out) if indicated.
4. Instruct the woman to void every several hours and after meals to keep her bladder empty. An undistended bladder may help decrease uterine cramping.

C. *Promoting Proper Bowel Function*
1. Teach the woman that bowel activity is sluggish because of decreased abdominal muscle tone, anesthetic effects, effects of progesterone, decreased solid food intake during labor, and prelabor diarrhea.
2. Inform the woman that pain from hemorrhoids, lacerations, and episiotomies may cause her to delay her first bowel movement.
3. Review the woman's dietary intake with her.
4. Encourage daily adequate amounts of fresh fruit, vegetables, fiber, and at least eight glasses of water.
5. Encourage frequent ambulation.
6. Administer stool softeners as indicated.

D. *Preventing Infection*
1. Observe for elevated temperature above 38°C.
2. Evaluate episiotomy/perineum for redness, ecchymosis, edema, discharge (color, amount, odor) and approximation of the skin.
3. Assess for pain, burning, and frequency on urination.
4. Administer antibiotics as ordered.

E. *Reducing Fatigue*
1. Provide a quiet and minimally disturbed environment.
2. Organize nursing care to keep interruptions to a minimum.
3. Encourage the woman to minimize visitors and phone calls.
4. Encourage the woman to sleep while the baby is sleeping.

F. *Minimizing Pain*
1. Instruct the woman to apply ice packs to the perineal area for the first 24 hours for perineal trauma or edema.

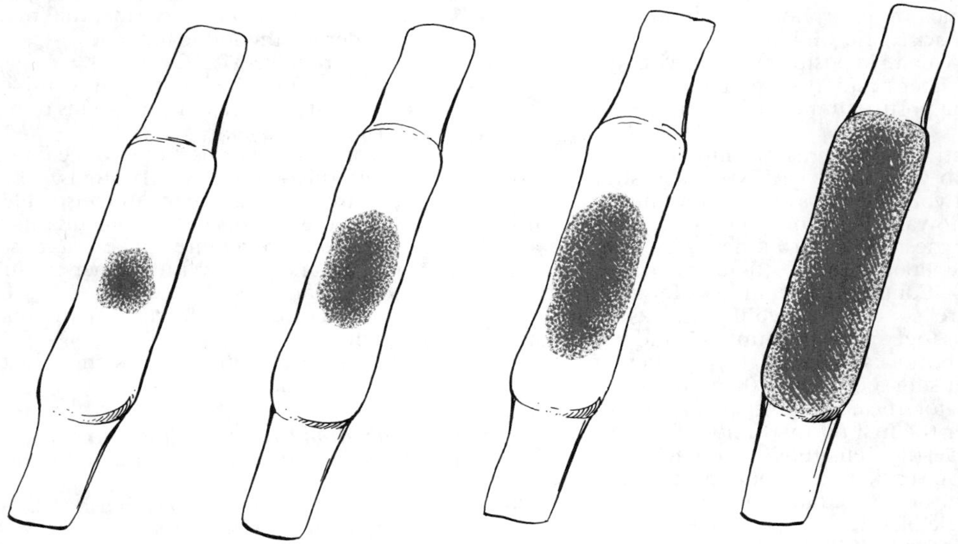

| **Scant amount** | **Light amount** | **Moderate amount** | **Heavy amount** |
| Blood only on tissue when wiped or less than 1-inch stain on peripad. | Less than 4-inch stain on peripad. | Less than 6-inch stain on peripad. | Saturated peripad within 1 hour. |

FIGURE 36-1 Assessing the volume of lochia by peri-pad saturation.

a. Take breaks between applications to prevent tissue damage.
b. Commercial or handmade packs of ice chips in a glove may be used.
c. Place a thin barrier between ice pack and skin.

2. Initiate the use of sitz baths for perineal discomfort after the first 24 hours
a. Use three times a day for 15 to 20 minutes

3. Instruct the woman to contract her buttocks before sitting to reduce perineal discomfort.

4. Assist the woman in the use of positioning cushions and pillows while sitting or lying.

5. Teach the woman to use a perineal bottle and squirt warm water against her perineum while voiding.

6. Provide pads such as Tucks or topical creams or ointments as indicated.

7. Administer pain medication as indicated.

8. Check the breasts for signs of engorgement (swollen, tender, tense, shiny breast tissue).
a. If breasts are engorged and the woman is breast-feeding:
   (1) Allow warm-to-hot shower water to flow over the breasts to improve comfort.
   (2) Hot compresses on the breasts may improve comfort.
   (3) Express some milk manually or by breast pump to improve comfort and make nipple more available for infant feeding.
   (4) Nurse the infant.
   (5) A mild analgesic may be used to enhance comfort.
b. If breasts are engorged and the mother is bottle-feeding:

   (1) Teach the woman to wear a supportive bra night and day.
   (2) Teach the woman to avoid handling her breasts, because this stimulates more milk production.
   (3) Suggest ice bags to the breasts to provide comfort.
   (4) Moderately strong analgesics may be needed to provide comfort.

G. *Promoting Postpartum Health Maintenance*
1. Teach the woman to perform perineal care—warm water over the perineum after each voiding and bowel movement routinely several times a day to promote comfort, cleanliness, and healing.

2. Promote sitz baths for the same purpose.

3. Teach the woman to apply perineal pads by touching the outside only, thus keeping clean the portion that will touch her perineum.

4. Assess the condition of the woman's breasts and nipples. Inspect nipples for reddening, erosions, or fissures. Reddened areas may be improved with A & D ointment, a lanolin cream, and air drying for 15 minutes several times a day.

5. Teach the woman to wash her breasts with warm water and NO soap, which prevents the removal of the protective skin oils.

6. Teach the woman to wear a bra that provides good support night and day.

7. Instruct the breast-feeding woman to add between 500 and 750 additional calories daily for milk production. Inform her that she also needs 2 to 3 quarts of liquid per day, 20 g more protein than before pregnancy, and

additional calcium; phosphorus; vitamins D, A, C, E, B, and B2; niacin; zinc; and iodine.

8. Instruct the woman in postpartum exercises for the immediate and later postpartum period.
   a. Immediate postpartum exercises can be performed in bed.
      (1) Toe stretch (tightens calf muscles)—While lying on your back, keep your legs straight and point your toes away from you, then pull your legs toward you and point your toes toward your chest. Repeat 10 times.
      (2) Pelvic floor exercise (tightens perineal muscles)—Contract your buttocks for a count of 5 and relax. Contract your buttocks and press thighs together for a count of 7 and relax. Contract buttocks, press thighs together, and draw in anus for a count of 10 and relax.
   b. Exercises for the later postpartum period can be done after the first postpartum visit.
      (1) Bicycle (tightens thighs, stomach, waist)—Lie on your back on the floor, arms at sides, palms down. Begin rotating your legs as if you were riding a bicycle, bringing the knees all the way in toward the chest and stretching the legs out as long and straight as possible. Breathe deeply and evenly. Do the exercises at a moderate speed and do not tire yourself.
      (2) Buttocks exercise (tightens buttocks)—Lie on your stomach and keep your legs straight. Raise your left leg in the air, then repeat with your right leg (feel the contraction in your buttocks). Keep your hips on the floor. Repeat 10 times.
      (3) Twist (tightens waist)—Stand with legs wide apart. Hold your arms at your sides, shoulder level, palms down. Twist your body from side to front and back again. Feel the twist in your waist.

H. Promoting Health Maintenance of the Newborn
1. Encourage the parents to participate in daily care of the infant.
2. Advise the parents to attend parenting and baby care classes offered during their stay at the birth facility.
3. Teach the parents to bathe and diaper the infant, perform circumcision care, and initiate either breast or bottle feeding (Table 36-1).
4. Foster bonding by encouraging skin-to-skin contact with the infant, eye contact, and talking to and touching the infant.

5. Instruct the parents to contact the infant's health care provider for the following:
   a. Fever above 37.2°C (100°F).
   b. Loss of appetite for two consecutive feedings.
   c. Inability to awaken baby to his or her usual activity state.
   d. Vomiting all or part of two feedings.
   e. Diarrhea—three watery stools.
   f. Extreme irritability or unconsolable crying.
6. Inform the parents that by law infants and young children in cars are required to be in a car safety seat. Demonstrate and review the proper technique for use of the car seat.
7. Provide positive reinforcement and reassurance to the parents.
8. Provide written instructions and educational material on discharge.

I. Promoting Breast-Feeding
1. Assist the woman and infant in the breast-feeding process.
   a. Have the mother wash her hands before feeding to help prevent infection.
   b. Encourage the mother to assume a comfortable position, such as sitting upright, tailor sitting, lying on her side.
   c. Have the woman hold the baby so that he or she is facing the mother. Common positions for holding the baby are the "cradle hold," with the baby's head and body supported against the mother's arm with buttocks resting in her hand; the "football hold," in which the baby's legs are supported under the mother's arm while the head is at the breast resting in the mother's hand; lying on the side with the baby lying on his/her side facing the mother.
   d. Teach the woman to bring the baby close to her, to prevent back, shoulder, and arm strain.
   e. Have the woman cup the breast in her hand in a "C" position with bottom of the breast in the palm of her hand and the thumb on top.
   f. Have the woman place her nipple against the baby's mouth, and when the mouth opens, guide the nipple and the areola into the mouth.
      (1) If the baby has "latched on" to the nipple only, take the baby off the breast by putting the tip of the mother's finger in the corner of the baby's mouth to break the suction, and then reposition on the breast to prevent nipple pain and trauma.

TABLE 36-1 Typical Pattern of Infant Feedings

Age of Infant	Number of Feedings	Volume per Feeding	Total
Birth–2 wk	6–10	2–3 oz (60–90 mL)	12–30 oz (360–900 mL)
2 wk to 1 mo	6–8	3–4 oz (90–120 mL)	18–32 oz (540–960 mL)
1–3 mo	5–6	5–6 oz (150–180 mL)	25–36 oz (750–1080 mL)
3–7 mo	4–5	6–7 oz (180–210 mL)	25–36 oz (750–1080 mL)
7–12 mo	3–4	7–8 oz (210–240 mL)	25–36 oz (750–1080 mL)

Taken from May, K. A., and Mahlmeister, L. R. Maternal and Neonatal Nursing—Family Centered Care (3rd Ed.). Philadelphia: J.B. Lippincott, 1994.

g. Encourage the woman to alternate the breast she begins feeding with at each feeding to ensure emptying of both breasts and stimulation for maintaining milk supply.

h. Advise the mother to use each breast at each feeding. Begin with about 5 minutes at each breast, then increase the time at each breast, allowing the infant to suck until he or she stops sucking actively. Pinning a safety pin to the bra as a reminder of which breast to start with at the next feeding is helpful.

i. Have the mother breast-feed frequently and on demand (every 2 to 4 hours) to help maintain the milk supply.

j. Have the mother air dry her nipples for about 15 to 20 minutes after feeding to help prevent nipple trauma.

k. Have the mother burp the infant at the end or midway through the feeding to help release the air in the stomach and make the infant less fretful.

2. Alert the mother that uterine cramping may occur, especially in multiparous women, due to the release of oxytocin, which can be worse in women with lessened uterine tone.

3. Teach the mother to provide for adequate rest and to avoid tension, fatigue, and a stressful environment, which can inhibit the letdown reflex and make breast milk less available at feeding.

4. Advise the woman to avoid taking medications and drugs, because many substances pass into the breast milk and may affect milk production or the infant.

Evaluation

A. Vital signs within normal limits; decreasing color and amount of lochia
B. Voids freely and without discomfort
C. Lack of constipation; eats high-fiber foods and uses stool softeners
D. Afebrile, no abnormal redness of perineum, no purulent discharge or foul odor of lochia
E. Verbalizes feeling rested
F. Verbalizes decreased pain
G. Incorporates postpartum care into activities of daily living
H. Demonstrates confidence in performing infant care; shows signs of maternal–child bonding
I. Demonstrates successful breast-feeding; breasts and nipples intact and without redness or cracks

Postpartum Patient Education

1. Advise the woman that healing occurs within 2 to 4 weeks; however, evaluation by the health care provider during the follow-up visit is necessary.

2. Inform the woman that intercourse may be resumed when perineal and uterine wounds have healed. Review methods of contraception.

3. Inform the woman that menstruation usually returns within 4 to 8 weeks if bottle-feeding; if breast-feeding, menstruation usually returns within 4 months, but may return between 2 and 18 months postpartum. Nursing mothers may ovulate even if experiencing amenorrhea, so a form of contraception should be used if pregnancy is to be avoided.

4. Counsel the woman to rest for at least 30 minutes after she arrives home from the hospital and to rest several times during the day for the first few weeks.

5. Advise the woman to confine her activities to one floor if possible and to avoid stair climbing as much as possible for the first several days at home.

6. Counsel the woman to provide quiet times for herself at home, and help her establish realistic goals for resuming her own interests and activities.

7. Encourage the couple to provide times to reestablish their own relationship and to renew their social interests and relationships.

Nursing Care of the Newborn

◆ PHYSIOLOGY OF THE NEWBORN

The first 24 hours of life constitute a highly vulnerable time, during which the infant must make major physiologic adjustments to extrauterine life.

Transitional Stages

During the period of postnatal transition, six overlapping stages have been identified:

Stage 1. Receives stimulation (during labor) from the pressure of the uterine contractions and from changes in pressure when the membranes rupture.
Stage 2. Encounters a variety of foreign stimuli—light, cold, gravity, and sound.
Stage 3. Initiates breathing.
Stage 4. Changes from fetal to neonatal circulation.
Stage 5. Undergoes alteration in metabolic processes, with activation of liver and gastrointestinal tract for passage of meconium.
Stage 6. Achieves a steady level of equilibrium in metabolic processes (production of enzymes, increased blood oxygen saturation, decrease in acidosis associated with birth, and recovery of the neurologic tissues from the trauma of labor and delivery).

Respiratory Changes

A. *Factors Initiating Respiration*
1. Physical—pressure changes from intrauterine to extrauterine life produce stimulation to initiate respirations.
2. Chemical—changes in the blood as a result of transitory asphyxia include:
   a. Lowered oxygen level.
   b. Increased carbon dioxide level.
   c. Lowered pH—if asphyxia is prolonged, depression of the respiratory center (rather than stimulation) occurs, and resuscitation is necessary
3. Sensory—light, sound, and tactile stimulation when the infant is touched and dried contribute to the initiation of respiration.
4. Thermal—a drop in temperature from 37°C (98.6°F) to 21° to 24°C (70° to 75°F).

5. First breath—maximum effort is required to expand the lungs and fill the collapsed alveoli.
   a. Surface tension in the respiratory tract and resistance in the lung tissue, the thorax, the diaphragm, and the respiratory muscles must be overcome.
   b. First active inspiration comes from a strong contraction of the diaphragm, which creates a high negative intrathoracic pressure, causing a marked retraction of the ribs and distention of the alveolar space. (Any remaining fluid is reabsorbed rapidly if the pulmonary capillary blood flow is adequate, because the fluid is hypotonic and passes easily into the capillaries.)

B. **Character of Normal Respirations**
1. The infant begins life with intense activity; diffuse, purposeless movements alternate with periods of relative immobility.
2. Respirations are rapid, as frequent as 80 breaths/minute, accompanied by tachycardia, 140 to 180 beats/minute.
3. Relaxation occurs and the infant usually sleeps; he or she then awakes to a second period of activity. Oral mucus may be a major problem during this period.
4. Respirations are reduced to 35 to 50 breaths/minute and become quiet and shallow; respiration is carried out by the diaphragm and abdominal muscles.
5. Period of dyspnea and cyanosis may occur suddenly in an infant who is breathing normally; this may indicate an anomaly or a pathologic condition.
6. Apnea is normal in the neonatal period and lasts 10 to 15 seconds.

Circulatory Changes

A. **Anatomic Changes (see p. 988)**

B. **Blood Volume**
Blood volume is 85 to 100 mL/kg at birth.
Factors that influence blood volume:
1. Maternal blood volume (affected by maternal diseases and iron intake).
2. Placental function.
3. Uterine contractions during labor.
4. Amount of blood loss associated with delivery.
5. Placental transfusion at birth—increase in blood volume of 60% if cord is clamped and cut after pulsation ceases.

C. **Peripheral Circulation**
Residual cyanosis in hands and feet for 1 to 2 hours after birth because of sluggish circulation.

D. **Pulse Rate**
1. Generally follows pattern similar to that of respiration.
2. Apical pulse rate is more accurate.
3. Normal rate 120 to 150 beats/minute.
4. May rise to 180 beats/minute when the infant is crying or drop to 70 beats/minute during deep sleep.

E. **Blood Pressure**
1. Blood pressure is 70/45 at birth; 100/50 by 10th day.
2. Blood pressure rises with crying.
3. Blood pressure in the leg will be slightly higher.

F. **Blood Coagulation**
Coagulability is temporarily diminished because of lack of bacteria in the intestinal tract that contributes to the synthesis of vitamin K.
1. Coagulation time, 3 to 4 minutes.
2. Bleeding time, 2 to 4 minutes.
3. Prothrombin, 50%, decreasing to 20% to 30%.

G. **Blood Elements**
Values for blood components in the neonate:
1. Hemoglobin, 16 to 22 g.
2. Reticulocytes, 2.5% to 6.5%.
3. Leukocytes, 15,000 to 20,000 mm^3.

Temperature Regulation

1. Mechanism not fully developed; heat production low.
2. Infant responds readily to environmental heat and cold stimuli.
3. Heat loss of 2° to 3°C may occur at birth by evaporation, convection, conduction, and radiation.
4. Infant develops mechanisms to counterbalance heat loss.
   a. Vasoconstriction—blood directed away from skin surfaces.
   b. Insulation—from subcutaneous adipose tissue.
   c. Heat production—by nonshivering thermogenesis elicited by the sympathetic nervous system's response to decreased temperatures; activated by adrenaline.
   d. Fetal position—by assuming a flexed position.

Basal Metabolism

1. Surface area of infant is large in comparison to weight.
2. Basal metabolism per kilogram of body weight is higher than that of an adult.
3. Calorie requirements are high—117 calories per kilogram of body weight per day.

Renal Function

Low arterial blood pressure and increased renal vascular resistance lead to the following effects:
1. Decreased ability to concentrate urine because of low tubular resorption rate and low levels of antidiuretic hormone.
2. Limited ability to maintain water balance by excretion of excess water or retention of needed water.
3. Decreased ability to maintain acid–base mechanism; slower excretion of electrolytes, especially sodium and the hydrogen ions, results in accumulation of these substances, which predisposes the infant to dehydration, acidosis, and hyperkalemia.
4. Excretion of large amount of uric acid during newborn period—appears as "brick dust" stain on diaper.

Hepatic Function

Function limited because of lack of gastrointestinal tract activity and limited blood supply; consequences include the following:

1. Decreased ability to conjugate bilirubin (rationale for physiologic jaundice).
2. Decreased ability to regulate blood glucose concentration (rationale for neonatal hypoglycemia).
3. Deficient production of prothrombin and other coagulation factors that depend on vitamin K for synthesis (rationale for neonate's predisposition to hemorrhage).

Endocrine Function

Endocrine glands are better organized than other systems: disturbances are most often related to maternally provided hormones.

This can cause the following:

1. Vaginal discharge (and/or bleeding) in female infants.
2. Enlargement of mammary glands in both sexes—related to increased estrogen, luteal, and prolactin activity. Milky secretions may be present.
3. Disturbances related to maternal endocrine pathology (eg, diabetic mother or mother with inadequate iodine intake).

Gastrointestinal Changes

The newborn's intestinal tract is proportionately longer than the adult's; however, elastic tissue and musculature are not fully developed, and neurologic control is variable and inadequate.

1. Most digestive enzymes are present, with the exception of pancreatic amylase and lipase. Protein and carbohydrates are easily absorbed, but fat absorption is poor.
2. Limitations relate primarily to anatomic structures and neutrality of the gastric contents.
3. Imperfect control of the cardiac and pyloric sphincters and immaturity of neurologic control cause mild regurgitation or slight vomiting.
4. Irregularities in peristaltic motility slow stomach emptying.
5. Peristalsis increases in the lower ileum, resulting in stool frequency—one to six stools per day. Absence of stool within 48 hours after birth is indicative of intestinal obstruction.

Neurologic Changes

Neurologic mechanisms are immature; they are not fully developed anatomically or physiologically, and as a result, uncoordinated movements, labile temperature regulation, and poor control over musculature are characteristic of the infant. Reflexes are important indicators of infant neural development (see p. 1095).

◆ NURSING ASSESSMENT

Pertinent Maternal History

1. Mother's age, socioeconomic status, ethnic or cultural group, educational level, marital status.
2. Mother's/family's past medical history.
3. Mother's past obstetric history.
4. Mother's prenatal history with this pregnancy.
5. Labor and delivery.

Physical Assessment Findings and Physiologic Functioning

A. Posture
1. Full-term newborn assumes symmetric posture; face turned to side; flexed extremities; hands tightly fisted with thumb covered by fingers.
2. Asymmetric posture may be caused by fractures of clavicle or humerus or by nerve injuries commonly of the brachial plexus.
3. Infants born in breech position may keep knees and legs straightened or in frog position, depending on the type of breech birth.

B. Length
Average length of full-term newborn is 51 cm (20 in.); range, 46 to 56 cm (18 to 22 in.).

C. Weight
Average weight of male infants is 3,400 g ($7\frac{1}{2}$ lb); female infants, 3,200 g (7 lb). Range of 80% of full-term newborns is 2,900 to 4,100 g (6 lb 5 oz–9 lb 2 oz).

D. Skin
Examine under natural light for:

1. Hair distribution—term infant will have some lanugo over back; most of the lanugo will have disappeared on extremities and other areas of the body.
2. Turgor—term infant should have good skin turgor.
3. Color
   a. Cyanosis—*acrocyanosis*, bluish color in hands and feet, is common due to immature peripheral circulation.
   b. Pallor—may indicate cold, stress, anemia, or cardiac failure.
   c. Plethora—reddish coloration may be due to excessive red blood cells from intrauterine intravascular transfusion (twins), cardiac disease, or diabetes in the mother.
   d. Jaundice—physiologic jaundice due to immaturity of liver is common beginning on day 2, peaking at 1 week and disappearing by the 2nd week. First appears in skin over face or upper body, then progresses over larger area; can also be seen in conjunctivae of eyes.
   e. Meconium staining—staining of skin, fingernails, and umbilical cord indicates compromise in utero, unless infant was in breech position.
4. Dryness/peeling—marked scaliness and desquamation are signs of postmaturity.
5. Vernix—in full-term infants, most vernix is found in skin folds under the arms and in the groin.
6. Nails—should reach end of fingertips and be well developed in the full-term infant.

7. Edema—some edema may be present over buttocks, back, and occiput if the infant has been supine; pitting edema may be due to erythroblastosis, heart failure, electrolyte imbalance.
8. Ecchymoses—may appear over the presenting part in a difficult delivery; may also indicate infection or bleeding problem.
9. Petechiae—pinpoint hemorrhages on skin due to increased intravascular pressure, infection, or thrombocytopenia; regresses within 48 hours.
10. Erythema toxicum ("newborn rash")—pink to red papular rash appearing on trunk and diaper areas; regresses within 48 hours.
11. Hemangiomas—vascular lesions present at birth; some may fade, but others may be permanent.
12. Telangiectatic nevi (stork bites)—flat red or purple lesions most often found on back of neck, lower occiput, upper eyelid, and bridge of nose; regress by 2 years of age.
13. Milia—enlarged sebaceous glands found on nose, chin, cheeks, and forehead; regress in several days to a week or two.
14. Mongolian spots—blue pigmentation on lower back, sacrum, and buttocks; common in blacks, Asians, and infants of southern European heritage; regress by 4 years of age.
15. Café-au-lait spots—brown macules, usually not significant; large numbers may indicate underlying neurofibromatosis.
16. Harlequin color change—when on side, dependent half turns red, upper half pale; due to gravity and vasomotor instability.
17. Abrasions or lacerations can result from internal monitoring and instruments used at birth.

E. Head
1. Examine head and face for symmetry, paralysis, shape, swelling, movement.
    a. *Caput succedaneum*—swelling of soft tissues of the scalp because of pressure; swelling crosses suture lines.
    b. *Cephalohematoma*—subperiosteal hemorrhage with collection of blood between periosteum and bone; swelling does not cross suture lines.
    c. *Molding*—overlapping of skull bones caused by compression during labor and delivery (disappears in a few days).
    d. Examine symmetry of facial movements.
2. Measure head circumference—33 to 35 cm (13–14 in.), approximately 2 cm (1 in.) larger than chest. Measure just above the eyebrows and over the occiput.
3. Fontanelles—area where more than two skull bones meet; covered with strong band of connective tissue; also called "soft spot."
    a. Enlarged or bulging—may indicate increased intracranial pressure.
    b. Sunken—often indicates dehydration.
    c. Size—posterior may be obliterated because of molding; generally closes in 2 to 3 months. Anterior is palpable; generally closes in 12 to 18 months.
4. Sutures—junctions of adjoining skull bones.
    a. Overriding—due to molding during labor and delivery.
    b. Separation—extensive separation may be found in malnourished infants and with increased intracranial pressure.

F. Face
1. Eyes—examine the following:
    a. Color—sclerae in most full-term infants are white; eye color usually gray-blue in white infants, brown in dark-skinned infants; final eye color is evident by 6 to 12 months.
    b. Hemorrhagic areas—subconjunctival hemorrhages may appear as a red band from pressure during delivery; regress within 2 weeks.
    c. Edema—edema of the eyelids may be caused by pressure on the head and face during labor and delivery.
    d. Conjunctivitis or discharge—may be due to instillation of silver nitrate or infections from organisms such as staphylococcus or gonococcus.
    e. Jaundice—may be seen in sclera because of physiologic jaundice or, if severe, blood group incompatibility.
    f. Pupils—equal in size and should constrict equally in bright light.
    g. Infant can see and discriminate patterns; limited by imperfect oculomotor coordination and inability to accommodate for varying distances.
    h. Red reflex—red-orange color seen when light from an ophthalmoscope is reflected from the retina. Absence of the red reflex indicates cataracts.
    i. Brushfield's spots—white or yellow pinpoint areas on iris that may indicate trisomy 21.
2. Nose—examine the following:
    a. Patency—necessary because infants breathe through the nose, not the mouth.
    b. Nasal flaring—may indicate respiratory distress.
    c. Discharge—due to congestion or possibly infection.
    d. Sense of smell—infants will turn toward familiar odors and away from noxious odors.
3. Ears—examine the following:
    a. Formation—large, flabby ears that slant forward may indicate abnormalities of kidney or other parts of urinary tract.
    b. Position in relation to eye—helix (top of ear) on same plane as eye; low-set ears may indicate chromosomal or renal abnormalities.
    c. Cartilage—full-term infant has sufficient cartilage to make ear feel firm.
    d. Hearing—auditory canals may be congested for a day or 2 after birth; the infant should hear well in a few days.
4. Mouth—examine the following:
    a. Size—small mouth found in trisomy 18 and 21; corners of mouth turn down ("fish mouth") in fetal alcohol syndrome.
    b. Palate—examine hard and soft palate for closure.
    c. Size of tongue in relation to mouth—normally does not extend much past the margin of gums. Excessively large tongue seen in congenital anomalies such as cretinism and trisomy 21.
    d. Teeth—predeciduous teeth are found on rare occasions; if they interfere with feeding, they may be removed.
    e. Epstein's pearls—small white nodules found on sides of hard palate (often mistaken for teeth); regress in a few weeks.
    f. Frenulum linguae—thin ridge of tissue running from base of tongue along undersurface to tip of tongue, formerly believed to cause tongue tie; no treatment necessary.
    g. Sucking blisters (labial taberales)—thickened areas on midline of upper lip; no treatment necessary.
    h. Infections—thrush, caused by *Candida albicans*, may appear as white patches on tongue that do not wash away with fluids; treated with nystatin suspension.

G. Neck
Examine the following:

1. Mobility—infant can move head from side to side; palpate for lymph nodes; palpate clavicle for fractures, especially after a difficult delivery.
2. Torticollis—appears as a spasmodic, one-sided contraction of neck muscles; generally from hematoma of sternocleidomastoid muscle; usually no treatment required.
3. Excessive skin folds may be associated with congenital abnormalities, such as trisomy 21.
4. Stiffness and hyperextension may be due to trauma or infection.
5. Clavicle—for intactness.

H. Chest

1. Circumference and symmetry—average circumference is 30 to 33 cm (12–13 in.), approximately 2 cm smaller than head circumference.
2. Breast
   a. Engorgement—may occur at day 3 because of withdrawal of maternal hormones, especially estrogen; no treatment required—regresses in 2 weeks.
   b. Nipples and areolae—less formed and pronounced in preterm infants.

I. Respiratory System
1. Rate—normally between 40 and 60 breaths/minute; influenced by sleep–wake status, when last fed, drugs taken by mother.
2. Rhythm—respirations may be shallow with irregular rhythm.
   a. Respiratory movements are mainly diaphragmatic because of weak thoracic muscles.
   b. Periodic breathing—resumption of respiration after 5- to 15-second period without respiration; decreases over time; more common in preterm infants.
   c. Observe for abnormal respiratory signs.
3. Breath sounds—determined by auscultation.
   a. Bronchial sounds are heard over most of the chest.
   b. Rales may be heard immediately after birth.

J. Cardiovascular System
1. Rate—ranges between 100 and 160 beats/minute; influenced by behavioral state, environmental temperature, medication; take apical count for 1 minute.
2. Rhythm—common to find periods of deceleration followed by periods of acceleration.
3. Heart sounds—second sound higher in pitch and sharper than first; third and fourth sounds rarely heard; murmurs common, majority are transitory.
4. Pulses—examine for presence of brachial, radial, pedal, and femoral pulses; lack of femoral pulses indicative of inadequate aortic blood flow.
5. Cyanosis—examine for cyanosis. Acrocyanosis of distal extremities is common; record location of any cyanosis, color changes over time, and when crying.
6. Blood pressure—newborns weighing more than 3 kg have systolic blood pressure between 60 and 80 mm Hg; diastolic, between 35 and 55 mm Hg.

K. Abdomen
1. Shape—cylindrical, protrudes slightly, moves synchronously with chest in respiration.
2. Distention may be due to bowel obstruction, organ enlargement, or infection.
3. Palpate abdomen for masses; gap between rectus muscles is common; palpate liver and spleen.
   a. Liver has decreased ability to conjugate bilirubin (rationale for physiologic jaundice).
   b. Liver has decreased production of prothrombin and factors that depend on vitamin K for synthesis (rationale for neonate's predisposition to hemorrhage).
4. Auscultate abdomen for bowel sounds; usually bowel sounds are present an hour after delivery.
5. Kidneys—palpate kidneys for size and shape.
   a. Infant has decreased ability of kidney to concentrate urine, excrete a solute load, maintain water and electrolyte balance.
   b. Urine may contain uric acid crystals, which appear on diaper as reddish blotches; uric acid crystals may yield false-positive result when the infant's urine is tested for protein.
6. Umbilical cord
   a. Normally contains two arteries, one vein; single artery associated with renal and other congenital abnormalities.
   b. Signs of infection around insertion into abdominal wall—redness, discharge.
   c. Meconium staining—associated with intrauterine compromise or postmaturity.
   d. By 24 hours, becomes yellowish brown; dries and falls off in about 7 to 10 days.
   e. Umbilical hernia—defect in abdominal wall.
7. Genitalia
   a. Female
      (1) Labia majora cover labia minora in full-term female infants.
      (2) Hymenal tag (tissue) may protrude from vagina—regresses within several weeks.
      (3) Vaginal discharge—white or pink discharge may be present because of the drop in maternal hormones; no treatment necessary.
   b. Male
      (1) Full-term—testes in scrotal sac; scrotal sac markedly wrinkled.
      (2) Edema may be present in scrotal sac if the infant was born in breech presentation; a frank collection of fluid in the scrotal sac is a *hydrocele*—regresses in about a month.
      (3) Examine glans penis for urethral opening—normally central; opening ventral (*hypospadias*); opening dorsally (*epispadias*); abnormally adherent foreskin (*phimosis*).

L. Back
1. Examine spinal column for normal curvature, closure, and presence of pilonidal dimple or sinus.
2. Examine anal area for anal opening, response of anal sphincter, fissures.

M. Musculoskeletal System
1. Examine extremities for fractures, paralysis, range of motion, irregular position.
2. Examine fingers and toes for number and separation: extra digits, *polydactyly*; fused digits, *syndactyly*.
3. Examine hips for dislocation—with the infant in supine position, flex knees and abduct hips to side and down to table surface; clicking sound indicates dislocation.

N. Neurologic System
1. Neurologic mechanisms are immature anatomically and physiologically; as a result, uncoordinated move-

ments, labile temperature regulation, and lack of control over musculature are characteristic of the infant.
2. Examine muscle tone, head control, and reflexes.

Behavioral Assessment

A. *Response to Stimulation*
1. Newborns exhibit predictable, directed responses when in social interactions with nurturing adults or in response to attractive auditory or visual stimuli.
2. Newborn responses are influenced by states of consciousness, such as:
   a. Quiet, deep sleep—no spontaneous activity, eyes closed, respirations regular.
   b. Light, active sleep—random startles, eyes closed, rapid eye movements, frequent change of state with response to stimulation.
   c. Drowsy awake—eyes open or closed, eyelids flutter, variable activity level, mild startles periodically, delayed response to stimulation.
   d. Quiet alert—eyes open, little motor activity, focuses on source of stimulation.
   e. Alert active—eyes open, much motor activity, increase in startles in response to stimulation.
   f. Crying—intense crying that is difficult to interrupt with stimulation.

B. *Sleeping Pattern*
1. Length of sleep cycles (rapid eye movement, active and quiet sleep) changes normally with maturation of the central nervous system.
2. Quiet sleep should increase over time in relation to rapid eye movement sleep.
3. Newborns usually sleep 20 hours per day.

C. *Feeding Pattern*
1. Most newborns eat six to eight times per day with 2 to 4 hours between feedings; establish fairly regular feeding patterns in about 2 weeks.
2. Caloric requirements are high—110 to 130 calories/kg of body weight daily.
3. Most digestive enzymes are present at birth.
4. Imperfect control of cardiac and pyloric sphincters; immaturity results in regurgitation.

D. *Pattern of Elimination*
1. Stool
   a. Meconium is usually passed in 24 hours.
   b. Passage of meconium (tarry green-black stools) continues for 48 hours, followed by transitional stools (combination of meconium and yellow or milk stools). Milk stools (yellow) are passed by day 5.
   c. Newborn has up to six stools per day in the first weeks after birth.
2. Voiding
   a. Newborn voids within first 24 hours.
   b. After first few days, infant voids from 10 to 15 times a day.

E. *Temperature Regulation*
1. Infant's body responds readily to changes in environmental temperature.
2. Heat loss at birth may occur through evaporation, convection, conduction, and radiation.
3. Physiologic mechanisms to avoid heat loss include:
   a. Vasoconstriction.
   b. Nonshivering thermogenesis elicited by sympathetic nervous system in response to decreased temperature.
   c. Adipose tissue and brown fat—the latter contains many small blood vessels, fat vacuoles, and mitochondria and is a site of heat production. Brown fat is found between scapulae, around neck and thorax, behind sternum, and around kidneys and adrenals.
   d. Flexed position of full-term newborn.

Metabolic Screening Tests

1. *Phenylketonuria (PKU)*—inability of the infant to metabolize phenylalanine; scheduled after 48 hours of protein feedings.
2. *Galactosemia*—inborn error of carbohydrate metabolism, in which galactose and lactose cannot be converted to glucose.
3. *Hypothyroidism*—thyroid hormone deficiency.
4. *Maple sugar urine disease (MSUD)*—inability to metabolize leucine, isoleucine, and valine.
5. *Homocystinuria*—inborn error of sulfur amino acid metabolism.
6. *Sickle cell anemia*—abnormally shaped red blood cells with lower oxygen solubility.

◆ NURSING MANAGEMENT

See Procedure Guidelines 36-1: Newborn Care.

In caring for the newborn, the nurse establishes an ongoing plan of care for the infant and the family until discharge. The nurse's assessment of the newborn includes observing and recording vital signs, daily weight gain or loss, bowel and bladder function, activity and sleep patterns, and thermoregulation. Observation for potential problems in the newborn, ensuring safety, and the prevention of infection are main goals of nursing care.

Another main component of caring for the newborn is to assist with establishing a healthy family unit. Because so much of the baby's time is spent with the parents, the nurse has the opportunity to assist them with promoting health maintenance by teaching feeding methods and by demonstrating baby care techniques, such as diapering, bathing, and circumcision care. The nurse provides health counseling and education and answers questions to enable the parents to gain confidence, control, and satisfaction in caring for their child at home.

PROCEDURE GUIDELINES 36-1 ◆ Newborn Care

EQUIPMENT

Cotton balls or disposable washcloths
Neutral soap
70% alcohol

Petrolatum gauze
Protective ointment
Glucose reagent strips

PROCEDURE	NURSING ACTION	RATIONALE

WEIGHT, TEMPERATURE, AND BLOOD PRESSURE

NURSING ACTION	RATIONALE
1. Weigh infant and record weight.	1. Infant may lose 5%–10% of birth weight because of minimal intake of nutrients and fluid and loss of excess fluid.
2. Take axillary temperature by placing thermometer in axilla and pressing infant's arm gently but firmly against it for 10 minutes. Prevent undue exposure; provide warm environment (24°–27°C [75°–80°F])	2. Use of rectal thermometer predisposes to irritation of rectal mucosa.
3. Take blood pressure.	3. Hypotension may be present and require remedial action.

BATHING TECHNIQUE (BATH WATER (37°–38°C [98°–100°F])

NURSING ACTION	RATIONALE
1. Use cotton balls or soft, disposable washcloths to wipe eyes, face, and outer ears. Eyes are wiped from inside corner outward.	1. Start from cleanest areas to most soiled.
2. Use a neutral soap—check pH. Clear water may be used if infant's skin is dry.	2. Prevents irritation of skin. The use of hexachlorophene to prevent staphylococcal infection is controversial. Hexachlorophene may cause brain damage if a sufficient quantity is absorbed through the skin.
3. Wash infant's head, using gentle circular motions.	3. Prevents cradle cap from forming, especially over the frontal areas.
4. Tilt head back to cleanse neck.	4. Exposes neck folds for more thorough cleansing.
5. Bathe torso and extremities quickly.	5. Prevents unnecessary exposure and chilling.
6. Inspect umbilical cord. Check area for bleeding or foul odor. A drying agent such as 70% alcohol or merthiolate is applied several times daily. Do not cover with diaper. Dressings are not used.	6. Minimizes colonization by bacteria.
7. Cleanse genital area of male infants.	
a. Retract foreskin gently for cleaning, and replace quickly.	7. a. Replacing foreskin quickly prevents edema.
b. Circumcision care—keep area clean. Place sterile petrolatum gauze over area for first 24 hours; change after voiding. Observe hourly for bleeding. Position infant and diaper to avoid friction.	b. Prevents infection and promotes healing. Bleeding can be controlled by pressure or by application of adrenaline solution. Prevents discomfort.
8. Cleanse genital area of female infants.	
a. Gently separate folds of the labia and remove secretions.	8. a. Vaginal discharge and smegma must be removed.
b. Wipe vaginal area with cotton ball, using 1 stroke in a front-to-back direction.	b. Front-to-back cleansing prevents contamination of vagina.
9. Bathe buttocks, using a gentle, patting motion. Keep area clean and dry to prevent diaper rash. If rash does occur, protective ointment (zinc oxide or A & D) may be used. Exposure of buttocks to air or heat lamp is helpful.	9. Area is susceptible to skin breakdown because of acid reaction of urine and feces.

STOOL OBSERVATION

NURSING ACTION	RATIONALE
1. Observe stool pattern—meconium during first 2–3 days.	1. Material composed of epithelial and epidermal cells, lanugo, and bile pigments.
2. Transitional stools—change from tarry black to greenish black, to greenish brown to brownish yellow to greenish yellow.	2. Changes reflect intake of milk—stools are composed of both meconium and milk stools.

(continued)

PROCEDURE GUIDELINES 36-1 ◆ Newborn Care *(continued)*

PROCEDURE *(cont'd)*	NURSING ACTION	RATIONALE

NURSING ACTION

3. Number, color, and consistency are recorded daily.

RATIONALE

3. For early identification of abnormalities.
   a. No stool within 48 hours indicates an intestinal obstruction.
   b. Passage of meconium only (without other stool) suggests obstruction in the ileum.
   c. Thick, putty-like meconium may indicate cystic fibrosis.
   d. Diarrhea may be caused by overfeeding or by gastroenteritis.
   e. Blood in the stool is an indication of intestinal bleeding.

NUTRITIONAL CONSIDERATIONS

NURSING ACTION

1. Provide for nutritional intake.
2. Promote feeding method of choice.

3. Test urine glucose using reagent strip test and blood glucose using enzymatic strip test.
4. First feeding is sterile water. If retained, formula is given at next feeding.

5. Instruct the parent in technique of bottle-feeding.
   a. Hold baby in semi-upright position.
   b. Position bottle so that neck of bottle is filled.
   c. Insert nipple into baby's mouth so that baby's tongue is under nipple.
   d. Burp during feeding by holding infant upright.

RATIONALE

1. Infants vary in their readiness to feed.
2. Although recommendations may be made, family decisions should be respected and continuity of care provided.
3. Infant may be hypoglycemic and require feeding sooner than usual 4–6-hour wait.
4. Glucose water, if aspirated, is dangerous to lung tissue. Most hospitals use prepared milk mixture in disposable containers. Various formulas are available.

5. a. Gravity assists flow of milk into stomach.
   b. Prevents the baby from swallowing air.
   c. Sucking and swallowing reflexes are used in feeding.

   d. Allows air to escape from stomach, preventing distention or milk regurgitation.

DISCHARGE PLANNING

NURSING ACTION

1. Preparation for home care: instruction is given concerning infant bathing and care, preparation of formula, and infant feeding. Written formula with instructions for preparation is provided to parents.
2. Provide ample opportunity for parent contact.

RATIONALE

1. Instruction for infant care is a combined responsibility of the medical and nursing staffs.

2. Early attachment results in improved parent–child relationships.

Selected References

Avery, G., et al. (1994). *Neonatology pathophysiology and management of the newborn* (4th ed.). Philadelphia: J.B. Lippincott.

Bear, K., et al. (1993). Management strategies for promoting successful breastfeeding. *Nursing Practice, 18*(6), 50, 53-54, 56-58 passim.

Faller, H. S., et al. (1993). Sibling visitation: How far should the pendulum swing? *Journal of Pediatric Nursing, 8*(2), 92-99.

Furmon, L. (1993). Breastfeeding and fulltime maternal employment: Does the baby lose out [editorial]? *Journal of Human Lactation, 9*(1), 1-2.

Gowie, T. M., et al. (1994). *Foundations of maternal newborn nursing*. Philadelphia: W.B. Saunders.

Hadson, P. (1992). Health visitors, preventing postnatal illness. *Nursing Times, 88*(43), 68, 70.

Hall, W. A., et al. (1993). Managing the early discharge experience: Taking control. *Journal of Advanced Nursing, 18*(4), 574-582.

May. K. A., & Mahlmeister, L. R. (1994). *Maternal and neonatal nursing: Family centered care* (3rd ed.). Philadelphia: J.B. Lippincott.

Parkin, P. C., et al. (1993). Randomized controlled trial of three interventions in the management of persistent crying of infancy. *Pediatrics, 92*(2), 197-201.

Watters, N. E., et al. (1995). The evaluation of combined mother/infant versus separate postnatal nursing care. *Research in Nursing, 18* (1), 17–26.

CHAPTER 37

Complications of the Childbearing Experience

Obstetric Complications

> **NURSING ALERT:**
> Many obstetric complications involve the possibility of hemorrhage requiring blood replacement. Determine the patient's feelings and beliefs regarding the possibility of transfusions and notify health care providers if transfusion is refused.

◆ ECTOPIC PREGNANCY

Ectopic pregnancy is any gestation located outside the uterine cavity.

Pathophysiology/Etiology

1. The fertilized ovum implants outside of the uterus.
   a. The most common site of implantation is the fallopian or uterine tube (Fig. 37-1).
   b. Other sites include the abdomen and the ovaries.
2. Structural factors that prevent or delay the passage of the fertilized ovum include adhesions of the tube, salpingitis, congenital and developmental anomalies of the fallopian or uterine tube, previous ectopic pregnancy, current use of an intrauterine device, and multiple induced abortions.
3. Functional factors include menstrual reflux and decreased tubal motility.
4. Contributing factors may include:
   a. History of pelvic inflammatory disease (PID)
   b. Endometriosis
   c. Previous tubal surgery

Clinical Manifestations

1. Abdominal or pelvic pain
2. Amenorrhea—in 75% of the cases
3. Vaginal bleeding—usually scanty and dark

4. Uterine size is usually similar to what it would be in a normally implanted pregnancy.
5. Abdominal tenderness on palpation
6. Nausea, vomiting, or faintness may be present.
7. Pelvic examination reveals a pelvic mass, posterior or lateral to the uterus, and cervical pain on movement of the cervix.

Note: Pain may become severe if a tubal rupture occurs and clinical presentation will be that of shock.

Diagnostic Evaluation

1. Serum β-human chorionic gonadotropin (β-hCG)—when done serially, will not show characteristic rise as in intrauterine pregnancy
2. Ultrasound—may identify tubal mass, absence of gestational sac within the uterus
3. Culdocentesis—bloody aspirate from the cul-de-sac of Douglas indicates intraperitoneal bleeding from tubal rupture
4. Laparoscopy—visualization of tubal pregnancy
5. Laparotomy—indication for surgery if there is any question about the diagnosis

Management

1. Preserve maternal life through removal of the pregnancy and reconstruction of the tube, if possible. The surgical procedure depends on the extent of tubal involvement and if rupture has occurred. Surgeries range from removal of ectopic pregnancy with tubal resection, salpingostomy, salpingectomy, and possibly salpingo-oophorectomy.
2. Treat shock and hemorrhage if necessary.

Nursing Assessment

Evaluate the following to determine pregnancy and to monitor for changes in patient's status, such as rupture or hemorrhage:

CAUSES

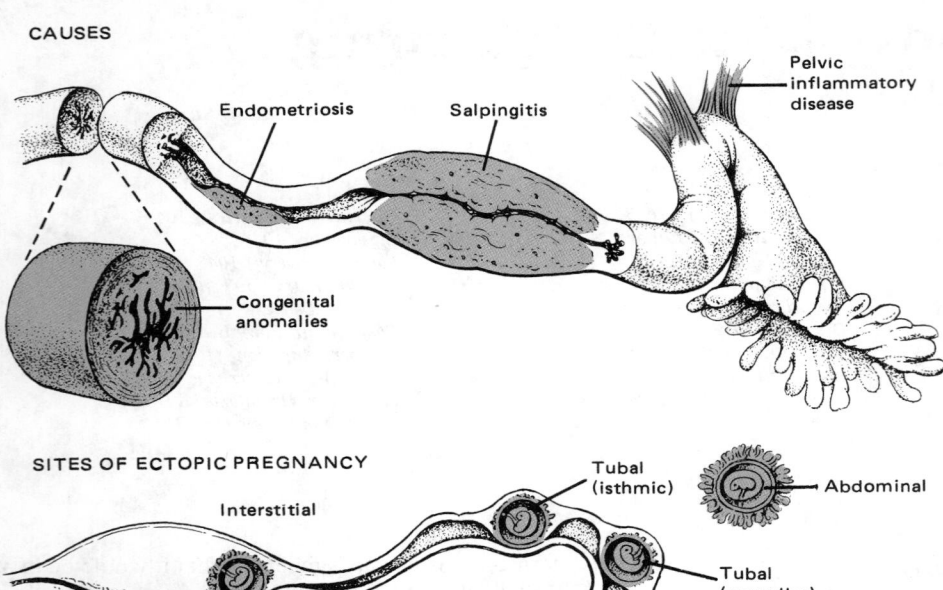

SITES OF ECTOPIC PREGNANCY

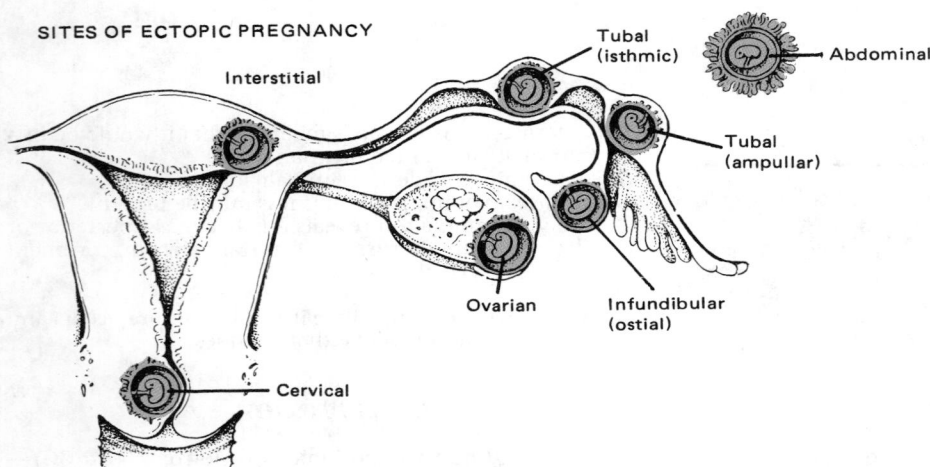

FIGURE 37-1 Ectopic pregnancy.

1. Maternal vital signs
2. Presence and amount of vaginal bleeding
3. Amount and type of pain
4. Presence of abdominal tenderness on palpation
5. Date of last menstrual period
6. Presence of positive pregnancy test

Nursing Diagnoses

A. Risk for Fluid Volume Deficit related to blood loss from ruptured tube
B. Pain related to ectopic pregnancy or rupture and bleeding into the peritoneal cavity
C. Anticipatory Grieving related to loss of pregnancy and potential loss of childbearing capacity

Nursing Interventions

A. *Maintaining Fluid Volume*
1. Establish an intravenous (IV) line with a large-bore catheter and infuse fluids and blood products as prescribed.
2. Obtain blood samples for complete blood count (CBC) and type and screen for whole blood, as directed.
3. Monitor vital signs and urine output frequently, depending on condition.

B. *Promoting Comfort*
1. Administer analgesics as needed and prescribed.
2. Encourage the use of relaxation techniques.

C. *Providing Support During Grief*
1. Be available to patient and provide emotional support.
2. Listen to concerns of patient and significant others.
3. Be aware that family may be experiencing denial or other stage of grieving.
4. Suggest referrals such as social worker, psychiatry, and clergy, as appropriate.

Note: The term "family" may refer to a nontraditional group of persons, such as the patient and significant other, friend, sibling, parent, or grandparent.

Patient Education/Health Maintenance

1. Teach signs of postoperative infection including fever, abdominal pain, and increased or malodorous vaginal discharge.

2. Reinforce that chances of another ectopic pregnancy are increased and that subsequent conception potential may be decreased, based on health care provider's explanation.
3. Discuss contraception.
4. Teach signs of recurrent ectopic pregnancy—abnormal vaginal bleeding, abdominal pain, menstrual irregularity.

Evaluation

A. Vital signs stable
B. Verbalizes pain relief
C. Patient and support person express sorrow over their loss

◆ HYDATIDIFORM MOLE

Hydatidiform mole is an abnormal pregnancy resulting from a developmental anomaly of the placenta. It is characterized by the conversion of the chorionic villi into a mass of clear vesicles. There may be no fetus or a degenerating fetus may be present.

Pathophysiology/Etiology

1. It is believed to be derived from the paternal haploid, X-carrying set of chromosomes that reaches 46 XX by its own duplication. Not all moles have the 46 XX chromosomal makeup.
2. It arises in fetal rather than maternal tissue.
3. Large amounts of hCG are present secondary to the proliferation of chorionic tissue. Assay values of β-hCG are elevated in the condition.
4. Contributing factors may include chromosomal abnormalities, malnutrition, hormonal imbalance, age under 20 or over 40, and low economic status.

Clinical Manifestations

1. First trimester bleeding
2. Absence of fetal heart tones and fetal structures
3. Rapid enlargement of the uterus; size greater than dates
4. β-hCG titers greater than expected for gestational age
5. Expulsion of the vesicles
6. Hyperemesis
7. Signs of pregnancy-induced hypertension (PIH) prior to 20 weeks' gestation

Diagnostic Evaluation

1. β-hCG levels—elevated
2. Ultrasound—shows a characteristic picture of the mole in most cases

Management

1. Suction curettage is the method of choice for immediate evacuation of the mole with possibility of laparotomy.

2. Follow-up for detection of malignant changes because a complication is the development of choriocarcinoma of the endometrium.

Nursing Assessment

1. Monitor maternal vital signs; note presence of hypertension.
2. Assess the amount and type of vaginal bleeding; note the presence of any other vaginal discharge.
3. Assess the urine for the presence of protein.
4. Palpate uterine height; if above the umbilicus, measure the fundal height.
5. Determine date of last menstrual period and date of positive pregnancy test.

Nursing Diagnoses

A. Potential for Fluid Volume Deficit related to maternal hemorrhage
B. Anxiety related to loss of pregnancy and medical interventions

Nursing Interventions

A. **Maintaining Fluid Volume**
1. Obtain blood samples for type and screen and have 2 to 4 units of whole blood available for possible replacement.
2. Establish and maintain IV line; start with a large needle to accommodate possible transfusion and large quantities of fluid.
3. Assess maternal vital signs and evaluate bleeding.
4. Monitor laboratory results to evaluate patient's status.

B. **Decreasing Anxiety**
1. Prepare the patient for surgery. Explain preoperative and postoperative care along with intraoperative procedures.
2. Educate patient and family on the disease process.
3. Allow the family to grieve over the loss of the pregnancy.

Patient Education/Health Maintenance

1. Advise the woman on the need for continuous follow-up care.
2. Provide reinforcement of follow-up procedures:
   a. Measure hCG levels every 1 to 2 weeks until normal—then begin monthly testing for 6 months, then every 2 months for a total of 1 year.
   b. Consider chemotherapy or hysterectomy if β-hCG levels rise or begin to plateau or there is evidence of metastasis.
3. Encourage ongoing discussion of care with health care provider.
4. Avoid pregnancy for a minimum of 1 year.

Evaluation

A. Vital signs stable; laboratory work within normal limits
B. Verbalizes concerns about self and related procedures; describes follow-up care and its importance

◆ SPONTANEOUS ABORTION

Spontaneous abortion is the unintended termination of pregnancy at any time before the fetus has attained viability (20 weeks' gestation or fetal weight of 500 g [1.1 lb]). See Table 37-1. For a discussion of therapeutic or voluntary abortion see Box 37-1.

Pathophysiology/Etiology

1. Cause frequently unknown, but 50% are due to chromosomal anomalies
2. Exposure or contact with teratogenic agents
3. Poor maternal nutritional status
4. Maternal illness with virus such as rubella, cytomegalovirus (CMV), active herpes, and toxoplasmosis, or specific bacterial microorganisms that put the pregnancy at risk.
5. History of diabetes, thyroid disease, anticardiolipin antibodies, or lupus erythematosus.
6. Smoking or drug abuse or both
7. Immunologic factor by which the mother and father are genetically similar, with similar major antigens, that cause the maternal immune system to reject the embryo
8. Luteal phase defect
9. Postmature sperm or ova
10. Structural defect in the maternal reproductive system (including an incompetent cervix)
11. Imperfect sperm or ova

Clinical Manifestations

1. Uterine cramping, low back pain
2. Vaginal bleeding usually begins as dark spotting, then progresses to frank bleeding as the embryo separates from the uterus.
3. β-hCG levels may be elevated for as long as 2 weeks after loss of the embryo.

Diagnostic Evaluation

1. Ultrasonic evaluation of the gestational sac or embryo
2. Visualization of the cervix; presence of dilation or tissue evaluated

TABLE 37-1 Types of Spontaneous Abortions

Classification	Clinical Manifestations	Management
1. Threatened	Vaginal bleeding or spotting Mild cramps Tenderness over uterus, simulates mild labor or persistent low backache with feeling of pelvic pressure Cervix closed or slightly dilated Symptoms subside or develop into an inevitable abortion	Vaginal examination Bed rest (some clinicians, citing the abnormal number of embryos that are aborted, will not limit activity in belief that the embryo will be aborted anyway) Pad count
2. Inevitable	Bleeding more profuse Cervix dilated Membranes rupture Painful uterine contractions	Embryo delivered, followed by dilatation and curettage (D&C)
3. Habitual	Spontaneous abortion occurs in successive pregnancies (3 or more)	D&C Treatment of possible causes: hormonal imbalance, tumors, thyroid dysfunction, abnormal uterus, incompetent cervix; with treatment, 70–80% carry a pregnancy successfully Hysterogram to rule out uterine abnormalities, infections Surgical suturing of the cervix if incompetent cervix is a causative factor
4. Incomplete	Fetus usually expelled Placenta and membranes retained	D&C
5. Missed	Fetus dies in utero and is retained Maceration No symptoms of abortion, but symptoms of pregnancy regress (uterine size, breast changes)	Real time ultrasound, and if second trimester, fetal monitoring to determine if fetus is dead If fetus is not passed after diagnosis, oxytocin induction may be used. Retained dead fetus may lead to development of disseminated intravascular coagulation or infection Fibrinogen concentrations should be measured weekly

BOX 37-1 *Therapeutic or Voluntary Abortion*

Therapeutic abortion is the termination of pregnancy before fetal viability for the purpose of safeguarding the woman's health.

Voluntary abortion is the termination of a pregnancy before fetal viability as a choice of the woman.

Procedures
1. First trimester abortions can be managed by dilation and curettage (D&C) or dilation and suction.
2. Second trimester abortions can be managed using prostaglandin E_2 vaginal suppositories or by IM injection of F_2 analogs. Laminaria or magnesium sulfate tents may be used prior to prostaglandin induction to "soften" the cervix and assist with dilatation.
3. Late second trimester abortions can be done using intra-amniotic saline injection, hysterotomy, or hysterectomy.

Complications
1. Retained products of conception
2. Hemorrhage
3. Prostaglandin complications including fever, diarrhea, nausea and vomiting, tachycardia, and bronchoconstriction
4. Surgical complications including uterine perforation, bowel trauma, cervical laceration

Nursing Considerations
1. Review the woman's knowledge of her choice and the options available in regard to childbearing to allow for informed decision-making.
2. Ensure patient understands the possible benefits and risks of a therapeutic or voluntary abortion.
3. Encourage patient to have support person accompany her and drive her home after the procedure.
4. Teach that cramping and bleeding, similar to a regular menstrual period, can be expected. Length of bleeding varies, but usually subsides in 3–4 days.
5. Discuss the need for contraception and advise when to begin again.
6. Inform that a normal menstrual cycle should resume in 4–6 weeks.
7. Discuss the need for pelvic rest, as ordered (usually 2–3 weeks), to prevent infection, consisting of avoidance of sexual intercourse, douching, inserting tampons, etc.
8. Teach signs of infection (fever, pelvic pain, increased bleeding) and advise to report them to provider immediately.
9. Arrange for follow-up appointment and counseling, if necessary.

Complications

1. Hemorrhage
2. Uterine infection
3. Septicemia
4. Disseminated intravascular coagulation (DIC) in a missed abortion

Nursing Assessment

1. Evaluate the amount and color of blood that is present; determine the time the bleeding began and any precipitating factors.
2. Determine if a positive pregnancy test has previously been obtained, also the date of the last menstrual period.
3. Monitor maternal vital signs for indications of complications such as hemorrhage, infection.
4. Evaluate any blood or clot tissue for the presence of fetal membranes, placenta, or fetus.

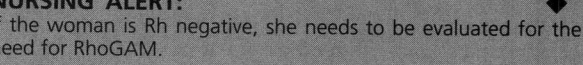

NURSING ALERT:
If the woman is Rh negative, she needs to be evaluated for the need for RhoGAM.

Nursing Diagnoses

A. Risk for Fluid Volume Deficit related to maternal bleeding
B. Anticipatory Grieving related to loss of pregnancy, cause of the abortion, future childbearing
C. Risk for Infection related to dilated cervix and open uterine vessels
D. Pain related to uterine cramping and possible procedures

Nursing Interventions

A. *Maintaining Fluid Volume*
1. Report any tachycardia, hypotension, diaphoresis, or pallor, indicating hemorrhage and shock.
2. Draw blood for type and screen for possible blood administration.
3. Establish and maintain an IV with large-bore catheter for possible transfusion and large quantities of fluid replacement.
4. Inspect all tissue passed for completeness.

B. *Providing Support Through the Grieving Process*
1. Assess the reaction of patient and support person and provide information regarding current status, as needed.
2. Encourage the patient to discuss feelings about the loss of the baby; include effects on relationship with the father.
3. Do not minimize the loss by focusing on future childbearing; rather acknowledge the loss and allow grieving.
4. Provide time alone for the couple to discuss their feelings.
5. Discuss the prognosis of future pregnancies with the couple.
6. If the fetus is aborted intact, provide an opportunity for viewing, if parents desire.
7. Refer to chaplain or social worker if indicated or requested.

C. *Preventing Infection*
1. Evaluate temperature every 4 hours if normal, and every 2 hours if elevated.
2. Check vaginal drainage for increased amount and odor, which may indicate infection.

3. Instruct on and encourage perineal care following each urination and defecation to prevent contamination.

D. *Promoting Comfort*
1. Instruct patient on the cause of pain to decrease anxiety.
2. Instruct and encourage the use of relaxation techniques to augment analgesics.
3. Administer pain medications as needed and as prescribed.

Patient Education/Health Maintenance

1. Provide the names of local support groups for couples who have experienced an early pregnancy loss: Resolve, Inc.; 1310 Broadway; Somerville, MA 02144-1731; 617-623-0744.
2. Discuss with the couple the methods of contraception to be used.
3. Explain the need to wait at least 3 to 6 months before attempting another pregnancy.
4. Teach the woman to observe for signs of infection (fever, pelvic pain, change in character and amount of vaginal discharge), and advise to report them to provider immediately.
5. Provide information regarding genetic testing of the products of conception if indicated; send the specimen according to policy.

Evaluation

A. Vital signs remain normal; minimal blood loss
B. Expresses feelings regarding the loss of the pregnancy
C. No signs of infection, temperature normal, performs perineal care
D. Verbalizes relief of pain

◆ HYPEREMESIS GRAVIDARUM

Hyperemesis gravidarum is exaggerated nausea and vomiting during pregnancy persisting past the first trimester.

Pathophysiology/Etiology

1. Cause unknown but may possibly result from high levels of hCG or estrogen.
2. Psychological factors including neurosis or altered self-concept may be contributory.
3. Seen in molar pregnancies, multiple gestation, and history of hyperemesis in previous pregnancies.
4. Slowed gastric motility occurs.
5. The persistent vomiting may result in fluid and electrolyte imbalances, dehydration, jaundice, and elevation of serum transaminase.

Clinical Manifestations

1. Persistent vomiting; inability to tolerate anything by mouth
2. Dehydration—fever, dry skin, decreased urine output

3. Weight loss (up to 5–10% of body weight)
4. Severity of symptoms increases as the disease progresses.

Diagnostic Evaluation

1. Tests may be done to rule out other conditions causing vomiting (cholecystitis, appendicitis).
2. Liver function studies—elevated aspartate aminotransferase up to four times normal in severe cases
3. Prothrombin time, partial thromboplastin time usually normal
4. Blood urea nitrogen (BUN) and creatinine—may be slightly elevated
5. Serum electrolytes—may be hypokalemia, hypo- or hypernatremia
6. Urine for ketones—positive

Management

1. Try withholding food and fluid for 24 hours, or until vomiting stops and appetite returns; then restart small feedings.
2. Control of vomiting may require antiemetic such as prochlorperazine (Compazine) in injectable or rectal suppository form.
3. Control of dehydration through IV fluids—often 1 to 3 liters of dextrose solution with electrolytes and vitamins, as needed. Bicarbonate may be given for acidosis.
4. Most women respond quickly to restricting oral intake and giving IV fluids, but repeated episodes may occur.
5. Rarely, total parenteral nutrition is needed.
6. Rarely, complications of hepatic or renal failure or coma could result from disease progression.

Nursing Assessment

1. Evaluate weight gain or loss pattern.
2. Evaluate 24- or 48-hour dietary recall.
3. Evaluate environment for factors that may affect the woman's appetite.
4. Monitor vital signs for tachycardia, hypotension, and fever due to dehydration.
5. Assess skin turgor and mucous membranes for signs of dehydration.

Nursing Diagnoses

A. Risk for Fluid Volume Deficit, Electrolyte Imbalance related to prolonged vomiting
B. Altered Nutrition (Less than Body Requirements) related to prolonged vomiting
C. Ineffective Individual Coping related to stress of pregnancy and illness

Nursing Interventions

A. *Maintaining Fluid Volume*
1. Establish an IV line and administer IV fluids as prescribed.

2. Monitor serum electrolytes and report abnormalities.
3. Medicate with antiemetics as prescribed.
   a. Administer intramuscularly or by rectal suppository to avoid loss of dose through vomiting.
4. Maintain NPO status except for ice chips until vomiting has stopped.
5. Assess intake and output, vital signs, skin turgor, and fetal heart tones as indicated by condition.

B. *Encouraging Adequate Nutrition*
1. Advise the woman that oral intake can be restarted when emesis has stopped and appetite returns.
2. Begin small feedings. Suggest or provide bland solid foods; serve hot foods hot and cold foods cold; do not serve lukewarm.
   a. Avoid greasy, gassy, and spicy foods.
   b. Provide liquids at times other than meal times.
3. Suggest or provide an environment conducive to eating.
   a. Keep room cool and quiet before and after meals.
   b. Keep emesis pan handy, yet out of sight.

C. *Strengthening Coping Mechanisms*
1. Allow patient to verbalize feelings regarding this pregnancy.
2. Encourage patient to discuss any personal stress that may have a negative effect on this pregnancy.
3. Refer to social service and counseling services as needed.

Patient Education/Health Maintenance

1. Educate the woman about proper diet and nutrition in pregnancy.
2. Educate the woman about healthy weight gain in pregnancy.
3. Maintain support for the woman with health care from referral services, as appropriate.

Evaluation

A. Urine output adequate; blood pressure stable
B. Tolerates small, bland feedings without vomiting
C. Verbalizes concerns and stresses related to pregnancy

◆ PLACENTA PREVIA

Placenta previa is the development of the placenta in the lower uterine segment, partially or completely covering the internal cervical os (Fig. 37-2).

Pathophysiology/Etiology

1. The cause is unknown.
2. One possible theory states that the embryo will implant in the lower uterine segment if the decidua in the uterine fundus is not favorable.
3. About 80% of placenta previa episodes occur in multiparas.
4. Seen more often with history of abortion, cesarean section, uterine scarring

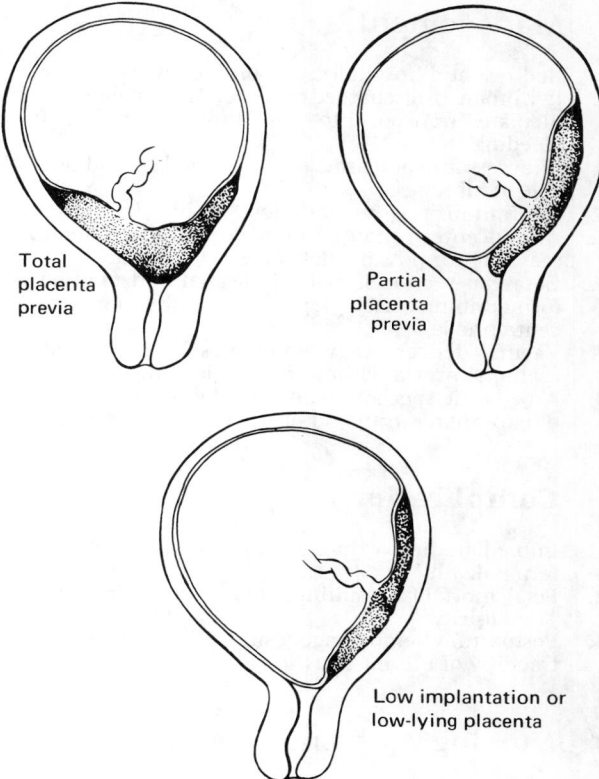

FIGURE 37-2 *Variations of placenta previa. (From Danforth, D. N. & Scott, J. R. Obstetrics and Gynecology (7th ed.). Philadelphia: J. B. Lippincott, 1994.)*

Clinical Manifestations

1. Characteristic sign is painless vaginal bleeding, which usually appears near the end of the second trimester or later.
2. Initial episode is rarely fatal and usually stops spontaneously, with subsequent bleeding episodes occurring spontaneously; each episode is more profuse than the previous one.
3. Bleeding from placenta previa may not occur until cervical dilation occurs and the placenta is loosened from the uterus.
4. With a complete placenta previa the bleeding will occur earlier in the pregnancy and be more profuse.

Diagnostic Evaluation

1. Ultrasound is the method of choice to show location of the placenta.
2. If findings are questionable, transvaginal ultrasound can improve the accuracy of diagnosis. Due to bleeding tendencies, however, this must be done by a highly skilled technician.

Management

1. Bed rest and hospitalization until delivery are usual.
2. If woman is discharged, she needs availability of immediate transport to the hospital for recurrent bleeding.
3. IV access and at least 2 units of blood should be available at all times.
4. Continuous maternal and fetal monitoring
5. Amniocentesis may be done to determine fetal lung maturity for possible delivery.
6. Cesarean section is often indicated and may be performed immediately depending on the degree of placenta previa.
7. Vaginal delivery may sometimes be attempted in a marginal previa without active bleeding.
8. A pediatric specialty team may be needed at delivery due to prematurity and other neonatal complications.

Complications

1. Immediate hemorrhage, with possible shock and maternal death
2. Fetal mortality resulting from hypoxia in utero and prematurity
3. Postpartum hemorrhage resulting from decreased contractility of uterine muscle

Nursing Assessment

1. Determine the amount and type of bleeding; also, review any history of bleeding throughout this pregnancy.
2. Inquire as to the presence or absence of pain in association with the bleeding.
3. Record maternal and fetal vital signs.
4. Palpate for the presence of uterine contractions.
5. Evaluate laboratory data on hemoglobin and hematocrit status.

> **NURSING ALERT:**
> Never perform a vaginal examination on anyone who is bleeding. This may puncture the placenta.

Nursing Diagnoses

A. Altered Tissue Perfusion, Placental, related to excessive bleeding
B. Fluid Volume Deficit related to excessive bleeding
C. Risk for Infection related to excessive blood loss and open vessels near cervix
D. Anxiety related to excessive bleeding, procedures, and possible maternal–fetal complications

Nursing Interventions

A. *Promoting Tissue Perfusion*
1. Frequently monitor mother and fetus.
2. Administer IV fluids, as prescribed.

3. Position on side to promote placental perfusion.
4. Administer oxygen by face mask, as indicated.

B. *Maintaining Fluid Volume*
1. Establish and maintain a large-bore IV line, as prescribed, and draw blood for type and screen for blood replacement.
2. Position in a sitting position to allow the weight of fetus to compress the placenta and decrease bleeding.
3. Maintain strict bed rest during any bleeding episode.
4. If bleeding is profuse and delivery cannot be delayed, prepare the woman physically and emotionally for a cesarean delivery.

C. *Preventing Infection*
1. Use aseptic technique when providing care.
2. Evaluate temperature every 4 hours unless elevated; then, evaluate every 2 hours.
3. Evaluate white blood cell (WBC) and differential count.
4. Teach perineal care and handwashing.
5. Assess odor of all vaginal bleeding or lochia.
6. Instruct on perineal care and handwashing techniques.

D. *Decreasing Anxiety*
1. Explain all treatments and procedures and answer all related questions.
2. Encourage verbalization of feelings by patient and family.
3. Provide information on a cesarean delivery and prepare patient emotionally.
4. Discuss the effects of long-term hospitalization or prolonged bed rest.

Patient Education/Health Maintenance

1. Educate the woman and her family about the etiology and treatment of placenta previa.
2. Educate the woman to inform medical personnel about her diagnosis and not to have vaginal examinations.
3. Educate the woman who is discharged from the hospital with a placenta previa to avoid intercourse or anything per vagina, to limit physical activity, to have an accessible person in the event of an emergency, and to go to the hospital immediately for repeat bleeding.

Evaluation

A. Fetal condition stable
B. Absence of shock, stable vital signs, absence of bleeding
C. Does not develop any symptoms of an infection
D. Verbalizes concerns and understanding of procedures and treatments

> **NURSING ALERT:**
> Women who have had a placenta previa are at risk for postpartum hemorrhage because of the decreased contractility of the lower uterine segment and the large space the placenta occupied.

◆ ABRUPTIO PLACENTAE

Abruptio placentae is premature separation of the normally implanted placenta. There are two types of abruptio placentae: concealed hemorrhage and external hemorrhage.

With a concealed hemorrhage the placenta separates centrally, and a large amount of blood is accumulated under the placenta. When an external hemorrhage is present, the separation is along the placental margin, and blood flows under the membranes and through the cervix (Fig. 37-3).

Pathophysiology/Etiology

1. Frequently, the etiology is unknown.
2. Women at risk for developing abruptio placentae include those with history of hypertension or previous abruptio placentae, or those who have rapid decompression of the uterine cavity, short umbilical cord, or presence of a uterine anomaly or tumor.
3. Additional risk occurs in existing pregnancies complicated by trauma, hypertension, alcohol, cigarette smoking, and cocaine abuse.
4. Hemorrhage occurs into the decidua basalis.
5. The decidua basalis then forms a hematoma.
6. This hematoma can expand as the bleeding increases, causing the hematoma to increase in size and further detach the placenta from the uterine wall.

Clinical Manifestations

1. Concealed hemorrhage—results in a change in maternal vital signs, but no visible signs of hemorrhage are present.
2. External hemorrhage—hemorrhage is evident along with a change in maternal vital signs.

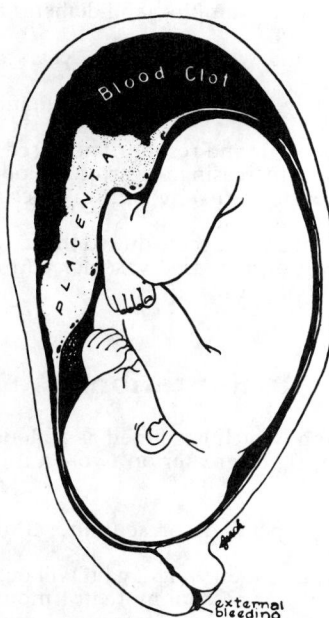

FIGURE 37-3 *Abruptio placentae with large blood clot between placenta and uterine wall.*

3. Fetal heart rate may change, depending on the degree of hemorrhage.
4. Abdominal pain is often present.

Diagnostic Evaluation

1. Based on signs and symptoms, including vaginal bleeding, abdominal pain, uterine contractions, uterine tenderness, fetal distress. Not all may be seen in every case.
2. Ultrasound is done but is not always sensitive enough to rule out the diagnosis.

Management

1. Hospitalization, bed rest, and continuous fetal monitoring
2. Management of hemorrhagic shock
3. Severe abruptions and fetal distress necessitate immediate delivery by cesarean section.
4. If the woman's status is stable, and there is no fetal distress, then a vaginal delivery may be considered.
5. A pediatric specialty team may be necessary at delivery due to prematurity and neonatal complications.

Complications

1. Maternal shock
2. DIC
3. Amniotic fluid embolism
4. Postpartum hemorrhage
5. Prematurity
6. Maternal/fetal death

Nursing Assessment

See Table 37-2.

1. Determine the amount and type of bleeding and the presence or absence of pain.
2. Monitor maternal and fetal vital signs.
3. Palpate the abdomen.
   a. Note the presence of contractions and relaxation between contractions (if contractions are present).
   b. If contractions are not present, assess the abdomen for firmness.
4. Measure and record fundal height to evaluate the presence of concealed bleeding.

Nursing Diagnoses

A. Altered Tissue Perfusion, Placental, related to excessive bleeding
B. Fluid Volume Deficit related to excessive bleeding
C. Fear related to excessive bleeding, procedures, and unknown outcome

Nursing Interventions

A. *Maintaining Tissue Perfusion*
1. Evaluate amount of bleeding by weighing all pads. Monitor CBC results and vital signs.
2. Position in the left lateral position, with the head elevated to enhance placental perfusion.

TABLE 37-2 Characteristics of Abruptio Placentae and Placenta Previa

Characteristic	Abruptio Placentae	Placenta Previa
Onset	Third trimester	Third trimester (commonly in eighth month)
Bleeding	May be concealed, external dark hemorrhage, or bloody amniotic fluid	Mostly external, small to profuse in amount, bright red
Pain and uterine tenderness	Usually present; irritable uterus, progresses to boardlike consistency	Usually absent; uterus soft
Fetal heart tone	May be irregular or absent	Usually normal
Presenting part	May or may not be engaged	Usually not engaged
Shock	Moderate to severe depending on extent of concealed and external hemorrhage	Usually not present unless bleeding is excessive
Delivery	Immediate delivery, usually by cesarean section	Delivery may be delayed, depending on size of fetus and amount of bleeding

3. Administer oxygen through a face mask.
4. Evaluate fetal status with continuous external fetal monitoring.
5. Encourage relaxation techniques.

B. **Maintaining Fluid Volume**
1. Establish and maintain large-bore IV line for fluids and blood products as prescribed.
2. Evaluate coagulation studies.
3. Monitor maternal vital signs and contractions.
4. Monitor vaginal bleeding and evaluate fundal height to detect an increase in bleeding.

C. **Decreasing Fear**
1. Inform the woman and her family about the status of both herself and the fetus.
2. Explain all procedures in advance when possible or as they are performed.
3. Answer questions in a calm manner, using simple terms.
4. Encourage the presence of a support person.

Patient Education/Health Maintenance

1. Provide information to the woman and her family regarding etiology and treatment for abruptio placentae.
2. Encourage involvement from the neonatal team regarding education related to fetal/neonatal outcome.

Evaluation

A. Fetal heart rate within normal range, without a loss of variability
B. Absence of shock, demonstrated by stable maternal vital signs
C. Demonstrates concern; asks questions

◆ PREGNANCY-INDUCED HYPERTENSION

Pregnancy-induced hypertension (PIH, preeclampsia, eclampsia) is a disorder occurring during pregnancy after the 20th week of gestation and involving edema, proteinuria, and hypertension. Eclampsia is diagnosed when convulsions occur in the absence of an underlying neurologic condition in the presence of hypertension, edema, and proteinuria.

Note: Eclampsia was previously referred to as toxemia because it was thought to be caused by toxins. Currently, the term eclampsia is more commonly used.

Pathophysiology/Etiology

1. Actual cause is unknown.
2. Theories of the etiology include the exposure to chorionic villi for the first time, or in large amounts, along with immunologic, genetic, and endocrine factors.
3. The disease is primarily seen in primagravidas.
4. Chronic hypertension, hydatidiform mole, multiple gestation, polyhydramnios, and diabetes mellitus may predispose to PIH.
5. Adolescents and women over 35 years of age are at higher risk.
6. Approximately 6% to 8% of pregnancies may be affected.
7. Vasospasms occur and result in increased resistance in vascular flow, increasing the arterial blood pressure.
8. Increased sensitivity to angiotensin II occurs before the onset of hypertension.
9. Hemoconcentration occurs due to the vasoconstriction or as a result of increased vascular permeability or a combination of both.

Clinical Manifestations

1. Hypertension, which is defined as a blood pressure of 140/90 mm Hg or greater on two occasions at least 6 hours apart
2. Proteinuria
3. Edema, nondependent, present after 8 to 12 hours of bed rest
4. Frequently, a sudden weight gain will occur, of 2 lb or more in 1 week, or 6 lb or more in 1 month. This often occurs before the edema is present.
5. Altered level of consciousness, visual changes, headache
6. Oliguria

7. Epigastric pain, chest pressure
8. Hyperreflexia with or without clonus

Diagnostic Evaluation

1. A 24-hour urine for protein of 300 mg or greater
2. Serum BUN and creatine to evaluate renal function
3. Sonogram, nonstress testing to evaluate placenta and fetus

Management

1. Directed toward decreasing the maternal blood pressure through the use of bed rest and antihypertensive medications along with increase in dietary protein and an increase in calories, if indicated
2. Hospitalization and seizure prevention/treatment may be necessary.
   a. Magnesium sulfate (MgSO$_4$) may be given either IV or intramuscularly.
   b. A 4- to 6-g loading dose is usually given IV followed by a maintenance dose of 1 to 4 g/h.
   c. Intramuscular injection of 10 g (5 g in each buttock) as a loading dose is usually given, followed by 5 g every 4 hours.
3. Antihypertensive drug therapy may be used when the diastolic pressure is above 110 mm Hg or when cerebrovascular accident is impending.
   a. Hydralazine (Apresoline) is the drug of choice. Hydralazine relaxes the arterioles and stimulates cardiac output.
   b. Side effects include tachycardia, palpitations, dizziness, faintness, headache.
4. Diazepam (Valium) and amobarbital sodium (Amytal Sodium) may be used if convulsions occur that respond to MgSO$_4$.
5. β-Adrenergic blockers are used by some to control acute hypertension. These drugs will rapidly lower the blood pressure; however, further studies are needed on these drugs and their use in pregnancy.
6. If symptoms are uncontrollable, delivery is planned.

Complications

1. Abruptio placentae
2. DIC
3. HELLP syndrome (Box 37-2)
4. Prematurity
5. Intrauterine growth retardation (IUGR) from decreased placental perfusion
6. Maternal/fetal death

Nursing Assessment

1. Evaluate blood pressure with patient in a sitting position and in the left lateral position.
2. Check the protein level of a spot urine specimen.
3. Evaluate edema, carefully noting the presence after 12 hours or more of bed rest. Measure weight.
4. Evaluate deep tendon reflexes and clonus.

BOX 37-2 *HELLP Syndrome*

HELLP syndrome is a severe complication of pregnancy-induced hypertension. It is comprised of *H*emolysis, *E*levated *L*iver enzymes, and *L*ow *P*latelets.
1. These findings are frequently associated with DIC and in fact may be diagnosed as DIC.
2. The hemolysis of erythrocytes is seen in the abnormal morphology of the cells.
3. The elevated liver enzyme measurement is associated with the decreased blood flow to the liver as a result of fibrin thrombi.
4. The low platelet count is related to vasospasm and platelet adhesions.
5. Treatment is similar to treatment for PIH with close monitoring of liver function and bleeding.
6. These women are at increased risk for postpartum hemorrhage.

Nursing Diagnoses

A. Fluid Volume Excess related to IV fluid overload
B. Altered Tissue Perfusion, Fetal Cardiac and Cerebral, related to altered placental blood flow
C. Risk for Injury related to convulsions
D. Anxiety related to concern for self and fetus

Nursing Interventions

A. *Maintaining Fluid Balance*
1. Control IV fluid intake using a continuous infusion pump.
2. Monitor intake and output strictly; notify health care provider if urine output is less than 30 mL/h.
4. Monitor hematocrit levels to evaluate intravascular fluid status.
5. Monitor vital signs every hour.
6. Auscultate breath sounds every 2 hours and report signs of pulmonary edema (wheezing, crackles, shortness of breath, increased pulse rate, increased respiratory rate).

B. *Promoting Adequate Tissue Perfusion*
1. Position on side, preferably the left side to promote placental perfusion.
2. Monitor fetal activity.
3. Evaluate nonstress tests to determine fetal status.
4. Increase protein intake to replace protein lost through kidneys.

C. *Preventing Injury*
1. Instruct on the importance of reporting headaches, visual changes, dizziness, and epigastric pain.
2. Instruct to lie down on left side if symptoms are present.
3. Keep the environment quiet and as calm as possible.
4. If hospitalized, side rails should be padded and remain up to prevent injury if seizure occurs.
5. If hospitalized, have oxygen and suction setup, along with a tongue blade and emergency medications immediately available for treatment of seizures.

D. *Decreasing Anxiety*
1. Explain the disease process and treatment plan.
2. Explain that PIH does not lead to chronic hypertension.
3. Explain that PIH usually does not occur with subsequent pregnancies.
4. Discuss the effects of all medications on the mother and fetus.
5. Allow time to ask questions and discuss feelings regarding the diagnosis and treatment plan.

Patient Education/Health Maintenance

1. Teach the woman the importance of bed rest in helping to control symptoms.
2. Encourage the support of family and friends while on bed rest.
3. Provide and suggest diversional activities while on bed rest.
4. Provide information on tests and procedures to evaluate maternal–fetal status, such as laboratory tests, sonogram, nonstress tests.
5. Include support of the neonatal team for discussion of fetal prognosis with the woman and her family.

Evaluation

A. No evidence of pulmonary edema; urine output adequate
B. Fetal heart rate within normal range; reactivity present
C. No seizure activity
D. Expresses concern for self and the fetus

◆ HYDRAMNIOS (POLYHYDRAMNIOS)

Hydramnios (polyhydramnios) is caused by an excessive amount of amniotic fluid. At 36 weeks of pregnancy there is usually about a liter of fluid present. The amount of amniotic fluid normally decreases after this time. The amount of amniotic fluid present is controlled in part by fetal urination, swallowing, and breathing.

Pathophysiology/Etiology

1. The etiology is often unclear.
2. Anomalies causing impaired fetal swallowing or excessive micturition may contribute to the condition.
3. It is associated with maternal diabetes, multiple gestation and Rh isoimmunization. Other associated factors are anomalies of the central nervous system including spina bifida and anencephaly or anomalies of the gastrointestinal tract including tracheoesophageal fistula.
4. In chronic hydramnios the fluid volume gradually increases; in the acute type the volume increases rapidly over a few days.

Clinical Manifestations

1. Excessive weight gain, dyspnea
2. Abdomen may be tense and shiny.

3. Edema of the vulva, legs, and lower extremities
4. Increased uterine size for gestational age usually accompanied by difficulty in palpating fetal parts and in auscultation of fetal heart

Diagnostic Evaluation

1. A diagnosis is made based on the present symptoms and ultrasound evaluation.
2. Ultrasound evaluation will show large pockets of fluid between the fetus and uterine wall or placenta.

Management

1. Depends on the severity of the condition and the cause; hospitalization is indicated for maternal distress or for intervention regarding fetal prognosis.
2. If impairment of maternal respiratory status occurs, amniocentesis for removal of fluid may be performed.
   a. The amniocentesis is performed under ultrasound for location of the placenta and fetal parts.
   b. The fluid is then slowly removed.
   c. Rapid removal of the fluid can result in a premature separation of the placenta.
   d. Usually 500 to 1,000 mL of fluid is removed.

Complications

1. Preterm labor
2. Dysfunctional labor with increased risk for cesarean section
3. Postpartum hemorrhage due to uterine atony from gross distention of the uterus

Nursing Assessment

1. Evaluate maternal respiratory status.
2. Inspect abdomen and evaluate uterine height and compare with previous findings.

Nursing Diagnoses

A. Ineffective Breathing Pattern related to pressure on the diaphragm
B. Altered Tissue Perfusion, Placental, related to pressure from excess fluid
C. Impaired Physical Mobility related to edema and discomfort from the enlarged uterus
D. Anxiety related to fetal outcome

Nursing Interventions

A. *Promoting Effective Breathing*
1. Position to promote chest expansion with head elevated.
2. Provide oxygen by face mask, if indicated.
3. Limit activities and plan for frequent rest periods.
4. Maintain adequate intake and output.

B. Promoting Placental Tissue Perfusion
1. Position on left side if possible, with head elevated. If unable to position on side, use a wedge to displace the uterus to the left.
2. Encourage passive or active assisted range of motion to the lower extremities.
3. Monitor fetal heart rate as directed.
4. Provide a diet adequate in protein, iron, and fluids.

C. Promoting Mobility
1. Assist the woman with position changes and ambulation as needed.
2. Advise on alternating activity with rest periods for legs.
3. Instruct the woman to wear loose fitting clothing and low-heeled shoes with good support.

D. Decreasing Anxiety
1. Explain the cause of hydramnios, if known.
2. Encourage the patient and family to ask questions regarding any treatment or procedures.
3. Encourage expression of feelings.
4. Prepare patient for the type of delivery that is anticipated and for the expected finding at the time of delivery.
5. Encourage presence of support person.

Patient Education/Health Maintenance

1. Instruct the woman to notify her health care provider if she experiences respiratory distress.
2. Teach the woman signs of preterm labor and the need to report them to health care provider.

Evaluation

A. Respirations 20 and unlabored
B. Fetal heart rate within normal limits
C. Verbalizes improved comfort; moves freely
D. Discusses realistically the pregnancy outcome; questions regarding treatment for self and fetus

◆ OLIGOHYDRAMNIOS

Oligohydramnios is caused by a marked decrease in the amount of amniotic fluid. Usually the fluid is extremely concentrated. Cord compression and fetal distress may occur and lead to a poor outcome. Often the infant will suffer from pulmonary hypoplasia due to a lack of fluid in the terminal air sacs.

Pathophysiology/Etiology

1. Frequently related to fetal problems such as obstruction in the urinary tract, renal agenesis, and IUGR
2. Associated with premature rupture of membranes (PROM) and severe preeclampsia where there is a significant decrease in fetal vascular volume causing decreased urine output
3. Frequently seen in postdate pregnancies

Clinical Manifestations

1. Prominent fetal parts on palpation of the abdomen
2. Small-for-date uterine size

Diagnostic Evaluation

1. Ultrasound evaluation of the amniotic fluid index—amniotic pockets of 2 to 8 cm in any vertical plane in each of the four quadrants of the uterus are associated with lower perinatal mortality. Pockets less than 2 cm carry a higher mortality rate.

Management

1. Frequent evaluation of fetal status through nonstress test and stress test as indicated
2. Ultrasound is also done to further evaluate fetal renal and urinary systems along with fetal growth.
3. Saline amnioinfusion during labor
4. Delivery may be indicated for conditions such as IUGR or fetal distress.

Complications

1. Umbilical cord compression
2. Passage of meconium
3. Fetal/neonatal death

Nursing Interventions/Patient Education

1. Evaluate fetal status via fetal monitoring.
2. Evaluate maternal vital signs for signs of infection, especially if oligohydramnios is secondary to PROM.
3. Assist with an amnioinfusion as indicated.
4. Inform health care provider of fetal distress, assist the woman to a left side-lying position, and treat as indicated.

◆ MULTIPLE GESTATION

Multiple gestation or multifetal pregnancy results when two or more fetuses are present in the uterus at the same time.

Etiology

1. Types of twinning
   a. *Dizygotic*—occurs when two separate ova are fertilized. Dizygotic twins do not have the same genetic makeup and are as similar as other brothers and sisters.
   b. *Monozygotic*—occurs when one ovum divides early in gestation and two embryos develop. Monozygotic twins are identical in genetic makeup.
2. Artificially induced ovulation as well as in vitro fertilization where multiple embryos are transferred into the uterus increase the chances of multiple gestation.

3. Increasing maternal age and parity increase the chance of twinning.

Clinical Manifestations

1. Usually the uterus is large for gestational age during the second trimester.
2. Auscultation of two distinct and separate fetal hearts may occur with a doppler late in the first trimester or with a fetoscope after 20 weeks' gestation.
3. Ultrasound is the best screening test at present. It may identify separate gestation sacs.

Complications

1. Spontaneous abortion
2. IUGR
3. Prematurity
4. Polyhydramnios
5. PIH

Management/Nursing Interventions

1. Nutrition counseling—stress increased caloric and protein intake as well as vitamin supplements to meet the demands of multiple gestation.
2. Fetal evaluation—encourage follow-up for serial sonograms during the pregnancy to evaluate growth and development and to detect IUGR. Explain nonstress tests, biophysical profile, and amniocentesis for detection of fetal lung maturity. Percutaneous umbilical cord sampling may be used to establish fetal well being if twin-to-twin transfusion is suspected.
3. Evaluate the woman for signs and symptoms of PIH, which is more common in multiple gestation.
4. Preterm labor prevention—explain that hospitalization may be necessary for signs and symptoms of preterm labor.
   a. Encourage bed rest and hydration.
   b. Institute fetal monitoring and assist with tocolytic therapy, if ordered (see Tocolytic Therapy, in next section). This is controversial therapy.
5. Explain to the woman that mode for delivery depends on the presentation of the twins, maternal and fetal status and gestational age. Delivery of multiples other than twins is done by cesarean section.
6. Intrapartum management
   a. Establish IV access to be prepared for emergency birth or other complications.
   b. Provide for electronic fetal monitoring for each fetus.
7. Emotional support—encourage family to discuss feelings about multiple births and identify ways in which they will need help. Refer to resources such as: National Organization of Mothers of Twins Clubs, Inc.; 12404 Princess Jeanne NE; Albuquerque, NM 87112-4640; 505-275-0955.

Complications of Labor

◆ PRETERM LABOR

Preterm labor is defined as uterine contractions occurring after 20 weeks' gestation and before 37 completed weeks of gestation. Contractions are less than 10 minutes apart, resulting in progressive cervical changes or cervical dilation of 2 cm or effacement of 75%.

Pathophysiology/Etiology

The exact etiology for preterm labor remains unknown. However, certain changes in the body occur with the onset of spontaneous labor. Cervical "ripening" occurs, which includes softening and shortening of the cervix. Oxytocin receptors are present in the myometrium. Prostaglandin levels in the amniotic fluid are increased. A number of risk factors are associated with preterm labor:

1. Multiple gestation
2. History of previous preterm labor or delivery
3. Abdominal surgery during current pregnancy
4. Uterine anomaly
5. History of cone biopsy
6. History of abortions—more than two first trimester abortions or more than one second trimester abortion
7. Fetal or placental malformation
8. Diethylstilbestrol exposure
9. Bleeding after the first trimester
10. Maternal age of less than 18 or greater than 35 years
11. Poor nutritional status
12. Poor, irregular, or no prenatal care
13. Emotional stress
14. More than 10 cigarettes smoked in a day
15. Recreational drug use

Management

The focus of treatment is prevention of delivery of a preterm infant. The method depends on the cervical dilatation and contraction pattern. If contractions are detected early and treatment is begun early, there is a higher rate of stopping labor.

A. Conservative Treatment
1. Treatment is begun early with the use of bed rest in a left lateral position.
2. Hydration with IV fluids and continuous monitoring of fetal status and uterine contraction pattern are instituted.
3. If this stops the contractions, tocolytic therapy is not needed.

B. Tocolytic Therapy If conservative therapy is not successful, tocolytic therapy is instituted. These drugs should be used only when the potential benefit to the fetus outweighs the potential risk

1. Betamimetic agents such as ritodrine (Yutopar) and terbutaline (Bricanyl)
   a. These drugs stimulate the β_2 receptors, which causes uterine relaxation.

b. Ritodrine is administered IV or orally; terbutaline may be administered IV, subcutaneously, or orally.
c. Frequent monitoring is necessary to observe for side effects of increased pulse, shortness of breath, chest pain, decreased blood pressure, hypervolemia, decreased potassium concentration, hyperglycemia, and hyperinsulinemia.
d. Before beginning administration of these medications the following laboratory tests should be done and a baseline ECG should be obtained: CBC with differential, electrolytes, glucose, BUN, creatinine, prothrombin time and partial thromboplastin time.

2. $MgSO_4$
a. $MgSO_4$ interferes with smooth muscle contractility. The exact action is not clear.
b. Administration is IV on an infusion pump.
c. During administration the woman is monitored for pulmonary edema, loss of deep tendon reflexes, decreased respirations, hypotension.
d. Serum magnesium levels are monitored.
e. Calcium gluconate is the antidote for $MgSO_4$ and should be at the bedside.

3. Indomethacin (Indocin)
a. Indomethacin is a prostaglandin inhibitor that inhibits contractions.
b. Administration is oral or rectal.
c. It is usually well tolerated by the woman.

4. Nifedipine (Procardia)
a. Nifedipine is a calcium channel blocker that relaxes smooth muscle.
b. Administration is oral.
c. Side effects include headache, nausea, and flushing from vasodilatation.

Complications

1. Prematurity and associated neonatal complications, such as lung immaturity

Nursing Assessment

During tocolytic therapy assess the following:

1. Fetal status via electronic fetal monitoring
2. Contraction pattern
3. Respiratory status (pulmonary edema is a common side effect)
4. Muscular tremors
5. Palpations
6. Dizziness/light-headedness
7. Urinary output

Nursing Diagnoses

A. Anxiety related to medication and fear of outcome of pregnancy
B. Diversional Activity Deficit related to prolonged bed rest

Nursing Interventions

A. *Decreasing Anxiety*
1. Provide accurate information on the status of the fetus and labor (contraction pattern).

2. Allow the woman and her support person to verbalize their feelings regarding the episode of preterm labor and the treatment.
3. If a private room is not used, do not place the woman in a room with a woman who is in labor or who has lost an infant.
4. Encourage relationship with other patients who are also experiencing preterm labor.

B. *Promoting Diversional Activities*
1. Determine quiet craft activities that can be done in bed.
2. Provide radio, books, and television.
3. Encourage visits from family, especially other children and friends. If possible encourage them to bring in favorite foods for the woman and to dine as a family.
4. Encourage other family activities, such as helping with homework. This will assist on maintaining the family unit.

Patient Education/Health Maintenance

1. Educate the woman about the importance of continuing the pregnancy until term or until there is evidence of fetal lung maturity.
2. Encourage the need for compliance with a decreased activity level or bed rest, as indicated.
3. Teach the woman the importance of proper nutrition and the need for adequate hydration, at least 8 glasses of fluids a day.
4. Instruct the woman not to engage in sexual activity.
5. Teach the woman the signs and symptoms of infection and to report them immediately.

Evaluation

A. Demonstrates concern about treatment and pregnancy outcome
B. Participates in diversional activities

◆ PRETERM RUPTURE OF MEMBRANES

Preterm rupture of membranes (PROM) is defined as rupture of the membranes before the onset of spontaneous labor.

Pathophysiology/Etiology

1. The exact etiology of PROM is not clearly understood. PROM at term may result from stretching of the membranes and fetal movements that cause the membranes to weaken.
2. In preterm PROM, risk factors include:
a. Infection
b. Previous history of PROM
c. Hydramnios
d. Incompetent cervix
e. Multiple gestation
f. Abruptio placentae
3. PROM is manifested by a large gush of amniotic fluid or leaking of fluid per vagina, which usually persists.

Diagnostic Evaluation

1. Sterile speculum examination for identification of "pooling" of fluid in the vagina.
2. Nitrazine test—positive test will change pH paper strip from yellow-green to blue in the presence of amniotic fluid taken from the vaginal canal.
3. Fern test—positive test will reveal "ferning" on a slide viewed under a microscope. A swab of the posterior vaginal fornix is taken to obtain amniotic fluid.

Management

1. Once PROM is confirmed, the woman is admitted to the hospital and usually remains there until delivery.
2. The woman is evaluated to rule out labor, fetal distress, and infection and to establish gestational age. If all factors are ruled out, the woman is managed expectantly.
3. For PROM, tocolytics, corticosteroids (to decrease the severity of respiratory distress syndrome in the premature neonate) and prophylactic antibiotics are used, but remain controversial.
4. Management of PROM at 36 weeks' gestation or greater focuses on delivery.
5. Vaginal examinations are kept to a minimum to prevent infection.

Complications

1. Preterm labor
2. Prematurity and associated complications
3. Maternal infection—chorioamnionitis
4. Fetal/neonatal infection

Nursing Assessment

1. Evaluate maternal blood pressure, respirations, pulse, and temperature every 4 hours. If temperature or pulse are elevated take them every 1 to 2 hours as indicated.
2. Monitor the amount and type of amniotic fluid that is leaking and observe for purulent, foul-smelling discharge.
3. Evaluate daily CBC with differentials, noting any shift to the left (ie, increase of immature forms of neutrophils).
4. Evaluate fetal status every 4 hours or as indicated, noting fetal activity and heart rate.
5. Determine if uterine tenderness occurs on abdominal palpation.

Nursing Diagnoses

A. Risk for Infection related to ascending bacteria

Also see Preterm Labor, page 1036.

Nursing Interventions

A. *Preventing Infection*
1. Evaluate amount and odor of amniotic fluid leakage.
2. Do not perform vaginal examinations without consulting the primary health care provider.
3. Place patient on disposable pads to collect leaking fluid and change pads every 2 hours or more frequently as needed.
4. Review the need for good handwashing technique and hygiene after urination and defecation.
5. Monitor fetal heart rate and fetal activity every 4 hours or as indicated.
6. Monitor maternal temperature, pulse respirations, blood pressure, and uterine tenderness every 4 hours or as indicated.

Evaluation

A. Free from signs of infection

◆ INDUCTION OF LABOR

Induction of labor is the deliberate initiation of uterine contractions before their spontaneous onset.

Indications

When the woman's life or well-being is in danger, or if the fetus may be compromised by remaining in the uterus any longer.

1. Maternal hypertension, diabetes mellitus, renal disease
2. PROM, placental insufficiency
3. Fetal postmaturity, erythroblastosis
4. History of rapid labors and living a long distance from birth center
5. IUGR, intrauterine fetal death

Contraindications

1. Herpes outbreak in the genital area
2. Vaginal bleeding, known placenta previa
3. Abnormal fetal presentation
4. Previous uterine scar (horizontal scar may not be considered by all to be a contraindication)
5. Known cephalopelvic disproportion (CPD)
6. Severe fetal distress

Management

A. *Amniotomy (Artificial Rupture of Membranes)*
1. Vulva is cleansed, amniohook is inserted through the cervix, and membranes are ruptured after the fetal presentation is evaluated.
2. Should make contractions stronger
3. Fetal heart tones are assessed continually for at least the next 20 minutes.
4. Complications include umbilical cord prolapse or compression, maternal or fetal infection.

B. *Oxytocin*
1. Fetal monitoring is instituted. If membranes have ruptured, an intrauterine catheter and internal scalp electrode may be used.

2. An IV is mixed with 10 units of oxytocin and piggy-backed into the primary IV at the port of entry nearest the skin insertion.

3. The oxytocin is given only with an infusion pump and when constant monitoring of maternal and fetal status is available.

4. The dose is increased every 20 to 30 minutes by 1 to 2 μU/min. The total dose should not exceed 30 μU/min.

5. The goal is to establish a regular labor pattern— contractions occurring every 2 to 3 minutes lasting 45 to 60 seconds and an intensity of 50 mm Hg (moderate).

6. Complications include uterine hyperstimulation, fetal distress, increased rate of cesarean section, and neonatal hyperbilirubinemia possibly from red blood cell trauma from intense contractions or decreased maturity of the neonate.

C. *Prostaglandin E₂* (PGE_2)
1. PGE_2 is primarily used before induction of labor for cervical ripening.
2. If labor results from administration of PGE_2, it is similar to spontaneous labor.
3. Prostaglandins are administered intracervically or vaginally.
   a. May be inserted in tablet or gel form
   b. PGE_2 gel is given via a catheter in doses ranging from 0.5 to 5 mg.
4. Uterine hyperstimulation is a complication.

D. *Stripping the Membranes*
1. Separating the membranes from the lower uterine segment without rupturing the membranes
2. Usually done during vaginal examination
3. Membranes and amniotic fluid now act as a wedge to dilate cervix.
4. Maternal/fetal infection is a complication.

Nursing Assessment

A. *Before Induction*
1. Make sure that patient is aware of the procedures to be used and all questions have been answered.
2. Obtain a 30-minute strip for the fetal heart rate and uterine activity.
3. Evaluate maternal vital signs.
4. Evaluate the patency of the IV site, if IV ordered.

B. *After the Administration of Oxytocin*
1. Continuously monitor fetal heart rate and uterine activity.
2. Assess maternal vital signs every 15 minutes until a labor pattern is established, then every 30 minutes. Temperature is taken every 4 hours unless an amniotomy has been performed and then every 2 hours.
3. Limit vaginal examinations, especially after the membranes have ruptured.
4. Maintain intake and output records, and watch for signs of water intoxication.
5. Evaluate IV site for patency and rate control for correct rate at least hourly.

Nursing Diagnoses

A. Anxiety related to planned childbirth and outcome
B. Altered Tissue Perfusion, uteroplacental, related to strength of uterine contractions

Nursing Interventions

A. *Decreasing Anxiety*
1. Teach or review the use of relaxation and distraction techniques.
2. Before beginning any new procedure explain the procedure to the woman and her support person.
3. Answer questions that the family and woman may have.

B. *Promoting Tissue Perfusion*
1. Assess fetal status and uterine contractions continuously through the use of a monitor.
2. Position on the left side to enhance placental perfusion.
3. Have oxygen set up with a mask ready and administer as prescribed if decelerations occur.
4. If hyperstimulation of the uterus or fetal distress occurs, discontinue the infusion, maintain the primary IV, and notify the health care provider immediately.

Evaluation

A. Verbalizes understanding of the induction process
B. No evidence of hyperstimulation or fetal distress

◆ DYSTOCIA

Dystocia, or difficult labor, refers to abnormal progress in labor. Maternal psychological factors such as fear, anxiety, and exhaustion may play a role in dystocia. Often more than one cause exists at a time.

Pathophysiology/Etiology

A. *Contraction Abnormalities*
1. Contractions that are not strong enough or frequent enough to produce a normal labor pattern will not result in dilatation and effacement within a normal time frame.
2. Problems with the force of labor will result in ineffective contractions or ineffective bearing down (pushing) during the second stage of labor.
3. Etiology of abnormalities in the force of labor include:
   a. Early or excessive use of analgesia
   b. Overdistention of the uterus
   c. Excessive cervical rigidity
   d. Grand multiparity
   e. Mild pelvic contraction
   f. Postmature and large infants

B. *Passageway Abnormalities*
1. Abnormalities in the passageway may be the result of problems in the pelvis or soft tissues of the reproductive tract.
2. Most often problems with the passageway are a result of pelvic abnormalities that interfere with the engagement, descent, and expulsion of the fetus.
   a. The size and shape of the pelvis is important.
   b. Obstruction may result from problems of the soft tissue such as a uterine or ovarian fibromyoma.
3. Contractions of the inlet are noted when the anteroposterior diameter is less than 10 cm or the greatest transverse diameter is less than 12 cm. Contracted inlets may be of genetic origin or a result of rickets.

4. Midpelvic contractions occur when the distance between the ischial spines is less than 9 cm. Often this is not detected early in labor because the fetal head has engaged, and molding along with caput formation gives the suggestion that the head has descended further than it has.
5. A contracted pelvic outlet is diagnosed when the distance between the ischial spines is less then 8 cm. When the pelvis is contracted and the fetus cannot fit through the pelvis, CPD exists.

C. *Fetal Passage Abnormalities*
1. Normal fetal passage
   a. Normally the fetus enters the pelvic inlet transversely and then rotates to an occiput anterior position, allowing for the smallest diameter of the fetal head to pass through the pelvis.
   b. When the fetal head enters the pelvis posteriorly, it must rotate to the anterior position. This is done usually without problems if the fetus is of average size and well flexed and the contractions are a good quality.
3. If the fetus does not turn, then it remains in the posterior position and may slow down the progress of descent.
   a. If the pelvis is large enough, the baby can be born in the posterior position.
   b. If the pelvis is borderline and the contractions ineffective, a cesarean section may be necessary.
4. Breech presentations occur in approximately 3% of all deliveries.
   a. This presentation is more common in multiple gestations, increased parity, hydramnios, placenta previa, and preterm infants.
   b. Usually the method of choice for delivery is a cesarean section.
5. Shoulder presentation occurs when the infant lies crosswise in the uterus. The infant is delivered by cesarean section.
6. A large fetus has an increased risk of trauma in its attempt to fit through a normal size pelvis. A large infant may not fit through the pelvis and CPD may result.

Diagnostic Evaluation

1. Inadequate progress of cervical effacement, dilatation, or descent of the presenting part as determined by vaginal examination
2. Evaluation of labor progress by recording and assessing serial vaginal examinations using Freidman's curve
   a. Using Freidman's curve, a prolonged latent phase in the primigravida is greater than 20 hours and in the multigravida it is greater than 14 hours.
   b. During the active phase, the cervix of a primigravida will normally dilate at least 1.2 cm/h, and the multigravida 1.5 cm. In addition, the fetus should be descending through the birth canal. In the primigravida the rate of descent is 1 cm/h and 2 cm/h for the multigravida.

Management

1. Treatment for contraction abnormalities involves stimulation of labor through the use of oxytocin. An intrauterine pressure catheter may be used.

2. Management for maternal passageway or fetal passage problems involves delivery in the safest manner for the mother and fetus.
   a. If the problem is related to the inlet or midpelvis, a cesarean delivery is indicated.
   b. If the size of the outlet is the problem, a forceps delivery is usually performed.

Complications

1. Maternal exhaustion
2. Infection
3. Fetal distress
4. Postpartum hemorrhage

Nursing Assessment

1. Evaluate fetal presentation, position, and size.
2. Evaluate progress of labor, noting dilations and effacement in relation to time of labor along with descent of the fetal head.
3. Monitor fetal heart rate and contraction status at least every 30 minutes.
4. Monitor maternal vital signs at least every hour.
5. Assess bladder fullness.

Nursing Diagnoses

A. Pain related to physical and psychological factors of difficult labor
B. Anxiety related to threat of change in the health status of self and fetus

Nursing Interventions

A. *Promoting Comfort*
1. Review relaxation techniques.
2. Encourage use of breathing techniques learned in prenatal classes.
3. Encourage frequent change of position.
4. Encourage voiding every hour.
5. Provide back rubs and sacral pressure as needed.
6. Offer ice chips as needed to combat a dry mouth, if permitted.
7. Provide a quiet, darkened room.
8. Provide frequent encouragement to the woman and her support person.
9. Administer pain medication for analgesia, as ordered.
10. Assist with the administration of anesthesia, as indicated.

B. *Decreasing Anxiety*
1. Provide anticipatory guidance regarding the use of medication, equipment, and procedures.
2. Educate the woman about the administration of oxytocin (Pitocin).
3. Discuss with the woman the nature of the contractions associated with an induced labor (ie, short acceleration, intense plateau, short deceleration).
4. Prepare the family for cesarean delivery, if necessary.

Evaluation

A. Verbalizes increased comfort
B. Verbalizes understanding of procedures

◆ UTERINE RUPTURE

Uterine rupture is a spontaneous or traumatic rupture of the uterus.

Pathophysiology/Etiology

1. Rupture of the scar from a previous cesarean delivery or hysterotomy
2. Uterine trauma related to manipulation with instrumentation (ie, curet) or abdominal trauma resulting from sharp objects (ie, knives, bullets), or accidents
3. Uterine congenital anomaly
4. Oxytocin stimulation in the woman of high parity
5. Breech extraction
6. Difficult delivery involving forceps
7. Multiple gestation or polyhydramnios causing uterine overdistention
8. Perforation from placement of intrauterine pressure catheter

Clinical Manifestations

A. *Complete Rupture*
1. Sudden sharp abdominal pain during contractions
2. Abdominal tenderness
3. Cessation of contractions
4. Bleeding into the abdominal cavity and sometimes into the vagina
5. Fetus easily palpated; fetal heart tones cease
6. Signs of shock—rapid, weak pulse; cold, clammy skin; pale color; flaring of nostrils due to air hunger
7. Chest pain from diaphragmatic irritation due to bleeding into the abdomen

B. *Incomplete Rupture* Develops over a period of a few hours

1. Abdominal pain during contractions
2. Contractions continue, but cervix fails to dilate.
3. Vaginal bleeding may be present.
4. Rising pulse rate and skin pallor
5. Loss of fetal heart tones or fetal distress
6. Increase in uterine tone

Management

1. Immediate preparation for surgery, including blood and fluid replacement.
2. The uterus is repaired if possible.
3. A hysterectomy is done if bleeding cannot be controlled.
4. After surgery, additional blood and fluid replacement is continued along with antibiotic therapy.

Complications

1. Maternal—hypovolemic shock, peritonitis
2. Fetal—anoxia, death

Nursing Assessment

1. Continuously evaluate maternal vital signs; especially note an increase in the rate and depth of respirations, an increase in pulse or a drop in blood pressure indicating status change.
2. Observe for signs and symptoms of rupture related to a change in the contractions.
3. Assess fetal status via monitoring.
4. Speak with family and evaluate their understanding of the situation.

Nursing Diagnoses

A. Fluid Volume Deficit related to active fluid loss from hemorrhage
B. Altered Tissue Perfusion, Maternal Vital Organ and Fetal, related to hypovolemia
C. Fear related to surgical outcome for fetus and mother

Nursing Interventions

A. *Maintaining Fluid Volume*
1. Start or maintain an IV as prescribed. Use a large-gauge Intracath when starting the IV for blood and large quantities of fluid replacement.
2. Maintain central venous pressure and arterial lines, as indicated for hemodynamic monitoring.
3. Maintain bed rest to decrease metabolic demands.
4. Insert Foley catheter and monitor urine output hourly or as indicated.
5. Obtain and administer blood products as indicated.

B. *Maintaining Maternal and Fetal Tissue Perfusion*
1. Administer oxygen using a face mask at 10 L/min or as ordered to provide high oxygen concentration.
2. Apply pulse oximeter and monitor oxygen saturation as indicated.
3. Monitor arterial blood gases and serum electrolytes as indicated to assess respiratory status, observing for hypoventilation and electrolyte imbalance.
4. Continually monitor maternal and fetal vital signs to assess pattern because progressive changes may indicate profound shock.

C. *Reducing Fear*
1. Give a brief explanation to the woman and her support person before beginning a procedure.
2. Answer questions that the family and woman may have.
3. Maintain a quiet and calm atmosphere to enhance relaxation.
4. Remain with the woman until anesthesia has been administered; offer support as needed.
5. Keep the family members aware of the situation while the woman is in surgery and allow time for them to express feelings.

Patient Education/Health Maintenance

1. Provide information and support regarding the possibility for future pregnancies.

2. Encourage the support of family and friends.
3. Inform the woman that postoperatively, diet will be advanced with the return of bowel sounds.
4. Educate the woman about the importance of ambulation to prevent intestinal gas and other postoperative complications.

Evaluation

A. Vital signs stable; no evidence of shock
B. Arterial blood gases within normal limits; fetal heart rate within normal limits
C. Verbalizes concerns about self and her fetus

◆ AMNIOTIC FLUID EMBOLISM

Amniotic fluid embolism is the escape of amniotic fluid containing debris such as meconium, lanugo, and vernix caseosa into the maternal circulation, usually resulting in deposition of fluid or debris in the pulmonary arterioles, resulting rapidly in respiratory distress, shock, and the possible development of DIC. Amniotic fluid embolism is rare and usually fatal.

Pathophysiology/Etiology

1. The exact mechanism causing amniotic fluid embolism is unclear.
2. It usually occurs in the intrapartum period.
3. Myometrial vessels are exposed, usually at the placental site and contractions are especially forceful. A thromboplastin-like substance is found in amniotic fluid, which causes defibrination leading to DIC.
4. Predisposing conditions include abruptio placentae, uterine rupture, intrauterine fetal demise, and high parity.

Clinical Manifestations

1. Sudden dyspnea and chest pain
2. Cyanosis, tachycardia
3. Pulmonary edema
4. Profound shock due to:
   a. Anaphylaxis, which causes vascular collapse
   b. Uterine bleeding with development of hypofibrinogenemia

Diagnostic Evaluation

1. Based on presenting signs and symptoms
2. DIC confirmed by coagulation studies

Management

1. Endotracheal intubation
2. Administration of IV crystalloid fluids
3. Administration of blood products and heparin to combat DIC
4. Establishment of central venous pressure line

5. Immediate delivery of the fetus
6. Initiation of cardiopulmonary resuscitation, if needed

Complications

The maternal–fetal mortality rate is estimated to be greater than 80% due to DIC and cardiopulmonary collapse.

Nursing Assessment/Interventions

1. Be alert to signs and symptoms of potential amniotic fluid embolism.
2. Monitor maternal vital signs and fetal heart rate frequently to assess for signs of shock and fetal/maternal demise.
3. Administer oxygen via face mask to assist respiratory status.
4. Alert medical staff immediately and assist with emergency procedures such as delivery and with the cardiopulmonary resuscitation as needed.
5. Provide information and comfort to the family or support persons. If unable to do this personally due to the emergent needs of the woman, delegate another member of the staff to stay with the family or support persons.

◆ PROLAPSED UMBILICAL CORD

A prolapsed umbilical cord slips in front of or alongside the fetal presenting part. Types of cord prolapse include:

- *Complete*—the cord can be felt on vaginal examination and be seen in the vaginal canal.
- *Occult*—the cord cannot be felt on vaginal examination or be seen. The cord lies between the presenting part and the maternal pelvis. Changes in the fetal heart rate are evident.
- *Forelying*—the cord can be felt on vaginal examination, but cannot be seen. The cord lies in front of the presenting part.

Pathophysiology/Etiology

A fetal cord prolapse may occur when there is adequate room between the fetal parts and the maternal pelvis. Predisposing factors include:

1. Rupture of membranes, when the presenting part is not engaged in the pelvis
2. More common in shoulder and foot presentations
3. Prematurity—small fetus allows more space around presenting part
4. Hydramnios—causes greater amount of fluid to be released with greater force when membranes rupture

Clinical Manifestations

1. Cord may be seen protruding from vagina or palpated in the vagina or cervix.

2. With compression, fetal heart rate pattern may show variable decelerations with contractions or between contractions; often fetal bradycardia is present.
3. If the cord is exposed to cold room air, there may be a reflex constriction of the umbilical blood vessels that further restricts the oxygen flow to the fetus.

NURSING ALERT:
Prolapse should be suspected with fetal heart rate deceleration after rupture of the membranes.

Management

1. Delivery of the fetus as soon as possible
2. Relief of pressure from the umbilical cord

Complications

A. Maternal
1. Infection
2. Risk for increased blood loss from emergency delivery
3. Risk for increased perineal trauma from emergency vaginal forceps delivery

B. Fetal
1. Prematurity
2. Complications resulting from hypoxia
3. Fetal death

Nursing Assessment/Interventions

1. Observe fetal heart rate deceleration.
2. Identify complete or forelying cord prolapse with a vaginal examination by a qualified nurse or health care provider.
3. Explain procedures as much as possible to the woman during this emergent situation.
4. Administer oxygen by face mask at 8 to 10 L/min.
5. Relieve pressure from the presenting part of the fetus off the umbilical cord by manually pushing the presenting part upward with a gloved hand. Pressure must be relieved until the fetus is delivered via cesarean or vaginally.
6. Provide constant support to the woman and her support persons.
7. Encourage the woman to talk about her feelings regarding herself and the baby after delivery.

◆ INVERTED UTERUS

Inversion of the uterus—the uterus turns inside out during the third stage of delivery. Inversion may be:

* *Spontaneous*—occurs with increased abdominal pressure, as seen with forceful coughing or bearing down
* *Forced*—occurs with pulling on the umbilical cord
* *Complete*—uterus totally inverts into the vagina
* *Incomplete*—fundus of uterus partially inverts but not beyond the cervical os

Pathophysiology/Etiology

Inversion is more commonly seen with fundal placental implantation and with a thin uterine wall at the site of implantation. Predisposing factors include:

1. Excessive traction on the cord while the placenta is still attached to the uterine wall
2. Lax or thin uterine wall
3. Fundal pressure
4. Spontaneous inversion
5. Delivery of an infant with a short umbilical cord

Clinical Manifestations

1. Maternal bleeding and shock, with symptoms often seeming out of proportion for the blood loss.
2. A complete inversion may appear protruding from vagina.
3. Inability to palpate fundus in association with clinical manifestations
4. Confirmed with bimanual examination

Management

1. Goal is to restore the uterus to its normal position, manually.
2. Often involves the use of general anesthesia and tocolytic therapy (terbutaline or MgSO$_4$).
3. In addition, blood replacement therapy may be instituted to correct the shock.
4. After the uterus has been restored to its normal position, oxytocin is given to contract the uterus.

Complications

1. Infection, anemia
2. Potential for a hysterectomy if uterus cannot be returned to its normal position

Nursing Assessment/Interventions

A. Before Correction of the Inversion
1. Check maternal vital signs and evaluate for blood loss.
2. Place the woman flat in bed in Trendelenburg's position so that pelvis is higher than head.
3. Administer oxygen by face mask at 8 to 12 L/min.
4. Establish an IV line with a 16- or 18-gauge catheter for administration of fluids, blood products, and medications. Two IV lines will be needed.
5. Apply a pulse oximeter to determine oxygen saturation.
6. If replacement of the uterus is unsuccessful, prepare the woman and her support persons for emergency surgery.

B. After Correction of the Inversion
1. Check maternal vital signs and monitor CBC for signs of bleeding, infection.
2. Measure and record accurate intake and output.
3. Evaluate uterine fundus for position and firmness.
4. Evaluate lochia for amount of blood loss.

5. Evaluate for transfusion reactions (ie, itching, wheezing, anaphylaxis).
6. Administer oxytocin and other uterine tonics, as ordered.
7. Administer antibiotics, as ordered, to minimize risk of infection.
8. Provide support to the woman and encourage her to express her feelings.

Operative Obstetrics

◆ EPISIOTOMY

An *episiotomy* is an incision of the perineum during delivery to:

- Substitute a straight surgical incision for the laceration that may otherwise occur
- Facilitate repair of laceration and promote healing
- Spare the infant's head from prolonged pressure and pushing against the rigid perineum, which may result in brain damage, especially in the premature infant
- Shorten the second stage of labor

Types of Episiotomies

A. Median (Midline)
1. Incision is made in the middle of the perineum and directed toward the rectum (Fig. 37-4).
2. This method is believed to heal with few complications, is more comfortable for the woman during healing, is easy to repair, and is associated with minimal blood loss.
3. If a larger incision is needed during delivery, however, it may necessitate incision into anal sphincter.

B. Mediolateral
1. Incision is made laterally in the perineum.
2. This method avoids the anal sphincter if enlargement is needed.
3. Women find it extremely uncomfortable during healing.
4. Associated with increased blood loss
5. Necessitates longer wound healing time

Management

1. Pain relief
   a. The stretching of the perineum and pressure from the fetal head may provide a natural numbing effect.
   b. Local perineal infiltration with lidocaine provides anesthesia for performing and repairing the episiotomy.
   c. A pudendal block provides anesthesia to the lower two thirds of the perineum and vagina using lidocaine injection into the vaginal walls.
   d. Epidural anesthesia provides anesthesia from the level of of the umbilicus to the mid-thigh area.
2. The episiotomy is performed when the fetal head is about 3 to 4 cm visible with a contraction.
3. The repair of the episiotomy usually begins after the delivery of the placenta.

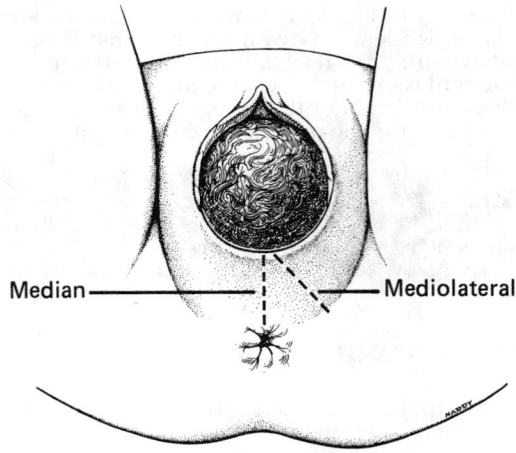

Median ——— Mediolateral

FIGURE 37-4 *Types of episiotomies.*

Complications

1. Infection
2. Increased risk of blood loss
3. Third and fourth degree lacerations
4. Episiotomy pain
5. Risk for hematoma
6. Dyspareunia (pain during intercourse), which may last up to 6 months

Nursing Assessment

During the recovery period the episiotomy should be evaluated every 15 minutes and three times a day after this.

1. Describe and document the degree of healing.
2. Assess for infection, which may be indicated by edema, redness, purulent drainage at the site; increased temperature.
3. Notify health care provider of bleeding at site, other than slight oozing.
4. Monitor for hematoma formation.

Nursing Diagnoses

A. Risk for Infection related to traumatized tissue
B. Pain related to surgical procedure

Nursing Interventions

A. Preventing Infection
1. Instruct the woman to cleanse from the front to the back.
2. Provide instructions on techniques used for perineal care.
   a. Provide a peri-bottle and teach the woman to squirt the water gently on her perineum after using the toilet.

3. Explain the importance of changing the perineal pad each time after urination and defecation and of not touching the inner surface of the pad.
4. Explain the importance of proper handwashing before and after perineal care.
5. Explain that perineal care should be carried out after urination and defecation and at least every 4 hours during the day.
6. Encourage a diet that is high in protein and vitamin C and encourage at least 2,000 mL of fluid each day.

B. **Promoting Comfort**
1. Apply ice packs to the perineal area for the first 24 hours after delivery. The ice packs should not remain in place longer than 30 minutes at a time to get the maximum benefit for the treatment.
2. Encourage sitz baths with either warm or cool water. The warm water is soothing, whereas the cool water helps to decrease pain sensation and edema.
3. Administer pain medication and topical anesthetics as ordered.
4. Instruct the woman to tighten her buttocks and perineal muscles before sitting in a chair and to release the muscles once seated.

Evaluation

A. No evidence of infection; afebrile
B. Demonstrates increase in comfort

◆ FORCEPS DELIVERY

Obstetric forceps (Table 37-3) are designed for rotating or extracting the fetal head. Forceps consist of two pieces: a right blade, which is slipped into the right side of the mother's pelvis, and a left blade, which is slipped into the left side. Each piece consists of four parts:

- Handle—used to hold the forceps
- Shank—the piece between the handle and the blade. It contributes to the length of the forceps.
- Lock—keeps the two pieces of forceps together
- Blade—fits around the fetal head

Types of Forceps Deliveries

A. **Outlet Forceps**
1. Scalp visible at the introitus; labia not separated
2. Fetal skull at pelvic floor
3. Sagittal suture in anteroposterior diameter or right to left occiput anterior or posterior position
4. Fetal head at or on perineum
5. Rotation not more than 45°

B. **Low Forceps**
1. Leading point of fetal skull is at station greater than or equal to +2 cm, and not on the pelvic floor.
2. Rotation less than or equal to 45° (left or right occiput anterior to occiput anterior, or left or right occiput posterior to occiput posterior)
3. Rotation greater than 45°

C. **Mid Forceps**   Station above +2 cm; head engaged

Indications for Forceps Delivery

A. **General Criteria**
1. Pelvis should be adequate, with no disproportion
2. Fetal head must be engaged—preferably deeply engaged
3. Cervix must be completely dilated
4. Accurate diagnosis of position and station must be made
5. Membranes must be ruptured
6. Some form of anesthesia should be used
7. Rectum and bladder should be empty

B. **Fetal Indications**
1. Fetal distress
2. Cord prolapse
3. Malposition of the head
4. Abruptio placentae

TABLE 37-3   Representative Types of Forceps*

Major Classifications	Use
1. Simpson—separated shanks (DeLee forcep is one example)	Extract fetus with elongated, molded head; commonly used with nulliparas who have long labors
2. Elliot—overlapping shanks (Tucker–McLean is one example)	Extract fetus with unmolded, rounder heads; commonly used with multiparas who have briefer labors
3. Specialized types a. Piper	Deliver aftercoming head in a breech presentation
b. Kielland	Rotate head from transverse or posterior position to an anterior position; used to deliver women with anthropoid pelves
c. Barton	Rotate head from transverse to an anterior position; designed for use in women with flat pelves

* There are more than 600 types of forceps.

C. *Maternal Indications*
1. Heart disease
2. Acute pulmonary edema
3. Intrapartum infections
4. Maternal hemorrhage
5. Maternal exhaustion
6. Eclampsia
7. Epidural or spinal anesthesia

Management

1. The woman is placed in the lithotomy position.
2. The bladder is usually emptied by catheterization.
3. Regional anesthesia is most frequently used.
4. The pediatric staff is in attendance at delivery.
5. An episiotomy is usually performed.

Complications

A. *Maternal*
1. Lacerations of the vulva, cervix and vagina
2. Extensions of the episiotomy to include the rectum
3. Bladder trauma, uterine rupture
4. Postpartum infection, postpartum hemorrhage

B. *Fetal*
1. Bruising from forceps application, cephalohematoma
2. From incorrect application of the forceps:
   a. Facial paralysis
   b. Brachial palsy
   c. Skull fracture
3. From incorrect application of the forceps or from compromised fetal status:
   a. Intracranial hemorrhage
   b. Brain damage
   c. Cord compression

Nursing Assessment

1. Following application of the forceps the fetal heart rate should be auscultated continuously or at least every 5 minutes for a full minute.
2. Evaluate maternal sensation.
3. Evaluate bladder fullness—bladder should be empty before the application of the forceps.

Nursing Diagnoses

A. Anxiety related to fetal outcome
B. Pain related to procedures

Nursing Interventions

A. *Decreasing Anxiety*
1. Explain how the forceps are applied.
2. Explain that a sensation of pressure rather than pain will be felt.
3. Answer any questions that the woman and her support persons might have.
4. Stay with the woman and provide guidance during the delivery process.

B. *Promoting Comfort*
1. Encourage use of breathing and relaxation techniques.
2. Make sure that bladder is completely empty.
3. Encourage relaxation between contractions and use of abdominal muscles and pushing with the contractions.
4. Use blankets and pillow supports when positioning the woman for delivery.

Evaluation

A. Verbalizes concerns regarding forceps; responds to instructions
B. Demonstrates increased level of comfort

◆ VACUUM EXTRACTION

A *vacuum extractor* applies suction to the fetal head, creating an artificial caput within the suction cup, thus allowing adequate traction for delivery of the infant's head. Classification is the same as for forceps delivery.

Indications

1. Indications for a vacuum delivery are the same as for a forceps delivery.
2. Contraindications for vacuum delivery include breech presentation, face or brow presentation, premature fetus, CPD.
3. Advantages include ease of application and ability to perform procedure without requiring extra space in birth canal, as with forceps.

Management

1. Fetus is in vertex presentation.
2. Membranes must be ruptured.
3. The woman is in the lithotomy position.
4. The bladder is usually catheterized.
5. Evaluate progress with suction.
6. Anesthesia may be indicated.
7. Unsuccessful extraction is followed by a cesarean section.
8. Pediatric staff is in attendance at delivery.

Complications

Complications are usually less frequent and less severe with vacuum extraction than with forceps.

A. *Maternal* Lacerations of the cervix or vagina

B. *Fetal*
1. Cephalohematoma
2. Caput succedaneum (head swelling) from the vacuum
3. From improper technique or from compromised fetal status:
   a. Intracranial hemorrhage
   b. Retinal hemorrhage

Nursing Assessment

1. Monitor the fetus continuously or at least every 5 minutes for a full minute.
2. Monitor the vacuum pressure of the equipment according to institution protocol.

Nursing Diagnoses/Interventions/ Evaluation

Same as for a forceps delivery.

◆ CESAREAN DELIVERY

Cesarean delivery is the surgical removal of the infant from the uterus through an incision made in the abdominal wall and an incision made in the uterus.

Types of Cesarean Delivery

A. Uterine Incisions
1. *Low segment transverse*—incision made transversely in lower segment of uterus; incision of choice
   a. Incision is made in thinnest portion so that blood loss is minimal and uterus is easier to open.
   b. Lower segment is area of least uterine activity.
   c. Postoperative convalescence is more comfortable.
   d. Possibility of later rupture is lessened.
   e. Incidence of postoperative adhesions and danger of intestinal obstruction are reduced.
   f. It is the incision of choice.
2. *Classical*—vertical incision is made directly into the wall of the body of the uterus; not frequently done.
   a. Useful when bladder and lower segment are involved in extensive adhesions
   b. Selected when anterior placenta previa exists
   c. Useful when fetus is in a transverse lie
3. *Low vertical*
   a. May be extended upward into a classical incision if extra room is needed for delivery
   b. May extend downward and cause trauma to the cervix, vagina, and bladder

B. Abdominal Incisions
1. *Pfannenstiel*—a horizontal incision right above the pubic hair line
   a. Cosmetic advantage of not being seen because pubic hair covers incision
   b. Decreased chance of dehiscence or hernia formation
2. *Vertical*—a vertical incision made in the midline of the abdomen below the umbilicus to the pubis
   a. Quicker procedure to perform
   b. Provides better uterine visualization
   c. Cosmetically less appealing
   d. Greater chance of wound dehiscence and hernia formation

Indications for Cesarean Delivery

1. CPD
2. Uterine dysfunction, inertia, inability of cervix to dilate
3. Neoplasm obstructing birth canal or pelvis

4. Malposition and malpresentation
5. Previous uterine surgery (cesarean delivery, myomectomy, hysterotomy) or cervical surgery—evaluated on an individual basis
6. Complete or partial placenta previa
7. Premature separation of the placenta
8. Prolapse of the umbilical cord
9. Fetal distress
10. Active herpes outbreak
11. Breech presentation
12. Indications for cesarean hysterectomy
    a. Ruptured uterus
    b. Intrauterine infection
    c. Hemorrhage due to uterine atony that does not respond to oxytocin, prostaglandin, or massage
    d. Laceration of major uterine vessel
    e. Severe dysplasia or carcinoma in situ of the cervix
    f. Placenta accreta
    g. Gross multiple fibromyomas

Management

1. NPO (except possibly ice chips) during labor
2. A blood sample should be typed and screened and available to be crossmatched if needed; a CBC is obtained.
3. Anesthesia, regional or general, depends on the indication for surgery.
4. A large-bore IV is established and Foley catheter is inserted.
5. An antacid is administered to reduce gastric acidity and the risk of aspiration pneumonia.
6. Antibiotics may be given prophylactically.
7. An abdominal prep is done and a grounding pad for electrocautery is applied.

Complications

1. Increase in morbidity and mortality compared with a vaginal birth
2. Hemorrhage, endometritis
3. Paralytic ileus, intestinal obstruction
4. Pulmonary embolism, thrombophlebitis
5. Increased chance of prematurity
6. Respiratory depression of the infant from anesthetic drugs
7. Possible delay in maternal-infant bonding

Nursing Assessment

A. Before Delivery
1. Assess knowledge of procedure.
2. Monitor maternal and fetal vital signs.
3. Determine maternal blood type and Rh.
4. Determine last time the woman ate.
5. Identify drug allergies.

B. After Delivery
1. Assess maternal vital signs every 15 minutes the first hour, every 30 minutes the second hour, and hourly until she is transferred to the postpartum unit or per facility protocol.
2. Evaluate fundal position and firmness along with vital signs.

3. Evaluate amount and type of lochia along with vital signs.
4. Assess condition of the incision line or dressing.
5. Monitor urinary output, presence of bowel sounds.
6. Assess level and presence of anesthesia or pain.
7. Auscultate lung sounds, maternal oxygen saturation.
8. Assess maternal-infant bonding.

Nursing Diagnoses

A. Anxiety related to cesarean delivery
B. Pain related to surgical procedure
C. Risk for Infection related to traumatized tissue
D. Risk for Altered Parenting related to interruption in bonding process

Nursing Interventions

A. *Relieving Anxiety*
1. Explain the reason for the cesarean delivery.
2. Answer any questions the woman and her support person may have regarding a cesarean delivery.
3. Explain all procedures before doing them.
4. Allow the support person to attend the birth.
5. Explain that a sensation of pressure will be felt during the delivery, but that little pain will occur. Instruct that any pain should be reported to the nurse.

B. *Promoting Comfort*
1. Encourage use of relaxation techniques after medication has been given for pain.
   Note: Do not administer parenteral narcotics if patient is receiving epidural narcotics unless ordered by anesthetist.
2. Monitor for respiratory depression up to 24 hours following epidural narcotic administration.
3. Use a back rub and a quiet environment to promote the effectiveness of the medication.
4. Support/splint the abdominal incision when moving or coughing and deep breathing.
5. Encourage frequent rest periods, and plan for them after activities; also, place a "Do Not Disturb" sign on the door during rest and sleep periods.
6. To reduce pain caused by gas, encourage ambulation and the use of a rocking chair.

C. *Preventing Infection*
1. If skin preparation includes shaving, shave skin carefully, avoiding any nicks in the skin. Then, carry out surgical skin preparation correctly.
2. Postoperatively, use aseptic technique when changing dressings.
3. Provide perineal care every 4 hours or as needed.
4. Provide routine postoperative care measures to prevent urinary or pulmonary infection.

D. *Promoting Effective Bonding*
1. Encourage the woman and her support person to discuss their feelings regarding the cesarean birth both before and after the delivery.
2. When talking of the birth, refer to it as a cesarean birth, to imply it is just another method of birth, not a surgical experience.
3. Encourage mother–child bonding as soon as possible.
4. Emphasize that adjustments to parenting under any circumstances are necessary and normal.

Patient Education/Health Maintenance

1. Teach the woman the "football hold" for breast-feeding so that the infant is not lying on her abdomen.
2. Teach the woman to observe for signs of infection (foul-smelling lochia, elevated temperature, increased pain, redness and edema at the incision site) and to report them immediately.
3. Assist the woman in planning for the assistance of friends, family, or hired help at home during the period immediately after discharge.

Evaluation

A. Verbalizes an understanding of the cesarean birth procedure and postdelivery care
B. Reports relief of pain
C. Has no signs of infection
D. Participates in care of self and infant

Postpartum Complications

◆ PUERPERAL INFECTION

Puerperal infection is a postpartum infection of the genital tract, usually of the endometrium, that may remain localized or may extend to various parts of the body.

Pathophysiology/Etiology

Bacterial organisms either are introduced from external sources or are normally present in the genital tract and are carried to the uterus. Predisposing factors include:

1. Prolonged labor or rupture of membranes, PROM
2. Number of vaginal examinations
3. Infection elsewhere in the body
4. Anemia, malnutrition
5. Size and number of perineal lacerations
6. Intrauterine manipulation
7. Retained placental fragments of membranes
8. Lapse in aseptic technique
9. Poor perineal hygiene
10. Cesarean section

Clinical Manifestations

Diagnosis is made by sustained fever of 38°C (100.4°F) or higher occurring on any two of the first 10 days postpartum, excluding the first 24 hours. Symptoms depend on site and extension of infection.

A. *Endometritis* Postpartum infection involving the endometrium

1. Uterus usually larger than expected for postdelivery day.
2. Lochia may be profuse, bloody, and foul smelling.

3. Chills and fever occur if lochial discharge is obstructed by clots.
4. Infection may spread to myometrium, parametrium, uterine (fallopian) tubes, peritoneum, and blood.

B. Parametritis (Pelvic Cellulitis) Infection of the pelvic connective tissue spread by the lymphatic system within the uterine wall. Often a result of an infected wound in the cervix, vagina, perineum, or lower uterine segment

1. Chills, fever (38.8°–40.0°C; 102°–104°F), tachycardia
2. Severe unilateral or bilateral pain in lower abdomen
3. Enlarged and tender uterus
4. Uterine position may become fixed as it is displaced by the exudate along the broad ligament.

Management

1. Antibiotic therapy is instituted after cultures are obtained and causative agent identified.
2. Supportive therapy is used to control pain and to maintain hydration and nutritional status.
3. Drainage is indicated for abscess development.

Complications

Thrombophlebitis may result from puerperal infection spread along the veins.

1. Femoral thrombophlebitis—appears 10 to 20 days after delivery as pain in calf, positive Homan's sign, fever, edema
2. Pelvic thrombophlebitis
   a. Infection of the veins of uterine wall and broad ligament usually caused by anaerobic streptococci
   b. Severe repeated chills and wide range of temperature changes occur about 2 weeks after delivery.
3. Strict bed rest, anticoagulants, and antibiotics are indicated.

Nursing Interventions/Patient Education

1. Perform postpartum assessment, noting uterine tenderness on palpation and the color, amount, and odor of lochia.
2. Monitor vital signs for signs of infection.
3. Assess knowledge and skill of perineal hygiene; teach proper technique and assist, if necessary.
4. Provide for adequate rest periods.
5. Position in high Fowler's position to promote drainage.
6. Administer antibiotics and analgesics, as ordered.
7. Explain the benefit of perineal washing or sitz baths and demonstrate setup.
8. Explain the need for good handwashing technique and how contamination of vagina from the rectum occurs.
9. Show how to place perineal pads and medications; encourage to change pads with each voiding, bowel movement, or every 4 hours while awake.
10. Encourage minimal separation from the infant and continuation of breast-feeding, as able.
11. Promote good handwashing technique for the mother before contact with the infant.

◆ POSTPARTUM HEMORRHAGE

Postpartum hemorrhage involves a loss of 500 mL or more of blood; it occurs most frequently in the first hour after delivery.

Pathophysiology/Etiology

1. Uterine atony—relaxation of the uterus secondary to:
   a. Multiple pregnancy—causes overdistention of uterus and a larger placental site
   b. Polyhydramnios (excessive amniotic fluid)
   c. High parity
   d. Prolonged labor with maternal exhaustion
   e. Deep anesthesia
   f. Fibromyomata—prevents uterus from contracting
   g. Retained placental fragments—result from manual removal of placenta, succenturiate (additional) lobe, abnormal adherent placenta (placenta accreta)
2. Laceration of the vagina, cervix, or perineum secondary to:
   a. Forceps delivery, especially rotation forceps
   b. Large infant
   c. Multiple pregnancy

Clinical Manifestations

1. With uterine atony uterus is soft or boggy, often difficult to palpate, and will not remain contracted; excessive vaginal bleeding occurs.
2. Hemorrhage usually occurs about the tenth postpartum day with retained placental fragments.
3. Lacerations of the vagina, cervix, or perineum cause bright red, continuous bleeding even when the fundus is firm.

Management

1. For uterine atony, oxytocin (Pitocin) or methylergonovine (Methergine) are prescribed.
2. Pain medication may be needed to counter uterine contractions.
3. If placental fragments have been retained, curettage of the uterus is indicated.
4. Lacerations may need to be repaired.

Nursing Assessment

1. Assess for hypotension, tachycardia, change in respiratory rate, decrease in urine output, and change in mental status—may indicate hypovolemic shock.
2. Assess location and firmness of uterine fundus.
3. Percuss and palpate for bladder distention, which may interfere with contracting of the uterus.
4. Monitor amount and type of bleeding or lochia present and the presence of clots.
5. Inspect for intactness of any perineal repair.

Nursing Diagnoses

A. Anxiety related to unexpected blood loss and uncertainty of outcome
B. Fluid Volume Deficit related to blood loss
C. Risk for Infection related to blood loss and vaginal examinations

Nursing Interventions

A. *Decreasing Anxiety*
1. Maintain a quiet and calm atmosphere.
2. Provide information about the situation and explain everything as it is done; answer questions that the woman and her family ask.
3. Encourage the presence of a support person.

B. *Maintaining Fluid Volume*
1. Maintain or start a large-bore IV line if vaginal bleeding becomes heavy.
2. Ensure that crossmatched blood is available.
3. Infuse oxytocin, IV fluids, and blood products at prescribed rate.
4. Monitor CBC for anemia.

C. *Preventing Infection*
1. Maintain aseptic technique.
2. Evaluate for symptoms of infection, chilling, and elevated temperature, changes in white blood cell count, uterine tenderness, and odor of lochia.
3. Administer antibiotics as prescribed.

Patient Education/Health Maintenance

1. Educate the woman about the cause of the hemorrhage.
2. Teach the woman the importance of eating a balanced diet and taking vitamin supplements.
3. Advise the woman that she may feel tired and fatigued and to schedule daily rest periods.
4. Advise the woman to notify her health care provider of increased bleeding or other changes in her status.

Evaluation

A. Verbalizes concerns about her well-being
B. Vital signs stable, urine output adequate, hematocrit stable
C. Remains afebrile, WBC count within normal limits

◆ POSTPARTUM HEMATOMAS

Postpartum hematomas are localized collections of blood in loose connective tissue beneath the skin that covers the external genitalia, beneath the vaginal mucosa, or in the broad ligaments.

Pathophysiology/Etiology

1. Trauma during spontaneous labor
2. Trauma during forceps application or delivery
3. Inadequate suturing of an episiotomy

Clinical Manifestations

1. Complaints of pressure and pain, often noting that the pain is excruciating
2. Discolored skin that is tight, full feeling, and painful to touch
3. Possible decrease in blood pressure, tachycardia

Management

1. Small hematomas are left to resolve on their own—ice packs may be applied.
2. Large hematomas may require evacuation of the blood and ligation of the bleeding vessel.
3. Analgesics and antibiotics may be ordered (due to increased chance of infection).

Complications

1. Hypovolemia and shock from extreme blood loss
2. Anemia, infection
3. Increased length of postpartum recovery period

Nursing Interventions/Patient Education

1. Inspect perineal and vulva area for signs of a hematoma when woman complains of pain or pressure after delivery.
2. Inspect the vaginal area for signs of a hematoma if woman is unable to void after anesthesia has worn off.
3. Monitor vital signs at least every 10 to 15 minutes and evaluate for signs of shock.
4. Relieve pain of a hematoma by applying an ice bag to perineal area, medicating with mild analgesics, and positioning for comfort to decrease pressure on the affected area.
5. Help relieve voiding problems by assisting to bathroom to void if able to ambulate. If patient is unable to ambulate, then assist her to sit on bedpan with legs hanging over side of bed. Provide privacy and run water while the woman is attempting to void.
6. If she is unable to void, catheterize.
7. Teach the woman the importance of eating a balanced diet and to include food high in iron.
8. Encourage the woman to take vitamin supplements and to take medications as ordered.
9. Instruct the woman in the use of the sitz bath to provide perineal comfort after the first 24 hours and at home.

◆ POSTPARTUM DEPRESSION

Postpartum depression may occur in the first 2 weeks after delivery and may be viewed as a normal developmental crisis related to the adjustments that are being made relative to the new role of parent, along with the added responsibilities, fatigue, and excitement that go with the birth. If a woman is unable to work through her feelings within about 2 weeks, and the symptoms continue, a more serious depression is indicated. Social, cultural, physiologic and psychological factors experienced may contribute to postpartum depression. Postpartum psychosis is a severe form of depression that occurs in a small percentage of women giving birth.

Clinical Manifestations

1. Exaggerated and prolonged periods of irritability, moodiness, hostility, fatigue
2. Ineffective coping
3. Withdrawal and inappropriate response to the infant or family
4. Loss of interest in activities
5. Insomnia

Management

Signs and symptoms may be overlooked, making the diagnosis of depression difficult. Counseling with a mental health professional, medication, and continuous support from family and friends may be helpful in managing the depressed patient. If untreated, the woman may not fully recover and possibly harm the infant or others.

Nursing Interventions/Patient Education

1. Listen to the woman regarding her adjustment to role of mother and observe for any clinical manifestations suggesting depression.
2. Ask the woman about the infant's behavior. Negative statements about the infant may suggest that the woman is having difficulty coping.
3. Refer regarding the woman's emotional status to health care provider and other resources as necessary.
4. Provide support and encourage family and friends to support and assist with the infant and mother. Physical support as well as emotional support may be indicated.
5. Educate the woman that treatment may help alleviate her symptoms and allow her to better care for herself and infant.

Selected References

Buckley, K., & Kulb, N. (1993). *High risk maternity nursing manual* (2nd ed.). Baltimore: Williams & Wilkins.

Burrow, G. N., & Ferris, T. F. (1995). *Medical complications during pregnancy* (4th ed.). Philadelphia: W. B. Saunders.

Creasy, R. K., & Resnik, R. (1994). *Maternal-fetal medicine principles and practice* (3rd ed.). Philadelphia: W. B. Saunders.

Danforth, D. N., & Scott, J. R. (1994). *Danforth's obstetrics and gynecology* (7th ed.). Philadelphia: J. B. Lippincott.

Dickason, E. J., et al. (1994). *Maternal-infant nursing care* (2nd ed.). St. Louis: Mosby-Year Book.

Gilbert, E. S., & Harmon, J. S. (1993). *Manual of high risk pregnancy and delivery*. St. Louis: Mosby-Year Book.

Gorrie, T. M., et al. (1994). *Foundations of maternal newborn nursing*. Philadelphia: W. B. Saunders.

James, D. K., et al. (1994). *High risk pregnancy management options*. Philadelphia: W. B. Saunders.

May, K. A., & Mahlmeister, L. R. (1994). *Maternal and neonatal nursing—family centered care* (3rd ed.). Philadelphia: J. B. Lippincott.

Mandeville, L. K., & Troiano, N. H. (1992). *NAACOG high-risk intrapartum nursing*. Philadelphia: J. B. Lippincott.

Queenan, J. T. (1994). *Management of high-risk pregnancy* (3rd ed.). Cambridge, MA: Blackwell Science.

PART IV ◆
Pediatric Nursing

UNIT 14

◆

General Practice Considerations

Pediatric Growth and Development

Growth and Development

◆ BASIC CONCEPTS

Growth and development begins with birth. Assessment of the newborn for appropriate development will primarily depend on a variety of reflexes.

Reflexes of the Newborn

1. *Pupillary reflexes*—ipsilateral (pertaining to the same side) and contralateral (pertaining to the other side) constriction to light.
2. *Rooting*—when corner of mouth is touched and object is moved toward cheek, infant will turn head toward object and open mouth.
3. *Palmar grasp*—pressure on palm of hand will elicit grasp.
4. *Plantar grasp*—pressure on the sole of foot behind toes will cause flexion of toes.
5. *Tonic neck reflex*—when head is turned to one side with leg and arm on that side extended, the extremities on the other side flex.
6. *Neck righting*—when head is turned to one side, the shoulder and trunk, followed by the pelvis, will turn to that side.
7. *Moro reflex*—response to sudden loud noise, causing body to stiffen and arms to go up and out, then forward and toward each other. Thumb and index finger will assume C shape.
8. *Positive-supporting reflex*—when held in an erect position, baby will stiffen lower extremities and support weight.
9. *Babinski's sign*—scratching sole of foot causes great toe to flex and toes to fan. After child begins to walk this sign cannot be elicited.
10. *Crossed extensor reflex*—when one leg is extended and the knee is held straight, while the sole of foot is stimulated, the opposite leg will flex.
11. *Landau's sign*—when baby is suspended horizontally with head depressed against trunk and neck flexed, legs will flex and be drawn up to trunk.
12. *Optical blink reflex*—when light is suddenly shone into open eyes, the eyes will close quickly with a quick dorsal flexion of head.
13. *Auditory blink reflex*—eyes quickly close if examiner loudly claps hands about 30 cm (11.5 inches) from infant's head.
14. *Recoil of arm*—when both arms are extended simultaneously by pulling outward and grasping wrists, both arms will flex at elbows when released.
15. *Withdrawal reflex*—pricking sole of foot will result in the baby's leg being flexed at hip, knee, and ankle.
16. *Stepping reflex*—when infant is held upright with dorsum of foot gently touching edge of table, will bend hips and knees and put foot on table. This will elicit stepping response in the opposite foot. Series of alternating stepping actions will result when infant is moved forward so that one foot at a time touches the firm surface.
17. *Parachute reflex*—while the infant is held prone and lowered quickly toward a surface, will extend arms and legs.
18. *Side-turning*—placing baby prone with head in midline will elicit the baby's turning head to the side.
19. Other characteristics of the newborn:
    a. Cries
    b. Sucks
    c. Has extremely sensitive skin
    d. Makes discriminating sounds
    e. Sleeps for long intervals
    f. Has little head control (head lag)

◆ INFANT TO ADOLESCENT GROWTH AND DEVELOPMENT

See table on pages 1057–1068.

Infant to Adolescent Growth and Development

Age and Physical Characteristics	Behavior Patterns	Nursing Implications/ Parental Guidance
Birth–4 weeks (1 month) Much neurologic disorganization Strong Moro reflex Sleep cycle disorganized Gastrointestinal system too immature for solid foods	**Motor Development** Momentary visual fixation on objects and adult face. Eyes follow bright moving objects. Lies awake on back with head averted. Immediately drops objects placed in hands. Responds to sounds of bell and other similar noises. Keeps hands fisted. **Socialization and Vocalization** Mews and makes throaty noises. Shows interest in human face. **Cognitive and Emotional Development** Reflexive. External stimuli are meaningless. Responses are generally limited to tension states or discomfort. Gains satisfaction from feeding and being held, rocked, fondled, and cuddled. Has an intense need for sucking pleasure. Quiets when picked up.	**Play Stimulation** Use human face—smile and talk. Dangle bright and moving object in field of vision (mobile). Hold, touch, caress, fondle, kiss. Rock, pat, change position. Play soft music or have infant listen to ticking clock, sing. Talk to infant, call by name. **Parental Guidance** Begin to expose infant to different household sounds. Change crib location in room. Use bright-colored clothing and linen. Keep infant nearby. Allow infant to sleep. Play with infant when awake. Hold during feeding.
8 weeks (2 months) Crossed extensor reflex disappears. Tonic neck reflex begins to fade.	**Motor Development** Reflexive behavior is slowly being replaced by voluntary movements. Turns from side to back. Begins to lift head momentarily from prone position. Shows eye coordination to light and objects. If bell is sounded nearby, infant will stop activity and listen. Eyes follow better, both vertically and horizontally. Focuses well. **Socialization and Vocalization** Begins vocalization—coos, especially to a voice. Crying becomes differentiated. Visually looks for sounds. May squeal with delight when stimulated by touching, talking, or singing. Begins social smile. Eyes follow person or object more intently. **Cognitive and Emotional Development** Recognizes familiar face. Becomes more aware and interested in environment. Anticipates being fed when in feeding position. Enjoys sucking—puts hand in mouth.	**Play Stimulation** Arrange mobile over crib so infant's movement will set it in motion. Hang wind chimes near infant. Hang bright-colored pictures on wall (yellow and red-colored stripes, for example). Use cradle gym and infant seat. Use rattles. Hold infant and walk around room. Allow freedom of kicking with clothes off. **Parental Guidance** Talk to infant and smile; get excited when baby coos. Place infant seat near mother's activities but where it cannot fall off or tip over. Put in prone position in bed or on floor. Expose infant to different textures. Exercise infant's arms and legs. Sing to infant. Provide tactile experience during bathing, diapering, feeding.

(continued)

Infant to Adolescent Growth and Development (continued)

Age and Physical Characteristics	Behavior Patterns	Nursing Implications/ Parental Guidance
12 weeks (3 months) Landau reflex appears at 3–4 months. Positive support reflex disappears. Posterior fontanelle closes. Increase in body fluids—real tears appear, drooling, and gastrointestinal juices increase.	**Motor Development** When prone, will rest on forearms and keep head in midline—makes crawling movements with legs, arches back, and holds head high; may get chest off surface. Indicates preference for prone or supine position. Discovers hands—strikes at objects while watching hands. Holds objects in hands and brings to mouth. Has fairly good head control. **Socialization and Vocalization** Smiles more readily. Babbles and coos. Stops crying when mother enters room or when caressed. Enjoys playing during feeding. Stays awake longer without crying. Turns head to follow familiar person. **Cognitive and Emotional Development** Shows active interest in environment. Recognizes familiar faces and objects. Focuses and follows objects. Shows repetitiveness in play activity. Is aware of strange situations. Derives pleasure from sucking—purposefully gets hand to mouth. Begins to establish routine preceding sleep.	**Play Stimulation** Encourage socialization, smiling, laughing. Place on mat on floor. Continue to introduce new sounds. **Parental Guidance** Take on daily outing as weather permits. Bounce on bed. Play with infant during feeding. Rattles can be used effectively for visual following and for hand play. Encourage older siblings to "make faces" and sing and talk to baby.
16 weeks (4 months) Moro reflex fades. Stepping reflex disappears. Rooting reflex disappears. By 4–5 months infant's weight approximately doubles birth weight. Average weekly weight gain, 140–200 g (4–7 oz). Average monthly height gain, 2.5 cm (1 inch). Pulse rate slows to 100–140 Respirations, 20–40/min Grasp becomes voluntary. Sucking becomes voluntary.	**Motor Development** Eyes focus on small objects; may pick a dangling ring. Holds head up (when being pulled to sitting position). Becomes more interested in environment. Hand comes to meet rattle. Listens—turns head to familiar sound. Sits with minimal support. Intentional rolling over, back to side. Reaches for offered objects. Grasps objects with both hands, and everything goes into mouth. **Socialization and Vocalization** Laughs and chuckles socially. Demands social attention by fussing. Recognizes mother. Begins to respond to "No, no." Enjoys being propped in sitting position. **Cognitive and Emotional Development** Actively interested in environment. Enjoys attention; becomes bored when alone for long periods of time. Recognizes bottle. More interested in mother. Indicates increasing trust and security. Sleeps through night; has defined nap time.	**Play Stimulation** Encourage mirror play. Provide soft squeeze toys in vivid colors of varying texture. Allow infant to splash in bath. Infant still enjoys holding and playing with rattles. Enjoys old-fashioned clothespins and playing pat-a-cake, peek-a-boo. **Parental Guidance** Be certain button eyes on toys and other small objects cannot be pulled off. Hold rattle and let infant reach and grasp it. When baby is in high chair, strap in. Let infant play with food; give finger foods. Move mobile out of reach—baby may grab it and cause injury. Repeat child's sounds. Talk in varying degrees of loudness. Begin looking at and naming pictures in book. Begin roughhousing play by both parents. Give space in playpen or on sheet on floor to practice rolling over.

Infant to Adolescent Growth and Development *(continued)*

Age and Physical Characteristics	Behavior Patterns	Nursing Implications/ Parental Guidance
26 weeks (7 months) By 5–6 months, tonic neck reflex disappears. By 6–7 months, palmar grasp disappears. By 7–9 months, develops eye-to-eye contact while talking; engages in social games. Two central lower incisors erupt. Spine "C shaped"—lacks lordotic and lumbar curves. Eustachian tube short and horizontal making baby prone to ear infections. Gastrointestinal system maturing enough for solid foods.	**Motor Development** Shows momentary sitting, with hand support. Bounces and bears some weight when held in standing position. Transfers and mouths objects in one hand. Discovers feet. Bangs objects together. Rolls over well. May begin some form of mobility. **Socialization and Vocalization** Discriminates between strangers and familiar figures. Crows and squeals. Starts to say "Ma," "Da." Self-play is self-contained. Laughs out loud. Makes "talking" sounds in response to others' talking. Begins fear of strangers, $8^{1}/_{2}$–10 months **Cognitive and Emotional Development** Secures objects by pulling on string. Searches for lost objects that are out of sight. Inspects objects; localizes sounds. Likes to sit in high chair. Drops and picks up objects. Displays exploratory behavior with food. Exhibits beginning fear of strangers. Becomes fretful when mother leaves. Shows much mouthing and biting.	**Play Stimulation** Enjoys social games, hide-and-seek with adult, toys, large blocks. Likes to bang objects. Plays in bounce chair, walker. Enjoys large nesting toys (round rather than square). Likes to drop and retrieve things. Likes metal cups, wooden spoons, and things to bang with. Loves crumpled paper. Enjoys squeeze toys in bath. Likes peek-a-boo, bye-bye, and pat-a-cake. **Parental Guidance** Will play as long as you can. Tie toys to chair with short string. Let play with extra spoon at feeding. Give soft finger foods. Because infant puts everything in mouth, *use safety precautions.* Keep small items away from infant; could choke on them. Show excitement at achievements. Supply kitchen items for toys.
40 weeks (10 months) 4 upper incisors erupt around 7–9 months. By 9–12 months, plantar reflex disappears. By 9–12 months, neck-righting reflex disappears. **6–12 months** Average weekly weight gain, 85–140 g (3–5 oz). Average monthly height gain, 1.25 cm ($^{1}/_{2}$ inch).	**Motor Development** Sits without support. Recovers balance. Manipulates objects with hands. Unwraps objects. Creeps. Pulls self upright at crib rails. Uses index finger and thumb to hold objects. Rings a bell. Can feed self a cracker and can hold bottle. Can control lips around cup. Does not like supine position. Can hold index finger and thumb in opposition. **Socialization and Verbalization** Claps hands on request. Responds to own name. Is very aware of social environment. Imitates gestures, facial expressions, and sounds. Smiles at image in mirror. Offers toy to adult, but does not release it. Begins to test parental reaction during feeding and at bedtime. Will entertain self for long periods of time.	**Play Stimulation** Encourage use of motion toys—rocking horse, stroller. Water play. Imitate animal sounds. Allow exploration outdoors. Provide for learning by imitation. Offer new objects (blocks). Child likes freedom of creeping and walking, but closeness of family is important. Good toys: milk carton; bean bag for tossing; fabric books; things to move around, fill up, empty out; pile-up and knock-down toys. **Parental Guidance** Do things with infant. Protect from dangerous objects—cover electrical outlets, block stairs, remove breakable objects from tables. Have child with family at mealtime. Offer cup.

(continued)

Infant to Adolescent Growth and Development (continued)

Age and Physical Characteristics	Behavior Patterns	Nursing Implications/ Parental Guidance
	Cognitive and Emotional Development Begins to imitate. Shows more interest in picture books. Enjoys achievements. Has strong urge toward independence—locomotion, feeding, dressing.	

12 months (1 year)
Developing lordotic and lumbar curves to make walking possible.
By 12–24 months, Landau reflex disappears.
Weight should approximately triple birth weight.
2 lower lateral incisors appear.
4 first molars appear by 14 months.
 	
Child Development Theories
Freudian: Behavior
  Birth–1 year—Oral Stage
Eriksonian: Emotion/Personality
  Birth–1 year—Sense of Trust vs. Mistrust
Piagetian: Intellectual Activity (Thought Process)
  Birth–2 years—Sensorimotor Period
	Motor Development
	Cruises around furniture.
	Beginning to stand alone and toddle.
	Turns pages in book.
	Tries tossing object.
	Shows hand dominance.
	Navigates stairs; climbs on chairs.
	Builds a tower of 2 blocks.
	Puts balls in box.
	May use spoon.
	Can release objects at will.
	Has regular bowel movements.
	
	Socialization and Verbalization
	Uses jargon.
	Points to indicate wants.
	Loves give-and-take game.
	Responds to music.
	Enjoys being center of attention and will repeat laughed-at activities.
	
	Cognitive and Emotional Development
	Shows fear, anger, affection, jealousy, anxiety, and sympathy.
	Experiments to reach new goals.
	Displays intense determination to remove barriers to action.
	Begins to develop concepts of space, time, and causality.
	Has increased attention span.
		Play Stimulation
		Ball play
		Cloth doll
		Motion objects and toys
		Transporting objects
		Name and point to body parts.
		''Put-in'' and ''take-out'' toys
		Sand box with spoons and other similar objects.
		Blocks
		Music
		
		Parental Guidance
		Allow self-directed play rather than adult-directed play.
		Continue to expose to foods of different textures, taste, smell, substance.
		Offer cup.
		Show affection and encourage child to return affection.

18 months *NOTE:* Between 1 and 3 years the child is called a ''toddler.'' Anterior fontanelle closes. Abdomen protrudes, arms and legs lengthen. Big muscles become well developed. 4 cuspids appear by 18 months. Fine muscle coordination begins to develop. Average yearly weight gain, 2–3 kg (4½–6½ lb). Average height gain during second year, 12 cm (4¾ inches).	**Motor Development** Walks up stairs with help, creeps downstairs. Walks without support and with balance. Falls less frequently. Throws ball. Stoops to pick up toys, look at bug. Turns pages of book. Holds and lifts cup. Builds 3-block tower. Picks up and places small beads in container. Begins to use spoon. **Cognitive and Emotional Development** Has vocabulary of 10 words that have meanings. Uses phrases, imitates words. Points to objects named by adult. Follows directions and requests. Imitates adult behavior. Retrieves toy from several hiding places.	**Play Stimulation** Allow unrestricted motor activity (within safety limits). Offer push-pull toys. Child selects favorite toy. Child likes blocks, pyramid toys, teddy bears, dolls, pots and pans, cloth picture books with colorful large pictures, telephone, musical top, nested blocks. **Parental Guidance** Begin to teach tooth brushing to establish good dental habits. Safety teaching: Child gets into everything within reach. Place medications in safe, locked place. Create a safe environment for child. Have ipecac syrup at home; stair guards; faucet protectors, drawer locks. Limits need to be set that give toddlers sense of security, yet encourage exploration. Identify behavior changes common in toddler.

Infant to Adolescent Growth and Development (continued)

Age and Physical Characteristics	Behavior Patterns	Nursing Implications/ Parental Guidance
	Psychosocial Development Develops new awareness of strangers. Wants to explore everything in reach. Plays alone, but near others. Is dependent on parents, but begins to reach out for autonomy. Finds security in a blanket, toy, or thumbsucking.	
2 years Protruding abdomen less noticeable. Landau reflex disappears. During first 2 years 35 cm (14–15 inches) are added to height. Slight bowing of legs with a wide-based walk. Handedness may become apparent.	**Motor Development** Walks up and down stairs. Opens doors; turns knobs. Has steady gait. Holds drinking cup well with 1 hand. Uses spoon without spilling food (may prefer fingers). Kicks a ball in front of him without support. Builds a tower of 4–6 blocks. Scribbles. Rides tricycle or kiddie car (without pedals). **Cognitive Development** Has 200–300 words in vocabulary. Begins to use short sentences. Refers to self by pronoun. Obeys simple commands. Does not know right from wrong. Begins to learn about time sequences. **Psychosocial Development** Uses word "mine" constantly. Is possessive with toys. Displays negativism—uses "no" as assertion of self. Routine and rituals are important. May begin cooperation in toilet training. Resists restrictions on freedom. Has fear of parents' leaving. Shows parallel play. Dawdles. Resists bedtime—uses transitional objects (blanket, toy). Vacillates between dependence and independence.	**Play Stimulation** Shows parallel play, although he enjoys having other children around. Has very short attention span. Enjoys same toys as child of 18 months. Likes doll play, ball. Imitates parents in domestic activities. Likes swing, hammering, paper, large crayons. **Parental Guidance** Has need for peer companionship, although displays immaturity by inability to share and take turns. A decrease in appetite normally occurs at this stage. Toilet training should be started (each child follows own pattern). Begin to have child eat meals with family if not already doing so. Begin to read to child; child likes storybooks with large pictures.
2–3 years Height approximates half adult height. Legs are about 34% of body length. Begins 2+ kg (5 lb) weight gain per year until 5 years old. At 2$\frac{1}{2}$ years has full set (20) of baby teeth. 4 second molars appear by 2$\frac{1}{2}$ years. Height gain, 6–8 cm (2$\frac{3}{8}$–3$\frac{1}{4}$ inches). Lordosis and protuberant abdomen of toddler disappear	**Motor Development** Throws objects overhead. Pedals tricycle. Walks backward. Washes and dries hands. Begins to use scissors. Can string large beads. Can undress himself. Feeds himself well. Tries to dance. Jumps in place. Builds tower of 8 blocks. Balances on one foot. Swings and climbs. Can eat an ice cream cone. Drinks from a straw. Chews gum without swallowing it.	**Play Stimulation** Plays simple games with other children. Enjoys story-telling and dress-up play. Plays "house." Colors. Uses scissors and paper. Rides tricycle. Read simple books to child. Will assist in developing memory skills, visual discrimination skills, and language.

(continued)

Infant to Adolescent Growth and Development (continued)

Age and Physical Characteristics	Behavior Patterns	Nursing Implications/ Parental Guidance
	Cognitive Development Shows increased attention span. Gives first and last name. Begins to ask "why." Is egocentric in thought and behavior. Beginning ability to reflect on own behavior. Talks in short sentences. Uses plurals. May attempt to sing simple songs. Has vocabulary of 900 words. Begins fantasy. Begins to understand what it means to take turns. Can repeat 3 numbers. Shows interest in colors.	**Parental Guidance** From 2–3 years, the child develops a seeming maturity; do not expect more than child is able to do. Arrange first visit to the dentist to have teeth checked. Be aware that negativistic and ritualistic behavior is normal. Be consistent in discipline. Control temper tantrums. Begin to teach traffic safety. Supervise outdoor play.

Child Development Theories
Freudian:
  1–3 years—Anal Stage
Eriksonian:
  1–3 years—Sense of Autonomy vs. Shame and Doubt
Piagetian:
  2–7 years—Preoperational Period; shows egocentrism and centering
	Psychosocial Development
	Negativism grows out of child's sense of developing independence—says "no" to every command.
	Ritualism is important to toddler for security (follows certain pattern, especially at bedtime).
	Temper tantrums may result from toddler's frustration in wanting to do everything for self.
	Shows parallel play as well as beginning interaction with others.
	Engages in associative play.
	Fears become pronounced.
	Continues to react to separation from parents but shows increasing ability to handle short periods of separation.
	Has daytime bladder control and is beginning to develop nighttime bladder control.
	Becomes more independent.
	Begins to identify sex (gender) roles.
	Explores environment outside the home.
	Can create different ways of getting desired outcome.	

3–4 years *NOTE:* Between 3 and 5 years, the child is called a "preschooler." May appear "knock kneed."	**Motor Development** Drawings have form and meaning, not detail. Copies a circle and a cross. Buttons front and side of clothes. Laces shoes. Bathes self, but needs direction. Brushes teeth. Shows continuous movement going up and down stairs. Climbs and jumps well. Attempts to print letters.	**Play Stimulation** Plays and interacts with other children. Shows creativity. Likes ring-around-the rosy. "Helps" adults. Likes costumes and enjoys dramatic play. Toys and games: record player, nursery rhymes, housekeeping toys, transportation toys (tricycle, trucks, cars, wagon), blocks, hammer and peg bench, floor trains, blackboard and chalk, easel and brushes, clay, crayon and finger paints, outside toys (sandbox, swing, small slide), books (short stories, action stories), drum, scrapbook.

Infant to Adolescent Growth and Development (continued)

Age and Physical Characteristics	Behavior Patterns	Nursing Implications/ Parental Guidance
	Cognitive Development Awareness of body is more stable; child becomes more aware of own vulnerability. Is less negativistic. Learns some number concepts. Begins naming colors. Can identify longer of 2 lines. Has vocabulary of 1500 words. Uses mild profanities and name-calling. Uses language aggressively. Asks many questions. May not be abstract enough to understand body parts that cannot be seen or felt. Can be given simple explanation as to cause and effect. Thinks very concretely; demonstrates irreversibility of thought. Immature concept of death—believes it is reversible. Has beginning understanding of past and future. Is egocentric in thought. **Psychosocial Development** Is more active with peers and engages in cooperative play. Performs simple tasks. Frequently has imaginary companion. Dramatizes experiences. Is proud of accomplishments. Exaggerates, boasts, and tattles on others. Can tolerate separation from mother longer without feeling anxiety. Is keen observer. Has good sense of "mine" and "yours." Behavior still frequently ritualistic. Becomes curious about life and sex. Often indulges in masturbation	**Parental Guidance** Base your expectations within child's limitations. Provide limited frustrations from environment to assist in coping. Give small errands to do around the house (putting silverware on table, drying a dish). Expand child's world with trips to the zoo, to the supermarket, to restaurant, etc. Prevent accidents. Provide for brief nonthreatening separation from parents and home. Reinforce correct use of language. Use opportunities for simple sexual education as child's needs arise. Accept masturbation as a normal phenomenon to be discouraged in public. Provide consistent discipline, motivated by love not anger. Consider nursery school.

4–5 years
By 2–5 years adds 25 cm (9–10 inches) to height.
At age 4, legs comprise about 44% of body length.
 	
Child Development Theories
Freudian:
  3–6 years—Phallic Stage
Eriksonian:
  3–6 years—Sense of Initiative vs. Guilt
Piagetian:
  2–7 years—Preoperational Period; shows egocentrism and centering
	Motor Development
	Hops 2 or more times.
	Dresses without supervision.
	Has good motor control—climbs and jumps well.
	Walks up stairs without grasping handrail.
	Walks backward.
	Washes self without wetting clothes.
	Prints first name and other words.
	Adds 3 or more details in drawings.
	Draws a square.
		Play Stimulation
		Demonstrates gross motor activity—likes to jump rope, skip, climb on jungle gyms, etc.
		Prefers group play and cooperates in projects.
		Plays simple letter, number, form, and picture games.
		Plays with cars and trucks.
		Still likes being read to.
		Continues to enjoy fantasy play.

(continued)

Infant to Adolescent Growth and Development (continued)

Age and Physical Characteristics	Behavior Patterns	Nursing Implications/ Parental Guidance
	Cognitive Development Has 2100-word vocabulary. Talks constantly. Uses adult speech forms. Participates in conversations. Asks for definitions. Knows age and residence. Identifies heavier of two objects. Knows weeks as time units. Names days of week. Begins to understand kinship. Knows primary colors. Can count to 10. Can copy a triangle. Has high degree of imagination. Questioning is at a peak. Begins to develop power of reasoning. **Psychosocial Development** May have an imaginary companion. Has a sense of order (likes to finish what was started). Is obedient and reliable. Is protective toward younger children. Begins to develop an elementary conscience with some influence in governing behavior. Has increased self-confidence. Accepts responsibility for acts. Is less rebellious. Has dreams and nightmares. Is cooperative and sympathetic. Shows generosity with toys. Begins to question parents' thinking. Identifies strongly with parent of same sex.	**Parental Guidance** Child no longer takes an afternoon nap. Prepare child for kindergarten. Tell him stories. Provide opportunities and reassurance for group play; have his friends visit for lunch and an afternoon of playing. Prevent accidents. Encourage child's participation in household activities.

Middle Childhood (5–9 years)
Growth rate is slow and steady.
Child gains an average of 3.18 kg (7 lb) per year. Height increases approximately 6.25 cm (2½ inches) per year.
Among children there is considerable variation in height and weight.
Child appears taller and slimmer.
Early lordosis disappears.
Child begins to lose baby teeth; permanent teeth appear at a rate of about 4 teeth per year from 7–14 years.
Neuromuscular and skeletal development allows improved coordination.
Eyes become fully developed; vision approaches 20/20.
Handedness should be well developed.
 	
Child Development Theories
Freudian:
  5–9 years—Beginning of Latency Period
Eriksonian:
  5–9 years—Industry vs. Inferiority
Piagetian:
  5–9 years—Enters stage of concrete operations
	Motor Development
	6 years
	  Is active and impulsive.
	  Balance improves.
	  Uses hands as manipulative tools in cutting, pasting, hammering.
	  Can draw large letters or figures.
	7 years
	  Has lower activity level.
	  Capable of fine hand movements; can print sentences.
	  Nervous habits such as nail biting are common.
	  Muscular skills such as ball throwing have improved.
	8 years
	  Moves with less restlessness.
	  Has developed grace and balance, even in active sports.
	  Has developed coordination of fine muscles, allowing child to write in script.
	9 years
	  Uses both hands independently
	  Has become skillful in manual activities because of improved eye–hand coordination.
		Parental Guidance
		Family atmosphere continues to have impact on child's emotional development and future response within the family.
		The child needs ongoing guidance in an open, inviting atmosphere. Limits should be set with conviction. Deal with only one incident at a time. When punishment is necessary, the child should not be humiliated. Child should know that it was the *act* that the adult found undesirable, not the child.
		Needs assistance in adjusting to new experiences and demands of school. Should be able to share experiences with family. Parents need to have communication with the teacher to work together for the health of the child.
		Convey love and caring in communication. The child understands language directed at feelings better than at intellect. Get down to eye level with the child.
		Focus attention on child's abilities and accomplishments rather than shortcomings and limitations.

Infant to Adolescent Growth and Development *(continued)*

Age and Physical Characteristics	Behavior Patterns	Nursing Implications/ Parental Guidance

	Cognitive Development
	6 years
	  Begins to learn to read. Defines objects in terms of use. Time sense is as much in past as present.
	  Is interested in relationship between home and neighborhood; knows some streets.
	  Uses sentences well; uses language to share others' experiences; may swear or use slang.
	  Distinguishes morning from afternoon.
	7 years
	
	  More reflective and has deeper understanding of meanings.
	  Interested in conclusions and logical endings. Begins to have scientific interests in cause and effect.
	  More responsible in relation to time, is more punctual. Sense of space is more realistic; child wants some space of own.
	  Knows value of coins.
	  Concept of death becoming mature—includes idea of irreversibility.
	8 years
	  Thinking is less animistic. Is aware of impersonal forces of nature. Begins to understand logical reasoning, conclusions, implications.
	  Less self-centered in thinking. Personal space is expanding; goes places on own. Aware of time; plans events of day. Understands right from left.
	9 years
	  Intellectually energetic and curious. Realistic; reasonable in thinking. Able to plan in advance. Breaks complex activities into steps.
	  Focuses on detail.
	  Sense of space includes the entire earth.
	  Participates in family discussions.
	  Likes to have secrets.
	
	Psychosocial Development
	(The following characteristics apply to the child in the 5–9-year group.)
	Still requires parental support, but pulls away from overt signs of affection.
	Peer groups provide companionship in widening circle of persons outside the home. Child learns more about self as he learns about others.
	"Chum" stage occurs at about 9–10 years of age. Child chooses a special friend of same sex and age in whom to confide. This is usually child's first love relationship outside of home, when someone becomes as important to him as himself.
	Play teaches the child new ideas and independence. Child progressively uses tools of competition, compromise, cooperation, and beginning collaboration.
		Child is sex-conscious. Child should be able to discuss questions at home rather than with friends. Requires simple, honest answers to questions.
		Common problems include teasing, quarreling, nail biting, enuresis, whining, poor manners, swearing, lying, cheating, stealing. These are usually fleeting phases and should not be handled negatively. The causes for such behavior should be investigated and dealt with constructively.
		
		The child needs order and consistency to help in coping with doubts, fears, unacceptable impulses, and unfamiliar experiences.
		Encourage peer activities as well as home responsibilities and give recognition to child's accomplishments and unique talents.
		Television may stimulate learning in several spheres, but should be monitored.
		Accidents are a major cause of disability and death. Safety practices should be continued. (Refer to section on safety, p. 1101).
		Exercise is essential to promote motor and psychosocial development. The child should have a safe place to play and simple pieces of equipment.
		A school health program should be available and concerned with the child's physical, emotional, mental, and social health. This should be augmented by information and example at home.
		Medical supervision should continue with yearly examination to detect developmental delay, disease. Appropriate immunizations should be administered.
		Child frequently has "quiet days"—periods of shyness, which should be tolerated as part of growing up and deciding who he or she is.
		Child may be subject to nightmares, a situation that requires reassurance and understanding.
		Parents, teachers, and health professionals should be available and able to provide information and answer questions about the physical changes that occur.

(continued)

Infant to Adolescent Growth and Development *(continued)*

Age and Physical Characteristics	Behavior Patterns	Nursing Implications/ Parental Guidance

	Body image and self-concept are fluid because of rapid physical, emotional, social changes.
	Latency-stage sexual drive is controlled and repressed. Emphasis is on the development of skills and talent.
	
	Patterns of Play
	6–7 years
	  Child acts out ideas of family and occupational groups with which he has contact.
	  Painting, pasting, reading, simple games, watching television, digging, running games, skating, riding bicycle, and swimming are all enjoyed activities.
	8 years
	  Child enjoys collections; loosely formed, short-lived clubs; table games; card games; books; television; records.	

Late Childhood (9–12 years)
Vital signs approach adult values.
Loses childish appearance of face and takes on features that will characterize individual as an adult.
Growth spurt occurs, and some secondary sex characteristics appear: in girls, at age 10–12 years; in boys, at age 12–14 years.
Physical changes of puberty:
  Increased height and weight, increased perspiration and activity of sebaceous glands; vasomotor instability; increased fat deposition.
Physical changes in girls:
  Pelvis increases in transverse diameter; hips broaden; tenderness in developing breast tissue; enlargement of areola diameter; appearance of pubic hair.
Physical changes in boys:
  Size of testes increases; scrotum color changes; breasts enlarge, temporarily; height and shoulder breadth increase
  Appearance of lightly pigmented hair at base of penis.
  Increase in length and width of penis.
 	
Child Development Theories
Freudian:
  9–12 years—Latency Period continues
Eriksonian:
  9–12 years—Industry vs. Inferiority continues
Piagetian:
  9–12 years—Stage of concrete operations continues
	Motor Development
	Energetic, restless, active movements such as finger-drumming or foot-tapping appear.
	Has skillful manipulative movements nearly equal to those of adults.
	Works hard to perfect physical skills.
	
	Cognitive Development
	10 years
	  Likes to reason, enjoys learning. Thinking is concrete, matter of fact. Wants to measure up to challenge. Likes to memorize, identify facts. Attention span may be short. Space is rather specific (ie, where things are).
	  Can write for relatively long time with speed.
	11 years
	  Likes action in learning.
	  Concentrates well when working competitively.
	  Can understand relational terms such as weight and size.
	  Perceives space as nothingness that goes on forever.
	  Able to discuss problems.
	  Can conceptualize symbolically enough to understand body parts.
	  Can describe some abstract terms.
	12 years
	  Enjoys learning.
	  Considers all aspects of a situation.
	  Motivated more by inner drive than by competition.
	  Able to classify, arrange, generalize.
	  Likes to discuss and debate.
	  Begins conceptual thinking.
	  Verbal, formal reasoning now possible.
	  Can recognize moral of a story.
	  Defines time as duration; likes to plan ahead.
	  Understands that space is abstract.
	  Can be critical of own work.
		Parental Guidance
		Continue appropriate interventions related to early childhood.
		Continue sex education and preparation for adolescent body changes. Understanding is important.
		Encourage participation in organized clubs, youth groups.
		Democratic guidance is essential as child works through a conflict between dependence (on parents) and independence. Child needs realistic limits set.
		Needs help channeling energy in proper direction—work and sports.
		Requires adequate explanation of body changes. Special understanding required for the child who lags in physical development.
		Continue consistent disciplinary style.

Infant to Adolescent Growth and Development (continued)

Age and Physical Characteristics	Behavior Patterns	Nursing Implications/ Parental Guidance
	Psychosocial Development Gang becomes important, and gang code takes precedence over nearly everything. Often gang codes are characterized by collective action against the mores of the adult world. Here, children begin to work out own social patterns without adult interference. Early gangs may include both sexes; later gangs are separated by sex. May strive for unreasonable independence from adult control. Often interested in religion, morality. Has increased interest in sexuality. May reach puberty; resurgence of sexual drives causes recapitulation of Oedipal struggle. **Patterns of Play** Continues to enjoy reading, TV, table games. More interested in active sports as a means to improve skills. Creative talents may appear; may enjoy drawing, modeling clay. By age 10, sex differences in play become profound. Occasional privacy is important. Begins to have vocational aspirations.	

Early Adolescence (12–14)
Phase of development begins when reproductive organs become functionally operative; phase ends when physical growth is completed.
Skeletal system grows faster than supporting muscles.
Hands and feet grow proportionately faster than rest of body.
Large muscles develop more quickly than small muscles.
Girls:
  Physical changes include appearance of menarche; growth of axillary and perineal hair; deepened voice; ovulation; further development of breasts.
Nutritional need for iron and calcium increase dramatically.
Boys:
  Physical changes include growth of axillary, perineal, facial, chest hair; deepening of voice; production of spermatozoa; nocturnal emissions.
 	
Child Development Theories
Freudian:
  12–14 years—Begins stage of sexuality
Eriksonian:
  12–14 years—Identity vs. Role Diffusion
Piagetian:
  12–14 years—Begins stage of formal operations
	Motor Development
	Often uncoordinated; has poor posture.
	Tires easily.
	
	Cognitive Development
	Mind has great ability to acquire and use knowledge.
	Abstract thinking is sufficient to learn multivariable ideas such as the influence of hormones on emotions.
	Categorizes thoughts into usable forms.
	May project thinking into the future.
	Is capable of highly imaginative thinking.
	
	Psychosocial Development
	Interest in opposite sex increases.
	Often revolts from adult authority to conform to peer-group standards.
	Continues to rework feelings for parent of opposite sex and unravel the ambivalence toward parent of same sex.
	Affection may turn temporarily to an adult outside of the family (for example, crush on family friend, neighbor, or teacher).
	Uses peer-group dialect—highly informal language or specially coined terminology.
	Peer groups are especially important and help adolescent to define own identity, to adapt to changing body image, to establish more mature relationships with others, and to deal with heightened sexual feelings.
	Cliques may develop.
		Parental Guidance
		Stresses frequently result from conflicting value systems between generations. Parents may need help to see that the adolescent is a product of the times and that actions reflect what is happening around the youngster.
		Parents' limits and rules should be realistic and consistent. They should convey the love and concern of parents and should be a source of comfort and reassurance, protecting the child from activities for which he is not ready.
		The home should be an accepting, emotionally stable environment.
		Continue sex education, including discussion of ovulation, fertilization, menstruation, pregnancy, contraception, masturbation, nocturnal emissions, and hygiene.
		Adolescents have an increased need for rest and sleep because they are expending large amounts of energy and are functioning with an inadequate oxygen supply.
		Recreational interests should be fostered. Favorite activities include sports, dating, dancing, reading, hobbies, and television. Talking on the telephone, listening to records are favorite pastimes.
		Adolescent health problems that require preventive education are accidents, obesity, acne, pregnancy, sexually transmitted disease, drug abuse.

(continued)

Infant to Adolescent Growth and Development *(continued)*

Age and Physical Characteristics	Behavior Patterns	Nursing Implications/ Parental Guidance
	Dating generally progresses from groups of couples to double dates and finally single couples. Teenage "hangouts" become important centers of activity. Begins questioning existing moral values.	Allow adolescent to handle own affairs as much as possible, but be aware of physical and psychosocial problems that may require help. Encourage independence but allow child to lean on parents for support when frightened or unable to attain goals. Adolescents with special problems should have access to specialists such as adolescent clinics and psychologists. Requires reassurance and help in accepting changing body image. Parents should make the most of child's positive qualities. Give gentle encouragement and guidance regarding dating. Avoid strong pressures in either direction. Understand conflicts as child attempts to deal with social, moral, and intellectual issues.

◆ DEVELOPMENTAL SCREENING TOOLS

Developmental screening tools have been created to determine the overall developmental age of the child or to detect specific areas of development that are lacking.

Goodenough–Harris Draw-a-Person Test

This test provides one of the methods of measuring the level of mental development of children between 3 and 10 years of age. It was originally described in 1926 and appears to be a sound one; there is a significant degree of correlation in the results of this test and IQ. Subsequently Harris brought the test up-to-date with specific scoring for drawings of a man or a woman.

1. *Procedure:* The child is supplied with a pencil (preferably a No. 2 with eraser) and a sheet of blank paper and instructed to "Draw a person," "Draw the best person you can." No additional directions are necessary. Encouragement may be supplied if necessary. Under no condition should the examiner suggest that the child's picture needs to be supplemented or changed in any way—the only exception being the drawing of the stick figure. In this case the examiner is permitted to encourage the child to "draw a whole person."
2. *Scoring:* The child receives one point for each detail present according to the following scoring guides:

Drawing of a Woman

1. Head present
2. Neck present
3. Neck, 2 dimensions
4. Eyes present
5. Eye detail: brow or lashes
6. Eye detail: pupil
7. Nose present (not round ball)
8. Nose, 2 dimensions
9. Bridge of nose (straight to eyes, narrower than base)

Drawing of a Man

1. Head present
2. Neck present
3. Neck, 2 dimensions
4. Eyes present
5. Eye detail: brow or lashes
6. Eye detail: pupil
7. Nose present
8. Nose, 2 dimensions (not round ball)
9. Mouth present

(continued)

Drawing of a Woman

10. Nostrils shown
11. Mouth present
12. Lips, 2 dimensions
13. Both nose and lips in 2 dimensions
14. Both chin and forehead shown
15. Hair I (any scribble)
16. Hair II (more detail)
17. Necklace or earrings
18. Arms present
19. Fingers present
20. Correct number of fingers shown
21. Opposition of thumb shown (must include fingers)
22. Hands present
23. Legs present
24. Feet (any indication)
25. Show "feminine" (any attempt such as high heels, open toe, strap)
26. Attachment of arms and legs I (to trunk anywhere)
27. Attachment of arms and legs II (to trunk at correct point)
28. Clothing indicated (any)
29. Sleeve
30. Neckline (any indication)
31. Trunk present
32. Trunk in proportion, 2 dimensions (length greater than breadth)

Drawing of a Man

10. Lips, 2 dimensions
11. Both nose and lips in 2 dimensions
12. Both chin and forehead shown
13. Bridge of nose (straight to eyes; narrower than base)
14. Hair I (any scribble)
15. Hair II (more detail)
16. Ears present
17. Fingers present
18. Correct number of fingers shown
19. Opposition of thumb shown (must include fingers)
20. Hands present
21. Arms present
22. Arms at side or engaged in activity
23. Feet; any indication
24. Attachment of arms and legs I (to trunk anywhere)
25. Attachment of arms and legs II (at correct point of trunk)
26. Trunk present
27. Trunk in proportion, 2 dimensions (length greater than breadth)
28. Clothing I (anything)
29. Clothing II (2 articles of clothing)

3. *Norms:* Minimum score for child to be within one standard deviation of age-appropriate mean.

	Drawing of Man		Drawing of Woman	
Age	By Boys	By Girls	By Boys	By Girls
3	4	5	4	6
4	7	7	7	8
5	11	12	11	14
6	13	14	13	16
7	16	17	16	19
8	18	20	20	23

(From Johns Hopkins Hospital: The Harriet Lane Handbook. 9th ed. Dennis L. Headings (ed). Copyright © 1981 by Year Book Medical Publishers, Inc., Chicago. Used with permission.)

Denver Developmental Screening Test

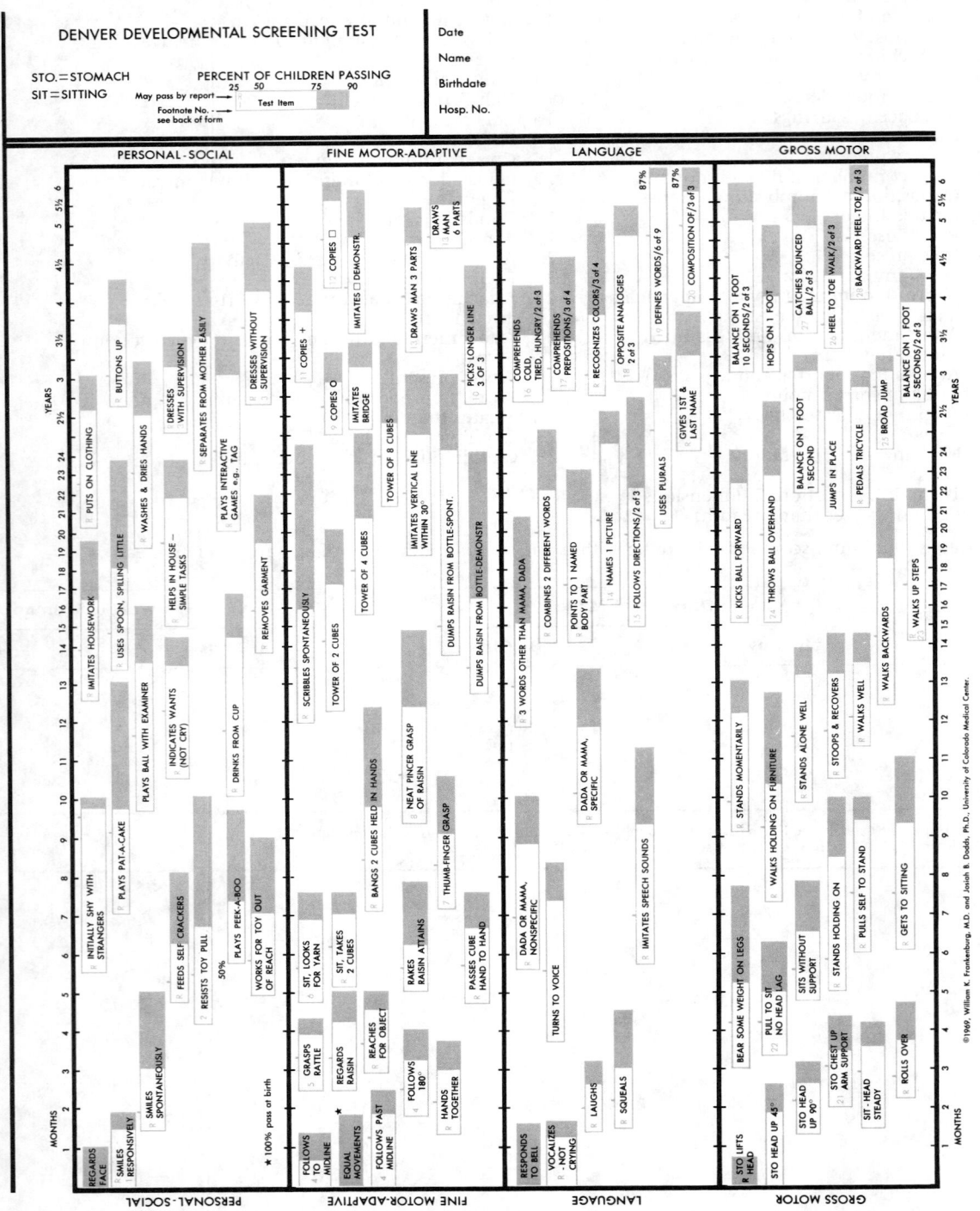

The Denver Developmental Assessment method developed by William K. Frankenburg, M.D., and his colleagues, is presented in a manual called Denver Developmental Screening Test. The test materials can be ordered from: Lodaco Project & Publishing Foundation, Inc., East 51st Avenue and Lincoln Street, Denver, Colorado 80216.

DIRECTIONS

1. Try to get child to smile by smiling, talking or waving to him. Do not touch him.
2. When child is playing with toy, pull it away from him. Pass if he resists.
3. Child does not have to be able to tie shoes or button in the back.
4. Move yarn slowly in an arc from one side to the other, about 6″ above child's face. Pass if eyes follow 90° to midline. (Past midline; 180°)
5. Pass if child grasps rattle when it is touched to the backs or tips of fingers.
6. Pass if child continues to look where yarn disappeared or tries to see where it went. Yarn should be dropped quickly from sight from tester's hand without arm movement.
7. Pass if child picks up raisin with any part of thumb and a finger.
8. Pass if child picks up raisin with the ends of thumb and index finger using an overhand approach.

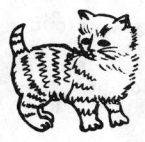   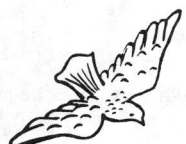   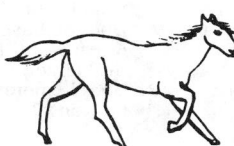   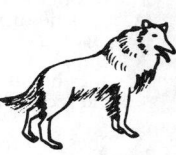

9. Pass any enclosed form. Fail continuous round motions.

10. Which line is longer? (Not bigger.) Turn paper upside down and repeat. ($^3/_3$ or $^5/_6$)

11. Pass any crossing lines.

12. Have child copy first. If failed, demonstrate.

When giving items 9, 11 and 12, do not name the forms. Do not demonstrate 9 and 11.

13. When scoring, each pair (2 arms, 2 legs, etc.) counts as one part.
14. Point to picture and have child name it. (No credit is given for sounds only.)

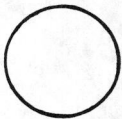   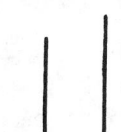   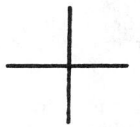   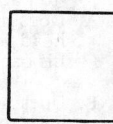

15. Tell child to: Give block to Mommie; put block on table; put block on floor. Pass 2 of 3. (Do not help child by pointing, moving head or eyes.)
16. Ask child: What do you do when you are cold? . . hungry? . . tired? . . Pass 2 of 3.
17. Tell child to: Put block *on* table; *under* table; *in front* of chair, *behind* chair. Pass 3 of 4. (Do not help child by pointing, moving head or eyes.)
18. Ask child: If fire is hot, ice is ?; Mother is a woman, Dad is a ?; a horse is big, a mouse is ?. Pass 2 of 3.
19. Ask child: What is a ball? . . lake? . . desk? . . house? . . banana? . . curtain? . . ceiling? . . hedge? . . pavement? Pass if defined in terms of use, shape, what it is made of or general category (such as banana is fruit, not just yellow). Pass 6 of 9.
20. Ask child: What is a spoon made of? . . a shoe made of? . . a door made of? (No other objects may be substituted.) Pass 3 of 3.
21. When placed on stomach, child lifts chest off table with support of forearms and/or hands.
22. When child is on back, grasp his hands and pull him to sitting. Pass if head does not hang back.
23. Child may use wall or rail only, not person. May not crawl.
24. Child must throw ball overhand 3 feet to within arm's reach of tester.
25. Child must perform standing broad jump over width of test sheet. ($8^1/_2$ inches)
26. Tell child to walk forward, 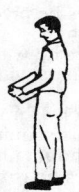 heel within 1 inch of toe. Tester may demonstrate. Child must walk 4 consecutive steps, 2 out of 3 trials.
27. Bounce ball to child who should stand 3 feet away from tester. Child must catch ball with hands, not arms, 2 out of 3 trials.
28. Tell child to walk backward, ← toe within 1 inch of heel. Tester may demonstrate. Child must walk 4 consecutive steps, 2 out of 3 trials.

DATE AND BEHAVIORAL OBSERVATIONS (how child feels at time of test, relation to tester, attention span, verbal behavior, self-confidence, etc.):

Developmental Assessment by Interview

A method of evaluation has been developed by using an interview technique asking parents a list of questions regarding milestones in achievements that most will remember. Developed by Drs. Capute and Biehl, it has been very successful in its use at the John F. Kennedy Institute for the Habilitation of Handicapped Children at John Hopkins Hospital.

Age	Gross Motor	Fine Motor	Language	Social
3 mo	A. Does he support himself on forearms when lying? B. Does he hold his head up steadily while on his stomach?	A. Are his hands usually open at rest? B. Does he pull at his clothing?	A. Does he laugh or make happy noises? B. Does he turn his head to sounds?	A. Does he smile at you? B. Does he reach for familiar people or objects?
6 mo	A. Does he lift his head when lying on his back? B. Does he roll from back to front?	A. Does he transfer a toy from one hand to the other? B. Does he pick up small objects	A. Does he "babble," repeat sounds together (ie, mum-mum-mum)? B. Is he frightened by angry noise?	A. Does he stretch his arms out to be picked up? B. Does he show his likes and dislikes?
9 mo	A. Does he sit for long periods without support? B. Does he pull up on furniture?	A. Does he pick up objects with his thumb and one finger? B. Does he finger-feed any foods?	A. Does he understand "no-no," "bye-bye"? B. Will he imitate any sounds or words if you make them first?	A. Does he hold his own bottle? B. Does he play any nursery games ("peek-a-boo," "bye-bye")?
12 mo	A. Is he walking (alone or with hand held)? B. Does he pivot when sitting?	A. Does he throw toys (objects)? B. Does he give you toys (let go) easily?	A. Does he have at least one meaningful word other than "mama," "dada"? B. Does he shake his head for "no"?	A. Does he cooperate in dressing? B. Does he come when you call him?
18 mo	A. Does he walk upstairs with help? B. Can he throw a toy while standing without falling?	A. Does he turn book pages (2 or 3 at a time)? B. Does he fill spoon and feed self?	A. Does he have at least 6 real words besides his "jargon"? B. Does he point at what he wants?	A. Does he copy you in routine tasks (sweeping, dusting, etc)? B. Does he play in the company of other children?
2 yr	A. Does he run well without falling? B. Does he walk up and down stairs alone?	A. Does he turn book pages one at a time? B. Does he remove his own shoes, pants?	A. Does he talk in short (2–3 word) sentences? B. Does he use pronouns ("me," "you," "mine")?	A. Does he ask to be taken to the toilet? B. Does he play in company of other children?
2½ yr	A. Does he jump, getting both feet off the floor? B. Does he throw a ball overhand?	A. Does he unbutton any buttons? B. Does he hold a pencil or crayon adult fashion?	A. Does he use plurals or past tense? B. Does he use the word "I" correctly most of the time?	A. Does he tell his first and last name if asked? B. Does he get himself a drink without help?
3 yr	A. Does he pedal a tricycle? B. Does he alternate feet (one stair per step) going upstairs?	A. Does he dry his hands (if reminded)? B. Does he dress and undress fully including front buttons?	A. Does he tell little stories about his experiences? B. Does he know his sex?	A. Does he share his toys? B. Does he play well with another child? Take turns?
4 yr	A. Does he attempt to hop or skip? B. Does he alternate feet going downstairs?	A. Does he button clothes fully? B. Does he catch a ball?	A. Does he say a song or a poem from memory? B. Does he know all his colors?	A. Does he tell "tall tales" or "show off"? B. Does he play cooperatively with a small group of children?
5 yr	A. Does he skip, alternating feet? B. Does he jump rope or jump over low obstacles?	A. Does he tie his own shoes? B. Does he spread with a knife?	A. Can he print his first name? B. Does he ever ask what a word means?	A. Is he a "mother's helper"—likes to do things for you? B. Does he play competitive games and abide by the rules?

(From Johns Hopkins Hospital: The Harriet Lane Handbook. 13th ed. Dennis L. Headings (ed). Copyright © 1993 by Year Book Medical Publishers, Chicago. Used with permission.)

Selected References

Bowers, A. C., & Thompson, J. M. (1991). *Clinical manual of health assessment* (4th ed.). St. Louis: C. V. Mosby.

Fuller, J., & Schaller-Ayers, J. (1994). *Health assessment: A nursing approach.* Philadelphia: J. B. Lippincott.

Gillis, A. J. (1990). Nurses' knowledge of growth and development principles in meeting psychosocial needs of hospitalized children. *Journal of Pediatric Nursing, 5,* 78.

Hoekelman, R. A., (ed.) (1991). *Primary pediatric care.* St. Louis: C. V. Mosby.

Jackson, D., & Saunders, R. (1993). *Child health nursing.* Philadelphia: J. B. Lippincott.

Kattner, I. (1991). Helpful strategies in working with preschool children in pediatric practice. *Pediatric Annals, 20,* 120.

Marino, B. L. (1991). Studying infant and toddler play. *Journal of pediatric nursing, 6,* 16.

Oski, F. A. (ed.) (1993). *Principles and practice of pediatrics.* Philadelphia: J. B. Lippincott.

Schuster, C. S., & Ashburn, S. S. (1992). *The process of human development.* Philadelphia: J. B. Lippincott.

Pediatric Physical Assessment

History

◆ OBTAINING A HISTORY

A history of the child is obtained to establish a relationship with the child and family; to assess what a family understands about their child's health; to formulate an individual plan of care; and to correct any misinformation the family may have.

Focus on specific topics in the history depending on the child's age, including:

Infant—stress prenatal and postnatal history, nutrition, development
Toddler—home environment, safety issues, development, parent's response
School age—school, friends, reaction to previous hospitalizations
Adolescent—alcohol, drugs, friends, sexual history, relationships with parents, identity

Identifying Information

A. *Type of Information Needed*
1. Date and time
2. Health care provider's name and telephone number, if known
3. Patient's name, address, telephone number, birth date
4. Referring health care source (eg, school, other health care provider, clinic
5. Insurance data

B. *Method of Collecting Data*
1. Identify the "care person" in charge of the patient by name and relationship to the patient; obtain relative's or care person's address, home and work telephone numbers, if different from those of the patient.
2. To make the informant feel more at ease, the questions should begin in a friendly, nonthreatening manner. Questions addressed to the parent should be phrased appropriately.
3. Casual, friendly responses or remarks on the part of the interviewer may also help break the ice.
   a. "Whoever takes care of this baby certainly does a good job."
   b. "That's a lovely outfit the baby is wearing." (Remember that families will often put a new dress or suit on a baby for a visit to a health care agency.)
4. Sometimes repeat the information to verify data. This will give you a better judgment of the care person's cooperation and reliability.
5. If age appropriate, get some data directly from child.

Chief Complaint

A. *Method of Recording*
1. Write an exact description of the complaint.
2. Use quotation marks to clearly indicate that the informant's words are being used. It is helpful to explain:
   a. "I'll write it down so there will be no mistake."
   b. "Let me read this back to you to be sure it is correct."
3. Quotation of the care person's exact words may give an indication of how he or she feels about the symptoms; may reflect fear, guilt, defensiveness, etc.

B. *Method of Collecting Information*
1. Begin with a helpful open-ended question. That is the first overture made to this patient.
   a. "How have things been going?"
   b. "Please tell me the reason for your coming here today."
   c. "What do you think is wrong with the baby?"
2. Then proceed to more specific questions.

C. *Duration of Complaint*
1. The information obtained may indicate the natural history of the disease, if one is present, and its gradual evolution. Pursue the information with a series of probing questions.
   a. "How long has the baby (child) had this problem?"
   b. If the informant cannot remember, try another route:
   "When did he (or she) last act well?"
   "Do you remember last Christmas? Did the baby have the trouble then?"
2. Write down the responses; try to assess, as more questions are asked, how accurate the informant's answers may be.

History of Present Illness

A. *Type of Information Needed*
When the patient is an infant or a preverbal child, information will consist mainly of what the informant has been able to observe. Having established what the chief complaint is, identify further problems, if any. Obtain the following information for each problem:

1. Body location—of pain, itching, weakness, etc.
2. Quality of complaint—both type (a burning pain) and severity (knifelike, comes and goes).
3. Degree of symptom—(eg, pain, how severe; cough, day and night; eye drainage, how much).

Sandra Nettina: *The Lippincott Manual of Nursing Practice, 6th ed.* © 1996 Lippincott-Raven Publishers

4. Chronology—indicate time sequence and whether problem is episodic (lasts for a while and then clears up completely).
5. Environment or setting—where and when the symptoms occur.
6. Aggravating and alleviating factors—what makes the pain worse or better?
7. Associated manifestations or symptoms—accompanied by vomiting, blurred vision, etc.

B. *Importance of Detail*
1. A carefully written description of a symptom will frequently be the source of a future diagnosis and will serve all who are involved in helping the patient.
2. Do not worry about large volume of notes at first.
3. You will be able to recheck this information when you do the review of systems.

Family History

1. Family members—Mother's age and state of health, father's age and health, siblings (who is at home with you?)
2. Family health history—Any of the following conditions:
   a. Eyes, ears, nose, throat—any nose bleeds, sinus problems, glaucoma, cataracts, myopia, strabismus, other problems related to eyes, ears, nose, throat
   b. Cardiorespiratory—tuberculosis, asthma, hay fever, hypertension, heart murmurs, heart attacks, strokes, anemia, rheumatic fever, leukemia, pneumonia, emphysema, other problems
   c. Gastrointestinal—ulcers, colitis, vomiting, diarrhea, other problems
   d. Genitourinary—kidney infections, bladder problems, congenital abnormalities
   e. Skeletomuscular—congenital hip or foot problems, muscular dystrophy, arthritis, other problems
   f. Neurologic—convulsions, seizures, epilepsy, nervous disorder, mental retardation, mental problems, comas, others
   g. Chronic disease—diabetes, jaundice, cancer, tumors, thyroid problems, congenital disorder
   h. Special senses—anyone deaf or blind?
   i. Miscellaneous—any other medical problem not mentioned
3. Family social history
   a. Residence—apartment or house, how large? Yard, stairs, proximity to transportation, shopping, playground, school, safe neighborhood? City water?
   b. Financial situation—who works, where, occupation, welfare, food stamps
   c. Outside help—baby sitters, day-care center
   d. Family interrelationships—happy, cooperative, antagonistic, chaotic, multiproblem, violent, etc

Past History

A. *Prenatal*
1. Pregnancy—planned or not; source of care; date (approximately) of seeking care; birth order of this pregnancy, including miscarriages. This area of the history may be one of great sensitivity. Try to make the questions gentle and supportive.
   a. "Did you plan a baby around this time?"
   b. "When did you manage to get your first checkup for the pregnancy?"
   c. "Were there any unusual problems related to your pregnancy or delivery?"
2. Maternal health—includes illnesses and dates, abnormal symptoms (eg, fever, rash, vaginal bleeding, edema, hypertension, urine abnormalities, sexually transmitted disease). Avoid technical words, if possible.
   a. "Were the doctors or nurses worried about your health?"
   b. "Were your rings tight?"
   c. "Do you know if your blood pressure went up?"
   d. "Did you have trouble with your urine?"
3. Weight gain—validate by trying to get a figure for nonpregnant weight and weight at delivery.
4. Medicines taken—eg, vitamins, iron, calcium, aspirin, cold preparations, tranquilizers ("nerve medicine"), antibiotics; use of ointments, hormones, injections during pregnancy, special or unusual diet; radiation exposure, sonography, amniocentesis.
5. Quality of the fetal movements: when felt?

B. *Natal*
1. Expected date of delivery and approximate duration of pregnancy
2. Place of delivery and who conducted the delivery
3. Labor—spontaneous or induced; duration and intensity
4. Analgesia or anesthesia
5. Presentation—vaginal, breech, or vertex; cesarean delivery, forceps
6. Complications (eg, need for blood transfusion, delay in delivery, etc.)

C. *Neonatal*
1. Condition of infant
2. Color (if seen) at delivery
3. Activity of infant
4. Crying heard
5. Breathing abnormality
6. Birth weight and length
7. Problems occurring immediately at birth

D. *Postnatal*
1. Duration of hospitalization of the mother and infant
2. Problems with baby's breathing or feeding
3. Need of supportive care (eg, oxygen, incubator, special care nursery, isolation, medications)
4. Weight changes, weight at discharge if known
5. Color—cyanosis or jaundice
6. Bowel movements—when
7. Problems—seizures, deformities identified, consultation required
8. Mother's contact with the baby and her first impression
   a. "What was it like when you first saw your baby?"
   b. "What did the baby do when you were first together?"

E. *Nutrition*
1. Breast or bottle fed; what formula? how prepared?
2. Amounts offered and consumed
3. Frequency of feeding; weight gain
4. Addition of juice or solid foods
5. Food preferences or allergies
6. Feeding problems—variations in appetite
7. Age of weaning
8. Vitamins—type, amount, regularity

9. Pattern of weight gain
10. Current diet; frequency and content of meals

F. **Growth and Development**
1. Past weights and lengths if available
2. Milestones—sat alone unsupported; walked alone; used words, then sentences
3. Teeth—eruption, difficulty, cavities, brushing, flossing
4. Toilet training
5. Current motor, social, and language skills
6. Sexual development
    a. Infant—swollen breast tissue, vaginal discharge, hypertrophy of the labia
    b. Toddler or school-aged child—early development of breasts or pubic hair
    c. Prepubertal or pubertal child—in girls, time of development of breasts, pubic hair; onset of menstruation. In boys, time of enlargement of testes, penis; development of pubic and facial hair; voice changes

G. **Health Maintenance**
1. Immunizations—rubella, rubeola, mumps, polio, diphtheria, pertussis, tetanus toxoid, bacille Calmette-Guérin (BCG), influenza, *Haemophilus influenzae* b (HIB), hepatitis B
   Indicate number and dates.
2. Screening procedures—hematocrit or hemoglobin, urinalysis tuberculin testing, visual and auditory acuity color vision; rubella antibodies, syphilis testing, gonorrhea screen, Papanicolaou smear
3. Dental care—source and frequency of care, dental hygienist visits, fillings or extractions

H. **Acute Infectious Diseases**
Rubella, rubeola, mumps, chickenpox, scarlet fever, rheumatic fever, hepatitis, infectious mononucleosis, sexually transmitted disease, tuberculosis. Recent exposure to communicable disease.

I. **Hospitalizations and Operations**
1. Dates, hospital, physician
2. Indications, diagnosis, procedures
3. Complications
4. Reactions to previous hospitalizations

J. **Injuries**
1. Emergency department visits—frequency and diagnosis
2. Fractures—location and treatment
3. Trauma, burns, bruises
4. Ingestions

K. **Medications**
1. For general use such as vitamins, antihistamines, laxatives
2. Special or fad diets
3. Recent antibiotics
4. Routine use of aspirin
5. Oral contraceptives—types and dose, duration
6. Drugs, narcotics, marijuana, hallucinogens, mood elevators, tranquilizers, alcohol
7. Determine when last dose of medication was taken; is medication with patient? How does the child take the medication?
8. Any medication allergy?

L. **Radiation**
1. Diagnosis requiring; number and occasion of exposures
2. Accidental exposure

3. Routine x-rays (chest, dental)
4. For injury, follow-up of fracture, etc.

B. **Method of Collecting Data**
1. Straightforward questions to a child (eg, "What grade are you in?" "Who are your friends?")
2. Three wishes offered to the child:
    a. "If Christmas were here, what would you ask for?"
    b. "If you had your way, who would you like to be?"
    c. "What would be the best thing that could happen to you?
3. "Who's your best friend?"
4. Questions to parents: "How does that seem to you?"
5. Adolescents—may want to interview without parents present, but parents must be included in some way.

School History

A. **Type of Information Needed**
1. Present and past schooling, grade, and performance
2. Favored and least favored subjects
3. School-related behavior—anxious to go, anxious to stay home
4. General attitude toward school and any career plans; attitude towards peer groups
5. Gang dress or behavior

B. **Method of Collecting Data**
Emphasize the positive (eg, "What's your best subject?" "Have you repeated a grade?" "Do you see your friends after school?")

Social History

A. **Type of Information Needed**
1. Environment—rural, urban
2. Housing—type, location, heating, sewage, water supply, family pets, other animal exposure
3. Parents' occupations (employment) and marital status
4. Number of individuals living in home, sleeping arrangements
5. Any religious affiliations
6. Utilization of social agencies previously
7. Health insurance and usual source of care

B. **Method of Collecting Data**
Parents are proud, so be careful with some of the questions. Ask permission.

1. "Can you tell me a little bit about your home?"
2. "I need to know more about how you live to help you with your child's problem."

Personal History

A. **Type of Information Needed**
1. Hygiene, exercise
2. Sleep habits
3. Elimination habits
4. Activities and hobbies, special talents
5. Friends, teacher relationships
6. Sibling and parent relationships
7. Expression of emotions
    a. Blows up easily
    b. Rather quiet

8. Idiosyncratic behavior and habits (eg, thumb sucking, nail biting, temper tantrums, head banging, pica, breath holding, rituals, tics, etc)

Review of Systems

A. *Type of Information Needed*
  1. General—activity, appetite, affect, sleep patterns, weight changes, edema, fever, behavior
  2. Allergy—eczema, hay fever, asthma, hives, food or drug allergy, sinus disorders
  3. Skin—rash or eruption, nodules, pigmentation or texture change, sweating or dryness, infection, hair growth, itching
  4. Head—headache, head trauma, dizziness
  5. Eyes—visual acuity, corrective lenses, strabismus, lacrimation, discharge, itching, redness, photophobia
  6. Ears—auditory acuity, earaches (frequency, ages, response to specific medications), infection, drainage
  7. Nose—colds and runny nose (frequency), infection, drainage
  8. Teeth—hygiene practices, general condition, cavities, maloclusions
  9. Throat—sore throat, tonsillitis, difficulty swallowing
  10. Speech—peculiarity of or change in voice; hoarseness, clarity, enunciation, stammering, development of articulation, vocabulary, use of sentences
  11. Respiratory—difficulty breathing, shortness of breath, chest pain, cough, wheezing, croup, pneumonia, tuberculosis or exposure, wheezing
  12. Cardiovascular—cyanosis, fainting, exercise intolerance, murmurs
  13. Hematologic—pallor, anemia, tendency to bruise or bleed
  14. Gastrointestinal—appetite (amount, frequency, cravings), nausea, vomiting, abdominal pain, abnormal size, bowel habits and nature of stools, parasites, encopresis (incontinence of feces), colic
  15. Genitourinary—age of toilet training, frequency of urination, straining, dysuria, hematuria (or unusual color or odor of infant's soiled diaper), previous urinary tract infection, enuresis (age of onset; day or nightime); urethral or vaginal discharge. Females: last menses, cramps, changes in interval and duration
  16. Musculoskeletal—deformities, fractures, sprains, joint pains or swelling, limitation of motion, abnormality of nails
  17. Neurologic—weakness or clumsiness, coordination, balance, gait, dominance, fatigability, tone, tremor. Seizures or paroxysmal behavior. Personality changes.

Physical Examination

General Principles

1. Establish the order of all data collection according to the needs of the patients. For example:
   a. An exhausted parent with a screaming baby will not give a careful, comprehensive history.
   b. Alternative care may not be available for preschoolers when the newborn comes in for the first checkup.
2. If the parent has come in with more than one child, try to organize some supervision of the other children so that you can have a little time with the parent alone.
3. Remember that the safest place for a young child is on the parent's knee. Privacy may not be possible because of the presence of other children.
4. Attempt to develop rapport with the young patient from the moment you first see or meet him or her.
5. Explain to the school-aged child or teenager what you are looking for as you proceed with the examination.

Approach to the Patient

1. Offer the young child a choice of being examined on parent's lap or your "special table."
2. To evaluate the chest properly, you need to listen through 10 heartbeats when the child is not screaming; therefore, the chest is a good place to begin the examination.
3. The part to be examined should be completely exposed, but if an apprehensive child objects to having clothes removed, slip your stethoscope under the shirt.
4. After listening to the heart, begin with parts of the body that are already exposed.
5. Start with either the head or the toes and work thoroughly and systematically toward the other end.
6. Gradually remove the child's clothes, look for asymmetry very carefully in the bodies of all children.
7. Develop a pattern appropriate to the patient's age.
   a. With infants it may be wise to leave the diaper area until last.
   b. Adolescents and school-aged children are often embarassed at the genital examination—and you may want to leave this until last.
8. Using a cold stethoscope may result in a frightened and screaming child, so warm the stethoscope before bringing it into contact with the child.
9. Some children are less frightened if able to hold the examining equipment first.
10. Show the child the procedure by demonstrating on the parent first.
11. Many young children, enjoy listening to their own hearts.
12. Toddlers and preschoolers enjoy blowing your otoscope light out.

Vital Signs

1. Obtain temperature, pulse rate, respiratory rate, and blood pressure as often as thought necessary, based on child's condition.

2. Measure core temperature, whenever possible, via rectal or ear route. Leave mercury thermometer in place 3–5 min. for rectal reading, longer for oral or axillary.
3. Obtain apical pulse rate on an infant or small child; radial, temporal, or carotid pulse may be measured with an older child. Pulse may be counted for 30 seconds and multiplied by two.
4. Count respirations on an infant for one full minute; observe the chest as well as the abdomen. Respirations may be counted for 30 seconds and multiplied by two in an older child.
5. Obtain blood pressure by auscultatory method, rather than palpation method, whenever possible. Make sure the cuff covers no less than ½ and no more than ⅔ the length of the upper arm or leg.

TECHNIQUE

Normal Vital Sign Ranges in Children

Temperature
Oral 36.4°–37.4°C. (97.6°–99.3°F.)
Rectal 36.2°–37.8°C. (97°–100°F.)
Axillary 35.9°–36.7°C. (96.6°–98°F.)

Pulse and Respiratory Rates

Age	Pulse	Respirations
Newborn	70–170	30–50
11 months	80–160	26–40
2 years	80–130	20–30
4 years	80–120	20–30
6 years	75–115	20–26
8 years	70–110	18–24
10 years	70–110	18–24
Adolescence	60–110	12–20

Blood Pressure
Varies with age, height, and weight of child

FINDINGS

Standing Height, Head Circumference, and Chest Circumference

1. Use tape measure to obtain accurate head circumference. Measure widest part of head.

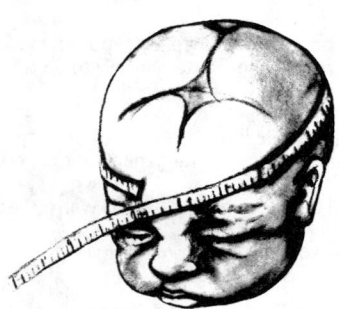

Head and Chest Circumference

Age Yr Mo	Head Circumference Inch	Cm.	Chest Circumference Inch	Cm.
Birth	13.8	35.0	13.0	33.0
3	15.9	40.4	15.8	40.2
6	17.1	43.4	17.1	43.4
9	17.8	45.3	18.0	45.7
1–0	18.3	46.6	18.6	47.3
1–6	18.9	47.9	19.4	49.2
2–0	19.3	48.9	19.8	50.4
3–0	19.6	49.8	20.6	52.5
3–6	—	—	20.8	52.8
4–0	19.8	50.4	21.0	53.4
5–0	20.0	50.8	21.5	54.6

(From Studies at Harvard School of Public Health.)

TECHNIQUE	FINDINGS

2. Record height and weight at each visit. Plot on growth chart.
3. Trends in growth are as important as the basic measurements.

General Appearance

1. Begin observations with the first contact with the patient, taking into account that there are at least two people to observe (child and parent).
2. The patient's interaction with the caretaker, whether it be the mother, father, a babysitter, an older sibling, or a friend of the family, is vital in the assessment of the child.

   As you observe for race, sex, general physical development, nutritional state, mental alertness, evidence of pain, restlessness, body position, clothes, apparent age, hygiene, and grooming, remember that many of these things are part of the parent's caretaking.

1. If the child is easily distracted or sleepy, it may be naptime.

2. Careful observation of the general state of the child will provide many clues about the child's relationship to the family and their response to the child.

Skin and Lymphatics

Examine as you move through each body region. (Include hair as well as skin.)

INSPECTION

Inspection of the skin is the same as for the adult (see p. 25).

1. Observe for skin color, pigmentation, lesions, jaundice, cyanosis, scars, superficial vascularity, moisture, edema, color of mucous membranes, hair distribution.
2. Describe any variation in color, particularly in children with increased pigmentation. Absence of pigment, or vitiligo, in darker children can be noted.
3. Birthmarks of any type are recorded. (May change as child grows older.)
4. Bruises or unusual marks of any kind, wounds or insect bites, scratch marks, scars, etc, may have particular significance.
5. Draw a picture of anything unusual like a scar, and measure the dimensions of the lesion when recording the findings.
6. To ascertain suspected jaundice, take the child to the window to get a true picture of the color of the skin. (A room with yellow walls and artificial lighting may create a wrong impression when jaundice is suspected.)

7. The skin of newborn infants will still be covered with vernix caseosa, the oily material that covers the fetus's body while in utero.
8. Postmature infants may have scaliness that persists for several weeks after birth, particularly around the feet. The color of the skin may change as the child gets a little older.
9. Note the presence of striae.
10. Dark skinned children may have Mongolian spots on base of spine or elsewhere.

1. In young babies, the skin is soft, smooth, and velvety in texture.

2. Pigmentations vary in children, depending on race, and will change as the child gets older.

3. A suntan, freckles, small, light-brown patches or café-au-lait spots may occur.

4. Bruises are particularly important because of the possibility of child abuse.

5. If you have difficulty in describing something, use ordinary words rather than inaccurate technical terms.

6. Carotenemia, which causes the nose and palms of the hands to have a yellowish tinge, may lead the parents to suspect jaundice; however, carotenemia is due to eating an excessive amount of yellow vegetables (carrots, sweet potatoes, squash, etc). In carotenemia, the sclerae are clear; this is not so in jaundice.

7. Swollen sebaceous glands over the nose and chin are frequently seen right after birth and are called *milia*.

8. The blotchy, pink patches over the eyelid, bridge of the nose, and the back of the neck may persist until the child is almost 2 years of age.

9. May indicate rapid weight gain.
10. Important to distinguish from child abuse.

TECHNIQUE	FINDINGS

PALPATION

1. Use the tips of the fingers to palpate—fingertips are more sensitive.
2. Feel the tension of the skin by pinching up a fold of skin—normal skin quickly falls back, but dehydrated skin remains in pinched position.

3. Feel the skin for texture, moisture, temperature, turgor, elasticity, masses, tenderness.

3. Skin that is rough and dry in texture may actually have a discrete rash that can be felt but not seen.

LYMPH

1. Observe and palpate for lymph node enlargement in lymph chain areas
   a. Neck
   b. Axilla
   c. Inguinal
   d. Epitrochlear
2. Note tenderness, size, and consistency

1. May be large or readily palpable, but should be nontender and spongy.

NAILS

1. Observe for color, shape, irregularities in surface, and general nail care; cleanliness, evidence of biting, etc.
2. Palpate the skin around the fingernails for firmness. Palpate any part that appears inflamed.

1. The nail beds should be pink, the nails convex.
2. General care of the child is frequently reflected in good care of the nails.

HAIR

1. Observe for color and distribution.
   a. Note according to the age of the child and race.
   b. Be aware that tufts of hair over the spine or sacral area may mark an underlying abnormality.
2. Note any change in pigmentation.

3. Palpate the hair for texture and thickness.

4. Examine to see if there are any patches where hair is missing on the head.

5. Separate thick hair on the head to get a good view of the scalp. Check for dandruff or scaliness in older children.
6. Check scalp for any signs of lice infestation.

7. Inspect in the axillae and over the pubis as well as the extremities for the presence and quantity of hair, to gauge the development and level of puberty.

1. *Newborn:* Normally varies from no hair to a thick bush. *Infant:* Consists of lanugo, a soft, downy covering frequently seen over the shoulders, back, arms, face, and sacral area, especially in dark-skinned children
2. Remember, children frequently experiment with mother's hair dye or rinse.
3. Texture may be thick or thin, coarse or fine, straight or curly.
4. May denote underlying skin infection; however, some children pull their hair out; sometimes the hair is braided so tightly that it falls out.
5. Look carefully for broken hairs, for scaliness on the scalp or cradle cap in infants.
6. Nits (louse eggs) appear on the hair as little white dots. Lice may be seen on the scalp; they move quickly and may jump.
7. The child need not be totally undressed; a prepubertal child will usually be embarrassed if all clothes are removed.

TECHNIQUE	FINDINGS

Head and Neck

1. Unless specifically requested to do otherwise, examine the eyes and ears at the very last, especially in the younger child.
2. Also, examine the throat toward the last, unless the child exhibits concern about the "throat stick." It is then best to examine the throat right away to "get it over with." If a child cries you may be able to avoid using a tongue blade.
3. To avoid frightening the child when palpating the head, make a game out of it—ask, "Where's your nose?" "Where are your eyes?"

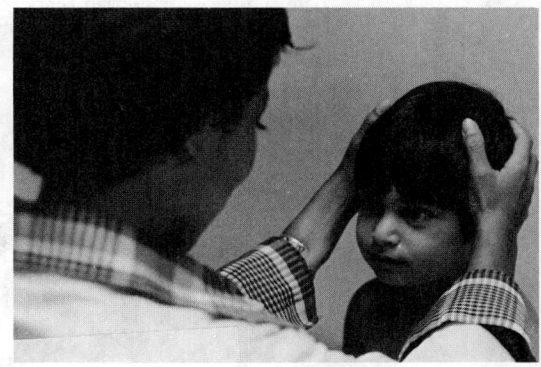

INSPECTION

1. Observe the face and skull for asymmetry, deformity, and abnormal or limited movements.

2. Closely observe facial expressions, blinking, etc, if the child is not crying. This may be one of your few moments to see the child when he or she is not crying.
   If you are examining a crying baby, watch particularly for asymmetry of the face.
3. Observe the movement of the head on the neck as the baby looks around. When turning an infant over, observe the head for control, position, and movement.
4. Because an infant's neck is often short and there are often several folds of skin under the chin, it is necessary to lift the chin a little to observe the skin completely—to see that it is clear and free of perspiration rash or irritation.

PALPATION

1. Palpate the skull for the suture lines. Feel the face for any masses, noting size, consistency, surface, temperature, and tenderness.

2. Palpate the anterior and posterior fontanelles.

1. A baby's head may be asymmetrical because of pressure during pregnancy and delivery. The rounded head of the baby born by breech delivery contrasts with the long, pointed head of a baby who is a firstborn and whose head was moulded during a prolonged labor.
2. In a baby born by forceps delivery, there may be signs of weakness of the facial nerve caused by pressure of the forceps over the front of the ear where the facial nerve emerges. When the baby cries, the involved side will show weakness and downturning of the mouth.
3. There should be very little head lag beyond the age of 3 months.

4. In the back, the neck should be free of webbing or extra folds of skin extending from just beneath the ear toward the shoulder.

1. The suture lines of the skull may be felt to override as a result of the pressure applied when contractions occurred during labor. This is usually most marked between the frontal and the parietal bone where the coronal suture is located.
2. The fontanelles are soft and flat. Tense or bulging fontanelles may indicate hydrocephalus. Depressed fontanelles are often a sign of dehydration. The fontanelles usually close by 18 months.

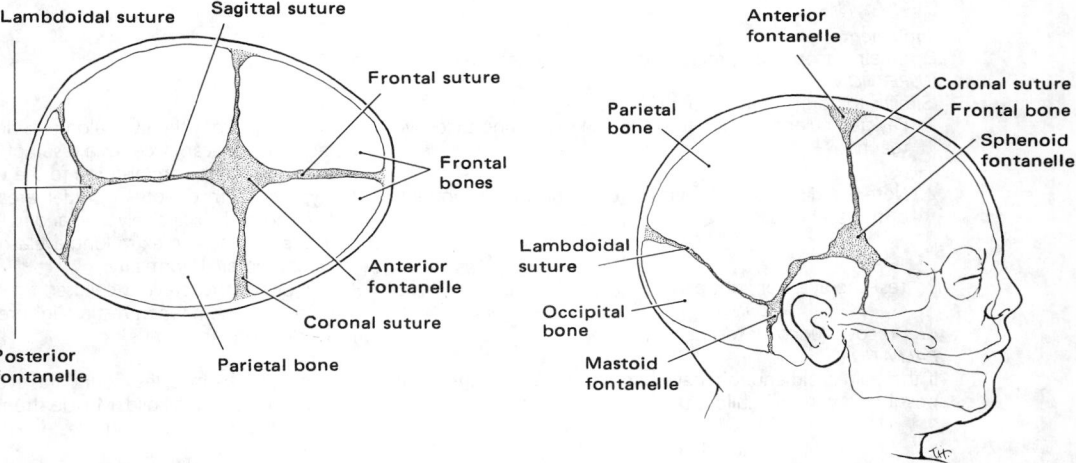

TECHNIQUE	FINDINGS

3. Palpate along the lambdoidal suture at the back of the head between the parietal bones and the occipital bone.
4. Palpate the neck for swollen lymph nodes, noting tenderness, mobility, location, and consistency.

4. Palpation of the lymph nodes may reveal slightly enlarged nodes in the anterior cervical chain secondary to sore throat.

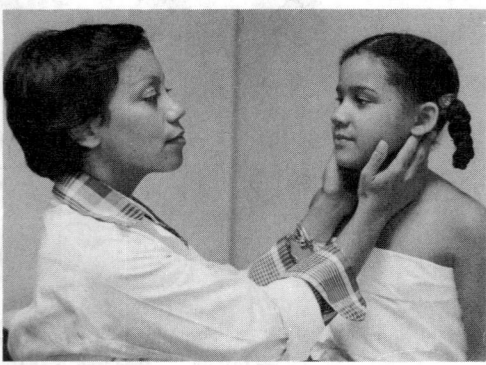

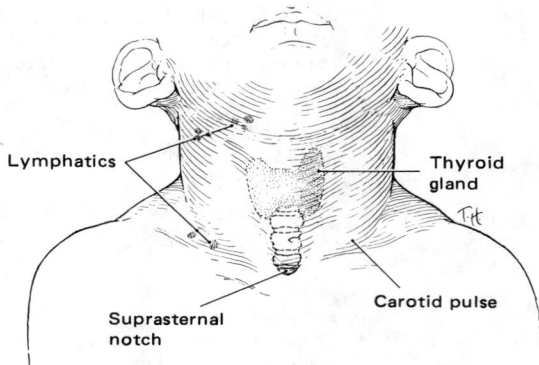

5. Note that there are other nodes, which are normally not palpable.

5. These include the pre- and postauricular, the posterior cervical (behind the sternomastoid), the submental and submandibular (under the jaw), and the occipital nodes (along the prominence of the occiput).

6. Feel the pulses in the neck for location, strength, and equality.
7. Check the thyroid for enlargement, position, texture, and tenderness.
8. Locate the trachea in the suprasternal notch for position in the center of the neck.
9. Palpate sternocleidomastoids making sure they are equal in size.

PERCUSSION

1. Percussion of the face may elicit tenderness over the sinuses.
2. Percuss over the head and neck directly with the fingertips, usually the middle finger of the right hand.

3. Percuss over the forehead for tenderness in the sinuses and across the zygoma, or cheekbone.

AUSCULTATION

Auscultate the skull and carotid arteries in the neck.

1. Tenderness may be due to a tooth cavity or sinus infection.
2. Gentle tapping over the skull elicits a typical noise when the sutures are open and a different sound when the sutures are closed.
3. This is to determine underlying tenderness in the frontal or maxillary sinus.

To determine presence of bruits.

Eyes and Vision

Equipment

Ophthalmoscope and penlight. Be sure batteries are new and lights are bright.

INSPECTION

(Similar to adult examination; p. 27)

1. Pay particular attention to the lacrimal duct and excessive tearing.

2. Note the distance between the eyes and the distribution of the eyebrows.

3. Test the eyes for light perception.

4. Do cover/uncover test.

PALPATION

If the child is old enough, have him squeeze eyes tightly (not possible in younger children).

1. Discharge from the eyes along the lower lid or from the lacrimal duct can occur as a result of infection or reaction to silver nitrate administered to the neonate.
2. Hypertelorism denotes a wider area between the eyes than normal. Excessively long and full eyebrows that meet in the midline and extra-long eyelashes may signify a developmental abnormality.
3. It is difficult to prevent children from blinking their eyes or closing them when testing light response.
4. To discover strabismus.

Weakness of the muscles around the eyes is difficult to demonstrate in the young child. Muscle strength or weakness can be evaluated when the child cries.

TECHNIQUE	FINDINGS

FUNDOSCOPIC EXAMINATION

1. Check to see that the child's eyes move in conjugate fashion.
   Ask the mother if she has noticed any signs of squinting, especially when the child is tired.
2. This is a difficult examination to conduct because children tend to watch the light and stare directly at you, which constricts their pupils. If the child cannot cooperate, it may be necessary to dilate the pupil to see the fundus.
   It is often not necessary to do a fundoscopic examination on children.
3. Start your examination at about ⅓ meter (1 foot) from the patient. Look for the red reflex, which should be readily observable.
4. Look for any opacities and then slowly approach the patient, turning the ophthalmoscopic dial to the smaller plus (+) numbers. Start originally at +8 to + 10.

5. To help guide your gaze, put your hand on top of the child's head, with your thumb at the corner of the eye at the outer edge. If you lose the fundus, you can return to your thumb and get your bearings by directing your gaze medial to the tip of your thumbnail.

1. Loss of vision can occur if the eyes are not working together properly. Squinting can indicate vision problems.

2. A picture can be pinned to the wall opposite the child, who is then instructed to look at the picture during the examination. If the child is examined while lying down, a picture can be placed on the ceiling.

4. The red reflex is diminished if there is something obstructing your view. A cataract or an opacity in the retina can cause this, as would a tumor filling the posterior chamber. If there is any paleness in the red reflex or difficulty in identifying it, a consultation should be sought immediately.

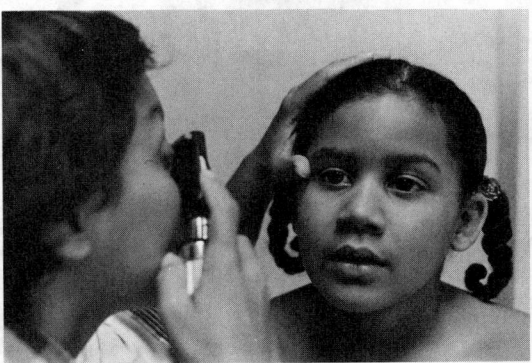

Ears and Hearing

Equipment
Tympanogram otoscope
Small speculum for child's ear

INSPECTION

1. When examining the external ear, the auricle, or the pinna, be sure to note the position of the ear.
   The top of the ear should cross an imaginary line drawn between the edge of the eye and the back of the occiput. If the ear is positioned more obliquely or is low-set, some underlying abnormality, particularly of the genitourinary system, may be present.

2. If you cannot get the child to cooperate by offering an explanation or by playing a game, the child will have to be restrained. Many children will enjoy watching the light on their leg or seeing the red glow of their finger with the light shining through or blowing the light out. If restraint is needed:

Fresh batteries to ensure a bright light

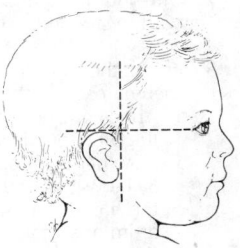

2. If the child is in a supine position, be sure to remove the shoes, because some children will kick when frightened.

TECHNIQUE	*FINDINGS*

a. The child can be seated on the parent's knee with the child's legs wedged between the parent's knees and the head held firmly with one hand while the baby's hands are controlled with the other hand.
b. An older child may be held in a supine position, with the parent holding the child's arms above the head and controlling the head.
c. If the child is very restless and apprehensive, examine the child from the top while the parent leans over the child's body, holds the arms down with her elbows, and at the same time grasps the child's head with her hands.

INSPECTION WITH OTOSCOPE

1. Hold the otoscope gently with the handle between the thumb and forefinger. This will enable you to control the head of the otoscope while keeping your hand steady on the child's head.

1. Small children will jerk about, so be careful not to push the speculum into the eardrum.

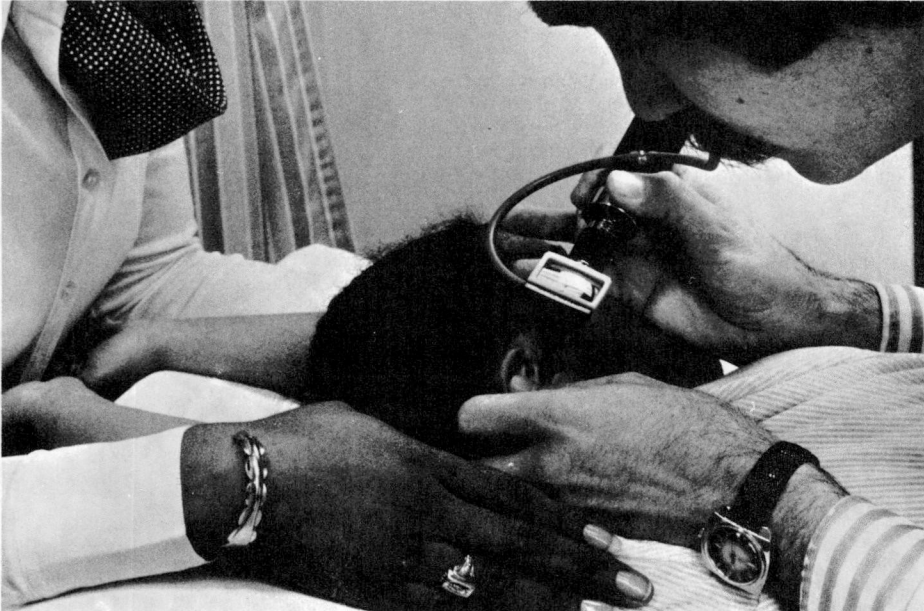

2. With your free hand, pull the pinna back and slightly upward to straighten the canal. Examine the canal.

3. Inspect the eardrum and test for mobility by means of the pneumatoscope (the tube attachment of the otoscope).
   a. Attach one end of the tube to the otoscope and place the other end in your mouth.
   b. Blow gently through the tube.
   By blowing through plastic tubing it is possible to see the normal eardrum move back and forth. If the eardrum does not move, this may be indicative of infection behind the drum (otitis media).
   c. This method is preferred to the squeeze bulb because it allows for greater control of the force with which the air is introduced into the ear.
   d. The best method of evaluation is the tympanogram.

PALPATION
Palpate behind the ear over the mastoid process.

2. Cerumen or wax may interfere with your view of the eardrum. You may need to remove the wax with a cureta syringe or hydrogen peroxide instillation.
3. The normal eardrum moves slightly when a soft breath is blown into the ear canal.

Tenderness behind the ear denotes infection.
Sometimes a lymph node can be felt in this area.

TECHNIQUE

FINDINGS

MECHANICAL

1. Most children will be able to respond to a test of gross hearing.

2. More specific tests using an electric screening device are used prior to school age.

1. A small bell, such as the kind found in the Denver kit, can be used to determine hearing ability by noting if the child stops moving when the bell is rung and turns head toward the sound.

Nose and Sinuses

Equipment
Nasoscope, small speculum

INSPECTION

1. Observe for general deformity.
2. With nasoscope, examine nasal septum, mucous membranes and turbinates, and for discharge and nasal obstruction (see Adult Physical Examination, p. 29).
3. Check for presence of any foreign body. Always remember that any child who has a "strange" odor may have a foreign body in the nose or ear. (In a female child, do not forget the vagina.)
4. Observe for nasal flaring.

PALPATION
Palpate the sinuses, remembering the order of development.

2. Dry mucous membranes may bleed and cause clots of blood to form in the nares. Scratches may also occur if child picks at nose or scratches when itching occurs.
3. A foreign body in the nose will cause a foul odor, purulent discharge, and may possibly cause bleeding.

Sinuses develop in a set order; the ethmoid and maxillary sinuses are present at birth. It used to be believed that the frontal sinus develops at around 7 years of age, and the sphenoid after puberty. These times of development are probably earlier than originally believed.

Mouth and Throat

Equipment

Penlight, tongue depressor

1. Shining the light into the mouth or around the lips and teeth is not a threatening gesture.
2. However, the tongue blade, which is used to press against the inside of the cheek to allow for examination of the mucous membranes and which is also used to push the tongue out of the way, is a threatening instrument.
3. When the tongue depressor is placed on the tongue, it can have the unpleasant effect of making the child gag.
4. To avoid this unpleasant occurrence, encourage the child to stick out his tongue, breath deeply, and say "ah." This may allow for easy visualization of the palate and uvula, without need for the "stick."

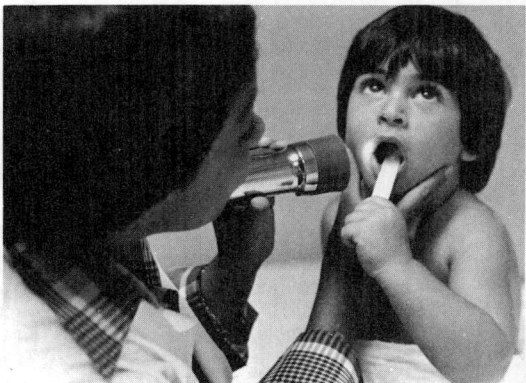

A child may also be allowed to place the tongue blade directly on own tongue while you guide with your hand.

5. If these steps are not feasible, then the child may need to be restrained. If such is the case, examining the throat should be left to last, so as not to frighten the child.

INSPECTION

1. Observe the lips, noting the color. (Remember that cyanosis is difficult to detect in a black child.)

2. Count the teeth (see p. 1086) and note any extra or missing teeth, and any evidence of caries, staining, tartar, and malocclusion.
3. Check the gums for swelling and signs of easy bleeding. Also note mouth odor.

1. *Infants:* There may be a protuberance on the upper lip, the so-called "sucking blister."
Children: May have dry lips and redness around the lips due to an allergy.

TECHNIQUE	*FINDINGS*
4. Check the tongue for movement, color, and the presence of taste buds on the surface. Check to see that the frenulum under the tongue is of the proper length.	4. If the frenulum is too short, the child may be tongue-tied (meaning that the baby cannot advance the tip of the tongue beyond the lips), although this is not thought to interfere with sucking or speech.
5. As the gag reflex is elicited, note how the palate moves upward and the uvula springs into view.	5. It should be midline and single, although occasionally it will be divided or bifid.
6. Examine the roof of the mouth.	6. The roof of the mouth at the junction of the hard and soft palate will frequently reveal whitish lesions, or Epstein's pearls, which persist through infancy.
7. Inspect the height of the arch of the palate.	7. With experience, an unusually high arch is easily recognizable.
8. Note the tonsils on each side of the uvula and immediately posterior to it for position, surface, size, equality, and color.	8. Any coating with pus or ulcers or a pocket or cryptic appearance should be recorded.
9. As the baby cries, note the odor of the breath and any hoarseness of the voice; note difficulty on inspiration, as in croup, or wheezing on expiration.	9. These signs may indicate throat and chest disturbances.
PALPATION	
1. Palpate the lips and cheeks manually using a finger cot or glove.	1. By comparing one side with the other, differences due to abnormality can be detected.
2. Note any evidence of swelling.	
3. Palpate for submucous cleft.	3. Submucous cleft may indicate a genetic disposition toward cleft palate.

Time of eruption of deciduous teeth

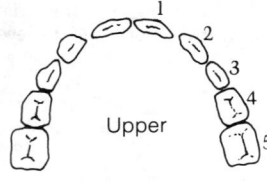

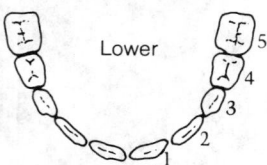

	(Upper)	(Lower)
1 Central incisor	8–12 mos.	5–9 mos.
2 Lateral incisor	8–12 mos.	12–18 mos.
3 Cuspid		18–24 mos.
4 First molar		12–18 mos.
5 Second molar		24–30 mos.

Time of eruption of permanent teeth

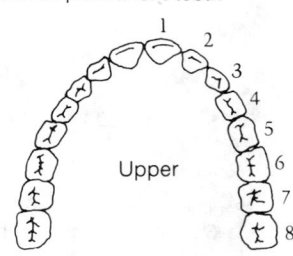

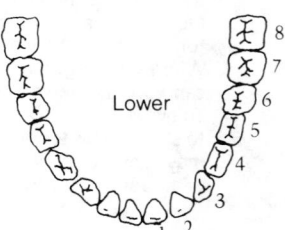

	(Upper)	(Lower)
1 Central incisor	6–7 yr.	7–8 yr.
2 Lateral incisor	7–8 yr.	8–9 yr.
3 Cuspid	9–10 yr.	11–12 yr.
4 First bicuspid	10–11 yr.	10–11 yr.
5 Second bicuspid	11–12 yr.	10–12 yr.
6 First molar	6–7 yr.	6–7 yr.
7 Second molar	11–13 yr.	12–13 yr.
8 Third molar	17 yr.	17–18 yr.

TECHNIQUE   FINDINGS

Breast and Thorax

1. Sometimes young children object to having their clothes removed.
2. The following approaches may overcome this problem:
   a. Distract the child by having him or her listen to a few heartbeats.
   b. Have the parent (while the child is on his or her knee) remove the underclothing while you stand by.
   c. For an older child entering puberty, provide an examining sheet, or gown.

BREAST

TECHNIQUE	FINDINGS
1. Check to see if there are any small extra nipples present.	1. These would appear along a line extending from the anterior axillary line through the normal nipple down toward the symphysis pubis.
2. In the newborn infant, the nipples appear a little darker than normal, and breast tissue underneath may form a small knot with occasional leakage of milk.	2. This leakage is a secondary effect of the hormone level in the mother; instruct the mother not to try to express the milk, because of the danger of infection.
3. In the child, a lump found under the nipple in either male or female may cause some concern for cancer.	3. Such lumps are usually secondary to hormone stimulation and occur toward puberty or during the newborn period.
4. Occasionally, the breasts begin to develop earlier than normal, at around 5 or 6 years.	4. This should be a reason for referral to a physician.

THORAX

INSPECTION

TECHNIQUE	FINDINGS
1. Observe the entire thorax as the child breathes; note symmetry and equal expansion of both sides as the lungs inflate.	1. In babies and young children (especially an infant lying on the parent's knee), diaphragm excursion is more marked than intercostal expansion. Thus the abdomen goes up and down more than the chest expands.
2. Confirm the respiratory rate as you observe the child with his shirt off.	
3. Observe for substernal, suprasternal, and intercostal retractions.	

PERCUSSION

Percussion of the child's chest is difficult. Because the underlying structures are crowded, not too much is elicited. The heart edge is difficult to outline.

Very light percussion is necessary; a hyperresonant note may be elicited over air, particularly of a stomach bubble that projects up into the left side of the chest.

PALPATION

TECHNIQUE	FINDINGS
1. Use warmed hands as you palpate the shape and angle of the sternum. Note if there is any depression of the sternum.	1. The shape of the sternum may vary although there may be a depression of the sternum (funnel sternum) that may cause subsequent trouble because of pressure on underlying structures. This should be referred to the pediatrician.
2. Palpate the costochondral junctions for tenderness and enlargement.	2. May suggest an underlying inflammatory response.
3. As you palpate, hoarse sounds (as in bronchitis) may be felt through your hands.	3. Normal inspiration and expiration do not give a sensation under the fingers, except for the expansion of the chest.
4. Vocal fremitus is difficult to elicit in the smaller child since it is difficult to have him make repetitive sounds on command.	4. In the older child, it is worth trying to obtain transmission of sound through the lung tissue

AUSCULTATION

TECHNIQUE	FINDINGS
1. Try to examine a baby before he or she begins crying.	1. Note, however, that crying increases lung expansion.
2. Warm the stethoscope before using by rubbing it between your hands.	2. A cold stethoscope will startle the child.
3. Be aware that breathing is louder in younger children with slightly increased length of inspiration, almost to the point of bronchovesicular breathing in the adult.	3. Bronchial breathing with equal inspiration and expiration is very loud and easy to hear if the patient has pneumonia.
4. Crackles (discontinuous; interrupted, explosive sounds) may be heard more easily in children.	4. Added coarse-quality sounds in the chest are commonly associated with mucus in the trachea or even in the back of the nose.
5. Wheezes	5. Recurrent airway disease is an important finding in children.

TECHNIQUE	*FINDINGS*

Heart

INSPECTION

In thin children, the apical beat or the point of maximal impulse (PMI) can easily be seen, particularly if you look obliquely across the chest wall.

As in all areas of the pediatric examination, measurement and documentation of the distance from the midline and the exact rib space are worth noting.

PALPATION

The apical beat may be felt in the 6th intercostal space about 5 cm (2 inches) from the midline in the school-aged child. It is more difficult to feel in the baby, particularly a plump child, and would not be so far out toward the anterior axillary line.

The apical beat will be deviated to the left with cardiac enlargement or a collapsed lung on that side.
The apical pulse could be pushed toward the right by a tumor or a collapsed lung on the right. Pneumothorax under tension will push the heart away from the side of the increased pressure.

AUSCULTATION

1. Identify the first heart sound (S_1) (occurs during systole).
   a. Locate the apical beat (closing of the mitral valve) by placing the stethoscope over the maximum impulse area, concentrating on the first heart sound. (As the ventricle on the left contracts, pushing the blood up into the aorta, the sound of the mitral valve closing is heard.)
   b. That sound can be identified by placing the thumb on the carotid pulse of the neck, which will coincide very closely with the heart sounds.

1. Consists of the "lub" portion of the "lub-dub" heart sound.

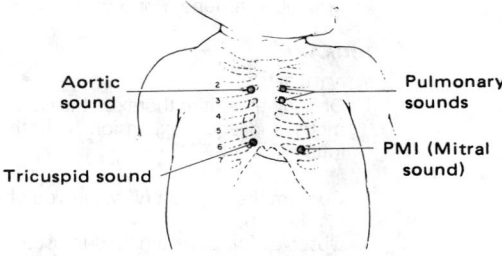

2. Identify the second heart sound (S_2).
   a. Move the stethoscope up toward the sternum and to the left.
   b. At the base of the heart, both over the aortic and pulmonic areas, S_2 is louder than S_1.

2. Represents the "dub" portion of the "lub-dub" heart sound.

   b. In a child, S_2 can be heard as two heart sounds because the two valves in the aorta and pulmonary vessels do not close at quite the same time. This split will increase with inspiration and decrease with expiration.

3. Move the stethoscope in small jumps from the apical area medially toward the sternum. Go up to the left side of the sternum, listening at each interspace next to the sternum.

3. This represents the area of maximum intensity of sound of the pulmonary vessels.

4. Move next to the patient's right second intercostal space—again next to the sternum.

4. It is at this area that you will hear the aortic sound best.

5. Listen to only one sound; concentrate on that to the exclusion of all others. Can you identify this sound? Is it clear? Compare it with your own heart sound or that of the parent.

5. The child will enjoy this comparison if he is allowed to listen.

6. If there is any question of a heart murmur or added sounds, refer to the physician.
7. As you listen to the heart sounds, you are also listening to the rhythm to confirm your findings on pulse.
   a. If child breathes in and out deeply, the sinus arrhythmia will be obvious.
   b. If a child holds his breath, the sinus arrhythmia will disappear.

7. The typical rhythm of a child is called *sinus arrhythmia.* As the heart speeds up, the child is breathing in; the heart slows down on expiration.

8. Be sure to count a rapid heart that is heard even when the child is quiet.
9. In the infant, heart sounds are just a series of taps; they occur so fast that it is impossible to make out which sound is S_1.

8. This may be indicative of a tachycardia that requires further investigation.
9. In the infant, the S_1 and S_2 are equal in intensity.

TECHNIQUE	*FINDINGS*

Abdomen

1. For examination of the abdomen, the child should be lying down, relaxed, and not crying. Placing a small child, particularly around the age of 1–3 years, on a high table on cold paper can be very frightening; as a result, the abdomen will not be relaxed.
2. Babies up to about 1 year do not seem to be perturbed and will often lie down and play very nicely as long as they can see the parent, who should be stationed at the head of the child while you examine the abdomen.
3. Having the child lie across the parent's knees with the legs dangling on one side and the head cradled in his or her arms, will enable you to feel the abdomen quite well.
   a. You may find that with the baby's head in the parent's left arm, you can use your left hand to examine the baby's abdomen on the right, feeling up under the right costal margin and into the right hypochondrium.
   b. You may need to turn the baby around and use your right hand to examine the left side of the child's abdomen.

INSPECTION

1. Observe the abdomen for contour and any markings both while the child is standing and when lying down. As you inspect, you may see some abdominal movement with respiration. (Remember that the diaphragm, as it goes up and down, will move the contents of the abdomen.)	1. Sometimes superficial veins are seen on the abdomen, particularly in a very blond infant. Striae are often noticed on the flank following rapid loss or gain of weight.
2. Check for early signs of puberty as evidenced by pubic hair over the symphysis pubis.	2. Early pubic hair in younger children (8–10 years) may appear long and silky. This will ultimately become curly toward the onset of puberty.
3. Carefully inspect the umbilicus for cleanliness and the presence of any scar tissue.	3. A deep umbilicus may be difficult to keep clean. Immediately after the cord has dropped off, a granuloma may occur.

AUSCULTATION

1. Because percussion and palpation will stimulate the small bowel and increase bowel sounds, auscultation should precede these two techniques.	1. Bowel sounds are heard as tinkling, irregular sounds that indicate that fluid is moving from one section of the bowel to the next.
2. To obtain the child's cooperation, you can conduct a running commentary as you listen, saying such things as, ''I can hear the Cheerios in there.''	2. In a quiet baby who has just eaten, not many bowel sounds will be heard. In a hungry child, noisy bowel sounds can be heard, even without a stethoscope.

PERCUSSION

1. On the right side, percuss for the liver. Confirm on palpation.	1. Liver dullness can frequently be outlined.
2. Percuss over the left upper quadrant.	2. Percussion over a gas-filled bowel or stomach gives a high-pitched, hollow sound.
3. Percuss the lower abdomen, particularly above the symphysis pubis.	3. Above the symphysis pubis, a filled bladder can produce a confusing sound, as does a pregnant uterus. (A mass in the abdomen of a girl over 10 years of age may be a fetus.)

PALPATION

1. Divide the abdomen into imaginary quadrants, palpating each with the fingertips.
2. In the right upper quadrant, palpate for the liver edge.
   a. Although the liver is easily palpable in most children, you may have to press quite firmly.
   b. The liver is frequently felt about 1 cm ($\frac{3}{8}$ inch) below the right costal margin and in some instances as low as 2 cm ($\frac{3}{4}$ inch). This is a common finding in the newborn and through the early school-age years.

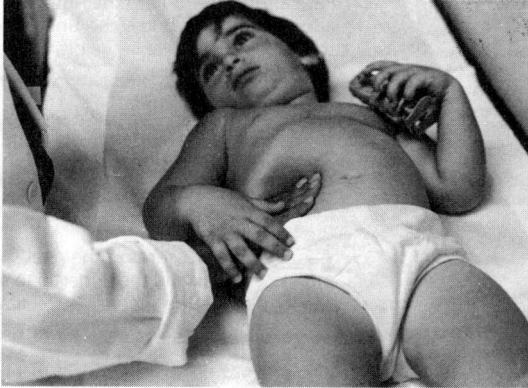

3. In the left upper quadrant, palpate for the spleen. Less resistance is encountered as you feel up under the left costal margin.	3. Only the tip of the spleen can be felt in the upper outer left quadrant, in the early months of life and in very thin children of preschool age.

TECHNIQUE	*FINDINGS*
4. In the upper quadrants also try to palpate for the kidneys. Deep palpation for both kidneys should routinely be a part of the examination to make sure there is no enlargement of the kidney. Normally, the kidney is not palpable.	4. Kidney palpation is difficult, but during the newborn period, the lower pole of the right kidney can frequently be felt and sometimes the left as well. (This applies to the period immediately following delivery, when the infant's abdomen is relaxed and the bowel is not distended.)
5. In the iliac fossa or the left lower quadrant, palpate for the descending bowel.	5. The descending colon can be felt, particularly if filled with firm stool. It may be slightly tender, but it should not cause severe pain on gentle palpation.
6. Palpate on the right lower quadrant (RLQ) where the appendix is located.	6. In the RLQ, usually the only sensation is that of gas-filled bowel. Tenderness in this area could be related to an inflamed appendix.
7. If the child has pain in any area or has pointed to the umbilicus when asked to show where the pain is, avoid the area demonstrated and leave it until last. Note whether the pain is with pressure or rebound.	7. If the painful area is palpated first, the child may tense up when the other areas of the abdomen are examined.
8. Palpate around the umbilicus for any masses that may indicate a hernia, especially in black children. As you press over the protruding hernia you can feel the sensation of gurgling under your fingers as the bowel returns to the abdomen.	8. Most of these hernias heal naturally by the age of 6 years. A hernia above the umbilicus can be revealed by asking the child to lift his head from the table. (Widening of the muscles above the umbilicus is called *diastasis recti*.)

Rectum and Anus

1. Rectal examinations are rarely necessary in infants and young children.
2. If the child will be examined by a health care provider, it is not necessary to duplicate this part of the examination.
3. Rectal examinations are embarrassing and uncomfortable for most children. Explain the procedure before performing the examination.
4. Positioning for a rectal examination:
   a. Infants can be placed on their abdomens, sides, or backs with the legs raised to the chest.
   b. Young children and teenagers can be positioned on their sides.

INSPECTION	
1. When examining a baby or toddler, place the child on a flat surface so that the weight is evenly distributed on the front of the pelvis. As the baby moves about on the abdomen, observe the entire back, the lower back, the upper thigh, and the tightening of the buttocks.	1. If one buttock is larger than the other, you will see that side projected above the other. Weakness of one side will be obvious as the baby moves around, although a child in the early stages of crawling will normally tend to use one knee as a predominant leader, dragging the other behind.
2. Notice particularly the lower part of the back for hairiness.	2. This may indicate an underlying abnormality of the vertebrae.
3. As the child moves away, part the buttocks and look at the cleft between them.	3. A pilonidal dimple or sinus may be seen over the lower back. This is a common finding, but parents should be told about it for cleaning purposes. Be sure there is no drainage.
4. Pay careful attention to the outer appearance of the anus and the perineal body, the underside of the scrotum in the male, and the labia majora in the female.	4. The anus is inspected for blood, fissures, or splitting in the external tissue, redness, swelling, or pads of extra flesh. On occasion, small white pinworms may be seen adhering to the anal skin.

PALPATION	
1. Consider the child's age and feelings; ask the mother to assist if need be. This part of the examination is not always necessary.	
2. Start by parting the buttocks with the left hand and introducing a well-lubricated finger (with finger cot) into the anus.	2. When an infant is being examined, the small finger should be used.
3. Gently apply pressure on the anal sphincter to allow the muscles to relax and the fingertip to slide into the rectum.	3. Apply pressure with pulp of the finger rather than jab at the anus with the fingertip.
4. Gently palpate the inner ring, feeling for areas of thickening and tenderness and simultaneously judging the sphincter tone.	4. As the perianal area is pressed on from the inside, tenderness will be elicited if a deep fissure exists or if an infection has occurred around a fissure.
5. If the rectum is full of feces, it will be impossible to feel any other mass.	5. In the young child, particularly the infant, dilatation provided by the finger may result in a bowel movement. In the older child, a suppository or even an enema may be required.
6. Palpate the walls of the rectum.	6. Within the rectum, the mucosal walls should be smooth, and deep palpation should elicit mild tenderness and no acute pain.

TECHNIQUE	*FINDINGS*

7. In the male, gently turn your finger through 180° and feel the posterior surface of the prostate. Note size, consistency, tenderness, and contour.
8. In the female, perform a bimanual examination and palpate the cervix.

Male Genitalia

1. This part of the examination requires a direct, matter-of-fact approach. Acknowledge that it is normal to feel embarrassed during an examination of the genitals. Explain what you are looking for as you proceed through the examination with a teenager.
2. Reassure the child after the examination that his genitals are normal. This decreases anxiety.
3. When examining the testes in a young child, you may need to block the canals to prevent them from retracting into the abdomen.

SCROTUM AND TESTES

INSPECTION

TECHNIQUE	FINDINGS
1. Before touching the child, determine by observation of the testes whether they are in the scrotum.	1. Retraction of the testes into the abdomen occurs very frequently in young children; the development of the scrotum depends on the presence of the testes.
2. Observe the skin over the scrotum for color and surface appearance, noting the presence of wrinkles, or rugae.	2. The skin over the scrotum varies in color, being a darker brown to black in the more pigmented races and reddish in the fair-skinned. The wrinkles, or rugae, are more developed as the child grows older.

PALPATION

TECHNIQUE	FINDINGS
1. Check the scrotum wall for swelling or sensitivity. Gently feel the testes, palpating across the upper pole and feeling for the epididymis. (Remember the scrotum is extremely sensitive to pressure.)	1. The epididymis is a ridge of soft, bumpy tissue extending from the superior pole and running down and behind the testis.
2. Estimate the size of the testes and identify the spermatic cord, tracing it from the testis up toward the groin.	2. The spermatic cord, with the vas deferens, feels firm and is accompanied by softer nerves, arteries, veins, and a few muscle fibers.

3. Make a special effort to locate the testis in a young child whose testes may be retracted into the abdomen via a hyperactive cremasteric reflex. You may have to have the child in a sitting or standing position. Occasionally you may have to ask a parent to check at home with the child sitting in a warm bathtub.
  a. If the testes cannot be felt in the scrotum, gently run the skin of the upper scrotum between your fingers, moving superiorly and approaching the external inguinal ring.
  b. Try to milk the testis down toward the scrotum from above with your hand.
  c. If this fails, have the child sit cross-legged to abolish the reflex of the cremaster muscle.
	3. The presence of the testes in the scrotum is vital in the preschool or early school-age child. Nondescent of the testes requires that the child be referred to a health care provider.
	
	During this period the testis is about 1.5–2 cm ($\frac{1}{2}$–$\frac{3}{4}$ inch) in length.
	In the quiescent period prior to puberty, the male genitalia remain fairly infantile.

4. When examining a boy in the early stages of puberty, it is important to note the size of the testis as well as the greater number of rugae on the scrotum and the appearance of pubic hair around the penis.	4. In early puberty, the testes start to grow. Onset of puberty varies, occurring in some boys by age 10 and in others as late as age 14. In most teenagers, the findings are similar to those in adults.

PENIS

TECHNIQUE	FINDINGS
1. Evaluate the penis on all sides by lifting up the shaft.	1. The shaft of the penis contains the urethra on the under, or ventral surface and is easily palpable.
2. If the child is not circumcised, partially retract the foreskin to observe the glans and meatus.	2. The foreskin may adhere to the glans for the first few years of life. It is not necessary for the parent to "stretch" the foreskin by retraction. Whitish discharge around the glans under the foreskin is normal and not a sign of infection. The foreskin should completely encircle the glans.
3. Observe the position of the meatus and evert the lips of the meatus to reveal an adequate orifice.	3. The meatus may be positioned off center. Refer the child to a health care provider if the meatus is located on the dorsal or ventral surface of the shaft.

TECHNIQUE	*FINDINGS*

4. In the older child, inspect the penis for ulcers, sores, or discharge from the meatus.

INGUINAL AREA

1. Palpate for hernia over the external inguinal ring. Have the child cough to enhance your observation.

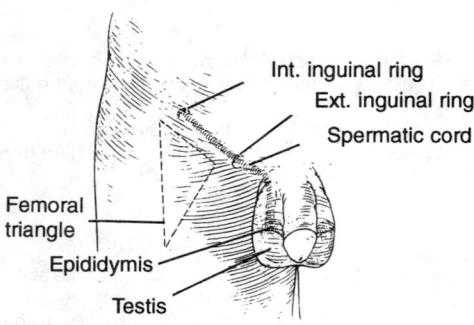

2. An increased cough reflex or swelling in the area should be checked by carefully placing the finger on the scrotal skin and invaginating the skin over your fingers toward the external ring. You are trying to follow the course of a hernia that would descend into the scrotum while you feel the external ring from below. A hernia in the inguinal region presents as a bulge that can be either seen or felt from below by placing the finger in the scrotum pointing up toward the external inguinal ring.
3. Also palpate for the inguinal lymph nodes.

FEMORAL AREA

Palpate the femoral triangle carefully for a hernia and for lymph nodes.

AUSCULTATION

If you are trying to reduce a mass, listen over the scrotum to see if there is a gurgling sound.

TRANSILLUMINATION

1. To locate the testis, darken the room and shine a bright light from behind the scrotum. In a normal child, the testis will stand out as the darker area.
2. Transilluminate any suspicious mass to help locate a hernia.

---

4. Consider sexually transmitted diseases in the older child and teenager.

1. Having the child stand either with the parent holding him or placing him against his or her knee will help you in locating a hernia in the inguinal area.

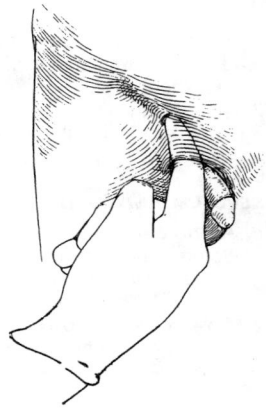

3. The inguinal lymph nodes in an infant are palpable as small and "shotty." Anything more than this should alert you to possible infection, since the perianal area drains into the superficial inguinal lymph nodes. Thus, any signs of diaper rash will explain enlargement of the lymph nodes, which should be noted and reported.

In the femoral area, a swelling that can be reduced with a gurgling sound is an unusual finding.

This will locate the bowel for you and confirm the presence of a hernia.

1. Testes that are swollen by fluid (hydrocele) will transilluminate. Fluid around the testes or cord must be differentiated from a hernia.
2. Any mass in this area must be reported to a health care provider immediately.

Female Genitalia

1. If the child will be examined by a health care provider, it is not necessary to duplicate this part of the examination.
2. Place the infant or toddler on the table or on the parent's knee while he or she holds the knees in an abducted and flexed position.
3. A preschool child can be allowed to lean over her parent's knee. However, remember that the structures are being visualized upside down.
4. The older child or teenager should be draped as an adult would and should be placed in a lithotomy position with the aid of stirrups.

TECHNIQUE	*FINDINGS*

EQUIPMENT
Disposable gloves, speculum, light source

1. Carefully inspect the perineal area for cleanliness, inflammation, and abnormality.
2. Fold back the labia majora and note the labia minora.

3. Part the labia and note the clitoris and the meatus at the anterior end. (The clitoris is a hook-like structure that extends over the opening of the urethral meatus.)
   The meatus appears as a slit that is slightly darker in color against the pink of the mucosa about 2 cm (¾ inch) posterior to the clitoris.
4. Having parted the labia, check for any signs of inflammation, discharge, tenderness, or infection. Include the urethral meatus, periurethral glands, the vagina, and the greater vestibular glands (Bartholin's). (Tenderness of these glands is unusual in young children, but may occur in adolescents.)

1. This includes the mons pubis, clitoris, labia, urethra, and perineal body.
2. The labia minora are seen as two slender folds of tissue inside the labia majora.
3. In some instances, adhesions of the labia minora occur because of the lack of natural hormones. The opening of the vagina is obscured by the two lateral flaps, which stick together, sometimes to the degree that urination is difficult because the urethral meatus is covered. This should be referred to a health care provider.
4. Inflammation and puslike discharge from the urethra may be noted on palpation. The periurethral glands may be tender because of infection—possibly due to gonococci. If discharge is collected from the vagina, it should be cultured.

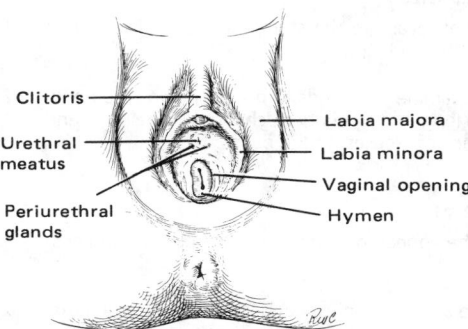

Clitoris — / Labia majora
Urethral meatus — / Labia minora
 / Vaginal opening
Periurethral glands — / Hymen

5. If the mother of a newborn infant has noted a bloody discharge from the infant's vagina during the first few days of life, reassure her that this is not an uncommon occurrence; the discharge will disappear, as will any swelling of the labia majora and clitoris and any enlargement of the infant's breasts.
6. Note the vaginal opening, which may vary in size because of the presence of a thin membrane, the hymen. The hymen varies in appearance according to the age of the child.

5. Hormone stimulation from the mother's body accounts for this occurrence. The discharge usually stops once the hormones are excreted. The bloody appearance on the diaper may be confused with the presence of urates, which are also orange-red and which appear quite normally in the urine.
6. The lack of an opening into the vagina may result in the retention of menstrual fluid when the child reaches puberty. In the sexually active adolescent, vestigial remains of the hymen may appear as small particles (caruncles) at the fringe of the vagina.
   If there is any possibility of sexual abuse, this examination should be referred to a specialist in sexual abuse.

7. In the young child, it is usually unnecessary to examine inside the vagina. Should you suspect the presence of a foreign body, insert a finger into the rectum and milk anteriorly to allow you to feel the lower part of the cervix and any firm foreign body within the vagina.
8. In an older child, the little finger can be inserted gently into the vagina and anterior pressure applied.

9. Turn the finger gradually, sweeping down the right side of the vagina, back over the rectum, and up on the left side of the vagina. Turn your finger, arm, and wrist so that undue pressure is not made on the child's tissues.
10. Once the genitalia are examined, lower the child's legs somewhat so that the femoral and inguinal areas can be palpated the same way as in the male.

7. A foreign body may be suspected if there is vaginal discharge (of any quantity) that is blood-tinged or has an odor. In the older child, vaginal discharge of this type may be due to gonorrhea.

8. Anterior pressure and milking downward palpates the urethra toward the meatus. The periurethral glands are located on each side of the urethra.

10. Enlargement of the lymph nodes in the presence of a hernia in the femoral triangle may be found. Similarly, enlargement of the inguinal nodes may occur.

TECHNIQUE	FINDINGS

Musculoskeletal System

1. Evaluation of the musculoskeletal system can be done both in an informal manner while watching the child at rest and at play and in a formal manner as specific findings are methodically checked.
2. In the newborn, observe the position of the extremities during sleep and the quality of movement when the infant is awake.
3. Various aspects of size, shape, and movement are evaluated as the baby is observed pushing up on arms and turning head towards mother.
4. The infant in the early stages of walking offers many opportunities for evaluation of muscle strength and movement.

   At the same time, rapport with the mother can be reinforced by your admiring the baby's ability and by inquiring if she is concerned about the manner in which the baby is walking.
5. A more mobile child can be evaluated as you watch him play and explore the room.
6. Having the older child reach for crayons, run after a ball, or walk around the room enables you to evaluate the musculoskeletal system and the child's sense of balance.

UPPER EXTREMITIES

1. In the infant, evaluate the status of the clavicles when examining the skull and neck.	1. During a difficult delivery, the clavicle that has been exposed to traction may snap. A lump can be felt on the bone at about 3 weeks of age.
2. Carefully examine the hands to note shape of the hand, shape and length of the fingers, changes in the nails, and the presence of creases on the palms.	2. Any variation in the hands or unusual length of the fingers should be noted. An incurved little finger or low-set thumb with the single simian crease may reflect Down syndrome.

LOWER EXTREMITIES

1. Examine the appearance of the infant's foot, noting arch formation.	1. The foot of an infant is usually flat and appears broad because the arch on the inside of the foot is covered by a fat pad. Parents may need reassurance in this regard.
2. Inspect the angle of the foot and lower leg and then manipulate the ankle to evaluate the range of motion.	2. Full flexibility of the foot (plantar flexion) rules out underlying abnormality. The foot should return to the neutral position after manipulation. Frequently, the foot will turn in, or adduct. Such a finding should be recorded.
3. Place the legs together and see how far the ankles and knees are separated.	3. The toddler has normally bowed legs, but with ankles touching, knees should be no more than 2 finger breaths apart. The preschooler has a normally knock-kneed walk, but with knees touching, ankles should be no more than 2 finger breaths apart.
4. Evaluate the baby's ability to walk, noting the appearance of the legs and foot placement. Remember to look at the child's shoes and see which side of the sole is worn down.	4. When babies first start to walk, their legs appear bowlegged. The feet are kept wide apart and turn slightly in so that the ankles seem curved when viewed from behind.

HIP

1. When examining children under 1 year of age, check to see if there are signs of hip dislocation.	1. Any difficulties with hip examination call for immediate medical consultation because of possible congenital dislocation of the hip. In the normal infant, the lateral aspect of each knee will touch the examining table without difficulty.

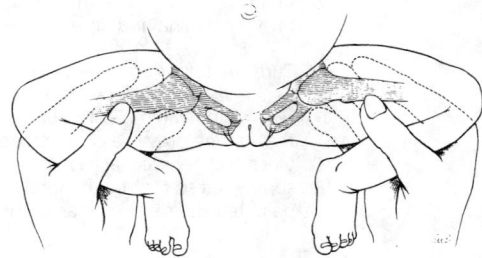

TECHNIQUE	FINDINGS

SPINE

1. Check the spine for any signs of abnormal curvature.

2. Observe the child from the side and back in the standing position to see forward curving of the shoulders.
3. Have the child bend forward with the arms hanging down. A unilateral rib prominence will be seen in children with scoliosis.

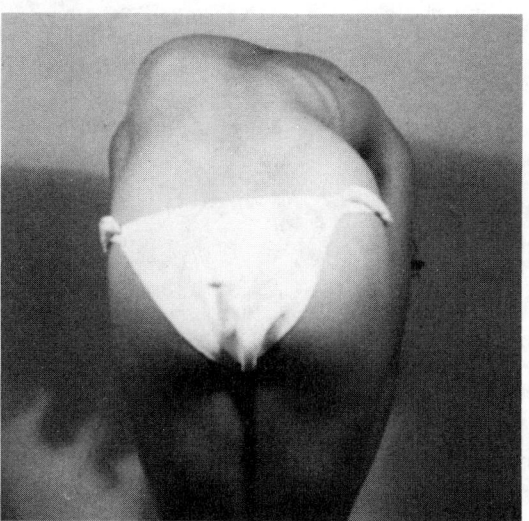

(O'Connor, B. J. Scoliosis: Classification and diagnosis in pediatric orthopedics. ONA J 3:84, Mar 1976)

1. The normal child has a curve inward at the lumbar region (lordosis), but this should not be exaggerated. It is normally more exaggerated in African American children. *Kyphosis:* Forward curvature of the shoulders. *Scoliosis:* Side-to-side curvature of the spine.
2. These appear most often during school years and adolescence.

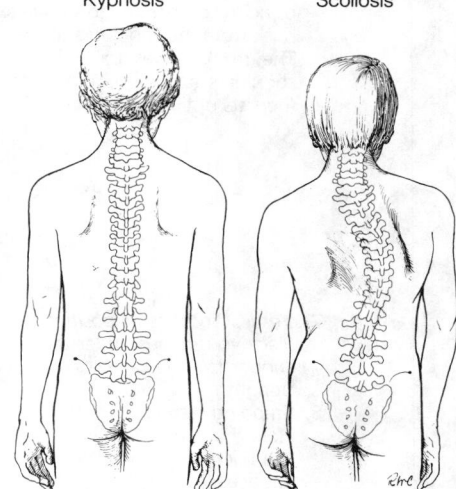

Scoliosis is more common in girls.

Neurologic Examination

1. The neurologic system at birth is different from that of the baby of a few months. There is an even greater contrast between the baby and children and adults.
2. The central nervous system at birth is underdeveloped and the functions tested are below the level of the cortex.

EQUIPMENT
Flashlight, noisemaker, ophthalmoscope, tongue depressor, tuning fork

Procedure for the Newborn and Young Infant
(See Guidelines: Nursing Care of the Newborn, p. 1021.)

1. Observe the newborn for general appearance, positioning, activity, crying, and alertness. Take note of the posture—including head, neck, and extremities.
2. Note the pitch, volume, and character of the cry.

3. Observe the infant's facial expression and the symmetry of the face when crying or sucking.

4. Most of the cranial nerves are difficult to check at this early age.

AUTOMATIC REFLEXES
1. *Blinking reflex due to loud noise*
   Clap your hands or produce a loud clicking noise, being careful not to clap near the baby so that a wave of air causes blinking of eyes anyway.
2. *Blinking reflex due to bright light*
   Shine a bright light into the infant's eyes to elicit blinking reflex.

1. Stiffness of the neck or marked attraction of the head will cause a position of opisthotonos and necessitates referral.

2. The high-pitched cry of the infant who has intracranial irritation is very distinctive.
3. Poor sucking, with dribbling, is abnormal. Transient weakness of the mouth due to 7th cranial nerve paralysis is frequently seen as a result of a forceps delivery in which the forceps is pressed on the facial nerve where it emerges from the ear.

1. Lack of a blink in response to a loud noise may indicate deafness.

2. Failure to blink may indicate blindness.

TECHNIQUE	*FINDINGS*

3. Cranial nerve 10 can be checked by using a tongue depressor to gag the infant.

4. *Palmar grasp reflex*
   Place your fingers across the baby's palm from the ulnar side. The baby needs to be in a relaxed position with his head in a central position. Reinforcement may be offered by having the baby suck on the bottle at the same time.

5. *Rooting reflex*
   Touch the edge of the baby's mouth.

6. *Incurving of the trunk*
   Hold the baby horizontally and prone in one arm while using the other hand to stimulate one side of the infant's back from the shoulders to the buttocks.
   The trunk curves toward the stimulated side as the shoulders and pelvis move toward the stroking hand (persists until infant is about 2 months old).

3. Palate moves.

4. Both hands will flex and can be compared for strength. Weakness on one side may be indicated by a failure to grasp when the palm is stimulated.

5. The baby's mouth will open, and the head will turn toward the side stimulated. This reflex is marked during the early weeks of life.

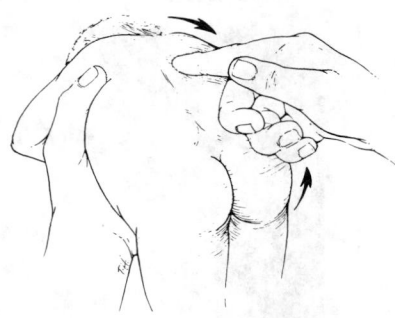

7. *Vertical suspension position*
   Place your hands under the baby's axillae with thumbs supporting the back of the head and hold the baby upright.

8. *Stepping response*
   Hold the baby under its axillae with thumbs supporting the back of the head. Allow baby's foot to touch firm surface.

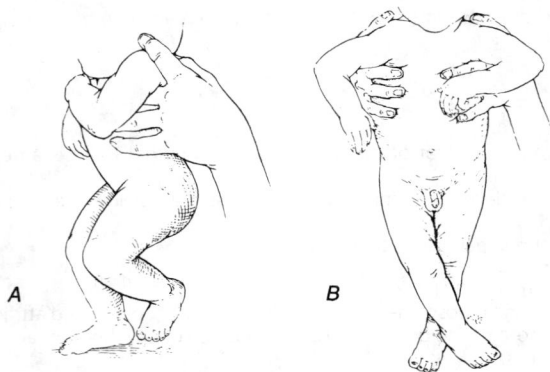

A   B

7. The legs flex at the hips and knees (persists for about 4 months).

8. Normally the baby responds by lifting one knee and hip into a flexed position and moving the opposite leg forward—making a series of stepping movements (*A*).

   a. Difficulty with the stepping reflex and stiffness or spasticity connected with crossing of the feet and scissoring (*B*) is indicative of spastic paraplegia or diplegia.
   b. It should be noted that the stepping response may be affected by breech delivery. (It may also be affected by weakness.)
   c. The stepping response is evident toward the end of the first week and persists for a variable time.

9. *Tonic neck reflex*
   Hold the baby in a supine position with the head turned to one side and the jaw held in place over the shoulder.

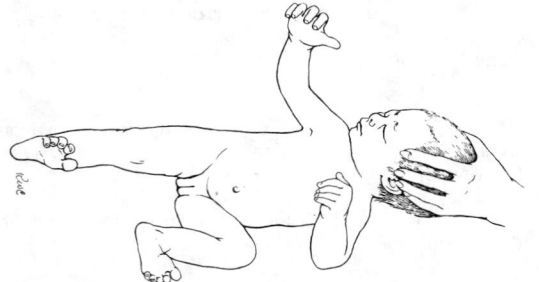

9. a. The arm and leg on the side to which the head is turned will extend, whereas those on the other side will flex (the so-called "bow and arrow position").
   b. This reflex persists for about 6 months; it may be present at birth or delayed until the baby is 6 or 8 weeks old.
   c. Persistence beyond 6 months suggests major cerebral damage.

TECHNIQUE	FINDINGS

10. *Mass reflexes* (Moro or startle reflex)
Hold the baby along your arm with the other hand below the lower legs. Lower the feet and body in a sudden motion.

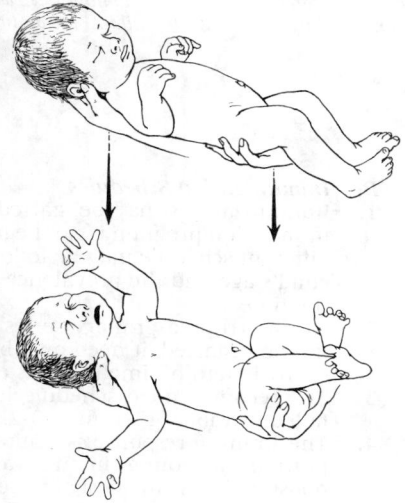

10. The arms will spring up and out, abducting and extending; the fingers are also extended. The arms then return forward over the body with a clasping motion. At the same time, the legs flex slightly and the hips abduct.
 a. The Moro reflex is present at birth and disappears at about the end of the third month. Persistence beyond 6 months is significant.
 b. Asymmetric response may be due to paralysis of the arm following a difficult delivery, tension and injury to the brachial plexus, or a fracture of the clavicle or humerus. A dislocated hip would produce an asymmetrical response in the lower extremities.

11. *Perez reflex*
Hold the baby in a prone position along your arm; place the thumb of the other hand on the sacrum and move it firmly toward the head, along the entire length of the spine.

11. The head and spine will extend and the knees will flex upward.

SUMMARY
1. Some of the jerking and shaking movements seen in infants are normal, but they should be rechecked frequently during the first few weeks of life.
2. Variants in the findings due to the baby's sleepiness or hunger should be taken into account and reevaluations should be carried out under different conditions.
3. Severe neurologic damage may be completely asymptomatic and impossible to detect during the first few weeks of life.

NEUROLOGIC EXAMINATION OF THE TODDLER AND EARLY SCHOOL-AGED CHILD
1. The neurologic examination for the toddler and the early school-aged child is similar to that for the adult.
2. The Draw-A-Person Test and the Denver Developmental Assessment are both excellent methods for testing areas in the development of the child (see p. 1068).
3. Beyond the newborn period, specific gross and fine motor coordination testing, accompanied by appropriate evaluation of the Denver test, will assist in assessing the child's level of development.
4. These tests also assess social and language development and are important screening devices.
5. Interview techniques can also be useful in assessing development in the preschool child (see p. 1072).

Selected References

Avery, M. E., & First, L. R. (Eds.). (1993). *Pediatric medicine* (pp. 3-22). Baltimore: Williams & Wilkins.

Bates, G. A. (1995). *A guide to physical examination* (6th ed.). Philadelphia: J. B. Lippincott.

Behrman, R. E., & Kliegman, R. (eds.) (1994). *Nelson essentials of pediatrics.* Philadelphia, W. B. Saunders.

Bowers, A. C., & Thompson, J. M. (1991). *Clinical manual of health assessment* (4th ed.). St. Louis: C. V. Mosby.

Engel, J. (1992). *Pocket guide to pediatric assessment.* St. Louis: C. V. Mosby.

Fuller, J., & Schaller-Ayers, J. (1994). *Health assessment: A nursing approach.* Philadelphia: J. B. Lippincott.

Gill, D., & O'Brien, N. (1993). *Paediatric clinical examination.* New York: Churchill Livingstone.

Green, M. (1992). *Pediatric diagnosis* (5th ed.). Philadelphia: W. B. Saunders.

Hoekelmann, R. A., (ed.) (1992). *Primary pediatric care.* St. Louis: C. V. Mosby.

Jackson, D., & Saunders, R. (1993). *Child health nursing.* Philadelphia: J. B. Lippincott.

Oski, F. A., (ed.) (1993). *Principles and practice of pediatrics.* Philadelphia: J. B. Lippincott.

Paradise, J. E., (1990). The medical evaluation of the sexually abused child. *Pediatric Clinics of North America, 37,* 839.

U.S. Preventive Services Task Force. (1990). The periodic health examination: Age-specific charts. *American Family Physician, 41*(1), 189-204.

Wilson, D., & Ratekin, C. (1990). Preparation for routine physical examination. *Children's Health Care, 19,* 178.

Pediatric Primary Care

Health Maintenance

Pediatric primary care involves all the health promotion and disease prevention needs of the child. The goal of pediatric primary care is the highest level of wellness attainable for each child. Health education, surveillance, and reassurance in the areas of immunizations, proper nutrition, dental care, and safety are basic components of health maintenance.

◆ IMMUNIZATIONS

With the dramatic effectiveness of routine immunizations, many childhood diseases have decreased in frequency. A number still cause significant morbidity in childhood. For immunizations to be successful and for diseases to be eradicated, children must receive their immunizations in a timely and complete manner. Nurses are in an ideal position to enhance the health of children by promoting immunizations. The child's immunization status should be reviewed at each health care visit and needed vaccines should be administered.

General Considerations

A. **Requirements of National Childhood Vaccine Injury Act (Effective 1988)**
1. Childhood-mandated vaccines (diphtheria tetanus toxoid, pertussis [DTP]; oral polio [OPV]; inactivated polio [IPV]; measles, mumps, rubella [MMR]; and *Haemophilus influenzae* type b [Hib] vaccines and any combination). Hepatitis B vaccine (HBV) is recommended. Varicella, pneumococcal, and influenzae vaccines are available but not part of the regular schedule at this time.
2. Patient, parent, or legal guardian should be informed about the benefits and risks of immunizations. They must be provided with pamphlets containing the appropriate information.
3. Health care provider must record in the patient's permanent medical record: month, day, and year of administration; vaccine or other biologic administered; manufacturer; lot number and its expiration date; site and route of administration; name, address, and title of the health care provider administering the vaccine.
4. Health care providers are required to report selected events occurring after vaccination to the Vaccine Adverse Events Reporting System (VAERS).

B. **Immunization Schedules**
1. Immunizations may be started at any age. If an immunization program is not begun in infancy, a slightly different schedule may be followed, depending on the child's age and the prevalence of specific infections at the time.
2. An interrupted primary series of immunization need not be restarted; it need only be continued, regardless of the length of time that has elapsed.
3. The recommended schedule for immunization is detailed in Tables 40-1 and 40-2.
4. The immunoresponse is limited in a significant proportion of young infants, and the recommended booster doses are designed to ensure and maintain immunity.

C. **Contraindications**
1. General for all vaccines
   a. Anaphylactic reaction to a vaccine
   b. Anaphylactic reaction to a vaccine constituent contraindicates the use of vaccines containing that substance.
   c. Moderate or severe illnesses with or without a fever
2. DTP/DTaP (diptheria, tetanus, acellular pertussis)
   a. Encephalopathy within 7 days of administration of previous dose of DTP
3. OPV
   a. Infection with human immunodeficiency virus (HIV) or household contact with HIV
   b. Known altered immunodeficiency
   c. Immunodeficient household contact
4. IPV
   a. Anaphylactic reaction to neomycin or streptomycin
5. MMR
   a. Anaphylactic reactions to egg ingestion and to neomycin
   b. Pregnancy
   c. Known altered immunodeficiency

D. **Misconceptions Concerning Vaccine Contraindications**
1. Some health care providers inappropriately consider certain conditions or circumstances to be contraindications to vaccination. Conditions most often inappropriately regarded as such include:
   a. Mild acute illness with low-grade fever or mild diarrheal illness in an otherwise well child
   b. Current antimicrobial therapy or the convalescent phase of illness
   c. Reaction to a previous DTP dose that involved only soreness, redness, swelling in the immediate vicinity of the vaccination site or temperature of less than 105°F (40.5°C).
   d. Prematurity

TABLE 40-1 Recommended Schedule for Immunization of Healthy Infants and Children*

Recommended Age†	Immunization(s)‡	Comments
Birth	HBV§	
1–2 mo	HBV§	
2 mo	DTP, Hib, OPV	DTP and OPV can be initiated as early as 4 wk after birth in areas of high endemicity or during outbreaks.
4 mo	DTP, Hib, OPV	2-mo interval (minimum of 6 wk) recommended for OPV.
6 mo	DTP, (Hib)‖	
6–18 mo	HBV,§ OPV	
12–15 mo	Hib, MMR	MMR should be given at 12 mo if age in high-risk areas. If indicated, tuberculin testing may be done at the same visit.
15–18 mo	DTaP or DTP	The fourth dose of DTP vaccine should be given 6–12 mo after the third dose of DTP and may be given as early as 12 mo of age, provided that the interval between doses 3 and 4 is at least 6 mo and DTP is given. DTaP is not currently licensed for use in children younger than 15 mo.
4–6 y	DTaP or DTP, OPV	DTaP or DTP and OPV should be given at entry to middle school or junior high school unless 2 doses were given at or after the 7th birthday.
5–12 y	MMR	MMR should be given at entry to middle school or junior high school unless 2 doses were given after 1st birthday.
14–16 y	Td	Repeat every 10 y throughout life.

* Table is not completely consistent with all package inserts. For products used, also consult manufacturer's package insert for instructions on storage, handling, dosage, and administration. Biologics prepared by different manufacturers may vary, and package inserts of the same manufacturer may change from time to time.
† These recommended ages should not be construed as absolute. For example, 2 mo can be 6–10 wk. However, MMR usually should not be given to children younger than 12 mo. If measles vaccination is indicated, monovalent measles vaccine is recommended, and MMR should be given subsequently, at 12–15 mo.
‡ Vaccine abbreviations: HBV, hepatitis B virus vaccine; DTP, diphtheria and tetanus toxoids and pertussis vaccine; DTaP, diphtheria and tetanus toxoids and acellular pertussis vaccine; Hib, *Haemophilus influenzae* type b conjugate vaccine; OPV, oral poliovirus vaccine (containing attenuated poliovirus 1, 2, and 3); MMR, live measles, mumps, and rubella viruses vaccine; Td, adult tetanus toxoid (full dose) and diphtheria toxoid (reduced dose), for children ≥7 y and adults.
§ An acceptable alternative to minimize the number of visits for immunizing infants of HBsAg-negative mothers is to administer dose 1 at 0–2 mo, dose 2 at 4 mo, and dose 3 at 6–18 mo.
‖ Hib: dose 3 of Hib is not indicated if the product for doses 1 and 2 was PedvaxHIB.

e. Pregnancy of mother or other household contact
f. Recent exposure to an infectious disease
g. Breast-feeding
h. History of nonspecific allergies or relatives with allergies
i. Allergies to penicillin or any other antibiotic, except anaphylactic reactions to neomycin or streptomycin
j. Allergies to duck meat or duck feathers
k. Family history of convulsions in persons considered for pertussis or measles vaccination
l. Family history of sudden infant death syndrome in children considered for DTP vaccination
m. Family history of an adverse event, unrelated to immunosuppression, after vaccination
n. Malnutrition

E. Preventive Considerations
1. Strict adherence to the manufacturer's storage and handling recommendation is vital. Failure to observe these precautions and recommendations may reduce the potency and effectiveness of vaccines.

2. Health care personnel administering vaccines should be immunized against measles, mumps, rubella, hepatitis B, influenza, tetanus, and diphtheria. Gloves are not required when administering vaccines unless the worker has open hand lesions or will contact potentially infectious body fluids. However, gloves can be worn as a recommended measure. Good handwashing technique is mandatory.
3. Sterile, disposable needles and syringes should be discarded promptly in appropriate biohazardous containers.
4. Parenteral vaccines should be administered in the anterolateral aspect of the upper thigh in infants and in the deltoid area of the upper arm in older children and adolescents. Recommended routes of administration are included in the package inserts of vaccines.
5. Before administering a subsequent dose of any vaccine, patients and parents must be questioned concerning side effects and possible reactions from previous doses.
6. Routine vaccines can be safely and effectively administered simultaneously.

TABLE 40-2 Recommended Immunization Schedules for Children Not Immunized in the First Year of Life

Recommended Time/Age	Immunization(s)*†	Comments
Younger Than 7 Years		
First visit	DTP, Hib, HBV, MMR, OPV	If indicated, tuberculin testing may be done at the visit. If a child is 5 y of age or older, Hib is not indicated.
Interval after first visit:		
1 mo	DTP, HBV	OPV may be given if accelerated poliomyelitis vaccination is necessary, such as for travelers to areas where polio is endemic.
2 mo	DTP, Hib, OPV	Second dose of Hib is indicated only in children whose first dose was received younger than 15 mo.
≥8 mo	DTP or DTaP,‡ HBV, OPV	OPV is not given if the third dose was given earlier.
4–6 y (at or before school entry)	DTP or DTaP,‡ OPV	DTP or DTaP is not necessary if the fourth dose was given after the 4th birthday; OPV is not necessary if the third dose was given after the 4th birthday.
11–12 y	DTP or DTaP,‡ OPV	At entry to middle school or junior high school
10 y later	Td	Repeat every 10 y throughout life.
7 Years and Older§‖		
First visit	HBV,§ OPV, MMR, Td	
Interval after first visit:		
2 mo	HBV,¶ OPV, Td	OPV may also be given 1 mo after the first visit if accelerated poliomyelitis vaccination is necessary.
8–14 mo	HBV,¶ OPV, Td	OPV is not given if the third dose was given earlier.
11–12 y	MMR	At entry to middle school or junior high.
10 y later	Td	Repeat every 10 y throughout life.

* If all needed vaccines cannot be administered simultaneously, priority should be given to protecting the child against diseases that pose the greatest immediate risk. In the United States, these diseases for children younger than 2 y usually are measles and *Haemophilus influenzae* type b infection; for children older than 7 y, they are measles, mumps, and rubella (MMR).
† DTP or DTaP, HBV, Hib, MMR, and OPV can be given simultaneously at separate sites if failure of the patient to return for future immunizations is a concern.
‡ DTaP is not currently licensed for use in children younger than 15 mo of age and is not recommended for primary immunizations (ie, first 3 doses) at any age.
§ If person is 18 y or older, routine poliovirus vaccination is not indicated in the United States.
‖ Minimal interval between doses of MMR is 1 mo.
¶ Priority should be given to hepatitis B immunization of adolescents.

Specific Immunization

A. DTP
1. A time lapse of 8 weeks is recommended between the first three DTP injections for desirable maximum effects.
2. The combination of depot antigens is preferred because it is more immunogenic.
3. Whole-cell DTP should be used for the first three doses in infants and children under 7 years of age.
4. Administration of acetaminophen at the time of immunization and at 4 and 8 hours after immunization decreases the incidence of febrile and local reactions.
5. Because of the increased risk of possible reactions to either diphtheria or pertussis antigen, Td (adult-type tetanus and diphtheria toxins) is recommended for children over 7 years of age.
6. For contaminated wounds, a booster dose of tetanus should be given if more than 5 years have elapsed since the last dose.
7. Protection of infants against pertussis should begin early.
8. In newborn infants, the best protection against pertussis is avoidance of household contacts by adequate immunization of older siblings.
9. Acellular pertussis vaccines are currently licensed in the United States for use only for the fourth and fifth doses for children aged 15 months and older.
10. Children who have recovered from culture-proven pertussis do not need pertussis immunization.
11. If the fourth dose of pertussis vaccine is given after the fourth birthday, no further doses are needed.

B. Tuberculin Test
1. It is recommended that the tuberculin test be given at the time of measles, mumps, and rubella (MMR).
   a. Measles vaccine can temporarily suppress tuberculin reactivity if given 4 to 6 weeks before a tuberculin test.
2. The frequency of repeated tuberculin testing depends on the following:

a. Risk of tuberculosis exposure to the child.
b. Prevalence of tuberculosis in the population group.
c. Presence of underlying host factors in the child (immunosuppressive conditions or HIV infection).

C. Measles Vaccine
1. Usually given at 12 to 15 months of age but should be given at 12 months in high-risk areas.
2. Second dose is recommended at 11 or 12 years of age unless local public health regulations require the second dose at school entry (age 4–6 years).
3. During an outbreak, infants as young as 6 months of age can be immunized. A second dose should be given at 12 to 15 months and again at age 11 or 12 years or at school entry.
4. Mild postimmunization symptoms include transient skin rashes and fever.
5. Immunoglobulin preparations interfere with the serologic response to measles vaccine for variable time periods depending on the dose.

D. Mumps Vaccine
1. Usually administered in combination with measles and rubella vaccine (MMR) at 12 to 15 months of age.
2. Second dose administered as MMR is important because a substantial number of cases have occurred in persons with previous immunizations.
3. Important to immunize susceptible children approaching puberty, adolescents, and adults.

E. Rubella Vaccine
1. Two doses of rubella vaccine are now recommended to avoid consequences such as congenital rubella syndrome.
2. Important to immunize postpubertal individuals, especially college students and military recruits.
3. Women should avoid pregnancy within 3 months of vaccine due to the theoretical risk to the fetus.

F. Polio Vaccine
1. Two types of trivalent vaccine are available—live oral polio virus vaccine (OPV) and inactivated polio virus vaccine (IPV), given parenterally. Both are effective in preventing poliomyelitis.
2. OPV is currently the vaccine of choice for most children because it induces intestinal immunity, is simple to administer, is well accepted by patients, results in immunization of some contacts of vaccinated persons, and has eliminated disease caused by wild polio viruses in the United States.
3. OPV should not be given to infants and children living in households with an immunodeficient person because OPV is excreted in the stool and can infect the person who may contract paralytic disease.
4. OPV primary series consists of three doses of vaccine given 6 to 8 weeks apart beginning at 6 to 8 weeks of age. Booster dose is given at 4 to 6 years of age.
5. IPV may be given to those who refuse OPV or in whom OPV is contraindicated. The first two doses are given at 4-8 week intervals beginning at 6-8 weeks of age. The third dose is given 6-12 months after. The booster dose is given at 4-6 years of age.

G. Hib Vaccine
1. Protects against *H. influenzae* type B bacteria.
2. Incidence of invasive disease caused by Hib has declined dramatically since the introduction of conjugate vaccine.
3. Four Hib conjugate vaccines and one combination Hib conjugate–DTP vaccine are licensed in the United States. Refer to package inserts for specific immunization guidelines.
4. Minimal adverse reactions (pain, redness, or swelling at immunization site for less than 24 hours).

H. HBV
1. Two vaccines currently available in the United States are produced by recombinant DNA technology.
2. Both are highly effective and safe.
3. Recommended for all infants born to HBsAg-negative mothers. Three-dose schedule is initiated in newborn period or by 2 months of age; second dose given 1 to 2 months later; third dose 6 to 18 months later.
4. Preterm infants weighing less than 2 kg may have lower seroconversion rates. Initiation of HBV should be delayed until just before hospital discharge if the infant weighs 2 kg or more or until approximately 2 months of age when other routine immunizations are given.
5. All infants born to HBsAg-positive mothers, including premature infants, should receive hepatitis B immunoglobulin and vaccine as soon as possible after birth.
6. All adolescents should be immunized against HBV infection to prevent the sexual transmission of HBV disease.

◆ NUTRITION IN CHILDREN

The nutritional status of the child is an important aspect of health maintenance. It has an impact on a child's general physical and psychosocial health. From early infancy through adolescence, growth and development are largely dependent on a balanced diet. Feeding provides emotional and psychological benefits in addition to nutritional needs. Table 40-3 presents complete nutritional guidelines throughout childhood.

◆ SAFETY

Safety is an area of major importance in the pediatric population. Injury is the leading cause of childhood morbidity and mortality. Although childhood deaths from other causes have decreased, injury death rates remain constant. Approximately one in five children requires medical care each year for an accidental injury.

Role of the Nurse

1. Identify environmental hazards and take action to reduce or eliminate them.
2. Identify behavioral characteristics of individual children that may be related to accidental liability and caution parents accordingly. Pay particular attention to children who show the following:
   a. Characteristics that increase exposure to hazards, such as excessive curiosity, inability to delay gratification, hyperactivity, and daringness
   b. Characteristics that reduce the child's ability to cope with hazards, such as aggressiveness, stubbornness, poor concentration, low frustration threshold, lack of self-control

TABLE 40-3 Nutrition in Children

Age and Developmental Influence on Nutritional Requirements and Feeding Patterns	Feeding Pattern/Diet	Nursing Implications/Parental Guidance

Neonate
Birth–4 wk
Newborn's rapid growth makes infant especially vulnerable to dietary inadequacies, dehydration, and iron deficiency anemia.
Feeding process is basis for infant's first human relationship, formation of trust. Feeding reinforces mother's sense of "motherliness."
Because of limited nutritional stores, neonates require vitamin and mineral supplements.
Neonates require more fluid relative to their size than do adults.
Sucking ability is influenced by individual neuromuscular maturity.
	Breast milk or formula is generally given in 6–8 feedings per day, spaced 2–4 h apart.
	Feeding schedules should be individualized according to infant's needs.
		Provide information to help parents make decision concerning breast- or bottle-feeding.
		Support parents in their decision.
		Breast-fed infant:
		1. Help mother assume comfortable and satisfying position for self and baby.
		2. Help mother to determine schedule, timing, and when infant is satisfied.
		3. Provide specific information about the following:
		  a. Feeding technique: position, "bubbling"
		  b. Care of breasts
		  c. Manual expression of milk from breast
		  d. Maternal diet
		Bottle-fed infant:
		1. Provide specific information concerning
		  a. Type of formula
		  b. Preparation of formula: measuring and sterilization
		  c. Equipment—types of bottles, nipples, etc.
		  d. Sterilization of equipment
		  e. Technique of feeding: position, "bubbling"
		2. Help mother to determine when infant is satisfied; develop schedule for feeding.
		Provide information concerning normal characteristics of stools, signs of dehydration, constipation, colic, milk allergy.
		Discuss need for vitamin supplements and how to administer.
		Discuss need for additional fluids during periods of hot weather, and with fever, diarrhea, and vomiting.
		Observe for evidence of common problems and intervene accordingly:
		1. Overfeeding
		2. Underfeeding
		3. Difficulty digesting formula because of its particular composition.
		4. Improper feeding technique; holes in nipples too large or too small; formula too hot or too cold; uncomfortable feeding position; failure to "bubble"; improper sterilization; bottle propping.
		5. Bottles should never be given to infants to take to bed.

Infant 3 mo–1 y Increased neuromuscular development allows infant to make transition from a totally liquid diet to a diet of milk and solid foods as well as to more active participation in the feeding process. 3–6 mo Sucking reflex becomes voluntary and chewing action begins; infant can approximate lips to rim of cup and may begin drinking from cup at 6 mo. 6–12 mo Eyes and hands can work together; infant is able to sit without support and has developed grasp; able to feed self a biscuit; bangs objects on table; able to hold own bottle at 9–12 mo; has "pincer" approach to food; able to be weaned as child becomes developmentally able to take sufficient fluids from the cup.	Number of feedings per day decreases through the first year. Most babies are ready to give up nighttime feedings by 4 mo of age. By 1 y of age, most infants are satisfied with 3 meals and additional fluids throughout the day. By 4–6 mo of age, the infant is generally ready to begin eating strained foods. The usual sequence of foods is cereal followed by fruits, and vegetables. Meats may be started at 8–9 mo. This sequence may vary according to individual preferences of pediatrician and family. Mashed table foods or junior foods generally are started at 6–8 mo, when infant begins chewing action. Infant begins to enjoy finger foods at 10–12 mo.	New foods should be offered one at a time and early in the feeding while the infant is still hungry. The person feeding should be calm, gentle, relaxed, and patient in approach. When the child is first offered puréed foods with a spoon, he expects and wants to suck. The protrusion of the tongue, which is needed in sucking, makes it appear that he is pushing the food out of mouth. This response should not be interpreted as dislike for the food; it is a result of immature muscle coordination and surprise at the taste and feel of the new food. The baby foods selected should be those that are high in nutrients without providing excessive calories. Personal and cultural preferences should be considered. Infants should be observed for allergic reactions when new foods are added. Common allergies are to citrus juices, egg white, cow's milk, and peanut butter. These foods should be avoided until 12 mo of age. Also avoid honey until 12 mo due to the risk of infantile botulism. Finger foods should be selected for their nutritional value. Good choices include teething biscuits, cooked vegetables, bananas, cheese sticks, and enriched cereals. Avoid nuts, raisins and raw vegetables, which can cause choking. Parents can be taught to prepare their own strained or junior foods using a commercial baby food grinder or blender.

(continued)

TABLE 40-3 Nutrition in Children *(continued)*

Age and Developmental Influence on Nutritional Requirements and Feeding Patterns	Feeding Pattern/Diet	Nursing Implications/Parental Guidance
Food provides the infant with a variety of learning experiences; motor control and coordination in self-feeding; recognition of shape, texture, color; stimulation of speech movement through use of mouth muscles. Mealtime allows the infant to continue development of trust in a consistent, loving atmosphere. The infant is forming lifetime eating habits; it is therefore important to make mealtime a positive experience.	The transition from iron-fortified formula or breast milk to cow's milk is usually advised at about 12 mo of age.	Weaning is a gradual process. 1. Assist parents to recognize indications of readiness. 2. Do not expect the infant to completely drop old pattern of behavior while learning a new one; allow overlap of old and new techniques. 3. Evening feedings usually the most difficult to eliminate, because the infant is tired and in need of sucking comfort. 4. During illness or household disorganization, the infant may regress and return to sucking to relieve his discomfort and frustration. SPECIAL CONSIDERATIONS: Hospitalized infant Obtain a thorough nursing history that includes the following: Feeding pattern and schedule; types of foods that have been introduced; likes and dislikes; breast or bottle fed, type of bottle; temperature at which infant prefers foods and fluids.
Toddler 1–3 y Growth slows at the end of the first year. The slower growth rate is reflected in a decreased appetite. The toddler has a total of 14–16 teeth, making him more able to chew foods. Increased self-awareness causes the toddler to want to do more for self. Refusals of food or of assistance in feedings are common ways in which the toddler asserts himself. Because body tissues, especially muscles, continue to grow quite rapidly, protein needs are high.	Appetite is sporadic, specific foods may be favored exclusively or refused from time to time. Child may be ritualistic concerning food preferences, schedule, manner of eating, etc. Diet should include a full range of foods: milk, meat, fruits, vegetables, breads, and cereals. Iron-fortified dry cereals (rice, barley) are an excellent source of iron during the second year of life. Older toddler can be expected to consume about one-half the amount of food that an adult consumes.	Provide foods with a variety of color, texture, and flavor. Toddlers need to experience the feel of foods. Offer small portions. It is fun for the child to ask for more. It is more effective to give small helpings than to insist that he eat a specific amount. Maintain a regular mealtime schedule. Provide appropriate mealtime equipment: 1. Silverware scaled to size. 2. Dishes—colorful, unbreakable; shallow, round bowls are preferable to flat plates. 3. Plastic bibs, placemats, and floor coverings permit a relaxed attitude toward child's self-feeding attempts. 4. Comfortable seating at good height and distance from table. Adults who help toddlers at mealtime should be calm and relaxed. Avoid bribes or force feeding because this reinforces negative behavior and may lead to a dislike for mealtime. Encourage independence, but provide assistance when necessary. Do not be concerned about table manners. Avoid the use of soda or "sweets" as rewards or between-meal snacks. Instead, substitute fruit, juice, or cereal. Toddlers who show little interest in eggs, meat, or vegetables should not be permitted to appease their appetite with carbohydrates or milk because this may lead to iron-deficiency anemia. Milk should be limited to approximately 16 oz/d. SPECIAL CONSIDERATIONS: Hospitalized toddler Nursing history should include the following: Feeding pattern and schedule; food likes and dislikes; food allergies; special eating equipment and utensils; whether or not child is weaned; what child is fed when ill.
Preschooler 3–5 y of age Increased manual dexterity enables child to have complete independence at mealtime. Psychosocially, this is a period of increased imitation and sex identification. The preschooler identifies with parents at the table and will enjoy what parents enjoy. Additional nutritional habits are developed that become part of the child's lifetime practices.	Appetite tends to be sporadic. Child requires the same basic 4 food groups as the adult, but in smaller quantities. Generally likes to eat one food from plate at a time. Likes vegetables that are crisp, raw, and cut into finger-sized pieces. Often dislikes strong-tasting foods.	Emphasis should be placed on the quality rather than the amount of food ingested. Foods should be attractively served, mildly flavored, plain, as well as being separated and distinctly identifiable in flavor and appearance. Nutritional foods (eg, crackers and cheese, yogurt, fruit) should be offered as snacks. Desserts should be nutritious and a natural part of the meal, not used as a reward for finishing the meal or omitted as punishment. Unless they persist, periods of overeating or not wanting to eat certain foods should not cause concern. The overall eating pattern from month to month is more pertinent to assess.

(continued)

TABLE 40-3 Nutrition in Children *(continued)*

Age and Developmental Influence on Nutritional Requirements and Feeding Patterns	Feeding Pattern/Diet	Nursing Implications/Parental Guidance
Slower growth rate and increased interest in exploring his environment may decrease the preschooler's interest in eating. Eating assumes increasing social significance. Mealtime promotes socialization and provides the preschooler with opportunities to learn appropriate mealtime behavior, language skills, and understanding of family rituals.		Frequent causes of insufficient eating: 1. Unhappy atmosphere at mealtime 2. Overeating between meals 3. Parental example 4. Attention-seeking 5. Excessive parental expectations 6. Inadequate variety or quantity of foods 7. Tooth decay 8. Physical illness 9. Fatigue 10. Emotional disturbance Measures to increase food intake: 1. Allow child to help with preparations, planning menu, setting table, and other simple chores. 2. Maintain calm environment with no distractions. 3. Avoid between-meal snacks. 4. Provide rest period before meal. 5. Avoid coaxing, bribing, threatening. SPECIAL CONSIDERATIONS: Hospitalized preschooler Consider cultural differences. Allow parents to bring in favorite foods or eating utensils from home. Encourage family members to be present at mealtime. Place children in small groups, preferably at tables during mealtime. Provide simple foods in small portions. Peanut butter and jelly sandwiches are often favorites. Allow and encourage children to feed themselves. Use nursing history. Do not punish children who refuse to eat. Offer alternative foods.
School-aged Child Slowed rate of growth during middle childhood results in gradual decline in food requirements per unit of body weight. The preadolescent growth spurt occurs about age 10 in girls and about age 12 in boys. At this time, energy needs increase and approach those of the adult. Intake is particularly important, since reserves are laid down for the demands of adolescence. The child becomes dependent on peers for approval and makes food choices accordingly. The child experiences increased socialization and independence through opportunities to eat away from home—for example, at school and homes of peers.	By this time, food practices are generally well-established, a product of the eating experiences of the toddler and preschool period. Many children are too busy with other affairs to take time out to eat. Play readily takes priority unless a firm understanding is reached and mealtime is relaxed and enjoyable.	Nutrition education should help the child to select foods wisely and to begin to plan and prepare meals. Parental attitudes continue to be important as the child copies parental behavior (eg, skipping breakfast, not eating certain foods). Most children require a nutritious breakfast to avoid lassitude in late morning. Mealtime should continue to be relaxed and enjoyable. Diversions such as television should be avoided. Calcium and vitamin D intake warrant special consideration. They must be adequate to support the rapid enlargement of bones. Parents and health professionals should be alert to signs of developing obesity. Intake should be altered accordingly. Table manners should not be overemphasized. The young child often stuffs his mouth, spills foods, and chatters incessantly while eating. Time and experience will improve his habits. Provide some companionship and conversation at the child's level during meals. Peers should be invited occasionally for meals. SPECIAL CONSIDERATIONS: Hospitalized child Nursing history should include the following: Food preferences; mealtime patterns and snacks; food allergies; food preferences when ill. Provide opportunities for children to eat in small groups at tables. Consider cultural differences. Allow parents to bring in favorite foods from home. Allow child to order own meal.

(continued)

TABLE 40-3 Nutrition in Children *(continued)*

Age and Developmental Influence on Nutritional Requirements and Feeding Patterns	Feeding Pattern/Diet	Nursing Implications/Parental Guidance
Adolescent 11–17 y of age Dietary requirements vary according to stage of sexual maturation, rate of physical growth, and extent of athletic and social activity. When rapid growth of puberty appears, there is a corresponding increase in energy requirements and appetite.	Previously learned dietary patterns are difficult to change. Food choices and eating habits may be quite unusual and are related to the adolescent's psychological and social milieu. Generally, a significant percentage of the daily caloric intake of the adolescent comes from snacking.	Continue nutrition education, with special emphasis on the following: 1. Selecting nutritious foods. 2. Nutritional needs related to growth. 3. Preparing favorite "adolescent foods." 4. Foods and physical fitness. Informal sessions are generally more effective than lectures on nutrition. Special problems requiring intervention: Obesity Excessive dieting Extreme fads—eccentric and grossly restricted diets Anorexia nervosa/bulimia Adolescent pregnancy Provide nutritious foods relevant to the adolescent's lifestyle Discourage cigarette smoking, which may contribute to poor nutritional status by decreasing appetite and increasing the body's metabolic rate. SPECIAL CONSIDERATIONS: Hospitalized adolescent Allow patient to choose own foods, especially if on a special diet. Provide a refrigerator in the recreation room for snacks, or utilize a snack cart. Serve foods that appeal to adolescents. Use a nursing history similar to that for the school-age child.

3. Provide anticipatory guidance about child development as it relates to accidents. Direct preventive teaching toward individuals or groups, toward children or adults.
4. Participate in policy setting for accident prevention with great emphasis on effective public health measures.

Principles of Safety

1. The child's developmental stage influences the types of accidents likely to occur. Potential accident situations may be foreseen by parents who have knowledge of their own child's typical patterns of growth and development.
2. Children are naturally curious, impulsive, and impatient. The young child needs to touch, feel, and investigate.
   a. Consistent adult supervision will enable children to learn what they want to know within limits of safety for their stage of growth and development.
   b. Young children should never be left alone at home.
3. Children copy the behavior of their parents and absorb parental attitudes. Parents and other adults should be certain that their ways of doing things are safe.
4. Children become less careful and less willing to listen to warnings and to observe routine safety precautions when they are tired or hungry.
5. An estimated 90% of all accidents are preventable.

General Areas of Adult Responsibility for Child Safety

A. Motor Vehicle
1. All automobiles should be maintained in good mechanical condition.
2. Seat belts or car seats should be used at all times.
3. Driver should look carefully in front of and in back of the car before accelerating.
4. All car doors should be locked when a child travels in the car.
5. Young children should never be left alone in a car.
6. Heavy or sharp objects should not be placed on the same seat with a child.

B. Sports and Recreation
1. Keep equipment in good condition and proper working order.
2. Wear appropriate clothing and safety equipment for the activity.
3. Do not attempt activities beyond one's physical endurance.
4. Keep firearms and ammunition locked up.

C. Electrical and Mechanical Equipment
1. Only underwriter-approved devices should be installed; they should be inspected periodically.
2. Dry hands before touching appliances. Keep radios, transportable heaters, and hair dryers out of the bathroom.
3. Disconnect appliances after each use and before attempting minor repairs.
4. Keep garden equipment and machinery in a restricted area. Teach proper use of the equipment as soon as the child is old enough.
5. Avoid overloading electrical circuits.
6. Discourage children from playing with or being in area where appliances or power tools (eg, washing machine, clothes dryer, saw, lawn mower) are in operation.

D. *Prevention of Falls*
1. Keep stairs well lighted and free from clutter.
2. Provide sturdy railings.
3. Anchor small rugs securely.
4. Use rubber mats in the bathtub and shower.
5. Use only sturdy ladders for climbing.

E. *Poisonings and Ingestions*
1. Do not mix bleaches with ammonia, vinegar, and other household cleaners.
2. See section on ingested poisons and pediatric poisoning (p. 1110).
3. Become familiar with telephone number for poison control centers where available.
4. Label poisonous household materials and keep them out of child's reach.

F. *Fire*
1. Maintain an adequate fire escape plan and routinely conduct home fire drills. Teach children escape routes as soon as they are old enough.
2. Keep a pressure-type hand fire extinguisher on each floor. Instruct all family members who are old enough in its use.
3. Fit fireplaces with snug fireplace screens.
4. Store gasoline and other flammable fluids in tightly covered containers that are clearly labeled and away from heat and sparks.
5. Dispose of paint- and oil-soaked cloth quickly.
6. Use flame-retardant sleepwear.
7. Mark children's rooms so they are obvious to firemen.
8. Teach children about the danger of smoke inhalation.
9. Teach children to stop, drop, and roll if their clothing catches fire.
10. Maintain smoke detectors in working order.
11. Keep lights and matches out of reach of children.
12. Keep children away from heated oven, stovetop, and outdoor grill.

G. *Swimming Pools*
1. Completely enclose pool with a fence that complies with local regulations. The gate should be self-closing and have a lock.
2. Indicate water depth with numbers on the edge of the pool. Place a safety float line where the bottom of the slope begins to deepen.
3. Install at least one ladder at each end of the pool. Ladders should have handrails on both sides, and the diameter of the rails should be small enough for a child to grasp.
4. Use nonslip materials on ladders, deck, and diving boards.
5. Install underwater lighting as well as outdoor lights if the pool is used at night. A ground fault circuit interrupter should be installed on the pool circuit to cut off electrical power and thus prevent electrocutions should electrical fault occur.
6. Instruct children about safety rules such as not swimming alone and not running around the pool or pushing others. Avoid using radios or other electrical appliances around the pool.
7. Keep essential rescue devices and first-aid equipment close to the pool.

H. *Emergency Precautions*
1. Record emergency telephone numbers in an obvious and easily accessible place.
2. Keep a well stocked first-aid kit immediately available for emergencies.

3. Give instruction in principles of first aid to all family members who are old enough.
   a. Responsible adults should enroll in first-aid courses offered by the American Red Cross, adult education programs, etc.
   b. Be aware of first-aid procedure for:
      • Burns
      • Electrical shock
      • Poisoning
      • Bites and stings
      • Cuts, scrapes and punctures
      • Drowning
      • Fractures
      • Cardiopulmonary arrest
   c. Teach children safety precautions concerning bicycles, answering telephone, door, strangers outside the home, being a pedestrian.
4. Know the location of gas, water, and electrical switches and how to turn them off in an emergency.
5. Teach children their address and telephone number and how to dial 911 in case of emergency.

I. *Miscellaneous*
1. Take advantage of preventive health care.
   a. Obtain recommended immunizations.
   b. Have regular physical and dental examinations.
2. Seek immediate treatment of all diseases and health problems.
3. Balance periods of work, rest, and exercise in daily living.

Pediatric Care Techniques

◆ NURSING MANAGEMENT OF THE CHILD WITH FEVER

Fever is any abnormal elevation of body temperature. Prolonged elevation of temperature above 40°C (104°F) may produce dehydration and harmful effects on the central nervous system. See Procedure Guidelines 40-1 for administration of a tepid water sponge bath.

Causes

1. Infection
2. Inflammatory disease
3. Dehydration
4. Tumors
5. Disturbance of temperature-regulating center
6. Extravasation of blood in the tissues
7. Drugs or toxins

Assessment

1. Consider basic principles related to temperature regulation in pediatric patients.
   a. Usually an infant's temperature does not stabilize before 1 week of age. A newborn's temperature varies with the temperature of the environment.
   b. The degree of fever does not always reflect the severity of the disease. A child may have a serious illness with a normal or subnormal temperature.

c. Febrile seizures may occur in some children when the temperature rises rapidly.
d. The range for normal temperature varies widely in children. A common explanation for "fever" is misinterpretation of a normal temperature reading. Review temperature measurement with parents.
e. The child's temperature is influenced by activity and by the time of day; temperatures are highest in late afternoon.
2. Be certain that accurate technique is used for temperature measurement. The mode should be appropriate for the child's age and condition, and the thermometer should be left in place for the required period of time.
3. Assist the health care provider in determining the cause of the illness.
   a. History
      • Age of the child
      • Pattern of the fever
      • Length of the illness
      • Change in normal patterns of eating, elimination, recreation, etc.
      • Other symptoms
      • Exposure to any illness
      • Recent immunizations or drugs
      • Treatment of fever and effectiveness of treatment
      • Previous experiences with fever and its control
   b. Physical examination
      • General appearance of the child
      • Inspection of the skin for rashes, sores, flushed appearance
      • Inspection of eyes, ears, nose, and throat for redness and drainage
      • Auscultation of lungs for abnormal sounds
      • Neurologic observation for changes in state of consciousness, pupillary reaction, strength of grip, abnormal muscle movement, or lack of movement
      • Inspection of the external genitals for redness and drainage
      • Presence of abdominal or flank pain
   c. Laboratory tests
      Initial tests frequently include complete blood count; urinalysis; cultures of the throat, nasopharynx, urine, blood, spinal fluid; and chest x-ray.
4. Attempt to identify the pattern of the fever. Take the child's temperature by the same method every hour until stable, then every 2 hours until normal, then every 4 hours for 24 hours.

Nursing Measures to Reduce Fever

Fever itself does not necessarily require treatment. The presence of fever should not be obscured by the indiscriminate use of antipyretic measures. However, if the child is uncomfortable or appears toxic because of fever, an attempt should be made to reduce it by any of the following nursing measures or by a combination of these measures:

1. Increase the child's fluid intake to prevent dehydration.
2. Expose the skin to the air by leaving the child lightly dressed in absorbent material. Avoid warm, binding clothing and blankets.
3. Administer antipyretic drugs.
4. Use tub or a hypothermia blanket.

◆ ADMINISTERING MEDICATIONS TO CHILDREN

Administration of medication is often traumatic for children. Proper approach to administration can facilitate the process and enhance the child's understanding of the importance of taking medications.

Important Considerations

1. The manner of approach should indicate that the nurse firmly expects the child to take the medication. This manner often convinces the child of the necessity of the procedure. Establishing a positive relationship with the child will allow expression of feelings, concerns, and fantasies regarding medications.
2. Explanation about medication should appeal to the child's level of understanding (ie, through play or comparison to something familiar).
3. The nurse must mask his or her own feelings regarding the medication.
4. Always be truthful when the child asks, "Does it taste bad?" or "Will it hurt?" Respond by saying, "The medication does not taste good, but I will give you some juice as soon as you swallow it," or "It will hurt for just a minute, like a mosquito bite."
5. It is often necessary to mix distasteful medications or crushed pills with a small amount of carbonated drink, cherry syrup, or applesauce.
6. Never threaten a child with an injection when refusing oral medication.
7. Medications should not be mixed with large quantities of food or with any food that is taken regularly (eg, milk).
8. Medications should not be given at mealtime unless specifically prescribed.
9. The nurse must know the following about each medication being administered: common usages and dosages, contraindications, side effects, and toxic effects.
10. When preparing intramuscular injections, draw 0.2 mL of air after the correct amount of solution is in the syringe. This clears all medication from the needle on injection and prevents backflow and the depositing of medication in subcutaneous fat when the needle is withdrawn.

Calculating the Pediatric Dosage

The nurse is responsible for knowing that medication being given is within the safe dosage range for children.

1. Know what factors determine the amount of drug prescribed.
   a. Action of the drug, absorption, detoxification, excretion are related to the maturity and metabolic rate of the child.
   b. Neonates and premature infants require a reduced dosage because of:
      (1) Deficient or absent detoxifying enzymes
      (2) Decreased effective renal function
      (3) Altered blood–brain barrier and protein-binding capacity

c. Dosage recommended according to age groups are not satisfactory because a child may be much smaller or larger than the average child in the age group.

d. Dosage calculations based on weight have limitations.

2. Be alert to a prescription that would be inappropriate for a child.

3. Consult drug literature for recommended dosage and other information.

Body Surface Area

The following formulas are used to estimate the pediatric dosage based on the child's body surface area (BSA). BSA calculations are generally preferred because many physiologic processes in the child (ie, blood volume, glomerular filtration) are related to BSA.

1. Surface area in square meters × Dose per square meter = Approximate child dose

2. Surface area of child/surface area of adult × Dose of adult = Approximate child dose

3. Surface area of child in square meters/1.75 × Adult dose = Child dose

Clark's Rule

The following rule may be used as an estimate of the pediatric dosage based on the child's weight in respect to the adult dose of the drug.

Child's weight in pounds/150 × Adult dose

= Approximate dose for child

Identifying the Patient

Always check a child's identification bracelet with medication card before administering a medication. Ask the older child his or her name.

Oral Medications

A. Infants

1. Draw up medication in a plastic dropper or disposable syringe.

2. Elevate infant's head and shoulders; depress chin with thumb to open mouth.

3. Place dropper or syringe on the middle of the tongue and slowly drop the medication on the tongue.

4. Release thumb and allow child to swallow.

5. Once the correct amount of medication has been measured, it can be placed in a nipple and the infant can suck the medication through the nipple.

6. If the nurse feels comfortable managing the infant in his or her lap, it is acceptable to hold the infant for medication administration.

B. Toddlers

1. Draw up liquid medications in syringe or measure into medicine cup. Medications may be placed in medicine cup or spoon after being measured accurately in a syringe.

2. Elevate the child's head and shoulders.

3. Squeeze cup and put it to the child's lips; or place the syringe (without needle) in the child's mouth, positioning the syringe tip in space between cheek mucosa and gum, and slowly expel the medicine. Child may prefer using a familiar teaspoon.

4. Allow the child time to swallow.

5. Allow the child to hold the medicine cup if able and to drink it at own pace. (This may be a more agreeable method.) Offer a favorite drink as a "chaser," if not contraindicated.

6. The small safe medicine cups can be given to the child for play.

C. School-aged Children

1. When a child is old enough to take medicine in pill or capsule form, teach the child to place the pill near the back of the tongue and immediately swallow fluid such as water or fruit juice. If swallowing of the fluid is emphasized, the child will no longer think about the pill.

2. Always praise a child after taking medication.

3. If the child finds it particularly difficult to take oral medications, express understanding of fear and displeasure and offer help.

Intramuscular Medications

A. General Considerations for Intramuscular Injections

1. After the medication is drawn from vial, draw up additional 0.2 to 0.3 mL of air into a syringe, thus clearing needle of medication and preventing medication seepage from the injection site.

2. When injecting less than 1 mL of medication, use a tuberculin syringe for accuracy.

3. Cleanse site thoroughly, using friction with an antiseptic solution; let site dry.

4. Establish anatomic landmarks (Fig. 40-1). Alternate injection site and keep record at bedside or on medication card.

5. After penetrating site, aspirate to check for blood vessel puncture. If this occurs, withdraw needle and discard medicine and start again.

6. Following injection, massage site (unless contraindicated). The complication of fibrosis and contracture of the muscle can be diminished by massage, warm soaks, and range-of-motion exercises to disrupt and stretch immature scar tissue when multiple injections are being administered.

B. Infants

1. Acceptable site selection includes rectus femoris (mid anterior thigh), vastus lateralis (middle third), or ventrogluteal. These are relatively free of major nerves and blood vessels. The gluteus maximus and deltoid muscles are underdeveloped in the infant and use of these sites can result in nerve damage.

2. Administration

  a. Rectus femoris

    (1) Place the child in a secure position to prevent movement of the extremity.

    (2) Do not use a needle more than 2.5 cm (1 inch).

    (3) Use upper quadrant of the thigh.

    (4) Insert needle at a 45° angle in a downward direction, toward the knee.

  b. Vastus lateralis

    (1) Place the child in a prone or supine position.

    (2) Area is a narrow strip of muscle extending along a line from the greater trochanter to lateral femoral condyle below.

    (3) Insert needle perpendicular to skin 2 to 4 cm deep—needle parallel to floor.

  c. Ventrogluteal—see below.

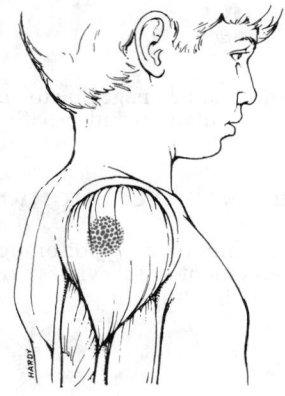

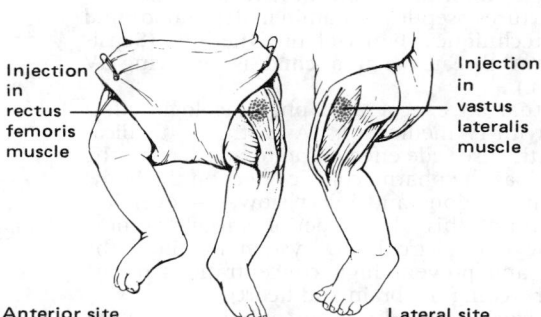

FIGURE 40-1 *Sites for IM injections in children.*

Arm for older child

Leg for small infant

3. Following administration of medication, hold and cuddle infant. The ventrogluteal site is also used on the older child who may be difficult to restrain.

C. **Toddlers and School-aged Children**
1. Site selection
   a. Posterogluteal—upper outer quadrant
      (1) Gluteal muscles do not develop until a child begins to walk; they should be used only when the child has been walking for 1 year or more. Complications include sciatic nerve injury or subcutaneous injury due to medication being injected, and poor absorption.
      (2) Upper outer quadrant of the young child's buttock is smaller in diameter than that of an adult; thus accuracy in determining the area comprising the upper outer quadrant is essential.
      (3) Administration
         (a) Do not use a needle longer than 2.5 cm (1 inch).
         (b) Position the child in a prone position.
         (c) Place thumb on the trochanter.
         (d) Place middle finger on the iliac crest.
         (e) Let index finger drop at a point midway between the thumb and middle finger to the upper outer quadrant of the buttock. This is the injection site.
         (f) Insert needle perpendicular to the surface on which the child is lying, not to the skin.
   b. Ventrogluteal
      (1) This site provides a dense muscle mass that is relatively free of the danger of injuring the nervous and vascular systems.
      (2) The disadvantage is that the injection site is visible to the child.
      (3) Administration
         (a) Place the child on back.
         (b) Place the index finger on the anterosuperior spine.
         (c) With the middle finger moving dorsally, locate the iliac crest; drop finger below the crest. The triangle formed by the iliac crest, index finger, and middle finger is the injection site.

         (d) Inject needle perpendicular to the surface on which the child is lying.
   c. Deltoid
      (1) May be used for older, larger children.
      (2) Determine injection site as with an adult.
      (3) Inject needle perpendicular to skin 2 to 3 cm deep.
   d. Lateral and anterior aspect of the thigh
      (1) Do not use a needle longer than 2.5 cm (1 inch).
      (2) Use the upper outer quadrant of the thigh.
      (3) Insert needle at a 45° angle in a downward direction, toward the knee.
2. Nursing support
   a. Explain to the child where you are going to give the injection (site) and why you are giving it.
   b. Allow the child to express fears.
   c. Carry out procedure quickly and gently. Have needle and syringe completely prepared and ready before contact with child.
   d. Numb site of injection by rubbing skin firmly with cleansing swab or with ice (older children may assist with this). Minimize pain of intramuscular injection by injecting needle into muscle with a quick, darting motion.
   e. Always secure the assistance of a second nurse to help immobilize the child and divert attention as well as to offer support and comfort.
   f. Praise the child for behavior after the injection. Often, allowing the child to assist with applying a Band-Aid will give some feeling of comfort.
   g. Also encourage activity that will use the muscle site of the injection—promotes dispersal of medication and decreases soreness. This can also be done by firmly massaging muscle following injection, unless contraindicated.
   h. Record accurately the injection site to ensure proper site rotation.

Intravenous Medications

1. Administration of intravenous (IV) medications may be done through a variety of techniques, including pig-

gyback, through a heparin lock, through a volume control set, or through an implantable port. See pages 1156–1160 for information on these techniques.

2. Prepare mixtures aseptically (laminar-flow hood) and use sterile technique when violating the line. (Sepsis is a constant threat when a child is receiving IV medications.)
3. Be aware that an exaggerated pharmacologic effect may exist with IV medications. As with any medication, know the use, side effects, and toxic effects of the drug, as well as the pharmacologic effect on the body.
4. Dilute IV medications and inject slowly—never less than 1 minute (this allows peripheral blood flow through the entire circulating system to dilute the medication and prevent high concentrations of the drug from reaching the brain and heart).
5. Be knowledgeable regarding compatibilities of drugs, electrolytes in IV solutions, and the fluid itself.
6. Observe IV site frequently. Restrain child, as needed, to prevent infiltration. Infiltration of fluids containing medications can cause rapid and severe tissue necrosis.

Special Considerations in Pediatric Primary Care

◆ ACUTE POISONING

Exposure to poisons can occur by ingestion, inhalation, or skin or mucous membrane contact. This section focuses on ingested poisonings because they are the most common type. Poisoning by ingestion refers to the oral intake of a harmful substance that, even in small amount, can damage tissues, disturb bodily functions, and possibly cause death. The substances may include medications, household products, and plants.

Etiology/Incidence

1. Improper or dangerous storage
2. Poor lighting—causes errors in reading
3. Human factors
   a. Failure to read label properly
   b. Failure to return poisons to their proper place
   c. Failure to recognize the material as poisonous
   d. Lack of supervision of the child
   e. Purposeful use of poison
4. Most often in children under 5 years of age with a peak incidence at 2 years of age
5. More than 80% of poisonings occur in the home
6. Poisoning accounts for approximately 10% to 20% of emergency department visits of which a high majority are pediatric patients.

Altered Physiology

Toxin is ingested and may have limited local effects or continue to a stage of absorption and interference with functioning of vital organ systems.

Complications

1. Arrhythmias
2. Permanent multiorgan damage due to initial loss of airway, breathing, circulation, and specific organ toxicity

Poisoning With Acetaminophen

Acetaminophen is a common drug poisoning agent in children due to its replacement of salicylates. Ingestion by adolescents is frequently intentional.

A. **Drug Action**
1. Antipyretic
2. Analgesic

B. **Clinical Manifestations**
1. Acetaminophen is toxic to the liver, resulting in cell necrosis and possibly cell death.
2. First 24 hours after ingestion
   a. May be asymptomatic
   b. Anorexia
   c. Nausea and vomiting
   d. Diaphoresis
   e. Malaise
   f. Pallor
3. Second 24 hours
   a. Above symptoms diminish or disappear.
   b. Right upper quadrant pain due to liver damage
   c. Elevated liver function tests
   d. Oliguria
4. Days 3 to 8
   a. Peak liver function abnormalities
   b. Anorexia, nausea, vomiting, and malaise may reappear.
5. Days 4 to 14
   a. Blood chemistry return to normal

C. **Diagnostic Measures**
1. Serum acetaminophen level 4 hours after ingestion

Note: Children under 6 years of age are unlikely to develop significant toxicity even with large doses of acetaminophen. Adolescents have higher incidences of toxic acetaminophen levels with markedly elevated liver enzymes.

D. **Treatment**
1. Syrup of ipecac
2. Gastric lavage
3. Charcoal
4. *n*-Acetylcysteine (Mucomyst) as antidote—if charcoal is given, lavage it out before giving Mucomyst.

Note: As with all treatments listed for poisons, airway, breathing, circulation, and treatment of shock are always the priority; see page 1160.

Iron Poisoning

This occurs frequently in childhood due to the prevalence of iron-containing preparations. The severity of iron poisoning is related to the amount of elemental iron absorbed. The range of potential toxicity is approximately 50 to 60 mg/kg.

A. *Drug Action*
1. Prevention of or treatment of iron deficiency anemia

B. *Clinical Manifestations*
1. 30 minutes to 2 hours after ingestion
   a. Local necrosis and hemorrhage of gastrointestinal tract
   b. Nausea and vomiting, including hematemesis
   c. Abdominal pain
   d. Diarrhea, often bloody
   e. Severe hypotension
   f. Symptoms subside after 6 to 12 hours.
2. 6 to 24 hours
   a. Period of apparent recovery
3. 24 to 40 hours
   a. Systemic toxicity with cardiovascular collapse, shock, hepatic and renal failure, seizures, coma, and possible death
   b. Metabolic acidosis
4. 2 to 4 weeks after ingestion
   a. Pyloric and duodenal stenosis
   b. Hepatic cirrhosis

C. *Diagnostic Evaluation*
1. Measurement of serum free iron
   a. Total serum iron
   b. Total serum iron-binding capacity
2. Abdominal x-ray to visualize iron tablets

D. *Treatment*
1. Administration of ipecac
2. Gastric lavage
3. Deferoxamine (Desferal) for severe cases. This drug binds with iron and is usually administered IV or intramuscularly.

Primary Assessment in Acute Poisoning

1. Use vital signs and neurologic assessment to determine a rough estimate of the child's status.

> **NURSING ALERT:** ❖
> It may be necessary to initiate emergency respiratory and circulatory support at this time. If needed, obtain venous access, maintain safety during seizure activity, and treat shock. Otherwise, continue with assessment.

2. Assess for symptomatic effects of poisoning by systems.
   a. Gastrointestinal—common in metallic acid, alkali, and bacterial poisoning. These may include nausea and vomiting, diarrhea, abdominal pain or cramping, and anorexia.
   b. Central nervous system (CNS)—may include convulsions (especially with CNS depressants such as alcohol, chloral hydrate, barbiturates) and behavioral changes. Dilated or pinpoint pupils may be noted.
   c. Skin rashes, burns to the mouth, esophagus and stomach, eye inflammation, skin irritations, stains around the mouth lesions of the mucous membranes. Cyanosis may be visible especially with cyanide and strychnine.

   d. Cardiopulmonary—dyspnea (especially with aspiration of hydrocarbons) and cardiopulmonary depression or arrest.
   e. Other—odor around the mouth
3. Identify the poison when possible.
   a. Determine the nature of the ingested substances from the child's history or by reading the label on the container. Nursing intervention may need to be implemented immediately after this assessment.
      (1) Call the nearest poison control center or toxicology section of the medical examiner's officer to identify the toxic ingredient and obtain recommendations for emergency treatment.
      (2) Save vomitus, stool, and urine for analysis once the child reaches the hospital.

Primary Interventions

A. *Assisting the Family by Telephone Management*
1. Calmly obtain and record the following information:
   a. Name, address, and telephone number of caller
   b. Evaluation of the severity of the ingestion
   c. Age, weight, and signs/symptoms of the child, including neurologic status
   d. Route of exposure
   e. Name of the ingested product, approximate amount ingested, and the time of ingestion
   f. Brief past medical history
   g. Caller's relationship to victim
2. Instruct the caller regarding appropriate emergency actions.
3. Direct the patient to the nearest emergency department. Dispatch an ambulance if necessary.
4. Instruct the caller to clear the child's mouth of any unswallowed poison.
5. Identify what treatments have already been initiated.
6. Instruct the parents to save vomitus, unswallowed liquid or pills, and the container and to bring them to the hospital as aids in identifying the poison.
7. Identify whether other children were involved in the poisoning to initiate treatment for them also.
8. If treatment is at home, follow-up phone calls should be made at $1/2$, 1, and 4 hours after exposure.

B. *Intervening Related to the Patient's Condition*
1. As described in Assessment, refer to previous section.
   a. Focus on airway, breathing, circulation.
   b. Identify the poison when possible.

C. *Removing the Poison From the Body*
1. Dilute with 6 to 8 oz of water if advised.
   a. For skin or eye contact, remove contaminated clothing and flush with water for 15 to 20 minutes.
   b. For inhalation poisons, remove from the exposed site.
2. Induce vomiting unless contraindicated.

> **NURSING ALERT:** ❖
> Do *not* induce vomiting if:
> 1. The child is convulsing, semiconscious, or comatose.
> 2. Poison is known to be a strong acid or alkali, strychnine, or a hydrocarbon (eg, lighter fluid, gasoline, kerosene, paint remover, or fingernail polish remover). Strong acids or alkalis may damage the esophagus for a second time during emesis, and hydrocarbons can cause severe pneumonia if aspirated.

a. For children over 6 months if age, administer syrup of ipecac according to the directions on the label.
b. If no vomiting occurs after 20 to 30 minutes, repeat this process one time only.

NURSING ALERT:
Do not use tincture of ipecac; it is much stronger than the syrup and is itself a poison.
Also, do not administer household neutralizing foods/products (unless physician recommended) because of the heat that is generated by the chemical reaction and the burn that could result (or exacerbation of the existing burn).

c. Position the child with head down or on his side to prevent aspiration of vomitus.
3. Administer gastric lavage. (This is indicated when vomiting is impossible because of the child's condition or age, when induction of vomiting has been unsuccessful, or when the poison is one that is rapidly absorbed, eg, cyanide.) See page 962.
4. Follow lavage with a cathartic and activated charcoal to hasten removal of the poison from the gastrointestinal tract.
a. Use cautiously with young children.
5. Be aware of the dangers associated with lavage.
a. Esophageal perforation—may occur in corrosive poisoning.
b. Gastric hemorrhage
c. Impaired pulmonary function resulting from aspiration
d. Cardiac arrest
e. Convulsions—may result from stimulation in strychnine ingestion.

D. *Reducing the Effect of the Poison by Administering an Antidote*
1. An antidote may either react with the poison to prevent its absorption or counteract the effects of the poison after its absorption.
2. Not all poisons have specific antidotes.
3. Information regarding appropriate antidotes for specific poisons is available through all poison control centers. Antidotes for the most common poisons should be listed in the emergency department of the hospital.
4. Effectiveness of the antidote usually depends on the amount of time that elapses between ingestion of the poisons and administration of the antidote.
5. Activated charcoal absorbs all poisons except cyanide, if given within 1 hour of poisoning and after vomiting has occurred, in a dose of 30 to 50 g in a child and 50 to 100 g in an adolescent in 175 to 250 mL (6–8 oz) of water with sweetener.

Note: Charcoal inactivates ipecac; therefore administer charcoal only *after* ipecac has induced vomiting.

E. *Eliminating the Absorbed Poison*
1. Force diuresis
a. Administer large quantities of fluid either orally or IV.
b. Carefully monitor intake and output.
2. Assist with kidney dialysis, which may be necessary if the child's own kidneys are not functioning effectively.
3. Assist with exchange transfusion if this method is indicated for removing the poison.

F. *Providing Emotional Support*
1. Remain calm and efficient while working rapidly.

2. Reassure child and family that therapeutic measures are being taken immediately.
3. Discourage anxious parents from holding, caressing, and overstimulating child.

Subsequent Nursing Assessment and Interventions

A. *Observing the Child for Progression of Symptoms*
1. CNS involvement
a. Observe for restlessness, confusion, delirium, seizures, lethargy, stupor, or coma.
b. Administer sedation with caution—to avoid CNS depression and masking of symptoms.
c. Avoid excessive manipulation of the child.
d. See nursing care of the child with seizures, page 1233.
e. See nursing care of the unconscious patient, Chapter 13.
2. Respiratory involvement
a. Observe for respiratory depression, obstruction, pulmonary edema, pneumonia, or tachypnea.
b. Have artificial airway and tracheostomy set available.
c. Be prepared to administer oxygen and provide artificial respiration.
d. Other nursing concerns:
(1) Nursing care for mechanical ventilation, page 1190.
(2) Procedures for administration of oxygen, page 1191.
(3) Procedure for cardiopulmonary resuscitation, page 942.
3. Cardiovascular involvement
a. Observe for peripheral circulatory collapse, disturbances of heart rate and rhythm, or cardiac failure.
b. Maintain IV therapy as directed to prevent shock. Assess for complications of overhydration.
c. Be prepared for cardiac arrest.
4. Gastrointestinal involvement
a. Observe for nausea, pain, abdominal distention, and difficulty swallowing.
b. Maintain IV therapy to replace water and electrolyte losses.
c. Offer a diet that is easily swallowed and digested.
(1) Begin with clear liquids.
(2) Progress to full liquids, soft foods, and then a regular diet as the child's condition improves.
5. Kidney involvement
a. Observe the child for decreased urine output. Record oral and IV intake and urine output exactly.
b. Observe for hypertension.
c. Insert indwelling catheter if necessary for urinary retention.
d. Administer appropriate amounts of fluids and electrolytes.
e. See nursing care of child with renal failure, page 1284.
f. Correct and monitor acid–base balance.
6. General considerations
a. Maintain adequate caloric, fluid, and vitamin intake. Oral fluids are preferable if they can be retained.
b. Avoid hypothermia or hyperthermia. (Control of body temperature is impaired in many types of poisoning.) Monitor the child's temperature frequently.

c. Observe closely for inflammation and tissue irritation.
 (1) This is especially important in ingestion of kerosene or other hydrocarbons, which cause chemical pneumonitis.
 (2) Isolate the patient from other children, especially those with respiratory infections.
 (3) Administer antibiotics as prescribed by the physician.
d. Counsel parents who often feel guilty about the accident.
 (1) Encourage parents to talk about the poisoning.
 (2) Emphasize how their quick action in getting treatment for the child has helped.
 (3) Discuss ways that they can be supportive to their child during the hospitalization.
 (4) Do not allow prolonged periods of self-incrimination to continue. Refer parents to a psychologist for assistance in resolving these feelings if necessary.
e. Involve the young child in therapeutic play to determine how he views the situation.
 (1) The child often sees nursing measures as punishments for misdeed involving the poisoning.
 (2) Explain treatment and correct misinterpretations in a manner appropriate for child's age.
f. Initiate a community health nursing referral. A home assessment should be made so that underlying problems are recognized and appropriate help is provided.

Note: Initiate patient and parental teaching only after the acute episode is over.

Health Education

A. Prevention
1. Information concerning poison prevention should be available on every hospital pediatric unit and during every child health care visit.
 a. Many free booklets and home safety checklists are available from sources such as insurance companies and drug companies.
 b. Teaching may be done with any parent regardless of the reason for the child's hospitalization or office visit.
2. Teach the following precautions:
 a. Keep medicines and poisons out of reach of children.
 b. Provide locked storage for highly toxic substances; select cabinet that is higher than child can reach or climb.
 c. Do not store poisons in the same areas as foods.
 d. Be certain all containers are properly marked and labeled. Keep medicines, drugs, and household chemicals in their original containers.
 e. Do not discard poisonous substances in receptacles where children can reach them, but *do* discard used containers of poisonous substances.
 f. Teach children not to taste or eat unfamiliar substances.
 g. Clean out medicine cabinets periodically.
 h. Keep medications in child-proof containers that are securely closed.
 i. Read all labels carefully before each use.
 j. Do not give medicines prescribed for one child to another.
 k. Never refer to drugs as candy or bribe children with such inducements.
 l. Never give or take medications in the dark.
 m. Encourage parents not to take medication in front of young children because children role-play adult behavior.
 n. Suggest that mothers *not* keep medications in their purses or on the kitchen table.
 o. Keep baby creams and ointments away from young children.
 p. Never puncture or burn aerosol containers.
 q. Store lawn and garden pesticides in a separate place under lock and key outside of the house; do not store large quantities of cleaning products, pesticides, etc.
 r. Keep a 30-mL (1-oz) bottle of ipecac syrup; be familiar with how to use it.
 s. Keep a list of emergency telephone numbers including the poison control center, physician's number, nearest hospital, and ambulance service.
 t. Reinforce the need for vigilance and consistent supervision of infants and young children due to their increased mobility, increased curiosity, and increased dexterity.

B. Emergency Actions to Teach Parents
1. Suspect poisoning with the occurrence of sudden, bizarre symptoms or peculiar behavior in toddlers and preschoolers.
2. Read label on the ingested product or call the health care provider, hospital, or poison control center for instructions regarding treatment for the poisoning. Give all relevant information about the child, condition, and substance taken.
3. Maintain an adequate airway in a child who is convulsing or who is not fully conscious.
4. Dilute the poison with 6 to 8 oz of water if advised.
5. Make the child vomit if so directed. Do not induce vomiting if any of the following occurs:
 a. The child is unconscious or convulsing.
 b. Ingested poison was a strong corrosive such as lye or drain cleaner.
 c. Ingested poison contains gasoline, kerosene, or other petroleum distillates.
6. Directions for making the child vomit:
 a. Administer 1 tablespoon of ipecac syrup with 250 mL (1 cup) of warm water.
 b. If vomiting does not occur in 20 minutes, this dose may be repeated once only.
7. Transport the child promptly to the nearest medical facility.
 a. Wrap the child in a blanket to prevent chilling.
 b. Bring the container and any vomitus or urine to the hospital with the child.
8. Avoid excessive manipulation of the child.
9. Act promptly but calmly.
10. Do not assume the child is safe simply because the emesis shows no trace of the poison or because the child appears well. The poison may have produced a delayed reaction or may have reached the small intestine where it is still being absorbed.

◆ LEAD POISONING

Lead poisoning (plumbism) results from the consumption of lead in some form. Lead poisoning is the best known of the environmental causes of illness in children. A small number of these children may die, but many are left with mental, emotional, and physical deficits.

Etiology/Incidence

1. Multiple episodes of chewing on, sucking, or ingestion of nonfood substances (pica)
   a. Toys, furniture, window sills, household fixtures, and plaster painted with lead-containing paint

   Note: Legislation stipulates that toys, children's furniture, and the interior of homes be painted with lead-free paint; however, the problem may continue if the deeper layers of paint and plaster are contaminated with lead. One paint chip contains much more lead than is considered safe.

   b. Cigarette butts and ashes
   c. Acidic juices or foods served in lead-based earthenware pottery made with lead glazes
   d. Colored paints used in newspapers, magazines, children's books, matches, playing cards, and food wrappers
   e. Water from lead pipes
   f. Fruit covered with insecticides
   g. Dirt containing lead fallout from automobile exhaust
   h. Antique pewter, especially when used to serve acidic juices or foods
   i. Lead weights (curtain weights, fishing sinkers)
   j. Continuous proximity to lead-processing center
   k. Occupations or hobbies that use lead
2. Inhalation of fumes containing lead (less common cause in children)
   a. Leaded gasoline
   b. Burning storage batteries
   c. Dust-containing lead salts
   d. Dust in the air at shooting galleries and in enclosed firing ranges with poor ventilation
   e. Cigarette smoke
3. Highest incidence in children between 1 and 6 years of age, especially those between 1 and 3 years
4. High incidence in individuals living in old homes or deteriorated housing conditions
5. No significant difference in incidence by sex
6. High incidence among siblings
7. Symptomatic lead poisoning occurs most frequently in summer months.
8. Recurrence rate is high, especially if lead is not removed from the home environment.

Epidemiologic Factors

1. Millions of children live in housing built before 1950, which contains the highest surface soil level and internal household dust contaminated with lead.
2. Normal hand-to-mouth activities of children may introduce leaded household dust, soil, and nonfood items into their gastrointestinal tract.
3. Pica (ie, leaded paint chips) is generally associated with more severe degrees of poisoning.

Altered Physiology

1. Lead absorption from gastrointestinal tract is affected by age, diet, and nutritional deficiency.
   a. Young children absorb 40% to 50% and retain 20% to 25 % of dietary lead.
2. It takes the body twice as long to excrete lead as it does to absorb it.
3. Lead is stored in two places in the body:
   a. Bone
   b. Soft tissue
4. Principle toxic effects occur in nervous systems, bone marrow, and kidneys.
5. Nervous system
   a. Brain—increased capillary permeability results in edema, increased intracranial pressure, and vascular damage; destruction of brain cells causes seizures, mental retardation, paralysis, blindness, and learning disabilities.
   b. Neurologic damage cannot be reversed.
   c. CNS of young children and fetuses is most sensitive to lead.
6. Bone marrow
   a. Lead attaches to red blood cells.
   b. Inhibition of a number of steps in the biosynthesis of heme, thus reducing the number of red blood cells, increasing fragility, and reducing half-life.
   c. The decreased production of hemoglobin results in anemia and respiratory distress.
7. Kidneys—injury to the cells of the proximal tubules, causing increased excretion of amino acids, protein, glucose, and phosphate.

Complications

1. Severe and often permanent mental, emotional and physical impairment
2. Neurologic deficits
   a. Learning disabilities
   b. Mental retardation
   c. Seizures
   d. Encephalopathy

Clinical Manifestations

Symptoms in young children may develop insidiously and may abate spontaneously.

1. Gastrointestinal—anorexia, sporadic vomiting, intermittent abdominal pain (colic), constipation
2. CNS—hyperirritability; decreased activity; personality changes; loss of recently acquired developmental skills; falling, clumsiness, loss of coordination (ataxia); local paralysis; peripheral nerve palsies
3. Hematologic—anemia, pallor
4. Cardiovascular—hypertension, bradycardia
5. Encephalopathy may occur 4 to 6 weeks following first symptoms:
   a. Sudden onset of persistent vomiting
   b. Severe ataxia
   c. Altered state of consciousness
   d. Coma
   e. Seizures
   f. Massive cerebral edema in younger children

Diagnostic Evaluation

1. Detailed history with emphasis on the presence or absence of clinical symptoms, evidence of pica, family history of lead poisoning, possible source of exposure to lead, recent change in behavior, developmental delay, or behavior problems, recent change of address, or recent renovations in the home.
2. Serum lead level (Table 40-4).
3. Hematologic evaluation for iron deficiency anemia.
4. Flat plate of abdomen—may reveal radiopaque material if lead has been ingested during the preceding 24 to 36 hours.
5. Erythrocyte protoporphyrin level—not sensitive enough for identifying lead levels below approximately 25 mg/dL. Can be used to follow levels after medical and environmental interventions for poisoned children have occurred. A progressive decline in erythrocyte protoporphyrin levels indicates management is successful.
6. 24-hour urine—more accurate than a single voided specimen in determining elevated urinary components that correspond with elevated blood lead levels.
7. Radiologic examination of long bones—unreliable for diagnosis of acute lead poisoning; may provide some indication of past lead poisoning or length of time poisoning has occurred.
8. Edetate disodium calcium provocation chelation test—used only in selected medical centers treating large numbers of lead-poisoned children, demonstrates increased lead levels in urine over an 8-hour period after injection of edetate disodium.

Treatment

A. **Removal of Lead From Environment**
1. Leaded paint/paint chips or objects containing lead must be removed from the child's environment.
2. Child should be away from environment during paint-stripping process.

B. **Low-Fat, High-Iron Diet**
1. To treat associated anemia
2. Iron supplements may be needed.

C. **Chelation Therapy**
1. Edetate calcium disodium (EDTA), British anti-Lewisite (BAL), and succimer (Chemet) bind with lead in the blood to form nontoxic compounds that are excreted by bowel and kidney.
2. Effectiveness of therapy depends on degree and duration of lead poisoning.
3. BAL is given first to decrease the chance of seizures.
   a. Used alone in patients with encephalopathy
   b. Do not give with iron supplements and avoid in patients with plant allergies.
   c. Avoid in patients with glucose-6-phosphate dehydrogenase (G6PD) deficiency due to hemolysis.
   d. Administered deep intramuscularly—results in pain and tissue necrosis at the injection site.
4. EDTA may be toxic to the kidneys.
   a. Monitor urinary output as well as kidney and liver function studies.
   b. Administer IV.
5. Chemet—approved for use in 1991.
   a. Not given to patients with encephalopathy
   b. Administer orally.
6. Dosage—depends on individual drug, the child's weight, severity of poisoning, prior history, and whether or not other chelating agents are being used simultaneously.
7. Chelating drugs are usually given every 4 hours for 5 days. A second course of therapy may be needed if there is a rebound in the blood lead level.
8. Increased oral and IV fluids are given to enhance excretion, except if increased intracranial pressure is present.

TABLE 40-4 Interpretation of Blood Lead Test Results and Follow-up Activities: Class of Child Based on Blood Lead Concentration

Class	Blood Lead Concentrations (μg/dL)	Comment
I	≤9	A child in class I is not considered to be lead poisoned.
IIA	10–14	Many children (or a large proportion of children) with blood lead levels in this range should trigger communitywide childhood lead poisoning prevention activities. Children in this range may need to be rescreened more frequently.
IIB	15–19	A child in class IIB should receive nutritional and educational interventions and more frequent screening. If the blood level persists in this range, environmental investigation and intervention should be done.
III	20–44	A child in class III should receive environmental evaluation and remediation and a medical evaluation. Such a child may need pharmacologic treatment of lead poisoning.
IV	45–69	A child in class IV will need both medical and environmental interventions, including chelation therapy.
V	≥70	A child with class V lead poisoning is a medical emergency. Medical and environmental management must begin immediately.

Source: Centers for Disease Control (1991). Preventing lead poisoning in young children. Atlanta, GA: U.S. Department of Health and Human Services, Public Health Service.

9. D-Penicillamine (Depen), another drug that chelates heavy metals, may be given for long-term chelation only if current exposure to lead is definitely excluded. If this drug is used, it should be given on an empty stomach, 2 hours before breakfast.

D. Additional Treatment
1. Supplemental calcium, phosphorus, and vitamin D to help lead move from the blood (where it is toxic) to the bones (where it is nontoxic)
2. For the child with encephalopathy, corticosteroids are given and intensive care management is maintained until acute stage is resolved.

Nursing Assessment

1. Early detection is key in preventing complications related to plumbism. All children should be assessed for early indicators of lead toxicity, including hyperactivity, developmental delay, constipation, anorexia, colicky abdominal pain, clumsiness, and pallor.
2. Inquire about presence of pica behavior in all children under 6 years of age.
   a. Observe and record the child's eating habits and food preferences.
   b. Report any attempted eating of nonfood substances.
   c. Provide regular meals and make mealtime a pleasurable time for the child.
   d. Discourage oral activity and substitute activity that contributes to play, social skills, and ego development.
   e. Refer the family for additional social or psychiatric casework if indicated to reduce the psychological or cultural factors that result in pica in the child.
3. Screen siblings and playmates of known cases immediately.
4. Screen all children from high-risk areas on a routine basis.
5. Asses the child's level of development. The Denver Developmental Screening Test (DDST) may be useful for this purpose (see p. 1070) and will help detect delays possibly caused by lead poisoning.

Nursing Diagnoses

A. Risk for Injury related to seizures and encephalopathy
B. Pain related to chelation therapy injections
C. Altered Growth and Development related to the effects of chronic lead exposure
D. Compromised Family Coping related to guilt and concern for child

Nursing Interventions

A. Preventing Seizures and Providing Supportive Care to the Child With Encephalopathy
1. Maintain seizure precautions.
   a. Crib or bed rails elevated and padded
   b. Tongue blade and suction equipment at bedside
2. Observe for signs of increased intracranial pressure:
   a. Rising blood pressure
   b. Papilledema
   c. Slow pulse
   d. Seizures
   e. Unconsciousness

3. Provide supportive care to maintain vital functions. Care is similar to that of child with Reye's syndrome (see p. 1241).

B. Reducing Pain Associated With Chelation Therapy
1. Plan appropriate play activities to prepare the child for the injections and as an outlet for pain and anger child feels.
2. Implement measures to decrease pain at injection site.
   a. Rotate sites of injection.
   b. Apply warm packs to site to decrease pain.
   c. Move painful areas slowly.
3. Provide diversional activities, fluids, and meals between injections.
4. Monitor intake and output and blood studies such as electrolytes and liver and kidney function tests as directed.

C. Promoting Growth and Development
1. Provide and encourage activities that will help the child to learn and progress from present developmental state to meet next appropriate milestone.
2. Initiate appropriate referrals in cases of obvious developmental delays or learning difficulties. Such referrals may be to such professionals as psychologists, psychiatrists, and specialists in early child education.
3. Share the results of developmental testing with the parent(s) and discuss ways to provide stimulation for the child at home.

D. Strengthening Family Coping
1. Use sensitivity in interviewing and teaching to avoid causing or increasing guilt feelings about the poisoning and to establish a positive, trusting relationship between the family and the health care facility.
2. Explain the treatment and its purpose because parents are frequently faced with putting asymptomatic child through painful treatments.
3. Encourage frequent visits by parents and siblings and facilitate involvement in child care.

Family Education/Health Maintenance

A. Long-term Follow-up
1. Teach the parents why long-term follow-up is important. Tell them that residual lead is liberated gradually after treatment and:
   a. May result in the renewal of symptoms
   b. May increase serum lead to a dangerous level
   c. Cause additional damage to the CNS, which may not become apparent for several months
2. Stress that acute infections must be recognized and treated promptly because these may reactivate the disease.
3. Teach that iron supplementation may be continued to treat anemia. Advise on administration and side effects and periodic complete blood count monitoring.

B. Preventing Reexposure of the Child to Lead
1. Advise parents that the single most important factor in managing childhood lead poisoning is reducing the child's re-exposure to lead.

NURSING ALERT: ◆◆◆
Children should not be discharged from the hospital until their home environment is lead free.

2. Instruct that parents regarding the seriousness of repeated lead exposure.
3. Initiate referrals to community outreach workers so that environmental case management is conducted. Lead abatement must be conducted by experts, not untrained parents, property owners, or contractors.
4. Suggest periodic, focused household cleaning to remove the lead dust; use a wet mop.
5. Encourage handwashing before meals and at bedtime to eliminate lead consumption from normal hand-to-mouth activity.
6. Make certain that the family is able to provide close supervision of the child or assist them to make arrangements to ensure that the child is adequately supervised at home.

C. *Community Education*
1. Initiate and support educational campaigns through schools, day-care centers, and news media to alert parents and children to hazards and symptoms of lead poisoning.
2. Provide in clinics, waiting rooms, and other appropriate settings literature stressing the hazards of lead, sources of lead, and signs of lead intoxication.
3. Support legislation to study the nature and extent of the lead poisoning problem and to eliminate the causes of lead poisoning.
4. Include the topic of pica and lead poisoning in nutritional teaching.
5. For additional information contact the state or local health department or Center for Disease Control and Prevention (CDC).

Evaluation

A. Seizure precautions maintained; no signs of increased intracranial pressure
B. Tolerating BAL injections; expressing anger through doll play
C. Parents providing appropriate play and stimulation for development
D. Family involved in care; providing support to the child

◆ COMMUNICABLE DISEASES

With the dramatic success of immunizations, many childhood diseases have decreased in frequency. However a number of communicable diseases still cause significant morbidity in children. See Table 40-5.

◆ CHILD ABUSE AND NEGLECT

Child abuse is any maltreatment of children or adolescents by their parents, guardians, or caretakers. Child abuse includes physical or emotional abuse, injury, trauma, neglect, or sexual abuse of a child that is intentional and nonaccidental. Abuse includes:

- Battering—physical injury
- Drug abuse—intentional administration of harmful drugs, especially during pregnancy
- Sexual abuse
- Sexual assault or molestation (nonfamily offender)
- Incest (family offender)
- Emotional abuse—scape-goating, belittling, humiliating, lack of mothering

Neglect is omission of certain appropriate behaviors, with such omission having detrimental physical or psychological effects on development. Neglect includes:

- Child abandonment
- Lack of provision of the basic needs of survival: shelter, clothing, stimulation, medical care, food, love, supervision, education, attention, emotional nurturing, and safety

Etiology/Incidence

Child abuse is not a uniform phenomenon with one set of causal factors, but is multidimensional. The abuse may be related to the combined presence of three factors: special kind of child, special kind of parent or caretaker, special circumstances of crisis. Abuse occurs in all ethnic, geographic, religious, educational, occupational, and socioeconomic groups.

1. Approximately 1% of all children are abused or neglected.
2. Each year, 4,000 children die from abuse.

Contributing Factors

1. Incidents of child abuse may develop as a result of disciplinary action taken by the abuser who responds in uncontrolled anger to real or perceived misconduct of the child. The parents may confuse punishment with discipline. "Good parenting" may be equated with physical contact to eradicate child behavior. The abuser may be a stern, authoritarian disciplinarian.
2. Incidents of child abuse may develop out of a quarrel between caretakers. The child may come to the aid of one parent, may find self in the midst of the quarrel; martial discord is common.
3. The abuser may be under a great deal of stress because of life circumstances (debt, poverty, illness) and may thus resort to child abuse. Crisis and stress may be ongoing. The abuser may have a low frustration tolerance level and may not have well developed means of coping with stress in general.
4. The abuser may be intoxicated with alcohol or drugs at the time of the abuse; only 10% of abusers have a history of mental illness.
5. Child abuse frequently occurs while the mother is away from the home and the child is left in the care of a babysitter or boyfriend.
6. Lack of effective parenting, inappropriate parent–child bonding, and punitive treatment as a child may contribute to the parent becoming an abuser.
7. Specific characteristics evident in many abusing parents include:
   a. Low self-esteem—a sense of incompetence in role, unworthiness, unimportance, have difficulty controlling aggressive impulses, and often live in social isolation

b. Unrealistic attitudes and expectations of child, little regard for the child's own needs and age appropriate abilities, lack of knowledge related to parenting skills

c. Fear of rejection—a deep need to feel wanted and loved, but a feeling of rejection when love is not obvious; a crying infant may elicit a feeling of rejection.

d. Inability to accept help—isolation from the community, loneliness

e. Unhappiness due to unsatisfactory relationships; may look to child for satisfaction of own emotional needs.

f. Child abusers are often the children of abuse or victims of spousal abuse.

8. Incidents of child abuse may develop from a general attitude or resentment or rejection on the part of the abuser toward the child.

9. Atypical child behavior (eg, hyperactivity or a technology-dependent child who needs additional care may unintentionally provoke the abuser)

10. The degree of the family crisis is not usually in proportion to the degree of abuse.

Clinical Manifestations

A. **Characteristics of the Child Used as an Index of Suspicion**

1. Child usually under 3 years of age. School-aged children and adolescents are also subject to abuse. The average age of a sexually abused child is 9 years.

2. General health of child indicates neglect (diaper rash, poor hygiene, malnutrition, unattended physical problem).

3. Characteristic distribution of fractures (scattered over many parts of body)

4. Disproportionate amount of soft tissue injury

5. Evidence that injuries occurred at different times (healed and new fractures, resolving and fresh bruises)

6. Cause of recent trauma in question

7. History of similar episodes in the past

8. No new lesions occurring during the child's stay in hospital

9. May show a wide range of reactions—may be either very withdrawn or overactive. The child may be anxious, tense, or nervous.

10. Child may show unusual affection for strangers or may be overly fearful of adults and avoid any physical contact with them.

11. For sexual abuse: child may fear no one will believe him or her; may experience self-blame; most know their abuser.

12. Children may not "tell" about abuse from parents, fearing loss of security; "a bad parent is better than no parent at all."

13. Behavior problems, depression, and acting-out behaviors may result.

14. For abuse that occurs in school or day care, the child may exhibit fear of the teacher, have nightmares, decrease school attendance, or develop psychosomatic illnesses.

B. **Injuries or Types of Abuse That May Occur**

1. Bruises, welts (linear or looplike)

2. Abrasions, contusions, lacerations (most common)

3. Wounds, cuts, punctures

4. Burns (cigarette, radiator, etc.) scalding—stocking or glove distribution

5. Bone fractures

6. Sprains, dislocations

7. Subdural hemorrhage or hematoma; "shaken baby syndrome"

8. Brain damage

9. Internal injuries

10. Drug intoxication

11. Malnutrition (deliberately inflicted)

12. Freezing, exposure

13. Whiplash-type injury

14. Eye injuries, periorbital injuries, ear bruises

15. Dirty, infected wounds or rashes

16. Unexplained coma in infant

17. Failure to thrive—developmental delay; malnutrition with decreased muscle mass; decreased interaction with environment and with others; dental caries; listless, behavior problems

18. Sexually transmitted diseases—genital trauma, recurrent urinary tract infection, pregnancy

Treatment

The goal of treatment is to ensure the physical and emotional safety of the child. Therefore, treatment is inclusive of other family members and caretakers.

1. It is estimated that 80% to 90% of abusing parents can be rehabilitated.

2. The ideal approach is to return the child to biologic parents.

3. Treatment is offered to help parents do the following:

a. Understand and redirect their anger

b. Develop an adequate parent–child relationship

c. See their child as an individual with own needs and differences

d. Enjoy the child

e. Develop realistic expectations of their child

f. Decrease their use of criticism

g. Increase their own sense of self-esteem and confidence

h. Establish supportive relationships with others

i. Improve their economic situation (if appropriate)

j. Show progress toward physical, emotional, and intellectual development of their child

Nursing Assessment

A. **Early Recognition of Potential Abuse**

1. Identify family or child at risk: alcohol/drug abuser, adolescent parent, low-income single-parent family, multiple births, or unwanted child; sickly and more demanding child or premature with long separation from mother at birth.

2. Use community resources and special programs (ie, "hot lines," crisis nurseries, self-help groups) to aid the parent in preventive support.

B. **Inspecting Every Child's Body for Evidence of Possible Abuse**

1. Describe completely on nursing records all bruises, lacerations, and similar lesions as to location and state of healing. Look carefully at areas generally covered with clothing (ie, buttocks, underarms, behind knees, bottom of feet). Be alert for abuse of the school-aged child.

2. Quote descriptions of the injury, including the date, time, and place of the event. Describe old, healing injuries; assess developmental level.

3. Collect any necessary specimens for identification of organisms, sperm, or semen.

4. Take color photographs.

5. Discuss with the health care provider the case of any child suspected of being abused.

C. *Observing for Behaviors Common in Abusing or Neglecting Parent(s)*

Be aware that not all abusing parents exhibit these behaviors but be alert for parent(s) who:

1. Anxiously volunteers information or withholds information related to an injury.

2. Gives explanation of the injury that does not fit the condition or gets story confused concerning the injury.

3. Shows inappropriate reaction or concern to severity of injury.

4. Becomes irritable about questions being asked.

5. Seldom touches or speaks to the child; does not respond to child. May be critical or indicate unreal expectations of child (or may be over solicitous to child).

6. Delays seeking medical help; refuses to sign permit for diagnostic studies; frequently changes hospitals or health care providers.

7. Shows no involvement in care of the hospitalized child; does not inquire about the child.

8. Obtains little or no prenatal care and shows inappropriate response to newborn; acts disinterested or unhappy with child.

D. *Observing the Parent–Child Relationship*

1. Do parents visit the child? Do parents become involved in caring for child?

2. How do(es) the parent(s) respond to the child? Does the parent talk to the child, touch, hold, and play with the child?

3. How does the child react to the parent? Is child excited when parent arrives? Does child appear frightened and withdrawn? Does child cry when parent leaves?

4. What does the parent expect of the child? Are expectations appropriate for the child? Is there role reversal between parent and child?

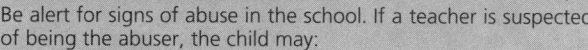

COMMUNITY-BASED CARE TIP:
Be alert for signs of abuse in the school. If a teacher is suspected of being the abuser, the child may:
1. Display increased fear of the teacher
2. Decrease school attendance
3. Develop psychosomatic symptoms during school days
4. Develop nightmares
5. Worry excessively over school performance

E. *Assessing for Sexual Abuse*

1. Asses for signs of sexual abuse. Sexual abuse should be suspected when the young, prepubertal child presents with:

a. Trauma not readily explained

b. Gonorrhea, syphilis, or other sexually transmitted organisms

c. Blood in urine or stool

d. Painful urination or defecation

e. Penile or vaginal infection or itch

f. Penile or vaginal discharge

g. Report of increased, excessive masturbation

h. Report of increased, unusual fears

2. Establish a relationship with the child based on mutual respect, empathy, and sensitivity to facilitate further investigation.

a. Consideration of the child's emotions in conjunction with a good relationship may encourage the child to express feelings either verbally or through drawings or play.

b. Prepare the child both physically and psychologically for the necessary physical and pelvic examination.

c. Talk with the child without the presence of the parents, especially when incest is possible.

F. *Reporting Suspicion of Child Abuse*

1. Be aware that all states (as well as the District of Columbia) have mandatory reporting laws based on Public Law 94-247 (Child Abuse and Neglect Act 1973). All states provide statutory immunity for those who report real or suspected child abuse. There is no immunity from civil or criminal liability for failure to report such. Notify the appropriate officials.

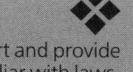

NURSING ALERT:
Every nurse is morally and legally responsible to report and provide protective services for the abused child. Become familiar with laws, procedures, and protective services in your community and state.

2. Prepare other children in family to be examined as soon as possible because they may be involved as well.

3. Establish and maintain a therapeutic relationship with the parents. Generally a team approach is recommended to assess family needs and determine the most effective use of community resources to protect the child and help the family. The parents are the focus of treatment. They are helped to develop a sense of self-esteem and confidence and to relinquish their abusive behavior.

Nursing Diagnoses

A. Fear of Adults related to experiences with abuse

B. Altered Parenting related to abusive treatment of child

A. *Relieving Fear and Fostering Trust*

1. Be aware that some of these children have never learned how to trust an adult; they are fearful of giving affection for fear of rejection.

2. Assign one nurse to care for the child over a period of time.

3. Make no threatening moves toward the child. The child will indicate readiness and awareness of the environment by verbal or facial expressions.

4. Touch the child gently.

5. Provide nonthreatening physical contact (hold and frequently cuddle child). Pick up and carry child around; encourage any exploration of your face, hair, etc.

6. Enlist the cooperation of volunteers to provide additional mothering.

7. Provide appropriate opportunities for play.

8. Set limits for child.

9. Provide therapeutic play to allow the child to express fears and anger in a nonverbal manner; be nonjudgmental and supportive with expression of feelings; correct misconceptions.

(text continues on page 1124)

TABLE 40-5 Childhood Diseases

Disease	Incubation (I) and Communicability (C) Periods	Symptoms
Chickenpox a. Varicella-zoster b. Highly communicable; acquired in direct contact, droplet spread and airborne transmission. c. 2–9 y; January to May Diagnostic tests: Tzanck smear shows multinucleated giant cells. Passive immunity: Best accomplished by varicella-zoster immunoglobin (VZIG) given within 72–96 hours of exposure.	I: 11–21 d after exposure C: Onset of fever (1–2 d before first lesion) until last vesicle is dried (5–7 d)	a. General malaise, low-grade fever and anorexia for 24 h b. Rash—macules to papules and vesicles to crusts within several hours c. Pruritis of lesions may be severe, and scratching may cause scarring Rash characteristics: Rash appears first on head and mucous membranes, then becomes concentrated on body and sparse on extremities, papulovesicular eruption.
Streptococcal pharyngitis a. β-Hemolytic streptococcus group A strain b. Direct or indirect contact with nasopharyngeal secretion of infected person or recently established carrier c. Rare under 3 y of age; 5–16 y; incidence higher in winter and spring. Diagnostic tests: nasopharyngeal (throat) culture; rapid diagnositic test.	I: 2–5 d C: Greatest during initial phase of illness	a. Onset is generally acute: high fever, headache, vomiting, chills b. After 12–24 h—some sore throat of varying degrees of severity, dry throat, anterior cervical lymphadenopathy, white tongue coating that becomes strawberry-red tongue, exudate on tonsils, scarlatina rash initially in axilla, groin, and neck area that becomes generalized.
Rubella (German 13-d measles) a. Rubella virus; RNA toga virus b. Oral droplet or transplacentally c. School age, young adults, spring, winter Diagnostic tests: tissue culture of throat, blood or urine, latex agglutination, enzyme immunoassay, passive hemagglutination, fluorescent immunoassay tests. Passive immunity: birth to 6 months of age from maternal antibodies.	I: 14–21 d after exposure C: Virus can be passed from 7 d before to 5 d after rash appears.	Enlarged lymph nodes in postanricular, auricular suboccipital, and cervical areas 24 h before rash develops. Eranthem: discrete rose spots on soft palate Exanthem: Variable, begins on face spreads quickly over entire body; usually maculopapular; clears by third day.
Roseola infantum (exanthem subitum) a. Human herpes virus-6 b. Transmission not known c. 6–18 months; late fall to early spring	I: 5–15 d C: Not known—believed not to be highly contagious	Fever of 39.4°–41.2°C (103°–106°F), either intermittent or sustained 3–4 d with no clinical findings. Fever suddenly drops and macular or maculopapular rash develops on trunk, spreading to arms and neck; mild involvement of face and legs; rash fades quickly.
Rubeola (hard, red, 7-d measles) a. Measles virus, RNA-containing paramyxovirus b. Direct contact with droplets from infected persons, respiratory route Diagnostic tests: serologic procedures not routinely done. Passive immunity: birth to 4–6 mo of age if mother is immune before pregnancy. c. 5–10 y, adolescents; spring.	I: 10–12 d C: 5th day of incubation to 4th day of rash	Fever, lethargy, cough, coryza, and conjunctivitis. 2–3 d later: Koplik's spots on buccal pharyngeal mucosa (grayish white spots with reddish areolae), which disappear within 12–18 h 2 d later: maculopapular rash appears at hairline and spreads to feet in 1 d; rash begins to clear after 3–4 d.
Mumps a. Mumps virus, paramyxovirus b. Direct contact, airborne droplets, saliva, and possibly urine. c. School age; all seasons but slightly more frequent in late winter and early spring. Diagnostic tests: cell culture from saliva, urine, spinal fluid or blood. Passive immunity: Birth to 6 mo of age if mother is immune before pregnancy	I: 14–21 d C: 7 d before to 9 d after swelling appears; virus in saliva greatest just before and after parotitis onset.	a. Headache, anorexia, generalized malaise; fever 1 d before glandular swelling; fever lasts 1–6 d. b. Glandular swelling, usually of parotid—one side or bilaterally. c. Enlargement and reddening of Wharton's duct and Stensen's duct d. Subclinical infection may occur.

Treatment	Complications	Special Considerations
Symptomatic: Shorten fingernails to prevent scratching Daily antiseptic baths Oral antihistamines to decrease pruritus Treatment of itching: Baking soda (sodium bicarbonate) or oatmeal baths, Calamine lotion to lesions Isolation until all lesions have crusted Acyclovir (Zovirax) PO within first 24 h Avoid salicylates	Complications are rare in normal children. Secondary bacterial infection of lesions Hemorrhagic varicella, pneumonia, encephalitis, and thrombocytopenia are not common, but they can occur. Reye's syndrome	Severe in neonate and pregnant women VZIG is available from American Red Cross for high-risk susceptible children who have been exposed to varicella zoster. High-risk children include those receiving corticosteroids or antimetabolites.

Isolation for 1 d while starting prescription
Antibiotic therapy:
    Penicillin G—IM
    Penicillin V—PO
Erythromycin (Pediazole)—if allergic to penicillin
Cephalosporins PO
	Acute glomerulonephritis, 1–2 wk after acute stage
	Rheumatic fever, 2–3 wk after acute stage
	Peritonsillar abscess, cervical adenitis
	Pneumonia, otitis media, meningitis, sinusitis, mastoiditis
	Erythrogenic toxin responsible for rash (scarlet fever). After 5–7 d rash may subside but desquamation of skin on face, trunks, hands, and feet may persist for 4–6 wk.
		Throat cultures are considered for entire household when: others are symptomatic concurrently or within past 3 wk; frequent or relapsing infections. Repeat throat cultures are recommended after treatment if child has history of rheumatic fever. Nonsymptomatic carriers have low risk for rheumatic fever and do not require treatment.

Symptomatic—isolation	In adolescent females: arthritis; arthralgias Encephalitis Thrombocytopenia	Exposure of nonimmune pregnant women in first trimester results in high percentage of affected fetuses and infants born with various birth defects: cataracts, deafness, growth retardation, congenital heart disease, mental retardation.
Symptomatic—antipyretic	Convulsions due to high fever Encephalitis (rare)	

Symptomatic:
    Sedatives
    Antipyretic
    Bed rest in humid, comfortably warm room
    Dark room for photophobia
    Adequate fluid
	Otitis media
	Pneumonia, laryngitis
	Mastoiditis, encephalitis
	Appendicitis	

Isolation until swelling has subsided
Symptomatic
    Analgesics
    Hydration
    Alimentation
    Antipyretics
    Rest
	Meningoencephalitis
	Orchitis, epididymitis
	Auditory nerve involvement, resulting in unilateral deafness	

(continued)

TABLE 40-5 Childhood Diseases *(continued)*

Disease	Incubation (I) and Communicability (C) Periods	Symptoms
Diphtheria a. *Corynebacterium diphtheriae* b. Acquired through secretions of carrier or infected individual by direct contact with contaminated articles and environment c. Incidence increased in autumn and winter Diagnostic tests: cultures of nose and throat	I: 2–4 d C: 2–4 wk untreated; 1–2 d with antibiotic treatment	Nasal diphtheria (1) Coryza with increasing viscosity, possibly epistaxis, low-grade fever (2) Whitish gray membrane may appear over nasal septum. Pharyngeal and/or tonsillar diphtheria: (1) General malaise, low-grade fever, anorexia (2) 1–2 d later, whitish gray membranous patch on tonsils, soft palate, and uvula (3) Lymph node swelling, fever, rapid pulse "bull neck" Laryngeal diphtheria (1) Usually spread from pharynx to larynx (2) Fever, harsh voice, strider barking cough; respiratory difficulty with inspiratory retraction Nonrespiratory diphtheria: affects eye, ear, genitals, or, rarely, skin
Pertussis (Whooping Cough) a. *Bordetella pertussis* b. Direct contact or respiratory droplet spread c. Infants and young children; females > males Diagnostic tests: culture of nasopharyngeal mucus	I: 5–21 d; mean of 7 d C: 7 d after exposure (greatest just before catarrhal stage) to 3 wk after onset of paroxysms or until cough has ceased.	Stage I (catarrhal stage) (1) Lasts 1–2 wk (2) Rhinorrhea, conjunctival injection, lacrimation, mild cough and low-grade fever Stage II (paroxysmal stage) (1) Lasts 2–4 wk or longer (2) Frequent severe, violent coughing attacks occurring in clusters leading to vomiting, cyanosis, and exhaustion Stage III (convalescent stage) (1) Lasts 2 wk to several months (2) Coughing attacks decrease, but may return with each respiratory infection Duration: 9 mo to 2 y
Staphyloccal Scaled Skin Syndrome (Ritter Disease) Group II phage type *Staphylococcus aureus* Disseminated from a primary infection site (usually nose or around eyes) Infants and children under 10 y Diagnostic tests: cultures of skin, conjunctiva, nasopharynx, stools and blood. Biopsy of exfoliated epidermis.	I: Few days C: Onset of rash until after antibiotics initiated	Malaise, fever, irritability or asymptomatic Rash develops in three phases: (1) Erythematous—macular involving face, neck, axilla, and groin (2) Exfoliative—upper layer of epidermis becomes wrinkled and can be removed by light stroking (Nikolsky sign); crusting around eyes, mouth, and nose produce characteristic "sunburst," radial pattern; irritable due to extreme tenderness of skin. (3) Desquamative—epidermis peels away leaving moist areas that dry quickly and heal in 10–14 d.
Poliomyelitis (polio) Virus serotypes 1, 2, and 3; incidence is higher in summer and fall Virus is harbored in gastrointestinal tract and is transmitted through saliva, vomitus, and feces Young children; peaks in August, September, and October, in temperate zones Diagnostic tests: isolation of polio virus from feces and throat	I: 7–14 d, paralytic or nonparalytic; 3–5 d for prodromal or minor illness C: Increases around onset when virus is in throat and is excreted in feces; virus is present in throat 1 wk after onset, in stool 3–4 wk after.	Nonparalytic polio (1) Headache, lethargy, anorexia, vomiting, fever (2) Muscle pain and stiffness of posterior muscles, neck, and limbs. Paralytic polio (1) Same as nonparalytic type, lasting about 1 wk (2) Then 1–2 d of CNS symptoms: loss of deep tendon reflexes, positive Kernig's and Brudzinki's signs, lethargy (3) 1–2 d later, weakening of muscles and paralysis

Treatment	Complications	Special Considerations
Diphtheria antitoxin IV Antibiotic therapy (penicillin, erythromycin) Supportive treatment: Respiratory support Isolation until three cultures are negative after antibiotic therapy is completed Bed rest for 2–3 wk Hydration Immunization with diphtheria toxoid after recovery	Myocarditis Neuritis Paralysis Toxic neurosis and hyaline degeneration of heart, liver, adrenal glands, and kidneys Gastritis, hepatitis Nephritis	

Specific:
  Erythromycin estolate
Supportive:
  Antipyretics
  Bed rest
  Quiet environment to reduce coughing
  Gentle suctioning
  Increase fluid intake
  Oxygen
	Respiratory: pneumonia, atelectasis, emphysema, aspiration pneumonia, pneumothorax
	CNS: convulsions, encephalopathy, coma
		Pertussis disease eliminates the need for pertussis immunization

Specific
  Therapy with penicillinase-resistant penicillin PO, IM, or IV
Symptomatic:
  Gentle cleansing of skin with compresses
	Excessive fluid loss, electrolyte imbalance
	Pneumonia, septicemia, cellulitis	

Nonparalytic: Supportive (ie, relief of pain)
  Analgesics, heat
  Enteric isolation
  Bed rest
Paralytic: Hospitalize
  Fluid and electrolytes
  Rest
  Relief of muscle pain and spasms
  Respiratory support
  Minimize skeletal deformity
	Respiratory paralysis
	Hypertension	

(continued)

TABLE 40-5 Childhood Diseases *(continued)*

Disease	Incubation (I) and Communicability (C) Periods	Symptoms
Erythema Infectiosum (Fifth Disease/Slapped Check) a. Parovirus B19 b. Respiratory route c. School-aged children Diagnostic tests: not widely available; IgM antibody test, polymerase chain reaction detection test	I: 6–14 d C: Until rash develops	Mild fever, chills, fatigue or asymptomatic rash develops in three stages: (1) Sudden appearance of bright erythema on cheeks (2) Erythematous, maculopapular rash on trunk and extremities (3) Rash on body fades with central clearing giving a lacy or reticulated appearance Rash lasts 2–39 d; frequently pruritic without desquamation. Occasional joint arthropathy
Rotavirus a. Reoviridae group A—most common agent responsible for infantile diarrhea b. Fecal–oral route c. 6 mo to 2 y of age; most common in winter in temperate climates Diagnostic tests: enzyme-linked immunosorbent assay	I: 36–48 h C: until 2–5 d after diarrhea	Fever Vomiting Profuse, watery, non–foul-smelling diarrhea
Oral fluid and electrolyte rehydration solutions.	Isotonic dehydration with acidosis Malnourished infants may develop malabsorption dehydration and die.	Excellent hygiene (handwashing) necessary to avoid spreading disease.

a. Agent
b. Mode of transmission
c. Age when most common

10. Provide additional help in the following areas:
    a. Having ambivalent feelings toward parent(s) or any adult caretaker
    b. Overcoming low self-image and the fear that something is wrong with him or her
    c. Fearing future abuse on return home or for misbehavior in the hospital

B. *Providing Support in Parenting*
 1. Assume a nonjudgmental attitude that is neither punitive nor threatening. The desire to help must be conveyed.
 2. Refrain from questioning them about the incident of abuse. (The suspected abuser will be interviewed by the health care provider, the social worker, and the authority who investigates the case.)
 3. Include the parents in the hospital experience (ie, orient them to the unit and to any procedure to be done to the child). Serve as a role model in the management of the child's behavior as well as their own. Try to give the parents as much information as possible about the care of their child. Listen to what they are saying.
 4. Refrain from challenging all the information they may give.
 5. Express appropriate concern and kindness. Remain objective yet empathic. This will help foster the parents' self-respect and improve their self-image and dignity.
 6. Discuss the reporting to the authorities with them because of the widespread nature of the problem and the need for education and assistance.

 7. Support the parents who may have feelings of guilt, anger, and helplessness. Explain to them the extent of trauma and educate them. Allow them to ventilate their feelings. Support their parental role in handling the child (ie, allow the child to talk about or play out the incident, but do not force it).
 8. Build a relationship by working with the parents' strengths rather than their weaknesses. Use compliments as positive reinforcement.
 9. Assist parents to learn safe and appropriate parenting skills.
    a. Remember that many of these parents were abused as children and have no role models or personal experience with nurturing behaviors.
    b. Foster attachment between child and parents, not between child and nurse, when the parents are present; the latter would increase their feelings of incompetence in the parenting role.
    c. Correct erroneous expectations as to what is appropriate behavior for a particular age group.
    d. Encourage parents to take time out from caring for their children to meet their own needs; assist them in identifying safe and appropriate resources for their child's care.
10. Provide the parent with psychological support and reinforcement for appropriate parenting behaviors that are exhibited.
11. Work with parent in planning for the child's future care.

Treatment	Complications	Special Considerations
No treatment is needed for healthy children Immunoglobulin for immunocompromised patients	Complications are rare among healthy children. Children with abnormal red blood cells (sickle cell disease, hereditary spherocytosis, thalassemia, etc) can develop transient aplastic anemia and may require multiple transfusions. Immunocompromised patients may develop severe, chronic anemia.	

12. Determine in what areas the parent needs help. Does the baby cry often? How does this make the parent feel? How does parent comfort child? Is there someone the parents can call for help?

C. *Understanding Your Own Feelings About Families of Child Abuse*
1. A critical part of working in this area is learning to recognize, examine, and work with your own feelings of anger, disgust, and contempt for the parents. It may help to do the following:
    a. Realize that most abusing parents do love their children and want the best for them despite their ambivalent feelings for the children.
    b. Understand the dynamics of child abuse and neglect. This crisis is due to the stress with which the parents are unable to cope and to the deprivations they have themselves suffered in the past.
    c. Focus on the needs of the parents rather than on the injuries of the child. Treatment is aimed at helping the parents reach their maximum potential as parents.
    d. Expect repeated rejection from the parents who lack self-esteem and trust.
    e. Understand that these parents are experiencing terror, guilt, and remorse; they are fearful and yet expect criticism and condemnation.
2. Before teaching or criticizing parenting behaviors, it is essential for the nurse to understand the culture of the client.

Family Education/Health Maintenance

A. *Teach the Parent About Normal Growth and Development*
(See Chapter 38 Growth and Development).
1. Give specific information about and examples of the types of behavior to expect at the various stages of development. Point out in a nonthreatening way normal behavior exhibited by their child.
2. Give specific information on dealing with this behavior.
3. Serve as a role model and teacher; minimize intensity when the parents become threatened.

B. *Teach the Parents How to Use Discipline Without Resorting to Physical Force*
1. Discipline must be consistent. Offer suggestions for alternative ways of handling undesirable behavior (time-out).
2. Rewards may be used for acceptable behavior (eg, a trip to the zoo, staying up later than usual for a special television show, a special treat).
3. Rewards are withheld for unacceptable behavior.

C. *Teach Children How to Avoid Being the Victim of Abuse*
1. Teach them about "good touch" and "bad touch."
2. Emphasize that they can say no to anyone who wants to touch their body.

3. Provide names or places where they can go if they feel they are being abused.

4. Assist them in dealing with their fears that their parents will be sent to jail or that they will be removed from the home.

D. *Support the Parents and Child in Preparation for Discharge to Home*

1. Both parents and child (if age is appropriate) need to know and understand any specific instructions relative to injury and follow-up care.

2. The parents need to be made aware of the most common posthospitalization behavior children may have (see p. 1127–1131).

3. Make known to parents your continued concern and your availability as a source of help. Stress the need for follow-up care. Help them to use community health nurse, therapy for parents, etc.

E. *Refer to Agencies and Organizations Dealing With Abuse*

National Committee to Prevent Child Abuse
332 South Michigan Ave., Suite 1600
Chicago, IL 60604
1-800-55NCPCA

National Clearinghouse on Child Abuse and Neglect Information
P.O. Box 1182
Washington, DC 20013-1182
1-800-FYI 3366

Evaluation

A. Child exhibiting affectionate behavior to primary nurse

B. Both parents participating in feeding and playing with child

Selected References

Barness, L. A. (1991). *Manual of pediatric physical diagnosis* (6th ed.). St. Louis: Mosby-Year Book

Behrman, R. E. (Ed.). (1992). *Nelson textbook of pediatrics* (14th ed.). Philadelphia: W. B. Sanders.

Bellack, J. P., & Edlund, B. J. (1992). *Nursing assessment and diagnosis* (2nd ed.). Boston: Jones & Bartlett.

Centers for Disease Control. (1991). *Preventing lead poisoning in young children.* Atlanta, GA: U.S. Department of Health and Human Services, Public Health Service.

Cohen, B. A. (1993). *Atlas of pediatric dermatology.* Baltimore: Wolfe.

Devlin, B. K. & Reynolds, E. (1994). Child Abuse: How to recognize it, how to intervene. *AJN, 94* (3), 26–31.

Green, M., & Haggerty, R. J. (Eds.). (1990). *Ambulatory pediatrics* (4th ed.). Philadelphia: W. B. Sanders.

Hathaway, W. E., Hay, W. W., Jr., Groothius, J. R., & Paisley, J. W. (Eds.). (1993). *Current pediatric diagnosis & treatment.* East Norwalk, CT: Appleton & Lange.

Hoekelmen, R. A. (Ed.) (1992). *Primary pediatric care* (2nd ed.). St. Louis: Mosby-Year Book.

Hofmann, A. D. (Ed.). (1983). *Adolescent medicine.* Reading, MA: Addison-Wesley.

Hurwitz, S. (1981). *Clinical pediatric dermatology.* Philadelphia: W. B. Saunders.

Neinstein, L. S. (1991). *Adolescent health care* (2nd ed.). Baltimore: Williams & Wilkins.

Peter, G. (Ed.). (1994). *1994 red book: Report of the Committee on Infectious Diseases* (23rd ed.). Elk Grove Village, IL: American Academy of Pediatrics.

Thomas, D. D. (1995). Fever in children: Friend or foe? *RN, 58* (4), 42–47.

CHAPTER 41

Care of the Sick or Hospitalized Child

General Principles of Care

◆ IMPACT OF HOSPITALIZATION ON STAGE OF DEVELOPMENT

The child has the same basic emotional and social needs during hospitalization as he or she does at home. Hospitalization can retard growth and development and cause adverse reactions in the child based on stage of development.

Neonate (Birth to 1 month)

A. Primary Concern
1. Bonding—hospitalization interrupts the early stages of the development of a healthy mother–child relationship, thus early stages of the development of trust are missing.
2. Sensory–motor deprivation—tactile, visual, auditory, kinesthetic
3. Sensory overload

B. Reactions
1. Impairment of mother–child attachment
2. Impairment of mother's ability to love and care for her baby
3. Risk of infant's emotional and physical well-being

C. Nursing Interventions
1. Provide for continual contact between baby and the parents (eye contact and touch).
2. Minimize isolation and strangeness by explaining and reexplaining equipment, procedures to parents.
3. Actively involve parents in caring for their baby—provide for rooming-in.
4. Foster neonate–sibling relationships as appropriate.
5. Identify areas of infant deprivation or overstimulation. Plan a schedule of appropriate stimulation (ie, hold and rock every 3–4 hours, eye contact).
6. Provide sensory–motor stimulation as appropriate.

7. Allow individuality to begin to emerge.
8. Provide consistent caretaker.

Young Infant (1–4 months)

A. Primary Concern
1. Separation—mother is learning to identify and meet the needs of her infant. Infant is learning to make his needs known and to trust his mother to meet them.
2. Sensory—motor deprivation.
3. Needs—security, motor activity, comforting measures.

B. Reactions
Separation anxiety is different from that of older child, because for the infant, the mother seems to be a part of him or her. Development of trust is disturbed when infant is separated from mother.

C. Nursing Interventions
1. Encourage mother to stay and care for her baby, thus minimizing separation. When mother is absent, give infant attention and frequent handling from a limited number of personnel.
2. Provide opportunity for sensory stimulation, motor development, and social responsiveness.
3. Help parents to work through their anxieties. Remember, a mother's touch communicates her comfort or discomfort to her infant.

Mid-age Infant (4–8 months)

A. Primary Concern
Separation from mother—infant now recognizes mother as a separate person from self. Infant rejects strangers.

B. Reactions
Separation anxiety—crying, terror, somatic upset, blank facial expression, extreme preoccupation

C. Nursing Interventions
1. Encourage mother to stay and care for her baby.
2. Attempt to adjust schedule to home routines.

3. Become friends with the infant through the mother.
4. The infant is beginning to develop purposeful activities and to strive toward independence. Provide opportunities and encouragement for this development to continue and provide ways for infant to use newly acquired skills.

Older Infant (8–12 months)

A. Primary Concern
Separation—infant becomes more possessive of mother and clings to her at the time of separation.

B. Reactions
Separation anxiety—tolerance is limited; fear of strangers, excessive crying, clinging, and overdependence on mother.

C. Nursing Interventions
1. Have the mother stay and care for her child.
2. Relieve some of tensions and loneliness with "transference" object (ie, blanket, toy).
3. Prepare the child for procedures. The procedures should be performed in another room or a treatment room and let the mother soothe the child afterward.
4. Provide for sensory stimulation and motor development appropriate for age. Provide opportunities for child to continue using acquired skills, such as feeding self and drinking from a cup.
5. Child needs opportunity to foster increased independence, curiosity and exploration, locomotion, and language skills. Use infant seats, swing; give room to move around in crib, playpen, or floor; use color, texture, and sound; physical stroking, rocking, and talking.

Toddler (1–3 years)

A. Primary Concerns
1. Separation anxiety—relationship with mother is intense. Separation represents the loss of family and familiar surroundings, resulting in feeling of insecurity, grief, anxiety, and abandonment. The toddler's emotional needs are intensified by the mother's absence.
2. Changes in rituals and routines, all of which are important to sense of security, become a source of concern.
3. Inability to communicate—beginning use and understanding of language affords child limited communication between self and the world. Child has limited capacity to understand reality, passage of time.
4. Loss of autonomy and independence—egocentric view of life helps child develop of a sense of autonomy. Child expresses self as a separate being with some potential control of own body and environment.
5. Body integrity—incomplete and inaccurate understanding of the body results in fear, anxiety, frustration, and anger.
6. Decrease in mobility—restricting mobility causes frustration. Child wants to keep moving for the pleasure it gives as well as for the feeling of independence, the opportunity to learn about the world, and the route it provides for coping with frustrations that cannot be verbally expressed. Physical interference with this freedom results in a sense of helplessness.

B. Reactions
1. Protest

a. Has urgent desire to find mother.
b. Expects that she will answer cries, "I want mommy."
c. Frequently cries and shakes crib.
d. Rejects attention of nurses.
e. When with mother, child shows signs of distrust with anger or tears.
2. Despair
a. Feels increasingly hopeless about seeing mother.
b. Becomes apathetic, anorectic, listless; looks sad.
c. May cry continuously or intermittently.
d. Uses comfort measures—thumbsucking, fingering lip, tightly clutching a toy.
3. Denial
a. Represses all feelings and images of mother.
b. Does not cry when she leaves.
c. May seem more attached to nurses—will go to anyone.
d. Finds little satisfaction in relationships with people.
e. Accepts care without protest.
4. Regression—temporarily ceases use of newly acquired skills in an attempt to retain or regain control of a stressful situation.

C. Nursing Interventions
1. Rooming-in, unlimited visiting. Parental visits provide:
a. Opportunity for child to express some of feelings about the situation
b. Assurance that parents are not abandoning or punishing child
c. Periods of comfort and reassurance that allow for the reestablishment of family bonds
2. Attempt to continue routines used at home, especially with regard to sleeping, eating, and bathing. Reestablish trust through body contact and comfort.
3. Set limits.
4. Obtain from parents key words in communicating with child. Find out about nonverbal behavior as well. Familiar toys, blankets, pillow cases, and family pictures can reinforce the child's sense of security.
5. Allow child to make choices when possible. Arrange physical setting to encourage independence. Allow child to explore environment.
6. A Band-Aid may give the child a security of wholeness after an injection.
7. Replace lost mobility with another form of motion: moving about in a wheelchair, cart, or bed. Exercise restrained extremity. Provide opportunity for the child to release energy suppressed by decreased mobility (ie, by pounding, throwing). Provide opportunity to continue learning about world through sensory modalities such as water play and diversional play.
8. Discharge—if rooming-in has not occurred during hospitalization, parents must be prepared for the possible posthospital behavior of their toddler. They will need support in understanding and handling these behaviors. The child may do any of the following.
a. Show lack of affection or resist close physical contact. Parents may interpret this as rejection.
b. Regress to an earlier stage of development.
c. Cling to mother, unable to tolerate any separation from her; show excessive need for love and affection.
9. Appropriate parental response to the child's behavior is vital if relationships are to be reestablished.
a. Extra love and understanding will help restore the child's trust.

b. Hostility and withdrawal of love will cause the child further loss of trust, self-esteem, and independence.

Preschool Child (3–5 years)

A. Primary Concerns
1. Separation—although cognitive and coping capabilities have increased and the child responds less violently to separation from parents, separation and hospitalization represent stress beyond the coping mechanisms and adaptive capabilities of the preschool child. Loneliness and insecurities are experienced.

   Language is important; although children may not verbally express what they are feeling, there is an attempt at this in 4- to 5-year olds.
2. Unfamiliar environment—this requires coping with a change in daily routine and represents a loss of control and security.
3. Abandonment and punishment—fantasies and thoughts may contain vengeful wishes for other persons, for which the child expects retribution. Illness may be interpreted as punishment for thoughts. Enforced parental separation may be interpreted as loss of parental love and represents abandonment by them.
4. Body image and integrity—hospitalization and intrusive procedures provide a multitude of threats of both bodily mutilation and loss of identity, which are just beginning to develop along with the acquisition of autonomy.
5. Immobility—mobility is the child's dominant form of self-expression and adaptation to the environment. The child has great urge for locomotion and exercise of large muscles. It represents the main expression of emotion and release of tension.
6. Loss of control—this influences the preschooler's perception of and reaction to separation, pain, and illness.

B. Reactions
1. *Regression*—child temporarily stops using newly acquired skills in an attempt to retain or regain control of a stressful situation. Preschooler may return to behavior of infant or toddler.
2. *Repression*—child may attempt to exclude the undesirable and unpleasant stresses from consciousness.
3. *Projection*—preschooler may transfer own emotional state, motives, and desires to others in environment.
4. *Displacement/sublimation*—emotions are permitted to be directed and expressed in other situations such as art or play.
5. *Identification*—the child assumes characteristics of the aggressor in an attempt to reduce fear and anxiety and to feel in control of the situation.
6. *Aggression*—hostility is direct and intentional; physical expression takes precedence over verbal expression.
7. *Denial and withdrawal*—the child is able to ignore interruptions and disavow any thought or feeling that would result in a painful experience.
8. *Fantasy*—a mental activity to help the child bridge the gap between reality and fantasy because of lack of experience.
9. The preschooler may simply show similar behaviors (protest, despair, denial) to those of the toddler although the stage of protest is usually less aggressive and direct.

C. Nursing Interventions
1. Minimize stress of separation by providing for parental presence and participation in care. Strive to shorten the hospital stay. Help parents understand what hospitalization means to the child.
2. Identify defense mechanisms apparent in the child and help child through the stressful situation by accepting, showing love and concern, and being alert to readiness to relinquish them.
3. Set limits for the child. Let child know that someone is there. Help the child become master of something in the situation.
4. Provide opportunity and encouragement for child to verbalize.
5. Careful preparation for all procedures should be done on the child's level of development and comprehension. Provide privacy during these procedures.
6. Be sure the child has opportunities for play. Play is one important medium through which the child can overcome fear and anxiety. A body outline, doll, and simple visual aids are appropriate teaching tools. Provide self-expression, role reversal through puppets, dolls, drawings.
7. Encourage activities with other children.
8. Provide consistency in nursing personnel and approach to care.
9. Encourage the child to participate in own care and hygiene as appropriate.
10. Deal specifically with castration and mutilation fears. If the child is having surgery, describe exactly which body part will be repaired.
11. Whenever appropriate, reassure the child that no one is to blame for the illness or hospitalization.
12. Discourage parents from reinforcing negative feelings to the child—"If you're not good I'll leave you here" or "I'll have the nurse give you a shot."

School-aged Children (5–12 years)

A. Concerns
1. Many fear loss of recently mastered skills.
2. Many worry about separation from school and peers. They may fear loss of former roles.
3. Mutilation fantasies are common.
4. Some may believe that they or their parents magically caused the illness merely by thinking that the event would occur.
5. Often they have increased concerns related to modesty and privacy.
6. The imposed passivity may be interpreted as punishment for being bad.
7. Children may feel their body no longer is their own but rather is controlled by doctors and nurses.

B. Reactions
1. Regression
2. Separation anxiety—especially early school-aged period
3. Negativism
4. Depression
5. Tendency to be phobic (normal)
   a. Fears include that of the dark, doctors, hospitals, surgery, medication, and death.
   b. Unrealistic fears are commonly attached to needles, x-ray procedures, and blood.
6. Conscious attempts at mature behavior.
7. Suppression or denial of symptoms.

C. Nursing Interventions
1. Help parents to prepare the child for elective hospitalizations.

2. Obtain a thorough nursing history, including information regarding health and physical developments, hospitalizations, social and cultural background, and normal daily activities. Use this information to plan care.
3. Provide order and consistency in the environment whenever possible.
4. Establish and enforce reasonable policies to protect the child and to increase sense of security in the environment.
5. Arrange the environment to allow for as much mobility as possible (ie, make sure articles are appropriately placed; move the bed if the child is immobilized).
6. Respect the child's need for privacy and respect modesty during examinations, bathing, and other activities.
7. Use treatment rooms whenever possible when performing painful or intrusive procedures. Keep the room as "safe" territory.
8. Help young children identify problems and questions (often through play). Then help them find the answers.
9. Provide information about the illness and hospitalization based on assessment of what facts the child needs and wants and how this information can be made readily understandable.
10. View all nursing care activities as teaching situations. Explain the function of equipment and allow the child to handle it. Teach scientific terminology for body parts, procedures, and equipment.
11. When explaining a procedure, make sure that the child knows its purpose, what will be done, and what will be expected. Reassure the child during the procedure by continuing the explanations and support.
12. Reassure the child having surgery; explain where the organ to be removed or repaired is located and that no other body part will be removed.
13. Carefully assess pain and provide appropriate relief.
14. Use play whenever appropriate to provide information about the hospital experience and to identify and decrease the child's fantasies and fears.
15. Reassure the child that he or she or parents are not to blame for illness.
16. Facilitate discharge of energy and aggression through appropriate play activities or through sharing aspects of ward management.
17. Encourage the child's participation in care and self-hygiene.
18. Support intellectual potential through the use of games, puzzles, school work, and drawings.
19. Assist the family to understand the child's reactions to illness and hospitalization so that family members can facilitate positive coping patterns.
20. Let the child know that his or her normal status as a family member remains intact during hospitalization. Encourage a consistent visiting pattern and allow sibling visits.
21. Help parents to deal with their own anxieties about hospitalization and assist them to help their child cope with the situation.
22. Encourage parental participation in the child's care when appropriate.
23. Encourage written communication with peers, and allow peer visiting when appropriate.
24. Begin discharge planning early, including plans for physical and emotional needs. Alert families to possible behavioral changes, including phobias, nightmares, regression, negativism, and disturbances in eating and learning.

Adolescent

A. *Concerns*
1. Physical illness, exposure, and lack of privacy may cause increased concern about body image and sexuality.
2. Separation from security of peers, family, and school may cause anxiety.
3. Interference with struggle for independence and emancipation from parents is a concern.
4. The adolescent may be threatened by helplessness and may see illness as a punishment for feelings not mastered or for breaking rules imposed by parents or physicians.

B. *Reactions*
1. Anxiety or embarrassment related to loss of control
2. Insecurity in strange environment
3. Intellectualization about disease details to avoid addressing actual concerns. They may know others with the same chronic type of illness who have died; may fear the future or feel guilty they have survived.
4. Rejection of treatment measures, even if previously accepted
5. Anger (may be directed toward parents or staff) because goals are being thwarted
6. Depression
7. Increased dependency or parents, staff
8. Denial or withdrawal
9. Demanding or uncooperative behavior (usually an attempt to assert control)
10. Capitalization on gains from illness or pain

C. *Nursing Interventions*
1. Help parents to prepare the adolescent for elective hospitalization.
2. Assess the impact of illness on the adolescent by considering factors such as timing, nature of illness, new experiences imposed, changes in body image, and expectations for the future. Be aware of misconceptions.
3. Introduce the adolescent to the hospital staff and to regular routines soon after admission.
4. Obtain a thorough nursing history that includes information about hobbies, school, family, illness, hospitalization, food habits, and recreation.
5. Encourage adolescents to wear their own clothes and allow them to decorate their beds or rooms to express themselves.
6. Have drawers and closets available to store personal items.
7. Allow the adolescent access to a telephone.
8. Allow adolescents control over appropriate matters (ie, timing of bath, selection of food, etc).
9. Respect their need for periodic isolation and privacy.
10. Have a supervised recreational and activities program available that is planned by a professional child care worker.
11. Accept adolescent's level of performance. Allow regression with expectation of growth.
12. Involve adolescent patients in planning care so that they will be more accepting of restrictions and receptive to health teaching. Focus on capabilities rather than limitations. Adolescent should be accepted as a vital member of the health care team. The adolescent's consent should be obtained for procedures and surgery.

13. Explain clearly all procedures, routines, expectations, and restrictions imposed by illness. If necessary, clarify the adolescent's interpretation of illness and hospitalization. Plan separate teaching sessions for parents.
14. Facilitate verbal rejection of treatment measures to protect the adolescent from harming himself physically by stopping treatment.
15. Assess the adolescent's intellectual skills and provide necessary information to allow for problem-solving to deal with illness and hospitalization.
16. Recognize positive and negative coping behaviors as attempts to adjust to a threatening situation. Attempt to deal with feeling that caused the behavior as well as with the behavior itself.
17. Be a good listener. Maintain a sense of humor. Be honest and respectful with the adolescent and family.
18. Provide opportunities such as writing, art work, and recreational activities to allow nonverbal adolescents to express themselves.
19. Foster interaction with other hospitalized adolescents and continuation of peer relationships with outside friends.
20. Establish regular group meetings to allow patients to meet with staff members and with each other to comment and ask questions about their hospital experiences.
21. Set necessary limits to encourage self-control and ensure the rights of others.
22. Help adolescents work through sexual feelings. Avoid behavior that could be interpreted as provocative or flirtatious. Masturbation, unless excessive, may be considered a psychologically healthy way to discharge sexual tension.
23. Describe and interpret the needs and reactions of hospitalized adolescents to parents. Emphasize the adolescent's need to be respected as a unique individual, separate from parents.
24. Assist parents to cope with the illness and hospitalization as well as to deal effectively with the adolescent's response to related stress.
25. Encourage continuation of education.
26. Stress the confidential nature of conversations between nurse and patient, physician and patient.

◆ FAMILY-CENTERED CARE

Family-centered care provides an opportunity for the family to care for the hospitalized child with nursing support.
The *goal* of family-centered care is to maintain or strengthen the roles and ties of the family with the hospitalized child to promote normality of the family unit.

Benefits for Parents and Child

1. Maintain close family interactions during stress.
2. Minimize separation anxiety.
3. Decrease reactions of protest, denial, and despair.
4. Increase sense of security for the child.
5. Fulfill family needs to care for their child physically and emotionally.
6. Allow parents to feel useful and important rather than making them dependent and destroying their confidence.
7. Decrease parental guilt feelings.

8. Increase parents' competence and confidence in caring for the sick child.
9. Comfort for the family provided by other families.
10. Greater absorption of staff teaching by the family.
11. Diminish posthospitalization reactions.

Implementation Strategies

Implementation of family-centered care will depend on regulations of the particular health care setting as well as the capabilities of the individual family unit. Examples of activities that can facilitate and strengthen family ties include:

1. Allowing rooming-in for parents of young children
2. Having parents participate in the child's physical care
3. Having flexible visiting regulations for family members, including siblings
4. Having pictures of family members available at the hospital
5. Encouraging telephone contact
6. Using family tape recordings

Role of the Nurse

1. To create an environment conducive to maintaining family integrity and unity. The nurse should:
   a. Help to maintain a healthy parent–child relationship. (Parents should not feel threatened by the nurse.)
   b. Facilitate a supportive marital relationship
   c. Include siblings in planning and intervention as appropriate
   d. Supplement the family in the common goal of the child's welfare
2. To assist parents to make decisions about when to stay with their child
   a. Parents' presence is especially important if the child is 5 years or younger, is especially anxious or upset, or is in medical crisis.
   b. The parents' decision is influenced by needs of other family members, as well as by job and home responsibilities.
   c. The nurse should try to alleviate guilty feelings of parents who are unable to stay with their child.
3. To develop trusting, goal-directed relationships with families
   a. Obtain a thorough nursing history that provides information to assess strengths, relationships, and concerns.
   b. Plan with the family toward mutual, realistic goals.
   c. Recognize good care that the child receives from parents.
4. To observe the parent–child relationship to be able to:
   a. Evaluate the degree of participation of the parents in physical and emotional care.
   b. Observe parents' attitudes, skills, and techniques and the child's behavior and response to them.
   c. Assess what teaching needs to be done.
   d. Detect problems in parent–child relationship.
5. To teach parents knowledge, understanding, and skills necessary to function effectively with the hospitalized child. The nurse should:
   a. Perform nursing techniques safely and efficiently.

b. Interpret the behavior of the hospitalized child to parents so that they can understand it and intervene as appropriate.

c. Interpret and reinforce what health care provider has told parents. Answer questions thoroughly and honestly as knowledge permits.

d. Interpret medical procedures and diagnostic tests.

e. Provide health teaching.

f. Offer anticipatory guidance.

6. To help parents adapt to the situation and to develop their own feeling of value by coping with the child's illness.

a. Be aware of common parental reactions to the stress experienced by families of children who have severe or chronic illness.

b. Be aware that defense mechanisms, if used in moderation, are constructive and may facilitate optimal coping.

c. Help parents recognize their own feelings.

d. Identify parental support systems as well as adaptive and maladaptive coping.

e. Be perceptive of parents' physical and emotional needs and limitations.

   (1) Do not allow parents to become fatigued.

   (2) Allow parents to leave and take a break.

7. To assist families as appropriate in dealing with normal family developmental tasks

a. Be aware that the child's hospitalization is often only one of many stresses a family experiences at a given time. Others may include:

   (1) Interpersonal problems

   (2) Debt, unemployment, job change

   (3) Recent changes in dwelling place and consequent disruption

   (4) Problems associated with child care and discipline

   (5) Concurrent illness of other family members

8. To ensure continuity of family-centered care between the hospital and home

◆ PEDIATRIC ACUTE CARE NURSING

Emotional Support to Child

1. Refer to the section on the impact of hospitalization on the developmental stage of the child (p. 1127). In addition to the stress of hospitalization and the illness itself, the child must deal with the noxious environment: high noise level, loss of sleep, bright lights, random and unpredictable procedures, and the drastic change from normal routine.

2. If possible, familiarize the child with the unit before admission.

3. Provide immediate physical care that communicates strength and facilitates trust.

4. Be alert to behavioral changes that may indicate physical distress.

5. Facilitate parent–child interaction—allow frequent family visits.

6. Question parents concerning the child's own way of responding to emotional stress. Use particular comforts that are most soothing to the child.

7. Support parents so that they will be best able to support their child.

8. Time activities; dim lights to allow for adequate sleep; whenever possible, cluster caregiving activities.

9. Do everything possible to reduce the amount of pain that the child must endure; provide comfort measures. Administer anxiety-reducing or pain-reducing medications as ordered and determine effectiveness.

10. Provide age-appropriate stimulation when indicated by the child's condition (TV, games, books, toys, etc).

11. Provide opportunities for the child to express fears and concerns.

12. If possible, avoid exposing an alert child to the death or resuscitation of another child. If the child is exposed, provide adequate explanation. The child must also be helped to express own feelings and work through the experience.

13. Prepare the child for transfer from the ICU by implementing a nursing care plan similar to one that the child will experience on a regular unit (eg, decrease frequency of monitoring of vital signs, encourage independence). Give a thorough report to the receiving nurse during transfer.

Emotional Support to Family

The parental role changes, once their child is admitted to the ICU, from that of parents of a well child to one of parents of a critically ill child. To ease this transition parents have the need to be informed about their child's current condition, plan of care, and the future. They also have the need to feel needed and vital in their child's recovery.

1. Orient parents to the unit and its waiting areas. Clarify visiting policies and hospital expectations.

a. If the admission to the ICU is expected, familiarize the parents with the ICU before the admission.

b. If the admission is unexpected and sudden, the experience can be traumatic for the family. Care to reduce fears, stress, and anxiety is of prime importance to the caretaker.

2. Encourage liberal visiting hours and unlimited phone calls from parents to the ICU.

3. Assure parents that everything possible is being done for their child. Whenever possible, allow them to see child receiving treatment.

4. Make certain that parents are informed of important changes in the child's clinical status. If parents are leaving the unit, exchange telephone numbers to ensure contact if needed. Reinforce medical interpretations.

5. Explain special equipment and changes in nursing management.

6. Provide opportunities for parents to ask questions and have them answered.

7. Encourage parents to keep a journal of their hospital experience. It is a very real way for parents to confront their feelings especially if they are not expressing them to the hospital team.

8. Encourage parents to interact verbally and physically with their child. Support them in this endeavor.

9. Facilitate expression of parental grief.

10. Provide opportunities for parents to talk to a person with whom they can share their concerns and fears. Be sure this person can see them as often as they require.

11. Provide opportunities for parents to meet together to share experiences and offer mutual support. Encourage parents not to compare progress of other patients to their child—it can set them up to be quickly disappointed. Focus on each child and situation as unique.

12. Be sensitive to parents' additional comments to family as well as to their need to remain with their child.

Whenever possible, allow visiting at mutually convenient time.
13. Help parents provide anticipatory guidance for siblings
and extended family members.
14. Refer parents to appropriate community resources for help
for financial, environmental, or psychological problems.
15. Offer follow-up contact to parents if appropriate.
16. For a complete list of references for families of sick,
hospitalized, or dying children, refer parents to: National Center for Education in Maternal and Child
Health; 2000 15th St. North, Suite 701; Arlington, VA
22201-2617; 703-524-7802.

◆ CHILD LIFE PROGRAMS

Play is a central mechanism in which children cope.
Through play, children can communicate, learn, and master a traumatic experience such as hospitalization.

Many hospitals have established programs with a specially trained staff whose job it is to concern themselves
solely with the social and emotional welfare of every pediatric patient. Such programs are called by a variety of
names, including "Child Life," "Children's Activities,"
"Recreational Therapy," "Play Therapy," and others.

Goals of Child Life Programs

1. To prevent some of the emotional pain and fear associated with illness and hospitalization
   a. Child life workers may assume primary responsibility
   or a supportive role in the preparation of patients for
   hospitalization, surgery, or particular procedures.
   b. In many hospitals, child life workers arrange pread-
   mission tours, puppet shows, and similar activities
   to which all children who are planned pediatric admissions are invited.
2. To provide a comfortable, accepting, and nonthreatening environment where the child may play and interact
with other children and with an adult who is not involved with health care
   a. Ideally, there is a separate child life playroom in
   every unit. However, there may be only an open
   area at the end of the corridor or in the middle of
   the ward.
   b. Generally, there is a specific regulation that no
   medical procedures (even a relatively benign one
   such as taking child's temperature) are to be carried
   out in the play area.
   c. In many settings, children are encouraged to have
   their meals in the playroom. Generally they not
   only enjoy the opportunity to eat with others, but
   also seem to eat better.
3. To provide the child with an opportunity for choice
   a. The child may choose whether or not he or she
   wishes to come to the playroom. Once there, child
   may choose what to do.
   b. A variety of craft and play materials, including real
   and miniature medical equipment, are available.
   c. Should the child choose to sit and watch or be held
   and rocked, these activities are seen as acceptable
   choices.
4. To provide a continuing educational program
   a. In some settings, teachers are paid by the hospital
   and are an integral part of the child life program. In
   others, teachers are provided by the local public

schools, and they work in close cooperation with
the child life department.
   b. In most hospitals, the educational program includes
   special activities for preschoolers and toddlers as
   well as a program of infant stimulation.

◆ THE CHILD UNDERGOING SURGERY

Preoperative Care

A. **Provide Emotional Support, Psychological
Preparation, and Preoperative Teaching**
Such preparation and support will minimize stress and will
help the child cope with fears.

1. Potential threats for the hospitalized child anticipating
surgery are:
   a. Physical harm—bodily injury, pain, mutilation, death
   b. Separation from parents
   c. The strange and unknown—possibility of surprise
   d. Confusion and uncertainty about limits and expected behavior
   e. Relative loss of control of world, loss of autonomy
   f. Fear of anesthesia
   g. Fear of the surgical procedure itself
   h. Misinterpretation of medical jargon (ie, dye–die)
2. All preparation and support must be based on the
child's age, developmental stage and level; personality;
past history and experience with health professionals
and hospitals; background—including religion, socioeconomic group, culture, and family attitudes.
   a. Inquire as to what information the child has already
   received.
   b. Determine what the child knows or expects.
   c. Additional guidelines in preparation include:
      (1) Using illustration of a child's body, concrete ex-
      amples, and simple terms (not medical jargon)
      (2) Identifying changes that may occur as a result of
      the procedure, both in body and daily routine
      (3) Giving the explanation slowly and clearly, sav-
      ing anxiety-producing aspects until the end
      (4) Making use of child's creative ability and logical
      thinking powers to aid in preparation for
      procedures
   d. Allow the child to participate as able.
   e. Suggest ways for the child to cope—crying is okay.
   f. Offer constant reassurance; speak in a calm manner.
3. Orient patient and family to the unit, room, location
of playroom, operating room, and recovery room and
introduce them to other children, parents, and some
personnel. Make arrangements for the child to meet
anesthesiologist as well as the operating room nurse
and recovery room nurse.
4. Allow and encourage questions. Give honest answers.
   a. Such questions will give the nurse a better understanding of the child's fears and perceptions of what
   is happening.
   b. Infants and young children need to form a trusting
   relationship with those who care for them.
   c. The older the child the more reassuring information
   can be.
5. Provide opportunity for child and parent to work out concerns and feelings (play, talk). Such supportive care should
result in less upset behavior and more cooperation.

6. Prepare child for what to expect postoperatively (ie, equipment to be used or attached to child, different location, how child will feel, what child will be expected to do, diet, new health caretakers).

B. Assist in Physical Preparation of Patient for Surgery
1. Assist with necessary laboratory studies. Explain to child what is going to happen before procedure and how he or she can respond. Give continual support during procedure.
2. See that patient has nothing by mouth (NPO). Explain to child and parents what NPO means and the importance of it.
3. Assist with fever reduction.
   a. Fever will result from some surgical diseases (ie, intestinal obstruction).
   b. Fever increases risk of anesthesia and need for fluids and calories.
4. Administer appropriate medications as prescribed. Sedatives and drugs to dry the secretions are often given on the unit.
5. Establish good hydration. Parental therapy may be necessary to hydrate the child, especially if child is NPO, vomiting, or febrile.

C. Support Parents During Time of Crisis
The attitudes of the parents toward hospitalization and surgery largely determine the attitudes of their child.

1. The experience may be emotionally distressing.
2. Parents may have feelings of fear or guilt.
3. The preparation and support should be integrated for parent, child, and family unit.
4. Give individual attention to parents; explore and clarify their feelings and thoughts; provide accurate information and appropriate reassurance.
5. Stress parents' importance to the child. Help mother understand how she can care for her child.

Postoperative Care

A. Immediate
1. Maintain a patent airway and prevent aspiration.
   a. Position the child on side or abdomen to allow secretions to drain and prevent tongue from obstructing pharynx.
   b. Suction any secretions present.
2. Make frequent observations of general condition and vital signs. Postoperative protocols may vary per procedure and facility.
   a. Take vital signs every 15 minutes until child is awake and condition is stable.
   b. Note respiratory rate and quality, pulse rate and quality, blood pressure, skin color.
   c. Watch for signs of shock.
      (1) All children in shock have signs of pallor, coldness, increased pulse, and irregular respirations.
      (2) Older children have decreased blood pressure and respirations.
   d. Change in vital signs may indicate airway obstruction, hemorrhage, or atelectasis.
   e. Restlessness may indicate pain or hypoxia. Medication for pain is not usually given until anesthesia has worn off.
   f. Check dressings for drainage or constriction and pressure.

3. See that all drainage tubes are connected and functioning properly. Gastric decompression relieves abdominal distention and decreases the possibility of respiratory embarrassment.
4. Monitor parenteral fluids as prescribed.
5. Be physically near as child awakens to offer soothing words and a gentle touch. Reunite parents and child as soon as possible after the child recovers from anesthesia. If a language barrier exists, the parents should be with the child during recovery from anesthesia.

B. After Recovery From Anesthesia
After undergoing simple surgery and receiving a small amount of anesthesia, the child may be ready to play and eat in a few hours. More complicated and extensive surgery debilitates the child for a longer period of time.

1. Continue to make frequent and astute observations in regard to behavior, vital signs, dressings or operative site, and special apparatus (intravenous [IV] lines, chest tubes, oxygen).
   a. Note signs of dehydration—dry skin and membranes; sunken eyes; poor skin turgor; sunken fontanelle in infant.
   b. Record any passage of flatus or stool, bowel sounds. Observe for intestinal ileus because crying children swallow air and even a minimal amount of ileus may cause gastric distention.
   c. Record vomiting time, amount, characteristics.
2. Assess behavior for signs of pain and medicate appropriately.
3. Record intake and output accurately.
   a. Parenteral fluids and oral intake
   b. Drainage from gastric tubes or chest tubes, colostomy, wound, and urinary output
   c. Parenteral fluid is evaluated and prescribed by considering output and intake. It is usually maintained until the child is taking adequate oral fluids.
4. Advance diet as tolerated, according to the child's age and the health care provider's directions.
   a. First feedings are usually clear fluids; if tolerated, advance slowly to full diet for age. Note any vomiting or abdominal distention.
   b. Because anorexia may occur, offer what the child likes, in small amounts and in an attractive manner.
5. Prevent infection.
   a. Keep the child away from other children or personnel with respiratory or other infections.
   b. Change the child's position every 2 to 4 hours; prop infants with a blanket roll.
   c. Encourage the child to cough and breathe deeply; let the infant cry for short periods of time, unless contraindicated.
   d. Keep operative site clean—change dressing as needed; keep diaper away from wound.
6. Provide good general hygiene, opportunities for exercise and diversional activity, and encourage sleep and rest.
7. Provide emotional support and psychological security. Reassure child that things are going well. Talk about going home, if appropriate.
8. Begin early to prepare for discharge: Teach special procedures, provide written instructions, and arrange for community nurse referral.

◆ THE DYING CHILD

The nursing role is to assist the child and family to cope with the experience in such a way that it will promote growth rather than destroy family integrity and emotional well-being.

Recognize the Stages of Dying

See Table 41-1.

1. Be aware that dying children, their families, and the staff will all progress through these stages, not necessarily at the same time.
2. Children experience the stages with much variation. They tend to pass more quickly through the stages and may merge some of these stages.
3. The nursing goal is to accept the child and family at whatever stage they are experiencing, not to push them through the stages.
4. Understand the meaning of illness and death at various stages of growth and development (Table 41-2).
5. Be aware of other factors that influence a child's personal concept of death. Of particular importance are:
   a. The amount and type of direct exposure a child has had to death
   b. Cultural values, beliefs, and patterns of bereavement
   c. Religious beliefs about death and an afterlife

Communicate With Child About Death

Research indicates that children generally can cope with more than adults will allow and that children appreciate the opportunity to know and understand what is happening to them. It is important that the child's questions be answered simply, but truthfully, and that they be based on child's particular level of understanding. The following responses have been suggested by Easom in *The Dying Child* and may be useful as a guide:

A. Preschool-aged Child
1. When the child at this age is comfortable enough to ask questions about illness, questions should be answered. When death is anticipated at some future time and the child asks, "Am I going to die?" a response might be, "We will all die someday, but you are not going to die today or tomorrow."
2. When death is imminent and the child asks, "Am I going to die?" the response might be, "Yes, you are going to die, but we will take care of you and stay with you."
3. When the child asks, "Will it hurt?" the response should be truthful and factual.
4. Death may be described as a form of sleep—a sleep where he will be secure in the love of those around. However, some children may fear sleep as the result of this type of explanation. Anesthesia is sometimes called a "special sleep" so it is *not* currently recommended to refer to death as "sleep."
5. Parents can express to the child the fact that they do not want child to go and that they will miss the child very much; they feel sad, too, that they are going to be separated.

B. School-aged Child
1. Responses to the school-aged child's questions about death should be answered truthfully. The child looks for support from those he or she trusts.
2. The school-aged child should be given a simple explanation of diagnosis and its meaning; child should also receive an explanation of all treatments and procedures.
3. The child should be given no specific time in terms of days or months because each individual and each illness is different.
4. When the school-age child asks, "Am I going to die?" and death is inevitable, child should be told the truth. The school-aged child does have the emotional ability to look to parents and those he or she trusts for comfort and support.
5. The school-aged child believes in parents. The child should be allowed to die in the comfort and security of family.

TABLE 41-1 Stages of Dying as Identified by Dr. Elizabeth Kübler-Ross

Stage	Nursing Implications
I. Denial, shock, disbelief.	Accept denial, but function within a reality sphere. Do not tear down the child's (or family's) defenses. Be aware that denial usually breaks down in the early morning when it may be dark and lonely. Be certain that it is the child or family who is using denial, not the staff.
II. Anger, rage, hostility.	Accept anger and help the child express it through positive channels. Be aware that anger may be expressed toward other family members, nursing staff, physicians, and other persons involved. Help families to recognize that it is normal for children to express anger for what they are losing.
III. Bargaining (from "No, not me." to "Yes, me, but . . .")	Recognize this period as a time for the child and family to regain strength. Encourage the family to finish any unfinished business with the child. This is the time to do things such as take the promised trip or buy the promised toy.
IV. Depression. (The child and/or family experiences silent grief and mourns past and future losses.)	Recognize this as a normal reaction and expression of strength. Help families to accept the child who does not want to talk and excludes help. This is a usual pattern of behavior. Reassure the child that you can understand his or her feelings.
V. Acceptance.	Assist families to provide significant loving human contact with their child and one another.

TABLE 41-2 Stages in the Development of a Child's Concept of Death

Age of Child	Stage of Development
Child up to 3 y	At this stage, the child cannot comprehend the relationship of life to death because child has not developed the concept of infinite time. The child fears separation from protecting and comforting adults. The child perceives death as a reversible fact.
Preschool child	At this age the child has no real understanding of the meaning of death; child feels safe and secure with parents. The child may view death as something that happens to others. The child may interpret the separation that occurs with hospitalization as punishment; the painful tests and procedures that child is subjected to support this idea. The child may become depressed because of not being able to correct these wrongdoings and regain the grace of adults. The concept may be connected with magical thoughts of mystery.
School-aged child	The child at this age sees death as the cessation of life; child understands that he or she is alive and can become "not alive"; child fears dying. The child differentiates death from sleep. Unlike sleep, the horror of death is in pain, progressive mutilation, and mystery. The child is vulnerable to guilt feelings related to death because of difficulty in differentiating death wishes and actual event. The child believes death may be caused by angry feelings or bad thoughts. The child learns the meaning of death from own personal experiences, such as pets, and the death of family members, political figures, etc. Television and movies have contributed to concept of death and understanding of the meaning of illness. There may be more knowledge in the meaning of the diagnosis and an awareness that death may occur violently.
Adolescent	The adolescent comprehends the permanence of death as the adult does although may not comprehend death as an event occurring to persons close to self. Adolescent wants to live—sees death as thwarting pursuit of goals: independence, success, achievement, physical improvement, and self-image. Adolescent fears death before fulfillment. The adolescent may become depressed and resentful because of bodily changes that may occur, dependency, and the loss of social environment. The adolescent may feel isolated and rejected because own adolescent friends may withdraw when faced with impending death of friend. The adolescent may express rage, bitterness, and resentment; especially resents the fact that fate is to die.

6. The school-aged child knows death means final separation and knows what will be missed. The child must be allowed to mourn this loss. The dying child may be sad and bitter and demonstrate aggressive behavior. The child must be allowed the opportunity to verbalize this if able to do so.

C. *Adolescent*
1. The adolescent should be given an explanation of illness and all necessary treatment and procedures.
2. The adolescent feels deprived and reasonably resentful regarding illness because he or she wants to live and reach fulfillment.
3. As death approaches, the adolescent becomes emotionally closer to family.
4. The adolescent should be allowed to maintain emotional defenses—including absolute denial. The adolescent will indicate by questions what kind of answers are desired.
5. If the adolescent states, "I am not going to die," he or she is pleading for support. Be truthful and state, "No, you are not going to die right now."
6. The adolescent may ask, "How long do I have to live?" Adolescents are able to face reality more directly and can tolerate more direct answers. No absolute time should be given because that blocks all hope. If an adolescent has what is felt to be a prognosis of approximately 3 months, the response might be, "People with an illness like yours may die in 3 to 6 months, but some may live much longer."

Support Parents' Adaptation to Child's Death

1. Develop a plan of care that includes the following approach:
   a. The primary responsibility for communicating with the parents should be designated to one nurse.
   b. Information regarding the parents' concerns should be communicated to all staff members.
2. Accept parental feelings about the child's anticipated death and help parents deal with these feelings.
   a. It is not unusual for parents to reach the point of wishing the child dead and to experience guilt and self-blame because of this thought.
   b. The parents may withdraw emotional attachments to the child if the process of dying is lengthy. This occurs because the parents complete most of the mourning process before the child reaches biologic death. They may relate to the child as if he or she were already dead.
3. Provide anticipatory guidance regarding the child's actual death and immediate decisions and responsibilities afterward.
   a. Describe what the death will probably be like and how to know when it is imminent. This is necessary to dispel the horrifying fantasies that many parents have. Reassure the parent that the child will be kept comfortable at the time of death.

b. Clarify the parents' wishes about being present at the child's death and respect their desires. See if they want to hold the child—before, during, or after the death.

c. If appropriate, allow the parents to discuss their feelings about issues such as autopsy and organ donation in order that they may make appropriate decisions. Do not make them feel guilty if they do not consent.

d. If necessary, assist the parents to think about funeral arrangements.

4. Be aware of factors that affect the family's capacity to cope with fatal illness, especially social and cultural features of the family system, previous experiences with death, present stage of family development, and resources available to them.

5. Contact the appropriate clergy if the family desires. Contact other extended family members for support if they wish.

6. During final hours, do not leave the family alone, unless they request it.

7. Encourage parents and siblings to share their thoughts with the dying child.

8. Provide information on bereavement support groups, usually available through hospital or church.

Pediatric Procedures

◆ RESTRAINTS

Protective measures to limit movement are mechanisms for restraining children (Fig. 41-1). They can be a short-term restraint to facilitate examination and minimize the child's discomfort during special tests, procedures, and specimen collections. Restraints can also be used for a longer period of time to maintain the child's safety and protection from injury.

Points to Consider

1. Protective devices should be used only when necessary and never as a substitute for careful observation of the child.

2. Protective devices cannot be used on a continuous basis without an order. Continuous use requires justification and full documentation of the type of restraint used, reason for use, and the effectiveness of the restraint used.

3. The reason for using the protective device should be explained to the child and parents to prevent misinterpretation and to ensure their cooperation with the procedure. Children often interpret restraints as punishment.

4. Any protective device should be checked frequently to make sure that it is effective. It should be removed periodically to prevent skin irritation or circulation impairment. Provide range of motion and skin care routinely.

5. Protective devices should always be applied in a manner that maintains proper body alignment and ensures the child's comfort.

6. Any protective device that requires attachment to the child's bed should be secured to the bed springs or frame, never the mattress or side rails. This allows the side rails to be adjusted without removing the restraint or injuring the child's extremity.

7. Any required knots should be tied in a manner that permits their quick release. This is a safety precaution.

8. When a child must be immobilized, an attempt should be made to replace the lost activity with another form of motion. For example, even though restrained, a child can be moved in a stroller, wheelchair, or in bed. When arms are restrained, the child may be allowed to play kicking games. Water play, mirrors, body games, and blowing bubbles are helpful replacements.

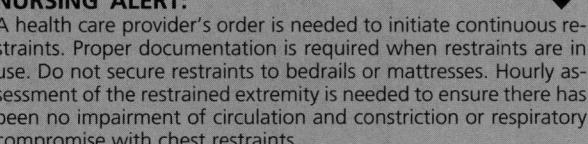

NURSING ALERT:
A health care provider's order is needed to initiate continuous restraints. Proper documentation is required when restraints are in use. Do not secure restraints to bedrails or mattresses. Hourly assessment of the restrained extremity is needed to ensure there has been no impairment of circulation and constriction or respiratory compromise with chest restraints.

Mummy Device

The mummy device involves securing a sheet or blanket around the child's body in such a way that the arms are held to the sides and leg movements are restricted (see Fig. 41-1). This short-term type of restraint is used on infants and small children during treatments and examinations involving the head and neck.

A. *Equipment*
Small sheet or blanket

B. *Nursing Action*
1. Place the blanket or sheet flat on the bed.
2. Fold over one corner of the blanket.
3. Place the child on the blanket with neck at the edge of the fold.
4. Pull the right side of the blanket firmly over the child's right shoulder.
5. Tuck the remainder of the right side of the blanket under the left side of the child's body.
6. Repeat the procedure with the left side of the blanket.
7. Separate the corners of the bottom portion of the sheet, and fold it up toward the child's neck.
8. Tuck both sides of the sheet under the infant's body.
9. Secure by crossing one side over the other in the back and tucking in the excess, or by pinning the blanket in place.

C. *Special Precautions*
Make certain that the child's extremities are in a comfortable position during this procedure.

Jacket Device

The jacket device is a piece of material that fits the child like a jacket or halter. Long tapes are attached to the sides of the jacket (see Fig. 41-1). Jacket device restraints are used to keep the child in a wheelchair, high chair, or crib.

A. *Nursing Action*
1. Put the jacket on the child so that the opening is in the back.
2. Tie the strings securely.
3. Position the child in high chair, wheelchair, or crib.

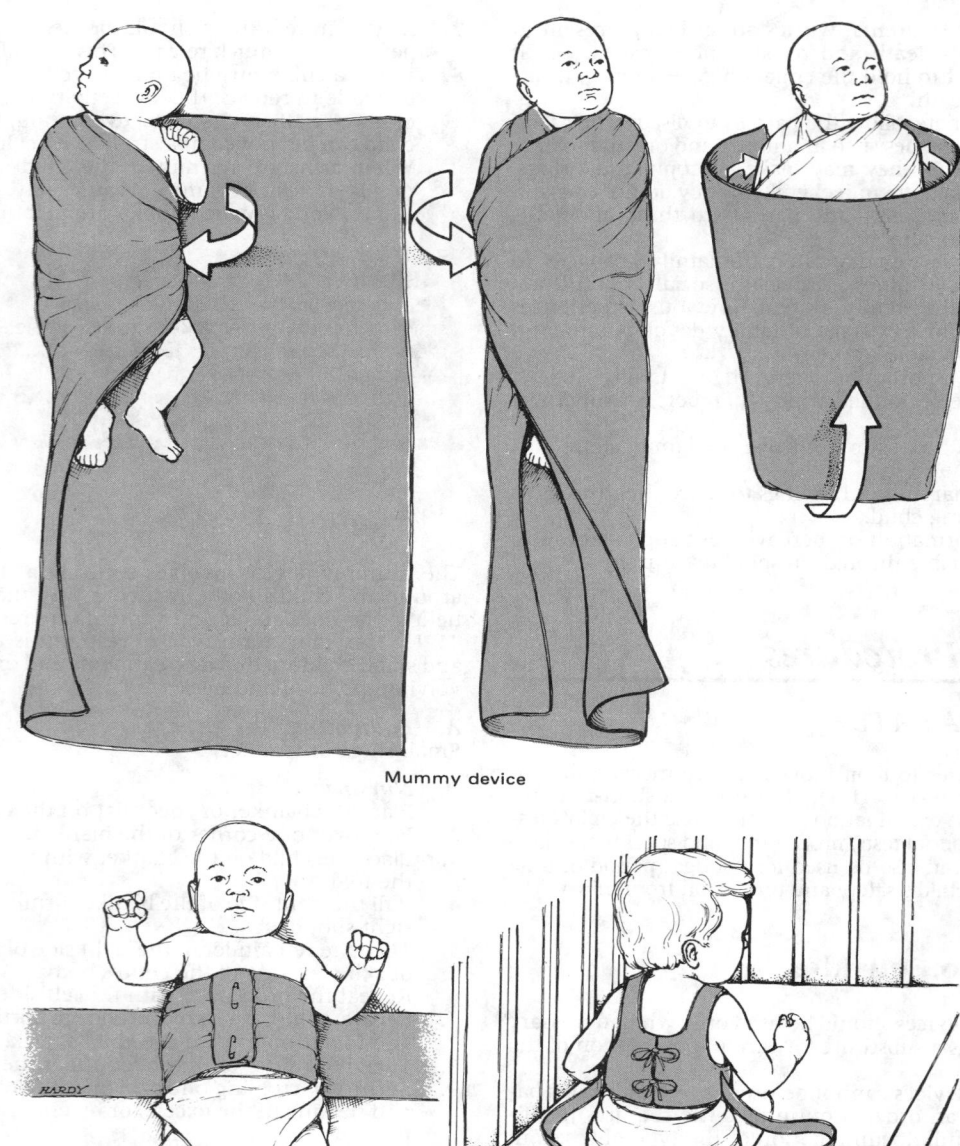

Mummy device

Belt device

Jacket device

FIGURE **41-1** *Types of restraints.*

4. Secure the long tapes appropriately:
 a. Under the arm supports of a chair
 b. Around the back of the wheelchair or high chair
 c. To the springs or frame of a crib

B. Special Precautions
Children in cribs must be observed frequently to make certain they do not become entangled in the long tapes of the jacket device.

Belt Device

The belt device is exactly like the jacket method of restraining, except that the material fits the child like a wide belt and buckles in the back (see Fig. 41-1).

Elbow Device

The elbow device consists of a piece of material into which tongue depressors have been inserted at regular intervals. It is especially useful for infants receiving a scalp vein infusion, those with eczema or cleft lip repair, and children having eye surgery. Some companies have plastic devices that fit around the arm at the elbow bend and are secured with Velcro straps. This type of restraint prevents flexion of the elbow.

A. Equipment
Elbow cuff
Tongue depressors
Safety pins, tapes, string or commercial plastic elbow restraint

B. Nursing Action
1. Insert tongue depressors into the appropriate places in the elbow cuff.
2. Place the child's arm in the center of the elbow cuff.
3. Wrap the cuff around the child's arm.
4. Secure the cuff with pins, tapes, or string.

C. Special Precautions
1. The tongue depressors should be cut to about 10 cm (4 inches) in length if the elbow cuff is to be used for an infant—for greatest comfort.
2. Additional security may be provided by dressing the child in long-sleeved shirt before the application of the elbow cuff. The ends of the shirt can then be turned back over the cuff and pinned securely.
3. If the plastic device is used, it may be applied over a shirt sleeve or padded to prevent sweating.

Devices to Limit Movement of the Extremities

Many different kinds of devices are available to limit motion of one or more extremities. One commercial variety consists of a piece of material with tapes on both ends to be secured to the frame of the bed. The material also has two small flaps sewn to it for securing the child's ankles or wrists. Similar devices are available that use sheepskin flaps. These should be used when the device will be necessary over a prolonged period or for children with sensitive skin. This restraining device may be used to restrain infants and young children for procedures such as IV therapies and urine collection.

A. Equipment
Extremity restraint of appropriate size for the child (small, medium, or large)
Several safety pins
Cotton wadding covered with gauze

B. Nursing Action
1. Secure the device to the crib frame.
2. Pad the extremities to be restrained with cotton wadding with gauze or other suitable material.
3. Pin the small flaps securely around the child's ankles or wrists.
4. Adjust the device by pinning a tuck in the center of the material if it is too large.

C. Special Precautions
1. The infant's fingers or toes should be observed frequently for coldness or discoloration and the skin under the device checked for signs of irritation.
2. The device should be removed periodically to provide skin care and range-of-motion exercises.

Abdominal Device

The abdominal device is used for restraining a small child in a crib. It operates exactly like the method described for limiting the movements of extremities. However, the strip of material is wider and has only one wide flap sewn in the center for fastening around the child's abdomen.

Clove-Hitch Device

The clove-hitch device is a mechanism for restraining an extremity by tying gauze strips or a diaper in a special way.

A. Equipment
Cotton wadding covered with gauze
Gauze bandage cut in lengths of 1.37 meters (1½ yards)

B. Nursing Action
1. Pad the extremity to be restrained with cotton wadding that is covered with gauze or other suitable material.
2. Spread out the gauze strip.
3. Make a figure 8 loop in the center of the gauze strip.
4. Place the child's wrist or ankle in the loop of the device.
5. Pull the ends of the device to the desired tightness.
6. Tie the ends to the crib springs or frame.
7. Check the device to make certain that it does not tighten when both ends are pulled taut or slip over the child's hand or foot.

Mitts

Mitts are used to prevent a child from injuring self with hands. They are especially useful for children with dermatologic conditions, such as eczema or burns. Mitts can be purchased commercially or made by wrapping the child's hands in Kling gauze.
Special Precaution: Mitts should be removed at least every 4 hours to permit skin care and to allow the child to exercise fingers.

Crib Top Device

A crib top device is used to prevent an infant or small child from climbing over the crib sides. Several types of commercial devices are available, including nets, plastic tops, and domes. A crib top device should be applied to the crib of an infant capable of climbing over the crib sides.

Special Precaution: In all instances, it is essential to be certain that the crib sides are kept all of the way up and latched securely. There should be no space between the top of the crib sides and the bottom of the crib top device.

◆ SPECIMEN COLLECTION

Evaluation of specimens such as blood, urine, and stool, is important in determining the status of the child. The nurse should be adept in the techniques for obtaining specimens, as well as meticulous in labeling and recording them.

For blood collection procedure, see Procedure Guidelines 41-1.

For urine specimen collection, see Procedure Guidelines 41-2.

For percutaneous suprapubic baldder aspiration, see Procedure Guidelines 41-3.

For stool collection, see Procedure Guidelines 41-4.

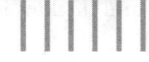

PROCEDURE GUIDELINES 41-1 ◆ Assisting With Blood Collection

EQUIPMENT No. 23–19-gauge short needle or scalp vein needle
Smaller volume or micro blood-collecting tubes
Smaller tourniquet (rubber band may be used with infant)
Gloves per universal precautions

PROCEDURE	*NURSING ACTION*	*RATIONALE*

PREPARATORY PHASE

1. Immobilize the child by placing in a mummy restraint if necessary (see p. 1137).

2. Position the patient.
   a. *Femoral venipuncture:* place the child on back with legs in froglike position. Nurse places hands on child's knees (see position for bladder puncture, p. 1142).
   b. *External jugular venipuncture:* place the child in mummy restraint and lower head over the side of the bed or table. Turn head to side and stabilize. Crying will make external jugular vein visible and causes blood to flow more readily.
   c. *Antecubital fossa venipuncture:* place the child in a supine position. The nurse stands on the side opposite the site to be used (across from the person drawing the specimen). The nurse positions right arm across the upper part of the child's chest and grasps the shoulder at the axilla position. Nurse's left arm is placed across the lower part of the child's chest and is used to extend the child's arm at the wrist (see figure).

1. Infants and young children squirm. Immobilizing them allows easier access to the venipuncture site. It also helps keep the infant warm.

2. These positions allow for optimal visualization and stabilization of the patient. Cover perineum to protect site and operator should infant void.

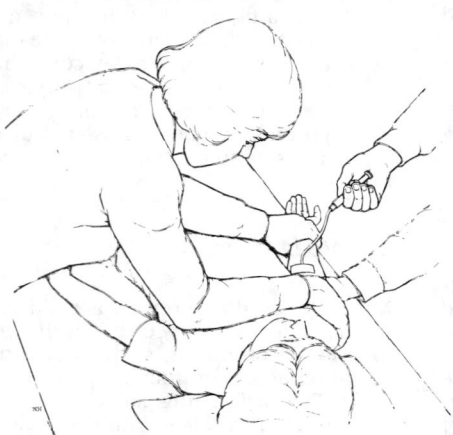

Assisting with antecubital fossa venipuncture.

PROCEDURE (cont'd)	NURSING ACTION	RATIONALE

d. *Infant—heel, toe, or digital puncture:* warm area with warm compress for 5–10 minutes.

d. This dilates vessels allowing blood to flow more freely.

PERFORMANCE PHASE

1. a. *Capillary:* clean area with antiseptic and dry with dry sterile 2 × 2 gauze. Hold heel firmly and with free hand quickly puncture with microlancet or sterile No. 21-gauge needle on most medial or lateral part of plantar surface. Puncture deeply enough to get free-flowing blood—never deeper than 2.4 mm. Discard first drop of blood; rapidly collect specimen in proper capillary tube.
2. After the specimen is collected and the needle is removed apply pressure to the site with dry gauze for 3–5 minutes.
   a. *Jugular venipuncture:* while applying pressure to the site, place the patient in an upright sitting position. Do not apply excessive pressure that may compromise circulation or respiration.
3. When the bleeding has been stopped, soothe and comfort the child before leaving.

1. Universal precautions. Both persons holding the infant and drawing the blood should wear gloves.

2. Both the femoral and jugular veins are large vessels. Since intravascular pressure is great, bleeding, oozing, and hematoma formation may result. External pressure prevents this from happening.

3. Crying and thrashing about may initiate bleeding.

FOLLOW-UP PHASE

1. Check the patient frequently for 1 hour after the procedure for oozing, bleeding, or evidence of a hematoma.
2. Record carefully and accurately:
   a. Site of venipuncture
   b. How the patient tolerated procedure
   c. Bleeding stopped or continued and for how long
   d. For what test the specimen was collected, time and place sent.

1. Reapply pressure and report if oozing continues.

PROCEDURE GUIDELINES 41-2 ◆ Collecting a Urine Specimen From the Infant or Young Child

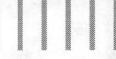

EQUIPMENT		

Collecting device—plastic, disposable urine bag or collector (Hollister, U-Bag, double chamber)
Cleansing agent
Wiping material—4 × 4s or cotton balls

Clean or sterile water
Containers for solutions
Specimen container
Gloves

PROCEDURE	NURSING ACTION	RATIONALE

PREPARATORY PHASE

1. Offer the young child choice of fluids to drink 30–60 min before procedure, if no contraindications.
2. Position the patient so that genitalia are exposed by placing on back with legs in froglike position. Assistance may be needed to hold the legs of the young child in proper position.
3. When small samples of urine are needed for pH, Clinitest, etc, to be done by the nurse, urine can be extracted from the diaper using a syringe or dropper.

1. To increase urine production.

2. Proper positioning will facilitate cleansing and allow for proper placement of collection device.

(continued)

PROCEDURE GUIDELINES 41-2 ◆ Collecting a Urine Specimen From the Infant or Young Child
(continued)

PROCEDURE (cont'd)

NURSING ACTION	RATIONALE
PERFORMANCE PHASE	
1. Wear gloves	1. Universal precautions.
2. Cleanse genital area.	2. This method of cleansing the female will prevent contamination of the genitalia from the anus, and will prevent contamination of the urine specimen obtained. During the cleansing be gentle to avoid any injury or possible stimulation of urination.
a. *Female:* using cotton balls, dip into cleansing agent, wipe labia majora from top to bottom (clitoris to anus) only once with each cotton ball. Repeat this once more. Wipe again with clear water. Then spread labia apart with one hand while wiping the labia minora in the same manner with other hand. Wipe area dry.	
b. *Male:* wipe tip of penis in circular motion down toward the scrotum. Be certain to retract foreskin if present. Wipe first with cleansing agent 2–3 times, then clear water. Dry the area.	
3. Apply collecting bag firmly so that the opening is exposed to receive urine.	3. If collecting bag is properly and securely placed, the procedure will not have to be repeated.
a. *Female:* stretch perineum taut during application. Attach bag to perineum first, then proceed up to symphysis.	a. This should ensure leak-proof contact.
Elevate head of bed or place the child in an infant seat, if appropriate.	To aid flow of urine by gravity.
b. *Male (small boys):* place penis inside bag.	
4. Apply diaper and comfort patient; possibly give additional clear fluids.	
5. Check the patient frequently (30–45 minutes) to see if he or she has voided. When the patient has voided, remove bag gently. Cleanse area and reapply diaper to the child. If child has not voided within 45 minutes, procedure must be repeated.	5. The adhesive on the collecting bag may tend to be sticky. Careful removal of the bag will prevent skin injury on and around genitalia. Also avoid spilling urine out of the bag during removal. Reapplication of bag will decrease the possibility of unreliable test results.
FOLLOW-UP PHASE	
1. Pour specimen into proper collecting container. Send specimen to the laboratory within 30 minutes or refrigerate.	1. Prompt delivery of specimen to the laboratory will prevent growth of organisms in an uncontrolled environment and distortion of the test results.
2. Accurately chart and describe the following in the nurse's notes:	2. Guideline for weighing diaper, excluding weight of dry diaper, 1 g = 1 mL urine.
a. Time specimen collection was started and ended	
b. Amount of urine voided	
c. Color of urine (cloudy, clear, any sediment)	
d. Type of test to be done	
e. Condition of skin of perineal area	

Note: If 24-hour urine collection is needed, use a collection bag that has a long tube attachment to facilitate frequent emptying of urine every 1–2 hours. Place urine in receptacle in refrigerator. Adherence of bag to skin can be improved by applying a thin coating of tincture of benzoin to skin and allowing this to dry before attaching collection bag.

EQUIPMENT   Antiseptic skin cleansing solution
Band-Aid
Sterile 4 × 4s
Gloves

Needle, No. 20-22 gauge, 3.7 cm (1½ inches) long
Syringe, 20 mL
Specimen container

NURSING ACTION	*RATIONALE*

PREPARATORY PHASE

1. Check diaper for wetness. If the child has just voided, report this or report last voiding time. At least 1 hour should pass without voiding.
2. Position the child on back on the examining table. Head should be toward nurse, feet toward the health care provider. Spread legs apart in a froglike position. Place hands on child's knees and thumbs along sides at the hip level (see accompanying figure).

1. To perform a successful bladder aspiration, enough urine must be present to distend the bladder up above the pubic symphysis—so that bladder is accessible.
2. This position allows the nurse to stabilize the child. It also gives a full view of the child, making it easier to observe, talk to him, and soothe the child.

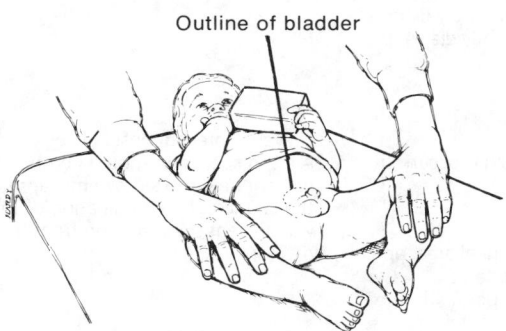

Outline of bladder

Assisting with percutaneous suprapubic bladder aspiration.

3. Ensure that the skin over the puncture site is cleansed in an antiseptic manner.

3. To prevent infection from being introduced into the bladder by inserting the needle through unclean skin, which would contaminate the specimen.

PERFORMANCE PHASE

1. Both the health care provider and nurse should wear gloves.
2. While the procedure is being performed, note the condition of the patient and any signs of distress. Comfort child by talking and smiling.

3. To prevent urination during procedure, compress the infant's urethra:
   a. *Male:* pressure on penis.
   b. *Female:* digital pressure upward on urethra from rectum.
4. When urine has been obtained or the procedure is discontinued and the needle is removed, apply pressure over the puncture site with a 4 × 4 and gloved fingers.
5. Apply a Band-Aid if necessary. Reapply diaper. Hold and comfort child for a few minutes.

1. Universal precautions.
2. Report any changes in color or respiration rate or other signs. Soothing the child will promote relaxation and decreased movement. Crying increases the muscle tone of the lower abdomen, making it more difficult to insert the needle.

4. This prevents any bleeding from occurring either internally or externally. Pressure should be maintained about 3 minutes or until oozing ceases and coagulation has taken place.
5. Holding the child will help to restore and maintain a good nurse–patient relationship and will help the child to relax after a frightening and painful procedure.

FOLLOW-UP PHASE

1. Check the child periodically for 1 hour after procedure to see that bleeding or oozing has not occurred.
2. Note time of first voiding after procedure. Note color of urine (it may be pink). Bloody urine should be reported to the health care provider.

3. Accurately describe and chart the procedure, including:
   a. Time of procedure
   b. Whether or not a specimen was obtained
   c. How the patient tolerated the procedure
   d. Description and amount of urine obtained
   e. Patient's condition and activity following the procedure.

1. This is not likely if pressure was applied properly after procedure and the patient was left quiet.
2. It is important to note any changes in voiding pattern following the procedure since change might indicate injury. The first voided urine may be bloody because of a small amount of local capillary bleeding at the time of the procedure.

PROCEDURE GUIDELINES 41-4 ◆ Collecting a Stool Specimen

EQUIPMENT   Diaper
Cellophane or plastic liner (used when stool is loose or watery)
Tongue blade
Specimen container
Gloves

Note: Collecting a stool specimen from an older child who is toilet-trained is the same as collecting such a specimen from an adult.

PROCEDURE	NURSING ACTION	RATIONALE

PREPARATORY PHASE

1. If a specimen is needed from a patient whose stools are loose or watery enough to be absorbed in the diaper, line the diaper with a piece of cellophane or plastic. Place this liner between the diaper and the skin. Then apply diaper to the child and position so that head is slightly elevated. If stools are soft or formed, apply diaper.

    1. The liner and position will allow the loose stool specimen to collect in the liner and not be absorbed by the diaper.

PERFORMANCE PHASE

1. Wear gloves.
2. Check the child frequently to see if stooling has occurred.

    1. Universal precautions.
    2. A fresh specimen should be obtained so that test results will not be distorted by time lapse. This will also decrease the chance of contamination of the stool with urine and will prevent skin irritation from the stool.

3. Remove soiled diaper from child. Clean perineal area, apply clean diaper, and leave the child comfortable.
4. Remove small amount of stool from diaper with the tongue blade and place it in the specimen container.
5. Send labeled specimen to the laboratory promptly.

    5. Prompt delivery to the laboratory will prevent changes from occurring in the specimen that could alter the test results.

FOLLOW-UP PHASE

1. Accurately describe and record the following:
   a. Time specimen was collected
   b. Color, amount, and consistency of stool (note any foul smell.)
   c. Type of specimen collected
   d. Nature of test for which the specimen was collected
   e. Condition of the skin

◆ FEEDING AND NUTRITION

Nutritional requirements of the infant or child may increase while ill, but the ability to feed naturally may be impaired by illness or the child's response to illness. If existing feeding patterns cannot be maintained, alternate methods may be necessary.

Breast-feeding

Refer to Procedure Guidelines 41-5.

1. Breast-feeding is the natural and ideal nourishment that will supply an infant with adequate nutrition as well as immunologic and anti-infection properties. With breast milk being at the proper temperature, it may prevent other gastrointestinal disturbances as well. The development of allergies is decreased in breast-fed babies.
2. Breast-feeding provides psychological and emotional satisfaction for the infant and mother and can promote bonding. The physical closeness may also provide comfort after a frightening or painful procedure.
3. Because breast milk is more easily and quickly digested, shorter periods of NPO both preoperatively and postoperatively may be necessary.
4. Hospitalization may interfere with the routine of breast-feeding; however the infant may nurse more frequently if the mother is available. In time of stress, the infant may cope with breast-feeding better than bottle-feeding. Do not attempt to wean if avoidable.

5. Stress of the child's hospitalization and illness experienced by the mother may decrease her milk supply and inhibit her "let down" reflex, as well as increase or decrease the infant's desire to suckle. Care may be initiated to help stimulate the mother's milk supply. Attempts should be made to maintain the breast-feeding bond and routines of the child and mother.

Artificial or Nipple-Feeding

Artificial or nipple-feeding is a method of supplying nutrition to the infant by oral feedings, using a bottle and nipple set-up. Nipple-feeding can provide the baby with adequate fluid and calorie intake appropriate for growth. Bottle-feeding can supplement breast-feeding with formula or water. Bottle-feeding can provide additional fluid intake between feedings. Refer to Procedure Guidelines 41-6.

Gavage Feeding

Refer to Procedure Guidelines 41-7.

1. Gavage feeding is a means of providing food via catheter passed through the nares or mouth, past the pharynx, down the esophagus, and into the stomach, slightly beyond the cardiac sphincter. Feedings may be continuous or intermittent.
2. Gavage feedings can provide a method of feeding or administering medications that require minimal patient effort when the infant is unable to suck or swallow adequately (ie, premature infants under 32 weeks' gestation or under 1560 g).
3. Gavage feedings provide a route that allows adequate calorie or fluid intake and they can provide supplemental or additional calories.
4. Gavage feedings can prevent fatigue or cyanosis that is apt to occur from bottle-feeding. They can provide supplement for an infant who is a poor bottle feeder.
5. Gavage feedings can provide a safe method of feeding a limp listless patient, a patient experiencing respiratory distress (respiratory rate greater than 60/min) or intubated patients, debilitated patients, or those with anomalies of the digestive tract.

Gastrostomy Feeding

Refer to Procedure Guidelines 41-8.

1. Gastrostomy feeding is a means of providing nourishment and fluids via a tube that is surgically inserted through an incision made through the abdominal wall into the stomach. It is the method of choice for those requiring tube feedings for an extended period of time.

2. Gastrostomy feedings provide a safe method of feeding a hypotonic patient or one who cannot tolerate alternative methods. Specific indications may include duodenal atresia, tracheoesophageal fistula, and omphalocele. Gastrostomy feedings may provide a route that allows adequate calorie or fluid intake in a child with chronic lung disease or in one who does not have continuity of the gastrointestinal tract such as in esophageal atresia, chronic reflux, or aspiration processes.
3. Gastrostomy tubes can also allow better decompression of the stomach (because of the large tube size) following a surgical procedure.

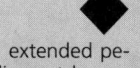

COMMUNITY-BASED CARE TIP:
Gastrostomy feedings often are maintained for an extended period of time. If a child is receiving these tube feedings at home, nurses need to:
1. Teach the child (if age appropriate) and family about gastrostomy feedings.
2. Teach the use of equipment: syringes, feeding bag, feeding tubing.
3. Teach the use of control pump (for continuous feedings).
4. Teach care of the gastrostomy tube—venting procedures, clamping procedures.
5. Stoma care.
6. Instruct about formula, need to refrigerate if opened, when to discard.
7. Teach measures to take in an emergency
a. Procedure to follow if the tube falls out
b. Cases of nonfunctioning equipment
c. Proper phone numbers available to have as a resource or to obtain assistance

Nasojejunal Feeding/Nasoduodenal Feedings

Refer to Procedure Guidelines 41-9.

1. Nasojejunal (N-J) or nasoduodenal (N-D) feedings are means of providing full enteral feedings via a catheter passed through the nares, past the pharynx, down the esophagus, bypassing the stomach through the pylorus into the duodenum or jejunum.
2. Duodenal or jejunal feedings decrease the risk of aspiration because the feeding bypasses the pylorus, can minimize regurgitation, and gastric distention.
3. N-D and N-J feedings provide a route that allows for adequate calorie or fluid intake (a full enteral feeding) via intermittent or continuous drip.
4. N-D or N-J feedings may also provide a route for administration of oral medications.
5. N-D or N-J feedings can provide a method of feeding that requires minimal patient effort when the child or infant is unable to tolerate alternative feeding methods (low birth weight, persistent respiratory effort in the intubated patient).

PROCEDURE GUIDELINES 41-5 ◆ Breast-Feeding the Ill or Hospitalized Infant

PROCEDURE	NURSING ACTION	RATIONALE

PREPARATORY PHASE

1. When an infant who is nursing is hospitalized, it is the nurse's responsibility to encourage the mother to continue breast-feeding if the infant's condition does not contraindicate it. Explain to the mother that:
    a. Supplemental artificial formula can be given to the infant if she is not available.
    b. She can pump her breasts and bring in her milk to be given to the infant via bottle when she is not available.
    c. Breast milk can be frozen for up to 6 months (check the facility's specific policy)
    d. Thaw frozen breast milk for use in tepid water. *Do not microwave for it may destroy vitamins and nutritional properties.*
2. When nursing is to be done in the hospital pediatric setting, the physical surroundings may need to be altered somewhat. Provide the mother and infant with a relatively quiet area that is as private as possible and free from interruption.
3. Provide the mother with a comfortable armchair or pillow so that she can assume a comfortable position during the feeding. A footstool should also be available so that she can support her feet and the infant.
4. The infant should be awake and dry before the feeding is started.
5. Dress the infant appropriately so that he or she is not too warm or too cool during the feeding. The infant should also be hungry.
6. Help position the baby at breast. Put in a semi-sitting position with face close to the breast and supported by one arm and hand. A pillow may be used under the baby for support.
    The breast may need to be supported by mother's other hand.

1. Some mothers have very strong feelings about wanting to nurse their baby. It gives them an emotional satisfaction that is vitally important to the mother–child relationship because it is an integral part of the total mothering process. The nurse must help to foster this relationship as much as she can, and offer suitable alternatives when appropriate.

2. This will provide the mother and infant with an opportunity to continue to develop their relationship during the crisis of illness and hospitalization.

3. Proper and comfortable position of the mother will enable her to hold the baby correctly and support baby while at the breast.

4. If awake and comfortable, infant will settle down and feed better.
5. If too warm, infant may fall asleep after the first few sucks of milk. A sleepy baby will not nurse well. If too cool, infant may be fussy and restless.
6. Proper positioning will provide the infant with comfort and security and make it easier to suck and swallow. This makes the nipple more easily accessible to the infant's mouth and prevents obstruction of nasal breathing.

PERFORMANCE PHASE

1. When the feeding is to start, let the breast touch the infant's cheek. Do not hold cheek and try to help infant find the nipple.

2. The infant's lips should be out over the areola and not just around the nipple before beginning to suck.

3. Note the presence or absence of the "let-down" reflex during the nursing period.

4. The length of feeding time may vary from 5 to 30 minutes. Let the infant nurse until satisfied.
5. Instruct the mother to burp the baby during and at the end of the feeding.

6. One or both breasts may be used at each feeding. It makes no difference as long as (a) baby is satisfied at the end of the feeding and (b) one breast is completely emptied at the feeding.
7. Once the infant has stopped sucking, he or she likes to cling to the breast. To break this suction, instruct mother to put her finger to the corner of the baby's mouth and gently pull.

1. The rooting reflex will take over and the infant will turn head toward the breast with mouth open. If cheek is touched with a hand, infant will become confused, perhaps turning toward the hand.
2. Because the nipple is so small, suction cannot be achieved merely by grasping it. The areola must be in the infant's mouth to establish suction and make the suck effective.
3. Milk flowing from the other breast during nursing is quite normal. It is not usually present when the mother is worried.
4. When the infant is satisfied and has nursed well he or she is relaxed and usually falls asleep. Infant will stop sucking.
5. When the infant is sucking, he or she swallows some air. Burping will help prevent abdominal distention and discomfort as well as regurgitation.
6. Regular and complete emptying of the breast is the only stimulation for the production of milk.

7. Gentle pulling will not hurt mother or infant.

PROCEDURE (cont'd)	NURSING ACTION	RATIONALE

FOLLOW-UP PHASE

1. When the infant has finished feeding, change diaper if it is wet or soiled.
2. Position infant on right side in bed.

3. Note if baby appears satisfied or still seems to be hungry.

4. Record descriptively and accurately.
   a. How baby fed—weight before and after may be helpful.
   b. How baby went to breast
   c. Satiety or hunger after feeding
   d. Breast or breasts used; which breast was emptied and which breast was nursed from thereafter.

5. For the new mother–infant nursing team:
   a. Provide the mother with anticipatory guidance for possible problems (ie, breast engorgement).
   b. Promote maternal confidence in handling and nursing her infant.
   c. Increase mother's knowledge about the mechanics of breast-feeding. Some facilities may have a Lactation Specialist to visit with the mother.
   d. Provide mother with literature and resources.
      The Womanly Art of Breast Feeding, 4th ed.
      LaLeche League International
      9616 Minneapolis Avenue
      Franklin Park, IL 60131

1. To provide comfort for a restful sleep and to prevent diaper rash
2. This facilitates emptying of the stomach and decreases the possibility of regurgitation.
3. Mother may not have enough milk to satisfy the baby. Supplemental formula may be necessary.

d. If both breasts were used, the second breast is not usually emptied and should be used first at the next feeding.
5. To help establish and maintain successful breast-feeding that will be continued following discharge. Encourage mother to continue to get adequate rest and nutrition during and after infant's discharge.

PROCEDURE GUIDELINES 41-6 ◆ Artificial or Nipple-Feeding

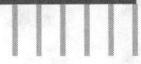

EQUIPMENT   Sterile nipple and bottle
Sterile formula or feeding fluid

PROCEDURE	NURSING ACTION	RATIONALE

PREPARATORY PHASE

1. Baby should be awake and hungry. Change wet or soiled diaper.

2. Check formula for correct type and amount.
3. Some babies prefer warmed formula *not* hot.

4. Sit in a comfortable chair. Cradle baby with one hand and arm, while supporting baby against your body or lap.

1. A sleepy baby will not feed well. A dry diaper will provide comfort so that the baby will settle down and eat more easily.
2. To prevent error.
3. Check temperature of formula on inner wrist before feeding.
4. Proper position will provide the baby with comfort and security and will make it easier to suck and swallow. Holding infant will enhance trust-building and provide sensory stimulation.

PERFORMANCE PHASE

1. Let the baby root for the nipple by touching the corner of mouth with the nipple. When infant opens mouth, insert the nipple.
2. Hold the bottle at an angle to completely fill the nipple with fluid.
3. NEVER prop the bottle or leave the baby unattended during feeding.

1. Place the nipple on top of the tongue and far enough in mouth so suction can be created when he sucks.

2. This prevents the baby from sucking and swallowing excessive amounts of air.
3. This is unsafe. Should vomiting occur, aspiration is more likely.

(continued)

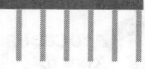

PROCEDURE GUIDELINES 41-6 ◆ Artificial or Nipple-Feeding *(continued)*

PROCEDURE (cont'd) NURSING ACTION	RATIONALE
4. The bottle should be handled so as not to contaminate the nipple or fluid.	4. Contamination will increase the chances of gastrointestinal disturbances.
5. Baby's feeding time will vary from 10 to 25 minutes. Position baby so eye contact can be established (en face) during feeding. Soothing talk and fondling can provide additional comfort to the baby.	5. The length of time will depend on the age of the baby and how vigorously he or she sucks.
6. Burp the baby at least once during the feeding and at the end of the feeding. a. Place the baby in sitting position in nurse's lap, tilt slightly forward, and gently rub or pat back or abdomen. b. Place the baby in prone position on nurse's shoulder and gently pat or rub back. c. Place the baby in prone position on nurse's lap and gently rub or pat back.	6. Most babies swallow some air during feeding. These positions aid in expelling air and thus prevent abdominal distention, discomfort, and regurgitation. Vigorous handling or patting may result in the infant spitting up or regurgitating feeding.

FOLLOW-UP PHASE

1. After final burping, change wet or soiled diaper and place baby in crib on right side.	1. This position aids in emptying the stomach and prevents regurgitation.
2. Check baby in a few minutes. If restless, pick baby up and burp. Note if any spitting-up has occurred.	2. Some babies relieve themselves of air when in the crib and also bring up small amounts of formula at the same time.
3. Accurate and descriptive recording: a. What was fed and amount b. How feeding was tolerated c. Any regurgitation or emesis—amount and material d. Length of time of feeding e. How baby sucked and took the feeding; behavior before, during, and following feeding.	

Note: When feeding a premature infant, the same principles apply. The premature infant, however, will tire more easily and fall asleep. Allow frequent rest periods and use a soft nipple so that less energy is needed to suck. To stimulate this infant to suck, the nurse can brush the infant's cheek with her finger, place thumb or finger under the infant's chin, or move the nipple slowly back and forth in mouth. Feeding time should not exceed 30 minutes. Keep the infant warm during feeding.

PROCEDURE GUIDELINES 41-7 ◆ Gavage Feeding

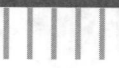

EQUIPMENT	
Sterile rubber or plastic catheter, rounded-tip, size 5–14 (French Argyle feeding tube) Clear, calibrated reservoir for feeding fluid Syringe Stethoscope	Water for lubrication Tape—hypoallergenic Feeding fluid, room temperature Pacifier

PROCEDURE NURSING ACTION	RATIONALE
PREPARATORY PHASE	
1. Position the infant on side or back with a diaper roll placed under shoulders. A mummy restraint may be necessary to help maintain this position.	1. This position allows for easy passage of the catheter, facilitates observation, and helps avoid obstruction of the airway.
2. Measure feeding catheter and mark with tape; measure distance from tip of nose to ear to xiphisternum.	2. Premeasuring the catheter provides a guideline as to how far to insert catheter.
3. Have suction apparatus readily available.	3. Suctioning clears the airway and prevents aspiration if vomiting occurs.

PERFORMANCE (cont'd)	NURSING ACTION	RATIONALE

PERFORMANCE PHASE

1. Lubricate catheter with sterile water or saline.
2. Stabilize the patient's head with one hand; use the other hand to insert catheter.
   Push nose up to widen nostril.
   a. *Insertion through nares:* slip the catheter into nostril and direct toward the occiput in a horizontal plane along floor of nasal cavity.
   b. *Insertion through the mouth:* pass the catheter through the mouth toward the back of the throat. Depress anterior portion of tongue with forefinger, insert catheter along forefinger, and tilt head slightly forward.
3. If the patient swallows, passage of the catheter may be synchronized with the swallowing.
   Do not push against resistance. Gently try rotating the tube if resistance is met.
4. If there is no swallowing, insert the catheter smoothly and quickly.
5. In the infant, especially, observe for vagal stimulation (ie, bradycardia [slow heart rate] and apnea).

6. Once the catheter has been inserted to the premeasured length, tape the catheter to the patient's face (see accompanying figure).

1. Do not use oil because of danger of aspiration.

   a. This direction will follow the nares passageway into the pharynx. Do not direct the catheter upward. Positioning in nares may cause partial airway obstruction; therefore, observe for respiratory distress. Avoid this route if there is critical airway compromise.

3. Swallowing motions will cause esophageal peristalsis, which opens the cardiac sphincter and facilitates passage of the catheter.
   Perforation occurs with very little pressure.
4. Because of cardiac sphincter spasm, resistance may be met at this point. Pause a few seconds, then proceed.
5. The vagus nerve pathway lies from the medulla through the neck and thorax to the abdomen. Above the stomach, the left and right branches unite to form the esophageal plexus. Stimulation of these nerve branches with the catheter will directly affect the cardiac and pulmonary plexus.
6. This prevents movement of catheter from the premeasured, preestablished correct position. Alternative method: loop narrow cloth tape around tube just below nostril, then secure it above lip or nose with tape. Some movement of tube may be seen with swallowing.

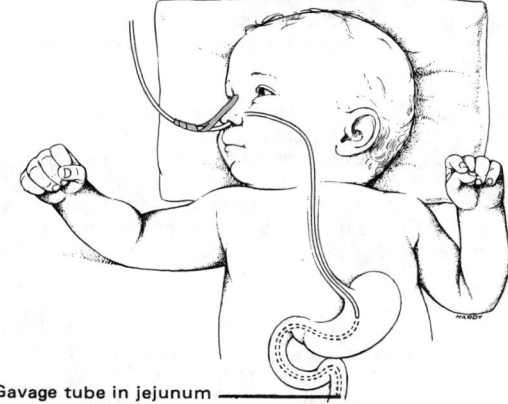

Gavage tube in jejunum

Gavage feeding.

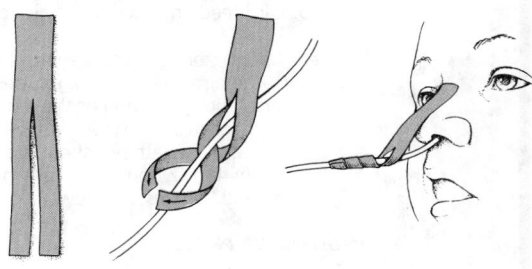

Steps in preparing adhesive tape to retain gavage tube

7. Test for correct position of the catheter in the stomach:
   a. Inject 0.5–5 mL air into the catheter and stomach. At the same time listen to the typical growling stomach sound with a stethoscope placed over the epigastric region.
   b. Aspirate injected air from the stomach.
   c. Aspirate small amount of stomach content and test acidity by pH tape.

   a. Aids in ensuring proper location of catheter.

   b. This prevents abdominal distention.
   c. Failure to obtain aspirate does not indicate improper placement; there may not be any stomach content or the catheter may not be in contact with the fluid.

(continued)

PROCEDURE GUIDELINES 41-7 ◆ Gavage Feeding *(continued)*

PERFORMANCE (cont'd)	NURSING ACTION	RATIONALE

NURSING ACTION

d. Observe and gently palpate abdomen for tip of catheter. Avoid inserting catheter into the infant's trachea. (An infant's anatomy makes it relatively difficult to enter the trachea because esophagus is behind the trachea.)

8. The feeding position should be right-side-lying, with head and chest slightly elevated. Attach reservoir to catheter and fill with feeding fluid. Encourage infant to suck on pacifier during feeding. Hold infant when possible.

9. Aspirate tube before feeding begins.
   a. If over half the previous feeding is obtained, withhold the feeding.
   b. If small residual of formula is obtained, return it to stomach and subtract that amount from the total amount of formula to be given.

10. The flow of the feeding should be slow. Do not apply pressure. Elevate reservoir 15–20 cm (6–8 inches) above the patient's head.

11. Food taken too rapidly will interfere with peristalsis, causing abdominal distention and regurgitation.

12. Feeding time should last approximately as long as when a corresponding amount is given by nipple, 5 mL/5–10 min or 15–20 minutes total time.

13. When the feeding is completed, the catheter may be irrigated with clear water. Before the fluid reaches the end of the catheter, clamp it off and withdraw it quickly or keep in place for next feeding.

14. Discard feeding tube and any leftover solution.

Note: Intermittent gavage feeding is often preferred to indwelling gavage feeding. An indwelling catheter may coil and knot, perforate the stomach, and cause nasal airway obstruction, ulceration, irritation of the mucous membranes, incompetence of esophageal–cardiac sphincter, and epistaxis. However, if intermittent intubation is not well tolerated and the indwelling method is used, the catheter should be clamped to prevent loss of feeding or entry of air and changed every 48–72 hours. (Use alternate sides of the nares.) Constant alertness to the above problems should be stressed. Indwelling method may be preferred with older infant or child.

FOLLOW-UP PHASE

1. Burp the patient.

2. Place the patient on right side for at least 1 hour.

3. Observe condition after feeding; bradycardia and apnea may still occur.
4. Note any vomiting or abdominal distention.

5. Note infant's activity.

6. Accurately describe and record procedure, including time of feeding, type of gavage feeding, type and amount of feeding fluid given, amount retained or vomited, how the patient tolerated feeding, and activity before, during, and following feeding.

RATIONALE

d. If improper placement occurs and the catheter enters the trachea, the patient may cough, fight, and become cyanotic. Remove the catheter immediately and allow the patient to rest before attempting to insert tube again.

8. This position allows the flow of fluid to be aided by gravity. The use of the pacifier will relax the infant, allowing for easier flow of fluid as well as provide for normal sucking needs. Sucking will help develop muscles and provide a positive association between sucking and relief of hunger.

9. This is done to monitor for appropriate fluid intake, digestion time, and overfeeding that can cause distention. Note an increase in gastric residual contents.

10. The rate of flow is controlled by the size of the feeding catheter; the smaller the size, the slower the flow. If the reservoir is too high, the pressure of the fluid itself increases the rate of flow.

11. The presence of food in the stomach stimulates peristalsis and causes the digestive process to begin. Also, when tube is in place, incompetence of the esophageal-cardiac sphincter may result in regurgitation.

13. Clamp the catheter before air enters the stomach and causes abdominal distention. Clamping also prevents fluid from dripping from the catheter into the pharynx, causing the patient to gag and aspirate.

1. Adequate expulsion of air swallowed or ingested during feeding will decrease abdominal distention and allow for better tolerance of the feeding.
2. To facilitate gastric emptying and minimize regurgitation and aspiration
3. Because of vagal stimulation as mentioned above

4. Due to overfeeding or too rapid feeding. Regurgitation of 1–2 mL may occur in the premature infant as the musculature of the sphincter of the gastrointestinal tract is relaxed and allows for easy reflex.
5. Fatigue or peaceful sleep offers insight as to tolerance of the feeding.
6. Observe for readiness of the infant to feed by nipple—note sucking activity and sleep–wake cycle in relation to feeding.

PROCEDURE GUIDELINES 41-8 ◆ Gastrostomy Feeding

EQUIPMENT
Warm feeding fluid
Pacifier
Reservoir syringe or funnel
Syringe for aspirating

PROCEDURE

NURSING ACTION	RATIONALE

PREPARATORY PHASE

1. Gastrostomy tube may be in one of three positions between feedings:
   a. Lowered and open to start drainage.
   b. Open, connected to reservoir (funnel, syringe) that is elevated 10–12 cm (4–4¾ inches).
   c. Clamped.

2. The nurse may be directed to check residual stomach contents before any feeding.
   a. Attach syringe and aspirate stomach contents.
   b. Measure.
   c. Residual fluid may be returned to stomach or discarded, depending on amount.
3. A Y-tube that is connected at the point where reservoir and gastrostomy tube join may be used during feeding.
4. When feeding is about to begin, infant/child should be placed in comfortable position in bed—either flat or with head slightly elevated. If condition permits, the nurse should hold the infant. A pacifier can be given.

Note: *Gastrostomy tube feeding button:*
The child may have a gastrostomy tube feeding button, in which case insert the special tube into the button and follow the feeding procedure in the Performance Phase.

PERFORMANCE PHASE

1. Attach reservoir syringe to tube (if not already open to continuous elevation) and fill reservoir with feeding fluid prior to unclamping tube.
2. Elevate tube and reservoir to 10–12 cm (4–4¾ inches) above abdominal wall. Do not apply any pressure to start flow.
3. Feed slowly, taking 20–45 minutes. Fill reservoir with remaining fluid before it is empty to avoid instillation of air.

4. Continue to provide infant with pleasant feelings associated with feeding.
5. When feeding is completed:
   a. Instill clear water (10–30 mL, or 0.3–1 oz) if tube is to be clamped. Apply clamp before water level reaches end of reservoir.
   b. Leave tube unclamped and open to continuous elevation.

6. Often when oral feedings are started, they are given simultaneously with gastrostomy feedings.

FOLLOW-UP PHASE

1. Check dressing and skin around point of tube entry for wetness. Clean skin and apply skin barrier (petrolatum, Maalox, aluminum paste, etc.). See that there is no pull on tube.

RATIONALE

a. Constant decompression.
b. To serve as safety valve outlet to prevent esophageal reflux and increased stomach pressure.
c. Most "normal" physiologic setup, preparation for home care or tube removal.
2. This is done to monitor for appropriate fluid intake, digestion time, and overfeeding that can cause distention.

3. To provide simultaneous decompression during feeding
4. When the infant/child is comfortable and relaxed, feeding fluid will flow more easily into stomach. Pacifier will satisfy normal sucking activity, provide exercise for jaw muscles, and relax musculature as well as provide pleasure normally associated with feeding.

1. Prevents air from entering tube (and then stomach), which may cause distention.
2. This elevation level will allow for slow, gravity-induced flow. Pressure may cause a backflow of fluid into the esophagus.
3. Too rapid a feeding will interfere with normal peristalsis and will cause abdominal distention and backflow into reservoir or esophagus.

a. This rinses tubing and will prevent clogging.

b. Feeding fluid is allowed to return to reservoir if infant cries or changes position, and thus decreases pressure on the stomach.
6. This allows the infant to learn or reestablish the sucking-swallowing process as well as to build up tolerance to eating without compromising nutritional intake.

1. Skin breakdown is caused by continued exposure to stomach contents that may be leaking out around tube causing excoriation and infection. Constant pulling on tube can cause widening of skin opening and subsequent leakage.

(continued)

PROCEDURE GUIDELINES 41-8 ◆ Gastrostomy Feeding (continued)

PROCEDURE (cont'd)	NURSING ACTION	RATIONALE
	2. Leave the infant dry and comfortable. If unable to hold infant during feeding, this may be a good time to hold, fondle, and provide warmth and love. Place on right side or in Fowler's position.	2. To promote relaxation and improved digestion of feeding.
	3. Accurately describe and record procedure, including time of feeding, type and amount of feeding fluid given, amount and characteristics of residual (if any) and what was done with it, how the patient tolerated feeding, any abdominal distention, and activity following feeding.	

Note: Should infant pull out gastrostomy tube, cover ostomy site with sterile dressing and tape, notify health care provider and accurately record events.

PROCEDURE GUIDELINES 41-9 ◆ Nasojejunal (N-J) and Nasoduodenal (N-D) Feedings

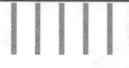

EQUIPMENT

Sterile radiopaque silicone or polyvinyl nasojejunal (N-J) or nasoduodenal (N-D) tube, 1 meter (39 inches) (appropriate size for child) may or may not have weighted tip
Tape
pH paper

Reservoir for feeding
Possibly an infusion pump
3-way stopcock
Syringe—0.5 mL normal saline or sterile water
Equipment for nasogastric (N-G) tube insertion; introducer catheter

NURSING ACTION	RATIONALE
PREPARATORY PHASE	
1. Attach cardiac monitor to infant.	1. To allow for continuous monitoring of heart rate and rhythm. The vagus nerve pathway lies from the medulla through the neck and thorax to the abdomen. Above the stomach, the left and right branches unite to form the esophageal plexus. Stimulation of these nerve branches with the catheter will directly affect the cardiac and pulmonary plexus.

2. Tube is generally inserted by a health care provider.
  a. Measure from glabella (prominent point between eyebrows) to the heel for estimated length.
  b. Measure and mark the remaining length of tubing and record.
	b. This serves as a double-check to ensure that tube has not advanced farther than intended.

3. Place the infant on right side with hips slightly elevated. Gentle restraint or soft mittens may have to be applied.	3. Facilitates passage of tube. Restraints prevent infant from pulling out tube before the tip passes the pylorus. Do not place on left side.
4. Tube is inserted by threading the N-J or N-D vinyl catheter into a No. 10 French feeding catheter and introducing both through the nostril into the stomach. The feeding tube is then withdrawn, and the ND/N-J feeding tube is allowed to advance through the pylorus.	4. Oral insertion may cause increased salivation, air swallowing, and regurgitation. The N-G acts as an introduction catheter and may not be needed because N-D or N-J catheters come with an internal guide wire to aid in placement.
5. Check intestinal aspirate for pH every 1–2 hours. Infant may be positioned on right side, back, or abdomen. Once the tube is past the pylorus, abdominal posteroanterior and lateral x-rays are taken to confirm that tip of catheter is at the ligament of Treitz. Remove the guide wire.	5. When aspiration fluid reaches a pH of 5–7 or bile-colored fluid is obtained, the tip of the tube has passed the pylorus and duodenum into the jejunum.
6. A small N-G feeding tube may be passed through the other nostril at this time and left indwelling. This is used to check stomach for residual fluid and regurgitation through the pylorus.	6. If gastric residual is significant, it will interfere with prescribed feeding. Notify health care provider. (4 mL/kg reflux in stomach is usually tolerated.) Do not remove N-G tube because it will adhere to N-J tube during withdrawal and pull out N-J tube also.

PROCEDURE (cont'd)	NURSING ACTION	RATIONALE

PROCEDURE (cont'd)

NURSING ACTION

7. N-D/N-J feedings can generally be started following this progression:
   a. D₅W initially
   b. ½ strength formula with low osmolality for 6–12 hours. Higher osmolarity formulas for older children.
   c. Full strength low osmolality formula for infants and high osmolarity formula for older children.
   d. The volume of feeding is increased at a slow rate until daily calorie and fluid requirements are being administered.
   e. Medications may be given via the N-D/N-J tube if prescribed. A 3-way stopcock will have to be placed at the connection of the N-J tube and the line from the feeding fluid. Alternative method for administering oral medications is by passing an oral–gastric or nasogastric feeding tube; in this way the stomach and process of digestion and absorption are not bypassed.

PERFORMANCE PHASE

1. N-J feedings can be given as follows:
   a. Intermittently (ie, q 1–3 h)
   b. In a continuous slow drip.

2. If intermittent feeding is the method used, the feeding techniques are the same as for nasogastric (gavage) feeding.

3. If slow continuous drip method is used, the set-up used is similar to the pediatric IV infusion using an infusion pump and small (100–250 mL) closed chamber for reservoir.
   a. Reservoir chamber and tubing should be changed q8–24 h.
   b. Record input every hour. Fill reservoir as needed, with no more than 3 hours worth of feeding fluid.

FOLLOW-UP PHASE

1. Be constantly alert for mechanical problems:
   a. Check for abdominal distention resulting from the infant's inability to handle ingested amount of fluid:
      • Palpate abdomen
      • Observe for ripple of intestines
      • Measure abdominal girth q3–8 h
      • Check residual formula in jejunum q3–8 h
      • Discard or refeed residual formula as prescribed.
   b. Check stools for occult blood and pH, and urine for glucose every voiding or 4–8 hours to determine tolerance of feeding fluid.
   c. Check emesis for blood and report to physician immediately—may be a sign of necrotizing enterocolitis.
2. Position child/infant in recumbent position.
3. Observe child/infant closely to avoid potential dangers as tube passes the pylorus.
   a. Close attention to amount, type, concentration, and osmolality of feeding fluid is stressed.
   b. Check heart rate and blood pressure.
4. Hold, fondle, and give positive stimulation to the child/infant if conditions permit
5. Accurately describe and record condition of infant and procedure, including type and amount of feeding given, amount of residual and characteristics, any signs of impending infant distress or problems.

RATIONALE

b. Low solute formulas include SMA, Similac, Enfamil (20 calories/30 mL).
c. Low osmolality formula is used to prevent loss of fluid into intestine and possible necrotizing enterocolitis.
d. 150 mL/kg fluid requirement is generally used (130–150 cal/kg).
e. Flush tubing with small amounts of normal saline solution or sterile water after medication is administered to ensure that infant receives entire dosage prescribed and to prevent any sediment from remaining in tubing or prevent tube clogging. Pills should be crushed finely.

b. Generally the preferred method to minimize the satiety–hunger cycle and large-volume instillation.
2. Feeding is given at room temperature. Avoid cold fluid, which may cause infant discomfort. If breast milk is used, gently rotate reservoir periodically to mix settled-out fat content.

a. To prevent growth of bacteria.

b. To ensure a constant flow and minimize overinfusion directly into the jejunum/duodenum.

1. Tube clogging due to inadequate rinsing. Tube advancing too far into jejunum; check protruding tube measurement. Fluid overload, causing aspiration.

2. Less likely for "dumping syndrome" to occur.
3. Diarrhea; as the tube passes through the pylorus, it (the tube) becomes stiff because of the change in pH. A stiff tube has been reported to cause intestinal perforation. If tube becomes clogged or dislodged, it must be removed.

4. This procedure limits the normal pleasures associated with feeding. Infant needs some attention to psychological needs to thrive.

◆ FLUID AND ELECTROLYTE BALANCE

Basic Principles

1. Infants and small children have different proportions of body water (Table 41-3) and body fat than do adults.
   a. The body water of a newborn infant approaches 80% of body weight compared to that of an average adult man, which approaches 60%.
   b. The normal infant demonstrates a rapid physiologic decline in the ratio of body weight to body water during the immediate postpartum period.
   c. Proportion of body water declines more slowly throughout infancy and reaches the characteristic value for adults by approximately 2 years of age.
2. Compared with adults, a greater percentage of the body water of infants and small children is contained in the extracellular compartment.
   a. Infants—approximately one-half of the body water is contained in the cell.
   b. Adults—approximately two-thirds of the body water is contained in the cell.
3. Compared with adults, the water turnover rate per unit of body weight is three or more times greater in infants and small children.
   a. The child has more body surface in relation to weight.
   b. The immaturity of kidney function in infants may impair their ability to conserve water.
4. Electrolyte balance depends on fluid balance and cardiovascular, renal, adrenal, pituitary, parathyroid, and pulmonary regulatory mechanisms (Table 41-4).
5. Infants and children are more vulnerable to disorders of hydration than are adults.
   a. The basic principles relating to fluid balance in children make the magnitude of fluid losses considerably greater in children than adults.
   b. Children are prone to severe disturbances of the gastrointestinal tract that result in diarrhea and vomiting.
   c. Young children cannot independently respond to increased losses by increased intake. They depend on others to provide them with adequate fluid.

Common Fluid and Electrolyte Therapy

1. Repair of preexisting deficits that may occur with prolonged or severe diarrhea or vomiting
   a. Deficits are estimated and corrected as soon and as safely as possible.

TABLE 41-3 Body Fluids Expressed as Percentage of Body Weight

Fluid	Adult		Infant (%)
	Male (%)	Female (%)	
Total Body Fluids	60	54	75
Intracellular	40	36	40
Extracellular	20	18	35

   b. Initial therapy is aimed at restoring blood and extracellular fluid volume to relieve or prevent shock and restore renal function.
   c. Intracellular deficits are replaced slowly over an 8- to 12-hour period after the circulatory status is improved.
2. Provision of maintenance requirements
   a. Maintenance requirements occur as a result of normal expenditures of water and electrolytes due to metabolism.
   b. Maintenance requirements bear a close relationship to metabolic rate and are ideally formulated in terms of caloric expenditure.
3. Correction of concurrent losses that may occur via the gastrointestinal tract as a result of vomiting, diarrhea, or drainage of secretions
4. Replacement should be similar in type and amount to the fluid being lost.
5. Replacement is usually formulated as milliliters of fluid and milliequivalents of electrolytes lost.

Intravenous Fluid Therapy

Intravenous therapy refers to the infusion of fluids directly into the venous system. This may be accomplished through the use of a needle or by venous cutdown and insertion of a small catheter directly into the vein (Fig. 41-2). IV therapy is used to restore and maintain the child's fluid and electrolyte balance and body homeostasis when oral intake is inadequate to serve this purpose. Refer to Procedure Guidelines 41-10.

1. Infusion pumps are often used in pediatrics to provide a controlled, constant rate of infusion.
2. Because infants and children are vulnerable to fluid shifts, the rates need to be controlled carefully.
3. During an IV infusion, every hour, check:
   a. Delivery rate
   b. Volume delivered
   c. For infiltration, because many pumps will continue to infuse solution even if infiltration has occurred.

TABLE 41-4 Common Abnormalities of Fluid and Electrolyte Metabolism

Substance	Major Function	Abnormality	Cause	Clinical Manifestation	Laboratory Data
Water	Medium of body fluids, chemical changes, body temperature, lubricant	Volume deficit	1. Primary—inadequate water intake 2. Secondary—loss following vomiting, diarrhea, gastrointestinal obstruction, etc.	Oliguria, weight loss, signs of dehydration including dry skin and mucous membranes, lassitude, sunken fontanelles, lack of tear formation, increased pulse rate, decreased blood pressure	Concentrated urine, azotemia, elevated hematocrit, hemoglobin and erythrocyte count
		Volume excess	1. Failure to excrete water in presence of normal intake such as in congestive heart failure, renal disease 2. Water intake in excess of output	Weight gain, peripheral edema, signs of pulmonary congestion	Variable urine volume, low specific gravity of urine, decreased hematocrit
Potassium	Intracellular fluid balance, regular heart rhythm, muscle and nerve irritability	Potassium deficit	1. Excessive loss of potassium due to vomiting, diarrhea, prolonged cortisone, ACTH or diuretic therapy, diabetic acidosis 2. Shift of potassium into the cells such as occurs with the healing phase of burns, recovery from diabetic acidosis	Signs and symptoms variable, including weakness, lethargy, irritability, abdominal distention, and eventually cardiac arrhythmias	Low plasma K^+ level (may be normal in some situations); hypochloremic alkalosis; ECG changes
		Potassium excess	Excessive administration of potassium-containing solutions, excessive release of potassium due to burns, severe kidney disease, adrenal insufficiency	Variable, including listlessness, confusion, heaviness of the legs, nausea, diarrhea, ECG changes, ultimately paralysis and cardiac arrest	Elevated potassium plasma level
Sodium	Osmotic pressure, muscle and nerve irritability	Sodium deficit	Water intake in excess of excretory capacity, replacement of fluid loss without sufficient sodium; excessive sodium losses	Headache, nausea, abdominal cramps, confusion alternating with stupor, diarrhea, lacrimation, salivation, later hypotension; early polyuria, later oliguria	Sodium plasma level may be high, low, or normal
		Sodium excess	Inadequate water intake especially in the presence of fever or sweating; increased intake without increased output; decreased output	Thirst, oliguria, weakness muscular pain, excitement, dry mucous membranes, hypotension, tachycardia, fever	Elevated Na^+ plasma level, high plasma volume
Bicarbonate	Acid–base balance	Primary bicarbonate deficit	Diarrhea (especially in infants), diabetes mellitus, starvation, infectious disease, shock or congestive heart failure producing tissue anoxia	Progressively increasing rate and depth of respiration—ultimately becoming Kussmaul respiration, flushed, warm skin, weakness, disorientation progressive to coma	Urine pH usually <6 Plasma bicarbonate <20 mEq/L Plasma pH <7.35
		Primary bicarbonate excess	Loss of chloride through vomiting, gastric suction, or the use of excessive diuretics, excessive ingestion of alkali.	Depressed respiration, muscle hypertonicity, hyperactive reflexes, tetany and sometimes convulsions.	Urine pH usually >7, plasma bicarbonate >25 mEq/L (30 mEq/L in adults), plasma pH >7.45

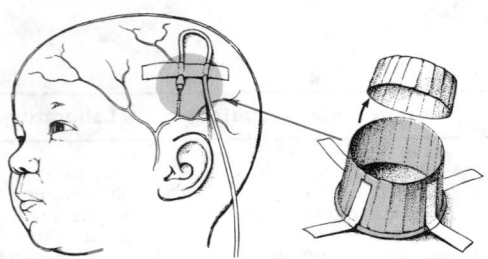

Venipuncture of scalp vein

Paper cup taped over venipuncture site for protection. A clear plastic cup may also be used.

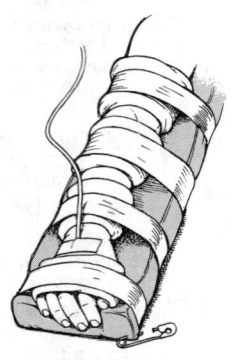

Restraint of arm when hand is site of infusion

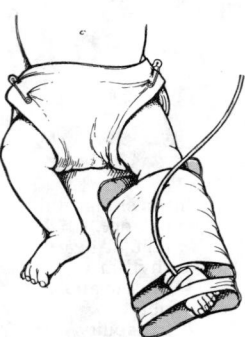

Infant's leg taped to sandbag for immobilization

FIGURE 41-2 IV fluid therapy.

PROCEDURE GUIDELINES 41-10 ◆ Intravenous Fluid Therapy

EQUIPMENT **A. NEEDLE METHOD**

IV solution
  The kind of solution is specified by the health care provider
  For small children, 250-mL bottles should be used for purposes of safety
IV pole, pump device
IV administration set, pump tubing
Micropore filter
Syringe, 5 or 10 mL—approximately ½–⅔ filled with normal saline
Butterfly needle or catheter of appropriate gauge
  The size of the needle depends on the age and size of the child and the type of fluid to be administered
Alcohol sponges, dry sponges
Betadine or other antibacterial cleansing solution
Normal saline
Small tourniquet or rubber band
Hypoallergenic tape, 1.2 cm (½ inch), 2.5 cm (1 inch), 5 cm (2 inches)
Padded armboard
Gauze bandage for securing the extremity to the armboard
Restraining devices—bath blanket, extremity restraint, covered sandbags
  The type of restraint depends on the child's age, his level of cooperation, and the kind of IV to be started.
Safety razor (if scalp vein is to be used)

B. CUTDOWN METHOD

IV solution, IV pole, IV administration set
Alcohol sponges
Hypoallergenic tape, 1.2 cm (½ inch), 2.5 cm (1 inch), 5 cm (2 inches)
Padded armboard

PROCEDURE (cont'd)	NURSING ACTION	RATIONALE

Dry sponges
Gauze bandage
Sterile cutdown tray
  The tray should include the following equipment: medicine cups, treatment towels, wound towel, syringe, No. 25 gauge 1.5-cm (⅝-inch) needle, No. 1-20 gauge 2.5-cm (1-inch) needle, knife handle and No. 15 blade, forceps, scissors, gauze sponges, 4-0 black silk suture, needle holder
Assorted sizes of sterile polyethylene tubing and Luer adapters
5-0 black silk suture with a straight eye needle
1%–2% procaine
Normal saline
Tourniquet
Sterile gloves
Restraining devices

PROCEDURE	NURSING ACTION	RATIONALE

PREPARATORY PHASE

1. Obtain the IV solution.

2. Check the IV fluid for sediment or contaminant by holding the container up to the light.

3. Check the container for cracks.

4. Attach a micropore filter to the end of the infusion tubing that attaches to the needle. Use aseptic technique.

5. Remove the metal seal from the IV container without touching the rubber top.

6. Following product information, insert the end of the administration set into the container's opening. Fill the tubing with solution.
7. Promote the cooperation of the child.
  a. *Infant:* provide with a pacifier.
  b. *Older child:* explain the procedure and its purpose.
8. Position the child for comfort.
9. Restrain the child as necessary.
  a. *Infant or young child:* restraints may include mummy wrappings, jacket or elbow restraints, or small sandbags.
  b. *Older child:* the extremity to be used should be comfortably restrained on the armboard. Free extremities may also require light restraints to remind the child not to move.

PERFORMANCE PHASE

1. The persons starting the IV and holding the infant should wear gloves.
2. Assist as necessary.
3. When applying the tourniquet, a second rubber band is placed crosswise under it. To remove the tourniquet, grasp the unstretched rubber band, pull up, and cut the tourniquet (see accompanying figure).

RATIONALE

1. Although the type of solution and the rate of flow are prescribed, the nurse should be aware of the composition of common parenteral solutions and should know how to calculate maintenance therapy.
2. Contaminant is most easily identified with the container in this position. If sediment is observed, the solution should be discarded.
3. If a flash of light can be seen through the bottle, it has a razor-thin crack and should be discarded.
4. A 0.45-μm filter prevents entry into the vein of larger particles, air emboli, and most bacterial and fungal organisms except some *Pseudomonas* organisms. A 0.22-μm filter prevents entry of any organisms but requires the use of an IV pump.
5. Do not use the solution if the seal has been broken. It is not necessary to cleanse the sterile, rubber top with alcohol unless it has been accidentally contaminated.

7. The procedure will be least traumatic if child is able to cooperate and is not frightened or resistant.

9. Protective devices may be necessary to prevent the child from dislodging the IV needle. The type and size of such devices should be appropriate for the child's age and the position of the IV.
  b. Toes and fingers should be visible to avoid compromising blood flow. The restraint board must be padded and the main pressure points (heel, palm) padded with gauze. Before strapping an extremity to the armboard, back the adhesive with tape or gauze wherever it touches the skin.

1. Universal precautions.

2. The nurse may insert the IV.

(continued)

PROCEDURE GUIDELINES 41-10 ◆ Intravenous Fluid Therapy *(continued)*

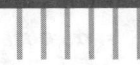

PROCEDURE (cont'd)	*NURSING ACTION*	*RATIONALE*

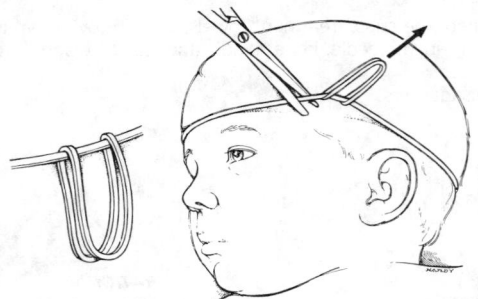

Applying the tourniquet for IV therapy.

4. Check the restraints at intervals and adjust them as necessary.

5. Comfort and reassure the child.

6. Regulate the IV rate via pump

7. Record:
   Type of solution being used
   Reading on the container or reservoir
   Rate of flow
   Time that the infusion began
   Name of the physician or nurse who started the IV
   Site of administration
   Reaction of the child to the procedure
8. Return the child to room.

FOLLOW-UP PHASE

1. Check the child at least hourly.
   a. Note the location of the IV.
   b. Note the color of the skin at the needle point.
   c. Check for swelling of the skin at the needle point.
      (1) If in a hand or foot, compare with the opposite extremity.
      (2) If in the head, look at the face to determine asymmetry.
   d. Feel the area around the IV site for sponginess or leakage.
   e. Check for blood return into the tube when the flow of fluid is stopped.
   f. Make certain that the child is adequately restrained.
   g. Check function of the pump—rate set versus amount infused.
2. Observe closely for complications.
   a. *Local reactions:*
      (1) Compromised circulation
      (2) Pressure sores
      (3) Thrombophlebitis

4. The restraints may become loose after a period of time and must be secured to ensure the child's safety. They may also become too tight and require loosening to maintain adequate circulation.
5. The procedure is usually disturbing for the child. This should be acknowledged. If crying and upset, the child should be reassured that his behavior is acceptable.
6. Pump infusion devices are more often than not used in IV rate regulation of infants and children.

1. The child must be observed frequently to make certain that the IV is not infiltrating and is functioning properly. Report any swelling, discoloration, or leakage.

2. Complications associated with the administration of intravenous fluids to infants and children are very serious and may have fatal consequences. Any signs of complications must be reported immediately.

PROCEDURE (cont'd)	NURSING ACTION	RATIONALE

NURSING ACTION

b. *Fluid and/or electrolyte disturbances:*
  (1) Maintain an accurate record of intake and output.
    (a) Total the intake and output q8h.
    (b) Describe carefully the amount and consistency of all stools and vomitus.
    (c) Collect all urine and weigh diapers if more accurate measurement of the child's output is necessary.
  (2) Weigh the child at regular intervals, using the same scales each time.

  (3) Monitor laboratory electrolytes.

  (4) Report:
    (a) Decreased skin turgor
    (b) Marked increase or decrease in urination
    (c) Fever
    (d) Sunken or bulging fontanelles in an infant
    (e) Sudden change in weight or vital signs
    (f) Diarrhea
    (g) Weakness, apathy, or lethargy
c. Pyrogenic reactions

3. Record essential information.
  a. Reading on the container or reservoir
  b. Amount of fluid absorbed in the hour
  c. Total amount of fluid absorbed (compare with the total amount of fluid intended to have been absorbed)
  d. Rate of flow
  e. Apparent condition of the child.
4. Irrigate the IV as necessary.
  a. Gather equipment:
    (1) Syringe with 1–3 mL normal saline solution
    (2) Several alcohol wipes
  b. Clamp off the IV solution.
  c. Disconnect the IV tubing at the needle insertion site. Keep it sterile.
  d. Remove the needle from the syringe.
  e. Connect the syringe to the tubing at the needle insertion site or stopcock.
  f. Slowly inject the normal saline solution.

  g. Disconnect the syringe and reconnect the IV tubing to the needle insertion site.
  h. Unclamp the IV and regulate the flow of the solution.
  i. Check frequently to make certain that the IV is functioning properly.
6. Change the IV container and tubing q24h or as per hospital policy.

7. If a catheter is used, check the dressing q4h and change according to policy.
8. Disconnect the IV when prescribed or if it has obviously infiltrated
  a. Gather equipment
    (1) Scissors
    (2) 4 × 4 gauze square
    (3) Band-Aid
  b. Explain the procedure to the child, depending on age.
  c. Clamp off the flow of the IV fluid.
  d. Determine the location of the needle.
  e. Loosen the tape around the needle, holding the needle firmly in position so that it does not slip out.

RATIONALE

b. Refer to Table 41-4, page 1135.

  (2) An increase or decrease of 5% within a relatively brief period of time is usually significant and should be reported.
  (3) Electrolyte imbalances can be corrected by replacement or changes in IV solution as ordered.

c. If severe, the IV should be discontinued. The solution should be saved for possible analysis.
3. Proper documentation should be followed.

4. Irrigation may be required to dislodge small clots in the needle or to maintain the infusion rate of a sluggish IV.

  f. Great force of injector should be avoided because this may cause the vein to rupture or the needle to become dislodged from the vein.

6. The IV set-up should be changed daily to maintain sterility and prevent contamination of the IV fluid during IV therapy.
7. This reduces the incidence of infection and other local complications.

(continued)

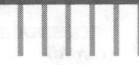

PROCEDURE GUIDELINES 41-10 ◆ Intravenous Fluid Therapy *(continued)*

PROCEDURE (cont'd)	NURSING ACTION	RATIONALE
	f. Hold the 4 × 4 lightly over the insertion site and re-move the needle quickly and carefully.	f. Inspect an Intracath or plastic needle to ensure that no portion has been left in the vein. If this is suspected, notify the physician. Alcohol sponges should not be used for removing IV needles because the stinging of alcohol on the puncture site causes unnecessary discomfort.
	g. Apply pressure to the site immediately and hold until bleeding stops.	
	h. Apply Band-Aid.	h. The Band-Aid should not be applied until all bleeding has stopped to minimize the possibility of prolonged or unnoticed bleeding.
	i. Remove the tape and armboard from the extremity.	
	j. Comfort the child as required.	
	k. Note the fluid level on the container or reservoir and complete recordings.	
	l. Record that the IV was discontinued.	

For additional information relating to IV therapy, including criteria for selecting a suitable vein for venipuncture, guidelines for administering an infusion using the antecubital fossa, and complications of intravenous therapy, refer to Chapter 4, IV Therapy, page 56.

◆ CARDIAC AND RESPIRATORY MONITORING

Cardiac and respiratory monitoring refers to electrical surveillance of heart and respiratory rates and patterns. It is indicated in all patients whose conditions are unstable.

Nursing Management

1. Select a monitor that is appropriate for the child's needs. This will depend on the child's age, ability to cooperate, purpose for monitoring, information desired, and equipment available.
2. Stabilize the device to reduce the amount of mechanical noise and for safety considerations.
3. Reduce the child's anxiety:
   a. Provide age-appropriate explanations of the equipment.
   b. When possible, involve the child in care, including change of electrodes.
4. Select lead placement sites according to equipment specifications.
   a. Cardiac monitors frequently use three leads located at:
      (1) Right upper lateral chest wall below clavicle
      (2) Left lower chest wall in the anterior axillary line
      (3) Upper left chest wall
   b. Respiratory monitors frequently use three electrodes located:
      (1) On either side of the chest (anterior axillary line in fourth or fifth intercostal space)
      (2) At a reference electrode placed on the manubrium or other suitable distal point
5. Apply electrodes by:
   a. Cleaning the appropriate areas on the chest with alcohol.
   b. Place pregelled, disposable electrodes.
   c. Apply the electrode firmly to completely dry skin.

6. Plug the leads into the lead cable at appropriate insertion points.
7. Be certain that the monitor alarms are in the "on" position. High and low alarm limits should be set according to the child's age and condition so that apnea, tachypnea, bradycardia, and tachycardia can be readily detected.
8. Avoid skin breakdown by changing lead placement sites as needed. Clean and dry old sites and expose them to air.
9. Check integrity of the entire system at least once each shift.
   a. Carefully inspect lead wires and cable for breaks and proper attachment.
   b. If malfunction is suspected, change equipment and notify the engineering department immediately.
10. Continue to count respiratory and apical rates at frequent intervals.
    a. Compare with monitor rates to verify accuracy of equipment.
    b. It must be remembered that monitors cannot substitute for close observation of the child.
11. Apnea mattresses or pads that use sensing devices may be used for infants, eliminating the need for electrodes.
    a. Although less susceptible to cardiovascular artifact, these devices may record physical impact, vibrations, or body movements as breaths.
    b. In addition, older infants can easily roll or crawl off the pad.

◆ CARDIOPULMONARY RESUSCITATION

Cardiopulmonary resuscitation (CPR) involves measures instituted to provide effective ventilation and circulation when the patient's respiration and heart have ceased to function. In children, more often the initial cause is of a respiratory nature.

Underlying Considerations

A. Cardiac Arrest
1. Signs—absence of heartbeat and absence of carotid and femoral pulses
2. Causes—asystole, ventricular fibrillation, or cardiovascular collapse related to arterial hypotension

B. Respiratory Arrest
1. Signs—apnea and cyanosis
2. Causes—obstructed airway, depression of the central nervous system, neuromuscular paralysis

C. Emergency Preparation
1. Every hospital should have a well defined and organized plan to be carried out in the event of cardiac or respiratory arrest.
2. Emergency carts should be placed in strategic locations in the hospital and checked daily to ensure that all equipment is available.

Equipment

Emergency cart—assembled and ready for use
Positive pressure breathing bag with nonrebreathing valve and universal 15-mm adapter
Mask (premature infant, child, adult sizes)
Oropharyngeal airways, sizes No. 0 to No. 4
Laryngoscope with blades of various sizes
Extra batteries and light bulbs for laryngoscope
Endotracheal tubes with connectors (complete sterile set, 25-8.0 mm inner diameter)
Portable suction equipment and sterile catheters of various sizes
Bulb syringe, DeLee trap
Oxygen source—portable supply gauge and tubing, masks of various sizes
Cardiac board (30 × 50 cm)
Emergency drugs:
  Sodium bicarbonate
  Epinephrine (Adrenalin)
  Isoproterenol (Isuprel)
  Saline solution (for dilution)
  Diphenhydramine hydrochloride (Benadryl)
  Diazepam (Valium)
  Hydrocortisone sodium succinate (Solu-Cortef)
  Digoxin (Lanoxin)
  Naloxone (Narcan)
  Calcium gluconate
  Calcium chloride 10%
  Dextrose 50%
  Lidocaine (Xylocaine)
  Atropine
  Phenytoin sodium (Dilantin)
  Insulin
  Procainamide (Pronestyl)
  Propranolol (Inderal)
  Dopamine (Intropin)
  Bretylium tosylate (Betylol)
  Volume expanders
  Ringer's lactate—Hespan
Intracardiac needles, No. 20 and 22 gauge, 6 to 8 cm ($2^{3}/_{8}$–$3^{1}/_{8}$ inches long)
IV equipment
  Fluids
  Infusion set
  Tourniquet
  Armboards

Tape
Scalp vein needles of various sizes
Nasogastric tubes of various sizes
Other equipment
  Syringes of various sizes
  Needles of various sizes
Intraosseous needles
Longdwell catheters of various sizes
3-way stopcock
Cutdown set
Pole
Labels
Alcohol wipes
Tongue blades
Sterile 4 × 4 gauze sponges
Sterile hemostat
Sterile scissors
Blood specimen tubes
Electrocardiograph and monitor
Lubricating jelly
Defibrillator and paddles (pediatric and adult)

Artificial Ventilation

A. Mouth to Mouth Technique
1. Infants and young children
   a. Slightly extend neck by gently pulling chin up and forward and the head back (chin lift or jaw thrust). Place a rolled towel or diaper under the infant's shoulder, or use one hand to support the neck in an extended position. Do not hyperextend the neck because this narrows the airway.
   b. Check the mouth and throat and clear mucus or vomitus with finger or suction, if necessary.
   c. Take a breath.
   d. Make a tight seal with your mouth over the infant's mouth and nose.
   e. Gently blow air from the cheeks and observe for chest expansion.
   f. Remove your mouth from infant's mouth and nose and allow the infant to exhale.
   g. If spontaneous respiration does not return, continue breathing at a rate and volume appropriate for the size of the infant (usually 20 times/min or 1 breath every 3 seconds).
2. Older children and adolescents
   a. Clear mouth of mucus or vomitus with fingers or suction.
   b. Hyperextend neck with one hand or a rolled towel (head tilt, chin lift, or jaw thrust).
   c. Clamp the nostrils with the fingers of one hand, which also continues to exert pressure on the forehead to maintain the neck extension.
   d. Take a deep breath.
   e. Make a tight seal with your mouth over the child's mouth.
   f. Force air into the lungs until the chest expansion is observed.
   g. Release your mouth from the child's mouth and release nostrils to allow the child to exhale passively.
   h. Repeat approximately 12 to 15 times/min or 1 breath every 4 to 5 seconds.

B. Hand-Operated Ventilation Devices
1. Remove secretions from mouth and throat and move mandible forward.

TABLE 41-5 Technique of Artificial Circulation

Size of Child	Preparatory Phase	Action Phase	Distance of Compression	Rate
Neonate, premature, or small infant	1. Place in supine position. 2. Encircle the chest with the hands, with thumbs over the midsternum *or* Use method for a larger infant, at a rate of 100–120/min.	1. Compress midsternum with both thumbs, gently but firmly.	2/3 distance to the spine or 1.3–1.8 cm ($\frac{1}{2}$–$\frac{3}{4}$ inch)	100–120/min
Larger infant	1. Place on a firm, flat surface. 2. Support the back with one hand or use a small blanket under the shoulders. 3. Place the tips of the index and middle fingers of one hand over the midsternum.	Compress the midsternum with the tips of the index and middle fingers.	1.3–2.5 cm ($\frac{1}{2}$–1 inch)	≥100/min
Small child	1. Place on a firm, flat surface. 2. Support the back by slipping one hand beneath it, or use a small blanket. 3. Place the heel of one hand over the midsternum, parallel with the long axis of the body.	1. Apply a rapid downward thrust to the midsternum, keeping the elbow straight. 2. Hold for approximately 0.4 seconds. 3. Instantly and completely release the pressure so the chest wall can recoil. 4. Do not remove the heel of the hand from the chest.	2.5–3.8 cm (1–1$\frac{1}{2}$ inches)	80–100/min
Larger child, adolescent	1. Place on a flat, firm surface or place a board under the thorax. 2. Place the heel of one hand on the lower half of the sternum, about 2.5–3.8 cm. (1–1$\frac{1}{2}$ inches) from the tip of the xiphoid process and parallel with the long axis of the body. 3. Place the other hand on top of the first one (may interlock fingers). 4. Place shoulders directly over child's sternum, in order to use own weight in application of pressure.	1. Exert pressure vertically downward to depress lower sternum, keeping elbows straight. 2. Hold for approximately 0.4 seconds. 3. Instantly and completely release the pressure so the chest wall can recoil. 4. Do not remove the hands from the chest.	3.8–5 cm (1$\frac{1}{2}$–2 inches)	80–100/min

2. Appropriately extend the neck with one hand or place a diaper roll behind the neck.
3. Select an appropriate size mask to obtain an adequate seal, and connect mask to bag.
4. Hold the mask snugly over the mouth and nose, holding the chin forward and the neck in extension.
5. Squeeze the bag, noting inflation of the lungs by chest expansion.
6. Release the bag, which will expand spontaneously. The child will exhale and the chest will fall.
7. Repeat 12 to 20 times/min (depending on size of the child).
8. Because this technique is often difficult to master, it should be practiced in advance, under supervision.

C. *Indications of Effective Technique*
1. Victim's chest rises and falls.

2. Rescuer can feel in own airway the resistance and compliance of the victim's lungs as they expand.
3. Rescuer can hear and feel the air escape during exhalation.
4. Victim's color improves.

D. *Management of Complications*
1. Gastric distention (occurs frequently if excessive pressures are used for inflation)
   a. Turn victim's head and shoulders to one side.
   b. Exert moderate pressure over the epigastrium between the umbilicus and the rib cage.
   c. A nasogastric tube may be used to decompress the stomach.
2. Vomiting
   a. Turn patient on side for drainage.
   b. Clear the airway with fingers or suction.
   c. Resume ventilations.

Artificial Circulation

A. ***General Principles Related to Artificial Circulation***
See Table 41-5 and Figure 41-3.

1. A backward tilt of the head lifts the back in infants and small children. A firm support beneath the back is therefore essential if external cardiac compression is to be effective.
2. A supine position on a firm surface is mandatory. Only in this position can chest compression squeeze the heart against the immobile spine enough to force blood into the systemic circulation.
3. External cardiac compression must always be accompanied by artificial ventilation for adequate oxygenation of the blood.
4. Compressions must be regular, smooth, and uninterrupted. Avoid sudden or jerking movements.
5. Relaxation must immediately follow compression; relaxation and compression must be of equal duration.
6. Between compression, the fingers or heel of the hand must completely release their pressure but should remain in constant contact with the chest.
7. Fingers should not rest on the patient's ribs during compression. Pressure with fingers on the ribs or lateral pressure increases the possibility of fractured ribs and costochondral separation.
8. Never compress the xiphoid process at the tip of the sternum. Pressure on it may cause laceration of the liver.
9. Indications of effective technique include:
   a. A palpable femoral or carotid pulse
   b. Decrease in size of pupils
   c. Improvement in the patient's color

B. ***Nursing Management in Cardiopulmonary Resuscitation***
1. Recognize cardiac and respiratory arrest.
2. Send for assistance and note time.
3. If alone:
   a. First ventilate the child's lungs rapidly two times, using appropriate technique, then palpate the carotid or brachial pulse. If a pulse is palpated, continue ventilatory support.
   b. If no pulse is felt, institute artificial circulation using appropriate technique.
   c. For an infant or child, interpose 1 breath after each series of 5 compressions. For an adolescent, interpose 2 breaths after each series of 15 compressions.
   d. Continue repeating this cycle until help arrives.
4. When help arrives:

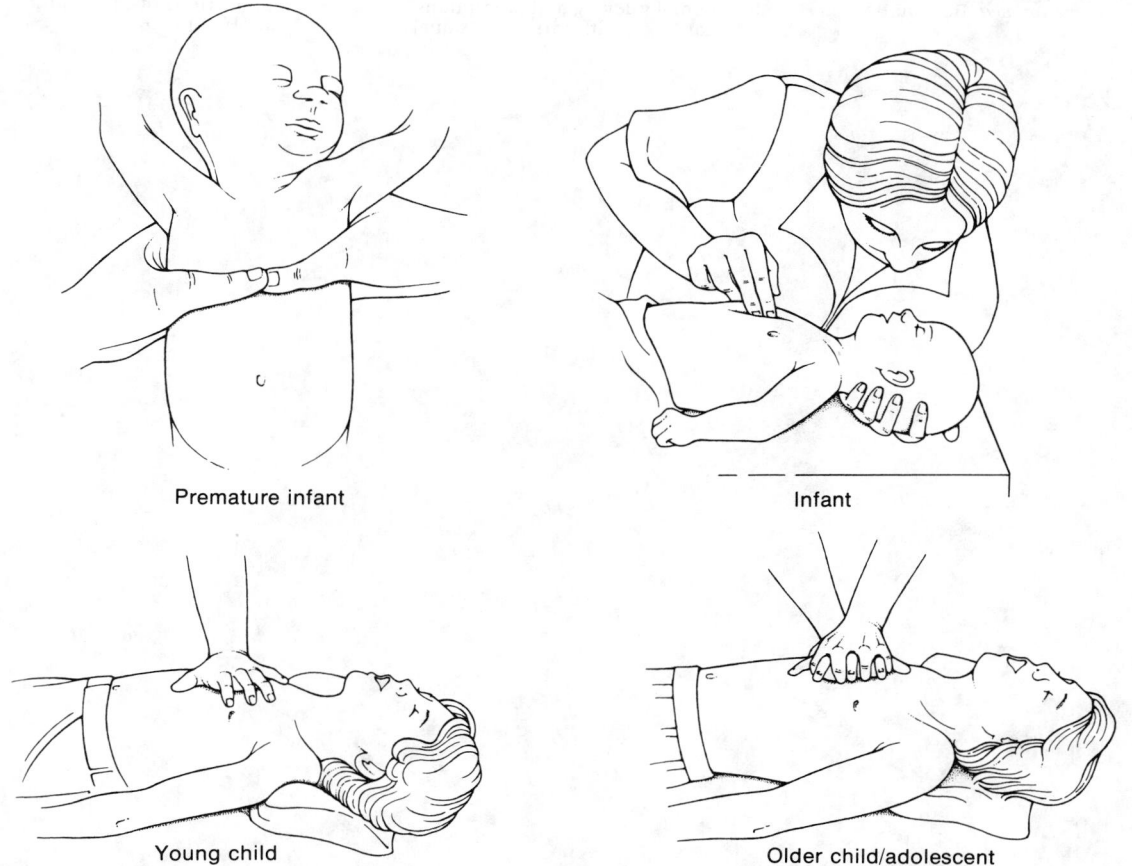

Premature infant

Infant

Young child

Older child/adolescent

FIGURE 41-3 *Cardiopulmonary resuscitation in children. In the young child, the heel of the hand is placed over the lower sternum. In older children and adolescents, both hands are used.*

a. One rescuer performs mouth-to-mouth resuscitation or institutes bag breathing.
b. Another rescuer performs cardiac compressions.
c. A ratio of 3 compressions to 1 breath is maintained for both infants and children (small) and 5 compressions to 1 breath for older children.
d. Cardiac compression should not be stopped for respiration. Breaths should be interposed on the upstroke of each fifth cardiac compression.
5. Anticipate and assist with emergency procedures and medications.

a. Assist with intubation, monitoring, placement of cutdown, administration of IV fluids, defibrillation, and other definitive measures.
b. Prepare and administer emergency medications as prescribed. Record dose and time.
6. After resuscitation:
a. Care for the child as required.
b. Determine if family members have been notified and are being cared for.
c. Record all events.
d. Restock emergency cart.

Selected References

Chameides, L. (ed.). (1990). *Textbook of pediatric advanced life support.* American Heart Association, American Academy of Pediatrics.

Davies, J. M. and Reynolds, B. M. (1992). The ethics of cardiopulmonary resuscitation: Background to decision making. *Archives of Disease in Childhood, 67*(12), 1498–1501.

Grollman, E. (1993). *Straight talk about death for teenagers—how to cope with losing someone you love.* Boston: Beacon Press.

Henden, D. (1973). *Death as a fact of life.* New York: WM Norton & Co., Inc.

Johnson, K. B. (ed.). (1993). *The Harriet Lane handbook.* St. Louis: Mosby.

Kenner, C. (1990). Caring for the NICU parent. *Journal of Perinatal Nursing, 4*(3), 78–87.

McIntier, T. M. (1995). Nursing the family when a child dies. *RN, 58*(2), 50–54.

Neidig, J. and Dalgas-Pelish, P. (1992). Parental grieving and preceptions regarding health care professionals interventions. *Comprehensive Pediatric Nursing, 14*(3), 179–191.

Slusher, I. and McClure, M. J. (1992). Infant stimulation during hospitalization. *Journal of Pediatric Nursing, 7*(4), 276–9.

Whaley, L. and Wong, D. (1991). *Nursing care of infants and children (4th ed.).* St. Louis: Mosby Yearbook.

Whittam, E. (1993). Terminal care of the dying child: Psychosocial implications of care. *Cancer, 71*(10 suppl), 3450–62.

UNIT 15

◆

Pediatric Disorders

CHAPTER 42

Pediatric Respiratory Disorders

The Disorders

◆ COMMON PEDIATRIC RESPIRATORY INFECTIONS

Respiratory tract infection is a frequent cause of acute illness in infants and children. Many pediatric infections are seasonal. The child's response to the infection will vary based on the age of the child, causative organism, general health of the child, existence of chronic medical conditions, and degree of contact with other children. Information about specific respiratory infections, including bacterial pneumonia, viral pneumonia, *Pneumocystis* pneumonia, *Mycoplasma pneumonia*, bronchiolitis, croup, and epiglottitis may be found in Figure 42-1 and Table 42-1.

Nursing Assessment

Determine the severity of the respiratory distress that the child is experiencing. Make an initial nursing assessment.

1. Observe the respiratory rate and pattern.
   a. Count the respirations for 1 full minute.
   b. Observe the child for retractions, and note severity and location.
   c. Listen to the chest with a stethoscope to determine if crackles are present and to evaluate the breath sounds.
2. Observe the child's color, and note any presence of cyanosis.
3. Observe for nasal flaring or grunting.
4. Evaluate the child's degree of restlessness, apprehension, and motor tone.
5. Note any wheezing, stridor, or hoarseness.

Nursing Diagnoses

A. Ineffective Airway Clearance related to inflammation, obstruction, secretions, or pain
B. Ineffective Breathing Pattern related to inflammatory process
C. Fluid Volume Deficit related to fever, decreased appetite, vomiting
D. Fatigue related to increased work of breathing

E. Anxiety related to respiratory distress and hospitalization
F. Parental Role Conflict related to hospitalization of the child

Nursing Interventions

A. **Promoting Effective Airway Clearance**
1. Provide a humidified environment enriched with oxygen to combat hypoxia and to liquefy secretions. See Procedure Guidelines 42-1, p. 1191.
   a. Use a croup tent with cool mist or ultrasonic mist in tent to moisten airway, minimize fluid loss from lungs, liquefy and mobilize respiratory secretions, and allow for oxygen therapy up to 40% concentration.
2. Advise parents to use ultrasonic nebulizer at home and encourage fluids as tolerated.

> **NURSING ALERT:** ◆
> At no time should the mist be allowed to become so dense that it obscures clear visualization of the patient's respiratory pattern.

B. **Improving Breathing Pattern**
1. Place the child in a comfortable position to promote easier ventilation.
   a. Semi-Fowler's—use pillows, infant seat, or elevate head of bed.
   b. Occasional side or abdominal position will aid drainage of liquefied secretions.
   c. Do not position the child in severe respiratory distress in a supine position—allow the child to assume a position of comfort.
2. Provide measures to improve ventilation of affected portion of the lung.
   a. Change position frequently.
   b. Provide postural drainage if prescribed.
   c. Relieve nasal obstruction that contributes to breathing difficulty. Instill saline solution or prescribed nose drops, and apply nasal suctioning.
   d. Quiet prolonged crying, which can irritate the airway, by soothing the child; however, crying may be an effective way to inflate the lungs.
   e. Realize that coughing is a normal tracheobronchial cleansing procedure, but temporarily relieve coughing by allowing the child to sip water; use extreme caution to prevent aspiration.

THE CHILD WITH EPIGLOTTITIS

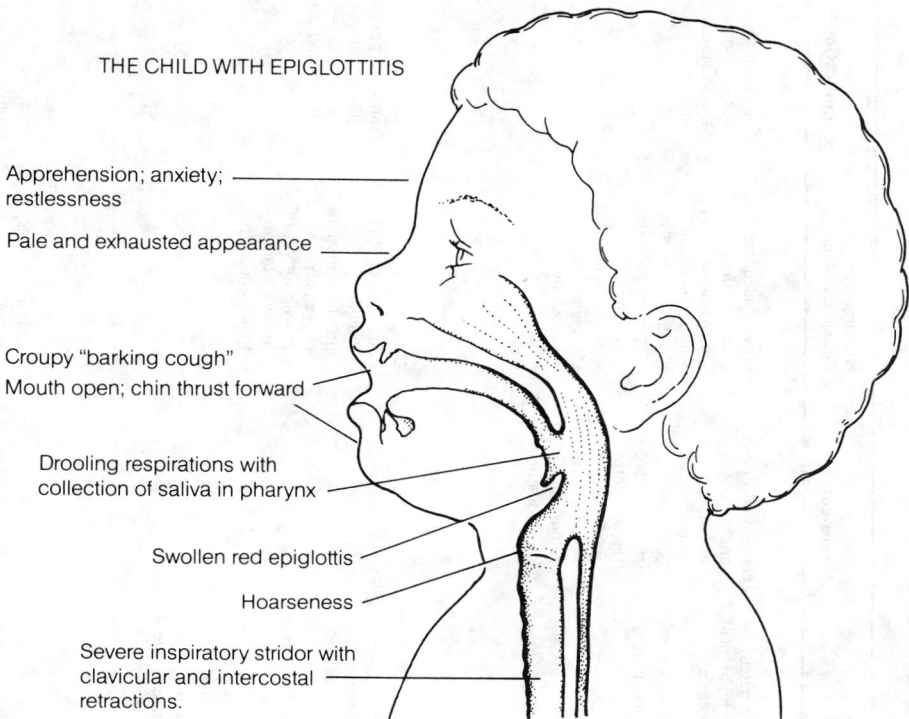

Apprehension; anxiety; restlessness

Pale and exhausted appearance

Croupy "barking cough"
Mouth open; chin thrust forward

Drooling respirations with collection of saliva in pharynx

Swollen red epiglottis

Hoarseness

Severe inspiratory stridor with clavicular and intercostal retractions.

FIGURE 42-1 *Epiglottitis.*

f. Insert a nasogastric tube as ordered to relieve abdominal distention, which can limit diaphragmatic excursion.

3. Ensure that compressed air or oxygen is supplied when using a mist tent to avoid excess CO_2 concentrations and increased respiratory rate.

4. Administer appropriate antibiotic therapy.
   a. Observe for drug sensitivity.
   b. Observe the child's response to therapy.

> **NURSING ALERT:**
> To minimize spasm and sudden blockage of airway, *avoid* the following: making the child lie flat, forcing the child to drink, and looking down the child's throat.

5. For cases of severe respiratory distress, assist with intubation or tracheostomy and mechanical ventilation.
   a. Traceostomy tubes are generally not cuffed for infants and small children because the tube itself is big enough relative to the size of the trachea to act as its own sealer.
   b. Position the infant with a trachesotomy with neck extended by placing a small roll under the shoulders to prevent occlusion of the tube by the chin. Support the head and neck carefully when moving the infant to prevent dislodgement of the tube.
   c. When feeding, cover the trachesotomy with a moist piece of gauze, or use a bib for older infants or young children.
   d. See p. 1190 in this chapter, as well as Chapter 8 for care of the patient on mechanical ventilation.

C. *Promoting Adequate Hydration*

1. Administer intravenous (IV) fluids at the prescribed rate.

2. To prevent aspiration, withhold all oral food and fluids if the child is in severe respiratory distress.

3. Offer the child small sips of clear fluid when the respiratory status improves.
   a. Note any vomiting or abdominal distention after the oral fluid is given.
   b. As the child begins to take more fluid by mouth, notify the health care provider and modify the IV fluid rate to prevent fluid overload.
   c. Do not force the child to take fluids orally, because this may cause increased distress and possibly vomiting. Anorexia will subside as the condition improves.

4. Assist in the control of fever to reduce respiratory rate and fluid loss.
   a. Give antipyretics as prescribed.
   b. Increase evaporation from skin with tepid sponges.

5. Record the child's intake and output, and monitor urine specific gravity.

D. *Promoting Adequate Rest*

1. Disturb the child as little as possible by organizing nursing care, and protect child from unnecessary interruptions.

2. Be aware of the age of the child, and be familiar with the level of growth and development as it applies to hospitalization.

3. Encourage the parents to stay with the child as much as possible to provide comfort and security.

(text continues on page 1172)

TABLE 42-1 Common Pediatric Respiratory Infections

Condition and Causative Agent	Age and Incidence	Clinical Manifestations	Diagnostic Evaluation	Treatment	Nursing Considerations	Complications
I. Bacterial Pneumonia Bacterial infection of the lung parenchyma A. Pneumococcal pneumonia— causative organism, *Streptococcus pneumoniae* (gram positive). This type of bacterial pneumonia is most frequent in children.	Birth–2 y Winter and spring (especially in patients with sickle cell disease or patients without spleens)	Mild upper respiratory infection (URI) with sudden symptom onset. Infants: refusal to eat, vomiting, diarrhea, hypothermia/ hyperthermia, tachypnea, grunting, retractions, nasal flaring Older children: prodromal URI, headache, anorexia, malaise, dry cough, fever, pleuritic pain, shallow, rapid respirations, abdominal pain	Chest x-ray: patchy area around bronchi Cultures: sputum, blood, nasopharyngeal Complete blood count (CBC): pronounced leukocytosis	Penicillin G or other antibiotics, including erythromycin, clindomycin, chloramphenicol, cephalosporins, ampicillin, trimethoprim-sulfamethoxazole Bronchodilators	Provide adequate rest with gradual increasing exercise. Monitor intake and output. Administer antipyretics. Provide humidification if oxygen is required. Change position frequently.	Complications are rare, but may include otitis media, sinusitis, empyema, bacteremia.
B. Streptococcal pneumonia— causative organism, Beta-hemolytic *Streptococcus* group A (gram positive)	3–5 y	Commonly superimposed on febrile respiratory infection in a child already ill with a viral infection. The child suddenly has an increased temperature, worsening cough, chills, pleuritic pain, and respiratory distress.	Chest x-ray: usually patchy, but may show disseminated infiltrate CBC: White blood cells (WBC) are increased (polymorphic leukocytosis), Erythrocyte sedimentation rate (ESR) increased Cultures: respiratory secretions, empyema fluid	Penicillin G	Administer antipyretics. Provide humidification if oxygen is required. Provide opportunities for rest. Monitor intake and output.	Empyema, pneumatocele, pneumothorax, permanent pulmonary fibrosis and pleural thickening
C. Staphylococcal pneumonia— causative organism, coagulase-positive *Staphylococcus aureus* (gram positive)	Birth–2 y October–May	History of predisposing factors, such as maternal infection, cystic fibrosis, immunodeficiency. Gradual onset with respiratory symptoms or sudden onset with systemic involvement (child presents appearing very sick). Presence of coarse, bubbly crepitations.	Chest x-ray: patchy consolidation of one or more lobes; pneumatocele, abcesses Cultures: sputum, gastric aspirate, lung aspirate, pulmonary fluid CBC: WBCs are elevated in older children; anemia	Methicillin, Chloramphenicol, Penicillin G, Ampicillin if organism is not resistant	Rapid treatment is important. Antibiotics should be given as soon as ordered. Monitor closely for signs of tension pneumothorax. Monitor fluid balance closely. Methicillin-resistant *S. aureus* poses a real threat to other hospitalized children. Care should be taken to prevent nosocomial infection.	Empyema, pneumothorax, lung abcess, osteomyelitis, staphylococcal pericarditis, bronchiectasis; infants with staphylococcal pneumonia should be tested for cystic fibrosis and screened for immunodeficiency disease.

D. *Haemophilus influenzae,* type B	6 mo–3 y Less common in healthy children	Similar to other lobar pneumonias and bronchopneumonia with spasmodic cough; "toxic appearance" (child looks very sick). Commonly associated infection: otitis media, meningitis, epiglottitis.	Chest x-ray: lobar consolidation; pleural effusion Culture: blood, nasal secretions CBC: increased WBC, lymphocytosis	Chloramphenicol, ampicillin, cephalosporins Cough suppressant	Administer antibiotics on time. Ensure adequate hydration. Monitor for signs of associated upper respiratory tract impairment (stridor, dusky color, drooling in the older child). Respiratory isolation should be instituted until 24 hours after appropriate antibiotic therapy is initiated.	Empyema
II. Viral Pneumonia Viral infection of lung parenchyma. Respiratory syncytial virus (RSV) most common; parainfluenza virus types 1,2,3; adenoviruses; influenza viruses	Birth–2 y; higher incidence in females than males Winter and early spring	Gradual onset following an upper respiratory infection. Infants with RSV have significant respiratory distress and may have apneic spells. Parainfluenza virus causes coryza, pharyngitis, cough; may develop after the child has had a bacterial pneumonia. Adenovirus causes pharyngitis and cervical adenitis; may develop after the child has had pneumonia.	Chest x-ray: one or more lobes infiltrated; x-ray more involved than clinical picture would suggest Culture: nasopharyngeal Antibody titer for suspected organism	Broad-spectrum antibiotic therapy initiated until confirmation of suspected organism established. Aerosolized Ribavirin for RSV	Monitor the infant closely to watch for signs of fatigue, indications that the infant requires supplemental oxygen or intubation for ventilatory support. RSV may be a life-threatening disease for the infant or young child with chronic cardiac or respiratory disease. Admission to intensive care unit may be required. Respiratory and contact isolation are instituted for the child with RSV.	
III. *Pneumocystis carinii* pneumonia *P. carinii* parasite presumed to be a sporozoan	Predisposing factors: prematurity, immature or debilitated infant, infectious disease, serious compromising disease (eg, cystic fibrosis); children receiving immunosuppressive medication; HIV-positive status; immunodeficiency disease	Onset is slow, peaks in 3–6 wk Presents as increasing tachypnea, grey to cyanotic color, dyspnea at rest, cough, decreased oxygen saturation.	Chest x-ray: bilateral diffuse alveolar densities, perihilar overdistension Open lung biopsy: cysts seen with special stain Needle aspiration of lung IgM-ELISA: elevated CBC: mild leukocytosis, moderate eosinophilia	Trimethoprim-sulfamethoxazole Supplemental oxygen as required Immunoglobulin administered IV Pentamidine may IV or through nebulization	Close monitoring of respiratory status, hydration, nutrition. Monitor for adverse reactions to therapy: hypoglycemia, nephrotoxicity, hypotension, hypocalcemia, nausea and vomiting, rash. Respiratory isolation should be instituted for 48 hours following initiation of therapy.	Pneumothorax from diagnostic tests; concomitant bacterial pneumonia; sepsis; death.

(continued)

TABLE 42-1 Common Pediatric Respiratory Infections *(continued)*

Condition and Causative Agent	Age and Incidence	Clinical Manifestations	Diagnostic Evaluation	Treatment	Nursing Considerations	Complications
IV. *Mycoplasma Pneumonia* *M. pneumoniae* microorganisms with properties between bacteria and viruses	10–15 y	Slow onset; 2 to 3-wk incubation period. Malaise, headache, low-grade fever, sore throat, irritating cough, vomiting, crepitation; subacute tracheobronchitis.	Chest x-ray: peribronchial infiltrate in lower lobes Complement fixation test: increased Cold agglutinins: increased Sputum culture: positive	Erythromycin, tetracycline for children older than 9 y	Children should be placed on secretion precautions. Monitor fever. Assess the need for medications to suppress cough.	May be fatal if the infection becomes systemic or if the child has a preexisting chronic lung disease.
V. Bronchiolitis Inflammation of the bronchioles. RSV, adenovirus, parainfluenza virus, type 1 or 3, influenza virus, *M. pneumoniae*	Most common in infants under 6 mo; may occur in children up to 2 y of age Greater incidence in males than females Winter–spring Increased incidence in day care centers	Onset gradual after exposure to individual with respiratory infection. Coryza of 1–3 d; tachypnea; retractions; expiratory ronchi or wheeze; dry, paroxysmal cough; fever; cyanosis; dehydration; tachypnea	Chest x-ray: hyperinflation of lungs Viral cultures nasopharyngeal Serologic studies for specific organism Arterial blood gases for children with significant respiratory distress	Broad-spectrum antibiotics until causative organism identified; humidified oxygen; ventilatory assistance as needed; bronchodilators through nebulization; ribavirin through aerosol for RSV	Avoid high-density humidity; may cause bronchospasm. Monitor fluid and electrolyte balance closely. Infants are obligate nose breathers; keep the nasal passages free of secretions. Position the child upright to facilitate effective breathing. Monitor the child closely for signs of impending respiratory failure. There is a high risk of cross contamination to noninfected children. Institute contact and respiratory isolation.	Exhaustion, resulting in the need for assisted ventilation Secondary bacterial infection Pneumothorax and pneumomediastinum Apneic episodes Life-threatening for the child with chronic respiratory or cardiac disease Dehydration

VI. Croup and Epiglottitis

	Age/Incidence	Clinical Manifestations	Diagnostic Findings	Treatment/Interventions	Complications
Viral infection of larynx and trachea. **A. Croup (subglottic)** Acute laryngotracheo-bronchitis (LTB); laryngotracheitis Parainfluenza virus 1,2,3 (most common virus) RSV Rhinovirus Adenovirus	3 mo–3 y; peak incidence is 18 mo Late fall, early winter Greater incidence in males than females	Onset is usually gradual and progresses slowly; occurs 1 to several days after an upper respiratory infection. Coryza; croupy, barking cough; inspiratory stridor; hoarseness; low-grade fever; apprehension, anxiety	Clinical evaluation and careful history; symptoms are often worse at night. A croup score may be assigned to grade severity. Lateral neck x-ray: subglottic edema with normal supraglottic structures	Cool humidified mist with supplemental oxygen as needed; hydration; nebulized racemic or L-epinephrine. Severe airway edema may require intubation and mechanical ventilation. Dexamethasone may be administered.	Airway obstruction Anorexia Dehydration Rebound upper airway obstruction may occur 2–3 h after administration of racemic epinephrine.
B. Bacterial tracheitis (pseudomembranous croup) Tracheal inflammation in the subglottic region *S. aureus* *H. influenzae* Streptococci	Age variable No seasonal variation	Rapid onset; child appears toxic. High fever; purulent, copious airway secretions; mucosal necrosis; stridor. Drooling is not present.	Lateral neck x-ray: severe narrowing of the airway; pseudomembrane in trachea Tracheal culture Laryngoscopy CBC: leukocytosis	Humidified oxygen as required. Antibiotic therapy (usually ampicillin), cephalosporins, oxacillin. Intubation and mechanical ventilation may be required. Tracheostomy may be required.	Tracheal stenosis in infants
C. Epiglottitis Inflammation of the epiglottis and surrounding structures (see Fig. 42-1) Bacterial agents: *H. influenzae* type B (most common); *S. pneumoniae* *S. aureus* Beta-hemolytic *Streptococcus*	3–10 y; 1–5 y peak ages Seasonal variation—increases in winter Incidence decreased significantly since *H. influenzae* vaccination has become routine	Onset and progression are rapid (6–24 h). May follow short duration of coryza. Severe inspiratory stridor with marked retractions; sore throat, refusal to eat, dysphagia; high fever; tachycardia; drooling; hoarseness. Tripod position: child sits erect, flexed forward at waist with hands on knees for support. Apprehension, anxiety, restlessness Absence of cough	Clinical evaluation and detailed history for onset of symptoms Lateral neck x-rays (epiglottic edema with normal trachea and larynx) Decreased oxygen saturation	Medical emergency: Initial treatment is based on avoiding agitation of the child and preparing to take the child to the OR for intubation by highly skilled personnel. Antibiotic therapy: usually chloramphenicol is used. Intubation and mechanical ventilation are required for 2–3 d. If epiglottitis is strongly suspected, nothing should be placed in the child's mouth. Temporary tracheostomy is sometimes required for cases of complete airway obstruction. Prior to OR: observe closely; keep emergency tracheostomy set at bedside. Allow the child to maintain position of comfort. Allow parents to hold, remain with the child. After intubation: Monitor for respiratory status closely. Administer antibiotics on schedule. Avoid agitation in the intubated child because this may cause increased airway edema.	Airway obstruction Death Bacteremia Pneumothorax

4. Provide opportunities for quiet play as the child's condition improves.

E. _Reducing Anxiety_
1. Explain procedures and hospital routine to the child as appropriate for age.
2. Provide a quiet, stress-free environment.
3. Observe the child's response to the oxygen therapy environment, and reassure the child.
   a. The child may experience fear of confinement or suffocation.
   b. Vision is distorted through the plastic.
   c. The environment is noisy and damp.
   d. Physical and diversional activities are restricted.
   e. Parental contact is decreased.
   f. The environment is often uncomfortable.
4. Provide frequent change of clothing and linen for a child in a tent to promote comfort; provide socks, booties, cap, if necessary, to keep child warm (temperature in mist tent is usually 6°–15°F below room temperature).

F. _Strengthening the Parents' Role_
1. Help parents understand the purpose of the mist tent and how to work with it.
2. Discuss their fears and concerns about the child's therapy.
3. Include the parents in planning for the child's care. Promote their participation in caring for the child.
4. Recognize that the parents will need rest periods. Encourage them to take breaks and eat on a regular basis.

Family Education/Health Maintenance

1. Teach the importance of good hygiene. Include information on handwashing and appropriate ways to handle respiratory secretions at home.
2. Teach methods to isolate sick from well children in the home. Teach the family when it is appropriate to keep the child home from school (any fever, coughing up secretions, significant runny nose in toddler or younger child).
3. Teach methods to keep the ill child well hydrated.
   a. Provide small amounts of fluids frequently.
   b. Offer clear liquids, such as Pedialyte.
   c. Avoid juices with a high sugar content.
4. Teach ways to assess the child's hydration status at home.
   a. Decreased number of wet diapers or number of times the child urinates in a day
   b. Decreased activity level
   c. Dry lips and mucous membranes
   d. No tears when the child cries
5. Teach parents when to contact their health care provider—signs of respiratory distress, recurrent fever, decreased appetite, and activity.
6. Teach about medications and follow-up.
7. If tracheostomy was required, teach care of the tracheostomy at home.

Evaluation

A. Breath sounds clear and equal
B. Easy, regular, unlabored respirations
C. Mucous membranes moist; urine output adequate
D. Bathing and feeding tolerated well
E. Child calm and interacting appropriately with family and staff
F. Parents participating in the child's care

◆ DISORDERS REQUIRING SURGERY OF THE TONSILS AND ADENOIDS

Tonsillectomy and _adenoidectomy_ are the surgical removal of the adenoidal and tonsillar structures, part of the lymphoid tissue that encircles the pharynx. These are the most frequently performed surgical procedures in the child. The most common disease processes that require tonsillectomy and adenoidectomy are obstructive sleep apnea, chronic persistent otitis media, and chronic, persistent tonsillitis or adenoiditis.

Etiology/Incidence

1. Obstructive sleep apnea
   a. Adenotonsillar hypertrophy causes airway obstruction during sleep.
   b. Peak incidence in children is 3 to 6 years.
   c. Incidence is increased in children with Down syndrome.
2. Tonsillitis/adenoiditis
   a. Infection is caused by bacterial or viral organisms, with viral organisms most commonly implicated.
   b. Group A beta-hemolytic _Streptococcus_ is the most common bacterial cause.
3. Otitis media
   a. Bacterial infection caused most commonly by _Streptococcus pneumoniae_ or _Haemophilus influenzae._

Altered Physiology

1. Function of tonsils and adenoids
   a. They are a first line of defense against respiratory infections.
   b. Because the growth of the tonsils and adenoids in the first 10 years of life exceeds general somatic growth, these structures appear especially large in the child.
   c. The natural process of involution of tonsillar and adenoidal lymphoid tissue in prepubertal years is associated with decreased frequency of throat and ear infections.
2. In obstructive sleep apnea, adenotonsillar hypertrophy results in obstruction of the airway and persistent hypoventilation during sleep.
3. In tonsillitis/adenoiditis, structures that are already large become inflamed due to an infectious agent and cause airway obstruction, decreased appetite, and pain.
4. Enlarged adenoids block drainage from the eustachian tubes, resulting in otitis media and are frequently associated with hearing loss.
   a. They also may block nasal passages, resulting in persistent mouth breathing.
   b. Chronic adenoiditis without tonsillitis is most often seen in children younger than 4 years.

Complications

1. If untreated, obstructive sleep apnea in the child may result in pulmonary hypertension, cor pulmonale, failure to thrive, respiratory failure, attention deficit disorders, cardiac arrhythmias.

2. Untreated chronic tonsillitis may result in difficulty swallowing, anorexia, failure to thrive, peritonsillar or retropharyngeal abscess.

3. Untreated chronic otitis media may result in hearing loss, scarring of the eardrum (tympanosclerosis), mastoiditis, meningitis.

4. Complications of surgery include hemorrhage, reactions to anesthesia, otitis media, bacteremia.

Clinical Manifestations

A. *Obstructive sleep apnea*
1. Loud snoring or noisy breathing in sleep
2. Excessive daytime sleepiness
3. Mouth breathing

B. *Chronic infection of tonsils and adenoids*
1. Mouth breathing or difficulty breathing
2. Frequent sore throat
3. Anorexia, decreased growth velocity
4. Fever

C. *Chronic otitis media*
1. Ear pain or general irritability in young children
2. Alterations in hearing
3. Fever
4. Enlarged lymph nodes
5. Anorexia

Diagnostic Evaluation

1. Thorough ear, nose, and throat examination and appropriate cultures to determine presence and source of infection

2. Preoperative blood studies to determine risk of bleeding—clotting time, smear for platelets, prothrombin time, partial thromboplastin time

Treatment

Appropriate antibiotics are given, and the decision to perform surgery is made. Tonsillectomy and adenoidectomy may be performed together or separately. Controversy exists over indications for and benefits of surgery.

A. *Indications for Tonsillectomy*
1. Conservative
   a. Recurrent or persistent tonsillitis with documented streptococcal infection four times in 1 year
   b. Marked hypertrophy of tonsils, which distorts speech, causes swallowing difficulties, and causes subsequent weight loss
   c. Tonsillar malignancy
   d. Diphtheria carrier
   e. Cor pulmonale due to obstruction
2. Controversial
   a. Peritonsillar abscess or retrotonsillar abscess
   b. Suppurative cervical adenitis with tonsillar focus
   c. Persistent hyperemia of anterior pillars
   d. Enlarged cervical lymph nodes

B. *Indications for Adenoidectomy*
1. Conservative
   a. Adenoid hypertrophy resulting in obstruction of airway leading to hypoxia, pulmonary hypertension, and cor pulmonale

   b. Hypertrophy with nasal obstruction accompanied by breathing difficulty and severe speech distortion
   c. Hypertrophy associated with chronic suppurative or serous otitis media and sensorineural or conductive hearing loss, chronic mastoiditis, or cholesteatoma
   d. Mouth breathing due to hypertrophied adenoids
2. Controversial
   a. Enlarged adenoids, chronic otitis media, and no evidence of complications

C. *Contraindications to Surgery*
1. Bleeding or coagulation disorders
2. Uncontrolled systemic disorders (ie, diabetes, rheumatic fever, cardiac or renal disease)
3. Child younger than 4 years, unless life-threatening situation
4. Presence of upper respiratory infection in child or immediate family
5. Specific for adenoidectomy—certain palate abnormalities (ie, cleft palate or submucous cleft palate)

Nursing Assessment

A. Preoperative assessment
   1. Assess child's developmental level.
   2. Assess parents' and child's understanding of the surgical procedure.
   3. Assess psychological preparation of the child for hospitalization and surgery.
     a. Does the child understand what will happen?
     b. Do the parents know the importance of telling the child the truth and have a good understanding of the procedure?
     c. Does the child have preconceived ideas from peers that may pose a threat?

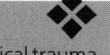

NURSING ALERT:
The preschool child is especially vulnerable to psychological trauma as a result of surgical procedures or hospitalization.

   4. Obtain thorough nursing history from the parents to obtain any pertinent information that would impact on the child's care.
     a. Has the child had a recent infection? It is desirable for the child to be free of respiratory infection for at least 2 to 3 weeks.
     b. Has the child recently been exposed to any communicable diseases?
     c. Does the child have any loose teeth that may pose the threat of aspiration?
     d. Are there any bleeding tendencies in the child or family?
   5. Assess the child's hydration status.
B. Postoperative assessment
   1. Assess pain on a frequent basis.
   2. Assess ability to maintain adequate oral intake.
   3. Assess frequently for signs of postoperative bleeding.
   4. Assess for indications of negative psychological sequelae related to the surgery and hospitalization.

Nursing Diagnoses

A. Fear related to painful procedure, unfamiliar environment

B. Parental Anxiety related to concept of surgery
C. Risk for Fluid Volume Deficit related to reduced intake postoperatively and blood loss
D. Ineffective Airway Clearance related to pain and effects of anesthesia
E. Pain related to surgical incision

Nursing Interventions

A. *Reducing Fear*
1. Prepare the child specifically for what to expect postoperatively, using techniques appropriate to the child's developmental level (books, dolls, drawings). Include the following:
    a. Where child will wake up
    b. Temporary sore throat, emesis of blood, position, foul taste and smell in mouth
    c. Ice collar, medications
    d. Fluid regimen
2. Talk to the child about the new things to be seen in the operating room, and clear up any misconceptions.

B. *Relieving Parental Anxiety*
1. Help the parents prepare the child by talking at first in general terms about surgery and progressing to more specific information.
2. Reassure parents that complication rates are low and that recovery is usually swift.
3. Encourage parents to stay with child and help provide care.

C. *Maintaining Adequate Fluid Volume*
1. Assess frequently for bleeding postoperatively. Indications of hemorrhage include the following:
    a. Increased pulse
    b. Frequent swallowing
    c. Pallor
    d. Restlessness
    e. Clearing of throat and vomiting of blood
    f. Continuous slight oozing of blood over a number of hours
    g. Oozing of blood in back of throat
2. Have suction equipment and packing material readily available in case of emergency.
3. Provide adequate fluid intake.
    a. Give ice chips 1 to 2 hours after awakening from anesthesia.
    b. When vomiting has ceased, advance to clear liquids cautiously.
    c. Offer cool fruit juices without pulp at first because they are best tolerated; then offer Popsicles, cool water for first 12 to 24 hours.
    d. There is some controversy regarding intake of milk and ice cream the evening of surgery: it can be soothing and can reduce swelling, but it does coat the mouth and throat, causing the child to clear throat more often, which may initiate bleeding.

D. *Promoting Effective Airway Clearance*
1. Assist the child in maintaining a patent airway by draining secretions and preventing aspiration of vomitus.
    a. Place the child prone or semiprone with head turned to side while still under the effects of anesthesia.
    b. Allow the child to assume a position of comfort when alert. (Parent may hold the child.)

c. The child may vomit old blood initially. If suctioning is necessary, avoid trauma to oropharynx.
    d. Remind the child not to cough or clear throat unless necessary.

E. *Improving Comfort*
1. Provide ice collar to neck, if desired. (Remove ice collar if child becomes restless.)
2. Give analgesics as ordered.
3. Rinse mouth with cool water or alkaline solution.
4. Keep child and environment free from blood-tinged drainage to help decrease anxiety.
5. Encourage the parents to be with the child when the child awakens. This is the most important comfort measure the nurse can provide for the child.
6. When parents must leave, reassure the child that they will return.

Family Education/Health Maintenance

1. Explain and write instructions concerning the care of the child at home after discharge.
    a. Diet should still consist of large amounts of fluids and soft, cool, nonirritating foods. (Supply list of suggestions.)
    b. Eating helps promote healing because it increases the blood supply to tissues.
    c. Bed rest should be maintained for 1 to 2 days and then daily rest periods for about 1 week. Resume normal eating and activities within 2 weeks following surgery.
    d. Avoid contact with people with infections.
    e. Discourage the child from frequent coughing and clearing of throat.
    f. Avoid gargling. Mouth odor may be present for a few days after surgery; only mouth rinsing is acceptable.
2. Advise when to call health care provider. (Ensure that parents have phone number of health care provider and emergency department.)
    a. Earache accompanied by fever
    b. Any bleeding, often indicated only by frequent swallowing; most common about fifth to 10th day when membrane sloughs from surgical site
3. Teach about medications prescribed or suggested for pain relief.
4. Discuss with the parents what results they can expect from the surgery.
    a. Decreased number of sore throats
    b. Lessened evidence of obstructive symptoms
    c. Decreased incidence of cervical lymphadenitis
    d. Improvement in nutritional status
    e. No improvement in nasal allergies
    f. No improvement in secretory otitis media
5. Guide parents in helping the child think of the experience as a positive one once surgery is over to make subsequent health care experiences easier.
    a. Talk about what happened and the positive outcomes.
    b. Let the child play out his or her feelings.

Evaluation

A. Child acting out surgery with dolls, asking questions
B. Parents interacting with the child, asking appropriate questions

C. Taking fluids well; no signs of bleeding
D. No vomiting; breathing without difficulty
E. Verbalizes reduced pain

◆ ASTHMA

Asthma is a recurrent, almost completely reversible condition of the lungs characterized by increased responsiveness or irritability of the trachea and bronchi. There is spasm of the bronchial smooth muscle, edema of the mucosa, and increased mucous secretions in the bronchioles as a response to various stimuli that change in severity either spontaneously or with treatment.

Etiology and Incidence

A. **Stimuli Responsible for Triggering Attacks**
1. Extrinsic—an antigen–antibody reaction, a positive reaction to certain allergens. Immunoglobulin E (IgE) or IgA antibodies are activated by allergens, resulting in bronchospasm, edema, and increased secretions of mucus (allergy to pollen, animal dander, feathers, foods, house dust, and mites).
2. Intrinsic—symptoms caused by other nonallergic factors. There is little evidence of IgE antibodies.
   a. Infection—respiratory syncytial virus, parainfluenza virus (types I and II), mycoplasmal pneumonia
   b. Physical factors—cold, humidity, sudden changes in temperature and barometric pressure
   c. Inheritable tendencies
   d. Irritants—chemicals, air pollutants (eg, sulfur dioxide, carbon monoxide, particulate matter, second-hand smoke)
   e. Psychic or emotional factors (ie, tension, fear, anxiety)
   f. Physical stress—fatigue, excessive exercise
   g. Endocrine factors—may worsen in relation to menses or improve at puberty

B. **Incidence**
1. Most common disease of childhood. Approximately 5% to 10% of school-age children have symptoms of asthma.
2. It may develop in infancy but is usually seen in children 3 years and older. Most children with asthma will have initial symptoms by 4 to 5 years.
   a. In younger children, the incidence is greater in boys.
   b. Incidence is equal in boys and girls during adolescence.
   c. Infants with eczema are at increased risk for developing asthma after the age of 10 years.
   d. Childhood asthma may decrease at puberty.
3. Prevalence is highest in African American males from urban settings.

C. **Classification of Asthma**
1. Mild, infrequent asthma—sporadic in nature, with varying intervals of freedom from difficulty breathing and with precipitating factors often readily defined
2. Moderate, chronic asthma—no outward signs or symptoms of asthma but some shortness of breath on occasion, transitory wheezing on strenuous exercise, and wheezy crackles heard during deep inspiration
3. Severe, chronic asthma—persistent wheezing requiring regular, daily medication to either control symptoms or to function

4. Status asthmaticus—severe attack in which the patient deteriorates despite adequate treatment with conventional methods
5. Exercise-induced asthma—bronchial obstruction occurs 5 to 15 minutes after cessation of strenuous exercise, especially in a cold, dry environment
6. Cough-variant asthma—most often seen in young children. Cough, most often occurring at night, is the principle symptom of asthma. The child may never wheeze.

Altered Physiology

1. Chemical mediators are released in asthma.
   a. Primarily involved are histamine and slow-reacting substance of anaphylaxis (SRS-A). SRS-A appears after histamine release and persists for a longer period. It is not inhibited by the action of the antihistamines.
   b. These materials are primarily responsible for changes in the blood vessels and mucous membranes in the bronchi and bronchioles and for the initiation of bronchospasm.
2. During an asthma attack, abnormal constriction of muscles surrounding the bronchioles (spasm) results in narrowed bronchiolar lumen and decreased oxygen supply in alveoli.
   a. In addition, edema, inflammation, and increased mucous production further compromise respirations.
   b. Hyper-resonance and decreased breath sounds may be observed (ominous sign).
3. Bronchial smooth muscle hypertrophy, bronchial spasms, mucus gland hypertrophy, edema of respiratory mucosa, and mucous plugging occur.

Complications

1. Infections—bronchiectasis, pneumonia, bronchiolitis
2. Atelectasis, pneumothorax, pneumomediastinum
3. Dehydration
4. Cardiac arrhythmias
5. Hypotension, hypertension
6. Emphysema, cor pulmonale
7. Respiratory failure and death (especially younger than 2 years)

Clinical Manifestations

1. The onset of an asthma attack may be gradual, with nasal congestion, sneezing, and a watery nasal discharge present before the attack, or sudden, often at night.
2. Asthma attacks are characterized by the following:
   a. Wheezing, which occurs primarily with expiration or may be absent due to minimal air movement
   b. Anxiety and apprehension
   c. Diaphoresis
   d. Uncontrollable cough
   e. Dyspnea, with increased effort during expiration
3. Severe, uncontrolled attacks may be characterized by the following:
   a. Increasing dyspnea, cyanosis
   b. Thick, tenacious mucus

c. Coarse and fine musical crackles
d. Nasal flaring, use of accessory muscles
e. Hypoxemia, respiratory alkalosis leading to respiratory acidosis and possibly metabolic acidosis
f. Increased heart and respiratory rates
g. Abdominal pain and vomiting from severe coughing
h. Extreme anxiety and apprehension, progressing to a decreased level of consciousness
4. Chronic signs of asthma include the following:
   a. Cough relieved by bronchodilators
   b. Nonspecific episodic dyspnea unrelated to exercise
   c. Recurrent lung infiltrates and atelectasis
   d. Anterior-posterior chest diameter may be increased
   e. Excessive nasal secretions and mouth gaping
   f. Inspiratory and expiratory wheeze

Diagnostic Evaluation

1. Eosinophilia in peripheral blood, nasal secretions, and sputum
2. Complete blood count—polymorphonuclear leukocytosis during infections
3. Pulmonary function studies—diminished maximal breathing capacity, tidal volume and timed vital capacity; spirometric picture of obstruction
4. Arterial blood gases—respiratory acidosis and later metabolic acidosis
5. Examination of sputum—bronchial casts and eosinophilia
6. Chest x-ray—hyperventilation during asthma attack; air trapping, atelectasis, pulmonary hypertension, bronchiolar edema
7. Routine skin testing to help determine allergic causes
   a. Serum IgE—elevated if allergic disease
   b. Radioallergosorbent test—assay for allergen-specific IgE

Treatment

A. Acute or Emergency Care
1. Goal is to relieve symptoms and increase ventilatory capacity.
2. Therapies are initiated in a stepwise fashion, with additional therapies added if the child fails to show improvement.
   a. Supplemental oxygen as needed to maintain oxygen saturation of more than 95%
   b. Administration of appropriate medications (Table 42-2).
      (1) Beta-agonists by inhalation or subcutaneous route
      (2) Methylxanthines
      (3) Anticholinergics
      (4) Corticosteroids by IV, oral route, or inhalation
3. Children in severe status asthmaticus unresponsive to above therapy may require the following:
   a. Intubation and mechanical ventilation
   b. Continuous infusion of isoproterenol (Isuprel) or terbutaline (Bricanyl)
   c. Pharmacologic paralysis to ventilate the child effectively
   d. Cardiorespiratory monitoring of the child's response to treatment and placement of an arterial line for monitoring arterial blood gases

B. Long-Term Care
1. Goals are prevention of acute asthmatic episodes and school absences, maximum control of symptoms with minimal medications and treatments, participation in normal activities, normalization of pulmonary function tests, and normal growth and development.
2. Education of the parents and child is crucial in aiding them to understand, accept, and manage asthma in a way that allows a fairly normal lifestyle.
   a. Removal of suspected stimuli—allergens, irritants, exercise, emotional factors
   b. Desensitization to build up the child's resistance to his or her allergens
   c. Drug therapy to control symptoms
      (1) Inhaled beta-agonists as needed
      (2) Inhaled anti-inflammatory agents (cromolyn sodium [Intal], corticosteroids)
      (3) Additional bronchodilators, such as theophylline (Slo-bid), oral albuterol (Proventil syrup)
   d. Supportive treatment
      (1) Adequate hydration
      (2) Adequate oxygenation
      (3) Appropriate treatment of any existing infection
      (4) Correction of acid–base imbalance
      (5) Relief of fatigue

Nursing Assessment

1. Make a baseline physical assessment of the child's condition to determine the severity of the attack and the degree of respiratory distress.
   a. Observe breathing pattern for prolonged expiratory phase of respiration, inspiratory and expiratory wheezing (may be audible from a distance in severe attacks), use of accessory muscles for breathing, and nasal flaring.
   b. Auscultate the chest with a stethoscope to identify crackles and wheezing and areas of decreased aeration.

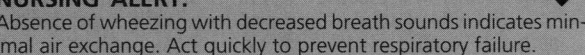

NURSING ALERT:
Absence of wheezing with decreased breath sounds indicates minimal air exchange. Act quickly to prevent respiratory failure.

   c. Assess level of anxiety and apprehension.
   d. Observe color of mucous membranes.
   e. Determine the heart and respiratory rates.
2. Obtain a nursing history to determine medication regimen at home and compliance, history of asthma exacerbations and hospitalization, and other medical conditions.

NURSING ALERT:
Be aware that the following demographic and history factors increase the risk of asthma-related death: adolescence, African American ethnicity, exacerbation requiring hospitalization within the last year, exacerbation requiring intubation, history of depression.

Nursing Diagnoses

A. Ineffective Breathing Pattern related to bronchospasm
B. Ineffective Airway Clearance related to thick secretions and airway narrowing

TABLE 42-2 Drugs Used in the Treatment of Pediatric Asthma

Drug	Available Forms	Action	Nursing Implications
Beta-Adrenergic Agonists			
Albuterol (Proventyl, Ventolin)	Metered-dose inhaler (MDI) Nebulizer solution Oral	Bronchodilator; relaxes airway smooth muscles May decrease release of substances that cause inflammatory response from MAST cells	This is drug of choice for initial treatment of acute exacerbation. It may be given as a continuous nebulization in status asthmaticus. Ensure that the drug is being delivered correctly (child is sitting upright; mask is applied correctly; child uses MDI correctly). Children older than 5 years can be taught to use an MDI. Use of a chamber or spacer may improve delivery of the drug to airways. Some recent research suggests that chronic regular use may result in development of tolerance or increased airway hyperresponsiveness. Children younger than 5 years should be given nebulized drug with compressed air or oxygen. Oxygen is generally used in acute exacerbations.
Metaproterenol (Alupent)	MDI Nebulizer solution Oral	Bronchodilator; relaxes airway smooth muscles	This has more cardiovascular effects than albuterol (increased heart rate is primary effect). Children younger than 5 years should be given nebulized drug with compressed air or oxygen. Oxygen is generally used in acute exacerbations.
Terbutaline (Brethine, Brethaire)	MDI Nebulizer solution Oral Subcutaneous, IV	Bronchodilator; relaxes airway smooth muscles	This has more cardiovascular effects than albuterol. Acute, severe exacerbations that do not respond to conventional treatment may be treated with subcutaneous injections or continuous IV infusion. See above for further information on administration.
Epinephrine (Susphrine)	Subcutaneous	Bronchodilator; relaxes airway smooth muscles	Sus-phrine is a longer acting form of subcutaneous epinephrine. It is given to children with acute, severe exacerbation not responding to inhaled bronchodilators. It may cause tachycardia, hypertension, palpitations, nervousness; it may potentiate theophylline toxicity.
Anticholinergics			
Atropine	Nebulizer solution	Causes bronchodilation through decrease in vagal tone to the airways	Systemic effects are frequently seen and include dry mouth, drying of respiratory secretions, blurred vision, tachycardia, anxiety, and agitation. Monitor the heart rate carefully, and notify the physician if heart rate exceeds a safe range.
Ipratropium (Atrovent)	MDI Nebulizer solution	Causes bronchodilation through decrease in vagal tone to the airways	Fewer systemic effects are seen with ipratropium.
Anti-inflammatories **Corticosteroids**			
Prednisone (Orasone) Prednisolone (Pediapred) Methylprednisolone (Medrol)	Parenteral (IM, IV) Oral	Thought to decrease inflammatory response by interfering with prostaglandin and arachadonic acid production; may increase responsiveness of airways to beta-agonists	A short (4–5 d) course of oral steroids is frequently used in acute exacerbations. A taper is not needed for a short oral course of the drug. Onset of action is about 3 h. Side effects may include increased appetite, increased activity or mood change, increased serum glucose levels. It is important to teach the parents about these potential side effects.

(continued)

TABLE 42-2   Drugs Used in the Treatment of Pediatric Asthma
(continued)

Drug	Available Forms	Action	Nursing Implications
Beclomethasone (Beclovent, Vanceril) Triamcinolone (Azmacort) Flunisolide (AeroBid)	Steroids available in MDL	Thought to decrease inflammatory response by interfering with prostaglandin and arachadonic acid production May increase responsiveness of airways to beta-agonists	Inhaled corticosteroids may cause oral candidiasis. This can be prevented by use of a chamber or spacer with the MDI. Patients also should be taught to rinse the mouth after corticosteroid MDI use. Cough due to upper airway irritation may be seen with use of corticosteroid MDIs.
Nonsteroidal anti-inflammatory drugs Cromolyn (Intal)	MDI Nebulizer solution Spinhaler dry powder for inhalation	Thought to stabilize MAST cell membranes, preventing the release of inflammatory substances	Administered prophylactically, especially for patients with exercise-induced asthma. It may take 4–6 wk before maximum benefit is seen. This drug is not used to treat acute exacerbation.
Methylxanthines Theophylline (Slo-bid, Theo-Dur)	Syrup Sustained-release tablets or capsules IV (aminophylline)	Bronchodilator May increase respiratory muscle contractions	Often used to treat nocturnal asthma. Aminophylline is a theophylline salt and is about 80% available theophylline. When the patient is converted from IV to oral theophylline, the dose must be adjusted and levels monitored. Metabolism is decreased in infants younger than 6 months and increased in children compared with adults. Metabolism of the drug is increased by administration of many antibiotics and decreased in fever. Many drugs have interactions with theophylline. Be aware of all drugs your patient is receiving. Levels should be monitored regularly. Signs and symptoms of theophylline toxicity include cardiac arrhythmias, restlessness, nausea and vomiting, and seizures. Many children experience GI upset with this drug.

C. Fluid Volume Deficit related to hyperventilation and decreased oral intake
D. Anxiety related to difficult breathing and medical intervention
E. Altered Family Processes related to chronic illness
F. Self Esteem Disturbance related to restrictions in activity and frequent medical follow-up

Nursing Interventions

A. *Promoting Effective Breathing Pattern*
1. Position the child in high Fowler's position to allow maximum lung expansion.
   a. Elevate the head of the bed 90 degrees.
   b. Place an overbed table padded with a pillow in front of the child to lean on to allow maximum use of accessory muscles for breathing.
2. Administer oxygen as directed.
   a. Do not wait for the appearance of cyanosis before administering oxygen. Give oxygen for oxygen saturation less than 94%.

   b. Institute pulse oximetry to monitor response to therapy.
3. Institute cardiac/respiratory monitoring, and assess vital signs frequently.
4. Obtain arterial blood gas samples frequently in the child with status asthmaticus.

B. *Facilitating Effective Airway Clearance*
1. Use humidity with or without oxygen to help liquefy secretions and reduce mucosal inflammation and edema. Reduce humidity if droplets are present; further bronchospasm may be triggered.
2. Use aerosolized bronchodilators or inhaler with spacer device with bronchodilators.
3. Notify health care provider if initial therapy is not effective so that further treatment can be added.

C. *Reducing Anxiety*
1. Provide a quiet room where the child can be closely observed.
2. Explain the purpose of the oxygen equipment before oxygen is administered, and allow the child to feel and touch the equipment.
3. Provide the child with maximum reassurance.

a. Encourage the parents to remain with the child.
b. Keep the parents informed of the child's progress—what is being done and why—to relieve their apprehension. Parental anxiety is readily transmitted to the child.
c. Talk calmly and quietly to the child, and reinforce that you are available.
d. Allow the child to have a favorite security object.
4. Organize care to avoid disturbing the child any more than necessary.

D. *Promoting Adequate Hydration*
1. Observe for signs of dehydration.
   a. Lack of skin turgor
   b. Lack of tears
   c. Dry, parched lips and mucous membranes
   d. Decreased urinary output, high specific gravity, and concentrated appearance of urine
2. Administer IV fluids as ordered.
3. Encourage moderate oral fluid intake.
   a. Determine the child's fluid preferences.
   b. Offer small sips of fluid frequently when respiratory effort improves.
   c. Avoid iced fluids, which may provoke bronchospasm.
   d. Avoid carbonated beverages when the child is wheezing (may contribute to acidosis).
4. Encourage a regular diet as soon as possible, and decrease IV fluids as oral intake increases.
5. Observe for signs of overhydration and pulmonary edema related to high negative pleural pressure generated during bronchospasm and accumulation of interstitial fluids.

E. *Normalizing Family Processes*
1. Assist the parents to develop a realistic attitude toward the child's illness.
2. Encourage parents and siblings to treat the child as a completely normal child who needs only a few additional restrictions because of illness.
3. Encourage parents to set consistent behavior limits and not provide secondary gains for asthma attack.
4. Encourage equal rights and responsibilities among all children in the family.
5. Provide the parents opportunities to discuss their fears and frustrations related to caring for a child with a chronic disease. Address problems such as loss of sleep, role conflicts, and financial difficulties, and provide referrals for counseling or social services as needed.

F. *Strengthening Self-esteem*
1. Encourage diversional activities while the child is ill that build on interests and skills.
2. Teach the child breathing exercises, modification of activity, and proper use of medications to promote control over asthma and sense of confidence.
3. Encourage the parents to make the child feel capable, loved, and respected.
4. Encourage participation in school and peer activities, especially programs such as art, music, and science, which are nonexertional.
5. Plan a team conference involving child, parents, school nurse, and teacher to discuss control of asthma attack at school.

Family Education/Health Maintenance

1. Instruct family on a well-balanced diet and increased fluid intake.

2. Advise adequate sleep, rest, and reasonable exercise; avoid fatigue and chilling.
3. Encourage parents to keep the child emotionally calm and at ease, and maintain an optimistic attitude.
4. Encourage regular medical follow-up, strict adherence to medication regimen, and prompt attention to infection or other illness.
5. Teach the child and parents proper breathing habits. Exercises strengthen the diaphragm so total lung capacity will be increased. Breathing exercises used with postural drainage may lessen the need for continuous medication and increase expectoration of mucus (see Box 42-1).

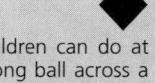
COMMUNITY-BASED CARE TIP:
Suggest fun breathing exercises that young children can do at home, such as blowing a cotton ball or ping pong ball across a table top and keeping score of the distance achieved or blowing large soap bubbles.

6. Teach the child the symptoms of an asthma attack and how to relax and use prescribed beta-agonist or other medication.
7. Teach the proper use of a peak flow meter to monitor condition, a metered-dose inhaler with spacer, or nebulizer for administration of medications.

COMMUNITY-BASED CARE TIP:
Have the child demonstrate use of metered-dose inhaler at regular visits to ensure proper technique and adequate treatment of asthma.

8. Encourage parents to keep a daily diary of symptoms, activity, environment, and any triggering factors.
9. Teach the importance of increasing fluid intake, especially during an asthma attack when fluid is lost through dyspnea and diaphoresis.
10. Teach about environmental control to avoid the offending allergen and control asthma attacks.
    a. Keep the child's bedroom as free from dust as possible by removing furniture that is not absolutely necessary; avoiding upholstered furniture, draperies, carpets, cloth items, and stuffed animals; and using cotton or synthetic washable curtains, throw rugs, blankets, and bedspreads (but not chenille or tufted types).
    b. Do not use insect or other sprays in the bedroom.
    c. Do not store outer clothing or household articles in bedroom closets.
    d. Enclose mattresses, box-springs, and pillows in dust proof covers.
    e. Blankets and clothing that have been stored should be thoroughly aired before use.
    f. Avoid irritating odors such as paint, tobacco smoke, insect powders, pine oils, jellies, and irritating cooking odors. No one should smoke in the home.
    g. If possible, use an exhaust fan in the kitchen to remove cooking odors.
    h. Consider removing all overstuffed furniture and rugs from the home.
    i. Avoid sitting and playing on overstuffed furniture and down pillows.
    j. Avoid carbonated drinks, such as ginger ale and colas (especially when wheezing).
    k. Avoid dusty and musty places (eg, basements, storerooms).

> **BOX 42-1** *Breathing Exercises for Asthma*

Many patients can abort asthma attacks entirely by doing simple breathing exercises. Should the child become short of breath or wheeze slightly during exercise, have him or her take single dose of bronchodilator, and wait several minutes. Exercise may produce coughing as mucus in the bronchial tubes becomes loosened, and the child may be able to cough it up with consequent relief of attack.

Encourage the child to do exercises in the morning before breakfast when well rested, at night to clear lungs before sleep, and at the first sign of an impending asthma attack. Instruct the child to clear nasal passages before beginning exercises and begin with a short, gentle inspiration through the nose, followed by a prolonged expiration through the mouth.

Exercise I—Abdominal Breathing
1. Lie on back with knees drawn up, body relaxed, and hands resting on upper abdomen.
2. Exhale slowly (through mouth); gently sink the chest and then upper abdomen until retracted at end of expiration.
3. Relax upper abdomen (bulges forward) while taking brief inspiration through nose (chest is not raised). Repeat 8–16 times; rest 1 minute; repeat set.

Exercise II—Side Expansion Breathing
1. Sit relaxed in a chair, and place palms of hands on each side of lower ribs.
2. Exhale slowly through mouth, contracting upper part of thorax. Lower ribs, and then compress palms against ribs. (This expels air from base of lungs.)
3. Inhale, expanding lower ribs against slight pressure from hands. Repeat 8–16 times; rest 1 minute; repeat set.

Exercise III—Forward Bending
1. Sit with feet apart, arms relaxed at sides.
2. Exhale slowly; drop head forward and downward to knees while retracting abdominal muscles.
3. Raise trunk slowly while inhaling, and expand upper abdomen.
4. Exhale quickly, sinking chest and abdomen, but remain erect.
5. Inhale, expanding upper abdomen.

Exercise IV—Elbow Arching
This exercise is performed between breathing exercises.
1. Sit leaning slightly forward, back straight, and fingers on shoulders.
2. Move elbows in circles forward, upward, backward, and downward. Repeat 4–8 times; rest; repeat set.

l. Avoid felt rug pads because of animal hair content.
m. Do not let dog or cat sleep in child's room or lay in child's play area.
n. Clean or replace furnace filters frequently.

Expected Outcomes

A. Respiratory rate within normal limits; minimal wheezing
B. Breath sounds clear with coughing
C. Taking fluids well; urine output adequate
D. Child verbalizing questions and concerns, interacting well with others
E. Family interacting well
F. Child describes interest in school and peer-related activities

◆ RESPIRATORY DISTRESS SYNDROME (HYALINE MEMBRANE DISEASE)

Respiratory distress syndrome (RDS) is a syndrome of immature infants that is characterized by a progressive and frequently fatal respiratory failure resulting from atelectasis and immaturity of the lungs.

Etiology and Incidence

1. The primary problem is pulmonary surfactant deficiency due to immaturity of the lungs.
2. Adequate pulmonary function at birth depends on the following:
   a. Adequate amount of surfactant (a lipoprotein mixture) lining the alveolar cells, which allows for alveolar stability and prevents alveolar collapse at the end of expiration
   b. Adequate surface area in air spaces to allow for gas exchange (ie, sufficient pulmonary capillary bed in contact with this alveolar surface area)
3. RDS is ultimately the result of decreased pulmonary surfactant, incomplete structural development of lung, and a highly compliant chest wall.
4. Contributing factors are any factor that decreases surfactant, such as the following:
   a. Prematurity and immature alveolar lining cells
   b. Acidosis
   c. Hypothermia
   d. Hypoxia
   e. Hypovolemia
   f. Diabetes
   g. Elective cesarean section
   h. Fetal or intrapartum stress that compromises blood supply to fetal lungs: vaginal bleeding, maternal hypertension, difficult resuscitation associated with birth asphyxia (Some situations, such as steroid therapy and heroin-addicted mother, result in the acceleration of surfactant.)
   i. unknown factors
5. RDS occurs most frequently in premature infants (primarily weighing between 1,000–1,500 g [2.2–3.3 lb]) and between 28 to 37 weeks' gestation; incidence increases with increased degree of prematurity.

Altered Physiology

1. Surfactant production is deficient by type II alveolar cells. (Although some surfactant may be present at birth, it may not be regenerated at adequate rate.) Surfactant production may be reduced due to the following:
   a. Extreme immaturity of alveolar lining cells
   b. Diminished or impaired production rate resulting from fetal or early neonatal stress

c. Impairment of release mechanism for phospholipid from type II alveolar cells

d. Death of many of these cells responsible for decreased surfactant production

2. Intra-aveolar surface tension is increased, and alveoli are unstable and collapse at the end of expiration. Functional reserve capacity—the amount of air left in the lungs after expiration—is decreased; thus, the next breath requires almost as much effort as the first breath after birth.

3. More oxygen and energy are required to expand the alveoli with each breath, causing fatigue.

4. The number of alveoli that expand progressively decreases, leading to alveolar instability and atelectasis.

5. Pulmonary vascular resistance increases, causing hypoperfusion of lung.

6. Persistence of fetal circulation right-to-left shunt results, leading to hypoxemia and hypercapnia, which lead to respiratory and metabolic acidosis.

7. Hypoxemia and pulmonary vascular pressure cause ischemia in the alveoli, leading to transudate into the alveoli and formation of membranous layer (Fig. 42-2).

8. Gas exchange becomes inhibited. Lungs become stiff (decreased compliance), requiring more pressure to expand them.

9. Airway obstruction leads to increased hypoxia and vasoconstriction, and the cycle continues.

10. RDS is usually a self-limited disease, and symptoms peak in about 3 to 4 days, at which time surfactant synthesis begins to accelerate, and pulmonary function and clinical appearance begin to improve.

a. Moderately ill infants or those who do not require assisted ventilation usually show slow improvement by about 48 hours and rapid recovery over 3 to 4 days with few complications.

b. Severely ill and very immature infants who require some ventilatory assistance usually demonstrate rapid deterioration. Ventilatory assistance may be required for several days, and chronic lung disease and other complications are common.

Complications

1. Complications related to respiratory therapy
   a. Air leak: pneumothorax, pneumomediastinum, pneumopericardium, and pneumoperitoneum
   b. Pneumonia, especially gram-negative organisms
   c. Pulmonary interstitial emphysema

2. Patent ductus arteriosus (PDA)

3. Intraventricular hemorrhage—most often seen in infants weighing less than 1,500 g (3.3 lb)

4. Disseminated intravascular coagulation (DIC)

5. Chronic problems associated with long-term use of oxygen
   a. Bronchopulmonary dysplasia (BPD)—cystic-appearing lungs with hyperinfiltration, obstructive bronchiolitis, dysplastic changes, and pulmonary fibrosis
   b. Chronic respiratory infections

6. Necrotizing enterocolitis

7. Tracheal stenosis

8. Retinopathy of prematurity (retrolental fibroplasia)

9. Other complications related to prematurity

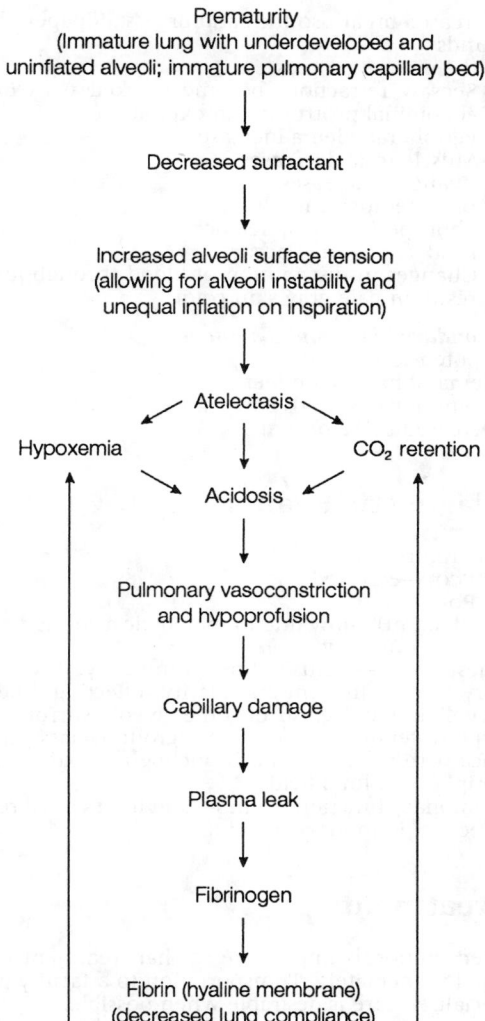

FIGURE 42-2 *Schematic outline of hyaline membrane disease.*

Clinical Manifestations

Symptoms are usually observed soon after birth and may include the following:

A. *Primary Signs and Symptoms*
1. Expiratory grunting or whining (when infant is not crying)
2. Sternal, suprasternal, substernal, and intercostal retractions progressing to paradoxical seesaw respirations
3. Inspiratory nasal flaring
4. Tachypnea
5. Hypothermia
6. Cyanosis when child is in room air (infants with severe disease may be cyanotic even when given oxygen), increasing need for oxygen

7. Decreased breath sounds and dry "sandpaper" breath sounds
8. As the disease progresses:
   a. Seesaw retractions become marked with marked abdominal protrusion on expiration.
   b. Peripheral edema increases.
   c. Muscle tone decreases.
   d. Cyanosis increases.
   e. Body temperature drops.
   f. Short periods of apnea occur.
   g. Bradycardia may occur.
   h. Changes in distribution of blood throughout body result in pale gray skin color.

B. *Secondary Signs and Symptoms*
1. Hypotension
2. Edema of hands and feet
3. Absent bowel sounds early in the illness
4. Decreased urine output

Diagnostic Evaluation

1. Laboratory tests
   a. PCO_2—elevated
   b. PO_2—low
   c. Blood pH—low due to metabolic acidosis
   d. Calcium—low
2. Chest x-ray—diffuse, fine granularity; "whiteout," very heavy, uniform granularity reflecting fluid-filled alveoli and atelectasis of some alveoli, surrounded by hyperdistended bronchioles; "ground glass" appearance with prominent air bronchogram extending into periphery of lung fields
3. Pulmonary function studies—stiff lung with a reduced effective pulmonary blood flow

Treatment

Early recognition is imperative so that treatment may be instituted immediately. Transportation to a facility providing specialized care is desirable when possible.

A. *Supportive*
1. Maintenance of oxygenation—PaO_2 at 60 to 80 mm Hg to prevent hypoxia; frequent arterial pH and blood gas measurements
2. Maintenance of respiration with ventilatory support if necessary—intermittent mandatory ventilations plus positive end-expiratory pressure (PEEP) or continuous positive airway pressure (CPAP)
3. Maintenance of normal body temperature
4. Maintenance of fluid, electrolyte, and acid–base balance—metabolic acidosis buffered with $NaHCO_3$
5. Maintenance of nutrition—IV dextrose 10% usually required
6. Antibiotics as needed to treat infection
7. Constant observation for complications—pneumothorax, DIC, PDA with heart failure, chronic lung disease
8. Care appropriate for small premature infant

B. *Aggressive (Offered in Tertiary Care Centers)*
1. Administration of exogenous surfactant into lungs early in the disease
   a. Especially beneficial in the very low birth weight (VLBW) infant
   b. May be given preventively to VLBW infants at birth

c. Available preparations: bovine (Survanta) and synthetic (Exosurf) surfactant
   d. Administered into the endotracheal tube; suction avoided for a few hours after instillation
2. High-frequency ventilation—mechanical ventilation that uses rapid rates (can be greater than 900 breaths/ min) and tidal volumes near and often less than anatomic dead spaces
   a. Jet ventilator delivers short burst of gases at high flow.
      (1) Exhalation is passive.
      (2) Necrotizing tracheitis is a significant complication.
   b. Oscillator ventilator delivers gases by vibrating columns of air.
      (1) Exhalation is active.
      (2) The child appears to shake on the bed, which may be frightening for parents.
3. Extracorporeal membrane oxygenation (ECMO)— modified heart-lung bypass machine used to allow gas exchange outside the body
   a. Blood is removed from the venous system by a catheter placed in the internal jugular vein or right atrium.
   b. Oxygen is added and carbon dioxide removed with a membrane oxygenator.
   c. Oxygenated blood is returned by way of the right common carotid (in venoarterial ECMO) or the femoral vein (in venovenous ECMO).
   d. The infant must be heparinized for the procedure, increasing the risk of intraventricular hemorrhage. For this reason, VLBW infants or infants of decreased gestational age are usually not candidates for the procedure.

Nursing Assessment

1. Review the birth history.
   a. Apgar scores 1 and 5 minutes after birth
   b. Type of resuscitation required
   c. Any treatment or medication administered
   d. Any medication or anesthesia the mother received during labor
   e. Estimated gestational age
   f. Maternal history—contributing factors or complications
2. Carefully assess the infant's respiratory status to determine the degree of respiratory distress.
   a. Determine the degree and severity of retractions.
   b. Count the respiratory rate for 1 full minute.
      (1) Determine if respirations are regular or irregular.
      (2) Identify any periods of apnea, their length, and what type of stimulation initiates breathing.
   c. Note the infant's activity at the time respirations are recorded (eg, crying, sleeping).
   d. Listen for expiratory grunting or whining sounds from the infant when not crying (indicates an attempt to maintain PEEP and prevent alveoli from collapsing).
   e. Note any nasal flaring.
   f. Note any cyanosis—location, improvement with oxygen.
   g. Auscultate chest for diminished breath sounds and presence of crackles.
3. Determine the infant's cardiac rate and rhythm.
   a. Count the apical pulse for 1 full minute.

b. Note any irregularity in the heart rate or bounding pulses.
4. Observe the infant's general activity.
  a. Lethargic or listless
  b. Active and responds to stimuli
  c. Infant's cry
5. Assess skin for cyanosis, jaundice, mottling, paleness or grayness, edema.

Nursing Diagnoses

A. Impaired Gas Exchange related to disease process
B. Altered Nutrition: Less than body requirements related to prematurity and increased energy expenditure on breathing
C. Ineffective Thermoregulation related to immaturity
D. Altered Parenting related to separation from the newborn due to hospitalization

Nursing Interventions

A. **Promoting Adequate Gas Exchange**
1. Have emergency equipment readily available for use in the event of cardiac or respiratory arrest.
2. Institute cardiorespiratory monitoring to monitor continuously heart and respiratory rates.
3. Administer supplemental oxygen.
  a. Incubator with oxygen at prescribed concentration
  b. Plastic hood with oxygen at prescribed concentration when using radiant warmer
  c. CPAP, if indicated, using nasal prongs or endotracheal tube
4. Assist with endotracheal intubation, and maintain mechanical ventilation as indicated.
5. Measure oxygen concentration every hour and record.
6. Monitor arterial blood gases as appropriate. Obtain sample through indwelling catheter (usually placed in the umbilical artery), arterial puncture, or capillary puncture.
7. Institute pulse oximetry, if available, for continuous monitoring of oxygen saturation of arterial blood (SaO_2) (see p. 152).
  a. Avoid using adhesive to secure the sensor when infant is active. Wrap it snugly enough to reduce sensitivity to movement but not tight enough to constrict blood flow.
  b. If transcutaneous PO_2 monitor ($TcPO_2$) is used, reposition the probe every 3 to 4 hours to avoid burns caused by heating the probe to achieve sufficient arterialization.
8. Observe the infant's response to oxygen.
  a. Observe for improvement in color, respiratory rate and pattern, and nasal flaring.
  b. Note response by improvement in arterial pH, PO_2, PCO_2, or capillary blood gas.
  c. Observe closely for apnea.
    (1) Stimulate infant if apnea occurs.
    (2) If unable to produce spontaneous respiration with stimulation within 15 to 30 seconds, initiate resuscitation.
9. Position the infant to allow for maximal lung expansion.
  a. Prone position provides for a larger lung volume because of the position of the diaphragm, decreases energy expenditure, and increases time spent in quiet sleep, but it may be contraindicated when umbilical artery catheter is in place.
  b. Change position frequently.

10. Suction as needed because the gag reflex is weak, and cough is ineffective.
11. Try to minimize time spent on procedures and interventions, and monitor effects on respiratory status. (Infants undergoing multiple procedures lasting 45 minutes to 1 hour have shown a moderate decrease in PO_2.)

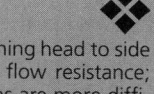

NURSING ALERT: Prone position may present several problems: turning head to side can compromise upper airway and increase air flow resistance; observation of chest is obstructed, and retractions are more difficult to detect; and abdominal distention is more difficult to recognize.

B. **Promoting Adequate Nutrition and Hydration**
1. Administer IV fluids or enteral feeding as ordered, and observe infusion rate closely to prevent fluid overload.
2. Observe IV sites for infiltration or infection; use meticulous technique to prevent sepsis.
3. If umbilical artery catheter is in place, observe for bleeding.
4. Provide adequate caloric intake (80–120 kcal/kg per 24 hours) through the following:
  a. Nasojejunal tube (best tolerated by VLBW infants)
  b. Nasogastric tube
  c. Parenteral nutrition—D10W or hyperalimentation fluid usually required
5. Monitor for hypoglycemia, which is especially common during stress. Maintain serum glucose >45 mg/dL.
6. Monitor intake and output closely.
  a. Include amount of blood drawn (small infants can become anemic due to frequent blood sampling).
  b. Apply urine collection bag to obtain sample of urine, and measure specific gravity periodically.
7. Weigh infant daily.

C. **Maintaining Thermoregulation**
1. Provide a neutral thermal environment to maintain the infant's abdominal skin temperature between 97° and 98°F (36° and 36.5°C) to prevent hypothermia, which may result in vasoconstriction and acidosis.
2. Adjust Isolette or radiant warmer to obtain desired skin temperature.
  a. For the infant weighing less than 1,250 g, the radiant warmer should be used with caution because of increased water loss and potential for hypoglycemia.
3. Prevent frequent opening of Isolette.
4. Ensure that O_2 is warmed to 87.6° to 93.2°F (32°–34°C) with 60% to 80% humidity.

D. **Encouraging Bonding**
1. If the infant has been transported to tertiary care center immediately after birth, send a photograph of the baby to the mother.
2. Call the parents daily to update them on the infant's condition until they are able to visit the child.
3. Refer to the child by his or her first name when speaking with the parents.
4. Prepare the parents for the neonatal intensive care unit (NICU) environment and how their child will appear prior to their first visit.
5. Assist the parents to participate in the child's care as appropriate.
6. Demonstrate for the parents how they can touch and speak to the child while the child is in an Isolette.

7. Allow the parents to hold the infant as soon as possible.
8. If the mother plans to breast-feed, assist her with pumping, and use the breast milk to feed the infant when enteral feedings are initiated.
9. If the infant has siblings, provide the parents with information on how to discuss the infant's illness with them.
10. If unit policies allow and the situation is appropriate, encourage sibling visitation with adequate preparation.
11. Provide the parents with information concerning the disease process, expected outcomes, and usual course of the NICU stay. Encourage the parents to ask questions and participate in the plan of care.
12. Help parents work through their grief at the birth of a premature child.

Family Education/Health Management

1. Prepare the family for long-term follow-up as appropriate. Infants with BPD may eventually go home on oxygen therapy.
2. Stress the importance of regular health care, periodic eye examinations, and developmental follow-up with the parents.
3. Ensure that the family receives information on routine well baby care.

Evaluation

A. Respiratory rate within norms for age; pattern regular and unlabored
B. Tolerating enteral feedings well; weight gain noted
C. Temperature maintained within normal limits
D. Parents interacting with infant, participating in care, and asking appropriate questions

◆ CYSTIC FIBROSIS

Cystic fibrosis is a generalized multisystem disorder affecting the exocrine glands so that the substances they secrete are abnormally viscous, affecting primarily pulmonary and gastrointestinal function.

Etiology and Incidence

1. Cystic fibrosis is inherited as an autosomal mendelian recessive trait.
2. Chloride channel functioning is affected, resulting in a decreased ability of cell membranes to transport water and electrolytes.
3. Incidence is estimated to be 1:1,600 to 1:2,500 in Caucasians, 1:17,000 in African Americans, and much lower in Asians.
   a. About 4% to 5% of the white population are carriers.
   b. Slightly more males than females are affected.
4. The average life expectancy for the cystic fibrosis patient is about 30 years.

Altered Physiology

1. The secretions of the exocrine glands are thick and sticky rather than thin and slippery.
2. Pulmonary involvement
   a. Decreased ciliary action
   b. Metaplasia and hyperplasia of squamous cells of mucus-secreting glands, leading to increased production of thick secretions (increased risk of infection)
   c. Plugged bronchi and bronchioles, resulting in bronchiectasis and bronchiolitis
   d. Atelectasis and hyperinfiltration of lungs
   e. Irreversible fibrotic changes in lungs
3. Gastrointestinal and pancreatic involvement
   a. Acini and ducts of pancreas become filled with thick mucus and are obstructed.
   b. Trypsin, chymotrypsin, lipase, and amylase do not reach the small intestine.
   c. Digestion is impaired. Interruption of the enterohepatic circulation of bile acids probably results in interference with normal pancreatic lipolysis and fat absorption through the intestinal wall.
   d. Stools are abnormal and indicate malabsorption syndrome.
   e. Meconium ileus often occurs in infant, indicating that bowel is obstructed by thick intestinal secretions.
   f. Biliary cirrhosis occurs because the intrahepatic biliary tract is obstructed by thick secretions.
4. Sweat gland involvement
   a. Secretions contain excessive amount of sodium and chloride, leading to excessive loss, especially with hot weather, fever, or exertion.
   b. Saliva also contains an excess of sodium and chloride.

Complications

1. Pulmonary infections
   a. Most frequently caused by *Pseudomonas aeruginosa*, *Staphylococcus aureus*, and *H. influenzae*. *Pseudomonas* is the most difficult organism to treat.
   b. Bronchiectasis and bronchiolitis
2. Other pulmonary complications, including emphysema, atelectasis, pneumothorax, and hemoptysis (primarily seen in adolescents)
3. Biliary cirrhosis, leading to portal hypertension, esophageal varices, and splenomegaly
4. Pancreatic fibrosis with islets of Langerhans involvement, resulting in glucose intolerance, diabetes mellitus
5. Cor pulmonale
6. Chronic sinusitis
7. Rectal polyps (3 months–3 years)
8. Rectal prolapse
9. Intussusception (younger than 2 years)
10. Pancreatitis
11. Nasal polyps
12. Heat prostration
13. Fibrosis of epididymis and vas deferens in male; aspermia
14. Growth retardation

Clinical Manifestations

1. Presentation usually occurs younger than 6 months of age but may occur at any age.
2. Meconium ileus is found in newborn.

3. Other presenting signs:
   a. Salty taste when parents kiss skin
   b. Cough (dry and hacking to loose and productive); wheezing
   c. Failure to gain weight or grow in the presence of a good appetite
   d. Frequent, bulky, and foul-smelling stools; excessive flatus
   e. Protuberant abdomen—pot belly
   f. Wasted buttocks
   g. Vomiting following coughing
   h. Recurrent pulmonary infections
   i. Clubbing of fingers in older child
   j. Increased anteroposterior chest diameter
   k. Decreased exertional endurance
   l. Maldigestion; steatorrhea (fatty stools, loss of fat-soluble vitamins)
   m. Hyperglycemia, glucosuria with polyuria, and weight loss

Diagnostic Evaluation

1. Sweat chloride test to measure sodium and chloride level in sweat
   a. Chloride level of more than 60 mEq/L is virtually diagnostic.
   b. Chloride of 40 to 60 mEq/L is borderline and should be repeated.
   c. Sodium level greater than 60 mEq/L is diagnostic.
2. Measurement of trypsin concentration in duodenal secretions; absence of normal concentration virtually diagnostic
3. Analysis of digestive enzymes (trypsin and chymotrypsin) in stool—reduced, used for initial screening for cystic fibrosis
4. Chest x-ray
   a. May be normal initially
   b. Later shows increased areas of infection, overinflation, bronchial thickening and plugging, atelectasis, and fibrosis
5. Analysis of stool for steatorrhea
6. BMC (Boehringer-Mannheim Corporation) meconium strip test for stool includes lactose and protein content; used for screening
7. Pulmonary function studies (after 4 years old)
   a. Decreased vital capacity and flow rates
   b. Increased residual volume or increased total lung capacity
8. Diagnosis made when a positive sweat test is seen in conjunction with one or more of the following:
   a. Positive family history for cystic fibrosis
   b. Typical chronic obstructive lung disease
   c. Documented exocrine pancreatic insufficiency

Treatment

A. **Pulmonary Interventions**
1. Antimicrobial therapy as indicated for pulmonary infection
   a. Oral antibiotics may be given prophylactically or when symptomatic.
   b. IV antibiotics are given when the child fails to respond to oral antibiotics; this may be inpatient or at home therapy.
   c. Inhaled antibiotics, such as gentamycin (Garamycin) or tobramycin (Nebcin), may be used for severe lung disease or colonization of organisms. Recently, some practitioners advocate using nebulized antibiotics earlier in therapy.
2. Bronchodilators and vasoconstrictors for relief of bronchospasm
3. Aerosol, expectorants, and mucolytic agents to decrease viscosity of secretions
4. Chest physical therapy for bronchial drainage, especially during acute exacerbations
   a. Postural drainage (see Procedure Guidelines 42-2, p. 1194)
   b. Coughing and deep breathing exercises
5. Bronchopulmonary lavage—treatment of atelectasis and mucoid impaction using large volumes of saline (used in some institutions in the United States)
6. Lobectomy—resection of symptomatic lobar bronchiectasis to retard progression of lesion to total lung involvement

B. **Gastrointestinal Interventions**
1. Pancreatic enzyme supplementation is provided with each feeding.
   a. Favored preparation is pancrelipase (Pancrease).
   b. Occasionally antacid is helpful to improve tolerance of enzymes.
   c. Favorable response to enzymes is based on tolerance of fatty foods, decreased stool frequency, absence of steatorrhea, improved appetite, and lack of abdominal pain.
2. Provide a high-energy diet by increasing carbohydrates, protein, and fat (possibly as high as 40%). Increases in dietary intake should consider growth and repair, infection, the work of breathing and energy expenditure for coughing, malabsorption, and physical activity.
3. Provide zinc and iron supplements.
4. Encourage daily intake of water-soluble vitamins.
5. Provide supplementary fat-soluble vitamins.
6. Ensure adequate fluid and salt intake.

C. **Controversial and Experimental Treatment**
1. Administration of aerosolized recombinant human deoxyribonuclease
   a. Enzyme that breaks down DNA in leukocytes is present in thick pulmonary secretions.
   b. The goal of treatment is to reduce viscosity of sputum, making the sputum easier to clear from the airways and decreasing the incidence of infection.
   c. Early trials show improvement in forced vital capacity and forced expiratory volume.
2. Heart-lung, double lung, or single-lung transplantation for end-stage lung disease
   a. This treatment is limited by availability of donor organs.
   b. Survival rate is similar to survival rates in patients without cystic fibrosis.
3. Gene therapy
   a. Phase 1 clinical trials in the United States were started in 1993.
   b. Therapy is based on somatic gene correction; an attempt to correct the defect in the cells of the individual is made by adding the correct gene sequence to the cells.
   c. One trial method will use a virus carrying DNA with the appropriate gene sequence, which will be introduced into the affected lung cells by nebulization.

d. A second method being investigated is the introduction into the lungs of DNA by nebulization with the appropriate gene sequence suspended in liposomes.

e. It is thought that the treatment will need to be repeated at regular intervals.

Assessment

1. Check for family history of cystic fibrosis, failure to thrive, and unexplained infant death; check the child's history and physical condition. Carefully listen for subtle information that may suggest cystic fibrosis.
2. Assess respiratory status.
   a. Increased work of breathing
   b. Quality of breath sounds by auscultation
   c. Child's perception of respiratory status
   d. Ability to participate in activities of daily living
3. Assess nutritional status and characteristics of stool.

Nursing Diagnoses

A. Ineffective Airway Clearance related to thick pulmonary secretions
B. Risk for Infection related to thick, tenacious secretions
C. Altered Nutrition: Less than body requirements related to decreased appetite or inadequate absorption
D. Body Image Disturbance related to chronic disease process
E. Altered Family Processes related to the child with a chronic disease

Nursing Interventions

A. *Promoting Airway Clearance*
1. Use intermittent aerosol therapy three to four times a day when child is symptomatic.
   a. Use prior to postural drainage.
   b. Administer bronchodilators and other medications, diluted in normal saline, in aerosol form to penetrate respiratory tract.

NURSING ALERT:
Mist therapy is no longer recommended because water droplets may cause bronchospasm in some patients, and the equipment required to deliver the therapy is frequently contaminated with opportunistic organisms.

2. Perform chest physical therapy three to four times a day following aerosol therapy; perform more frequently if infection is present.
   a. Perform 1 hour after eating to prevent vomiting or discomfort.
   b. Place child in position that gives greatest access to affected lobes of lung and facilitates gravity drainage of mucus from specific lung areas (Fig. 42-3).

3. Help the child to relax to cough more easily following postural drainage.
4. Suction the infant or young child when necessary if not able to cough.
5. Teach child breathing exercises using pursed lips to increase duration of exhalation.

B. *Preventing Infection*
1. Provide good skin care and position changes to prevent skin breakdown of malnourished child.
2. Change diapers promptly to prevent diaper rash and superimposed infection.
3. Provide frequent mouth care to reduce the chance of infection because mucus is present.
4. Restrict contact with people with respiratory infection.
5. Administer antibiotics as prescribed to treat specific organisms when child is symptomatic.

C. *Promoting Adequate Nutrition*
1. Encourage diet composed of foods high in calories and protein and moderate to high in fat because absorption of food is incomplete.
   a. Provide 120% to 150% of recommended dietary allowances because only 80% to 85% of intake is absorbed.
2. Administer fat-soluble vitamins in water-miscible solution in two to three times the normal dose, as prescribed, to counteract malabsorption.
   a. Give vitamins A, D, and E on a daily basis.
   b. Give vitamin K when the child has an infection or is being treated with antibiotics.
3. Administer pancreatic enzymes with each meal and snack.
   a. Mix capsule, granules, or powder with small portion of food for infant or small child; do not mix with formula (may not be finished).
   b. Offer the older child capsules or tablets.
   c. Withhold enzymes, as ordered, if child is taking only clear liquid diet or enteral feedings.
4. Increase salt intake during hot weather, fever, or excessive exercise to prevent sodium depletion and cardiovascular compromise.
5. To prevent vomiting, allow ample time for feeding if irritable because of not feeling well and coughing.
6. Monitor weight at least weekly to assess effectiveness of nutritional interventions.

D. *Enhancing Self-esteem*
1. Explain each procedure, medication, and treatment to the child as appropriate for age.
2. Allow child to show frustrations, fears, and feelings by talking, complaining, or crying.
3. Support and comfort the child by talking to and holding child.
4. Provide diversional activities related to child's interests, and praise child for accomplishments.
5. Encourage older child to take responsibility for treatments and be involved in care plan.
6. Help child to identify strengths and limitations and to feel good about self.
7. If child resists chest physical therapy due to anger, fear, or frustration, help to redirect those feelings.
8. Encourage regular exercise and activity to foster sense of accomplishment and independence and improve pulmonary function.

FIGURE 42-3 *Positions for postural drainage.* ▶

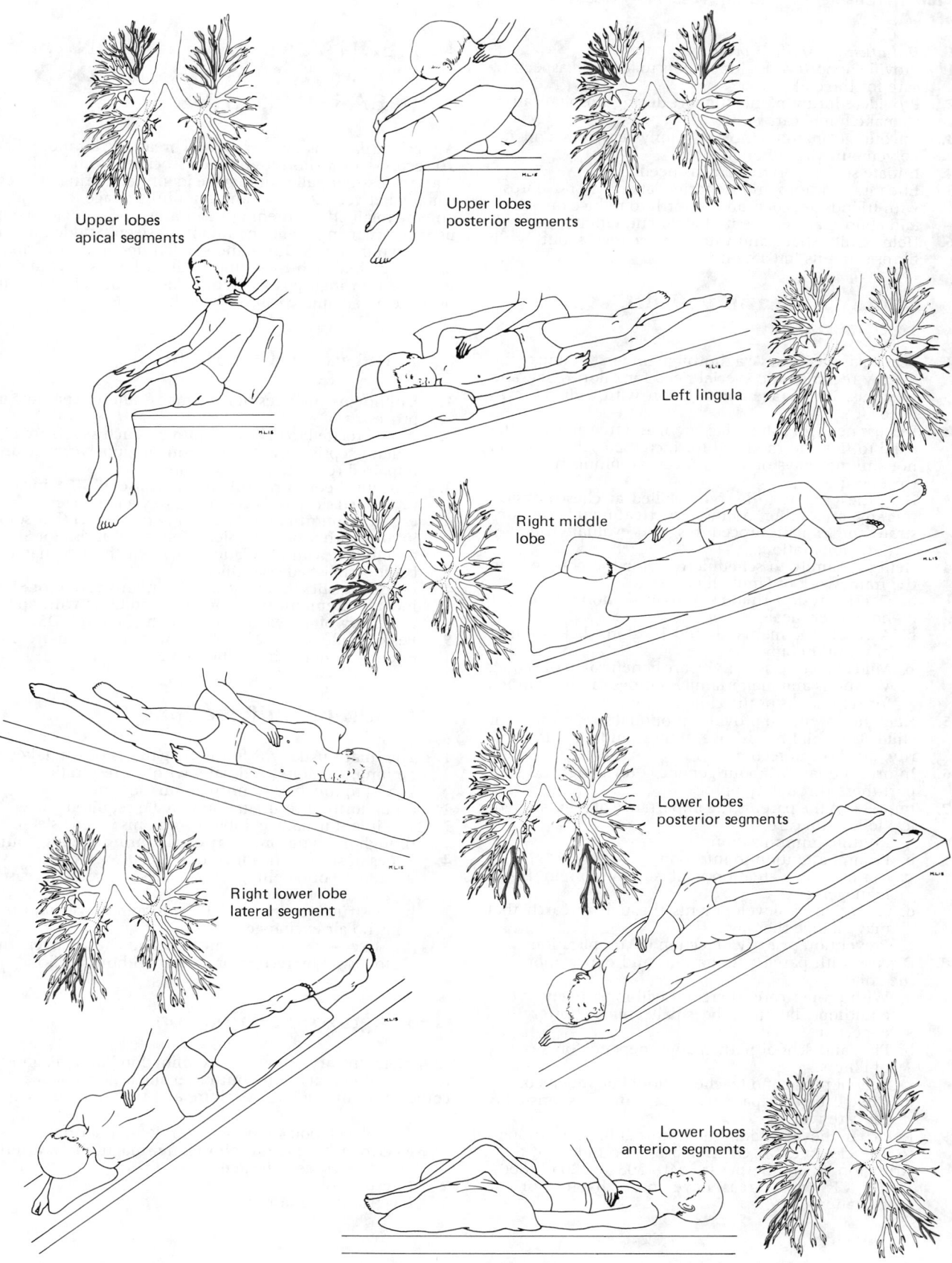

Upper lobes
apical segments

Upper lobes
posterior segments

Left lingula

Right middle
lobe

Lower lobes
posterior segments

Right lower lobe
lateral segment

Lower lobes
anterior segments

E. *Enhancing Family Processes*
1. Provide opportunities for parents to learn all aspects of care for the child.
2. Provide education and support during hospitalization to make home care easier.
3. Encourage maintenance of family activities and involvement with other children.
4. Initiate social work referral as needed.
5. Encourage information sharing about cystic fibrosis with friends, teacher, and so forth to reduce questions and abnormal treatment of child and family.
6. Help family share and interpret feelings about cystic fibrosis and its impact on them.

Family Education/Health Maintenance

1. Teach parents to have a thorough understanding of the dietary regimen and special need for calories, fat, and vitamins. Encourage consultation with a dietitian as needed.
2. Discuss need for salt replacement and free access of the child to salt and the need for increased salt intake on hot summer days or when fever, vomiting, and diarrhea occur.
3. Help the parents to become skilled at chest physical therapy and other pulmonary treatments. Demonstrate and explain procedures, and evaluate their return demonstration.
4. Help the family to schedule care for the child within the framework of family life.
   a. Chest physical therapy should be done at least 1 hour after meals.
   b. Aerosol treatments should be done before chest physical therapy.
   c. Mild exercise and activity are beneficial to the child.
   d. Vacations and major family outings can be planned for remissions of the child's symptoms.
5. Help the parents to provide emotional support to their child. The child needs love, understanding, and security, not overprotection.
6. Inform the family about genetic counseling, and support them through the process.
7. Impress on the parents the importance of regular medical follow-up care:
   a. Routine immunizations
   b. Prompt attention to infection
   c. Continued evaluation and supervision in home management
   d. Attention to developments through research that may change therapy
   e. Prevention or early detection of complications
8. Discuss with parents limitations and expectations for the child
   a. With proper care, the child will most likely live to adulthood but may be smaller and shorter than expected.
   b. Play and school participation depends on severity of illness.
   c. School nurse and teachers should be involved.
   d. Child can participate in and take over responsibility for care with age.
9. Refer families for additional information and support to agencies such as Cystic Fibrosis Foundation, 6931 Arlington Road, Bethesda, MD 20814-3205, (800)-FIGHT CF. Most areas have local chapters of the organization.

◆ NEONATAL OR PROLONGED SLEEP APNEA OR INFANCY (NEAR-MISS SIDS)

Apnea of infancy is the cessation of breathing for more than 20 seconds, or a shorter episode associated with bradycardia, cyanosis, or pallor. It may be identified during infancy, usually between 2 weeks and 6 months of age, because of an unexplained frightening respiratory or cardiac event, usually occurring while the infant is asleep. Sudden infant death syndrome (SIDS) is the sudden death of any infant or young child, which is unexplained by history, and in which a thorough postmortem examination fails to demonstrate an adequate cause of death.

Etiology and Incidence

1. Unknown—may result from many different pathologic processes.
2. Apnea related to organic disorders, such as seizure disorders, sepsis, severe infection, hyppoglycemia, and impaired regulation of breathing.
3. Current theories relating to the cause of SIDS include prolonged sleep apnea, chronic oxygen deficiency, and enzyme abnormalities. Although many feel that some infants with prolonged sleep apnea are at risk for SIDS, a definitive causal relation between the two has not been established scientifically.
4. Characteristics that may identify infants at risk for SIDS include prematurity, neonatal conditions with apnea or history of apnea, and familial history of SIDS.
5. Peak incidence is 2 to 4 months; occurs more frequently in males in a ratio of 3:2.

Clinical Manifestations

1. The infant usually is found by parents or caretaker to be limp, cyanotic, and pale, with no respiration. Skin is cool to touch with normal muscle tone.
2. Some form of resuscitation may be required.
3. The infant usually exhibits symptoms when asleep, although the syndrome may occur during waking hours.
4. Types of sleep apnea include:
   a. Central or diaphragmatic—chest movement ceases, absence of airflow.
   b. Obstructive—chest and diaphragm move, but there is no air exchange.
   c. Mixed—cessation of air flow and chest movement, followed by respiratory effort without air flow.

Diagnostic Evaluation

Complete history, physical examination, and diagnostic tests are aimed at ruling out other medical problems that could result in respiratory failure as a secondary cause.

1. Complete blood count with differential, serum glucose, electrolytes, calcium, phosphate, magnesium, arterial blood gases, as indicated
2. Chest x-ray
3. Electrocardiogram

4. Electroencephalogram (may not be routine) and neurologic examination
5. Respiratory studies—a 12- to 24-hour pneumogram recording of small changes in electrical resistance with each breath or respiratory pattern; multichannel sleep test with continuous printout
6. Continuous cardiac and apnea monitoring for recurrence of event, prolonged apnea, or bradycardia
7. Barium swallow for gastroesophageal reflex
8. Because of hypoxemia that may have occurred, child should be assessed for learning difficulties (hearing, eyesight), discrete neurologic impairments, personality disorders, etc.

Treatment

1. Cardiopulmonary monitoring is critical.
2. Specific treatment of the underlying cause.
3. Theophylline (Theolair) may be used to decrease apneic spells.
4. Long-term follow-up for physiologic and neurologic behavioral functions.

> **NURSING ALERT:**
> Infants who have experienced infant apnea may be at risk for recurrent apnea, hypoxia, and sudden death, and should be monitored closely. Research has shown that SIDS is more likely in infants sleeping prone. It is now recommended that all infants be put to sleep on their backs or sides.

Nursing Assessment

1. Obtain a nursing history, including the parents' description of the events that preceded the hospitalization, and their understanding of prolonged apnea.
   a. This information may provide clues for factors to observe during hospitalization and provides data for the development of a teaching plan.
   b. It allows for the correction of misinformation and misconceptions.
2. Have the parents describe sleep patterns, feeding habits, prior health problems, immunizations, and medications; this may provide data regarding possible influencing factors or causes of the condition.
3. Have the parents describe a typical day in the life of the infant and the family unit. This provides important data on how home monitoring may affect family life, and contributes to the effective development of home management and family teaching plans; it also provides a basis for continuity of care for the infant.

Nursing Diagnoses

A. Ineffective Breathing Pattern related to periods of apnea
B. Parental Anxiety related to life-threatening event
C. Knowledge Deficit regarding home monitoring

Nursing Interventions

A. *Maintaining Breathing Pattern*
1. Be prepared for the infant's admission and have all equipment, including apnea monitor, ready for use.

   a. Select a room that is clearly visible from the nursing station; the room should be quiet to reduce sensory stimulation, which may reduce the likelihood of a recurring episode.
   b. Be aware that the family has just experienced the extreme stress of feeling that their infant has almost died. Reassure them with empathy and efficiency at the time of admission.
2. Continuously monitor respirations. Document any apnea along with sleep status, color, position of infant, and intervention necessary (nothing, gentle stimulation, vigorous stimulation, resuscitation).
3. Administer theophylline, if prescribed. Observe for signs of toxicity: apical rate above 200, vomiting, and agitation.
4. Continue the infant's normal activities whenever possible (ie, holding him or her for feedings, playing with him or her, disconnecting from monitor for bathing); allow for continuation of usual eating or sleeping patterns. Simulating the home environment as much as possible will encourage deep-sleep patterns, which may stimulte apnea and provide valuable diagnostic information.

B. *Minimizing Anxiety*
1. Encourage parents to continue involvement in infant care during hospitalization.
2. Clarify any misconceptions about apnea and SIDS.
3. Allow ventilation of feelings and concerns.
4. Assess family dynamics for any conflicts or maladapted responses; intervene or refer as appropriate.
5. Use anticipatory guidance in preparing parents for emotional responses to home monitoring.
   a. Increased anxiety or tension
   b. Constant worry about the alarm even when it does not go off
   c. Fatigue
   d. Financial and emotional burdens encountered by the family
   e. Perceived loss of "normal, healthy chiild"; parents may grieve when given the diagnosis

C. *Improving Confidence in Home Monitoring*
1. Demonstrate operation and maintenance of the monitor. Reinforce teaching by equipment supplier. Provide information on contacting a monitor technician.
2. Describe how to record apnea in relation to activity and position and when to report apnea to health care provider.
3. Teach methods of responding to alarms; what to observe (ie, color, presence or absence of breathing) and how to respond (gentle versus vigorous stimulation, CPR).
4. Discuss adjustments in daily living that will be necessary. Identify a typical family day and discuss anticipated changes.
   a. Emphasize that responsibility must be shared by family members.
   b. Discuss the possible impact on siblings.
   c. Advise the parents to eliminate noises that would interfere with their ability to hear the alarm (ie, showering, vacuum cleaning). Someone must always be available to hear and respond to the alarm.
   d. Avoid traveling long distances alone with infant.
   e. Encourage the parents to maintain their relationship with one another by using another person trained in CPR to occasionally assume infant care.

5. Emphasize the healthy aspects of the infant. Encourage the parents to continue as many usual routines as possible. Provide specific things parents can do to encourage normal development and a healthy parent–child relationship.
6. Encourage the parents to provide total care for their infant 24 hours prior to discharge so they regain confidence in caring for their child.

Family Education/Health Maintenance

1. Educate about feeding precautions: frequent burping, no bottle in bed, upright position after feeding, postioning infant on back or side, not abdomen.
2. Have parents contact local emergncy service to inform them about their infant, and to be certain that they have infant resuscitation equipment. It may be possible to arrange for the power company to notify the parents if the power supply is to go off.
3. Instruct the parents in the administration of any new medications.
4. Teach CPR or arrange training to the parents as well as to any person responsible for the infant's care.
5. For further information and support, refer to agencies such as National Sudden Infant Death Syndrome Foundation (NSIDF); 1314 Bedford Avenue, Suite 210; Baltimore, MD 21208; 1-800-221-SIDS; New York City Information and Counselling Program for Sudden Infant Death; 520 First Avenue, Room 50; New York, NY 10016; (212) 686-8854.

Evaluation

A. Monitoring maintained; respirations regular without apnea
B. Parents verbalize concern over infant's well-being
C. Parents demonstrate correct operation of respiratory monitor and response to alarms

Pediatric Respiratory Procedures

◆ MECHANICAL VENTILATION

Available ventilators for pediatric use have a wide range of capabilities, versatility, and clinical application. Some are more suitable for use with infants, others with older children. Nurses must be well acquainted with the characteristics of the particular machine being used and the meaning of the settings and alarms on the machine.

Nursing Management

Refer to Guidelines for Managing the Patient Requiring Mechanical Ventilation (p. 191). In addition, the nurse who is caring for a pediatric patient should remember the following.

A. **Setting Controls**
In setting controls, inspiratory flow rate will be less, and the respiratory rate will be greater than in the adult patient. These depend on the patient's size and condition and are determined by the health care provider or respiratory therapist.

B. **Humidification**
1. Because of their small diameters, pediatric endotracheal tubes easily become obstructed by thickened secretions. Therefore, adequate humidification must be maintained to keep secretions loose.
2. During ventilation of an infant in an incubator, the amount of ventilator tubing outside the incubator should be kept to a minimum. The warm temperature inside the incubator helps decrease the amount of condensation in the tubing and thus provides higher water content in the inspired gas.

C. **Oxygen Concentration**
1. In infants inspired concentrations of oxygen should always be kept as low as possible (while still providing for physiologic requirements) to prevent the development of retrolental fibroplasia or pulmonary O_2 toxicity.
2. The oxygen concentration should be checked periodically with an analyzer.

D. **Blood Gases**
1. The arterialized capillary sample method is inaccurate for infants in respiratory distress because the constricted peripheral circulation may not reflect the arterial blood gases accurately.
2. An umbilical artery catheter is most frequently used to obtain arterial blood samples.

E. **Sterile Precautions**
The newborn has only those antibodies transferred across the placenta from the mother. Therefore, sterile precautions are essential.

1. Ventilator tubing should be changed every 24 hours.
2. Routine cultures should be taken after intubation; there should be daily Gram-staining of secretions.
3. Suctioning requires aseptic technique.

F. **Tubing Support**
1. Special frames are available to support ventilator tubing; this helps to prevent accidental decannulation in infants and small children.
2. Infants may require folded diapers or padding on either side and at the top of their heads to decrease mobility and take up space between the head and the frame.

G. **Monitoring the Ventilator**
1. Pressure gauges should be checked at frequent intervals because this gives an indication of changing compliance or increased airway resistance.
2. Volume measurements are difficult to obtain in infants because most spirometers incorporated into ventilators and meters do not read accurately at low volumes and flows. However, they are helpful with older children.
3. Measure respiratory rates of the machine and the patient at least every hour.

PROCEDURE GUIDELINES 42-1 ◆ Oxygen Therapy for Children

GENERAL NURSING RESPONSIBILITIES

NURSING ACTION	RATIONALE
1. Explain the procedure to the child and allow him or her to feel the equipment and the oxygen flowing through the tube, mask, and so forth.	1. The child will be reassured if he or she understands the procedure and knows what to expect.
2. Maintain a clear airway by suctioning, if necessary.	2. The delivery of oxygen requires a clear airway.
3. Provide a source of humidification.	3. Oxygen is a dry gas and requires the addition of moisture to prevent drying of the tracheobronchial tree and thickening and consolidating secretions.

4. Measure oxygen concentrations every 1–2 hours when a child is receiving oxygen through incubator hood, tent, or Croupette.
  a. Measure when the oxygen environment is closed.
  b. Measure the concentration close to the child's airway.
  c. Record oxygen concentrations and simultaneous measurements of the pulse and respirations.
	4. It is desirable to keep the oxygen concentration as low as possible while still providing for physiologic requirements. This minimizes the danger of the child's developing retrolental fibroplasia or pulmonary oxygen toxicity. (Desired oxygen concentrations are determined by the arterial oxygen tension measurement.) The oxygen analyzer itself should be calibrated daily on both room air and 100% oxygen. The concentration of oxygen within the space is determined by the liter flow, the efficiency of the equipment, and the frequency with which it is opened to the external environment.

5. Observe the child's response to oxygen.	5. Desired response includes
	  a. Decreased restlessness
	  b. Decreased respiratory distress
	  c. Improved color
	  d. Improved vital sign values

6. Organize nursing care so that interruption of therapy is minimal.	6. Interruption of therapy may result in the return of anoxia and defeat the goals of therapy.
7. Periodically check all equipment during each tour of duty.	7. For optimal functioning, the equipment should be clean, undamaged, and in good working order.
8. Clean equipment daily, and change it at least once each week. (Tubing and nebulizer jars should be changed daily.)	8. Unclean equipment may be a source of contamination.

9. Keep combustible materials and potential sources of fire away from oxygen equipment.
  a. Avoid using oil or grease around oxygen connections.
  b. Do not use alcohol or oils on a child in an oxygen tent.
  c. Do not permit any electrical devices in or near an oxygen tent.
  d. Avoid the use of wool blankets and those made from some synthetic fibers because of the hazards resulting from static electricity.
  e. Prohibit smoking in areas where oxygen is being used.
  f. Have a fire extinguisher available.
	9. Oxygen supports combustion.

10. Terminate oxygen therapy gradually.
  a. Slowly reduce liter flow.
  b. Open air vents in incubators.
  c. Open zippers or flip a section of the canopy over the top of the tent.
	10. This allows the child to adjust to normal atmospheric oxygen concentrations.

11. Continually monitor the child's response during weaning. Observe for restlessness, increased pulse rate, respiratory distress, cyanosis.	11. These are indications that the child is unable to tolerate reduced oxygen concentration.

(continued)

PROCEDURE GUIDELINES 42-1 ◆ Oxygen Therapy for Children (continued)

SPECIFIC METHODS FOR ADMINIS- TERING OXYGEN TO PEDIATRIC PATIENTS

NURSING ACTION	RATIONALE
OXYGEN BY NASAL CANNULA OR CATHETER	
1. Refer to Procedure Guidelines: Administering Oxygen by Nasal Canula, p. 178	
OXYGEN BY MASK	
1. Choose an appropriate size mask that covers the mouth and nose but not the eyes.	1. Extra space under the mask and around the face is added dead space and decreases the effectiveness of the therapy.
2. Use a mask that is capable of delivering the desired oxygen concentration.	2. Venturi masks, available for use in pediatrics, deliver low to moderate concentrations of oxygen: 24%, 28%, 35%, or 40%.
3. Place the mask over the child's mouth and nose so that it fits securely. Secure the mask with an elastic head grip.	3. Make sure that the mask is adjusted properly over the mouth and nose. Do not allow the oxygen to blow in child's eyes. Small pieces of cotton may be placed above the ears to help relieve pressure and discomfort caused by the head strap.
4. Remove the oxygen mask at hourly intervals; wash the face and dry.	4. Makes the patient feel more comfortable.
5. Do not use masks for comatose infants or children.	5. Such children are more likely to vomit. The risk of aspiration may be increased with mask therapy because of obstruction of the flow of vomitus.
6. For additional information, refer to Procedure Guidelines: Administering Oxygen by Venturi Mask (p. 181) and by Face Mask (p. 180).	
FACE TENT	
1. Face tents are available in the adult size only. They can be used effectively in pediatric patients if inverted to create a smaller reservoir and better fit.	1. Face tents combine the positive qualities of aerosol masks and mist tents. The child is accessible and may continue to play without feeling confined.
2. A flow of 8–10 L should be used to flush the system and provide a stable oxygen concentration.	2. Larger children will require higher flows.
T-BARS AND TRACHEOSTOMY MASKS	
1. These devices are used to deliver oxygen to intubated patients.	
2. The flow rate must be set to meet the minute volume requirements of the child and to provide a 100% source of gas.	2. T-bars require a short, flexible tube on the distal end to act as a reservoir and prevent room-air entrapment.
OXYGEN TENT	
1. Select the smallest tent and canopy that will achieve the desired concentration of oxygen and maintain patient comfort.	1. This increases the efficiency of the unit.
2. Pad the metal frame that supports the canopy.	2. This protects the child from injury.
3. Analyze and record the tent atmosphere every 1–2 hours. Concentrations of 30%–50% can be achieved in well-maintained tents.	3. The concentration varies with the efficiency of the tent, the rate of flow of oxygen, and the frequency with which the tent is opened to the outside environment.
4. Maintain a tight-fitting canopy. Whenever possible, provide nursing care through the sleeves or pockets of the tent.	4. This prevents oxygen leakage and disruption of the tent atmosphere. a. If the child is extremely restless or uncooperative, it may be useful to permit a parent to hold the child's hand through a small opening in the zipper of the canopy.

SPECIFIC METHODS FOR ADMINIS-TERING OXYGEN TO PEDIATRIC PATIENTS *(cont'd)*

NURSING ACTION	RATIONALE
5. Make certain that the crib sides are up.	5. The canopy, when tucked into the mattress, often gives the illusion of a safe, confined environment.
6. Select toys that retard absorption, are washable, and will not produce static electricity.	6. The child needs toys for stimulation and diversion. They should be safe and practical.

CROUPETTE

1. This is an oxygen tent equipped with a high-humidification system (refer to procedure under "Oxygen Tent" above).	1. If the child's condition requires high humidity but not oxygen, the unit can be operated with compressed air.
2. Change the child's clothing and bed linen when damp. Cover the child with a cotton blanket.	2. This prevents chilling in an environment of cooled, supersaturated, aerated mist.
3. Check the child frequently.	3. Condensation on the canopy may make it difficult to see the child.
4. If possible, remove the child from the mist periodically.	4. This prevents maceration of the skin. Mist may be delivered through nebulizer tubing or mask during these periods.
5. Promote postural drainage, and suction the child as necessary.	5. Rapid mobilization of secretions may follow initiation of mist tent therapy.
6. Observe the small infant for signs of overhydration.	6. This occasionally results from intensive use of an ultrasonic nebulizer, especially if a saline solution is nebulized.

CLOSED INCUBATORS/ISOLETTES

1. The incubator is used to provide a controlled environment for the neonate.	1. The unit is able to provide precise environmental control of temperature, oxygen, humidity, and isolation.
2. Adjust the oxygen flow to achieve the desired oxygen concentration.	2. Refer to Table PG 42-1, below.
a. An oxygen limiter prevents the oxygen concentration inside the incubator from exceeding 40%.	a. This is desirable because it reduces the hazard of the child's developing retrolental fibroplasia.
b. Higher concentrations (up to 85%) may be obtained by placing the red reminder flag in the vertical position.	b. This operates by reducing the air intake.

Incubator Oxygen Therapy

Red Flag in Horizontal Position		Red Flag in Vertical Position	
Flow of Oxygen (L/min)	Concentration of Oxygen (%)	Flow of Oxygen (L/min)	Concentration of Oxygen (%)
4	28–31	4	Flow not sufficient for high concentration
6	32–36	8	70–75
8	37–40	10	75–80
		12	80–85

From Lough, M. D., & Doershuk, C. F. Oxygen therapy. In M. D. Lough, C. F. Doershuk, & R. C. Stern. (1995). *Pediatric respiratory therapy.* Chicago; Year Book Medical Pub. Used with Permission.

3. Secure a nebulizer to the inside wall of the incubator if mist therapy is desired.	3. This should be cleaned and autoclaved daily. Sterile solutions are used to keep the bacteria count at a minimum.
4. Keep sleeves of incubator closed to prevent loss of oxygen.	4. When incubator or sleeves are opened, supply supplemental oxygen with oxygen mask to face and nose.
5. Periodically analyze the incubator atmosphere.	5. Be certain that the child is receiving the desired concentration of oxygen.

(continued)

PROCEDURE GUIDELINES 42-1 ◆ Oxygen Therapy for Children *(continued)*

*SPECIFIC
METHODS FOR
ADMINIS-
TERING
OXYGEN TO
PEDIATRIC
PATIENTS
(cont'd)*

NURSING ACTION	RATIONALE
OXYGEN HOOD	
1. Warmed, humidified oxygen is supplied through a plastic container that fits over the child's head.	1. This is especially useful when high concentrations of oxygen are desired. The hood may be used in an incubator or with a warming unit. Oxygen should not be allowed to blow directly into the infant's face.

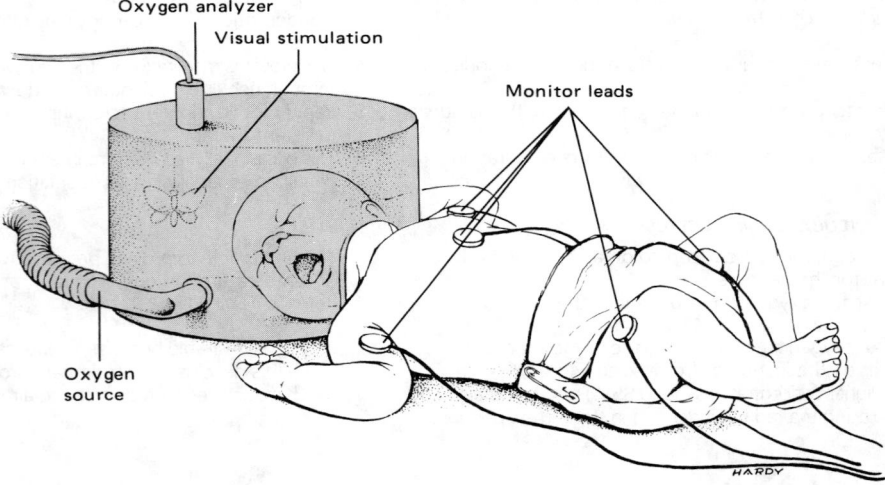

Oxygen hood.

2. Continuously monitor the oxygen concentration, temperature, and humidity inside the hood.	2. Oxygen should be warmed to 31°–34°C. (87.8°–93.2°F) to prevent a neonatal response to cold stress, including oxygen deprivation, metabolic acidosis, rapid depletion of glycogen stores, and reduction of blood glucose levels.
3. Open the hood or remove the baby from it as infrequently as possible.	3. This prevents fluctuations of heat and oxygen, which may further debilitate the young infant.
4. Several different designs are available for use. The manufacturer's directions should be carefully followed.	4. This is a safety consideration.

PROCEDURE GUIDELINES 42-2 ◆ Promoting Postural Drainage in the Pediatric Patient

Postural drainage is the positioning of the patient so that gravity will assist in the movement of secretions from the smaller bronchial airways to the main bronchus and trachea, from which the secretions can be removed by coughing or suctioning.

PROCEDURE	
NURSING ACTION	**RATIONALE**

PREPARATORY PHASE

1. Assess the child's respiratory status.
    a. Obtain a baseline respiratory rate.
    b. Observe for respiratory distress, retractions, nasal flaring, and so forth.
2. Identify the involved portion(s) of the lung by auscultation, percussion, or review of the x-ray report.
3. Explain the procedure to the child or the parent.

4. Make the child comfortable.
    a. Remove constricting clothes.
    b. Flex the child's knees and hips.
    c. Have tissues and an emesis basin available.
    d. Have several pillows available.
5. Provide bronchodilator or nebulization therapy prior to the procedure if indicated.

1. This is necessary to evaluate the effectiveness of the therapy.

2. The positions selected for drainage will depend on what portion of the lung is involved.
3. This allays anxiety and helps to secure the child's cooperation.
    b. To assist in relaxing and decreasing strain on the abdominal muscles during coughing.

    c. To collect mucus.
    d. To facilitate positioning.
5. It is easier to raise mucus mechanically after the bronchi are dilated and the secretions are thinned.

PERFORMANCE PHASE

1. Place the child in a series of appropriate positions.
    a. The area to be drained should be elevated and its respective bronchus placed in a vertical position.

    b. The spine should be as straight as possible to permit optimal expansion of the rib cage.

2. Unless contraindicated, cup the chest wall for 1–2 minutes.
3. Have the child inhale deeply; then, as he exhales, vibrate the chest wall during three to five exhalations.
4. Encourage the child to cough.
5. Allow the child to rest for a minute, then repeat cupping, vibration, and coughing until no more mucus is produced or the child's condition indicates that the procedure should be stopped.

1. The positions are selected and modified according to the lung area involved, the child's age and general condition, and equipment such as IV, tracheostomies, monitors, ventilators.
    b. Infants are positioned on the nurse's lap, in the Isolette, or in the crib; older children may be treated on a tilt board or in bed.
2. More secretions can be raised in a shorter period of time when cupping and vibration are added to posturing.

4. Infants and young children may require suctioning.
5. Total treatment time should generally not exceed 20–30 minutes.
    a. In acute conditions such as atelectasis, postural drainage may be done for 5 minutes of every hour.
    b. In chronic conditions such as cystic fibrosis, postural drainage may be done two to five times per day for 15–30 minutes.

NURSING ALERT:
Postural drainage should not be done immediately after meals because it may induce vomiting.

6. Provide for patient safety.

6. Stay with the child during the procedure, especially when he or she is in a head-down position.

Selected References

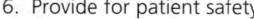

Avery, M. E., & First, L. R. (Eds.) (1993). *Pediatric medicine* (2nd ed.). Philadelphia: Williams and Wilkins.
Avery, G. B., Fletcher, M. A., & MacDonald, M. G. (Eds.) (1994).

Neonatology: Pathophysiology and management of the newborn (4th ed.). Philadelphia: J.B. Lippincott.
Barnes, L. P. (1992). Tracheostomy care: Preparing parents for discharge. *MCN:*

American Journal of Maternal Child Nursing, 17(6), 293.
Briars, G., & Warner, J. (1993). Cystic fibrosis. *Practitioner, 237*(1531), 765–769.

Coutelle, C., Caplen, N., Hart, S., Huxley, C., & Williamson, R. (1993). Gene therapy for cystic fibrosis. *Archives of Disease in Childhood, 68*(4), 437–439.

Custer, J. R. (1993). Croup and related disorders. *Pediatrics in Review, 14*(1), 19–29.

Faris, M. A., & Steele, P. H. (1993). Airway support management: A teaching module. *Journal of Pediatric Nursing, 8*(4), 265–268.

Geller, G. (1995). Cystic fibrosis and the pediatric caregiver: Benefits and burdens of genetic technology. *Pediatric Nursing, 21* (1), 57–61.

Gunkel, J. H., & Banks, P. L. (1993). Surfactant therapy and intracranial hemorrhage: Review of the literature and results of new analysis. *Pediatrics, 92*(6), 775–786.

Hazinski, M. F. (Ed.) (1992). *Nursing care of the critically ill child* (2nd ed.). Philadelphia: Mosby-Yearbook.

Holberg, C. J., Wright, A. L., Martinez, F. D., Ray, C. G., Taussig, L. M., & Lebowitz, M. D. (1991). Risk factors for respiratory syncytial virus associated with lower respiratory illness in the first year of life. *American Journal of Epidemiology, 133*(11), 1135–1151.

Horner, S. D. (1995). A family care approach for managing childhood asthma. *Journal of the American Academy of Nurse Practitioners, 7* (5), 221–227.

Janal, H. K., Stutman, H. R., Zaleska, M., Rob, B., Eyzaguirre, M., Marks, M. I., & Nussbaum, E. (1993). Ribavirin effect on pulmonary function in young infants with respiratory syncytial virus bronchiolitis. *Pediatric Infectious Diseases Journal, 12*(3), 214–218.

Kelly, H. W. (1993). Current controversies in asthma treatment. *American Pharmacy, NS33*(10), 48–54.

Larter, N. L., Kieckhefer, G., & Paeth, S. T. (1993). Content validation of standards of nursing care for the child with asthma. *Journal of Pediatric Nursing, 8*(1), 15–21.

Littlewood, J. M., Smye, S. W., & Cunliffe, H. (1993). Aerosol antibiotics in cystic fibrosis. *Archives of Disease in Childhood, 68*(6), 788–792.

Loughlin, G. M., & Eigen, H. (Eds.) (1994). *Respiratory disease in children: Diagnosis and management.* Baltimore, MD: Williams and Wilkins.

Loutzenhiser, J. K., & Clark, R. (1993). Physical activity and exercise in children with cystic fibrosis. *Journal of Pediatric Nursing, 8*(2), 112–119.

Majer, L. S. (1993). Managing patients who have asthma: The peidatrician and the school. *Pediatrics in Review, 14*(10), 391–394.

McGee, R. S. (1993). Pulmonary surfactant: A historical perspective of how it came to be used in the treatment of respiratory distress syndrome in the neonate. *North Carolina Medical Journal, 54*(9), 447–451.

Merenstein, G. B., & Gardner, S. L. (1993). *Handbook of neonatal intensive care* (3rd ed.). Philadelphia: Mosby-Yearbook.

National Heart, Lung and Blood Institute (1991). *Executive summary: Guidelines for the diagnosis and management of asthma.* Publication Number 91-304A. Washington, DC: U.S. Department of Health and Human Services.

O'Donnell, A. C. (1993). Children can control their own asthma. *American Pharmacy, NS33*(8), 39–40.

Pencharz, P. B., & Durie, P. R. (1993). Nutritional management of cystic fibrosis. *Annual Review of Nutrition, 13,* 111–136.

Rachelefsky, G., Fitzgerald, S., Page, D., & Santamaria, B. (1993). An update on the diagnosis and management of pediatric asthma. *Nurse Practitioner, 18*(2), 51–62.

Ramsey, B. W., Astley, S. J., Aitken, M. L., et al. (1993). Efficacy and safety of short-term administration of aerosolized recombinant human deoxyribonuclease in patients with cystic fibrosis. *American Review of Respiratory Disease, 148*(1), 145–151.

Skolnik, N. (1993). Croup. *The Journal of Family Practice, 37*(2), 165–169.

Wilsher, M. L., Kolbe, J. (1995). Association of mycoplasma pneumonia antigen with initial onset of bronchial asthma. *American Journal of Respiratory and Critical Care Medicine, 15* (2 part I), 579–580.

Wiswell, T. E., & Mendiola, J., Jr. (1993). Respiratory distress syndrome in the newborn: Innovative therapies. *American Family Physician, 47*(2), 407–414.

Wung, J. T. (1993). Respiratory management for low-birth-weight infants. *Critical Care Medicine, 21*(9 Suppl.), S364–S365.

Zimmerman, J. L., Dellinger, R. P., Shah, A. N., & Taylor, R. W. (1993). Endotracheal intubation and mechanical ventilation in severe asthma. *Critical Care Medicine, 21*(11), 1727–1730.

CHAPTER 43

Pediatric Cardiovascular Disorders

Congenital Heart Disease

Congenital heart disease (CHD) is a structural malformation of the heart or great vessels present at birth, but not necessarily detected at that time. CHD may represent an individual heart defect or a combination of defects. Children with CHD also are more likely to have extracardiac defects, such as tracheoesophageal fistula, renal agenesis, and diaphragmatic hernia.

Etiology/Incidence

1. Approximately 32,000 infants are born each year with congenital heart disease (8 in 1,000 live births).
2. As a category, CHD is the most common form of cardiac disease in children.
3. Exact cause is unknown in about 90% of cases.
4. CHD results from abnormal embryonic development or the persistence of fetal structure beyond the time of normal involution.
5. Associated factors include the following:
   a. Fetal and maternal infection occurring during first trimester (primarily rubella)
   b. Teratogenic effects of drugs and alcohol
   c. Maternal dietary deficiencies
   d. Genetic factors (trisomies)
   e. Maternal age greater than 40
   f. Maternal insulin-dependent diabetes

Common Congenital Heart Malformations

Congenital cardiac anomalies are generally classified by the presence or absence or cyanosis. However, there may be variations in the clinical presentation due to the degree of defect and individual response (Table 43-1).

A. Acyanotic
1. Obstructive lesions (normal pulmonary blood flow)
   a. Aortic valvular stenosis
   b. Pulmonic stenosis
   c. Coarctation of the aorta
2. Left-to-right shunts (increased pulmonary blood flow)
   a. Patent ductus arteriosus (PDA)
   b. Atrial septal defect (ASD)
   c. Ventricular septal defect (VSD)

B. Cyanotic
1. Right-to-left shunts (decreased pulmonary blood flow)
   a. Tetralogy of Fallot
   b. Tricuspid atresia
2. Mixed blood flow
   a. Transposition of great arteries
   b. Total anomalous pulmonary venous return
   c. Truncus arteriosus
   d. Hypoplastic left heart syndrome

◆ AORTIC VALVULAR STENOSIS

Aortic valvular stenosis occurs when there is obstruction to the left ventricular outflow at the level of the valve. This is the most common form of aortic stenosis, others being hypertrophic subvalvular stenosis and supravalvular stenosis. This accounts for 6% of all congenital heart defects.

Altered Physiology

1. Blood flows from the left ventricle through the obstructed aortic valve into the aorta.
2. Left ventricular pressure increases to overcome the resistance of the obstructed valve.
3. Myocardial ischemia may occur as a result of an imbalance between the increased oxygen requirements of the hypertrophied left ventricle and the amount of oxygen that can be supplied to the myocardium.
4. Left ventricle may fail, resulting in pulmonary edema.

Complications

1. Congestive heart failure (CHF)
2. Syncope
3. Bacterial endocarditis (increased incidence with age)
4. Sudden death

Clinical Manifestations

1. Rarely symptomatic during infancy; evidence of decreased cardiac output, such as faint peripheral

TABLE 43-1 Congenital Heart Abnormalities*

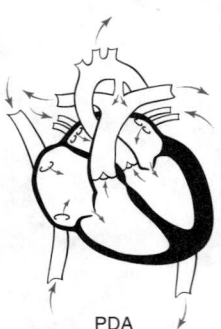

PDA

Patent Ductus Arteriosus (PDA)

The PDA is a vascular connection that, during fetal life, short circuits the pulmonary vascular bed and directs blood from the pulmonary artery to the aorta. Functional closure of the ductus normally occurs soon after birth. If the ductus remains patent after birth, the direction of blood flow in the ductus is reversed by the higher pressure in the aorta.

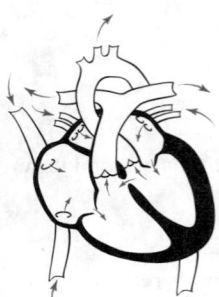

VSD

Ventricular Septal Defect (VSD)

A VSD is an abnormal opening between the right and left ventricle. VSDs vary in size and may occur in either the membranous or muscular portion of the ventricular septum. Due to higher pressure in the left ventricle, a shunting of blood from the left to right ventricle occurs during systole. If pulmonary vascular resistance produces pulmonary hypertension, the shunt of blood is then reversed from the right to the left ventricle, with cyanosis resulting.

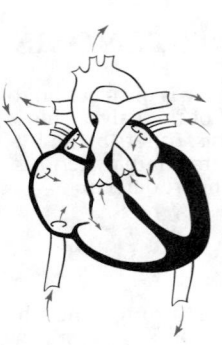

PS

Pulmonary Stenosis

Pulmonary stenosis refers to any lesion that obstructs the blood flow from the right ventricle to the pulmonary artery. The right ventricular pressure increases and can cause right ventricular hypertrophy and eventual right-sided heart failure.

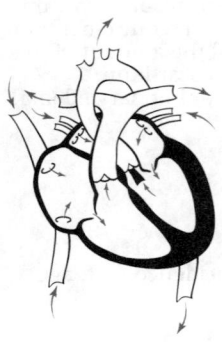

SS

Subaortic Stenosis

In many instances, the stenosis is valvular with thickening and fusion of the cusps. Subaortic stenosis is caused by a fibrous ring below the aortic valve in the outflow tract of the left ventricle. At times, both valvular and subaortic stenosis exist in combination. The obstruction presents an increased workload for the normal output of the left ventricular blood and results in left ventricular enlargement.

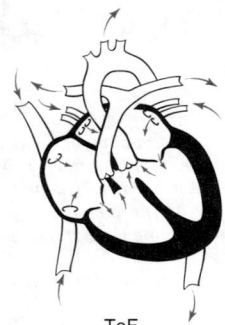

ToF

Tetralogy of Fallot

Tetralogy of Fallot is characterized by the combination of four defects: 1) pulmonary stenosis, 2) ventricular septal defects, 3) overriding aorta, 4) hypertrophy of right ventricle. It is the most common defect causing cyanosis in patients surviving beyond 2 years of age. The severity of symptoms depends on the degree of pulmonary stenosis, the size of the ventricular septal defect, and the degree to which the aorta overrides the septal defect.

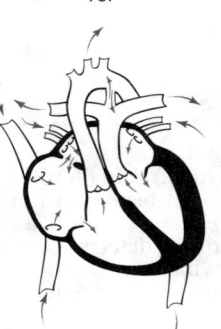

ToGV

Complete Transposition of Great Vessels

This anomaly is an embryologic defect caused by a straight division of the bulbar trunk without normal spiraling. As a result, the aorta originates from the right ventricle and the pulmonary artery from the left ventricle. An abnormal communication between the two circulations must be present to sustain life.

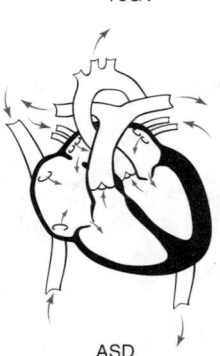

ASD

Artial Septal Defects (ASD)

An ASD is an abnormal opening between the right and left atria. Basically, three types of abnormalities result from incorrect development of the atrial septum. An incompetent foramen ovale is the most common defect. The high ostium secundum defect results from abnormal development of the septum secundum. Improper development of the septum primum produces a basal opening known as an ostium primum defect, frequently involving the atrioventricular valves. In general, left-to-right shunting of blood occurs in all ASDs.

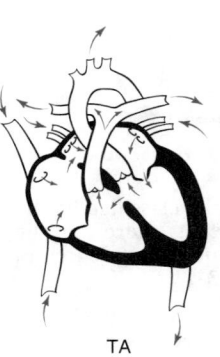

TA

Tricuspid Atresia

Tricuspid valvular atresia is characterized by a small right ventricle, large left ventricle, and usually a diminished pulmonary circulation. Blood from the right atrium passes through an ASD into the left atrium, mixes with oxygenated blood returning from the lungs, flows into the left ventricle, and is propelled into the systemic circulation. The lungs may receive blood through one of three routes: 1) a small VSD, 2) PDA, 3) bronchial vessels.

(continued)

TABLE 43-1 Congenital Heart Abnormalities* (continued)

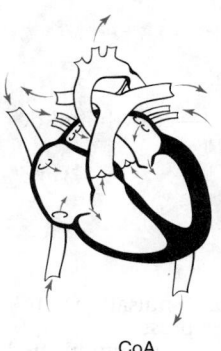

CoA

Coarctation of the Aorta

Coarctation of the aorta is characterized by a narrowed aortic lumen. It exists as a preductal or postductal obstruction, depending on the position of the obstruction in relation to the ductus arteriosus. Coarctations exist with great variation in anatomic features. The lesion produces an obstruction to the flow of blood through the aorta causing an increased left ventricular pressure and workload.

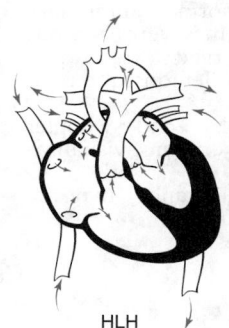

HLH

Hypoplastic Left Heart

A collection of complex congenital heart lesions results in the abnormal development of the left side of the heart. The right ventricle pumps blood through the pulmonary and systemic circulations. A patent foramen ovale allows a left-to-right shunt, and blood is shunted from left atrium back to right atrium. A PDA is the sole supply of blood to the system.

* Courtesy, Ross Laboratories.

pulses and pale, gray, cool skin, in infants with severe cases
2. Chest pain, dyspnea, fatigue, and shortness of breath with exertion in older children
3. Narrow pulse pressure
4. Weak peripheral pulses
5. Fainting spells
6. Exercise intolerance

Diagnostic Evaluation

1. Auscultation
   a. Harsh, low-pitched systolic ejection murmur, maximal at the second right intercostal space, radiating to apex, back, neck
   b. Ejection click at fourth interspace to the left of the sternum (mild or moderately severe cases)
   c. Single or narrowly split second heart sound
2. Chest x-ray detects dilated ascending aorta and varying degrees of left ventricular enlargement.
3. Electrocardiogram (ECG)—normal or left ventricular hypertrophy. Strain pattern (T-wave inversion) is evidence of severe stenosis. ST segment depression indicates myocardial ischemia (poor correlation between ECG and degree of aortic stenosis).
4. Echocardiography and Doppler measurements determine peak flow velocity and can accurately identify the level of obstruction.
5. Cardiac catheterization and angiography may be needed to evaluate the condition fully.

Treatment

A. Medical Management
1. Treatment of CHF
2. Exercise restriction
3. Precaution against bacterial endocarditis

B. Surgical Management
1. Aortic valvulotomy
2. Prosthetic valve replacement
3. Balloon dilatation

◆ PULMONIC STENOSIS

Pulmonic stenosis refers to any lesion that obstructs the flow of blood from the right ventricle. It accounts for 8% of congenital heart defects; 90% of obstruction occurs at the level of the pulmonary valve. Others include subvalvular or supravalvular.

Altered Physiology

1. Blood flows from the right ventricle through the obstructed pulmonary valve into the pulmonary artery.
2. Right ventricular pressure increases to maintain normal cardiac output.
3. Right ventricular hypertrophy develops.
4. Right-sided heart failure occurs in severe cases.

Complications

1. Anoxic spells in infants with severe lesions
2. Bacterial endocarditis
3. CHF
4. Sudden death at any age

Clinical Manifestations

1. The child is generally asymptomatic but may have decreased exercise tolerance with fatigue and dyspnea.
2. With severe obstruction, the child may have dyspnea, generalized cyanosis.
3. The child may complain of precordial pain.

Diagnostic Evaluation

1. Auscultation
   a. Systolic ejection murmur occurs over pulmonic area.

b. Often an ejection click and a widely split second sound can be heard.

2. Chest x-ray shows right ventricular enlargement, main pulmonary artery enlargement, normal pulmonary vascularity, and normal left side. In severe stenosis, right atrial hypertrophy also is observed.
3. On ECG, moderate or severe cases demonstrate right ventricular hypertrophy.
4. Two-dimensional echocardiography and Doppler study with color flow mapping can enhance visualization of the level of obstruction.
5. Cardiac catheterization and angiography may be needed to evaluate the condition fully.

Treatment

A. Medical Management
1. Treat CHF.
2. Take precautions with bacterial endocarditis.
3. Prostaglandin E_1 (PGE_1) maintains patency of ductus arteriosus until surgical correction.
4. Asymptomatic children with moderate pulmonic stenosis should be evaluated at regular intervals for progression of the lesion.

B. Surgical Management (Symptomatic Patients)
1. Valvulotomy
2. Balloon dilatation of pulmonic obstruction
3. Blalock-Taussig (BT) shunt (palliative)

◆ COARCTATION OF THE AORTA

Coarctation of the aorta is a narrowing or constriction of the vessel at any point. Most commonly, the constriction is located just distal to the origin of the left subclavian artery in the vicinity of the ductus arteriosus. It accounts for 6% of congenital heart defects. Types of coarctation of the aorta include the following:

1. Juxtaductal—most common, narrowing in vicinity or ductus arteriosus
2. Preductal—narrowing of aorta proximal to ductus arteriosus and associated with other defects such as VSD, PDA, transposition of the great arteries (TGA); seen in neonates
3. Postductal—narrowing of aorta distal to ductus arteriosus; found in older children

Altered Physiology

1. The narrowing of the aorta obstructs blood flow through the constricted segment of the aorta, thus increasing left ventricular pressure and workload.
2. Collateral vessels develop, arising chiefly from the branches of the subclavian and intercostal arteries, bypassing the coarcted segment of the aorta and supplying circulation to the lower extremities.

Complications

1. CHF
2. Cerebral hemorrhage

3. Infective endocarditis
4. Rupture of the aorta
5. Cerebrovascular accident (CVA)

Clinical Manifestations

1. Usually asymptomatic in childhood—growth and development normal
2. May demonstrate
   a. Occasional fatigue
   b. Headache, dizziness
   c. Nosebleeds
   d. Leg cramps
   e. Cold feet
3. Absent or greatly reduced femoral pulsations; full bounding carotid pulses; wide pulse pressure
4. Hypertension in upper extremities and diminished blood pressure in lower extremities
5. Symptoms secondary to hypertension (rare in children)
6. Severe anomalies that cause symptoms in infants and include poor feeding, growth failure, tachypnea, dyspnea, peripheral edema, acidosis (low cardiac output state), and severe CHF

Diagnostic Evaluation

1. Auscultation—nonspecific systolic murmur heard along the left sternal border
2. Chest x-ray
   a. Prominent aorta can occur.
   b. Rib notching is a common finding in children older than 8 to 10 years.
   c. Seriously ill infants demonstrate significant cardiomegaly with increased pulmonary vascularity.
3. ECG—normal or varying degrees of left ventricular hypertrophy; right ventricular hypertrophy frequently present
4. Ultrasound, two-dimensional echocardiogram, Doppler studies with color flow mapping to determine extent of obstruction and hypertrophy
5. Barium esophagogram to detect associated defects
6. Cardiac catheterization and angiography frequently not needed but helpful to diagnose associated anomalies

Treatment

A. Medical Management
1. Treatment of CHF
2. PGE_1 infusion to maintain ductal patency and maintain blood flow below the coarctation

B. Surgical Management
1. Indicated for infants who present in the first 6 months of life with heart failure
2. Surgical resection recommended for children between the ages of 2 and 4 years with significant coarctation

◆ PATENT DUCTUS ARTERIOSUS

PDA is the persistence of a fetal connection (ductus arteriosus) between the pulmonary artery and the aorta, resulting in a left-to-right shunt. PDA accounts for 10% of congenital heart defects; 15% of infants with PDA have other heart defects.

Altered Physiology

1. During fetal life, the ductus arteriosus allows most of the right ventricular blood to bypass the nonfunctioning lungs by directing blood from the pulmonary artery to the aorta.
   a. It is maintained open by endogenous production of PGE, which relaxes ductal smooth muscle in the low-oxygen intrauterine environment.
2. After birth, with the initiation of respiration, the ductus arteriosus is no longer necessary. It should functionally close within several hours after birth and anatomically close within several weeks after birth.
   a. The smooth muscle in the wall of the ductus arteriosus contracts to obliterate the lumen within 24 hours of birth.
   b. Within several weeks after birth, degenerative changes occur in the ductus arteriosus, and it becomes a cord of fibrous connective tissue (ligamentum arteriosum).
3. When the ductus arteriosus remains patent, oxygenated blood from the higher pressure systemic circuit (aorta) flows to the lower pressure pulmonary circuit (pulmonary artery) through the PDA.
4. The volume of blood that the heart must pump to meet the demands of the peripheral tissues is increased. A greater volume burden is placed on the lungs and eventually on the left heart.

Complications

1. CHF
2. Infective endocarditis

Clinical Manifestations

1. Small PDA—usually asymptomatic
2. Large PDA—may develop symptoms in very early infancy
   a. Slow weight gain
   b. Feeding difficulties; decreased exercise tolerance
   c. Frequent respiratory infections
   d. Dyspnea

Diagnostic Evaluation

1. Auscultation—continuous machinery-like murmur at the left intraclavicular area is heard in most older children. Neonates with PDA have a variety of murmurs.
2. The child may have a wide pulse pressure or bounding posterior tibial and dorsalis pedis pulses.
3. Chest x-ray shows the following:
   a. X-ray is normal with small PDA.
   b. Large PDA shows left-sided hypertrophy, a prominant ascending aorta, and dilation of the proximal pulmonary arteries.
4. ECG may be normal or may demonstrate left ventricular hypertrophy.

5. Echocardiography and Doppler study with color flow mapping allow for visualization of PDA and blood flow across PDA: from right to left, left to right, or both directions.
6. Cardiac catheterization and angiography may not be necessary.

Treatment

A. Medical Management
1. Treat CHF.
2. Indomethacin (Indocin) appears to trigger the natural closing of the ductus. It is the treatment of choice for many preterm infants.

B. Surgical Management
Division of the PDA (closed heart surgery through lateral thoracotomy incision to ligate the ductus) may be done in early infancy if CHF develops and connot be controlled or electively by 1 to 2 years.

◆ ATRIAL SEPTAL DEFECT

ASD is an abnormal opening in the septum between the left atrium and the right atrium. ASD accounts for 9% of congenital heart defects.

1. Ostium secundum type—located in the center of the atrial septum at the site of the foramen ovale (most common)
2. Ostium primum type—large gap at the base of the atrial septum frequently associated with deformities of the mitral and tricuspid valves or a small, high VSD (endocardial cushion defects)

Altered Physiology

1. The pressure in the left atrium is greater than the pressure in the right atrium and promotes the flow of oxygenated blood from the left atrium to the right atrium (a left-to-right shunt).
2. The oxygenated blood that flows through the defect enters the right atrium and mixes with the systemic venous blood returning to the lungs. The blood flow through the shunt recirculates through the lungs, thus increasing the total blood flow through the lungs.
3. The major hemodynamic abnormality is volume overload of the right ventricle, resulting in hypertrophy of the right ventricle.
4. Eventually, if the pulmonary resistance is great, this may increase right atrial pressure, thus causing a reversal of the shunt, with unoxygenated blood flowing from the right atrium to the left atrium. (This situation will produce cyanosis.)

Complications

These are rare in children.

1. Infective endocarditis
2. Cardiac failure
3. Pulmonary hypertension
4. Coronary artery disease

5. Atrial fibrillation
6. Mitral valve prolapse

Clinical Manifestations

1. Ostium secundum type—generally asymptomatic even when this defect is large
2. Ostium primum type—generally asymptomatic, although the following may occur:
   a. Slow weight gain
   b. Easily fatigued
   c. Dyspnea with exertion
   d. History of frequent respiratory infections
   e. CHF
   f. Hypertension related to pulmonary edema

Diagnostic Evaluation

1. Auscultation
   a. Systolic, medium-pitched ejection murmur heard best at the second left interspace
   b. Fixed widely split second sound
   c. May have mid-diastolic filling sound at the lower left sternal border
2. Chest x-ray—prominent main pulmonary artery, right atrial and right ventricular enlargement, increase in vascular markings of the lungs
3. ECG—possible right ventricular hypertrophy and right axis deviation (ostium secundum defect); left axis deviation, P wave changes indicating atrial enlargement, and prolonged PR interval common in ostium primum defects
4. Two-dimensional echocardiogram, Doppler study, and color flow mapping to fully evaluate blood flow and hypertrophy
5. Cardiac catheterization, angiography, and magnetic resonance imaging (MRI) to evaluate condition further

Treatment

1. Spontaneous closure in small percentage
2. Medical management—treatment of CHF, precautions for bacterial endocarditis
3. Surgical management—closure by open-heart surgery through medial sternotomy incision with cardiopulmonary bypass by suture or patch

◆ VENTRICULAR SEPTAL DEFECT

VSD is an abnormal opening in the septum between the right and left ventricles. It may vary in size from very small defects to very large defects and may occur in either the membranous or muscular portion of the ventricular septum. VSD accounts for 25% to 29% of all congenital heart defects.

Altered Physiology

1. The pressure in the left ventricle is greater than the pressure in the right ventricle and promotes the flow of oxygenated blood from the left ventricle to the right ventricle (a left-to-right shunt).
2. The oxygenated blood that flows through the defect mixes with the blood returning from the right atrium. The blood flow through the shunt recirculates through the lungs, thus increasing the total blood flow through the lungs.
3. The major hemodynamic abnormalities follow:
   a. Increased right ventricular and pulmonary arterial pressure
   b. Increased blood flow to the right ventricle, pulmonary arteries and lungs
4. If the pulmonary vascular resistance is great, this may increase right ventricular pressure, thus causing a reversal of the shunt with unoxygenated blood flowing from the right ventricle to the left ventricle. (This situation, termed Eisenmenger's complex, will produce cyanosis.)

Complications

1. Infective endocarditis
2. CHF

Clinical Manifestations

1. Small VSDs—usually asymptomatic (many close spontaneously)
2. Large VSDs—may develop symptoms as early as 1 to 2 months of age
   a. Slow weight gain, failure to thrive
   b. Feeding difficulties; increased fatigue
   c. Pale, delicate-looking, scrawny appearance
   d. Frequent respiratory infections
   e. Tachypnea, excessive sweating, CHF

Diagnostic Evaluation

1. Auscultation produces harsh holosystolic murmur, heard best at the fourth interspace to the left of the sternum. Elevated pulmonary resistance is manifested by a loud, banging, pulmonic component of the second sound.
2. Chest x-ray ranges from normal (small defect) to enlargement, pulmonary artery enlargement, and increased pulmonary vascular markings.
3. ECG is normal or shows biventricular hypertrophy.
4. Two-dimensional echocardiography, Doppler, and color flow mapping studies identify presence, size, and location of defects and associated chamber enlargement.
5. Cardiac catheterization and angiography may be done to evaluate the condition further.

Treatment

A. Medical Management
Treat CHF if this occurs in early infancy.

B. Surgical Management
1. Patch closure is required if CHF is intractable to medical management.

2. Patients with pulmonary arterial hypertension require early surgery (before 2 years of age) to avoid irreversible pulmonary bed changes.
  a. This is pulmonary artery banding around the pulmonary artery to decrease pulmonary blood flow and control CHF and prevent pulmonary arteriolar disease.
  b. Later, deband and do patch closure.
3. Surgery is contraindicated in patients with Eisenmenger's complex.

◆ TETRALOGY OF FALLOT

Tetralogy of Fallot is a cyanotic heart defect consisting of four abnormalities: 1) pulmonary stenosis, 2) VSD, 3) overriding of the aorta (dextraposition of the aorta), and 4) right ventricular hypertrophy. It accounts for 6% to 10% of all congenital heart defects.

Altered Physiology

1. Obstruction of the blood flow from the right ventricle to the pulmonary circulation is caused by obstruction at the pulmonary valve level or the infundibular area of the right ventricle below the pulmonary valve.
2. Unoxygenated blood is shunted from the right ventricle through the VSD directly into the aorta (a right-to-left shunt).
3. The right ventricle is hypertrophied because of high right ventricular pressure.
4. Unoxygenated blood is shunted back through the body.

Complications

1. CHF—may occur in newborn but is uncommon beyond infancy
2. Infective endocarditis
3. CVA (due to thrombosis caused by increased blood viscosity or severe hypoxia)
4. Brain abscess

Clinical Manifestations

1. Clinical manifestations are variable and depend on the size of the VSD and the degree of right ventricular outflow obstruction
2. Cyanosis
  a. Initially, the shunt through the VSD may be from left to right. Many infants with this defect are not cyanotic at birth, but they develop cyanosis as they grow and as the stenosis becomes relatively more severe.
  b. Cyanosis may at first be observed only with exertion and crying, but during the first few years of life, the child may become cyanotic even at rest.
  c. Infundibular stenosis may be minimal so that cyanosis never develops ("pink tetralogy").
  d. Polycythemia results in increased hematocrit.
3. Clubbing of the fingers and toes

4. Squatting (a posture characteristically assumed by children with this defect once they have reached the walking stage)
  a. Used to deflect blood flow from extremities and keep oxygenated blood in the trunk and head
  b. Increases systemic resistance and aids in venous return
5. Slow weight gain; failure to thrive
6. Dyspnea on exertion
7. Hypoxic spells ("tet" spells); transient cerebral ischemia
  a. Common in children younger than 2 years
  b. Especially initiated by crying
  c. Commonly seen with cyanosis, irritability, pallor, tachypnea, flaccidity, and possible loss of consciousness
  d. Occurrence of attacks in morning after awakening from sleep, during or after crying, during or after defecation, or during or immediately following feeding

> **NURSING ALERT:**
> Once a "tet" spell is recognized, call for assistance, and immediately place child in knee-chest position with head of bed elevated; administer oxygen by mask. Be prepared to administer medications as prescribed, and assume a calm, reassuring attitude.

Diagnostic Evaluation

1. Auscultation
  a. Single second sound (aortic component)
  b. Systolic ejection murmur at the second and third interspaces to the left of the sternum
  c. Prominent ejection click immediately after the first heart sound
2. Chest x-ray
  a. Heart size normal
  b. Pulmonary segment small and concave ("boot-shaped heart")
  c. Diminished pulmonary vascular markings
3. ECG—right axis deviation; right ventricular hypertrophy
4. Two-dimensional echocardiography, Doppler study, and color flow mapping to identify VSD and blood flow across VSD
5. Cardiac catheterization may be helpful in evaluating heart function
6. Magnetic resonance imaging (MRI) to detect structural abnormalities
7. Complete blood cell count—increased hematocrit and red blood cells (polycythemia)
  a. Increased hematocrit

Treatment

The goal is to improve oxygenation of arterial blood.

1. Palliative (for some)
  a. Blalock-Taussig shunt—anastomosis between the right or left subclavian artery and the right pulmonary artery (preferred method); creates an artificial ductus arteriosus

b. Waterston shunt—anastomosis between the posterior lateral aspect of the ascending aorta and the right pulmonary artery
2. Total correction (treatment of choice)
   a. Shunt is removed if previously performed.
   b. With cardiopulmonary bypass, VSD is repaired with patch closure, and right ventricular outflow obstruction is relieved.
   c. Total correction is increasingly being advocated for all infants in whom pulmonary arteries are of sufficient size.

◆ TRANSPOSITION OF THE GREAT ARTERIES

TGA occurs when the pulmonary artery originates posteriorly from the left ventricle and the aorta originates anteriorly from the right ventricle. It accounts for 5% to 10% of congenital heart defects.

Altered Physiology

1. This defect results in two separate circulations; the right heart manages the systemic circulation (unoxygenated), and the left heart manages the pulmonary circulation (oxygenated).
2. To sustain life, there must be an accompanying defect that provides for the mixing of oxygenated and unoxygenated blood between the two circulations.
3. The mixing of oxygenated and unoxygenated blood occurs through one or more of the following shunts: ASD, VSD, PDA, patent foramen ovale.

Complications

1. CHF
2. Infective endocarditis
3. Brain abscess
4. CVA (due to thrombosis or severe hypoxia)

Clinical Manifestations

Influenced predominantly by the extent of intercirculatory mixing.

1. Cyanosis, usually developing shortly after birth (degree depends on the type of associated malformations)
2. Low Apgar score at birth
3. Easily fatigued
4. Slow weight gain, although birth weight normal or above normal
5. Clubbing of the fingers and toes
6. Coexistence of CHF, manifested by tachypnea, cardiomegaly, hepatomegaly

Diagnostic Evaluation

1. Auscultation—murmurs possibly absent in infancy; may be a murmur of an associated defect

2. Chest x-ray—cardiomegaly, narrow mediastinum, egg-shaped cardiac silhouette, increased vascular markings (decreased vascular markings in children with associated pulmonary stenosis); neonatal x-ray often normal
3. ECG—right axis deviation, right or biventricular hypertrophy; variable findings depending on age and anatomic factors
4. Two-dimensional echocardiogram, Doppler study, cardiac catheterization, MRI, and radionuclide angiography to further evaluate the condition
5. Laboratory tests—polycythemia, low PaO_2 or metabolic acidosis

Treatment

A. Medical Management
Treat CHF vigorously.

B. Surgical Management
1. Palliative procedures to allow improved interatrial mixing
   a. Rashkind procedure—creation of an ASD with a balloon catheter during cardiac catheterization
   b. Blalock-Hanlon procedure—surgical creation of an ASD
   c. Medical use of PGE to keep PDA open
2. Complete correction—redirection of blood flow
   a. Mustard procedure—with cardiopulmonary bypass, the atrial septum is removed and a baffle of Dacron velour or pericardium is sutured in place in such a way that the pulmonary venous blood is directed toward the right ventricle, and the systemic venous blood is directed toward the left ventricle.
   b. Senning procedure—with cardiopulmonary bypass, the systemic and pulmonary returns are rerouted by arranging flaps of the interatrial septum and right atrial free wall to form the new venous channels.
   c. Rastelli procedure is the surgery of choice for transposition with VSD and left ventricular outflow tract obstruction. With cardiopulmonary bypass, the VSD is closed in such a way that the left ventricle communicates with the aorta. The pulmonary artery is ligated, and the right ventricle is connected to the distal portion of the pulmonary artery by means of a valve-bearing tubular graft.
   d. Recent procedures have been developed for anatomic correction of TGA by direct contraposition of the transposed vessels. Arterial switch is gaining popularity and may become the preferred treatment.
   e. As with other types of congenital cardiac surgery, the question of optimum timing for surgery is controversial. Increasingly, total correction is recommended when feasible.

◆ TRICUSPID ATRESIA

Tricuspid atresia is a condition in which there is 1) atresia of the tricuspid valve so that there is no communication between the right atrium and right ventricle, 2) interatrial septal defect (or patent foramen ovale), and 3) a hypoplastic right ventricle.

Altered Physiology

1. Blood from the systemic circulation is shunted from the right atrium through an interatrial communication (patent foramen ovale or ASD) to the left atrium and then to the left ventricle.
2. Pulmonary blood flow is established either through a PDA, bronchial circulation, or a VSD.

Complications

1. CVA
2. Brain abscess
3. Bacterial endocarditis

Clinical Manifestations

1. Severe cyanosis in the neonatal period
2. Respiratory distress (exertional dyspnea)
3. Clubbing
4. Hypoxic spells
5. Delayed weight gain
6. Right heart failure (may occur)
7. Easily fatigued

Diagnostic Evaluation

1. Auscultation shows the following:
   a. Pansystolic murmurs are audible along the left sternal border.
   b. The second heart sound is single.
2. Chest x-ray—patients with diminished pulmonary blood flow have a normal to mildly increased cardiac silhouette, concavity in the region of the main pulmonary artery, and diminished pulmonary vascular markings; those with increased pulmonary flow have cardiac enlargement and plethoric pulmonary vasculature (less common).
3. ECG shows right atrial, left atrial, left ventricular hypertrophy, left axis deviation.
4. Two-dimensional echocardiogram demonstrates diminutive right ventricular chamber and no tricuspid valve. Color flow mapping can identify right-to-left shunt at atrial level and presence of VSD or PDA.
5. Cardiac catheterization and angiography may be done to evaluate condition further.
6. Laboratory tests—polycythemia, normal PH and PCO_2, PaO_2—may vary from near normal (with VSD or PDA) to extremely low with limited shunting.

Treatment

A. Medical Management
Treat CHF; PGE_1 infusion maintains ductal patency.

B. Surgical Management
1. Palliative procedures to increase pulmonary blood flow
   a. Balloon septostomy to improve intra-atrial mixing
   b. Waterston shunt—anastomosis between the ascending aorta and right pulmonary artery
   c. Glenn procedure—side-to-end anastomosis of the superior vena cava to the right pulmonary artery

   d. Blalock-Taussig shunt—subclavian to pulmonary artery anastomosis
2. Complete correction
   a. Fontan procedure involves placement of tubular conduit with a valve between the right atrium and main pulmonary artery. The atrial defect is closed, and the main pulmonary artery is ligated just above the pulmonary valve.
   b. This procedure has been successful in a growing number of older, symptomatic patients with diminished blood flow.

◆ AORTIC VALVE/HYPOPLASTIC LEFT HEART SYNDROME

Hypoplastic left heart syndrome is a condition in which there is 1) mitral atresia or stenosis; 2) a diminutive or absent left ventricle; and 3) failure of the aortic valve to develop, resulting in aortic atresia, a severe hypoplastic ascending aorta, and aortic arch (severe coarctation of aorta).

Altered Physiology

1. The left ventricle is not functional.
2. The right ventricle has to pump blood through both pulmonary and systemic circulations.
3. A patent foramen ovale allows a left-to-right shunt, because blood is shunted from the left atrium back to the right atrium.
4. A PDA is the sole supply of blood to the system until it begins to close.

Complications

1. Severe CHF
2. Shock
3. Death in more than half of the cases in the first few months of life

Clinical Manifestations

1. May appear normal at birth; increasing signs shortly afterward
2. CHF, dyspnea, hepatomegaly
3. Low cardiac output
   a. Pallor, mild to moderate cyanosis, or a grayish color
   b. Weak peripheral pulses
   c. Decreased blood pressure

Diagnostic Evaluation

1. Auscultation
   a. Nondescript systolic murmur
   b. Single second sound, representing closure of only the pulmonary valve
2. Chest x-ray—cardiomegaly and increased pulmonary vascularity
3. ECG—normal or right axis deviation and right ventricular hypertrophy

4. Echocardiography, Doppler study, and color flow mapping—increased right atrium and right ventricle, a diminutive left ventricle, and a poorly functioning or absent mitral valve
5. Cardiac catheterization

Treatment

A. *Medical Management*
Treat CHF; PGE$_1$ infusion maintains patency of ductus arteriosus until surgery.

B. *Surgical Management*
1. Staged approach—Norwood procedure—to establish systemic and pulmonary circulations
2. Fontan procedure
3. Arterial switch
4. Cardiac transplantation

◆ NURSING CARE OF THE CHILD WITH CONGENITAL HEART DISEASE

Nursing Assessment

1. Obtain a thorough nursing history to become familiar with the child and family to recognize normal and abnormal patterns (eg, color, respirations, murmur; feeding schedule, amount, and method; skin temperature of the extremities; exercise tolerance).
2. Discuss plan of care with the healthcare provider for both child and family.
3. Observe and record information relevant to the child's growth and development (motor coordination, muscular development, cognitive abilities, psychosocial skills).
   a. Compare data with those for siblings, other family members, and children of the same chronologic age.
   b. Plot appropriate information on growth chart.
4. Observe and record the child's level of exercise tolerance.
   a. Observe the child at play:
      (1) Is play interrupted to rest?
      (2) How does child play compared with peers?
      (3) Does child squat during play? (Squatting is a characteristic position a cyanotic child assumes when resting after exertion.)
   b. Observe infant while feeding. Does the infant stop feeding to rest or fall asleep during feeding? Assess pulse and respiratory rate of children during feedings.
5. Observe the child's skin and mucous membranes for color and temperature changes.
   a. Skin—Color changes vary from pink, dusky, mottled, to cyanotic. Earlobes are good indicators of the degree of oxygen saturation. Circumoral cyanosis occurs with oxygen deprivation. Nail beds are good indicators of color change.
   b. Mucous membranes—Lips and tongue indicate color change because they are vascular areas and contain superficial blood vessels; mucous membranes are the best places to observe for cyanosis.

   c. Extremities—Are extremities cool? Is there a difference between upper and lower extremities? Check quality of pulses in all four extremities. Check edema in extremities.
   d. Record where cyanosis was observed (localized or generalized), when it was observed, and the duration (continuous or intermittent, whether variable with exercise).
6. Observe for clubbing (increase in soft tissue around terminal phalanges) of fingers, especially the thumbnails; this may occur in cyanotic children by 2 to 3 months of age.
7. Observe for chest deformities: visible pulsations; left- or right-sided prominence.
8. Observe respiratory pattern.
   a. Remove any clothing or covers that obscure visualization of the chest.
   b. Count respirations for at least 30 seconds.
   c. Count respirations while child is at rest; if unable to soothe the child, document crying, irritability, and so forth.
   d. Observe for increased respiratory rate, grunting, retractions, nasal flaring, irregularity of respirations.
   e. Record all signs of respiratory distress, including change from usual pattern, when it occurred, duration, and so forth.
   f. Ascultate for crackles, rhonchi, stridor, congestion, and so forth.
   g. Assess quality of the cry.
9. Palpate the child's pulses in all extremities.
   a. Radial or dorsalis pedis is difficult to feel in the newborn.
   b. Femoral pulsations are easily felt in the inguinal region and can be compared with brachial pulsations.
   c. Record the strength of the pulse (full, bounding, weak, or faint).
   d. When a pulse is difficult to locate, mark its location with a pen to facilitate locating it the next time.
10. Ausculate the child's heart:
   a. Count apical pulse rate for 1 full minute.
   b. Determine cardiac rhythm or change in rhythm.
   c. Become familiar with a known murmur.
   d. Determine the presence of new murmurs.
11. Record vital signs (apical pulse, blood pressure, respirations).
   a. Keep child quiet for baseline vital signs.
   b. Record quality and quantity of pulse and blood pressure in all extremities.
   c. Record which extremity is used for blood pressure measurement. Note: Make sure that blood pressure cuff is the appropriate size for the child—either 1.5 times the diameter of the extremity being used or no less than $\frac{1}{2}$ and no more than $\frac{2}{3}$ of the part of the extremity being used.

Nursing Diagnoses

A. Impaired Gas Exchange related to altered pulmonary blood flow or oxygen deprivation
B. Decreased Cardiac Output related to the specific anatomic defect
C. Activity Intolerance related to decreased oxygenation in blood and tissues
D. Altered Nutrition: Less than body requirements related to the excessive energy demands required by increased cardiac workload

E. Risk for Infection related to cardiac dysfunction, poor nutritional status, and reduced body defenses

F. Fear related to life-threatening illness

Nursing Interventions

A. *Relieving Respiratory Distress*
1. Determine the degree of respiratory distress.
   a. Infants—respirations greater than 60 breaths/min indicate respiratory difficulty.
   b. Young children—respirations greater than 40 breaths/min indicate respiratory difficulty.
   c. Observe the regularity of the respiratory pattern.
   d. Observe for retractions (drawing in of soft tissue in the rib interspaces, below the costal margin, or above and below the sternum with each inspiration; may be barely visible, mild, or severe).
   e. Observe for nasal flaring; listen for grunting.
2. Include specific information in nursing record.
   a. Number of respirations per minute
   b. Regularity of respirations
   c. Type and severity of retractions
   d. Presence of nasal flaring, grunting
   e. Response to oxygen therapy
   f. Response to positioning
   g. Color changes
   h. Irritability or anxiety observed
3. Position the child at a 45-degree angle (orthopnic position) to decrease pressure of the viscera on the diaphragm and increase lung volume.
   a. Infant (depending on the child)—place in an infant seat or prone, propped on knees.
   b. Children—elevate head of the bed and support the arms with pillows.
4. Pin diapers loosely; provide loose-fitting pajamas for older children.
5. Feed slowly, allowing frequent rest periods.
   a. Rapid respirations and frequent coughing predispose the child to aspiration.
   b. Child may require gavage feeding.
   c. Observe for abdominal distention, which may increase respiratory difficulty.
6. Tilt the infant's or child's head back slightly.
7. Suction the nose and throat if the child is unable to cough up secretions adequately.
8. Provide oxygen therapy as indicated.
9. Administer medications as ordered to help reduce lung congestion.
   a. Diuretics
      (1) Monitor effectiveness.
      (2) Monitor intake and output; weigh diapers.
      (3) Measure specific gravity of urine.
      (4) Weigh daily with same scale at same time each day.
      (5) Restrict fluids as ordered.
      (6) Monitor serum electrolytes, and replace electrolytes as ordered.

B. *Improving Cardiac Output*
1. Organize nursing care to provide periods of uninterrupted rest.
2. Avoid unnecessary activities, such as frequent, complete baths and clothing changes; avoid excessive handling.
3. Prevent excessive crying; anticipate needs.
   a. Use pacifier.

   b. Hold the infant.
   c. Feed when hungry.
   d. Keep the infant comfortable.
4. Explain to the child the need for rest.
5. Provide diversional activities that require limited expenditures of energy; provide passive play.
6. Avoid discussing the child's condition or the condition of other children in the presence of the patient to prevent unnecessary anxiety.
7. Avoid temperature excesses; maintain normothermia.
8. Prevent constipation.
9. Administer cardiac support medications as ordered.
   a. Digoxin (Lanoxin)
      (1) Check heart rate for 1 full minute before dose.
      (2) Do not give with meals in case of emesis, and do not repeat if child has emesis.
      (3) Watch for signs of digoxin toxicity—bradycardia, nausea, vomiting, anorexia.
      (4) Give at same time each day to maintain therapeutic levels.
      (5) Monitor serum drug level and serum electrolytes.
   b. Afterload-reducing medications
      (1) Check blood pressure before and after dose.
      (2) Hold medication according to ordered parameters.
      (3) Watch for signs of hypotension, such as pale, cool skin; faint pulses; delayed capillary refill.

C. *Improving Oxygenation and Activity Tolerance*
1. Provide a safe, effective oxygen environment (refer to procedure on oxygen therapy, p. 1191).
2. Explain to the child how oxygen will help; orient child to equipment before it is used.
3. Observe the child's response to oxygen therapy.
   a. Improvement of color
   b. Change in rate and character of respirations
   c. Change in anxiety level
4. Observe the child's response while being weaned from oxygen.
   a. Reduce liter flow gradually, and observe response after each reduction.
   b. Measure oxygen saturation with pulse oximeter.

D. *Providing Adequate Nutrition*
1. Feed slowly in a semierect position; burp infants after each ounce to decrease compression of stomach on heart and lungs.
2. Use soft nipples with large holes, which make it easier for the infant to suck.
3. Provide small, frequent feedings; provide foods easy to chew and digest.
4. Feeding should generally be completed within 45 minutes or sooner if the infant tires.
5. Provide foods that have high nutritional value.
   a. Add needed calories for healing to promote maximal growth.
   b. Provide foods high in iron and potassium levels if needed.
6. Determine the child's likes and dislikes, and plan meals with the dietitian, taking into consideration the child's preferences.
7. Observe the child at mealtime; does a poor appetite represent a lack of interest in food, or does the child become fatigued while eating?
8. Report vomiting, and specify the amount, type, and relationship to feeding or to medications.
9. Report diarrhea, and specify type and amount.

10. Maintain adequate hydration in the cyanotic child when he or she is vomiting, has diarrhea or fever, or is exposed to high environmental temperatures because polycythemia predisposes to thrombosis.
11. Be alert for dyspnea and tachycardia during feedings and the need for nasogastric feedings.
12. Maintain strict intake and output.
13. Maintain ordered low sodium or fluid restriction in children with CHF.
14. Monitor daily weight (same scale, same time of day, same attire) to check fluid retention/diuresis or physical growth.

E. *Preventing Infection*
1. Prevent exposure to communicable diseases, including exposure to children with upper respiratory infections, diarrhea, wound infections, and so forth.
2. Check with the parents to be certain the child's immunizations are up to date.
3. Practice careful handwashing technique, and teach this to the child.
4. Report temperature elevation, diarrhea, vomiting, and upper respiratory symptoms promptly; take axillary temperature.
5. Be certain that the child receives prophylactic antibiotics for infective endocarditis before genitourinary instrumentation or dental work.
6. Prevent cold stress.

F. *Reducing Fear*
1. Explain the cardiac problem to child and parents.
   a. Discuss with the parents the importance of being truthful with the child about heart condition.
   b. The time to tell the child is generally when the child begins asking questions as to why he or she visits the doctor so frequently and why the doctor listens to the child's heart so closely.
   c. Answer questions truthfully and simply.
   d. Clarify misconceptions.
   e. Support positive coping mechanisms.
2. Prepare the child for diagnostic and treatment procedures.
   a. Explain to the child what is going to be done in simple, age-appropriate terms (refer to section on hospitalized child, pp. 1127–1131).
   b. Encourage the child to express fears and fantasies verbally or through play.
3. Prepare child and family for corrective surgery.
   a. Explain the procedure in simple terms.
   b. Diagrams are helpful.
   c. Allow time for child and parent to ask questions and express concerns.
4. Refer the family to appropriate resources concerned with the financial or emotional aspects of caring for a child with CHD.
   a. Social worker
   b. Other parents and organized support groups
   c. American Heart Association: 772 Greenville Avenue, Dallas, Texas 75231, 214-373-6300

Family Education/Health Maintenance

1. Instruct the family in necessary measures to maintain the child's health:
   a. Complete immunization
   b. Adequate diet and rest
   c. Prevention and control of infections
   d. Regular medical and dental checkup. The child should be protected against infective endocarditis when undergoing certain dental procedures (refer to American Heart Association Protocol).
   e. Regular cardiac checkups
2. Teach the family about the defect and its treatment.
   a. Signs and symptoms of CHF (below)
   b. Signs of hypoxic spells associated with cyanotic defects (p. 1203) and need to place child in knee-chest position and administer oxygen
   c. Need to prevent dehydration which increases risk of thrombotic complications
   d. Emergency precautions related to hypoxic attacks, pulmonary edema, cardiac arrest (if appropriate)
   e. Special home care equipment, monitors, O_2, and so forth
3. Encourage the parents and other people (eg, teachers, peers) to treat the child in as normal a manner as possible.
   a. Avoid overprotection and overindulgence.
   b. Avoid rejection.
   c. Promote growth and development with modifications. Facilitate performance of the usual developmental tasks within the limits of the child's physiologic state.
   d. Prevent adults from projecting their fears and anxieties onto the child.
   e. Help family deal with their anger, guilt, and concerns related to their disabled child.
4. Initiate a community health nursing referral if indicated.
5. Stress the need for follow-up care.

Evaluation

A. Improved oxygenation evidenced by easy, comfortable respirations
B. Improved cardiac output demonstrated by stable vital signs and adequate peripheral perfusion
C. Improved oxygenation as child exhibits comfortable rest periods and improved objective respiratory measurements
D. Maximal nutritional status demonstrated by weight gain and growth toward the normal curve
E. Prompt treatment sought for signs of infection
F. Parents discussing diagnosis and treatment honestly with child

◆ CONGESTIVE HEART FAILURE

CHF occurs when the cardiac output is inadequate to meet the metabolic demands of the body and results in accumulation of excessive blood volume in the pulmonary or systemic venous system. It is a symptom related to underlying cardiac disease.

Etiology/Incidence

1. CHD, especially left-to-right shunts (primary cause in the first 3 years of life)
2. Acquired heart disease—rheumatic heart disease, endocarditis, myocarditis

3. Noncardiovascular causes—acidosis, pulmonary disease, various metabolic diseases, anemias

Altered Physiology

1. For any number of reasons, cardiac output is inadequate to meet the oxygenation and nutritional requirements of vital organs.
2. Various compensatory mechanisms occur.
   a. Stroke volume increases, and cardiomegaly develops.
   b. Tachycardia occurs in an effort to maintain adequate stroke volume.
   c. Catecholamines are released by the sympathetic nervous system that increase systemic vascular resistance and venous tone and decrease cutaneous, splanchnic, and renal blood flow.
   d. Glomerular filtration decreases, and tubular reabsorption increases, causing diminished urinary output and sodium retention.
   e. Diaphoresis occurs.
3. Cardiac output decreases further as compensatory mechanisms fail.
4. The pulmonary vascular bed is not emptied efficiently, causing engorgement of the pulmonic system with subsequent pulmonary hypertension and edema.
5. There is diminished blood return to the heart, with venous congestion and a rise in venous pressure.

Complications

1. Respiratory infections
2. Pulmonary edema
3. Intractable CHF
4. Myocardial failure

Clinical Manifestations

1. Impaired myocardial function
   a. Tachycardia, restlessness
   b. Weak cry, easily fatigued
   c. Pallor, cool extremities, diaphoresis
   d. Decreased urine output
   e. Feeding difficulties or anorexia
2. Pulmonary congestion
   a. Dyspnea, tachypnea, orthopnea
   b. Nonproductive, irritating cough
   c. Retractions, nasal flaring, grunting, cyanosis
3. Systemic venous congestion
   a. Hepatomegaly/abdominal discomfort
   b. Peripheral, orbital, scrotal edema
   c. Neck vein distention
   d. Weight gain, oliguria

Diagnostic Evaluation

1. Palpation
   a. May have weak peripheral pulses
   b. Hepatomegaly (feature of right-heart failure) related to blood backing up in venous system
   c. Abnormal precordial activity
2. Auscultation
   a. Gallop rhythm (frequent)

b. Cardiac murmurs (may or may not be present)
   c. Crackles (infrequent in infants)
3. Chest x-rays—cardiomegaly, pulmonary congestion
4. Laboratory data—increased sodium (dilutional), decreased chloride, increased potassium

Treatment

1. Digoxin therapy to slow conduction through the atrioventricular node and increase cardiac contractility
2. Diuretic therapy to reduce intravascular fluid volume
3. Afterload reducing medications such as angiotensin-converting enzyme (ACE) inhibitors

Nursing Assessment

See CHF, p. 310.

1. Focus on parameters discussed in the section, Clinical Manifestations (ie, tachycardia, dyspnea).
2. Auscultate heart, lungs, abdomen; expect variable results, depending on severity of disease.
3. Palpate abdomen, and measure abdominal girth.
4. Assess urinary output and specific gravity.
5. Assess psychosocial status by observation and interview of child and family.

Nursing Diagnoses

A. Decreased Cardiac Output related to myocardial dysfunction
B. Fluid Volume Excess related to the inability of the heart to pump blood from the ventricle(s) and decreased blood flow to the kidney
C. Impaired Gas Exchange related to pulmonary engorgement
D. Activity Intolerance related to fatigue
E. Risk for Infection related to pulmonary congestion and decreased body defenses
F. Altered Nutrition: Less than body requirements related to decreased energy for feeding
G. Anxiety of child or parent related to their perception(s) of the child's condition and potential for death

Nursing Interventions

A. *Improving Myocardial Efficiency*
1. Administer digoxin as prescribed by the healthcare provider.
   a. Carefully calculate dosage *daily* based on child's daily weight; digoxin is given to infants and children in very small amounts.
   b. Give at same time each day to maintain therapeutic levels.
   c. Count apical pulse for 1 full minute before administering. Be aware of the heart rate at which the healthcare provider wants the medication withheld (usually 90–100 for infants and 70 for older children). Contact healthcare provider if two consecutive doses are held.

d. Report vomiting, which may occur following administration of digoxin, to determine if healthcare provider desires dose to be repeated.

e. Observe for the development of premature ventricular contractions when digoxin is initially started; report this to healthcare provider.

f. Be aware of signs of digitalis intoxication: anorexia, bradycardia, dysrhythmias, nausea, vomiting, diarrhea, altered emotional status ("digitalis blues"—not as evident in young children)

NURSING ALERT: ❖❖

Hypokalemia can contribute to the development of digitalis toxicity even in the presence of low serum digoxin levels. Hypomagnesemia and hypercalcemia also may aggravate digitalis toxicity.

---

2. Administer afterload-reduction medications such as captopril (Capoten) as ordered.
   a. Check blood pressure before and after administering.
   b. Hold medication according to blood pressure parameters ordered by healthcare provider.
   c. Notify healthcare provider if two consecutive doses are held.
   d. Watch for hypotension.

B. *Maintaining Fluid and Electrolyte Balance*
1. Administer diuretics as prescribed by the healthcare provider.
   a. Be aware of the side effects of the prescribed medication.
   b. Weigh the child at least daily to observe response (same time of day, same scale, same attire).
   c. Maintain an accurate record of intake and output (weigh diapers). Record urine-specific gravity.
   d. Encourage foods such as bananas and orange juice that have a high potassium content to prevent potassium depletion associated with many diuretics.
   e. Monitor serum electrolytes. Hypokalemia may cause weakened myocardial contractions and may precipitate digitalis toxicity.
   f. Administer oral potassium supplements as ordered when a child is on diuretics for an extended period of time.
2. Restrict sodium intake.
   a. The child may be placed on a low-sodium diet.
   b. Be aware of the prescribed diet and the amount of sodium in foods and fluids offered to the child.
   c. Question the child about likes and dislikes so that the diet can be made as appealing as possible.
   d. Interpret the diet and its purpose to the child and parents.
   e. Infants may require low-sodium formulas.
3. Monitor fluid restriction.
   a. Check child's dietary trays.
   b. Remember to count fluids used for medication administration intake.
   c. Do not leave fluids at the bedside.
   d. Put fluids in small cups to make them appear more than they are.
   e. Allow more fluid to be consumed during wakeful hours.

C. *Relieving Respiratory Distress*
1. Refer to section on CHD, p. 1206.
2. Provide measures to improve tissue oxygenation.

a. Administer oxygen therapy; refer to procedure, pp. 1191 to 1194.
b. Maintain the infant in a neutral thermal environment.
c. Elevate head of bed.
d. Do not use constricting clothing.

D. *Reducing Energy Requirements*
1. Organize nursing care to provide periods of uninterrupted rest.
2. Avoid unnecessary activities, such as frequent complete baths and clothing changes.
3. Prevent excessive crying; anticipate needs.
   a. Use pacifier.
   b. Hold baby.
   c. Eliminate source of distress (eg, hunger, wet diapers).
4. Avoid overheating or chilling.
5. Explain to the child the need for rest.
6. Provide diversional activities that require limited expenditure of energy.
7. Provide small, frequent meals with foods easy to chew and digest.
8. Avoid constipation.

E. *Decreasing the Danger of Infection*
1. Practice careful handwashing technique.
2. Avoid exposure to other children with upper respiratory infections, diarrhea, and so forth.
3. Report changes, such as temperature elevation, diarrhea, vomiting, and upper respiratory symptoms, promptly.

F. *Providing Adequate Nutrition*
1. Provide foods that the child enjoys in small amounts, because child may have a poor appetite due to liver enlargement.
2. For infant feeding, feed frequently in small amounts.
   a. Feed slowly in a sitting position, allowing frequent rest periods.
   b. Administer supplemental oral feedings with gavage feeding if the infant is unable to take an adequate amount of formula by mouth. Consider tube feeding during sleeping hours.
   c. Record the amount of formula taken.
   d. Use high-calorie formulas.
   e. Place the child in an infant seat following feeding to prevent pressure of the viscera on the diaphragm.
   f. Observe for distention and vomiting following feeding.

G. *Reducing Anxiety*
1. Use terminology that the child and parents can understand.
2. Correct misinterpretations; parents and children frequently interpret CHF to be synonymous with myocardial infarction, or they may fear that the heart is about to stop beating.
3. Allow parent and child to ask questions and express concerns.

Family Education/Health Maintenance

1. Teach signs and symptoms of CHF.
2. Teach home medications, including side effects, withholding parameters, toxic effects. Reinforce need to maintain schedule.

3. Teach home management if signs and symptoms develop (ie, oxygen therapy, fluid restriction, extra dose of diuretics as ordered by healthcare provider).
4. Reinforce appropriate time to seek medical help. Teach home cardiopulmonary resuscitation (CPR).
5. Explain dietary or activity restrictions.
6. Explain methods to prevent infection.
7. Initiate a community health nursing referral if indicated.
8. Stress need for continued follow-up care.

Evaluation

A. Lungs clear, abdominal girth stable, urine output adequate
B. Decreased edema; serum sodium and potasssium within normal limits
C. Maintains oxygenation, evidenced by normal color, decreased cyanosis, and improved arterial blood gas (ABG) values
D. Conserves energy and rest in accordance with needs
E. Remains infection free
F. Nutritional intake adequate for age
G. Parents discussing their concerns about the child's condition with one another; adequate coping mechanisms

Acquired Heart Disease

◆ ACUTE RHEUMATIC FEVER

Acute rheumatic fever (ARF) is a systemic disease characterized by inflammatory lesions of connective tissue and endothelial tissue. It is a primary type of acquired heart disease.

Etiology/Incidence

1. The pathogenesis is thought to be an autoimmune response to group A beta-hemolytic *Streptococcus.*
2. Most first attacks of ARF are preceded by an untreated streptococcal infection of the throat or upper respiratory tract at an interval of 2 to 6 weeks.
3. ARF is *not* caused by direct infection by the organism.
4. ARF is commonly seen in children 5 to 15 years of age, during winter months, and in poorer living conditions.
5. Incidence is greater in underdeveloped countries, although it is on the rise in the United States.

Altered Physiology

1. There is a cross-reactivity between cardiac tissue antigens and streptococcal cell wall components.
2. The *Streptococcus* may no longer be present, but autoantibodies attack one's heart (myocardium, pericardium, or valves).
3. The unique pathologic lesion of rheumatic fever is the Aschoff body, a collection of reticuloendothelial cells surrounding a necrotic center on some structure of the heart.

4. The inflammatory process involves the heart, joints, skin, and central nervous system. The inflammation may involve the leaflets or chordae tendinae of the heart valves, most frequently the mitral or aortic valves, resulting in sclerosis and fusion of valve margins.
5. Valvular incompetence results.
6. There is a high recurrence rate.
7. Of those with AFR, 75% progress to rheumatic heart disease in adulthood.
8. ARF is a preventable condition with penicillin treatment of the primary infection. Erythromycin is treatment for those with penicillin sensitivities.

Complications

1. Significant CHF
2. Pericarditis, pericardial effusions
3. Aortic/mitral valve regurgitation
4. Permanent cardiac damage

Clinical Manifestations and Diagnostic Evaluation

No single clinical or laboratory finding is characteristic of ARF. The diagnosis is based on a combination of manifestations characteristic of this disease and in the absence of other diseases that may mimic it. For this reason, the Jones criteria, as established by a committee of the American Heart Association, are used. The presence of two major criteria, or one major and two minor criteria, plus evidence of a preceding streptococcal infection are required to establish a diagnosis.

A. *Major Manifestations*
1. Carditis—manifested by significant murmurs, signs of pericarditis, cardiac enlargement, or CHF.
2. Polyarthritis—almost always migratory and is manifested by swelling, heat, redness and tenderness or by pain and limitation of motion of two or more joints. (The synovial fluid is sterile.)
3. Chorea, a CNS disorder that lasts 1 to 3 months—purposeless, involuntary, rapid movements often are associated with muscle weakness, involuntary facial grimaces, speech disturbances, and emotional lability.
4. Erythema marginatum—an evanescent nonpruritic, pink rash. The erythematous areas have pale centers and round or wavy margins, vary greatly in size, and occur mainly on the trunk and extremities. Erythema is transient, migrates from place to place, and may be brought out by the application of heat.
5. Subcutaneous nodules—firm, painless nodules seen or felt over the extensor surface of certain joints, particularly elbows, knees, and wrists, in the occipital region, or over the spinous processes of the thoracic and lumbar vertebrae; the skin overlying them moves freely and is not inflamed.

B. *Minor Manifestations*
1. History of previous rheumatic fever or evidence of preexisting rheumatic heart disease
2. Arthralgia—pain in one or more joints without evidence of inflammation, tenderness to touch, or limitation of motion
3. Fever—temperature in excess of 38°C (100.4°F)

4. Elevated erythrocyte sedimentation rate (ESR)
5. Positive C-reactive protein
6. ECG changes—mainly PR interval prolongation
7. Elevated white blood cell count (leukocytosis)

C. **Supporting Evidence of Streptococcal Infection**
1. Increased titer of streptococcal antibodies (antistreptolysin O or ASO titer)
2. Positive throat culture for group A beta-hemolytic streptococci
3. Recent scarlet fever

Treatment

1. Treatment of streptococcal infection—generally intramuscular (IM) penicillin G (Bicillin L-A); erythromycin (Eryc) for patients with penicillin allergy
2. Prevention of permanent cardiac damage—corticosteroids for patients with carditis
3. Palliative management of other symptoms—salicylates prescribed for patients with arthritis (but not while on high-dose corticosteroids due to risk of gastrointestinal bleeding); antipyretics after diagnosis has been established
4. Prevention of recurrences of ARF

Nursing Assessment

1. Listen to the child's chest with a stethoscope to become familiar with the murmur or to determine the presence of a murmur not previously heard; listen for a friction rub.
2. Ask whether the child is experiencing any pain or discomfort. (Also observe the child's facial expression as child moves because children may deny pain, thinking they will be able to go home or resume activity.)
3. Describe the pain as to location, when it occurs, and whether there is any heat, swelling, redness, or tenderness.
4. Examine the knees, elbows, wrists, occipital region, and spine for nodules; describe location.
5. Determine whether the child has any muscle weakness or rapid, purposeless movements.

Nursing Diagnoses

A. Risk for Infection related to ARF progression
B. Decreased Cardiac Output related to heart damage
C. Pain related to polyarthritis and bed rest
D. Risk for Injury related to progression of ARF and chorea
E. Activity Intolerance related to muscle weakness and inflamed joints

Nursing Interventions

A. **Controlling Infection**
1. Administer medication as prescribed by the healthcare provider.

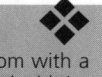

NURSING ALERT:
Before administering penicillin, elicit a history for possible drug allergy.

2. Administer salicylates with milk or antacids.
   a. Observe for gastrointestinal upset, ringing in the ears, headaches, bleeding, and disturbances in the mental state.
   b. Report side effects promptly.
   c. Monitor salicylate blood levels as ordered.
   d. Withhold antipyretics during the diagnostic period as requested.
3. Prepare the child and family for the expected side effects of steroid therapy, such as rounding facial contour, acne, excessive hair, weight gain.
   a. Watch for mental and emotional disturbances, which may necessitate discontinuing the medication.
   b. Hypertension and the tendency to retain water and sodium may result from steroid therapy. Restrict sodium and fluids, and obtain daily weights as indicated.
   c. Be aware that steroids diminish the child's resistance to infection and may mask symptoms of infection.

NURSING ALERT:
Do not place a child with an infectious disease in a room with a child with rheumatic fever. Restrict visitors and personnel with infectious diseases from contact with the child on steroid therapy.

   d. Make the family aware that a combination of steroid therapy and stress may lead to the development of gastric ulcers.
4. Administer antipyretics; alternating schedule of different antipyretics may be required to provide relief of child's fever.
5. Administer medications punctually and at regular intervals to achieve constant therapeutic blood levels.
6. Report signs of increased rheumatic activity as salicylates or steroids are being tapered.
   a. Observe for the development or disappearance of any major or minor manifestations of the disease.
   b. Monitor carditis by careful documentation of the child's pulse (sleeping pulse counted for 1 full minute), respirations, and blood pressure.

B. **Maintaining Cardiac Output**
1. Explain to the child the need for rest (usually prescribed for 4–12 weeks, depending on the severity of the disease and healthcare provider's preference).
2. Assure the child that bed rest will be imposed no longer than necessary. This is usually until the ESR returns to normal.
3. Organize nursing care to provide periods of uninterrupted rest.
4. Assure the child that needs will be met by reviewing call light and answering calls promptly.
5. Assist the child to resume activity very gradually once asymptomatic at rest and indicators of acute inflammation have become normal.
6. Continue to monitor the pulse rate carefully after periods of activity to assess the degree of cardiac compensation.
7. Provide nursing care for the child with CHF if symptomatic (see p. 1208).

C. *Maintaining Comfort*

1. Use bed cradle.
2. Reassure that arthritis is *not* destructive.
3. Change positions in bed often to decrease stiffness and decrease skin breakdown.
4. Support inflamed joints; handle gently.
5. Provide meticulous skin care.
6. Position the legs in good body alignment; use a foot board.
7. Elevate the back of the bed, and support the arms with pillows when child is dyspneic.

D. *Providing Safe, Supportive Care for the Child With Chorea*

1. Place the child in a bed with padded side rails, especially if uncontrolled body movements are severe.
2. Feed the child slowly and carefully because of uncoordinated movements of the head, mouth, and swallowing muscles. Avoid the use of sharp eating utensils, and do not use straws.
3. Provide frequent feedings that are high in calories, protein, vitamins, and iron, because constant movements cause the child to burn calories at a rapid rate.
4. Spend time talking with the child even though speech may be defective. If severe, use other methods of communication.
5. Administer sedative, if prescribed.
6. Reassure the child about the cause of instability and that symptoms will subside.
7. Encourage positive parent–child relationships that may have been strained if the onset of symptoms was insidious (eg, lack of concentration at school, mood swings, deteriorating handwriting, irritability).
8. Help the child regain former skills once symptoms begin to subside.
   a. Support the child during periods of ambulation.
   b. Provide activities that require the use of large muscles, and progress to materials that require fine coordination.
9. Keep the environment calm, and provide increased periods of rest because movements increase with fatigue and increased excitement.

E. *Maintaining Bed Rest*

1. Complete or partial bed rest is encouraged.
2. Help the child understand the restrictions and that progress may be slow.
3. Initiate appropriate measures to help the child maintain level of development during the lengthy hospitalization.
   a. Refer to care of the hospitalized child, p. 1127.
   b. Arrange for continuation of school and tutors.
   c. Facilitate interaction with family, including siblings.
   d. Provide diversional activities that will help the child feel a sense of achievement or satisfaction.
   e. Offer quiet play, such as board games, television, radio, reading, and drawing.
   f. Involve child life groups and physical and occupational therapy.
   g. Facilitate contact with peers through writing, tape recording, telephone, or selected visitation.

F. *Reducing Anxiety for Child and Parent*

1. Explain ARF and its progression and management, such as the need for intravenous (IV) line and follow-up laboratory work.
2. Use honest, simple, age-appropriate explanations.
   a. Give the child information about rheumatic fever in understandable terms; for example, "Rheumatic fever is a hard thing to understand because you can't see it. When you scratch yourself, you can see the mark, and you can see the scratch heal. Rheumatic fever is something like that—only you can't see the healing because it happens to the tissue underneath the skin (and sometimes it happens to the valves in the heart)."
   b. Assure the child that healthcare providers know how to treat rheumatic fever.
   c. Communicate information about the child's reactions to all staff members to provide consistent information.
   d. Children may be concerned that they have had a heart attack; reassure that their heart is functioning by letting them listen to it.
3. Allow the child and parent time to ask questions and express their concerns.
4. Allow the child to participate in decision making when possible.

Family Education/Health Maintenance

1. Initiate specific preventive teaching to prevent a recurrence or an additional case of rheumatic fever within the family.
   a. Have all family members screened for *Streptococcus* by referring them for throat cultures.
   b. All people with positive cultures should be treated.
   c. Teach the specific symptoms of streptococcal infections and the need for antibiotics.
2. Prevent a recurrent attack of rheumatic fever by reinforcing the need for prophylactic antimicrobial therapy.
   a. Penicillin is the drug of choice—either IM benzathine penicillin G every 28 days, oral penicillin V (Pen-Vee K) or G (Pentids) twice daily, or one daily dose of sulfadiazine (Microsulfon).
   b. Continuous prophylaxis is recommended throughout the childhood years and well into adult life, often indefinitely.
   c. Use creativity in recommending methods to remind families about administering the medication.
      (1) The child should be taught to assume responsibility for own medication at an early age so that it becomes habitual.
      (2) Some children profit from the use of a calendar or special chart. Others find it useful to associate their medication schedule with other routine tasks, such as brushing their teeth.
   d. Encourage administration of prophylactic medication on schedule.
   e. Advise on additional prophylaxis for prevention of infective endocarditis. The American Heart Association's recommendations for the prevention of endocarditis should be observed for children undergoing certain dental procedures and for surgery or instrumentation of the upper respiratory tract, genitourinary tract, or lower gastrointestinal tract.
3. Begin to prepare for discharge early enough with the parents that sufficient adjustments and preparations may be made.
   a. The child should have own bed and preferably own room.

b. A responsible adult must be in the home to care for child.

c. Provide information about activity restrictions, medications (dosage, schedule, side effects), dietary instructions, symptoms to report (pain, malaise, anorexia, tachycardia, tachypnea, weight gain), telephone number of healthcare provider, follow-up appointment.

d. Initiate a community nursing referral; this may be done prior to discharge if a home evaluation is desired or if home care nursing is needed.

e. Offer financial consultation as available.

4. Instruct in additional measures to maintain health.
   a. Complete immunization schedules
   b. Regular medical and dental care
   c. The need to seek immediate medical care for signs of streptococcal infections

Evaluation

A. Reduction in symptoms; no serious symptoms of medications

B. Stable vital signs; no signs of CHF

C. Patient comfortable as evidenced by unlabored respirations and no complaints

D. Neurologic status improving and no injuries reported

E. Child coping effectively with activity restrictions

F. Anxiety reduced as evidenced by family cooperation and appropriate discussion of disease management

◆ CARDIOMYOPATHY

Cardiomyopathy is an abnormality of the myocardium impairing the cardiac muscle to contract. It is rare in children. Of the three types of cardiomyopathy, dilated congestive cardiomyopathy is the most common seen in children. See Chapter 11 for a discussion of the other types of cardiomyopathy.

Etiology/Altered Physiology

1. Most cardiomyopathies are primary or idiopathic and not related to CHD or other systemic diseases. In most cases, the cause is unknown.

2. Secondary cardiomyopathies may develop as a result of systemic disease, infection, deficiency states, metabolic disorders, and collagen vascular diseases, or after a surgical correction for a congenital heart defect where severe ventricular dysfunction has developed.

3. Dilated cardiomyopathy involves large ventricular dilation with greatly decreased contractility.

Complications

1. Intraatrial/intraventricular thrombi
2. Systemic or pulmonary emboli
3. Severe malignant arrythmias
4. Sudden death

Clinical Manifestations

1. Tachycardia, dyspnea
2. Fatigue, lethargy, exercise intolerance

3. Poor growth
4. Chest pain, syncope
5. Hepatosplenomegaly
6. Dysrhythmias, murmur

Diagnostic Evaluation

1. ECG—usually abnormal with ST segment changes, dysrhythmias
2. Chest x-ray—cardiomegaly, congested lung fields
3. Echocardiogram—poor ventricular contractility, dilated left or right ventricle, asymmetric septal hypertrophy, increased left ventricular wall thickness with small left ventricular cavity
4. Cardiac catheterization/angiography—assists with diagnosis; identifies possible infectious causes; evaluates ventricular function

Treatment

1. Correct underlying cause of the disease, although cardiomyopathy is usually not a reversible disease.
2. Congestive myopathy
   a. Decrease workload of the heart with drugs for arterial dilation and relaxation.
   b. Anticoagulants prevent emboli.
   c. Treatment is mostly palliative.
3. Hypertrophic cardiomyopathy
   a. Beta-blockers and calcium channel-blockers lower heart rate and contractile force.
4. Restrictive cardiomyopathy
   a. Similar to congestive myopathy in reducing workload of heart
   b. Palliative measures

Nursing Assessment

Perform a thorough assessment, similar to nursing assessment for CHD, p. 1206.

Nursing Diagnoses

A. Decreased Cardiac Output related to ventricular dysfunction

B. Altered Nutrition: Less than body requirements related to poor feeding from fatigue and dyspnea

C. Powerlessness related to debilitating condition with poor prognosis

Nursing Interventions

A. *Maximinizing Cardiac Output*
1. Use continuous ECG monitoring.
   a. Observe and immediately report dysrhythmias.
   b. Monitor electrolytes—imbalances may depress cardiac output and cause increased dysrhythmias.
2. Provide supplemental oxygen therapy.
3. Administer medications as ordered by healthcare provider.

a. Administer anticoagulants, and observe bleeding precautions (ie, no IM injections, no rectal temperatures, urine and stool tests for blood).
b. Administer diuretics, and monitor intake and output, urine-specific gravity, and improvement of symptoms.
4. Use mechanical ventilation to lessen the workload of the heart for severely ill and dyspneic children.
a. Maintain comfort; sedation may be necessary.
b. Maintain a calm, reassuring attitude and environment.
5. Maintain bed rest to lessen cardiac workload.
6. Also see nursing interventions for CHF, p. 1209.

B. Providing Maximal Nutritional Support
1. Include child and dietary services in choices.
2. Include high calorie supplements (eg, milk shakes).
3. Provide frequent, small meals.
4. Maintain accurate calorie count.
5. Consider supplemental tube feedings if nutritional requirements are not met.
6. Administer hyperalimentation, intralipids as necessary.

C. Promoting Decision Making and Control Within the Family Unit
1. Organize a patient care conference using a network of support services. Include the family and child if age appropriate.
a. Review outside support services, such as clergy, community support groups, financial counselors, extended family.
b. Explain available treatment options, including cardiac transplantation.
c. Refer to other centers for additional treatment options.
d. Initiate a plan of care.
2. Allow family and child to voice concerns, fears, and questions. Involve them in the decision-making process of this life-threatening disease.
a. Discuss the possibility of ventilatory support.
b. Share information with family regularly.

Family Education/Health Maintenance

1. Teach about medications, side effects, and special precautions, such as bleeding precautions for child on anticoagulant therapy.
a. Protect child from bruising and other trauma.
b. Use soft toothbrush, no sharp knives or forks.
c. Observe urine and stool for blood.
d. Report for periodic blood work to evaluate prothrombin time.
2. Advise on symptoms to report, such as worsening shortness of breath, fatigability, irregular pulse, syncope.
3. Teach CPR to caregivers.

Evaluation

A. Maximal cardiac support as evidenced by stable vital signs and relief of symptoms of CHF
B. Maximal nutritional status as evidenced by weight gain and growth
C. Family and child involved in the decisions of care

Cardiac Procedures

◆ CARDIAC CATHETERIZATION

Cardiac catheterization involves introducing a radiopaque catheter into a vein or artery in the groin or in the arm, either percutaneously or by means of a cutdown. The catheter is advanced into the cardiac chambers and vessels, where pressures are measured and samples for oxygen concentration are obtained. The procedure is usually done in conjunction with angiography, the injection of radiopaque material into various chambers of the heart. Cardiac catheterization may be diagnostic, interventional, or electrophysiologic. Also see cardiac catheterization of the adult, p. 253.

Purposes

1. To establish diagnosis of a cardiovascular defect
2. To identify the severity of the defect
3. To evaluate the effects of the defect on cardiovascular function or to evaluate dysrythmias
4. An alternative to surgery in some cases

Complications

1. Dysrhythmias—generally catheter induced
2. Hemorrhage at site of insertion
3. Arterial blockage—loss of pulse in extremity used for cannulation; cold, pale mottled extremity
4. Infection
5. Allergic reaction to the dye—low-grade fever, nausea, vomiting, flushing

Preoperative Nursing Interventions

A. Prepare the Child and Parents Emotionally
1. Reinforce explanations of the procedure to the child and parents. Provide specific information.
a. Time of the test
b. Preparation for the procedure (eg, nothing by mouth [NPO], sedation)
c. Site of the venipuncture (if known)
d. What the child will see (atmosphere of the catheterization room)
e. What will be expected of the child during the procedure
f. Routines after the procedure
2. Provide the appropriate detail, length, and timing of explanations for the child's age and level of cognitive development.
a. Photographs or a miniature replica of the cardiac laboratory and equipment may facilitate understanding of explanations.
b. Older children and parents may benefit from an opportunity to see the room where the procedure will be done.
c. It is helpful for some children to handle the mask and other equipment that will be used.

d. Describe sensations with careful choice of words and with appropriate timing based on the age of the child. With injection of the dye, child may experience warmth, nausea, headache, restlessness, and chest pains.

e. In preparing the child, do not use the word "dye" for the injectable substance; use "special medicine."

3. Provide parents with an opportunity for private discussion of the anticipated procedure.

B. **Prepare the Child Physically**
1. Maintain adequate hydration (especially important for children with cyanotic heart disease). Offer fluids just prior to NPO period.
2. Cleanse proposed catheterization site thoroughly. Clean fingernails or toenails.
3. Obtain baseline set of vital signs just prior to the time of catheterization.
   a. Blood pressure in all four extremities
   b. Color and temperature of all extremities
   c. Activity level of child
   d. Child's weight
   e. Quality of pulses in all extremities
   f. Baseline oximetry level
4. Administer sedation if prescribed.
   a. Raise and secure side rails after the child has been medicated.
   b. Observe the child closely for depressed respirations.

Postoperative Nursing Interventions

A. **Observe for and Prevent Complications**
1. Monitor vital signs frequently and report:
   a. Sudden drop in blood pressure
   b. Changes in pulse rate or rhythm
   c. Increased or depressed respirations
   d. Faintness, weakness
   e. Elevated temperature
   f. Decreased temperature in the extremity used for the catheterization
   g. Hemorrhage or hematoma at the injection site
   h. Inflammation at the site or other signs of infection
2. Observe for complications resulting from damage to the vessels through which the catheter was passed.
   a. Check the dressing or puncture site for bleeding.
   b. Observe site for redness, swelling, pain, or induration.
   c. Observe for numbness, pallor, decreased temperature, decreased motion, cyanosis, or mottling of affected extremity.
   d. Palpate pulses in affected extremity, and compare with pulses in the opposite extremity.
3. Keep the child warm to avoid the risk of hypothermia. This is especially important for small infants and children who may already be hypoxic because of their cardiac condition.
4. Maintain the child in a reclining position for several hours after catheterization to avoid the following:
   a. Possibility of sudden drop in blood pressure that may accompany an abrupt assumption of an upright position
   b. Bleeding at the site of catheter entry
5. Offer fluids as soon as the child is able to take them to avoid dehydration. This is especially important for cyanotic children who are polycythemic and prone to thrombus formation.

6. Make security objects and favorite toys available to child in recovery room.

B. **Prepare the Child and Parents for Discharge**
1. Reinforce discharge information. Parents should be informed about the following:
   a. Care of the incision, puncture site
   b. Dressing change (if any)
   c. Activity limitations (if any)
   d. Observing for and reporting late complications (especially infection—redness, swelling, drainage from catheter site)
   e. Follow-up medical care
2. If the child is a candidate for surgery, use appropriate opportunities to prepare family for the experience.
   a. Explain the surgical procedure in honest, simple, age-appropriate terms.
   b. Use diagrams when possible.
   c. Allow time for child and parents to ask questions and express concerns.
   d. Encourage contact with children who are convalescing from surgery; provide support for both child and parent.
   e. Refer to cardiac surgery preoperative section, p. 1217.

◆ CARDIAC SURGERY

The ultimate goal of the treatment of cardiovascular disease is the restoration of the normal structure and function of the heart. It is now possible to operate on most patients with CHD because of advances in medical and surgical techniques. Generally, nursing care of children who require cardiac surgery is similar to that of adults (refer to pp. 283–285). In addition, the nurse who works with pediatric patients should remember the following.

Procedures and Indications

Pediatric surgery involves more intracardiac reconstruction than adults.

A. **Closed Heart Surgery Through a Lateral Thoracotomy**
1. Pulmonary artery banding
2. PDA ligation
3. Coarctation repair
4. Palliative surgery for shunt provisions
5. Surgery for vascular rings

B. **Open Heart Surgery Through a Midsternal Incision**
This can involve cardiopulmonary bypass (extracorporeal circulation) enabling surgeons to operate inside the heart, or it can be accomplished by deep hypothermia (25°C, 77°F) to lower metabolic demands and reduce needs for oxygen.

1. ASD, VSD
2. Tetralogy of Fallot
3. Pulmonary stenosis, aortic stenosis
4. TGA
5. Tricuspid atresia
6. Hypoplastic left heart syndrome
7. Truncus arteriosus
8. Anomalous venous return
9. Complex congenital defects

Cardiac Transplantation

1. This technique has been successful since 1967 and has been gaining popularity in neonates, infants, and children during the last 10 years.
2. This is considered a treatment option for the following:
   a. Infants and children with end-stage congenital heart defects, such as hypoplastic left heart syndrome, single ventricle, complex cyanotic heart disease
   b. Infants and children with acquired heart disease, such as cardiomyopathy unresponsive to maximum medical or surgical management
3. Preoperative and postoperative care is quite extensive and involves many physical, emotional, and psychosocial aspects for the patient and family.
4. Many questions are raised, including ones of ethics, scarcity of donors, the painful waiting process, donor allocation, and financial issues.

Complications of Specific Surgeries

1. PDA (rare)—laryngeal nerve damage, phrenic nerve damage, diaphragmatic paralysis, thoracic duct injury
2. Coarctation of the aorta—paradoxical hypertension; abdominal pain, distention; aneurysm at synthetic patch site; bacterial endocarditis; thoracic duct injury
3. ASD—atrial dysrhythmias, transient or permanent heart block, left ventricular failure
4. VSD—conduction disturbance, complete heart block, residual VSD, impaired cardiac output
5. Tetralogy of Fallot—low cardiac output, rhythm disturbances, complete heart block, residual VSD
6. Transposition of great arteries—dysrhythmias, low cardiac output, hemorrhage leading to cardiac tamponade, thoracic duct injury
7. Aortic stenosis—aortic insufficiency, altered renal function, endocarditis
8. Tricuspid atresia (Fontan procedure)—increased pulmonary vascular resistance, resulting in decreased pulmonary blood flow; systemic venous hypertension; dsyrhthmias and heart block; left ventricular dysfunction; thoracic duct injury
9. Hypoplastic left heart—altered pulmonary flow, hemorrhage

Preoperative Nursing Interventions

A. *Preparing the Child Emotionally*
1. Be prepared for questions that parents frequently ask.
   a. What to tell the child
   b. When to begin preparation
   c. What to bring to the hospital
   d. Anticipated sequence of events
   e. Separation—rooming-in, whether or not to leave at night, and so forth.
2. Be honest, and base teaching on the child's age.
3. Consult with the parents prior to beginning explanation. Their desires regarding how much information to give the child should be respected, and they should be active participants in preparing the child.
4. Provide information about preparation for surgery.
   a. Diagnostic tests
   b. Antibacterial skin preparation or baths

c. NPO period
d. Injections—antimicrobials or sedatives
e. Time of surgery
f. Transportation to the operating room (OR)
g. Sensations in the OR (sounds, temperature, colors, dress, and masks worn by OR staff)
5. Provide information abut postoperative expectations; use careful choice of words based on age.
6. Provide detail, length, and time of explanations that are appropriate to the child's age and level of cognitive development.
   a. Photographs or a miniature replica of the intensive care unit may facilitate understanding of explanations.
   b. Older children and parents often benefit from an opportunity to see the intensive care unit.
   c. It is helpful for some children to have an opportunity to manipulate some of the equipment that will be used (eg, try on mask, OR cap, sterile gloves, and scrub suit; experience blood pressure cuff, oxygen mask, cardiac leads).
   d. Use a model of the heart to explain what will be done. Pictures and diagrams also are helpful
   e. Demonstrate on a doll the site of the incision, dressings, and tubes.
7. Test the child's comprehension of teaching by asking simple questions, having child place equipment on a doll, demonstrating coughing and deep breathing, and other similar activities.
8. Allow opportunity for the child to express concerns, either verbally or in play situations.
9. Provide parents with the same type of information as their child, as well as where to wait, usual length of surgery, intensive care unit expectations, policies.
10. Provide emotional support to the parents and answer their questions so that they are in the best position to support their child.

D. *Making Baseline Assessments*
1. Obtain height and weight.
2. Measure vital signs.
3. Observe sleep/wake patterns.
4. Assess elimination patterns and toileting words.
5. Evaluate normal intake and special feeding routines.
6. Observe for any indications that surgery may need to be canceled.
   a. Signs of infection or inflammation (eg, upper respiratory infection, hoarseness, elevated temperature, vomiting, diarrhea, skin lesions).
   b. Signs of CHF (see p. 1209)
   c. Anemia—check complete blood cells
7. Send the nursing history and care plan to the intensive care unit, and relay information about the child and family to appropriate personnel.

Postoperative Nursing Interventions

A. *Observing for and Preventing Complications*
1. Observe for respiratory distress.
   a. Provide patent airway—ventilation is supported by oral or nasal endotracheal tubes and mechanical ventilation.
   b. Suction endotracheal tube to maintain patency.
   c. Auscultate chest for breath sounds in all lung fields; atelectasis, pneumothorax, pleural effusion, hemothorax may present with decreased breath sounds.

d. Assess child's color, peripheral perfusion, capillary refill frequently to determine effectiveness of cardiac and respiratory function.

e. Sedate adequately, per healthcare provider's orders, to help the child tolerate the ventilator.

f. Perform chest percussion and postural drainage as ordered.

g. Assess chest tubes for drainage, and notify healthcare provider of amount.

h. Extubate as condition stabilizes.

i. After extubation, provide high humidity oxygen by hood, mask, or cannula, and assess respiratory status frequently.

2. Assess for cardiac overload.
   a. Maintain continuous ECG monitoring.
   b. Maintain intracardiac lines (may be used postoperatively to provide information on cardiac function and output).
   c. Provide rest; organize care.
   d. Decrease stress.
   e. Decrease pain; initially medicate on regular schedule and not PRN.

3. Assess for fluid overload.
   a. Monitor intake and output. Include all access lines and drains (ie, chest tubes).
   b. Monitor specific gravity of urine.
   c. Monitor results of fluid bolus or diuretic therapy.

4. Watch for chylothorax (accumulation of chyle from the lymphatic system in the chest) following some surgeries that may cause injury or obstruction of thoracic ducts.
   a. Observe for creamy white drainage in the chest tubes.
   b. Maintain drainage of chest tubes (but may require eventual dietary restrictions and surgical ligation of the thoracic duct or sclerosis of chylothorax with antibiotics).

5. Monitor for neurologic deficits.
   a. Be aware that hypoperfusion may produce CNS damage after surgery.
   b. Observe for signs and symptoms of hypoxia, such as restlessness, confusion, headache, low blood pressure, cyanosis.
   c. Observe general neurologic status, such as level of responsiveness, response to verbal commands and painful stimuli, pupil sizes and reaction to light, extremity movements.

6. Watch for hemorrhage related to increased anticoagulants used while on heart-lung machine.
   a. Monitor vital signs.
   b. Monitor blood loss from all orifices and wounds.
   c. Handle gently.

7. Assess for acid–base imbalance through serum electrolyte and ABG results.

8. Be aware of specific complications that may occur following particular surgery for CHD (see p. 1217).

B. **Providing Emotional Support and Sense of Family**
1. Provide continuity of care as much as possible and support the parents during the time that the child is in the intensive care unit.

2. Explain emotional changes in children following surgery:
   a. Depression because of sleep deprivation and overstimulation
   b. Anger at their parents (for bringing them to the hospital)
   c. Regression—may become bed wetters
   d. Guilt in older children about their illness.
   e. Nightmares
   f. Fear of others (strangers)
   g. Reassure parents that these emotional changes resolve when the child returns to a more normal routine and environment such as home

Convalescent Nursing Interventions

A. **Preventing Late Complications**
1. Observe for respiratory complications, such as atelectasis, pneumothorax, and pulmonary edema.
   a. Continue coughing and deep breathing exercises.
   b. Ambulate child as tolerated.
   c. Note changes in character of respirations, dyspnea, chest pain, tachycardia, and cyanosis.
2. Be alert for infection, especially bacterial endocarditis.
   a. Monitor temperature at regular intervals.
   b. Observe incision sites for redness, swelling, drainage.
   c. Administer prophylactic antibiotics as indicated.
3. Monitor for CHF (see Nursing Interventions, pp. 1209–1210).
4. Check laboratory results for hematologic changes, such as anemia and thrombocytopenia, related to hemorrhage and heart-lung machine.

B. **Preparing for Discharge**
1. Encourage active parental participation in the child's care to facilitate discharge teaching.
2. Provide the family with oral and written discharge recommendations:
   a. Activity restrictions—not to focus on limitations but on what the child can do
   b. Care of incision
   c. Medications—exact amounts and times of administration, side effects; prophylactic medications
   d. Special diet (low sodium is often indicated)
   e. Emotional reactions, such as regression in toilet habits, feeding, and other learned skills; nightmares, increased dependency; decreased appetite; demanding behavior (need to set limits)
   f. Signs of complications, such as fever, increased heart rate, chest pain, shortness of breath, problems with the incision, vomiting or diarrhea, rash
3. Provide the parents with the names and telephone numbers of people to call for questions and emergencies.
4. Explain infective endocarditis precautions (see Chapter 11).
5. Stress need for follow-up care.
6. Initiate community referrals and supportive services.

Selected References

Branvon, M. E., & Neely, J. M. (1991). *Nursing the child and adult with congenital heart disease. Essentials of cardiovascular nursing.* Gaithersburg, MD: Aspen.

Catania, U. (1994). Monitoring coumadin therapy. *RN, 57*(2), 29–32.

Craig, J. (1991). The postoperative cardiac infant: Physiologic basis for neonatal nursing interventions. *Journal of Perinatal and Neonatal Nursing, 5*(2), 60–70.

Fink, B. (1991). *Congenital heart disease—A deductive approach to its diagnosis.* St. Louis: Mosby Yearbook.

Hazinski M. F. (1992). *Nursing care of the critically ill child* (2nd ed.). St. Louis: Mosby Yearbook.

Kirklin, J., & Barroth-Boyes, B. (1993). *Cardiac surgery* (2nd ed.). New York: Churchill Livingstone.

Rikard, D. H. (1993). Nursing care of the neonate receiving prostaglandin E(1) therapy. *Neonatal Network, 12*(4), 17–22.

Stillwell, S. (1992). *Mosby's critical care nursing reference.* St. Louis: Mosby Yearbook.

Whaley, L., & Wong, D. (1991). *Nursing care of infants and children* (4th ed.). St. Louis: Mosby Yearbook.

Zahr, L. K., & Boisvert, J. (1990). Hypoplastic left heart syndrome repair. Preventing complications. *Dimensions of Critical Care Nursing, 9*(2), 88–96.

CHAPTER 44

Pediatric Neurologic Disorders

Neurologic and Neurosurgical Disorders

◆ CEREBRAL PALSY

Cerebral palsy is a comprehensive diagnostic term used to designate a group of nonprogressive disorders resulting from malfunction of the motor centers and pathways of the brain. Although there are varying degrees and clinical manifestations of cerebral palsy, it is generally characterized by paralysis, weakness, incoordination, or ataxia.

Etiology and Incidence

A. Prenatal Factors (Most Common)
1. Infection, such as rubella, toxoplasmosis, herpes simplex, and cytomegalovirus
2. Maternal anoxia, anemia, placental infarcts, abruptio placentae
3. Prenatal cerebral hemorrhage, maternal bleeding, maternal toxemia, Rh or ABO incompatibility
4. Prenatal anoxia, twisting or kinking of the cord
5. Genetic factors
6. Miscellaneous—toxins, drugs

B. Perinatal Factors
1. Anoxia from any cause
   a. Anesthetic and analgesic drugs administered during labor
   b. Prolonged labor
   c. Placenta previa or abruptio placentae
   d. Respiratory obstruction
2. Cerebral trauma during delivery
3. Complications of birth
   a. "Small for date" babies, prematurity, immaturity, postmaturity, low birth weight (especially <1,500 g)
   b. Hyperbilirubinemia
   c. Hemolytic disorders
   d. Respiratory distress
   e. Infections
   f. Electrolyte disturbances (hypoglycemia, hypocalcemia)

C. Postnatal Factors
1. Head trauma
2. Infections
   a. Meningitis
   b. Encephalitis
   c. Brain abscess

3. Vascular accidents
4. Anoxia
5. Neoplastic and late neurodevelopmental defects

D. Incidence
Cerebral palsy occurs in approximately 2 per 1,000 live births. It is a major cause of disability among children in the United States.

Altered Physiology

A. Spastic Type
1. Defect in the cortical motor area or pyramidal tract causes abnormally strong tonus of certain muscle groups.
2. Attempt to move a joint causes muscles to contract and block the motion. Permanent contractures develop without muscle training.

B. Dyskinetic Type
Lesions of the extrapyramidal tract and basal ganglia cause involuntary, uncoordinated, uncontrollable movements of muscle groups.

C. Ataxia
Disturbances of balance result from cerebellar involvement.

Complications

1. Contractures

Clinical Manifestations (Table 44-1)

A. Early Signs
Early signs may include one or more of the following:

1. Asymmetric movements
2. Listlessness or irritability
3. Difficulty in feeding or swallowing or poor sucking with tongue thrust
4. Excessive, high-pitched, or feeble cry
5. Long, thin infants who are slow to gain weight
6. Poor head control

B. Late Signs
Late signs may include one or more of the following:

1. Failure to follow normal pattern of motor development. Delayed gross motor development is a universal manifestation of cerebral palsy.
2. Persistence of infantile reflexes

TABLE 44-1 Classification of Cerebral Palsy

Type	Characteristics
Classification by Clinical Type	

Spasticity—40%–50%; usually appears by 6 mo	1. Persistent primitive reflexes; delay of normal posture control, spastic paresis
	2. Arms pressed against body with forearm bent at right angle and hand flexed against forearm; in milder cases, fingers overextended and rotation of wrist on reaching
	3. Legs usually more involved than arms, but may be less involved
	  a. Mild cases—wide-based gait on walking
	  b. Moderate cases—slow and labored movements; walking jerky; balance poor
	  c. Severe cases—unable to sit or walk unsupported
	  d. Bilateral leg involvment—contractures cause scissoring (legs crossing and toes pointing out)

Dyskinesia—20%–25%; accentuated by emotional stress	1. Involuntary extraneous motor activity known as athetosis 2. Jerky, irregular, twisting movements of any or all extremities, especially the fingers and wrists, except when sleeping 3. Walk writhing, lurching, stumbling with incoordination of the arms 4. Improvement when well rested and calm
Ataxia—1%–10%	1. Difficulty achieving and maintaining balance, gross or fine motor incoordination 2. High-stepping, stumbling, or lurching gait 3. Nystagmus
Topographical Classification	
Hemiplegia—35%–40%	1. Findings limited to one side of the body 2. Arm usually involved more than leg
Diplegia—10%–20%	1. Similar parts of both sides of body involved 2. Legs usually involved more than arms
Paraplegia—10%–20%	1. Legs only involved
Quadriplegia—15%–20%	1. All four extremities involved 2. Upper and lower extremities affected equally
Monoplegia—rare	1. Only one extremity involved
Triplegia—rare	1. Three extremities involved
Classification by Degree of Severity	
Mild	1. Impairment of only fine precision movement
Moderate	1. Gross and fine movements and speech impaired 2. Able to perform usual activities of living
Severe	1. Inability to perform adequately the usual activities of living (walking, using hands, communicating verbally)

3. Weakness
4. Preference for one hand before the infant is 12 to 15 months old
5. Abnormal postures
6. Delayed or defective speech
7. Evidence of mental retardation

C. *Common Associated Findings*
1. Seizures
2. Hearing deficiency
3. Visual defect
4. Perceptual disorders
5. Mental retardation
6. Language disorders
7. Growth disorders
8. Gastroesophageal reflux
9. Behavioral problems

Diagnostic Evaluation

1. Thorough evaluation of prenatal, perinatal, and post-natal factors; APGAR scores

2. Laboratory data (computed tomography [CT] scan and blood testing) to rule out presence of toxins, infectious processes, neoplasms
3. Psychological testing to determine cognitive functioning

Treatment

1. Correction or alleviation of specific neuromotor deficits or associated disabilities
   a. Administration of antispasticity medications, such as dantrolene (Dantrium) or diazepam (Valium)
   b. Administration of antireflux medications, such as metoclopramide (Reglan) or bethanechol (Duvoid)
   c. Orthopedic management of scoliosis, contractures, dislocations
   d. Selective dorsal rhizotomy in an attempt to decrease spasticity
2. Developmental enrichment experiences
   a. Development of prevocational, vocational, and socialization skills
   b. Emotional, behavioral, and social adjustments

3. Family's ability to carry out supportive and participant roles in rehabilitation—key determinant of the success of any comprehensive management program

Nursing Assessment

1. Perform a functional assessment; determine ability to perform activities of daily living.
2. Perform a developmental assessment; use Denver developmental (p. 1070) or other screening tool.
3. Evaluate ability to protect airway—gag reflex, swallowing.
4. Assess nutritional status—growth, signs of deficiency.
5. Assess neuromuscular function and mobility—range of motion, spasticity, coordination.
6. Assess speech, hearing, vision.
7. Evaluate parent–child interactions.
8. Determine parents' understanding of and compliance with treatment plan.

Nursing Diagnoses

A. Impaired Physical Mobility related to altered neuromuscular functioning
B. Altered Growth and Development related to the nature and extent of the disorder
C. Altered Family Processes related to the nature of the defect, the demands of daily management, and resultant changes in family life
D. Risk for Injury related to deficit in motor activity and coordination

Nursing Interventions

A. **Increasing Mobility and Minimizing Deformity**
1. Carry out and teach the parents to carry out appropriate exercises under the direction of the physical therapist.
2. Use splints and braces to facilitate muscle control and improve body functioning.
   a. Apply as directed.
   b. Remove for recommended time.
   c. Inspect underlying skin for redness and irritation, signs of improper application, or poor fit.
3. Use assistive devices, such as adapted grooming tools, writing implements, and utensils, to enhance independence.
   a. Handles of toothbrushes, spoons, and forks can be built up with sponges or specially curved to make holding easier.
4. Encourage self-dressing with easy pull-on pants, large sweatshirts, and other loose clothing.
5. Use play, such as board games, ball games, peg boards, and puzzles, to improve coordination.
6. Maintain good body alignment to prevent contractures.
7. Provide adequate rest periods.
   a. Avoid exciting events before rest or bedtime.
   b. Administer or teach parents to administer muscle relaxants or anticonvulsants as prescribed.
   c. Schedule physical therapy after child has rested, and avoid stress and frustration during physical therapy.

B. **Maximizing Growth and Development**
1. Evaluate the child's developmental level and then assist with tasks within that level.
2. Provide for continuity of care at home, day care, therapy centers, and the hospital.
   a. Obtain a thorough history from the parents regarding the child's usual home routines, weaknesses and strengths, and likes and dislikes.
   b. Communicate with representatives from all disciplines involved in the child's care.
   c. Formulate a consistent care plan that incorporates the goals of all related disciplines and meets the needs of the child and family. Include in the care plan guidelines for the following:
      (1) Feeding
      (2) Sleeping
      (3) Physical therapy
      (4) Play
      (5) Other ways to foster growth and development
      (6) Special interests and emotional needs, such as use of security objects
3. During feeding, maintain a pleasant, distraction free environment.
   a. Provide a comfortable chair.
   b. Serve the child alone, initially. After the child begins to master the task of eating, encourage the child to eat with other children.
   c. Do not attempt feedings if the child is very fatigued.
   d. Find the eating position in which the child can be most self-sufficient.
   e. Allow the child to hold the spoon even if self-feeding is minimal.
   f. Stand behind and reach over the child's shoulder to guide the spoon from the plate to the child's mouth.
   g. Serve foods that stick to the spoon, such as thick applesauce or mashed potatoes.
   h. Encourage finger foods that the child can handle alone.
   i. Provide appropriate assistive devices for independent feeding, such as spoon and fork with special handles, plate and glass holders, and special feeding chair.
   j. Disregard "messy" eating; use a large plastic bib, smock, or towel to protect the child's clothes.
4. If the child must be fed, do so slowly and carefully. Be aware of any difficulty sucking and swallowing due to poor muscle control.
   a. Cut solid foods into small pieces.
   b. Place the food back on the tongue for ease in swallowing.
5. Be alert for associated sensory deficits that delay development and could be corrected.
   a. Hearing, speech, vision
   b. Squinting, failure to follow objects, or bringing objects very close to the face

C. **Strengthening Family Processes**
1. Encourage the parents to express their feelings about the child and cerebral palsy, and help them to deal with these feelings.
2. Assist the parents to appraise the child's assets so that they may capitalize on these positive features.
   a. Early recognition of the extent of the child's disability and realistic direction for obtainable goals are essential.
   b. Help the parents to recognize immediate needs and identify short-term goals that can be integrated into the long-range plan.

3. Acknowledge the numerous challenges of daily care of a child with cerebral palsy, and allow the parents to express frustration over the many demands and limited resources for such care.
4. Provide positive feedback for effective parenting skills and positive approaches to caring for the child.
5. Assist the parents to deal with siblings' responses to the disabled child.
   a. Encourage parents to find time to spend with each sibling separately.
   b. Encourage family to maintain contacts with friends and community and engage in outside activities as much as possible.
   c. Suggest family counselling.
6. Assist the parents to secure respite care to provide a break from the day-to-day care of the child with cerebral palsy when needed.
7. Assist parents to find local resources to help in the child's care.
   a. Look in phone book for county social service agency.
   b. Contact hospital social worker or discharge planner.
   c. Contact local United Way or Catholic Charities office.
   d. Visit public library to look up specific community service programs.

D. *Protecting the Child From Injury*
1. Evaluate the child's need for specific safety measures, such as suction machine, safety helmet, or seizure precautions, and modify the environment as appropriate to ensure the child's safety.
2. Select toys that are safe.

Family Education/Health Maintenance

1. Instruct the parents in all areas of the child's physical care.
2. Encourage regular medical and dental evaluations.
   a. The child should receive all regular immunizations.
   b. Dental visits should occur every 6 months, starting at the age of 2 years.
3. Advise parents that the child needs discipline to feel secure and relaxed.
   a. Set realistic limits within which the child can function successfully.
   b. Be firm but not rejecting.
4. Refer parents to agencies such as The United Cerebral Palsy Association of America, Inc.; 1660 L St. NW, Suite 700 Washington, DC, 20036; 1-800-872-5827.

Evaluation

A. Dressing and feeding independently; no contractures noted
B. Consistent growth curve maintained; sequential developmental milestones consistent with condition achieved
C. Participation in school and community activities; use of respite care once a week
D. Child wearing bicycle helmet while playing outdoors; no injury reported

◆ HYDROCEPHALUS

Hydrocephalus is a condition of altered production, flow, or absorption of cerebrospinal fluid. It is characterized by an abnormal increase in cerebrospinal fluid volume within the intracranial cavity and by enlargement of the head in infancy.

Etiology and Incidence

1. Obstruction in the system between the source of cerebrospinal fluid production (ventricles) and the area of its reabsorption (the subarachnoid space); noncommunicating hydrocephalus
   a. May be partial, intermittent, or complete
   b. Majority of cases
   c. Causes
      (1) Congenital defects, such as Arnold-Chiari malformation, Dandy-Walker cyst (etiology largely unknown)
      (2) Acquired conditions, such as infections, trauma, spontaneous intracranial bleeding, and neoplasms
2. Failure in the absorption system (communicating type)—cause unknown
3. Excessive production of cerebrospinal fluid (communicating type)—tumor or unknown causes (rare)
4. Approximately 3 to 4 cases per 1,000 births, including those associated with spina bifida

Altered Physiology

1. The ventricular system is greatly distended.
2. The increased ventricular pressure results in thinning of the cerebral cortex and cranial bones, especially in the frontal, parietal, and temporal areas.
3. The floor of the third ventricle commonly bulges downward, compresses the optic nerves, dilates the sella turcica, and often compresses the hypophysis cerebri.
4. The basal ganglia, brain stem, and cerebellum remain relatively normal but compressed.
5. The choroid plexus is usually atrophied to some degree.

Complications

1. Seizures
2. Herniation of the brain
3. Spontaneous arrest due to natural compensatory mechanisms, persistent increased intracranial pressure (IICP), and brain herniation
4. Developmental delays

Clinical Manifestations

May be rapid, slow and steadily advancing, or remittent. Clinical signs depend on the age of the child, whether or not the anterior fontanel has closed, whether the cranial sutures have fused, and the type and duration of hydrocephalus.

A. *Infants*
1. Excessive head growth (may be seen up to 3 years of age)
2. Delayed closure of the anterior fontanel
3. Fontanel tense and elevated above the surface of the skull
4. Signs of IICP
   a. Vomiting
   b. Restlessness and irritability
   c. High-pitched, shrill cry
   d. Alteration in vital signs—increased systolic blood pressure, decreased pulse, decreased and irregular respirations
   e. Pupillary changes
   f. Seizures
   g. Lethargy
   h. Stupor
   i. Coma
5. Alteration of muscle tone of the extremities
6. Later physical signs
   a. Forehead becomes prominent ("bossing").
   b. Scalp appears shiny with prominent scalp veins.
   c. Eyebrows and eyelids may be drawn upward, exposing the sclera above the iris.
   d. Infant cannot gaze upward, causing "sunset eyes."
   e. Strabismus, nystagmus, and optic atrophy may occur.
   f. Infant has difficulty holding head up.
   g. Child may experience physical or mental developmental lag.

B. *Older Children*
Older children have closed sutures and present with signs of IICP.

1. Headache, especially on awakening
2. Vomiting
3. Lethargy, fatigue, apathy
4. Personality changes
5. Separation of cranial sutures (may be seen in children up to 10 years of age)
6. Double vision, constricted peripheral vision, sudden appearance of internal strabismus, pupillary changes
7. Alteration in vital signs similar to those seen in infants
8. Difficulty with gait
9. Stupor
10. Coma
11. Papilledema

Diagnostic Evaluation

1. Infant's head transilluminates, indicative of abnormal fluid collection.
2. Percussion of the infant's skull may produce a typical "cracked pot" sound (Macewen's sign).
3. Ophthalmoscopy may reveal papilledema.
4. CT scan is the diagnostic tool of choice.
5. With ventriculography (rarely used), abnormalities are visualized in the ventricular system or the subarachnoid space.
6. Skull x-rays show widening of the fontanel and sutures and erosion of intracranial bone.

Treatment

Hydrocephalus can be treated through a variety of surgical procedures, including direct operation on the lesion causing the obstruction, such as a tumor; intracranial shunts for selected cases of noncommunicating hydrocephalus to divert fluid from the obstructed segment of the ventricular system to the subarachnoid space; and extracranial shunts (most common) to divert fluid from the ventricular system to an extracranial compartment, frequently the peritoneum or right atrium.

A. *Extracranial Shunt Procedures*
1. Ventriculoperitoneal shunt (V-P shunt)
   a. Diverts cerebrospinal fluid from a lateral ventricle or the spinal subarachnoid space to the peritoneal cavity.
   b. A tube is passed from the lateral ventricle through an occipital burr hole subcutaneously through the posterior aspect of neck and paraspinal region to the peritoneal cavity through a small incision in the right lower quadrant.
2. Ventriculoatrial shunt (V-A shunt)
   a. A tube is passed from the dilated lateral ventricle through a burr hole in the parietal region of the skull.
   b. It then is passed under the skin behind the ear and into a vein down to a point where it discharges into the right atrium or superior vena cava.
   c. A one-way pressure sensitive valve will close to prevent reflux of blood into the ventricle and open as ventricular pressure rises, allowing fluid to pass from the ventricle into the bloodstream.
3. Ventriculopleural shunt
   a. Diverts cerebrospinal fluid to the pleural cavity
   b. Indicated when the V-P or V-A route cannot be used
4. Ventricle-gall bladder shunt
   a. Diverts cerebrospinal fluid to the common bile duct
   b. Used when all other routes are unavailable
5. Most shunts have the following components:
   a. Ventricular tubing
   b. A one-way or unidirectional pressure sensitive flow valve
   c. A pumping chamber
   d. Distal tubing

B. *Shunt Complications*
1. Need for shunt revision frequently occurs because of occlusion, infection, or malfunction.
2. Shunt revision may be necessary because of growth of the child. Newer models, however, include coiled tubing to allow the shunt to grow with the child.
3. Shunt dependency frequently occurs. The child rapidly manifests symptoms of IICP if the shunt does not function optimally.
4. Children with ventriculoatrial shunts may experience endocardial contusions and clotting, leading to bacterial endocarditis, bacteremia, and ventriculitis or thromboembolism and cor pulmonale.

C. *Prognosis*
1. Prognosis is dependent on early diagnosis and prompt therapy.
2. With improved diagnostic and management techniques, the prognosis is becoming considerably better.
   a. Many children experience normal motor and intellectual development.
   b. The severity of neurologic deficits is directly proportional to the interval between onset of hydrocephalus and the time of diagnosis.
3. Hydrocephalus due to meningitis might spontaneously resolve due to gradual disappearance of adhesions.

4. Approximately two-thirds of patients will die at an early age if they do not receive surgical treatment.

Nursing Assessment

A. Infants
1. Assess head circumference.
  a. Measure at the occipitofrontal circumference—point of largest measurement.
  b. Measure the head at approximately the same time each day.
  c. Use a centimeter measure for greatest accuracy.
2. Palpate fontanel for tenseness, bulging.
3. Assess pupillary response.
4. Assess level of consciousness.
5. Evaluate breathing patterns and effectiveness.
6. Assess feeding patterns and patterns of emesis.
7. Assess motor activity.
8. Determine attainment of developmental milestones.

B. Older Child
1. Measure vital signs for signs of IICP.
2. Assess patterns of headache, emesis.
3. Determine pupillary response.
4. Evaluate level of consciousness.
5. Assess motor function.
6. Evaluate attainment of milestones, school performance.
7. Obtain parents' report of recent behavior.

Nursing Diagnoses

A. Altered Cerebral Tissue perfusion related to IICP prior to surgery
B. Altered Nutrition: Less than body requirements related to reduced oral intake and vomiting
C. Risk for Impaired Skin Integrity related to alterations in level of consciousness and enlarged head
D. Anxiety (of parents) related to child undergoing surgery
E. Risk for Injury related to malfunctioning shunt
F. Risk for Fluid Volume Deficit related to cerebrospinal fluid drainage, decreased intake postoperatively
G. Risk for Infection related to bacterial infiltration of the shunt
H. Ineffective Family Coping related to diagnosis and surgery

Nursing Interventions

A. Maintaining Cerebral Perfusion
1. Observe for evidence of IICP, and report immediately.

> **NURSING ALERT:**
> Brain stem herniation can occur with IICP and is manifested by opisthotonic positioning (flexion of head and feet backward). This is a grave sign and may be followed by respiratory arrest. Obtain help, and prepare for ventricular tap. Have emergency equipment on hand for resuscitation.

2. Assist with diagnositic procedures to determine cause of hydrocephalus and indication for surgical intervention.

a. Explain the procedure to the child and parents at their levels of comprehension.
b. Administer prescribed sedatives 30 minutes before the procedure to ensure their effectiveness.
c. Organize activities so that the child is permitted to rest after administration of the sedative.

> **NURSING ALERT:**
> Sedatives are contraindicated in many cases because IICP predisposes the child to hypoventilation or respiratory arrest. If they are administered, the child should be observed very closely for evidence of respiratory depression.

  e. Observe the child closely following ventriculography:
    (1) Leaking of cerebrospinal fluid from the sites of subdural or ventricular taps. These tap holes should be covered with a small piece of gauze or cotton saturated with collodion.
    (2) Reactions to the sedative, especially respiratory depression
    (3) Changes in vital signs indicative of shock
    (4) Signs of IICP, which may occur if air has been injected into the ventricles

B. Providing Adequate Nutrition
1. Be aware that feeding is often a problem because the child may be listless, anorectic, and prone to vomiting.
2. Complete nursing care and treatments before feeding so that the child will not be disturbed after feeding.
3. Hold the infant in a semisitting position with head well supported during feeding. Allow ample time for bubbling.
4. Offer small, frequent feedings.
5. Place the child on side with head elevated after feeding to prevent aspiration.

C. Maintaining Skin Integrity
1. Prevent pressure sores (pressure sores of the head are a frequent problem) by placing the child on a sponge rubber or lamb's wool pad or an alternating-pressure or egg crate mattress to keep weight evenly distributed.
2. Keep the scalp clean and dry.
3. Turn the child's head frequently; change position at least every 2 hours.
  a. When turning the child, rotate head and body together to prevent strain on the neck.
  b. A firm pillow may be placed under the child's head and shoulders for further support when lifting the child.
4. Provide meticulous skin care to all parts of the body, and observe skin for the effects of pressure.
5. Give passive range-of-motion exercises to the extremities, especially the legs.
6. Keep the eyes moistened with artificial tears if the child is unable to close the eyelids normally. This prevents corneal ulcerations and infections.

D. Reducing Anxiety
1. Prepare the parents for their child's surgery by answering questions, describing what nursing care will take place postoperatively, and explaining how the shunt will work.
2. Encourage the parents to discuss all the risks and benefits with the surgeon. Help them to understand the prognosis and what to expect of the child's neurologic and cognitive development.

3. Prepare the child for surgery by using dolls or other forms of play to describe what interventions will occur.

E. *Improving Cerebral Tissue Perfusion Postoperatively*
1. Monitor the child's temperature, pulse, respiration, blood pressure, and pupillary size and reaction every 15 minutes until stable; then monitor every 1 to 2 hours.
2. Avoid hypothermia or hyperthermia.
   a. Provide appropriate blankets or covers, an Isolette or infant warmer, or hypothermia blanket.
   b. Administer a tepid sponge bath or antipyretic medication for temperature elevation.
3. Aspirate mucus from the nose and throat as necessary to prevent respiratory difficulty.
4. Turn the child frequently.
5. Promote optimal drainage of cerebrospinal fluid through the shunt by pumping the shunt and positioning the child as directed.
   a. If pumping is prescribed, carefully compress the valve the specified number of times at regularly scheduled intervals.
   b. Report any difficulties in pumping the shunt.
   c. Gradually elevate the head of child's bed to 30 to 45 degrees as ordered. Initially the child will be positioned flat to prevent excessive cerebrospinal fluid drainage.
6. Assess for excessive drainage of cerebrospinal fluid.
   a. Sunken fontanel, agitation, restlessness (infant)
   b. Decreased level of consciousness (older child)
7. Assess closely for IICP, indicating shunt malfunction.
   a. Note especially change in level of consciousness, change in vital signs (increased systolic blood pressure, decreased pulse rate, decreased or irregular respirations), vomiting, pupillary changes.
   b. Report these changes immediately to prevent cerebral hypoxia and possible brain herniation.
8. Prevent excessive pressure of skin overlying shunt by placing cotton behind and over the ears under the head dressing and avoiding positioning the child on the area of the valve or the incision until the wound is well healed.

F. *Maintaining Fluid Balance*
1. Accurately measure and record total fluid intake and output.
2. Administer intravenous (IV) fluids as prescribed; carefully monitor infusion rate to prevent fluid overload.
3. Use a nasogastric tube if necessary for abdominal distention.
   a. This is most frequently used when a ventriculoperitoneal shunt has been performed.
   b. Measure the drainage, and record the amount and color.
   c. Monitor for return of bowel sounds after nasogastric suction has been disconnected for at least 30 minutes.
4. Give frequent mouth care while the child is to have nothing by mouth (NPO).
5. Begin oral feedings once the child is fully recovered from the anesthetic and displays interest.
   a. Begin with small amounts of 5% dextrose water.
   b. Gradually introduce formula.
   c. Introduce solid foods suitable to the child's age and tolerance.
   d. Encourage a high-protein diet.

e. Observe for and report any decrease in urine output, increased urine specific gravity, diminished skin turgor, dryness of mucous membranes, or lethargy, indicating dehydration.

G. *Preventing Infection*
1. Assess for fever (temperature normally fluctuates during the first 24 hours after surgery), purulent drainage from the incision, or swelling, redness, and tenderness along the shunt tract.
2. Administer prescribed prophylactic antibiotics.

H. *Strengthening Family Coping*
1. Begin discharge planning early, including specific techniques for care of the shunt and suggested methods for providing daily care.
   a. Turning, holding, and positioning
   b. Skin care over shunt
   c. Exercises to strenghten muscles—incorporated with play
   d. Feeding techniques and schedule
   e. Pumping the shunt
2. Accompany all instructions with reassurance necessary to prevent the parents from becoming anxious or fearful about assuming the care of the child.
3. Encourage the parents to treat the child as normally as possible, providing him or her with appropriate toys and love.
4. Help the parents to assist siblings to understand hydrocephalus and the child's special needs. Encourage parents to spend individual time with siblings and not to neglect their needs as well. Suggest family counselling if needed.
5. Assist parents in locating additional resources.
   a. Social worker, discharge planner, or department of social services
   b. Visiting or home health nurses or aides
   c. Parent groups
   d. Community agencies
   e. Special programs at school

Family Education/Health Maintenance

1. Stress the importance of recognizing symptoms of IICP and reporting them immediately.
2. Advise parents to report shunt malfunction or infection immediately to prevent IICP.
3. Teach parents that illnesses that cause vomiting and diarrhea or that prevent an adequate fluid intake are a great threat to the child who has had a shunt procedure. Advise parents to consult with the child's healthcare provider about immediate treatment of fever, control of vomiting and diarrhea, and replacement of fluids.
4. Tell the parents that few restrictions are required for children with shunts and to consult with the healthcare provider about specific concerns.

Evaluation

A. No changes in vital signs, level of consciousness, or head size; no vomiting; pupils equal and responsive
B. Feeding every 4 hours without vomiting
C. No erythema, blanching, or skin breakdown

D. Parents verbalizing purpose and type of operative procedure, risks, and benefits
E. Shunt pumping without resistance; stable level of consciousness and vital signs
F. Urine output less than intake; skin turgor normal; electrolytes within normal limits
G. Afebrile; no drainage from shunt site
H. Parents actively seeking resources, showing affection for patient and siblings

◆ SPINA BIFIDA

Spina bifida, also called spinal dysraphia, refers to a malformation of the spine in which the posterior portion of the laminae of the vertebrae fails to close. Several types of spina bifida are recognized, of which the following three are most common (Fig. 44-1):

1. *Spina bifida occulta*, in which the defect is only in the vertebrae. The spinal cord and meninges are normal.
2. *Meningocele*, in which the meninges protrude through the opening in the spinal canal. This forms a cyst filled with cerebrospinal fluid and covered with skin.
3. *Myelomeningocele* (or meningomyelocele), in which both the spinal cord and cord membranes protrude through the defect in the laminae of the vertebral column. Myelomeningoceles are covered by a thin membrane.

Etiology and Incidence

1. Unknown but generally thought to result from genetic predisposition triggered by something in the environment.
2. Involves an arrest in the orderly formation of the vertebral arches and spinal cord that occurs between the fourth and sixth week of embryogenesis.
3. Theories of causation follow:
   a. There is incomplete closure of the neural tube during the fourth week of embryonic life.
   b. The neural tube forms adequately but then ruptures.
4. Geographic distribution and incidence vary widely.
5. Condition occurs in approximately 1 per 1,000 live births in the United States.
6. It is the most common developmental defect of the central nervous system (CNS).
7. It is more common in white than in nonwhite people.
8. The condition may have other congenital anomalies associated with it.
9. Women who have spina bifida and parents who have one affected child have an increased risk of producing children with neural tube defects.

Altered Physiology

A. *Spina Bifida Occulta (Most Common)*
1. The bony defect may range from a very thin slit separating one lamina from the spinous process to a complete absence of the spine and laminae.
2. A thin, fibrous membrane sometimes covers the defect.
3. The spinal cord and its meninges may be connected with a fistulous tract extending to and opening onto the surface of the skin.

B. *Meningocele*
1. The defect may occur anywhere on the cord. Higher defects (from thorax and upward) are usually meningoceles.
2. Surgical correction is necessary to prevent rupture of the sac and subsequent infection.
3. Prognosis is good with surgical correction.

C. *Myelomeningocele (Meningomyelocele)*
1. Occurs four to five times more frequently than meningocele.
2. The lesion contains both the spinal cord and cord membranes. A bluish area may be evident on the top because of exposed neural tissue.

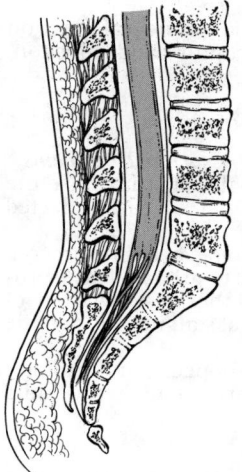 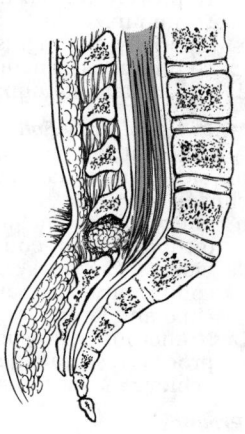 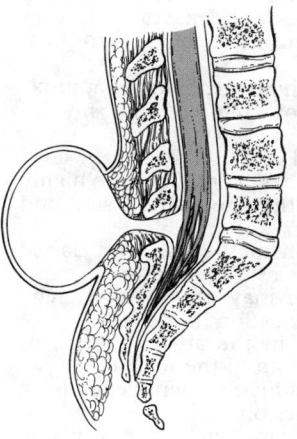 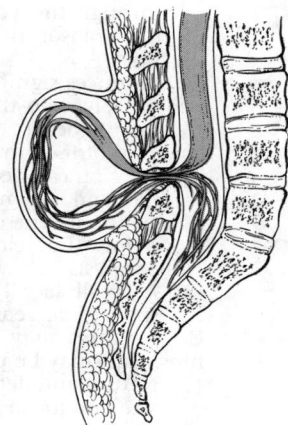

A B C D

FIGURE 44-1 Spina bifida. **(A)** Normal spine. **(B)** Spina bifida occulta. **(C)** Spina bifida with meningocele. **(D)** Spina bifida with myelomeningocele.

3. The sac may leak in utero or may rupture after birth, allowing free drainage of cerebrospinal fluid. This renders the child highly susceptible to meningitis.

Complications

1. Hydrocephalus associated with meningocele; may be aggravated by surgical repair
2. Scoliosis, contractures, and joint dislocation
3. Skin breakdown in sensory denervated areas and under braces

Clinical Manifestations

A. *Spina Bifida Occulta*
1. Most patients have no symptoms.
   a. They may have a dimple in the skin or a growth of hair over the malformed vertebra.
   b. There is no externally visible sac.
2. With growth, the child may develop foot weakness or bowel and bladder sphincter disturbances.

B. *Meningocele*
1. An external cystic defect can be seen in the spinal cord, usually in the center line.
   a. The sac is composed only of meninges and is filled with cerebrospinal fluid.
   b. The cord and nerve roots are usually normal.
2. There is seldom evidence of weakness of the legs or lack of sphincter control.

C. *Myelomeningocele*
1. A round, raised, and poorly epithelialized area may be noted at any level of the spinal column. However, the highest incidence of the lesion occurs in the lumbosacral area. Clinical problems due to myelomeningocele include the following:
   a. Arnold-Chiari malformation
      (1) Associated malformation involving the brain stem and cerebellum
      (2) Causes a block in the flow of cerebrospinal fluid through the ventricles and leads to failure in the reabsorption mechanism of cerebrospinal fluid
      (3) Produces significant hydrocephalus in approximately two-thirds of children with myelomeningocele
   b. Loss of motor control and sensation below the level of the lesion can occur. These conditions are highly variable and depend on the size of the lesion and its position on the cord.
      (1) A low thoracic lesion may cause total flaccid paralysis below the waist.
      (2) A small sacral lesion may cause only patchy spots of decreased sensation in the feet.
   c. Contractures may occur in the ankles, knees, or hips. Hips may be pulled out of the sockets.
      (1) Nature and degree of involvement depends on size and location of lesion.
      (2) This occurs because some fibers of innervation do get through. One side of a hip, knee, or ankle may be innervated while the opposing side may not be. The unopposed side then becomes pulled out of position.
   d. Clubfeet are a common accompanying anomaly.
      (1) This anomaly is thought to be related to the position of paraplegic feet in the uterus.
   e. Bladder dysfunction can occur.
      (1) Almost all lesions affect the sacral nerves that innervate the bladder.
      (2) The bladder fails to respond to normal messages that it is time to void and simply fills and overflows, causing incontinence and susceptibility to urinary tract infections because of incomplete emptying.
   f. Fecal incontinence and constipation are caused by poor innervation of the anal sphincter and bowel musculature.
2. Developmental disabilities include the following:
   a. Most children have average intellectual ability despite hydrocephalus.
   b. Most children are able to learn in a "mainstreamed" school environment, provided they are able to overcome other barriers (architectural and attitudinal).
   c. The most significant problems are secondarily handicapping conditions that develop when a child has a disability of this degree.

Diagnostic Evaluation

1. Prenatal detection is now possible through amniocentesis and measurement of alpha-fetoprotein. This testing should be offered to all women at risk (women who are affected or have had other affected children).
2. Diagnosis is primarily based on clinical manifestations.
3. CT scan and magnetic resonance imaging may be performed to evaluate further the brain and spinal cord.

Treatment

A. *Surgical Intervention*
1. Procedure
   a. Laminectomy and closure of the open lesion or removal of the sac usually can be done soon after birth.
2. Purpose
   a. To prevent further deterioration of neural function
   b. To minimize the danger of rupture and infection, especially meningitis
   c. To improve cosmetic effect
   d. To facilitate handling of the infant

B. *Multidisciplinary Follow-up for Associated Problems*
1. A coordinated team approach will help maximize the physical and intellectual potential of each affected child.
   a. The team may include a neurologist, neurosurgeon, orthopedic surgeon, urologist, primary care provider, social worker, physical therapist, a variety of community-based and hospital staff nurses, and the child and family.
   b. Numerous neurosurgical, orthopedic, and urologic procedures may be necessary to help the child achieve maximum potential.

C. *Prognosis*
1. Influenced by the site of the lesion and the presence and degree of associated hydrocephalus. Generally, the higher the defect, the greater the extent of neurologic deficit and the greater the likelihood of hydrocephalus.

a. In the absence of treatment, most infants with meningomyelocele die early in infancy.
b. Surgical intervention is most effective if it is done early in the neonatal period, preferably within the first few days of life.
c. Even with surgical intervention, infants can be expected to manifest associated neurosurgical, orthopedic, or urologic problems.
d. New techniques of treatment, intensive research, and improved services have increased life expectancy and have greatly enhanced the quality of life for most children who receive treatment.

Nursing Assessment

1. Assess sensory and motor response of lower extremities.
2. Assess ability to void spontaneously, retention of urine, symptoms of urinary tract infection.
3. Assess usual stooling patterns, need for medications to facilitate elimination.
4. Assess mobility and use of braces, casts, and other special equipment.

Nursing Diagnoses

Preoperative: Neonatal Period

A. Risk for Impaired Skin Integrity related to impaired motor and sensory function
B. Risk for Infection related to contamination of the myelomeningocele site
C. Altered Urinary Elimination related to neurologic deficits
D. Altered Cerebral Tissue Perfusion related to potential hydrocephalus
E. Fear (parents) related to neonate with neurologic disorder and to surgery

Postoperative: Infancy and Childhood

F. Ineffective Thermoregulation following surgery
G. Reflex Incontinence related to sacral denervation
H. Bowel Incontinence/Constipation related to impaired innervation of anal sphincter and bowel musculature
I. Body Image Disturbance related to the child's appearance, difficulties with locomotion, and lack of control over excretory functions

Nursing Interventions

Preoperative: Neonatal Period

A. **Protecting Skin Integrity**
 1. Avoid positioning on the infant's back to prevent pressure on the sac. Check position at least once every hour.
 2. Do not place a diaper or other covering directly over the sac.
 3. Observe the sac frequently for evidence of irritation or leakage of cerebrospinal fluid.
 4. Use prone positioning with hips only slightly flexed to decrease tension on the sac.

5. Place a foam rubber pad covered with a soft cloth between the infant's legs to maintain the hips in abduction and to prevent or counteract subluxation. A diaper roll or small pillow may be used in place of the foam rubber pad.
6. Allow the infant's feet to hang freely over the pads or mattress edge to prevent aggravation of foot deformities.
7. Provide meticulous skin care to all areas of the body, especially ankles, knees, tip of nose, cheeks, and chin.
8. Provide passive range-of-motion exercises for muscles and joints that the infant does not use spontaneously. Avoid hip exercises because of common hip dislocation, unless otherwise recommended.
9. Use a foam or fleece pad to reduce pressure of the mattress against the infant's skin.
10. Avoid pressure on infant's back during feeding by holding the infant with your elbow rotated to avoid touching the sac, or feeding while infant is lying on side or prone on your lap. Encourage parents to use these positions to provide infant stimulation and bonding.

B. **Preventing Infection**
 1. Be aware that infection of the sac is most commonly caused by contamination by urine and feces.
 2. Keep the buttocks and genitalia scrupulously clean.
   a. Do not diaper the infant if the defect is in the lower portion of the spine.
   b. Use a small plastic drape taped between the defect and the anus to help to prevent contamination.
 3. Apply a sterile gauze pad or towel or a sterile, moistened dressing over the sac as directed.
   a. When the sterile covering is used, it should be changed frequently to keep the area free of exudate and to maintain sterility.
   b. Care must be taken to prevent the covering from adhering to and damaging the sac.
 4. Monitor and report immediately any signs of infection.
   a. Oozing of fluid or pus from the sac
   b. Fever
   c. Irritability or listlessness
   d. Seizure

C. **Promoting Urinary Elimination**
 1. Use the Credé method for emptying the bladder (unless contraindicated by vesicoureteral reflux), and teach parents the technique.
   a. Apply firm, gentle pressure to the abdomen, beginning in the umbilical area and progressing toward the symphysis pubis.
   b. Continue the procedure as long as urine can be manually expressed.
 2. Ensure fluid intake to dilute the urine.
 3. Administer prescribed prophylactic antibiotics.
 4. Monitor and report concentrated or foul-smelling urine.

D. **Maintaining Cerebral Tissue Perfusion**
 1. Monitor for signs of hydrocephalus, and report immediately.
   a. Irritability
   b. Feeding difficulty, vomiting, decreased appetite
   c. Temperature fluctuation
   d. Decreased alertness
   e. Tense fontanel
   f. Increased head circumference

E. **Reducing Fear**
 1. Encourage parents to express feelings of guilt, fear, lack of control, or helplessness.

2. Provide accurate information about spina bifida and what to expect postoperatively.

3. Include the parents in all of infant's care, and encourage private bonding time.

Postoperative: Infancy and Childhood

F. *Preventing Complications*

1. Frequently monitor temperature, pulse, respirations, color, and level of responsiveness postoperatively, based on the infant's stability.

2. Use an Isolette or infant warmer to prevent temperature fluctuation.

3. Prevent respiratory complications
  a. Periodically reposition the infant to promote lung expansion.
  b. Watch for abdominal distention, which could interfere with breathing.
  c. Have oxygen available.

4. Maintain hydration and nutritional intake.
  a. Administer IV fluids as ordered; keep accurate intake and output log.
  b. Administer gavage feedings as ordered.
  c. Begin bottle feeding when infant is responsive and tolerating feedings. Give small, frequent feedings slowly so that air can be expelled naturally without bubbling.

5. Keep the surgical dressing clean and dry, and observe for drainage. Avoid pressure to the area and diapers that cover the incision until well healed.

6. Monitor for and teach parents to recognize signs of hydrocephalus. Report immediately.

7. Be aware that children with spina bifida have a far greater risk for latex allergy than the general population, estimated at up to 20% of spina bifida patients.
  a. Symptoms include hives, itching, wheezing, and anaphylaxis.
  b. Incidence increases with time and may be related to repeated exposure to products containing latex.
  c. Limit or prevent direct contact of the child to products routinely used that contain latex, such as blood pressure cuffs, tourniquets, tape, foley catheters, gloves, and IV tubing injection ports. Develop protocols specifying modification of care for children at risk for latex allergy.

COMMUNITY-BASED CARE TIP:
Toys and equipment for children, such as nipples, pacifiers, and elastic on the legs of disposable diapers, also contain latex. The home environment should be surveyed for latex and substitute products obtained, if possible. Teach the parents how to recognize latex allergy and to notify the child's healthcare provider.

G. *Achieving Continence*

1. Teach parents that continence can usually be achieved with clean, intermittent self-catheterization.
  a. Children can generally be taught to catheterize themselves by the age of 6 to 7 years.
  b. Parents can catheterize younger children.

2. Teach the following procedure:
  a. Gather equipment: catheter, water-soluble lubricant, soap and water, urine collection container.
  b. Wash hands.
  c. Clean the area around the urethral meatus.
  d. Lubricate the catheter tip.
  e. Insert the catheter until urine starts to flow.
  f. Remove catheter when urine is drained from bladder.
  g. Clean off any lubricant from child.
  h. Dispose of urine.
  i. Wash hands.

COMMUNITY-BASED CARE TIP:
The family can be taught to clean and reuse urinary catheters. The catheter should be washed in warm, soapy water and rinsed well in warm water. The catheter should be air dried and when completely dried, placed in a clean jar or plastic bag. A catheter should be replaced when it becomes dry, cracked, stiff, or if the child develops a urinary tract infection.

3. Teach about the action of medications, such as imipramine hydrochloride (Tofranil) and ephedrine sulfate (Ephed II), if prescribed, which are used to help children retain urine rather than dribbling. When used with self-catheterization, many children can stay dry for 3 to 4 hours at a time.

4. Teach the signs of urinary tract infection (concentrated, foul-smelling urine; burning; and fever) and the proper administration of antibiotics either prophylactically or when prescribed for infection.

5. For children who cannot achieve urinary continence through intermittent catheterization, provide information about options, such as surgically implanted mechanical urinary sphincters and bladder pacemakers, indwelling catheters or external collecting devices, or urinary diversion (may be necessary in some cases).

H. *Achieving Regular Bowel Elimination*

1. Assist with bowel training program to compensate for decreased sacral sensation.
  a. Children are placed on a toileting schedule and are taught to push.
  b. Medications, such as stool softeners, suppositories, or enemas, may be used initially to help determine scheduling.

2. To prevent constipation and enhance fecal control, encourage intake of high-fiber, high-fluid diet. Medications such as psyllium (Metamucil) may be used to increase bulk or soften stool.

I. *Fostering Positive Body Image*

1. Emphasize rehabilitation that makes use of the child's strengths and minimizes disabilities.

2. Continually reassess functional abilities, and offer suggestions to increase independence. Periodically consult with physical or occupational therapists to help maximize function.

3. Encourage the use of braces and specialized equipment to enhance ambulation while minimizing the appearance of the equipment. For example, wear pants instead of dresses or shorts to cover leg braces; choose a compact wheelchair that can be decorated or personalized for the child.

4. Encourage participation with peer group and in activities that build on strengths, such as cognitive abilities, interest in music, or art.

5. Periodically reassess bowel and bladder programs. The ability to stay dry for reasonable time intervals is one of the greatest factors in enhancing self-esteem and positive body image.

Family Education/Health Maintenance

1. Prepare the parents to feed, hold, and stimulate their infant as naturally as possible.
2. Teach the parents the special techniques that may be required for holding and positioning, feeding, caring for the incision, emptying the bladder, and exercising muscles.
3. Alert the parents to safety needs of the child with decreased sensation, such as protection from prolonged pressure, the risk of burns due to bath water that is too warm, and avoidance of trauma from contact with sharp objects.
4. Instruct the parents to notify the healthcare provider for signs of associated problems, such as hydrocephalus, meningitis, urinary tract infection, and latex sensitivity.
5. Urge continued follow-up and health maintenance, including immunizations and evaluation of growth and development.
6. Advise parents that children with paralysis are at risk for becoming overweight due to inactivity, so they should provide a low-fat, balanced diet; control snacking; and encourage as much activity as possible.
7. For additional resources, refer families to agencies such as The Spina Bifida Association of America; 4590 MacArthur Blvd. NW, Suite 250; Washington, DC 20007; 800-621-3141.

Evaluation

A. No signs of meningeal sac or skin breakdown
B. Afebrile, alert, and active
C. Voiding at intervals; clear urine without odor
D. Fontanel soft; head circumference stable
E. Parents asking questions about surgery, showing affection for infant
F. Vital signs stable; incisional dressing dry and intact
G. Parents/child demonstrate proper catheterization technique
H. Passing stool once a day
I. Child verbalizes participation in chorus, girl or boy scouts, or school activities

◆ BACTERIAL MENINGITIS

Bacterial meningitis is an inflammation of the meninges that follows the invasion of the spinal fluid by a bacterial agent.

Etiology and Incidence

1. The proportion of cases due to a specific organism varies from year to year; there also is considerable geographic difference.
2. The organisms most commonly causing bacterial meningitis in different age groups follow:
   a. Birth to 3 months
      (1) *Escherichia coli*
      (2) *Streptococcus*, group B
      (3) *Listeria monocytogenes*
   b. 3 months to 6 years
      (1) *Haemophilus influenzae*
      (2) *Streptococcus pneumoniae*
      (3) *Neisseria meningitidis*
   c. 6 to 16 years
      (1) *S. pneumoniae*
      (2) *N. meningitidis*
      (3) *Mycobacterium tuberculosis*
3. Most cases are seen in children younger than 5 years.

Altered Physiology

1. Bacterial meningitis is frequently preceded by an upper respiratory infection, which is complicated by bacteremia.
2. Bacteria in the circulating blood then invade the cerebrospinal fluid.
3. Less commonly, bacterial meningitis may occur as an extension of a local bacterial infection, such as otitis media, mastoiditis, or sinusitis.
4. Bacteria also may gain direct entry through a penetrating wound, spinal tap, surgery, or anatomic abnormality.
5. The infective process results in inflammation, exudation, and varying degrees of tissue damage in the brain.

Complications

1. Acute—seizures, cerebral edema and IICP, shock, syndrome of inappropriate antidiuretic hormone secretion (SIADH)
2. Long-term—sensorineural hearing loss, hydrocephalus, blindness, learning disabilities/developmental delays

Clinical Manifestations

1. Signs and symptoms are variable, depending on the patient's age, the etiologic agent, and the duration of the illness when diagnosed.
   a. Infants younger than 2 months usually display irritability, lethargy, vomiting, lack of appetite, seizures, high-pitched cry, fever, or hypothermia.
   b. Infants up to 2 years of age manifest symptoms similar to those of the young infant and may have altered sleep patterns, fever, tenseness of the fontanel, nuchal rigidity, positive Kernig's or Brudzinski's signs.
   c. Children older than 2 years initially have vomiting, headache, mental confusion, lethargy, and photophobia. Later symptoms include nuchal rigidity within 12 to 24 hours after onset, positive Kernig's or Brudzinski's sign, seizures, and progressive decline in responsiveness.
2. Onset may be insidious or fulminant.
3. Petechiae or purpura may develop.
   a. Characteristic skin lesions are most often observed in cases of meningococcal or *Pseudomonas* infection.
   b. Hemorrhagic rashes may occur in any child with overwhelming bacterial sepsis because of disseminated intravascular coagulation.
4. Septic arthritis suggests either meningococcal or *H. influenzae* infection.

Diagnostic Evaluation

1. Diagnosis is usually established by performance of a lumbar puncture and examination of the cerebrospinal fluid.
   a. Cloudy or turbid appearance

b. Elevated cerebrospinal fluid pressure
c. High cell count with mostly polymorphonuclear cells
d. Low glucose level
e. Elevated protein level (also may be normal)
f. Positive Gram stain and cultures (identifies the causative organism)
2. Additional laboratory studies include the following:
a. Complete blood count—total white blood cell count often increased, with a preponderance of young neutrophils in the differential blood count
b. Blood, urine, and nasopharyngeal cultures to look for source of infection
c. Platelet count, serum electrolytes, glucose, blood urea nitrogen (BUN) and creatinine, and urinalysis usually done to monitor critically ill patient

Treatment

1. IV administration of the appropriate antimicrobial agents to promote rapid destruction of the bacteria and to suppress the emergence of resistant strains. The first dose of antibiotics should be administered as soon as possible.
2. Recognition and treatment of hyponatremia caused by SIADH
3. Supportive management of the comatose child or the child with seizures
4. Appropriate prophylactic treatment provided for contacts when indicated

Nursing Assessment

1. Obtain a history from the parents about recent upper respiratory or other infection.
2. Assess level of consciousness and neurologic status.
a. Evaluate for *Kernig's sign*—With the child in the supine position and knees flexed, flex the leg at the hip so that the thigh is brought to a position perpendicular to the trunk. Attempt to extend the knee. If meningeal irritation is present, this cannot be done, and attempts to extend the knee result in pain.
b. Evaluate for *Brudzinski's sign*—Flex the patient's neck. Spontaneous flexion of the lower extremities indicates meningeal irritation.
3. Monitor breathing pattern and circulatory status.

Nursing Diagnoses

A. Altered Cerebral Tissue Perfusion related to endotoxin release into the cerebrospinal fluid
B. Hyperthermia related to infectious process
C. Pain related to neurologic effects from the disease process
D. Risk for Infection Transmission related to bacterial agents
E. Altered Cerebral Tissue Perfusion related to complications of infectious process
F. Anxiety of parents related to severity of illness and hospitalization

Nursing Interventions

A. **Maintaining Cerebral Tissue Perfusion**
1. Administer antimicrobial agents at specified time intervals to obtain optimal serum levels. Obtain bloodwork for peak and trough levels as ordered.
2. Maintain patent IV line for medication administration; observe for signs of infiltration and phlebitis.
3. Monitor closely for signs of complications affecting cerebral perfusion.
a. Monitor vital signs, level of consciousness, and neurologic status at frequent intervals.
b. Monitor intake and output, weight, and head circumference daily to assess for hydrocephalus.
c. Be especially alert for lethargy or subtle changes in condition, which may indicate cerebral edema.
d. Accurately chart child's behavior and clinical signs.

B. **Reducing Fever**
1. Administer antipyretics, tepid sponge baths, and hypothermia blanket as ordered to reduce fever.
a. Fever increases metabolic rate and energy requirements by the brain; this may lead to hypoxemia and brain damage in the child with cerebral vascular compromise.
2. Monitor for seizures and use seizure precautions in the febrile child.
a. There is an increased potential for seizures in the febrile child.
b. Ensure safety by using padded bed or crib rails and having an airway and suction equipment on hand.

C. **Relieving Pain and Irritability**
1. Reduce the general noise level around the child, and prevent sudden loud noises.
2. Organize nursing care to provide for periods of uninterrupted rest.
3. Keep general handling of the child at a minimum. When necessary, approach the child slowly and gently.
4. Maintain subdued lighting as much as possible.
5. Speak in a low, well-modulated tone of voice.
6. Medicate for pain as ordered, avoiding narcotics that cause CNS and respiratory depression.

D. **Preventing Transmission of Infection**
1. Use precautions until at least 24 hours after initiation of appropriate antibiotic therapy.
2. Practice careful handwashing technique.
3. Ensure that personnel with colds or other infections avoid contact with infants with meningitis, and wear a mask when it is necessary to enter the nursery.
4. Teach parents and other visitors proper handwashing and gown technique.
5. Maintain sterile technique for procedures when indicated.
6. Identify close contacts of the child with meningitis caused by *H. influenzae* or *N. meningitidis* who might benefit from prophylactic treatment.

E. **Avoiding Complications**
1. Monitor for and report any of the following:
a. Decreased respirations, decreased pulse rate, increased systolic blood pressure, pupillary changes, or decreased responsiveness, which may indicate IICP
b. Decreased urine volume and increased body weight, which may indicate SIADH

c. Sudden appearance of a skin rash and bleeding from other sites, which may indicate disseminated intravascular coagulation
d. Persistent or recurring fever, bulging fontanel, signs of IICP, focal neurologic signs, seizures, or increased head circumference, which may indicate subdural effusion
e. Hearing disturbances and apparent deafness, indicating cranial nerve involvement
2. Observe for episodes of apnea, and initiate measures to stimulate respiration.
   a. Institute respiratory monitoring.
   b. Stimulate the infant when apnea does occur.
      (1) Pinch feet and provide more vigorous stimulation if necessary.
      (2) When spontaneous respiration does not occur within 15 to 20 seconds, provide bag, valve, or mask ventilation.
   c. Report any periods of apnea.
   d. Record length of apnea episode and response to stimulation

F. *Allaying Parental Anxiety*
1. Encourage the parents to engage in quiet activities with their child, such as reading or listening to soft music.
2. Provide the parents with an opportunity to express their concerns and answer questions they may have regarding the child's progress and care.
3. Engage the parents in the supportive care of the child so that they may feel some control over the situation.

Family Eduction/Health Maintenance

1. Provide parents with appropriate information if they and other family members are to receive antibiotic prophylaxis, usually one dose of rifampin (Rifadin).
2. Discuss symptoms for which the parents should watch as signs of possible latent complications, especially hydrocephalus.
3. Give specific instruction regarding medications to be administered at home.
4. Encourage regular health maintenance visits to chart growth and development and assess for any delays.

Evaluation

A. Alert without signs of IICP
B. Fever below 101°F (38.4°C)
C. Resting comfortably, verbalizing reduced pain
D. Pecautions maintained
E. Vital signs stable; breathing pattern regular without apnea
F. Parents participating in child's care, asking questions

◆ SEIZURE DISORDERS (CONVULSIVE DISORDERS, EPILEPSY)

Seizure disorders is a term used to encompass a number of varieties of episodic disturbances of brain function. Seizures should not be regarded as one specific disease, but as a symptom of an underlying disorder. They are relatively common in children, being more prevalent during the first 2 years than at any other time in life.

Etiology and Incidence

Seizure disordes are idiopathic or related to a variety of contributing factors.

A. *Prenatal Factors*
1. Genetic predisposition
2. Congenital structural anomalies
3. Fetal infections
4. Maternal diseases

B. *Perinatal Factors*
1. Trauma
2. Hypoxia
3. Jaundice
4. Infection
5. Prematurity
6. Drug withdrawal

C. *Postnatal Factors*
1. Primary infection of the CNS
2. Infectious diseases of childhood with encephalopathy
3. Head trauma
4. Circulatory diseases
5. Toxic encephalopathy
6. Allergic encephalopathy
7. Metabolic encephalopathy
8. Degenerative diseases
9. Cerebral neoplasms
10. Renal disease
11. Anoxia

D. *Incidence*
1. Incidence of epilepsy is estimated at 15 cases per 100,000 population.
2. Of individuals with seizure disorders, 90% are diagnosed before the age of 20.

Altered Physiology

1. The basic mechanism for all seizures appears to be prolonged depolarization, causing brain cells to become overactive and to discharge in a sudden, violent, disorderly manner.
2. This paroxysmal burst of electrical energy spreads to adjacent areas of the brain or may jump to distant areas of the CNS, resulting in a seizure.
3. The biochemical basis of seizures is incompletely understood, but some seizures appear to occur under the influence of a triggering factor.
   a. Hormonal factors, such as those related to the menstrual period, menarche, and menopause
   b. Nonsensory factors, such as hyperthermia, hyperventilation, metabolic disorders, sleep deprivation, emotional disturbances, and physical stress
   c. Sensory factors, such as those related to vision, hearing, touch, the startle reaction, and those that are self-induced

Complications

1. Apnea/hypoventilation
2. Hypoglycemia (status epilepticus)

Clinical Manifestations: Types of Seizures

A. Generalized Seizures (Convulsive and Nonconvulsive)
1. Onset
   a. Onset is abrupt.
   b. May occur at night.
   c. An aura (peculiar sensation, often dizziness) occurs in about one-third of epileptic children prior to a generalized seizure.
2. Tonic spasm
   a. The child's entire body becomes stiff.
   b. The child loses consciousness.
   c. The face may become pale and distorted.
   d. The eyes are frequently fixed in one position.
   e. The back may be arched with head held backward or to one side.
   f. Arms are usually flexed and hands clenched.
   g. If standing, the child falls to the ground.
   h. The child may utter a peculiar, piercing cry.
   i. The child is often unable to swallow saliva.
   j. Breathing is ineffective, and cyanosis results if spasm includes the muscles of respiration.
   k. The pulse may become weak and irregular.
3. Clonic phase
   a. Characterized by rhythmic, jerking movements that follow the tonic state.
   b. Usually start in one place and become generalized, including the muscles of the face.
   c. The child may be incontinent and may bite the tongue or cheek. (This occurs because of sudden forceful contraction of the jaw and abdominal muscles.)
4. Duration
   a. Varies from a few seconds to 30 minutes or longer.
   b. Usually seizures cease after a few minutes.
5. Postictal (postconvulsive) state
   a. Usually is sleepy or exhausted
   b. May complain of headache
   c. May appear to be in a dazed state
   d. Often performs relatively automatic tasks without being able to recall the episode

B. Status Epilepticus
1. State of continuing or recurring seizures that last longer than 30 minutes or occur in a series without the patient's regaining consciousness between attacks.
2. Transient postictal signs and symptoms include ataxia, aphasia, and mental sluggishness.
3. Damage to cerebral tissue may occur secondary to prolonged cerebral hypoxia or hypoglycemia, not the seizure itself.
4. This condition should be treated as a medical emergency.

C. Absence Seizures
1. Onset
   a. Rarely appears before 5 years of age
   b. Previously referred to as petit mal seizures
2. Clinical signs
   a. The child will lose contact with the environment for a few brief seconds.
   b. The child may appear to be staring or daydreaming.
   c. If reading or writing, the child will suddenly discontinue the activity and may resume it when the seizure has ended.
   d. Atypical absence seizure—minor manifestations include rolling of the eyes, nodding of the head, slight hand movements, and smacking of the lips.
3. Duration
   a. Usually 5 to 10 seconds
4. Frequency
   a. Varies from one or two per month to several hundred each day
5. Precipitating factors
   a. Hyperventilation, fatigue, hypoglycemia, and stress
6. Postseizure state
   a. Child appears normal.
   b. Child is not aware of having had a seizure.

D. Partial Seizures
1. Psychomotor
   a. Occur most frequently in children 3 years through adolescence.
   b. Seizure discharge usually originates in the temporal lobe and may be referred to as "temporal lobe seizures."
   c. Clinical signs include the following:
      (1) The child frequently experiences a sense of fullness rising from the abdomen to the thorax.
      (2) Aura, if present, often includes bad odor or taste.
      (3) The child may experience complex auditory or visual hallucinations, déjà vu feeling, or strong sense of fear and anxiety.
      (4) Perceptual alterations may occur.
      (5) Dysphagia or aphasia may be present.
      (6) Most common motor symptom is drawing or jerking of the mouth and face.
      (7) The child may perform coordinated but inappropriate movements repeatedly in a stereotypical manner (eg, clutching, kicking, picking at clothes, walking in circles, chewing, licking, spitting).
      (8) Consciousness may be impaired but is rarely completely lost.
   d. Duration is brief, usually from 30 seconds to 5 to 10 minutes.
   e. Postictal state is usual after an attack. Confusion and amnesia are common.
2. Focal motor
   a. Clinical signs
      (1) Sudden jerking movements occur in a particular area of the body, such as the face, thumb, or toe.
      (2) Consciousness may or may not be disturbed.
      (3) Clonic movements occasionally begin in one area of the body and spread to adjacent areas on the same side in a fixed progression (Jacksonian seizures).
   b. Prognosis
      (1) Seizures may become more extensive as the child matures, leading to generalized seizures.
3. Focal sensory (rare in children)—sensations occur, such as numbness, tingling, and coldness, in the part of the body controlled by the area of the brain cell overactivity.

E. Infantile Spasms (Myoclonic Seizures, Massive Myoclonic Spasms)
1. These seizures occur in infants; they are second in incidence only to generalized seizures in this age group.
2. Peak incidence is in children between 3 and 6 months; onset after 2 years is rare.

3. Clinical signs include the following:
   a. Sudden, forceful, myoclonic contractions involving the musculature of the trunk, neck, and extremities.
      (1) Flexor type—the infant adducts and flexes the extremities, drops the head, and doubles on himself or herself.
      (2) Extensor type—the infant extends neck, spreads arms out, and bends body backward in a position described as "spread eagle."
   b. A cry or grunt may accompany severe attacks.
   c. The infant may grimace, laugh, or appear fearful during or after the attack.
4. Duration is momentary (usually less than 1 minute).
5. Frequency varies from a few attacks per day to hundreds per day.
6. The prognosis follows:
   a. It is almost always associated with cerebral abnormalities.
   b. Usually this type of seizure disappears spontaneously by the time the child reaches 4 years of age.
   c. Subsequent generalized or other types of seizures often develop.
   d. Mental retardation usually accompanies this disorder.

Diagnostic Evaluation

A. Electroencephalogram
The electroencephalogram (EEG) shows characteristic abnormalities during seizures and with generalized seizures, between seizures as well.

C. Laboratory studies
1. Serum electrolytes—Hyponatremia may cause seizures.
2. Toxicology screen—Drug overdoses may cause seizures.
3. Blood cultures—Fever and CNS infections may cause seizures.
4. Lumbar puncture may be done if fever is present.
5. Serum levels of seizure medications should follow therapy.

Treatment

A. General Principles Related to the Administration of Medications
1. Selection of the most effective drug(s) depends on correct identification of the clinical seizure type.
2. A desirable drug level is one that will prevent seizures without producing undesirable side effects.
3. Dosages are adjusted according to blood level and clinical signs.
4. Accurate timing is essential to prevent seizures. This is especially true when the child tends to have seizures at a certain time each day.
5. Enteric-coated tablets, which have a delayed effect, should be used for children who are prone to attacks during sleep.
6. Most anticonvulsants are available in liquid form and in capsules or tablets. Some drugs are less well absorbed in liquid form.
7. It may take several months to find the best combination of medications and the best dosages of each to control the child's seizures. Single drug therapy is attempted initially. If this is not successful, a second drug may be tried or added on.

8. Symptoms may not be controlled 100% in every patient.
9. Dosage adjustment may be required from time to time because of the child's growth.
10. Blood counts, urinalyses, and liver function studies are done at regular intervals in children receiving certain anticonvulsants.
11. Medication is often not discontinued until 2 to 3 years after the last attack.
12. Weaning from medication should always be gradual, with stepwise reduction of dosage and withdrawal of one drug at a time.
13. There is some evidence to suggest that long-term use of some antiepileptic agents may cause intellectual impairment in children with epilepsy.

B. Drugs Commonly Used for the Control of Seizures in Children
See Table 44-2.

C. Surgical Management
1. Surgical removal is the appropriate treatment for an identified lesion, such as a hematoma or brain tumor.
2. Surgical treatment, such as hemispherectomy, nontemporal lobe resection, or corpus callostomy, may be performed in children with severe, medically intractable seizure disorders.

D. Diet Therapy
1. The ketogenic diet may be used for seizure control and consists of precisely calculated portions of protein and fat without carbohydrates. This diet causes the child to become ketotic because fats are used for fuel rather than carbohydrates. It is thought that ketones may inhibit seizures.
   a. Children on this diet should not be given IV fluids with dextrose.
   b. All medications should be in sugar-free suspensions.
   c. The child will be on strict fluid restriction.
2. The mechanism of action of this treatment is unknown.

E. General Prognosis
1. General prognosis depends on type and severity of seizure disorder, coexisting mental retardation, organic disorders, and the type of medical management.
2. Medically treated seizures—spontaneous cessation of seizures may occur. Drugs may be gradually discontinued when the child has been free from attacks for an extensive period and the EEG pattern has reverted to normal.
3. Nontreated epilepsy—seizures tend to become more numerous.

Nursing Assessment

1. During a seizure, assess the following:
   a. Any indications of difficulties with airway or breathing
   b. Significant preseizure events, such as noise, excitement, lethargy
   c. Behavior before the seizure, aura
   d. Types of movements observed
   e. Time seizure began and ended
   f. Site where twitching or contraction began
   g. Areas of the body involved
   h. Movements of the eyes and changes in pupil size

TABLE 44-2 Drugs Used to Treat Seizures in children

Drugs and Dosage	Advantages	Adverse Reactions	Special Considerations
Phenobarbital (Luminal) Maintenance dosage: 3–8 mg/kg per day given qd or bid Status epilepticus: 10–20 mg/kg, may repeat to maximum 40 mg/kg	Relatively safe and inexpensive	Excitement, hyperactivity, rash, gastrointestinal (GI) distress, dizziness, ataxia, worsening of psychomotor seizures, drowsiness; toxicity causing respiratory depression, circulatory collapse, and renal impairment	This is contraindicated in hepatic or renal dysfunction, hypersensitivity. IM or IV loading dose can be given. IV rate should not exceed 1 mg/kg per minute.
Phenytoin (Dilantin) Loading dose: 15 mg/kg Maintenance: 4–7 mg/kg per day given qd or bid	Safest drug for psychomotor seizures; does not cause drowsiness	Hypertrophy of gums, hirsutism, rickets, nystagmus, ataxia, rash; may accentuate absence seizures; toxicity may cause blood dyscrasias and liver damage	May interact with a wide variety of drugs due to extensive protein binding. Daily gum massage may prevent gum disease. Avoid IM administration If given IV, do not exceed rate of 1 mg/kg per minute. Drug must be given with normal saline to prevent precipitation.
Ethosuximide (Zarontin) Maintenance: 20–40 mg/kg per day given qd by oral route only	Used for absence seizures	Drowsiness, GI distress, lethargy, euphoria; may aggravate generalized seizures; toxicity causes blood dyscrasias and psychiatric symptoms	This is contraindicated in hepatic or renal disease. Dosage should not be increased more often than every 4–7 d.
Primidone (Mysoline) children younger than 8 years: 10–25 mg/kg per day given tid or qid Children older than 8 years: 750–1,500 mg/d tid or qid by oral route only	May control generalized seizures not responsive to treatment by other drugs	Ataxia, vertigo, GI symptoms; megaloblastic anemia as a rare idiosyncratic reaction; drowsiness in breastfed infants of treated mothers; Stevens-Johnson syndrome, gum hypertrophy, night terrors	This is contraindicated in those hypersensitive to phenobarbital and those with porphyria. It is often used with other drugs for mixed seizures. Dosage increases are usually done weekly until effect is seen.
Diazepam (Valium) IV dosage: 0.2–0.3 mg/kg to maximum of 10 mg Rectal dosage: 0.5 mg/kg	Used IV, IM, or rectally for status epilepticus or as adjunct therapy	Ataxia, drowsiness, fatigue, venous thrombosis or phlebitis at injection site, confusion, depression, headache; tonic status epilepticus when given IV for absence seizures; toxicity may cause somnolence, confusion, diminished reflexes, hypotension, coma, apnea, cardiac arrest	If administered IV, give no faster than 1 mg/min. Drug used cautiously in children with limited pulmonary reserve. Monitor respirations closely.
Carbamazepine (Tegretol) 20–30 mg/kg per day tid or qid Maximum dose of 1,000 mg/d	Especially useful for major motor and psychomotor seizures	Most likely to occur during initiation of therapy: dizziness, drowsiness, nausea and vomiting; toxicity may cause bone marrow depression (fever, sore throat, oral ulcers, easy bruising)	Administration with phenytoin reduces half-life of phenytoin; higher dose of phenytoin may be needed. This is contraindicated in previous bone marrow depression and is used cautiously in patients with cardiac, hepatic, or renal problems. Erythromycin increases plasma levels. Give with food.
Lorazepam (Ativan) 0.05–0.15 mg/kg per dose Maximum dose: 4 mg and may be repeated once	Used IV or rectally for status epilepticus; longer acting; may cause less respiratory depression	Sedation, dizziness, respiratory depression, hypotension, ataxia, weakness	Use with caution in patients with hepatic or renal dysfunction. Monitor respiratory status closely.

i. Incontinence
j. Color change—pallor, cyanosis, flushing
k. Mouth—teeth clenched, abnormal movements, tongue bitten
l. Apparent degree of consciousness during the seizure
2. After a seizure, assess the following:
a. Degree of memory for recent events
b. Types of speech
c. Coordination, paralysis or weakness
d. Length of time the child is postictal
e. Pupillary reaction
f. Vital signs

Nursing Diagnoses

A. Risk for Injury during a seizure
B. Ineffective Breathing Pattern related to spasms of respiratory musculature
C. Social Isolation related to the child's feelings about seizures or public fears and misconceptions
D. Self Esteem Disturbance related to lack of control over seizures

Nursing Interventions

A. *Ensuring Safety During a Seizure*
1. Use preventive measures.
a. Remove hard toys from the bed.
b. Pad the sides of the crib or side rails of the bed.
c. Have a suction machine available to remove secretions during a seizure.
d. Have an emergency oxygen source in the room in case of sudden respiratory difficulty.
2. Make sure the child can be readily observed.
3. During a seizure, monitor vital signs and assess neurologic status frequently.
4. Following a seizure, check the child frequently and report the following:
a. Behavior changes
b. Irritability
c. Restlessness
d. Listlessness

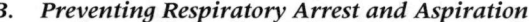

COMMUNITY-BASED CARE TIP:
Ensure that the home environment is safe, especially where the child sleeps and plays. Remove toys with sharp edges or parts or small pieces the child could choke on if they are put in the mouth, and cover very hard surfaces, such as the floor, against which the child could fall.

B. *Preventing Respiratory Arrest and Aspiration*
1. During a seizure take the following emergency actions:
a. Clear the area around the child.
b. Do not restrain the child.
c. Loosen the clothing around the neck.
d. Turn the child on side so that saliva can flow out of the mouth.
e. Place a small, folded blanket under the head to prevent trauma if the seizure occurs when the child is on the floor.
2. Suction the child, and administer oxygen as necessary.
3. Do not give anything by mouth or attempt to place anything in the mouth.
4. After the seizure, place the child in a sidelying position.

C. *Promoting Socialization*
1. Advise the parents that the child should be in an environment that is as normal as possible.
2. Encourage regular attendance at school after the school nurse and teachers have been notified, and emergency treatment of seizures is understood.
3. Encourage the child to participate in organizations and outside activities with limited restrictions.
a. Each child must be treated individually; the kind of activity depends on the degree of control.
b. Generally, children with seizure disorders should not be allowed to climb in high places or to swim alone.
c. Responsible adults should be made aware of the child's disorder.

D. *Strengthening Self-Esteem*
1. Offer reassurance and praise to the parents and child for coping effectively with seizures.
2. Observe the parent–child interactions for evidence of rejection or overprotection.
a. Tell the parents that the child should not be made to feel that he or she can never be left alone.
b. Advise the parents that the child needs to be disciplined as any other child and should not gain attention directly or indirectly by having seizures.
3. Help the child gain more control by providing education about seizure disorders.
a. Include the child in treatment planning.
b. Allow the opportunity to ask questions, and answer them honestly.
c. Make sure the child is aware of restrictions and can deal with them.
d. Encourage parents gradually to give the child responsibility for taking medications.
4. Help the older child or adolescent to achieve independence.
a. Encourage the parents to give the older child the opportunity for privacy to discuss concerns with the physician.
b. Encourage parents to allow the older child to use his or her own judgment in making decisions.
c. Help the older child to develop realistic educational and career goals.
5. Help parents deal with a noncompliant child. Fantasies that "there is nothing wrong with me" or the refusal to take medications requires prompt intervention. This is most often seen during adolescence. Family counseling may be necessary.

Family Education/Health Maintenance

1. Describe completely any examinations, evaluations, treatments that the child is receiving.
2. Provide information regarding the disease itself.
a. Epilepsy is *not* contagious, is seldom dangerous, and does *not* indicate insanity or mental retardation.
b. Most children with epilepsy have infrequent seizures and with medications can completely control their convulsions.
c. The child may have normal intelligence and can live a useful and productive life.
d. The child's medication is not addicting when used as prescribed. It should in no way cause him or her to become a drug addict.

e. It is impossible to predict accurately the possibility of the seizure disorder appearing in siblings or offspring of the affected child.

3. Prepare the parents for the fact that it may take several months of regulating drug dosages before adequate control is obtained.

4. Encourage parents and older children to obtain genetic counseling.
   a. People with epilepsy can marry and have children.
   b. There is no proof that epilepsy is hereditary, although there may be a tendency to transmit a low convulsive threshold.

5. Teach the parents and child factors that may precipitate a seizure.
   a. The child should be kept in optimal physical condition with routine immunizations, medical care, dental care, and eye care, and should receive prompt evaluation and treatment of infections.
   b. Excessive fatigue, overhydration, and hyperventilation should be avoided.
   c. Irregular, fluctuating schedules are detrimental. A routine of daily living should be encouraged.

6. For additional resources, refer families to agencies such as The Epilepsy Foundation of America; 4351 Garden City Drive; Landover, MD, 20785-2267; 800-332-1000.

Evaluation

A. Padded bed rails in place; suction machine and airway at bedside; only stuffed animals in crib
B. Breathing unlabored following seizure with lungs clear
C. Parents and child verbalize understanding of child's ability to participate in activities
D. Child participating in treatment plan, taking medications as ordered without reminders

◆ FEBRILE SEIZURES

Febrile seizures refer to seizures that occur in the context of a febrile illness in a previously normal child. The seizures are brief and generalized. They should be distinguished from focal or prolonged seizures, which occur in a child with an underlying seizure disorder that is exacerbated by fever.

Etiology and Incidence

1. Seizures accompany intercurrent infections, especially viral illness, tonsillitis, pharyngitis, and otitis.
2. They appear to occur in a familial pattern, although exact pattern of inheritance is incompletely understood. Children with a positive family history of febrile seizures have a greater risk of recurrent febrile seizures.
3. It is unclear whether the seizure is triggered by a rapid rise in temperature or the actual temperature attained.
4. Febrile seizures occur in approximately 3% to 5% of all children.
5. Most first febrile seizures occur in children between the ages of 6 months and 3 years and are unusual after 5 years.
6. Boys are more likely to have febrile seizures than girls.

Altered Physiology

1. Most febrile seizures consist of generalized tonic-clonic seizures. See altered physiology for seizure disorders, above.

Clinical Manifestations

1. Seizures generally last less than 15 minutes.
2. Fever is usually more than 101.8°F (38.8°C) rectally.
3. Seizures usually occur near the onset of fever rather than after prolonged fever.

Complications

1. Injury may occur during seizure.

Diagnostic Evaluation

Measures are directed toward delineating the cause of any seizure as precisely as possible so that its implications and prognosis may be discussed with the parents. Diagnostic methods may include the following:

1. Cerebrospinal fluid examination to detect CNS infection
2. Complete blood count and urinalysis to detect signs of infection
3. Cultures of nasopharynx, blood, or urine as appropriate to determine cause of fever
4. Blood glucose, calcium, and electrolyte levels to detect abnormalities that may cause seizures
5. EEG
   a. Demonstrates mild, postictal slowing soon after the attack
   b. Pattern is generally normal after a few days

Treatment

The goals of treatment are to control seizures and decrease temperature.

1. Administration of antipyretics and other cooling measures
2. Administration of medications to control seizures
   a. The advisability of long-term anticonvulsant medications in normal children with simple febrile seizures is controversial. Recommendations vary among healthcare providers from no medication to maintenance therapy with phenobarbital (Luminal).
   b. Intermittent therapy with phenobarbital during febrile episodes is apparently of no value because of the length of time required to achieve therapeutic serum levels of the drug.
3. Airway management as required
4. Prognosis
   a. The likelihood of febrile seizure recurrence is about 40% to 50% for a second febrile seizure.
   c. The younger the child is at the time of the first seizure, the greater the risk for additional febrile seizures.

d. The risk for development of nonfebrile seizures is relatively low (about 3%). At risk are children who demonstrate the following characteristics:
    (1) Multiple febrile seizures during 1 day
    (2) Prolonged febrile seizures
    (3) Persistent EEG abnormalities
    (4) CNS infection

Nursing Assessment/Interventions

Nursing assessment and interventions are the same as for seizure disorders, p. 1235.

Family Education/Health Maintenance

1. Reinforce realistic, reassuring information, such as the following:
    a. A seizure does not necessarily imply that the underlying disease is serious.
    b. The prognosis depends on the cause of the seizure.
        (1) A single febrile seizure does not indicate later chronic epilepsy.
        (2) Children who have a tendency to develop febrile seizures usually lose it as they grow older.
        (3) Occasional, brief seizures have no adverse effects on the child's ultimate development.
2. Discuss and demonstrate emergency management of seizures.
3. Stress that medical evaluation is indicated as soon as the child develops a fever.
    a. Review technique of temperature measurement.
    b. Prompt administration of antipyretic measures is necessary when the child is febrile but may not prevent a febrile seizure.
4. Review administration schedule, adverse reactions, and appropriate follow-up in regard to anticonvulsant therapy.

◆ SUBDURAL HEMATOMA

Subdural hematoma refers to an accumulation of fluid, blood, and its degradation products within the potential space between the dura and arachnoid (subdural space). Subdural hematomas are classified as acute or chronic, depending on the time between injury and the onset of symptoms.

Etiology and Incidence

A. Causes
1. Direct or indirect trauma to the head
    a. Birth trauma
    b. Accidental causes
    c. Purposeful violence, as in cases of child abuse
2. Meningitis

B. Classification
1. Acute syndrome
    a. Presents as an acute problem, closely related to the time of presumed injury

2. Chronic
    a. Signs and symptoms are nonlocalizing and subacute.
    b. This is the most common type of subdural hematoma in children.
    c. It is often difficult to delineate the exact time and type of injury, because the precipitating episode may appear relatively insignificant.

Altered Physiology

1. Trauma to the head causes tearing of the delicate subdural veins, resulting in small hemorrhages into the subdural space. (Bleeding may be of arterial origin in cases of acute subdural hematoma.)
2. As the blood breaks down, there is an increased capillary permeability and effusion of blood cells and protein into the subdural space.
3. The breakdown products of blood stimulate the growth of connective tissue and capillaries largely from the dura.
4. A membrane is formed that usually extends frontally and laterally over the hemispheres, surrounding the clot.
5. Fluid accumulates within the membrane and increases the width of the subdural space.
6. Further hemorrhages occur.
7. The lesion enlarges, compressing the brain and expanding the skull and if unrelieved, ultimately causes cerebral atrophy or death from compression and herniation.
8. The lesion may arrest spontaneously at any point.
9. Further bleeding may occur into an already existing sac and may increase symptoms.
10. In long-standing subdural hematoma, the fluid may disappear, leaving a constricting membrane that prevents normal brain growth.

Complications

1. Mental retardation
2. Ocular abnormalities
3. Seizures
4. Spasticity
5. Paralysis

Clinical Manifestations

A. Acute
1. Often present with continuous unconsciousness from the time of injury, but child may present with a lucid interval.
2. Ensuing manifestations include deterioration of level of consciousness, progressive hemiplegia, focal seizures, and signs of brain stem herniation (pupillary enlargement, changes in vital signs, decerebrate posturing, and respiratory failure).

B. Chronic
This has a slow, gradual onset; symptoms are variable and are related to the age of the child.

1. Infants—early signs
    a. Anorexia
    b. Difficulty feeding

   c. Vomiting
   d. Irritability
   e. Low-grade fever
   f. Retinal hemorrhages
   g. Failure to gain weight
2. Infants—later signs
   a. Enlargement of the head
   b. Bulging and pulsation of the anterior fontanel
   c. Tight, glossy scalp with dilated scalp veins
   d. Strabismus, pupillary inequality, ocular palsies (rare)
   e. Hyperactive reflexes
   f. Seizures
   g. Retarded motor development
3. Older children—early signs
   a. Lethargy
   b. Anorexia
   c. Symptoms of IICP (vomiting, irritability, headache)
4. Older children—later signs (also may occur immediately if bleeding takes place rapidly)
   a. Seizures
   b. Coma

Diagnostic Evaluation

1. CT scan is the procedure of choice for diagnosing subdural hematomas.
2. Bilateral subdural taps may provide the diagnosis and immediate relief of IICP.
3. Skull films may be obtained if abuse is suspected.

Treatment

A. *Acute Subdural Hematoma*
This requires evacuation of the clot through a burr hole or craniotomy.

B. *Chronic Subdural Hematoma*
1. Repeated subdural taps are done to remove the collecting fluid.
   a. In infants, the needle can be inserted through the fontanel or suture line.
   b. In older children, burr holes into the skull are necessary before the needle can be inserted.
   c. The subdural taps may be the only treatment required if the fluid disappears entirely, and symptoms do not recur.
   d. Concurrently, treatment is instituted to correct anemia, electrolyte imbalance, and malnutrition.
2. Shunting procedure may be indicated if repeated taps fail to reduce significantly the volume or protein content of the subdural collections. Shunting is usually to the peritoneal cavity.

C. *Prognosis*
1. Treatment is usually successful when the diagnosis is made before cerebral atrophy and a fixed neurologic deficit have occurred. In such cases, subsequent development is normal.
2. Prognosis depends on the effect of the initial trauma on the brain and the effect of continued fluid collection.
3. Mortality in massive, acute subdural bleeding is very high, even if promptly diagnosed.

Nursing Assessment

Assess the child's neurologic status to evaluate the effectiveness of treatment or to identify disease progress.

1. Observe general behavior, especially irritability, lethargy, and evidence of personality changes. It is important to obtain a thorough history from the parents regarding normal behavior and level of functioning so that abnormalities can be more easily recognized.
2. Evaluate appetite and feeding difficulties, including vomiting.
3. Assess for signs of IICP.
   a. Vital signs, including pulse, respiration, and blood pressure, should be monitored frequently.
   b. Be alert for the following:
     (1) Increased systolic blood pressure
     (2) Widened pulse pressure
     (3) Decreased pulse or irregularities
     (4) Changes in respiratory rate or difficulty breathing
4. Assess level of consciousness; describe response explicitly, including what type of stimulus was required to elicit a response.
5. Asses pupillary and visual changes, especially dilated pupil, double vision, lack of response to light, alterations in visual acuity, and nonsymmetrical or abnormal eye movements.
6. Monitor for seizures.
7. Evaluate motor function, including ability to move all extremities. The ability to grasp should be checked and compared bilaterally.
8. Inspect for drainage of cerebrospinal fluid from the nose or ears.

Nursing Diagnoses

A. Altered Cerebral Tissue Perfusion related to disease process
B. Impaired Physical Mobility related to decreased level of consciousness
C. Altered Nutrition: Less than body requirements related to decreased level of consciousness
D. Ineffective Family Coping: Compromised related to hospitalization of child

Nursing Interventions

A. *Maintaining Cerebral Tissue Perfusion*
1. Avoid additional increase in intracranial pressure.
   a. Maintain a quiet environment.
   b. Avoid sudden changes in position.
   c. Organize nursing activities to allow for long periods of uninterrupted rest.
   d. Carefully regulate fluid administration to avoid danger of fluid overload.
   e. Measure urine output, and record specific gravity.
   f. Administer laxatives or suppositories to prevent straining during a bowel movement.
2. Assist with subdural taps.
   a. Protect and restrain the child as needed (see p. 1137).
   b. Hold the child securely to avoid injury caused by sudden movement.

c. Apply firm pressure over the puncture site(s) for a few minutes after the tap has been completed to prevent fluid leakage along the needle tract.
d. Observe the child frequently after the procedure for shock, drainage from the site of the tap.
e. Note whether there is serous drainage or frank blood.
f. Reinforce the dressing as needed to prevent contamination of the wound.
g. Monitor temperature frequently, and monitor for signs of developing infection.
h. Report purulent drainage from the site of the subdural tap.

3. Avoid discussing the child's condition near the bed. Even though comatose, the child may be able to hear.
4. Have emergency equipment available for resuscitation.

B. Preventing Complications of Immobility
1. Change the child's position frequently, and provide meticulous skin care to prevent hypostatic pneumonia and decubitus ulcers.
2. Prevent contractures.
a. Apply passive range of motion exercises to all extremities.
b. Place pillows appropriately to support the child's body in good alignment.
c. Use splints designed by physical therapy as instructed.
3. Suction the child as necessary to remove secretions in the mouth and nasopharynx.
4. Observe for signs of respiratory or urinary infection related to stasis.
5. Keep the child's eyes well lubricated to prevent corneal damage.

C. Maintaining Nutritional Status
1. Provide nutrition and fluids through nasogastric feedings as ordered. Observe for gastric distention.
2. Monitor urine output and specific gravity daily.
3. Monitor electrolyte and protein levels on laboratory work.
4. Do not neglect mouth care, even if child is not eating.

D. Strengthening Family Coping
1. Encourage the parents to hold and cuddle the infant as much as possible.
2. Encourage the parents to bring diversional activities from home.
a. Infants—mobiles or musical toys
b. Older children—quiet games, books, dolls
3. Provide emotional support to the parents.
a. Encourage as much parental participation in the child's care as possible.
b. Reassure the parents that the prognosis is favorable with adequate treatment.
4. Act nonjudgmental in cases caused by intentional or accidental trauma.
a. Attempt to alleviate their guilt feelings if present.
b. Ensure that cases of suspected child abuse have been reported to the appropriate agency and that parents have been referred for counseling.
5. Encourage visitation by siblings.

Family Education/Health Maintenance

1. Reinforce explanations in the following areas:
a. The condition

b. The causes of the child's specific symptoms
c. The need and rationale for treatment
d. Postoperative and recovery expectations
2. Encourage parents to keep all follow-up appointments for medical evaluation and physical and occupational therapy.
3. Teach parents safety measures to prevent injuries in the future.
4. Assist parents in seeking additional support and resources through social work department, church groups, community agencies, or private counseling.

Evaluation

A. Drowsy but responsive to verbal stimuli; pupils equal and reactive to light; vital signs stable; ventricular tap site without drainage
B. Skin without signs of erythema or breakdown; full range of motion of all joints; functional position maintained
C. Tolerating nasogastric feedings without distention; urine output sufficient
D. Parents participating in child's care, holding and reading to child; parents receiving counseling

◆ REYE'S SYNDROME

Reye's syndrome in children is a multisystem disease clinically characterized by a complex of signs and symptoms, including encephalopathy and fatty degeneration of the viscera, mainly affecting the liver, brain, and kidneys.

Etiology and Incidence

1. Etiology is unknown.
2. Most consistent single factor is an antecedent viral infection.
a. Influenza B—clustered geographically, occurring in older children (mean age is 11 years)
b. Varicella—sporadic occurrence in younger children (mean age is 6 years)
c. Gastroenteritis
d. Upper respiratory tract infection
3. Other related viruses include adenovirus, coxsackievirus, echovirus, herpes simplex and zoster, reovirus, and polio type I.
4. Other possible contributing factors include the following:
a. Genetic makeup of child that increases susceptibility, triggered by virus, toxins, drugs, or endogenous factors
b. Environmental factors—chemical toxins (ie, pesticides or fertilizers).
c. Drugs—salicylates and phenothiazines, acetaminophen
d. May have an autoimmune component.
5. Occurs more commonly in white children living in rural or suburban areas younger than 16 years. Occurs more frequently in African American infants from lower socioeconomic urban areas than white infants.
6. Peak seasonal occurrences are in winter and spring.

Altered Physiology

1. Mitochondrial injury or change is primary in all tissues. Mitochondrial damage results in decreased enzymes for proper functioning of specific metabolic pathways.
2. Liver is enlarged and bright yellow; fatty infiltration takes the form of small lipid droplets; mitochondria are large and swollen with some decrease of enzymatic activity, particularly for ammonia detoxification, resulting in hyperammonemia.
   a. Liver function studies are elevated—SGOT, SGPT.
   b. Clotting disturbances result in decreased clotting factor and prolonged prothrombin time (PT) and partial prothrombin time (PTT).
   c. Dysfunction of gluconeogenetic enzymatic pathway and depleted supply of glycogen stores. Hypoglycemia leads to the increased production of ammonia and fatty acidemia. Hypoglycemia seen in younger children is related to less liver reserve of glycogen and a higher metabolic rate.
3. Brain shows cerebral edema with small ventricles, possible neuronal necrosis; findings are consistent with hypoxia. Inflammatory reaction is absent; grossly enlarged mitochondria and pervasive watery blebs occur.
   a. Hypoxia or hypoglycemia are evidenced by neuronal degeneration.
   b. Cerebrospinal fluid is usually normal, except in later stages of disease when pressure is elevated.
   c. Loss of autoregulation leads to decrease in cerebral blood flow, tissue hypoxia, and neuronal death.
4. Kidney shows fatty degeneration of loop of Henle and proximal convoluted tubules with a few lipid droplets in distal tubular cells.
   a. Renal vasculature and glomeruli are normal.
   b. Renal insufficiency occurs. Edema, decreased urinary output, increased BUN and creatinine occur.
5. Heart shows fatty accumulation in muscle fibers, bundle of His, and bundle branches.

Complications

1. Developmental delays
2. Motor impairment
3. Mental retardation
4. Posthospital anxiety and apprehension
5. SIADH
6. Diabetes insipidus
7. Coma and death

Clinical Manifestations

NURSING ALERT:
Early diagnosis is critical because of the rapidly fatal course of the disease.

1. Prodromal illness (see etiology) that is usually improving
2. Sudden onset of intractable vomiting—fever usually not present
3. Irrational behavior
4. Altered sensorium—from mild lethargy to progressive stupor and coma
5. Hyperventilation, tachypnea

6. Hepatomegaly
7. Stages
   a. Children with Reye's syndrome advance through definite stages of progression. After diagnosis is made, the child should be categorized as fitting within one of the stages, with any progression noted. Generally, the more rapid the progression through these stages, the poorer the prognosis. A consensus conference sponsored by the National Institutes of Health developed the following staging system:
      (1) Stage I: Lethargy, follows verbal commands, normal posture, purposeful response to pain, brisk pupillary light reflex, normal oculocephalic reflex (doll's eye sign)
      (2) Stage II: Combative or stuporous, inappropriate verbalizing, normal posture, purposeful or nonpurposeful response to pain, sluggish pupillary reflexes, conjugate deviation on doll's eye maneuver
      (3) Stage III: Comatose, decorticate posture, decorticate response to pain, sluggish pupillary response, conjugate deviation on doll's eye maneuver
      (4) Stage IV: Comatose, decerebrate posture and decerebrate response to pain, sluggish pupillary reflexes, inconsistent or negative oculocephalic reflex (absent doll's eye sign)
      (5) Stage V: Comatose, flaccid, no response to pain, no pupillary response, negative oculocephalic reflex

Diagnostic Evaluation

1. General condition and appearance of child: History of prodromal illness—mild upper respiratory infection or other infection with sudden development of intractable vomiting, presence of other symptoms
2. Differential diagnosis—acute toxic encephalopathy, hepatic coma, hepatitis, meningitis, or encephalitis; history to rule out ingestion of medications or toxic materials
3. Laboratory data
   a. Elevated serum ammonia
   b. Elevated liver enzymes (SGOT, SGPT)
   c. Prolonged clotting factors (PT and PTT)
   d. Decreased serum glucose
   e. Elevated creatinine
   f. Elevated BUN
   g. Elevated amino acids, free fatty acids
   h. Acid–base status—acidemia
   i. Serum levels for salicylates, acetaminophen, phenothiazines, toxins to rule out other cause
   j. Complete blood count, electrolytes, serum osmolality, urinalysis, urine electrolytes, and urine osmolality to monitor condition
4. Lumbar puncture if cerebrospinal fluid is needed to rule out other diagnoses. If symptoms of IICP exist, the lumbar puncture should not be done until a CT scan is obtained to identify the potential for rapid decompression resulting in herniation of the brain.
5. Liver biopsy—if done, shows microvesicular fatty degeneration of liver

Treatment

A. General Considerations
1. Although this is a multisystem disease, maintaining adequate cerebral tissue perfusion is the priority, and

if the brain can be supported through the course of the illness, the chance of the other organs escaping injury is very high.

2. Treatment is supportive: The goal is to maintain adequate levels of circulating glucose and cerebral perfusion while preventing or controlling IICP. Treatment is aimed toward normalization of organ function and protection of the brain from irreversible damage.

B. Supportive Interventions
1. Admission to an intensive care unit is recommended for any child in stage II or greater. Invasive monitoring, including intracranial pressure monitoring and direct arterial pressure monitoring, may be instituted.
   a. It takes many hours to several days after control of the disease process is achieved to begin withdrawal therapy without having recurring symptoms of IICP.
2. General supportive care includes the following:
   a. Correction of hypoglycemia
   b. Correction of fluid and electrolyte imbalance
   c. Correction of acidosis to ensure optimal cerebral blood flow
   d. Prevention or correction of hypoxia
   e. Prevention of or treatment of IICP
   f. Correction of metabolic abnormalities
   g. Continuous monitoring of cardiopulmonary and neurologic status
   h. Evaluation of laboratory data

Nursing Assessment

1. Identify history that suggests Reye's syndrome.
2. Assess the child's stage of presentation by thorough neurologic assessment. Use the Glasgow Coma Scale to assess level of consciousness (Table 44-3).
3. Assess effectiveness of breathing patterns and circulatory status.
4. Assess the child for signs and symptoms of hypoglycemia and dehydration.

Nursing Diagnoses

A. Altered Cerebral Tissue Perfusion related to cerebral edema
B. Risk for Fluid Volume Deficit or Excess related to disease process and therapy
C. Ineffective Family Coping: Compromised related to severity and rapid course of illness
D. Fear related to intensive care experience and parental separation

Nursing Interventions

A. Improving Cerebral Perfusion
1. Provide supportive care of the child in stage I or II (noncomatose).
   a. Provide hourly neurologic checks using Glasgow Coma Scale.
   b. Administer sedation as ordered to decrease anxiety, restlessness, and potential for IICP.

TABLE 44-3 Glasgow Coma Scale

Eyes open	Spontaneously	4
	To speech	3
	To pain	2
	No response	1
Best verbal response	Oriented	5
	Confused	4
	Inappropriate words	3
	Incomprehensible sounds	2
	None	1
Best motor response	Obeys commands	5
	Localizes pain	4
	Flexion to pain	3
	Extension to pain	2
	None	1

Add the best score obtained in each area to obtain a final score.

2. Provide intensive care management of the child in stage III, IV, or V (comatose).
   a. If an intraventricular catheter or subarachnoid bolt is inserted, monitor intracranial pressure frequently. Goal is to maintain intracranial pressure within normal range of 10 to 15 mm Hg and to maintain cerebral perfusion pressure of at least 50 mm Hg.
   b. Provide routine care for a child who is intubated and mechanically ventilated to correct acidosis and provide optimal cerebral blood flow. Monitor arterial blood gases to maintain $PaCO_2$ about 25 mm Hg and PaO_2 at 100 to 150 mm Hg.
   c. Administer muscle relaxants and short-acting barbiturates as ordered.
   d. Monitor and maintain core body temperature at 97.7°F to 98.6°F (36.5°–37°C).
   e. Position supine with head of bed elevated 30 degrees; keep head midline to promote intracranial venous drainage.
   f. Provide chest physical therapy as tolerated to prevent infection, atelectasis, and increased intrathoracic pressure, thus increasing intracranial pressure. The risk of IICP must be weighed against the benefit of the procedure.
   g. Maintain continuous EEG monitoring if instituted.
   h. Monitor nursing activities that may cause IICP: suctioning, turning, chest physical therapy, painful (intrusive) procedures, conversation at bedside about diagnosis.
3. Administer drugs to control IICP.
   a. Muscle relaxant—pancuronium bromide (Pavulon) while on mechanical ventilator
   b. Sedative—diazepam (Valium), chloral hydrate (Noctec)
   c. Osmotic diuretic—mannitol (Osmitrol), glycerol
   d. Barbiturate therapy—thiopental (Pentothal), phenobarbital (Luminal)
   e. Analgesia as appropriate
4. Show a constant awareness of any activity, noise, and distractions that increase intracranial pressure.
5. For children in stage I or II, monitor serum glucose to maintain at 150 to 200 mg/dL. IV hypertonic glucose solution is usually required.
6. For children in stage III, IV, or V, monitor and administer IV glucose to maintain serum glucose at 200 to 300 mg/dL and serum osmolality at 300 to 310 mOsm/L.

7. Insert a nasogastric tube, and measure drainage. Give an antacid every 2 to 4 hours to maintain gastric pH above 4. Neomycin may be given through nasogastric tube to aid in reduction of ammonia.

B. **Maintaining Fluid Balance**
1. Administer nothing by mouth.
2. Keep strict intake and output record, and monitor weight at least daily. Measure urine-specific gravity every 4 hours.
3. Administer vitamin K (AquaMEPHYTON) as needed to combat coagulation defects and prevent bleeding.
4. For children in stage III, IV, or V, maintain an arterial line for pressure monitoring and blood sampling.
5. Limit fluid intake; peripheral IV fluids are given at a rate of $^2/_3$ maintenance because of potential cerebral edema and IICP. Calculate administered medications as part of fluid intake.
6. Observe for fluid volume defect—hemoconcentration, decreased urinary output, decreased mean arterial pressure.
7. Observe for fluid overload—elevated central venous pressure (6–8 cm H_2O), decreased urine output (less than 2 mL/kg per hour), edema.

C. **Strengthening Family Coping**
1. Prepare the parents for the intensity and invasiveness of the medical interventions surrounding their child. Accompany them to the bedside, and assist them to touch and comfort their child despite equipment and tubing.
2. Explain the routine of the intensive care unit, the purpose of procedures and equipment, and how to obtain information at any time about their child so that they will not feel completely out of control in the hospital environment.
3. Help the parents and siblings express feelings, such as guilt about what has happened and how it is affecting them.
4. Assess their coping mechanisms, family bonding, and other support systems.
5. Initiate referrals to the chaplain, social worker, and other resources as needed.

D. **Reducing Fear**
1. Tell the family that although the child may be heavily sedated, comatose, or paralyzed from muscle relaxants,

he or she perceives in varying degrees what is happening in his or her environment. Therefore, family members should continue to show love, affection, and support to the child.
2. Encourage parents to bring in a favorite toy or security object or tape recording of family members' voices.
3. Because parental separation may increase anxiety, support as necessary.
4. Explain all procedures to the child even if comatose.
5. Be aware that when a sedated or comatose child awakens, the child may be disoriented and have amnesia. Provide explanations and reassurance as appropriate.

Family Education/Health Maintenance

1. Ensure that the parents understand the importance of medical follow-up, especially related to any complications associated with the illness. The child recovering from Reye's syndrome without any neurologic sequelae should recover fairly rapidly; however, when the child has experienced sequelae or complications, a multidisciplinary team approach to treatment will ensure optimal rehabilitation.
2. Encourage parents to become involved in community education to help caretakers recognize early signs and symptoms that suggest Reye's syndrome.
3. For additional resources and support, refer parents to agencies such as The National Reye's Syndrome Foundation; PO Box 829; Bryan, Ohio, 43506; 800-233-7393.

Evaluation

A. Glasgow Coma Scale score of 15; briskly reactive pupils; normal posture
B. Urine output 1 mL/kg or greater per hour; vital signs stable
C. Parents verbalizing fears and appropriate questions about child's condition
D. Child resting comfortably without tachycardia or restlessness

Selected References

Berg, A. T. (1993). Are febrile seizures provoked by a rapid rise in temperature? *American Journal of Diseases of the Child, 147*, 1101–1103.

Eicher, P. S., & Batshaw, M. L. (1993). Cerebral palsy. *Pediatric Clinics of North America, 40*(3), 537–551.

Fisher, R. S. (1993). Emerging anitepileptic drugs. *Neurology, 43*(Supplement 5), S12–S18.

Fleisher G. R. & Ludwig, S. (Eds.) (1993). *Textbook of pediatric emergency medicine* (3rd ed.). Philadelphia: Williams & Wilkins.

Greif, L., & Miller, C. L. (1991). Shunt lengthening: A descriptive review. *Journal of Neuroscience Nursing, 23*(2), 120–124.

Hickey, J. V. (1992). *The clinical practice of neurological and neurosurgical nursing* (3rd ed.). Philadelphia: J.B. Lippincott.

Holmes, G. L. (1993). Surgery for intractable seizures in infancy and early childhood. *Neurology, 43*(Supplement 5), S28–S35.

Johnson, K. B. (Ed.) (1993). *The Harriet Lane handbook* (13th ed.). Philadelphia: Mosby-Yearbook.

Kinsman, S. L., Vining, E. P. G., Quaskey, S. A., Mellits, D., & Freeman, J. M. (1992). Efficacy of the ketogenic diet for intractable seizure disorders: Review of 58 cases. *Epilepsia, 33*(6), 1132–1136.

Kirk, E. A., White, C., & Freeman, S. (1992). Effects of a nursing education intervention on parents' knowledge of hydrocephalus and shunts. *Journal of Neuroscience Nursing, 24*(2), 99–103.

Kurtz, L. A., & Scull, S. A. (1993). Rehabilitation for developmental disabilities. *Pediatric Clinics of North America, 40*(3), 629–643.

Lipton, J. D., & Schafermeyer, R. W. (1993). Evolving concepts in pediatric bacterial meningitis-part I: Pathophysiology and diagnosis. *Annals of Emergency Medicine, 22*(10), 1602–1613.

McLone, D. G. (1992). Continuing concepts in the management of spina bifida. *Pediatric Neurosurgery, 18*, 254–256.

Michaud, L. J. (1993). Traumatic brain injury in children. *Pediatric Clinics of North America, 40*(3), 553–565.

Oski, F. (Ed.), *Principles and practice of pediatrics* (2nd ed.). Philadelphia: J.B. Lippincott.

Paneth, N. (1993). The causes of cerebral palsy. Recent evidence. *Clinical and Investigative Medicine, 16*(2), 95–101.

Piatt, J. H., Jr. (1992). Physical examination of patients with cerebrospinal fluid shunts: Is there useful information in pumping the shunt? *Pediatrics, 89*(3), 470–473.

Pohl, C. A. (1993). Practical approach to bacterial meningitis in childhood. *American Family Physician, 47*(7), 1595–1603.

Polivka, B. J., Nickel, J. T., & Wilkins, J. R. III (1993). Cerebral palsy: Evaluation of a model of risk. *Research in Nursing and Health, 16,* 113–121.

Rose, B. A. (1993). Neurologic therapies in critical care. *Critical Care Nursing Clinics of North America, 5*(2), 237–246.

Sackett, C. K. (1993). Spina bifida, Part 1: Physical effects. *Urologic Nursing, 13*(2), 58–61.

Selzman, A. A., Elder, J. S., & Mapstone, T. B. (1993). Urologic consequences of myelodysplasia and other congenital abnormalities of the spinal cord. *Urologic Clinics of North America, 20*(3), 485–504.

Sood, B. A., Kim, S., Ham, S. D., Canady, A. I., & Greninger, N. (1993). Useful components of the shunt tap test for evaluation of shunt malfunction. *Child's Nervous System, 9,* 157–162.

Staudt, C. A. & Peacock, W. J. (1995). Dorsal rhizotomy for spasticity. *Western Journal of Medicine, 162* (3), 260.

Thomas, G. H., Thomas, B., & Trachtenberg, S. W. (1993). Growing up with Patricia. *Pediatric Clinics of North America, 40*(3), 675–683.

Vessy, J. A., Holland, C. V., McVay, C. J., Williams, S. D., & McNatt, S. (1993). Latex allergy: A threat to you and your patients? *Pediatric Nursing, 19*(5), 517–519.

White, M., & Williams, J. (1992). A good start to a full life. Managing continence in children with spina bifida and hydrocephalus. *Professional Nurse, 7*(7), 474–477.

Williams, E. M., Galbraith, J. G., & Duncan, C. C. (1995). Neuroendoscopic laser-assisted ventriculostomy for the third ventricle. *AORN Journal, 61* (2), 345–348.

CHAPTER 45

Pediatric Gastrointestinal and Nutritional Disorders

◆ CLEFT LIP AND PALATE

Cleft lip and palate are congenital anomalies resulting in structural facial malformation. They are usually apparent at birth.

Etiology and Incidence

1. Failure of embryonic development—cause not known
2. Hereditary factor
3. May be related to mutant genes, chromosomal abnormalities, teratogens
4. Cleft lip—approximately 1 in 1,000 births; more frequent in boys (with or without cleft palate)
5. Cleft palate—approximately 1 in 2,500 births; more frequent in girls
6. Combination of cleft lip and palate, approximately 50%; cleft lip, about 25%; and cleft palate, about 25%

Altered Physiology

A. *Types of Defect*
1. Development of lip and palate independent; thus, can have any combination of defects and degree of involvement
2. Cleft lip—prealveolar cleft
   a. Varies from a notch in the lip to complete separation of the lip into the nose
   b. May be unilateral or bilateral
   c. Failure of maxillary process to fuse with nasal elevations on frontal prominence; normally occurs during fifth and sixth week of gestation
   d. Merging of upper lip at midline complete between seventh and eighth week of gestation
3. Isolated cleft palate—postalveolar cleft
   a. Cleft of uvula
   b. Cleft of soft palate
   c. Cleft of both soft and hard palate through roof of mouth
   d. Unilateral or bilateral
   e. Failure of mesodermal masses of lateral palatine process to meet and fuse; normally occurs between seventh and 12th week of gestation
4. Submucous cleft
   a. Muscles of soft palate not joined
   b. Not recognized until child talks; cannot be seen at birth

5. Pierre Robin syndrome—cleft palate, glossoptosis (tongue back on pharynx), and micrognathia (underdeveloped mandible)
   a. This causes feeding difficulties, potential airway obstruction by tongue, slow weight gain, and ear infections.
   b. By 3 to 4 months of age, the mandible has grown enough to accommodate the tongue, and respiratory difficulty is greatly diminished.

Complications

1. Speech and hearing impairment
2. Improper tooth placement
3. Recurring otitis media
4. Faulty social adjustment: poor self-concept and abnormal speech
5. Possible intellectual deficits

Clinical Manifestations

1. Physical appearance of cleft lip or palate
   a. Incompletely formed lip
   b. Opening in roof of mouth felt with examiner's finger on palate
2. Eating difficulty
   a. Suction cannot be created for effective sucking
   b. Food returns through the nose
3. Nasal speech

Diagnostic Evaluation

1. Photography to document the abnormality
2. Serial x-rays before and after treatment
3. Magnetic resonance imaging to evaluate extent of abnormality before treatment
4. Dental impressions for expansion prosthesis

Treatment

1. General management is focused on closure of the cleft(s), prevention of complications, habilitation, and facilitation of normal growth and development of the child.

2. The cleft lip is generally repaired before the palate defect.
   a. Immediate repair—several hours to several weeks after birth
   b. Intraoral or extraoral prosthesis to prevent maxillary collapse, stimulate body growth, and aid in feeding and speech development; may be used before surgical repair
   c. Later repair when infant is 6 to 12 weeks old, hemoglobin 10 g/dL, steady weight gain seen—10 lb or 10,000 mm³ white blood cells (WBC)
3. Cleft palate repair may be done anytime between 6 months and 5 years; it is based on degree of deformity, width of oropharynx, neuromuscular function of palate and pharynx, and surgeon's preference.
   a. Repair at 12 to 24 months may be preferred because speech patterns have not been set, yet growth of involved structures allows for improved surgical repair.
   b. If repair is delayed to age 4 or 5 years, a special denture palate is used to help occlude the cleft and aid in establishing speech patterns.

Nursing Assessment

1. If cleft lip is visualized, assess for cleft palate by direct visualization and palpation with finger.
2. Obtain family history of cleft lip or palate.
3. Evaluate feeding abilities.
   a. Effectiveness of suck and swallow
   b. Amount taken

Nursing Diagnoses

A. Altered Nutrition: Less than body requirements related to eating difficulties
B. Risk for Infection related to open wound created by malformation
C. Impaired Adjustment to infant related to malformation and special care needs
D. Risk for Aspiration related to tongue and palate deformities in Pierre-Robin syndrome
E. Knowledge Deficit related to home management of infant with cleft malformation

Nursing Interventions

A. *Maintaining Adequate Nutrition*
1. Administer gavage feedings if nipple feeding is to be delayed to prevent spread of a cleft lip.
2. If sucking is permitted, use a soft nipple with enlarged holes to facilitate feeding.
3. If sucking is ineffective due to inability to create a vacuum, try alternate oral feeding methods.
   a. Feeding devices include regular nipple with enlarged holes: Lamb's nipple, Duckey nipple, Brecht feeder, and Premi nipple.
   b. A soft base or disposable bottle can be helpful by applying gentle, constant pressure to maintain flow. Note: Lamb's nipple may evoke gagging.
   c. Rubber-tipped asepto syringe or dropper; the rubber extension should be long enough to extend back into the mouth to prevent regurgitation through the nose. Direct tip to side of mouth, and feed slowly.

4. Feed baby in an upright, sitting position to decrease possibility of fluid being aspirated or returned through the nose or back to the auditory canal.
   a. Feed slowly; place the nipple in the infant's mouth so that it can be compressed between the existing palate and tongue.
   b. Bubble frequently during feeding to decrease amount of air swallowed.
   c. Avoid repeated removal of nipple due to fear of choking. This may only frustrate the infant, causing crying and increasing chances of aspiration.
   d. Smaller but more frequent feedings may be necessary if the infant tires or requires extended time to eat.
5. Advance diet as appropriate for age and needs of baby. Eating often improves when solids are introduced because they are easier for the baby to manipulate.
6. Encourage the mother to begin feeding the baby as soon as possible to enhance bonding.
7. Assist mother with breast-feeding if this is preferred. Suggest the use of a breast pump before nursing to stimulate the let-down reflex.

B. *Preventing Infection*
1. Protect child from infection so that surgery will not be delayed.
   a. Use and teach good handwashing practice.
   b. Avoid patient contact with anyone who has an infection.
2. Change the baby's position frequently.
3. Clean the cleft after each feeding with water and a cotton-tipped applicator.
4. Observe for fever, irritability, redness, or drainage around cleft, and report promptly.

C. *Promoting Acceptance and Adjustment*
1. Show acceptance of the baby; maintain composure, and do not show negative emotion when handling the infant. The manner in which the nurse handles the baby can make a lasting impression on the parents.
2. Support parents when showing a newborn baby for the first time. Demonstrate acceptance of both the baby and the parents' feelings. Parents may be grieving about the infant's cosmetic imperfections and may harbor ambivalent feelings about this baby.
3. Be aware that the sequence of normal parental responses may include shock and disbelief, sadness, anxiety and anger, and then proceed to a state of equilibrium and reorganization.
4. Be supportive of the parents by reassuring them that successful reparative surgery can be done.
5. Encourage parental involvement in infant's care: frequent holding, cuddling, and playing.

D. *Preventing Aspiration and Airway Obstruction*
1. When feeding the infant with Pierre Robin syndrome, consideration must be given to respiratory effort, flaccid tongue, and cleft palate. Generally, feeding can be done with a nursing bottle (feeding techniques similar to those used for cleft palate).
   a. Use orthopneic position—vertical and slightly forward; this allows infant to push jaw forward to suck and allows the feeder a clear view of the infant.
   b. Use gentle finger pressure at mandibular attachment to bring the jaw forward.
   c. Feed slowly.

2. Prevent respiratory obstruction by the tongue, especially on inspiration and when the infant is quiet.
   a. Place the infant in prone position so that tongue and jaw fall forward.
   b. Tilt head back as tolerated by the infant, and slightly elevate upper trunk.
   c. Place stockinette cap on infant's head, and suspend from an overhead support to assist the infant to maintain a position for easy ventilation.
   d. Suction nasopharynx as needed.
   e. If the tongue is sutured to pull it forward, observe for slipping, cut tongue, and infection.
3. Observe closely for respiratory compromise.

E. *Preparing for Home Management*
 1. Prepare family for home feedings by providing several days to practice feeding and to become familiar with the baby's feeding pattern.
 2. Alert caregiver to difficulties with feeding and how to manage them.
   a. Formula returning through the nose: Feed in more upright position.
   b. Respiratory distress: Feed slowly, and observe for aspiration.
   c. Longer feeding times: Feed more frequently so infant does not tire.
 3. Suggest that about 1 week prior to scheduled admission for surgery, the mother begin using feeding techniques preferred by surgeon for postoperative feeding.
   a. Side of spoon
   b. Rubber-tipped dropper
   c. Toddler cup
 4. Encourage the parents to prepare siblings at home for the arrival of this baby. Suggest a picture of the new baby.
 5. Initiate a community nurse referral to continue emotional support and teaching progress at home.
 6. Offer parents available literature about children with cleft lip and palate.
 7. Describe and reinforce surgical treatment plans to the parents to promote communication and hope.
 8. Initiate referrals, as indicated, for additional support and financial assistance.
 9. Make sure the parents realize the complex and long-term care in which they will be involved with their child, including visits to a variety of specialists (eg, pediatrician, plastic surgeon, dentist, orthodontist, prosthodontist, speech therapist).
 10. Stress compliance with follow-up care to prevent chronic otitis media, hearing loss, speech impairment, and emotional problems.

Nursing Care of the Child Undergoing Surgery

A. *Preoperative Care*
 1. Prepare the infant or toddler for the postoperative experience to decrease fear and increase cooperation.
   a. Practice the feeding measure that will be used postoperatively—cup, side of spoon, or syringe.
   b. Use elbow restraints for short periods of time; allow the child to play with them and the caregiver to use them.
   c. Explain that jacket restraint may be necessary in older child to prevent rolling over and rubbing suture line against sheets.

   d. Place child on back or side to familiarize with these positions.
   e. Demonstrate and practice mouth irrigation as it will be done postoperatively for cleft palate repair; allow the child to assist if age appropriate.
 2. Prepare the parents emotionally for the postoperative appearance of the child.
   a. Explain the use of the Logan bow (a curved metal wire that prevents stress on the suture line) and restraints.
   b. Encourage a parent to be with the child, especially when awakening from anesthesia, to offer security and comfort.

B. *Postoperative Care*
 1. Apply elbow restraints to prevent hands from reaching the mouth while still allowing some freedom of movement.
   a. Pad restraint and place it from the axilla to inner aspect of the wrist.
   b. Remove restraints occasionally, one at a time, to exercise the arms.
   c. Consider pinning restraints or cuff of shirt to the bed to decrease chances of the infant rubbing lip with his upper arm.
 2. Check Logan bow, butterfly-type adhesive, or Band-aid placed cheek-to-cheek across top of lip to prevent lateral tension on cleft lip incision.
   a. Prevent wetting tape, or it will loosen.
   b. Observe for and report bleeding.
 3. Prevent the child from crying, blowing, sucking, talking, and laughing, which increase tension on the suture line.
   a. Encourage the mother to hold and cuddle the child.
   b. Keep the child dry, fed, and comfortable.
 4. Position the child on back or propped on side to keep from rubbing lip on the sheets. An infant seat may be useful for variation of position, comfort, entertainment, and to prevent interference with suture line.
   a. Provide for appropriate diversional activity, hanging toys, mobiles, and so forth.
   b. If only cleft palate was repaired, child may lie on abdomen.
 5. Do not allow child to put anything in mouth, such as straw, eating utensils, or fingers.
 6. Monitor respiratory effort following cleft palate repair.
   a. Be aware that breathing with a closed palate is different from the child's customary way of breathing; the child also must contend with increased mucus production.
   b. Provide for croup tent with mist to decrease occurrence of respiratory problems and provide moisture to mucous membranes that may become dry from mouth breathing.
 7. Clean suture line after every feeding.
   a. Gently wipe lip incision with cotton-tipped applicator and solution of choice, such as water, saline, or hydrogen peroxide. Gently pat dry and apply antibiotic ointment or petroleum if ordered.
   b. Rinse the mouth with water, or offer a drink of water after each feeding.
   c. Irrigate the mouth with normal saline solution or water following cleft palate repair. Direct a gentle stream over the suture line using an ear bulb syringe with the child in a sitting position with head forward.
   d. Keep the mouth moist to promote healing and provide comfort.

8. Accomplish feeding without tension on the suture line for several days following lip repair.
   a. Use dropper or syringe with a rubber tip, and insert from the side to avoid suture line or to avoid stimulating sucking.
   b. Use side of spoon. Never put spoon into the mouth.
   c. Perform nasogastric gavage; usually this is last treatment of choice.
   d. Advance slowly to nipple feeding as directed. The infant should be able to suck more efficiently with the lip repaired.
9. Following palate repair, feed the child in the manner used preoperatively (cup, side of spoon, or rubber-tipped syringe). Never use straw, nipple, or plain syringe.
   a. Diet progresses from clear liquids to full liquids to soft foods.
   b. Soft foods are usually continued for about 1 month after surgery, at which time a regular diet is started, excluding hard food.
10. Check weight periodically to see if adequate nutrition is being maintained.
11. Administer antibiotics as prescribed because the mouth and suture line are constantly contaminated.

Family Education/Health Maintenance

1. Instruct on continued protection of the mouth following surgery. Child cannot put anything in mouth, including lollipops.
2. Demonstrate how to rinse mouth following eating.
3. Advise on increased risk of ear infections and need to seek medical attention for colds, ear pain, fever, or other signs and symptoms. Routine ear examinations and hearing tests should be done to reduce the risk of hearing deficits.
4. Stress the importance of speech therapy and the parents practicing exercises with the child as directed by speech therapist.
5. Help the parents realize that even though rehabilitation of the child is long and expensive, the child can live a normal life.
6. Advise the parents to discuss the child's problem with the school nurse, teacher, and other responsible adults who will have close contact with the child.
7. For additional information and support, Prescription Parents Inc.; P.O. Box 426 Quincy, MA, 02269; 617-479-2463.

Evaluation

A. Infant feeding with Lamb's nipple in small amounts every 1 to 2 hours
B. No signs of infection
C. Parents holding and talking to infant
D. Prone position maintained; no airway obstruction
E. Parents demonstrate proper feeding technique

◆ ESOPHAGEAL ATRESIA WITH TRACHEOESOPHAGEAL FISTULA

Esophageal atresia is failure of the esophagus to form a continuous passage from the pharynx to the stomach during embryonic development. Tracheoesophageal fistula (TEF) is the abnormal connection between the trachea and esophagus.

Etiology and Incidence

1. Failure of embryonic development
2. Cause unknown in most cases
3. Possible influences
   a. Inheritable genetic factor
   b. Teratogen
   c. Environmental factors
4. Occurs in 1 in 3,500 births
5. Frequently associated with prematurity and low birth weight
6. No sex differences

Altered Physiology

Failure of proper separation of the embryonic channel into the esophagus and trachea occurring during the fourth and fifth weeks of gestation.

A. **Classification of Esophageal Atresia (Fig. 45-1)**
1. Type I (10%–15% of cases; second most common): Proximal and distal segments of esophagus are blind; there is no connection to trachea.
2. Type II (very rare): Proximal segment of esophagus opens into trachea by a fistula; distal segment is blind.
3. Type III (80%–90% of cases; most common; discussion is limited to this type): Proximal segment of esophagus has blind end; distal segment of esophagus connects into trachea by a fistula.
4. Type IV (very rare): Esophageal atresia with fistula between both proximal and distal ends of trachea and esophagus.
5. Type V (not usually diagnosed at birth): Both proximal and distal segments of esophagus open into trachea by a fistula; no esophageal atresia (H-type).

B. **Tracheoesophageal Fistula**
1. Child is unable to swallow effectively.
2. Saliva or formula accumulates in upper esophageal pouch and is aspirated into airway.
3. Gastric acid is regurgitated through distal fistula.
   a. Abdominal distention occurs as a result of air entering the lower esophagus through the fistula and passing into the stomach, especially when the child is crying.
   b. Gastric distention may be severe enough to cause respiratory distress by elevation of the diaphragm.

Complications of Tracheoesophageal Fistula

1. Pneumonitis secondary to
   a. Salivary aspiration
   b. Gastric acid reflux
2. Concomitant lesions (approximately 40%–50%)
   a. Congenital heart disease
   b. Gastrointestinal (GI) anomalies, particularly imperforate anus
   c. Skeletal and muscular deformities

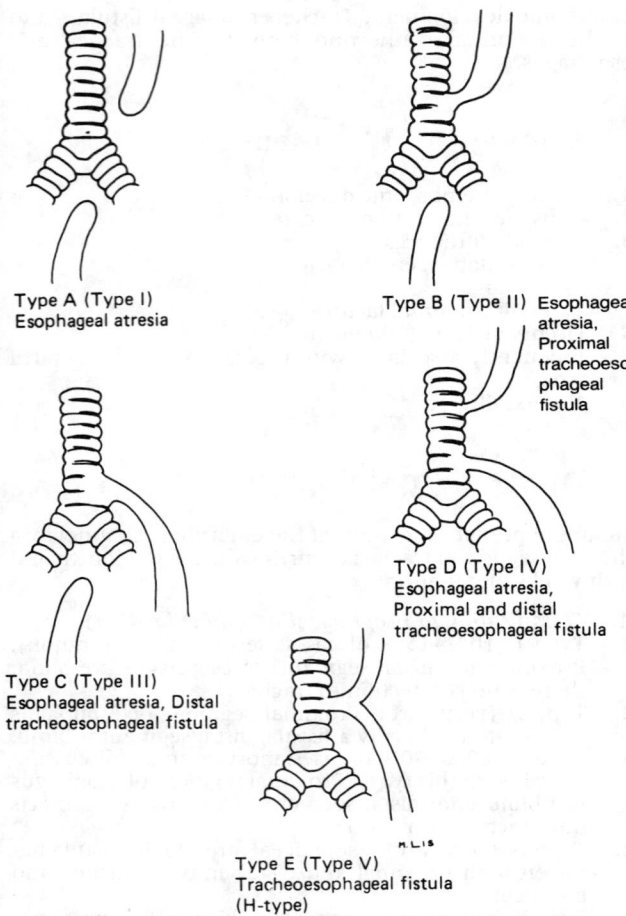

Type A (Type I)
Esophageal atresia

Type B (Type II) Esophageal
atresia,
Proximal
tracheoeso-
phageal
fistula

Type C (Type III)
Esophageal atresia, Distal
tracheoesophageal fistula

Type D (Type IV)
Esophageal atresia,
Proximal and distal
tracheoesophageal fistula

Type E (Type V)
Tracheoesophageal fistula
(H-type)

FIGURE 45-1 *Types of esophageal atresia: Esophageal atresia and tracheoesophageal fistula (TEF).*

    d. Renal anomalies
    e. Vertebral defects (possibility of Vater syndrome—vertebral defects, anal atresia, TEF, and radial limb dysfunction)
3. Prematurity
4. Dehydration and electrolyte imbalance

Clinical Manifestations

These appear soon after birth.

1. Excessive secretions
    a. Constant drooling
    b. Large amount of secretions from nose
2. Intermittent unexplained cyanosis; laryngospasm caused by aspiration of accumulated saliva in blind pouch
3. Abdominal distention
4. Violent response after first or second swallow of feeding
    a. The infant coughs and chokes.
    b. Fluid returns through nose and mouth.
    c. Cyanosis occurs.

    d. The infant struggles.
5. Inability to pass catheter through nose or mouth into stomach; tip of catheter stops at blind pouch, or atresia. Note: Be aware of coiling of catheter; coiling may make catheter appear to be descending into stomach.
6. Infant often premature and pregnancy complicated by polyhydramnios

Diagnostic Evaluation

1. Ultrasound scanning techniques enable TEF to be identified in utero for some infants.
2. A stiff, radiopaque 8- to 10-Fr catheter is unable to pass into stomach through nose or mouth.
3. X-ray flat plate of abdomen and chest may reveal presence of gas in stomach and tip of catheter in blind pouch.
4. Electrocardiogram and echocardiogram are performed because there is a high association with cardiac anomalies.

Treatment

A. Immediate Treatment
1. Propping infant at 30-degree angle to prevent reflux of gastric contents
2. Suctioning of upper esophageal pouch with Replogle tube or sump drain
3. Gastrostomy to decompress stomach and prevent aspiration; later used for feedings
4. Nothing by mouth (NPO), intravenous (IV) fluids

B. Appropriate Treatment of Any Existing Pathologic Processes
These processes are either acquired complications, such as pneumonitis, or complications from concomitant lesions, such as congestive heart failure.

C. Supportive Therapy
Supportive therapy includes meeting nutritional requirements, IV fluids, antibiotics, respiratory support, maintaining thermally neutral environment.

D. Surgery
1. Prompt primary repair: Fistula is divided followed by esophageal anastomosis of proximal and distal segments if infant is greater than 2,000 g and is without pneumonia.
2. Short-term delay: Subsequent primary repair is used to stabilize infant and prevent deterioration when the patient's condition contraindicates immediate surgery.
3. Staging: Initially, fistula division and gastrostomy are performed with later secondary esophageal anastomosis. Approach may be used with a very small, premature infant or a very sick neonate or when severe congenital anomalies exist.
4. Circular esophagomyotomy may be performed on proximal pouch to gain length and allow for primary anastomosis at initial surgery.
5. Cervical esophagostomy: When ends of esophagus are too widely separated, esophageal replacement with segment of intestine is done at 18 to 24 months of age.
6. Postoperative complications occur in 5% to 10%.
    a. Leak at anastomosis site
    b. Recurrent fistulas
    c. Esophageal strictures

d. Abnormal function of distal esophagus sphincter (gastroesophageal reflux [GER]) and esophagitis
e. Tracheomalacia
f. Feeding problems with the older child

Nursing Assessment

Assessment begins immediately after birth.

1. Be alert for risk factors of polyhydramnios and prematurity.
2. Suspect in infant with the following:
   a. Excessive amount of mucus
   b. Difficulty with secretions
   c. Cyanotic episodes (unexplained)
3. Report suspicion to healthcare provider immediately.

Nursing Diagnoses

For Preoperative Care:

A. Risk for Aspiration related to structural abnormality
B. Risk for Fluid Volume Deficit related to inability to take oral fluids
C. Anxiety of parents related to critical situation of newborn

For Postoperative Care:

A. Ineffective Airway Clearance related to surgical intervention
B. Altered Nutrition: Less than body requirements related to restricted oral intake and increased nutritional needs for healing
C. Pain related to surgical procedure
D. Impaired Tissue Integrity related to postoperative drainage

Preoperative Nursing Interventions

A. *Preventing Aspiration*
1. Position the infant with head and chest elevated 20 to 30 degrees to prevent or decrease reflux of gastric juices into the tracheobronchial tree.
   a. This position also may ease respiratory effort by dropping the distended intestines away from the diaphragm.
   b. Prone position will allow gastric juices to pool anteriorly away from the esophagus.
   c. Turn frequently to prevent atelectasis and pneumonia.
2. Perform intermittent nasopharyngeal suctioning or maintain indwelling Replogle tube (double-lumen tube) or sump tube with constant suction to remove secretions from esophageal blind pouch.
   a. Tip of tube is placed in the blind pouch.
   b. Replogle or sump tube allows air to be drawn in through a second lumen and prevents tube obstruction by mucous membrane of pouch.
   c. Maintain indwelling tube patency by irrigating with 1 mL normal saline solution frequently.

d. Ensure that indwelling tube is changed as needed and at least once every 12 to 24 hours (by the healthcare provider); alternate nostrils. Prevent necrosis of nostrils from pressure by catheter.
3. Place the infant in an Isolette or under a radiant warmer with high humidity to aid in liquefying secretions and thick mucus. Give mouth care.
4. Administer oxygen as needed.
5. Suction mouth to keep clear of secretions and prevent aspiration.
6. Be alert for indications of respiratory distress.
   a. Retractions
   b. Circumoral cyanosis
   c. Restlessness
   d. Nasal flaring
   e. Increased respiration and heart rate
7. Maintain NPO status.
8. Administer antibiotics as ordered to prevent or treat associated pneumonitis.

B. *Preventing Dehydration*
1. Administer parenteral fluids and electrolytes as prescribed (see p. 1154).
2. Monitor vital signs frequently for changes in blood pressure and pulse, which may indicate dehydration or fluid volume overload.
3. Record intake and output, including gastric drainage (if gastrostomy tube for decompression is present).

C. *Reducing Parental Anxiety*
1. Explain procedures and necessary events to parents as soon as possible.
2. Orient parents to hospital and intensive care nursery environment.
3. Allow family to hold and assist in caring for infant.
4. Offer reassurance and encouragement to family frequently. Provide for additional support by social worker, clergy, and counselor as needed.

D. *Providing Additional Nursing Care*
1. Observe infant carefully for any change in condition; report changes immediately.
   a. Check vital signs, color and amount of secretions, abdominal distention, and respiratory distress.
   b. Evaluate for complications that can occur in any neonate or premature infant.
2. Be available and recognize need for emergency care or resuscitation.
   a. Have resuscitation equipment on hand.
   b. Accompany the infant to other departments and the operating room in Isolette with portable oxygen and suction equipment.
3. Monitor for signs or symptoms that may indicate additional congenital anomalies or complications.
4. Maintain the infant's temperature in thermoneutral zone, and ensure environmental isolation to prevent infection by using Isolette.
5. Gastrostomy tube may be placed prior to definitive surgery to aid in gastric decompression and prevention of reflux. Maintain gastrostomy tube to straight gravity drainage, and do not irrigate before surgery.

Postoperative Nursing Interventions

A. *Maintaining Patent Airway*
1. Request that the surgeon mark a suction catheter, indicating how far the catheter can be safely inserted

without disturbing the anastomosis.
a. Suction frequently; every 5 to 10 minutes may be necessary, but at least every 1 to 2 hours.
b. Observe for signs of obstructed airway.
2. Administer chest physiotherapy as prescribed.
a. Change the infant's position by turning; stimulate crying to promote full expansion of lungs.
b. Elevate head and shoulders 20 to 30 degrees.
c. Use mechanical vibrator 2 to 3 days postoperatively (to minimize trauma to anastomosis), followed by more vigorous physical therapy after the third day.

> **NURSING ALERT:** ❖
> Care should be taken not to hyperextend the neck, causing stress to the operative site.

3. Continue use of Isolette or radiant warmer with humidity.
4. Be prepared for an emergency: Have emergency equipment available, including suction machine, catheter, oxygen, laryngoscope, endotracheal tubes in varying sizes.

B. Providing Adequate Nutrition
Feedings may be given by mouth, by gastrostomy, or (rarely) by a feeding tube into the esophagus, depending on the type of operation performed and the infant's condition. The gastrostomy is generally attached to gravity drainage for 3 days postoperatively, then elevated and left open to allow for air to escape and gastric secretions to pass into the duodenum before feedings are begun.

1. Administer IV solutions until gastrostomy feedings can be started.
2. Begin gastrostomy feedings as soon as ordered because adequate nutrition is an important factor in healing.
a. Give the infant a pacifier to suck during feedings, unless contraindicated.
b. Use care to prevent air from entering the stomach, thereby causing gastric distention and possible reflux.
c. Continue gastrostomy feedings until the infant can tolerate full feedings orally.

C. Providing Comfort Measures
1. Position comfortably.
2. Avoid restraints when possible.
3. Administer mouth care frequently.
4. Offer pacifier frequently.
5. Administer analgesics as ordered.
6. Hold and cuddle infant frequently.

D. Maintaining Chest Drainage
1. Assess type of chest drainage present (determined by surgical approach).
a. Retropleural—small tube in posterior mediastinum; may be left open for drainage
b. Transthoracic—chest tube placed in pleural space and connected to suction
2. Keep tubing patent: free from clots, unkinked, and without tension.
3. If a break occurs in the closed drainage system, immediately clamp tubing close to the infant to prevent pneumothorax.

E. Observing for Complications
1. Inspect for leak at the anastomosis, causing mediastinitis, pneumothorax, and saliva in chest tube: hypo-

thermia or hyperthermia, severe respiratory distress, cyanosis, restlessness, weak pulses
2. Continue to monitor for complications during the recovery process.
a. Stricture at the anastomosis: difficulty in swallowing, vomiting, or spitting up of ingested fluid; refusing to eat; fever secondary to aspiration and pneumonia
b. Recurrent fistula: coughing, choking, and cyanosis associated with feeding; excessive salivation; difficulty in swallowing associated with abnormal distention; repeated episodes of pneumonitis; general poor physical condition (no weight gain)
c. Atelectasis or pneumonitis: aspiration, respiratory distress

F. Caring for Cervical Esophagostomy
This is an artificial opening in the neck that allows for drainage of the upper esophagus.

1. Keep the area clean of saliva.
a. Wash with clear water.
b. Place an absorbent pad over the area.
2. As soon as possible, allow the infant to suck a few milliliters of milk at the same time gastrostomy feeding is being done. Advance the infant to solid foods as appropriate if esophagostomy is maintained for a few months.
a. Encourage sucking and swallowing.
b. Familiarize the infant with food so that when able to eat orally, infant will be used to it.

G. Beginning Oral Feedings
Oral feedings may begin 10 to 14 days postoperatively following anastomosis.

1. Feed slowly to allow the infant time to swallow.
2. Use upright sitting position.
3. Bubble frequently.
4. Use demand feedings rather than strictly scheduled feeding.
5. Do not allow the infant to become overtired at feeding time. Note cardiac rate.
6. Try to make each feeding a pleasant experience for the infant. Use a consistent approach and patience. Encourage parental involvement.

H. Providing Infant Stimulation and Parent–Infant Bonding
The extent of hospitalization and long-term care puts a strain on the normal opportunities in these areas.

1. Hold and cuddle the infant for feedings and after feedings.
2. Encourage parents to cuddle and talk to the infant.
3. Provide for visual, auditory, and tactile stimulation as appropriate for the infant's physical condition and age.
4. Provide opportunities for the parents to learn all aspects of care of their infant.
5. Encourage the parents to talk about their feelings, fears, and concerns.
6. Help to develop a healthy parent–child relationship through flexible visiting, frequent phone calls, and encouraging physical contact between child and parents.

Family Education/Health Maintenance

1. Teach carefully and thoroughly all procedures to be done at home. Show the parents how to do them, and

then watch return demonstration of the following procedures:
a. Gastrostomy feedings and care
b. Esophagostomy care with feeding technique
c. Suctioning
d. Identifying signs of respiratory distress
2. Help the parents understand the psychological needs of the infant for sucking, warmth, comfort, stimulation, and affection. Suggest that activity be appropriate for age.
3. Encourage the parents to continue close medical follow-up and help them learn to recognize possible problems.
   a. Eating problems may occur, especially when solids are introduced.
   b. Repeated respiratory tract infection should be reported.
   c. Occurrence of stricture at site of anastomosis weeks to months later may be recognized by difficulty in swallowing, spitting of ingested fluid, and fever.
   d. Dilatation of esophagus may be necessary to treat stricture at the site of the anastomosis.
   e. Signs of fistula leakage are dusky color or choking with feeding.
4. Help the parents understand the need for good nutrition and the need to follow the diet regimen suggested by the healthcare provider.
5. Reassure parents that an infant's raspy cough is normal and will gradually diminish as the infant's trachea becomes stronger over 6 to 24 months (most infants have some tracheomalasis).
6. Teach parents to guard against the child swallowing foreign objects. Cutting food into small pieces and chewing food well will help avoid potential esophageal obstruction.
7. For additional information and support, refer parents to Association of Birth Defects in Children; 827 Irma Ave.; Orlando, FL, 32806; 407-245-7035 or 1-800-313-2232.

Evaluation

A. No cyanosis or respiratory distress
B. Hydrated; urine output adequate
C. Parents holding infant; expressing concerns
D. Postoperatively, tolerating gastrostomy feedings without distention or regurgitation

◆ GASTROESOPHAGEAL REFLUX

Gastroesophageal reflux (GER) is a malfunction of the distal end of the esophagus, antireflux barrier, permitting return of acid stomach content into the esophagus.

Etiology and Incidence

1. Cause undetermined in most patients
2. Possible causes
   a. Delayed neuromuscular development
   b. Cerebral defects
   c. Obstruction at or just below the pylorus
   d. Physiologic immaturity
   e. Complication of esophageal surgery

3. Mechanisms of GER may involve an interplay of
   a. Esophageal motility
   b. Lower esophageal sphincter activity
   c. Gastric emptying
   d. Physiologic immaturity
   e. Complication of esophageal surgery
4. Associated conditions that cause reflux include
   a. Coughing and wheezing from cystic fibrosis, bronchopulmonary dysplasia, asthma
   b. Indwelling oronasogastric feeding tube
   c. Medications: theophylline, which affects lower sphincter and increases gastric acidity
   d. Position: supine, chest physical therapy positions
5. Common problem during first year of life; about 3% of newborns
6. Males affected 3% more frequently than females

Altered Physiology

1. The lower esophageal sphincter is a physiologic rather than an anatomic segment that forms an antireflux barrier.
   a. The segment is 2 to 5 cm in length.
   b. The segment is characterized by a pressure greater than that found proximally in the esophagus or distally in the stomach.
   c. Constitutes an effective barrier to protect the esophageal mucosa from damage by gastric contents (acid, pepsin, bile salts).
2. GER is a consequence of incompetence or malfunctioning of this lower esophageal sphincter.
   a. Filling of the esophagus from the stomach on inspiration, leading to vomiting
   b. Increased intra-abdominal pressure

Complications

Complications result from frequent and sustained reflux of gastric contents into lower esophagus.

1. Recurrent pulmonary disease; aspiration pneumonia
2. Chronic esophagitis
3. Failure to thrive
4. Anemia
5. Cynanotic episodes may be associated with choking
6. Apnea
7. Near-miss sudden infant death syndrome
8. Esophageal stricture from scarring; esophagitis
9. Asthma
10. Hiatal hernia frequently associated with a chalasia (reflux; relaxation or incompetence of lower esophageal sphincter)

Clinical Manifestations

A. *Infant*
1. Vomiting (unexplained)
   a. Immediately after feeding, especially when the infant is placed in a prone position
   b. Usually regurgitation rather than projectile vomiting
2. Onset usually soon after birth
3. Weight loss or failure to gain weight; rumination

4. Dehydration
5. Recurrent pulmonary symptoms
6. Colic, excessive crying
7. Sleep disturbances

B. *Older Child*
1. Substernal burning
2. Upper abdominal discomfort; pressure or "squeezing" feeling
3. Persistent pulmonary problems
4. Dysphagia as evidenced by irritability during eating
5. Anemia
6. Hematemesis or melena (blood in stools)

Diagnostic Evaluation

1. History of infant or child's feeding habits
2. Upper GI barium x-ray with fluoroscopy—shows reflux into esophagus
3. pH in esophagus—extended 18 to 24 hours (appears to be most useful procedure)
4. Serum studies
   a. Calcium level may be lowered.
   b. Alkalosis shows pH greater than 7.45.
   c. Hemoglobin and hematocrit may be decreased.
5. Fiberoptic esophagoscopy—may show presence of gastric folds above the diaphragm and esophageal biopsy for tissue sample

Treatment

Goal of treatment is to reduce reflux and associated complications. May be treated medically or surgically.

A. *Medical Management*
1. Positioning—based on premise that gravity will help reduce amount of reflux; should be maintained as much as possible
   a. Infants younger than 6 months
      (1) Prone: Elevated infant with folded blankets or towels under mattress.
      (2) Position infant in harness at 30-degree angle, 60 minutes to constant 24 hours.
      (3) Infant also may be held upright.
      (4) When positioned in infant seat, infant will probably slump, causing increased intra-abdominal pressure and increased GER.
   b. Older infant—placement in a walker with parental instruction about safety and continuous monitoring of infant
   c. Older child—head of bed raised with blocks to maintain 30- to 45-degree angle
2. Feeding
   a. Infant
      (1) Thickened feedings, such as dry rice cereal or commercial thickening agent
      (2) May cause a decrease in the number of episodes; however, the duration of reflux episodes is increased, thus increasing the risk of complications
      (3) Small, frequent feedings followed by positioning
   b. Older child
      (1) Nothing to eat 2 hours before bedtime
      (2) Possible avoidance of certain foods
      (3) Should remain upright while awake

3. Medication
   a. Medication to stimulate lower esophageal sphincter pressure (tone) and increase peristaltic wave amplitude and clearance rate, such as metoclopramide (Reglan), bethanechol (Duvoid), and domperidone (Motilium).
   b. H_2 blockers, such as cimetidine (Tagamet), when esophagitis has been documented
   c. Antacid between feedings if esophagitis is present (forms a floating barrier)

B. *Surgical Management*
1. Surgical reconstruction of esophagogastric junction (fundoplication) may be necessary if conservative management does not improve condition or if recurrent severe respiratory disease and apnea or refractory esophagitis with stricture occur. Fundoplication recreates a valve by wrapping the fundus of the stomach around the lower part of the esophagus; any defects in diaphragm are reported.
2. Gastropexy is surgical fixation of stomach in the abdomen below the diaphragm.
3. Temporary gastrostomy may be performed to decompress the stomach, avoiding gastric distention.
4. Complications include retching with feeding, watery diarrhea, growth retardation, small bowel obstruction, and dumping syndrome. Dumping syndrome usually occurs 30 minutes after meal and includes symptoms such as diaphoresis, palpitations, weakness, syncope, abdominal fullness, nausea, and diarrhea.
5. Nursing care is similar to care of child after surgery for pyloric stenosis.

Nursing Assessment

1. Obtain history of infant's or child's eating habits.
2. Observe infant's or child's feeding behaviors.
3. Assess general appearance, skin integrity, and growth and development.

Nursing Diagnoses

A. Risk for Aspiration related to reflux of gastric contents
B. Altered Nutrition: Less than body requirements related to decreased oral intake
C. Risk for Fluid Volume Deficit related to frequent vomiting

Nursing Interventions

A. *Preventing Aspiration*
1. Administer medications such as metoclopromide 30 minutes prior to feeding and before sleep for best effect.
2. Maintain infant or child upright 30 to 40 degrees at all times whether awake or asleep. Gravity will help reduce reflux and help clear esophagus more readily.

NURSING ALERT:
Avoid slouching position because this may change angle of esophagus in relation to stomach, increase intra-abdominal pressure, and facilitate reflux of stomach contents.

3. Use infant "antireflux" saddle—covered, padded wedges with a sling designed for infant to straddle face down at elevated angle.
   a. Observe for lower leg edema, flattening of parietal skull, and torticollis (muscle contraction of neck).
   b. Turn infant's head frequently.
   c. Elevate infant's legs prior to eating or bathing.
4. Use cardiac and apnea monitors for infants and children with severe reflux.
   a. Observe for apneic periods of more than 20 seconds or accompanied by cyanosis, pallor, or bradycardia.
   b. Document apnea episodes, associated symptoms, and recovery efforts.

B. *Maintaining Adequate Nutrition*
1. Thicken formula for each feeding.
   a. Add 1 teaspoon to 1 tablespoon of rice cereal to each ounce of formula.
   b. Enlarge nipple hole so that formula can be more easily extracted by cross-cutting it.
2. Prop infant upright.
3. Reduce crying before and after meals, which increases intra-abdominal pressure and swallowing of air, increasing the likelihood of reflux.
4. Use a pacifier for non-nutritive sucking after eating only when infant is seated upright, because use of pacifier while prone increases reflux.
5. Handle the infant gently, with minimal movement during and after feeding.
6. Bubble frequently during and after feeding.
7. Record accurately activity of infant.
   a. Amount of feeding taken; whether retained
   b. Emesis; estimated amount, type, occurrence in relation to feeding
   c. Any change in behavior as a result of feeding technique
8. If breast-feeding, feeding modifications must be made (ie, express milk and thicken with cereal).
9. Ensure that older children avoid caffeine-containing food and beverages (such as chocolate) to reduce gastric acid production. Also maintain a low-fat diet because fat delays gastric emptying, and discourage eating 2 to 4 hours before bedtime.
10. Monitor weight frequently to evaluate progress.

C. *Maintaining Fluid and Electrolyte Balance*
1. Monitor vital signs, and assess skin turgor for signs of dehydration.
2. Observe and record accurately urinary output.
   a. Amount, frequency, color, and concentration
   b. Specific gravity
3. Monitor IV therapy if ordered.
4. Monitor serum electrolytes, and replace sodium and potassium as ordered.
5. Promote good skin care to prevent lesions of dry and delicate tissues.
   a. Change position frequently.
   b. Change soiled diapers often.
   c. Apply lotion, and gently massage any reddened areas.

Family Education/Health Maintenance

1. Plan a program of intensive parental teaching on how to handle and care for the infant. Explain rationale to parents. Ensure that they have proper equipment for propping the infant. Help the parents understand that it is not necessary to keep infant in infant seat or propped at all times.
   a. Bathe or play with the infant prior to feeding.
   b. Change position about 1 hour after feeding.
   c. During the night after feeding, the infant can sleep in an upright position.
   d. Expect occasional small amounts of vomiting.
2. Offer clear, concise instructions. Focus on parental fears. Discuss techniques to promote developmental tasks of infants while facilitating bonding and normal parental behavior.
3. Help parents to understand that chalasia is self-limited; symptoms usually disappear within 12 months.
4. If a temporary gastrostomy is done, ensure that the parents know how to use, clear, and replace the tube. Tube and vent should be elevated to avoid gastric distention.
5. Help the parents understand the importance of follow-up of weight gain and development.
6. Assist with community resource planning (ie, education, advocacy, and financial assistance). Identify support groups.
7. Instruct parents and caregivers in cardiopulmonary resuscitation training prior to discharge of infant, if indicated.
8. Provide written and verbal instructions as to medications and side effects.
9. Encourage family to contact their healthcare provider immediately with treatment concerns or problems.

Evaluation

A. Mild regurgitation immediately following feeding; no apnea or cyanosis noted
B. Taking 3 to 4 oz thickened formula every 2 hours; weight gain
C. Urine output adequate

◆ HYPERTROPHIC PYLORIC STENOSIS

Hypertrophic pyloric stenosis is congenital, progressive hypertrophy of the muscle of the pylorus, causing partial or total obstruction of the stomach outlet (pyloric sphincter). It is the second most common condition requiring surgery during the first 2 months of life (after inguinal hernia).

Etiology and Incidence

1. Unknown cause
2. Possibly, immature pyloric ganglion cells—environmental, partial genetic basis
3. Incidence—1 in 150 male births and 1 in 750 female births
4. Less frequently seen in African American and Asian than in Caucasian infants

Altered Physiology

1. Increase in size of the circular musculature of the pylorus with thickening (size and shape of an olive). The

pylorus muscle becomes elongated and thickened and is enlarged to about twice the usual size.
2. Hypertrophy of the pylorus musculature occurs with narrowing of the pyloric lumen.
3. Constriction of the lumen of the pyloric canal (at the distal end of the stomach) causes the stomach to become dilated.
4. Gastric emptying is delayed; vomiting after feeding and obstruction also occurs.

Complications

1. Starvation
2. Dehydration
3. Severe electrolyte imbalance
4. Hematemesis

Clinical Manifestations

Onset is within the first 2 months after birth, usually about 3 weeks of age.

1. Vomiting—onset may be gradual and intermittent or sudden and forceful, with the following characteristics:
   a. Occasional, nonprojectile vomiting at first, gradually increasing in frequency and intensity
   b. Projectile vomiting, not bile stained
2. Constipation—decreased quantity of stools
3. Loss of weight or failure to gain weight
4. Visible gastric peristaltic waves, left to right
5. Excessive hunger—willingness to eat immediately after vomiting
6. Dehydration—electrolyte disturbance with alkalosis
7. Decreased urinary output
8. Palpable pyloric mass in upper right quadrant of abdomen, to the right of the umbilicus and best felt during feeding or immediately after vomiting

Diagnostic Evaluation

1. Palpation of pyloric mass ("olive") in conjunction with persistent, projectile vomiting with associated alkalosis
2. Tests for metabolic alkalosis due to loss of hydrochloric acid and potassium from vomiting
   a. Decreased serum sodium
   b. Decreased serum chloride
   c. Decreased serum potassium
   d. Increased serum pH above 7
   e. Increased Serum CO_2
3. Urinalysis—urine alkaline and concentrated
4. Blood hematocrit and hemoglobin—elevated due to hemoconcentration
5. Flat film of abdomen—dilated, air-filled stomach; non-dilated pyloric canal
6. X-ray examination with barium—narrowing of pyloric canal, delayed gastric emptying, enlarged stomach, increased peristaltic waves, and gas distal to stomach
7. Ultrasound evaluation—thick hypoechoic ring in the region of the pylorus

Treatment

1. Initial treatment
   a. Rehydrate to correct electrolytes
   b. Correct alkalosis

2. Surgical—pyloromyotomy (Fredet-Ramstedt procedure)
   a. Hypertrophy of the pyloric muscle regresses to normal size by about 12 weeks postoperatively.
   b. GER may be a complication of surgery.

Nursing Assessment

1. Obtain a thorough history of infant's feeding behaviors and history of vomiting.
2. Assess and chart growth and development parameters.

Nursing Diagnoses

A. Fluid Volume Deficit related to frequent vomiting
B. Altered Nutrition: Less than body requirements (failure to thrive) related to vomiting
C. Pain related to gastric distention
D. Anxiety of parents related to illness, hospitalization, and impending surgery of child

Preoperative Nursing Care

A. *Maintaining Fluid and Electrolyte Balance*
1. Administer IV therapy as ordered to treat dehydration, metabolic alkalosis, and electrolyte deficiency.
2. Carefully observe output, including amount, and characteristics of urine (check specific gravity), vomiting, and stools.
3. Accurately measure daily weight as a guide for calculating need for parenteral fluid.
4. Monitor laboratory data for serum electrolytes.
5. Apply appropriate restraints on infants to prevent interference with fluid therapy.
6. Provide pacifier for infants who are NPO.
7. Monitor vital signs as indicated by condition. Watch for tachycardia, hypotension, change in respirations.

> **NURSING ALERT:**
> Irregular respiratory rate with apnea is a sign of severe alkalosis.

B. *Maintaining Nutrition*
1. Emphasize rehydration, electrolyte balance, and replacement of body fat and protein stores. This depends on severity of depletion and may require total parenteral nutrition for several days or weeks prior to surgery to improve surgical risk.
2. Maintain NPO status with indwelling nasogastric tube (inserted to remove any residual barium and retained formula) as ordered. Ensure proper functioning of tube, and note drainage.
3. If oral feedings are to be continued, do the following:
   a. Provide small, frequent feedings, given slowly.
   b. Bubble frequently before, during, and after feeding.
   c. Thicken formula if ordered.
   d. Allow breast-feeding as tolerated.
4. Prop the patient in upright position (Fig. 45-2).
   a. Elevate head of bed, mattress, or infant seat at a 75- to 80-degree angle.
   b. Place slightly on right side to aid in gastric emptying.
   c. Handle gently and minimally after feeding.

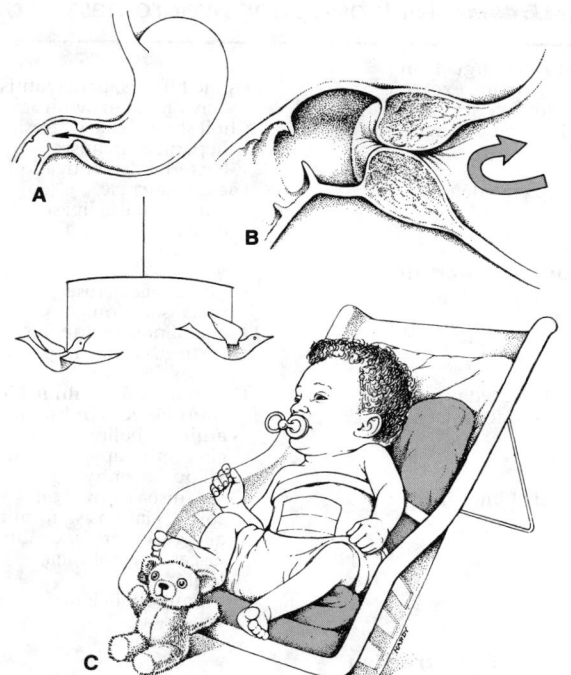

FIGURE 45-2 *Pyloric stenosis.* **(A)** *Normal passage through pyloric sphincter.* **(B)** *Stoppage of flow due to stenotic sphincter.* **(C)** *Postoperative treatment: Child propped upright, slightly on right side aids in gastric emptying.*

Postoperative Nursing Care

A. Preventing Complications
1. Assess vital signs to evaluate for fluid and electrolyte imbalances.
2. Assess skin and mucous membranes for hydration status.
3. Weigh daily to assess gain or loss.
4. Elevate head slightly.
5. Maintain patent nasogastric tube to prevent gastric distention. Record losses.
6. Monitor blood glucose levels to prevent hypoglycemia.

B. Maintaining Hydration
1. Administer IV fluids until adequate intake has been established.
2. Resume oral feeding 2 to 8 hours after surgery when infant is alert or as ordered.
3. Start with small, frequent feedings of glucose water, and slowly advance to full-strength formula and regular diet as tolerated.
4. Report any vomiting—the amount and characteristics. Feeding schedule may be withheld 4 hours and then restarted.
5. Feed slowly and bubble frequently.
6. Note how feeding is taken and if it is retained.
7. Increase the amount of feeding as the time interval between feedings is lengthened.
8. Allow breast-feeding to resume as tolerated, beginning with limited nursing of 5 to 8 minutes and gradually increase.
9. Continue to elevate the infant's head and shoulders after feeding for 45 to 60 minutes for several feedings after surgery. Place on right side to aid gastric emptying.
10. Expect that regurgitation may continue for a short period after surgery. Nasogastric tube may be maintained for length of time, as determined by provider.

C. Other Nursing Responsibilities
1. Administer analgesics as ordered and as indicated by behavior of infant.
2. Provide additional comfort measures, such as a pacifier, rocking, and other soothing stimulation.
3. Involve parents in care of infant postoperatively to prepare them for care after discharge.
4. Observe for drainage or signs of inflammation at incision site, and provide care to incision as ordered.
5. Note that poor nutritional status may delay wound healing.

Family Education/Health Maintenance

1. Teach proper care of the operative site.
   a. Check for signs and symptoms of inflammation.
   b. Observe for drainage.
   c. Provide specific care of site as ordered by provider.
2. Teach feeding technique to be continued at home; length of feeding technique varies depending on wound healing, nutritional status, and growth.
3. Provide written and verbal instructions as to infant's care and follow-up schedule.
4. Review with family when medical attention is needed and appropriate resource:
   a. Signs of infection

C. Providing Comfort
1. Provide mouth care, and wet lips frequently if NPO.
2. Let the infant suck on a pacifier.
3. Provide for physical contact or nearness without excessive stimulation.
4. Provide for audio and visual stimulation that may be soothing.
5. Do not palpate pyloric "olive" to decrease risk of postoperative wound infection from bruising abdominal wall and excoriating tissue in operative site.
6. Administer analgesics as ordered.

D. Alleviating Parental Anxiety
1. Assess understanding of diagnosis and plan of care.
2. Help minimize guilt feelings by providing adequate, specific information and clarifying any misconceptions.
3. Prepare the parents for the surgery of their child.
   a. Be honest with them.
   b. Prepare them for the expected postoperative appearance of the infant.
   c. Show them where the operating room and recovery room are located and where to wait during surgery.
4. Allow them to hold the infant to maintain bonding.
5. Encourage them to rest to care better for the infant postoperatively.
6. Accept and explore negative displays of emotion, which may be due to fatigue and frustration because of the extensive care given to the child prior to hospitalization.
7. Reassure them that surgery is considered curative, and normal feeding should resume shortly afterward.

b. Frequent vomiting or poor feeding with signs of dehydration
c. Abdominal distention

Evaluation

A. Vital signs stable; urine output adequate
B. Tolerating 1- to 2-oz feedings in upright position without vomiting
C. Quietly resting with pacifier
D. Parents verbalizing understanding of surgery and postoperative care

◆ CELIAC DISEASE

Celiac disease, also called gluten-sensitive enteropathy or celiac sprue, is a disease of the small intestines characterized by a permanent inability to tolerate dietary gluten. Celiac disease is classified as a malabsorption syndrome. Characteristics of malabsorption syndromes are 1) steatorrhea (fatty, frothy, foul-smelling, bulky stool); 2) general malnutrition; 3) abdominal distention; and 4) secondary vitamin deficiencies. Other causes of malabsorption syndromes are listed in Table 45-1.

Etiology and Incidence

1. The cause is unknown; although the relationship of gluten to mucosal abnormalities is established, the mechanism of these mucosal changes is unclear.
2. Genetics include the following:
   a. Familial incidence
   b. Mode of inheritance not clear; probably autosomal recessive with incomplete penetrance
3. Environmental inference is likely; role of other "allergens" is unclear.
4. Current theories being investigated include the following:
   a. Immunologic (autoimmune versus specific immune abnormality, aberrant immunologic response to gluten)
   b. Search to identify deficient enzymes that digest gluten or possible lack of intestinal enzymes that detoxify glutens; altered epithelial cell surfaces, which allow gluten or gluten-fragment binding with resultant cellular toxicity
5. Highest incidence is reported in western Ireland and other countries of northwestern Europe.
6. Male to female ratio is 1:1.2 to 1.4.

Altered Physiology

1. Characteristics of celiac disease include the following:
   a. Impaired intestinal absorption
   b. Histologic abnormalities of the small intestine
   c. Clinical and histologic improvement with wheat- and rye-free (possibly also barley- and oat-free) diet
   d. Recurrence of clinical manifestations and histologic changes after reintroduction of dietary gluten

TABLE 45-1   Malabsorption Syndromes

Reduced Digestion	
Pancreatic exocrine deficiency	Cystic fibrosis, pancreatitis, Schwachman syndrome
Bile salt deficiency	Cholestasis, biliary atresia, hepatitis, cirrhosis, bacterial deconjugation
Enzyme defects	Lactase, sucrase, enterokinase, lipase deficiences
Reduced Absorption	
Primary absorption defects	Glucose—galactose malabsorption, abetalipoproteinemia, cystinuria, Hartnup disease
Decreased mucosal surface area	Crohn disease, malnutrition, short bowel syndrome, antimetabolite chemotherapy, familial villous atrophy
Small intestinal disease	Celiac disease, tropical sprue, giardiasis, immune/allergic enteritis, Crohn disease, lymphoma, acquired immunodeficiency syndrome
Lymphatic Obstruction	
	Lymphangiectasia, Whipple disease, lymphoma, chylous ascites
Other	
Drugs	Antibiotics, antimetabolites, neomycin, laxatives
Collagen vascular	Scleroderma
Infestations	Hookworms, tapeworm, giardiasis, immune defects

2. Histologic changes in mucosa of small bowel, especially duodenum and jejunum, resulting from dietary gluten include the following:
   a. Irregularity of epithelial cells
   b. Loss of normal villous pattern
   c. Obliteration of intervillous spaces that are infiltrated with plasma cells and eosinophils
   d. Loss of epithelial cell brush border
3. Mucosal damage results in the following:
   a. Disaccharidase deficiency
   b. Depression of peptidase activity
4. Subsequent malabsorption probably results from the following:
   a. Decreased area of absorption in small bowel
   b. Impaired enzyme activity
5. The body is unable to absorb fats, fat-soluble vitamins (A, D, E, and K), minerals, and some protein and carbohydrates.
6. The severity of symptoms of the disease depends on the extent of intestine with histologic changes.
   a. The extent of affected intestine is variable.
   b. Generally, proximal small intestine mucosal damage is most severe, and condition decreases in severity distally.

Complications

1. Possible predisposition to malignant lymphoma of small intestine at later age if dietary restrictions are terminated
2. Refractory sprue
3. Associated disorders
   a. Dermatitis herpetiformis
   b. Insulin-dependent diabetes mellitus
   c. Cystic fibrosis
4. Impaired growth, inability to fight infection, electrolyte disturbances, and blood clotting

Clinical Manifestations

The age and mode of presenting signs and symptoms are extremely variable. Diagnosis is most commonly made by 6 to 24 months of age; however, it can be made in the adult.

A. *3 to 9 Months of Age*
1. Acutely ill; severe diarrhea and vomiting
2. Possibly failure to thrive

B. *9 to 18 Months of Age*
"Typical" celiac appearance is seen.

1. Impaired growth
   a. Normal growth during early months of life
   b. Slackening of weight followed by weight loss
2. Abnormal stools
   a. Pale
   b. Soft
   c. Bulky
   d. Offensive odor
   e. Greasy—steatorrhea
   f. May increase in number
3. Abdominal distention
4. Anorexia
5. Muscle wasting—most obvious in buttocks and proximal parts of extremities
6. Hypotonia
7. Mood changes—ill humor, irritability, temper tantrums, shyness
8. Mild clubbing of fingers
9. Vomiting—often occurring in evening

C. *Older Child*
1. Signs and symptoms often related to nutritional or secondary deficiencies resulting from disease
2. May have abnormal stools and growth impairment
3. May have colicky abdominal pain with constipation and large, pale stools

D. *Manifestations Secondary to Malabsorption*
1. Anemia, vitamin deficiency
2. Hypoproteinemia with edema
3. Hypocalcemia, hypokalemia, hypomagnesemia
4. Hypoprothrombinemia resulting from impaired vitamin K absorption
5. Disaccharide intolerance—with acid sugar-containing stools (secondary to the altered small bowel mucosa)

E. *Celiac Crisis*
This is rare and most often seen in very young children and toddlers.

1. Profound anorexia
2. Severe vomiting and diarrhea
3. Weight loss
4. Marked dehydration and acidosis (secondary to intractable diarrhea and vomiting)
5. Immobility
6. Grossly distended abdomen
   a. Fluid rattle is present
   b. Abdomen flattens with passage of large, liquid stool
7. Patient shocklike and profoundly depressed

Diagnostic Evaluation

1. Thorough history, including dietary patterns, and general status of the child
2. Small bowel biopsy—abnormal mucosa
3. Diagnostic criteria
   a. Severely damaged or flat, villous lesions
   b. Clinical response to gluten elimination
   c. Histologic recovery following gluten elimination
   d. Histologic recurrence of villous injury within 2 years of gluten reintroduction
4. D-Kylose absorption—less than 20 to 25 mg/dL at 60 minutes
5. Red blood count smear—hypochromia
6. Serum iron and folate—folic acid reduced
7. Immunoglobulin determination—immunoglobulin A may be increased in acute stage of disease
8. 24-hour stool collection for fecal fat times three—increased
9. Measurement of hemoglobin levels—may be reduced
10. Prothrombin time—may be decreased (done before intestinal biopsy)
11. Radiologic studies—skeletal x-rays
    a. Demineralization
    b. Retarded bone age
12. Sweat test and pancreatic function studies to rule out cystic fibrosis

Treatment

A. *Dietary Modifications*
1. Lifelong gluten-free diet
   a. Avoid all foods containing wheat or rye gluten. The exclusion of barley and oats is controversial; however, it is often wise to err on the safe side or to offer specific challenges and to test with biopsy.
   b. The small intestinal mucosa will always respond abnormally to dietary gluten, even though clinical signs may not be immediately evident.
   c. Biopsy reverts to normal with appropriate diet.
   d. Clinical signs of improvement should be seen 1 to 4 weeks after proper diet is initiated.
2. Adequate caloric intake
3. Supplemental vitamins and minerals
   a. Folic acid for 1 to 2 months
   b. Vitamins A and D because not absorbed
   c. Iron for 1 to 2 months if anemic
   d. Vitamin K if evidence of hypoprothrombinemia and bleeding
   e. Calcium if milk is restricted
4. Reduction of fat intake (rare)
5. Possible elimination of lactose from diet for 6 to 8 weeks based on reduced disaccharidase activity

B. *Treatment of Celiac Crisis*
1. IV restoration of electrolyte balance and fluids for replacement of blood volume

2. Corticosteroids
3. Parenteral hyperalimentation with amino acids, medium chain triglycerides, and glucose for short periods of time
4. Initial oral feedings disaccharide- or completely sugar-free

Nursing Assessment

1. Obtain family dietary history as it relates to onset of symptoms.
2. Assess child's nutritional status.
3. Check for signs of infection.
4. Assess growth and development.

Nursing Diagnoses

A. Altered Nutrition: Less than body requirements related to malabsorption of nutrients, diarrhea, and vomiting
B. Risk for Infection related to malnourishment and anemia
C. Fluid Volume Deficit related to celiac crisis
D. Altered Parenting related to inability to control behavioral problems

Nursing Interventions

A. *Providing Adequate Nutrition and Dietary Restrictions*
1. Ensure that initial diet is high in protein, relatively low in fat, and free of starch
   a. Provide mild protein or skim milk that is sweetened with sucrose or banana powder.
   b. Watch for fat intolerance in infants and young children.
2. Advise adding proteins and sugars gradually.
   a. Add individual foods one at a time at several day intervals, such as lean meat, cottage cheese, egg white, and raw ground apple.
   b. Add starchy foods to diet last.
3. Restrict wheat and rye from diet.
4. Maintain NPO status during the initial treatment of celiac crisis or during diagnostic testing; Take special precautions to ensure proper restriction if the child is ambulatory.
5. Encourage small, frequent, appetizing meals, but do not force eating if the child has anorexia.
6. Note the child's reaction to food. Close observation of the child's responses to food may reveal other intolerances. Note and record the following:
   a. Foods taken and those refused
   b. Appetite
   c. Change in behavior after eating
   d. Characteristics and frequency of stools
   e. General disposition—behavior improvement often seen within 2 to 3 days after diet control is initiated
7. Be prepared to temporarily eliminate new food introduced if symptoms increase.
8. Assist with gluten-challenge diet if used to evaluate histologic and clinical response during therapy.
   a. Be aware that after an extended time on dietary regimen, the child may dislike gluten-containing foods.

   b. Assess for mild GI symptoms (eg, loose stools, vague abdominal pain) that may be related to anxiety rather than gluten intolerance.
   c. Support the family, and provide reassurance. The gluten-challenge diet may last 3 to 4 months before bowel biopsy is repeated.

B. *Preventing Infection*
1. Advise parents to avoid exposing the child to anyone with an infection.
2. Teach parents that the child usually perspires freely and has a subnormal temperature with cold extremities; prevent dampness and chilling and encourage appropriate clothing.
3. Prevent upper respiratory infection by position changes, good hygiene, and clearance of secretions.
4. Teach and practice good handwashing.
5. Assess for fever, cough, irritability, or other signs of infection.

C. *Replacing Fluid Volume in Celiac Crisis*
1. Replace fluids and electrolytes by parenteral therapy as ordered.
2. Give nothing by mouth, especially if child is vomiting. Nasogastric tube may be prescribed; monitor drainage and patency.
3. Observe the child carefully for shock.
4. Monitor respirations for increased rate and depth, indicating acidosis.
5. Monitor serum electrolytes and arterial pH levels to detect intolerances and help guide therapy.

D. *Promoting Effective Parenting*
1. Teach the parents to develop an awareness of the child's behavior; recognize changes and care for child accordingly.
2. Explain that diet and eating have a direct effect on behavior and that behavior may indicate how the child is feeling.
3. Help the parents recognize and understand mood swings, from having temper tantrums to being very timid, nervous, or unstable.
4. Advise the parents to allow the child to express feelings freely through safe and age-appropriate media.
   a. Encourage parents to define limits of behavior for the child and convey them to all family members.
   b. Avoid conflict or emotional upset in the child's presence when possible. These may precipitate diarrhea, vomiting, and celiac crisis.
5. Encourage patience, routines, and consistency.
6. Advise parents to record changes in behavior, especially in relation to eating and diet to document effectiveness of therapy.
7. Help the parents to maintain a balance between the child with celiac disease, the other family members, and additional rules and responsibilities.
8. If the child is withdrawn, advise providing opportunity for play with other children, especially when the child begins to feel better.
9. Explain that the toddler may cling to infantile habits for security. Allow this behavior; it may disappear as physical condition improves.
10. Suggest offering the child other sensory stimulation to compensate for lack of eating pleasure.
11. Help the parents to understand that after initial rapid weight gain, further improvement may be slow.
12. Provide emotional support for the child and parents.
13. Refer for counseling if indicated.

Family Education/Health Maintenance

1. Teach parents about celiac disease and how it is controlled by diet.
   a. Provide a specific list of restricted and acceptable foods.
   b. Teach the parents how to read labels on foods to identify those containing wheat and rye glutens, thus avoiding them.
   c. Provide substitutes for wheat, rye, barley, and oats, such as corn, rice, soybean flour, and gluten-free starch.
   d. Help the parents become comfortable in situation problem solving (ie, supplying gluten-free cupcakes for birthday party to which child has been invited).
   e. Initiate referral with dietitian.
   f. Emphasize the importance of the vitamin regimen.
   g. Discuss the importance of continued adherence to diet, even though the child is feeling well, eating well, and has normal stools. Advancing diet too rapidly may result in a setback. Encourage child to become involved in diet.
   h. Adolescent compliance may be variable. Encourage support and understanding.
   i. Alteration in diet may have significant cultural, ethnic, and religious implications. Help parents identify how adjustments can be made.
2. Impress on the parents the importance of regular medical follow-up.
   a. Encourage the parents to seek prompt medical attention if the child has an upper respiratory infection that might trigger celiac crisis if untreated.
   b. Ensure that the parents understand measures to prevent celiac crisis—dietary control, dangers of prolonged fasting, informing unfamiliar healthcare provider of celiac disorder, and use of anticholinergic drugs that may decrease GI motility and precipitate celiac crisis.
3. Encourage the parents to practice good hygiene to prevent infection because this child is especially prone to infection because of malnutrition and anemia.
4. Help the parents to understand that the emotional climate in the home and around the child is vitally important in maintaining the child's medical and physical stability.
5. Stress that the disorder is lifelong; however, changes in the mucosal lining of the intestine and the general clinical condition of their child are reversible when dietary gluten is avoided.
6. A reference for parents entitled "Pointers for Parents: Coping with Celiac Sprue" is available from Clinical Nutrition Dept. #23, Children's Memorial Hospital, 2300 Children's Plaza, Chicago, IL, 60614, 312-880-4000.
7. For additional information and support, refer to Celiac Sprue Association; P.O. Box 31700; Omaha, NE, 68131-0700; 402-558-0600.

Evaluation

A. Tolerating starch-free diet well without pain or vomiting
B. No signs of infection
C. Vital signs stable; remains NPO

D. Parents setting limits with child and documenting behavior in relation to meals

◆ DIARRHEA

Diarrhea is an excessive loss of water and electrolytes that occurs with passage of one or more unformed stools. It is a symptom of many conditions and may be caused by many diseases (Table 45-2).

Etiology and Incidence

Often the cause is difficult to determine; occasionally it is unknown. The numerous causes of diarrhea in infants and young children include the following:

A. *Infectious Factors*
1. Bacterial
   a. Enteropathogenic *Escherichia coli*
   b. *Salmonella*
   c. *Shigella*
   d. *Yersinia enterocolitica*
   e. *Campylobacter fetus*
2. Viral
   a. Enteroviruses—echoviruses
   b. Adenoviruses
   c. Human reovirus-like agent
   d. Rotovirus—frequent during winter months
3. Normal intestinal tract inhabitants that act as pathogens in certain circumstances (ie, after ingestion of antibiotics)
4. Fungal—*Candida* enteritis
5. Parasitic—*Giardia lamblia*
6. Protozoal

B. *Noninfectious Factors*
1. Allergy to certain foods—milk, wheat protein
2. Metabolic disorders
   a. Celiac disease
   b. Cystic fibrosis of pancreas
3. Disaccharidase deficiencies
4. Infant exposed to overfeeding; displaying emotional excitement and fatigue
5. Direct irritation of GI tract by foods
6. Inappropriate use of laxatives and purgatives

C. *Mechanical Disorders*
1. Malrotation
2. Incomplete small bowel obstruction
3. Intermittent volvulus

D. *Congenital Anomalies (ie, Hirschsprung's disease)*

E. *Acute Diarrhea*
1. Sudden change in frequency of stools
2. Usually self-limited, but can result in dehydration

F. *Chronic Diarrhea*
1. Passage of loose stools with increased frequency of more than 2 weeks' duration
2. Associated with disorders of malabsorption, anatomic defects, abnormal bowel motility, hypersensitivity reaction, or a long-term inflammatory response

TABLE 45-2 Differential Diagnosis of Diarrhea

	Infant	Child	Adolescent
Acute			
Common	Gastroenteritis Systemic infection Antibiotic associated Overfeeding	Gastroenteritis Food poisoning Systemic infection Antibiotic associated	Gastroenteritis Food poisoning Antibiotic associated
Rare	Primary disaccharidase deficiency Hirschsprung toxic colitis Adrenogenital syndrome	Toxic ingestion	Hyperthyroidism
Chronic			
Common	Postinfectious secondary lactase deficiency Cow's milk/soy protein intolerance Chronic nonspecific diarrhea of infancy Celiac disease Cystic fibrosis AIDS enteropathy	Postinfectious secondary lactase deficiency Irritable bowel syndrome Celiac disease Lactose intolerance Giardiasis Inflammatory bowel disease AIDS enteropathy	Irritable bowel syndrome Inflammatory bowel disease Lactose intolerance Giardiasis Laxative abuse (anorexia nervosa)
Rare	Primary immune defects Familial villous atrophy Secretory tumors Acrodermatitis enteropathica Lymphangiectasia Abetalipoproteinemia Eosinophilic gastroenteritis Short bowel syndrome Intractable diarrhea syndrome Autoimmune enteropathy	Acquired immune defects Secretory tumors Pseudo-obstruction	Secretory tumor Primary bowel tumor Gay bowel disease

AIDS = acquired immunodeficiency syndrome.

COMMUNITY-BASED CARE TIP:
Infants and young children in day care centers may be at increased risk for diarrhea due to *Shigella*, *Salmonella*, rotovirus, endopathogenic *E. coli*, and giardiasis. This is known as "day care diarrhea," and handwashing is the major preventive measure.

G. Predisposing Factors
1. Age—The younger the child, the greater the susceptibility and severity.
   a. Extracellular fluid volume is proportionately larger in the infant and young child.
   b. Nutritional reserves are relatively smaller in the young child.
2. Impaired health—Susceptibility is increased in the malnourished or debilitated child.
3. Climate—Susceptibility is increased in warm weather.
4. Environment—Frequency is increased where there is overcrowding, poor sanitation, inadequate refrigeration of food, and inadequate healthcare and education.
5. Virulence of a potential pathogen affects severity.

Altered Physiology

A. Mechanisms of Diarrhea
1. Secretory—decreased absorption, increased secretion
2. Osmotic—maldigestion, transport defects, ingestion of unabsorbable solute
3. Increased motility—decreased transit time or stasis (bacterial overgrowth)
4. Decreased surface area—decreased functional capacity
5. Mucosal invasion (motile or secretory)—inflammation, decreased colonic reabsorption, increased motility

B. Physiologic Effects of Diarrhea
1. Dehydration (extracellular fluid loss)
   a. Large loss of fluid and electrolytes in watery stools
   b. Losses with repeated vomiting; decreased fluid intake
   c. Increased insensible fluid losses from skin and lungs resulting from fever and rapid respirations
   d. Continued urine excretion
2. Electrolyte imbalance
   a. Potassium—varies
   b. Chloride; sodium; hypotonic, isotonic, or hypertonic dehydration
3. Acid–base imbalance—metabolic acidosis
   a. From large losses of potassium, sodium, and bicarbonate in stools
   b. From impaired renal function
4. Monosaccharide intolerance and protein hypersensitivity

Complications

1. Severe dehydration and acid–base derangements with acidosis
2. Shock

Clinical Manifestations

Symptoms vary with severity, specific cause, and type of onset (gradual versus sudden).

1. Low-grade fever to 41.1°C (100°F)
2. Anorexia
3. Mild and intermittent to severe vomiting
4. Stools
   a. Appearance of diarrhea from a few hours to 3 days
   b. Loose and fluid consistency
   c. Greenish or yellow-green
   d. May contain mucus, pus, or blood
   e. Frequency varies from 2 to 20 per day
   f. Expelled with force; may be preceded by pain
5. Behavioral changes
   a. Irritability and restlessness
   b. Weakness
   c. Extreme prostration
   d. Stupor and convulsions
   e. Flaccidity
6. Physical changes
   a. Little to extreme loss of subcutaneous fat
   b. Up to 50% total body weight loss
   c. Poor skin turgor and dry skin
   d. Pallor
   e. Sunken fontanels and eyes
7. Vital sign/output changes
   a. Low blood pressure
   b. High pulse
   c. Respirations rapid and hyperpneic
   d. Decreased or absent urinary output
   e. Collapse imminent

Diagnostic Evaluation

A. Studies to Evaluate Condition
1. Electrolyte and kidney function tests—serum sodium, chloride, potassium, and blood urea nitrogen variable
2. Acid–base balance—serum CO_2; arterial pH and CO_2 possibly abnormal
3. Complete blood count to determine plasma volume by hematocrit; infection by WBC and differential
4. Sedimentation rate—elevated in infection and inflammation

B. Studies to Determine Cause
1. Stool and rectal swab cultures and stool for ova and parasites can detect specific pathogens.
2. Stool pH, reducing substances—Decreased pH may indicate various noninfectious causes; acid stool containing sugar is characteristic of disaccharide intolerance.
3. Blood cultures can rule out septicemia.
4. Serologic studies can detect viral pathogens.
5. Breath hydrogen test can determine carbohydrate malabsorption and bacterial overgrowth.
6. Urinalysis can exclude urinary tract infection as cause of nonspecific diarrhea.

Treatment

1. Prevent spread of disease; suspect disease to be communicable until proven otherwise. Use enteric isolation precautions.

2. Provide supportive care. Maintain hydration and electrolyte balance; record IV fluids, weights, fluid loss from diarrhea, urine, and vomiting.
3. Administer specific antimicrobial therapy.
   a. Complications include dehydration, protracted diarrheal state, transient lactose intolerance.

Nursing Assessment

1. Obtain accurate history of signs and symptoms: nature and frequency of stools, type of onset, length of illness, associated symptoms.

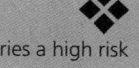

NURSING ALERT:
Severe diarrhea with sudden onset in the infant carries a high risk of mortality.

2. Assess state of hydration: overall general appearance, sunken eyes, and fontanels, skin turgor, abdominal appearance, condition of mucous membranes.
3. Assess vital signs for hypotension and tachycardia.
4. Obtain weight and compare with most recent weight.
5. Observe for activity level of infant or child; determine if changes in behavior and activity level occurred with onset of illness.

Nursing Diagnoses

A. Fluid Volume Deficit related to diarrhea and extracellular fluid loss
B. Risk for Infection transmission related to infectious diarrhea
C. Risk for Impaired Skin Integrity related to irritation by frequent stools
D. Altered Nutrition: Less than body requirements related to malabsorption
E. Anxiety and Fear related to hospitalization and illness

NURSING ALERT:
Assess child's behavior to determine comfort level. Crying or legs drawn up to abdomen usually indicates pain.

Nursing Interventions

A. Restoring Fluid Balance
1. Monitor amount and rate of IV fluid therapy, which have been calculated by the healthcare provider. Fluid needs are based on fluid deficit, ongoing losses, and body weight.
2. Prevent overload of circulatory system:
   a. Check flow rate and amount absorbed hourly and totally.
   b. Adhere to prescribed volume carefully when oral feedings are given in conjunction with IV fluid.
   c. Observe for signs of fluid overload: edema, increased blood pressure, bounding pulse, labored respirations, and crackles in lung fields.
3. Check IV site for infiltration or improper flow so site can be changed as necessary.

4. Use appropriate protective devices to prevent the child from injuring involved extremity or causing IV to malfunction.
5. Weigh the patient daily as a guide for fluid needs and patient status.
6. Monitor urine output, and keep accurate intake and output record, including vomitus and liquid stools.
7. If NPO, provide frequent mouth care and non-nutritive sucking with a pacifier. Continue to bubble infant to expel air swallowed while crying or sucking.
8. Mild or moderate diarrhea may be managed with oral electrolyte rehydration solutions, such as Lytren, Pedialyte, and Rehydralyte.
   a. Do not advance too quickly; base administration of solution on number of stools.
   b. Gradual resumption of previous diet is recommended after oral rehydration solutions are given.
   c. Breast-feeding may be resumed.

NURSING ALERT:
Diluted fruit juices and soft drinks are not recommended. High carbohydrate content aggravates diarrhea by osmotic effect.

B. *Preventing Spread of Infection*
1. Ensure adherence to good handwashing and gown technique protocols for all people having contact with infant or child.
2. Follow policy as to care of diapers.
3. Handle specimens collected using universal precautions, and transport to laboratories in appropriate containers per policy.
4. Teach good hygiene measures to older children.

COMMUNITY-BASED CARE TIP:
Assess sanitation and hygiene practices in the home for overcrowding, number of working toilets in the home for number of people, availability of working sinks with soap and towels in the bathrooms and their proximity to food preparation areas, disposal of diapers, and handwashing practices of caregivers and children.

C. *Preventing Skin Impairment*
1. Protect infant's diaper area from becoming excoriated by making frequent diaper changes.
2. Expose to air and light as much as possible.
3. Avoid commercial baby wipes, which contain alcohol and may sting inflamed or excoriated diaper area. Use mild soap and water, or place infant in tub of water for cleaning.
4. Prevent scratching or rubbing of irritated area. Holding infant on parent's protected lap may provide comfort and stimulation for parent and infant.
5. Use protective barrier creams, such as zinc oxide (Desitin) or karaya powder; completely remove after each stool for thorough cleansing.
6. Leave diaper area open to air until thoroughly dried.
7. Be aware and advise parents that antidiarrheal medications are seldom used; they have little effect on the course of infantile diarrhea and may cause toxicity.

D. *Resuming Adequate Nutritional Intake*
1. After rehydration, give lactose-free oral feedings, and advance slowly from clear liquids, such as gelatin-flavored water, to half-strength formula, to regular diet.
   a. Older child may advance more rapidly.
   b. If infant or young child is well hydrated, regular formula may not be omitted.

2. As diet is advanced, note any vomiting or increase in stools, and report it immediately. Oral feedings should not be resumed too early or advanced too rapidly, because diarrhea may recur.
3. Advise family to avoid milk products and lactose-containing formulas for at least 1 week for children with severe diarrhea. Nutramigen or Progestimal may be substituted.

E. *Reducing Fear and Anxiety*
1. Acknowledge that hospitalization is frightening, especially when it is sudden, as with diarrhea.
2. Many treatments and procedures may be painful. Give reassurance to the child before, during, and after treatment.
   a. Talk to the child.
   b. Hold and comfort child after the procedure.
   c. Explain in age-appropriate language.
   d. Include family in care and treatments when possible.
3. Explain to family that intermittent abdominal cramps may be painful, and provide support.
4. Provide some means of pleasant stimulation, entertainment, or diversion, especially while child remains in bed.
   a. Infant—mobile, musical toy
   b. Young child—books, tapes
   c. Older child—television, videos
5. Provide physical closeness to provide comfort, if child displays interest.
   a. Petting, stroking
   b. Holding, rocking

Family Education/Health Maintenance

1. After the cause of the diarrhea is determined, it may be necessary to teach proper hygiene, formula or food preparation, handling, and storage.
   a. Use handwashing before bottle and food preparation.
   b. Use disposable bottles, or sterilize or use dishwasher for reusable bottles.
   c. Refrigerate reconstituted formula and all other fluids between uses. Milk may become contaminated within 1 hour if left out at room temperature; juice becomes contaminated within several hours.
   d. Discard small amounts of food or fluid from containers already used.
2. Explain the fecal–oral mode of transmission of infectious diarrheal illnesses.
3. Explain the early symptoms of a diarrheal illness and of dehydration, which requires notification of the healthcare provider.
4. Help the parents understand the importance of medical care and general good hygiene.
5. For additional information and support, refer to Child Health Foundation; 10630 Little Patuxent Pkwy., Suite 325; Columbia, MD, 21044; 301-596-4514.

Evaluation

A. Vital signs stable; urine output adequate
B. Family, staff members handwashing properly and frequently

C. No redness or excoriation of diaper area
D. Tolerating small feedings of clear liquids without diarrhea or vomiting
E. Child listening to tapes; has stopped crying

◆ HIRSCHSPRUNG'S DISEASE

Hirschsprung's disease (congenital aganglionic megacolon) is a congenital absence of the parasympathetic ganglion nerve cells from within the muscle wall of the intestinal tract, usually at the distal end of the colon.

Etiology and Incidence

1. An arrest in embryologic development affecting the migration of parasympathetic nerves (innervation) of the intestine, occurring prior to the 12th week of gestation
2. Unknown cause; may be familial
3. 1 in 8,000 live births—white infants, 90%; African Americans infants, less than 10%
4. Three times more common in males
5. Higher incidence in children with Down syndrome

Altered Physiology

1. The parasympathetic ganglion cells in Auerbach's plexus within the intestinal tract muscle wall are absent or reduced in number, usually at the distal end of the colon and the rectum. Most commonly affected site is the rectosigmoid colon.
2. No peristalsis occurs in the affected portion of intestine (ie, spastic and contracted).
   a. This section is usually narrow; therefore, no fecal material passes through it.
   b. The intestine above the affected section has an accumulation of fecal material.
3. Proximal to the narrow affected section the colon is dilated.
   a. Filled with fecal material and gas.
   b. Hypertrophy of muscular coating.
   c. Ulceration of mucosa may be seen in newborn.
4. The internal rectal sphincter fails to relax, and evacuation of fecal material and gas is prevented. Abdominal distention and constipation result.

Complications

1. Prior to primary surgery
   a. Enterocolitis—a major cause of death
   b. Hydroureter or hydronephrosis
   c. Water intoxication from tap water enemas
   d. Cecal perforation
2. Postoperative
   a. Enterocolitis
   b. Leaking of anastomosis and pelvic abscess
   c. Temporary sudden inability to evacuate colon
   d. Long-term: intestinal obstruction from adhesions, volvulus, intussusception
3. Postoperative—colostomy
   a. Abdominal distention
   b. Respiratory distress

c. Infection
d. Hemorrhage, shock

Clinical Manifestations

Clinical manifestations vary depending on degree of involved bowel.

1. Newborn—symptoms appearing at birth or within first weeks of life
   a. No meconium passed
   b. Vomiting—bile-stained or fecal
   c. Abdominal distention
   d. Constipation—occurs in 100% of patients
   e. Overflow-type diarrhea
   f. Anorexia
   g. Temporary relief of symptoms with enema
2. Older child—symptoms not prominent at birth
   a. History of obstipation at birth
   b. Distention of abdomen—progressive enlarging
   c. Thin abdominal wall—progressive enlarging
   d. Peristaltic activity observable
   e. Constipation—no fecal soiling; relieved temporarily with enema
   f. Ribbonlike, fluidlike, or in pellet stools
   g. Failure to grow—loss of subcutaneous fat; appears malnourished; perhaps has stunted growth
   h. Anemia

Diagnostic Evaluation

1. Rectal examination, which exhibits absence of fecal material
2. X-ray examination with barium enema
   a. Narrow segment of intestine proximal to anus
   b. Dilated intestine proximal to narrow segment
3. Rectal biopsy—absence or reduced number of ganglion nerve cells
4. Anorectal manometry—records the reflex response of sphincter
5. Ultrasonogram—shows dilated colon

Treatment

Definitive treatment is removal of the aganglionic, nonfunctioning, dilated segment of the bowel, followed by anastomosis, and improved functioning of internal rectal sphincter.

1. Initially a colostomy or ileostomy is performed to decompress intestine, divert fecal stream, and rest the normal bowel.
2. Definitive surgery includes the following:
   a. Abdominoperineal pull-through
   b. Endorectal pull-through, rectorectal pull-through
   c. May be delayed until 9 to 12 months old or until child is 6.8 to 9 kg (15–20 lb)
3. In older child when symptoms are chronic but not severe, treatment may consist of isotonic enemas, stool softeners, and low-residue diet.

Nursing Assessment

1. Careful observation in the neonatal period for constipation

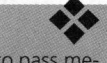

> **NURSING ALERT:**
> Diagnosis should be suspected in any infant who fails to pass meconium within the first 24 hours and requires repeated rectal stimulation to induce bowel movements.

2. Obtain parents' history, especially on infant's bowel and feeding habits.
   a. Onset of constipation
   b. Character of stools (ribbonlike or fluid-filled)
   c. Frequency of bowel movements
   d. Enemas needed
3. Observe for irritability, distended abdomen, and signs of malnutrition (pallor, muscle weakness, thin extremities, fatigue).

Nursing Diagnoses

A. Ineffective Breathing Pattern related to abdominal distention
B. Pain related to intestinal obstruction
C. Altered Nutrition: Less than body requirements related to poor intake

Preoperative Nursing Care

A. *Improving Breathing Pattern*
1. Monitor for respiratory embarrassment that may result from abdominal distention; watch for rapid, shallow respirations; cyanosis; sternal retractions.
2. Elevate head and chest of infant by tilting mattress.
3. Administer oxygen as ordered to support respiratory status.

B. *Relieving Pain*
1. Note degree of abdominal tenderness.
   a. Legs of infant drawn up
   b. Chest breathing
2. Note color of abdomen and presence of gastric waves; take sequential measurements of abdominal girth for evidence of changes.
3. Assist in emptying the bowel by giving repeated enemas and colonic irrigations.
   a. Procedure for enema in an infant is similar to that in an adult, except that less fluid and pressure are used.
   b. Physiologic saline solution (warmed) should be used for irrigations. Tap water may result in large quantities of water being absorbed and in water intoxication.
4. Administer medications (antibiotics) to reduce the bacterial flora of the bowel.
5. Note any change in degree of distention before and after irrigation. Record if location of distention changes (ie, upper or lower abdomen).
6. Record all intake and output of irrigant and drainage. Report marked discrepancies in retention or loss of fluid.

7. Insert rectal tube for escape of accumulated fluid and gas as ordered.
8. If abdominal distention is not relieved by enemas and discomfort is significant, insert a nasogastric tube as ordered.
   a. Note drainage from nasogastric tube, and chart characteristics.
   b. Check for patency; saline irrigations may be requested. Carefully record intake and output.
   c. Give frequent mouth care.
   d. Alternate nares when changing nasogastric tube every 24 hours, and use minimal amount of tape to prevent skin irritation.
9. Offer pacifier for non-nutritive sucking if on parenteral fluids.
10. Encourage parents to hold and rock infant.
11. Maintain position of comfort with head elevated. Offer soothing stimulation (eg, music, touch, play therapy).

C. *Providing Adequate Nutrition*
1. Obtain a dietary history regarding food and eating habits.
   a. This will contribute to planning dietary alterations.
   b. Explain to parents that eating problems are common with Hirschsprung's disease.
2. Monitor IV fluids appropriately. Measure all output.
3. Offer small, frequent feedings. (Low-residue diet will aid in keeping stools soft.)
   a. Feed child slowly.
   b. Provide as comfortable a position as possible for child during feedings.
4. Inform parents that defect can be corrected, but it may take some time for their child's physical status and feeding habits to improve.
   a. Feeding may cause additional discomfort because of distention and nausea.
   b. Parenteral nutrition may be necessary.

D. *Caring for the Older Child*
1. Be aware that older children who present with milder forms of the disorder may be treated medically (rare).
2. Note and record frequency and characteristics of stools. (Obstipation is likely to occur.)
3. Provide demonstration and written and verbal instructions to family for saline enema administration and use of stool softeners.
4. Obtain dietary consultation for teaching of low-residue diet.

Postoperative Nursing Care

A. *Preventing Complications*
1. Monitor vital signs and respiratory status closely.

> **NURSING ALERT:**
> Prevent injury to rectal mucosa by taking axillary or external ear temperature.

2. Monitor for proper functioning of colostomy, if present.
   a. Note drainage from colostomy: characteristics, frequency, fecal material, or liquid drainage.
   b. Note abdominal distention.
   c. Measure fluid loss from colostomy because the amount will affect fluid replacement.

3. Report signs of obstruction from peritonitis, paralytic ileus, handling bowel, or swelling.
   a. No output from colostomy
   b. Increased tenderness
   c. Irritability
   d. Vomiting
   e. Increased temperature

B. Preventing Infection
1. Change wound dressing using sterile technique.
2. Prevent contamination from diaper.
   a. Apply diaper below dressing.
   b. Change diaper frequently.
3. Prevent perianal and anal excoriation by thorough cleansing, and use ointments after the infant soils.
4. Use careful handwashing technique.
5. Report any wound redness, swelling or drainage, evisceration, or dehiscence immediately.
6. Suction secretions frequently to prevent infection of the tracheobronchial tree and lungs.
7. Encourage frequent coughing and deep breathing to maintain respiratory status.
8. Allow the infant to cry for short periods to prevent atelectasis.
9. Change infant's position frequently to increase circulation and allow for aeration of all lung areas.
10. Take axillary temperatures to avoid injury.

C. Preventing Abdominal Distention
1. Maintain patency of nasogastric tube immediately postoperatively.
   a. Watch for increasing abdominal distention; measure abdominal girth.
   b. Measure fluid loss because amount will affect fluid replacement.
2. Maintain NPO status until bowel sounds return and the bowel is ready for feedings as determined by provider.
3. Administer fluids to maintain hydration and replace lost electrolytes.
4. Provide frequent oral hygiene while NPO.
5. Begin oral feedings as ordered.
   a. Avoid overfeeding.
   b. Bubble frequently during feeding.
   c. Turn head to side or elevate after feeding to prevent aspiration.

D. Supporting the Parents
1. Acknowledge that even a temporary colostomy can be a difficult procedure to accept and learn to manage.
   a. Initiate ostomy referral.
   b. Support the parents when teaching them to care for the colostomy.
   c. Include them soon after surgery in dressing changes and any other appropriate activities.
   d. Assist and encourage them to treat the baby or child as normally as possible.
   e. Reassure parents that colostomy will not cause delay in the child's normal development.
2. Encourage the parents to talk about their fears and anxieties. Anticipating future surgery for resection may be confusing and frightening.
3. Initiate community-nurse referral to help the parents care for the child at home away from the comforting situation of the hospital, and obtain necessary equipment.

Ostomy Care in Children

Care of the colostomy and ileostomy in the infant and young child is based on the same principles and is essentially the same as that for an adult (see Chapter 16), with the following exceptions:

1. Colostomy irrigation is not part of management in small children. Irrigation is primarily for the purpose of regulating the colostomy to empty at regular intervals. Because children have bowel movements at more frequent intervals, this type of control is not feasible. Irrigation should be done only in preparation for tests or surgery and occasionally for the treatment of constipation.
2. Dehydration occurs quickly in the infant or small child; therefore, it is particularly important to observe drainage for amount and characteristics. Drainage should be measured to provide an accurate basis for computation of fluid replacement.
3. Prevention and treatment of skin excoriation around the stoma is of primary concern. With the advent of better skin shields and equipment designed especially for the pediatric patient, keeping an ostomy appliance in place is now less difficult. Through careful application and trying different types of pouches until a proper fit is obtained, most children can be kept clean and dry for at least 24 hours between changes. This is a significant factor in preventing skin breakdown and subsequent infections in the peristomal area. Remember, however, that infant dressings must be checked frequently.
   a. Dressings and collection bags may not adhere well or stay in place.
   b. Skin breakdown is more frequent.
   c. Infant elimination is more frequent than in the older child.
4. Helping agency for parents:
   a. United Ostomy Association; 36 Executive Park, Suite 120; Irvine, CA, 92714-6744; 800-826-0826
5. Some companies manufacture pediatric size ostomy equipment:
   a. United Surgical (Division of Howmedia, Inc.); Largo, FL, 33540
   b. Coloplast, C. R. Bard Inc.; 713 Central Avenue; Murray Hill, NJ, 07974
   c. Hollister, Inc.; 211 E. Chicago Avenue; Chicago, IL, 60611

Family Education/Health Maintenance

1. Begin early teaching about the colostomy, how it works, and how to care for it and the child. Explanations should be thorough and in accordance with family readiness. Encourage care of the ostomy as part of normal activities of daily living.
   a. Involve the entire family in teaching colostomy care to enhance acceptance of body change of the child.
   b. An older child should become totally responsible for own colostomy care.
   c. Procedures need to be thoroughly understood and practiced, including preparation of skin, application of collecting appliance, care of appliance, and control of odor.

d. Signs of stomal complications include ribbonlike stool, diarrhea, failure of evacuation of stool or flatus, bleeding.

e. Dilatation of stoma with finger may need to be taught and practiced.

f. Increased fluid intake is needed because colon absorption is decreased; low-residue food is needed to decrease bulk of stool.

g. Prepare parents and older child for colostomy closure as appropriate.

2. Review gastrostomy feeding techniques and procedures for care and dilation of anus as indicated.

3. Allow the parents to learn and practice these procedures long before the infant is to be discharged.

4. Emphasize the importance of treating the child as normally as possible to prevent behavior problems later.

5. Parents need to understand about good nutrition and diet prior to the child's discharge. Involve the dietitian as necessary.

6. Encourage close medical follow-up and general good health and hygiene.
a. Nutrition
b. General growth and development
c. Immunizations

7. For additional information and support, refer to American Pseudo-Obstruction and Hirschsprung's Disease Society; P.O. Box 772; Medford, MA, 02155; 617-395-4255.

Evaluation

A. Respiratory rate normal for age and unlabored; no cyanosis

B. Abdominal girth decreased; resting comfortably

C. Tolerating 1- to 2-oz feedings every hour

◆ INTUSSUSCEPTION

Intussusception is the invagination or telescoping of a portion of the intestine into an adjacent, more distal section of the intestine.

Etiology and Incidence

1. Cause usually unknown
2. May be due to increased mobility of intestine and hyperperistalsis present in young children
3. Lymphoid hyperplasia (Peyer patches) lead point of the proximal intussusception segment
4. Possible contributing causes in older child
a. Meckel's diverticulum
b. Polyps, cysts in the bowel
c. Malrotation of intestines
d. Acute enteritis
e. Abdominal injury
f. Abdominal surgery; intestinal intubation
g. Cystic fibrosis
h. Celiac disease
5. Most common cause of bowel obstruction in first year of life
6. Twice as common in male infants as in female infants
7. Most common in 6- to 18-month age group

Altered Physiology

1. Mesentery pulled into intestine when invagination occurs
2. Progression to obstruction
a. Intestine becomes curved, sausagelike; blood supply is cut off.
b. Bowel begins to swell; hemorrhage may occur.
c. Complete intestinal obstruction results; necrosis of involved segment occurs.
3. Classification of location
a. Ileocecal (most common): Ileum invaginates into ascending colon.
b. Ileocolic: Ileum invaginates into colon.
c. Colocolic: Colon invaginates into colon.
d. Ileo-ileo (enteroenteric): Small bowel invaginates into small bowel.

Complications

1. Perforation
2. Peritonitis

Clinical Manifestations

1. Paroxysmal abdominal pain
2. Currant jellylike stools
a. Blood and mucus present in stool
b. One or more stools with this characteristic
c. Presence of bloody mucus on finger following rectal examination
d. Hemoccult positive
3. Vomiting
4. Increasing absence of stools
5. Increasing abdominal distention and tenderness
6. Sausage-like mass palpable in abdomen
7. Unusual looking anus; may look like rectal prolapse
8. Dehydration and fever
9. Shocklike state with rapid pulse, pallor, marked sweating

Diagnostic Evaluation

1. X-ray examination
a. Flat plate of abdomen reveals staircase pattern. (Invagination appears like stair steps on x-ray—"coiled spring.")
b. Barium enema under fluoroscopy shows coil-like appearance of bowel.
2. Ultrasonogram to locate area of telescoped bowel

Treatment

1. Hydrostatic reduction of telescoped bowel with barium enema used during first 48 hours after onset may reduce intussusception in 75% of patients.
2. Intussusception can be surgically reduced; resection may be necessary if bowel is gangrenous.

Nursing Assessment

1. Obtain careful history of infant's or child's physical and behavioral symptoms.

> **NURSING ALERT:**
> Report of episodic, severe, colicky abdominal pain combined with vomiting suggests intussusception.

2. Perform physical examination, which may reveal a well-developed, well-nourished, afebrile infant with abdominal tenderness and distention.
3. Observe for mild dehydration.

Nursing Diagnoses

A. Pain related to paroxysmal abdominal pain, fever, and treatments
B. Risk for Fluid Volume Deficit related to vomiting
C. Ineffective Breathing Pattern related to abdominal distention
D. Anxiety related to hospitalization, surgery, and treatments

Preoperative Nursing Care

A. *Minimizing Pain*
1. Observe behavior as indicator of pain; the infant may be irritable and very sensitive to handling or lethargic or unresponsive. Handle very gently.
2. Encourage family to participate in comfort measures. Explain cause of pain, and reassure parents as to purpose of diagnostic tests and treatments.
3. Administer medications as prescribed.

B. *Maintaining Fluid and Electrolyte Balance*
1. Monitor fluids, and maintain NPO status.
2. Restrain infant as necessary for IV therapy.
3. Monitor intake and output.

C. *Promoting Effective Breathing*
1. Be alert for respiratory distress because of abdominal distention. Watch for grunting or shallow and rapid respirations if in shocklike state.
2. Insert nasogastric tube if ordered to decompress stomach.
   a. Irrigate at frequent intervals.
   b. Note drainage and return from irrigation.
3. Maintain NPO status as ordered.
   a. Wet lips, and give mouth care.
   b. Give infant pacifier to suck.
4. Continually reassess condition because increased pain and bloody stools may indicate perforation.

> **NURSING ALERT:**
> Passage of one normal brown stool may occur, clearing the colon distal to the intussusception. Passage of more than one normal brown stool may indicate that the intussusception has reduced itself. Report any stools immediately to the provider.

D. *Preparing for Surgery*
1. Offer support to the parents during time of crisis and fear.
2. Prepare the patient for surgery if shocklike or febrile.
   a. Administer blood or plasma to restore circulating blood volume, and observe for transfusion reactions.
   b. Monitor pulse rate carefully, and know appropriate pulse range for age of child. Report tachycardia, indicating shock.
   c. Reduce temperature because fever increases metabolism and makes oxygenation during anesthesia more complicated.

Postoperative Nursing Care

Care of the child following reduction of intussusception by hydrostatic barium enema involves careful monitoring of vital signs and general condition, especially abdominal tenderness, bowel sounds, lethargy, and tolerance to fluids. Care following surgical reduction or resection is similar to general postabdominal surgical care. Additionally, administer antipyretics and cooling measures to reduce fever. Fever is usually present from absorption of bacteria through the damaged intestinal wall.

Family Education/Health Maintenance

1. Explain that recurrences are rare and usually occur within 36 hours after reduction. Review signs and symptoms with parents.
2. Review activity restrictions with parents (eg, positioning on back or side, quiet play, and avoidance of water sports until wound heals).
3. Encourage follow-up care.
4. Provide anticipatory guidance for developmental age of child.

Evaluation

A. Less irritable, dozing
B. Urine output adequate
C. Respirations unlabored; abdominal distention relieved
D. Postoperative vital signs stable; good skin turgor; audible bowel activity; passes stool on fourth postoperative day; abdominal distention relieved

◆ IMPERFORATE ANUS (ANORECTAL MALFORMATIONS)

The term imperforate anus is used to describe all congenital abnormalities of the anorectal canal or in the location of the anus within the perineum.

Etiology and Incidence

1. An arrest in embryologic development of the anus, lower rectum, and urogenital tract at the eighth week of embryonic life

2. Cause unknown
3. 1 in 4,000 to 1 in 5,000 incidence; slight male predominance
4. Closely associated with other congenital deviations, including
   a. Congenital heart disease—6%
   b. Esophageal atresia with TEF—10%
   c. Spinal malformations—30%
   d. Genitourinary anomalies—38%
   e. Low birth weight, central nervous system anomalies—9%
5. Increased incidence associated with Down syndrome

Altered Physiology

Anorectal malformations result from a defect or arrest in embryologic development of the terminal hindgut.

Types (Fig. 45-3)

1. Anal stenosis
   a. Anal opening is very small.
   b. Defecation is difficult.
   c. Stools may be ribbonlike.
   d. This accounts for 10% of anomalies.
2. Imperforate anal membrane
   a. Infant fails to pass meconium.
   b. Greenish, bulging membrane is seen.
   c. Bowel and sphincter return to normal after excision.
3. Anal agenesis
   a. Anal dimple is present.
   b. Stimulation of the perianal area leads to puckering (indicative of external sphincter).
   c. Intestinal obstruction occurs if no associated fistula.
   d. Fistulas may be perineal or vulvar in the female and perineal or urethral in male.
4. Rectal agenesis
   a. Fistulas are usually present.
   b. Fistulas in male may communicate with posterior urethra; in females, fistula ends high in vagina.
   c. Associated major congenital malformations are common.
   d. Accounts for 75% of anomalies.

Complications

1. Infection
2. Intestinal obstruction
3. Loss of sphincter control

Clinical Manifestations

Condition is usually discovered immediately after birth or within several hours.

1. No anal opening is present.
2. Thermometer or small finger cannot be inserted into rectum.
3. Meconium stool is absent.
4. Green-tinged urine is present if fistula is present (high, male).
5. Progressive abdominal distention occurs.
6. Fistula is likely to be present.

Diagnostic Evaluation

1. Urine examination for presence of meconium and epithelial debris indicates presence of fistula.
2. Voiding cystourethrogram shows abnormality.
3. Wangensteen-Rice x-ray (upside-down position)
   a. Limited accuracy in locating rectal pouch
   b. Useful only after infant is 24 hours of age
4. Sonography locates rectal pouch.

Treatment

1. Low—female
   a. Decompression of bowel with catheter irrigations
   b. Dilatation of fistula for 8 to 12 months thereafter
   c. Definitive repair
2. Low—male
   a. Rectal cutback anoplasty or Y-V plasty
   b. Local dilatation of fistula
3. High—male
   a. Colostomy for decompression
   b. Definitive pull-through surgery; deferred until about 1 year of age or when child attains 6.75 to 9 kg (15–20 lb)

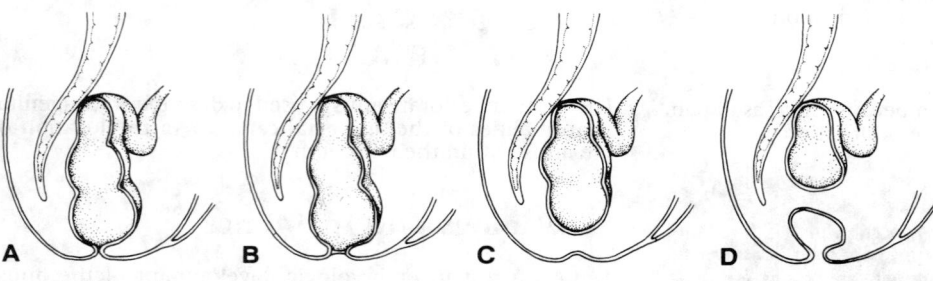

A	B	C	D
Anal stenosis	Imperforate anal membrane	Anal agenesis	Rectal agenesis

FIGURE 45-3 Anorectal malformations.

4. High—female
   a. Colostomy
   b. Definitive repair done when infant is 1 year of age or 6.75 to 9 kg (15–20 lb)

Nursing Assessment

1. Perform physical assessment of newborn for abnormalities.

> **NURSING ALERT:** ❖
> A newborn who does not pass a stool in the first 24 hours after birth requires further assessment.

   a. Presence of perineal fistula
   b. Meconium coming from vagina or presence of meconium-stained urine
   c. No anal opening or inability to pass thermometer into rectum
2. Perform thorough examination for other congenital anomalies.

Preoperative Nursing Care

A. Maintaining Stability Prior to Surgery
1. Withhold feedings. Note any vomiting: color and amount.
2. Maintain nasogastric tube passed to decompress the stomach. Measure abdominal girth.
3. Observe the patient carefully for any signs of distress and report. Check vital signs frequently.
4. Use an Isolette or radiant warmer to maintain temperature stability.
5. Keep fistula area clean.

Postoperative Nursing Diagnoses

A. Risk for Infection related to surgical incision of anoplasty
B. Risk for Impaired Skin Integrity related to ostomy
C. Risk for Fluid Volume Deficit related to restricted intake
D. Family Coping: Potential for Growth related to increased needs of infant

Postoperative Nursing Care

Depending on the location, type of imperforate anus, and sex of child, one of three surgical approaches may be used: 1) anoplasty, 2) temporary colostomy with definitive pull-through at a later time when the child is older and larger, or 3) abdominal or sacroperineal pull-through. Give good postoperative care, and observe for possible postoperative complications. Especially note any vomiting or stooling.

A. Preventing Infection of Suture Line
1. Following anoplasty, do not put anything in rectum.
2. Expose perineum to air.
3. Position the infant for easy access to perineum for cleansing and minimal irritation to site (ie, place the infant on abdomen, possibly with hips elevated, to prevent pressure on perineal surfaces; turn side-to-side)
4. Observe for redness, drainage, poor healing.

B. Preventing Skin Breakdown (see Ostomy Care, Chapter 16)

C. Maintaining Fluid and Electrolyte Balance
1. Start oral feedings as ordered (usually within hours after an anoplasty).
2. Monitor for return of peristalsis. When primary repair is done, nasogastric suction may be maintained until feedings are started.
3. Monitor parenteral fluids, and discontinue when oral intake is sustained.

D. Strengthening Coping
1. Ensure the parents that colostomy is temporary.
2. Encourage the parents to participate in care of the child and to provide emotional security for the child.
3. Provide thorough teaching program for special care needed at home.
   a. Colostomy care
   b. Anal dilatation to prevent a stricture at site of anastomosis from scar tissue (after instructions by healthcare provider)
4. Initiate referral to community nurse, especially if the parents are particularly anxious about caring for the child at home.
5. Encourage the parents to talk about their concerns.
6. Enlist help of enterostomal therapy, enterostomal therapy nurse, or provide support for anticipated home care needs.

E. Providing Appropriate Care for Definitive Pull-Through Surgery
1. Carry out perineal care as stated previously.
2. Provide proper care of gastrostomy or nasogastric tube used to decompress the GI tract until peristalsis returns.
3. Provide proper care of bladder catheter, if used, and measure urinary output accurately.
4. Observe carefully for abdominal distention, bleeding from perineum, and respiratory embarrassment.

Family Education/Health Maintenance

1. Review special care and procedures to be continued at home. Involve parents and other caregivers in teaching.
2. Help the parents to understand situations that may be encountered as a result of imperforate anus as the baby gets older.
   a. Fecal impaction due to lack of sensation to defecate
   b. Future surgery if primary repair was not done
   c. Toilet training—may be delayed, especially following a pull-through procedure
   d. Inability to control fecal seepage from rectum
3. Provide some practical guidelines to help parents cope.
   a. Fecal control may not be achieved until age 10 years; however, about 80% of children achieve normal or socially acceptable continence.
   b. Encourage bowel habit training or patterning of defecation (eg, after breakfast).
   c. Promote diet modifications; teach foods that produce laxative effect (plums, prunes, chocolate, nuts, corn) and foods that have binding effect (peanut butter, hot cereal, cheese).

d. Stool softeners and at other times antidiarrheal medications may be effective, especially Imodium.

e. Rectal inertia may cause fecal impaction in rectosigmoid colon with soiling from fluid overflow. Bisacodyl suppository or cleansing enema provides assistance in management.

4. Encourage mutual support from other families who have a child with an anorectal malformation.

Evaluation

A. No signs of infection of suture line
B. Skin intact surrounding ostomy
C. Bowel sounds present; oral feeding tolerated without vomiting
D. Family discussing plans for home care with enterostomal therapist

Selected References

Behrman, R., & Kleigman R. (1994). *Nelson essentials of pediatrics* (2nd ed.). Philadelphia: W.B. Saunders.

Ellett, M. L., Fitzgerald, J. F., & Winchester, M. (1993). Dietary management of chronic diarrhea in children. *Gastroenterology Nursing, 15*(9), 170–177.

Fennerty, M. B., et al. (1993). Gastroesophageal reflux disease. *Hospital Medicine, 29*(4), 28, 32–34, 37–40.

Frost, G. (1992). Hirschsprung disease in infants and children. *Gastroenterology Nursing, 15*(1), 45–48.

Hamilton, H. (1993). Care improves while costs reduce: The clinical nurse specialist in total parenteral nutrition. *Professional Nurse, 8*(9), 592–594, 596.

Ladebauche, P. (1992). Pediatric update—Intussusception in pediatric patients. *Journal of Emergency Nursing, 18*(3), 175–177.

Kurdahl Zahr, L., Heflin, H., La Rosa, P., & Damian, F. (1992). The short bowel syndrome: An update and a case study. *Journal of Pediatric Nursing, 7*(3), 189–195.

Shannon, R. (1993). Gastroesophageal reflux in infancy: Review and update. *Journal of Pediatric Health Care, 7*(2), 71–76.

Sherkin-Langer, F., Langer, J. C., Zupancic, J., Winthrop, A. L., & Issenman, R. M. (1993). Home esophageal self-dilation in children. *Gastroenterology Nursing, 16*(1), 5–8.

Sterling, C. E., et al. (1991). Nursing responsibility in the diagnosis, care and treatment of the child with gastroesophageal reflux. *Journal of Pediatric Nursing, 6*(6), 435–440.

Trier, J. S. (1992). Clinical clues to malabsorption. *Emergency Medicine, 24*(6), 122–124.

Wirt, S. W., et al. (1992). Cleft lip and palate. *Plactic Surgery Nursing, 12*(4), 140–147, 162.

Wise, B. (1992). Neonatal short bowel syndrome. *Neonatal Network, 11*(7), 9–15.

Worman, S., & Ganiats, T. (1995). Hirschsprung's disease: A cause of chronic constipation in children. *American Family Physician, 51*(2), 487–494.

Yeo, H. M. (1992). Surgical intervention for oesophageal atresia with tracheo-oesophageal fistula. *Professional Nurse, 8*(1), 50–52.

CHAPTER 46

Pediatric Renal and Genitourinary Disorders

Acute Disorders

◆ ACUTE GLOMERULONEPHRITIS

Acute glomerulonephritis is a broad term used to describe a number of disease processes resulting in glomerular injury. The glomerular injury is the result of antigen–antibody deposits within the glomeruli.

Etiology/Incidence

1. Presumed cause—antigen–antibody reaction secondary to an infection elsewhere in the body
2. Initial infection
   a. Usually either an upper respiratory infection or a skin infection
   b. Most frequent causative agent—nephritogenic strains of group A β-hemolytic streptococcus
3. More common in boys than girls (2:1)
4. Most common in early school-age group
5. Rare in children under 2 years of age
6. Incidence varies with the prevalence of nephritogenic strains of streptococci. This is most common in the southern United States and Caribbean.

Altered Physiology

1. It is speculated that the streptococcal infection is followed by the release of a membranelike material from the organism into the circulation.
2. Antibodies produced to fight the invading organism also react against the glomerular tissue, forming immune complexes.
3. The immune complexes become trapped in the glomerular loop and cause an inflammatory reaction in the affected glomeruli.
4. Changes in the glomerular capillaries reduce the amount of the glomerular filtrate, allow passage of blood cells and protein into the filtrate, and reduce the amount of sodium and water that is passed to the tubules for reabsorption.
5. General vascular disturbances, including loss of capillary integrity and spasm of arterioles, are secondary.

Complications

(Occur infrequently)

1. Hypertensive encephalopathy
2. Congestive heart failure
3. Uremia
4. Anemia

Clinical Manifestations

A. Onset
1. Usually 1 to 2 weeks after the onset of the initiating infection
2. May be abrupt and severe or mild and detected only by laboratory measures

B. Signs and Symptoms
1. Urinary symptoms
   a. Decreased urine output
   b. Bloody or brown-colored urine
2. Edema
   a. Present in most patients
   b. Usually mild
   c. Often manifested by periorbital edema in the morning
   d. May appear only as rapid weight gain
   e. May be generalized and influenced by posture
3. Hypertension
   a. Present in over 50% of patients
   b. Usually mild
   c. Rise in blood pressure may be sudden
   d. Usually appears during the first 4 to 5 days of the illness
4. Malaise
5. Mild headache
6. Gastrointestinal disturbances, especially anorexia and vomiting

Diagnostic Evaluation

1. Urinalysis
   a. Decreased output—may approach anuria
   b. Microscopic or gross hematuria
   c. Specific gravity—moderately elevated
   d. Proteinuria (3+ to 4+)
   e. Microscopic—red blood cells, leukocytes, epithelial cells, and casts
2. Serum complement level—usually reduced
3. Blood urea nitrogen (BUN) and creatinine—often mildly to moderately elevated
4. Antistreptolysin-O (ASO) titre—elevated
5. DNAase B antigen titer—elevated
6. Erythrocyte sedimentation rate (ESR)—elevated
7. Complement C3—depressed
8. Chest x-ray—may show pulmonary congestion, cardiac enlargement during the edematous phase
9. Renal function studies—normal in 50% of the patients

Treatment

1. Antibiotic therapy if streptococci still present
2. Other management is mostly symptomatic; in most patients spontaneous recovery is expected.
3. Salt and fluid restriction early in course of illness may prevent hypertension.
4. Therapy for rapidly progressive glomerulonephritis (child does not recover from apparent acute poststreptococcal glomerulonephritis and continues to have abnormalities in the urine) may include high doses of glucocorticoids.

Nursing Assessment

1. Obtain history regarding recent streptococcal infection.
2. Obtain culture and assess for current infection.
3. Measure urine output and degree of hematuria.
4. Weigh child and document areas and extent of edema.

Nursing Diagnoses

A. Altered Urinary Elimination related to glomerular dysfunction
B. Fluid Volume Excess related to kidney failure
C. Diversional Activity Deficit related to focus on fluid restriction
D. Knowledge Deficit related to lack of information of acute glomerulonephritis and its management

Nursing Interventions

A. *Promoting Normal Urinary Pattern*
1. Monitor daily intake and output.
2. Test and record urine for specific gravity and proteinuria as ordered. Note color of urine.
3. Monitor daily weights.

B. *Reducing Excess Fluid Volume*
1. Provide a regular diet, as ordered, without added salt during the acute phase.

2. Restrict protein and potassium if any degree of renal failure is exhibited.
3. Restrict fluids in children with hypertension, edema, congestive failure, or renal failure.
4. Place a sign indicating dietary restrictions on the child's bed so that staff and visitors will be aware of special needs.
5. With fluid restrictions, offer small amounts of fluids spaced at regular intervals throughout the day and evening. Use an appropriate size of cup for the amount of fluid being offered.
6. Check blood pressure as ordered or needed and observe for signs of hypertension. Administer antihypertensive drugs as ordered by health care provider.

C. *Promoting Diversional Activity*
1. Explain the restriction at an age-appropriate level and direct the child's focus away from restrictions.
2. Provide the child with diversional activity/play therapy.
3. Play nonexertional games to prevent excessive fluid requirements.

D. *Providing Information*
1. Explain all aspects of the diagnostic tests and treatment in terms the family can understand.
2. Explain the purpose of all medications and the restricted diet, including a review of high-sodium foods to avoid, and sample menus.
3. Encourage family participation in the child's care.
4. Help the family plan for adaptation of the child's nursing care to the home environment.
5. Arrange for appointments for continued medical supervision and initiate referrals when appropriate.

Family Education/Health Maintenance

1. Reinforce medical explanation of the disease process.
   a. Emphasize the need for medical evaluation and culture of all sore throats for all family members.
   b. Alert the family to signs and symptoms of disease recurrence.
2. Advise that tonsillectomy or other oral surgery is not recommended for several months after the acute phase of glomerulonephritis.
   a. If this type of surgery is necessary, penicillin may be recommended before and after the procedure to prevent bacterial infection.
   b. Obtain information regarding drug allergies before administering penicillin.

Evaluation

A. Output remains adequate
B. Weight remains stable
C. Child is able to read, listen to music, and does not complain of thirst
D. Parents and child are able to state rationale for treatment

◆ NEPHROTIC SYNDROME

Nephrotic syndrome refers to a grouping of clinical and laboratory abnormalities caused by a variety of renal injuries. There are many types of nephrotic syndrome; disease with minimal changes occurs most frequently, in 80% of children.

Etiology/Incidence

1. Underlying defect—increased permeability of glomerular capillary wall to circulating plasma proteins, mainly albumin
2. Large losses of albumin are far more than the body can replenish with albumin syntheses.
3. Annually afflicts about 2 to 3 children per 100,000 under the age of 8 years in the United States.
4. Mean age at onset is 3.5 + 2.1 years
5. More common in boys than in girls (2:1)

Altered Physiology

1. For unknown reasons, the glomerular membrane, usually impermeable to large proteins, becomes permeable.
2. Protein, especially albumin, leaks through the membrane and is lost in the urine.
3. Plasma proteins decrease as proteinuria increases.
4. The colloidal osmotic pressure that holds water in the vascular compartments is reduced because of the decrease in amount of serum albumin. This allows fluid to flow from the capillaries into the extracellular space, producing edema.
5. The shift of fluid from the plasma to the interstitial spaces reduces the vascular fluid volume (hypovolemia), which in turn stimulates the renin–angiotensin system and the secretion of antidiuretic hormone and aldosterone.
6. Tubular reabsorption of sodium and water is increased in an attempt to increase intravascular volume.
7. The loss of proteins, particularly immunoglobulins, predisposes the child to infection.

Complications

1. Patients are prone to infections:
   a. Septicemia
   b. Pneumonia
   c. Peritonitis
   d. Urinary tract infection (UTI)
   e. Lymphangitis

Clinical Manifestations

A. Onset
1. Insidious—often follows mild upper respiratory infection

B. Signs and Symptoms
1. Edema is often the presenting symptom.
   a. Edema may be minimal or massive.
   b. Edema is usually first apparent around the eyes.
   c. Ascites may be severe.
   d. Intense scrotal and labial edema is common.
   e. Peripheral edema is dependent and shifts with the child's position.
   f. Striae may appear on the skin from overstretching.

2. Profound weight gain; the child may actually double normal weight.
3. Decreased urine output during the edematous phase—urine appears dark, opalescent, and frothy.
4. Irritability and fatigue
5. Gastrointestinal disturbances, including vomiting and diarrhea due to edema of intestinal mucosa
6. Anorexia—malnutrition may become severe.
7. Recurrent infections
8. Wasting of skeletal muscles may occur because of the continuous drain of plasma protein nitrogen into the urine.

C. Severity and Duration of the Clinical Course Variable and affects the prognosis although prognosis for ultimate recovery in most cases is good

Diagnostic Evaluation

1. Urinalysis
   a. Protein—2+ or greater
   b. Casts—numerous
   c. Blood—absent or transient
2. 24-hour urine
   a. Protein—frequently greater than 2 g/m^2 per day
   b. Creatinine clearance—variable, often normal
3. Blood
   a. Total protein—reduced
   b. Albumin—less than 2 g/dL
   c. Cholesterol—greater than 200 mg/dL in the presence of edema
4. Renal biopsy is indicated if patient is steroid resistant (has failed to achieve remission).

Treatment

1. Most children experience remission after the initial course of treatment.
   a. Of these responders, most will relapse once or not at all during the subsequent 6 months.
   b. About one-third of the responders experience multiple relapses after the initial remission.
   c. Approximately 10% of children with nephrotic syndrome will be resistant to all forms of therapy.
   d. Many of these children will progress to chronic renal failure.
2. Steroid therapy is the preferred approach to treatment because steroids appear to affect the basic disease process in addition to controlling edema.
   a. Prednisone (Orasone) is usually the drug of choice because it is less likely to induce salt retention and potassium loss and is the least expensive. There is no standard program of therapy, but most children receive 2 mg/kg until the urine is free from protein and remains negative on urine dipstick for 1 to 2 weeks. This is followed by a steroid taper over several weeks while monitoring urine dipsticks for protein.
   b. Children with nephrotic syndrome may respond to steroid therapy in several ways.
      (1) Steroid sensitive—children respond to a single short course of steroids without evidence of relapse after cessation of therapy.
      (2) Steroid dependent—children respond incompletely or tend to relapse on lowered dosages

of steroids and require additional supportive treatment.

    (3) Steroid resistant—children become resistant to steroid therapy or cannot be maintained in remission without developing serious side effects of treatment.

3. Immunosuppressive drug therapy
   a. Cyclophosphamide (Cytoxan) is the drug of choice.
   b. This therapy is generally reserved for treatment with steroid-dependent or steroid-resistant nephrosis because of severe side effects.
4. Intravenous (IV) albumin 25% to shift fluid from interstitial space into the vascular system. This is only a temporary treatment to relieve edema but may be used in severe cases of edema causing respiratory distress or severe discomfort.
5. Diuretic therapy—used in combination with IV albumin to help relieve edema. In cases of hypovolemia, diuretics may not be indicated.

Nursing Assessment

1. Obtain history of onset of illness and symptoms.
   a. Precipitating events
   b. Recent immunizations
   c. Recent upper respiratory tract infections
   d. Presence of flulike symptoms
   e. Time of onset and location of edema
   f. Urinary pattern changes
2. Perform physical examination focusing on vital signs; auscultation of breath sounds to determine presence of adventitious sounds; areas and extent of edema, especially periorbital region, extremities, genitalia, abdomen; and peripheral perfusion pulses, color, warmth of extremities.

Nursing Diagnoses

A. Fluid Volume Excess related to fluid accumulation in tissues
B. Risk for Infection related to chronic steroid use
C. Altered Nutrition (Less than Body Requirements) related to loss of proteins through urine and anorexia
D. Altered Family Processes related to childhood illness

Nursing Interventions

A. *Relieving Excess Fluid*
1. Administer corticosteroids as recommended by the health care provider.
   a. Observe for evidence of side effects and complications of therapy such as Cushing's syndrome—increased body hair (hirsutism), rounding of the face ("moon face"), abdominal distention, striae, increased appetite with weight gain, and aggravation of adolescent acne.
   b. Provide child with access to a mirror so that child can observe gradual physical changes.
   c. Stress that these physical changes are not harmful or permanent and will disappear after the steroid treatment is stopped.
   d. Observe for serious side effects and uncommon complications of corticosteroids (see p. 711).

NURSING ALERT:
No vaccinations or immunizations should be given during active episodes of nephrosis or while the child is receiving immunosuppressive therapy.

2. Administer immunosuppressive drugs as prescribed.
   a. Ensure that patient and parents understand the desired and adverse effects of therapy.
   b. Observe for complications of therapy such as decreased white blood count and increased susceptibility to infection, hair loss, cystitis, and sterility (may result in both sexes from long-term use).

NURSING ALERT:
Administer cyclophosphamide in the morning with large volumes of fluid to prevent concentration of the drug in the urine and increased susceptibility to cystitis.

3. Administer diuretics as prescribed.
   a. Be aware of those diuretics that may cause potassium depletion.
   b. Offer foods high in potassium, such as orange juice, bananas, grapes, and milk.
   c. Administer supplemental potassium chloride as ordered and if the urine output is adequate.
4. Maintain the child on bed rest during periods of severe edema.
5. Provide a diet low in sodium and ensure that moderate sodium restriction is followed, as indicated.
   a. Exclude excessively salty foods and eliminate extra salt.
6. Restrict fluids as ordered (usually only during the extreme edematous phases).
   a. Restriction is carefully calculated at frequent intervals, based on the urine output of the previous day plus estimated insensible losses.
   b. Offer small amounts of fluids spaced at regular intervals throughout the day and evening. Use a cup of appropriate size for the amount of fluid being offered.
   c. Measure fluids accurately in graduated containers. Do not estimate fluid intake or output.
   d. Place a sign on the child's bed to ensure that no urine is accidentally discarded and that all intake is recorded.
   e. Determine total intake and output every 8 hours. In children who are not toilet trained, a fairly accurate record of output can be obtained by weighing diapers before and after voiding.
   f. Record other causes of fluid loss such as the number of stools per day, perspiration, etc.
7. Assist with abdominal paracentesis; this may be required because of marked ascites. During the procedure, fluid is withdrawn from the peritoneal cavity to relieve pressure symptoms and respiratory distress.

B. *Protecting the Child From Infection*
1. Monitor complete blood count for decreased white cell count and neutropenia.
2. Closely observe the child taking corticosteroids for signs of infection. Be aware that fever and other symptoms may be masked.
3. Provide meticulous skin care to the edematous areas of the body.
   a. Bathe the child frequently and apply powder. Areas of concern are moist parts of the body and edema-

tous male genitalia. Support the scrotum with a cotton pad held in place by a T-binder, if necessary, for the child's comfort.

    b. Position the child so that edematous skin surfaces are not in contact. Place a pillow between the child's legs when lying on side, etc.

    c. Irrigate swollen eyes and cleanse the surrounding area several times daily to remove exudate.

    d. Elevate the child's head to reduce edema.

4. If possible, avoid invasive procedures such as femoral venipunctures and intramuscular injections to decrease the chance of introducing pathogens. Venipuncture of the lower extremities may also predispose the child to thromboembolism because of the hypovolemia, stasis, and increased plasma concentration of clotting factors.

C. *Providing Protein to Restore Losses*

1. Offer a high-protein, high-calorie diet. Maintain salt restrictions during periods of edema and hypertension.

2. Obtain a complete history of dietary preferences and patterns so that the child's meals can be as acceptable as possible.

3. Place a sign on the child's bed indicating any dietary restrictions, so that everyone will be aware of special needs.

4. Permit additional amounts of food at the child's discretion.

D. *Providing Emotional Support*

1. Encourage frequent visiting and allow as much parental participation in the child's care as possible.

2. Allow the child as much activity as tolerated.

    a. Bed rest should be enforced during periods of hypertension.

    b. Balance periods of rest, recreation, and quiet activities during the convalescent phase.

    c. Allow the child to eat meals with family or other children.

3. Encourage the child and family to verbalize fears, frustrations, and questions.

    a. Be aware that young children frequently fear abandonment by their parents or loss of integrity. (The boy who is unable to visualize his penis because of extensive edema may think he has been castrated and needs reassurance that his body is intact.)

    b. Allow parents to express frustrations regarding the uncertainties associated with the cause of the disease, the clinical course, and prognosis.

    c. Explain the difference between nephritis and nephrosis if parents have questions.

4. Help the child adjust to changes in body image, such as cushingoid appearance and hair loss, by explaining changes ahead of time.

    a. Encourage the use of scarves and hats as desired.

    b. Provide the child with access to a mirror to watch the change in physical appearance gradually.

5. Discuss the problems of discipline with the parents. Encourage them to set consistent limits and reasonable expectations of their child's behavior.

6. Begin discharge planning early.

    a. Have the dietitian discuss special diets with the parents. Encourage them to plan sample menus.

    b. Encourage the parents to administer the child's medication before discharge.

    c. Instruct the parents about urine testing.

    d. Provide suggestions regarding activity restriction at home.

    e. Initiate a community health nursing referral if necessary for reassessment and reinforcement of teaching.

Family Education/Health Maintenance

1. Stress the importance of attention to the details of the child's care and continued medical supervision.

2. Emphasize the necessity of taking medication according to the prescribed schedule and for an extended time. Discuss complications encountered with steroid therapy.

3. Provide written instructions concerning:

    a. Diet

    b. Prevention of infection

    c. Skin care

    c. Administration of medications

    d. Activity restrictions

    e. Urine testing

    f. Symptoms of relapse

    g. Follow-up appointments

Evaluation

A. Shows reduction in edema and ascites; urine output adequate; fluid restriction maintained

B. Exhibits no signs of infection

C. Consumes high-protein diet

D. Engages in play activities; family verbalizing feelings and frustrations with one another and nursing staff

◆ URINARY TRACT INFECTION

A UTI is defined as the presence of bacteria anywhere between the renal cortex and the urethral meatus. Because it is often difficult to determine the exact location of the infection, the term UTI is used to explain the presence of microorganisms anywhere within the urinary tract.

Etiology/Incidence

1. Causative organisms—*Escherichia coli* (80%)

2. Route of entry

    a. Ascent from the urethra (most common)

    b. Circulating blood

3. Contributing causes

    a. Urinary stasis

    b. Obstruction, usually congenital

    c. Vesicoureteral reflux

    d. Infections elsewhere in the body—upper respiratory; gastrointestinal, diarrhea

    e. Poor perineal hygiene

    f. Short female urethra

    g. Catheterization and instrumentation

    h. Entrance of an irritant into the bladder

    i. Inherent defect in the ability of the bladder mucosa to protect it from microbial invasion

    j. Chronic or intermittent constipation

    k. Local inflammation

    l. Antimicrobials

4. Infection is more common in male infants during the neonatal period due to congenital renal anomalies

5. The female-to-male ratio of UTI incidence during childhood is 10:1.

Altered Physiology

1. Inflammatory changes occur in the affected portions of the urinary tract.
2. Clumps of bacteria may be present.
3. Inflammation results in urinary retention and stasis of urine in the bladder. There may be backflow of urine into the kidneys through the ureters.
4. There are inflammatory changes in the renal pelvis and throughout the kidney when this organ is involved.
5. Scarring of the kidney parenchyma occurs in chronic infection and interferes with kidney function, particularly with the ability to concentrate urine.
6. Eventually, the kidney becomes small, tissue is destroyed, and renal function fails.

Complications

1. There is a tendency for recurrent infection.
2. Children with obstructive lesions of the urinary tract and those with severe vesicoureteral reflux are at highest risk for kidney damage.

Clinical Manifestations

A. *Onset*
1. May be abrupt or gradual
2. May be asymptomatic

B. *Signs and Symptoms*
 1. Fever
    a. May be moderate or severe
    b. May fluctuate rapidly
    c. May be accompanied by chills or convulsions
 2. Anorexia and general malaise
 3. Urinary frequency, urgency, dysuria, dribbling
 4. Daytime or nocturnal enuresis
 5. Foul odor or change in the appearance of urine
 6. Abdominal or suprapubic pain
 7. Tenderness over one or both kidneys
 8. Irritability
 9. Vomiting
10. Failure to thrive in infancy

Diagnostic Evaluation

1. Urine culture
   a. Documentation of pathogenic organisms in the urine is the only means of definitive diagnosis.
   b. A urine culture demonstrating more than 100,000 bacteria per milliliter indicates significant bacteriuria.
   c. A catheterized urine specimen with growth greater than 100 colonies of bacteria per milliliter is considered significant.
2. Urinalysis
   a. Pus is present in abnormal amounts.
   b. Casts, especially white cell casts, may be present and are indicative of intrarenal infection.
   c. Hematuria—occurs occasionally
3. Renal concentrating ability—decreased
4. Urologic and radiologic studies to identify anatomic abnormalities or renal changes stemming from recurrent

infections—renal ultrasound, voiding cystourethrogram, intravenous pyelogram (IVP), and dimercaptosuccinic acid scan.

Treatment

See Table 46-1.
1. Oral antibiotic therapy for uncomplicated UTI
2. Repeat culture may be necessary before treatment is discontinued.

Nursing Assessment

1. Obtain history to determine if UTI is initial or recurrent, and to determine if there may be other disease processes contributing to this infection.
2. Focus assessment on identifying clinical manifestations and determining location of infection, such as presence and appearance of urethral discharge; high-grade fever (more common with upper UTI); low-grade fever (more common with lower UTI).
3. Determine urinary pattern (ie, amount and frequency) and associated discomfort.

Nursing Diagnoses

A. Altered Urinary Elimination related to infection
B. Pain related to inflammatory changes and fever
C. Self-Esteem Disturbance related to exposure and manipulation of the genitourinary tract

Nursing Interventions

A. *Promoting Urinary Elimination*
1. Obtain a clean urine specimen for urinalysis or culture.
   a. Obtain freshly voided early morning specimen, if possible (most accurate). This urine is usually acid and concentrated, which tends to preserve the formed elements.
   b. Provide fluids to help the child void.
   c. Perform catheterization if necessary to obtain a sterile specimen; however, this procedure may cause emotional trauma and the accidental introduction of additional bacteria.
   d. Send urine to the laboratory immediately or refrigerate to avoid a falsely high bacterial count.
2. Administer antibiotics as ordered by the health care provider (after specimen has been obtained for culture).
   a. Antibiotic therapy is generally determined by the results of the urine cultures and sensitivities and by the child's response to therapy; however, empirical therapy may be started before culture results are back.
   b. Become familiar with toxic effects of antimicrobial agents and assess the child regularly for any of the signs and symptoms.

B. *Maintaining Comfort and Providing Symptomatic Relief*
1. Administer analgesics and antipyretics as ordered.
2. Maintain child on bed rest while febrile.
3. Encourage fluids to reduce the fever and dilute the concentration of the urine.
4. Administer IV fluids if necessary.

TABLE 46-1 Antimicrobial Agents Commonly Used in the
Management of Childhood Urinary Tract Infection

Drug	Adverse Effects	Nursing Considerations
Amoxicillin (Amoxil)	Occasional nausea, vomiting, diarrhea Hypersensitivity reactions of skin	Readily absorbed May be taken with food
Ampicillin (omnipen)	Diarrhea, urticaria Anaphylactic reaction	Contraindicated in penicillin-sensitive children. Package insert should be consulted regarding reconstitution, administration, and storage of IM and IV preparations. Absorption of oral preparations may be decreased with food. Dose must be repeated q6h to ensure therapeutic blood levels.
Cephalexin (Keflex)	Diarrhea, nausea, vomiting	May be taken with food. Dose should be reduced if renal function is impaired.
Gentamicin (Garamycin)	Renal and auditory toxicity; respiratory paralysis	Toxic effects can be minimized by slow IV infusion (over 1 h).
Nitrofurantoin (Macrodantin)	Fever, nausea, vomiting, peripheral neuropathy	Recommended for prolonged use. Give with food or milk to decrease gastrointestinal side effects. May cause urine to be amber or brown in color. Contraindicated in renal failure and in infants under 3 mo of age
Sulfasoxazole	Nausea, vomiting, drug fever, rashes, photosensitivity	Keep the child well hydrated to avoid crystallization of the drug in the urine. Contraindicated if known drug sensitivity and in infants under 2 mo of age
Trimethoprim-sulfamethoxazole (Bactrim, Septra)	Same as with other sulfonamides	Commonly used if bacterial resistance is anticipated or the child fails to respond to initial therapy.

C. *Protecting Self-Esteem*
1. Reinforce medical explanations of the disease and its therapy.
2. Explain all diagnostic tests and procedures to the child, allowing time for questions and answers.
3. Encourage verbalizing. Correct any misconceptions and particularly address concerns about the functioning of the urinary tract and sexual function. Reassure the child that he or she did not cause the problem.
4. Maintain privacy for the child as much as possible.
5. Provide an environment that is as close to normal as possible during hospitalization. Include opportunities for the child to play.
6. Prepare the child and family for discharge and begin discussions of rest, fluids, and medications.

Family Education/Health Maintenance

1. Review long-term antibiotic therapy, if prescribed, to prevent recurrence of UTI. Schedules for prolonged therapy vary from several months to continuous prophylaxis.
2. Encourage scheduled follow-up because of the possibility of disease recurrence.
   a. Emphasize that even though this disease may have few symptoms, it can lead to very serious, permanent disability.
   b. Advise family that periodic urine cultures are indicated for 2 years after the acute infection.
3. Teach measures of prevention:

   a. Minimize spread of bacteria from the anal and vaginal areas to the urethra in female children by cleansing the perianal area from the urethra back toward the anus.
   b. Avoid bubble baths because of the bladder-irritant effect of these solutions.
   c. Encourage adequate fluid intake, especially water.
   d. Avoid carbonated beverages because of their irritative effect on bladder mucosa.
   e. Encourage the child to void frequently and to empty the bladder completely with each voiding.

Evaluation

A. Voiding less frequently in adequate amounts
B. No complaints of pain during or after voiding; afebrile
C. Shows less anxiety about hospitalization; appears more relaxed about appearance, body image, tests

Abnormalities of the Genitourinary Tract That Require Surgery

◆ EXSTROPHY OF THE BLADDER

Exstrophy of the bladder is a part of a spectrum of anomalies involving the urogenital tract and the musculoskeletal system and sometimes the intestinal tract.

Etiology/Incidence

1. Results from failure of the abdominal wall and its underlying structures to fuse in utero
2. Occurs once in about every 30,000 deliveries
3. The male-to-female ratio is 3:1.
4. The condition is fairly familial.

Altered Physiology

In exstrophy of the bladder, the anterior surface of the bladder lies open on the lower part of the abdomen, allowing constant passage of urine to the outside.

Complications

1. Skin excoriation
2. Infection
3. Trauma to bladder mucosa

Clinical Manifestations

1. Urine dribbles constantly.
2. Infection and ulceration of the bladder mucosa may occur.
3. Genitalia may be ambiguous.
4. Affected children walk with a waddling or unsteady gait.

Diagnostic Evaluation

1. Inspection is often the most important tool in evaluation. The obvious anomaly may involve multiple systems.
2. Diagnostic procedures such as radiography, ultrasound, cystoscopic examination, urodynamic testing, and IVP determine extent of the anomaly.

Treatment

1. Surgical closure of bladder within first 48 hours
2. Complete correction by school age by means of staged reconstructive and orthopedic surgery
3. Urinary diversion may be necessary.

Nursing Management

A. *Preoperative Care*
1. Protect the bladder area from trauma and infection.
   a. Position the infant on back or side.
   b. Cleanse the area frequently with mild soap and water. Pat the area dry or use a hair dryer on the lowest setting.
   c. Keep the infant in an Isolette to avoid irritation from clothing and blankets.
   d. Expose the area to warm, dry air, sunlight, or artificial light at least once or twice each day.
   e. Cover the defect with sterile gauze to which a moisture barrier or skin sealant has been applied.
   f. Change the gauze covering and the infant's diaper frequently to prevent contamination.
2. Observe the infant closely for signs of infection.
3. Collect urine specimens by holding the infant over an emesis basin in a position that allows urine to drip into the container.
4. Assist the parents in dealing with their emotional reactions regarding the child's defect.
5. Prepare child and parents for the proposed surgery (see p. 1282).

B. *Postoperative Care*
1. Provide care for the ureteral and urethral catheters. Observe and record the amount of urinary drainage, catheter positions, and occurrence of bladder spasms.
2. The child may be placed in a body cast for several weeks (see p. 1365) or a traction system (see p. 1366).
3. An ileal conduit may be necessary (see p. 606).
4. Observe for complications.
   a. Urinary or incisional infections
   b. Fistulae in the suprapubic or penile incisions
5. Long-term support will be necessary for many children and families to help them deal with such fears as appearance of genitalia, potential inability to procreate, and rejection by peers. Ongoing discussion groups for parents and children may be helpful.
6. Teach the parents how to care for the child at home and make appropriate referrals.

C. *Resources*
Association for Bladder Extrophy Children
13823 Shavano Downs
San Antonio, TX 78230
(210) 492-6062

◆ OBSTRUCTIVE LESIONS OF THE LOWER URINARY TRACT

The effect of obstruction on ureteral and renal function depends on the degree and duration of obstruction, on the rate of urine formation, and on the presence or absence of infection.

Types of Obstruction

1. Urethral valves
   a. Filamentous valves that obstruct urine flow
   b. Most commonly found in urethra
2. Congenital narrowing of the urethra
3. Bladder neck obstruction—most common site of lower urinary tract obstruction
4. Meatal stricture
5. Neuromuscular dysfunction
6. Severe phimosis (rare)
7. Inflammatory processes
8. Neoplasia
9. Urolithiasis (calculi)
   a. Occurs more in adult life
   b. Affects men more than women
10. Trauma

Altered Physiology

1. Urinary tract becomes distended proximal to the point of obstruction.
2. The bladder dilates and hypertrophies.
3. Stasis of urine occurs.
4. The ureters become elongated, dilated, and tortuous.
5. Hydronephrosis and destruction of kidney tissue inevitably result.

Complications

1. Urinary stasis
2. Renal dysfunction
3. UTI

Clinical Manifestations

1. Abnormal urination
   a. Dysuria
   b. Frequency
   c. Enuresis
   d. Dribbling
   e. Reduced force of urine stream
   f. Difficulty starting urine stream
   g. Straining during urination
   h. Abrupt cessation during urination

Diagnostic Evaluation

1. Physical examination may reveal abdominal mass.
2. Laboratory findings depend on the degree that renal function is compromised.
3. IVP may show hydronephrosis.
4. Renal and bladder ultrasound
5. Radionuclide scanning
6. Endoscopic examination
7. Ureteroscopy
8. Urodynamic examination

Treatment

1. Prevention or eradication of infection
2. Dilation of urethral stenosis or stricture
3. Surgical relief of the obstruction

◆ OBSTRUCTIVE LESIONS OF THE UPPER URINARY TRACT

Obstructive lesions of the upper urinary tract primarily involve the ureters and often are congenital.

Types of Obstruction

1. Ureteropelvic junction obstruction
2. Stricture of a ureter
3. Congenital absence of one ureter

4. Duplication of the ureter of one kidney
5. Compression of a ureter by a blood vessel

Clinical Manifestations

1. Hydronephrosis may present as an abdominal mass.
2. Often asymptomatic (there is seldom any problem with voiding).
3. Vague symptoms such as failure to thrive may be present.
4. UTIs may be frequent.
5. Hypertension may occur.

Treatment

Treatment involves prevention or eradication of infection and surgical correction of the obstruction.

◆ HYPOSPADIAS

Hypospadias is a malposition of the urethral opening.

Etiology/Incidence

1. It is frequently associated with other urogenital tract anomalies.
2. Although rare, it is the most common disorder involving the penis.
3. Possibly due to decreased testosterone production in early gestation
4. Increased chance for incidence with future male siblings
5. Rare in girls

Altered Physiology

A. *Males*
1. The urethra opens on the ventral aspect of the penis.
2. In severe cases, the urethra may open on the shaft of the penis and deflects the penis downward.

B. *Females*
The urethra opens into the vagina (rare).

Complications

1. Undescended testicle may be associated.
2. Inguinal hernia

Clinical Manifestations

1. Inability to void with the penis in the normal elevated position.
2. Severe forms interfere with the ability to procreate.

Diagnostic Evaluation

1. Usually not difficult to diagnose due to visual anomaly
2. Severe cases require genotypic/phenotypic sex determination, chromosomal and hormonal studies.
3. Renal ultrasound, IVP, voiding cystourethrography to determine associated defects

Treatment

Surgical reconstruction beginning before 1 year of age

◆ CRYPTORCHIDISM (UNDESCENDED TESTICLE)

Cryptorchidism refers to the failure of one or both testes to descend through the inguinal canal to the normal position in the scrotum.

Etiology/Incidence

1. Possibly caused by delayed descent, prevention of descent by mechanical lesion, or endocrine disorder (rare)
2. More common in premature infants
3. Most common surgical problem in pediatric urologic practice

Altered Physiology

1. Testicular and ductal development are abnormal. It is unclear whether this is due to congenital dysplasia or underdevelopment.
2. Degeneration of the sperm-forming cells occurs after puberty because of the higher temperatures of the abdomen compared with normal location in the scrotum.

Complications

1. Testicular torsion
2. Associated hernias
3. Emotional disturbances
4. Significant increase in sterility and malignancy later in life

Clinical Manifestations

1. Undescended testicle not felt within the scrotum

Diagnostic Evaluation

1. Ultrasonography reveals undescended testis.
2. Serum testosterone measurements may be decreased.

Treatment

1. Orchiopexy surgery to achieve permanent fixation of the testis in the scrotum. Surgery should be performed between the ages of 1 and 3 to prevent damage to the tissues and to lessen emotional concerns related to body image.
2. Plastic surgery in patients with an absent testicle
3. Administration of human chorionic gonadotropin (HCG) has produced descent of the testes in some children. Testes may have descended spontaneously in many of these cases.

Nursing Management

A. *Preoperative Care*
1. Encourage the child and his parents to express their feelings about the condition.
2. Discuss the condition and surgery frankly, in terms the child can understand, and clarify any misunderstandings.

B. *Postoperative Care*
1. Prevent contamination of the suture line.
2. Maintain traction.
   a. A suture is placed in the lower portion of the scrotum and is attached to a rubber band that is fastened to the upper aspect of the inner thigh by a piece of adhesive.
   b. This traction anchors the testicle to the scrotum and is removed in 5 to 7 days.
3. Administer antibiotics as prescribed to prevent infection.

◆ CARE OF THE CHILD REQUIRING UROLOGIC SURGERY

See also Chapter 19 for a discussion of kidney surgery and urinary diversion.

Nursing Assessment

1. Obtain history from prenatal and birth record, family, and child.
2. Ask and observe about:
   a. Feeding and crying patterns indicating potential obstruction or abdominal pain
   b. Urinary elimination pattern to determine degree of disorder
   c. Nausea and vomiting
   d. Associated congenital defects
   e. Failure to thrive
   f. Family's response to body image changes
      (1) Expect anxieties regarding sterility and homosexuality and perceptions of the child as defective or inadequate.
3. Measure and record vital signs, height, weight, abdominal girth and compare with previous measurements if available. Renal insufficiency may alter growth. Fever may be indicative of infection.

4. Visually and manually inspect genitalia and record abnormalities (ie, if bladder mucosa is visible, describe signs of irritation).
5. Palpate abdomen; note masses.
6. Obtain urine for culture and sensitivity. Note color, amount, odor, degree of cloudiness.
7. Review results of all laboratory and diagnostic procedures.

Nursing Diagnoses

A. Knowledge Deficit related to surgery
B. Altered Urinary Elimination related to the condition and surgical intervention
C. Body Image Disturbance related to appearance of genitalia
D. Risk for Infection related to surgical incision and drainage tubes
E. Risk for Fluid Volume Deficit related to surgical losses
F. Pain related to surgical incision and drainage tubes

Nursing Interventions

A. *Promoting Understanding of Surgical Treatment*
1. Determine the child's expectation regarding illness and hospitalization through discussion and play therapy.
2. Explain the anatomy and physiology of the urinary system in terms the child can understand.
   a. Use a body outline appropriate for the age of the child.
   b. Explain how the child differs from the normal. Relate defect to symptoms whenever possible.
3. Explain all diagnostic test before their occurrence. These may include urinalysis, 24-hour urine collections, IV and retrograde pyelography, angiography, and cystoscopy. Descriptions should include such information as:
   a. Preparation required—fasting, enemas, etc
   b. Location of the test—operating room, radiology department, etc
   c. Appearance and attire of personnel
   d. Positioning
   e. Anesthesia
   f. Pain or discomfort
   g. Expectations after the procedure—diet, rest, urine collections, etc
4. Determine the child's understanding of the procedure.
   a. Ask simple, direct questions.
   b. Allow child to perform the procedure on a doll or demonstrate it on a diagram.
5. Explain the surgical procedure, including:
   a. Preparation required—fasting, enemas, etc.
   b. Description of the operating room, including the appearance of the personnel
   c. Anesthesia
   d. Postoperative appearance—urinary drainage tubing and collection devices, appearance of urine, sutures, bandages, IV infusion
6. Determine the child's understanding of surgery and reinforce teaching when necessary.
7. Emphasize additional points:
   a. The child is in no way to blame for illness.
   b. No other part of the body will be operated on.

B. *Promoting Normal Urinary Pattern*
1. Monitor daily intake and output.
2. Monitor daily weights.
3. Care for all catheters and urinary tubes according to hospital policy. Maintain appropriate position of tubes.
4. Observe and record amount and appearance of urinary drainage, occurrence of bladder spasms, symptoms of urinary or incisional infection.

C. *Providing Emotional Support Regarding Body Image*
1. Continue reassurance about appearance of genitalia.
2. Maintain discussions regarding reactions. This may need to be done with patient and family alone as well as a family unit.
3. Discuss plans for interim period from initial surgery until secondary or reconstructive procedures can be performed.
4. Initiate independence of care.
5. Focus on activities the child can perform and accomplish.

D. *Preventing Infection*
1. Administer antibiotics and IV fluids as ordered.
2. Maintain patency of catheter(s). Provide catheter care as directed.
3. Administer wound care using aseptic technique. Inspect incision for drainage or signs of infection.

E. *Maintaining Fluid Volume*
1. Administer fluids as ordered.
2. Monitor vital signs for hypotension or tachycardia.
3. Assess patient's skin turgor and mucous membranes for signs of dehydration.
4. Measure and record accurate intake and output.

F. *Promoting Comfort*
1. Administer analgesics as ordered and according to assessment of complaints of pain, restlessness, crying, or withdrawal.
2. Administer antispasmodics as ordered for bladder spasm.

Evaluation

A. Child and family verbalizing understanding of surgery
B. Clear urine draining via catheter
C. Child and family verbalizing relief that defects can be surgically repaired and reconstructed
D. Incision without drainage or signs of infection
E. Vital signs stable; urine output adequate
F. Decreased crying and increased restful periods and sleep noted

Renal Failure and Dialysis

◆ ACUTE RENAL FAILURE

Acute renal failure is a sudden, usually reversible deterioration in normal renal function. This results in fluid and electrolyte imbalance and accumulation of metabolic toxins. Nursing care of children with acute renal failure is generally the same as that of adults (see p. 611) although there are special considerations for pediatric patients.

Etiology/Incidence

1. Prerenal causes
   a. Often due to hypovolemia leading to decreased perfusion to a normal kidney (dehydration, shock, trauma, burns)
   b. No preexisting kidney defect
2. Postrenal causes
   a. Uncommon, except for obstructive uropathies in the first year of life
   b. Renal function is restored with relief of the obstruction.
3. Intrarenal causes (the largest group to require extended medical management)
   a. Vascular diseases (hemolytic uremic syndrome, thrombosis)
   b. Tubular nephropathies (myoglobulinuria, hemoglobulinuria, toxins)
   c. Interstitial nephritis (penicillins, allergies)

Altered Physiology

1. The exact pathophysiology of acute renal failure is not always known. Three phases of acute renal failure are recognized in children (Table 46-2).
2. Mechanical obstructions and other conditions, such as hypovolemia and hypotension, reduce blood flow to kidney. This leads to a reduction in glomerular filtration rate (GFR), renal ischemia, and tubular damage.
3. Trauma, burns, and nephrotoxic agents may cause acute tubular necrosis and temporary cessation of renal function. Myoglobin (a protein released from muscle when injury occurs) and hemoglobin are released, causing renal toxicity, ischemia, or both.
4. Severe transfusion reactions may result in hemoglobin filtering through the kidney glomeruli. This becomes concentrated in the kidney tubules. Resulting precipitation interferes with the excretion of urine.
5. Nonsteroidal anti-inflammatory drugs interfere with prostaglandins that normally protect renal blood flow, decreasing GFR.

Complications

1. Fluid and electrolyte imbalance, especially hyperkalemia— when glomerular filtration rate is reduced, patient is unable to excrete potassium.
2. Metabolic acidosis due to decreased acid excretion and bicarbonate regeneration

TABLE 46-2   Phases of Acute Renal Failure in Children

1. Initiating phase—begins when kidney is injured and lasts from hours to days. Signs and symptoms of renal impairment are present.
2. Oliguric phase—usually lasts 5–15 days, but can persist for weeks. Shorter in infants and children (3–5 days). Longer in older children and adolescents (10–14 days)
3. Diuretic phase—highly variable, from mild and lasting only a few days, to profound

3. Insufficient nutritional intake due to metabolic abnormalities and symptoms such as nausea and vomiting

Clinical Manifestations

1. Nausea and vomiting
2. Diarrhea
3. Decreased tissue turgor
4. Dry mucous membranes
5. Lethargy
6. Difficulty in voiding; changes in urine flow
7. Steady rise in serum creatinine
8. Fever
9. Edema

Diagnostic Evaluation

1. Serum creatinine level—the most reliable measure of the GFR, found to be rising
2. Radionuclide studies to evaluate GFR and renal blood flow and distribution
3. Urinalysis—reveals proteinuria, hematuria, casts
4. Ultrasonography to determine anatomic abnormalities

Treatment

1. 75% of children with acute renal failure attain complete recovery.
2. Treatment is directed toward the underlying cause.
3. Correction of any reversible cause of acute renal failure (ie, surgical relief of obstruction)
4. Correction and control of fluid and electrolyte imbalances
5. Restoration and maintenance of stable vital signs
6. Maintenance of nutrition with low-sodium, low-potassium, low-phosphate, moderate-protein diet
7. Initiation of dialysis for patients with life-threatening complications

◆ CHRONIC RENAL FAILURE

Chronic renal failure is irreversible destruction of nephrons so that they are no longer capable of maintaining normal fluid and electrolyte balance. Nursing care of children with chronic renal failure is similar to that of adults (see p. 613). The following considerations are important for pediatric patients.

Etiology/Incidence

1. Congenital renal and urinary tract abnormalities (most common cause under 5 years of age).
2. Most common causes from 5 to 15 years:
   a. Glomerular disease
   b. Hereditary renal disease
   c. Renal vascular disorders

Altered Physiology

1. Similar progression regardless of cause
2. Nephron damage resulting in hypertrophy and hyperplasia of remaining nephrons

3. Overload results in decreased ability for nephrons to excrete effectively.
4. Results in azotemia and clinical uremia
5. Severity of chronic renal failure is indicated by GFR. The lower the GFR the greater the loss of renal function.

Complications

1. Azotemia/uremia—nitrogen waste products accumulating in blood. Toxic levels manifest themselves in many ways such as coma, headache, gastrointestinal disturbances, neuromuscular disturbances.
2. Metabolic acidosis—as a result of decreasing GFR
3. Electrolyte imbalance
4. Severe anemia—kidneys unable to stimulate erythropoietin; uremic toxins deplete erythrocytes; nutritional deficiencies.
5. Hypertension—renal ischemia stimulates renin–angiotensin system.
6. Congestive heart failure

Clinical Manifestations

Variable and not chronological

1. Decreased appetite and energy level
2. Increased urinary output and fluid intake
3. Bone or joint pain
4. Delayed or absent sexual maturation
5. Growth retardation
6. Dryness and itching of skin
7. Anemia
8. Markedly elevated BUN and creatinine

Diagnostic Evaluation

Determine extent of disease; monitor progression.

1. Serum studies
   a. Decreased hematocrit, hemoglobin, Na^+, Ca^{++}; increased K^+, phosphorous
   b. As renal function declines, BUN, uric acid, and creatinine values continue to climb.
2. Urine studies
   a. Specific gravity—increased or decreased
   b. 24-hour urine for creatinine clearance is decreased (increased creatinine in urine) reflecting decreased GFR
   c. Changes in total output
3. Many other tests may be ordered to evaluate other systems and extent of disease (ie, chest x-ray, electrocardiogram)

Treatment

1. Correction of calcium phosphorous imbalance. Administer activated vitamin D to increase calcium absorption and calcium phosphate binders with meals to bind phosphate in the gastrointestinal tract.
2. Correction of acidosis with buffers such as Bicitra

3. Diets should meet caloric needs of the child containing adequate protein for development (1.0–1.5 g/kg per day).
4. Correction of anemia through the use of erythropoietin (Epogen) administered subcutaneously at home
5. Growth retardation should be evaluated for possible use of growth hormone.
6. Treatment options for end-stage renal disease are hemodialysis, peritoneal dialysis, or transplantation.
7. Institute dialysis therapy while transplant work-up is in progress.

Nursing Assessment

A comprehensive, multisystem assessment is warranted and will help in planning care for the child. Physical assessment should focus on the clinical manifestations and complications of chronic renal failure.

Nursing Diagnoses

Children with chronic renal failure are in multisystem physiologic crises. The nursing diagnoses throughout the chapter are applicable, but focus may be:
A. Fluid Volume Excess related to renal failure
B. Altered Nutrition (Less than Body Requirements) related to gastrointestinal disturbances and diet restrictions
C. Risk for Infection related to decreased immunity
D. Risk for Injury related to neuromuscular abnormalities
E. Activity Intolerance related to fatigue and anemia
F. Grieving related to changes in lifestyle and body image, dialysis
G. Powerlessness related to hospitalization, separation, treatment, and prognosis

Nursing Interventions

As with the assessment and diagnoses, many detailed interventions are listed elsewhere in chapter that may apply. Additionally, provide the following care.

A. **Ensuring Safety**
1. Protect the child from the effects of decreased level of consciousness and involuntary movements by maintaining crib or bed side rails up and padded, as necessary.
2. Monitor for any seizure activity and have airway or tongue blade and suction equipment on hand.

B. **Educating About Chronic Renal Failure**
1. Because numerous issues may interfere with the child's psychological and social development and education, help the child and family to cope with:
   a. Uncertainty regarding the course of the disease and ultimate prognosis
   b. Abnormal lifestyle necessitated by dialysis
   c. Burden of dialysis and continuous administration of medications
   d. Problems of adjustment related to growth failure
   e. Fear of death, present in most children, adolescents, and family members

f. Possible kidney transplantation involving major surgery, prolonged hospitalization; followed by altered body image due to high-dose steroids and potential for rejection, which may threaten survival

2. Advise the family about support services and media resources available. For example, ''It's Just a Part of My Life—a Kid's View of Dialysis'' by the National Kidney Foundation; 30 E. 33rd Street; New York, NY, 10016; 212-889-2210.

◆ RENAL TRANSPLANT

Renal (kidney) transplantation is the optimal therapeutic modality for end-stage renal disease in the pediatric age group. With transplantation, there is a greater likelihood of complete rehabilitation than with any form of dialytic therapy. The potential for normal growth and pubertal development is significantly increased after transplantation. However, it should be noted that posttransplant growth is variable related to caloric intake, corticosteroid dosage, bone age at transplantation, and rejection episodes. Nursing care of children experiencing kidney transplantation is similar to that of adults (see p. 604).

Evaluation of Recipient

The major issues that must be evaluated when considering renal transplantation in children are:

1. Patient age
2. Primary renal disease
3. Psychological status
4. Live versus cadaveric donor allograft
5. Optimal immunosuppressive regimen
6. Maximization of growth and pubertal development

Donor Selection (by Priority)

1. Identical twin sibling
2. Sibling—it is important to note that siblings cannot be used as donors until they are of legal age to give consent for removal of a kidney.
3. Parent
4. Aunt or uncle
5. Unrelated live donor (seldom used) or cadaver donor

Operative Procedure

Small children may require replacement within the abdomen with vessel anastomosis to the aorta and superior vena cava.

Potential Emotional Concerns of Children With Transplants

1. The concept of a foreign body, especially a cadaver kidney, inside one's own body may be disturbing.

2. Fear that the kidney may wear out sooner if it is from an older person
3. Altered body image due to growth failure and the effects of steroid therapy
4. Guilt feelings if a live donor transplant fails, especially a family donor

Nursing Care

Refer to sections on:

1. Chronic renal failure, page 613.
2. Care of the child requiring urologic surgery, page 613.
3. Kidney transplantation, page 606.

◆ THE CHILD UNDERGOING DIALYSIS

Dialysis is the passage of a solute through a semipermeable membrane. The purpose of dialysis is to preserve life by replacing some of the normal kidney functions. See Procedure Guidelines 46-1.

Nursing Care

In addition to understanding the types and principles of dialysis (see p. 600), the following principles should be considered by the nurse working with pediatric patients:

1. Peritoneal dialysis
   a. Because of the child's small size, the volume of dialysate is 40 mL/kg or 1,100 mL/m^2.
   b. Because the child may be unable to hold still, it may be necessary to apply protective measures to limit motion to avoid contamination of the sterile field or injury to the child (see p. 1137) for acute peritoneal dialysis.
   c. For patients on chronic peritoneal dialysis allow the child to participate at an age-appropriate level with his or her own care.
2. Hemodialysis
   a. When possible, avoid giving subcutaneous or intramuscular injections because the child is anticoagulated with heparin at least twice weekly
   b. Blood pressure cuff and tourniquets should not be applied to a limb with a fistula.
3. Specific care for the child during dialysis is generally provided by specially trained personnel in a dialysis unit. However, the following considerations should be noted.
   a. Choice for vascular access depends on patient size and availability of peripheral blood vessels of suitable size.
   b. Extracorporeal blood volume (blood outside of the body at any given time) should be as small as possible. It should not exceed 8% to 10% of the child's total blood volume.
   c. Efficiency or adequacy of the dialyzer relative to the child's weight should be noted.
   d. Secure external catheter or restrain patient to ensure catheter is not manipulated.

PROCEDURE GUIDELINES 46-1 ◆ Caring for the Child Undergoing Dialysis

PROCEDURE	
NURSING ACTION	**RATIONALE**

1. Prepare the child for the procedure.
   a. Explain the procedure in terms that child can understand.
      (1) Allow the child to handle equipment similar to that which will be used during dialysis.
      (2) Encourage the child to express fears so that misinterpretations can be corrected.
      (3) Provide simple pictures and diagrams, if appropriate.
      (4) Allow the child to talk with peers who have undergone dialysis.
   b. Explain the procedure to the family and answer questions so that they will be in the best position to support their child.
2. Protect the child from infection.
   a. Keep the dressings and area around the catheter clean and dry.
   b. Use aseptic technique throughout the dialysis procedure.
   c. Provide supplemental vitamins since a protein-restricted diet is poor in vitamins.
   d. Provide meticulous daily hygiene.
3. Maintain appropriate diet restrictions with sodium, potassium and fluids if patient is on hemodialysis. Because anorexia is often seen in chronic renal failure, provide small frequent meals.
4. Provide liberal protein in diet, as desired, and no restrictions if patient is on peritoneal dialysis.
5. Maintain careful records of intake and output, vital signs, blood pressure, and daily weights.
6. Support the child during the dialysis procedure.
   a. Provide symptomatic relief of nausea, vomiting, malaise, or headache. Notify the health care provider if these symptoms are severe.
   b. Be alert to clues from the child for helpful methods of offering support.
      (1) Young children often cling to stuffed toys or blankets or depend on parents' presence at the bedside.
      (2) Older children may benefit from radio, television, magazines, or contact with peers.
7. Provide an environment that is as normal as possible.
   a. Encourage the family to bring in articles that will make the child's room appear more homelike (ie, pictures, posters, etc.)
   b. Encourage the child to be as independent as possible in daily care.
   c. Provide for age-appropriate recreation and diversion.
   d. Help the child to keep up with school work by initiating a referral to a tutor, providing study times, etc.

1. Dialysis is threatening to most children and may evoke fears of pain, mutilation, immobilization, helplessness, and dependency. Many children have fears of losing all of their blood in this process. A child who is well prepared will be less frightened and better able to cooperate during the procedure.

2. These children are prone to infection because of their general debilitated state and because of protein loss and anemia.

3. Fluids and sodium are restricted to prevent fluid overload. Potassium is limited to prevent complications related to hyperkalemia. The child may see dietary restrictions as a punishment and must be helped to realize the purpose of restrictions.
4. Peritoneal dialysis is a continual treatment and therefore is able to constantly dialyze metabolic waste and fluids off. Protein is not restricted because it is vital to allow for normal growth and development.
5. These provide valuable information about the effectiveness of the therapy.

7. Although life is preserved, it is by no means normal during the time on dialysis or between dialyses. These measures may increase the child's feeling of self-esteem and diminish regression and social isolation. By serving as role models, health professionals may encourage parents to recognize and foster the normal, healthy aspects of the child's daily life.

(continued)

PROCEDURE GUIDELINES 46-1 ◆ Caring for the Child Undergoing Dialysis *(continued)*

PROCEDURE (cont'd)	NURSING ACTION	RATIONALE

	8. Offer appropriate support to the family.
	  a. Provide opportunity for family members to discuss their feelings, fears, and frustrations and to ask questions.
	  b. Allow family members to become involved in the child's care to the extent that they wish and that is helpful for the child and family.
	  c. Provide for continuity of personnel.
	  d. Initiate appropriate referrals. These may include referrals to a social worker, psychiatrist, dietitian, community health agency, or other families who are coping with dialysis.
	9. Teach the child and family about all of the important aspects of renal failure and dialysis, including:
	  a. Signs and symptoms of uremia
	  b. Shunt care and protection.
	  c. Protection from infection
	  d. Dietary restrictions and recommendations; ways of incorporating the special diet into the family meal plan
	  e. Dialysis schedule
	  f. Medications
	  g. Emergency procedures
		8. Families often need extensive support from many health professionals to cope with the physical psychological, financial, and logistical aspects of renal failure and dialysis. Attention must be focused on siblings as well as parents because sibling relationships are often strained and difficult.
		
		9. The family should be prepared to care for the child at home well before the day of discharge. Learning about the child's care also helps restore some sense of control in a frightening situation.

Selected References

Erickson, P. (1993). Idiopathic glomerulonephritis: Is it IgA nephropathy. *ANNA Journal, 20*(2), 127-132.

Graham-MaCaluso, M. M. (1991). Complications of peritoneal dialysis: Nursing care plans to document teaching. *ANNA Journal, 18*(5), 479-483.

Hazinski, M. F. (1992). *Nursing care of the critically ill child* (2nd ed.). St. Louis, MD: Mosby-Year Book.

Kelalis, P. P., King, L. R., & Belman, A. B. (1992). *Clinical pediatric urology.* Philadelphia: W. B. Saunders.

Knight, F., Gorynski, L., Genston, M., & Harmon, W. (1993). Hemodialysis of the infant or small child with chronic renal failure. *ANNA Journal, 20*(3), 315-323.

Oski, F. A., DeAngelis, C. D., Ferguin, R. D., & Warshaw, J. B. (1994). *Principles and practice of pediatrics.* 2nd ed. Philadelphia: J. B. Lippincott.

Wiserman, K. (1991). Nephrotic syndrome: Pathophysiology and treatment. *ANNA Journal, 18*(5), 469-476.

Pediatric Metabolic and Endocrine Disorders

Assessment

◆ COMMON NURSING ASSESSMENT FOR GROWTH AND DEVELOPMENT

Endocrine dysfunction in children frequently leads to altered growth and development. Accurate nursing assessment can help detect variations in growth and developmental patterns, identify factors such as diet and medications that may have an impact on growth and development, and obtain information about compliance and understanding of treatment.

Evaluation of Growth Patterns

1. Perform frequent and accurate measurements of both height and weight.
2. Accurately plot measurements on growth curve for absolute chronologic age.
3. Assess growth pattern for any deviation from the child's percentile or from the parallel of the growth curve for age (includes both an upward as well as downward deviation).
4. Report any child whose pattern deviates from the expected pattern for age to health care provider.

> **COMMUNITY-BASED CARE TIP:** ◆
> The school nurse who measures the child on an annual basis is the best source for detecting a growth disorder. Height percentiles should accompany absolute measurements. Changes in percentiles on consecutive measurements indicate need for a closer evaluation of growth.

History of General Health

1. Dietary history—what is the child's meal frequency, volume and food preferences? Be especially critical in the history of a child where anorexia may be possible—growth velocity will usually be low in addition to poor weight gain.

2. Clothing—outgrowing clothing and shoes?
3. Social history relative to friendships
   a. Academic/school performance—recent changes?
   b. Activity—activities the child participates in? Intensity and type of exercise?

Medication History/Compliance

1. Is child on any steroidal medications (such as prednisone) that would suppress growth?
2. Does child have access to any gonadal steroids where pubertal signs are present on physical examination (ie, birth control pills, anabolic steroids)?
3. Are child and family compliant with treatment medications according to dose, frequency, and route? Is medication stored properly?
4. Do child and family know what the medications are and their indications?
5. If taking oral medication, is it being taken with food if indicated? If pills are being chewed, are teeth being brushed soon after, which could be rinsing out the medications?
6. If injectable—are injection sites being rotated appropriately? Review technique.

Physical Examination Relative to Development

1. Dental development—eruption of teeth and presence of permanent teeth (see p. 1056)
2. Pubertal development—Tanner staging of pubic hair and gonadal development (Table 47-1).
3. Presence of genetic dysmorphology—such as short-limbed dwarfism and various atypical stigmata

Disorders of the Anterior Pituitary

The anterior pituitary is under the control of the hypothalamus and secretes six specific hormones: growth hormone (GH), thyroid-stimulating hormone (TSH), adrenocortico-

TABLE 47-1 Tanner Staging of Puberty

Boys' Genital Development	Girls' Breast Development	Both Sexes: Pubic Hair
Stage I Preadolescent. Testes, scrotum, and penis are of about the same size and proportion as in early childhood. 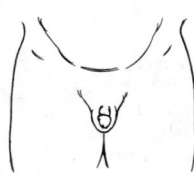	Preadolescent. Elevation of papilla only. 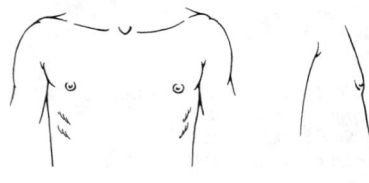	Preadolescent. The vellus over the pubis is not further developed than that over the abdominal wall, ie, no pubic hair. 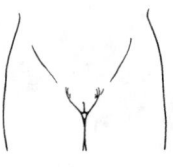 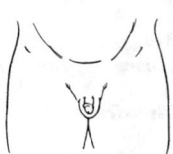
Stage 2 Enlargement of scrotum and testes. Skin of scrotum reddens and changes in texture. Little or no enlargement of penis at this time. 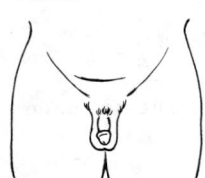	Breast bud stage. Elevation of breast and papilla as small mound. Enlargement of areola diameter. 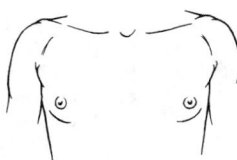	Sparse growth of long, slightly pigmented downy hair. Straight or slightly curled at base of penis or along labia. 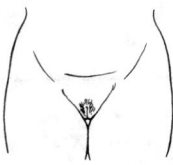 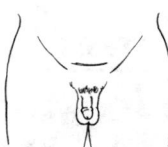
Stage 3 Enlargement of penis that occurs at first mainly in length. Further growth of testes and scrotum. 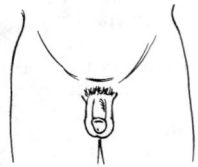	Further enlargement and elevation of breast and areola with no separation of their contours. 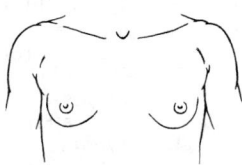	Considerably darker, coarser, and more curled. The hair spreads sparsely over the symphysis of the pubes. 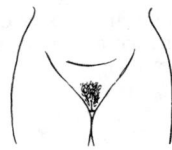 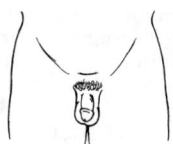
Stage 4 Increased size of penis with growth in breadth and development of glans. Testes and scrotum larger; scrotal skin darkened. 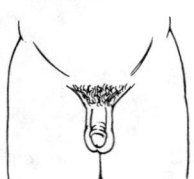	Projection of areola and papilla to form a secondary mound above level of the breast. 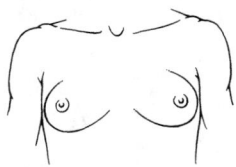	Hair now adult in type, but area covered is still considerably smaller than in adult. No spread to medial surface of thighs. 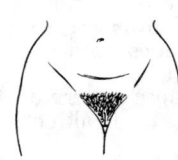 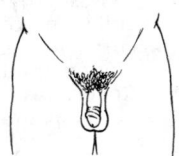
Stage 5 Genitalia adult in size and shape. 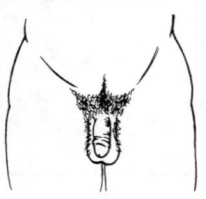	Mature stage: projection of papilla only, due to recession of the areola to the general contour of the breast. 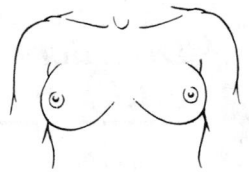	Adult in quantity and type; distribution of the horizontal (or classically ''feminine'') pattern. Spread to medial surface of thighs or above base of the inverse triangle occurs late (stage 6). 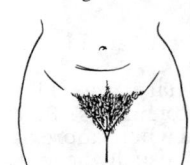 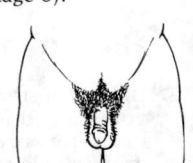

Adapted from: Tanner, J. M. (1975). Growth and endocrinology of the adolescent. In: Gardner, L. (Ed.). *Endocrine and genetic diseases of childhood and adolescence* (2nd ed.). Philadelphia: W. B. Saunders.

tropic hormone (ACTH), luteinizing hormone (LH), follicle-stimulating hormone (FSH), and prolactin. GH is the only hormone that does not have a target gland to induce further hormonal secretion. Hypopituitarism is a deficiency of one, some, or all of the hormones secreted by the pituitary gland. With the exception of GH, decreased secretion results in hypofunction of the consequential target gland. GH insufficiency is discussed below; see hypothyroidism (p. 715) and adrenal insufficiency (p. 729) for other manifestations of hypopituitarism.

◆ GROWTH HORMONE INSUFFICIENCY

Insufficient secretion of GH is caused by the lack of pituitary production or hypothalamic stimulation on the pituitary.

Etiology/Incidence

1. Incidence is approximately 1 in 3,500 for classic GH insufficiency, unknown for varying degrees of insufficiency
2. Organic etiology
   a. Intracranial cyst
   b. Central nervous system (CNS) tumor (adenoma)
   c. Craniopharyngioma
   d. CNS irradiation
   e. Exogenous (head trauma, infection)
   f. Histiocytosis X
   g. Septo-optic dysplasia (abnormal forebrain development)
2. Idiopathic
   a. Isolated GH deficiency
   b. Traumatic birth or breech delivery
   c. Genetic (GH gene deletion)
   d. Aplasia

Altered Physiology

1. The lack of GH impairs the body's ability to perform the following functions:
   a. Protein metabolism—growth through increased protein synthesis; nitrogen, phosphorous and potassium storage
   b. Fat metabolism—increases lipolysis and oxidation of fat
   c. Carbohydrate metabolism—decreases conversion of glucose to fat in adipose tissue

Complications

1. Altered carbohydrate, protein, and fat metabolism
2. Hypoglycemia—seizures/death in newborns

Clinical Manifestations

1. Hypoglycemia (usually in the newborn)
2. Growth velocity usually less than the 5th percentile for chronologic age

3. Delayed skeletal maturation—bone age at least 1 year delayed from chronologic age
4. "Pudgy" where the weight age (50% for weight) exceeds the height age (50% for height)
5. Frequently delayed eruption of primary and secondary teeth (not as severe as in hypothyroidism)
6. Delayed or lack of sexual development

Diagnostic Evaluation

1. Rule out organic, nonendocrine causes of short stature (ie, chronic illness, nutritional deficiencies, genetic disorders, psychosocial factors)
2. Calculate growth velocity (does growth pattern parallel or deviate from the growth curve?)
3. Bone age assessment—ascertain age of physical development—it is usually delayed.
4. General physical examination—physical development that of a younger appearing child?
5. Thyroid function tests to rule out hypothyroidism
6. GH secretion laboratory indicators: IGF-1, IGF-binding protein 3 are decreased.
7. Subnormal secretion of GH in response to two provocative stimuli
8. In the newborn with hypoglycemia, GH release is reduced at time of documented hypoglycemia.
9. Computed tomography (CT) scanning or magnetic resonance imaging (MRI) of head to rule out lesion etiology

Treatment

1. Goal of treatment is to restore normal growth and development as well as to maximize growth potential and prevent hypoglycemia.
2. Replacement of deficiency uses recombinant DNA-derived GH given as subcutaneous injection.
3. Typical dose is 0.2 to 0.3 mg/kg per week divided in 3, 6 or 7 doses weekly until final height is achieved.

Nursing Assessment

1. See common nursing assessment for growth and development, page 1289.
2. Obtain family history related to parental heights and ages of pubertal maturation.

Nursing Diagnoses

A. Altered Growth and Development related to lack of GH
B. Social Isolation related to short stature and peer acceptance
C. Self-Esteem Disturbance related to discordant expectations by peers and adults

Nursing Interventions

A. *Promoting Child's Own Pattern of Growth and Development*
1. Teach method of injecting GH through written and verbal instructions. Give demonstration and encourage return demonstration.

2. Encourage rotation of sites in the subcutaneous tissue of the upper arms or thighs if irritation occurs.
3. Document growth at regular intervals.

B. *Encouraging Social Interaction*
1. Encourage the child to verbalize feelings regarding short stature.
2. Have the child describe what he or she likes about certain people to help the child understand that friendships and social value are based on personality traits rather than absolute height.
3. Suggest involvement in activities that do not use height as an advantage, such as music, art, and gymnastics.
4. Ask the child to identify behaviors that may deter socialization (may or may not be related to short stature) and find ways to change behavior.

C. *Strengthening Self-Esteem*
1. Help child and parents to identify age-appropriate behaviors and develop a plan for maintaining consistent behaviors both in the home and socially.
2. Make sure parents have realistic expectations of child.
3. Encourage the use of positive feedback rather than punishment.

Family Education/Health Maintenance

1. Tell child and family that short stature is not a "disease." It is the symptom of growth failure.
   a. Growth catch-up to peers usually occurs when peers have stopped growing.
   b. After initial start-up of treatment, growth rate should be in the 2- to 3-inch/year rate.
   c. Treatment is not to make child tall—it is to restore normal growth that is reflected in height achievement.
2. Review medication dosage and injection technique periodically.
3. Tell family to think of GH as a replacement rather than a medication; therefore, it should always be given regardless of illness or other medication therapies.
4. Encourage regular follow-up for growth evaluation and maintenance of therapy.

Evaluation

A. Child demonstrates appropriate injection technique; 1 inch growth over past 6 month.
B. Child reports interest in school activities and playing with friends.
C. Parents report more positive behavior.

Disorders of the Posterior Pituitary

The posterior pituitary is under the control of the hypothalamus and secretes two hormones, vasopressin (antidiuretic hormone—ADH) and oxytocin. Abnormality of ADH function is the most common disorder seen in children. The function of ADH is to conserve water at the distal tubules and collecting ducts of the kidney and to act on smooth muscle to increase blood pressure.

◆ DIABETES INSIPIDUS

Diabetes insipidus (DI) is failure of the body to conserve water due to a deficiency of ADH, decreased renal sensitivity to ADH, or suppression of ADH secondary to excessive ingestion of fluids (primary polydipsia).

Etiology/Incidence

A. *Central DI*   Low levels of ADH

1. Congenital causes—CNS defects (septo-optic dysplasia), hereditary (X-linked recessive)
2. Acquired causes—CNS tumors, head trauma, infections, vascular disorders, idiopathic

B. *Nephrogenic*   Renal unresponsiveness to vasopressin

1. Congenital—rare
2. Chronic renal disease

Altered Physiology

1. The function of water metabolism in the body is to maintain a constant plasma osmolality near the mean level of 287 mOsm/kg.
2. Intake and output of water are governed by the centers in the hypothalamus to control thirst and synthesis of ADH.
3. Thirst ensures adequate intake of water and ADH prevents water loss through the kidney.
4. Patients with DI are unable to produce appropriate levels or action of ADH, leading to polyuria, increased plasma osmolality, and increased thirst.

Complications

1. Dehydration
2. Hypernatremia

Clinical Manifestations

1. Sudden onset of excessive thirst and polyuria
2. In infants:
   a. Excessive crying—quieted with water more than milk feeding
   b. Rapid weight loss—caloric loss due to water preference over feedings
   c. Constipation
   d. Growth failure—failure to thrive
   e. Sunken fontanel with dehydration
3. In children:
   a. Excessive thirst and drinking
   b. Polyuria with nocturia and enuresis
   c. Pale dry skin with reduced sweating

Diagnostic Evaluation

Tests document inability to produce ADH in the face of hyperosomolality of plasma.

1. Urine specific gravity, sodium, and osmolality are decreased.
2. Serum osmolality and sodium are elevated.
3. Serum measurement of ADH is low in conjunction with high plasma osmolality.
4. Water deprivation test—(potentially dangerous)
   a. Fluids are restricted and the urinary volumes and concentrations are monitored hourly along with the child's weight.
   b. Test is terminated if child loses more than 3% to 5% of body weight. Serum sodium and osmolality are measured at completion of test and are high; urine osmolality remains lower.
   c. Test is completed by giving the child a dose of ADH, which should stop the abnormal diuresis. If it does not, child may have nephrogenic DI (renal unresponsiveness).
5. Assess for underlying cause
   a. MRI or CT scan of hypothalamic-pituitary region
   b. High incidence of associated anterior pituitary disorders

Treatment

1. Daily replacement of ADH using desmopressin (DDAVP)—a synthetic analogue
2. Available as a metered nasal spray or a measured insufflation (nasal) tube. In children with cleft lip and palate, sublingual administration has been shown to be effective.
3. Thiazide diuretics in nephrogenic DI

Nursing Assessment

1. Assess children with complaints or behaviors of polyuria and polydipsia for dehydration.
2. Obtain a thorough history of symptoms and behaviors—specific attention to changes in sleep patterns (may be caused by enuresis), choices of fluids including sources of water (eg, does child drink from toilet bowls or dog dishes).
3. Evaluate height and weight—assess for weight loss related to possible decrease in calories due to excessive drinking, which cuts appetite.
4. For the child on treatment, assess for hydration status. Obtain history of fluid intake and output from the parents to assess appropriate dosage, frequency, and administration of medication.

Nursing Diagnoses

A. Fluid Volume Deficit related to disease process
B. Altered Nutrition (Less than Body Requirements) due to fluid preference over food
C. Sleep Pattern Disturbance related to nocturia and enuresis

Nursing Interventions

A. *Regaining Fluid Balance*
1. Assess for and teach parents assessment of dehydration—dry mucous membranes, weight loss, increased pulse, listlessness or irritability, sunken fontanelle in infants, fever, poor skin turgor
2. Administer intravenous (IV) fluid as ordered if acutely dehydrated.
3. Teach parents to maintain record of fluid intake and output in child. Reduced output may require restriction of fluids if overdosage of DDAVP is suspected.

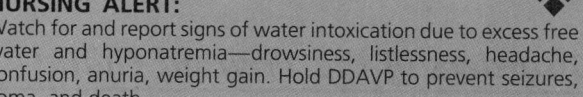

NURSING ALERT:
Watch for and report signs of water intoxication due to excess free water and hyponatremia—drowsiness, listlessness, headache, confusion, anuria, weight gain. Hold DDAVP to prevent seizures, coma, and death.

4. Administer and teach proper administration of DDAVP. Proper management should eliminate symptoms.
5. Teach parents to provide free access to fluid (water) sources at all times. However, caution parents that child is unprotected from water excess.
6. Calculate rough estimated total daily fluid requirements based on body size to assess fluid replacement versus excess: 100 mL/kg for first 10 kg of body weight, 50 mL/kg for second 10 kg of body weight, 20 mL/kg for each additional kilogram.

B. *Maintaining Adequate Nutrition*
1. Ensure that adequate formula is ingested between plain water bottles.
2. For older child, provide liquid nutritional supplements.
3. Stress to parents or caregivers the importance of providing nutritional requirements with fluids to ensure meeting caloric demands for growth.
4. Consult with dietitian about need for vitamin or other supplements.
5. Monitor length and weight and developmental milestones at regular intervals.

C. *Normalizing Sleep Pattern*
1. Ensure adequate evening administration of DDAVP to prevent nighttime water craving and enuresis.
2. Suggest the use of diapers at night and plastic padding on bed to make bedwetting easier until optimum management of condition is attained.
3. Encourage easy access to fluids and toilet or commode for older child during night.

Family Education/Health Maintenance

1. Teach family about administration of medication.
   a. Demonstrate insufflation method for infants and young children, inhalation for older children.
   b. Nostrils should be as clear as possible before administration of dose.
   c. Advise that medication must remain cool/refrigerated.
   d. If dose is thought to be swallowed, do not readminister due to potential overdosage. Split the dose into both nares if swallowing is occurring.

2. Advise parents that children should wear Medic Alert bracelet for DI.
3. Tell parents that school personnel should be aware of condition and symptoms needing attention.
4. Advise routine follow-up; treatment may be temporary or lifelong depending on cause.

Evaluation

A. No signs of dehydration, intake equals output
B. No weight loss, growth curve maintained
C. Two diaper changes during night reported, falls back to sleep easily

Disorders of the Thyroid Gland

Under hypothalamic-pituitary regulation, the thyroid gland secretes thyroxine (T4) and triiodothyronine (T3). The action of these hormones promotes cellular growth and differentiation, protein synthesis, and lipid metabolism (cholesterol turnover). Disorders of the thyroid gland are broadly classified as hypothyroidism and hyperthyroidism.

◆ HYPOTHYROIDISM

Hypothyroidism is low circulating level of thyroid hormone (T_4).

Etiology/Incidence

A. **Congenital** 1 in 4,000 live births

1. Thyroid agenesis or dysgenesis
2. Hormone synthesis defect
3. Maternal thyroid antibodies crossing placenta
4. Iodine deficiency
5. Drug-induced destruction (thionamides for treatment of hyperthyroidism, iodide excess)
6. Peripheral T_4 resistance

B. **Acquired (Postnatal)**
1. Autoimmune thyroiditis (Hashimoto or chronic lymphocytic thyroiditis)
2. Radiation
3. Surgical ablation (thyroidectomy)
4. Antithyroid drugs
5. Iodine deficiency
6. Central hypothyroidism (TRH/TSH deficiency)

Altered Physiology

1. Circulating levels of T4 are dependent on hypothalamic-pituitary stimulation (TRH/TSH) of the thyroid gland.
2. Low levels of T4 cause a rise in TSH.
3. Absent or decreased levels of T4 result in abnormal development of the CNS of the newborn.
4. In older children, hypothyroidism results in a decrease in metabolism, growth, and physical maturation.

Complications

1. Mental retardation in newborn who is undiagnosed or untreated
2. Short stature, growth failure, and delayed physical maturation and development in the older child

Clinical Manifestations

A. **Newborn**
1. Very subtle physical signs, if any
2. Markedly open posterior fontanelle
3. Prolonged physiologic jaundice
4. Feeding difficulties
5. Skin cool to touch/mottled
6. Poor muscle tone—hypotonia, umbilical hernia

B. **After 6 Months**
1. Growth failure
2. Large protruding tongue
3. Coarse facial features
4. Poor feeding and constipation

C. **Acquired**
1. Growth retardation—slow growth rate
2. Lethargy—obedient, nonaggressive, somnolent
3. Cold intolerance
4. Possible poor school performance

Diagnostic Evaluation

1. Neonatal screening of T4 and TSH. Elevation of TSH or a low T4 may indicate congenital hypothyroidism.
2. Thyroid nuclear scan—reduced uptake
3. Abnormal growth rate
4. Bone age x-ray; delayed
5. Blood studies
   a. T_4, T_3 resin uptake may be decreased; TSH elevated
   b. Thyroid antibodies—elevated in autoimmune thyroiditis

Treatment

1. Replacement of thyroid hormone: levothyroxine (Synthroid, Levothroid)
2. Treatment must not be delayed.
3. Therapy goal is to maintain normalcy of thyroid function tests (T_4 and T_3 concentrations).

Nursing Assessment

1. Assess newborn for clinical manifestations listed above.
2. Perform behavioral assessment to include sleeping, eating, bowel patterns, and level of alertness, school performance.
3. Assess growth patterns: growth velocity (rate of growth over time), weight gain, and head circumference.

Nursing Diagnoses

A. Altered Growth and Development related to effects of hypothyroidism

B. Anxiety related to lack of knowledge regarding hypothyroidism and its treatment

Nursing Interventions

A. *Promoting Growth and Development*
1. Administer or teach parents to administer thyroid hormone replacement daily.
2. Discourage mixing thyroid medication with liquid in bottle that may not be completely finished during a feeding; instead mix with small amount of fluid and give with dropper or syringe.
3. If thyroid pill is being chewed, rather than swallowed, have patient avoid brushing teeth immediately after to protect against rinsing away dose.
4. Monitor growth and developmental milestones at regular intervals.

B. *Reducing Anxiety*
1. Encourage parents to verbalize feelings about child and the condition.
2. Educate the parents as to the importance of the therapy so child will grow and develop normally.
3. Stress that with replacement therapy, the child can participate in all usual activities.

Family Education/Health Maintenance

1. Encourage follow-up for blood studies and evaluation of neurologic development to ensure adequate treatment and prevent mental retardation.
2. Make sure the family understands that therapy is lifelong.
3. Support the parents and refer child for special testing and therapy if mental retardation is suspected.

Evaluation

A. Parents claim compliance with medication administration; growth curve maintained.
B. Parents verbalize understanding and acceptance of therapy.

◆ HYPERTHYROIDISM

Hyperthyroidism is a disorder of the thyroid gland in which a high circulating level of T4 results in abnormally increased body metabolism (thyrotoxicosis).

Etiology/Incidence

1. Autoimmune—thyrotropin receptor antibodies of a stimulating nature are produced.
   a. Graves' disease—most common cause of hyperthyroidism in children; 1% to 2% of school-aged children
   b. Chronic thyroiditis—Hashimoto's; usually short-term hyperthyroidism before developing hypothyroidism
2. Ingestion or overdosage of thyroid medication
3. Pituitary adenoma—TSH initiated

Altered Physiology

1. Autoantibodies stimulate thyroid gland to produce and secrete T_4.
2. Elevated circulating thyroid hormone increases the body's metabolic rate causing an increase in excitability of the neuromuscular, cardiovascular, and sympathetic nervous system.

Complications

1. Development of a goiter (glandular enlargement due to overstimulation)
2. Cardiac problems of tachycardia and hypertension
3. Exophthalmos—abnormal protrusion of the eyeball

Clinical Manifestations

1. Thyromegaly—enlargement of the thyroid, possibly with a bruit
2. Polyphagia with weight loss
3. Exophthalmos, proptosis, lid retraction
4. Hyperactivity—restlessness, nervousness, hand tremors, sleeping disturbances, emotional lability
5. Heat intolerance, excessive diaphoresis
6. Fatigue, muscle weakness
7. Tachycardia, wide pulse pressure
8. Tall stature, underweight for height

Diagnostic Evaluation

1. Serum thyroid function tests—elevated T_4, T_3 resin uptake with a suppressed TSH
2. Microsomal antibodies—positive
3. Thyroid radionuclide scan of goiter—rule out cold nodules that could indicate thyroid carcinoma

Treatment

1. Propranolol (Inderal), a β-adrenergic blocking agent, for cardiac effects
2. Inorganic iodide preparation, such as propylthiouracil (PTU), methimazole (Tapazole), or carbimazole, to block release of thyroid hormone
3. Radioactive ablation of thyroid gland using radioiodine—preferred over thyroidectomy. This is chosen when medical management is ineffective. Results in permanent hypothyroidism that requires treatment.

Nursing Assessment

1. Perform physical assessment to include temperature, heart rate, blood pressure, height, and weight.
2. Obtain history of symptoms specific to onset and subsequent development of symptoms.
3. Elicit history of any changes in behavior, emotions, or sleep patterns.
4. Assess for presence of goiter—pain with swallowing or talking, palpation of thyroid.

Nursing Diagnoses

A. Activity Intolerance related to effects of excessive metabolic activity
B. Altered Nutrition (Less than Body Requirements) due to increased metabolic demand
C. Sleep Pattern Disturbance related to high metabolic rate
D. Fear related to radioiodine ablation of gland if therapy choice

Nursing Interventions

A. *Improving Activity Tolerance*
1. Administer and teach parents to administer medications and comply with treatment to gradually lower the metabolic rate and improve activity tolerance.
2. Assess activity tolerance periodically. Ascertain if fatigue is present at rest, with activities of daily living, or with excercise.
3. Avoid overactivity.

B. *Ensuring Adequate Diet*
1. Encourage high-calorie, nutritious diet to try to maintain weight.
2. Advise parents that effective treatment will lower metabolic rate and facilitate appropriate weight gain.
3. Periodically assess growth and development parameters.

C. *Normalizing Sleep Pattern*
1. Assess sleep pattern including naps, sleeping through the night.
2. Adjust schedule to allow maximum amount of rest until sleeping through the night.

D. *Reducing Fear*
1. Encourage parents and child to verbalize fears related to the thyroid ablation.
2. Teach them about the procedure and clear up misconceptions.
   a. Ablation is accomplished through radioactive destruction of thyroid tissue by administration of a radioactive iodine pill.
   b. The thyroid gland is the only tissue in the body that absorbs iodine; therefore, the radiation only destroys thyroid tissue.
   c. Radiation will be eliminated through the child's urine and feces; precautions for disposal must be followed according to nuclear medicine department policies.
3. Tell them that the resultant effect will most likely be hypothyroidism, which can be managed with lifelong treatment of T_4 replacement.

Family Education/Health Maintenance

1. Review prescribed medications and their function. Stress the importance of compliance.

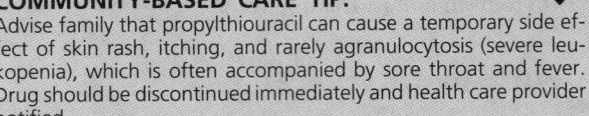

COMMUNITY-BASED CARE TIP:
Advise family that propylthiouracil can cause a temporary side effect of skin rash, itching, and rarely agranulocytosis (severe leukopenia), which is often accompanied by sore throat and fever. Drug should be discontinued immediately and health care provider notified.

2. Educate family for side effects of oversuppression where hypothyroidism could develop.
3. Encourage follow-up to monitor treatment through blood tests, growth and development evaluation, and size of thyroid gland.

Evaluation

A. Plays for 1 hour without fatigue
B. No weight loss noted
C. Sleeping 8 hours with 2-hour nap
D. Parents and child verbalize understanding of radiation procedure and its rationale.

Disorders of Calcium Metabolism

Calcium and phosphorous homeostasis depends on the function of parathyroid hormone (PTH) and vitamin D.

Parathyroid hormone is secreted by the parathyroid glands primarily for regulation of calcium. The target tissues are bone for mobilization of calcium and phosphorus and kidney for excretion of phosphorus and reabsorption of calcium.

Vitamin D is absorbed from the intestine or produced in the skin through sunlight ultraviolet photochemical conversion primarily for regulation of phosphorus. Target tissues are the intestine for absorption of calcium from the diet; bone for normal growth and mineralization via incorporation of intestinal calcium into bone matrix; and kidney for absorption of phosphorus and inverse regulation of calcium.

Disorders of calcium metabolism are caused by dysfunction of the parathyroid glands or a target organ. Hypoparathyroidism is impaired synthesis and secretion of PTH or target organ resistance to the effects of PTH (pseudohypoparathyroidism). Management is similar to that of adults (see p. 724). Hyperparathyroidism is overactivity of the parathyroid glands resulting in excess secretion of PTH. Management is similar to that of adults (see p. 722).

◆ RICKETS

Rickets is undermineralization of the cartilaginous epiphyseal growth plate and reduction in mineralization of bone (osteomalacia).

Etiology/Incidence

1. Vitamin D deficiency
   a. Nutritional deprivation/malabsorption
   b. Inadequate sun exposure

c. Anticonvulsant therapy that causes increased hepatic elimination of vitamin D
d. Renal disease
2. Hypophosphatemic rickets
   a. Primary hypophosphatemic rickets—proximal renal tubular phosphate wasting
   b. Fibrous tumors or dysplasias of bone
   c. Fanconi syndrome—complex proximal renal tubular dysfunction
3. Accumulation of acid
   a. Distal renal tubular acidosis
4. End organ resistance to vitamin D
5. Decreased synthesis of vitamin to metabolites

Altered Physiology

1. Reduced serum phosphate concentration either due to vitamin D deficiency or renal wasting
2. Results in lower than needed optimal mineralization for bone development
3. Lack of vitamin D impairs function of PTH at bone

Complications

1. Hypocalcemia
2. Secondary hyperparathyroidism
3. Hypophosphatemia

Clinical Manifestations

1. Develop osseous manifestations: proliferation of uncalcified cartilage, frontal bossing, thickening of the wrist, palpable swelling of the costochondral junction (rachitic rosary), bowing of the legs (genu varum)
2. Walking problem in toddlers
3. Latent signs of hypocalcemia if severe enough

Diagnostic Evaluation

1. Growth evaluation
2. Reduced serum phosphate concentration
3. Irregular mineralization on x-ray

Treatment

1. Primary hypophosphatemia
   a. Phosphate supplementation (Neutra-Phos, Neutra-Phos-K, or K-Phos)
   b. Active vitamin D metabolite, calcitriol (Rocaltrol)
2. Vitamin D deficiency
   a. Vitamin D or one of the metabolites with varying doses, depending on the condition

Nursing Assessment

1. Assess growth and development—important to include measurement of head circumference.

NURSING ALERT:
If child has leg bowing, standing heights may exaggerate bowing and thus decrease absolute height. Recumbent measurements may be more accurate even in the older child.

2. Determine familial history of rickets.
3. Assess for rachitic deformities, leg bowing, flaring of wrists, frontal bossing.

Nursing Diagnoses

A. Impaired Physical Mobility related to skeletal deformities
B. Noncompliance related to difficult dosage schedule for phosphorous
C. Diarrhea related to phosphorous replacement

Nursing Interventions

A. *Promoting Mobility*
1. Along with growth and developmental evaluation, assess walking ability in young child at regular intervals.
2. Encourage referral for orthopedic evaluation and bracing if bowing is severe or interferes with functional ability.
3. Stress to parents and child the importance of investing in their therapy now to prevent future leg and mobility problems. Encourage and support a child in braces.
4. Share with parents the x-ray findings of the skeletal deformities—specifically the "roughened" epiphyseal plates and the correction if present due to their therapeutic management at home.

B. *Improving Compliance*
1. Teach the physiology of bone growth and maturation with respect to phosphorous, calcium, and vitamin D to family and explain the chronicity of the condition.
2. Stress to caregivers that early growth and bone formation is critical in the young child. Constantly reinforce that treatment is prevention.

C. *Controlling Diarrhea*
1. Advise family that phosphorous replacement upsets gastrointestinal function. Stress need to give medication with food.
2. Assess frequency and consistency of stools. Assess for dehydration indicating inadequate fluid replacement.
3. Suggest alternative supplementation if diarrhea persists.

Family Education/Health Maintenance

1. Continue to stress that the focused compulsive treatment with respect to the medication replacement will prevent future skeletal problems.
2. Encourage follow-up to evaluate bone growth and proper development.
3. Advise parents that treatment is usually lifelong with close follow-up through the growth years.

Evaluation

A. Walking effectively with leg braces
B. Parents report compliance with medication
C. Loose, formed stools no more than 3 times a day

Disorders of the Adrenal Glands

The adrenal glands are responsible for the life-sustaining production of mineralocorticoids (aldosterone) for sodium retention, glucocorticoids (cortisol) for blood glucose regulation, and androgens (DHEA, androstenedione) for phallic and secondary sex characteristic development (adrenarchy).

Adrenocortical insufficiency is the inability of the adrenal gland to produce aldosterone and cortisol due to adrenal failure or lack of adrenal stimulation. With the exception of congenital adrenal hyperplasia (discussed below), pediatric adrenocortical insufficiency is similar in adults (see p. 729).

Hyperadrenalism, although rare in children, does occur, causing tissue to be exposed to excessive glucocorticoids (cortisol). This is commonly called Cushing's syndrome. Additionally, hyperfunction of the adrenal medulla in which epinephrine, norepinephrine, and other catecholamines are secreted is commonly seen in the disorder of pheochromocytoma. See pages 727 and 730 for a discussion of these conditions.

◆ CONGENITAL ADRENAL HYPERPLASIA

Congenital adrenal hyperplasia (CAH) is the most common type of adrenocortical insufficiency in children. Adrenal dysfunction is a result of an enzyme deficiency in the steroid pathway to aldosterone, cortisol, or androgen production. The most common form of the condition is life threatening and requires diagnosis and treatment soon after birth.

Etiology/Incidence (Most Common Forms)

1. Deficiency of 21-hydroxylase (90–95% of CAH cases)—insufficiency in cortisol and usually aldosterone production
2. 11-β-Hydroxylase (5–8%)—insufficiency of cortisol and aldosterone; however, precursor block to aldosterone is a potent mineralocorticoid.
3. 3-β-Hydroxysteroid dehydrogenase (5%)—insufficiency in cortisol, aldosterone, and androgen production

Altered Physiology

1. Production of adrenal mineralocorticoids and glucocorticoids is blocked by an enzyme deficiency in the steroid pathway. "Blocks" may be severe or partial. Due to lack of feedback suppression, ACTH and renin are secreted to stimulate adrenal gland production causing hyperplasia of the gland.

2. Aldosterone insufficiency
  a. Diminished production results in fluid and electrolyte imbalance. Loss of sodium at the kidney results in loss of fluid and an increase in serum potassium (cation exchange).
  b. Depletion of extracellular fluid leads to decreased blood pressure.
  c. Low blood pressure stimulates renin in the kidney to activate the adrenal aldosterone pathway.
3. Cortisol insufficiency—diminished hepatic gluconeogenesis and tissue glucose uptake
  a. Diminished production/secretion results in low blood sugar levels—more pronounced in times of stress
  b. Low blood sugar, stress, or low cortisol stimulates feedback to hypothalamic-pituitary axis to release ACTH to stimulate adrenal activity, which also stimulates the release of melanocyte-stimulating hormone (MSH).
  c. Constant ACTH stimulation of gland causes overproduction and "backup" of blocked steroid pathways resulting in "spillover" production of adrenal androgens.
4. Depending on etiology, overproduction of androgens will virilize female external genitalia or underproduction of androgens will block virilization of male external genitalia.

Complications

1. Aldosterone insufficiency
  a. Hyponatremia, hyperkalemia
  b. Hypotension
  c. Shock
  d. Hypertension in 11-β-hydroxylase where aldosterone precursor is potent mineralocorticoid
2. Cortisol insufficiency
  a. Hypoglycemia

Clinical Manifestations

1. Ambiguous female genitalia—varying degrees of virilization due to exposure of androgens during development in utero
  a. Clitoromegaly (may be penile shaped)
  b. Labial fusion (partial or complete)
  c. Rugated labia appearing scrotal
  d. Vagina may be incomplete ending in blind pouch.
2. Ambiguous male genitalia (3-β-dehydrogenase)—incomplete virilization development of external genitalia
  a. Small phallic development
  b. Incomplete scrotal fusion
3. Hyperpigmentation (due to MSH secretion)
4. Dehydration
5. Vomiting/poor feeding
6. Shock
7. Latent signs—basal cortisol levels are normal due to compensated chronic ACTH stimulation.
  a. Weakness, fatigue
  b. Anorexia, nausea, diarrhea
  c. Weight loss (failure to thrive)
  d. Hyperpigmentation—no bathing suit lines
  e. Hypotension/postural dizziness

f. Rapid growth rate—adrenal androgen effect
g. Premature adrenarche—pubic hair, axillary hair, acne, body odor

Diagnostic Evaluation

A. Newborns
1. Pelvic ultrasound for identification of uterus, ovaries, or testes to determine true sex (internal development of gender-specific organs depends on presence or absence of Y chromosomal activity—the outer genital development depends on the presence or absence of androgens).
2. Karyotype
3. Serum electrolytes—sodium depletion
4. Serum glucose levels—hypoglycemia
5. Serum 17-hydroxyprogesterone (most common precursor to 21-hydroxylase)—elevated

B. Latent Diagnosis
1. Rapid growth velocity, premature adrenarche
2. Advanced bone age x-ray for chronologic age
3. Elevated serum 17-hydroxyprogesterone
4. Elevated plasma renin activity—compensated prevention of salt loss

Treatment

1. Glucocorticoid replacement—physiologic production of cortisol is 15 to 20 mg/m² per day. Doses are individually dependent. Replacement is with hydrocortisone (Cortef) twice or three times a day; or prednisone (Orasone) once daily when final growth has been achieved.
2. Mineralocorticoid replacement—aldosterone is replaced with fludrocortisone (Florinef) tablets at 0.05 to 0.20 mg daily
3. Added salt to the diet of newborns if salt loss is severe
4. Surgical correction of ambiguous genitalia—can require multiple corrections over time

Nursing Assessment

A. Newborns
1. Assess genitalia for ambiguity.

NURSING ALERT:
In male-appearing genitals, at least one testis must be palpated; if not, assumption must be that child is female with severe virilization. Notify health care provider so diagnostic evaluation can be initiated.

2. Assess for signs of hypoglycemia, hyponatremia, and hyperkalemia (Table 47-2)
3. Assess feeding pattern of newborn
4. Look for hyperpigmentation—may be subjective

B. Latent Diagnosis or Child on Treatment
1. Assess growth and development.
2. Monitor vital signs—include sitting and recumbent blood pressure for orthostatic changes.
3. Assess skin for hyperpigmentation.

TABLE 47-2 Manifestations of Hyponatremia and Hyperkalemia

Hyponatremia	Hyperkalemia
Caused by dilution of Na when water intake exceeds output. Signs and symptoms occur when Na level falls below 120 mEq/L.	Caused by a shift of K out of cells to compensate for decreased Na caused by an oliguric state. Usually asymptomatic except for ECG changes.
Gradual fall: anorexia, apathy, mild nausea and vomiting	ECG characteristics: (progressive) shortened QT interval tall, peaked T waves, ventricular arrhythmias, degeneration of QRS complex, ventricular asystole or fibrillation
Rapid fall: headache, mental confusion, muscular irritability, delerium, convulsions	

4. Obtain history to include level of activity/fatigue, dietary history, salt craving, behavior, and school performance.

Nursing Diagnoses

A. Fatigue related to hypoglycemia and electrolytic imbalances
B. Risk for Fluid Volume Deficit related to aldosterone deficiency
C. Risk for Injury related to stress and deficiency of corticosteroids
D. Anxiety of Parent related to gender, sexual ambiguity, and chronic illness

Nursing Interventions

A. Minimizing Fatigue
1. Administer glucocorticoids and emphasize compliance to increase energy level.
2. Encourage frequent rest periods and prevent overactivity.
3. Assess activity tolerance to determine adequacy of replacement therapy.

B. Maintaining Fluid Balance
1. Assess for fluid status and review history of fluid intake and output for appropriate volumes. Assess hydration status of child.
2. If vomiting and unable to take oral fluids and mineralocorticoids, administer IV fluids. Start with D₅NS and monitor serum sodium level.

NURSING ALERT:
No less than 0.5% NS should be infused in the child who is aldosterone deficient due to the inability to retain mineralocorticoid replacement.

3. Emphasize compliance with mineralocorticoid replacement.

C. *Preventing Acute Adrenocortical Insufficiency*
1. Identify times of stress such as acute infections, surgical procedures, or extreme emotional stress that require increased corticosteroid replacement.
2. Teach the parents how to use and give intramuscular injection of hydrocortisone (Solucortef) for stress management when oral supplementation is not possible due to vomiting.
3. Ensure that child is evaluated by the primary care provider and treated for the cause of stress.

D. *Reducing Anxiety*
1. Encourage parents to verbalize feelings regarding diagnosis, gender decisions or changes, and treatment plans.
2. Describe to the parents that the ambiguity is a result of the development process just not being completed rather than being a "mistake."

Family Education/Health Maintenance

1. Stress and reinforce the function and need for constant replacement of adrenal steroid therapy to maintain normal daily activities.
2. Encourage parents to obtain a Medic Alert bracelet, which indicates steroid dependency, for the child.

Evaluation

A. Parents report child is more active.
B. No signs of dehydration
C. Mother demonstrates correct technique for hydrocortisone injection.
D. Parents verbalize understanding of disorder and need for reconstructive surgery.

Disorders of Gonadal Function

Proper gonadal function is necessary for developing sexual maturation (puberty). The process involves the hypothalamic release of gonadotropin-releasing hormone (GnRH), which in turn stimulates the pituitary to release LH and FSH. In turn, these stimulate the gonads to produce and release the gonadal steroids of testosterone from the testes in males or estrogen from the ovaries in females. The actions of these steroids lead to the development of secondary sexual characteristics and maturation.

◆ DELAYED SEXUAL DEVELOPMENT

Delayed sexual development is the lack of pubertal development or progression.

Etiology/Incidence

A. *Primary* Absence or dysfunction of the gonads

1. 45 XO Turner syndrome (chromosomal variants)
   a. Occurs in 1 of 2,000 girls

2. Sporadic gonadal dysgenesis
3. Bilateral gonadal failure
   a. Radiation
   b. Chemotherapy
   c. Infection
   d. Defect in gonadal steroid synthesis
   e. Trauma

B. *Secondary* Lack of hypothalamic-pituitary stimulation to gonads

1. Hypothalamic lesions due to infections, trauma, irradiation or isolated deficiency of GnRH (Kallmann's syndrome)
2. Pituitary lesions—lesions due to infection, trauma, or irradiation; also hypopituitarism or isolated LH and FSH deficiencies

C. *Other Causes*
1. Chronic illness
2. Anorexia nervosa
3. Autoimmune atrophy
4. End organ lack of receptors—androgen insensitivity.

Altered Physiology

1. Lack of production or secretion of gonadal steroids from the testes (testosterone) or ovaries (estrogen) either due to the lack of pituitary stimulation or gonad dysfunction
2. Failure of end organs to respond to circulating gonadal steroid
3. Resultant effect is failure to achieve sexual maturity.

Complications

1. Sterility
2. Ambiguity—in androgen insensitivity, male genital development does not respond to circulating level of testosterone from testes—may result in mistaken gender assignment.
3. Potential for dysfunctional dormant gonad to become malignant

Clinical Manifestations

1. Females—lack of breast development by age 13 to 13.5 years or failure to progress through puberty
2. Males—lack of testicular enlargement by age 13.5 to 14 years or failure to progress through puberty
3. Emotional lability

Diagnostic Evaluation

1. Bone age x-ray to determine physical age—pubertal delay is not consistent with bone age
2. Laboratory measurement of sex steroids (testosterone and estrogen) and gonadotropins (LH, FSH)
   a. Gonadal failure will show elevated LH and FSH with low estrogen.
   b. No good test is available to distinguish isolated gonadotropin deficiency (LH or FSH).

c. End organ insensitivity (lack of gonadal steroid receptor)—both sex steroid and gonadotropins will be elevated. Hypothalamic receptors for feedback inhibition are the same as the end organ receptors, therefore no hypothalamic "shut-off."

4. Abdominal ultrasound to view internal organ structure and development

Treatment

1. Replacement of gonadal steroid—should be as close to the physiologic level as possible; however, maximal adult height may become compromised due to potential side effect of acceleration of skeletal maturation.
   a. Boys—testosterone enanthate (Testone LA); 50 to 100 mg monthly by injection until final height is achieved, then 200 mg monthly
   b. Girls—conjugated estrogen (Premarin); 0.3 to 0.625 mg daily by oral tablet. When appropriate, a progestational agent is added to the therapy for normal periods to occur.
2. There is no pituitary or hypothalamic agent for use in secondary gonadal failure.

Nursing Assessment

1. Assess growth and development, particularly height and sexual development at regular intervals.

Nursing Diagnoses

A. Altered Growth and Development related to lack of sexual development
B. Body Image Disturbance related to delayed sexual maturation
C. Self-Esteem Disturbance related to delayed sexual maturation

Nursing Interventions

A. *Promoting Sexual Development*
1. Administer or teach self-administration of medication as prescribed.
2. Teach technique for intramuscular injections of testosterone enanthate (Testone LA). Watch return demonstration.
3. Stress compliance with prescribed dose and not to exceed recommended dose. Excessive use of testosterone will stunt potential statural growth.

B. *Improving Body Image*
1. Discuss strategies for improving appearance through hair style, clothing, makeup, and minimizing delay in sex characteristics.
2. Stress the importance of cautious therapy to prevent loss of potential height, therefore making sexual development a slow process.

C. *Improving Self-Esteem*
1. Encourage child to discuss self-concept; list positive and negative characteristics.

2. Explore ways to strengthen and add to positive characteristics.
3. Encourage participation in age-appropriate activities and social functions.

Family Education/Health Maintenance

1. Teach the patient about side effects of testosterone replacement—possible behavioral changes (aggressiveness, moodiness) and an increase in acne.
   a. Suggest over-the-counter acne products or referral to dermatologist if indicated.
   b. Alert family to report behavioral changes to the health care provider.
2. Teach the patient taking estrogen replacement the importance of daily compliance. Missed doses could result in break-through bleeding/spotting due to drop in circulatory estrogen levels.
   a. Alert patient to notify health care provider if spotting does occur with estrogen replacement.
3. In both treatments, stress to child not to exceed prescribed dose to prevent loss of final adult height.

Evaluation

A. Increase in height, progression of sexual development
B. Child verbalizing improved feelings of body image
C. Lists more positive concepts of self

◆ ADVANCED SEXUAL DEVELOPMENT/PRECOCIOUS PUBERTY

Advanced sexual development is secondary sexual development earlier than the normal timing for a child's maturation.

Etiology/Incidence

A. *Central Precocious Puberty (CPP)*
1. Early activation of the hypothalamic-pituitary gonadotropin axis
2. May be idiopathic or caused by:
   a. Tumors of hypothalamus/pituitary
   b. Cranial irradiation
   c. Trauma
   d. Infection—meningitis
   e. Hydrocephalus
3. Most common form of precocious puberty

B. *Peripheral Precocious Puberty (PPP)*
1. Sex hormone production at the glandular level independent of central stimulation
2. Ovarian PPP caused by estrogen-producing tumors or cysts
3. Testicular PPP caused by androgen- and estrogen-producing tumors or autonomous production of testosterone
4. Adrenal PPP caused by enzyme defects (CAH) or androgen- and estrogen-producing tumors

C. *Other Causes*
1. Hypothyroidism
2. Exogenous estrogen or androgen exposure

Altered Physiology

1. Abnormal early production and secretion of the gonadal steroids or adrenal androgens
2. Normal pubertal development abnormally early
3. Skeletal maturation is advanced under presence of sex steroids and adrenal androgens

Complications

1. Complications of underlying tumor
2. Behavioral problems
3. Short stature for final height due to early epiphyseal closure

Clinical Manifestations

1. Boys
   a. Testicular enlargement (4 mL): under age 8.5 years
   b. Tanner stage II pubic hair: under age 9.0 years
   c. Tanner stage III pubic hair: under age 10.0 years
2. Girls
   a. Breast bud (stage II): under age 8.0 years
   b. Tanner stage III pubic hair: under age 8.5 years
   c. Menarche: under age 9.5 years
3. In both sexes, rapid growth (increased growth velocity) is evident.

Diagnostic Evaluation

1. Physical assessment: Tanner staging
   a. If adrenarche is present without thelarche (breast development) or testicular enlargement, adrenal cause is likely.
   b. In girls, if thelarche is only present, ovarian or exogenous estrogen involvement likely.
   c. If both adrenarche and pubarche (gonadal signs) are present, central cause is likely.
2. Skeletal x-ray for bone age—usually advanced. Pubertal stage development is often commensurate with bone age maturation.
3. Laboratory analysis:
   a. Gonadal steroids—may be elevated; however, secretion is diurnal early in development.
   b. Elevated gonadotropins to GnRH (Factrel) stimulation if CPP. Basal levels are frequently unreliable. Lack of elevation of gonadotropins may indicate peripheral source.
   c. Thyroid function to rule out hypothyroidism
4. MRI and CT of head to rule out central etiology
5. Ultrasound of abdomen, pelvis, testes for presence of cysts or tumors

Treatment

(For CPP, most common form of advanced sexual development in children)

1. Inhibit puberty to preserve psychosocial well-being and to delay epiphyseal closure to maximize adult height.
   a. GnRH agonist—downregulates GnRH receptors of the pituitary against endogenous GnRH
      (1) Nafarelin (Synarel)—intranasal spray, twice daily
      (2) Leuprolide (Lupron)—daily subcutaneous injection
      (3) Depot-leuprolide (Lupron Depot, Lupron Depot-Ped)—monthly intramuscular injection
      (4) Histrelin (Supprelin)—subcutaneous daily injection
   b. Progestins
      (1) Medroxyprogesterone injections (Depo-Provera)—biweekly intramuscular injections
      (2) Medroxyprogesterone tablets (Cycrin)—oral daily dosing

Nursing Assessment

1. Assess sexual development using Tanner scale.
2. Obtain history of when signs and symptoms began with specific attention to chronology of events.
3. Perform psychosocial assessment relative to peer relations.
4. While child is on treatment, perform ongoing assessment of height and sexual characteristics.

Nursing Diagnoses

A. Body Image Disturbance related to early presence of secondary sexual characteristics
B. Fear related to knowledge deficit regarding maturing body and sexuality
C. Personal Identity Disturbance due to societal height expectations versus appropriate age-related expectations

Nursing Interventions

A. *Fostering Positive Body Image*
1. Encourage the child to verbalize concerns regarding body development changes.
2. Stress to child that the changes are normal events that peers will go through; however, they are occurring abnormally early.
3. Teach the child that therapy will halt the process and soon peers will catch up.

B. *Reducing Fear*
1. Teach and encourage the parents to teach the child about sexual development to reduce fear of the unknown.
2. Encourage proper hygiene practices for body odor, hair growth, and menses.
3. Teach administration techniques for medication treatment, including intranasal, intramuscular, or subcutaneous administration as indicated.
4. In GnRH agonist treatment in girls, instruct child and parents that it takes 10 to 12 days to fully downregulate the pituitary receptors. The suppression results in a fall of estrogen and thus may cause breakthrough bleeding or even a period to occur. This will only happen once if child remains suppressed on therapy.

C. *Promoting Sense of Identity*
1. Encourage the child and parents to discuss normal age-related behaviors and identify inappropriate behaviors that are associated with society's expectations of advanced height and development.
2. Encourage the child to wear age-appropriate clothing, participate in age-appropriate activities, and socialize with peers.
3. Suggest counseling as needed.

Family Education/Health Maintenance

1. Encourage follow-up at regular intervals while on treatment, and if condition is not treated, to monitor progress and address behavioral issues.

Evaluation

A. Child accepting body changes
B. Adequate return demonstration of intramuscular injection; verbalizes understanding of sexual development
C. Participating in school activities and socializing with peers

Disorder of the Pancreas

The pancreas manufactures powerful enzymes for digestion as well as the hormones insulin and glucagon. These hormones are manufactured and secreted from cell clusters called the islets of Langerhans. Both glucagon and insulin regulate the amount of sugar that is present in the bloodstream. Glucagon is a potent conterregulatory hormone that raises the blood sugar by fostering the release of glucose from stores in the liver. Insulin stimulates glucose uptake by peripheral tissues, inhibits lipolysis, and inhibits hepatic glucose production.

◆ DIABETES MELLITUS

Diabetes mellitus is a disorder of glucose intolerance caused by a deficiency in insulin production and action resulting in hyperglycemia, and abnormal carbohydrate, protein, and fat metabolism.

Etiology/Incidence

1. In pediatrics, over 98% of the cases are type I or insulin-dependent diabetes mellitus (IDDM).
2. Annual incidence is 15/100,00 under age 20
3. Etiology suggests genetic and environmental or acquired factors, association with certain HLA types, and abnormal immune responses, including autoimmune reactions.

Altered Physiology

Same as for adults (see p. 743).

Complications

A. *Acute*   Usually reversible

1. Diabetic ketoacidosis (DKA) accounts for 70% of diabetes-related deaths in children less than 10 years of age.
2. Cerebral edema—related to treatment correction. Thought to be due to a rapid decline in blood glucose causing a fluid shift.
3. Hyperglycemia (untreated or undertreated)
4. Hypoglycemia (insulin reaction)

B. *Subacute*   Develops over short period of time

1. Lipohypertrophy—repeated injections in the same area—can cause abnormal absorption
2. Skeletal and joint abnormalities—limited joint mobility
3. Growth failure and delayed sexual maturation due to underinsulinization

C. *Chronic*   Very rarely seen in children

1. Retinopathy—cataracts/blindness
2. Neuropathy—impaired nerve conduction
3. Nephropathy—proteinuria/renal failure
4. Cardiopathy—congestive cardiac failure

Clinical Manifestations

1. Rapid onset (usually over a period of a few weeks)
2. Major symptoms
   a. Increased thirst
   b. Increased urination, enuresis
   c. Increased food ingestion
   d. Weight loss
   e. Fatigue
3. Minor symptoms
   a. Skin infections
   b. Dry skin, poor wound healing
   c. Monilial vaginitis in adolescent girls
4. DKA
   a. Precomatose state
      (1) Drowsiness
      (2) Dryness of skin
      (3) Cherry red lips
      (4) Increased respirations
      (5) Nausea
      (6) Vomiting
      (7) Abdominal pain
   b. Comatose state
      (1) Extreme hyperpnea (Kussmaul breathing)
      (2) Acetone breath
      (3) Soft, sunken eyeballs
      (4) Rigid abdomen
      (5) Rapid, weak pulse
      (6) Decreased temperature
      (7) Decreased blood pressure
   c. Circulatory collapse and renal failure may follow, resulting from the combination of lowered pH, electrolyte deficiency, and dehydration.

Diagnostic Evaluation

1. Presence of symptoms
2. Glycosuria on routine examination
3. Random blood glucose higher than 200 mg/dL
4. Ketonuria
5. Metabolic acidosis (pH less than 7.3 and bicarbonate less than 14 mEq/L)

Treatment

1. Fluid therapy in DKA—treat dehydration, increase peripheral perfusion, and replace sodium and potassium loss due to osmotic diuresis
2. Insulin therapy—to reduce hyperglycemia, inhibit lipolysis and ketogenesis (Table 47-3)
   a. Subcutaneous insulin may be given twice a day at a dose usually of a 2:1 ratio of NPH to regular, and a 2:1 ratio for morning to evening dose.
   b. Dosage needs are based on the child's size, diet, and level of activity. Dosages are adjusted through daily monitoring of blood glucose levels.
   c. DKA treatment—low dose continuous IV infusion of regular insulin only (Box 47-1)

Nursing Assessment

1. Prediagnosis/treatment
   a. Obtain history of onset of signs and symptoms of clinical manifestations.
   b. Assess for levels of dehydration and weight loss with level of appetite.
   c. Check for sores that are slow to heal.
   d. Identify any fruity smell to breath—acetone breath due to ketosis.
   e. Assess abdominal pain—may mimic appendicitis.
2. Initial diagnosis/treatment (DKA)
   a. Assess for potential cerebral edema (diminished level of consciousness) when fluid replacement is initiated.
   b. Assess cardiac function—tachycardia with dehydration, arrhythmias related to potassium imbalances.
   c. Assess renal function—urinary output with intake and output, ketonuria, glucosuria.
   d. Watch for hypoglycemia—overtreatment of insulin—glucose level correction should be slow. IV replacements frequently contain glucose to prevent large osmotic fluid shifts leading to cerebral edema.
3. On treatment/routine follow-up

TABLE 47-3 Types of Insulin and Their Effects

Type of Insulin	Onset (hours)	Maximal Activity (hours)	Duration (hours)
Regular	$1/2$–1	2–4	6–8
Semi-Lente	$1/2$–1	2–4	10–12
NPH	2	4–12	24
Lente	2	8–10	24
Ultralente	4–8	14–20	36

BOX 47-1 *Treatment of Diabetic Ketoacidosis*

A. Initiate IV Fluids
1. Start with 0.9% NS.
2. Estimate fluid deficit by amount of weight loss (1 kg [2.2 lb] equals 1 liter fluid).
3. Infuse fluids to replace one-half of estimated loss plus maintenance needs (10–20 mL/kg) over first 8–12 h; second half plus maintenance needs over next 16–36 h.

NURSING ALERT:
Avoid infusion of hypotonic solutions and replace fluids slowly to prevent rapid decline in serum osmolarity, which may precipitate cerebral edema.

4. When blood glucose falls below 250 mg/dL, change to 5% glucose in 0.9 or 0.45% NS.
5. Closely monitor vital signs, ECG, and intake and output, and obtain laboratory values including urine and blood glucose, electrolytes, BUN and creatinine, serum osmolarity, arterial or venous pH, serum and urine ketones, calcium and phosphorous 1–4 h as condition warrants.

B. Administer Insulin
1. Give IV bolus of 0.1 unit/kg of regular insulin if no intermediate-acting insulin has been given in the last 6–8 h.
2. Provide continuous IV drip of regular insulin at rate of 0.1 unit/kg/h.

NURSING ALERT:
Flush IV tubing with insulin solution before infusion because insulin will bind to the plastic tubing.

3. Continue IV insulin until metabolic acidosis is corrected (pH greater than 7.3 and bicarbonate greater than 13–15) and bowel sounds have returned and can take oral fluids.
4. When meals are tolerated, begin subcutaneous regular insulin dose of 0.25–1 unit/kg divided in four doses, before meals and at bedtime.
5. When stabilized, return to previous insulin regimen or determine twice daily dosing of NPH and regular insulin.

C. Potassium and Bicarbonate Replacement
1. Initial serum K levels will be normal or high even though intracellular levels are low. Serum levels will fall as insulin therapy drives K into the cells.
2. Begin replacement of K when urine output and renal function have been established.
3. Add KCl 30–40 mEq to each liter of fluid.
4. Monitor T waves on ECG for peaking (hyperkalemia) or flattening (hypokalemia).
5. Bicarbonate administration is controversial in correcting acidosis but may be indicated for respiratory depression, decreased myocardial contractility, or refractory, severe acidosis.

Adapted from: Wheeler, M.D. (1991). Care of the child in diabetic ketoacidosis. In: *Proceedings of the 7th Annual Conference on Pediatric Critical Care Nursing* (pp. 210–216). Danville, CA: Contemporary Forums.

a. Assess growth parameters—excessive weight gain may indicate overtreatment of insulin (child eats due to constant hunger). Loss or lack of weight gain may indicate underinsulinization (losing calories that are not metabolized).

b. Review blood glucose diaries for level of control and need for insulin adjustments (check for appropriate adjustments of insulin made by parents).

c. Obtain history of any hypoglycemic reactions—be specific to time of day, dietary record, and exercise/activity.

d. Assess injection sites—look for signs of lipohypertrophy (localized tissue build-up from giving injections in the same site).

e. Assess for signs of hyperglycemia—polyuria, polydipsia. Does child need to get up in the night to go to the bathroom?

Nursing Diagnoses

A. Fluid Volume Deficit related to osmotic diuresis and vomiting

B. Altered Nutrition (Less than Body Requirements) due to metabolic catabolism due to lack of insulin

C. Knowledge Deficit related to insulin management

D. Knowledge Deficit related to blood glucose monitoring

E. Risk for Injury related to hypoglycemia

F. Fear/Anxiety of Child and Family related to diagnosis, treatment, and management procedures

Nursing Interventions

A. *Restoring Fluid Balance*
1. Administer IV fluids as ordered.
2. Monitor intake and output, blood pressure, serum electrolyte results, and daily weights.

B. *Meeting Nutritional Requirements*
1. Provide an adequate diet for the child and teach the family about the diet.
   a. Most prescribed diets are of the unmeasured type. The diet plan eliminates concentrated sweets and follows recommended allowances from all of the four basic food groups, but otherwise does not require measuring or rigidity.
   b. Occasionally a more rigid, strictly controlled diet is necessary.
   c. The diet should be composed of approximately 55% carbohydrate, 30% fat, and 15% protein.
      (1) Most diets are restricted in carbohydrates, saturated fats, and cholesterol, and may be based on the exchange method as recommended by the American Diabetes Association.
      (2) Approximately 70% of the carbohydrate content should be derived from complex carbohydrates such as starch.
      (3) Foods with high fiber content should be encouraged.
      (4) All diets must supply sufficient caloric intake for activity and growth, sufficient protein for growth, and the required vitamins and minerals.
   d. Foods are distributed throughout the day to accommodate varying peak action of insulin. Distribution may be adjusted for increased or decreased amounts of exercise.

2. Determine the child's usual dietary habits so that adherence to the controlled diet will be easier.
3. Include the child and parents in meal planning as soon as possible.
4. Allow the child normal activity while hospitalized so that the observed result of the dietary control will be valid. Because the child's activity level usually decreases during the hospital stay, the child and family must understand that the insulin and dietary needs will alter on discharge.
5. Allow the child to eat with other children.
6. Make certain that the child adheres to the prescribed diet and understands the rationale for this.
7. Refer family to a dietitian for additional planning and education.

C. *Increasing Knowledge About Insulin Administration*
1. Insulin should be given one-half hour before breakfast. If split-dose insulin is prescribed, it should be given one-half hour before breakfast and one-half hour before the evening meal.
2. Be aware of the major types of insulin and their effects.
3. Develop a systematic plan for injections that emphasizes rotation of sites (Fig. 47-1).
   a. The upper arms and thighs are the most acceptable sites for injection in children, but the outer areas of the abdomen or hips may also be used.
   b. Subsequent injections are given about 2.5 cm (1 inch) apart.
   c. Guidelines for site location:
      (1) Arms—begin below the deltoid muscle and end one hand breadth above the elbow. Begin at the midline and progress outward laterally using the external surface only.
      (2) Thighs—begin one hand breadth below the hip and end one hand breadth above the knee. Begin at the midline and progress outward laterally, using only the outer, anterior surface.
      (3) Abdomen—avoid the beltline and 1 inch around the umbilicus.
      (4) Buttocks—use the upper outer quadrant of the buttocks.
4. Be certain that the measuring scale of the syringe matches the unit strength on the bottle of insulin.
   a. Insulin is available in strengths of 40, 80, and 100 units/mL.
   b. U-100 insulin is preferred because it allows the smallest possible amount to be given.
5. Use insulin that is at room temperature.
   a. The bottle in use may be kept at room temperature without losing appreciable strength.
   b. Extra bottles should be stored in the refrigerator.
6. Mix the solution by rotating the vial between the hands. Do not shake vigorously.
7. Administer insulin subcutaneously.
8. Observe the skin closely for signs of irritation. Avoid the injection site for several weeks if signs of local irritation are observed.
9. Observe the skin for a rash indicating an allergic reaction to the insulin. Notify the health care provider immediately if there is an allergic reaction.
10. Be aware of factors that vary the need for and utilization of insulin, particularly exercise and infection.
    a. Exercise
       (1) Tends to lower the blood sugar level.
       (2) Encourage normal activity, regulated in amount and time.
    b. Infection or illness

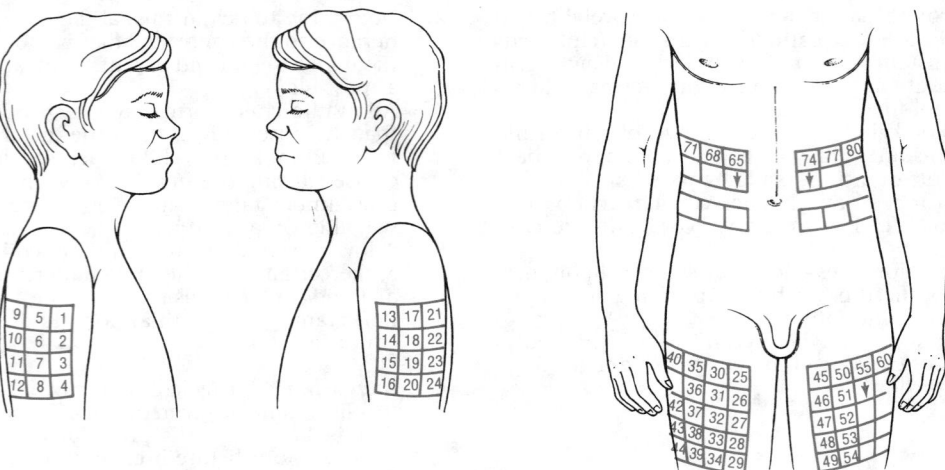

FIGURE 47-1   *Rotating injection sites for insulin in the pediatric patient.*

(1) Increases the child's insulin requirement (insulin still administered during illness)
(2) Be alert for signs of infection and dehydration.
11. Encourage the child to express feelings about the injections. The child may be helped to master fear of injections by gaining control of the situation through play and active participation in the procedure.

D. *Providing Information About Blood Glucose Monitoring*
1. Teach child and parents the chosen method for blood glucose monitoring.
2. The procedure requires a drop of blood, obtained by finger stick, a reagent strip, and a reflectance meter.
3. Specific instructions for performing the procedure vary with the equipment being used and must be followed explicitly.
4. Blood glucose measurements are usually made four times a day, before meals and at bedtime.
5. Additional blood tests are helpful during episodes of hypoglycemic symptoms or other problem situations.
6. Urine tests for ketones should be continued if the child is ill or if blood glucose level is greater than 240 mg/ 100 mL.
7. Record the results of blood glucose testing accurately.
   a. Use a standard form for recording so that the information will be clear and readily available.
   b. Help the child to understand how the disease is controlled by teaching the child to test his or her own blood, record results, and report information to health care personnel or parents.

E. *Identifying and Controlling Hypoglycemia*
1. Have glucagon available for injection if hypoglycemic reaction occurs. Administer 0.5 to 1 mg intramuscularly or subcutaneously and assess response.
2. Teach family the causes, signs and symptoms, and treatment for hypoglycemia.
   a. Common causes
      (1) Overdose of insulin
      (2) Reduction in diet or increased exercise without sufficient caloric coverage
   b. Symptoms
      (1) Trembling

(2) Shaking
(3) Sweating
(4) Apprehension
(5) Tachycardia
(6) Hunger
(7) Drowsiness
(8) Odd behavior
(9) Mental confusion
(10) Seizures
(11) Coma
   c. Be prepared to give orange juice or other food containing readily available simple sugars.

COMMUNITY-BASED CARE TIP
Suggest a simple, convenient source of sugar that can be easily carried by the child or parents in a pocket, purse, or backpack to have available for hypoglycemic symptoms. A good example is cake decorating gel that comes is a tube, such as Cake Mate.

3. Watch for a pattern of activity or time of day that precedes hypoglycemic reactions and work with family to alter behavior to prevent reactions.
4. If prescribed, teach the child and family how to use an emergency glucagon injection kit.

F. *Reducing Fear and Anxiety*
1. Explain the need and purpose of every test to child and parent. Allow child to vent feelings and cry if fearful. When appropriate, demonstrate procedures on yourself first (eg, finger sticks for glucose testing, allowing parent to give saline injection for practice of insulin injection).
2. Teach family the pathophysiology of diabetes. Understanding the disease process aids in understanding the treatment, signs, and symptoms. Assess knowledge level of teaching by having family verbalize knowledge of disease management.
3. Allow parent to verbalize feelings related to the expectations of their performance. Stress that the learning is through the actual "hands-on" management. Assist the parent in performing the needed tasks (finger sticks, insulin injections) to build their confidence.

Give the parent clear objectives and directions for home management.

4. Stress that the child's condition is now the family's condition as well. Only the foods appropriate for the child should be in the home.

5. Caution the parents that the focus on the child may cause sibling rivalry. Encourage involvement by all family members in making the home a healthy one and urge the parents to give individual attention to the nondiabetic children as well.

6. Explain to child that he or she did not cause the disease to occur—young children often blame themselves for "bad" things that happen to them. Help the child understand that good management is the key to participating in all usual activities. The perspective should be that he or she is a "child with diabetes," not a "diabetic child."

Health Education/Health Maintenance

Patient or parental education is one of the most important aspects in the nursing care of the child with diabetes. Thorough instruction is essential in the following areas:

1. Influence of exercise, emotional stress, and other illnesses on both insulin and diet needs
2. Recognition of the symptoms of insulin shock and diabetic acidosis and knowledge of related emergency management
3. Prevention of infection
   a. Attend to regular body hygiene with special attention to foot care.
   b. Report any breaks in the skin. Treat them promptly.
   c. Use only properly fitted shoes; do not wear vinyl or plastic, which do not permit ventilation. Avoid calluses and blisters.
   d. Dress the child appropriately for the weather.
   e. See that the child receives regular dental checkups and maintenance every 6 months.

f. Follow routine immunizations according to the recommended schedule.

4. Precautionary measures
   a. Have the child cary an identifying card that states the he or she has diabetes and includes name, address, telephone number, and health care provider's name and telephone number.
   b. See that the child has orange juice, a lump of sugar, or a bar of candy available in case of an insulin reaction.
   c. Have the family discuss the child's disease with the school nurse and with other responsible adults who are in close contact with the child (teachers, Scout leaders, etc).
   d. Advise parents that vials of insulin should be kept on one's person when traveling because baggage may be subjected to extreme temperatures and pressures incompatible with the stability of insulin. If necessary, a thermos can be used to keep the insulin at the appropriate temperature.

5. For additional information and support, refer to agencies such as: American Diabetes Association; 1660 Duke Street; Alexandria, VA 22314; 1-800-232-3472; and Juvenile Diabetes Foundation; 120 Wall Street, 19th floor; New York, NY 10005; 1-800-JDF-CURE.

Evaluation

A. Intake equals output, blood pressure stable, sodium and potassium within normal limits
B. Parents and child describe balanced low concentrated carbohydrate diet.
C. Child and parents demonstrate correct insulin administration technique.
D. Child and parents demonstrate correct glucose monitoring technique.
E. Child and parents verbalize causes, signs and symptoms, and treatment for hypoglycemia.
F. Child and parents speak openly about diabetes, ask appropriate questions, display no crying.

Selected References

Aarskog, D. (1991). Rickets and growth. Growth—Genetics & Hormones, 7(4), 1-3.

August, G. P. (1993). Hypogonadism and cryptorchidism. In: A current review of pediatric endocrinology—April 28–May 2, 1993 (pp. 57-64). Norwell, MA: Serono Symposia, USA.

Cappy, M. S., Blizzard, R. M., Migeon, C. J. (Eds.). (1994). Wilkins—The diagnosis and treatment of endocrine disorders in childhood and adolescence (4th ed.). Springfield, IL: Charles C. Thomas.

Carpenter, T. O. (1993). Vitamin D metabolism and phosphate homeostasis: Physiology and clinical application. In: A current review of pediatric endocrinology—April 28–May 2, 1993 (pp. 213 -222). Norwell, MA: Serono Symposia, USA.

Chrousos, G. P. (1993). Adrenal insufficiency. In: A current review of

pediatric endocrinology—April 28–May 2, 1993 (pp. 73-84). Norwell, MA: Serono Symposia, USA.

Clemons, R. D., Kappy, M. S., Stuart, T. E., Perelman, A. H., & Hoekstra, F. T. (1992). Long-term effectiveness of depot gonadotropin-releasing hormone analogue in the treatment of children with central precocious puberty. American Journal of Diseases of Children, 147, 653-657.

Howie, J. (1991). Congenital adrenal hyperplasia. In: The Fourth Annual Conference of the Pediatric Endocrinology Nursing Society (pp. 9-14). Norwell, MA: Serono Symposia, USA.

Jackson, D. B., & Saunders, R. B. (Eds.) (1993). Child health nursing—A comprehensive approach to the care of children and their families. Philadelphia: J. B. Lippincott.

Kaplan, S. L. (Ed.) (1990). Clinical pediatric and adolescent

endocrinology. Philadelphia: W. B. Saunders.

Lawson Wilkins Pediatric Endocrine Society (1995). A current review of pediatric endocrinology. Norwell, MA: Serano Symposia USA, Inc.

Moore, W. V. (1993). Disorders of growth hormone secretion and action. In: A current review of pediatric endocrinology—April 28–May 2, 1993 (pp. 9-14). Norwell, MA: Serono Symposia, USA.

Rosenfeld, R. L. (1993). Precocious puberty. In: A current review of pediatric endocrinology—April 28–May 2, 1993 (pp. 51-56). Norwell, MA: Serono Symposia, USA.

Strowig, S. (1995). Insulin therapy. RN, 58(6), 30-36.

Wheeler, M. D. (1991). Care of the child in diabetic ketoacidosis. In: Proceedings of the 7th Annual Conference on Pediatric Critical Care Nursing. Danville, CA: Contemporary Forums.

CHAPTER 48

Pediatric Oncology

Introduction to Pediatric Oncology

Cancer is the second leading cause of death from disease in children from 1 to 14 years of age. It affects approximately 14/100,000 children annually in the United States. The incidence of specific cancers is related to age, sex, and ethnic background.

Common types of cancer in children (in order of frequency) include leukemia, central nervous system (CNS) cancers, lymphoma, neuroblastoma, rhabdomyosarcoma, Wilms' tumor, bone cancer, and retinoblastoma. Treatment modalities include surgery, radiation, and chemotherapy, much like treatment of cancer in the adult (see p. 102).

Pediatric Oncology Disorders

◆ ACUTE LYMPHOCYTIC LEUKEMIA

Acute lymphocytic leukemia (ALL) is a primary disorder of the bone marrow in which the normal marrow elements are replaced by immature or undifferentiated blast cells. When the quantity of normal marrow is depleted below the level necessary to maintain peripheral blood elements within normal ranges, anemia, neutropenia, and thrombocytopenia occur.

Etiology/Incidence

1. The exact cause of ALL is unknown.
2. Environmental causes, infectious agents (especially viruses), genetic factors, and chromosomal abnormalities are suspected in some cases.
3. ALL is the most common malignancy in children, occurring in nearly 4/100,000 children under 15 years of age.
4. ALL is classified according to the cell type involved: T cell, B cell, early pre-B, and pre-B.
5. The incidence of ALL is more common among Caucasian children.
6. The incidence of ALL is higher in boys than girls, with the greatest difference during puberty.

Altered Physiology

1. ALL results from the growth of an abnormal type of nongranular, fragile leukocyte in the blood-forming tissues, particularly in the bone marrow, spleen, and lymph nodes.
2. The abnormal lymphoblast has little cytoplasm and a round, homogeneous nucleus (Fig. 48-1).
3. Normal bone marrow elements may be displaced or replaced in this type of leukemia.
4. The changes in the blood and bone marrow result from the accumulation of leukemic cells and from the deficiency of normal cells.
   a. Red blood cell precursors and megakaryocytes from which platelets are formed are decreased, causing anemia, prolonged and unusual bleeding, tendency to bruise easily, and petechiae.
   b. Normal white blood cells are markedly decreased, predisposing the child to infection.
   c. The bone marrow is hyperplastic with a uniform appearance due to the presence of leukemic cells.
5. Leukemic cells may infiltrate into lymph nodes, spleen, and liver, causing diffuse adenopathy and hepatosplenomegaly.
6. Expansion of marrow or infiltration of leukemic cells into bone causes joint pain.
7. Invasion of the CNS by leukemic cells may cause headache, vomiting, cranial nerve palsies, convulsions, coma, papilledema, and blurred or double vision.
8. Weight loss, muscle wasting, and fatigue may occur when the body cells are deprived of nutrients because of the immense metabolic needs of the proliferating leukemic cells.

Complications

1. Infection—most frequently occurs in the lungs, gastrointestinal tract, or skin.
2. Hemorrhage—usually due to thrombocytopenia
3. CNS involvement
4. Bony involvement
5. Testicular involvement
6. Urate nephropathy
7. Late effects of treatment

Clinical Manifestations

1. Manifestations depend on the degree to which the bone marrow has been compromised and the location and extent of extramedullary infiltration.
2. Presenting symptoms
   a. Fatigability
   b. General malaise, listlessness
   c. Persistent fever of unknown cause
   d. Recurrent infection

Sandra Nettina: *The Lippincott Manual of Nursing Practice, 6th ed.*   © 1996 Lippincott-Raven Publishers

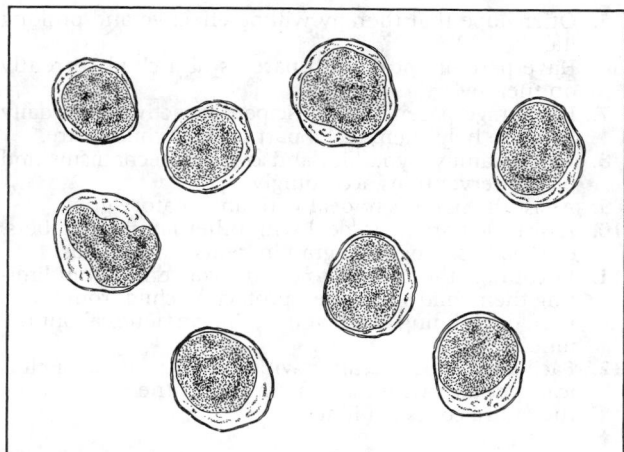

FIGURE 48-1 *Abnormal lymphoblast in acute lymphocytic leukemia (ALL).*

e. Petechiae, purpura, and ecchymoses after minor trauma
f. Pallor
g. Generalized lymphadenopathy
h. Abdominal pain due to organomegaly
i. Bone and joint pain
j. Headache and vomiting (with CNS involvement)
3. Presenting symptoms may be isolated or in any combination or sequence.

Diagnostic Evaluation

1. May have altered peripheral blood counts. Blood studies may show the following:
   a. Low hemoglobin, red blood cell count, hematocrit, and platelet count
   b. Decreased, elevated, or normal white blood cell count
2. Stained peripheral smear and bone marrow examination show large numbers of lymphoblasts and lymphocytes.
3. Lumbar puncture—to determine if there is CNS involvement
4. Renal and liver function studies—to determine any contraindications or precautions for chemotherapy
5. Chest x-ray to determine if a mediastinal mass or pneumonia is present
6. Varicella and cytomegalovirus titer to determine risk of infection

Treatment

A. Supportive Therapy To control disease complications such as hyperuricemia, infection, anemia, and bleeding

B. Specific Therapy To eradicate malignant cells and to restore normal marrow function

1. Chemotherapy is used to achieve complete remission with restoration of normal peripheral blood and physical findings.
2. There is no universally accepted standard therapy for the treatment of children with ALL, but most centers have similar protocols that use a combination of drugs.
3. Components of therapy
   a. Induction—the initial course of therapy designed to achieve a complete remission. It usually includes a combination of vincristine (Oncovin) and prednisone (Orasone). A third drug, such as 6-mercaptopurine (Purinethol), L-asparaginase (Elspar), daunorubicin (Cerubidine), doxorubicin (Adriamycin), or cytosine arabinoside (Cytosar-U), may be added.
   b. CNS prophylaxis—generally consists of intrathecal administration of methotrexate (Mexate) alone or in combination with hydrocortisone (Cortef) and cytarbine (Ara-C). Craniospinal irradiation may also be used.
   c. Consolidation treatment—a period of intensified treatment immediately after remission induction to attempt total eradication of leukemic cells. It usually includes a combination of methotrexate (Mexate), 6-mercaptopurine (Purinethol), teniposide (M-26, Vumon), etoposide (VP-16, VePesid), cytosine arabinoside (Cytosar-U), cyclophosphamide (Cytoxan), prednisone (Orasone), vincristine (Oncovin), and doxorubicin (Adriamycin) or daunorubicin (Cerubidine).
   d. Maintenance or continuation therapy—to prevent reappearance of the disease (usually continued for about 2.5 to 3 years). It usually includes daily oral administration of 6-mercaptopurine (Purinethol) and weekly oral or intramuscular administration of methotrexate (Mexate) with intermittent administration of other drugs such as vincristine (Oncovin), prednisone (Orasone), cyclophosphamide (Cytoxan), cytosine arabinoside (Cytosar-U), or daunorubicin (Cerubidine).
   e. Reinduction therapy—to induce remissions if relapse occurs; usually includes the same initial drugs. Sometimes additional agents are added.
   f. If testicular relapse occurs, radiation therapy to the testicles is administered.
4. An indwelling central venous catheter or implantable port is usually inserted to administer chemotherapy.
5. Research is continuing to determine the optimal method of inducing and maintaining remission with the least risk to the patient.
6. Bone marrow transplantation has been used successfully for treating children who fail to respond to conventional treatment.

C. Prognosis
1. At least 95% of children with ALL can be expected to achieve an initial remission if treated in a specialized center.
2. At least 70% of children with ALL will survive more than 5 years.
3. Children with good prognostic features have an 80% chance of long-term survival.
4. The prognosis becomes poorer with each relapse the child experiences.
5. Relapse is rare after 7 years from diagnosis.
6. Prognosis is related to the child's age and white blood cell count on diagnosis and the type of leukemia.

Nursing Assessment

1. Obtain a history.
   a. When taking the history, focus on symptoms that led to the diagnosis and previous symptoms for the past couple of weeks. For example, inquire about headache, nausea, vomiting, pallor, bleeding, pain, or fever.
   b. Ask about past history of varicella zoster infection (chickenpox), which could lead to disseminated infection if acquired during immunosuppression.
2. Perform a physical examination, including:
   a. Examination of skin for petechiae, purpura, and ecchymoses
   b. Palpation of lymph nodes for enlargement, tenderness, and mobility
   c. Palpation of spleen and liver for enlargement
   d. Examination of fundi to detect papilledema with CNS disease
   e. Inspection of skin for areas of infection, including indwelling catheter sites
   f. Auscultation of lungs for presence of rales or rhonchi indicative of pneumonia
   g. Temperature for presence of fever

NURSING ALERT:
Report changes in behavior or personality, persistent nausea, vomiting, headache, lethargy, irritability, dizziness, ataxia, convulsions, or alterations in state of consciousness. These may be signs of CNS disease or relapse.

Nursing Diagnoses

A. Anxiety of Parents related to learning of diagnosis
B. Risk for Infection and Hemorrhage related to bone marrow suppression due to chemotherapy and disease
C. Body Image Disturbance related to alopecia associated with chemotherapy
D. Altered Nutrition (Less than Body Requirements) related to anemia, anorexia, nausea, vomiting, and mucosal ulceration secondary to chemotherapy or radiation
E. Pain related to diagnostic procedures and progression of the disease
F. Activity Intolerance related to fatigue resulting from the disease and treatment
G. Anxiety of Child related to hospitalization and diagnostic and treatment procedures

Nursing Interventions

A. *Decreasing Parental Anxiety*
1. Be available to the parents when they feel that they want to discuss their feelings.
2. Offer kindness, concern, consideration, and sincerity toward the child and parents; be a source of consolation.
3. Contact the family's clergyman or the hospital chaplain.
4. Obtain the services of a social worker as appropriate to help the family use appropriate community resources.

5. Offer hope that therapy will be effective and prolong life.
6. Have parents speak with parents of a child currently on therapy.
7. Encourage parents to participate in activities of daily living to help them feel a part of their child's care.
8. Assess family dynamics and coping mechanisms and plan interventions accordingly.
9. Assist the parents to deal with anticipatory grief.
10. Assist the parents to deal with other family members, especially siblings and grandparents, and friends.
11. Encourage the parents to discuss concerns about limiting their child's activities, protecting child from infection, disciplining child, and having anxieties about the illness.
12. Facilitate communication with the clinic nurse or clinical specialist who may interact with the child during the entire course of illness.

B. *Preventing Infection and Hemorrhage*
1. Monitor complete blood count (CBC) as ordered.
2. Provide adequate hydration.
   a. Maintain parenteral fluid administration.
   b. Offer small amounts of oral fluids if tolerated.
3. Observe renal function carefully.
   a. Measure and record urinary output.
   b. Check specific gravity.
   c. Observe the urine for any evidence of gross bleeding.
   d. Use labsticks to determine if occult urinary bleeding is present.
4. Protect the child from sources of infection.
   a. Family, friends, personnel and other patients who have infections should not visit or care for the child.
   b. Do not place a child with an infection in the room with a child with leukemia.
   c. Good handwashing is the most important way to control infection.
   d. Observe the child closely and be alert for signs of impending infection.
      (1) Observe any area of broken skin or mucous membrane for signs of infection.
      (2) Report any fever over 101°F (38.4°C).
   e. Administer growth factors, such as granulocyte colony-stimulating factor (G-CSF), to stimulate the production of neutrophils and decrease the incidence of severe infections in the child after undergoing intense chemotherapy.
   f. Administer intravenous (IV) antibiotics as ordered.
   g. Administer trimethoprim-sulfamethoxazole (Bactrim), if ordered, twice daily three times per week to prevent infection with *Pneumocystis carinii*.
5. Record vital signs and report any changes that may indicate hemorrhage.
   a. Tachycardia
   b. Lowered blood pressure
   c. Pallor
   d. Diaphoresis
   e. Increasing anxiety and restlessness
6. Observe for gastrointestinal bleeding and hematest all emesis and stool.
7. Move and turn the child gently because hemarthrosis may occur and cause movement to be painful.
   a. Handle the child in a gentle manner.
   b. Turn frequently to prevent pressure sores.
   c. Place the child in proper body alignment, in a comfortable position.

d. Allow the child to be out of bed in a chair if this position is more comfortable.

8. Avoid intramuscular injections if possible.
9. Handle catheters as well as drainage and suction tubes carefully to prevent mucosal bleeding.
10. Protect the child from injury by monitoring activities and environmental hazards.
11. Be aware of emergency procedures for control of bleeding:
    a. Apply local pressure carefully so as not to interfere with clot formation.
    b. Administer leukocyte-poor packed red blood cells and platelets as ordered.

C. Promoting Acceptance of Body Changes

1. Prepare the patient for potential changes in body image (alopecia, weight loss, muscle wasting, etc) and help child cope with related feelings.
2. Contact the school nurse and teacher to help them prepare for the child's return to school. Discuss the bodily changes that have occurred and that may happen in the future.

D. Promoting Optimal Nutrition

1. Provide a highly nutritious diet as tolerated by the child.
   a. Determine the child's likes and dislikes.
   b. Offer frequent, small meals.
   c. Offer supplemental feedings high in calories and protein.
   d. Encourage the parents to assist at mealtime.
   e. Allow the child to eat with a group at a table if condition allows this.
   f. Avoid foods high in salt while child is taking steroids.
2. Give careful oral hygiene; the gums and mucous membranes of the mouth may bleed easily.
   a. Use a soft toothbrush.
   b. If the child's mouth is bleeding or painful, clean the teeth and mouth with a moistened cotton swab or toothette.
   c. Use a nonirritating rinse for the mouth (no alcohol-containing mouthwash or hydrogen peroxide).
   d. Apply petrolatum to cracked, dry lips.

E. Relieving Pain

1. Position the child for comfort. Water beds and bean bag chairs are often helpful.
2. Administer medications on a preventive schedule before pain becomes more intense. Continuous infusion pumps for narcotic administration are used.
3. Manipulate the environment as necessary to increase the child's comfort and minimize unnecessary exertion.
4. Prepare the child for treatment and diagnostic procedures.
   a. Use knowledge of growth and development to prepare the child for procedures such as bone marrow aspirations, spinal taps, blood transfusions, and chemotherapy.
   b. Provide a means for talking about the experience. Play, storytelling, or role playing may be helpful.
   c. Convey to the child an acceptance of fears and anger.
   d. Use Emla cream for local anesthesia at spinal tap, injection, and bone marrow sites to decrease pain.
   e. Administer conscious sedation before procedures and monitor pulse, blood pressure, respirations, and pulse oximetry during and after procedures.

F. Conserving Energy

1. Assess the child's energy level and space needed activities accordingly. Allow the child to rest in between if necessary.
2. Encourage the child to lie down and rest after diagnostic procedures, such as bone marrows and spinal taps.

G. Reducing the Child's Anxiety

1. Provide for continuity of care.
2. Encourage family-centered care (see p. 1131).
3. Facilitate play activities for the child and use opportunities to communicate through play.
4. Maintain some discipline, placing calm limitations on unacceptable behavior.
5. Provide appropriate diversional activities.
6. Encourage independence and provide opportunities that allow the child to control the environment.
7. Explain the diagnosis and treatment in terms the child can understand.

Family Education/Health Maintenance

1. Teach parents about normal CBC values and expected variations due to therapy.
2. Instruct parents about leukemia and side effects of chemotherapy.
3. Inform parents to call if child has a temperature of over 101°F (38.4°C), any bleeding, any signs of infections, and any exposure to chickenpox if the child has not had it. Immunosuppressed children are in danger of developing disseminated varicella and may be treated prophylactically with varicella immune globulin.

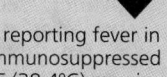

COMMUNITY-BASED CARE TIP:
Teach parents the importance of detecting and reporting fever in the child with leukemia. Unlike other children, immunosuppressed children rarely develop fever. A fever over 101°F (38.4°C) may indicate overwhelming infection and impending septic shock.

4. Teach preventive measures, such as handwashing and isolation from children with communicable diseases.
5. Ensure that parents can demonstrate the proper technique for care of venous access.
6. Refer parents to agencies, such as: Leukemia Society of America; 1-800-955-4572.

Evaluation

A. Parents discussing their feelings about the child's diagnosis and treatment
B. Afebrile, no signs of localized infection or bleeding
C. Maintains a positive body image; does not become overly self-conscious or shy about appearance
D. Eats at mealtime; takes between meal feedings
E. Experiences relief from pain (no crying or expression of pain)
F. Resting at intervals
G. Child acting out feelings in play; participating in age-appropriate activities

◆ BRAIN TUMORS IN CHILDREN

Brain tumors are expanding lesions within the skull. About 20% of the malignant tumors that occur in children are brain tumors.

There are four main types of brain tumors in children. *Cerebellar astrocytoma* is a slow-growing, often cystic type of tumor of the cerebellum. *Medulloblastoma* is a highly malignant, rapidly growing tumor, usually found in the cerebellum. *Brain stem glioma* is a tumor of the brain stem. *Ependymoma* is a tumor derived from the ependyma, or lining of the central canal of the spinal cord and cerebral ventricles. It frequently arises on the floor of the fourth ventricle, causing obstruction of the flow of cerebrospinal fluid (CSF).

Etiology/Incidence

1. The etiology of brain tumors is unknown.
2. Cerebellar astrocytoma accounts for about 10% to 20% of all pediatric brain tumors.
3. Medulloblastoma is the single most common tumor of the CNS in children. About 65% of medulloblastomas occur in boys.
4. Brain stem glioma accounts for approximately 15% of brain tumors in children.
5. Ependymomas represent about 5% to 10% of all primary childhood CNS tumors.

Altered Physiology

1. Cerebellar astrocytoma produces slowly increasing intracranial pressure. It is classified according to its malignancy, from grade I (least malignant) to grade IV (most malignant).
2. Medulloblastoma grows rapidly and produces evidence of increased intracranial pressure progressing over a period of weeks. As the tumor grows, it seeds along CSF pathways.
3. Through its growth, brain stem glioma interferes early with the function of cranial nerve nuclei, pyramidal tracts, and cerebellar pathways.
4. Ependymomas grow with varying speed. Because of location, tumors can invade the cardiorespiratory center, cerebellum, and spinal cord. They are graded according to degree of differentiation, as are the astrocytomas.

Complications

1. Brain stem herniation
2. Hydrocephalus

Clinical Manifestations

A. **Cerebellar Astrocytoma**   Insidious onset and slow course

1. Evidence of increased intracranial pressure—especially headache, visual disturbances, papilledema, and personality changes
2. Cerebellar signs—ataxia, dysmetria (inability to control the range of muscular movement), nystagmus
3. Behavioral changes

B. **Medulloblastoma**
1. Similar to manifestations of cerebellar astrocytoma, but condition develops more rapidly
2. The child may present with unsteady gait, anorexia, vomiting, and early morning headache, and later develop ataxia, nystagmus, papilledema, drowsiness, and increased head circumference.

C. **Brain Stem Glioma**
1. Cranial nerve palsies
   a. Strabismus
   b. Weakness, atrophy, and fasciculations of the tongue
   c. Swallowing difficulties
2. Hemiparesis
3. Cerebellar ataxia
4. Signs of increased intracranial pressure (rare)

D. **Ependymoma of the Fourth Ventricle**
1. Nausea or vomiting
2. Headache
3. Unsteady gait/ataxia; dysmetria
4. Signs of increased intracranial pressure
5. Focal motor weakness, visual disturbances, seizures

Diagnostic Evaluation

Determined by the type of tumor that is suspected; usually includes many or all of the following procedures to localize and determine extent of the tumor:

1. Computed tomography (CT)
2. Angiography
3. Magnetic resonance imaging (MRI)
4. Myelogram
5. Positron emission tomography (PET)
6. Lumbar puncture
7. Electroencephalogram—of limited value, but possibly useful when seizures are manifested

Treatment

1. Surgery is performed to determine the type of the tumor, to assess the extent of invasiveness, and to excise as much of the lesion as possible.
2. Radiation therapy is usually initiated as soon as the diagnosis is established and the surgical wound is healed.
3. Chemotherapy is used in children under age 4 with medulloblastoma to avoid early radiation and in children with ependymomas.
4. A ventriculoperitoneal shunt is often necessary for children who develop hydrocephalus.
5. Prognosis is improved in cases involving early diagnosis and adequate therapy. Five-year survivors are increasing, especially in children with low-grade astrocytomas or ependymomas.

Nursing Assessment

Assess the child's neurologic status to help locate the site of the tumor and the extent of involvement; identify signs of disease progress.

1. Obtain a thorough nursing history from the child and parents—particularly data related to normal behavioral patterns and presenting symptoms.
2. Perform portions of the neurologic examination as appropriate. Assess muscle strength, coordination, gait, and posture.
3. Observe for the appearance or disappearance of any of the clinical manifestations previously described. Report these to the health care provider and record each of the following in detail:
   a. Headache—duration, location, severity
   b. Vomiting—time occurring, whether or not projectile
   c. Seizures—activity before seizure, type of seizure, areas of body involved, behavior during and after seizure
4. Monitor vital signs frequently, including blood pressure and pupillary reaction.
5. Monitor ocular signs. Check pupils for size, equality, reaction to light, and accommodation.
6. Observe for signs of brain stem herniation—should be considered a neurosurgical emergency.
   a. Attacks of opisthotonos (Fig. 48-2)
   b. Tilting of the head; neck stiffness
   c. Poorly reactive pupils
   d. Increased blood pressure; widened pulse pressure
   e. Change in respiratory rate and nature of respirations
   f. Irregularity of pulse or lowered pulse rate
   g. Alterations of body temperature

NURSING ALERT:
Signs of brain stem herniation, especially opisthotonus, are ominous. The health care provider should be called immediately and the child prepared for ventricular tap to relieve pressure. Have resuscitation equipment on hand.

Nursing Diagnoses

A. Anxiety of Parents related to the nature of the diagnosis and the need for surgery
B. Anxiety of Child related to hospitalization and to diagnostic and treatment procedures
C. Pain related to increased intracranial pressure and surgery
D. Altered Nutrition (Less than Body Requirements) related to nausea and vomiting associated with increased intracranial pressure, chemotherapy, and radiation
E. Risk for Infection postoperatively
F. Disturbance of Body Image related to appearance of the incision, shaved head, or changes due to radiation, chemotherapy, and steroids

Nursing Interventions

A. **Reducing the Parents' Anxiety**
See also page 1310.

1. Encourage the parents to ask questions and to understand fully the risks and benefits of surgery.
2. Prepare the parents for the postoperative appearance of their child and for the fact that he or she might be comatose immediately following surgery.
3. Continue supporting the parents during the postoperative period. They may be frightened and upset by the appearance of their child and necessary emergency procedures.
4. Facilitate the return of normal parent–child relationships.
   a. The parents may be overprotective.
   b. Help the parents to see the child's increasing capabilities and encourage them to foster independence.

B. **Reducing the Child's Anxiety**
See also page 1311.

1. Prepare the child for surgery in realistic terms but at the appropriate developmental level.
2. Determine the plan regarding shaving of the child's head, bandages, and other procedures. Prepare the child accordingly.
3. Prepare the child for postoperative expectations (ie, may feel sleepy or have a headache and will need to remain flat).

C. **Reducing Pain Postoperatively**
1. Administer narcotics as ordered in the immediate postoperative period, assessing the child's level of consciousness before administration.
2. Keep the child as comfortable as possible by repositioning.

D. **Maintaining Nutritional Status**
1. Feed the child after he or she vomits. (Vomiting is not usually associated with nausea.)
2. Allow the child to participate in the selection of foods and the preparation of tray.
3. Maintain IV hydration or hyperalimentation and intralipids if indicated.
4. As the child recovers, encourage child to eat progressively larger meals.
5. If the child is unable to eat, provide tube feedings. A gastrostomy tube may be inserted.

E. **Preventing Infection and Other Complications Postoperatively**
1. Position the child according to surgeon's request—usually on unaffected side with head level.
   a. Raising the foot of the bed may increase intracranial pressure and bleeding.
   b. Post a sign above the bed noting the exact position of the head.
2. Check the dressing for bleeding and for drainage of CSF.

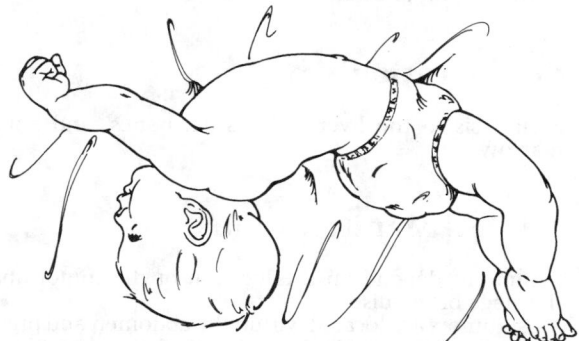
FIGURE 48-2 Opisthotonos, a sign of brainstem herniation.

3. Monitor the child's temperature closely.
   a. A marked rise in temperature may be due to trauma, to disturbance of the heat-regulating center, or to intracranial edema.
   b. If hyperthermia occurs, administer antipyretics and sponge baths as ordered. Temperature should not be reduced too rapidly.
4. Observe child closely for signs of shock, increased intracranial pressure, and alterations in level of consciousness.
5. Assess the child for edema of the head, face, and neck.
6. Carefully regulate fluid administration to prevent increased cerebral edema.
7. Change the child's position frequently and provide meticulous skin care to prevent hypostatic pneumonia and pressure sores.
   a. Move the child carefully and slowly, being certain to move the head in line with the body.
   b. Support paralyzed or spastic extremities with pillows, rolls, or other means.
8. Have equipment readily available for cardiopulmonary resuscitation, respiratory assistance, oxygen inhalation, blood transfusion, ventricular tap, and other potential emergency situations.
9. Report any elevated temperature or sign of infection.
10. If the child is receiving chemotherapy or radiation, instruct the parents to call if child has a fever of over 101°F (38.4° C) or nausea and vomiting unrelated to chemotherapy.

F. *Promoting Acceptance of Body Changes*
1. Encourage the child to express feelings regarding the threat to body image.
2. Reassure the child that a wig or a hat can be worn after recovery.
3. If the child's hair has not been totally shaved, comb it so that the area of baldness is not evident.
4. Reassure the child that hair will grow back.

Family Education/Health Maintenance

1. Provide parents with written information regarding the child's needs—medications, activity, care of the incision, and follow-up appointments.
2. Teach the parents about radiation and chemotherapy and their side effects.
3. If a child has a ventriculoperitoneal shunt, teach parents to report fever, nausea, vomiting, irritability, or a bulging anterior fontanelle.
4. Initiate a referral to a community health nurse to reinforce teaching and to maintain therapeutic support for the family.
5. Encourage parents to contact the child's teacher and the school nurse before the child returns to school so that they can prepare classmates for child's return and help them to deal with their feelings.
6. Provide the parents with the phone number of the clinic or nursing unit so that they may call if questions occur to them after discharge.
7. For additional resources refer family to agencies such as: American Brain Tumor Association; 2720 River Road; Des Plaines, IL 60018; 708-827-9910.

Evaluation

A. Parents discussing feelings about the child's diagnosis and surgery
B. Child demonstrating lessened anxiety through verbalization, play, or other age-appropriate activities
C. Child verbalizing relief from pain
D. Eating three meals, no weight loss noted
E. Afebrile, lungs clear, vital signs stable
F. Child verbalizing acceptance of appearance with hat, desire to visit with friends

◆ NEUROBLASTOMA

Neuroblastoma refers to a malignant tumor arising from the sympathetic nervous system.

Etiology/Incidence

1. Etiology is unknown.
2. Most common extracranial solid tumor of childhood
3. Annual incidence is less than 1/10,000 children.
4. Primarily affects infants and young children
5. Occurs slightly more frequently in boys

Altered Physiology

1. Tumors arise from embryonic neural crest cells anywhere along the craniospinal axis.
2. Histologic picture varies greatly from tumor to tumor and even within the same tumor.
3. Tumors are staged primarily on the basis of the extent of disease.
   a. Evans staging system
      (1) Stage I (tumor confined to the organ or structure of origin) to stage IV (remote disease involving the skeleton, parenchymal organs, soft tissue, distant lymph nodes, or bone marrow)
      (2) Stage IV-S refers to cases that would otherwise be stage I or II, but who have remote disease confined to one or more sites, either the liver, skin, or bone marrow, without evidence of skeletal metastasis.
   b. Pediatric Oncology Group Staging Stages A–D—examine regional lymph nodes for presence of disease.
4. Neuroblastoma is one of the few tumors that may demonstrate spontaneous remission.

Complications

1. Metastasis to the liver, soft tissue, bones, and bone marrow

Clinical Manifestations

1. Symptoms depend on the location of the tumor and the stage of the disease.
2. Most tumors are located within the abdomen and present as firm, nontender, irregular masses that cross the midline.

3. Other common signs:
   a. Bowel or bladder dysfunction resulting from compression by a paraspinal or pelvic tumor
   b. Neurologic symptoms because of compression by the tumor on nerve roots or because of tumor extension
   c. Supraorbital ecchymosis, periorbital edema, and exophthalmos resulting from metastases to the skull bones and retrobulbar soft tissue
   d. Lymphadenopathy, especially in the cervical area
   e. Bone pain with skeletal involvement
   f. Swelling of the neck or face and cough with thoracic masses
   g. General symptoms of pallor, anorexia, weight loss, and weakness with widespread metastasis

Diagnostic Evaluation

Work-up done to document the extent of the disease throughout the body:

1. Chest and skeletal x-rays
2. Bone scan
3. Bone marrow aspiration and possible biopsy
4. CBC, platelet count, ferritin
5. 24-hour urine collection—elevated excretion of homovanillic acid (HVA) and vanillylmandelic acid (VMA)
6. Liver and kidney function tests
7. Histologic confirmation
8. Additional studies
   a. CT scan of primary site and chest
   b. Ultrasound examination
   c. Liver/spleen scan
9. N-*myc* oncogene—multiple copies associated with a poor prognosis

Treatment

1. Surgery
   a. Role is both diagnostic and therapeutic.
   b. Either primary (before chemotherapy or radiation) or delayed/secondary (after therapy).
2. When complete surgical resection of a stage I tumor is possible, this may be the only treatment required.
3. Children with other than stage I disease generally receive a combination of surgery, radiation therapy, and chemotherapy. Drugs of choice include vincristine (Oncovin), dacarbazine (DTIC-Dome), cyclophosphamide (Cytoxan), doxorubicin (Adriamycin), cisplatin (Platinol), carboplatin (Paraplatin), and ifosfamide (Ifex).
4. Overall survival rate is about 30% to 35%, with almost all recurrences or deaths occurring within the first 2 years after diagnosis.
5. Influencing factors for prognosis:
   a. Stage of disease—the earlier the stage, the better the prognosis.
   b. Age—infants under 1 year of age demonstrate the best survival.
   c. Pattern of metastasis—children with metastases to the bone marrow, liver, and skin have better prognoses than those with radiographic bone involvement.
   d. Site of primary tumor—children with tumors of the thorax, pelvis, or neck appear to do better than children with abdominal tumors.

6. Neuroblastoma is one of few childhood tumors that has not responded dramatically to modern antitumor therapy.
7. The use of newer chemotherapy drugs and other techniques, such as immunotherapy and bone marrow transplant, may improve survival rates for these children.

Nursing Assessment

1. Obtain a history.
   a. Inquire about when symptoms began. Focus on decrease in appetite, weakness, pain, abdominal distention, or change in bowel and bladder function.
   b. Symptoms exhibited depend on the location of the primary tumor.
2. Perform a physical examination, including:
   a. Examination of skin for signs of increased bruising or petechiae
   b. Palpation of liver and spleen for enlargement
   c. Palpation of abdominal mass or other primary site of tumor
   d. Auscultation of lungs
   e. Palpation of lymph nodes
   f. Blood pressure for detection of hypertension
   g. Temperature for presence of fever due to infection or disease
   h. Assessment of bones and joints for pain or swelling
   i. Neurologic examination for signs of compression by tumor. Nerves involved depend on location of tumor.

Nursing Diagnoses

A. Anxiety of Parents related to learning of diagnosis
B. Fear of Child related to diagnostic procedures and surgery or biopsy
C. Activity Intolerance related to fatigue from tumor growth and bone marrow suppression
D. Potential Constipation or Bowel and Bladder Incontinence related to pressure of tumor
E. Risk for Infection related to bone marrow suppression from chemotherapy and radiation
F. Pain related to presence of tumor, surgery, or progression of disease
G. Disturbance in Body Image related to hair loss

Nursing Interventions

A. *Reducing the Parents' Anxiety*
See page 1310.

B. *Reducing the Child's Fear*
See page 1311.

C. *Increasing Activity Tolerance*
See page 1311.

D. *Regaining Normal Bowel and Bladder Function*
1. Assess normal elimination patterns the child had before the illness began.
2. Keep careful intake and output records.
3. Assess for urinary overflow incontinence and loss of bowel function depending on the age of the child.

E. *Preventing Infection*
See also page 1310.

1. Observe the surgical incision for erythema, drainage, or separation of the incision. Report any of these changes.

F. *Relieving Pain*
See page 1311.

G. *Promoting Acceptance of Body Changes*
See page 1311.

Family Education/Health Maintenance

1. Teach parents about the laboratory tests and x-rays needed at diagnosis and periodically throughout therapy.
2. Instruct parents about chemotherapy medications used and their potential side effects.
3. Inform parents about potential treatment methods, such as radiation therapy and bone marrow transplant.
4. Advise parents to use good handwashing and to prevent exposure to children with communicable diseases.

Evaluation

A. Parents and child discussing their feelings about diagnosis and treatment
B. Child participating in play and expressing feelings through play
C. Activity level normal
D. Voiding and stooling according to normal pattern
E. Afebrile, lungs clear, no signs of localized infections
F. Child resting without crying or guarding surgical incision
G. Child interacting with others, seems comfortable with self

◆ RHABDOMYOSARCOMA

Rhabdomyosarcoma is a highly malignant soft tissue tumor that arises from the embryonic mesenchymal cells that form striated muscle.

Etiology/Incidence

1. Etiology is unknown.
2. Genetic and environmental factors have been implicated.
3. Most common soft tissue tumor in persons under age 21.
4. Accounts for 5% to 8% of all malignant disease in children under 15 years of age.
5. Peak incidence is during the first decade of life.
6. Sixth most common form of cancer.

Altered Physiology

1. Classified in six pathologic categories based on histologic characteristics.

2. Tumor spreads either by local extension or by metastasis via the venous and lymphatic system.
3. Frequent sites of metastasis include the regional lymph nodes, lungs, bone marrow, bones, and brain.
4. Tumor staging is on the basis of the extent of the disease:
   a. Stage I: localized tumor, completely resected
   b. Stage II: regional disease, resected
   c. Stage III: localized disease, not completely resected
   d. Stage IV: metastatic disease at diagnosis

Clinical Manifestations

1. Often presents as an asymptomatic lump noted by the patient or parent.
2. Signs and symptoms are variable and reflect the location of the tumor and metastases.
   a. Orbit—ptosis, ocular paralysis, exophthalmos
   b. Nasopharynx—epistaxis, pain, dysphagia, nasal voice, airway obstruction
   c. Sinuses—swelling, pain, discharge, sinusitis
   d. Middle ear—pain, chronic otitis, facial nerve palsy
   e. Neck—hoarseness, dysphagia
   f. Truncal, extremities, testicular areas—enlarging soft tissue masses
   g. Prostate, bladder—urinary tract symptoms
   h. Retroperitoneal tumors—gastrointestinal and urinary tract obstruction, weakness, paresthesia, pain
   i. Vaginal—abnormal vaginal bleeding or mass

Diagnostic Evaluation

To document the extent of the disease and provide objective criteria for measuring response to therapy:

1. CBC, liver and renal function tests, electrolytes, serum calcium and phosphorus, uric acid
2. Urinalysis
3. Chest x-ray
4. Bone scan or skeletal survey
5. Bone marrow aspiration and biopsy
6. Liver scan
7. CT scan of the chest and primary lesion
8. Lumbar puncture—for children with cranial lesions
9. Open biopsy of the primary tumor—definitive diagnostic procedure
10. Ultrasound
11. MRI

Treatment

1. Surgery—to biopsy the lesion, determine the stage of the disease, and completely remove or reduce the primary tumor. Increasingly, chemotherapy/radiation therapy is used before surgery to avoid the disability associated with radical surgery for selected anatomic sites (head, neck, and pelvis).
2. Radiation—high-dose radiation is generally recommended for the primary tumor and metastasis.
3. Chemotherapy
   a. Used for all patients, usually in combination with irradiation

b. Commonly used drugs include dactinomycin (Actinomycin D), vincristine (Oncovin), cyclophosphamide (Cytoxan), doxorubicin (Adriamycin), cisplatin (Platinol), and etoposide (VP-16, VePesid).

c. Other agents under investigation include ifosfamide (Ifex), methotrexate (Mexate), and melphalan (Alkeran).

4. Survival rates have improved considerably in recent years and overall survival is approximately 70%.

5. Prognosis is related to the stage of the disease at diagnosis and the location of the primary tumor.

Nursing Assessment

1. Obtain a history.
   a. Inquire about recent illness history and when the child became symptomatic.
   b. Obtain review of systems, can help identify the primary tumor and any metastases present.
2. Perform a physical examination, including:
   a. Palpation of lymph nodes for enlargement, tenderness, and mobility
   b. Palpation of the liver and spleen to detect hepatosplenomegaly
   c. Palpation of primary site of tumor and suspected areas of metastasis
   d. Auscultation of lungs to assess breath sounds or abnormality due to the spread of the tumor

Nursing Diagnoses

A. Anxiety of Parents related to learning of diagnosis
B. Anxiety of Child related to diagnostic procedures and surgery or biopsy
C. Altered Nutrition (Less than Body Requirements) related to anemia, anorexia, nausea, vomiting, and mucosal ulceration secondary to chemotherapy or radiation
D. Pain related to surgery or possible progression of disease
E. Body Image Disturbance related to alopecia associated with chemotherapy
F. Risk for Infection related to bone marrow suppression from chemotherapy or radiation

Nursing Interventions

A. *Reducing the Parents' Anxiety*
See page 1310.

B. *Reducing the Child's Anxiety*
See page 1311.

C. *Improving Nutritional Intake*
See page 1311.

D. *Relieving Pain*
See page 1311.

E. *Maintaining Positive Body Image*
See page 1311.

F. *Preventing Infection*
See page 1310.

Family Education/Health Teaching

1. Teach parents about laboratory diagnostic tests done initially and that will be done periodically to follow-up the child's condition.
2. Instruct parents about treatment methods including chemotherapy and radiation protocols postoperatively and their side effects.
3. Stress the importance of follow-up so that any recurrence can be detected early and appropriate treatment instituted.

Evaluation

A. Parents verbalizing understanding of diagnosis
B. Child playing, interacting with others and asking questions
C. Eating three small meals and snacks
D. Child verbalizing reduced pain
E. Child verbalizing acceptance of self; looks in mirror
F. Afebrile, no signs of localized infection

◆ WILMS' TUMOR

Wilms' tumor is a malignant renal tumor.

Etiology/Incidence

1. The etiology of Wilms' tumor is not known.
2. Genetic inheritance has been documented in a small percentage of cases.
3. Wilms' tumor is the most common renal neoplasm in children.
4. It constitutes approximately 30% of all pediatric renal masses and 7% of all childhood tumors.
5. Seventy-five percent of cases occur before the child is 5 years of age.
6. One child in 10,000 develops a Wilms' tumor.

Altered Physiology

1. Wilms' tumor has a capacity for rapid growth and usually grows to a large size before it is diagnosed.
2. The effect of the tumor on the kidney depends on the site of the tumor.
3. In most cases, the tumor expands the renal parenchyma, and the capsule of the kidney becomes stretched over the surface of the tumor.
4. The tumor is often exceedingly vascular, soft, mushy, or gelatinous in character.
5. Wilms' tumors present various histologic patterns.
6. The neoplasms metastasize, either by direct extension or by way of the bloodstream. They may invade perirenal tissues, lymph nodes, the liver, the diaphragm, abdominal muscles, and the lungs. Invasions of bone and brain are less common.
7. Staging of Wilms' tumor is done on the basis of clinical and anatomic findings. It ranges from group I (tumor is limited to the kidney and is completely resected) to group IV (metastases are present in the liver, lung, bone, or brain). Group V includes those cases in which there is bilateral involvement either initially or sequently.

Clinical Manifestations

1. A firm, nontender upper quadrant abdominal mass is usually the presenting sign; it may be on either side. (It is frequently observed by the parents.)
2. Abdominal pain, which is related to rapid growth of the tumor, may occur. As the tumor enlarges, pressure may cause constipation, vomiting, abdominal distress, anorexia, weight loss, and dyspnea.
3. Less common are hypertension, fever, hematuria, and anemia.
4. Associated anomalies:
   a. Hemihypertrophy of the vertebrae
   b. Aniridia (absence of the iris)
   c. Genitourinary anomalies

Diagnostic Evaluation

1. Abdominal ultrasound—to demonstrate the tumor and to assess the status of the opposite kidney
2. Radiography of chest and chest CT to identify metastases
3. CBC and peripheral smear—for baseline data
4. Urinalysis for hematuria
5. Blood chemistries, especially serum electrolytes, uric acid, renal function tests (blood urea nitrogen and creatinine), and liver function tests (bilirubin, alanine aminotransferase [ALT], aspartate aminotransferase [AST], lactic dehydrogenase [LDH], total protein, albumin, and alkaline phosphatase) may show abnormalities.
6. Urinary VMA and HVA to distinguish from neuroblastoma
7. MRI or CT scan of the kidney to evaluate local spread to lymph nodes

Treatment

1. Determined by the stage of the tumor
2. Includes a combination of surgery, chemotherapy, and radiation therapy
3. Radiation therapy is given to the tumor bed postoperatively to render nonviable all cells that have escaped locally from the excised tumor. It is usually indicated for children who have stage III and IV Wilms' tumor or an unfavorable histology.
4. Whole lung radiation is used to treat stage IV tumors with lung metastasis.
5. Late effects of radiation therapy to the abdomen include scoliosis and underdevelopment of soft tissues.
6. Chemotherapy is initiated postoperatively to achieve maximal killing of tumor cells.
7. Overall survival rates for Wilms' tumor are the highest among all childhood cancers, greater than 85%.
8. Prognosis is best in children whose tumor is classified as stage I or II and who receive both surgery and chemotherapy.

Nursing Assessment

1. Obtain a history.
   a. Inquire about how tumor was first discovered.
   b. Ask whether the child has history of any other genitourinary anomalies or whether there is a family history of any type of cancer.
   c. Determine whether the child has had hematuria, dysuria, constipation, abdominal pain, decreased appetite, or fever before hospitalization and ask how these were treated.
2. Perform a physical examination, including:
   a. Assessment for presence of associated anomalies: aniridia, hemihypertrophy of the spine, or cryptorchidism
   b. Palpation of lymph nodes for enlargement, tenderness, and mobility
   c. Palpation of the liver and spleen for enlargement
   d. Palpation of the abdomen to determine the size and location of the tumor
   e. Auscultation of the lungs to assess breath sounds or abnormality due to spread of tumor

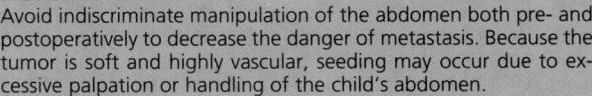

NURSING ALERT:
Avoid indiscriminate manipulation of the abdomen both pre- and postoperatively to decrease the danger of metastasis. Because the tumor is soft and highly vascular, seeding may occur due to excessive palpation or handling of the child's abdomen.

Nursing Diagnoses

A. Anxiety of Parents related to learning of diagnosis
B. Anxiety of Child related to surgery and diagnostic tests
C. Risk for Fluid Volume Deficit postoperatively
D. Pain related to surgery and possible progression of the disease.
E. Altered Nutrition (Less than Body Requirements) related to anemia, anorexia, nausea, vomiting, and mucosal ulceration secondary to chemotherapy or radiation
F. Body Image Disturbance related to alopecia associated with chemotherapy
G. Activity Intolerance related to fatigue resulting from the size of the tumor and treatment
H. Risk for Infection and Hemorrhage related to bone marrow suppression due to chemotherapy

Nursing Interventions

A. *Reducing Parental Anxiety*
See page 1310.

B. *Reducing the Child's Anxiety*
See page 1311.

C. *Preventing Fluid Volume Deficit and Other Complications*
1. Insert a nasogastric tube as ordered. Many children require gastric suction postoperatively to prevent distention or vomiting.
2. Monitor gastric output accurately and replace it with the appropriate IV fluids as ordered.
3. When bowel sounds have returned, begin with small amounts of clear fluids.
4. Keep accurate intake and output record.
5. Monitor vital signs as the child's condition warrants and check the surgical dressing frequently for drainage.

D. Controlling Pain
See page 1311.

E. Promoting Adequate Nutrition
See page 1311.

F. Promoting Acceptance of Body Changes
See page 1311.

G. Increasing Activity Tolerance
See page 1311.

H. Preventing Infection
See page 1310.

Family Education/Health Maintenance

1. Teach parents that children who have only one kidney should not play rough contact sports to avoid injuring the remaining kidney.
2. Inform parents to call if child has a temperature of over 101°F (38.4°C), any bleeding, any signs of infections, or any exposure to chickenpox if the child has not had it.
3. Teach measures to prevent infection such as handwashing and isolation from children with communicable disease.

Evaluation

A. Parents discussing their feelings about diagnosis and treatment
B. Child expressing feelings during play and participating in playroom activities
C. No abdominal distention or vomiting, vital signs stable
D. Child verbalizing relief from pain
E. Eating three meals, nausea relieved by antiemetics
F. Child playing with others without notice to alopecia
G. Participating in all normal daily activities without fatigue
H. Afebrile, no signs of local infection

◆ OSTEOGENIC SARCOMA

Osteogenic sarcoma is a malignant tumor of the bone.

Etiology/Incidence

1. Etiology is unknown.
2. Most frequent malignant bone cancer in children, with approximately 11 cases per million adolescents.
3. Peak incidence between 10 and 25 years of age.
   a. Most common at the peak of the adolescent growth spurt.
   b. The male-to-female ratio is 1.5:1.

Altered Physiology

1. Presumably arises from bone-forming mesenchyme tissue

2. Produces malignant spindle-cell stroma, which gives rise to malignant osteoid tissue
3. Common sites of occurrence—distal femur, proximal tibia, and proximal humerus. Less common sites include the pelvis, phalanges, and jaw.
4. Most commonly metastasize to lungs and other bones

Clinical Manifestations

1. Pain in the affected site, frequently causing limp or limitation of motion
2. Palpable, tender, fixed bony mass
3. Additional symptoms related to site of metastasis, if present

Diagnostic Evaluation

1. Radiographic examination of lesion—to visualize the tumor
2. Serum alkaline phosphatase—often elevated but does not correlate reliably with extent of disease
3. Bone scan—helpful in detecting initial extent of malignancy, planning therapy, and evaluating effects of treatment
4. Biopsy of lesion—to confirm the diagnosis and provide histologic date for the selection of a treatment plan
5. Chest x-ray or CT scan of chest—to identify lung metastasis and to evaluate extent of primary tumor
6. Renal and liver function tests—to screen for problems before initiating chemotherapy
7. MRI—to evaluate site of tumor

Treatment

1. Surgery
   a. Radical amputation of the affected extremity, and often the joint proximal to the involved area, is required in most cases.
   b. Newer techniques include transmedullary amputation and limb-salvaging surgery, such as total femur replacement.
2. Chemotherapy is advocated for 1 to 3 years after surgery. It is also used preoperatively for patients undergoing resectional surgery and for metastatic disease.
3. Survival has greatly improved with the aggressive use of multimodal therapy.
4. Approximately 50% to 60% of patients who undergo surgery followed by chemotherapy can expect to be disease-free after 3 years.
5. Limb-saving surgery has improved the quality of life for many survivors.

Nursing Assessment

1. Obtain a history.
   a. Inquire about how symptoms first presented and the duration of symptoms.
   b. Determine whether the child has any pain or limitation of motion in the affected area.
2. Perform a physical examination, including:

a. Palpation of the mass to determine the size and location. Determine whether the mass is tender or
fixed to the bone.
b. Palpation of other bones to check for metastases
c. Auscultation of the lungs to assess breath sounds or
other abnormalities due to spread of tumor

Nursing Diagnoses

A. **Anxiety of Parents** related to learning of diagnosis
B. **Anxiety of Child or Adolescent** related to surgery, diagnostic tests, and treatment
C. **Disturbance in Body Image** related to surgery and possible amputation and alopecia associated with chemotherapy
D. **Pain** related to surgery and possible progression of the
disease
E. **Altered Nutrition (Less than Body Requirements)** related to anemia, anorexia, nausea, vomiting, and mucosal ulceration due to chemotherapy
F. **Risk for Infection** related to surgery or bone marrow
suppression secondary to chemotherapy

Nursing Interventions

A. *Reducing the Parent's Anxiety*
See page 1310.

B. *Reducing the Adolescent's Anxiety*
1. Incorporate the adolescent's developmental level and
develop a teaching program to include diagnostic tests
and postoperative care.
2. Support and prepare the child for routine surgical care
or care of the amputated limb. Involve the parents in
teaching plan and make sure they all know what to
expect before going to surgery.
3. If an amputation is going to be done, teach the child
about the need for physical therapy for exercises and
to learn crutch walking and the need for a prosthesis.
4. Nursing care of the adolescent with osteogenic sarcoma
is the same as the care of the adult (see p. 880).

C. *Promoting Acceptance of New Self-Image*
1. Understand that adolescents need time and support to
accept the diagnosis and surgery and to grieve for their
lost body part if an amputation is done.
2. Try to introduce the adolescent to another adolescent
with the same diagnosis who has undergone similar
treatment.
3. Suggest the selection of clothing that will camouflage
the prosthesis and is fashionable and appealing.
4. Suggest wigs, scarves, or hats for adolescents experiencing hair loss due to chemotherapy.
5. Encourage visits by peers and help the child to deal
with questions and reactions from peers.

D. *Relieving Pain*
See page 1311.

E. *Promoting Adequate Nutrition*
See page 1311.

F. *Preventing Infection and Hemorrhage*
See page 1310.

Family Education/Health Maintenance

1. Encourage the parents to contact the school system to
arrange for a tutor for students who need to remain
out of school for lengthy periods of time.
2. Assist the parents in contacting the school nurse to facilitate reentry into the classroom.
3. Educate parents about changes that may need to be
made in the home due to handicaps.
4. Teach adolescent and parents about infection control
measures, such as good handwashing and preventing
exposure to children with communicable diseases because chemotherapy is usually long term.
5. Parents and adolescents should be instructed about
chemotherapy medications used and their potential
side effects.

Evaluation

A. Parents discussing feelings about surgery and chemo-
therapy treatments
B. Child verbalizing feelings about surgery and asking
questions
C. Child looking in mirror, touching amputation site
D. Child verbalizing relief from pain
E. Eating pattern adequate, nausea relieved by antiemetics
F. Afebrile, vital signs stable, no signs of bleeding

◆ RETINOBLASTOMA

Retinoblastoma is a malignant, congenital tumor arising in
the retina of one or both eyes.

Etiology/Incidence

1. Unknown etiology
2. Nonhereditary somatic mutations:
a. Account for approximately 60% of all retinoblastomas
b. Always demonstrate unilateral involvement
3. Hereditary germinal mutations:
a. Account for approximately 40% of all retinoblastomas
b. May be bilateral or unilateral
c. Mode of inheritance is autosomal dominant.
4. Can be associated with chromosomal aberrations
5. The incidence is relatively rare, usually diagnosed in
patients before 2 years of age.
6. Occurs in approximately 11 per million children under
5, or approximately 200 children in the United States
each year.
7. Incidence is increasing because of prolonged survival
of affected children, with transmission of the tumor to
their offspring, and increased exposure to mutagenic
agents.

Altered Physiology

1. Retinoblastomas are malignant neuroblastic tumors that may arise in any of the nucleated retinal layers.
2. Usually arise in multiple foci rather than a single tumor
3. Some tumors (endophytic type) arise in the internal nuclear layers of the retina and grow forward into the vitreous cavity.
4. Some tumors (exophytic type) arise in the external nuclear layer and grow into the subretinal space, with detachment of the retina.
5. Most tumors have a combination of endophytic and exophytic growth.
6. Extension of the tumor may occur into the choroid, the sclera, and optic nerve.
7. Hematogenous spread of the tumor may occur to the bone marrow, skeleton, lymph nodes, and liver.
8. Tumor staging reflects the extent of the disease and the probability of preserving useful vision in the affected eye, from group I (very favorable) to group V (very unfavorable).

Clinical Manifestations

1. Signs and symptoms of an intraocular tumor depend on its size and position.
2. "Cat's eye reflex"—whitish appearance of the pupil, represents visualization of the tumor through the lens as light falls on the tumor mass—most common sign.
3. Strabismus—second most common presenting sign
4. Other occasional presenting signs:
   a. Orbital inflammation
   b. Hyphema
   c. Fixed pupil
   d. Heterochromia iridis—different colors of each iris or in the same iris
5. Vision loss is not a symptom because young children do not complain of unilaterally decreased vision.
6. Symptoms of distant metastasis—anorexia, weight loss, vomiting, headache

Diagnostic Evaluation

1. Bilateral indirect ophthalmoscopy under general anesthesia
2. CT scan or MRI of head and eyes to visualize tumor
3. Bone marrow aspiration and lumbar puncture under anesthesia to determine metastasis

Treatment

1. Depends on the stage of the disease at the time of diagnosis
2. Unilateral tumors in stages I, II, or III are usually treated with external beam irradiation.
   a. Goal of treatment is to eradicate the tumor(s) and preserve useful vision.
   b. Radiation is usually administered over a period of 3 to 4 weeks.

3. Surgery (enucleation) is the treatment of choice for advanced tumor growth, especially with optic nerve involvement.
4. Bilateral disease often requires enucleation of the severely diseased eye and irradiation of the least affected eye.
   a. Every attempt is made to salvage whatever vision there may be.
   b. Bilateral enucleation is indicated with extensive bilateral retinoblastoma where there is no hope of vision.
5. Radioactive applicators, light coagulation, and cryotherapy are sometimes used to treat small, localized tumors.
6. Chemotherapy is used for cases of extraocular disease: regional or distant metastases. Drugs commonly used include cyclophosphamide (Cytoxan), vincristine (Oncovin), dactinomycin (Actinomycin D), doxorubicin (Adriamycin), ifosfamide (Ifex), methotrexate (Mexate), cisplatin (Platinol), and teniposide (VM-26, Vumon).
7. Overall survival rate is high (90%).
8. Heritable retinoblastoma and bilateral retinoblastoma are associated with a high incidence of spontaneous and radiation-related new tumors, particularly sarcomas.

Nursing Assessment

1. Obtain a history.
   a. Ask about a family history that is positive for retinoblastoma or other types of cancer.
   b. Inquire about when symptoms began and presence of strabismus, "cat's eye reflex" (leukocoria), any orbital inflammation, vomiting, or headache.
2. Perform a physical examination.
   a. Assess pupils for reactivity of light, size, and presence of leukocoria.
   b. Evaluate the presence of strabismus when checking muscle balance.
   c. Assess eyes for presence of associated signs, such as erythema, inflammation of the orbit, hyphema, and heterochromia iridis.

Nursing Diagnoses

A. Parental Anxiety related to the diagnosis, treatment, and genetic implications of the diagnosis
B. Impaired Tissue Integrity related to skin changes, loss of lashes, fat atrophy, impaired bone growth, and dry eye due to radiation
C. Fear of the Child related to hospitalization and to diagnostic and treatment procedures
D. Disturbance in Body Image and Ineffective Coping related to enucleation and need for an eye prosthesis
E. Sensory/Perceptual Alteration (Vision) related to disease process or enucleation

Nursing Interventions

A. **Decreasing Parental Anxiety and Guilt**
1. Listen to the parental feelings of guilt about transmitting the disease to the child or because they did not notice symptoms earlier.

2. Discuss the benefit of consultation about the probability of having another affected child.
   a. Risk ranges from approximately 1% to 10%, depending on family history and whether the affected child had unilateral or bilateral disease.
   b. The reportedly high lifelong cancer burden among retinoblastoma patients may also be important to parents in making informed decisions.
   c. Support parental decisions regarding future pregnancies.
3. Encourage the parents to seek genetic counseling for the affected child when he or she reaches puberty.
   a. The risk to offspring is from 1% to 50%, depending on family history and whether disease was unilateral or bilateral.
   b. Among affected offspring, there is a high probability (greater than 50%) of bilateral disease.

B. Preserving Tissue Integrity
1. Sedate the child for radiation, if necessary.
   a. Administer the medication in a timely manner so that sedation is adequate for positioning of the child.
2. Observe for possible side effects of irradiation and prepare the parents for their occurrence.
   a. Skin changes at the temples
      (1) Use soap sparingly in these areas.
      (2) Avoid exposure to the sun.
      (3) Apply a nonirritating lubricant.
   b. Loss of lashes
   c. Fat atrophy with ptosis
   d. Delayed wound healing
   e. Dry eye
   f. Permanent radiation dermatitis
   g. Impaired bone growth

C. Allaying the Child's Fear
See also page 1311.

1. Encourage the parents to "room-in" and participate in the child's care to minimize separation anxiety.
2. Prepare the child and parents for all diagnostic procedures.
3. Describe the surgery and anticipated postoperative appearance of the child. Draw pictures or use a doll if available.
   a. A surgically implanted sphere maintains the shape of the eyeball.
   b. The child's face may be edematous and ecchymotic.
4. Offer the family the opportunity to talk with another parent who has gone through the experience or to see pictures of another child with an artificial eye.
5. See nursing management of eye enucleation on page 431.

D. Promoting Acceptance of Prosthesis
1. Explain to child the changes in terms of losing diseased eye, having a bandaged orbit until it is healed after surgery, and then receiving a prosthetic eye.
2. Explain that the prosthesis will be made for him or her and will look like the removed eye.
3. Tell parents to expect the child to grieve the loss and to help the child by talking about it, but treating the child as the same person.

E. Minimizing Effects of Vision Loss
1. Maintain a safe, uncluttered environment for the child.
2. Hold the child frequently and stand close, within child's field of vision, while speaking or providing care.
3. Encourage the use of touch and other senses for exploring.
4. Set environmental limits so the child feels safe and can obtain help easily.

Family Education/Health Maintenance

1. Teach care of the orbit.
2. Teach care of the prosthesis—initial instructions are provided by the ocularist and should be reinforced by the nurse.
3. Advise protection of the remaining eye from accidental injury, such as wear safety glass for sports, do not put sharp objects near eye, treat eye infections promptly.
4. Encourage maintenance of routine check-ups for eye and medical care.
5. Stress need to have subsequent children carefully evaluated for retinoblastoma.
   a. An ophthalmologic examination under anesthesia is usually recommended at about 2 months of age.
   b. The child should receive frequent examinations thereafter until judged safe from developing retinoblastoma, usually about age 3 years.

Evaluation

A. Parents discussing their feelings openly, show affection to the child
B. Parents describing possible side effects of radiation and how to care for skin around eyes
C. Child demonstrating lessened anxiety by participating in age-appropriate activities
D. Child showing acceptance of the presence of the prosthesis and not inhibited in behavior
E. Child moving about environment with ease

Selected References

Albright, A. (1993). Pediatric brain tumors. *CA A Cancer Journal for Clinicians, 34*(5), 272-288.

Altman, A. J., & Quinn, J. J. (1995). Cancer in infancy. *Contemporary Pediatrics, 12* (2), 39-63.

Berg, S., et al. (1991). Principles of treatment of solid tumors. *Pediatric Clinics of North America, 38*(2), 249-267.

Betcher, D., et al. (1991). Granulocyte-macrophage colony-stimulating factor.

Journal of Pediatric Oncology Nursing, 8(3), 134-135.

Brandt, B. (1990). Nursing protocol for the patient with neutropenia. *Oncology Nursing Forum, 17*(1), 9-15.

Cohn, S. (1991). Advances in treatment

of neuroblastoma. *Contemporary Oncology,* September-October, 44-50.

Feinbach, D., & Vietti, T. (1991). *Clinical pediatric oncology.* St. Louis: Mosby-Year Book.

Fletcher, B., & Pratt, C. (1991). Evaluation of the child with a suspected malignant solid tumor. *Pediatric Clinics of North America, 38*(2), 223-248.

Goede, I., & Betcher, D. (1994). EMLA. *Journal of Pediatric Oncology Nursing, 11*(1), 38-41.

Meyer, W., & Malawer, M. (1991). Osteosarcoma: Clinical features and evolving surgical and chemotherapeutic strategies. *Pediatric Clinics of North America, 38*(2), 317-348.

Nichols, M. L. (1995). Social support and coping in young adolescents with cancer. *Pediatric Nursing, 21* (3), 235-240.

Pizzo, P., & Poplach, D. (1993). *Principles and practice of pediatric oncology* (2nd ed.). Philadelphia: JB Lippincott.

Schonfeld, D. (1993). Talking with children about death. *Journal of Pediatric Health Care, 7*(6), 269-274.

Servodidio, C. et al. (1991). Retinoblastoma. *Cancer Nursing, 14*(3), 117-123.

Shiminski-Maher, T. (1993). Brain tumors in childhood: Implications for nursing practice. *Journal of Pediatric Health Care 4* (3), 122-130.

Zelter, L. (1990). Report of the subcommittee on the management of pain associated with procedures in children with cancer. *Pediatrics, 86*(5), 826-831.

Pediatric Hematologic Disorders

◆ ANEMIA

Anemia refers to a deficit of red blood cells (RBC) or hemoglobin in the blood resulting in decreased oxygen-carrying capacity. It is the most frequent hematologic disorder encountered in children.

Etiology/Incidence

1. Blood loss related to:
   a. Trauma and ulceration
   b. Decreased production of platelets
   c. Increased destruction of platelets
   d. Decreased number of clotting factors
2. Impairment of RBC production
   a. Nutritional deficiency
      (1) Iron deficiency—most common type of anemia in all age groups; about 3% of all children
      (2) Folic acid deficiency
      (3) Vitamin B_{12} deficiency
      (4) Vitamin B_6 deficiency
3. Decreased erythrocyte production
   a. Pure RBC anemia
   b. Secondary hemolytic anemias associated with chronic infection, renal disease, and drugs
   c. Bone marrow depression—leukemia, aplastic anemias, transient erythocytopenia of childhood
4. Increased erythrocyte destruction
   a. Extrinsic factors
      (1) Drugs and chemicals
      (2) Infections—parovirus (fifth disease)
      (3) Antibody reactions—passively acquired antibodies against Rh, A or B isoimmunization, autoimmune hemolytic anemia, burns, poisons (including lead poisoning)
   b. Intrinsic factors
      (1) Abnormalities of the RBC membrane
      (2) Enzymatic defects—glucose-6-phosphate dehydrogenase deficiency (G6PD)
      (3) Abnormal hemoglobin synthesis—sickle cell disease, thalassemia syndromes

Altered Physiology

1. RBCs and hemoglobin are normally formed at the same rate at which they are destroyed.
2. Whenever formation of RBCs or hemoglobin is decreased or their destruction is increased, anemia results.

3. The ability of hemoglobin to carry oxygen to the tissues and remove carbon dioxide for excretion by the lungs is decreased.
4. In anemia of chronic infection and inflammation, the life span of the RBC is moderately decreased and the ability of the bone marrow to produce RBCs is significantly decreased. (This is the principal factor in determining the degree of anemia.)
5. In hemolytic anemias:
   a. The RBCs are destroyed at abnormally high rates primarily by the spleen.
   b. The activity of the bone marrow increases to compensate for the shortened survival time of the RBCs.
   c. Bone marrow hypertrophies and occupies a larger than normal share of the inner structure of bones.
   d. Products of RBC breakdown increase with hemolysis.
   e. Jaundice results when the liver is unable to clear the blood of the pigment resulting from the breakdown of hemoglobin from destroyed RBCs.
   f. Iron builds up (hemosiderosis) and may deposit on body tissues.

Complications

1. Mental sluggishness as a result of decreased oxygen and energy for normal neural activity usually associated with a decreased attention span, deceased intelligence, and lethargy
2. Growth retardation related to anorexia and decreased cellular metabolism
3. Delayed puberty related to growth retardation
4. Cardiac enlargement related to muscle hypertrophy due to increased strain on the heart attempting to compensate for increased oxygen demand by the tissues; eventually results in congestive heart failure
5. Death from cardiac failure related to circulatory collapse and shock

Clinical Manifestations

1. Condition may be acute or chronic.
2. Early symptoms
   a. Listlessness
   b. Fatigability
   c. Anorexia related to decreased energy
3. Late symptoms
   a. Pallor
   b. Weakness
   c. Tachycardia
   d. Palpitations
   e. Tachypnea; shortness of breath on exertion
   f. Jaundice (with hemolytic anemias)

Diagnostic Evaluation

1. Complete blood count (CBC) with indices and reticulocytes—vary with types of anemia (Table 49-1)
2. Serum iron and total iron-binding capacity—ratio of less than 0.2
3. Serum ferritin–less than 12 $\mu g/dL$
4. Lead—greater than 20 $\mu g/dL$
5. Free erythrocyte protoporphyrin—greater than 35 $\mu g/dL$
6. B_{12}, B_6, folate levels—may be decreased
7. Hemoglobin electrophoresis—may show hemoglobin S or other abnormality
8. Parovirus B19 titer—may be elevated in transient erythroblastopenia

Treatment

A. Iron Deficiency Anemia
1. Oral iron at a dose of 6 mg elemental iron per kilogram per day given between meals
2. Dietary: decrease milk intake to 16 oz/day; include iron-fortified cereals and bread products; increase consumption of red meat.
3. Rarely is iron given intramuscularly at present due to high incidence of allergic reactions. If administered intramuscularly, it is given by Z-track method.

B. Lead   (see page 1113)

1. Administration of chelating agents ethylenediaminetetraacetic acid (EDTA) or dimercaprol (BAL) according to recommendations of the Centers for Disease Control and Prevention
2. Use of lead-free paints, gasoline, etc.
3. Testing of the house and soil
4. Removal of individuals from unsafe environment

C. Megaloblastic Anemia
1. Folate deficiency—administration of folic acid orally
2. B_{12} deficiency—administration of B_{12} (cyanocobalamin [Cyanoject]) intramuscularly

D. Hemoglobinopathies
1. Sickle cell anemia (see p. 1327)
2. Thalassemia (see p. 1332)

E. Transient Erythroblastopenia of Childhood
1. For hemoglobins of under 5 g or cardiac failure, usually a transfusion of packed RBCs
2. Unless there is cardiac failure, there is usually no therapy, but supportive care is provided.

Nursing Assessment

1. Obtain history of potential causes.
   a. Dietary history including the amount of milk and meat consumed
   b. Medications
   c. Persistent infection, fever, or chronic disease
   d. Exposure to drugs, poisons, etc.
   e. Pica—craving and consuming nonfood items (ie, paint chips, ice, paper, etc.)
2. Obtain a baseline assessment.
   a. Observe skin and mucous membranes for pallor.
   b. Obtain height and weight and plot on growth curve.
   c. Measure vital signs including blood pressure.
   d. Assess child's functional level—level of exercise tolerance, mental functioning.
   e. Assess attainment of developmental milestones.
3. Observe for fatigue, listlessness, irritability, etc.
4. Observe for blood loss: bruising, bleeding, hematuria, or hematochezia (blood in stool).

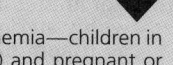

COMMUNITY-BASED CARE TIP:
Be alert for children at risk for iron deficiency anemia—children in rapid growth stages (toddlers and adolescents) and pregnant or lactating adolescents.

Nursing Diagnoses

A. Fatigue related to decreased ability of blood to transport oxygen to the tissues
B. Altered Nutrition (Less than Body Requirements) of recommended daily dietary allowances
C. Risk for Infection related to debilitated state
D. Anxiety related to hospitalization and painful diagnostic procedures (venipunctures, finger sticks, etc.)
E. Altered Growth and Development related to decreased energy

TABLE 49-1   Blood Tests in Anemia by Cause

	MCV	MCHC	Reticulocyte	Ferritin	FEP
Iron deficiency	Low	Low	Low	Low	High
Lead poisoning	Low	Low	Low	Normal	High
β-Thalassemia	Low	Low	Low	Normal	Normal
Folate deficiency	High	Normal	Low	Normal	Normal
B_{12} deficiency	High	Normal	Low	Normal	Normal
Sickle cell disease	Normal	Normal	High	Normal	Normal

FEP, free erythrocyte protoporphyrin; MCHC, mean corpuscular hemoglobin concentration; MCV, mean corpuscular volume

Nursing Interventions

A. *Minimizing Fatigue*
1. Plan nursing care to allow for lengthy periods when the child is not disturbed by hospital routines, procedures, treatments, etc.; set priorities.
2. Observe for early signs of fatigue such as irritability, hyperactivity, listless, etc.
3. Encourage sedentary rather than active projects.
4. Administer oxygen and position upright if dyspnea present.
5. Do not always encourage self-care.
6. Provide finger foods that are easy to chew to conserve energy.

B. *Providing Adequate Nutritional Intake*
1. Be aware of the child's food preferences and plan diet accordingly.
2. Offer small amounts of food at frequent intervals.
3. Reward the child for positive attempts to eat.
4. Allow the child to participate in selection of foods and in preparation of meal tray.
5. Avoid tiring activities and unpleasant procedures at mealtime.
6. Make mealtime as pleasurable as possible.
7. Provide iron-rich food and vitamins when necessary.
8. If iron is ordered, give between meals and with orange juice (iron is absorbed best in acidic environment).
9. Limit milk and milk products to 16 to 24 oz/day. Milk products inhibit the absorption of oral iron.
10. Administer liquid iron with a dropper or straw or dilute with water or fruit juice to prevent staining of the teeth.
    a. If administered by dropper, ensure the liquid iron is deposited in the back of the mouth.
    b. Dental stains can be removed by brushing the teeth with sodium bicarbonate or hydrogen peroxide and then rinsing with water after each administration.
11. Be alert for side effects of iron supplements—gastric distress, colic pain, diarrhea, or constipation—may call for decreased dose.
12. Advise family that child's stool may turn dark green or black.
13. Stress the importance of continuing iron therapy according to health care provider's directions even though the child may not appear to be ill.

C. *Preventing Infection*
1. Teach and assist with good hygiene practices such as handwashing and mouth care.
2. Avoid exposure to others with colds, infections, etc.
3. Ensure that staff, family, and visitors always wash hands thoroughly.
4. Report any temperature elevation or other signs of infection.

D. *Reducing Anxiety*
1. Allow the child to handle equipment used for tests and procedures (tourniquets, syringes, etc.).
2. Explain all procedures and the treatment plan to the child in a way that child can understand.
3. Allow the older child to look through a microscope at a blood smear, if interested and appropriate for child's age.
4. Permit the child to cleanse the area for a venipuncture or finger stick and to choose the finger.

E. *Promoting Normal Growth and Development*
1. Ensure that nutrition is adequate for age and activity level.

2. Encourage participation in age-related activities.
3. Encourage doing homework and tutored activities.
4. Encourage peer socialization.
5. Promote age-appropriate play and therapeutic play.

COMMUNITY-BASED CARE TIP:
Perform periodic developmental testing and set goals for parents if child is falling behind. Share results with parents and explain the association between diet/anemia and growth and development.

Family Education/Health Maintenance

1. Stress to the parents the importance of continuing the iron therapy according to the provider's directions even though the child may not appear ill.

NURSING ALERT:
There is a great deal of variation in the elemental iron content of the commercially available liquid preparations containing iron. To avoid confusion, the dosage should be expressed in terms of elemental iron and then converted to the proper amount of the therapeutic agent selected.

2. Initiate and reinforce good dietary habits.
   a. Foods rich in iron include dark green leafy vegetables, fortified cereals, dried fruits, nuts, and red meats.
   b. Do not allow the child to drink excessive quantities of milk to the exclusion of other foods that contain more iron. Limit milk intake to 16 to 24 oz/day.
   c. Provide vitamin supplements if necessary. Vitamin C appears to enhance the absorption of iron.
   d. Explain the reasons for diet change to parents in language they can understand. Visual aids and pictures may be helpful.
   e. Assist the parents to select iron-rich foods that are acceptable to the child, within the family's food budget, and culturally acceptable.
3. Discuss with parents any of the social, economic, and environmental problems that may contribute to the child's disease.
4. Emphasize to the parents the benefits of a referral to a community health nurse if it appears that the family will need support in dealing with the child's chronic disease.
5. Discuss general health measures, including adequate rest, diet, sunshine, and fresh air activity.
6. Encourage regular medical and dental evaluations. Emphasize the need for appropriate follow-up.
7. Explain that infection may be prevented by dressing the child according to the weather and keeping away from persons with colds, sore throats, and other infections.
8. Teach the parents how to administer medication.
9. Alert the parents to signs of disease progress.

Evaluation

A. Increasing activity noted
B. Eating frequent small feedings of cereal, bread, red

meat, vegetables; tolerating iron supplement without side effects
C. Remaining free of infection; normal temperature
D. Cooperating with frequent blood sampling
E. Maintaining growth curve; managing age-appropriate developmental activities

◆ SICKLE CELL DISEASE (SICKLE CELL ANEMIA)

Sickle cell disease is a severe, chronic, hemolytic anemia occurring in persons who are homozygous for the sickle gene. The clinical course is characterized by episodes of pain due to the occlusion of small blood vessels by sickled RBCs. Persons heterozygous for the sickling gene are said to possess sickle cell trait, which is associated with a benign clinical course.

Etiology/Incidence

1. Genetically determined, inherited disease—autosomal recessive
2. Each person inherits one gene from each parent, which governs the synthesis of hemoglobin (Table 49-2).
3. Found almost entirely in African Americans and persons of Arabic northern Mediterranean ancestry.
4. Approximately 8% of African Americans have sickle cell trait.
5. Approximately 1 of every 600 African American infants born in the United States has sickle cell anemia.

Altered Physiology

1. Normally each hemoglobin molecule consists of four molecules of heme folded into one molecule of globin. Each globin molecule consists of two α chains and two β chains.
2. The amino acid sequence on the β chain is altered in sickle cell hemoglobin—valine is substituted for glutamic acid in the sixth position of the 574 amino acids that make up the globin fraction of hemoglobin.
3. Sickle cell hemoglobin aggregates into elongated crystals under conditions of low oxygen concentration, acidosis, and dehydration.

TABLE 49-2 Transmission of Sickle Cell Disease

Genotype of Parents	Probability of Abnormal Hemoglobin in Offspring		
	Normal	Trait	Disease
1 parent with trait	50%	50%	0
Both parents with trait	25%	50%	25%
1 parent with trait; 1 parent with disease	0	50%	50%
Both parents with disease	0	0	100%

4. This distorts the membrane of the RBC, causing it to assume a crescent or sickle shape. The cells easily become entangled and enmeshed leading to increased blood viscosity, vessel occlusion, and tissue necrosis.
5. Sickled RBCs are fragile and are rapidly destroyed in the circulation; they live 6 to 20 days versus 120 days for normal RBCs.
6. Anemia results when the rate of destruction of RBCs is greater than the rate of production.
7. Increased sequestration of RBCs occurs in the spleen.

Complications

1. Chronic hemolytic anemia
2. Greatest risk of death is in children under 5 years of age, mainly from overwhelming sepsis or sequestration.
3. Episodes of splenic sequestration, hemolysis, aplasia, vaso-occlusion
4. Life expectancy is variable; however, it is improving with new forms of treatment.

Clinical Manifestations

Children are rarely symptomatic until late in the first year of life, related to increased amounts of fetal hemoglobin (HgF). Clinical manifestations are sporadic; the child may be asymptomatic for several months. Periods of crisis occur at variable intervals.

A. *Signs of Anemia* May last 1 to 2 weeks and subside spontaneously

1. Hemoglobin—6 to 9 g/dL
2. Loss of appetite
3. Paleness
4. Weakness
5. Fever
6. Irritability
7. Jaundice; increased hemolysis results in hemosiderosis (increased iron storage in the liver)

B. *Precipitating Factors of Crisis*
1. Dehydration
2. Infection
3. Trauma
4. Strenuous physical exertion
5. Extreme fatigue
6. Cold exposure
7. Hypoxia
8. Acidosis

C. *Vaso-occlusive Crisis* Most common form of crisis

1. Small blood vessels are occluded by the sickle-shaped cells, causing distal ischemia and infarction.
2. Extremities
   a. Bony destruction—related to erythroid hyperplasia of marrow leading to osteoporosis or ischemic necrosis
   b. Bone pain; painful and swollen large joints
   c. Dactylitis ("hand–foot" syndrome)—aseptic infarction of metacarpals and metatarsals causing symmetrical swelling and pain; often first vaso-occlusive seen in infants and toddlers

3. Spleen
   a. Abdominal pain
   b. Splenomegaly—initially increases in size due to increased activity as site of RBC hemolysis; increased size results in discomfort.
   c. After multiple episodes of splenic vaso-occlusion, the spleen becomes fibrotic and atrophied.
   d. Decreased splenic function increases the risk of infection.
4. Cerebral occlusion
   a. Strokes
   b. Hemiplegia
   c. Retinal damage leading to blindness
   d. Seizures
5. Pulmonary infarction
6. Altered renal function: enuresis, hematuria
7. Impaired liver function
8. Priapism—abnormal, recurrent, prolonged, painful penile erection

D. **Splenic Sequestration Crisis**
1. Large amounts of blood become pooled in the spleen.
2. Spleen becomes massively enlarged.
3. Great decrease in RBC mass occurs within hours.
4. Signs of circulatory collapse develop rapidly.
5. Frequent cause of death in infant with sickle cell disease

E. **Aplastic Crisis**
1. Bone marrow ceases production of RBCs, only.
2. Results in low reticulocyte counts

F. **Chronic Symptoms**
Chronic organ damage results in organ dysfunction.

1. Jaundice
2. Gallstones
3. Progressive impairment of kidney function
4. Fibrotic spleen resulting in high susceptibility to *Haemophilus influenzae* and *Streptococcus pneumoniae* infections, osteomyelitis, and pneumococcal septicemia.
5. Growth retardation of the long bones and spine deformities
6. Delayed puberty
7. Cardiac decompensation related to chronic anemia
8. Chronic, painful leg ulcers related to decreased peripheral circulation and unrelated to injury; may take months to heal or may not heal without intense therapy including blood transfusions and grafting.
9. Decreased life span
10. Altered bony structures—aseptic necrosis of the bones, especially the femoral and humoral heads

Diagnostic Evaluation

NURSING ALERT:
In 1987, the National Institutes of Health issued guidelines for all infants born in the United States to be mandatorily tested for sickle cell disease. This is done before discharge using the sickle cell prep from a heel stick.

1. Sickle cell prep (sickling test)
   a. Done by finger or heel stick
   b. Oxygen is removed from a drop of blood.
   c. The blood is observed under the microscope for the presence of sickle-shaped cells.

   d. Test does not distinguish between persons with sickle cell trait and disease or other sickle hemoglobinopathies.
2. Sickledex
   a. Done by finger stick
   b. A small amount of blood is placed in a solution containing a chemical reducing agent.
   c. The presence of sickle hemoglobin is indicated if the solution turns cloudy.
   d. Test also does not distinguish between persons with sickle cell trait and disease or other sickle hemoglobinopathies.
3. Hemoglobin electrophoresis
   a. Requires venipuncture
   b. Hemoglobin is subjected to an electric current that separates the various types and determines the amounts present.
   c. Test is used to diagnose both sickle cell trait and sickle cell disease if two types of hemoglobin are demonstrated in approximately equal amounts.
   d. A person is diagnosed as having sickle cell anemia if the majority of hemoglobin is sickle hemoglobin. This may also diagnose other sickle hemoglobinopathies including sickle C, sickle–β-thalassemia, or other hemoglobin variants.
4. Antenatal diagnosis is available to the high-risk group through amniocentesis and gene mapping.

Treatment

A. **Prevent Sickling**
1. Promote adequate oxygenation and hemodilution.
   a. Encourage increased intake of fluids—150 mL/kg per day or 2,250 mL/m² per day.
   b. Avoid high altitudes and other low-oxygen environments.
   c. Avoid strenuous physical exertion.
   d. Administer oxygen for pulse oximetry of 90% or less.

B. **Crisis Episodes**
Supportive and symptomatic care depend on type.

1. Aplastic episode—usually requires a blood transfusion starting at 10 mL/kg
2. Splenic sequestration—usually requires a blood transfusion to release trapped RBCs in severe cases. Plasma volume expanders may also be used to correct hypovolemia. One or more episodes may require splenectomy.
3. Hemolytic episode—usually requires only hydration. May occur with splenic sequestration, aplastic, and painful episodes, which are then treated accordingly. Transfusions are required if there is a significant drop in hemoglobin.
4. Vaso-occlusive or painful episode—must be individualized; must determine if the painful event is a manifestation of an underlying illness (infection) or inflammatory condition. Most often due to increased sickling resulting from hypoxia and acidosis.
   a. Hydration—to reverse dehydration that may have been caused by decreased fluid intake, increased insensible loss, hyposthenuria, and hyperthermia (fever). This is accomplished by increased oral and parenteral fluid intake of up to one and a half or twice fluid maintenance needs.

b. Electrolyte and pH balance must be closely monitored.
c. Analgesics—administered on fixed schedule, not to extend beyond the duration of the pharmacologic effect. Intravenous (IV) narcotics such as morphine (Duramorph) are preferred for severe pain, either as a continuous infusion or on a patient-controlled analgesia (PCA) pump to reach desired effects. Other agents such as nonsteroidal anti-inflammatory drugs (NSAIDs) and acetaminophen (Tylenol) are used for milder pain or to increase the analgesic effects of narcotics.
d. Alternative pain management techniques—behavior modification programs, relaxation therapy, hypnosis, and transcutaneous electrical nerve stimulation (TENS)
e. New research on α-butyrate and hydroxyurea (Hydrea), which increase fetal hemoglobin and prevent sickling, is being conducted.
3. Infection—major cause of morbidity and mortality
a. Most serious include *S. pneumoniae*, *H. influenzae*, *Neisseria meningitidis*, *Salmonella* species, *Mycoplasma pneumoniae*, *Staphylococcus aureus*, *Escherichia coli*, and *Streptococcus pyogenes*.
b. Infection of any type is more difficult to eradicate in patients with sickle cell and often exacerbates crises such as aplastic episodes caused by parovirus (fifth disease), increases the rate of hemolysis, and precipitates vaso-occlusive episodes.
c. Prevention is most important—give usual primary immunizations as well as pneumococcal, *Haemophilus* b conjugate, hepatitis, meningococcal, and trivalent influenza vaccines.
d. Antibiotic prophylaxis—prevents bacteremia and reduces nasopharyngeal colonization.
e. Fever of 102°F (38.9°C) with minimal clinical signs should be treated with broad-spectrum antibiotics such as cefuroxime (Kefurox) 100 mg/kg per day to prevent septicemia. The choice of subsequent antibiotics can be guided by results of cultures and clinical course.

Nursing Assessment

1. Obtain history for possible dehydration, hypoxia, infection, or other precipitating event.
2. Obtain history and characterization of pain.
3. Observe for pallor and jaundice, changes in vital signs (elevated temperature, tachycardia, hypotension, tachypnea), change in mental status, swelling of extremities, ulcers or skin lesions, or signs of dehydration (decreased elasticity of skin, dry mucous membranes, decreased urine output, increased urine concentration and specific gravity).
4. Examine for enlarged liver and spleen, tenderness of hands or feet.
5. Evaluate growth and development.

Nursing Diagnoses

A. Pain related to tissue anoxia from disease process
B. Altered Tissue Perfusion related to increased blood viscosity

C. Risk for Infection related to fibrotic changes in the spleen
D. Impaired Gas Exchange related to effects of narcotics, anesthesia, and blood loss of surgery
E. Activity Intolerance related to anemia
F. Altered Family Process related to frequent medical care, hospitalization, and chronic illness

Nursing Interventions

Also see Nursing Care Plan 49-1: Painful Vaso-occlusive Crisis

A. *Relieving Pain*
1. Identify and use effective measures to alleviate pain such as:
a. Carefully position and support painful areas.
b. Hold or rock the infant; handle gently.
c. Distract the child by singing, reading stories, providing play activities.
d. Provide familiar objects; encourage visits by familiar persons.
e. Bathe the child in warm water, applying local heat or massage.
f. Give prescribed medications. *Do not* give aspirin because it enhances acidosis.
g. Maintain bed rest during crisis.
2. Share effective methods of reducing pain with other staff members and family.

B. *Increasing Tissue Perfusion*
1. Administer blood for severe anemia and vaso-occlusion.
2. Administer oxygen via tent, face mask, or nasal cannula, depending on age.

C. *Reducing Infection*
1. Administer antibiotics as prescribed.
2. Give meticulous care to leg ulcers and other open wounds.
3. Use good handwashing and meticulous technique in all procedures.

D. *Preventing Hypoxia*
1. Monitor for and prevent respiratory depression due to narcotics.
a. Check respiratory rate and depth frequently.
b. Encourage coughing and deep breathing.
c. Use incentive spirometry.
d. Obtain pulse oximetry reading as indicated.
e. Raise side rails and supervise ambulation if drowsiness occurs.
2. Help reduce the risks of anesthesia and blood loss during surgery.
a. Administer preoperative blood transfusion(s) as prescribed to suppress the formation of new sickle cells and to reduce the threat of anoxia.
b. Maintain adequate hydration before and after surgery.
c. Observe the child closely for signs of infection, especially of the respiratory tract.
d. Inform anesthesia department of child's disease status.
e. Monitor vital signs frequently and obtain pulse oximetry readings.

E. *Improving Activity Tolerance*
1. Maintain bed rest during crisis, then increase activity gradually to increase endurance.
2. Encourage rest periods alternating with activity.
3. Encourage good eating habits, sleep, and relaxation.

F. *Normalizing Family Processes*
1. Encourage parents to talk about their child, the illness, and how they feel about it.
2. Expect such feelings as guilt, shock, frustration, depression, and resentment.
3. Accept negative feelings but try to build on positive coping mechanisms.
4. Provide factual information to child and parents about their concerns.
5. Encourage role playing and play activities to identify fears.
6. Assure adolescents that although sexual development is delayed, they will eventually catch up with their peers.
7. Stress the normalcy of the child despite sickle cell.
   a. Sickle cell disease does not affect intelligence; the child should go to school and keep up with class work while stable.
   b. Between periods of crisis the child can usually participate in peer group activities with the exception of some strenuous sports.
   c. The child needs discipline and limit setting as do other children in family.

Family Education/Health Maintenance

1. Discuss the genetic implications of sickle cell disease and offer genetic counseling to the family.
2. Instruct the parents in ways that they can help their child to avoid sickling episodes.
   a. Do not allow the child to become chilled or to wear tight clothing that might impede circulation.
   b. Provide adequate fluids and notify health care provider if excessive fluids are lost through vomiting, diarrhea, fever, excessive sweating.
3. Instruct parents how to recognize signs of dehydration (dry skin and mucous membranes, decreased urine output; irritability or listlessness in the infant).
4. Encourage parents to seek prompt treatment of cuts, sores, mosquito bites, etc. and to notify the health care provider if the child is exposed to a communicable disease.
5. Encourage good dental hygiene and frequent dental checkups to avoid dental infections.
6. Instruct on preventive care including all the normal childhood immunizations and a tuberculin test every 2 to 3 years. In addition, children over age 2 should receive the pneumococcal, *Haemophilus* type b, meningococcal, recombinant hepatitis B (series of 3), varicella, and trivalent influenza (yearly) vaccines.
7. Teach the child to avoid undue emotional stress.

8. Warn against trips to the mountains or in unpressurized airplanes that will decrease oxygen concentration.
9. Provide sexually active adolescents with information on contraception and sexually transmitted disease.
10. Teach signs of a mild crisis:
    a. Fever
    b. Decreased appetite
    c. Irritability
    d. Pain or swelling in abdomen, extremities, back
    e. Teach parents to palpate spleen.
11. Instruct on home management of mild crisis.
    a. Push fluids.
    b. Administer antipyretic medications, as directed by health care provider familiar with condition.
    c. Encourage rest.
    d. Keep the child warm.
    e. Apply warm compresses to the painful area.
    f. Hospitalization may be required for the child if pain becomes severe or if IV hydration is required.
12. Teach the signs of severe crises and who to notify:
    a. Pallor
    b. Lethargy and listlessness
    c. Difficulty in awakening
    d. Irritability
    e. Severe pain
    f. Fever of 102°F (38.9°C)—report immediately
13. Instruct the parents to have emergency information available to those involved in the child's care (school nurse, teacher, babysitter, family members, etc.).
    a. Name and phone number of health care provider or clinic
    b. Closest emergency facility and ambulance phone number
    c. Child's blood type, allergies, medications, and medical records number
    d. Name of informed neighbor or relative to be notified in an emergency
14. Stress the benefit of wearing a Medic Alert tag.
15. For additional information and support refer to Sickle Cell Foundation; 4401 Crenshaw Blvd., Suite 208; Los Angeles, CA 90043; 213-299-3600.

Evaluation

A. Appears more comfortable and does not cry or complain of pain
B. Less pallor noted with oxygen use
C. Afebrile with no signs of infection
D. No change in respirations; using incentive spirometer hourly

---

NURSING CARE PLAN 49-1 ◆ *Painful Vaso-occlusive Crisis*

You are assigned Danielle, a 6-year-old with sickle cell anemia who has been admitted with a fever of 38.9°C (102°F), chest pain, bilateral leg pain, and an oxygen saturation of 90%.

Subjective Data: Danielle complains of bilateral leg pain, states that it hurts to breathe, and she has the chills. She felt tired and had a great deal of pain yesterday and was unable to go to school. Mom was giving her some pain medication at home, but when she spiked a fever, she was brought to the emergency room and admitted to your unit.

(continued)

NURSING CARE PLAN 49-1 ◆ *Painful Vaso-occlusive Crisis* (continued)

Objective Data: Vital signs—temperature of 38.2°C (100.7°F), pulse 120, BP 90/52, and respirations of 34. You notice that her legs are warm and swollen, tender to touch. Respiratory evaluation reveals bilateral crackles at the lung bases, labored respirations with O_2 mask on, and pallor.

Laboratory data:
1. CBC—WBC, 15.4; HgB, 6.5; Hct, 20.1; and platelets, 636,000
2. Pulse oximetry—90%
3. Chest x-ray—bilateral lower lobe pneumonia
4. Electrolytes—Na, 131; Cl, 110; K, 4.8
5. Blood, urine, and throat cultures are pending.

You know that hypoxia, dehydration, and acidosis may have been caused by the underlying respiratory infection and can all precipitate vaso-oclusive crisis. You develop your plan of care to focus on resolution of these factors and to support the patient through crisis.

NURSING DIAGNOSIS: Impaired Gas Exchange related to pneumonia

GOAL: Oxygenation will be enhanced and respiratory acidosis will be prevented.

NURSING INTERVENTIONS	RATIONALE	EVALUATION
1. Administer oxygen via face mask to relieve dyspnea and promote oxygenation. a. Obtain pulse oximetry reading frequently and correlate with arterial blood gas results. b. Assess respiratory rate, use of accessory muscles and depth of respirations.	1. Secretion-filled aveoli impair gas exchange leading to hypoxemia a. Pulse oximetry serves as guide to improving or worsening oxygenation. Arterial blood gases should be done for correlation and to evaluate acid–base status. b. Increasing rate, decreasing depth, and increased effort of breathing may lead to respiratory failure.	1. Respirations 34, shallow, and with sternal retractions on face mask. Pulse oximetry 88%. Changed to Venturi mask at 40%.
2. Administer bronchodilator nebulization treatments q3h, followed by cough and deep breathing exercises. Auscultate lungs hourly.	2. Will promote opening of airways and expectoration of secretions. Frequent auscultation of lungs will help evaluate effectiveness of therapy and determine the need for corticosteroids to reduce inflammation and open the airways further.	2. Lungs clearer following nebulization and coughing.
3. Administer IV antibiotics, as ordered.	3. To resolve pneumonia.	3. Antibiotic infusing via peripheral line.

NURSING DIAGNOSIS: Pain related to tissue anoxia due to abnormal hemoglobin and clumping of sickled cells within the small vessels

GOAL: Pain will be relieved.

NURSING INTERVENTIONS	RATIONALE	EVALUATION
1. Use nonpharmacologic strategies to help manage pain: distraction, relaxation, guided imagery, positive self-talk, cutaneous stimulation (warm soaks, massage, etc), behavioral contracting. a. Involve parent and child in selecting strategies. b. Institute and teach selected strategies before pain becomes severe.	1. Will limit the amount of analgesia, which may depress respirations. a. Child will be more receptive to own choices and allows participation in care. b. If pain is severe, child may not be able to concentrate on these strategies if not practiced.	1. Child uses blowing, looks at magic wand, listens to relaxation tapes and videos; states that they help.
2. Administer prescribed analgesia around the clock. Avoid PRN orders when pain is predictable and continuous.	2. To maintain a steady state of analgesia and prevent clock watching.	2. Receives medication q4h without breakthrough pain reported.

(continued)

NURSING CARE PLAN 49-1 ◆ *Painful Vaso-occlusive Crisis* (continued)

NURSING ALERT:
Avoid IM analgesia if possible because children associate great deal of pain with shots and may deny pain to avoid getting shot.

3. Assess pain relief and increase or decrease dose or time interval of medication for adequate control.
   a. Avoid placebo.
   b. Assess for respiratory depression, hypotension, and drowsiness with narcotics.

3. To maximize analgesia with minimal side effects.
   a. If expected effect is not received by placebo, child may lose trust in caretakers.
   b. Narcotics may cause CNS depression, shallow respirations, and hypotension in large or frequent dosing.

3. No breakthrough pain with increased time interval (6 h) between doses.
   b. Alert, respirations 24 and deep, BP 96/56

NURSING DIAGNOSIS: Fluid Volume Deficit related to fever, insensible loss through mouth breathing and increased respiratory rate, and increased blood viscosity

GOAL: Hydration will be promoted.

NURSING INTERVENTIONS	RATIONALE	EVALUATION
1. Administer IV fluids as ordered based on calculation of recommended daily fluid intake requirements plus estimated loss.	1. Child should consume approximately 1,500 mL/m². Loss may be established by decrease in body weight (1 kg equals 1 liter of fluid).	1. D₅NS infusing via peripheral IV volumetric pump.
2. Encourage child to drink by providing fluids preferred.	2. Intake will be enhanced by using preferences.	2. Sipping juices at intervals.
3. Monitor intake and output. Monitor urine specific gravity.	3. To determine fluid balance and hydration status.	3. Intake and output equal; urine specific gravity 1.020.
4. Administer acetaminophen for fever over 38°C (100.4°F) and maintain bed rest.	4. To reduce fluid loss through perspiration due to fever or exertion.	4. Temperature 37.5°C (99.5°F).

E. Ambulating 20 minutes four or five times a day
F. Parents verbalizing concerns about chronic illness

◆ THALASSEMIA MAJOR (COOLEY'S ANEMIA)

Thalassemia major is the most severe of the β-thalassemia syndromes and represents the homozygous form of the disease. *Beta-thalassemia* (*β-thalassemia*) refers to an inherited hemolytic anemia characterized by a reduction or absence of the β-globulin chain in hemoglobin synthesis.

This RBC has a decreased amount of hemoglobin resulting in a fragile RBC with a short life span.

Etiology/Incidence

1. Genetically determined, inherited disease
2. Autosomal recessive pattern of inheritance
3. Homozygous form of the disease
4. Most prevalent in the Mediterranean basin, Middle East, Southeast Asia, and Africa
5. In the United States, it is most common in children of Italian, Greek, and Southeastern Asian ancestry.
6. About 1,400 people in the United States are affected.

Altered Physiology

1. Insufficient β-globin chain synthesis allows large amounts of unstable α chains to accumulate.
2. The precipitates of α chains that form cause RBCs to be rigid and easily destroyed, leading to severe hemolytic anemia and resultant chronic hypoxia.
3. Erythroid activity is markedly increased in an attempt to overcome the increased rate of destruction, resulting in enormous expansion of bone marrow, thinning of bony cortex leading to:
   a. Skeletal deformities: frontal and maxillary bossing
   b. Growth retardation
   c. Pathologic fractures
4. Rapid destruction of defective RBCs, decreased production of hemoglobin, and increased absorption of dietary iron due to the body's response to anemia result

in an excess supply of available iron (hemosiderosis), which deposits iron on organ tissues resulting in decreased function (especially cardiac).

5. In response to the low level of adult hemoglobin, large concentrations of HgF, which does not contain β chains, are produced; HgF does not hold oxygen well.

Complications

1. Splenomegaly—usually requires splenectomy; overwhelming postsplenectomy infection rate seen in 25% of these patients
2. Growth retardation in second decade
3. Endocrine abnormalities
   a. Delayed development of secondary sex characteristics—the majority of boys fail to undergo puberty; most girls experience alteration in menstruation.
   b. Diabetes mellitus is often seen in older patients, related to iron deposits on the pancreas.
   c. Hypermetabolic rate results in increased temperature and lethargy.
4. Skeletal complications—becoming less common because of early transfusion therapy and keeping hemoglobin levels above 10 g/dL.
   a. Frontal and parietal bossing (enlarging)
   b. Maxillary hypertrophy leading to malocclusion
   c. Broad ribs
   d. Premature fusion of epiphyses of long bones
   e. Generalized skeletal osteoporosis
   f. Pathologic fractures of the long bones and vertebral collapse
5. Cardiac complications
   a. Fibrosis and hypertrophy
   b. Pericarditis
   c. Congestive heart failure—usual cause of death
6. Liver enlargement—fibrosis, coagulation abnormalities, and eventually cirrhosis
7. Gallbladder disease—gallstones are common by late adolescence; may require cholecystectomy
8. Megaloblastic anemia—due to sporadic folic acid deficiency from increased use by hyperplastic marrow
9. Skin—bronze pigmentation due to iron deposits in the dermis; jaundice
10. Leg ulcers

Clinical Manifestations

1. Onset is usually insidious, with symptoms noted toward the end of the first year of life.
2. Symptoms are primarily related to the progressive anemia, expansion of the marrow cavities of the bone, and the development of hemosiderosis
3. Early symptoms often include progressive pallor, poor feeding, and lethargy.
4. Further signs of progressive anemia include headache, bone pain, exercise intolerance, jaundice, and protuberant abdomen due to hepatosplenomegaly.

Diagnostic Evaluation

1. Hemoglobin level—decreased
2. RBCs—increased number

3. Low mean corpuscular volume (MCV) and mean corpuscular hemoglobin (MCHC) concentration—microcytosis and hypochromia
4. Peripheral blood smear—many anisopoikilocytes, nucleated RBCs
5. Reticulocyte count—low, usually less than 10%
6. Hemoglobin electrophoresis—elevated levels of HgF and HgA$_2$; limited amount of HgA

Treatment

1. Frequent and regular blood transfusions of packed RBCs to maintain hemoglobin levels above 10 g/dL
   a. Washed, packed RBCs are usually used to minimize the possibility of transfusion reactions. If unavailable, leukofiltered cells can be substituted.
   b. The frequency and amount of transfusions depend on the size of the child, usually 10 to 15 mL packed RBC per kg body weight every 2 to 3 weeks.
2. Iron chelation therapy with deferoxamine (Desferal) reduces the toxic side effects of excess iron; increases iron excretion through urine and feces.
   a. IV infusion of 100 to 150 mg/kg per day given in hospital during blood transfusion or for child with very high ferritin level and poor compliance with home chelation therapy
   b. Subcutaneous infusion of 50 mg/kg per day usually infused over 12 hours during night for home therapy
3. Splenectomy
4. Supportive management of complications
5. Bone marrow transplants are a possibility; however, the survival rate is poor. Young patients with few complications are good candidates.
6. Prognosis is poor because there is no known cure; often fatal in late adolescence or early adulthood.

Nursing Assessment

1. Obtain family history of β-thalassemia or unexplained anemia or heart failure.
2. Perform whole body examination to assess for anemia and systemic complications of thalassemia.
3. Measure growth and development parameters.

Nursing Diagnoses

A. Altered Tissue Perfusion related to abnormal hemoglobin
B. Chronic Pain related to progression of disease in bone
C. Activity Intolerance related to bone pain, cardiac dysfunction, and anemia
D. Risk for Infection related to progressive anemia and splenectomy
E. Knowledge Deficit related to iron chelation therapy
F. Body Image Disturbance related to endocrine and skeletal abnormalities
G. Ineffective Family Coping related to poor prognosis

Nursing Interventions

A. *Maximizing Tissue Perfusion*
1. Administer blood transfusions as ordered.
   a. Observe for signs of transfusion reaction (increased chance due to frequency) including allergic, febrile, septic, circulatory overload, and hemolytic reactions.

b. Allergic reactions usually occur within 15 to 20 minutes of start of the transfusion.
c. Be aware that delayed reactions may occur up to several months later.

2. Monitor cardiovascular status for complications.
   a. Monitor apical pulse, blood pressure, and respirations.
   b. Assess for edema.
   c. Auscultate heart sounds for gallop and lungs for rales.
   d. Assess extremities for ulcer formation.
3. Refer to care of the child with congestive heart failure (see p. 1208).

B. Relieving Bone Pain
1. Monitor CBC as ordered and report hemoglobin levels of less than 10 g/dL.
2. Elevate lower extremities.
3. Provide warm baths or soaks.
4. Administer or teach proper administration of NSAIDs such as ibuprofen (Motrin) or naproxen (Naprosyn).
   a. Use carefully and monitor liver enzymes in patients with liver complications.

C. Minimizing Activity Intolerance
1. Encourage participation in activities that do not require significant strenuous activity. Full participation in some activities, especially with peers, will increase self-esteem.
2. Facilitate physical and occupational therapy consultation to develop an acceptable exercise plan.
3. Assist the parents in contacting the child's school and develop a plan of gym activities, classes, and rest periods that allow the greatest level of participation and slowly develop endurance. Advise parents that during week for the scheduled transfusion, the fatigue will be greatest so gym and other exertional activities should be modified.
4. Suggest that driving the child to school and providing adequate rest at home will provide the child with more energy for school activities.
5. Discourage participation in contact or other sports that increase the child's risk for a fracture (skateboarding, football, soccer, etc.).

D. Preventing Infection
1. Explain to parents that after splenectomy, child has increased susceptibility to infection and should be maintained on oral penicillin prophylaxis.
2. Ensure that child has been vaccinated against *H. influenzae*, pneumococcal, and meningococcal infections before splenectomy and encourage yearly trivalent influenza vaccination.
3. Encourage prompt medical attention for fever or signs of infection. Fever of 102°F (38.9°C) should be reported immediately and IV broad-spectrum antibiotics such ceftriaxone (Rocephin) started.

E. Promoting Understanding and Compliance
1. Explain to family that deferoxamine (Desferal) is used as a chelating (binding) agent to decrease iron deposits in tissues and to increase iron excretion through urine and feces.
2. Administer IV deferoxamine as ordered.
   a. Infuse slowly, over 8 to 24 hours, through peripheral line or implanted infusion device, via volumetric pump.
   b. Have emergency resuscitation equipment nearby in case severe allergic reaction occurs.
3. Teach administration of subcutaneous deferoxamine and initiate referral for home infusion therapy.

a. Infuse over 12 hours, usually overnight.
b. Pick a site in the subcutaneous tissue in the abdomen, thigh, or arm and insert a small subcutaneous needle attached to a syringe pump.
c. Emla, a topical anesthetic, may be used to decrease pain at the insertion site.
d. Infusion site may become red, hard, and painful. Must rotate sites. Warm soaks to area are helpful.
e. Because allergic reaction may occur, instruct parents to give antihistamine and if necessary, epinephrine.
4. Be alert for visual and hearing deficits associated with use of deferoxamine and encourage follow-up for periodic visual and audiometric testing.

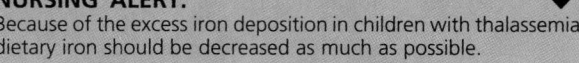

NURSING ALERT:
Because of the excess iron deposition in children with thalassemia, dietary iron should be decreased as much as possible.

F. Improving Body Image
1. Explore the child's feelings of being different from other children.
2. Encourage the child to express feelings through the use of play: art, role playing, etc.
3. Give positive reinforcement regarding appearance.
4. Encourage socialization and peer interaction.
5. Suggest endocrine consultation for delayed growth and puberty and craniofacial specialist for bony abnormalities.
6. Encourage the use of makeup, clothing, hair styles that will make the adolescent appear older.
7. Suggest support group or individual counseling as needed.

G. Improving Family Coping Strategies
1. Alleviate the child's anxieties about illness by providing explanation in a way the child can understand.
2. Use role playing and play activities to identify concerns.
3. Assist parents in strengthening coping mechanisms such as support network, problem solving, and planning ahead.
4. Help identify resources for financial support, medical supplies, respite care, etc.
5. Encourage parents to continue education of child and obtain vocational planning, if realistic.
6. Encourage parents to set limits and provide discipline for child consistent with other children in family.
7. Provide supportive care to the dying child (see p. 1134).
8. Encourage bereavement support for parents, siblings, and family.

Family Education/Health Maintenance

1. Discuss the genetic implications of thalassemia and refer for genetic counseling.
2. Provide detailed instruction regarding:
   a. Prevention and prompt treatment of infections
   b. Medications
   c. Home chelation therapy
   d. Dietary modifications to limit iron intake

e. Activity restrictions including avoidance of activities that increase the risk of fractures

f. Signs of complications

3. Encourage parents to provide information about the child's condition to significant adults who are involved with the child (teacher, school nurse, babysitter, Scout leader, etc.).

4. For additional information and support refer to Cooley's Anemia Foundation 129-09 26th Ave., Room 203; Flushing, NY 11354; 718-321-2873.

Evaluation

A. Blood pressure stable; no edema; no leg ulcers

B. Verbalizes better tolerance of pain

C. Reports increased participation in activity, less fatigue

D. Afebrile; immunizations current

E. Parents verbalizing purpose of chelation therapy, treatment of allergic reaction, how to treat site; demonstrating correct technique for infusion

F. Verbalizing interest in appearance and positive statements about self

G. Parents seeking help from support group and social worker; discussing illness with child and siblings

◆ HEMOPHILIA

Hemophilia is usually an inherited, congenital bleeding disorder characterized by a lack of blood clotting factors, especially factors VIII and IX. It appears primarily in males but is transmitted by females.

Etiology/Incidence

1. Hereditary (about 80% of patients)
   a. Sex-linked, recessive trait—caused by a gene carried on the X chromosome
   b. Transmitted by asymptomatic females (Table 49-3)
   c. Appears in males who have the hemophilic gene on their only X chromosome
   d. Affected males may pass the gene to female offspring, making them carriers.
   e. May appear in females if a female carrier bears offspring with a male hemophiliac

2. Spontaneous mutations may cause the condition when the family history is negative for the disease (about 20% of patients).

3. Occurs in 1/5,000 males
   a. Eighty to 85% have factor VIII deficiency or hemophilia A (classic hemophilia).
   b. Fifteen to 20% have factor IX deficiency or hemophilia B (Christmas disease).
   c. Very few have factor XI deficiency or hemophilia C.

4. There is no racial predilection and hemophilia is found in all ethnic groups.

Altered Physiology

1. Hemophilia results from the absence or malfunction of any one of the blood clotting factors from the plasma. The basic defect is in the intrinsic phase of the coagulation cascade.

2. The blood clotting factors are necessary for the formation of prothrombin activator, which acts as a catalyst in the conversion of prothrombin to thrombin.
   a. The rate of formation of thrombin from prothrombin is almost directly proportional to the amount of prothrombin activator available.
   b. The rapidity of the clotting process is proportional to the amount of thrombin formed.

3. The result is an unstable fibrin clot.

4. Platelet number and function are normal; therefore, small lacerations and minor hemorrhages are usually not a problem.

Complications

1. Airway obstruction due to hemorrhage into the neck and pharynx

2. Repeated hemorrhages may produce degenerative joint changes with osteoporosis and muscle atrophy.

3. Intestinal obstruction due to bleeding into intestinal walls or peritoneum

4. Compression of nerves with paralysis due to hemorrhaging into deep tissues; known as compartment syndrome

5. Intracranial bleeding resulting in serious neurologic impairments

6. Death may result from from exsanguination after any serious hemorrhage such as intracranial, airway, or other highly vascular areas.

7. Contaminated cryoprecipitate, fresh frozen plasma, and concentrates have resulted in chronic active hepatitis and secondary cirrhosis.

TABLE 49-3 Transmission of Hemophilia

| | Probability of Abnormality in Offspring | | | | |
| | Female | | | Male | |
Genotype of Parents	Normal	Carrier	Hemophiliac	Normal	Hemophiliac
Female carrier/normal male	50%	50%	0	50%	50%
Noncarrier female/hemophiliac male	0	100%	0	100%	0
Female carrier/hemophiliac male	0	50%	50%	50%	50%

8. Acquired immunodeficiency syndrome (AIDS) and human immunodeficiency virus (HIV)-related infections in patients receiving transfusions before 1985 with nontested HIV-contaminated blood products
9. Uncertain life span for many hemophiliacs as a result of complications from hemorrhage or blood-borne viruses (hepatitis/AIDS). However, as a result of advances in therapy, viral inactivation of human plasma-derived factor concentrates and the new recombinant factor VIII concentrate, a normal life span is now possible.
10. It has been estimated that 20% of the patients with hemophilia will develop an inhibitor or an autoantibody to the infused factor replacement. This results in more serious hemorrhages as a result of the difficulty in treating these patients to control the hemorrhage.

Clinical Manifestations

1. Seldom diagnosed in infancy unless excessive bleeding is observed from the umbilical cord or after circumcision
2. Usually diagnosed after the child becomes active
3. Varies in severity depending on the plasma level of the coagulation factor involved
   a. Level of less than 1% of normal—severe hemophilia; often severe clinical bleeding with a tendency for spontaneous bleeds
   b. Level of 1% to 5% of normal—moderately afflicted; may be free of spontaneous bleeding and may not manifest severe bleeding until after trauma
   c. Level of 6% to 30% of normal—mildly afflicted; usually lead normal lives and bleed only with severe injury or surgery
   d. Degree of severity tends to be constant within a given family.
4. Signs and symptoms of abnormal bleeding include:
   a. History of prolonged bleeding episodes, such as after circumcision
   b. Easily bruised
   c. Prolonged bleeding from the mucous membranes of the nose and mouth from lacerations
   d. Spontaneous soft tissue hematomas
   e. Hemorrhages into the joints (hemarthrosis)—especially elbows, knees, and ankles causing pain, swelling, limitation of movement
   f. Spontaneous hematuria
   g. Gastrointestinal bleeding
   h. Cyclic bleeding episodes may occur with periods of little bleeding followed by periods of severe bleeding.
   i. Head trauma resulting in intracranial hemorrhage

Diagnostic Evaluation

1. Prothrombin time and bleeding time are normal
2. Partial thromboplastin time—prolonged
3. Prothrombin consumption—decreased
4. Thromboplastin—increased
5. Assays for specific clotting factors—abnormal
6. Gene analysis—to detect carrier state, for prenatal diagnosis

Treatment

1. Prompt early appropriate treatment is the key to preventing most complications.
2. Must replace missing coagulation factor (VIII or IX) through the administration of type-specific coagulation concentrates during bleeding episodes
   a. Factor VIII—made from cryoprecipitate that has been viral inactivated, monoclonal or solvent detergent purified. The monoclonal concentrates are the cleanest because most viruses and extraneous proteins have been removed. Since 1993, recombinant factor VIII concentrates are available for use. The factor VIII molecule has been sequenced and placed in a mammalian cell culture to produce recombinant factor VIII, which is free of all viruses.
   b. Factor IX—made from fresh frozen plasm that has been viral inactivated, by solvent detergent, monoclonal, heptane vapor, or affinity chromatography. The purest factor IX products are those that have gone through the monoclonal process or the affinity chromatography process that removes most viruses and any other extraneous proteins and other factors. These are known as factor IX coagulation concentrates.
3. No viral inactivated concentrate exists for hemophilia C; fresh frozen plasma is given to supply factor XI.
4. Mild and moderate factor VIII-deficient hemophiliacs may respond to desmopressin (DDAVP), which causes the release of factor VIII from the endothelial stores. It is given in a dose of 0.3 μg/kg per dose, usually every 24 hours.
5. Antifibrinolytics such as aminocaproic acid (Amicar) and tranexamic acid (Cyklokapron) are given as adjunctive therapy for mucosal bleeding to prevent clot breakdown by salivary proteins.
6. Activated prothrombin complex concentrates that have activated factors VII, X, and IX are used when inhibitors (autoantibodies) have developed, to bypass factor VIII or IX. In the case of factor VIII inhibitors, porcine factor VIII may also be given.
7. Supportive therapies
   a. NSAIDs are used to decrease inflammation and arthritic-like pain associated with chronic hemarthroses. Must be used with caution because some types and higher doses interfere with platelet adhesion.
   b. Physical therapy to prevent contractures and muscle atrophy. This includes exercise, whirlpool, and icing.
   c. Orthotics to prevent injury to affected joint and help to resolve hemorrhages
8. Synovectomy—orthopedic surgical intervention to remove damaged synovium in chronically involved joints
   a. Open procedure provides direct visualization of joint and removal of damaged tissue.
   b. Arthroscopic—visualization and removal of the joint synovium through the use of an arthroscope
   c. Radionucleotide—instillation of ^{32}P that removes damaged synovium; usually done through a needle
9. Research into gene therapy—genetic copies of sequenced factor VIII and IX molecules are inserted into the body via some type of vector cell to find their way into the human host genetic machinery and begin to produce either factor VIII or factor IX in deficient patients.

Nursing Assessment

1. Obtain history of and observe for unusual bleeding—eccyhmosis, prolonged bleeding from mucous membranes and lacerations, hematomas, hemarthroses, hematuria, rectal and gastrointestinal bleeding.
2. Assess joints for swelling, warmth, tenderness, range of motion, contractures, and surrounding muscle atrophy.

Nursing Diagnoses

A. Risk for Fluid Volume Deficit related to hemorrhage
B. Altered Protection related to inability of blood to clot
C. Impaired Physical Mobility related to repeated hemarthroses
D. Pain related to bleeding into joints and muscles
E. Ineffective Family Coping related to disabling and life-threatening disease

Nursing Interventions

A. *Preventing Hypovolemia Through Control of Bleeding*
1. Provide emergency care for bleeding.
   a. Apply pressure and cold on the area for 10 to 15 minutes to allow clot formation. This should especially be done after any venipuncture or injection.
   b. Place fibrin foam or absorbable gelatin foam in the wound.
   c. Suturing and cauterization should be avoided.
2. Immobilize the affected part and elevate above the level of the heart.
3. Administer recombinant factor VIII or factor IX coagulation concentrate.
   a. Avoid rapid administration to minimize the possibility of transfusion reaction; usually 2 to 3 mL/min; consult package inserts.
   b. Cryoprecipitate and fresh frozen plasma are not recommended due to their lack of viral inactivation treatment.
   c. Stop the transfusion if hives, headaches, tingling, chills, flushing, or fever occurs.
4. Apply fibrinolytic agents to wound for oral bleeding.
5. Keep child quiet during treatment to decrease pulse and rate of bleeding.
6. Monitor vital signs and treat for shock if child becomes hypotensive (see p. 952).

B. *Providing Protection Against Bleeding*
1. Avoid rectal temperatures; insert thermometer probe gently and use axillary, oral (if age appropriate), or external ear route.
2. Avoid injections if possible.
   a. Administer medications orally whenever possible.
   b. Subcutaneous route is preferred over intramuscular.
   c. Apply pressure to injection site for 10 to 15 minutes. Then apply a pressure dressing with self-adhesive gauze (Coban).

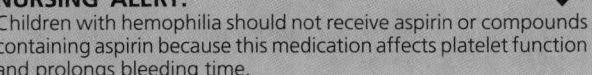

NURSING ALERT:
Children with hemophilia should not receive aspirin or compounds containing aspirin because this medication affects platelet function and prolongs bleeding time.

3. Maintain a safe environment and teach parents safety measures.
   a. Pad crib or bed rails.
   b. Inspect toys for sharp or rough edges.
   c. Offer finger foods and fluids in plastic or paper containers.
   d. Supervise small children when they are ambulatory.
   e. Use protective devices that the child brings from home. (Many children wear helmets, knee and elbow pads.)
   f. Continually assess environment for potential hazards.
   g. No straws or sharp eating utensils
   h. No hard candy, suckers, or candy canes

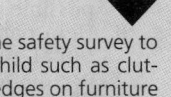

COMMUNITY-BASED CARE TIP:
Perform or encourage parents to perform a home safety survey to identify potential hazards to the hemophiliac child such as cluttered furniture the child may bump into, sharp edges on furniture or other objects, loose rugs that promote falls, slippery tub or floor surfaces, rocks or holes in backyard, or concrete play areas.

C. *Preserving Mobility*
1. Treat hemarthrosis or muscle bleed as soon as possible.
2. Provide supportive care for hemarthrosis.
   a. Immobilize the joint in a position of slight flexion.
   b. Elevate the affected part above the level of the heart.
   c. Apply ice packs. Later, after active bleeding has stopped, apply heat to promote absorption of blood.
3. For severe hemarthroses, continue immobilization through casting, if necessary, and prevent weight bearing on the affected limb.
4. For less severe hemarthroses, begin gentle, passive exercise 48 hours after the acute phase to prevent joint stiffness and fibrosis. Progress to active exercises.
5. Administer short course of corticosteroids as ordered to relieve inflammation.
6. Refer for physical therapy if persistent deformity or if crutches, braces, splints, or specialized treatments are needed.

D. *Relieving Pain*
1. Be aware that increased pain usually means that there is continuing bleeding and further replacement therapy may be needed.
2. Assess for further swelling of joints and limitation of movement.
3. Administer or teach administration of acetaminophen (Tylenol) during acute phase. NSAIDs may be used for chronic pain, but cautiously to prevent interference with platelet function.
4. Administer narcotics sparingly, as ordered for severe, acute pain.
5. For chronic pain consider alternatives such as hypnosis, biofeedback, relaxation techniques, and TENS.

E. *Enhancing Family Coping*
1. Help parents understand that no one is to blame.
2. Allow the child and other family members to handle equipment used in care.
3. Use play to help the young child and siblings adjust to illness by "transfusing" teddy bear, etc.
4. Encourage the parents to allow the child to participate in as many normal activities as possible within the realm of safety.

5. Encourage the child's continuing education. Parents fear sending the child to school, but safety issues can be addressed through discussions with the school nurse, teachers, and principal. Home or hospital tutoring should be continued while child is away from school.
6. Refer to social worker for counseling and identification of resources for financial concerns, etc.
7. Encourage avoidance of overprotection—this can be more disabling than the disease itself.
   a. Promote a sense of independence and self-care within the patient's limitations.
   b. Encourage healthful activity and reasonably aggressive pursuits. Reinforce self-judgment of child or teenager in selection of safe physical activities.
   c. Participate in as many age-appropriate activities as possible.
   d. Help parents understand the importance of vocational guidance for their child—emphasis given to occupations using intellect or skills rather than physical effort.
8. Encourage involvement in support group.

Family Education/Health Maintenance

1. Review safety measures to prevent or minimize trauma.
2. Encourage education by parents to teachers, babysitters, and others involved of child's care so that they can be responsive in an emergency.
3. Advise wearing a Medic Alert bracelet.
4. Remind parents not to administer aspirin to the child.
5. Teach emergency treatment for hemorrhage.
   a. Immobilize the part with splints or an elastic compression bandage. (These materials should be immediately available in the home.)
   b. Apply ice packs. Parents should keep two or three plastic bags of ice immediately available in the freezer.
   c. Consult the child's health care provider and initiate additional recommended therapy.
6. Encourage regular medical and dental supervision.
   a. Preventive dental care is important. Soft-bristled or sponge-tipped toothbrushes should be used to prevent bleeding. Factor replacement therapy is necessary for extensive dental work and extractions.
   b. Hepatitis B vaccine is necessary to protect against hepatitis from blood transfusions.

7. Teach healthy diet to avoid overweight, which places additional strain on the child's weight-bearing joints and predisposes to hemarthroses. Also, teach child to avoid sharp utensils, hard candy, suckers, and other foods with sharp edges that may cause mucosal lacerations.
8. Assist the parents in teaching the child to understand the exact nature of the illness as early as possible. Special attention should be given to the signs of hemorrhage, and the child should be told of the need to report even the slightest bleeding to an adult immediately.
9. Provide teaching and referrals to initiate a home care program—parents and child administer infusion therapy at home when hemorrhage begins. Assist with teaching the following:
   a. How to assess the child to determine if and what treatment is needed
   b. Storage and preparation of replacement factors
   c. Venipuncture technique
   d. Transfusion management
   e. Record keeping
   f. Awareness of signs of transfusion reaction and its management
   g. Recognition of indications of need for subsequent transfusions
10. Advise families that genetic counseling and family planning are available for parents and adolescent patients.
11. Educate regarding hepatitis B and C and HIV disease, risks of treatment.
12. For additional information and support, refer to National Hemophilia Foundation; 104 East 40th St., Suite 506; New York, NY 10016; 212-682-5510; National Center for Education in Maternal and Child Health; 2000 15th Street North, Suite 701; Arlington, VA 22201-2617; 703-524-7802.

Evaluation

A. Bleeding controlled; blood pressure stable
B. Needle sticks avoided; staff and parents observing safety precautions
C. Performing passive range of motion without pain
D. Verbalizing relief of pain with acetaminophen
E. Parents participating in care, playing with child

◆ HYPERBILIRUBINEMIA

See Box 49-1.

BOX 49-1 *Hyperbilirubinemia*

Hyperbilirubinemia (jaundice) in the newborn is an accumulation of serum bilirubin above normal levels. It results from increased load of bilirubin from RBC destruction and/or decreased clearance of bilirubin from plasma.

Causes
1. Increased bilirubin load
   a. Hemolytic disease—Rh and ABO incompatibility
   b. Morphologic abnormalities of red blood cells
   c. Red blood cell enzyme defects
   d. Physiologic jaundice
2. Extravascular blood—cephalohematoma; pulmonary or cerebral hemorrhage; any enclosed occult blood

Management/Nursing Care
1. Phototherapy—to allow for utilization of alternate pathways for bilirubin excretion; effectiveness depends on intensity of illumination; area of skin exposed; and effect on bilirubin in skin.
   a. Check light intensity for therapeutic range daily (425–475 nm).
   b. Ensure that light is 45–60 cm from infant and that plexiglass shield is in place
   c. Make sure that infant is under the light for prescribed time daily

BOX 49-1   *Hyperbilirubinemia* (continued)

3. Decrease or inhibition of bilirubin conjugation
   a. Inherited bilirubin conjugation defect: Crigler-Najjar syndrome (deficiency of glucuronyl transferase).
   b. Acquired bilirubin conjugation defect: breast-milk jaundice, Lucey-Driscoll syndrome, infant of diabetic mother, asphyxiated infant with respiratory distress
4. Increased extrahepatic circulation—intestinal obstruction
5. Polycythemia—twin-twin transfusion; maternofetal transfusion; infant of diabetic mother; small-for-gestational-age infant
6. Mixed jaundice—increased bilirubin load and decreased clearance resulting in elevated indirect and direct bilirubin levels
   a. Sepsis
   b. Severe hemolytic disease
   c. Intrauterine transfusion
   d. Galactosemia
   e. Biliary atresia—absence of extrahepatic ducts or presence of cordlike structures without a lumen
7. Hypothyroidism
8. Familial, transient—associated with inhibiting factor in plasma
9. Unknown

Clinical Manifestations

Onset of clinical jaundice seen when serum bilirubin levels are 5–7 mg/100 dL.
1. Sclerae appearing yellow before skin appears yellow
2. Skin appearing light to bright yellow
3. Lethargy
4. Dark amber, concentrated urine
5. Poor feeding
6. Dark stools

d. Have the infant completely undressed so entire skin surface is exposed to light
e. Keep the infant's eyes covered to protect them from the constant exposure to high-intensity light which may cause retinal injury.
f. Develop a systematic schedule of turning infant so all surfaces are exposed (ie, every 2 hours).
g. Shield gonads of newborn
h. Maintain thermo-neutrality (phototherapy may rise the ambient temperature)

NURSING ALERT:
If priapism occurs, turn the infant on abdomen for short periods of time and this will cease.

2. Exchange transfusion—to mechanically remove bilirubin
3. Enzyme induction agents such as phenobarbital or ethanol to reduce bilirubin levels by inducing hepatic enzyme system involved in bilirubin clearance
4. Maintain hydration—the amount of fluid intake determines the excretion rate of bilirubin. Early feeding is a good preventive measure for hyperbilirubinemia and will enhance its treatment
5. Close monitoring for complications
   a. Kernicterus—encephalopathy hearalded by poor feeding, vomiting, lethargy, high-pitched cry, hypotonia, decreased reflexes such as Moro reflex. Later may have opisthotonos, spasticity, apnea, seizures, deafness
   b. Nephrotoxicity

Selected References

Brewin-Wilson, D. (1989). Transient erythroblastopenia of childhood: Implications for nurse practitioners. *Journal of Pediatric Health Care, 3,* 200-202.

Hoyer, L. (1994). Hemophilia A. *New England Journal of Medicine, 330,* 38-47.

Jacobs, R. F. & Schutze, G. E. (1995). What's causing the hyperbilirubinemia? *Patient Care, 28* (20), 127–128.

Kleinert, D., et al. (1990). Hemophilia patients in surgery. *AORN, 25*(4), 743-752.

Lusher, J., & Warrier, I. (1991). Hemophilia. *Pediatrics in Review, 12*(9), 275-281.

Lusher, J., Arkin, S., Abildgard, C., & Schwartz, R. (1993). Blood coagulation factor 8. *New England Journal of Medicine, 328*(7), 453–459.

Martin, M., & Butler, R. (1993). Understanding the basics of B-thalassemia major. *Pediatric Nursing, 19*(2), 143-145.

Mills, D. (1992). When blood won't clot. *RN, November,* 28-32.

Nathan, D., & Oski, F. (1993). *Hematology of infancy and childhood* (3rd ed.). Philadelphia: W. B. Saunders.

Ogamdi, S., & White, G. (1993). Sickle cell disease: Detection and management. *Clinician Reviews, February,* 65-84.

Quintero, C. (1993). Blood administration in pediatric Jehovah's Witnesses. *Pediatric Nursing, 19*(1), 46-48.

Riske, B. (1995). *Hemophilia nursing handbook.* New York: Hemophilia Foundation.

Rivers, R., & Williamson, N. (1990). Sickle cell anemia-complex disease, nursing challenge. *RN, June,* 24-28.

Selekman, J. (1993). Update: New guidelines for the treatment of infants with sickle cell disease. *Pediatric Nursing, 19*(6), 600-605.

Sickle Cell Disease Guidance Panel. (1994). *Sickle cell disease: comprehensive screening and management in newborns and infants.* Washington, DC: US Department of Health and Human Services.

Wimberley, T., & Parks, B. (1991). Iron preparations: It's elementary, my dear. *Pediatric Nursing, 17*(3), 274-275.

CHAPTER 50

Pediatric Immunologic Disorders

Immunodeficiency

◆ PEDIATRIC HIV DISEASE

Pediatric human immunodeficiency virus (HIV) disease is represented by a continuum of health conditions ranging from nonsymptomatic disease to conditions that define the child as having acquired immunodeficiency syndrome (AIDS). A child infected with HIV will, over time, show signs of impaired immune function although the severity of the impairment can vary widely from mildly abnormal laboratory markers of immune function to full-blown AIDS-defining illnesses.

Etiology/Incidence

1. The causative agent is a retrovirus that damages the immune system by infecting and depleting the CD4 lymphocytes (T4-helper cells). These CD4 lymphocytes play a central role in the regulation of the immune system.
2. There are also abnormalities in the function of the B cells, CD8 cells, natural killer cells, monocytes, and macrophages.
3. With loss of the immune function, the disease becomes clinically manifested.
4. HIV is transmitted by sexual contact, through exposure to blood and blood components, perinatally from an infected mother to the child, and through breast-feeding from an HIV-infected mother to her infant.
5. Perinatal transmission accounts for at least 90% of all pediatric HIV disease in the United States.
6. In the United States, the perinatal transmission rate is about 20% to 30% (varying rates are reported from different centers in the United States).
7. Transmission can be in utero, intrapartum, or postpartum (through breast milk).
8. An HIV-infected mother can have a child who is also infected and have future children who are not infected. Likewise, one twin or triplet can be infected while the other is not.
9. It is estimated that in the United States, by the mid-1990s, there will be 9,000 children, under the age of 5 years, infected with HIV.
10. Currently, only those children who have developed an AIDS-defining condition are reported to the Centers for Disease Control and Prevention (CDC).
11. Fifty percent of HIV-infected children, over the age of 3 years, are only mildly or moderately symptomatic and lead quite normal lives. As more is learned about this disease and measures that help minimize the effects of an impaired immune system are instituted, these children will have much longer life spans.

Altered Physiology

1. Progressive destruction of the immune system leading to increased incidence of serious bacterial infections (bacteremias, bacterial pneumonias, osteomyelitis), more aggressive forms of viral infections (such as severe varicella, disseminated zoster, cytomegalovirus pneumonitis), opportunistic infections (ie, *Pneumocystis carinii* pneumonia [PCP]), and cancers, especially lymphomas
2. Multisystem organ damage by HIV resulting in cardiomyopathies, nephropathies, neurologic impairment, gastrointestinal dysfunction, and hematologic disorders

Complications

1. Repeated, overwhelming infections and certain cancers, particularly lymphomas
2. Cardiac disease, renal disease, neurologic impairment, developmental delays and regression, anemias, thrombocytopenia
3. Death

Clinical Manifestations

1. Generalized lymphadenopathy, especially in less common sites such as epitrochlear and axillary areas
2. Persistent, recurrent oral candidiasis
3. Failure to thrive
4. Developmental delays or loss of previously acquired milestones
5. Hepatomegaly
6. Splenomegaly
7. Persistent diarrhea
8. Hyper- or hypogammaglobulinemia (elevated IgG, IgM, IgA)
9. Parotitis
10. Low CD4 counts for age
11. Unexplained anemias, thrombocytopenia
12. Unexplained cardiac or kidney disease
13. Recurrent serious bacterial infections

Diagnostic Evaluation

1. Neonatal testing with enzyme-linked immunosorbent assay (ELISA) is *not* indicated because this is only testing for the presence of circulating maternal antibodies to HIV and not an indication of the child's infection status.

2. Newer diagnostic tests such as polymerase chain reaction (PCR) and P24 antigen will allow for earlier confirmation of infection status (by 2–3 months of age). These tests are just now becoming commercially available.

3. After 15 months of age, ELISA can be used for testing. As with adults, a reactive ELISA must be followed by a confirmatory Western blot test.

4. CD4 lymphocyte counts are essential to determine an at-risk infant's need for PCP prophylaxis. These should be done by 1 month of age and then every 2 to 3 months thereafter until the child is known to be not infected with HIV.

5. For a known infected child, complete blood counts (CBC), platelet counts, and serum chemistries should be done every 3 to 6 months (depending on previous results and the stage of disease). In addition, a baseline echocardiogram and chest x-ray should be done and repeated yearly.

6. In known infected children, or at-risk infants (infants born to an HIV-infected mother but still indeterminate as to their own status), computed tomography scanning or magnetic resonance imaging of the head is indicated if there is evidence of neurologic impairment, falling rate of head growth, or developmental delays or regression.

Treatment

1. Initiation of PCP prophylaxis when indicated by low CD4 counts (Table 50-1). The first drug of choice is trimethoprim-sulfamethoxazole (Bactrim). Pentamidine and dapsone are alternate choices.

2. In a known infected child, initiation of antiretroviral therapy when the child becomes symptomatic or has CD4 count 250 cells/mm³ *above* the threshold for initiation of PCP prophylaxis. Currently only zidovudine (AZT, ZDV, Retrovir) and didanosine (ddI, Videx) are licensed for use in children. Other drugs, including dideoxycytidine (ddC, zalcitabine, HIVID) are available through clinical treatment trials and "compassionate use" protocols. As with adults, there is no conclusive evidence that early intervention with antiretroviral agents alters the course of the disease, but anecdotal findings seem to suggest some benefits.

3. Use of intravenous immune globulin (IVIG) in infected children who have had two or more serious bacterial infections within 1 year or for the treatment of HIV-related thrombocytopenia

TABLE 50-1 Guidelines for *Pneumocystis carinii* Pneumonia Prophylaxis

Age	Percent CD4 Cells	Absolute Number CD4 Cells
1–12 mo	≤20%	≤1,500/mm³
12–24 mo	≤20%	≤750/mm³
24–72 mo	≤20%	≤500/mm³
>6 y	≤20%	≤200/mm³

Any age: Prior episode of *Pneumocystis carinii* pneumonia

4. Use of antifungal drugs such as nystatin, ketoconazole (Nizoral), fluconazole (Diflucan), clotrimazole (Mycelex) for persistent or recurrent oral candidiasis

5. Aggressive, *prompt* assessment and treatment of febrile illnesses

6. Nutritional support

7. Evaluation and treatment of developmental delays and regression

8. Adequate pain management in advanced or end-stage disease

9. Support and interventions for both the child and family around disclosure issues, parental guilt issues, long-term care issues (including caretakers for the child in the event of maternal death)

NURSING ALERT:
Families can find out about clinical treatment trials available for their child by calling 1-800-TRIALS-A.

Nursing Assessment

1. Review maternal records to identify newborn infants who may be at risk for HIV disease.

2. Review records of at-risk or known infected children to determine nutritional status, growth and development, frequency of serious bacterial infections, presence of or risk for opportunistic infections, laboratory values, and immunization status.

3. Assess growth, development, lymph nodes, hepatomegaly, splenomegaly, and presence of oral candidiasis.

4. Assess the family's understanding of the child's condition, care needs, prognosis, and medical plan of care.

5. Assess the family's coping mechanisms, comfort with disclosure issues, long-term plans for care (including plans for alternate caretakers).

6. Assess the child's understanding of health condition.

7. In children with advanced or end-stage disease, assess the level of pain and discomfort.

8. Assess the child's coping and response to the frequent painful and invasive procedures experienced as part of the ongoing diagnosis and management of the disease.

Nursing Diagnoses

A. Risk for Infection related to immunodeficiency, neutropenia

B. Altered Nutrition (Less than Body Requirements) related to malabsorption, anorexia, and pain

C. Altered Oral Mucous Membranes related to candidiasis

D. Diarrhea related to enteric pathogens, disease process, and medications

E. Hyperthermia related to HIV infection and secondary infection

F. Altered Growth and Development related to HIV cerebral infection

G. Ineffective Family Coping related to parental guilt and nature of disease

H. Ineffective Individual Coping by Child related to unresolved issues around disclosure

I. Pain related to advanced or end-stage HIV disease

J. Fear related to frequent invasive procedures

Nursing Interventions

A. Preventing Infection
1. Have a high index of suspicion for secondary infection even when clinical manifestations are subtle or absent.
2. Administer or teach caretaker to administer prescribed pharmacologic agents that may help prevent serious bacterial infections, prevent opportunistic infections, and treat infections that occur.
3. Monitor absolute neutrophil counts, which may drop to very low levels from antiretroviral drug therapy.
4. Maintain cleanliness of the environment and teach family members the essentials of environmental sanitation.
5. Use aseptic techniques when performing invasive procedures.
6. Administer and teach the family good skin care—a break in the skin is a source of secondary infection.
7. Teach the family the importance of safe food preparation to avoid introducing pathogens through contaminated or undercooked food.
8. Monitor immunization status and advise families of the need to complete all recommended childhood immunizations. Currently, it is advised that all HIV-infected children follow the recommended schedule of pediatric immunizations with the *addition* of yearly influenza vaccine (after age 6 months) and pneumococcal vaccine (after age 2 years).

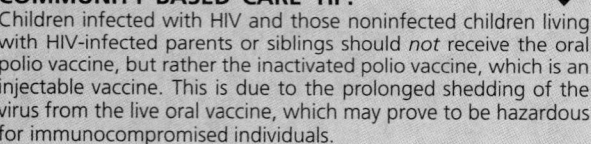

COMMUNITY-BASED CARE TIP:
Children infected with HIV and those noninfected children living with HIV-infected parents or siblings should *not* receive the oral polio vaccine, but rather the inactivated polio vaccine, which is an injectable vaccine. This is due to the prolonged shedding of the virus from the live oral vaccine, which may prove to be hazardous for immunocompromised individuals.

B. Maintaining Adequate Nutrition
1. Carefully monitor growth parameters (height, weight, head circumference).
2. Consult with a dietitian to develop strategies for nutritional care including additional calories and nutritional supplements.
3. Teach the family to prepare high-calorie, nutritious meals that are pleasing and acceptable to children.
4. As age appropriate, involve the child in meal planning.
5. Encourage small, frequent meals if the child is experiencing absorption problems.

C. Maintaining Oral Mucosa Integrity
1. Include regular examinations of the oral mucosa in the physical assessment of the child.
2. Administer prescribed antifungal therapy.
3. Offer fluids and blenderized foods to minimize chewing and facilitate swallowing.
4. Avoid highly seasoned or acidic foods.

D. Minimizing Effects of Diarrhea
1. Monitor for the presence or development of diarrhea.
2. Monitor daily weights when diarrhea is present.
3. Monitor intake and output and assess skin and mucous membranes for turgor and dryness.
4. Use enteric precautions.
5. Avoid foods that increase intestinal motility.
6. Plan a regimen of skin care including cleansing/blot drying of the anal area and application of ointment or skin barrier cream.

7. Teach the family safe food preparation techniques to minimize contamination of food.

E. Detecting and Controlling Fever
1. Monitor for fever and report any core temperature over 101°F (38.4°C).
2. Institute comfort measures such as sponge baths, dry clothing and linens, and antipyretics as ordered.
3. Teach the family how to accurately monitor the child's rectal temperature.
4. Teach the family to promptly report any febrile episode over 101°F (38.4°C) rectally.

F. Promoting Developmental Goals
1. Assess the child's developmental status on a regular basis.
2. Report any regression or delay in achieving developmental milestones.
3. Make appropriate referrals for more in depth developmental evaluation when delays and regression are noted.
4. Teach the family appropriate developmental stimulation activities for their child.
5. Implement any recommendations for developmental stimulation and assist the family in doing likewise.

G. Promoting Effective Family Coping
1. Assess the family's coping mechanisms, strengths, and weaknesses.
2. Provide emotional support to the family.
3. Refer the family to appropriate community resources for grief counseling, legal assistance (such as with wills, custody issues).
4. Help the family set realistic goals and expectations for the child.
5. Maintain a nonjudgmental attitude and nonprejudicial approach.
6. Allow the family to use denial as a protective mechanism—this gives them some sense of control.
7. Explain all care and treatment plans to the family.
8. Involve the family in planning for the care and management of their child.

H. Strengthening Coping Skills of the Child
1. Introduce the subject of disclosure of diagnosis to the child with the family. Offer the family guidelines as to age-appropriate approaches.
2. Accept that some families may not be able to disclose the nature of the disease to their child—even after much support and guidance.
   a. Explore with these families how they want you to address questions the child may present to you, the nurse.
   b. The illness and the impact of the illness can be effectively dealt with without actually telling the child that he or she has HIV disease or AIDS, if the family refuses to disclose.
3. Answer the child's questions as honestly as possible within parental constraints that may be present.
4. Actively involve the child in as much of the care as possible—such as having the child decide where to place the intravenous (IV) line, cleaning off their skin for needle insertion, and so forth.
5. Use therapeutic play techniques (age appropriate) such as drawings, play with dolls, play with medical equipment, and storytelling to allow the child to express self in less verbal ways.

6. Refer the child and family for counseling if the child's coping skills do not progress or there appears to be regression in how the child is handling the issue of illness and chronic health care needs. Signs indicating possible need for additional in depth interventions include more acting out by the child, withdrawn behavior, and difficulty in school (either behaviorally or academically).

I. *Minimizing Discomfort*
1. Assess for signs of pain in the child. In the infant or nonverbal child such signs include restlessness, crying, withdrawn behavior, and changes in vital signs.
2. Discuss concerns over pain issues with the primary health care provider and team providing care for the child. Initiate or request referral to a pain management team if the child does not experience relief.
3. Stress with the parent or guardian the need for adequate pain management in children because many people do not acknowledge that infants or children suffer from pain and that this needs to be alleviated.
4. Use appropriate techniques to assess the level of pain or discomfort a child is experiencing.

J. *Minimizing Fear*
1. Ensure all painful and invasive procedures are done in a location other than the child's bed.
2. Monitor central line if used for venous access. A central line access may be less traumatic over time than repeated peripheral access attempts. Many children with HIV will need long-term, probably lifelong, IV therapies and blood monitoring and a central line greatly eliminates the pain and anxiety associated with these procedures.
3. Ensure that the parent/caregiver realizes that most clinic visits will involve blood tests so that they do not falsely reassure the child that "no needle sticks" will occur.
4. Use diversionary techniques, such as bubble blowing, for distraction during painful procedures. Practice first with the child and tell him or her this is an activity that you will help with during the procedure. Children can also be taught other relaxation techniques.
5. Offer small rewards (such as stickers, small toy items, etc) after painful procedures to reduce anxiety. Such rewards should be given regardless of how the child reacted. The reward is not for "not crying" but acknowledges difficulty in going through painful and invasive procedures on a regular basis.
6. Involve the child in the procedure as much as possible (age appropriate). Such involvement can include selecting a possible site for accessing or receiving IV medications, cleaning the site, selecting a special bandage for after procedure, etc.

Family Education/Health Maintenance

1. Teach families and other caretakers of the child universal precautions. In caring for HIV-infected infants and children, gloves are recommended when handling potentially contaminated body fluids (such as blood), but not considered necessary for routine diaper changing *unless* bloody diarrhea or hematuria exists.
2. Facilitate access of adequate numbers of latex gloves to families to use as indicated.

3. Offer guidance as to how to initiate discussion of their child's HIV status with schools and day-care settings. The "need to know" principle serves as a guideline when deciding to whom disclosure should be made (generally the principal, school nurse, and classroom teacher). It is not currently *required* that schools and day-care centers be advised but is generally encouraged because this alerts the school to notify the parent promptly in the event of an outbreak of infectious disease that could pose a threat for the HIV-infected child (such as varicella).
4. Give families concrete guidelines as to when to notify health care providers about their child's condition. Signs and symptoms of illnesses require prompt notification, all fevers over 101°F (38.4°C) should be reported, and any adverse experiences or suspected adverse experiences with medications need prompt reporting.
5. Assess if the parents are receiving care for themselves. Many times parents will neglect their own care to provide for their child. As a result, the parents' immune status may become more quickly compromised.
6. Refer families to a social worker or social services agency. Children with HIV may qualify for certain entitlement programs that help with their health care and the family's financial situation. Many states have initiated case management programs for people with HIV.
7. Provide guidance in dealing with chronic illness in children. As a chronic illness, HIV is growing in incidence and involves all the same issues, plus some additional ones (especially in the area of disclosure and parental guilt) as any chronic childhood disease.
8. Assist parents in obtaining the latest information regarding treatment protocols of pediatric HIV. Such information can be obtained by calling: 1-800-TRIALS-A.

Evaluation

A. Absolute neutrophil count within normal limits; aseptic technique maintained
B. Eating small meals and snacks; growth curve maintained
C. Oral mucous membranes without ulceration
D. Two to three loose stools per day; perianal skin without irritation
E. Afebrile; mother demonstrates accurate monitoring of temperature
F. Assessment using Denver developmental tool appropriate for age
G. Mother assisting with care and seeking help through social services
H. Child asking questions and participating in care
I. Child reporting increase in comfort level
J. Child practicing distraction techniques during procedures

Connective Tissue Disorders

◆ JUVENILE RHEUMATOID ARTHRITIS

Juvenile rheumatoid arthritis (JRA) is a chronic inflammatory, generalized, systemic disease that involves a wide spectrum of manifestations, including joint, connective tissue, and visceral lesions throughout the body.

Etiology/Incidence

1. The cause of JRA is unknown.
2. Current hypotheses
   a. Infection from an unidentified organism
   b. Autoimmune process or hypersensitivity to unknown stimuli
   c. Some subtypes have genetic predisposition.
3. Affects about 250,000 children in the United States

Altered Physiology

1. In the early stages, one or more joints show signs of inflammation.
2. The inflammation is initially localized in a joint capsule, primarily in the synovium. The tissue becomes thickened from congestion and edema.
3. A characteristic inflammatory response develops in the interior of the joint.
4. The articular cartilage may become adherent and deprived of nutrition.
5. By starvation and invasion, this inflammatory tissue slowly destroys the articular cartilage.
6. Inflamed and overgrown synovial tissue eventually fills the joint space, leading to narrowing, fibrous ankylosis, and bony fusion.
7. Growth centers next to inflamed joints may undergo either premature epiphyseal closure or accelerated epiphyseal growth.
8. Tendons and tendon sheaths may develop inflammatory changes similar to the synovial tissues.
9. Inflammation of muscle may occur.
10. Eventually there is deformity, subluxation, and fibrous or bony ankylosis (fusion) of joint(s).

Complications

1. Bony deformities—crippling from progressive polyarthritis
   a. Growth disturbance
   b. Failure to thrive—short stature
   c. Cervical spine and temporomandibular jaw problems (micrognathia—receding chin)
   d. Leg length discrepancies
2. Psychological and social reactions to this chronic illness
3. Iridocyclitis—leading to cataracts, glaucoma, or blindness
4. Pericarditis

Clinical Manifestations

1. Characterized by exacerbations and remissions. Infections, injuries, or surgical procedures often precipitate exacerbations (Table 50-2).
2. Involved joints become inflamed with morning stiffness (gelling), swelling, warmth, pain, and impaired movement. This may occur gradually or suddenly and lead to joint destruction, dislocation, deformity, or fusion.
3. Symptoms of iridocyclitis include eye redness, pain, photophobia, decreased visual acuity, and nonreactive pupil(s). It can be unilateral or bilateral.
4. Rheumatoid nodules are uncommon in children.

Diagnostic Evaluation

(Of limited value; however, helps to differentiate subtypes)

1. Elevated erythrocyte sedimentation rate (ESR)
2. Leukocytosis
3. High total serum proteins
4. Positive C-reactive protein
5. Possible positive serum antinuclear antibodies (ANA) and rheumatoid factor
6. Possible alteration in serum proteins (increased α and γ; decreased albumin)
7. Changes in bone, demonstrated by x-rays—initially nonspecific
8. Slit-lamp examinations of eye to rule out iridocyclitis

Treatment

1. Although this is a painful disease of long duration, the outlook for remission is good (70%).
2. There is no specific cure; treatment is supportive.
3. The goal of drug therapy is to reduce inflammation and relieve pain.
   a. Nonsteroidal anti-inflammatory drugs (NSAIDs) such as aspirin, tolmetin sodium (Tolectin), ibuprofen (Motrin), and naproxen (Naprosyn)
      (1) Daily dose usually divided into two to four doses.
      (2) Aspirin is the drug of choice, preferably enteric-coated to avoid gastrointestinal complications.
      (3) Serum levels of aspirin are monitored (keep at 20–30 mg/dL) for anti-inflammatory effectiveness and to avoid toxicity. Therapeutic response may take weeks or even months.
      (4) Signs of toxicity may include rapid or deep breathing or tinnitus.

COMMUNITY-BASED CARE TIP:
Because of the increased association of aspirin treatment during a viral illness and the development of Reye's syndrome, advise the family to contact the health care provider when the child has a viral illness. Aspirin may be discontinued and another treatment for JRA substituted until the viral illness is over.

   b. Disease-modifying antirheumatic drugs (DMARDs) such as gold sodium thiomalate (Myochrysine) or aurothioglucose (Solganal); D-penicillamine (Depen); or hydroxychloroquine (Plaquenil) may be added to the regimen when NSAIDs have been ineffective.
      (1) Injectable gold salts are used sparingly because of the high risk of toxic side effects (skin rash, nephritis with hematuria or proteinuria, thrombocytopenia, neurotoxicity, gastric upset, leukopenia, anemia, and mucosal ulcers).
      (2) An oral gold, auranofin (Ridaura), is being studied for use in children.
      (3) Hydroxychloroquine (Plaquenil) or chloroquine (Aralen), used mainly for polyarticular disease, may cause gastric upset, retinal toxicity, and corneal and retinal changes leading to blindness.

TABLE 50-2 Clinical Manifestations of Juvenile Rheumatoid Arthritis by Subgroups

	Polyarticular (−) RF	Polyarticular (+) RF	Pauciarticular Type 1	Pauciarticular Type II	Systemic-Onset
Percentage of JRA Patients	20–25	5–10	35–40	10–15	20
Age at Onset	Throughout childhood	Late childhood	<10	>10	1–3 and 8–10
Sex	90% girls	80% girls	80% girls	90% boys	60% boys
Joints Involved	>4; any joints—usually affects small joints of fingers and hands symmetrically	>4; any joints—usually affects small joints symmetrically	<5 (usually large joints: knee, ankle, elbow) nonsymmetrical	<5 (few large joints—hip) nonsymmetrical	Any joints
Lab Tests:					
CRP/ESR	Elevated	Elevated	Elevated	Elevated	Elevated with severe anemia and leukocytosis
RF	Negative	Positive	Negative	Negative	Negative
Serum ANA	25% positive	75% positive	90% positive	Negative	Negative
HLA studies	?	+HLA DR4	+HLA DRW5, DRW6, DRW8	+HLA B27	?
Other Symptoms	Minimal systemic signs such as low-grade fever, malaise, lymph adenopathy.	Minimal systemic signs such as low-grade fever, malaise, lymph-adenopathy	Chronic iridocyclites (eye inflammation) low-grade fever, malaise	Sacroilitis, iridocyclitis, few systemic manifestations	High intermittent fever (102°), malaise, macular rash, pleuritis, pericarditis, splenomegaly, hepatomegaly, lymphadenopathy.
Prognosis	10–15% severe arthritis; 1:4 remission	>50% severe arthritis; 1:4 remission	Blindness (10%) Polyarthritis (20%) 2:3 remission	Ankylosing spondylitis 2:3 remission	25% severe arthritis; 1–2% mortality

ANA, antinuclear antibody; CRP/ESR, C-reactive protein and erythrocyte sedimentation rate; HLA, human leukocyte antigen (indicating genetic predisposition); RF, rheumatoid factor.

c. Immunosuppressant cytotoxic drugs, such as cyclophosphamide (Cytoxan), azathioprine (Imuran), chlorambucil (Leukeran), and methotrexate (Mexate), are reserved for patients with severe debilitating disease and those who have responded poorly to NSAIDs and DMARDs.
d. Corticosteroids—the most potent anti-inflammatory agents available; used for life-threatening disease, incapacitating systemic disease that has been unresponsive to other anti-inflammatory therapy, and iridocyclitis
  (1) Administered in the lowest effective dose, on alternate days (rather than daily). Their use does not prevent complications of severe arthritis or influence ultimate prognosis.
  (2) Tuberculin test should be done before starting steroid therapy because corticosteroids can blunt skin test results.
  (3) Monitor for glucosuria and other side effects such as weight gain, edema, acne, and fatigue.
e. Gamma globulin and monoclonal antibodies are being investigated.
4. Exercise program to promote joint movement
5. Surgery
a. Synovectomy—to maintain function when extensive synovitis develops, especially around wrists
b. Joint replacement—with severe destructive arthritis (ankylosing spondylitis)

Nursing Assessment

1. Focus history on child's general health, onset of symptoms, activity impairment, level of pain, and treatments used at home.
2. Focus physical examination on the clinical manifestations that differentiate the subtypes of JRA, such as extent of joint involvement, as well as vital signs and growth and development.
3. Gather data for psychosocial assessment about impact of this chronic painful disease on the child and family.

Nursing Diagnoses

A. Pain related to joint inflammation
B. Impaired Physical Mobility related to joint destruction and pain
C. Self-Care Deficit related to pain and immobility
D. Altered Family Processes related to caring for a child with a chronic/painful illness

Nursing Interventions

A. *Minimizing Discomfort*
1. Administer and teach parents to administer analgesic and anti-inflammatory drugs as prescribed and based on child's response.
2. Provide daytime heat to joints through the use of tub baths, whirlpools, paraffin baths, warm moist pads, and soaking; and nighttime warmth through the use of a sleeping bag, thermal underwear, or heated waterbed.
3. Immobilize any acutely inflamed joints with pillows, splints, or slings.

B. *Preserving Joint Mobility*
1. Encourage compliance with physical therapy regimen to strengthen muscles and mobilize joints. Assist with range-of-motion exercises as indicated.
2. Splint joints to maintain proper position (joint extension), decrease pain and deformity.
3. Encourage prone position with thin or no pillow and firm mattress.
4. Encourage therapeutic play (swimming, throwing, riding bike).
5. Encourage child to do own activities of daily living to maintain joint mobility.

C. *Promoting Self-Care*
1. Refer to occupational therapy for provision of adaptation devices to facilitate completion of daily activities (Velcro closures, utensils and self-care implements with enlarged handles).
2. Positively reward child for task completion.
3. Schedule rest periods to maximize energy; discourage bed rest and lengthy inactivity because they increase stiffness.
4. Offer pain medications and treatments before daily activities (tub baths, dressing, feeding).

D. *Normalizing Family Processes*
1. Refer to community resources and support groups.
2. Encourage child and family to verbalize feelings.
3. Encourage attendance in school as much as possible, participation in activities, and socialization with peers.
4. Remind parents to devote time to other children, themselves, and each other because this disease affects the whole family.

Family Education/Health Maintenance

1. Educate and motivate parents and child in continuing program of treatment at home. This is a chronic disease and has an unpredictable course; however, compliance with prescribed treatment will minimize crippling and allow the child to grow and develop to full potential. Avoid unorthodox and unproven treatments.
2. Teach the family that daily exercise such as swimming helps to maintain full range of motion. Avoid exercises that cause overtiring and joint pain.
3. Urge the parents to keep the school nurse informed of child's condition so that there will be continuity of care even at school. Tell the parents to inform child's teacher of need for hourly movement, side effects of medications, and application of special equipment.
4. Teach the family about a nutritionally balanced diet to prevent obesity that puts additional stress on joints.
5. Stress the need for routine follow-up care, ophthalmologic evaluation, and prompt attention to infections or other illness that may prompt exacerbations.

COMMUNITY-BASED CARE TIP:
Review immunization record for completeness because specialty focus may have caused parents and health care providers to overlook primary care needs. Advise child to get flu vaccine each year to decrease stress caused by the flu and the chance of Reye's syndrome from salicylate intake.

6. Refer family to agencies such as American Juvenile Arthritis Foundation;1314 Spring Street, NW; Atlanta, GA 30309; 404-872-7100.

Evaluation

A. Child demonstrates improved comfort.
B. Range of motion of all joints intact
C. Child completes self-care with minimal assistance
D. Parents seek additional resources

◆ SYSTEMIC LUPUS ERYTHEMATOSUS

Systemic lupus erythematosus (SLE) is a chronic inflammatory disease of the connective tissue with vascular and perivascular fibrinoid changes that may involve any organ or system. A number of clinical variants of SLE have been identified, including discoid lupus (usually affects only the skin), subacute cutaneous lupus erythematosus (skin and mild systemic manifestations), neonatal lupus (transient skin lesions, heart block, and hematologic abnormalities), and drug-induced lupus (lupuslike syndrome resolves when drug is discontinued).

Etiology/Incidence

1. Incidence higher in females than in males (8:1); most common during the childbearing period (15–44 years). However, it can affect children 5 to 15 years of age. It is generally more acute and severe in children than in adults. It is more prevalent in African American, Hispanic, or Asian populations.
2. Cause is unknown.
3. General theory of etiology is altered immune regulation. Possible causes include:
   a. Genetic predisposition—genetic markers within human leukocyte antigen (HLA) system have been demonstrated.
   b. Viral—nonspecific antibody rise as part of general immunologic hyperactivity
4. Possible factors that trigger or unmask initial symptoms:
   a. Exposure to sunlight; snow on bright day
   b. Injury, infection
   c. Stress, extreme fatigue
   d. Radiation therapy
   e. Vaccination
   f. Antioxidants
   g. Other drugs such as anticonvulsants, sulfonamides

Altered Physiology

1. Connective tissue in different organs develops nonspecific aberrations such as fibrinoid change in collagen and cellular infiltration, either in the walls of small blood vessels or elsewhere.
2. Alteration of collagen and subendothelial thickening of small blood vessels obstruct the flow of blood. These changes may be widespread or limited in distribution.

Complications

1. Sepsis—primarily resulting from steroid and immunosuppressive therapy
2. Renal failure
3. Cardiac complications
4. Growth retardation related to steroids and immunosuppressive therapy

Clinical Manifestations

1. Onset may be gradual with vague symptoms or acute with significant manifestations.
2. General characteristic signs and symptoms may include:
   a. Malar erythema (butterfly rash), which usually spreads over bridge of nose; rash may vary from a faint blush to scaly erythematous papules and may be photosensitive. Rash spreads from face and scalp to neck, chest, and extremities.
   b. Acute polyarthritis, arthralgia
   c. Fever
   d. Fatigue, malaise
   e. Anorexia, weight loss
3. Cardiac involvement—pleurisy or pericarditis most diagnostic
4. Nephritis—at onset or during course of disease
   a. Hematuria, proteinuria, hypertension
5. Central nervous system (CNS) involvement—during course of disease
   a. Behavior disturbances, convulsions, coma
6. Splenomegaly, hepatomegaly, lymphadenopathy
7. Anemia, thrombocytopenia, hypoglobulinemia
8. Raynaud's phenomenon
9. Pulmonary involvement with pleural effusion and lupus pneumonitis

Diagnostic Evaluation

1. Diagnosis made largely by clinical manifestations (Table 50-3).
2. Antibody studies

TABLE 50-3 American Rheumatism Association Criteria for Diagnosis of Systemic Lupus Erythematosus

The presence of four or more criteria must be documented to diagnose SLE.
1. Malar rash
2. Discoid rash
3. Photosensitivity
4. Oral ulcers
5. Arthritis of two or more joints
6. Serositis—pleuritis or pericarditis
7. Renal disorder—persistent proteinuria or cellular casts
8. Neurologic disorder—seizures or psychosis
9. Hematologic disorder—hemolytic anemia, leukopenia, lymphopenia, or thrombocytopenia
10. Immunologic disorder—positive lupus erythematosus preparation or anti-DNA antibody or anti-Sm antibody or false-positive serologic test for syphilis
11. Positive antinuclear antibody (ANA)

a. ANA—nonspecific but positive in 90% of people with SLE
b. Other antibodies such as anti-dsDNA, anti-ssDNS, anti-nRNP, anti-Ro, and anti-La if diagnosis is unclear or to identify clinical variant
3. ESR—elevated
4. Serum complement studies—lowered
5. CBC—leukopenia and mild to moderate anemia; can be hemolytic anemia, thrombocytopenia
6. Serologic test for syphilis—false positive
7. Serum chemistry and urine studies to detect kidney and other body system involvement
8. Renal biopsy—verifies lupus nephritis
9. Evaluation of the special situation when a neonate is born to a known SLE mother
a. Positive ANA and lupus erythematosus factor transmitted transplacentally
(1) Infant may have clinical or nonclinical evidence of lupus erythematosus. Discoid lesions may be present.
(2) Other infants may have no clinical symptoms.
b. Symptoms usually resolve in 3 to 4 months; however, the child has a small chance of developing SLE later in life.

Treatment

1. Course is unpredictable, often progressive, and may terminate in death if untreated. Therapy is based on the extent and severity of disease. To simplify therapy, SLE is classified as mild (fever, arthritis, pleurisy, pericarditis, or rash) or severe (hemolytic anemia, thrombocytopenic purpura, massive pleural or pericardial involvement, significant renal, gastrointestinal, or CNS involvement).
2. Control of symptoms with medication to decrease inflammation
a. Salicylates and NSAIDs to relieve joint symptoms, fever, fatigue, pain
b. Antimalarials such as hydroxychloroquine (Plaquenil) to relieve joint symptoms and skin rash
c. Steroids such as prednisone (Orasone)—used when there is renal or neurologic involvement or hemolytic anemia
d. Immunosuppressive agents such as azathioprine (Imuran), cyclophosphamide (Cytoxan), and chlorambucil (Leukeran)—used in severe disease, especially with nephritis or steroid-resistant patients
3. Dialysis and renal transplantation as adjunctive therapy for severe lupus nephritis
4. Supportive
a. Rest
b. Adequate nutrition; avoid obesity because of joint problems
c. Treatment of existing complications with antibiotics, antihypertensives, and anticonvulsants
d. Early identification and treatment of opportunistic infection
e. Topical steroid preparations—may help suppress cutaneous lesions

Nursing Assessment

1. Obtain a review of systems to determine involvement of other body systems.

2. Perform a complete physical examination, focusing on vital signs that might indicate renal or cardiac involvement, auscultation of the chest for heart and lung involvement, abdominal examination, and evaluation of the skin and extremities for vascular or cutaneous lesions.
3. Assess psychosocial status to evaluate child and family coping with chronic illness, school performance, and socialization.

Nursing Diagnoses

A. Fatigue related to disease process
B. Pain related to arthritis
C. Hyperthermia related to disease process
D. Risk for Injury related to seizures
E. Altered Urinary Elimination related to kidney involvement
F. Altered Nutrition (Less than Body Requirements) related to anorexia and oral ulcers
G. Body Image Disturbance related to manifestations of disease or drugs

Nursing Interventions

A. *Minimizing Fatigue*
1. Intersperse periods of rest between activities.
2. Provide opportunities for nonexertional therapeutic play.
3. Schedule procedures and activities after rest.

B. *Promoting Comfort*
1. Administer or teach parents to administer analgesics, NSAIDs, or steroids as prescribed and according to child's response.
2. For child on steroids, monitor for glycosuria and check blood test results for hyperglycemia and hypokalemia.
3. Provide diversional activities such as listening to music and quiet games.

C. *Controlling Fever*
1. Monitor temperature every 4 hours and document pattern.
2. Administer or teach parents to administer antipyretics as prescribed; note results.
3. Give tub or sponge bath to help reduce fever if necessary.
4. Encourage increased fluids by mouth when feverish.
5. Monitor for signs of dehydration such as dry skin and mucous membranes, poor skin turgor, decreased urine output, and thirst.
6. Administer IV fluids as ordered if dehydration develops.

D. *Avoiding Injury Related to Seizures*
1. Institute seizure precautions if indicated.
a. Padded crib or bed rails
b. Safe play area with no sharp toys or surfaces
c. Airway and suction equipment on hand
2. Encourage protective environment and equipment such as bicycle helmet if prone to seizures.
3. Monitor condition during seizure and behavior after seizure.

E. *Maintaining Urinary Elimination*
1. Monitor laboratory work for signs of renal abnormalities (blood urea nitrogen [BUN], creatinine, urine specific gravity, proteinuria, etc).

2. Monitor intake and output.
3. Monitor blood pressure; watch for development of edema.

F. *Maintaining Weight*
1. Allow child to help in selecting and preparing foods. Give finger foods to smaller children.
2. Encourage small meals with snacks in between.
3. Apply topical medication to oral ulcers or give analgesics before meals.
4. Monitor food intake and weight.

G. *Improving Self-Image*
1. Encourage contact with peers and family.
2. Allow child to ventilate feeling about bodily changes and chronic illness.
3. Allow child to be involved in planning care and making decisions.
4. Structure play therapy to reduce fears and anxiety, promote interaction with other children, and allow child to gain control and master some tasks.

Family Education/Health Maintenance

1. Teach ways to prevent exacerbations and complications of the disease:
   a. Important "do's"
      (1) Get enough rest.
      (2) Avoid anxiety and tension.
      (3) Follow treatment plan and medication schedule; understand medication side effects (especially salicylates and steroids).
      (4) Avoid contact with persons with infectious diseases, get pneumococcal and flu vaccine and keep routine immunizations up to date.
      (5) Follow prescribed diet, especially when receiving steroids.
      (6) Seek medical attention at times of illness or stress.
      (7) Recognize warning signs of exacerbation such as chills, anorexia, fever, and fatigue.
      (8) Become knowledgeable about SLE.
   b. Important "don't's"
      (1) Do not overexert.
      (2) Do not alter prescribed medications.
      (3) Do not use over-the-counter drugs.
      (4) Do not alter treatment plan.
      (5) Do not expose self to sun and reflected sun through clouds, on snow, water, or white concrete, or fluorescent lighting. When exposure cannot be avoided use sunscreen with PABA.
      (6) Do not use unorthodox or unproven therapies.
2. Teach parents about normal growth and development, emphasizing normal problems such as adolescent body image and peer relationships and how chronic illness can affect the child and the family.
3. Teach the importance of continual medical follow-up.
   a. Disease progress needs reevaluation, especially renal function, and drug therapy and laboratory results need frequent monitoring to prevent complications. Prognosis varies widely depending on the organ involvement and the intensity of the inflammatory reaction. Some children have milder SLE with little organ involvement. Prolonged spontaneous remission is unusual in children. The 5-year survival rate is 90%.

   b. Keep school nurse informed of condition so individual educational plan can be updated.
   c. Reevaluate need for physical and occupational therapy.
   d. Child on hydroxychloroquine (Plaquenil) requires frequent ophthalmologic evaluation for corneal and retinal changes to prevent blindness.
4. Refer to agencies such as The American Lupus Society; 260 Maple Court, Suite 123; Ventura, CA 93003; 805-339-0443; and Lupus Foundation of America, Inc.; 4 Research Place, Suite 180; Rockville, MD 20850-3226; 301-670-9292 and 1-800-558-0121.

Evaluation

A. Plays for 45 minutes without fatigue
B. Reporting reduced level of pain
C. Afebrile
D. Seizure precautions maintained
E. Urine output adequate
F. Eating three small meals and two snacks; weight stable
G. Interacting with siblings and peers

◆ HENOCH-SCHÖNLEIN PURPURA

Henoch-Schönlein purpura (anaphylactoid purpura, Schönlein-Henoch vasculitis) is a diffuse disease resulting from inflammatory reaction around capillaries and arterioles involving the skin, intestines, joints, kidneys, and nervous system.

Etiology/Incidence

1. Higher incidence in boys than in girls (2:1). Onset is between ages 2 and 8 years.
2. Seen most often in winter and can occur in clusters
3. Cause is unknown; however, theories include an allergic reaction to a variety of antigenic stimuli such as infection (eg, β streptococci), airborne allergens, insect bites, food, and drugs.

Altered Physiology

1. Acute vasculitis
   a. Swelling and edema of capillaries, small venules, and arterioles
   b. Fibrin is deposited in the glomeruli of the kidney.
2. Vasculitis results in skin manifestations (nonthrombocytopenic purpura), arthritis, and gastrointestinal symptoms.

Complications

1. Acute nephritis or nephrosis that may lead to chronic nephritis
2. Intussusception
3. Neurologic vasculitis with headaches, seizures, and neuropathies

Clinical Manifestations

1. Rash—sudden onset may precede or follow other manifestations
   a. Typical rash begins with itching, urticarial wheals, and then proceeds to maculopapular erythematous lesions.
   b. These lesions become less raised and more petechial or purpuric in character and do not fade with pressure. They blanch initially, then progress to ecchymotic areas until they fade.
   c. Several stages of the rash may be present at one time.
   d. Rash appears primarily on buttocks, lower back, extensor aspects of arms, legs, and face, then disappears.
2. Arthritis of knee and ankle joint develops.
   a. The condition is moderately severe, with painful swelling due to periarticular edema and migrating arthritis.
   b. Movement is limited, but there is no permanent damage or deformity.
3. Angioedema—especially of scrotum
4. Colicky abdominal pain—from submucosal hemorrhage
5. Nausea, vomiting, malaise, low-grade fever
6. Proteinuria
7. Microscopic hematuria
8. Symptoms may appear acutely or gradually and vary in intensity and duration.

Diagnostic Evaluation

1. Blood studies (not diagnostic, but support clinical evidence)
   a. IgA may be elevated.
   b. Coagulation studies and platelet count are normal in presence of purpura.
   c. ESR and white blood cell count are elevated.
   d. Anemia possible
   e. Elevated BUN and creatinine with severe kidney involvement
2. Urine studies show proteinuria, microscopic hematuria, and casts.
3. Stools show occult or gross blood.

Treatment

Treatment is primarily symptomatic and supportive.

1. Encourage bed rest until the child is able to ambulate and can do so without increasing edema of feet.
2. Remove allergen if it is known.
3. Give antibiotic therapy if acute episode was preceded by infection, especially streptococcal.
4. Manage complicating abdominal or renal involvement and arthritis.
   a. Steroids such as prednisone (Orasone) may relieve abdominal symptoms and prevent intussusception from bowel edema.
   b. Immunosuppressive therapy such as azathioprine (Imuran) or cyclophosphamide (Cytoxan) may be given to stabilize persistent renal involvement.
5. Provide comfort measures and analgesics. Salicylates are not particularly effective; NSAIDS are given.

Nursing Assessment

1. Obtain a complete history, checking for recent upper respiratory infection, medications, and allergen exposure.
2. Perform physical assessment of renal, integumentary, musculoskeletal, and gastrointestinal systems.
3. Determine impact of illness on the psychosocial well-being of the child and family.

Nursing Diagnoses

A. Pain related to arthritis and abdominal pain
B. Activity Intolerance related to fatigue and pain
C. Risk for Impaired Skin Integrity related to rash and itching
D. Altered Urinary Elimination related to renal involvement
E. Fear related to discomfort, hospitalization, and lack of knowledge

Nursing Interventions

A. *Reducing Discomfort*
1. Monitor pain level and location. Nonverbal behavior may be the most important source of information in the small child.
2. Administer pain or teach parents to administer medications as prescribed and according to the child's response.
3. Apply warm or cool compresses to joints or abdomen for 30-minute periods to help soothe painful areas.
4. Provide diversional activities such as listening to music, coloring, or quiet games.
5. Place in position of comfort; elevate affected limbs.
6. Observe for signs of intussusception—sudden onset of paroxysmal abdominal pain, currant jellylike stools, vomiting, increasing abdominal distention and tenderness—and report immediately.

B. *Increasing Participation in Activities*
1. Monitor completion of daily and diversional activities.
2. Alternate activities with rest periods.
3. Allow child to choose activities.
4. Modify play to be nonexertional and done while sitting.

C. *Maintaining Skin Integrity*
1. Assess skin condition and turgor.
2. Maintain adequate fluids.
3. Provide loose, comfortable clothing.
4. Administer, or teach parents to administer, antipruritics such as hydroxyzine (Atarax) by mouth, or topical products as needed.
5. Avoid soap, scratching, or dry skin that may exacerbate rash.

D. *Maintaining Urinary Output*
1. Record intake and output, vital signs, weight, specific gravity, and level of edema.
2. Check urine for protein, hematuria, and color.
3. Report, or teach parents to report, changes promptly.

E. *Alleviating Fear*
1. Allow child and family to verbalize feelings about hospitalization and illness.
2. Monitor anxiety level of child and family.
3. Offer realistic encouragement. The long-term outlook is good when renal involvement is minimal.
4. Encourage family and peer visitation of the hospitalized child and bringing in of familiar articles from home.
5. Allow child to make some age-appropriate decisions and become involved in planning care.

Family Education/Health Maintenance

1. Reassure the parents that symptoms are self-limiting.
2. Ensure that parents and child understand the disease and need to report changes in urine or signs of intussusception.
3. Encourage the parents to comply with follow-up. Urinalysis will be evaluated 6 and 12 months following the acute episode because of possible delayed renal damage.

Evaluation

A. Child demonstrating relief of pain
B. Child participating in activity for longer period each day
C. Rash resolved, skin intact
D. Urine output adequate, negative protein
E. Child playing, interacting with others

◆ KAWASAKI DISEASE

Kawasaki disease (mucocutaneous lymph node syndrome) is a multisystem vasculitis identified by a febrile illness with several distinguishing features that compromise vital body systems. It is the leading cause of acquired heart disease in children in the United States.

Etiology/Incidence

1. Cause is unknown. Streptococcal toxins, fumes from carpet shampoos, and other agents have been implicated.
2. Peak age of occurrence is in the toddler; 80% are under age 5. Seldom occurs in children over 8 years old. Boy-to-girl ratio is 1.5:1. Most frequently seen in Japan and children of Japanese heritage.
3. Seasonal epidemics usually occur in late winter, early spring.
4. Long-term prognosis is still unknown.

Altered Physiology

1. Although vasculitis is a multisystem disease, the cardiovascular system seems to be primarily involved.
2. Initially: stage I

a. Perivasculitis of arterioles, venules, and capillaries
b. Coronary arteries are included—pancarditis
3. As disease progresses: stages II and III
a. Panvasculitis and perivasculitis of coronary arteries
b. Aneurysm formation, pericarditis, myocarditis, endocarditis, and phlebitis may result.
4. Stage IV
a. Coronary arterial scarring, stenosis, calcification
b. Myocardial fibrosis and endocardial fibroelastosis
c. Healing begins

Complications

1. Fifteen to 20% develop cardiac complications (coronary arteritis, aneurysmal thrombosis or rupture, myocardial infarction, congestive heart failure, coronary insufficiency, and ischemia)
2. Aspirin toxicity
3. Mortality rate is less than 0.3%.

Clinical Manifestations

A. *Acute Febrile Phase—Stage I*
1. The child appears severely ill and irritable (days 1–11).
2. Major criteria according to CDC as diagnostic of Kawasaki disease:
a. High, spiking fever, 5 or more days
b. Bilateral conjunctival injection
c. Oropharyngeal erythema, "strawberry" tongue, red and dry lips
d. Indurative edema of hands and feet; or erythema of palms and soles; or general edema; or periungual desquamation
e. Erythematous rash
f. Cervical lymphadenopathy greater than 1.5 cm
3. Carditis—pericarditis, myocarditis, cardiomegaly, congestive heart failure, coronary thrombosis
4. Iridocyclitis and aseptic meningitis

B. *Subacute Phase—Stage II*
1. Acute symptoms of stage I subside as temperature returns to normal. The child remains irritable and anorectic (days 11–21).
2. Dry, cracked lips with fissures
3. Desquamation of toes and fingers
4. Arthralgia, arthritis (temporary)
5. Coronary thrombosis, aneurysms

C. *Convalescent Phase—Stage III*
1. The child appears well (days 21–60.)
2. Transverse grooves of fingers and toenails (Beau's lines)
3. Coronary thrombosis; aneurysms (may occur)

Diagnostic Evaluation

1. The CDC requires that fever and four of the six major criteria listed above in stage 1 be demonstrated.
2. Electrocardiogram, echocardiogram, cardiac catheterization, and angiocardiography may be required to diagnose cardiac abnormalities.
3. Although there are no specific laboratory tests, the following may help support diagnosis or rule out other diseases:
a. CBC—leukocytosis during acute stage

b. ESR—elevated during acute stage
c. Erythrocytes and hemoglobin—slight decrease
d. C-reactive protein—positive
e. Platelet count—increased during second to fourth week of illness
f. IgM, IgA, IgG, and IgF—transiently elevated
g. Urine—protein and leukocytes present

Treatment

1. Although treatment is considered controversial, goals are amelioration of symptoms and prevention of coronary thrombosis, coronary aneurysm, and death
2. Immune globulin (gamma globulin) IV therapy—IVGG (2 g/kg per day) is initiated during stage 1 in one 10- to 12-hour infusion to reduce the incidence of coronary artery abnormalities.

> **NURSING ALERT:**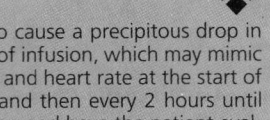
> Infusion of IVGG has been known to cause a precipitous drop in blood pressure, possibly due to rate of infusion, which may mimic anaphylaxis. Monitor blood pressure and heart rate at the start of infusion, after 30 minutes, 1 hour, and then every 2 hours until infusion is complete. Slow the infusion and have the patient evaluated for any drop in blood pressure. Keep epinephrine on hand to use for an anaphylactic reaction.

3. Aspirin therapy
   a. Anti-inflammatory dose (80–100 mg/kg per day) during acute stage of illness
   b. Antiplatelet dose (3–5 mg/kg per day) after fever is controlled and continued for 2 to 3 months after illness (when the echocardiogram is normal) or until ESR and platelet count are normal, to reduce risk of spontaneous coronary thrombosis. It may be continued indefinitely if there are coronary abnormalities.
4. Thrombolytic therapy may be required during the acute phase or during convalescence. Dipyridamole (Persantine) may be given as a platelet aggregation inhibitor if aneurysms are present.
5. Supportive measures
   a. Maintain fluid and electrolyte balance; give nutritional support.
   b. Provide comfort.
6. Cardiac follow-up by pediatric cardiologist with serial two-dimensional echocardiograms, angiography, and cardiac isoenzymes

Nursing Assessment

1. Focus history on gathering data that support the diagnosis of Kawasaki disease such as fever and skin manifestations.
2. Perform physical examination concentrating on the cardiovascular system.

Nursing Diagnoses

A. Pain related to conjunctival inflammation and arthritis
B. Decreased Cardiac Output related to vasculitis and aneurysms
C. Altered Oral Mucous Membrane related to disease process

D. Risk for Impaired Skin Integrity related to edema, dehydration, desquamation, and bed rest
E. Fluid Volume Deficit related to hyperthermia, anorexia, and oral ulcers
F. Fear of Parents and Child related to severity of illness and hospitalization

Nursing Interventions

A. *Reducing Discomfort*
1. Allow the child periods of uninterrupted rest. Offer pain medication routinely rather than PRN during acute phase.
2. Perform comfort measures related to the eyes.
   a. Conjunctivitis can cause photosensitivity so darken the room, offer sunglasses.
   b. Apply cool compresses.
   c. Discourage rubbing eyes.
   d. Instill artificial tear drops to soothe conjunctiva.
3. Perform comfort measures related to joint pain and tender lymph nodes.
   a. Use passive range-of-motion exercises every 4 hours while the child is awake because movement may be restricted.
   b. Allow and encourage the child to move about freely under supervision.
   c. Provide soft toys and quiet play and encourage use of hands and fingers.
   d. Monitor pain level and child's response to analgesics.
4. Provide quiet, peaceful environment with diversional activity such as listening to music.

B. *Maintaining Cardiac Output*
1. Institute continual cardiac monitoring and assessment for complications.
   a. Take vital signs and blood pressure every 2 hours; report abnormalities.
   b. Ensure proper functioning of cardiac monitor; observe for and report any arrhythmia.
   c. Assess the child for signs of myocarditis (tachycardia, gallop rhythm, chest pain).
   d. Monitor the child for congestive heart failure (dyspnea, nasal flaring, grunting, retractions, cyanosis, orthopnea, crackles, moist respirations, distended neck veins, edema).
2. Closely monitor intake and output and administer oral and IV fluids as ordered.
3. Prepare the child for cardiac surgery or thrombolytic therapy as indicated (see p. 1216).

C. *Preserving Oral Mucous Membranes*
1. Offer cool liquids (ice chips and popsicles).
2. Progress to soft, bland foods.
3. Give mouth care every 1 to 4 hours with special mouth swabs; use soft toothbrush only after healing has occurred.
4. Apply petroleum to dried, cracked lips.
5. Observe the mouth frequently for signs of infection.

D. *Improving Skin Integrity*
1. Avoid use of soap because it tends to dry skin and makes it more likely to break down.
2. Elevate edematous extremities.
3. Use sheepskin, egg-crate mattress, and smooth sheets.
4. If clothes are used, encourage use of soft flannel or terry cloth that fits loosely.
5. Apply emollients to skin, as ordered.
6. Protect peeling skin; observe for signs of infection.

E. Maintaining Fluid Balance
1. Monitor temperature every 4 to 8 hours, every 2 hours if elevated. Give tub or sponge baths for temperature over 101°F (38.3°C), or use a cooling blanket for higher temperatures not responsive to antipyretics.
2. Offer clear liquids every hour when child is awake.
3. Encourage the child to eat meats and snacks to prevent nutritional deficit.
5. Monitor hydration status by checking skin turgor, weight, urinary output, presence of tears, and specific gravity.
6. Infuse IV fluids through a volume control device if dehydration is present and check the site and amount hourly.

F. Reducing Fear
1. Use play therapy (both passive and active) to help the child express feelings.
2. Explain all procedures to the child and family.
3. Provide respite for parents during irritable stage of illness when child may be inconsolable.
4. Encourage the parents and child to verbalize their concerns, fears, and questions.
5. Practice relaxation techniques with child such as relaxation breathing, guided imagery, and distraction.
6. Keep family informed of progress and reinforce information about stages and prognosis.

Family Education/Health Maintenance

1. Ensure that the family understands the medications, follow-up tests, and level of physical activity that has been prescribed for the child based on specific categories. For long-term follow-up care children can be categorized into one of three groups: those with no cardiac involvement, those with small coronary aneurysms, and those with aneurysms greater than 8 mm.

2. Teach parents that long-term care after discharge is critical because complications can occur during period of convalescence or months following acute illness.
3. Provide written instructions about cardiac complications and stress the need to report the development of symptoms.
4. Teach family members cardiopulmonary resuscitation.
5. Teach parents to report the possible development of salicylate toxicity—tinnitus, nausea and vomiting, gastrointestinal distress, blood in stool, increased respirations.
6. Provide anticipatory guidance about child's behavior.
   a. Do not overprotect the child. Discuss with parents the grief and mourning process of denial, anger, bargaining, depression, and acceptance they may be going through because of the chronic illness.
   b. Allow child to be as active as desired unless the stress test is abnormal or the child is on anticoagulants. Try to protect the child from injury if taking anticoagulants (no sharp toys, no contact sports).
   c. Discuss regression that might occur as a result of hospitalization or the disease process and how to deal with these changes.
7. Refer for additional information to agencies such as American Heart Association; 7272 Greenville Ave.; Dallas, TX 75231-4596; 214-373-6300.

Evaluation

A. Child reporting less pain; minimal crying noted
B. Vital signs stable, no edema noted
C. Taking fluids by mouth well; no signs of oral infection
D. Mild peeling of skin, no signs of infection
E. Skin and mucous membranes moist, urine output adequate

Selected References

Applegate, B. (1995). Kawasaki syndrome: An important consideration in the febrile child. *Postgraduate Medicine, 97*(2), 121–126.

Baumeister, L. & Nicol, N. H. (1994). Pediatric lupus and the role of sun protection. *Pediatric Nursing, 20*(4), 371–375.

Behrman, R. E., & Kliegman, R. M. (Eds.). (1992). *Nelson textbook of pediatrics* (14th ed.). Philadelphia: W. B. Saunders.

Centers for Disease Control and Prevention (1993, July). HIV/AIDS surveillance report.

Centers for Disease Control and Prevention. (1986). Classification system for human T-lymphotropic virus type III/lymphadenopathy associated virus infection. *MMWR, 35*, 334–339.

Centers for Disease Control and Prevention. (1991). Guidelines for prophylaxis against *Pneumocystis carinii* pneumonia for children infected with human immunoddficiency virus. *MMWR, 40*(RR-2), 1-13.

Driscoll, S. W. et al. (1994). Juvenile rheumatoid arthritis. *Physical Medicine and Rehabilitation Clinics of North America, 5*(4), 763–783.

Feigin, R. D., & Cherry, J. D. (1992). *Textbook of pediatric infectious diseases* (3rd ed.). Philadelphia: W. B. Saunders.

Gregory, E., & Blair, C. (1993). Nursing practice management. . .develop a health care plan for a student with a chronic health problem, Systemic Lupus Erythematosus (SLE). *Journal of School Nursing, 9*(2), 40-42.

Harris, J. A., et al. (1991). Psychosocial effects of juvenile rheumatic disease: The family and peer systems as a context for coping. *Arthritis Care and Research, 4*(3), 123–130.

Kellinger, K. G. (1994). Providing primary care to the HIV at risk and infected child. *The Nurse Practitioner, 19*(8), 48-52.

Lux, K. M. (1991). New hope for children with Kawasaki disease. *Journal of Pediatric Nursing, 16*(3), 159-165.

Lynch, J., & Potter M. (1990). Henoch-Schönlein purpura: A case study. *Pediatric Nursing, 16*(6), 561-566.

National Institute of Child Health and Human Development Intravenous Immunoglobulin Study Group. (1991). Intravenous immune globulin for the prevention of bacterial infections in children with symptomatic HIV infection. *The New England Journal of Medicine, 325*, 74-80.

National Pediatric HIV Resource Center. (1992). *A resource manual for enhancing services to HIV-affected children in Head Start.* Newark: Author.

Sundel, R. P., et al. (1993). Gamma globulin re-treatment in Kawasaki disease. *Journal of Pediatrics, 123*, 657-659.

Tsubata, S. et al. (1995). Successful thrombolytic therapy using tissue-type plasminogen activator in Kawasaki disease. *Pediatric Cardiology, 16*, 186–189.

U.S. Department of Health and Human Services, Public Health Service, Agency for Health Care Policy and Research. (1994, January). Clinical Practice Guideline, Number 7, pp. 81-93.

Whaley, L. F., & Wong, D. L. (1991). *Nursing care of infants and children.* St. Louis: C. V. Mosby.

CHAPTER 51

Pediatric Orthopedic Problems

Common Orthopedic Disorders in Children

◆ FRACTURES

A fracture is a break or disruption in the continuity of bone. Fractures in children differ from those in adults. The anatomy, biomechanics, and physiology of the child's skeleton is different than that of the adult.

Etiology and Incidence

1. Most fractures in children are a result of low velocity trauma, such as a fall.
2. Up to age 2, most fractures are sustained as a result of the child being injured by another person.
3. Violent or severe accidental trauma can occur at any age.
4. Epiphyseal injuries:
   a. More frequent in boys.
   b. More common at the distal physis.
   c. Represent 30% to 50% of all long bone fractures in children.
5. Forearm fractures:
   a. Common in children after the age of 2 years.
   b. Forty-five percent of all fractures in children.
   c. Sixty-two percent of all upper extremity fractures.
   d. Eighty-one percent of fractures after the age of 5 years.
   e. Most common cause is from a fall.
   f. Peak incidence in the months from April through September.
6. Humerus fractures:
   a. Supracondylar fractures are most common, representing nearly 60% of all humerus fractures.
7. Spinal fractures—are rare in children.
8. Pelvis and hip fractures:
   a. True incidence is difficult to determine.
   b. Studies indicate a range of 0.5% to 7.5% of pediatric musculoskeletal admissions.
9. Femur fractures:
   a. Usually diaphyseal and result from accidental trauma.
10. Tibia fractures:
    a. Nonphyseal injuries are usually from accidental trauma.

Altered Physiology

A bone fractures when the force applied to it exceeds the amount the bone can absorb.

A. Classification
1. Open fractures—underlying fracture in bone communicates directly with an external wound.
2. Closed fractures—underlying fracture with no open wound.
3. Plastic deformation—a bending of the bone in such a manner as to cause a microscopic fracture line that does not cross the bone. When the force is removed, the bone remains bent. Unique to children and most common in the ulna.
4. Buckle (torus)—fracture on the tension side of the bone near the softer metaphyseal bone; crosses the bone and buckles the harder diaphyseal bone on the opposite side, causing a bulge.
5. Greenstick—the bone is bent and the fracture begins but does not entirely cross through the bone.
6. Complete:
   a. Spiral—from a rotational force.
   b. Oblique—diagonal across the diaphysis.
   c. Transverse—usually diaphyseal.
   d. Epiphyseal—through the physis.

B. Specifics of Children's Bones
1. Thickened periosteum.
2. Open epiphyseal plates—injuries to these areas are unique to children; the plate is weaker than surrounding ligaments, tendons, and joint capsules and is disrupted before these tissues are injured.
3. More often treated by closed reduction and immobilization.
4. Usually heal very rapidly.

Complications

1. Vascular injuries—intimal tears, arterial spasm
2. Compartment syndromes
3. Nerve injuries—palsies
4. Malunion
5. Nonunion
6. Epiphyseal arrest—deformities in angulation or limb length
7. Ectopic bone formation—higher incidence in head injury and burn victims, those in a coma, or those having spasticity.

8. Hypercalcemia
9. Deep vein thrombosis—rare in children
10. Refracture—highest in young males
11. Cast syndrome
12. Cast sores
13. Synostosis—rare joining of two bones by osseous material
14. Fat embolism

Clinical Manifestations

1. Pain
2. Obvious deformity
3. Crepitus or gross motion at injured site—loss of skeletal integrity
4. Swelling
5. Ecchymosis
6. Muscle spasm

Diagnostic Evaluation

1. X-rays of suspected limb fractures should include joint above and below injured part.
   a. Should always include a minimum of two views at 90-degree angles to one another.
   b. Comparison views of opposite extremity are frequently needed.
2. Further radiologic studies may be indicated in certain instances to evaluate fracture: tomograms, computed tomography (CT) scan, magnetic resonance imaging (MRI), bone scan, myelogram, fluoroscopy.
3. Vascular assessment may include:
   a. Doppler studies.
   b. Compartment pressure monitoring.
   c. Angiography.

Treatment

Dependent on type of fracture, location, and age of child.

1. Basic treatment may consist of:
   a. Closed reduction followed by a period of immobilization in a cast or splint.
   b. Open reduction with or without internal fixation and usually followed by a period of immobilization in a cast or splint (see p. 1365).
   c. Closed reduction and percutaneous fixation followed by a period of immobilization.
   d. Closed/open reduction and application of external fixation.
   e. Traction (skin, skeletal) followed by a period of immobilization (see p. 1366).
2. Most children's fractures heal in 12 weeks or less. Simple fractures that are closed and nondisplaced can heal enough to be free from immobilization in 3 weeks.

Nursing Assessment

1. Follow the basic assessment for the trauma victim.
2. Obtain history from child or others to include accident or trauma details, noting the position of the extremity at impact.

3. Perform physical exam for location of deformity, swelling, ecchymosis, and pain; vital signs; and neurovascular assessment.
4. Assess child's support mechanisms/social situation with consideration of discharge needs.

Nursing Diagnoses

A. Pain related to injury process
B. Altered Peripheral Tissue Perfusion related to swelling and/or immobilization
C. Impaired Skin Integrity related to immobilization
D. Ineffective Coping related to injury, hospitalization, and or rehabilitation
E. Impaired Physical Mobility related to injury or immobilization
F. Self Care Deficit related to injury or immobilization
G. Risk for infection related to open fractures or treatment

Nursing Interventions

A. *Promoting Comfort*
1. Monitor and assess pain level.
2. Properly position, align, and support affected body part.
3. Administer analgesics as indicated.
4. Use nontraditional relief methods—music therapy, diversionary activities, relaxation techniques.

B. *Maintaining Tissue Perfusion*
1. Frequently assess perfusion to limb by checking temperature, color, sensation, and pulses.
2. Elevate extremity to prevent edema.
3. Encourage movement of digits.

C. *Maintaining Skin Integrity*
1. Assess for and relieve pressure caused by tight bandages, casts, splints.
2. Provide periodic cleansing, thorough drying, and lubrication to pressure points if in traction.
3. Encourage frequent position changes as allowed.

D. *Promoting Effective Coping*
1. Assess child's and parents' response to events.
2. Explain condition, treatment, and rehabilitation goals as indicated.
3. Reassure as necessary.
4. Refer to community-based support agencies (eg, social services, United Way), if indicated.

E. *Promoting Mobility*
1. Encourage exercise of uninvolved limbs.
2. Teach appropriate ambulation techniques using aids, such as crutches, walkers, or wheelchairs, as indicated.

F. *Attaining Independence*
1. Assess family situation for ability to care for child at home.
2. Allow child to care for self when able.
3. Encourage parents and siblings to assist only as needed.

G. *Preventing Infection*
1. Assess wounds frequently for warmth, erythema, swelling, tenderness, or purulent drainage.
2. Report signs of infection.

3. Provide appropriate wound care for open injuries and surgical wounds.
4. Administer antibiotics as ordered.

Family Education/Health Maintenance

1. Teach proper care of casts, splints, and immobilization devices (see p. 1365).
2. Teach safety measures and prevention of further injuries.
   a. Advise use of bicycle helmets and knee, elbow, and wrist pads.
   b. Emphasize importance of supervising young children while playing.
   c. Teach safety measures, such as gates at stairs and top-opening windows on second story.

Evaluation

A. Child reports acceptable level of comfort
B. Extremity warm with good color, sensation, pulses, and capillary refill
C. No skin breakdown noted
D. Parents comforting child, child responding appropriately
E. Using aids and ambulating independently
F. Bathing and feeding self with minimal assistance
G. No signs of infection surrounding wound

◆ OSTEOMYELITIS

Osteomyelitis is a pyogenic infection of the bone and/or surrounding soft tissues.

Etiology and Incidence

1. Usually bacterial in origin; isolated organisms include:
   a. *Staphylococcus aureus*
   b. *Escherichia coli*
   c. *Pseudomonas*
   d. *Klebsiella*
   e. *Salmonella*
   f. *Proteus*
2. Inoculation
   a. Hematogenous infection—through the bloodstream.
      (1) Occurs often in children after blunt trauma to long bones.
   b. Contiguous infection—direct spread from adjacent tissue.
      (1) After surgery.
      (2) From a primary infection.
   c. Direct inoculation—through puncture or stab wounds.
      (1) Open fractures.
      (2) Surgical wounds.
3. Occurs at any age.
   a. More common in children younger than the age of 12 years.
   b. Males more frequently than females.

c. Increased if other risk factors are present:
   (1) External fixation device.
   (2) Urinary drainage—Foley catheters
   (3) Central or peripheral IV lines.

Altered Physiology

1. Site is inoculated.
2. Inflammatory and immunologic response:
   a. Pus formation
   b. Edema
   c. Vascular congestion
3. Vascular occlusion leads to:
   a. Ischemia
   b. Bone necrosis
4. Infection spreads through bone via Volkmann's and haversian canals, causing further vascular occlusion.
5. Ischemia allows necrotic bone to separate from living bone, forming sequestra.
6. Sequestra enlarge, spreading toward and breaching the cortex, forming a subperiosteal abscess, further interfering with the vascular supply.
7. Vascular supply may remain sufficient to maintain life of bone tissue.
   a. New bone is created.
   b. Bone healing occurs.
8. If vascular supply is diminished below that necessary to maintain life of bone tissue:
   a. Bone dies and becomes inert. Small pieces of dead bone may be completely destroyed by granulation tissue from contiguous living tissue.
   b. Large pieces of dead bone cannot be completely destroyed.
      (1) Central residual remains as a sequestrum composed of cancellous or cortical bone or combination.
      (2) New bone is laid down beneath the elevated periosteum and tends to form an encasement (involucrum) around the sequestrum.
      (3) The involucrum is punctured by numerous channels through which pus may escape from the inside.
      (4) Pockets of infection are walled off in which organisms can lie dormant for long periods.
      (5) Chronic sinuses may form that eventually reach the surface and drain.
      (6) Drainage continues until infection quiets once more. Channels become plugged with granulations and remain closed until the pressure of the pus builds up and causes the sinuses to re-open or reach the surface through new channels (chronic osteomyelitis).
      (7) Complete healing takes place only when all the dead bone has been destroyed, discharged, or excised.

Complications

1. Chronic osteomyelitis
2. Pathologic fracture
3. Joint destruction
4. Skeletal deformities
5. Limb length discrepancy
6. Life threatening if unrecognized and untreated

Clinical Manifestations

1. Localized pain
2. Swelling
3. Erythema
4. Elevated temperature
   Note: Above signs may be masked in early stages of process.
5. Malaise
6. Irritability
7. Generalized signs of sepsis

Diagnostic Evaluation

1. Blood cultures should be obtained before initiation of antibiotic therapy to help make definitive diagnosis.
2. Needle aspiration of bone may be done if necessary to identify the causative agent.
   a. Gram stain, culture, and sensitivity of specimen, once obtained.
   b. Negative aspirate does not always rule out infection.
3. Complete blood count—marked leukocytosis, low hemoglobin.
4. Erythrocyte sedimentation rate (ESR)—elevated.
5. X-ray may be negative in early stages.
   a. Rules out fracture.
   b. Will eventually demonstrate changes.
6. Bone scan to rule out multiple lesions.
7. Gallium scan to rule out soft tissue involvement is sometimes indicated.
8. MRI to differentiate soft tissue from bone marrow involvement.

Treatment

1. Intravenous antibiotics.
   a. Broad-spectrum antibiotics until organism sensitivity obtained.
   b. Intravenous antibiotics for 4 to 8 weeks.
   c. Usually requires placement of a central intermittent infusion catheter.
   d. Additional 4 to 8 weeks of oral antibiotics at completion of IV therapy is recommended.
2. If abscessed, surgical incision and drainage is performed.

Nursing Assessment

1. Obtain a detailed history to include recent infections (ear, tonsils, urinary), trauma, onset of symptoms.
2. Obtain history of current or recent antibiotic therapy to help determine resistance of organism.
3. Perform physical assessment for signs of primary infection as well as osteomyelitis.

Nursing Diagnoses

A. Pain related to disease process
B. Hyperthermia secondary to inflammatory response
C. Impaired Physical Mobility related to pain of affected limb
D. Risk for Infection related to invasive procedures, surgical drainage
E. Ineffective Management of Therapeutic Regimen related to long-term antibiotics

Nursing Interventions

A. *Maintaining Comfort*
1. Assess pain characteristics.
2. Maintain rest and immobilization of affected part.
3. Administer analgesics as indicated.

B. *Reducing Temperature*
1. Assess temperature every 4 hours.
2. Increase fluid intake to prevent dehydration.
3. Administer antipyretics as indicated.

C. *Preventing Complications of Immobility*
1. Instruct on allowable activities—generally no weight bearing on affected limb and bed rest during acute phase.
2. Encourage usage or exercise of unaffected limbs and joints through play.

D. *Preventing Additional Infection*
1. Inspect and cleanse surgical wounds every 4 to 8 hours.
2. Instruct patient and/or family in proper care of surgical wounds.
3. Teach proper IV catheter and site care.

E. *Promoting Therapeutic Regimen*
1. Instruct patient and family on need for maintaining serum levels of antibiotics after discharge, even after signs and symptoms improve.
2. Initiate appropriate home care referrals for reinforcement and monitoring of IV therapy.
3. Encourage evaluation of response to treatment through periodic laboratory tests (ESR, serum drug levels) and follow up.

Family Education/Health Maintenance

1. Instruct in signs and symptoms of recurrent or chronic infection.
2. Stress the importance of compliance with treatment.
3. Encourage early medical intervention for subsequent infections.

Evaluation

A. Reports reduced pain
B. Afebrile
C. Exercising unaffected limbs
D. Surgical wounds without signs of infection
E. Child/parents demonstrate proper techniques for IV therapy

◆ DEVELOPMENTAL DYSPLASIA OF THE HIP

Previously referred to as congenital dislocation of the hip, this term is now the accepted means of describing those conditions involving the abnormal development of the proximal femur and/or acetabulum. The variability in presentation has spawned the need for a more accurate way of referring to this group of disorders.

Etiology and Incidence

1. Exact etiology is unknown.
2. Suggested contributing factors include:
   a. Hereditary component, higher risk with family history and in identical twins.
   b. Increased ligamentous laxity secondary to maternal hormones.
   c. Breech presentation.
   d. First-born children.
   e. In utero restrictions to fetal movement.
   f. Swaddling in the postnatal period, where the hips are in adduction and extension.
3. Incidence:
   a. Hip instability: 10 per 100 live births.
   b. True dislocation: 1 per 100 live births.
   c. Left hip more frequently than right.
   d. Bilateral involvement in 20% of cases.
   e. More frequent in Caucasians.
   f. Associated with other congenital anomalies.
   g. Females more frequently than males.

Altered Physiology

1. Acetabulum tends to be shallow and extremely oblique.

2. Head of the femur tends to be smaller than normal.
3. Ossification centers are delayed in appearance.
4. Dysplasia—shallow acetabulum, acetabular roof slants upward.
5. Subluxation—acetabular surface of the femoral head is in contact with shallow dysplastic acetabular surface, but the head slides laterally and superiorly.
6. Dislocation—articular cartilage of completely displaced femoral head does not contact acetabular articular cartilage.

Complications

1. Avascular necrosis of the femoral head
2. Loss of range of motion
3. Leg length inequality
4. Early osteoarthritis
5. Recurrent dislocation or unstable hip

Clinical Manifestations

Physical findings change as child ages; the presence of one or more of the following should be noted:

1. Asymmetry of thigh or gluteal folds
2. Limitation in abduction of the hip
3. Leg length inequality
4. Ortolani's sign and positive Barlow's test (Fig. 51-1)
5. Abnormal gait pattern

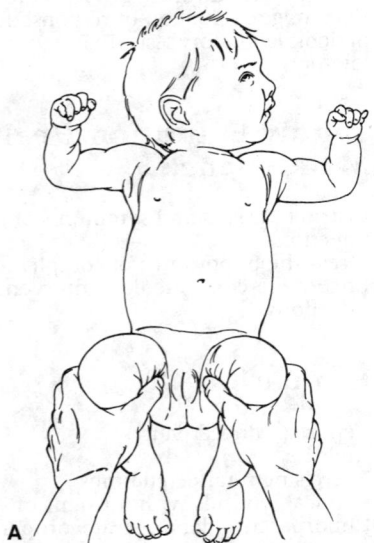 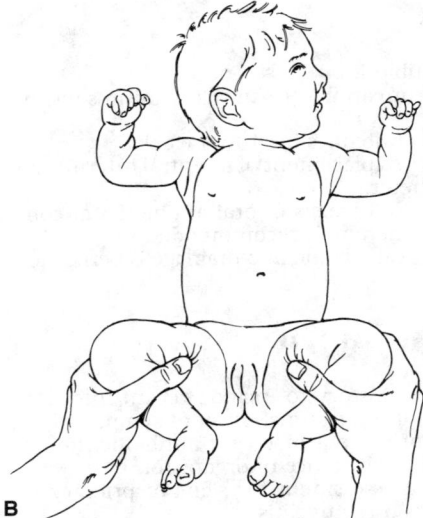

FIGURE 51-1 *Assessing for Barlow's and Ortolani's signs Place the child supine on a firm surface. Be gentle, not forceful. **(A)** Barlow's test—used to detect hip instability. The located hip is subluxed or dislocated during the maneuver. The examiner's fingers are placed over the child's greater trochanters. Holding the hips and knees at 90 degrees of flexion, a backward pressure is applied while adducting the hips. The femoral head is felt slipping out of the acetabulum postereolaterally when the test is positive. **(B)** Ortolani's Sign—present when the hip is dislocated. The maneuver relocates the femoral head. With the examiner's fingers on the child's greater trochanters, the hips and knees are flexed to 90 degrees. The hips are then abducted while applying upward pressure over the greater trochanter. A positive sign is detected when a "clunk" is felt as the femoral head reenters the acetabulum.*

6. Trendelenburg's sign—downward tilt of the pelvis on the affected side
7. Pain in the older child

Diagnostic Evaluation

1. X-rays—cartilaginous femoral head is difficult to visualize in the newborn. As the child ages, the ossification center can be better viewed and the efficiency of this exam increases. It can be useful in ruling out other pelvic, spinal, and femoral anomalies.
2. Ultrasound examination—yields a high degree of accuracy in diagnosing dysplasia with a skilled technician.
3. CT—helpful after operative intervention, such as reduction and casting, because plain x-rays have difficulty penetrating the casting material and visualizing the femoral head.
4. Arthrograms—can be useful to outline the cartilaginous portions of the acetabulum and femoral head.
5. MRI—is costly, often requires the child to be sedated, and provides little in the way of additional information.

Treatment

Goal: To restore as closely as possible the anatomic alignment of the hip. Methodology depends on the age of the child at presentation.

A. *Birth to Age Three Months*
1. Splinting or bracing the hips in flexion and abduction. With devices such as the Pavlik harness (treatment of choice), Frejka pillow, von Rosen splint, or Camp orthosis (Fig. 51-2).
2. The length of time varies with the stability of the hip at exam. If the hip remains unstable, progression to a more aggressive management approach ensues.

B. *Age Three Months to Two Years*
1. Closed reduction and placement of the child in a hip spica cast is the preferred treatment.
   a. There is usually a period of preoperative traction to increase the chances of reducing the hip as well as decreasing the chances of avascular necrosis after reduction.
   b. Closed reduction is usually performed under a general anesthetic.
   c. The cast is maintained for a period of 2 to 6 months based on clinical exam.
2. Open reduction of the hip with or without femoral shortening is decided on if the hip is not reducible in traction or at the time of attempted closed reduction.
   a. Followed by a period of immobilization, usually in a hip spica cast.
3. Cast immobilization is usually followed by an abduction splint or orthosis that is usually rigid.

C. *After Age Two Years*
1. Treatment is almost always surgical.
   a. Open reduction of the hip is usually accompanied by any combination of femoral or pelvic osteotomies designed to restore the anatomic alignment of the hip and prevent the progression of joint destruction.

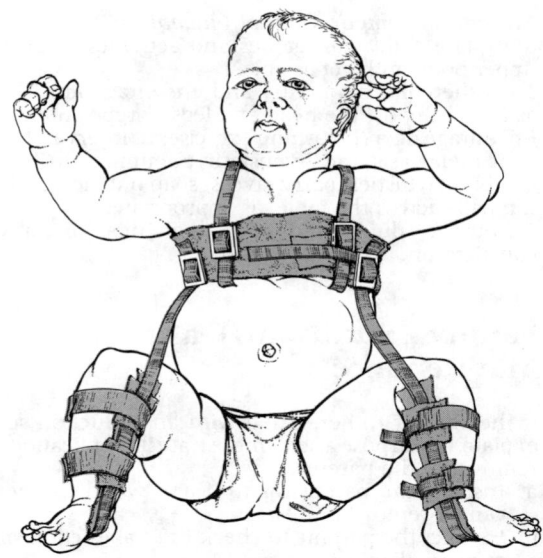

FIGURE 51-2 *Pavlik harness.*

   b. As the child ages, the risks of surgery increase. Risks may outweigh benefits, especially if the condition is bilateral.

Nursing Assessment

1. Obtain a family history, including hip pathology.
2. Obtain an obstetric history for presence of risk factors, such as breech presentation, first-born status.
3. Perform a physical assessment for range of motion, appearance of Trendelenburg's sign, Barlow's test, Ortolani's sign, and asymmetrical thigh folds.

Nursing Diagnoses

A. Altered Parenting related to diagnosis and treatment
B. Risk for Impaired Skin Integrity related to perineal soiling (cast immobilization)
C. Physical Immobility related to lengthy treatment

Nursing Interventions

A. *Promoting Effective Parenting*
1. Explain the condition and treatment in terms the family can understand.
2. Encourage holding of the child with abduction of the hips while handling and avoidance of swaddling as an infant.
3. Reassure parents that effective outcome depends on early intervention and compliance.

B. *Maintaining Skin Integrity*
See p. 1355.

C. *Preventing Complications of Immobility*
1. Stimulate child with games and activities to exercise upper body and feet as able.
2. Turn the child frequently and encourage ambulation as able. Support the head and legs to reposition.
3. Encourage deep-breathing exercises at intervals to prevent atelectasis and hypostatic pneumonia. Children can blow whistles, party favors, soap bubbles, and cotton balls across the table, as appropriate.
4. Encourage fluids and high-fiber diet to prevent constipation.

Family Education/Health Maintenance

1. If the child is to be treated with an abduction splint, explain its purpose and demonstrate its application and removal to the parents.
   a. Instruct the parents as to if and when the device can be removed.
   b. Instruct the parents to check fit of abduction splint at every diaper change.
   c. Allow the parents to demonstrate their ability to properly place the device on the child.
   d. Follow this with written instructions whenever possible.
2. Instruct on skin care and reporting any skin breakdown or disruption of the cast, brace, or splint.
3. Encourage regular follow-up evaluations and regular health maintenance visits.

Evaluation

A. Parents holding child and participating in care
B. No perineal skin breakdown
C. Child exercising and performing deep-breathing exercises

◆ CONGENITAL CLUBFOOT (TALIPES EQUINOVARUS)

Clubfoot is a congenital anomaly characterized by a three-part deformity of the foot, consisting of inversion of the heel (varus), adduction and supination of the forefoot, and ankle equinus. Other congenital disorders of the foot and ankle occur, but are less common.

Etiology and Incidence

1. Exact etiology is unknown.
2. Suggested contributing factors include:
   a. Intrauterine positioning.
   b. Primary arrest in fetal development.
   c. Familial tendency.
3. Incidence:
   a. 1 to 2 per 100 live births.
   b. Males more frequently than females.
   c. Fifty percent are bilateral.
   d. Unilateral cases, right slightly more frequent than left.

Altered Physiology

1. Foot is plantar flexed at the ankle and subtalar joints.
2. Hind foot is inverted.
3. Midfoot and forefoot are adducted and inverted.
4. Contractures of the soft tissues maintain the malalignments.

Complications

1. "Rocker bottom" deformity from excessive dorsiflexion and a "breaking through" the midtarsal bones.
2. Deformity becomes fixed if untreated, which can lead to:
   a. Child bearing weight on lateral border of foot.
   b. Gait is awkward.
   c. Callosities and bursae may develop over the lateral side of the foot.
3. Disturbances in epiphyseal plates from overaggressive manipulations.
4. Recurrent or residual deformity.

Clinical Manifestations

1. Deformity usually obvious at birth, with varying degree of rigidity and ability to correct position.

Diagnostic Evaluation

1. Clinical presentation and physical examination are usually diagnostic.
2. X-rays have been used to determine bony anatomy and assess treatment efficiency.

Treatment

Should begin as soon after birth as is possible, with the goal to establish a functional, painfree foot that can be fit with standard footwear.

A. *Initial—Nonoperative*
1. Serial manipulations followed by immobilization in a plaster cast, taping or strapping started at the time of diagnosis
   a. Done daily as an inpatient or weekly as an outpatient procedure.
   b. After the initial period (age 2 to 6 months), evaluation will determine the need to continue with manipulation and casting, proceeding to corrective shoes or solid ankle orthotics or a definitive surgical correction.
2. Corrective footwear consists of a reverse last or outflare shoe with or without a Dennis-Browne bar or the more recent Wheaton brace or Bebax shoe.

B. *Surgical Treatment*
1. Usually performed at 4 to 9 months of age so that the child is free of postoperative immobilization before the beginning of walking.

2. The child who presents late or has a recurrent or residual deformity may require an aggressive surgical procedure to stabilize the bony structures and balance the muscle and tendons by a combination of fusions, releases, lengthenings, and transfers.
3. Postoperative routines usually include a period of cast immobilization of up to 12 weeks followed by a brace (ankle foot orthosis) or corrective shoe for a period of 2 to 4 years.

Nursing Assessment

1. Obtain a family history of foot deformities.
2. Obtain an obstetric history for risk factors.
3. Perform a physical assessment for presence of other anomalies and classic foot position and range of motion. If late presentation, perform thorough neurologic exam to rule out causative factors.

Nursing Diagnoses

A. Altered Parenting related to guilt and grief over child with a deformity
B. Risk for Impaired Skin Integrity related to treatment method
C. Altered Peripheral Tissue Perfusion related to postoperative edema or casting
D. Pain related to surgical procedure

Nursing Interventions

A. *Promoting Effective Parenting*
1. Provide an accurate description of deformity and the importance of treatment in terms the parents can understand.
2. Provide opportunity for parents to verbalize questions and concerns.
3. Reinforce causative factors and the fact that it was not one's fault.
4. Encourage parents to hold and play with child and participate in care.

B. *Protecting Skin Integrity*
1. Assess fit of cast, splint, orthotic device, or special shoes. Teach parents that due to rapid growth rate of infant, device may need to be replaced to prevent blistering.
2. Assess and teach assessment of excessive pressure on skin—redness, excoriations, foul odor from underneath cast, or pain.

C. *Preserving Tissue Perfusion*
1. Perform frequent neurovascular assessments after surgery, including color, warmth, sensation, capillary refill, pulses, and presence of pain.
2. Elevate the extremity to prevent edema.
3. Place ice packs over casts for the first 24 hours.
4. Stimulate movement of toes to promote circulation.

D. *Relieving Pain*
1. Assess for signs of discomfort, such as irritability, crying, poor feeding and sleeping, tachycardia, increased blood pressure.
2. Administer analgesics regularly for 24 to 48 hours after surgery.
3. Provide comfort measures, such as soft music, pacifier, teething ring, rocking.

Family Education/Health Maintenance

1. Teach parents to remove cast at home before weekly manipulation and recasting by soaking in water and vinegar mixture to avoid anxiety and possible abrasions from using cast saw.
2. Teach the parents when orthotic devices may be removed—usually for bathing. Stress that devices must be worn as prescribed.
3. Advise parents that infant's sleep may be disturbed initially due to wearing brace at night and may be irritable while awake due to fatigue.
4. Instruct parents on providing a safe environment for the ambulatory child.
5. Discuss the importance of long-term and frequent follow-up and assist the parents with special needs, such as transportation, flexible appointment times, and financing orthotic equipment.

Evaluation

A. Parents holding infant, participating in care
B. No signs of skin breakdown
C. Neurovascular status of affected foot intact
D. Resting and feeding well

◆ LEGG-CALVÉ-PERTHES DISEASE

Legg-Calvé-Perthes disease is a self-limiting condition of the proximal femur characterized by avascular necrosis of the femoral head.

Etiology and Incidence

1. Exact etiology is unknown.
2. Onset is between 2 and 12 years of age.
3. Peak incidence from 4 to 8 years of age.
4. Males are affected four times more frequently than females.
5. Highest incidence in Japanese, Mongolian, Eskimo, and Central European descent.
6. Lowest incidence in Australians, native Americans, Polynesian, and African Americans.
7. Bilateral in 12% to 20% of cases.

Altered Physiology

Interruption of the vascular supply to the femoral head leads to the death of bone. Deformity can occur with loss of the spherical nature of the femoral head during the disease process. The disease progresses through identifiable stages.

A. Stage I (Avascularity)
1. Spontaneous interruption of the blood supply to the upper femoral epiphysis.
2. Bone-forming cells in the epiphysis die and bone ceases to grow.
3. Slight widening of the joint space.
4. Swelling of the soft tissues around the hip.

B. Stage II (Revascularization)
1. Growth of new vessels supplies the area of necrosis; bone resorption and deposition take place.
2. The new bone lacks strength, and pathologic fractures may occur.
3. Abnormal forces on the weakened epiphysis may produce progressive deformity.

C. Stage III (Reossification)
1. The head of the femur gradually reforms.
2. Nucleus of the epiphysis breaks up into a number of fragments with cystlike spaces between them.
3. New bone starts to develop at the medial and lateral edges of the epiphysis, which becomes widened.
4. Dead bone is removed and is replaced with new bone, which gradually spreads to heal the lesion.

D. Stage IV (Postrecovery)
1. Without treatment:
   a. Head of the femur flattens and becomes mushroom shaped.
   b. Incongruity between the head of the femur and the acetabulum persists and worsens.
2. With treatment:
   a. Head of the femur remains near spherical.
   b. Acetabulum appears normal.
   c. Width of the neck of the femur is normal.

Complications

1. Early degenerative joint disease.
2. Loss of motion and or function of involved hip.
3. Persistent pain and gait disturbance.

Clinical Manifestations

1. Synovitis causing limp and pain in the hip (may be intermittent initially).
2. Referred pain to knee, inner thigh, and groin.
3. Limited abduction and internal rotation of the hip.
4. Mild to moderate muscle spasm.

Diagnostic Evaluation

1. Early X-ray findings may be normal.
2. X-ray findings are related to the stage of the disease process.
3. MRI has been useful in demonstrating the pathologic process.
4. Bone scans can detect avascular state early.
5. Arthrograms may be useful to evaluate sphericity of femoral head.

Treatment

Goal is to maintain as normal a shape to the femoral head as is possible.

1. Restore motion—initial relief of synovitis, muscle spasm, and pain in the joint.
   a. Salicylates/antiinflammatories.
   b. Limitation of activities, bed rest with or without skin traction.
2. Prevent deformity—primarily of femoral head by containing it within the acetabulum.
   a. Non-weight-bearing abduction cast or brace (Petrie casts).
   b. Weight-bearing abduction brace (Scottish Rite orthosis).
   c. Surgical intervention by means of an osteotomy of the proximal femur or acetabulum (Salter innominate) or a combination of these.

Nursing Assessment

1. Obtain a detailed history, including onset of symptoms and characteristics of pain.
2. Perform a physical assessment to include evaluation of gait, range of motion, and presence of any contractures.

Nursing Diagnoses

A. Pain related to disease process
B. Impaired Physical Mobility related to immobilization and/or disease process
C. Self Care Deficit related to immobilization and/or disease process
D. Body Image Disturbance related to disease process and/or treatment

Nursing Interventions

A. Promoting Comfort
1. Monitor and assess pain level.
2. Instruct child and parents as to which activities can be continued and which to avoid (eg, contact sports, high-impact running).
3. Administer analgesics as indicated.

B. Promoting Mobility
1. Encourage activities to maintain range of motion (swimming, bicycle riding).
2. Encourage parents to allow activities that involve unaffected body parts within restriction guidelines.
3. Provide equipment to assist with mobility (eg, wheelchair, walker).

C. Achieving Independence
1. Assess parents' ability to care for child at home. Provide community-based referral to assist if indicated.
2. Teach parents/siblings to assist only as needed.
3. Allow child to care and participate for self as able.

D. Maintaining a Positive Self-Image
1. Reinforce to child that he or she is only temporarily restricted. Stress remaining positive aspects of activity.
2. Provide an opportunity for child to express fears and emotions. Offer support when needed.
3. Encourage participation in prior activities within restriction guidelines.

Family Education/Health Maintenance

1. Teach proper care of casts/braces and the need to remain compliant with usage.
2. Stress need to remain active within restrictions and to promote positive body image.

Evaluation

A. Child free from pain
B. Child participating in self-care
C. Parents understand disease process and assist child as needed
D. Range of motion and function maintained

◆ STRUCTURAL SCOLIOSIS

Structural scoliosis is a lateral curvature of the spine with vertebral body rotation.

Etiology and Incidence

1. Idiopathic scoliosis—exact etiology is unknown. Classified into three groups:
   a. Infantile—presentation before age 3 years.
   b. Juvenile—presentation between the ages of 3 and 10 years.
   c. Adolescent—presentation after age 10 years.
      (1) Most common age of presentation.
      (2) A right thoracic curve predominates.
      (3) Progressive curvatures appear to favor females over males.
      (4) Overall incidence is less than 1%.
2. Congenital scoliosis—exact etiology is unknown. Represented as a malformation of one or more vertebral bodies.
   a. Failure of vertebral body formation (hemivertebra).
   b. Failure of segmentation (block vertebrae).
3. Neuromuscular scoliosis—child has a definite neuromuscular condition that directly contributes to the deformity.
   a. Includes cerebral palsy, spinal muscle atrophy, syringomyelia, neurofibromatosis, and spina bifida.
   b. Myopathic conditions such as muscular dystrophy and arthrogryposis have a similar presentation.
4. Additional but less common causes of scoliosis are osteopathic conditions, such as fractures, bone disease, arthritic conditions, and infections.
5. Miscellaneous conditions that can cause a scoliosis include spinal irradiation, endocrine disorders, postthoracotomy, and nerve root irritation.

Altered Physiology

1. Vertebral column develops lateral curvature.
2. The vertebrae rotate to the convex side of the curve, which rotate the spinous processes toward the concavity.
3. Vertebrae become wedge shaped.

4. Disk shape is altered, as are the neural canal and posterior arch of the vertebral body.
5. As the deformity progresses, changes in the thoracic cage become worsened, with eventual respiratory and cardiovascular compromise.
6. Changes in the thoracic cage, ribs, and sternum lead to further characteristic deformities, such as the "rib hump."
7. Neurologic compromise in idiopathic scoliosis is rare.

Complications

1. Untreated progressive scoliosis can cause a significant deformity.
2. Cardiopulmonary compromise
3. Shortened life expectancy
4. Increased back pain

Clinical Manifestations

1. Physical characteristics:
   a. Poor posture
   b. Uneven shoulder height
   c. One hip appears more prominent
   d. Crooked neck
   e. Lump (rib hump) on back
   f. Uneven waistline (pelvis) or hemline
   g. Uneven breast size
2. Visualization of the deformity.
3. Back pain may be present but is not a routine finding in idiopathic scoliosis. The adolescent who presents with back pain and a scoliosis warrants close consideration to rule out a distinct pathologic condition, such as a tumor, disk disease, or intraspinal anomalies.

Diagnostic Evaluation

1. X-rays of the spine in the upright position, preferably on one long (36 in.) cassette—show characteristic curvature.
2. MRI, myelograms, tomograms, CT with or without three-dimensional reconstruction may be indicated for those children with severe curvatures who have a known or suspected spinal column anomaly before management decisions are made.
3. Pulmonary function tests for compromised respiratory status.
4. Clinical photographs to assist with documenting the appearance of the spine over time. (*Note:* Consent for photographs must be obtained from the child's legal guardian.)
5. Workup for associated renal abnormalities with a congenital scoliosis due to a high correlation between the two.

Treatment

Goal: To stop progression of the existing curve with nonoperative management. When this fails, the goal of operative management should be to correct the scoliosis as much as is possible and stabilize the spine with a fusion to prevent further progression.

A. Medical Management

1. Observation—periodic physical and radiographic examinations to detect curve progression.
2. Brace management—goal is to prevent progression of the curve.
   a. Requires faithful compliance on the part of the child for success.
   b. Some curves progress despite brace wear.
   c. Recommended wearing time is 23 hours per day.
3. Types of braces include:
   a. Boston orthosis for low thoracic and thoracolumbar curves. This is an underarm molded orthosis.
   b. Milwaukee brace for thoracic or double major curves. Standard brace has neck ring with chin rest.
   c. Charleston bending brace has been tried for nighttime usage in selected patients. Results have been positive in some centers, but widespread acceptance has not occurred.
4. Exercise therapy has been promoted to help maintain flexibility in the spine and prevent muscle atrophy during prolonged bracing.

B. Surgical Correction

1. Stabilization of the spinal column is the goal. This is usually accomplished with a spinal fusion and one of several methods of instrumentation.
2. Indications for surgical correction vary, but generally accepted principles are:
   a. Progression of the curve over a short period in a curve greater than 45 degrees despite bracing.
   b. Skeletal immaturity.
   c. Bracing is not possible.
3. Preoperative traction or casting may be used to help gain correction and increase flexibility.
4. Postoperative protection of the fusion mass by means of a cast or brace is usually required.
5. Surgical approach and techniques may be anterior or posterior with various instrumentation methods, such as:
   a. Harrington instrumentation and posterior spinal fusion.
   b. Multiple-level (segmental fixation) systems, such as the Texas Scottish Rite Hospital (TSRH) system, or Cotrel-Dubousset system.
   c. Luque technique, which includes dual rods with sublaminar wire segmental fixation (usually reserved for those children with a neurologic compromise already existing due to the increased risk of neurologic damage with the use of sublaminar wires).
   d. Anterior procedures, which include staple and cable or rod systems, such as the Dwyer or anterior TSRH.

Nursing Assessment

1. Assess respiratory, cardiovascular, and neurologic systems.
2. Perform a physical exam in the upright and forward-bending positions to include observation of physical characteristics as well as leg lengths, gait, and overall development.

Nursing Diagnoses

A. Self Esteem Disturbance related to deformity or brace wear
B. Impaired Skin Integrity related to brace or cast wear

Nursing Interventions

A. Strengthening Self-Esteem

1. Promote comfort with proper fit of brace/cast.
2. Provide opportunity for the child to express fears and ask questions about deformity and/or brace wear.
3. Instruct as to which previous activities can be continued in the brace. Usually all but collision sports and certain gymnastic activities.
4. Provide a peer support person when possible so the child can associate positive outcomes and experiences from others.

B. Preserving Skin Integrity

1. Assess skin integrity and fit of brace at every follow-up appointment.
2. Assess for proper fit of brace/cast.
3. Teach proper skin care to patient and/or family.
4. Instruct patient to wear cotton shirt under brace to avoid rubbing.

Family Education/Health Maintenance

1. Provide adequate information on condition and treatment.
2. Instruct to examine brace daily for signs of loosening or breakage. Instruct to contact orthotist when repairs are needed.

Evaluation

A. Child maintaining social activities
B. Skin without signs of breakdown

Orthopedic Procedures

◆ IMMOBILIZATION: CASTS, BRACES, AND SPLINTS

Casting, bracing, and splinting are all means of immobilizing an injured or diseased body part. The length of time can vary from a few days to several months depending on the nature of the problem. The management of children who are immobilized differs little from that of the adult, however, age appropriate changes must be considered. See Procedure Guidelines 51-1: Care of the Child With a Cast, Splint, or Brace.

Complications of Immobilization

1. Peripheral neurovascular compromise.
2. Alteration in skin integrity due to pressure or friction.
3. Loss of efficient use of affected extremity due to noncompliance.

PROCEDURE GUIDELINES 51-1 ◆ Care of the Child With a Cast, Splint, or Brace

EQUIPMENT   Casting materials or immobilization device
Cotton padding material, plastic padding

NURSING ACTION	RATIONALE
1. Prepare child for procedure by showing materials to be used and describing the procedure in age-appropriate terms.	1. Reduces fear and enlists cooperation.
2. Assess the need for pain medication, sedation, distraction techniques, or restraint and administer as ordered.	2. Manipulation of the affected part may be painful, so pharmacologic preparation is often necessary.
3. Obtain baseline neurovascular assessment, including discoloration or cyanosis, impaired movement, loss of sensation, edema, absent pulses, and pain disproportionate to injury or not relieved by analgesics.	3. Will serve as a baseline to compare subsequent assessments after immobilization.
4. Assist with application of the immobilization device as indicated.	

5. If a cast or plaster splint was applied, help facilitate drying.
  a. Keep the child and/or affected part still until thoroughly dry.
  b. Support the curves of the cast with pillows.
  c. Avoid excessive handling of the cast, and use palms of hands when handling it.
	5. About 24–48 hours are required for drying. Dries from the outside inward, so may appear dry but is still moldable with movement or pressure.

6. Assess the skin around edges of the device daily for signs of skin irritation. Teach child or parents to look for and report redness, skin breakdown, localized pain, foul odor that may indicate open wounds under device.	6. Pressure or friction may disrupt skin integrity. May be readily visible or occur under the device and not detected until advanced. Braces can be altered if skin irritation becomes apparent.
7. Try to prevent skin breakdown by padding edges of device and telling child to avoid placing anything inside the device.	
8. Assess neurovascular status frequently after application of device, then daily to detect compromise.	8. Initial swelling from the injury may contribute to vascular insufficiency and/or nerve compression.

9. If child is in hip spica cast, prevent skin breakdown from frequent soiling around perineum.
  a. Line cast edges around the perineum with a plastic covering to prevent soiling of cast.
  b. Use a fracture bedpan or urinal to facilitate toileting.
  c. If not toilet trained, use a small diaper or perineal pad tucked under the edges of the cast, covered by a larger diaper, and change diapers as soon as soiled.
  d. Wash the perineum frequently and dry thoroughly.
  e. If the cast is synthetic and becomes soiled, clean it with a damp cloth and small amount of detergent.
	9. Soiled edges of the cast may contribute to skin irritation or begin to disintegrate.
	
	  e. Plaster casts cannot be washed because they absorb water and soften.

CAST REMOVAL

1. Prepare the child for cast removal by describing the sensation (warmth, vibration) and demonstrating the cast cutter by touching it lightly to your palm.	1. Children are frightened by the loud noise and believe that the cast cutter will cut through their skin or extremity.

2. Provide and teach care of skin after cast, brace, or splint removal.
  a. Wash with soapy warm water.
  b. Soak the area daily with warm water to facilitate removal of desquamated skin and secretions.
  c. Advise child to avoid scratching; instead apply lotion or oil to relieve itching.
  d. Encourage exercise as prescribed to regain strength and function.
	2. An accumulation of dead skin and sebaceous secretions causes the skin to appear brown and flaky.
	
	  c. Excessive rubbing may cause trauma.
	
	  d. May initially be weak and stiff due to lack of use.

◆ TRACTION

Traction is the application of a pulling force to an injured or diseased part of the body or an extremity while a countertraction pulls in the opposite direction. Traction may be used to reduce fractures or dislocations, maintain alignment and correct deformities, decrease muscle spasms and relieve pain, promote rest of a diseased or injured body part, and promote exercise. See Procedure Guidelines 51-2: Care of a Child in Traction.

Types of Traction

1. Manual—direct pulling on the extremity or body part.
   a. Usually used to reduce fractures before treatment or immobilization.
2. Skin—force is applied directly to the skin by means of traction strips or tapes secured by Ace bandages or by means of traction boots.

   a. Usually of short-term duration and often used in children where small amounts of force are required.
3. Skeletal—force is applied to the body part through fixation directly into or through bone by means of a traction pin or screw.
   a. Allows for greater force over longer periods of time or when skin traction is not feasible, as in soft tissue injury or damage.
4. Continuous or intermittent—traction forces should only be disrupted in accordance with the health care provider's orders.

Complications of Traction

1. Neurovascular compromise to extremity.
2. Skin and soft tissue injury.
3. Pin or screw tract infection, osteomyelitis (with skeletal traction).

PROCEDURE GUIDELINES 51-2 ◆ Care of a Child in Traction

EQUIPMENT	Traction tapes Adhesive tape Elastic bandages	Tincture of Benzoin/other adhesive agent Spreader blocks, ropes, weights, pulleys Traction bars, slings

PROCEDURE	NURSING ACTION	RATIONALE
	1. Explain the procedure to the child and parents.	1. If the traction is to be effective, it is essential that the parents understand and cooperate while the child is in traction.
	2. Maintain even, constant traction.	2. Traction must be kept constant to achieve the desired results.
	a. Do not add or remove weights unless ordered. b. Allow the weights to hang free at all times. c. Be certain that the ropes are in the wheel grooves of the pulleys. d. Keep the weights out of the child's reach. e. Wrap knotted areas of the ropes with adhesive tape to prevent slipping. f. Do not elevate the head or foot of the bed without consulting health care provider. g. Supervise the child's position so that the purpose of the traction is accomplished.	d. To prevent loosening or undoing of traction knots. f. May disrupt traction forces.
	3. Check for disturbance of circulation by observing the following: a. Skin color—for redness, pallor, cyanosis b. Joint motion restriction c. Skin temperature—warmth d. Tingling, numbness e. Swelling, edema	3. Compare the affected extremity with the unaffected one. a. May indicate neurovascular compromise.
	4. Provide skin care.	4. Immobilized children readily develop areas of pressure unless meticulous skin care is provided.
	a. Pad bony prominences (ankles) with cotton padding before wrapping with elastic bandages. b. Wash and dry all exposed areas thoroughly. c. Massage the child's back and sacral area frequently. d. Inspect the heels, ankles, popliteal space, and top of the foot for signs of pressure from elastic bandages. e. Keep the linen free from wrinkles and food crumbs.	a. Protects skin from injury. c. Stimulates microcirculation. d. These are the areas most prone to breakdown. e. This prevents undue pressure areas.

PROCEDURE (cont'd)	NURSING ACTION	RATIONALE

NURSING ACTION

f. Do not allow the traction cords to dig into the child's skin.
g. Use a fracture bedpan.

5. Plan for short periods of muscle exercise every day.

   a. Encourage use of unaffected extremity.
   b. Assist the child to exercise unaffected joints.
   c. Provide for diversionary activities that require movement of unaffected joints and muscles.

6. Encourage deep breathing exercises.

7. Record the intake and output.

8. Encourage a diet high in fiber and fluids.

9. Provide daily diversion and encourage family visitation.

   a. Suspend or place favorite toys within easy reach of child.
   b. Provide for continuing education for school-age children.
   c. Encourage activities that will allow for diversion: drawing, coloring, videogames.
   d. Immobilized patients should be roomed together if possible.

10. If not contraindicated, provide the child with an overhead trapeze.

11. Document the following:

   a. Color, temperature and appearance of the affected limb
   b. Skin condition
   c. Body alignment

   d. Functioning of traction system
   e. Response of child to treatment.

12. Ensure countertraction is provided.
   a. Foot of bed may need to be raised or placed on "shock blocks" to prevent child from being pulled to foot of bed.

13. Do not alter the traction system.
14. Avoid sudden movement or jarring of bed.
15. Do not allow weights to hang over the child's bed.

SKIN TRACTION

1. Do not apply over an open wound or over damaged skin.

2. Prepare the skin with an adhesive agent before application of traction tapes.

SKELETAL TRACTION

1. Treat all entry sites as surgical wounds.

   a. Cleanse entry site according to institutional policy or guidelines. This should be done at least once per shift.
   b. Assess the entry site every shift for indications of infection or slippage.

2. Protect the exposed ends of skeletal traction pins.

RATIONALE

f. This is a safety measure.

g. This is less awkward and more comfortable for the child.

5. Disuse of muscles can result in atrophy, contractures, and deformities.

6. Prevents respiratory complications of prolonged immobilization.

7. Prolonged immobilization renders the child prone to urinary retention and renal calculi.

8. Helps to prevent constipation and urinary calculi.

9. This helps prevent boredom and assists the child to cope with immobilization.

   b. Length of immobilization in traction may be considerable.
   c. Activities that can be done while remaining in traction.
   d. Encourages peer support.

10. This will assist with movement and self-help.

11. Proper documentation facilitates communication between health care providers.

   c. Proper alignment facilitates proper extremity positioning and maintains proper traction force.

12. The child's body is the usual counterweight.
   a. Frequently the child's weight is insufficient to maintain proper alignment of the extremity.

13. Notify the health care provider if adjustment is indicated.
14. This can cause pain to the child and disturb alignment.
15. This is a safety precaution.

1. The skin must be intact for the pull of the traction to be effective. Prevents contamination of the wound and further skin breakdown.

2. Adhesive agents allow the traction tapes to adhere better, preventing friction on the skin surface.

1. Reduces the chance of infection along the pin or screw tract.
   a. Policies vary. Cleansing the pin site prevents infection, promotes comfort by preventing skin from adhering to pin.
   b. Notify health care provider if either of these conditions exists.

2. Protects the health care provider as well as the child from injury.

(continued)

PROCEDURE GUIDELINES 51-2 ◆ Care of a Child in Traction (continued)

PROCEDURE (cont'd)	NURSING ACTION	RATIONALE

SPECIFIC TRACTION TYPES: BRYANT'S *(SEE ACCOMPANYING FIGURE)*

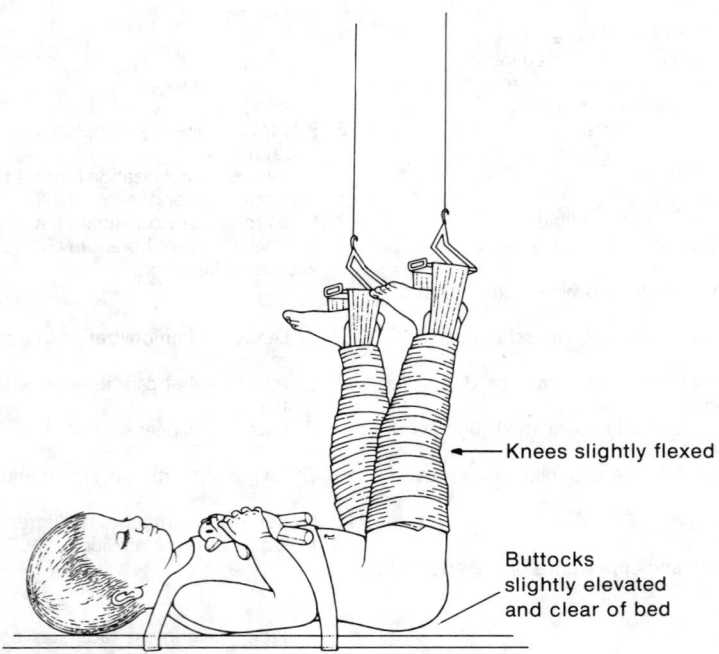

←Knees slightly flexed

Buttocks slightly elevated and clear of bed

Bryant's traction.

Indications:
1. To reduce fractures of the femur in children younger than age 2 or weighing less than 30 lb (14 kg).
2. Also used to stabilize the hip joint when casting is not indicated.
3. Preoperatively to attempt reduction of a congenitally dislocated hip in the same age group.

Mechanism of Action:
Involves the bilateral vertical extension of the child's legs. The child's weight serves as the countertraction. Skin traction is applied to both limbs to minimize potential trauma and maintain stability and alignment of child.

1. Maintain appropriate position:
   a. The legs are extended at right angles to the body.
   b. The hips are elevated slightly from the bed.
   c. The buttocks are elevated slightly from the bed.
   d. The heels and ankles are free from pressure.
2. Check condition and position of elastic bandages every shift. Rewrap as indicated and permitted by the health care provider.

1. Proper positioning is needed to achieve desired results.

   c. This ensures proper traction pull.
   d. Prevents skin breakdown.
2. Elastic bandages can cause compression and compromise circulation. In addition, force across skin surfaces needs to be constant and free from constriction to prevent skin breakdown and ensure adequate traction force.

PROCEDURE (cont'd)	*NURSING ACTION*	*RATIONALE*

RUSSEL'S TRACTION *(SEE ACCOMPANYING FIGURE)*

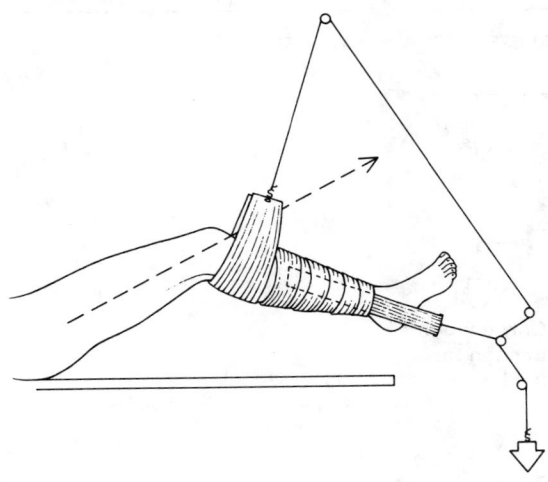

Russel's traction.

Indications:
1. To reduce fractures of the femur or hip.
2. Treatment of specific types of knee injuries or contractures.

Mechanism of Action:
Traction force is applied to the limb through application of skin traction. This can be accomplished with traction tapes or a traction boot in older individuals.

NURSING ACTION	RATIONALE

1. Application of elastic bandages:
  a. Wrap bandages from ankle to thigh on patients younger than 2 years of age.
  b. Older patients should have bandages wrapped from ankle to the knee.
	1. Proper application of the tapes prevents neurovascular compromise and ensures proper and adequate pull on the extremity.

2. Place foot support against both feet.	2. This prevents footdrop.
3. Keep the heel free from the bed.	3. Prevents pressure sores and ensures continuous traction pull.
4. Carefully assess the popliteal space for signs of pressure from the knee sling.	4. Prevents pressure sores.
5. Assess the neurovascular status of limb at least every 2 hours.	5. Early detection can prevent injury to patient.
6. Make certain that the footplate or spreader block is wide enough.	6. Prevents pressure sores and circulatory compromise.

(continued)

PROCEDURE GUIDELINES 51-2 ◆ Care of a Child in Traction *(continued)*

PROCEDURE (cont'd)	NURSING ACTION	RATIONALE

90-DEGREE–90-DEGREE TRACTION (90–90) *(SEE ACCOMPANYING FIGURE)*

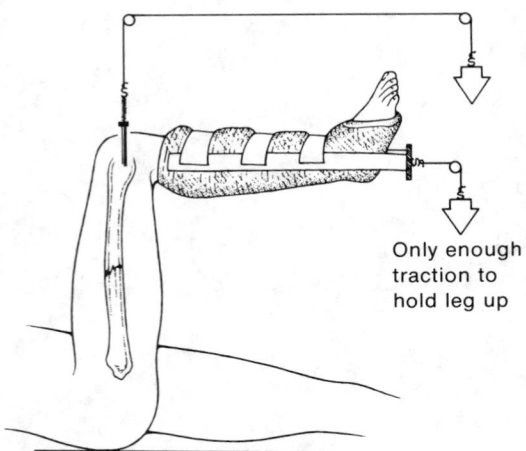

Only enough traction to hold leg up

90–90 traction.

Indications:
To reduce fractures of the femur when skin traction is inadequate.

Mechanism of Action:
Traction force is applied through skeletal traction pin placed through the distal femur. A short leg cast or foam boot may be used to help suspend the lower leg. Traction force is only applied to femur through pin. Only enough weight should be used to hold lower limb suspended.

BUCK'S EXTENSION

Indications:
Used to correct or prevent knee and hip contractures, to rest the limb, to prevent spasm of injured muscles or joints, or to temporarily immobilize a fractured limb.

Mechanism of Action:
The traction force is delivered through a traction boot or skin traction in a straight line. See p. 857.

BALANCED SUSPENSION WITH THOMAS SPLINT AND PEARSON ATTACHMENT

Indications:
Used in older children and adolescents for fractured femurs, to rest an injured lower extremity or joint.

Mechanism of action:
Thomas splint suspends the thigh; Pearson attachment applied to the splint allows knee flexion and supports the leg below the knee. See p. 854.

| PROCEDURE (cont'd) | *NURSING ACTION* | *RATIONALE* |

DUNLOP'S TRACTION (OVERHEAD 90–90) *(SEE ACCOMPANYING FIGURE)*

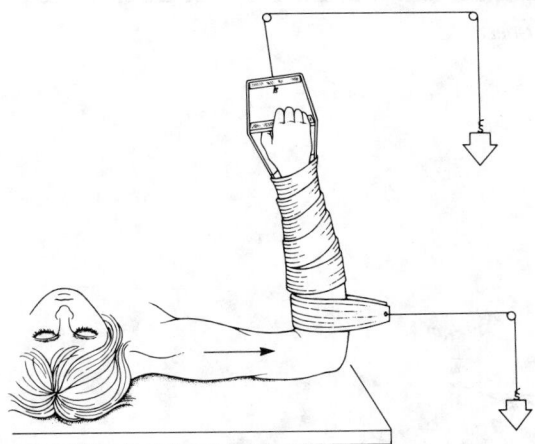

Dunlop's traction.

Indications:
Used to treat fractures of the humerus and injuries in or around the shoulder girdle.

Mechanism of Action:
Traction force is applied usually through skin traction on the upper arm only. Occasionally, skeletal traction through an olecranon screw or pin in the distal humerus may be indicated. The lower arm is held in balanced suspension only. The elbow is maintained at 90 degrees of flexion or slightly more.

1. Be certain that the traction tapes are properly adhered and wrapped.
2. Assess the neurovascular status of the extremity every 2 hours.

1. Prevents damage to the skin and ensures proper pull.
2. Elastic bandages can cause circulatory or neurologic compromise. Early detection can prevent patient harm.

(continued)

PROCEDURE GUIDELINES 51-2 ◆ Care of a Child in Traction *(continued)*

PROCEDURE (cont'd)	*NURSING ACTION*	*RATIONALE*

CERVICAL TRACTION *(SEE ACCOMPANYING FIGURE)*

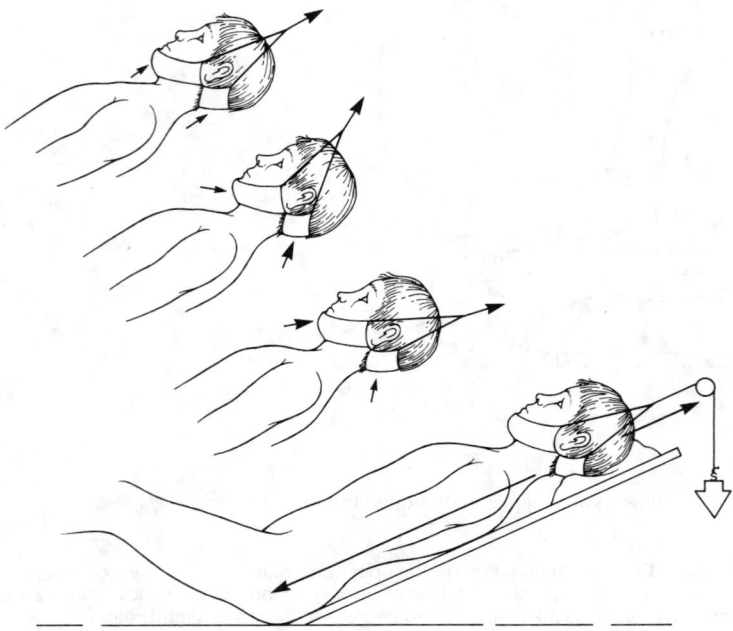

Cervical traction.

Indications:
Used for stabilization of spinal fractures or injuries, muscle spasms, muscle contractures.

Mechanism of Action:
Traction force applied through a head halter (skin traction) or directly to the skull by means of Crutchfield tongs or halo apparatus.

1. Head halter must be assessed for proper positioning. It should not place pressure on ears, skin, or throat.	1. Prevents pressure sores.
2. Maintain flat bed position.	2. Proper spinal alignment is critical to prevention of further injury.
3. Keep the child in proper position and alignment.	
4. Crutchfield tongs or halo pin sites should be treated as skeletal traction sites.	4. Prevents infection.
5. If permissible, place the child on a Stryker frame or specially equipped bed.	5. Allows the child to be repositioned without disrupting spinal alignment.

HALO-FEMORAL

Indications:
Used to correct severe spinal curvatures either before surgery or after a spinal release before final correction.

Mechanism of Action:
A halo is affixed to the skull. A traction pin is placed in each distal femur. Traction force is applied upward to the halo and downward to the femurs, pulling the spine into alignment.

PROCEDURE (cont'd)	NURSING ACTION	RATIONALE
	1. General traction considerations must be followed.	
	2. Assess the child carefully every 2 hours for any increased complaints of pain, respiratory difficulty, or nerve injury.	2. Complaints should not be ignored, because alteration in any of these can indicate neurologic or spinal injury. Notification of health care provider is vital to prevent further harm.
	3. Be alert for symptoms of injury to cranial nerves: a. Lateral gaze paralysis b. Difficulty in swallowing. c. Difficulty in coughing. d. Voice changes. e. Tongue weakness.	3. Common cranial nerve injuries: a. Abducens nerve palsy (most common injury). b. Vagus nerve. d. Glossopharyngeal nerve. e. Hypoglossal nerve.
	4. Be alert for symptoms of injury to spinal cord: a. Weakness, numbness in legs. b. Loss of bladder function. c. Upturning or downturning of toes. d. Clonus of ankles or knees.	4. These complaints may indicate lower spinal nerve root or cauda equina damage and should be reported promptly.
	5. Be alert for symptoms of brachial plexus injuries: a. Difficulty in moving hand, shoulder, or arm. b. Numbness or weakness in hand.	5. These complaints or findings may indicate damage to upper extremity and should be reported promptly.
	6. Assess all pin sites for loosening every shift.	6. Loose pins can cause harm to the child as well as prevent proper traction pull.
	7. Keep the torque wrench for the halo pins at the bedside at all times.	7. The halo or pins may have to be removed or adjusted in an emergency or to ensure proper tension on the pins.

Selected References

Green, N. E., & Swiontkowski, M. F. (1994). *Skeletal trauma in children.* Philadelphia: W.B. Saunders.

Hayes, M. A. (1995). Traction at home for infants with developmental dysplasia of the hip. *Orthopedic Nursing, 14*(1), 33–40.

Lonstein, J. E., Bradford, D. S., Winter, R. B., & Ogilvie, J. W. (1995). *Moe's textbook of scoliosis and other spinal deformities.* Philadelphia: W. B. Saunders.

Maher, A. E., Salmond, S. W., & Pellino, T. A. (1994). *Orthopedic nursing.* Philadelphia: W.B. Saunders.

Newman, D. M. & Fawcett, J. (1995). Caring for a young child in a body cast: Impact on the care giver. *Orthopedic Nursing, 14*(1), 41–46.

Styrcula, L. (1994). Traction basics: Part III, Types of traction. *Orthopedic Nursing, 13*(4), 34–43.

Tachdjian, M. O. (1990). *Pediatric orthopedics* (2nd ed.). Philadelphia: W.B. Saunders.

Wiesel, S. W., Delahay, J. N., & Connell, M. C. (1993). *Essentials of orthopedic surgery.* Philadelphia: W.B. Saunders.

CHAPTER 52 ◆

Pediatric Integumentary Disorders

Burns

◆ MANAGEMENT OF BURNS IN CHILDREN

Burns are a frequent form of childhood injury. They may be caused by heat, electrical energy, or chemicals. The effects of burns are not limited to the burn area. Very serious burns may include:

1. Second-dregree burn of 10% or more of body surface.
2. Burns of face, hands, feet, perineum, or joint surfaces.
3. Electrical burns.
4. Burns in the presence of other injuries.
5. When home situation is not adequate for optimal care.

Incidence and Etiology

1. Burns are the second leading cause of accidental deaths in childhood, with the highest incidence of burns occurring in children younger than 5 years of age.
2. Children at high risk are of lower socioeconomic status and of single parents. However, any child, supervised or unsupervised, is at risk for a burn injury.
3. Scalds are the leading cause of injury in children, followed by flame burns.
4. Burns from hot liquid are most common in children younger than age 3 years.
   a. Child (left unsupervised in tub) turns on hot water tap.
   b. Tap water temperature above 125°F (at 130°F it takes only 30 seconds to produce a full-thickness injury in adult skin; less time in the very young).
   c. Child placed in tub of hot water that has not been tested.
   d. Spilling of hot coffee or tea on child. Spilling occurs especially when pot handles stick out on top of stove, when hot liquids and foods are removed from microwave oven, and when child grabs or pulls items from surfaces.
   e. Ingestion and aspiration of hot foods and liquids from microwave oven as well as scald burns to skin and palate from hot formula.
5. Burns from open flames:
   a. House fires.
   b. Child climbing on stove, resulting in ignited clothing.
   c. Children playing with lighters, especially 3- to 10-year-olds.
   d. Playing or working with gasoline.
   e. Automobile accidents with subsequent fire.
   f. Juvenile fire setters.
6. Electrical burns are most common in toddlers and adolescents and may be caused by:
   a. Child playing with electrical outlets or appliances.
   b. Child playing with extension cords; often bite through the cord.
   c. Child playing on railroad tracks; climbing trees and touching high tension wires, lightning.
7. Other causes:
   a. Caustic acid or alkali burns of mouth and esophagus.
   b. Chemical burns of the skin—child playing with gasoline that comes in contact with skin (often gasoline ignites).
   c. Burns inflicted on the child as a result of neglect or abuse (an estimated 30% of all burns brought to a hospital; immersion and contact burns most common).
   d. Smoke inhalation and inhalation from products of combustion of synthetics, that is, plastics, rayons; may yield cyanide, formaldehyde.
   e. Radiation burns—sunburn most common, may be secondary to cancer radiation therapy.
   f. Contact burns from touching hot surfaces, such as radiators or wood-burning stoves.
   g. Fireworks burns, often as a result of misuse and lack of adult supervision; may be combined with explosive hand injuries.

> **NURSING ALERT:** ◆
> With combined injury, the trauma takes precedence over the burn.

Altered Physiology

See Burns in Adults, page 906.

Complications

Depend on severity of burn injury; commonly occur, especially with severe burn injury.

A. **Acute**
1. Infection; burn wound sepsis, pneumonia, urinary tract infection, phlebitis, toxic shock syndrome.
2. Curling's (stress) ulcer, gastrointestinal hemorrhage; rarely seen now that histamine 2 (HZ) blockers are commonly used prophylactically, especially in burns greater than 20% total body surface area (TBSA).

Sandra Nettina: *The Lippincott Manual of Nursing Practice, 6th ed.* © 1996 Lippincott-Raven Publishers

3. Acute gastric dilation, paralytic ileus; occurs especially in child younger than 2 years of age with greater than 20% injury and develops early in postburn period, lasting 2 to 3 days.
4. Renal failure.
5. Respiratory failure; severe inhalation injury is the insult most likely to cause death.
6. Postburn seizures.
7. Hypertension.
8. Central nervous system dysfunction.
9. Vascular ischemia.
10. Anemia and malnutrition; may resolve once burn area is covered.
11. Fecal impaction.
12. Depression secondary to hospitalization and changing body image.

B. Long-term
1. Growth and development delays secondary to malnutrition.
2. Scarring, disfigurement, and contractures.
3. Psychological trauma.

Clinical Manifestations

A. Characteristics of Burn Wounds
1. See page 906 for characteristics of first-, second-, and third-degree burns.
2. *Electrical burns.*
   a. Especially of the mouth in child younger than age 2 years; may chew or suck on live wire.
   b. Are progressive and may take up to 3 weeks to fully declare the full extent of injury.

B. Symptoms of Shock
Symptoms of shock appear soon after the burn.

1. Rapid pulse, low blood pressure.
2. Subnormal temperature.
3. Pallor, cyanosis, prostration.
4. Failure to recognize familiar people.
5. Poor muscle tone; may become flaccid.

C. Symptoms of Toxemia
Symptoms may develop 1 to 2 days after burn.

1. Prostration, fever, rapid pulse

> **NURSING ALERT:**
> The fever of toxemia is not to be confused with expected "burn fever," which may be as high as 103°F (39.5°C), because of the hypermetabolic state.

2. Glucosuria, decreased urinary output
3. Vomiting, edema
4. These symptoms may progress to coma or death.

D. Upper Respiratory Tract Injury
Causes inflammation or edema of the glottis, vocal cords, and upper trachea and is characterized by symptoms of upper airway obstruction.

1. Dyspnea, tachypnea, hoarseness
2. Stridor, substernal and intercostal retractions, nasal flaring
3. Restlessness, drooling, cough

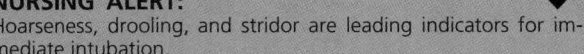

> **NURSING ALERT:**
> Hoarseness, drooling, and stridor are leading indicators for immediate intubation.

E. Smoke Inhalation
May cause no initial symptoms other than mild bronchial obstruction during the initial phase after the burn. Within 6 to 48 hours, the child may develop sudden onset of the following conditions:

1. Bronchiolitis
2. Pulmonary edema (adult respiratory distress syndrome)
3. Severe airway obstruction
4. Delayed damage: up to 7 days after the burn injury

Diagnostic Evaluation

A. Calculation of the Burn Area
1. "Rule of Nines" (used in assessment of extent of burns in adults) has not proven to be exact when applied to young children. May be acceptable to use in child older than 10 years of age. It is not recommended for hospital use; the Lund and Browder chart is recommended. Total body surface area is based on age, thus compensating for changes is percentages resulting from growth (Fig. 52-1).
   a. During infancy and early childhood, the relative surface area of different parts of the body varies with age.
   b. The younger the child, the greater the proportion of the surface area is constituted by the head and the lesser the proportion of the surface area is constituted by the legs.
2. A rough estimate can be obtained by using the child's hand, which is equal to 1%.

B. Categorization of Severity of Burn
1. Total area injured, depth of injury, location of injury
2. Age of child
3. Condition of patient (ie, level of consciousness)
4. Medical history (ie, chronic disease)
5. Additional injuries

C. Schematic Classification of Burn Severity
1. Minor burn—10% TBSA, first- and second-degree burn.
2. Moderate burn:
   a. Ten percent to 20% TBSA, second-degree burn.
   b. Two percent to 5% TBSA, third-degree burn not involving eyes, ears, face, genitals, hands, or feet or circumferential burns.
3. Major burn:
   a. Twenty percent TBSA, second-degree burn.
   b. All third-degree burns greater than 10%; depending on age of child, 5% is sometimes used.
   c. All burns involving hands, face, eyes, ears, feet, and/or genitals.
   d. All electrical burns.
   e. Complicated burn injuries involving fracture or other major trauma.
   f. All poor-risk patients (ie, head injury, cancer, lung disease, diabetes).

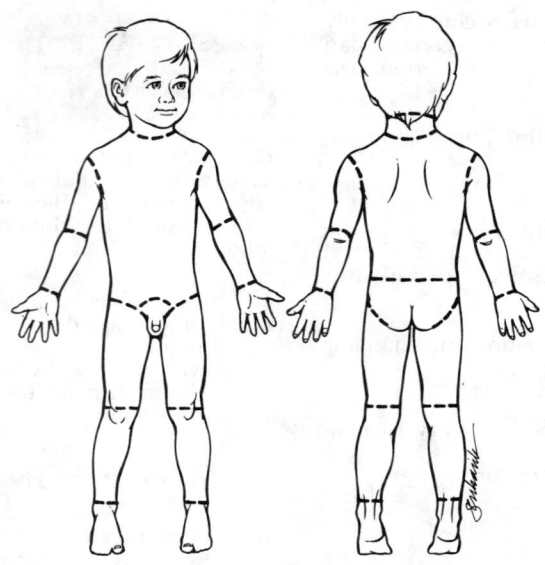

Age-Years

Area	0–1	1–4	5–9	10–15	Adult	% 2	% 3	% Total
Head	19	17	13	10	7			
Neck	2	2	2	2	2			
Ant. Trunk	13	13	13	13	13			
Post. Trunk	13	13	13	13	13			
R. Buttock	2	2	2	2	2			
L. Buttock	2	2	2	2	2			
Genitalia	1	1	1	1	1			
R. U. Arm	4	4	4	4	4			
L. U. Arm	4	4	4	4	4			
R. L. Arm	3	3	3	3	3			
L. L. Arm	3	3	3	3	3			
R. Hand	2	2	2	2	2			
L. Hand	2	2	2	2	2			
R. Thigh	5	6	8	8	9			
L. Thigh	5	6	8	8	9			
R. Leg	5	5	5	6	7			
L. Leg	5	5	5	6	7			
R. Foot	3	3	3	3	3			
L. Foot	3	3	3	3	3			
					Total			

FIGURE 52-1 *Lund and Browder chart for determining extent of burns. Adapted with permission from Franklin H. Martin Memorial Foundation. (1944). Surgery, Gynecology, and Obstetrics, 79, 352. From: Jackson and Saunders. Child Health Nursing-Lippincott 1993.*

Treatment

A. Fluid Resuscitation: Intravenous Fluid Replacement
Note: Controversy exists regarding fluid resuscitation solution and amount.

1. Fluid loss from transcapillary leakage is greatest during the first 12 hours after injury and diminishes to almost zero 12 to 24 hours after injury. Fluid loss after 48 hours is due to vaporization of water from wound.
2. Replacement usually consists of Ringer's solution—an isotonic electrolyte solution.
3. The Parkland formula is commonly used to determine the fluid needed for resuscitation for burns greater than 15% to 20% TBSA (see page 910).

B. Burn Treatment
Burns may be treated by the open or closed methods or combination technique.

Children appear to be more mobile when burn injury is covered, because they experience less pain.

Hydrotherapy is treatment of choice for cleansing of wounds. Isotonic saline may be needed for large wounds and small children, rather than water.

Gaining popularity is the use of a shower to facilitate the loosening and removal of sloughing tissue, eschar, exudate, and topical medications. The child is suspended over a tub in a fine-mesh nylon sling. The shower, water about 32°C (90°F), flows over the child; then debridement is done.

See pages 911–915 for wound cleansing and debridement, hydrotherapy, topical antimicrobials, surgical management, and burn wound grafting.

Nursing Assessment

1. Initially, perform emergency assessment of the burn patient to determine priorities of care.
   a. Airway, breathing, and circulation: airway may be compromised with inhalation injury.
   b. Extent of burn injury.
   c. Additional injuries.
2. Obtain a history of the injury; for example, ask if the child was involved in an automobile accident or dropped from a window for rescue to help establish if additional injuries may exist.
3. Obtain a complete medical history, including childhood diseases, immunizations (especially tetanus status), current medications, allergies, recent infections.
4. Subsequently, focus assessment on fluid volume balance, condition of the burn wounds, and signs of infection (burn wound, pulmonary, urinary).
5. Assess level of comfort and emotional status; provide reassurance while performing assessment and determining priorities.

Nursing Diagnoses

A. Decreased Cardiac Output related to fluid loss and hypermetabolic state
B. Risk for Infection related to altered skin integrity, decreased circulation and immobility
C. Impaired Gas Exchange related to inhalation injury, pain, and immobility
D. Risk for Injury related to paralytic ileus and stress
E. Altered Nutrition, Less Than Body Requirements, related to hypermetabolic state and poor appetite
F. Impaired Physical Mobility related to dressings, pain, and contractures
G. Pain related to burn wound and associated treatments
H. Body Image Disturbance related to pain, scarring, and disfigurement
I. Fear and Anxiety related to pain, treatments, procedures, and hospitalization
J. Altered Parenting related to crisis situation, prolonged hospitalization, and disfigurement

Nursing Interventions

A. Supporting Cardiac Output
1. Be alert to the symptoms of shock that occur very shortly after a severe burn—tachycardia, hypothermia, hypotension, pallor, prostration, shallow respirations, anuria.
2. Monitor the administration of intravenous fluid, because major burns are followed by a reduction in blood volume due to outflow of plasma into the tissues.
3. Maintain and record intake and output to provide an accurate measure of volume.
   a. Record time and amount of all fluids given.
   b. Measure accurately urinary output every hour and report diminished output as ordered (usually, 0.5 cc/kg/hour is considered minimally acceptable urinary output).
   c. Check specific gravity to determine urine concentration or dilution.
4. With severe burn injuries, insert an indwelling catheter.
5. Weigh daily to help evaluate fluid balance.
6. Monitor sensorium, pulse, pulse pressure, capillary filling, and blood gases.
7. Provide a rich oxygen environment to combat hypoxia, as necessary.
8. Monitor electrolyte and hematocrit results as a guide to fluid replacement.
9. Maintain a warm, humidified ambient environment (especially with burns >20% TBSA) to maintain body temperature and decrease fluid needs.

B. Preventing Infection
1. Provide scrupulous skin care to prevent infection and promote healing.

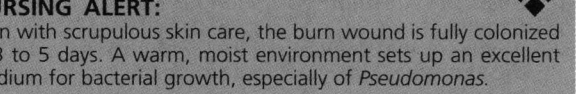

NURSING ALERT:
Even with scrupulous skin care, the burn wound is fully colonized in 3 to 5 days. A warm, moist environment sets up an excellent medium for bacterial growth, especially of *Pseudomonas*.

2. Prevent child from scratching by administering antipruritics and applying protective devices to hands.
3. Obtain serial wound biopsy and cultures as ordered.
4. Observe burn wounds with each dressing change: assess drainage for color, odor, and amount; necrosis; increase in pain; and surrounding erythema, warmth, swelling, and tenderness, which may indicate infection.
5. Administer topical antimicrobials and systemic antibiotics as ordered.

6. Observe for signs of toxemia, such as fever, prostration, tachycardia, vomiting, oliguria, and report immediately.
7. Be alert for the development of pneumonia or urinary tract infection related to immobility and invasive procedures. Encourage coughing, turning, deep breathing, ambulation, and early discontinuation of indwelling catheter to minimize the complications.
8. Administer tetanus prophylaxis based on immunization history.
   a. If primary series complete (or at least three doses of tetanus toxoid obtained) and last injection within past 5 years, it is not necessary.
   b. If at least three doses obtained and last injection greater than 5 years, give tetanus toxoid.
   c. If two or fewer doses obtained, give tetanus immunoglobulin and tetanus toxoid.
9. Obtain urine, sputum, and blood cultures for two or more consecutive temperatures of 103°F (39.5°C) or a single temperature of 104°F (40°C).

C. **Optimizing Gas Exchange**
1. Be alert for and report symptoms of respiratory distress—dyspnea, stridor, tachypnea, restlessness, cyanosis, coughing, increasing hoarseness, drooling.
2. Administer supplemental humidified oxygen.
3. Monitor arterial blood gases.
4. Evaluate the carboxyhemoglobin on arterial blood gases (due to inhalation of carbon monoxide, a product of combustion) and be prepared to support ventilation if signs of hypoxemia and respiratory failure develop.
5. Assist with pulmonary function and bronchoscopy as indicated.
6. Have intubation supplies immediately available. If unable to intubate the child, then tracheostomy may be necessary. If unable to extubate in 14 to 21 days, then may be converted to tracheostomy for continuous pulmonary management.

D. **Relieving Gastric Dilation and Preventing Stress Ulcer**
1. Be alert for the development of gastric distention, especially with burns greater than 20% TBSA, associated injury, or tachypnea.
2. Maintain nothing-by-mouth status if distention or decreased bowel sounds develop.
3. Insert nasogastric tube as indicated to prevent vomiting, aspiration, and paralytic ileus.
4. Monitor the return of bowel sounds after nasogastric extubation and before reinstituting oral feeding.
5. Administer H2 blockers, such as cimetidine (Tagamet), to prevent Curling's ulcer development.

E. **Ensuring Adequate Nutrition for Healing and Growth Needs**
1. Be aware that hypernutrition is important because of the extreme hypermetabolism related to large burn injuries.
   a. Twice the predicted basal metabolic rate in calories, based on ideal weight, may be necessary. Caloric recommendation is 1,800 kcal/m² body surface for maintenance, plus 2,000 kcal/m² of burned surface area.
   b. Hypermetabolic state generally subsides when the majority of the wounds are grafted or healed.
   c. High caloric intake to support hypermetabolic state; protein synthesis; calories should come from carbohydrates.

d. High-protein intake to replace protein lost by exudation; support synthesis of immunoglobulins and structural protein; prevent negative nitrogen balance.
   e. Vitamin and mineral supplement needed, particularly vitamins B and C, iron, and zinc.
2. Maintain ambient temperature, 28°C to 32°C (90°F) to minimize metabolic expenditure by maintaining core temperature.
3. Minimize anorexia to increase caloric intake.
   a. Offer small amounts of food, perhaps four to five feedings rather than three per day.
   b. Give choice of foods; determine favorites.
   c. Provide high-calorie, high-protein oral or nasogastric supplementation as necessary.
   d. Make meals a pleasant time, unassociated with treatments or unpleasant interruptions.
4. Monitor dietary compliance with dietary goals and adjustment as needed.
5. Administer total parenteral nutrition if necessary.
6. Administer serum albumin or fresh frozen plasma to combat hypoalbuminemia when burn area exceeds 20% TBSA.
7. Monitor nutritional status through weight gain, wound healing, serum transferrin, and serum albumin.

F. **Preserving Mobility**
1. Ensure that physical and occupational therapy are begun early to facilitate rehabilitation.
2. Encourage range-of-motion exercises, ambulation, and positioning to minimize joint and skin complications.
3. Position joint in opposite direction of expected contracture.
4. Apply splints to aid joint positioning and decrease skin contractures and hypertrophy.
5. Apply pressure garments to aid circulation, protect newly healed skin, and prevent and treat hypertrophic scar formation by promoting dermal collagen fiber growth in parallel direction. Encourage use of pressure garments for as long as 12 to 18 months after injury, until the healed skin has matured.
6. Medicate for pain before therapy or exercise to minimize discomfort.
7. Use play opportunities to help the child accept the therapy program (eg, tricycle riding may be used as form of exercise).

G. **Controlling Pain**
1. Assess for signs of pain, such as irritability, crying, increased blood pressure, tachycardia, decreased mobility, and inability to sleep.
2. Administer analgesics and/or sedatives to relieve pain.
   a. Analgesia may include, but is not limited to, acetaminophen (Tylenol), acetaminophen with codeine (Tylenol #2 or #3), meperidine (Demerol), morphine (Duramorph), hydroxyzine (Vistaril), and ibuprofen (Motrin).
   b. In severe burns, analgesia should be given intravenously because of lack of absorption of intramuscular injections during the emergency phase.
3. Use an alternating water or sand bed to relieve pressure and provide comfort.
4. Maintain warmth and prevent chilling.
5. Provide diversional activities appropriate for age to distract from focus on pain.
6. Teach simple relaxation techniques, such as relaxation breathing and guided imagery.

7. Recognize that fear may exaggerate discomfort; provide reassurance and empathy.

H. Preventing Negative Body Image
1. Encourage the child to talk about the way he or she feels and looks.
   a. The child may feel guilty and think that the burn is punishment for some wrong deed.
   b. Small children may be fearful of the appearance of bandages, scars, or pressure garments; offer reassurance.
   c. Encourage the use of play with dolls or puppets, role playing, or picture drawing to help child express feelings and fears.
2. Treat child with warmth and affection and encourage parents to continually point out their love even though child has a bad burn.
3. Support child in viewing self in mirror when ready and encourage presence of family members.
4. Encourage early contact with other children.
5. Suggest psychiatric consultation for:
   a. Refusing to eat.
   b. Resisting all nursing procedures.
   c. Resisting socialization.
6. Advise parents that separation from the hospital environment, caregivers, and other patients can produce excessive anxiety. Short-time home passes (overnight, weekend) are helpful before final discharge.
7. If the child is school age, help prepare for school reentry—contact teacher or discuss with parents the need to prepare peers for what to expect.
8. Discuss issues of social reentry, such as responding to questions and stares from strangers, and perceived rejection by friends.
   a. Refer to a support group and/or have a child who has recovered from burns visit child.
   b. Refer to a burn camp—often this may be the first opportunity for the child to wear a swimsuit after the injury.
9. Initiate family consult with plastic surgeon about future scar revision.
10. Encourage older child to experiment with clothing and consult with a burn cosmetic specialist to enhance appearance and body image.

I. Reducing Fear and Anxiety
1. Explain procedures, surgeries, and treatments to the child according to age and level of understanding.
2. Allow the child to express fears through puppets, dolls, water play, clay, and drawings.
3. Expect regression due to the physical pain and psychological trauma the child is going through.
4. Encourage parents to stay with a young child as much as possible.
5. Try to involve child in group play and unit activities.
6. Encourage involvement with treatment plan and self-care activities.

J. Promoting Effective Parenting
1. Be alert to signs that parents may react to the situation with depression and/or stress syndromes, and encourage counseling for them to promote a healthier family.
2. Encourage parents to assess the effects on siblings at home; they may have needs that are unrecognized or neglected as a result of this crisis.
3. Attempt to have parents become actively involved in the child's care when they are ready to do so.

a. Advise parents that their visits and involvement can have a positive effect on the child's survival and recovery.
b. If the parents are unable to visit, telephone calls and family photographs are helpful.
4. Give the parents the opportunity to discuss their feelings.
   a. Parents frequently express guilt regarding their lack of supervision when the accident occurred.
   b. Frequently, burn injury is associated with actual or perceived parental neglect. Remember that this type of injury is sudden and acute, placing the family in a state of crisis.
5. Keep the parents informed of the child's progress.
   a. Begin initial teaching at admission with supportive words and limited technical information.
   b. Education and orientation to the facility and the burn injury will decrease some anxiety and begin to build rapport on which future support can be based.
   c. Encourage meetings with other parents who have coped with trauma.

Family Education/Health Maintenance

1. Teach that special skin care is necessary after burn injury.
   a. Avoid exposure to sunlight; use sunscreen of sun protective factor 24 or higher and apply frequently.
   b. Use pressure garments to prevent hypertrophic scar and keloid formation; worn 23 of 24 hours for effectiveness.
   c. Use lotions and creams to prevent skin from drying, cracking, and itching.
   d. Burn area has decreased sensation to touch, heat, and pressure; take precautions to prevent injury to area.
2. Advise that adjustment after burn is often prolonged and painful. Encourage ongoing family and individual psychological support.
3. Encourage continued physical therapy to prevent contractures and preserve function.
4. Ensure that parents are able to:
   a. Discuss and demonstrate treatments, procedures, and dressing changes.
   b. Obtain equipment necessary to perform treatment at home.
   c. Understand reason for and side effects of medications as well as dietary requirements.
   d. Follow up at appropriate intervals with the designated health care provider.
5. Initiate home health, financial assistance, and other referrals as necessary.
6. Teach parents and children the prevention of burn injury as well as other safety measures (see p. 1101).
7. Teach first-aid emergency care for burn injury (ie, cool burned area with cool water; remove clothing, seek medical assistance).
8. Teach children how to stop, drop, and roll if their clothes catch on fire and how to crawl to safety if a fire occurs in the house.

COMMUNITY-BASED CARE TIP:
Encourage the use of smoke alarms on every floor in homes, fire extinguisher, and an emergency fire escape plan.

Evaluation

A. Absence of shock: stabilization of vital signs, normal serum and electrolyte values
B. Absence of infection: normal laboratory values, clean wound, and normal temperature
C. No respiratory distress: stable vital signs, respiratory status, and arterial blood gases
D. No gastrointestinal complications: normal bowel sounds and ability to tolerate oral feeding
E. Adequate nutritional status: weight gain and wound healing
F. Improved mobility: involvement in play and other activities
G. Minimal discomfort: stable vital signs, verbalization, and involvement in play
H. Positive body image: verbalization, socialization, and ability to look in mirror
I. Relief of fear: able to play, participates in care
J. Effective parenting: involvement in child's care, accurate discussion of child's progress and treatment plan

Dermatologic Disorders

◆ ATOPIC DERMATITIS (INFANTILE AND CHILDHOOD ECZEMA)

Atopic dermatitis, the most common cause of eczema in childhood, is a characteristic inflammatory response of the skin. The major features include pruritus, a typical morphology and distribution, chronic or chronically relapsing nature, and a personal or family history of atopy (asthma, hay fever, and atopic dermatitis). There is a tendency toward dry skin and a lower threshold to itching.

Etiology and Incidence

1. Atopic dermatitis affects 10% to 15% of the childhood population.
2. It usually starts after 2 months of age. By age 5, 90% of the patients who will develop atopic dermatitis have already manifested the disease. It may stop after an indefinite period of time or it may progress from infancy to adulthood with little or no relief. It is rare for adults to develop atopic dermatitis without a history of eczema in childhood.
3. The etiology is unknown but has familial tendencies. Almost 75% of patients with this form of eczema have a family history of atopic dermatitis, hay fever, or asthma. One-third to one-half of children with eczema will develop hay fever or asthma themselves.

Altered Physiology

1. Atopic dermatitis involves immunologic abnormalities, such as elevated immunoglobulin E levels and increased rates of sensitization to common contact allergens and to intradermal skin tests. Although exact cause is unknown, there is a constitutional predisposition to develop pruritus. In general, the skin of patients with atopic dermatitis is different from that of healthy patients in the following respects:
   a. Increased tendency toward dryness.
   b. Lowered threshold for pruritus from minor irritants, such as soap, wool, perspiration, cold weather, and heat.
   c. Tendency toward lichenification (leathery thickening of skin) and production of a rash when the skin is rubbed or scratched

Complications

1. Common—secondary infection (pyoderma), usually associated with group A beta-hemolytic streptococci and/or *S. aureus*.
2. Rare—eczema vaccinatum (eczema herpeticum or Kaposi's varicelliform eruption) after exposure of an eczematoid child to a smallpox vaccination or a person recently vaccinated with smallpox.

Clinical Manifestations

A. Age and Distribution of Lesions
Atopic dermatitis is divided into three phases based on the age of the patient and the distribution of the lesions. These are referred to as the infantile, childhood, and adult phases.

1. Infantile (2 months to 2 years)
   a. The onset is between 2 and 6 months of age. Half of affected infants have spontaneous resolution by age 2 or 3.
   b. Characterized by intense itching, erythema, papules, vesicles, oozing, and crusting.
   c. The rash usually begins on the cheeks, forehead, or scalp and then extends to the trunk or extremities in scattered, often symmetrical patches. The perioral, perinasal, and diaper areas are usually spared (Fig. 52-2).
2. Childhood (4 to 10 years)
   a. Affected persons in this age group are less likely to have exudative and crusted lesions. Eruptions are characteristically more dry and papular and often occur as circumscribed scaly patches. There is a greater tendency toward chronicity and lichenification.
   b. The typical areas of involvement are the face, with the perioral and perinasal areas affected; neck; antecubital and popliteal fossae; and wrists and ankles.
3. Adult (puberty to old age)
   a. Predominant areas of involvement include the flexor folds, face, neck, upper arms, back, dorsa (back) of the hands, feet, fingers, and toes.
   b. The eruption is characterized by dry, thick lesions; confluent papules; and the formation of large lichenified plaques. Weeping, crusting, and exudation can occur, but they are usually the result of superimposed external irritation or infection.

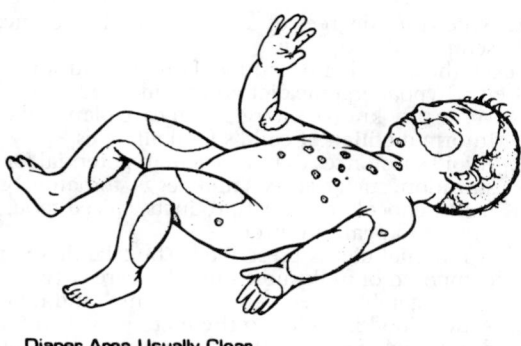

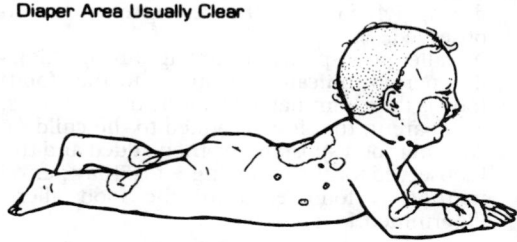

Diaper Area Usually Clear

FIGURE 52-2 *Infantile atopic eczema occurs primarily on the face, but may develop on symmetrical areas of the body. (From Sauer GC. Manual of Skin Diseases. 5th ed. Philadelphia, JB Lippincott, 1986)*

B. Clinical Appearance

Atopic dermatitis is also divided into three stages based on the clinical appearance of the lesions. The acute, subacute, and chronic stages can occur in infants, children, and adults.

1. Acute
   a. Moderate to intense erythema, vesicles, a wet surface, and severe itching.
2. Subacute
   a. Erythema and scaling are present in various patterns with indistinct borders. The redness may be faint or intense. The surface is dry. There are varying degrees of pruritus.
   b. The subacute stage may be an initial stage or may follow an acute inflammation or exacerbation of a chronic stage. Irritation, allergy, or infection can convert a subacute process into an acute one.
3. Chronic
   a. The inflamed area thickens and the surface skin markings become more prominent. Thick plaques with deep parallel skin markings are said to be lichenified. The surface of the skin is dry and the border of the lesion well defined. There is moderate to intense itching.

Diagnostic Evaluation

Atopic dermatitis is usually a clinical diagnosis based on the evaluation of the aggregate of signs, symptoms, stigmata, course, and associated familial findings. The major features include pruritus, a characteristic morphology and typical distribution for the age of the patient, a chronic or chronically relapsing nature, and a personal or family history of atopic disease. When the diagnosis is in doubt, a skin biopsy may be performed.

Treatment

A. Acute
1. Open wet dressings for 1 to 3 days.
2. Avoidance of any known allergen.
3. Topical corticosteroids.
4. Oral medications to relieve itching—hydroxyzine hydrochloride (Atarax), diphenhydramine hydrochloride (Benadryl), promethazine hydrochloride (Phenergan).
5. Management of secondary infection, if present, with oral antibiotics.
6. Initiation of a hypoallergenic diet to eliminate any responsible food for infants and children with severe, recalcitrant atopic dermatitis.

B. Subacute and Chronic
1. Prevention of dry skin
   a. Diminish the frequency and duration of bathing.
   b. Use mild soap or hydrophilic lotion.
   c. Lubricate the skin with emollients.
   d. Add tar preparations to the bath water.
   e. Maintain environmental humidity above 40% in winter months.
2. Same as for acute stage with exception of dressings.

Nursing Assessment

1. Take a nursing history focusing on clinical manifestations:
   a. Onset and duration of rash.
   b. Location, course, and distribution of lesions.
   c. Change in morphology of lesions.
   d. Local and systemic symptoms.
   e. Exposure to possible allergens.
   f. Previous episodes of rashes.
   g. Personal history of allergies, asthma, or hay fever.
   h. Family history of eczema, allergies, or hay fever.
   i. Medications, treatments tried, and their effect.
2. Perform a physical assessment.
   a. Examine the entire skin in an orderly fashion with specific attention to the type of lesion (eg, macule, papule, vesicle), its appearance (shape, border, color, texture, and surface), and its distribution (areas of the body involved).
   b. Note any associated symptoms, such as scratching, fever, or drainage.
3. Document findings.
   a. Describe skin findings using dermatologic terminology.
   b. Draw pictures to facilitate communication.

Nursing Diagnoses

A. Impaired Skin Integrity, high risk for impairment, related to skin pathology and scratching
B. Sensory/Perceptual Alterations (Tactile), related to skin pathology
C. Risk for infection related to increased bacterial colonization of skin and possible break in defensive barrier

Nursing Interventions

The nurse may perform the following interventions or teach the patient or family to do the following.

A. *Improving Skin Integrity*
1. Reduce inflammation during the acute stage with the topical application of open wet dressings.
   a. Use a soft lightweight cloth, such as a handkerchief, a thin diaper, or strips of bed sheeting. Do not use gauze (adheres to skin), washcloths, or towels (too heavy).
   b. Open wet dressings should be clean. In certain situations, they should be sterile to prevent contamination.
   c. Solutions should be lukewarm or body temperature to soothe and prevent chilling.
   d. Compresses should be moderately wet, not dripping, and removed after 20 minutes, unless otherwise directed. They should be reapplied three to four times a day to promote skin hydration.
   e. After the compress, a topical corticosteroid may be applied to reduce itching and inflammation.
   f. Observe the skin for changes in response to therapy.
2. Prevent dry skin during the subacute and chronic stage.
   a. Decrease the frequency and duration of bathing. Long, hot tub baths are to be avoided.
   b. Avoid hot water and harsh soaps. Patients should bathe in lukewarm water using mild soap (Dove, Neutrogena); avoid bubble bath; rinse well and pat skin dry with towel.
   c. If bath water stings, add 1 cup of table salt.
   d. Apply unscented emollients (eg, Eucerin, Keri, Lubriderm) within 3 minutes of bathing, when the skin is slightly moist. Creams and ointments are more effective than lotions because they are better at preventing the evaporation of water from the skin. Bathing will dry and damage the skin unless an emollient is applied immediately after exiting the bath.
   e. Some patients may benefit from soaking in a tar bath for 15 to 20 minutes daily, preferably in the evening. Add to bath water as directed. Tar preparations can stain the skin and clothing and may cause sunlight sensitivity.
   f. For patients with extremely dry skin, cleanse with a hydrophilic lotion (eg, Cetaphil). Apply without water until light foam occurs. Remove by wiping with soft cotton cloth or cleansing tissue.
   g. Keep environmental humidity above 40% in winter months. Use a humidifier.
   h. Observe the skin for changes in response to therapy.

B. *Controlling Pruritus*
1. Apply topical corticosteroids.
   a. Use a thin layer of topical corticosteroids to the affected skin two to four times a day as directed. Use only for the duration prescribed.
   b. Avoid very potent (Group 1) topical corticosteroids in children younger than 12 years of age because of greater skin absorption.
   c. Observe for possible side effects from long-term use of topical corticosteroids (eg, striae, cutaneous atrophy, telangiectasia, acne, growth retardation).
   d. Note any scratching and intervene as necessary.
2. Administer oral antipruritic medications.
   a. Give medications exactly as prescribed.
   b. Diphenhydramine hydrochloride (Benadryl) and promethazine hydrochloride (Phenergan) cause more sedation than hydroxyzine hydrochloride (Atarax). Mild sedation may be desirable.
   c. Note the degree of sedation and presence of scratching.
3. Teach the caretaker or family of infants and small children a hypoallergenic diet when indicated.
   a. Write any known allergens on care plan and chart. Inform dietitian of child's food allergies.
   b. Avoid substances that have a high potential for sensitization, such as cow's milk, eggs, tomatoes, citrus fruits, chocolate, wheat products, spiced food, fish, nuts, and peanut butter.
   c. A minimal diet is prescribed. The trial diet may be composed of milk substitute, rice cereal, two fruits, two vegetables, beef, a multivitamin, and no eggs.
   d. A new food is added to the diet every 3 to 5 days, during which time the response to the food is observed.
   e. An allergic response occurring during this 3-to-5-day period indicates sensitivity to that food. That food is then eliminated from the diet. If no response is apparent, that food is added to the child's diet.
   f. Another food substance is then added and the child is observed for the following 3-to-5-day period. This method is followed until the food allergen is determined.

C. *Preventing Infection*
1. Assess and/or treat secondary infection:
   a. Observe the skin for signs of bacterial infection (discharge, oozing, crusts). Report positive findings.
   b. Administer antibiotics as prescribed.
   c. Loosen exudate and crusts with water or wet dressings, unless otherwise specified.
   d. Note changes in the skin in response to therapy.

Family Education/Health Education

1. Teach the patient or family to avoid potential precipitants, including:
   a. Exposure to excessive heat and cold, windy weather, and rapidly changing temperatures.
   b. Wool and occlusive synthetic fabrics which promote sweating and pruritus. Soft, lightweight cotton fabrics are the preferred wearing apparel.
   c. Strenuous athletic activities that provoke sweating. Activities should be modified according to the needs of the child. Swimming is permitted if the child showers after pool swimming and applies a lubricant and/or other topical medications.
   d. Soaps, perfumes, detergents, and certain chemicals.
   e. Stress—stressful situations should be avoided when possible.
   f. Any foods that are associated with skin reactions.

Evaluation

A. Skin intact with minimal erythema and lichenification
B. Verbalizes less itching; less scratching observed
C. No signs of secondary infection

◆ OTHER DERMATOLOGIC DISORDERS

See Table 52-1.

TABLE 52-1 Common Pediatric Skin Problems

Disorder/Organism	Clinical Manifestations	Treatment/Prevention	Nursing/Patient Care Considerations

Impetigo
Bacterial infectious disease affecting the superficial layers of the skin and characterized by the formation of vesicles, crusts, or bullae.
 	
Etiology and Incidence
1. Caused by *Staphylococcus aureus* and *Streptococcus pyogenes*.
2. Occurs most frequently when personal hygiene is poor.
3. Common in children under 10 years of age.
4. Spread by close contact—easily conveyed from person to person via hands, nasal discharge, shared towels, toys, etc.; plastic wading pools in summer—when water is replaced and no disinfectant is used. Very contagious.
5. Any abrasion of skin may serve as portal of entry.
 	
Diagnosis
1. Usually clinical.
2. Rarely, culture of lesion exudate is indicated to confirm the diagnosis.
	1. Incubation period of 1–10 days.
	2. Lesion first appears as pink-red macules that quickly change to vesicles that, in turn, rupture, develop crusts, and leave temporary superficial erythematous area
	   a. Bullous (newborn and older child)—broken blisters form thin, light brown, liquorlike crust. Lesions are more prominent in axillae and groin.
	   b. Crusted (preschool-age—seen more often in summer on exposed body parts)—lesions appear with thick, yellow crusts; skin around crusts is red and weeping with satellite lesions.
	3. Regional lymphadenopathy—common with secondary infection of insect bites, eczema, poison ivy, scabies.
	4. Autoinoculation is major cause of spreading.
	5. Pruritus may occur.
		Based on etiology and type of infection
		1. Removal of crusts, and debris from the affected area by soaking or wet compresses. Use tap water, normal saline tap water, or 1:20 Burrow's solution. Remove crusts when softened.
		2. Topical antibacterial medication such as Bacitracin or mupirocin ointment (Bactroban).
		3. Systemic antibiotic—when severe, or recurrent (cephalosporins, erythromycin, or dicloxacillin).
		4. Prevention—close contact with other children should be avoided until 24 hours after treatment is initiated.
			1. Assess the child's skin condition and document the location and appearance of lesions.
			2. Initiate and teach measures to prevent the spread of infection.
			   a. Engage in frequent hand washing.
			   b. Observe drainage/secretion precautions for 24 hours after the start of therapy.
			   c. Isolate the child from direct contact with other children (school/day-care) until 24 hours after treatment has started.
			3. Provide or teach comfort measures.
			   a. Engage child in diversional activities.
			   b. Administer topical or systemic medications to relieve itching.
			   c. Trim fingernails and toenails and apply mittens to discourage scratching and itching.
			4. Teach child and family general measures to improve health and hygiene.
			5. Be aware that the patient with streptococcal impetigo has an increased risk for acute glomerulonephritis.

Ringworm of the Scalp (tinea capitis)
A fungal infection of the scalp and hair follicles.
 	
Etiology and Incidence
1. Most ringworm of the scalp is caused by *Trichophyton tonsurans. Micosporum canis* and *Micosporum audovinti* are also causative agents.
2. Seen primarily in children before puberty; most commonly in ages 3–10 years.
3. The infection may be spread through child-to-child contact as well as through the common use of towels, combs, brushes, hats. Cats and dogs may be the source of the infection.
	1. Lesions usually develop in the occipital, temporal, and parietal areas of the scalp.
	2. Pruritus usually occurs in the area.
	3. The involved areas of the scalp appear as patches, rounded or oval in outline, covered by scales and lusterless, irregularly broken hairs.
	4. Single or multiple patches of alopecia may occur.
	5. *Kerion,* an acute inflammation that produces edema, pustules, and granulomatous swelling, may occur.
		1. Griseofulvin (Grisactin)—an antifungal antibiotic that is administered orally, 10–20 mg/kg/ dose b.i.d. × 4–8 weeks.
		2. Topical agents—applied b.i.d. Antifungals are not effective
		3. Selenium sulfide lotion 2.5% (Selsun Rx) used twice weekly decreases fungal shedding and may curb infection.
			1. Assess the scalp for characteristic lesions.
			2. Administer or teach patient/family to administer topical or oral medications as prescribed.
			   a. Be aware of side effects, such as headache, heartburn, nausea, epigastric discomfort, diarrhea, urticaria, photosensitivity, and possible granulocytopenia caused by griseofulvin.
			   b. A diet high in fat may enhance intestinal absorption of griseofulvin. Give after a meal with peanut butter or ice cream.

(continued)

TABLE 52-1 Common Pediatric Skin Problems *(continued)*

Disorder/Organism	Clinical Manifestations	Treatment/Prevention	Nursing/Patient Care Considerations

Diagnosis
 1. Wood's lamp evaluation causes *Microsporum* infections to fluoresce. *Trichophyton* infections will not fluoresce.
 2. Microscopic evaluation of skin scrapings and fungal culture.
			3. Teach the child and family methods to prevent further episodes.
			   a. Teach general hygiene measures—regular shampooing and bathing.
			   b. Advise them to avoid the sharing of hats, combs, brushes, etc.
			   c. All family members and close contacts should be screened for infection. The child's school should be notified.
			 4. Temporary hair loss may occur. Provide emotional support and suggest the use of scarves.
			 5. Child may attend school once treatment has been initiated.

Pediculosis
 The infestation of human beings by lice
 Etiology
 1. Three types of lice affect human beings.
   a. *Pediculosis capitis*—head louse
   b. *Pediculosis corporis*—body louse (rare in U.S.)
   c. *Phthirus pubis*—pubic louse/ crab louse (seldom found in children) can attach only to curly hair—pubes, axillae, eyebrows.
 2. Each type of louse generally remains in the area designated by its name, but it may occasionally be seen in other areas of the body
 3. Lice are transmitted by personal contact with people harboring them or through contact with articles that temporarily harbor them (clothing, bed linen)
	1. Severe itching in the area affected is the primary symptom of pediculosis; scratch marks will be evident in these areas.
	 2. Infested scalp areas may become secondarily infected from scratching.
	 3. Crusts, pediculi (lice), nits (eggs), and dirt may combine to cause a foul odor and matted hair.
	 4. Body lice may produce minute red lesions.
	 5. The lice on the skin produce itching; the longer the infestation persists, the more severe the skin reaction becomes and the more severe the lesions appear.
		1. *Pediculosis capitis* may be treated with permethrin (NIX), natural pyrethrin-based products (A-2OO, RID, R&C), lindane 1% (Kwell), or malathion 0.5% (Ovide). Natural pyrethrin-based products and lindane may be reapplied 7–10 days later. Lindane should be avoided in children under 2 years of age.
		 2. For infestations of eyelashes by crab lice, petroleum jelly applied twice daily for 8–10 days is effective.
		 3. *Pediculosis corporis* is treated by thorough washing of all clothing and linens where lice may be harboring.
			1. Administer or teach administration of antiparasitic as directed.
			 2. Use of a fine-toothed comb aids in the mechanical removal of nits. Soaking the hair in white vinegar and water can facilitate the removal of nits with combing.
			 3. Provide appropriate teaching for the family to prevent recurrences.
			   a. Wash clothing and linens in water temperature above 52°C (120°F) for 10 minutes or store in a closed plastic bag for 10 days.
			   b. Caution against using same hairbrush and comb. Do not wear one another's hats or head gear (ie, helmets)
			   c. Disinfect combs and brushes by soaking in hot water for 10 minutes or washing with a pediculocide shampoo.
			   d. Screen the whole family for parasitic infection. Notify the child's school or day-care center.
			   e. Children should be allowed back to school or day care the morning after their first treatment.

Scabies

A disease of the skin produced by the burrowing action of a parasite mite resulting in irritation and the formation of vesicles or pustules.

Etiology
1. Scabies is caused by the itch mite, *Sarcoptes scabiei*.
2. Scabies occurs in persons of all socioeconomic levels, regardless of personal hygiene standards.
3. Scabies occurs as a result of direct contact with infected persons or by indirect contact through soiled bed linen, clothing, etc.

Diagnosis
Presence on skin of female mite, ova, and feces from skin scrapings.

1. Itching, particularly at night, is the primary symptom. The itching is usually very severe.
2. Scratching frequently produces secondary skin infection.
3. Systemic manifestations are absent, unless they result from the secondary infection (ie, fever, leukocytosis).
4. The burrows may occur in any part of the body in infants and small children
5. The burrow is seen most commonly in older children and adults between the fingers, but may occur in any natural fold of the skin or in pressure areas (eg, heel of palm, axillary and buttock folds, male genitalia, female breasts).
6. Incubation period in child without previous exposure is 4–6 weeks.

1. Application of a scabicide to the skin:
   a. The drug of choice is 5% permethrin (Elimite). Alternative drugs are lindane 1% (Kwell) and crotaminton (Eurax). Permethrin should be removed by bathing after 8–14 hours, lindane after 8–12 hours, and crotaminton after 48 hours.
   b. Lindane can cause neurotoxicity from absorption through the skin. It should be avoided in children under 2 years of age, pregnant women, lactating women, and persons with extensive dermatitis.
   c. Infected children and adults should apply the scabicidal lotion or cream on the entire body from the neck down. The entire head, neck, and body of infants and young children should be treated.

1. Persons caring for affected children should wear gloves.
2. Contagion unlikely 24 hours after treatment; may return to school or day care.
3. Teach the patient and family to launder all clothing and bedding with hot water and hot drying cycle to kill mites. Clothing that cannot be laundered can be stored in a plastic bag for 1 week. Further environmental disinfection is rarely necessary.
4. Itching may continue 2–3 weeks after destruction of mites due to allergic reaction. This can be controlled by using a topical antipruritic.
5. Household contacts should be treated prophylactically. Caretakers with prolonged skin-to-skin contact with infected patients may also benefit from prophylactic treatment.

Oral Candidiasis (Thrush)/Candidal Diaper Dermatitis

Oral candidiasis is a mycotic stomatitis characterized by the appearance of white plaques on the oral mucous membrane, the gums, and the tongue.

Thrush
1. The infant develops small plaques on the oral mucous membrane, tongue, or gums; these plaques appear like curds of milk but cannot be wiped out of the mouth.
2. Thrush often appears to cause the infant no pain or discomfort, unless the case is severe and there is erosion and ulceration of the mucosa.
3. The mouth may be dry.
4. Occasionally, the infant may appear to have some difficulty in swallowing or eat less vigorously.
5. Enteric infection is frequently associated with oral thrush.

Thrush
1. Oral administration of nystatin (Mycostatin) in suspension 3–4 times daily (treatment of choice). Apply over affected surfaces or oral cavity after feeding, allowing the child to swallow any medication to treat any lesions along the gastrointestinal tract.
2. Amphotericin B (Fungizone), clotrimazole (Lotrimin), or ketoconazole (Nizoral) is used for candidiasis resistant to nystatin.

Thrush
1. Recognize the appearance of thrush and be aware of the infant who is particularly susceptible to the development of the condition.
2. Teach parents to inspect mouth *before* every feeding for presence of thrush and report the appearance of thrush.
3. Practice and teach the family measures that prevent the development and spread of thrush.
   a. Practice careful hand-washing techniques.
   b. Practice techniques that ensure that nipples, bottles, or any other objects that come into direct or indirect contact with the infant's mouth are clean.

(continued)

TABLE 52-1 Common Pediatric Skin Problems *(continued)*

Disorder/Organism	Clinical Manifestations	Treatment/Prevention	Nursing/Patient Care Considerations
Candidal diaper dermatitis is a rash characterized by red, scaly, sharply circumscribed but moist patches with pustular satellite lesions. *Etiology* 1. Caused by *Candida albicans*, which is plentiful in humans and the environment 2. Most frequently seen in newborns, but may be seen in older infants, usually as a complication of antibiotic therapy or underlying disease (malignant neoplasm, immune deficiency disorders). 3. Maternal vulvovaginal candidiasis is the primary source of neonatal thrush.	*Diaper dermatitis* 1. Buttock rash consisting of erythematous maculopapular eruption with perianal distribution. 2. Generally causes discomfort, especially with wetting and cleanings. Lesions last approximately 2 weeks, desquamate, and resolve without scarring.	*Diaper dermatitis* 1. Keep dry and clean. 2. Topical application of nystatin (Mycostatin) or miconazole nitrate (Monistat) cream or ointment. 3. Nystatin may be given orally if rash is persistent. 4. Burow's solution compress for severe inflammation or vesiculation.	*Diaper dermatitis* 1. Recognize and teach the parents to recognize the appearance of candidal diaper dermatitis and report to health care provider. 2. Allow the infant to go without a diaper for short periods to leave area open to air. 3. Teach parents the general principles of preventing diaper dermatitis. a. Change diaper as soon as possible after wetting or soiling. Check diaper every hour in newborn. Disposable diapers are useful. b. Wash entire diaper area with warm water thoroughly and dry area before applying clean diaper. Commercial wiping agents may cause burning. c. Use a second hot rinse when washing diapers to neutralize ammonia produced when infant urinates; use vinegar, Borax, or Diaparene in wash. d. Avoid powder and oil, which tend to clog pores and cake on skin, retaining bacteria. e. Avoid occlusive plastic coverings, tightly pinned or double diapers, all of which tend to increase production and retention of body heat and moisture.

Selected References

Hahn, M. (1995). "My child has a rash": A direct approach to pediatric dermatology. *Advance for Nurse Practitioners, 3*(5), 47–48.

Hanifen, J. M. (1991). Atopic dermatitis in infants and children. *Pediatric Clinics of North America, 38*(4), 763-789.

Hildreth, M. A., Herndon, D. N., Desai, M. H., & Broemeling, L. D. (1993). Caloric requirements of patients with burns under one year of age. *Journal of Burn Care and Rehabilitation, 14*(1), 108-112.

Hogan, D. J., Schachner, L., & Tanglertsampan, C. (1991). Diagnosis and treatment of childhood scabies and pediculosis. *Pediatric Clinics of North America, 38*(4), 941-957.

Hurwitz, S. (1993). *Clinical pediatric dermatology* (2nd ed.). Philadelphia: W.B. Saunders.

Kelly, H. (1994). Initial nursing assessment and management of burn injured children. *British Journal of Nursing, 3*(2), 54-56.

Leyden, J. J. (1992). Review of mupirocin ointment in the treatment of impetigo. *Clinical Pediatrics, 31*(9), 549-553.

Puffenbarger, N. K., Tuggle, D. W., & Smith, E. (1994). Rapid isotonic fluid resuscitation in pediatric thermal injury. *Journal of Pediatric Surgery, 29*(2), 339-341.

Report of the Committee of Infectious Diseases (23rd ed.). (1994). Elk Grove Village, IL: American Academy of Pediatrics.

Reynolds, E. M., Ryan, D. P., & Doody, D. P. (1993). Mortality and respiratory failure in a pediatric burn population. *Journal of Pediatric Surgery, 28*(10), 1326-1330.

Rodheaver, G., Baharestani, M. M., Brabec, M. E., Byrd, H. J., Salzberg, C. A., Scnerer, P., & Vogelpohl, T. S. (1994). Wound healing and wound management: Focus on debridement. An interdisciplinary round table, September 18, 1992, Jackson Hole, Wy. *Advances in Wound Care, 7*(1), 22-24, 26-29, 32-36.

Ruddy, R. M. (1994). Smoke inhalation injury. *Pediatric Clinics of North America, 41*(2), 317-336.

CHAPTER 53 ◆

Pediatric Eye and Ear Disorders

Conditions of the Eye

◆ INFECTIOUS PROCESSES

Infectious processes of the eye are characterized by inflammation and tissue damage caused by microbes, such as bacteria, viruses, or *Chlamydia trachomatis*.

Etiology and Incidence

1. Infectious conjunctivitis is a common problem, affecting almost all children at some time or another.
2. Because the infecting agents are easily spread from person to person, the disease may occur in outbreaks in which several children in the same family, classroom, or community are affected.
3. Common etiologic agents include *Staphylococcus, Streptococcus, Pneumococcus,* and *Haemophilus influenzae*.

Altered Physiology

1. Microbes are usually introduced into the eye or surrounding tissues by direct contact with infected objects.
2. This initiates an inflammatory response that includes dilation of blood vessels, swelling, antibody production, and destruction of the offending agent by white blood cells.

Complications

1. Spread of infection to surrounding tissues.
2. Extensive tissue damage may result in permanent visual impairment.

Clinical Manifestations

These depend on the part of the eye that is infected. Infection of one area may spread to involve surrounding tissues.

A. *Conjunctivitis*
See Table 53-1.

1. Redness of the eye caused by dilation of the blood vessels of the conjunctiva.
2. Excessive tearing and/or exudate.
3. Photophobia.
4. Impaired vision.

B. *Orbital Cellulitis*
1. Swelling and inflammation of soft tissues surrounding the eye.
2. Tenderness/pain.
3. Increased temperature of affected areas.
4. Impaired vision.

C. *Hordeolum (Stye)*
1. Pustule in area of eyelash follicle.
2. Tenderness/pain.
3. Localized swelling.

Diagnostic Evaluation

1. Culture of exudate for bacteria or virus or antigen testing for *Neisseria gonorrheae* or *C. trachomatis*. Different media are required for each. The most likely agents are tested for based on historic and physical findings.

NURSING ALERT:
A child who has a painful red eye should be referred immediately for medical evaluation, because this may indicate herpetic infection or damage to the cornea.

Treatment

1. Antibiotic eye drops or ointment, such as erythromycin (Ilosone) or sulfacetamide (Sulamyd), will shorten the course of bacterial conjunctivitis and make the child more comfortable.
2. Systemic antibiotic treatment is indicated for orbital cellulitis. These children may be admitted to the hospital for close observation and aggressive management.
3. Hordeolums will usually resolve spontaneously without antibiotic treatment.

Nursing Assessment

1. Assess nature and extent of symptoms and their effect on function and activities of daily living.
2. Assess visual acuity.
3. Determine resources available to patient for treatment and coping, and refer as necessary.

Nursing Diagnoses

A. Risk for Infection (transmission) related to hand-to-hand or hand-to-object contact
B. Pain related to tissue swelling, inflammation, and light sensitivity

TABLE 53-1 Common Causes of Eye Redness in Children

Cause	Associated Symptoms	Management
Conjunctivitis		
Viral	Often associated with other symptoms of generalized viral illness	Hygiene, rest
Bacterial	Yellow, green, or white pus, photophobia	Antibiotic eye drops or ointment, hygiene
Chlamydial	Cough, history of maternal infection	Systemic antibiotic
Herpetic	Pain, photophobia, skin lesions	Evaluation by specialist, antiviral agents
Allergic	Itching, seasonal onset of symptoms, other allergic symptoms, watery discharge	Antihistamine, eye drops, avoidance of allergens
Chemical	Watery discharge, onset of symptoms when exposed to cigarettes or other irritants	Avoidance of irritating substances
Trauma	Pain, photophobia, increased tear production	Eye patch, referral to specialist
Congenital Glaucoma	Increased tear production, cloudiness of cornea	Referral to specialist

Nursing Interventions

A. Preventing Infection
1. Perform or teach proper cleansing of drainage.
   a. Use warm water or saline and a disposable applicator, such as cotton balls or gauze.
   b. Use a separate applicator for each eye.
   c. Wipe from inner to outer canthus to avoid contamination.
2. Teach self-care measures to prevent spread of disease to others.
   a. Observe good hand-washing practices.
   b. Do not share washcloths or towels.
   c. Avoid swimming until infection is resolved.
   d. Dispose of contaminated items in proper receptacles.
3. Administer and teach proper instillation of eye drops or ointment (see p. 421).

B. Minimizing Pain
1. Apply warm compresses to affected area.
2. Suggest darkened room for photophobic patients.

Family Education/Health Maintenance

1. Advise parents of indications for reevaluation by health care provider.
   a. Lack of response to antibiotic treatment.
   b. Increase in swelling and tenderness.
   c. Eye pain.
   d. Worsening of visual acuity.
   e. Development of additional symptoms, for example, fever.
2. Encourage routine follow-up.

Evaluation

A. Parents performing treatment correctly; hygiene procedures followed.
B. Patient verbalizes less pain; tolerates bright light.

◆ CONGENITAL PROBLEMS

Congenital problems of the eye include structural defects present at birth or developing soon thereafter. These are often genetically transmitted. They include cataract, glaucoma, ptosis, and strabismus.

Etiology/Incidence

A. Congenital Cataract
1. Not well understood, but possible causes include:
   a. An abnormal developmental event.
   b. Infection during pregnancy.
   c. Disturbance of carbohydrate metabolism.
   d. Metabolic disorders (eg, diabetes mellitus).
   e. Retinopathy of prematurity.
   f. Genetic factors.
2. Approximately 1 in 250 newborns are affected.

B. Dacryostenosis (Obstruction of Nasolacrimal Duct)
1. This relatively common condition may occur at any time but is most common during the 3rd through 6th months of life.
2. May be unilateral or bilateral.

C. Glaucoma
1. A developmental abnormality or acquired obstruction that impairs the outflow of aqueous humor from the eye, resulting in increased intraocular pressure.
2. Occurs in 0.05% of all neonates.
3. Symptoms are present at birth in approximately 35% of those affected.

D. Ptosis
1. May be caused by a congenital or acquired condition either of the muscle itself or of the nerve that innervates it.

E. Strabismus
1. A muscle imbalance or paralysis that causes malalignment of the eyes.
2. Occurs in approximately 3% of the population

Altered Physiology

A. *Congenital Cataract*
1. Trauma or metabolic changes cause the protein of the eye lens to become opaque, rather than clear. This reduces the ability of the lens to transmit light and clear visual images to the retina.

B. *Dacryostenosis*
1. The affected lacrimal duct(s) may be unusually small or clogged with cellular debris.
2. Tears produced are not carried from the eye to the nasal cavity and spill over onto the cheek.

C. *Glaucoma*
1. The balance between aqueous fluid production and flow out of the anterior chamber is disrupted. Fluid builds up in the anterior chamber.
2. The resulting pressure damages the retina, cornea, and other delicate eye structures.

D. *Ptosis*
1. A weakness or paralysis of the superior levator palpebrae muscle or, less frequently, Müller's muscle. This causes one or both eyelids to droop and cover part of the iris and/or pupil.
2. Vision is impaired, because part of the visual field is obstructed.

E. *Strabismus*
1. Malalignment of the eyes prevents both eyes from focusing correctly on the same object.
2. Double images are perceived and depth perception is impaired.

Complications

1. Loss of visual acuity (most likely with cataracts or glaucoma).
2. Unilateral conditions (cataract, glaucoma, strabismus, or ptosis) may result in amblyopia, because the less clear image is suppressed and, with time, the neural pathways of the unused eye become nonfunctional.
3. Nasolacrimal sac infection (dacryostenosis).

Clinical Manifestations

A. *Congenital Cataract*
1. Lack of red reflex.
2. Visible clouding of the lens.
3. Decrease in visual acuity.

B. *Dacryostenosis*
1. Excessive tearing, spilling of clear tears from eye to cheek.
2. Normal-appearing eyes without redness, swelling, or pus.

C. *Glaucoma*
1. Haziness of the cornea.
2. Photophobia.
3. Excessive tearing.
4. Decrease in visual acuity.

D. *Ptosis*
1. Drooping of affected eyelid.

2. Impairment of visual acuity if the eyelid covers all or part of the pupil.

E. *Strabismus*
1. Asymmetrical pupillary light reflexes.
2. Asymmetrical extraocular movements.
3. Diplopia.
4. Tendency to close one eye or tilt the head during acuity testing.

Diagnostic Evaluation

1. Thorough ophthalmologic examination, including visual acuity for visual assessment.
2. Tonometry for glaucoma to determine presence and extent of intraocular pressure.

Treatment

A. *Cataract*
1. Surgical removal of the lens as soon as possible after birth.
   a. Sedation for first 24 hours postoperatively to prevent crying and vomiting, protecting sutures from increased intraocular pressure.
   b. Antibiotic and steroid eye ointments to prevent postoperative infection.
   c. A patch and shield are often in place for several days after surgery for eye rest and protection.
2. Eyeglasses or contact lenses are used to correct vision.

B. *Dacryostenosis*
1. May resolve without treatment.
2. Parents may be instructed to massage the nasolacrimal sac several times a day to help remove cellular debris and promote opening of the duct.
3. Surgical probing to open the lacrimal duct may be indicated if the problem persists beyond age 6 months.

C. *Glaucoma*
1. Surgical intervention may be necessary to normalize intraocular pressure.
   a. A patch and shield are often in place for several days after surgery to rest and protect the eye.

D. *Ptosis*
1. Surgical correction to raise the eyelid and increase the visual field.

E. *Strabismus*
1. Patching of the stronger eye may correct latent strabismus by exercising the muscles of the weaker eye.
2. Surgical repositioning of the extraocular muscles may be required for fixed or severe deviations.
   a. Antibiotic ointment to prevent infection after surgery.
   b. No eye patch is required after surgery.

Nursing Assessment

1. Assess for red light reflex, especially in newborns. Absence of the red light reflex may indicate congenital cataract or an intraocular tumor.

2. Inspect the eyes for redness of conjunctiva, cloudiness of the cornea, excessive tearing, eyelids that partially occlude the pupil, or obvious misalignment; provides clues to congenital eye problems.

3. Assess visual acuity routinely in children who can cooperate sufficiently. Changes in acuity may be the first manifestation of a problem or indication of effectiveness of treatment.

4. Perform Hirschberg's test for symmetry of the pupillary light reflexes to help detect strabismus. Normally, the light reflexes are in the same position in each pupil, but will not be with strabismus (positive Hirschberg's test).

5. Perform the cover–uncover test to detect latent strabismus due to weak eye muscles. When covered, the "lazy" eye drifts out of position and snaps back quickly when uncovered.

Nursing Diagnoses

A. Sensory/Perceptual Alterations (Visual), related to reduction in visual acuity
B. Body Image Disturbance related to the need for patch or glasses
C. Risk for Injury related to reduced visual acuity and modified depth perception
D. Altered Growth and Development related to altered visual stimulation and possible overprotective behavior of parents

Nursing Interventions

A. *Minimizing Effects of Vision Loss*
1. Visual acuity problems will be identified and treated promptly to minimize functional impairment.
   a. Newborns should be examined in the nursery to detect congenital eye problems.
   b. All children should be screened for visual acuity and strabismus. In very young children, this is accomplished by physical examination and assessment of developmental milestones (ie, looking at mother's face, responsive smile, reaching for objects). By 3 to 5 years of age, most children can cooperate for performance of accurate visual acuity screening tests.
2. Encourage and assist parents in obtaining corrective lenses for child.
3. Encourage and assist parents in providing normal experiences for child to achieve maximum potential:
   a. Assist parents in locating and accessing resources, such as financial assistance, special education in braille, or parent support groups.
   b. Advise parents of their child's right to a public education.

B. *Minimizing Body Image Disturbance*
1. Encourage parents to focus on normalization, rather than on overprotection. This means having expectations based on the child's abilities rather than disabilities, providing opportunities for interaction with peers, and making the child's life as normal as possible.
2. Encourage acceptance of appearance and emphasize the positive aspects of treatment.

C. *Preventing Injury*
1. Encourage the family to be aware of safety in the home, school, and community.
   a. Suggest the use of impact-resistant eyeglasses and devices to keep eyeglasses from falling off.
   b. Advise the family to maintain an uncluttered furniture arrangement that remains consistent; notify child of planned changes.
   c. Instruct child in the use of a cane or other assistive device.
   d. Teach traffic safety and personal security measures.

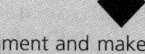

COMMUNITY-BASED CARE TIP:
Perform a safety inspection of the home environment and make changes as necessary to help prevent falls or other injuries.

2. Orient visually impaired children in the hospital to the placement of furniture and other objects in their room.
   a. Orient child to food placement on meal trays.
   b. Assist child with ambulation and use side rails on bed or crib to prevent falls.

D. *Promoting Normal Growth and Development*
1. Encourage parents to provide many sensory opportunities, such as manipulating objects, hearing a variety of sounds, noting the smells in the environment, and tasting an assortment of substances.
2. Allow child to perform activities of daily living as independently as possible.

Family Education/Health Maintenance

1. Teach about instillation of medications, use of eye shield, and any activity restrictions after surgery.
   a. Teach about activity restrictions that follow glaucoma surgery. Bed rest may be required immediately postoperatively, and older children should not engage in strenuous activity or contact sports for 2 weeks.
   b. Advise that activity is usually not restricted for surgery for strabismus.
   c. Encourage behaviors to reduce the risk of damage to sutures from increased intraocular pressure initially after cataract surgery, for example, avoid overfeeding to prevent vomiting and minimize crying.
2. Advise of indications for reevaluation by health care provider:
   a. Worsening of visual acuity.
   b. Evidence of infection, such as, pain, redness, swelling, drainage, increased temperature.
3. Refer family for information on eye disease and safety measures: Prevent Blindness America, 500 East Remington Road; Schaumburg, IL 60173; 800-331-2020.

Evaluation

A. Child wearing glasses as prescribed; vision improved
B. Parents and child report involvement in activities, satisfactory school performance, and positive peer interactions
C. No injuries reported
D. Age-appropriate developmental milestones achieved

◆ EYE TRAUMA

Eye trauma causes structural damage to the eye and is produced by mechanical force or contact with a corrosive chemical. Some common types of eye trauma are corneal abrasions, blunt trauma, perforating injuries, and chemical injuries.

Etiology/Incidence

1. Eye injuries are common among children and are usually related to their involvement in vigorous play activities.
2. Most childhood injuries are not severe and will resolve spontaneously with no adverse long-term consequences. It is important, however, to identify and obtain prompt treatment for significant injuries.

Altered Physiology

A. *Corneal Abrasion*
1. Produced when an area of the cornea is scratched.
2. This may happen when a foreign object becomes lodged in the eye, a contact lens rubs against the eye because of inadequate tear production, or a fingernail or other sharp object enters the eye and scrapes the cornea.

B. *Blunt Trauma*
1. This occurs when the eye and/or surrounding tissues are struck by a blunt object, such as a ball.
2. The resulting injury includes tissue swelling and seepage of blood into the surrounding tissues.
3. The bony structures surrounding the eye may be fractured.
4. The lens may become dislodged or the retina may separate from the back of the eye.

C. *Perforating Injury*
1. When an object penetrates the eyeball, there may be loss of vitreous material and/or damage to the internal structures of the eye.
2. Bacteria may also be introduced into the interior of the eye, causing infection.

D. *Chemical Injuries*
1. Corrosive chemicals burn the delicate tissues of the cornea and may penetrate into deeper layers of the eye.
2. Healing may occur with scarring.

Complications

1. Infection.
2. Extensive tissue damage may result in permanent visual impairment.
3. Disfigurement may result from severe or extensive tissue damage.

Clinical Manifestations

1. Pain—due to the delicate tissues of the eye containing many nerve endings.

> **NURSING ALERT:**
> At times, the presence of pain may be useful in distinguishing a serious eye problem from a self-limiting condition.

2. Increased tear production—one of the eye's defenses against injury or irritation.
3. Injection of the blood vessels of the cornea—Increase of blood flow to the cornea is another protective mechanism; most likely to be seen with foreign bodies, abrasions or chemical burns affecting the cornea.
4. Impaired visual acuity due to:
   a. Swelling of the cornea, reducing its clarity.
   b. Swelling of the soft tissues surrounding the eye, causing the eye to partially or completely close.
   c. Excessive tear production, impairing vision.
   d. Damage to internal structures of the eye, altering or obstructing visual pathways.
5. Visible signs of injury—bruising, swelling, or a foreign object visible in the eye.

Diagnostic Evaluation

1. Thorough inspection of the eye, including eversion of the upper lid to inspect for a foreign object.
2. Fundoscopic examination may detect abnormalities, such as a dislodged lens, retinal hemorrhage, retinal detachment, or increased intraocular pressure.
3. Staining with fluorescein dye will reveal lesions of the cornea, such as abrasions.
4. Assessment of eye function, including near and far acuity, extraocular movements, and visual fields.

Treatment

A. *Corneal Abrasion*
1. If the abrasion was caused by a contact lens or foreign body, removal of the offending body is indicated.
2. Patching of the affected eye will control pain.
3. Antibiotic eye drops or ointment to prevent infection.

B. *Blunt Trauma*
1. Application of cold compresses may help control pain and swelling.
2. The head should be elevated 30 degrees to avoid increased intraocular pressure.
3. Surgery may be required if there is damage to underlying bones or eye structures.

C. *Perforating Injury*
1. Surgery is usually necessary to remove the object and reconstruct damaged tissues.

> **NURSING ALERT:**
> Never remove a penetrating object from the eye. It should be stabilized and the eye shielded with no pressure applied. The other eye should be patched and the patient transported by stretcher. The head should be elevated 30 degrees to avoid increased intraocular pressure, and the child should be kept on nothing-by-mouth orders in preparation for surgery.

D. *Chemical Injuries*
1. Gentle flushing of the affected eye(s) with water will help remove the offending chemical. This should be done from inner aspect of eye to outer to prevent contaminated water from flowing into the other eye.
2. Antibiotics may be prescribed to prevent infection.
3. Further management depends on the nature and extent of the injury.

Nursing Assessment

1. Obtain history of injury, including the child's account of how the injury occurred, and a description of symptoms experienced by the child.
2. Inspect for location and extent of swelling and/or bruising, any asymmetry, or abnormality in appearance of any part of the eye.
3. Assess visual acuity and compare with baseline. This should include near and far acuity in each eye. If the patient cannot see well enough to read a Snellen chart, assess ability to count fingers or perceive light.

Nursing Diagnoses

A. Pain related to inflammation, photophobia, or trauma to eye tissue
B. Risk for Injury related to impaired vision and side effects of pain medications
C. Self Care Deficit related to impaired vision and side effects of pain medications

Nursing Interventions

A. *Minimizing Pain*
1. Apply cold compresses to the affected area to help reduce swelling and discomfort.
2. Keep the child's room as dark as possible to help reduce pain for photophobic patients.
3. Administer or teach parents to administer analgesics as prescribed.

B. *Preventing Injury*
1. Enforce safety measures:
   a. Use of side rails.
   b. Assistance with ambulation.
   c. Observe closely.

C. *Maintaining Activities of Daily Living*
1. Provide assistance with eating, bathing, toileting, and other activities of daily living, as needed.
2. Teach child location of self-care items and positioning of food on tray to promote independence.
3. Encourage child to attempt self-care, and offer praise even if unsuccessful.

Family Education/Health Maintenance

1. Teach indications for reevaluation by health care provider.
   a. Increase in swelling, tenderness, discoloration, or pain.

b. Worsening of visual acuity.
c. Development of additional symptoms, for example, fever, alteration in sensorium, or other indications of neurologic injury
2. Provide families with information and support as they cope with having a visually impaired child in the home. Refer to such agencies as the Blind Children's Center, 800-222-3566.

Evaluation

A. Demonstrates decreased pain
B. No injuries reported
C. Dressing and feeding self with minimal assistance

◆ FUNCTIONAL PROBLEMS

Functional problems of the eye involve impairment of the vision due to refractive errors or disuse of visual pathways.

Etiology/Incidence

1. Approximately 1 in 500 schoolchildren in the United States have partial vision (acuity between 20/70 and 20/200).
2. Another 35,000 children have visual acuity between 20/200 and total blindness.
3. Refractive errors are usually caused by a genetic predisposition to have shortened or elongated eyeballs or by individual variations in growth.
4. Amblyopia affects 2% to 3% of the population.
5. Amblyopia may result from any condition that causes the two retinas to receive different images.
   a. Diplopia due to strabismus.
   b. Significant difference in acuity of the two eyes.
   c. Cataract.
   d. Unilateral ptosis.

Altered Physiology

A. *Refractive Errors*
1. In an elongated or shortened eyeball, the visual image is focused either in front of or behind the retina, resulting in unclear images.
2. The nearsighted (myopic) child is able to see near objects, such as print in schoolbooks, but is unable to focus clearly on far objects, such as writing on the blackboard.
3. The farsighted (hyperopic) child can see far objects clearly, but has difficulty seeing near objects.
4. The problem may be unilateral or bilateral.

B. *Amblyopia*
1. When there is a discrepancy between images received on the two retinas, the more unclear image is suppressed.
2. Over time, a young child will become permanently unable to use the visual pathways of the suppressed eye.
3. Although the visual pathways are structurally normal, the child is blind in that eye.

Complications

1. Increased incidence of accidental injuries due to inability to read warning signs and possible lack of depth perception.

Clinical Manifestations

Children often do not complain of being unable to see well, but may exhibit other signs of vision problems, including:

1. Poor academic performance or behavioral problems in school.
2. Dislike for reading.
3. Head tilting.
4. Squinting.
5. Sitting close to the television or holding reading materials close to the face.
6. Refusal or resistance to covering one eye during vision screening.

Diagnostic Evaluation

1. Standardized vision screening tests, such as the Snellen chart, the Titmus machine, or the H:O:T:V matching symbol test, may be used for distance acuity screening.
   a. Tests can be administered to children as young as 3 years of age.
   b. Each eye should be tested separately.
2. Near vision may be tested by having the child read or by standardized vision screening tests, such as the Titmus machine.
   a. Each eye should be tested separately.
3. Muscle balance can be tested using the cover test and the Titmus machine.

Treatment

1. Most visual acuity problems can be treated by the use of corrective lenses.
2. Amblyopia is not treatable, but can be prevented by early identification and treatment of problems that may cause it.

Nursing Assessment

1. Begin visual acuity screening early, in the preschool years, and whenever a child displays behaviors suggestive of acuity problems.
2. Assess Hirschberg's test for symmetry of the pupillary light reflexes routinely beginning at birth.
3. Perform the cover–uncover test as part of routine eye assessment as soon as the child is able to cooperate (as young as 3 years of age).
4. Assess the effect of the functional deficit on the child's overall function, including academic progress, self-esteem, and safety.

Nursing Diagnoses

A. Sensory/Perceptual Alterations (Visual) related to reduced acuity or inability to use one eye
B. Risk for Injury related to impaired visual acuity or lack of depth perception
C. Self Esteem Disturbance related to lowered performance caused by poor vision

Nursing Interventions

A. *Minimizing Effects of Sensory Deficits*
1. Assist the patient and family with effective coping mechanisms to promote family stability.
2. Encourage the consistent use of corrective lenses as prescribed.
3. Teach the parents ways to help develop the child's skills in interpreting information through the senses of hearing, smell, and touch.
   a. Familiarize the child with common sounds and smells in the environment. Also orient the child to traffic sounds and sounds associated with danger, for example, animals and speeding vehicles, and instruct the child how to respond.
   b. Use voice or touch, rather than facial expressions or gestures, to express emotion.
   c. Speak to the child before touching to reduce startling.
   d. Allow the child to touch and handle unfamiliar objects to learn about them.
   e. Have the child practice such things as retelling stories and giving the home telephone number and address.
   f. Explain unfamiliar sounds and smells to the hospitalized child.

B. *Preventing Injury*
1. Recommend the use of shatterproof eyeglasses with flexible frames.
2. Recommend the use of eye protection on a routine basis, because eye trauma can occur unexpectedly. This is especially important for children who rely on only one eye.
3. Suggest extra protection, such as shatterproof goggles or shields, when participating in contact or ball sports and activities.
4. Maintain a stable arrangement of furniture in the home, adequate lighting, and an uncluttered environment to minimize falls.
5. Orient hospitalized children to the hospital room and offer assistance when walking.

C. *Promoting a Positive Sense of Self-Esteem*
1. Provide opportunities for mastery of developmentally appropriate activities.
2. Encourage interactions with sighted children to decrease feelings of isolation. Also suggest interactions with children with similar alterations in vision.
3. Encourage the child to discuss feelings and strategies for coping with negative peer reactions, for example, teasing.
4. Encourage independence in self-care activities to promote autonomy, such as dressing, feeding, and use of bathroom.

Family Education/Health Maintenance

1. Inform families of their child's right to a public education and assist them in locating appropriate educational resources.
2. Refer families for financial assistance in obtaining eyeglasses, if indicated.
3. Refer families of blind children to community resources that can help their child learn special skills, such as reading braille, using a cane, or developing self-care skills. Information can be obtained from agencies such as the American Council of the Blind, 800-424-8666; and the National Association of Parents of the Visually Impaired, PO Box 317, Watertown, MA 02272-0317, 800-562-6265.

Evaluation

A. Child identifies common sounds
B. No injury reported; wears protective eyeglasses
C. Reports good school performance and participation in extracurricular activities; able to eat and dress independently

Conditions of the Ear

◆ EUSTACHIAN TUBE DYSFUNCTION

Eustachian tube dysfunction comprises disorders arising from closure of the eustachian tube, which ventilates the middle ear to equalize pressure on both sides of the tympanic membrane.

Etiology/Incidence

1. Serous otitis and otitis media are two of the most common health problems seen in childhood.
2. Approximately 75% of children experience one or more episodes of otitis media by the time they are 10 years of age. Some children experience multiple episodes.
3. Children between the ages of 6 and 24 months are predisposed to the development of acute otitis media because their short, relatively straight eustachian tubes more easily allow the passage of infected nasal secretions into the middle ear cavity.
4. Other etiologic factors include:
   a. More frequent episodes of upper respiratory tract infections in younger children.
   b. Nasal allergies.
   c. Genetics—in some families, children's eustachian tubes tend to be "floppy" and close easily.
   d. Native American or Eskimo heritage.
   e. Craniofacial abnormalities.
   f. Down's syndrome.
   g. Lower socioeconomic status.

Altered Physiology

1. Swelling of the eustachian tube lining is caused by an acute upper respiratory tract infection or by an allergic response.
2. At this time, infected secretions may pass through the tube from the nasal area into the middle ear.
3. When swelling causes the eustachian tube to close, the passage of air into and out of the middle ear is prevented.
4. The air in the middle ear is absorbed into the middle ear lining and a vacuum is created.
5. The vacuum is filled by serous fluid that seeps out of the middle ear lining.
6. The warm, moist environment of the middle ear and the presence of nutrients in the serous fluid are conducive to the growth of viruses and/or bacteria that may be present in the middle ear cavity.
7. Barotrauma, caused by rapid changes in atmospheric pressure, may also lead to closure of the eustachian tube and development of serous otitis.
   a. This is less likely to involve introduction of microorganisms through infected nasal secretions; development of acute otitis media is less common.

Complications

1. Temporary conductive hearing loss; usually resolves when tympanic membrane mobility is restored.
2. Permanent hearing loss; perforations of the tympanic membrane, scarring due to healed perforations, or damage to the ossicles of the middle ear.
3. Delayed speech and language development.
4. Mastoiditis, meningitis, lateral sinus thrombosis, or intracranial abscess; spread of bacterial infection.

Clinical Manifestations

1. Decreased hearing.
2. Sensation of fullness in the affected ear(s).
3. Popping sensations in the affected ear(s) may be experienced as the eustachian tube begins to open and admit air into the middle ear cavity.
4. Ear pain.
5. Signs of infection—fever, irritability, or decreased appetite.

Diagnostic Evaluation

1. Otoscopic Examination
   a. Serous otitis—yellowish, prominent bony landmarks, a diffuse light reflex, and decreased mobility of tympanic membrane.
   b. Acute otitis media—inflamed tympanic membrane with decreased or absent mobility; bulging of the tympanic membrane may obscure the bony landmarks and light reflex.
2. Tympanometry—quick and simple way to assess tympanic membrane mobility (Fig. 53-1).
   a. A probe occludes the ear canal while pressure is varied and a test sound is emitted. The test produces a graphic display showing the mobility of the tympanic membrane at various air pressures.

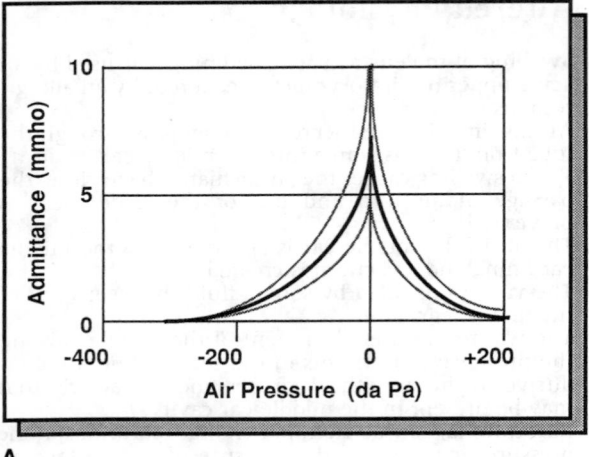

A

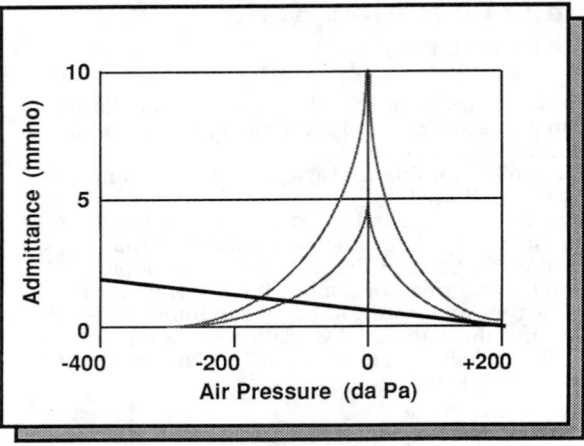

B

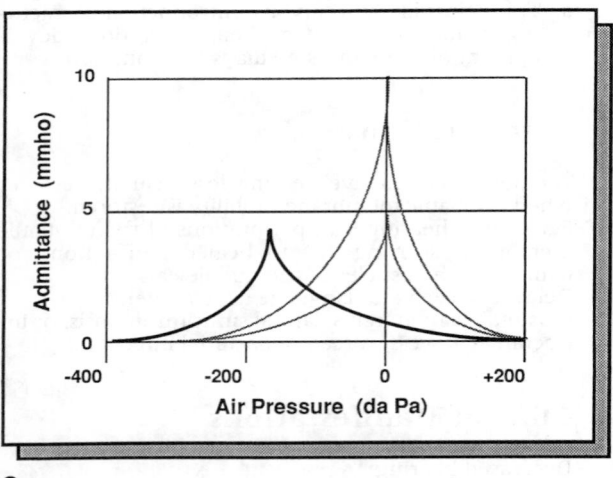

C

FIGURE 53-1 **(A)** Type A Tympanogram: This is the normal pattern showing mobility of the tympanic membrane with a peak mobility at the 0 point (the point at which there is neither positive nor negative pressure in the external ear canal). **(B)** Type B Tympanogram: This pattern shows a low level of mobility with no peak. It is characteristic of impaired mobility due to the presence of fluid in the middle ear. **(C)** Type C Tympanogram: This pattern shows a distinct peak in the mobility level of the tympanic membrane, but the peak occurs when there is negative pressure in the external ear canal. This indicates eustachian tube dysfunction causing negative pressure in the middle ear cavity. Negative pressure in the external ear canal equalizes pressure on both sides of the tympanic membrane and allows for maximum mobility. Dershewitz, R.A. (1988) Ambulatory Pediatric Care. Philadelphia: J.B. Lippincott Company. p. 372.

b. A normal reading has a distinct peak in the middle of the graph (see Figure 53-1A).
c. A flat tympanogram (no peak) indicates lack of mobility of the tympanic membrane, usually caused by serous otitis or acute otitis media (see Figure 53-1B).
d. A peak to the left of the center indicates negative pressure in the middle ear (see Figure 53-1C).

Treatment

A. Serous Otitis
1. Usually resolves spontaneously.
2. Antihistamines or decongestants sometimes used, although not always effective.
3. Corticosteroids may be used.
4. If the effusion persists for up to 30 days, antibiotics may be given for presence of bacteria.
5. Effusions persisting for 3 or more months are often managed by placement of ventilating tubes.
6. Adenoidectomy may benefit some children.

B. Acute Otitis Media
1. Systemic antibiotic treatment.
    a. Usually an oral preparation taken for 10 days.
    b. May include amoxicillin (Trimox), ampicillin (Omnipen), cefaclor (Ceclor), erythromycin-sulfisoxazole combinations (Pediazole), amoxicillin/clavulanate potassium (Augmentin), or trimethoprim-sulfamethoxazole (Bactrim).

Nursing Assessment

1. Assess for etiologic factors contributing to eustachian tube dysfunction.
2. Assess for symptoms of serous otitis and acute otitis media to identify and document the nature and severity of the illness.
3. Assess hearing after the middle ear effusion is resolved. Promptly identify any hearing loss which may have social and educational consequences.

4. Assess speech and language development in children experiencing recurrent or prolonged infections to determine deficits; initiate referrals, as needed.

> **NURSING ALERT:**
> Prompt identification of speech and language delays is important in young children, because speech and language development is quite rapid at this time. Young children may demonstrate rapid regression or failure of progression.

5. Assess for effects of illness on family, such as sleep deprivation of parents due to staying up with child at night, decreased attendance at work due to keeping child out of school.

Nursing Diagnoses

A. Pain related to increased pressure in the middle ear
B. Sensory/Perceptual Alterations (Auditory), related to reduced sound wave conduction
C. Impaired Verbal Communication due to conductive hearing loss

Nursing Interventions

The nurse may perform interventions and teach family to participate.

A. Minimizing Discomfort
1. Administer antibiotics. Provide instruction in:
   a. Measurement of correct dosage.
   b. Time of doses.
   c. Importance of administering all doses.
   d. Proper storage and disposal of unused medication.
   e. Side effects.
2. Administer acetaminophen as directed for pain or fever.
3. Apply warm compresses to the external ear.
4. Administer analgesic otic drops, if prescribed; usually indicated when there is no perforation of the tympanic membrane.
5. Advise elevation of head to facilitate drainage of fluid from the middle ear into the pharynx.
6. Teach older children to open their eustachian tubes by yawning or performing the Valsalva's maneuver.

B. Minimizing Hearing Loss
1. Teach parents to recognize early signs of otitis and to seek prompt treatment.
2. Stress the importance of the follow-up visit to ensure that otitis has resolved.

C. Facilitating Verbal Communication
1. Assess hearing, speech, and language development regularly.
2. Alert parents to immediately report signs of hearing difficulty or delayed speech to ensure early intervention.
3. Refer to a specialist for evaluation and treatment, if necessary.

Family Education/Health Maintenance

1. Teach parents that episodes of otitis may be minimized by:
   a. Breast-feeding.
   b. Holding bottle-fed infants in a sitting position during feeding.
   c. Using specially designed bottles to allow upright feeding.
   d. Identifying and eliminating allergens, such as particular foods, molds, dust.
2. If ventilation tubes are placed, instruct parents to do the following:
   a. Avoid water or other fluids from entering the ear canal. Encourage use of earplugs when the child is bathing or swimming.
   b. Discourage instillation of eardrops or other medications in the external ear.
   c. Tubes will come out of the ear spontaneously, usually in 6 to 12 months.

Evaluation

A. Demonstrates improved comfort; family states proper treatment regimen
B. Follow-up visits maintained; effusion resolved
C. Speech and language development appropriate for age; reports regular assessment; receives therapy from specialist, if indicated

◆ EXTERNAL OTITIS

External otitis is inflammation in the external ear canal. It is frequently unilateral, but may be bilateral.

Etiology/Incidence

1. Children who frequently get water in their ears are at high risk.
2. Occurs most frequently in summer, when water activities are popular.
3. Caused by bacteria or fungi.

Altered Physiology

1. When water remains in the external ear canal, a warm, moist environment is created.
2. Skin lining the canal is irritated, causing breakdown of its protective barrier.
3. Bacteria or fungi overgrow in the conducive environment and cause symptoms of inflammation and infection in 1 to 2 days.
4. Breakdown of protective barrier and introduction and proliferation of infectious organisms can also occur through trauma to the ear canal, such as cleaning the ear with an inappropriate object or technique.

Complications

1. Temporary hearing loss caused by occlusion of the canal.

Clinical Manifestations

1. Ear pain, itching, and white, yellow, or greenish drainage.
2. Inflammation of the external ear canal and structures.
3. Pain when the ear pinna is manipulated.

Diagnostic Evaluation

1. Otoscopic examination; may be difficult due to severe pain and swelling; shows redness, swelling, and drainage in canal; tympanic membrane appears normal.
2. Cultures usually not necessary.

Treatment

1. Acetic acid solution (VoSol) to dry and modify the pH of the ear canal.
2. Topical antibiotic solution, possibly combined with a steroid to reduce significant discomfort and swelling.
3. Ear canal may need to be irrigated to remove drainage.
4. A medication-soaked wick may be applied to facilitate medication administration.

Nursing Assessment

1. Assess severity of symptoms and need for pain relief.
2. Assess ear hygiene and the need for earplugs.

Nursing Diagnosis

A. Pain related to inflammation and irritation of drainage

Nursing Interventions

The nurse may perform interventions or teach family the techniques.

A. *Relieving Pain*
1. Administer eardrops as prescribed.
   a. Have child lie on side with affected ear upward.
   b. Instill drops, using caution not to contaminate dropper.
   c. Have child maintain position for 5 minutes to facilitate penetration of medication into ear canal.
   d. Repeat on other side if ordered.
2. Administer analgesics, such as acetaminophen (Tylenol), as directed.
3. Suggest application of warm or cold compresses to outer ear to relieve discomfort.
4. Frequently cleanse drainage from area surrounding opening of ear canal to relieve irritation.

Family Education/Health Maintenance

1. Teach proper ear hygiene.
   a. Insert nothing into ear canal for cleaning or scratching.
   b. Cleanse the outer area with a washcloth only.
   c. Drain water promptly from ear by leaning the child over and pulling auricle slightly downward and outward.
2. Instruct in the use of well-fitting earplugs, if necessary.
3. Instruct in the use of routine acetic acid solution instillation after water activity, if prescribed.

Evaluation

A. Reports pain relieved; uses compresses and analgesics, if necessary

◆ FUNCTIONAL HEARING DISORDERS

These conditions arise from problems in the function of the ear. In a quiet environment, the healthy child can hear tones between 0 and 25 decibels. Categories of hearing impairment are slight, 15 to 25 decibels; mild, 25 to 40 decibels; moderate, 40 to 65 decibels; severe, 65 to 95 decibels; profound, 95 or higher decibels.

Etiology/Incidence

1. Hearing impairment is the most common disorder causing long-term disability in children.
2. Congenital hearing loss occurs in approximately 1:600 live births.
3. Transient episodes of impaired hearing associated with problems such as otitis media or external otitis are very common.
4. Hearing loss may be conductive or sensorineural.
   a. Conductive loss occurs when there is impaired transmission of sound through the outer and/or middle ear.
   b. Conductive loss may be caused by impaction of cerumen in the external ear canal, the presence of fluid in the middle ear cavity, and reduced mobility of the tympanic membrane due to scarring.
   c. Sensorineural hearing loss results from damage to the cochlea or auditory nerve and congenital defects of the cochlea. Examples include damage caused by ototoxic drugs, damage resulting from prenatal infections, and damage caused by prolonged exposure to loud noise.

Altered Physiology

1. In conductive hearing loss, a variety of mechanisms may occur:
   a. A mechanical obstruction, such as the presence of cerumen or a foreign object blocking the external ear canal, may block the passage of sound waves to the tympanic membrane.

b. With otitis media or serous otitis, fluid in the middle ear cavity does not transmit sound as well as air.
c. A scarred or perforated tympanic membrane has lost its normal mobility and does not transmit sound as well as a normal one.
d. Most cases of conductive hearing loss in children are reversible and produce no permanent effect.
2. Sensorineural problems are usually irreversible.
a. Damage to the auditory nerve prevents transmission of sound impulses to the brain for interpretation.
b. Damage to the hair cells of the cochlea may be caused by prolonged exposure to loud noise, resulting in hearing loss. This is especially pronounced for high-pitched sounds.

Complications

1. Speech and language delays.
2. Inadequate social development.

Clinical Manifestations

Children often do not complain of being unable to hear well. They may exhibit other signs of hearing problems, including:

1. Poor academic performance or behavior problems in school.
2. Lack of response to sounds.
3. Delayed language development.
4. Listening to the television or radio at a loud volume.
5. Speaking loudly.

Diagnostic Evaluation

1. Routine audiometric screening should be done beginning as soon as the child can cooperate and follow instructions (between ages 3 and 5 years).

Treatment

1. Treatment of the underlying problem, such as impacted cerumen or otitis media.
2. Hearing aids may be helpful for both conductive and sensorineural hearing loss.
3. Cochlear implants help some children with sensorineural hearing loss.
a. Consists of an external microphone and speech processor, which sends radio signals to an internal electrode array implanted in the cochlea.
b. Most effective in young child who has had shorter hearing deprivation, but requires long period of rehabilitation.
4. If problem cannot be corrected, the focus of treatment is on development of adaptive skills through special education, sign language, or technical devices for the hearing impaired.

Nursing Assessment

1. Assess hearing periodically in the child with an identified hearing impairment to follow up promptly on changes in ability to hear.

2. Assess speech and language development frequently so that children may obtain special assistance, as indicated.
3. Assess social development and academic progress periodically so that counseling and intervention can be instituted.

Nursing Diagnoses

A. Sensory/Perceptual Alterations (Auditory), related to limited ability to hear
B. Impaired Verbal Communication related to inability to hear and imitate speech sounds
C. Risk for Injury related to inability to hear warning sounds of impending danger
D. Self Esteem Disturbance related to social and academic difficulties

Nursing Interventions

A. *Minimizing Effects of Hearing Loss*
1. Face the child, use appropriate facial expressions, and make sure the child can see your face clearly when communicating.
2. Approach the child so that you can be seen; touch the deaf child on the shoulder to get attention.

B. *Promoting Effective Communication*
1. Determine usual method of communication; ability to write, use verbal cues, or read lips. Do not depend on gestures to communicate with child or with a third party who does not know sign language.
2. Obtain an interpreter when necessary for children who communicate using sign language. Adequate communication is especially important when providing health education or treating children who may have been abused.
3. Help the parents of a young child to stimulate and communicate with the child.
a. Teach them to use gestures, mime, and nonverbal communication.
b. Teach them to help the baby develop "watching behavior" by rewarding baby with pleasure and praise.
c. Teach them to talk to child while looking directly into child's eyes and using appropriate facial expressions.

C. *Preventing Injury*
1. Advise parents that home safety devices, such as smoke detectors, may need to have visual or tactile alarms (flashing lights or vibration) rather than auditory alarms.
2. Encourage the use of other senses to compensate for inability to hear. For example, the child should be especially careful to look in all directions when crossing the street.
3. Do not leave child alone in unfamiliar environment without means of communication.
4. Provide close surveillance and frequent visual contact for the hospitalized child.

D. *Increasing Self-Esteem*
1. Inform families of their child's right to a public education.

2. Encourage interaction with hearing and nonhearing children to promote integration.
3. Encourage mastery of developmental milestones and skills through self-care activities and play.
4. Help parents understand that child may not be able to express anxiety or frustration and may act out instead. Teach them to be consistent in their use of discipline and to provide alternative ways for child to gain attention or relieve stress.
5. Praise the child for accomplishments and attempts at social interaction.

Family Education/Health Maintenance

1. Encourage families to learn sign language and alternate methods of communication along with child.

2. Advise on proper cleaning and maintenance of hearing aids.
3. Encourage attention to health maintenance needs, such as immunizations and well-child visits.
4. For additional support and information, refer to agencies such as the American Speech-Language-Hearing Association, 10801 Rockville Pike, Rockville, MD 20852 (800-638-TALK).

Evaluation

A. Responds appropriately to environmental stimuli
B. Communicates effectively through sign language, interpreter, and visual cues
C. No injuries reported
D. Reports adequate progress in school and participation in extracurricular activities

Selected References

Behrman, R. E., & Kleigman, R. M. (1994). *Nelson essentials of pediatrics* (2nd ed.). Philadelphia: W.B. Saunders.

Castiglia, P. T., & Harbin, R. E. (1992). Child health care: Process and practice. Philadelphia: J.B. Lippincott.

Hoekelman, R. A. (1992). *Primary pediatric care* (2nd ed.). St. Louis: Mosby Year Book.

Huddleston, K. R. (1994). Strabismus repair in the pediatric patient. *AORN Journal, 60*(5), 754–760.

Jackson, C. B. (1990). Primary health care for deaf children, Part II. *Journal of Pediatric Health Care, 4*(1), 39–41.

Jewell, G., Reeves, B., Saffin, K. & Crofts, B. (1994). The effectiveness of vision screening by school nurses in secondary school. *Archives of Disease in Childhood, 70*(1), 14–18.

Kelly, J. S. (1994). Topical ophthalmic drug administration: A practical approach. *British Journal of Nursing, 3*(10), 518–520.

Owens, T. (1992). *Ear disease: A school nurse manual.* Houston: Peanut Publishing.

Schwartz, M. W., Charmey, E. B., Curry, T. A., & Ludwig, S. (1990). *Pediatric primary care: A problem-oriented approach* (2nd ed.). Chicago: Year Book Medical Publishers.

Terris, M. H., Magit, A. E. & Davidson, T. M. Otitis media with effusion in infants in children. *Postgraduate Medicine, 97*(1), 137–151.

Young, N. (1994). Cochlear implants in children. *Current Problems in Pediatrics, 24,* 131-138.

CHAPTER 54 ◆

Genetic and Developmental Disorders

Human Genetics

Human genetics is the study of the human condition as it is influenced by inherited factors that affect and determine growth and development and that can be transmitted from generation to generation.

◆ UNDERLYING PRINCIPLES

Biologic and Genetic Principles

See Figure 54-1.

1. Cell—basic unit of biology.
   a. Cytoplasm—contains functional structures important to cellular functioning, including mitochondria, which contain extranuclear deoxyribonucleic acid (DNA) important to mitochondrial functioning.
   b. Nucleus—contains 46 chromosomes in each somatic (body) cell, or 23 chromosomes in each germ cell (egg or sperm).
2. Chromosomes
   a. Each somatic cell with a nucleus has 22 pairs of autosomes (the same in both sexes) and 1 pair of sex chromosomes.
   b. Females have two X sex chromosomes; males have one Y sex chromosome and one X sex chromosome.
   c. Normally, at conception, each individual receives one copy of each chromosome pair from the maternal egg cell and one copy of each chromosome pair from the paternal sperm cell, for a total of 46 chromosomes.
   d. Karyotype is the term used to define the chromosomal complement of an individual, for example, 46, XY, as is determined by laboratory chromosome analysis
   e. Each chromosome contains about 2,000 genes.
3. Genes
   a. The basic unit of inherited information.
   b. Each human nucleated somatic cell has about 100,000 genes.
   c. Alternate forms of a gene are termed *alleles*.
   d. An individual receives one gene from each parent for the same trait, thus has two alleles for each gene on the autosomes and also on the X chromosomes in females.
   e. Males have only one X chromosome and therefore only one allele for all genes on the X chromosome; they are hemizygous for all X-linked genes.

   f. At any autosomal locus, or gene site, an individual can have two identical alleles and be termed homozygous for that trait or can have two different alleles at a particular locus, for example, for eye color, and be termed heterozygous.
   g. Genotype refers to the gene constitution of an individual; for practical purposes it is commonly used to address a specific gene pair, for example, the gene for sickle cell disease or that for cystic fibrosis.
   h. Phenotype refers to the physical or biochemical characteristics an individual manifests regarding expression of presence of a particular feature, or set of features, associated with a particular gene.
   i. Each gene is composed of a sequence of DNA bases.
4. DNA
   a. Human DNA is a double-stranded helical structure comprised of four different bases, the sequence of which code for the assembly of amino acids to make a protein, or enzyme. These proteins are important to body characteristics, such as eye color; for cellular functioning, such as the gene for the digestion of phenylalanine; or for body structure, such as a collagen gene important to bone formation.
   b. The four DNA bases are adenine, guanine, cytosine, and thymine—A, G, C, and T.
   c. A change, or mutation, in the coding sequence, such as a duplicated or deleted region, or even a change in only one base, alters the production or functioning of the gene or gene product, thus affecting cellular processes, growth and development, etc.
   d. DNA analysis can be done on almost any body tissue (blood, muscle, skin, etc.) using molecular techniques (not visible under a microscope) for mutation analysis of a specific gene with a known sequence or for DNA linkage of genetic markers associated with a particular gene.
5. Normal cell division
   a. Mitosis occurs in all somatic cells, which under normal circumstances results in the formation of cells identical to the original cell, with the same 46 chromosomes.
   b. Meiosis, or reduction division, occurs in the germ cell line, resulting in gametes (egg and sperm cells) with only 23 chromosomes, one representative of each chromosome pair.
   c. During the process of meiosis, parental homologous chromosomes (from the same pair) pair and undergo exchanges of genetic material, resulting in recombinations of alleles on a chromosome and thus variation in individuals from generation to generation.

From the Whole to the (Microscopic) Parts

| The human body contains 100 trillion **cells** | There is a **nucleus** inside each human cell (except red blood cells) | Each nucleus contains 46 **chromosomes**, arranged in 23 pairs | One **chromosome** of every pair is from each parent | The chromosomes are filled with tightly coiled strands **of DNA** | **Genes** are segments of DNA that contain instructions to make proteins the building blocks of life |

FIGURE 54-1 *Cells, chromosomes, DNA, and genes.*

◆ GENETIC DISORDERS

Presentations warranting genetic consideration include mental retardation, birth defects, biochemical or metabolic disorders, structural abnormalities, and multiple miscarriages.

Disorders that result from abnormalities of chromosomes or genes, or that are at least in part, influenced by genetic factors, are described in Table 54-1.

Classification of Genetic Alterations

A. Chromosomal
1. Entire chromosome or part of chromosome is affected.
   a. Numerical—abnormal number of chromosomes due to nondisjunction (error in chromosomal separation during cell division).
   b. Structural—abnormality involving deletions, additions, or translocations (rearrangements) of parts of chromosomes.
   c. Fragile sites—regions susceptible to chromosomal breakage.
2. May involve autosomes or sex chromosomes.

B. Genetic: Involving a Single Gene or Pair of Genes
1. Autosomal dominant—presence of a single copy of an abnormal gene results in phenotypic expression.
   a. Can be inherited from one parent, whose physical manifestations can vary, depending on specific disorder and the gene's penetrance and expressivity.
   b. Can arise as result of a new mutation in that gene in the affected individual.
   c. Individual with an autosomal dominant gene has a 50% risk of transmitting that gene to all offspring.
2. Autosomal recessive—requires that both alleles at a gene locus be abnormal for an individual to be affected.
   a. Generally, both parents are considered obligate carriers (unaffected) of one copy of the abnormal gene.
   b. Such a carrier couple has a 25% risk, with each pregnancy, to have an affected child, a 50% chance for the child to be an unaffected carrier, and a 25% chance for the child to be an unaffected noncarrier.

3. X-linked recessive—due to an abnormal gene, or genes, on the X chromosome.
   a. Recessively inherited, in most cases, meaning that two abnormal genes are required to be affected; however, only one abnormal gene needs to be present in a male to be affected, because males are hemizygous for all X-linked genes.
   b. Females are typically only carriers of X-linked recessive disorders because the presence of a corresponding normal gene on the other X chromosome in a female produces enough gene product for normal functioning; females can be affected in certain circumstances.
   c. A carrier has a 25% risk, with each pregnancy, to have an affected son, a 25% risk to have a carrier daughter, a 25% chance to have an unaffected son, and a 25% chance to have an unaffected noncarrier daughter.
   d. A male with an abnormal X-linked gene who has children will transmit that gene to all of his daughters, who will be carriers of that gene (usually unaffected); none of his sons will inherit his abnormal X-linked gene, because they receive his Y chromosome.
4. Mitochondrial—genes whose DNA is within the mitochondria, which are located in the cytoplasm, not in the nucleus, and therefore do not follow mendelian laws of inheritance.
   a. Essentially are maternally inherited, because the egg cell contains the cytoplasmic material that is involved in the zygote; the sperm cell contributes mainly only nuclear DNA.
   b. Varying phenotypes, depending on the number and distribution of abnormal mitochondrial genes.
   c. Can affect males or females, but males transmit few, if any, mitochondrial genes.

C. Multifactorial
1. Caused by several genetic factors in addition to other nongenetic influences (eg, environmental).
2. Because of the genetic components, affected individuals or close relatives are at an increased risk, compared with the general population, to have an affected child; that risk is generally 2% to 5%.

3. Elimination of known nongenetic risk factors, or proactive treatment regimen, in some conditions, can reduce risk for occurrence (eg, diet modification to manage hypercholesterolemia, cessation of smoking to reduce risk of cancer or weight control and exercise to prevent type II diabetes in susceptible individuals).

◆ GENETIC COUNSELING

Genetic counseling is a communication process that deals with human problems associated with the occurrence, or recurrence, of a genetic disorder in a family. There is a specific concern about risk associated with a certain problem or because of the relationship to someone who is affected, the *proband*. Several steps occur in the genetic evaluation, including obtaining and reviewing the medical history and records of the affected; eliciting the family history with special attention to factors pertinent to the diagnosis in the proband; evaluating and examining the affected (if available and indicated); ordering appropriate tests and interpreting results; and then meeting with the person seeking consult and/or proband.

Goals of Genetic Counseling

Assist the proband and/or consultant to:
1. Comprehend the medical facts, including the diagnosis, the possible course of the disorder, and the available management.
2. Understand the inheritance of the disorder and the risk of recurrence in specified relatives.
3. Understand the options for dealing with the risk of recurrence.
4. Choose the course of action that seems appropriate to individuals involved in view of their risk, family goals, and religious beliefs and act in accordance with that decision.
5. Make the best possible adjustment to that disorder.

Identify Persons in Need of Genetic Counseling

1. Parent(s) of a child with a birth defect(s), mental retardation, or known/possible genetic disorder.
2. Any individual with a genetic or potentially genetic disorder.
3. Persons with a family history of mental retardation, birth defect/s, or genetic disorder.
4. Pregnant women who will be 35 or older at the time of delivery.
5. Couples of ethnic origin known to be at an increased risk for a specific genetic disorder.
6. Couples who have experienced two or more miscarriages.
7. Women who have had an elevated or low alpha-fetoprotein maternal serum screening test result.
8. Women who have been exposed to drugs or infections during pregnancy.
9. Couples who are related to each other.
10. Persons who are concerned about risk for a genetic disorder.

Genetic Screening and Testing

1. Screening—level of testing offered to large populations (eg, newborn) or high-risk segments of the population (eg, African Americans, Ashkenazi Jews, Mediterranean peoples) to identify individuals with a genetic disorder, increased risk for abnormality, or carrier of a genetic disorder.
   a. Criteria include that the test itself must be reliable, appropriate to the designated population, and cost-effective and that the condition being tested for must be treatable or that early identification will enhance health.
   b. Newborn screening varies among states, testing for disorders such as phenylketonuria (PKU), hypothyroidism, maple syrup urine disease (MSUD), and histidinemia.
   c. Prenatal screening—maternal serum alpha-fetoprotein (AFP) or triple screen (includes measurement of maternal serum alpha-fetoprotein, beta–human chorionic gonadotropin (bHCG), and estriol).
2. Testing
   a. Biochemical—measurement of enzyme levels, activity.
   b. DNA—for gene mutation or DNA linkage study.
   c. Chromosomal—for detection of various conditions, such as extra, missing, deleted, duplicated, or rearranged chromosomes.
3. Prenatal testing
   a. Chorionic villus sampling (CVS)—for chromosomal, biochemical, and DNA testing; done at 9 to 12 weeks gestation.
   b. Amniocentesis—for chromosomal, biochemical and DNA testing at 13 weeks (early amniocentesis); and AFP can be done at 14 to 18 weeks gestation.
   c. Ultrasound—for dating pregnancy and assessment of fetal structures, placenta, and amniotic fluid; done throughout pregnancy, but fetal structures best visualized after 12 weeks.
   d. AFP—for maternal serum levels, tested after 14 weeks' gestation.
   e. Fetoscopy—for obtaining fetal blood samples or visualizing details of fetal structures; done during second trimester.
   f. Percutaneous umbilical blood sampling (PUBS)—for obtaining fetal blood, done during second trimester.

Nursing Responsibilities

1. Recognize or suspect genetic disorders by their physical characteristics and clinical manifestations.
2. Explain/review those aspects of diagnosis, prognosis, and treatment that affect a child's growth and development and that the parents need to know to plan for the care of their child.
3. Clear up misconceptions and allay feelings of guilt.
4. Assist with the diagnostic process by exploring medical and family history information by using physical assessment skills, by obtaining blood samples and/or assisting with CVS or amniocentesis, as indicated.
5. Enhance and reinforce self-image and self-worth of parents and child.
6. Encourage interaction with family and friends; offer referrals, phone numbers of support groups.

(text continues on page 1409)

TABLE 54-1 Genetic Disorders Presenting in the Pediatric Population

Disorder and Incidence	Characteristics	Etiology and Recurrence Risks	Considerations and Comments
Chromosomal Disorders **Autosomal** *Down syndrome (trisomy 21)* 1 in 700 newborns; incidence increases with advanced maternal age (eg, risk at maternal age 25 is 1 in 1350; at age 35, 1 in 384; at age 45, 1 in 28)	Brachycephaly; oblique palpebral fissures; epicanthal folds; Brushfield spots; flat nasal bridge; protruding tongue; small, low-set ears; clinodactyly; simian crease; congenital heart defects; hypotonia; mental retardation; growth retardation; dry, scaly skin	Extra copy of number 21 chromosome (total of three copies): 94%—trisomy Down syndrome (karyotype 47, +21)—three distinct number 21 chromosomes due to nondisjunction, (failure of chromosomal separation during meiosis); recurrence risk 1%, plus maternal age-related risk if over 35. 4%—translocation Down syndrome—extra number 21 attached to another chromosome, usually a number 13 or number 14: half of these translocations are new occurrences, the other half are inherited from a parent. 2%—mosaic Down syndrome—affected has two different cell lines, one with the normal number of chromosomes and the other cell line trisomic for the number 21 chromosome; due to a postconception error in chromosomal division during mitosis.	• Recurrence risk for parents of affected are dependent on one or more of the following: chromosomal type of disorder, maternal age, parental karyotype, family history, and sex of transmitting parent and other chromosome involved (if translocation). • May demonstrate nuccal thickening prenatally on ultrasound examination. • Associated with moderate mental retardation. • No phenotypic differences between trisomy Down syndrome and translocation Down syndrome. • Chromosome analysis should be performed on all persons with Down syndrome.
Trisomy 13 (Patau syndrome) 1 in 5,000 live births	Holoprosencephaly; cleft lip or palate, or both; abnormal helices; cardiac defects; rocker-bottom feet; overlapping positioning of fingers; seizures; severe mental retardation	Extra number 13 chromosome (total of three copies): Either trisomy form, due to nondisjunction, with less than a 1% recurrence risk; or translocation form, with recurrence risk less than that of translocation Down's syndrome and dependent on other factors, including chromosomes involved.	• 44% die within the 1st month; 18% survive 1st year of life.
Trisomy 18 (Edwards syndrome) 1 in 6,000 live births	Small for gestational age (may be detected prenatally); feeble fetal activity; weak cry; prominent occiput; low-set, malformed ears; short palpebral fissures; small oral opening; overlapping positioning of fingers (fifth digit over fourth, index over third); nail hypoplasia, short hallux; cardiac defects; inguinal or umbilical hernia; cryptorchidism in males; severe mental retardation	Extra number 18 chromosome (total of three copies): Majority due to trisomy with less than 1% recurrence risk.	• Most trisomy 18 conceptions miscarry; 90% of liveborn die within 1st year of life.
Sex Chromosome *Klinefelter syndrome* 1 in 700 males 47, XXY abnormality in 90%;	Body habitus may be tall, slim, and underweight; long limbs; gynecomastia; small testes;	Due to nondisjunction during meiosis, except for cases of mosaicism, which are due to mitotic	• No distinguishing features prenatally. Diagnosis may not be suspected or pursued before puberty.

Microdeletion/Microduplication

Condition/Incidence	Clinical Features	Cause	Comments
other 10% have more than two X chromosomes in addition to the Y chromosome or have mosaicism (about 20%)	inadequate verilization; azoospermia or low sperm count; cognitive defects; behavioral problems	nondisjunction.	• Diagnosis in childhood is beneficial in planning for testosterone replacement therapy, in addition to accurate understanding of learning or behavioral problems. • Tend to be delayed in onset of speech, have difficulty in expressive language; may be relatively immature; may have history of recurrent respiratory infections.
Turner syndrome (45, X) 1 in 2,500 female births	Webbing of neck and short stature; lymphedema of hands and feet as newborn; congenital cardiac defects (especially coarctation of the aorta); low posterior hairline; cubitus valgus; widely spaced nipples; underdeveloped breasts; immature internal genitalia (eg, streak ovaries); primary amenorrhea; learning disabilities	About 50% due to a nondisjunctional error during meiosis (karyotype 45, X); 20% are mosaic due to nondisjunction during mitosis; 30% have two X chromosomes but one is functionally inadequate (eg, due to presence of abnormal gene); generally a sporadic occurrence.	• Webbing of neck and short stature may be detected prenatally by ultrasound. • Early diagnosis enhances optimal health care management, eg, planning for administration of growth hormone therapy, estrogen replacement. • Psychosocial implications associated with short stature, delayed onset of puberty. • Infertility associated with ovarian dysgenesis; adoption is generally the only option for having children.
Fragile X 1 in 1,200 males; 1 in 2,500 females	Motor delays; hypotonia; speech delay and language difficulty; hyperactivity; classic features including long face, prominent ears, and macroorchidism manifest around puberty; autism (about 7% of males); mental retardation in most males; learning disabilities in most affected females	Mutation in the fragile X mental retardation gene (FMR-1), represented as a large DNA expansion of a normally present trinucleotide. Carrier mother of an affected male has a 50% risk for future affected males and 50% risk to transmit the FMR-1 X chromosome to a daughter who would be a carrier, may be unaffected, or manifest features associated with the Fragile X syndrome and has a 50% risk to transmit that gene to future offspring	• Both cytogenetic testing for expression of the fragile X site and DNA analysis for the expansion is available, but the latter is superior. • Phenotypic expression of this gene in males and females is variable; genetic mechanisms determining expression of this gene are very complicated. • Fragile X should be considered in the differential diagnosis of any mentally retarded male who is undiagnosed; it is the most common mental retardation in males.
Prader-Willi syndrome Estimated incidence 1 in 25,000	Hypotonia and poor sucking ability in infancy; almond-shaped palpebral fissures; small stature; small, slow growth of hands and/or feet; small penis, cryptorchidism; insatiable appetite, behavioral problems onsetting in childhood; below-normal intelligence or mental retardation	Cytogenetic microdeletion in chromosome 15 q11–13 identified in 50–70% of cases; deletion associated with paternally inherited number 15 chromosome. Generally sporadic occurrence; empiric recurrence risk 1.6%.	• Consider diagnosis in infants presenting with hypotonia and sucking problems where etiology is unknown. • Associated with lack of a functioning paternal gene at this locus; presents clinical evidence for the necessity of two functioning genes, *both a* maternal and paternal contribution. • Another distinct entity, termed Angelman syndrome, is associated with a deletion of the *maternal* contribution in this same cytogenetic region; it is also associated with mental deficiency, but with a different phenotypic presentation.

(continued)

TABLE 54-1 Genetic Disorders Presenting in the Pediatric Population
(continued)

Disorder and Incidence	Characteristics	Etiology and Recurrence Risks	Considerations and Comments
Mendelian Disorders—Single Gene **Autosomal Dominant**			
Achondroplasia 1 in 10,000 live births Increased incidence associated with advanced paternal age (>40)	Megalocephaly; small foramen magnum and short cranial base with early spheno-occipital closure; prominent forehead; low nasal bridge; midfacial hypoplasia; small stature; short extremities; lumbar lordosis; short tubular bones; incomplete extension at the elbow; normal intelligence	Autosomal dominant inheritance; 80–90% are due to a new mutation. In those cases that are inherited, the affected parent has a 50% risk to transmit the gene to each child.	• Hydrocephalus can be a complication of achondroplasia and may be masked by megalocephaly. • Risk for apnea secondary to cervical spinal cord and lower brain stem compression due to alterations in shape of cervical vertebral bodies; respiratory problems are also a risk because of the small chest and upper airway obstruction. • Can be diagnosed prenatally by ultrasound.
Osteogenesis imperfecta (Type 1) 1 in 15,000 live births	Blue sclerae; fractures (variable number); deafness may occur	Defect in the procollagen gene associated with decreased synthesis of a constituent chain important to collagen structure. Can occur as a new mutation in that gene or can be inherited from a parent who has a 50% recurrence risk to transmit the gene; most severe cases represent a sporadic occurrence within a family.	• There are at least four general classifications of osteogenesis imperfecta, each with varying clinical severity, presentation, and pattern of genetic transmission. • Treatment with calcitonin and fluoride may be beneficial in reducing the number of fractures.
Autosomal Recessive			
Sickle cell disease 1 in 400 live births of African American ancestry	Physically normal in appearance at birth; hemolytic anemia and the occurrence of acute exacerbations (crises), resulting in increased susceptibility to infection and vascular occlusive episodes	Point mutation in the sickle cell gene resulting in an altered gene product; red blood cells susceptible to sickling at times of low oxygen tension. Parents of an affected individual are both unaffected carriers of one abnormal copy of the sickle cell gene (sickle cell trait) and together have a 25% risk for recurrence in any offspring.	• 1 in 10 African Americans is a carrier of the sickle cell gene; population screening is indicated for these individuals. • Unaffected siblings of an affected individual have a 2/3, or 67%, risk to have the sickle cell trait and should be screened. • See p. 1327 for nursing care. • Prenatal testing is available through DNA analysis from specimen obtained during chorionic villus sampling or amniocentesis.

Cystic fibrosis (CF) 1 in 2,000 live births (predominantly Caucasian)	Phenotypically normal at birth; may present with meconium ileus (10%) as neonate or later with persistent cough, recurrent respiratory problems, gastrointestinal complaints, abdominal pain, or infertility	Mutation in the cystic fibrosis transmembrane conduction regulator gene on chromosome 7 results in an abnormality of a protein integral to the cell membrane. Parents of an affected individual are both considered obligate carriers of one copy of the abnormal CF gene; thus, together they have a 25% recurrence risk with each conception.	• 1 in 20 whites is a carrier of a CF gene mutation. • Several different mutations have been identified within the CF gene, the most common of which is ΔF508, which accounts for about 70% of CF mutations. CF screening can identify about 85% of all CF mutations (95% in Jewish population); it is not yet being used for general population screening. • DNA analysis of the CF gene is advised for affected individuals and relatives of persons with CF. • See p. 1184 for nursing care.
Tay-Sachs disease 1 in 3,600 Ashkenazic Jews	Normal at birth; progressive neurodegenerative manifestations, including loss of developmental milestones and lack of central nervous system (CNS) maturation; cherry-red spot on macula	Mutation in the gene for hexosaminidase A, an enzyme important to cellular metabolic processes, results in accumulation of metabolic by-products within the cell (especially brain), impairing functioning and causing the neurodegenerative effects. Parents of an affected individual are both considered unaffected obligate carriers of one copy of the Tay-Sachs disease gene; together they have a 25% risk of recurrence in their offspring.	• About 1 in 25 Ashkenazic Jews is a carrier of the Tay-Sachs gene; about 1 in 17 French Canadians is a carrier of an abnormal Tay-Sachs gene (different mutation from that of the Jewish ancestry); persons of these ancestries should be screened. • No treatment available; results in death in childhood. • Prenatal testing is available.
X-Linked Recessive *Duchenne's muscular dystrophy (DMD)* 1 in 3,500 males	Phenotypically normal a birth; dramatically elevated creatinine phosphokinase (CPK) level (detectable as early as 2 days of age); hypertrophy of the calves; history of tendency to trip and fall (at about 3 years of age); Gowers' sign (tendency to push off oneself when getting up from a sitting position)	DNA mutation, generally a deletion, detectable in 70% of affected males. Carrier females have a 25% risk with each pregnancy to have an affected male, a 25% risk to have a carrier female, a 25% chance to have a healthy male, and a 25% chance to have a healthy noncarrier female.	• 1 in 1,750 females is a carrier of the DMD gene. • In the case of an isolated affected male, the mother has a $^2/_3$ statistical risk that she is a carrier of the DMD gene and a $^1/_3$ chance that her affected son arose as the result of a new mutation in that gene (she is not a carrier). • DNA testing is recommended for affected males, and once one type of gene mutation is known in that family, prenatal diagnosis and evaluation of potential female carriers can be carried out. • DNA analysis may provide clues as to expected clinical severity.

(continued)

TABLE 54-1 Genetic Disorders Presenting in the Pediatric Population

(continued)

Disorder and Incidence	Characteristics	Etiology and Recurrence Risks	Considerations and Comments
Hemophilia A 1 in 7,000 males	Phenotypically normal at birth; bleeding tendency (ranging from frequent spontaneous bleeds associated with the severe form to bleeding only after trauma associated with the mild form)	Deficiency of Factor XIII (antihemophilic factor) due to abnormality in this gene located on the X chromosome. Carrier females have a 25% risk with each pregnancy to have an affected son, a 25% risk for a carrier daughter, and a 25% chance each for a healthy unaffected daughter or son.	• Frequency of carrier females is about 1 in 3500. • The severe form occurs in about 48% of cases. • Moderate cases account for 31% • The mild form accounts for 21% of cases. • See p. 1335 for nursing care.
Glucose 6-phosphate dehydrogenase (G6PD) 10–14% of male live births of African American origin	Phenotypically normal at birth; many remain asymptomatic through life; may manifest acute hemolysis associated with exposure to outside factors, eg, certain medications	Abnormality of the G6PD gene on the X chromosome. Carrier females have a 25% risk with each pregnancy to have an affected male and 25% risk to have a carrier female.	• Be aware of drugs, such as antimalarial drugs or sulfonamides; or chemicals, such as phenylhydrazine (used in silvering mirrors, photography, soldering) associated with hemolysis in G6PD deficient individuals.
Multifactorial Disorders			
Neural tube defects 1 in 1,000 live births	Abnormalities of neural tube closure, ranging from anencephaly to myelomeningocele to spina bifida occulta	Probably several genetic factors may predispose certain individuals, or families, to susceptibility, but certain environmental (eg, prolonged hyperthermia) and other unknown factors play an additive role in surpassing an arbitrary threshold, placing the developing fetus at risk. Recurrence risk for isolated neural tube defects range between 1% and 5%.	• Recurrence risk for isolated neural tube defects is dependent on the severity of the defect, ie, a defect in the neurulation (the cranial end of the neural tube) versus cannulation (the development of the caudal end) and if there is a positive family history. • Maternal screening can be performed prenatally (after 14 weeks' gestation) through alpha-fetoprotein levels in maternal serum. • Can be associated with chromosomal or genetic disorders.
Cleft lip and/or cleft palate 1 in 1,000 live births	Unilateral or bilateral; cleft lip and cleft palate may occur together or in isolation	Failure of migration and fusion of the maxillary processes during embryogenesis. Recurrence risk for first-degree relatives of a person with an isolated cleft lip and/or cleft palate ranges between 2% and 6%.	• Clefting can occur as an isolated congenital abnormality or be one component of a syndrome, genetic defect, or chromosome abnormality, these latter three of which are associated with a recurrence risk specific to that disorder. • Recurrence for isolated cleft lip and/or palate are dependent on the type of cleft, the sex of the affected individual, and the family history.

7. Refer and prepare family for genetic counseling.
   a. Inform that prenatal testing does not mean termination of pregnancy (eg, it may confirm that the fetus is not affected, thus eliminating worry throughout pregnancy, although the determination of an abnormality is also a possibility).
   b. Encourage the parents to allow adequate time to deliberate on course of action (eg, do not rush into a tubal ligation, because in a few years they may want more children).
   c. Remain nonjudgmental.
8. Refer for further information and support to: March of Dimes Birth Defects Foundation; 1275 Mamaroneck Avenue; White Plains, NY 10605 (for educational materials and information on location of genetic services); and National Clearinghouse for Maternal and Child Health; 3520 Prospect Street, NW, Suite 1; Washington, DC 20057 (for genetic and child health information and material); International Society of Nurses in Genetics; c/o 5586 Main St., Suite 210; Buffalo, NY 14221 (genetics resource, network, and professional organization for nurses; Alliance of Genetic Support Groups; 38th and R Streets NW; Washington, DC 20057 (resource and advocate for national and local genetic support groups; for lay persons and professionals).

Developmental Disabilities

Developmental disabilities are a group of closely interrelated chronic, nonprogressive neurologic handicaps occurring in childhood. They include mental retardation, cerebral palsy, learning disabilities, language disorders, autism, and impairments of vision and hearing. When discussing development, four major areas are usually considered; gross motor, fine motor, language (expressive and receptive), and social adaptive. Language is considered to be the best predictor of future intellectual functioning.

Development of the child begins with the embryo and continues throughout a person's life. It is a step-by-step process related to the maturation of the central nervous system and dependent on a variety of environmental factors. The most common presentation of a developmental disability is failure to achieve age-appropriate developmental skills in any one or more of the four major areas.

◆ MENTAL RETARDATION

Mental retardation (cognitive developmental delay) refers to the most severe, general lack of cognitive and problem-solving skills. The American Association on Mental Deficiency defines mental retardation as a significant subaverage general intellectual functioning existing concurrently with deficits in adaptive behaviors and manifested during the developmental period. There are may causes and a wide range of impairments.

Etiology and Incidence

1. Three percent of the U.S. population, 6.6 million people, are considered mentally retarded.
2. Of every 1,000 babies born, 30 will be classified as mentally retarded before they reach the age of 18.
3. The more severe types of mental retardation tend to be diagnosed in early infancy, especially when they coexist with an identifiable syndrome or congenital anomalies.
4. Milder forms of mental retardation tend to be diagnosed in preschool years, when language and behavioral concerns call attention to slower development.
5. No identifiable organic or biologic cause can be found for 50% of children.
6. Identifiable causes include:
   a. Genetic causes, such as Down syndrome, fragile X syndrome, or inborn errors of metabolism, such as PKU.
   b. Congenital anomalies, including brain malformations, hydrocephalus, and microcephaly.
   c. Intrauterine influences, such as congenital infections, drug exposure, and teratogens.
   d. Perinatal trauma—birth anoxia, intracranial hemorrhage.
   e. Postnatal trauma—head injuries from falls, motor vehicle accidents.
   f. Postnatal infections (meningitis, sepsis).
   g. Environmental exposure to toxins, such as lead; environmental deprivation; and neglect.

Altered Physiology

1. The malfunctioning brain is poorly understood in most cases, but physiologic alterations identified in some cases include:
   a. Congenital brain malformations, brain tissue damage, or underdevelopment of the brain as shown by abnormal results of computed tomography scan or magnetic resonance imaging.
   b. Biochemical or errors of metabolism, in which an absence of an enzyme or hormone produces abnormal brain function or formation, as in PKU or hypothyroidism.
2. Intelligence quotient (IQ) is 75 or below; classification has been recently changed to *mild* and *severe* and includes both cognitive and functional ability.
3. Limitations in adaptive ability occur in communication, self-care, home living, social skills, community use, self-direction, health and safety, functional academics, leisure, and work.

Complications/Associated Findings

1. Seizures
2. Cerebral palsy
3. Sensory deficits
4. Communication disorders (speech and language)
5. Neurodegenerative disorders
6. Psychiatric illness

Clinical Manifestations

Developmental delays (failure to achieve age-appropriate skills) are evident to some degree in almost all areas.

A. *Infancy*
1. "Poor feeder"—a weak or uncoordinated suck results in poor breast- or bottle-feeding, resulting in poor weight gain.
2. Delayed or decreased visual alertness and curiosity with poor visual tracking of face or objects.
3. Decreased or lack of auditory response.
4. Decreased spontaneous activity.
5. Delayed head and trunk control.

NURSING ALERT:
Although 75% of individuals with mental retardation have no physical signs, they often achieve motor milestones at a slower rate.

6. Floppy (hypotonia) or spastic muscle tone

B. *Toddler*
1. Delayed independent sitting, crawling, pull to stand, and independent ambulation.
2. Delayed communication—failure to develop receptive and expressive language milestones. Almost half of children with mental retardation are identified after the age of 3 years, when speech delays manifest themselves.
3. Failure of the child to make progress or show interest in the area of independence in self-feeding, dressing, and toilet training may reflect cognitive impairment.
4. Short attention span and distractibility.
5. Behavioral disturbances.
6. Clumsiness.

Diagnostic Evaluation

No single test can diagnose mental retardation. The multi-disciplinary evaluation should be individually tailored to the child.

1. Rule out sensory deficits by assessment of vision and hearing.
2. Medical evaluation should include developmental history, sequential developmental assessments, family history, and physical examination. The positive findings determine the direction of the individual evaluation.
   a. Unusual appearance (dysmorphic features) warrant genetic workup.
   b. History consistent with loss of developmental milestones and positive family history warrants workup for presence of an inborn error of metabolism (diagnosed by blood and urine analysis).
   c. Children with macrocephaly, microcephaly, or neurologic abnormalities may require a computed tomography scan or magnetic resonance imaging.
   d. Electroencephalogram is necessary for children with seizures.
3. Psychological testing
   a. The Bayley Scales are used to assess fine motor, gross motor, and language skills and visual problem solving in infants of developmental age of 2 months to 3 years (this test is weighted on nonlanguage items).
   b. The McCarthy Scale offers a "general cognitive index" that is roughly equivalent to an IQ score.
   c. The Stanford-Binet Intelligence Scale is used to test children with mental abilities of 2 years and older.
   d. The Wechsler Preschool and Primary Scale of Intelligence (WPPSI) 1991 measures mental age of 3 to 7 years.
   e. The Wechsler Intelligence Scale for Children (WISC) III 1991 for children whose functional age is above a 6-year level.
   f. The Vineland Scale tests social-adaptive abilities—self-help skills, self-control, interaction with others, cooperation; the Adaptive Behavior Scale is similar to Vineland but also measures adjustment.

Treatment

1. An interdisciplinary team evaluation by a developmental pediatrician, clinical psychologist, and counselor is usually the initial step in the management of mental retardation. This type of evaluation can be obtained through a state or private diagnostic and evaluation center, public school, or university-affiliated program.
2. If a treatable cause is identified, such as an inborn error of metabolism, a therapeutic diet can be instituted. Hypothyroidism can be treated with thyroid hormone.
3. Associated medical problems, such as seizures, poor nutrition, sensory deficits, or dental problems must be treated to allow the child to maximize his or her potential.
4. A family assessment is essential to address:
   a. Financial stressors—financial aid may be available through Social Security Income, Medicaid, or state and local programs to help families with children with mental retardation.
   b. Family coping abilities.
   c. Support for siblings.
   d. Respite services.
   e. Support groups.
   f. Recreational programs, for example, Special Olympics, summer camps.
   g. Identification of other affected or at risk persons.
5. The initial evaluation often leads to recommendations for more targeted evaluations, such as physical therapy, occupational therapy, social work assessment.
6. Public laws are in place to ensure that individuals with disabilities receive the help that they need to function. In 1993, Public Law 102-119 was passed to provide for assessment and treatment of all children from birth to age 3 years. It encompasses support that the family might require to meet the needs of the child, for example, drug counseling, transportation, parent support, teaching or counseling. After all of the above assessments are completed, an individualized family service plan is devised and a case manager appointed to ensure that the program is implemented. The plan is reviewed and revised annually.
7. Agencies that may provide information, support, and additional resources include:
   The ARC (formerly, Association for Retarded Citizens of the United States), 500 East Border Street, Suite 300, Arlington, TX 76010 (1-800-433-5255).
   The Joseph P. Kennedy, Jr., Foundation, 1325 G Street, Suite 500, Washington, DC 20005-4709 (202-393-1250).
   National Information Center for Children and Youth With Disabilities; 1-800-695-0285.

◆ DOWN SYNDROME

Down syndrome, or trisomy 21, is the most common identifiable cause of mental retardation and a condition associated with a variety of congenital anomalies. The most common life experience of a child with Down syndrome is to live with the family, participate in infant stimulation and preschool programs, and attend school while receiving some support for special education. Adults with Down syndrome can function in supported employment programs and live in small groups. Their life expectancy depends on the presence of medical complications; when there are no complications, life expectancy is slightly shorter than average. Down syndrome is one of the most widely known syndromes associated with mental retardation.

Etiology and Incidence

See page 1404.

Associated Problems

Table 54-2 provides a comprehensive list of potential problems that occur with Down syndrome. Some are identified at birth, others arise and cause difficulties later in the life cycle. Percentages are listed that represent occurrence within the Down syndrome population.

Diagnosis and Treatment

1. An interdisciplinary and multispecialty team is essential to evaluate physiologic and psychosocial functioning.
2. Medical and surgical interventions are carried out as indicated for associated problems.
3. Physical, speech, and occupational therapists; social workers; mental health counselors; and special education teachers are all involved to provide and carry out necessary training and treatment, along with the parents, to optimize functioning.
4. Agencies that provide support, information, and additional resources are:
   National Down Syndrome Congress, 1605 Chantilly Drive, Suite 250; Atlanta, GA 30324 (800-232-6372) (publishes Down Syndrome News, booklets, bibliographies).
   National Down Syndrome Society, 666 Broadway, New York, NY 10012 (800-221-4602).
   Parents of Down's Syndrome Children—local groups listed in phone book or community services directory.

◆ FRAGILE X SYNDROME

Fragile X is the second most common identifiable cause of mental retardation and the most common cause among males. Chromosome analysis reveals that the long arm of the X chromosome is constricted and appears fragile, but cannot be detected in all cases, thus DNA analysis is preferred for diagnosis. This anomaly produces an individual (more commonly males, but females can be symptomatic) with similar facial features, degrees of mental retardation, communication disorders, and behavioral alterations, such as hyperactivity, attention deficit, and self-stimulating and self-injurious behaviors.

Etiology and Incidence

See page 1414.

Associated Problems

Associated problems include mitral valve prolapse, seizures, hypotonia, and feeding problems. See Table 54-3 for a thorough discussion of problems.

Diagnosis and Treatment

1. Physical/speech therapy evaluation for feeding techniques may be indicated for poor feeders. Special attention should be given to see that intake is adequate, because the infant will sleep excessively and seem content with lack of stimulation.
2. Neurologic evaluation is indicated for development of seizures.
3. All children with fragile X should be evaluated for mitral valve prolapse.
4. Behavioral/social/discipline problems are the greatest issue and should be addressed consistently through planned behavior modification techniques.
5. Functional capacity varies with severity of disorder. Ability to attend school, perform self-care, and obtain vocational training is based on frequent assessment.
6. Genetic consultation and evaluation is indicated because the mother may be a carrier and others in family may be affected or at risk.
7. Resources include:
   National Fragile X Foundation, 1441 York Street, Suite 303, Denver CO 80206 (800-688-8765; 303-333-6155).

◆ ATTENTION DEFICIT HYPERACTIVITY DISORDER AND LEARNING DISABILITIES

Attention deficit hyperactivity disorder (ADHD) is characterized by a cluster of symptoms, including developmentally inappropriate short attention span, impulsivity, and distractibility. Hyperactivity does not always occur along with attention deficit. It is a diagnosis of exclusion; other disorders associated with these symptoms must be ruled out before a diagnosis of ADHD can be made. Hearing and visual impairments, seizures, mental retardation, learning disabilities, side effects of medications, and psychiatric disorders are just a few that need to be ruled out.

The term "learning disabilities" (LD) is defined as a "heterogeneous group of disorders manifested by significant difficulties in the acquisition of listening, speaking, reading, writing, reasoning, or mathematical abilities, or of social skills" (Interagency Committee of Learning Disabilities, 1987). Learning disabilities and ADHD often occur together (Fig. 54-2).

Manifestations and treatment are discussed in general terms together in this text; however, ADHD and LD are separate but overlapping problems and may need specific approaches based on the nature of the disability.

Etiology and Incidence

Multiple hypotheses exist because the exact causes are unknown.

1. Genetic
   a. A family trait—other members of the family often have similar difficulties.

TABLE 54-2 Down Syndrome

Potential Problems	Evaluation	Management
Congenital heart malformations (ie, AV canal, VSD, and tetralogy of Fallot) (40%)	Observe for color changes, pulse, and respiratory rate at rest and with stress. Assess tolerance of feeding for early tiring or frequent interruptions in feeding. Echocardiogram usually done during newborn period on all infants with DS.	Early identification and treatment can prevent congestive heart failure and decompensation or poor growth. Medical or surgical correction is possible to repair the defect.
Congenital gastrointestinal malformations (12%): Pyloric stenosis Duodenal atresia, tracheoesophageal fistula	Observe for coughing or vomiting, especially with feeding: bile-stained vomitus suggests lower tract abnormalities; partially digested contents suggest upper tract problem. Observe bowel movements and for distention of abdomen. Radiographic studies are done.	Spillage of material from esophagus into the trachea can cause aspiration and pneumonia. Surgical intervention occurs in early newborn period.
Hypothyroidism (10–20%)	Monitor for weight gain, hair loss, lethargy, short stature, voice changes, and depression (can develop at any time over life cycle). Newborn screening includes T_3, TSH, T_4 biannually.	Thyroid hormone replacement.
Visual defects: Refractive errors (70%) Strabismus (50%) Nystagmus (35%) Cataracts (3%)	Use Teller activity as a visual screen tool for those who cannot cooperate with Snellen chart. Positive findings in first year of life warrant immediate referral to ophthalmologist. All individuals should be seen by an ophthalmologist at 1 year of age, and vision screening should continue throughout life.	Undetected visual deficits can cause failure to achieve developmental milestones and cause permanent loss of vision.
Hearing defects (60–90%): Mild–moderate conductive hearing loss Enlarged adenoids Sleep apnea	Assess for curiosity and response to sounds of varying quality. Auditory brain stem response assesses hearing in infants. Sound field testing for children over 1 year of age. Tympanometry to assess middle ear function.	Narrow ear canals and subtle immune deficiencies can cause chronic middle ear infections. Enlarged adenoids can cause upper airway obstruction especially during sleep. Treatment can range from antibiotics for simple otitis media to myringotomy tubes, adenoidectomy, or hearing loss.
Hypotonia of infants:	Observe for floppiness, poor head control, poor oral motor function. Infant should be placed on abdomen periodically while being observed and monitored for potential for suffocation.	Physical, occupational, and speech therapy. Adaptive equipment gives extra support to head and neck when handling newborn. Always keep head elevated for at least 1 hour after meals. Change position regularly.
Atlanto-occipital and atlano-axial subluxation (dislocation of the upper spine due to joint laxity) 15%	Assess for head tilt; increasing clumsiness, limping, or refusal to walk; weakness of arms. X-ray of spine at age 2 years and then every 5 years during childhood. Precise measurements are taken to document alignment of the skull and vertebrae. Shifting of the two causes compression and neurologic damage.	If present, participation in contact sports and gymnastics is contraindicated. In severe cases, surgery to fuse the vertebrae and occiput and stabilize spinal column.
Gait abnormalities (15%)	Monitor for onset of limp, leg length discrepancy. Hip X-rays can document dislocation or subluxation.	Physical therapy and sometimes orthopedic surgery are necessary.
Failure to thrive	Monitor growth on Down syndrome growth chart. Monitor feedings for length of feeding, feeding schedule, loss of feeding by vomiting or poor seal on nipple. Monitor type of formula and caloric content.	Nutritionist can advise on formula adjustments. Therapists can help with positioning types of nipples used to counteract effects of weak sucking reflex and large, protruding tongue.
Short stature 100%	Plot growth on Down syndrome growth chart. Monitor stages of puberty. Delayed puberty may warrant further investigation.	Use of human growth hormone may be considered; this is still controversial.

(continued)

TABLE 54-2 **Down Syndrome** *(continued)*

Potential Problems	Evaluation	Management
Obesity 50%	Monitor thyroid hormone levels. Serial monitoring of weight. Monitor for amount of exercise, caloric intake.	Overindulgence by adults or use of food in behavior management increases risk of overeating. Lack of social involvement lead to decreased activity. Behavior modification is necessary.
Malocclusions 60–100%	Assess for malocclusions, periodontal disease, delayed eruption of teeth. Regular dental checkups begin at age 2.	Encourage good oral hygiene with proper teeth brushing.
Mental retardation 100% with varying degrees from mild to moderate	Routine developmental assessment using standardized tools of measurement.	Special education and training.
Alzheimer's disease after the age of 40 years 15–30%	Assess for decreased cognitive function and loss of memory. MRI or CT scan shows areas of plaque.	Increased supervision is needed.
Other problems: Communication Disorders Alopecia 10% Seizures 6% Leukemia 1%		

VSD: ventricular septal defect; AV: atrioventricular; DS: Down syndrome; T_3: triiodothyronine; TSH: thyroid stimulating hormone; T_4: levothyroxine; MRI: magnetic resonance imaging; CT: computed tomography.

---

   b. Characteristics of inborn errors of metabolism.
   c. Sex chromosome abnormalities often exhibit these traits.
2. Not shown to be associated with history of birth trauma or brain damage.
3. Exposure to prenatal and postnatal factors that might adversely affect brain development and function—lead, alcohol, cocaine, central nervous system infections, low birth weight, and prematurity.
4. May coexist with other handicapping conditions, such as spina bifida, cerebral palsy, or seizure disorders.
5. An estimated 5% to 10% of children (ranging up to 30%) have ADHD; LD is reportedly present in 12.6% of children by the end of the second grade.
6. Males are diagnosed twice as frequently as females (girls may go undiagnosed, because they are less likely to exhibit disruptive behaviors).

Altered Physiology

1. Mechanisms are not completely understood.
2. Attention deficit hyperactivity disorder—alteration in response-inhibition mechanisms of brain controlled by the frontal cortex and reticular activating system; alteration in neurotransmitter.
3. Learning disabilities—authorities are investigating abnormalities in the parietal lobe of the brain and in the central visual pathways located in the occipital lobe.

Clinical Manifestations

1. See Table 54-4 for diagnostic criteria for ADHD; child must have at least 8 of the 14 symptoms for more than 6 months.

2. Symptoms of ADHD may vary slightly based on the age of the child.
   a. Toddlers— constant movement, described as "into everything"; may have focused attention in highly motivated situations.
   b. School age—fidgety, easily distracted, does not finish tasks, loses things; school achievement is below child's potential.
3. Symptoms of LD:
   a. School achievement is significantly lower than potential.
   b. Perceptual-motor impairments.
   c. Emotional lability.
   d. Speech and language disorders.
   e. Coordination deficits.
4. There can be a wide range of cognitive ability from mild retardation to above-average intelligence.

Diagnostic Evaluation

1. Complete medical review, family history, and physical examination, including vision and hearing assessment and neurologic evaluation to rule out other disorders.
2. Psychological testing to determine the exact nature of cognitive and perceptual dysfunctions.
3. Behavioral and social assessment.
4. Assessment of academic performance.
5. Magnetic resonance imaging, electroencephalogram, positron-emission tomography to determine underlying neurologic abnormality.

NURSING ALERT:
Historically, preschool and kindergarten screening tools have not been accurate in predicting LD; newer tests of language and memory appear to be better predictors.

TABLE 54-3 Fragile X Syndrome

Potential Problems	Evaluation	Management
Hypotonia of infancy	Assess ability to control head and assume upright posture. Assess feeding for efficient suck and coordination of suck/swallow.	Physical therapy, stimulation program, feeding adaptations.
Seizures (20% of cases)	Assess for muscle tremors, deviation of eyes to one side, rhythmic jerking of the body, and loss of consciousness.	Referral to neurologist for diagnosis and anticonvulsants to treat seizures.
Mitral valve prolapse (80% of males)	Assess dyspnea, cyanosis, murmur. Echocardiogram to evaluate valve function.	Antibiotics for prophylaxis before invasive procedures to prevent endocarditis. Treatment of congestive heart failure; surgical repair may be necessary.
Self-stimulating behavior	Rule out any source of pain (ie, otitis media, tooth pain) that may be causing behavior. Rule out sensory deficits.	Behavior management techniques: Focus on replacing undesirable behaviors with purposeful, meaningful substitutes, with emphasis on positive reinforcement and extinguishing negative reinforcement.
Hyperactivity attention deficits	Assess activity of attention span within the context of the developmental age of the child.	Behavior management and special educational techniques.
Discipline problems	Assess social skills.	Boys tend to do best in self-contained classrooms for children with similar degrees of mental retardation.
Communication disorders	Assess language development (often weakest area of development).	Speech–language therapy can be beneficial.
Poor auditory memory; auditory reception	Assess how child lets needs be known: cries, gestures, single words, and/or sentences.	Speech therapy, behavior modification.
Cognitive dysfunction: Short-term memory deficits Poor problem-solving skills Functional limitations in self-care	Assess for appropriateness of educational placement and child's reaction to situation.	Specialized training and education, assisted living.

Treatment

Multidisciplinary approach, including environmental and behavioral approaches, is treatment of choice.

A. *Pharmacologic Treatment*
1. Central nervous system stimulants work for 70% to 75% of ADHD children (reserved for children older than 7 years of age)
   a. Effective in decreasing motor activities and increasing attention span and concentration, thereby allowing child to be more available to learn.
   b. Medications commonly used: methylphenidate (Ritalin), dextroamphetamine (Dexadrine), and pemoline (Cylert).
2. Side effects of stimulants:
   a. Insomnia may result from increased dosage or if administered too late in the day.
   b. Anorexia and temporary growth retardation
   c. Increased pulse and respiratory rates, nervousness, nausea, and stomachache.
   d. Liver dysfunction (pemoline): periodic liver function tests are required.
   e. Altered effects of many antiseizure drugs and tricyclic antidepressants.
   f. Do not cause euphoric effect or addiction in children.

3. Nursing responsibilities/patient teaching points:
   a. Administer before breakfast and lunch (sustained-release forms do not require a lunch dose).
   b. Work with school system to ensure that lunch dose is given.
   c. Consider "drug holidays" during vacations and on weekends to monitor effectiveness and the need for change; this is especially recommended at the start of each academic school year.
   d. Stimulant medications are not usually given to children younger than 6 years of age.
   e. The child is usually started on a small dose, which is gradually increased until the desired response is achieved.
   f. Evaluate the child's response to medication by direct observation and consultation with others, such as parent and teachers.

B. *Special Teaching Strategies*
1. For visual perceptual deficit—present material verbally; use hands-on experience; tape record teaching sessions.
2. For auditory perceptual deficit—provide materials in written form; use pictures; provide tactile learning.
3. For integrative deficit—use multisensory approaches; print directions while you verbalize them; use calendars and lists to organize tasks and activities.

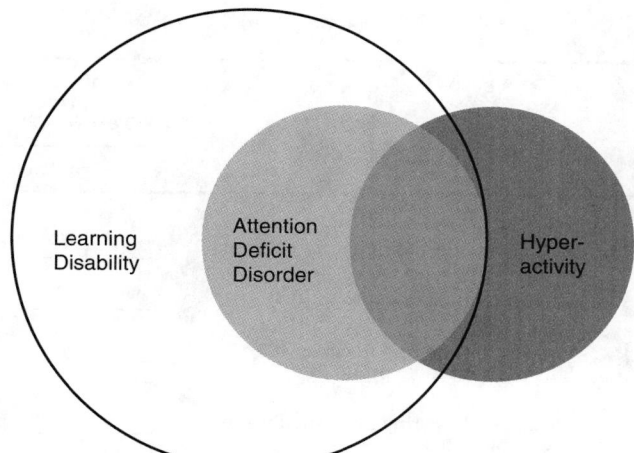

FIGURE 54-2 *Interrelationships among attention deficit disorder, learning disabilities, and hyperactivity. Children with attention deficit disorder tend to have learning disabilities; some are also hyperactive (ADHD). However, not all children with hyperactivity or learning disabilities have attention deficit disorder. From: Batshew M and Perret Y. Children with Disabilities: A Medical Primer 3rd. Ed. Paul Brooks Publishing Co., Baltimore, MD, 1992.*

4. For motor/expressive deficits—break down skills and projects into their multiple component parts; verbally describe the component parts; provide extra time to perform; allow child to type work rather than using cursive writing.
5. For highly distractible child—provide a structured environment; have child sit in front of class; place child away from doors or windows; decrease clutter on desk.

TABLE 54-4 Diagnostic Criteria for Attention Deficit Hyperactivity Disorder*

- Does the child often fidget with hands or feet or squirm in seat?
- Does the child have difficulty remaining seated when required to do so?
- Is the child easily distracted by extraneous stimuli?
- Does the child have difficulty awaiting his or her turn in games or group situations?
- Does the child often blurt out answers to questions before they have been completed?
- Does the child often have difficulty following instructions from others?
- Does the child have difficulty sustaining attention in tasks or play activities?
- Does the child often shift from one uncompleted activity to another?
- Does the child have difficulty playing quietly?
- Does the child often talk excessively?
- Does the child often interrupt or intrude on others?
- Does the child often not seem to listen to what is being said to him or her?
- Does the child often lose things necessary for tasks or activities at school or at home?
- Does the child often engage in physically dangerous activities without considering possible consequences?

---

* The child must experience a disturbance for at least 6 months and exhibit 8 of the 14 symptoms.
Source: American Psychiatric Association (1994).

C. *Resources*
1. Resources include:
    Learning Disability Association of America; 4156 Liberty Road: Pittsburgh, PA 15234; 412-341-1515.
    Attention Deficit Disorder Association; 1-800-487-2282.
    Council for Learning Disabilities, PO Box 40303, Overland Park, KS 66204 (913-492-8755).

◆ NURSING PROCESS OVERVIEW: THE CHILD WITH A DEVELOPMENTAL DISABILITY

Nursing Assessment

1. Review the child's record to determine prior existing health problems that may cause or affect the developmental disability. Always rule out a vision or hearing impairment.
2. Assess the family's understanding of the diagnosis and its ramifications. The parents' experiences, cultural biases, cognitive ability, stage of grief, and physical condition affect their ability to assimilate information provided. It will be necessary to repeat the information. (For example, a woman who has just given birth to a child with Down syndrome will not be able to retain much information until her body returns to a state of homeostasis.)
3. Determine the developmental age of the child. The pediatric nurse should be familiar with normal developmental milestones (Chapter 38, p. 1056), noting the areas of strengths and weaknesses of the child in each area of development, for example, the communication skills are at a 12-month level and the gross motor skills are at a 36-month level. Children who are found to be functioning at one-half or less of their chronologic age have a moderate to severe developmental problem.
    The use of the Clinical Adaptive Test–Clinical Linguistic Auditory Milestone Scales (CAT–CLAMS) is a reliable tool that nurses can be trained to use to assess cognitive and communicative development in children at the 1- to 36-month developmental level. It has been found to be more sensitive than the Denver Developmental Screening Scale, because language development is the best early predictor of cognitive abilities (Table 54-5).
4. Assess the functional level of the child. The WeeFIM is a tool used to track functional independence in children. It uses the following categories to describe function: completely dependent, needs some physical assistance, is physically able to perform the task but needs verbal cues and coaching, and completely independent. Functional areas to assess include:
    a. Feeding
    b. Grooming and bathing
    c. Dressing
    d. Mobility
    e. Problem solving
    f. Communication
5. Assess parents' perception of the child's development level and the appropriateness of parental expectations. Use questions such as, "What age child does your child act like?" or "In the area of communication, how does your child's ability compare with other children the same age?"

TABLE 54-5 The CAT and CLAMS

	Clinical Linguistic Auditory Milestone Scales (CLAMS)			Clinical Adaptive Test (CAT)	
	Yes	No	Age (mos)	Yes	No
1 month Alerts to sound (0.5).	___	___	___		
Soothes when picked up (0.5).	___	___	___		
2 months Social smile (1.0).	___	___	___		
3 months Cooing (1.0).	___	___	___		
4 months Orients to voice (0.5).	___	___	___		
Laughs aloud (0.5).	___	___	___		
5 months Orients toward bell laterally (0.3).	___	___	___		
Ah-goo (0.3).	___	___	___		
Razzing (0.3).	___	___	___		
6 months Babbling (1.0).	___	___	___		
7 months Orients toward bell (1.0), upwardly indirectly (90°).	___	___	___		
8 months Says "Dada" inappropriately (0.5).	___	___	___		
Says "Mama" inappropriately (0.5).	___	___	___		
9 months Orients toward bell upward directly (180°) (0.5).	___	___	___		
Gesture language (0.5).	___	___	___		
10 months Understands "no" (0.3).	___	___	___		
Uses "dada" appropriately (0.3).	___	___	___		
Uses "mama" appropriately (0.3).	___	___	___		
11 months 1 word (other than "mama" & "dada") (1.0).	___	___	___		
12 months 1-step command with gesture (0.5).	___	___	___		
2-word vocabulary (0.5).	___	___	___		
14 months 3-word vocabulary (1.0).	___	___	___		
Immature jargoning (1.0).	___	___	___		

CAT items (right column):

	Yes	No
1 month Visually fixates momentarily upon red ring (0.5).	___	___
Lifts chin off table in prone (0.5).		
2 months Visually follows ring in circle (0.5). Lifts chest off table prone (0.5).	___	___
3 months Visually follows ring horizontally and vertically (0.5). Supports on forearms in prone (0.3). Visual threat (0.3).	___	___
4 months Unfisted (0.3). Manipulates fingers (0.3). Supports on wrists in prone (0.3).	___	___
5 months Pulls down rings (0.3).	___	___
Transfers (0.3). Regards pellet (0.3).	___	___
6 months Obtains cube (0.3). Lifts cup (0.3). Radial rake (0.3).	___	___
7 months Attempts pellet (0.3). Pulls out peg (0.3). Inspects ring (0.3).	___	___
8 months Pulls ring by string (0.3).	___	___
Secures pellet (0.3).	___	___
Inspects bell (0.3).	___	___
9 months 30-finger scissor grasp (0.3).	___	___
Rings bell (0.3). Over the edge for toy (0.3).	___	___
10 months Combines cube-cup (0.3). Uncovers bell (0.3). Fingers pegboard (0.3).	___	___
11 months Mature overhand pincer movement (0.5). Solves cube under cup (0.5).	___	___
12 months Releases 1 cube in cup (0.5).	___	___
Crayon mark (0.5).	___	___
14 months Solves glass frustration (0.6). Out-in with peg (0.6). Solves pellet-bottle with demonstration (0.6).	___	___

(continued)

TABLE 54-5 The CAT and CLAMS (continued)

	Clinical Linguistic Auditory Milestone Scales (CLAMS)				Clinical Adaptive Test (CAT)	
	Yes	No	Age (mos)		Yes	No
16 months Four- to six-word vocabulary (1.0).	___	___	___	**16 months** Solves pellet-bottle spontaneously (0.6).	___	___
One-step command without gesture (1.0).	___	___	___	Round block in formboard (0.6).	___	___
				Scribbles in imitation (0.6).	___	___
18 months Mature jargoning (0.5). 7-to-10-word vocabulary (0.5).	___	___	___	**18 months** 10 cubes in cup (0.5).	___	___
Body parts (0.5).	___	___	___	Solves round hole in formboard reversed (0.5).	___	___
Points to one picture (0.5).	___	___	___	Spontaneous scribbling with crayon (0.5).	___	___
				Pegboard completed spontaneously (0.5).	___	___
21 months 20-word vocabulary (1.0).	___	___	___	**21 months** Obtains object with stick (1.0).	___	___
2-word phrases (1.0).	___	___	___	Solves square in formboard (1.0).	___	___
Points to two pictures (1.0).	___	___	___	Tower of 3 cubes (1.0).	___	___
24 months 50-word vocabulary (1.0).	___	___	___	**24 months** Attempts to fold paper (0.7).	___	___
2-step command (1.0).	___	___	___	Horizontal 4-cube train.	___	___
Pronouns (I, you, me) inappropriately (1.0).	___	___	___	Imitates stroke with pencil (0.7).	___	___
				Completes formboard (0.7).	___	___
30 months Uses pronouns appropriately (1.5).	___	___	___	**30 months** Horizontal-vertical stroke with pencil (1.5).	___	___
Concept of one (1.5).	___	___	___	Formboard reversed (1.5).	___	___
Points to 7 pictures (1.5).	___	___	___	Folds paper with definite crease (1.5).	___	___
2 digits forward (1.5).	___	___	___	Train with chimney (1.5).	___	___
36 months 250-word vocabulary (1.5).	___	___	___	**36 months** 3-cube bridge (1.5).	___	___
3-word sentence (1.5)	___	___	___	Draws circle (1.5).	___	___
3-digits forward (1.5).	___	___	___	Names 1 color (1.5).	___	___
Follows 2 prepositional commands (1.5).	___	___	___	Draw-a-person with head plus 1 other body part (1.5).	___	___
Reliability of informant (0 = unreliable; 1 = reliable).	___					

6. Assess parent–child interaction. Observe and explore bonding and attachment, ability to set appropriate limits, management of behavioral problems, and methods of discipline.
7. Assess the need for additional resources, such as financial aid, transportation, and counseling, for long-term support of child and family.

Nursing Diagnoses

A. Impaired Adjustment related to birth/diagnosis of developmentally disabled child
B. Altered Parenting related to multiple needs of child and difficult bonding
C. Ineffective Infant Feeding Pattern related to protruding tongue, poor muscle tone, and weak sucking
D. Altered Growth and Development related to disability
E. Social Isolation related to developmental differences from other children
F. Risk for Injury related to developmental age

Nursing Interventions

A. *Promoting Adjustment*
1. Allow the parents access to the baby at all possible times to promote bonding when parents appear ready.
2. Focus on the positive aspects of the baby and serve as a role model for handling and stimulating.
3. Be cognizant of the grieving process (loss of the "normal child") that families experience when a diagnosis is made, and be aware that spouses can be at different stages.

4. Accept all questions and reactions nonjudgmentally, offering verbal and written explanations.
5. Provide the family a quiet place to discuss their questions with each other and someone knowledgeable about the condition (primary care provider, clinical nurse specialist) to support them in grieving.
6. Offer the family the option to take advantage of counseling. A social worker or psychologist can assist families to deal with immediate reactions. Many parents benefit from continuous or periodic support of counseling professionals.

NURSING ALERT:
Children with developmental disabilities and chronic illness are at greater risk of experiencing divorce, child abuse, and neglect than the general population.

B. Strengthening the Role of Parents
1. Help the family to realize what strengths they have in caring for their child. The role of the parents is critical; a nurturing, loving environment gives the child the best chance at maximizing potential. Individuals who grow up at home have markedly higher adaptive abilities and increased life spans compared with children raised in institutions.
2. Enlist the help of family and siblings who can offer valuable support to the parents and child and assist with stimulation activities. Including siblings in the care can help them feel needed and involved, thus strengthening the family.
3. If sibling issues arise, suggest counseling.
4. Identify resources available to the family, such as parent support groups, early intervention programs, specialty clinics, pediatrician/primary health care provider, financial support programs, and advocacy groups for individuals with developmental disabilities.
5. For those parents concerned with their ability to care for the child, explore with them their options of adoption or institutionalization in a nonjudgmental manner.

C. Establishing Effective Feeding Techniques
1. Be aware of the poor neurologic development of children with Down syndrome and of infants with other developmental disabilities and how that interferes with sucking and swallowing.
2. Demonstrate proper feeding positioning, with head elevated, and encourage the parents to always hold the infant during feedings with head elevated and supported in arms.
3. Try different nipples and bottles to determine which is easiest for infant to use without leakage or danger of aspiration.
4. Allow adequate time for feeding, and increase frequency of feedings if infant tires easily.
5. Offer support and guidance for breast-feeding.
6. If feeding remains difficult, consider referral to a speech therapist, who is knowledgeable in the area and may be beneficial.

D. Promoting Optimum Growth and Development
1. Help the parents to understand the concept of developmental age, and identify the functional level of the child.
2. Determine if there is consistency between the developmental age of the child and degree of independence. Cognitive and physical limitations may interfere with emerging independence, however, parents may "baby" or over indulge a child who has a disability.

3. Work with parents to set reasonable expectations and to break tasks down into simple, achievable steps. Care should be taken not to address too many areas at one time so as not to overwhelm the family.
4. Use appropriate behavior modification techniques, such as extinction, time-out, and reward, to achieve cooperation and success.
5. Demonstrate and encourage play with the child at the appropriate level to provide stimulation, and work toward achieving developmental milestones.
6. Refer parents to the Early Intervention Program administered by their county so that they can take advantage of the educational and support services available for infants from birth to 3 years of age.
7. If condition is identified after the age of 3 years, refer parents for help through the Pupil Personnel Department of the school system in which they reside.

E. Providing Meaningful Social Interaction
1. Make parents aware that recreational and leisure-time experiences are valuable in building social skills and self-esteem.
2. Offer suggestions that will be enjoyable and developmentally appropriate for child. In general, individuals with developmental delays do better in small groups. Interaction with both developmentally delayed and non-developmentally delayed peers is desirable. The Special Olympics is one example of an adaptive program. Local programs are available in many areas. Social outings, such as sight-seeing, camping, dances, and dating opportunities, are also important for older children.
3. Praise child for participation in activities, regardless of whether the child succeeds or fails.

F. Maintaining Safety
1. When handling the infant, provide adequate support with a firm grasp, because infant may be very floppy due to poor muscle tone.
2. Position the infant so that if vomiting should occur, aspiration will be prevented.
   a. Prop infant with a diaper roll so that position will be maintained.
   b. Change position frequently, because the infant is not usually very active.
   c. Continuously check environment for safety needs for this child.

COMMUNITY-BASED CARE TIP:
Teach caregivers to base safety needs on the developmental, not the chronologic, age of the child.

3. Advise the parents to:
   a. Maintain constant surveillance of the child when cooking or exposing child to other potential hazards that child may be able to get into but not understand.
   b. Help child read words such as "danger" and "stop."
   c. Teach child how to call and ask for help.
   d. Teach child to say no to strangers.
   e. Provide sex education in a way the child can understand.

Family Education/Health Maintenance

1. Remind the parents to recognize the child's routine health care needs and maintain regular follow-up with a primary care provider.

a. Immunizations.
b. Regular dental checkups.
c. Visual and hearing examinations.
2. Teach parents to provide a therapeutic home environment.
   a. Maintain regular sleeping, eating, working, and playing routines.
   b. Ensure adequate nutrition.
   c. Divide tasks and expectations into small, manageable parts. Give only one or two instructions at a time.
   d. Set firm but reasonable limits on behavior and carry through with consistent discipline.
   e. Avoid situations that cause excessive excitement, stimulation, or fatigue.
   f. Provide energy outlet through physical activity, vocal outlet, and outdoor play.
   g. Channel need for movement into safe, appropriate activities.
3. Discuss preparation for independent living.
   a. Help the parents identify areas of home responsibilities that may be delegated to the retarded child.
   b. Teach habits that are essential to later vocational life, such as getting to places on time, cooperating, focusing on the task at hand, and establishing acceptable interpersonal relationships.
   c. Help the child to develop a set of attitudes and behaviors that will increase motivation.
   d. Refer for vocational assistance to ARC or other rehabilitative agencies.

4. Refer for genetic consultation for information about genetics of the disorder, risk in subsequent pregnancies (parents), or risk to offspring (patient), or risk to other relatives.
5. Encourage compliance with the multidimensional treatment plan, and make sure parents know who to contact when problems arise. Encourage parents to develop a system (such as notebook with calendar) to keep track of all agencies, subspecialists, and professionals who will be involved with their child. It should include names, addresses, phone numbers, appointment dates, health providers' orders, insurance information.

Evaluation

A. Parents holding infant frequently and seeking information from health care provider
B. Parents and siblings feeding and assisting with care of infant
C. Infant feeding for 15 to 20 minutes every 1 to 2 hours; taking 50 to 100 mL
D. Parents describe developmental level of child and realistic goals for attainment of next milestones
E. Parents seeking information about Special Olympics
F. Child describes concept of stranger and appropriate response if approached

Selected References

Ad Hoc Committee on Genetic Counseling of the American Society of Human Genetics. (1975). Genetic counseling. *American Journal of Human Genetics, 27*, 240-242.

Batshaw, M., & Perret, Y. (1992). Children with disabilities: A medical primer (3rd ed.). Baltimore: Paul Brooks Publishing.

Briggs, G. G., Freeman, R. K., & Yaffe, S. J. (1990). *Drugs in pregnancy and lactation* (3rd ed.). Baltimore: Williams & Wilkins.

Briskin, H., & Liptak, G. S. (1995). Helping families with children with developmental disabilities. *Pediatric Annals, 24* (5), 262-266.

Capute, A. J., & Accardo, P. J. (1980). *Developmental disabilities in infancy and childhood.* Baltimore: Paul Brooks Publishing.

Darras, B. T., Koenig, M., Kunkel, L. M., et al. (1988). Direct method for prenatal diagnosis and carrier detection in Duchenne/Becker muscular dystrophy using entire dystrophin cDNA. *American Journal of Medical Genetics, 29*, 713-726.

Emery, A. E. H., & Rimoin, D. L. (eds.). (1990). *Principles and practice of medical genetics* (2nd ed.). Edinburgh: Churchill Livingstone.

Epps, S., & Kroeker, R. (1995). Effects of child age and level of developmental delay on family practice physicians' diagnostic impressions. *Mental Retardation, 33* (1), 35-41.

Erbe, R. W. (1994). Medical genetics. *Scientific American, 4*, 1-54.

Farrell, C. D. (1989). Genetic counseling: The emerging reality. *Journal of Perinatal and Neonatal Nursing, 2*(4), 21-33.

Harper, P. S. (1991). *Practical genetic counseling* (4th ed.). Bristol: Wright.

King, R. C., & Stansfield, W. D. (1992). *A dictionary of genetics* (4th ed.). New York: Oxford University Press.

Mange, E. J., & Mange, A. P. (1994). *Basic human genetics.* Sunderland, MA: Sinauer Associates.

McKusick, V. A. (1994). *Mendelian inheritance in man* (11th ed.). Baltimore: Johns Hopkins University Press.

Msall, M. E., Digaudio, K., Duffy, L. C.,

LaForest, S., & Granger, C. V. (In press). WeeFimm: Normative sample of an instrument for tracking functional dependence in children. *Clinical Pediatrics, 33* (7), 431-438.

Prows, C. A. (1992). Utilization of genetic knowledge in pediatric nursing practice. *Journal of Pediatric Nursing, 1*, 58-62.

Scriver, C. R., Beaudet, A. L., Sly, W. S., et al. (1994). *Metabolic and molecular bases of inherited disease* (7th ed.). New York: McGraw-Hill Information Services.

Seideman, R., & Kleine, P. (1995). A theory of transformed parenting: Parenting a child with developmental delay/mental retardation. *Nursing Research, 44* (1), 38-44.

Shepard, T. H. (1992). *Catalog of teratogenic agents* (7th ed.). Baltimore: Johns Hopkins University Press.

Simko A, Hornstein L, Soukup S, et al. Fragile X syndrome: Recognition in young children. *Pediatrics, 83*, 547-552.

Thompson, M. W. (1991). *Thompson and Thompson genetics in medicine* (5th ed.). Philadelphia: W.B. Saunders.

PART V ◆
Psychiatric Nursing

CHAPTER 55 ◆

Psychiatric Disorders

Anxiety-Related Disorders

◆ ANXIETY, SOMATOFORM, AND DISSOCIATIVE DISORDERS

The anxiety-related disorders include disturbances in which subjective (feeling) or objective (expressed) anxiety is the primary or focal symptom.

Anxiety is a subjective feeling of apprehension and tension that is manifested by psychophysiologic arousal and a variety of behavioral patterns. The common theme among all the anxiety-related disorders is that affected persons experience a level of anxiety that interferes with functioning in personal, occupational, or social spheres as well as with psychophysiologic well-being.

Classification

Diagnostic and Statistical Manual, 4th Edition—defined anxiety-related disorders include the following:

A. Anxiety Disorders
1. Panic disorder without agoraphobia
2. Panic disorder with agoraphobia
3. Agoraphobia without history of panic disorder
4. Special phobia
5. Social phobia
6. Obsessive-compulsive disorder
7. Posttraumatic stress disorder
8. Acute stress disorder
9. Generalized anxiety disorder
10. Anxiety disorder due to a general medical condition
11. Substance-induced anxiety disorder
12. Anxiety disorder not otherwise specified

B. Somatoform Disorders
1. Somatization disorder
2. Undifferentiated somatoform disorder
3. Conversion disorder
4. Pain disorder
5. Hypochondriasis
6. Body dysmorphic disorder
7. Somatoform disorder not otherwise specified

C. Dissociative Disorders
1. Dissociative amnesia
2. Dissociative fugue
3. Dissociative identity disorder
4. Depersonalization disorder
5. Dissociative disorder not otherwise specified

Pathophysiology/Etiology

The underlying etiology of anxiety disorders is difficult to define. Therefore, it is essential to examine the following factors: (1) biochemical, (2) genetic, (3) psychosocial, and (4) sociocultural.

A. Biochemical Factors
1. Locus ceruleus in the pons is examined because of its noradrenergic function.
2. Limbic system, which may generate anticipatory anxiety.
3. Prefrontal cortex, which may be responsible for phobic avoidance.
4. The brain's gamma-aminobutyric acid (GABA) functions as an inhibitor or a "brake" on anxiety. GABA and its receptors have a role in producing a general inhibition of neuronal function by opening chloride channels across cell membranes.
5. Positron-emission tomographic scans have identified abnormal blood flow to the frontal lobes and basal ganglia in persons diagnosed with obsessive-compulsive disorder.
6. Obsessive-compulsive disorder has been associated with an excessive level of serotonin.
7. Persons who have panic attacks have been reported to have higher levels of norepinephrine, suggestive of a catecholamine system abnormality.
8. Studies of persons diagnosed with somatoform disorders have not demonstrated conclusive evidence of neurophysiologic etiology.
9. Some individuals might be predisposed to pain disorder related to abnormalities in brain chemical balance or limbic or sensory system structural abnormalities.
10. Pain disorder may also be related to deficiency in serotonin and endorphins.
11. Some clinicians propose that conversion disorder is related to central nervous system arousal disturbances. There may be an association with inhibition of afferent sensorimotor impulse, which produces a high arousal.
12. Dissociative disorders do not seem to have strong biologic foundations. Depersonalization disorder is the only one that has a significant biologic link.

B. Genetic Factors
1. An 80% to 90% concordance of panic disorder has been demonstrated in identical twins and a 10% to 15% concordance rate for fraternal twins.

2. Approximately 20% of first-degree relatives of persons with agoraphobia also have agoraphobia.
3. Approximately 3% to 7% of persons with obsessive-compulsive disorder have first-degree relatives with the same disorder.
4. Approximately 25% of the first-degree relatives with generalized anxiety disorder are also affected by generalized anxiety disorder.
5. Somatoform disorders have not been identified as being genetically transmitted.

C. Psychosocial Factors
1. Unconscious childhood conflicts, which may form the basis for symptom development of anxiety disorders.
2. Emotional distress of unmet (early) needs.
3. Learned response that can be unlearned.
4. Distortions in the way the person thinks and perceives.
5. Dissociative disorders can be learned as a method for avoiding stress and anxiety.
6. Dissociative disorders can also represent attempts to use repression to block a traumatic event from one's awareness and to avoid the anxiety-producing memory. Therefore, dissociation of certain mental processes takes place to protect the person from specific painful and anxiety-producing memories.

D. Sociocultural Factors
1. Anxiety disorders and ritualistic behaviors are commonly seen in high-technology societies.
2. There is higher incidence of anxiety disorders in urban communities versus rural communities.
3. Somatoform disorders have a higher incidence among persons from lower socioeconomic groups.

Clinical Manifestations

See Table 55-1.

Diagnostic Evaluation

1. Measurement tools for anxiety:
   a. Manifest Anxiety Scale
   b. Institute for Personality and Ability Testing (IPAT) Anxiety Scale Questionnaire
   c. Sheehan Anxiety Scale
   d. Total Anxiety Scale
   e. Yale-Brown Obsessive-Compulsive Scale
2. Measurement tools for dissociation:
   a. Dissociation Experiences Scale
3. Sodium lactate infusion or carbon dioxide inhalation will likely produce a panic attack in a person with panic disorder.
4. Increased arousal may be measured through studies of autonomic functioning (ie, heart rate, electromyography, sweat gland activity) in a person with posttraumatic stress disorder.

Management

1. Determine the level and place of care to be provided: psychiatric inpatient or outpatient, psychiatric home care.
2. Psychoeducational strategies:
   a. Relaxation techniques

   b. Progressive muscle relaxation
   c. Guided imagery
3. Psychotherapy
   a. Psychodynamic: Assist persons in understanding their experiences by identifying unconscious conflicts and developing effective coping behaviors.
   b. Behavioral: Focus on the individual problematic behavior and work to modify or extinguish the behavior. One form of behavioral therapy effective in management of anxiety disorders is systematic desensitization.
   c. Hypnotherapy can be used as part of therapy for those suffering dissociative disorders.
4. Somatic therapies
   a. Biofeedback: Relaxation through biofeedback is achieved when a person learns to control physiologic mechanisms that are not ordinarily within his or her awareness. Awareness and control are accomplished by monitoring body processes, including muscle tone, heart rate, and brain waves.
   b. Psychopharmacologic intervention directed at targeted symptoms with specific desired outcomes to prevent polypharmacy.
   c. Narcotherapy: Sodium amobarbital or intravenous sodium thiopental may assist the therapist in gaining access to a patient's repressed memories and buried conflicts. In a person experiencing dissociative amnesia or dissociative fugue, the therapist may explore dissociated events. If the person is diagnosed with dissociative identity disorder, this type of interview may facilitate the access of other personalities.

Complications

1. Undiagnosed medical reasons for anxiety could lead to physical deterioration and a delay in obtaining appropriate medical care.
2. If panic and phobic disorders are left untreated, these disorders can lead to increasing social withdrawal and isolation, which may severely impair the person's social and work life.
3. Untreated obsessive-compulsive disorder can lead to aggressive behavior toward self or others as well as depression, skin breakdown from obsessive washing, and possible infection.
4. Undiagnosed or untreated posttraumatic stress disorder or acute stress disorder can lead to substance abuse or dependence, aggressive/violent behavior, and possibly suicide.
5. If a person with a dissociative disorder goes untreated, he or she may develop aggressive behavior toward self or others. Such behaviors may include assaults, depression, posttraumatic stress disorder, psychoactive substance abuse disorder, rape, self-mutilation, and suicide attempts.

Nursing Assessment

1. Assess psychological processes.
   a. Defense mechanisms used.
   b. Mood.
   c. Suicide potential.
   d. Thought content and process.
   e. Usual coping ability.
   f. Understanding of illness.

TABLE 55-1 Diagnostic Criteria for Anxiety-Related Disorders

A. Anxiety Disorders

Panic Disorder
1. Recurrent unexpected anxiety attacks.
2. Sudden onset with intense apprehension and dread.
3. At least four of the following symptoms:
   - Dyspnea
   - Chest discomfort
   - Dizziness
   - Hot or cold flashes
   - Tingling of hands or feet
   - Feelings of unreality
   - Palpitations
   - Syncope
   - Diaphoresis
   - Trembling
   - Fear of losing control, going crazy, or dying

Posttraumatic Stress Disorder
1. After experiencing a psychologically traumatic event outside the range of usual experience (eg, rape, combat, bombings, kidnapping), the person reexperiences the event through recurrent dreams and flashbacks.
2. Emotional numbness, detachment, and estrangement may be used to defend against anxiety.
3. May experience sleep disturbance, hypervigilance, guilt about surviving, poor concentration, and avoidance of activities that trigger memory of the event.

Phobias
1. Irrational fear of an object or situation that persists, although the person may recognize it as unreasonable.
2. Types include:
   Agoraphobia: Fear of being alone in open or public places where escape might be difficult; may not leave home.
   Social phobia: Fear of situations in which one might be seen and embarrassed or criticized; fear of eating in public, public speaking, or performing.
   Specific phobia: Fear of a single object, activity, or situation (eg, snakes, closed spaces, and flying).
3. Anxiety is severe if the object, situation, or activity cannot be avoided.

Obsessive-Compulsive Disorder
1. Preoccupation with persistent intrusive thoughts (obsessions), repeated performance of rituals designed to prevent some event (compulsions), or both.
2. Anxiety occurs if obsessions or compulsions are resisted and from feeling powerless to resist the thoughts or rituals.

Substance-Induced Anxiety Disorder
1. Prominent anxiety, panic attacks, or obsessions or compulsions predominate.
2. Symptoms developed within 1 month of substance intoxication or withdrawal.
3. Medication use is related to disturbance.
4. The disturbance doesn't occur exclusively during the course of delirium.
5. Significant distress or impairment in social and occupational functioning results.

Generalized Anxiety Disorder
1. Persists for at least 6 months.
2. Symptoms present from three of the four categories:
   - Motor tension (eg, trembling, restlessness, inability to relax, and fatigue).
   - Autonomic hyperactivity (eg, sweating, palpitations, cold clammy hands, urinary frequency, lump in throat, pallor or flushing, increased pulse, and rapid respirations).
   - Apprehensiveness (eg, worry, dread, fear, rumination, insomnia, and inability to concentrate).
   - Hypervigilance (eg, feeling edgy, scanning the environment, and distractibility).

Acute Stress Disorder
1. Person has been exposed to a traumatic event either witnessed or experienced.
2. Develops three or more of these dissociative symptoms:
   - Subjective sense of numbing
   - Absence of emotional responsiveness
   - Feeling dazed
   - Derealization
   - Depersonalization
   - Dissociative amnesia
3. Duration of 2 days to 4 weeks.

B. Dissociative Disorders

Dissociative Amnesia
1. One of more episodes of inability to recall important information—usually of a traumatic or stressful nature.
2. Other psychological (eg, multiple personality disorder) and physical (eg, substance-induced) disorders are ruled out.

Dissociative Identity Disorder
1. Presence of two or more distinct identities, each with its own patterns of relating, perceiving, and thinking.
2. At least two of these identities take control of the person's behavior.
3. Inability to recall important personal information too extensive to be explained by ordinary forgetfulness.
4. Other causes ruled out.

Dissociative Fugue
1. Sudden, unexpected travel away from home or one's place of work with inability to remember past.
2. Confusion about personal identity or assumption of new identity.

Depersonalization Disorder
1. Persistent or recurrent experience of feeling detached from and outside one's mental processes or body.
2. Reality testing remains intact.
3. The experience causes significant impairment in social or occupational functioning or causes marked distress.
4. Does not occur exclusively during course of another mental disorder.

C. Somatoform Disorders

Somatization Disorder
1. History of many physical complaints before age 30, occurring over a period of years, resulting in change of lifestyle.
2. Complaints must include all of the following:
   - History of pain in at least four different sites or functions.
   - History of at least two GI symptoms other than pain.
   - History of at least one sexual or reproductive symptom.
   - History of at least one symptom defined as or suggesting a neurologic disorder.

Hypochondriasis
1. Preoccupation with fears of having or the idea that one has a serious disease.
2. Preoccupation persists despite appropriate medical tests and assurances to the contrary.
3. Other disorders are ruled out, eg, somatic delusional disorders.
4. Preoccupation causes significant impairment in social or occupational functioning or causes marked distress.

Body Dysmorphic Disorder
1. Preoccupation with some imagined defect in appearance in a normal-appearing person (if the defect is present, concern is excessive).
2. Preoccupation causes significant impairment in social or occupational functioning or causes marked distress.

(continued)

TABLE 55-1 Diagnostic Criteria for Anxiety-Related Disorders *(continued)*

Conversion Disorder
1. Development of a symptom or deficit suggesting:
   - Neurologic disorder (blindness, deafness, loss of touch, or pain sensation)
   - Involuntary motor function (aphonia, impaired coordination, paralysis, seizures, etc.)
2. Not due to malingering or factitious disorder and not culturally sanctioned.
3. Causes impairment in social or occupational functioning, causes marked distress, or requires medical attention.

Pain Disorder
1. Pain in one or more anatomic sites is a major part of the clinical picture.
2. Causes significant impairment in occupational or social functioning or causes marked distress.
3. Psychological factors are thought to cause onset, severity, or exacerbation.
4. If a medical condition is present, it plays a minor role in accounting for pain.

Undifferentiated Somatoform Disorder
1. One or more physical complaints:
   - Fatigue
   - Loss of appetite
   - Gastrointestinal symptoms
   - Urinary symptoms
2. No physiologic explanation after an investigation.
3. Symptoms cause clinically significant distress or impairment in social or occupational areas of functioning.
4. Duration of the disturbance is at least 6 months.

Adapted from the American Psychiatric Association DSMIV 1994. Washington, D.C. APA

---

2. Explore social functioning.
   a. Ability to function in social and work situations.
   b. Degree of strain in relationships.
   c. Diversional and recreative behavior.
   d. Identification of stressors or threats to self-concept, role performance, life values, social status, and support systems.
   e. Usual relationship patterns.
   f. Benefits and risks of the presenting symptoms.

Nursing Diagnoses

A. Anxiety related to unexpected panic attacks or related to re-experiencing traumatic events
B. Altered Thought Processes related to severe anxiety
C. Social Isolation related to avoidance behavior or related to embarrassment and shame associated with symptoms
D. Self Care Deficit related to physical disability
E. Personal Identity Disturbance related to a traumatic event

Nursing Interventions

A. *Reducing Symptoms of Anxiety*
1. Help patient identify anxiety-producing situations and plan for such events.
2. Assist patient to develop assertiveness and communication skills.
3. Practice stress-reduction techniques with patient.
4. Monitor for objective and subjective manifestations of anxiety.
   a. Tachycardia, tachypnea.
   b. Verbalization of feelings of anxiety.
   c. Signs and symptoms associated with autonomic stimulation—perspiration, difficulty concentrating, insomnia.

B. *Improving Concentration*
1. Use short, simple sentences when communicating with patient.
2. Maintain a calm, serene manner.
3. Use adjuncts to verbal communication, such as visual aids and role playing, to stimulate memory and retention of information.
4. Teach relaxation techniques to diminish distress that interferes with concentration ability.
5. Administer prescribed anxiolytics to decrease anxiety level.

C. *Increasing Social Interaction*
1. Encourage discussion of reasons for and feelings about social isolation.
2. Help patient identify specific causes/situations that produce anxiety that inhibits social interaction.
3. Recommend participation in programs directed at specific conflict areas or skill deficiencies. Such programs may focus on assertiveness skills, body awareness, managing multiple role responsibilities, and stress management.

D. *Encouraging Independence*
1. Identify secondary benefits, such as decreased responsibility and increased dependency, that inhibit patient's move to independence.
2. Provide experiences in which patient can be successful.
3. Explore alternative methods of meeting dependency needs.
4. Explore beliefs that support a helpless or dependent mode of behavior.
5. Teach and role-play assertive behaviors in specific situations.
6. Assist patient to improve skills based on performance.

E. *Strengthening Identity*
1. Develop an honest, nonjudgmental relationship with the patient.
2. Try to establish communication between patient's alters.
3. Do not overwhelm patient with information or memories.
4. Assist patient to incorporate dissociated material into conscious memory by encouraging the sharing of painful, repressed memories.

Patient Education/Health Maintenance

1. Teach patient and family members about anxiety.
   a. Define anxiety and differentiate it from fear.
   b. Explain causes of anxiety.
   c. Identity events that can trigger anxiety.
   d. Identify the relevant signs and symptoms of anxiety.
2. Describe the medication regimen.
3. Identify, describe, and practice deep-muscle relaxation techniques, relaxation breathing, imagery, and other relaxation therapies.
4. Teach family to give positive reinforcement for use of healthy behaviors.
5. Teach family not to assume responsibilities or roles normally assigned to the patient.
6. Teach family to give attention to the patient, not to the patient's symptoms.
7. Teach alternative ways to perform activities of daily living (ADLs) if physical disability inhibits function and performance.
8. For additional information and support, refer to agencies such as: Agoraphobics in Motion; 1729 Crooks; Royal Oak, MI 48067; 810-547-0400; Anxiety Disorders Association of America; 6000 Executive Boulevard, Suite 513; Rockville, MD 20852; 301-231-9350; Obsessive-Compulsive Disorder Foundation; Box 60; Vernon, CT 06066; Phobia Society of America; 133 Rollins Avenue, Suite 4B; Rockville, MD 20852; International Society for the Study of Multiple Personality and Dissociation; 5700 Old Orchard Road, 1st Floor; Skokie, IL 60077-1024; and Multiple Personality Clinic; Department of Psychiatry, Rush University; 600 South Paulina; Chicago, IL 60612.

Evaluation

A. Identifies stressors and demonstrates normal heart rate, respirations, sleep pattern, and subjective feelings of anxiety
B. Demonstrates improved concentration and thought processes through improved ability to focus, think, and problem solve
C. Reports increased participation in family- and community-related events
D. Reports independently performing ADLs; clean, appropriately dressed appearance noted
E. Reports absence of other identities or thoughts of depersonalization

Mood Disturbances

◆ DEPRESSIVE DISORDERS

Depressive disorders are considered mood disorders. A mood is a sustained emotion that, when extreme, colors the person's view of the world. A depressive illness is painful and can be psychophysiologically debilitating. Depression is much more than just sadness; it affects the way one feels about the future and can alter basic attitudes about the self. A depressed person can become so despairing that he or she expresses hopelessness. When moods become severe or prolonged or interfere with a person's interpersonal or occupational functioning, this alteration in mood may signal a mood disorder.

Etiology/Pathophysiology

A. *Biologic Factors*
1. Twin studies have consistently demonstrated that genetic factors play a role in the development of depressive disorders.
2. Twin studies demonstrate that if one twin has a depressive disorder, the remaining twin has a 72% chance of likewise developing a depressive disorder.

B. *Biochemical Factors*
1. It is proposed that there are several central nervous system neurotransmitter abnormalities that can cause depression.
2. Neurotransmitter abnormalities may be the result of environmental or inherited factors or the presence of coexisting medical conditions.
3. The main neurotransmitters related to mood disorders are serotonin, norepinephrine, and dopamine.

C. *Neuroendocrine Factors*
1. The most predominantly studied neuroendocrine system related to depression is the hyperactivity of the limbic-hypothalamic-pituitary-adrenal axis.
2. Some individuals with depression have a hypersecretion of cortisol.

D. *Sleep Abnormalities*
1. Abnormalities of sleep architecture are among the most significant biologic markers of depression.
2. Decreased rapid eye movement (REM) latency (the time between falling asleep and the first REM period) is seen in two-thirds of depressed patients.
3. There is an increased length of the first REM period.
4. Increased early morning awakening is common, as are multiple nighttime awakenings.

E. *Psychosocial Factors*
1. Life events and environmental stress: There has been a positive correlation between the loss of a parent before age 11 or the loss of a spouse with major depression.
2. Premorbid personality factors.
   a. Dependent personality.
   b. Obsessive-compulsive personality.
   c. Narcissistic personality.
3. Psychoanalytic factors: The two central themes significant to the development of depression are loss and aggression. Depression is triggered by a loss, and the depressive mood is the result of aggression turned against the self.

4. Learned helplessness: A person who internalizes the belief that an unwanted event is his or her fault and that nothing can be done to avoid or change it is prone to developing depression.
5. Cognitive theories: Cognitive interpretations include negative distortions of life experiences that produce negative self-evaluation, pessimistic thinking, and eventual helplessness.

Clinical Manifestations

See Table 55-2.

Diagnostic Evaluation

1. Rating scales of depression—to determine presence and severity of the problem.
   a. Zung Self-Rating Scale
   b. Raskin Severity of Depression Scale
   c. Hamilton Depression Scale
   d. Beck Depression Inventory
2. Laboratory studies:
   a. Thyroid function tests and thyrotropin-releasing hormone stimulation test—to detect underlying hypothyroidism, which may cause depression.
   b. Dexamethasone suppression test—to evaluate depression that may be responsive to antidepressant or electroconvulsive therapy (ECT).
   c. Twenty-four hour urinary 3-methoxy-4-hydroxy-phenylglycol (MHPG)—may show slightly lower level in unipolar depression than in bipolar depression.
3. Polysomography—an increase in the overall amount of REM sleep and shortened REM latency period in patients with major depression.
4. Additional diagnostic tests to evaluate physical conditions, such as computed tomography (CT) scan or magnetic resonance imaging (MRI), complete blood count (CBC), chemistry panel, rapid plasma reagin (RPR), human immunodeficiency virus (HIV) test, electroencephalogram (EEG), vitamin B_{12} and folate levels, toxicology studies.

Management

1. Decision is made for the patient to be treated on an inpatient or outpatient basis.
2. Inpatient treatment is required for those with the following conditions:
   a. Suicidal
   b. Severely disabled
   c. In crisis
   d. Require a complex diagnostic evaluation
   e. Require high-risk treatments
   f. Require electroconvulsive therapy (ECT)
3. Goals of treatment for depression are symptom reduction, improved function, and recurrence prevention.
4. Psychotherapy for depressive disorders:
   a. Interpersonal psychotherapy
   b. Cognitive therapy
   c. Behavioral therapy
   d. Marital therapy
   e. Family therapy
5. Antidepressant psychopharmacologic therapy (see Table 55-3).

TABLE 55-2 Characteristics of Depressive Disorders

Major Depressive Disorder
1. Occurs over a 2-week period.
2. Represents a change in previous functions.
3. Impairs social and occupational functioning.
4. Five or more of the following occur nearly every day for most waking hours:
   - Depressed mood
   - Anhedonia
   - Significant weight loss or gain (more than 5% of body weight per month)
   - Insomnia or hypersomnia
   - Increased or decreased motor activity
   - Anergy (fatigue or loss of energy)
   - Feelings of worthlessness or inappropriate guilt (may be delusional)
   - Decreased concentration or indecisiveness
   - Recurrent thought of death or suicidal ideation (with or without plan)

Specifiers
1. Severity
2. Psychotic features
3. Remission—chronic
4. Seasonal affective disorder related to either winter or summer
5. Catatonic features
6. Melancholic features
7. Atypical features
8. Postpartum onset

Dysthymic Disorder
1. Occurs over a 2-year period (1 year for children and adolescents), presence of depressed mood
2. Still able to function in social and occupational spheres
3. Presence of some of the following:
   - Decreased or increased appetite
   - Insomnia or hypersomnia
   - Anergy or chronic fatigue
   - Anhedonia
   - Decreased self-esteem
   - Poor concentration or difficulty making decisions
   - Perceived inability to cope with routine responsibilities
   - Feelings of hopelessness or despair
   - Pessimistic about the future, brooding over the past, or feeling sorry for self
   - Recurrent thoughts of death or suicide

Adapted from APA DSMIV 1994–Washington, DC

6. Additional somatic therapies:
   a. ECT
   b. High-intensity artificial light therapy
   c. Sleep deprivation therapy
7. Exercise program.

Complications

1. An undiagnosed medical condition causing depressive symptoms could lead to physical deterioration and/or delay in obtaining appropriate treatment.
2. Potential for suicide or death from other undetected medical conditions.
3. Potential for suicide attempt with significant physical illness or injury.

TABLE 55-3 Pharmacology of Antidepressant Medications

Medication: Class/Generic/Trade Name	Therapeutic Dosage Range (mg/day) in Adults	Adverse Reactions
Tricyclic Agents		
Amitriptyline (Elavil, Endep)	75–300 mg	For all tricyclic and tetracyclic agents:
Clomipramine (Anafranil)	75–300 mg	Possibility of enduring a manic episode in bipolar patients.
Desipramine (Norpramin, Pertofrane)	75–300 mg	Anticholinergic effects. Dry mouth, constipation, blurred vision, urinary retention.
Doxepin (Adapin, Sinequan)	75–300 mg	Sedative effects.
Imipramine (Tofranil, Tofranil-PM, Janimine, SK-pramine)	75–300 mg	Autonomic effects: orthostatic hypotension, sweating, palpitations, and increased blood pressure.
Nortriptyline (Aventyl, Pamelor)	40–200 mg	Cardiac effects: tachycardia, T-wave flattening, prolonged QT interval.
Protriptyline (Vivactil)	20–60 mg	Neurologic effects: delirium tremors, twitch.
Trimipramine (Surmontil)	75–300 mg	
Tetracyclic Agent		
Maprotiline (Ludiomil)	100–225 mg	
Bicyclic Agent		
Venlafaxine (Effexor)	375 mg	Sedation, weight gain, drowsiness, hypotension.
Selective Serotonin Reuptake Inhibitors (SSRIs)		
Fluoxetine (Prozac)	10–40 mg	Delayed orgasm, headache, nervousness, insomnia, anxiety, tremor, dizziness, nausea, diarrhea, anorexia, dry mouth.
Paroxetine (Paxil)	20–50 mg	Nausea, dry mouth, headache, somnolence, insomnia, diarrhea, constipation, tremor.
Sertraline (Zoloft)	50–150 mg	Insomnia, diarrhea, nausea, weight loss.
Fluvoxamine (Luvox)	50–300 mg	Nausea, vomiting, drowsiness, anorexia, constipation, tremor, insomnia.
Monoamine Oxidase Inhibitors (MAOIs)		
Isocarboxazid (Marplan)	30–50 mg	For all MOAIs:
Phenelzine (Nardil)	45–90 mg	Orthostatic hypotension, weight gain, edema, insomnia, sexual dysfunction, myoclonus, muscle pains, parethesias.
Tranylcypromine (Parnate)	20–60 mg	
Pargyline (Eutonyl)	150 mg	
Selegiline (Eldepryl, Deprenyl)	10 mg	
Dibenzoxazepine Agent		
Amoxapine (Asendin)	100–600 mg	Dizziness, postural hypotension, reflex tachycardia, extrapyramidal movement disorders.
Unicyclic Agent		
Bupropion (Wellbutrin)	225–450 mg	Dry mouth, constipation, headache, insomnia, restlessness, agitation, menstrual irregularities.
Triazolopyridine Agent		
Trazodone (Desyrel)	150–600 mg	Sedation, orthostatic hypotension, dizziness, headache, nausea.
Phenylipiperazine Agent		
Nefazodone (Serzone)	200–600 mg	Postural hypotension, anxiety, nervous tremor, agitation.

4. Use of alcohol or drugs to "feel better" or numb dysphoric feelings.

Nursing Assessment

1. Assess posture and affect for:
   a. Poor/slumped posture
   b. Appearance of being older than stated age
   c. Facial expression of sadness, dejection
   d. Episodes of weeping
   e. Anhedonia—inability to experience pleasure
2. Assess thought processes.
   a. Identify the presence of suicidal thoughts
   b. Poor judgment, indecisiveness
   c. Impaired problem solving, poor concentration
   d. Negative thoughts
3. Explore feelings for:
   a. Anger and irritability

  b. Anxiety, guilt
  c. Worthlessness
  d. Helplessness, hopelessness
4. Assess physical behavior for:
  a. Psychomotor agitation or retardation
  b. Vegetative signs of depression
    (1) Change in eating patterns
    (2) Change in sleeping patterns
    (3) Change in elimination patterns
    (4) Change in level of interest in sex
5. Assess for evidence of "masked depression"
  a. Hypochondriasis
  b. Psychosomatic disorders
  c. Compulsive gambling
  d. Compulsive overwork
  e. Accident proneness
  f. Eating disorders
  g. Addictive illnesses

Nursing Diagnoses

A. Hopelessness related to depressive thoughts
B. Risk for Injury related to hopelessness and impaired problem solving
C. Self Care Deficit related to lack of motivation and poor concentration
D. Sleep Pattern Disturbance related to insomnia

Nursing Interventions

A. *Strengthening Coping and Sense of Hope*
1. Initiate interaction with the patient at a regularly scheduled time.
2. Be clear and honest about your own feelings related to the patient's behavior.
3. Encourage verbal expression of feelings.
4. Validate feelings that are appropriate to the situation.
5. Explore with the patient what is producing and maintaining the feeling of depression.
6. Encourage the patient to identify events that cause unpleasant emotional responses.
7. Assess significant losses the patient has experienced.
8. Identify cultural and social factors that may contribute to how the patient copes with loss and feelings.
9. Assess the patient's support network.

B. *Maintaining Safety*
1. Assess current suicide risk.
2. Implement appropriate level of observation based on a focused suicide assessment (ie, constant observation or 15-minute checks).
3. Explain observation precautions to the patient.
4. Remove harmful objects from the patient's possession, and assess environmental safety of the patient's room and unit.
5. Encourage the patient to negotiate a no self-harm/no suicide agreement with the staff.
6. Monitor need to revise level of observation.
7. Provide additional structure by keeping the patient involved in therapeutic and psychorehabilitative activities.

C. *Encouraging Participation in Activities of Daily Living*
1. Collaborate with occupational and physical therapists to determine patient's functional capacity to accomplish ADLs.

2. If patient is unable to accomplish ADLs independently, provide hygiene activities in collaboration with patient.
3. Acknowledge and reinforce the patient's efforts to maintain appearance; do not rush the patient when self-care is slow.
4. Reinforce what the patient can do rather than what he or she cannot do without assistance.
5. Remain with the patient during mealtime to determine the level of need for assistance or cuing in the ability to eat.

D. *Facilitating Sleep*
1. Determine the patient's past and current sleep patterns and sleep hygiene.
2. Ask what strategies the patient has already used to improve sleep, and elicit which ones have been successful.
3. Consider decreasing the amount of daytime sleep by encouraging participation in an activity.
4. Discuss alternative methods for facilitating sleep:
  a. Avoid caffeine.
  b. Avoid emotionally charged or upsetting discussions before bedtime.
  c. Avoid exercise $1/2$ to 1 hour before bed.
  d. Increase physical activity within functional limits.
  e. Use relaxation techniques.
  f. Try a warm bath or warm milk.

Patient Education/Health Maintenance

1. Instruct patient and family members about biologic symptoms of depression.
2. Instruct patient and family members about purpose of antidepressant medication, effects, side effects and their management, and how to recognize early signs and symptoms of relapse.
3. Instruct patient and family members about the effect of a depressive disorder on the family system.
4. Provide patient and family members with written material on coping with depression.
5. Provide patient and family members with information about appropriate community-based programs and support groups, such as the National Foundation for Depressive Illness; PO Box 2257; New York, NY 10116; 800-248-4344.

Evaluation

A. Patient identifies ineffective coping behaviors and consequences
B. Remains safe from self-harm
C. Eats, bathes, and dresses with verbal cues
D. Obtains a minimum of 5 hours of uninterrupted sleep

◆ BIPOLAR DISORDERS

The bipolar disorders, also considered mood disorders, include the occurrence of depressive episodes and one or more elated mood episodes. An elated mood can include a range of affect, from normal mood to hypomania to mania. In the most intense presentation, the person with a bipolar disorder experiences altered thought processes, which can produce bizarre delusions.

Pathophysiology/Etiology

A. *Genetic Basis*
1. There is a higher rate of bipolar disorder and cyclothymia in relatives of patients with bipolar disorders, compared with relatives of patients with major depression or the general population.
2. Twin studies support a genetic marker for the bipolar disorders.
3. The genetic defect may involve the "circadian pacemaker" or the systems modulating it.

B. *Biogenic Amines*
1. Patients with bipolar disorders may have lower plasma norepinephrine, urinary MHPG, and platelet serotonin uptake and higher red blood cell/plasma lithium rates than do unipolar populations.
2. Pathology of the limbic system, basal ganglia, and hypothalamus is proposed to contribute to the development of mood disorders.

C. *Psychosocial Factors*
1. Psychosocial stressors appear to have an important role early in the illness in concert with the electrical kindling and behavioral sensitization models.
2. Mania and hypomania have been viewed by psychoanalytic theorists as a defense against depression.

Clinical Manifestations

See Table 55-4.

Diagnostic Evaluation

1. Rating scale assessment tools:
   a. Mania Rating Scale
   b. Mini Mental Status Examination
2. There appear to be no laboratory features that distinguish major depressive episodes found in major depressive disorder from those in bipolar I or bipolar II disorder.
3. Complete psychophysiologic examination.
4. Complete assessment to rule out medical conditions.

Management

1. Psychotherapy
   a. Individual therapy
   b. Family therapy
2. Psychopharmacologic intervention for acute mania.
   a. Usually treated in the hospital to ensure a safe environment to initiate and stabilize medication.
   b. Lithium carbonate (Lithobid).
   c. Adjunctive treatment.
      (1) Neuroleptic agent such as haloperidol (Haldol).
      (2) Benzodiazepine such as clonazepam (Klonopin) or lorazepam (Ativan).
   d. Anticonvulsants for mood-stabilizing properties, such as carbamazepine (Tegretol) and valproate (Depakene).

TABLE 55-4 Characteristics of Bipolar Disorders

Bipolar I Disorder
1. Presence of only one manic episode.
2. No past major depressive episodes.
3. The manic episode is not accounted for by schizoaffective disorder.
4. Manic episode is not superimposed on schizophrenia, schizophreniform disorder, delusional disorder, or psychotic disorder.

Specifiers
- Mixed symptoms
- Severity/Psychotic
- Remission specifiers
- Catatonic features
- Postpartum onset

Bipolar II Disorder
1. Presence/history of one or more major depressive episodes.
2. Presence/history of at least one hypomanic episode.
3. There has not been a manic or mixed episode.
4. The symptoms cause clinically significant distress or impairment in social or occupational functioning.

Specifiers
- Hypomanic
- Depressed

Cyclothymic Disorder
- Over a period of 2 years, there are numerous periods without hypomanic symptoms and numerous periods with depressive symptoms that don't meet criteria for a major depressive episode.
- During the 2-year period, the client has not been without these symptoms for more than 2 months at time.
- No major depressive episode, manic episode, or mixed episode during the first 2 years of the disturbance.
- Symptoms are not due to physiologic aspects.
- Symptoms cause clinically significant distress or impairment in all aspects of functioning.

Adapted from APA DSMIV (1994), Washington, DC

   e. Combination therapy consisting of lithium and anticonvulsants.
3. Pharmacologic therapy for acute depression.
   a. Lithium.
   b. Combination therapy consisting of an antidepressant with lithium.
   c. Monoamine oxidase (MAO) inhibitors.
4. Maintenance therapy of psychopharmacologic agents.
5. Psychiatric home care nursing to facilitate compliance with medications and therapeutic interventions.
6. Community-based support group participation.

Complications

1. Untreated bipolar disorder can lead to physical exhaustion.
2. Poor judgment can lead to financial problems.
3. Alcohol and drug abuse problems can develop and cause disruption in the family.
4. Concurrent medical conditions may be exacerbated.

Nursing Assessment

1. Assess mood for stability; range of affect, from elation to irritability to severe agitation; laughing, joking, and talking continuously; uninhibited familiarity with interviewer.
2. Assess behavior for constant activity, starting many projects but finishing few, mild to severe hyperactivity, spending large sums of money, increased appetite, indiscriminant sex, minimal to no sleeping, outlandish or bizarre dress, poor concentration.
3. Assess thought processes for flight of ideas; pressured speech, often with content that is sexually explicit; clang associations (sound of word, rather than its meaning, directs subsequent associations); delusions; hallucinations.

Nursing Diagnoses

A. Altered Thought Processes related to biologic changes as demonstrated by agitation, hyperactivity, and inability to concentrate
B. Sleep Pattern Disturbance related to hyperactivity and perceived lack of need for sleep
C. Altered Family Processes related to role changes, economic strain, and lack of knowledge about the patient's illness
D. Altered Nutrition, Less Than Body Requirements, related to hyperactivity

Nursing Interventions

A. *Improving Thought Processes and Decreasing Sensory Overload*
1. Assess patient's degree of distorted thinking.
2. Redirect the patient when you are unable to follow his or her thought processes.
3. Use brief explanations.
4. Remain consistent in approach and expectations.
5. Frequently reality-orient the patient; speak in a clear, simple manner.
6. Provide the patient with a relaxing area with decreased environmental stimulation.
7. Assist the patient with a gradual and progressive integration into the social environment while observing for behavioral changes that indicate readiness for participation in further activities.

B. *Improving Sleep Pattern*
1. Establish a distraction-free environment at bedtime.
2. Help the patient avoid the intake of caffeine and nicotine.
3. Administer prescribed medications as ordered, and monitor the patient's response.

C. *Improving the Effect of Bipolar Illness on Family*
1. Assess the family's external support network, and encourage participation in family therapy and support groups.
2. Assess communication and boundaries within the family.
3. Observe and assess interaction patterns within the family and discuss their influence on the patient and his or her family functioning.

4. Provide the patient and family with information regarding bipolar disorder and the treatment plan, prognosis, and aftercare plan.

D. *Ensuring Adequate Nutrition*
1. Maintain accurate documentation of food and fluid intake.
2. Offer small, frequent meals of high-calorie foods. Include food that the patient likes and that can be eaten "on the move."
3. Serve the patient meals in a low-stimulus environment.
4. Monitor the patient's serum electrolyte and albumin levels and weigh every other day.
5. Monitor vital signs.

Patient Education/Health Maintenance

1. Instruct patient and family about bipolar illness, including symptoms of relapse.
2. Instruct patient and family members about psychopharmacologic treatment, including its purpose, effects, side effects, and management.
3. Advise patient and family members about community-based support groups or health care agencies that are relevant to their care.

Evaluation

A. Improved thought processes demonstrated by completion of simple tasks
B. Sleeping for 5 hours at night
C. Family members verbalize realistic, goal-directed thinking related to the patient's abilities, recovery, and control of condition
D. No weight loss noted

Thought Disturbances (Psychotic Disorders)

◆ SCHIZOPHRENIA, SCHIZOPHRENIFORM, AND DELUSIONAL DISORDERS

The disorders included in this section have defining features of psychotic symptoms. Psychotic symptoms are produced by a loss of ego boundaries and/or a gross impairment in reality testing, which includes prominent hallucinations and delusions, disorganized speech, and grossly disorganized or catatonic behavior.

Pathophysiology/Etiology

A. *Schizophrenia, Schizophreniform Disorder*
1. Genetic
   a. Identical twins and concordance rate for schizophrenia is 35% to 70% greater than for the general population.

b. Identical twin concordance rate is three times that of fraternal twins.

c. Studies using a broad-spectrum definition of schizophrenic illness have demonstrated that having an affected parent increased the risk of developing schizophrenia or a disorder within that spectrum, such as schizotypal personality.

d. Research continues to identify a schizophrenia gene.

2. Neurobiologic hypotheses

a. Dopamine hypothesis—hyperactivity in the dopaminergic system, possibly due to receptor neurons that are functionally hyperactive.

b. Norepinephrine, serotonin, glutamate, and GABA may also have a role in modulating the symptoms of schizophrenia.

c. Endogenous dysfunction of N-methyl-D-aspartate receptor-mediated neurotransmission could lead to the development of schizophrenia.

d. Neuroanatomic studies—cerebral ventricular enlargement; sulcal enlargement; cerebellar atrophy; decreased cranial, cerebral, and frontal size; abnormalities in basal ganglia; structural abnormalities at the cellular level, particularly in the limbic and periventricular regions.

e. Functional and metabolic studies—regional cerebral blood flow studies demonstrated hypofrontality: schizophrenic patients were unable to increase blood flow to their frontal lobes during a task thought to increase frontal lobe functions; positron-emission tomography (PET) studies also consistently found evidence for a relative hypofrontality.

f. Electrophysiologic studies—Electroencephalogram findings in schizophrenic patients demonstrated decreased alpha and increased delta activity; changes in evoked potentials and amplitude reduction may occur in responses reflecting selective attention and stimulus evaluation. P300 response (reduced amplitude to unexpected stimuli using auditory and visual parameters) is the most pronounced and is prolonged. This defect leads to information or sensory overload and an inability to "screen out" irrelevant stimuli.

3. Developmental hypotheses

a. The essential feature of schizophrenia as proposed by psychoanalytic theory is a defect in interpersonal relationships due to a withdrawal of the libido into the self.

b. Schizophrenia is proposed to be rooted in the early mother–child relationship.

c. Interpersonal theory of schizophrenia proposes that if a person lacks sufficient exposure to positive interpersonal relationships, a personality deficit or schizophrenia might develop.

d. Parental influences are no longer considered causative of schizophrenia. Research continues in the area of highly expressed emotion within the family.

e. Research in expressed emotion has included intervention trials to determine whether family therapy can lower expressed emotion and prevent schizophrenic patients from relapse situations.

4. Neurodevelopmental factors

a. Research evidence supports speculation that schizophrenia is a neurodevelopmental disorder resulting from brain injury occurring early in life and interfering with normal maturational events.

b. Schizophrenic patients are more likely than other psychiatric patients or normal control subjects to have a history of obstetric complications.

B. *Delusional Disorder*

1. Little has been established about the etiology of delusional disorder.

2. There is no demonstrated genetic linkage.

3. It is possible that psychosocial stressors have a role in the etiology of delusional disorder in some persons. This is illustrated in some of the more rare conditions, such as shared psychotic disorder.

Clinical Manifestations

See Tables 55-5 and 55-6.

Diagnostic Evaluation

1. Clinical diagnosis is developed on historical information and thorough mental status examination.

2. No laboratory findings have been identified that are diagnostic of schizophrenia.

3. Routine battery of laboratory tests may be useful in ruling out possible organic etiologies, including CBC, urinalysis, liver function tests, thyroid function tests, RPR, HIV test, serum ceruloplasmin (rules out Wilson's disease), PET scan, CT, and MRI.

4. Rating scale assessment

a. Scale for the Assessment of Negative Symptoms

b. Scale for the Assessment of Positive Symptoms

Management

A. *Schizophrenia/Schizophreniform Disorder*

1. Psychopharmacologic interventions:

a. Antipsychotics (neuroleptic)

b. Adjunctive pharmacologic agents: anxiolytics, lithium, antidepressants, propranolol (Inderal), carbamazepine (Tegretol).

2. ECT may be indicated for catatonic patients.

3. Psychosocial treatments

a. Supportive individual psychotherapy that is reality oriented and pragmatic.

b. Structured group psychotherapy.

c. Family therapy.

d. Psychoeducational group.

e. Support groups in community.

f. Community-based partial hospitalization programs.

g. Psychiatric home care nursing.

4. Vocational and social skills education.

B. *Delusional Disorder*

1. Neuroleptic agents have demonstrated some success in reducing the intensity of the delusion.

2. Individual psychotherapy.

3. Hospitalization for comprehensive assessment for diagnostic purposes or if suicidal or homicidal.

Complications

1. If left undiagnosed, untreated, or ineffectively treated, schizophrenia can lead to aggressive/violent behavior toward others.

2. Catatonic behavior can develop, which could render the person totally incapable of self-care.

TABLE 55-5 Characteristics of Schizophrenia, Schizophreniform, and Schizoaffective Disorders

Schizophrenia Subtypes	Schizophreniform Disorder	Schizoaffective Disorder
Paranoid 1. Dominant—hallucinations and delusions. 2. No disorganized speech, disorganized behavior, or disorganized affect present. **Disorganized** 1. Dominant—disorganized speech and disorganized behavior. 2. Delusions and hallucinations if present are not prominent or fragmented. **Residual** 1. No. longer has positive symptoms, eg, delusions, hallucinations, or disorganized speech or behaviors. 2. However, persistence of some symptoms is noted, eg, • Marked social isolation or withdrawal • Marked impairment in role function (wage earner, student, or homemaker) • Markedly peculiar behavior • Marked impairment in personal hygiene • Marked lack of initiative, interest, or energy • Blunted or inappropriate affect **Catatonic** 1. Motor immobility (waxy flexibility) 2. Excessive purposeless motor activity (agitation) 3. Extreme negativism or mutism 4. Peculiar voluntary movement • Posturing • Stereotyped movements • Prominent mannerisms • Prominent grimaces 5. Echolalia or echopraxia **Undifferentiated** 1. Has positive symptoms (does have hallucinations, delusions, and bizarre behaviors) 2. No one clinical presentation dominates, eg, • Paranoid • Disorganized • Catatonic	1. Two or more of the following symptoms: (1) Delusions (2) Hallucinations (3) Disorganized speech (4) Grossly disorganized or catatonic behavior • Affective flattening • Alogia • Avolition 2. Schizoaffective and mood disorders, chemical dependence, or a causative general medical condition is ruled out. 3. Lasts at least 1 month but less than 6 months.	1. An uninterrupted period of illness where there was either a major depressive, manic, or mixed episode. 2. Concurrent positive and negative symptoms of schizophrenia. 3. Disturbance not due to direct physiologic effects of a chemical or general medical condition.

Adapted from APA DSMIV 1994, Washington, DC

3. Depression and suicide.
4. Chemical use, abuse, or dependency.

Nursing Assessment

Assess for positive symptoms of schizophrenia. These symptoms reflect aberrant mental activity and are usually present early in the first phase of the schizophrenic illness.

A. *Alterations in Thinking*
1. Delusion: false, fixed belief that is not amenable to change by reasoning. The most frequent elicited delusions include:

a. Ideas of reference
b. Delusions of grandeur
c. Delusions of jealousy
d. Delusions of persecution
e. Somatic delusions
2. Loose associations: the thought process becomes illogical and confused.
3. Neologisms: made-up words that have a special meaning to the delusional person.
4. Concrete thinking: an overemphasis on small or specific details and an impaired ability to abstract.
5. Echolalia: pathologic repeating of another's words.
6. Clang associations: the meaningless rhyming of a word in a forceful way.

TABLE 55-6 Characteristics of Psychotic Disorders (Not Schizophrenic)

Delusional Disorder
1. Nonbizarre delusions of at least 1 month's duration.
2. No positive/negative symptoms of schizophrenia present.
3. Tactile/olfactory hallucinations may be present and are related to the delusional theme.
4. Functioning is not markedly impaired and behavior is not obviously bizarre or odd.
5. Only brief mood episodes, if any.
6. Not due to direct physiologic effects of a chemical or a general medical condition.

Psychotic Disorder Due to a General Medical Disorder
1. Prominent hallucinations or delusions.
2. Evidence from the history, physical examination, or lab studies that the disorder is due to physiologic consequences of a general medical condition.
3. Disturbance does not occur exclusively during the course of delirium.

Brief Psychotic Disorder
1. Presence of 1 or more of these symptoms:
   • Delusions
   • Disorganized speech
   • Grossly disorganized or catatonic behavior
   • Hallucinations
2. Duration of the disturbance is at least 1 day and less than 1 month.
3. Eventual return to premorbid level of functioning.

Specifiers:
   • With marked stressors
   • Without marked stressors
   • With postpartum onset

Shared Psychotic Disorder
1. Delusion develops in an individual who has an already established delusion in the context of a close relationship.
2. Delusion is similar in content to the other person's.
3. Disturbance doesn't meet criteria for other psychotic disorders.

Substance-Induced Psychotic Disorder
1. Prominent hallucinations or delusions.
2. There is evidence from the history or physical assessment of the following:
   • Symptoms developed during or within 1 month of substance intoxication/withdrawal.
   • Medication use is related to the disturbance.
3. Disturbance does not occur exclusively during the course of a delirium.

Specifiers
   • Specific substance
   • Onset during intoxication
   • Onset during withdrawal

Adapted from the APA DSMIV 1994 Washington, DC

7. Word salad: a mixture of words that is meaningless to the listener.

B. Alterations in Perceiving
1. Hallucinations: sensory perceptions that have no external stimulus. The most common are:
   a. Auditory
   b. Visual
   c. Gustatory

   d. Olfactory
   e. Tactile
2. Loss of ego boundaries: lack a sense of their body and how they relate to the environment.
   a. Depersonalization is a nonspecific feeling or sense that a person has lost his or her identity or is unreal.
   b. Derealization is the false perception by a person that the environment has changed.

C. Alterations in Behavioral Responses
1. Bizarre behavioral patterns
   a. Motor agitation/restlessness
   b. Automatic obedience/robotlike movement
   c. Negativism
   d. Stereotyped behaviors
   e. Stupor
   f. Waxy flexibility
2. Agitated or impulsive behavior

Assess for negative symptoms of schizophrenia that reflect a deficiency of mental functioning.

1. Alogia—inability to speak
2. Anergia—inability to react
3. Anhedonia—inability to experience pleasure
4. Avolition—inability to choose or decide
5. Poor social functioning
6. Poverty of speech
7. Social withdrawal
8. Thought blocking

Assess for associated symptoms of schizophrenia.

1. Chemical use/abuse/dependence
2. Depression
3. Fantasy
4. Violent or aggressive behavior
5. Water intoxication
6. Withdrawal

Nursing Diagnoses

A. Altered Thought Processes related to perceptual and cognitive distortions, as demonstrated by suspiciousness, defensive behavior, and disruptions in thought
B. Social Isolation related to an inability to trust
C. Risk for Activity Intolerance related to adverse reactions to psychopharmacologic medications
D. Ineffective Individual Coping related to misinterpretation of environment and impaired communication ability
E. Risk for Violence: Self-directed or directed at others, related to delusional thinking and hallucinatory experiences

Nursing Interventions

A. Strengthening Differentiation Between Delusions and Reality
1. Provide the patient with honest and consistent feedback in a nonthreatening manner.
2. Avoid challenging the content of the patient's behaviors.
3. Focus interactions on the patient's behaviors.

4. Administer medications as prescribed while monitoring and documenting the patient's response to the medication regimen (Table 55-7).
5. Use simple and clear language when speaking with the patient.
6. Explain all procedures, tests, and activities to the patient before starting them, and provide written or video material for learning purposes.

B. Promoting Socialization
1. Encourage the patient to talk about feelings.
2. Allow patient time to reveal delusions to you without engaging in a power struggle over the content or the reality of the delusions.
3. Use a supportive, empathic approach to focus on the patients feelings about troubling events and/or conflicts.
4. Provide opportunities for socialization and encourage participation in group activities.
5. Be aware of the patient's personal space and use touch judiciously.
6. Assist the patient to identify behaviors that alienate significant others and family members.

C. Improving Activity Tolerance
1. Assess the patient's response to prescribed antipsychotic medication.
2. Collaborate with the patient and occupational and physical therapy specialists to assess the patient's ability to perform activities of daily living.
3. Collaborate with the patient to establish a daily, achievable routine within physical limitations.
4. Teach strategies to manage side effects of antipsychotics that affect the patient's functional status, including the following:
   a. Change positions slowly.
   b. Gradually increase physical activities.
   c. Limit overdoing it in hot, sunny weather.
   d. Use sun precautions.
   e. Use caution in activities if extrapyramidal symptoms develop.

D. Improving Coping With Thoughts and Feelings
1. Encourage patient to express feelings.
2. Focus on patient's feelings and behavior.
3. Provide honest perceptions of reality and feedback about symptoms and behaviors.
4. Encourage the patient to explore adaptive behaviors that increase the patient's abilities and success in socializing and accomplishing activities of daily living.
5. Decrease environmental stimuli.

E. Ensuring Safety
1. Monitor the patient for behaviors that indicate increased anxiety.
2. Collaborate with the patient to identify anxious behaviors as well as the causes.
3. Tell the patient that you will help him or her maintain control.
4. Establish consistent limits on the patient's behaviors and clearly communicate these limits to the patient, family members, and health care providers.
5. Secure all potential weapons and articles that could be used to inflict an injury from the patient's room and the unit environment.
6. To prepare for possible continued escalation, form a psychiatric emergency assist team and designate a leader to facilitate an effective and safe aggression management process.

7. Determine the need for external control, including seclusion and/or restraints. Communicate the decision to the patient and put plan into action.
8. Frequently monitor the patient within the guidelines of the institution's policy on restrictive devices and assess the patient's level of agitation.
9. When the patient's level of agitation begins to decrease and self-control is regained, establish a behavioral agreement that identifies specific behaviors that indicate self-control against a reescalation of agitation.

Patient Education/Health Maintenance

1. Instruct the patient and family members in disease process and how to recognize and cope with relapse symptoms.
2. Instruct the patient and family members about the uses, actions, and side effects of any prescribed medications.
3. Instruct the patient and family in community resources, support groups and possible use of psychiatric home care nursing.
4. For additional information and support, refer to the National Alliance for Research on Schizophrenia and Depression (NARSAD); 60 Cutter Mill Road, Suite 200; Great Neck, NY 11021; 516-829-0091.

Evaluation

A. Exhibits improved reality orientation, concentration, and attention span
B. Exhibits improved interaction with staff, family members
C. Performing ADLs according to agreed plan
D. Expressing feelings and discussing behaviors
E. Remains free from harm or violent acts

Cognitive Impairment Disturbances

◆ DELIRIUM, DEMENTIA, AND AMNESIC DISORDER

Cognitive impairment disturbances encompass specific disorders that produce either temporary or permanent neuronal damage, resulting in psychological or behavioral dysfunction. Cognitive impairment disorders described in the *Diagnostic and Statistical Manual, 4th Edition*, include delirium, dementia, and amnesic disorder.

Delirium is a disturbance of consciousness and a change in cognition that develops over a brief time period. Dementia is a disturbance involving multiple cognitive deficits, including memory impairment. Amnesic disorder is characterized by memory impairment in the absence of other significant cognitive impairments.

Pathophysiology and Etiology

A. Delirium
Can be caused by numerous pathophysiologic conditions. Some of the major possibilities include:

TABLE 55-7 Management of Adverse Effects of Neuroleptic Medications

Orthostatic (postural) hypotension	Coping with dizziness: Assess for orthostatic blood pressure changes and teach the patient: • When rising from bed or chair, get up slowly. • Sit at side of bed for a few minutes, dangling legs. • Do ankle pumps before standing. • Once standing, move slowly. • Don't twist or turn quickly. • Use assistive devices, hand rails, canes, walkers when necessary for functional deficits. • Don't drive or operate machinery when dizzy.
Peripheral anticholinergic effects: dry mouth and nose, blurred vision, constipation, urinary retention	Dry mouth: Teach the patient: • Brush teeth after each meal with a fluoridated toothpaste. • Rinse mouth frequently. • Limit caffeinated or alcoholic drinks, because they can be dehydrating. • Stop smoking due to the irritation of oral mucosa. • Suck on sugarless candy or gum; avoid sugared candy to decrease the risk of fungal infections and dental caries. • Avoid dry or spicy foods. • Drink fluids between meals unless you are on a specific fluid restriction. • Avoid acidic beverages due to potential irritation. • Use dressing, juices, or sauces (if allowed) to moisten food. Constipation: Teach the patient: • Drink fluids (within prescribed limits set by health care provider). • Eat roughage: fruits, vegetables (raw leafy types) to increase bulk and help soften stool. • Eat dried fruits, such as prunes or dates, for laxative effect. • Maintain activity level within functional limits. • Consult with health care provider to determine appropriate use of over-the-counter laxatives (Metamucil, Citrucel) and/or prescribed stool softeners.
Extrapyramidal Side Effects: Short Term Akathisia—restless legs, jitters, nervous energy, motor agitation Akinesia—weakness (hypotonia), fatigue, painful muscles, anergy (lack of energy), absence of movement Dystonias, dyskinesias—grimacing, torticollis, intermittent spasms, opisthotonos, oculogyric crises, head–neck stiffness, myoclonic twitches, laryngeal-pharyngeal dystonia Parkinsonian effects—muscle stiffness, cog wheel rigidity, shuffling gait, stooped posture, drooling	• Reassure patient. • Differentiate between agitation and akathisia. • Consider reducing dosage. • Consider switching patient to another class of antipsychotic. • Assess functional ability. • Dose reduction or cessation should improve movement if problems are due to akinesia versus psychotic symptoms. • Consider prophylaxis with anticholinergic medications. • Treat with IM/IV anticholinergics, as prescribed. • Treat with anticholinergics, as prescribed. • Stop the antipsychotic, as directed.
Long-Term Effects of Neuroleptics Tardive dyskinesia—a delayed effect of neuroleptic agents usually occurring after 6 months of treatment involving abnormal, involuntary, irregular, choreoathetoid movements of the muscles of the head, limbs, and trunk.	• Complete regular objective rating/assessment of the movement disorder. • Reduce/stop neuroleptic as directed. • Consider clozapine or respiridol. • Comprehensive medical psychiatric assessment necessary with close monitoring of movement disorder.

IM: intramuscular; IV: intravenous.

1. CNS pathology: head trauma, hypertensive cerebral changes, seizures, tumors
2. Endocrinopathies: thyroidism, parathyroidism
3. Hypoxemia
4. Hypothermia/hyperthermia
5. Intoxication/abstinence and withdrawal states
6. Metals/toxins/drugs
7. Metabolic: diabetic acidosis, hypoglycemia, acid–base imbalances
8. Hepatic encephalopathy
9. Thiamine deficiency
10. Postoperative states

11. Psychosocial stressors: relocation stress, sensory deprivation/overload, sleep deprivation, immobilization

B. Dementia

Primary dementias—degenerative disorders that are progressive, irreversible, and not due to any other condition. Specific disorders are dementia of the Alzheimer's type and vascular dementia (formerly multiinfarct dementia).

1. Genetic: Family members of Alzheimer's patients have a higher risk of acquiring the disease than does the general population. Research into chromosomal defects is providing some explanation of early- versus late-onset forms.
2. Toxin model: There is speculation that high levels of aluminum in the blood may be related to Alzheimer's disease.
3. Additional areas of investigation:
   a. Slow viral infection
   b. Autoimmune processes
   c. Head trauma
   d. Decreased cerebral blood flow
4. Neuropathologic changes
   a. Neurofibrillary tangle (intraneuronal)
   b. Senile "neuritic" plaque (extraneuronal)
   c. Granulovascular degeneration (intraneuronal)
   d. Amyloid angiopathy (extraneuronal)

Secondary dementias—occur as a result of another pathologic process).

1. Infection-related dementias
   a. Acquired immunodeficiency syndrome
   b. Chronic meningitis
   c. Jakob-Creutzfeldt disease
   d. Progressive multifocal leukoencephalopathy
   e. Postencephalitic dementia syndrome
   f. Syphilis
   g. Subacute sclerosing panencephalitis
   h. Tuberculosis
2. Subcortical degenerative disorders
   a. Huntington's disease
   b. Parkinson's disease
   c. Wilson's disease
   d. Thalamic dementia
3. Hydrocephalic dementias
4. Vascular dementias
5. Traumatic conditions, such as posttraumatic encephalopathy and subdural hematoma
6. Neoplastic dementias
   a. Glioma
   b. Meningioma
   c. Meningeal carcinomatosis
   d. Metastatic deposits
7. Inflammatory conditions, such as sarcoidosis, systemic lupus erythematosus, temporal arteritis.
8. Toxic conditions, such as alcohol-related syndrome and iatrogenic dementias (anticonvulsants, anticholinergics, antihypertensives, psychotropic agents).
9. Metabolic disorders
   a. Anemias
   b. Deficiency states (minerals and vitamins)
   c. Cardiac/pulmonary failure
   d. Hepatic encephalopathy
   e. Porphyria
   f. Uremia

C. Amnestic Disorder

1. Posttraumatic amnesia: head trauma is the most common cause of amnesia
2. Poststroke amnesia: damage to the fornix or hippocampus

3. Neoplasms
4. Anoxic states
5. Herpes simplex encephalitis
6. Hypoglycemic states
7. Epileptic seizures
8. ECT
9. Substance-induced

Clinical Manifestations

See Table 55-8.

Diagnostic Evaluation

A wide variety of diagnostic tests may be done to determine cause. A comprehensive neuropsychiatric evaluation must be completed to make an accurate diagnosis.

1. Basic laboratory examination, including complete blood count with differential, chemistry panel (including blood urea nitrogen, creatine, and ammonia), arterial blood gasses, chest X-ray, toxicology screen (comprehensive), thyroid function tests, and serologic tests for syphilis.
2. Additional tests may include CT, MRI imaging, additional blood chemistries (heavy metals, thiamine, folate, antinuclear antibody (ANA), and urinary porphobilinogen), lumbar puncture, PET/single photon emission computer tomography scans
3. Mini Mental Status Examination
4. Blessed Dementia Scale
5. Physical examination
6. Vital signs

Management

A. Delirium

1. The goal is diagnosis to identify specific reversible causes of the delirium so that treatment is focused on ameliorating the causative factor(s).
2. Psychopharmacotherapy is dependent on underlying cause(s).
   a. Benzodiazepines such as lorazepam (Ativan) for abstinence withdrawal states.
   b. Neuroleptics such as haloperidol (Haldol) for agitation.
   c. Combined intravenous administration of haloperidol and lorazepam for agitated and psychotic symptomatology.
3. Environmental management
   a. Safe, structured environment.
   b. Orientation facilitated by accurate clocks and calendars.
   c. Family involvement.

B. Dementia

1. Effective treatment is based on:
   a. Diagnosis of primary illness and concurrent psychiatric disorders.
   b. Assessment of auditory and visual impairment.
   c. Measurement of the degree, nature, and progression of cognitive deficits.
   d. Assessment of functional capacity and ability for self-care.
   e. Family and social system assessment.
2. Environmental strategies.

TABLE 55-8 Clinical Manifestations: Cognitive Impairment Disorders

Disorder	DSMIV Diagnoses	Defining Characteristics
Delirium (severe impairment in functioning)	• Delirium due to a general medical condition. • Substance-induced delirium. • Delirium due to multiple etiologies.	• Fluctuating levels of awareness. • Clouding of consciousness (confused and disoriented). • Perceptual disturbances (illusions and hallucinations). • Memory, especially recent memory, is distrubed. • Alteration in sleep–wake cycle. • EEG changes. • Abrupt onset may last about 1 week. • Reversible when underlying cause has been treated.
Dementia (severe impairment in functioning)	• Dementia of the Alzheimer's type. • Vascular dementia. • Dementia due to a general medical condition. • Substance-induced persisting dementia. • Dementia due to multiple etiologies. • Substance-induced persisting dementia. • Dementia due to general medical conditions.	• Slow, insidious onset. • Impaired long- and short-term memory. • Deterioration of cognitive abilities—judgment, abstract thinking. • Often irreversible if untreatable. • Personality changes. • No or slow EEG changes.
Amnestic syndrome (moderate to severe impairment in functioning)	• Amnestic disorder due to a general medical condition. • Substance-induced persisting amnestic disorder.	• Impairment in short- and long-term memory. • Inability to learn new material. • Remote memory better than that of recent events. • Confabulation. • Apathy, lack of initiative. • Emotionally bland.

DSMIV: *Diagnostic and Statistical Manual, 4th Edition*, EEG: electroencephalogram.

3. Psychopharmacotherapy is used in the person with dementia for behavioral control and symptom reduction.
   a. Agitation management: neuroleptic agents
   b. Psychosis: neuroleptic agents
   c. Depression: antidepressants, ECT
   d. Cognitive dysfunction: ergoloid mesylates (Hydergine Germinal)
4. Hypertension management in vascular dementia.

Complications

1. Without accurate diagnosis and treatment, secondary dementias may become permanent.
2. Falls with serious orthopedic or cerebral injuries.
3. Self-inflicted injuries.
4. Aggression or violence toward self, others, or property.
5. Wandering events, in which the person can get lost and potentially suffer exposure, hypothermia, and even death.

Nursing Assessment

Assess factors such as onset, course, mood, perception, memory, and communication to help differentiate the cognitive impairment and provide proper care. See Table 55-9.

Nursing Diagnoses

A. Impaired Communication related to cerebral impairment as demonstrated by altered memory, judgment, and word finding
B. Self-Care Deficit related to cognitive impairment as demonstrated by inattention and inability to complete ADLs
C. Risk for Injury related to cognitive impairment and wandering behavior
D. Impaired Social Interaction related to cognitive impairment
E. Risk for Violence: Self-directed or directed toward others due to suspicion and inability to recognize people or places

Nursing Interventions

A. *Improving Communication*
1. Speak slowly and use short, simple words and phrases.
2. Consistently identify yourself, and address the person by name at each meeting.
3. Focus on one piece of information at a time. Review what has been discussed with patient.
4. If patient has vision or hearing disturbances, have patient wear prescription eyeglasses and/or a hearing device.
5. Maintain a well-lighted environment.

TABLE 55-9   Delirium/Dementia/Amnesic Disorder Nursing Assessment

Disorder	Delirium	Dementia	Amnestic Disorder
Onset	Acute	Slow, insidious	Sudden
Course	Usually brief	Progresses over years	Transient or chronic
Mood	Fearfulness, anxiety, irritability	Mood labile, personality traits accentuated	Apathy, agitation, emotional blandness, shallow range of affective expression
Perception	Auditory, visual, tactile hallucinations; illusions	Hallucinations not a prominent feature	No hallucinatory experiences
Memory	Short-term memory impaired	Short-term memory damage followed by long-term memory damage	Impaired ability to learn new information; unable to recall previously learned information or past events
Communication	Slurred speech; confabulation	Normal—early stage progressive aphasia and confabulation	Confabulation

6. Use clocks, calendars, and familiar personal effects in the patient's view.
7. If patient becomes verbally aggressive, identify and acknowledge how he or she is feeling.
8. If patient becomes aggressive, shift the topic to a safer, more familiar one.
9. If patient becomes delusional, acknowledge his or her feelings and reinforce reality. Do not attempt to challenge the content of the delusion.

B.   Promoting Independence in Self-Care
1. Assess and monitor the patient's ability to perform ADLs.
2. Encourage decision making regarding ADLs as much as possible.
3. Label clothes with patient's name, address, and telephone number.
4. Use clothing with elastic and Velcro for fastenings rather than buttons or zippers, which may be too difficult for the patient to manipulate.
5. Monitor food and fluid intake.
6. Weigh the patient weekly.
7. Provide food that patient can eat while moving.
8. Sit with the patient during meals and assist by cueing.
9. Initiate a bowel and bladder program early in the disease process to maintain continence and prevent constipation or urinary retention.

C.   Ensuring Safety
1. Discuss restriction of driving when recommended.
2. Assess home for safety: remove throw rugs, label rooms, and keep the house well-lit.
3. Assess community for safety.
4. Alert neighbors about the patient's wandering behavior.
5. Alert police, and have current pictures taken.
6. Provide patient with a Medic-Alert bracelet.
7. Install complex safety locks on doors to outside or basement.
8. Install safety bars in bathroom.
9. Closely observe patient if he or she is smoking.
10. Encourage physical activity during the daytime.
11. Give the patient a card with simple instructions (address and phone number) in case he or she is lost.
12. Use night-lights.
13. Install alarm/sensor devices on doors.

D.   Improving Socialization
1. Provide magazines with pictures as reading and language abilities diminish.
2. Encourage participation in simple, familiar group activities, such as singing, reminiscing, and painting.
3. Encourage participation in simple activities that promote the exercise of large muscle groups.

E.   Preventing Violence and Aggression
1. Respond calmly and do not raise your voice.
2. Remove objects that might be used to harm self or others.
3. Identify stressors that increase agitation.
4. Distract patient when an upsetting situation develops.

Patient Education/Health Maintenance

1. Instruct the family about the process of the disorder, whether delirium, dementia, or amnesic disorder.
2. Instruct the family about safety measures to be used when the patient is at home or in the hospital.
3. Instruct and refer family members to community-based group (adult day care centers, senior assessment centers, home care, respite care, and family support groups).
4. For additional information and support, refer to the Alzheimer's Association; 919 North Michigan Avenue, Suite 1000; Chicago, IL 60611-1676; 800-621-0379; or National Institutes of Health, National Institute on Aging, Alzheimer's Disease Education and Referral Center; 1-800-438-4380.

Evaluation

A. Patient cooperative and communicating needs
B. Performing basic bathing, dressing, and feeding activities with cues from staff
C. Safety precautions and close surveillance maintained
D. Increased interaction with staff and family members
E. No violence or aggression noted

Selected References

American Psychiatric Association. (Eds.). (1994). *Diagnostic and statistical manual of mental disorders* (4th ed.). Washington, DC: Author.

Andreasen, N. C., & Carpenter, W. T. (1993). Diagnosis and classification of schizophrenia. *Schizophrenia Bulletin, 19*, 199-214.

Andreasen, N. C., Flaum, M., et al. (1990). Positive and negative symptoms in schizophrenia: A critical reappraisal *Archives of General Psychiatry, 47*, 615-621.

Backlar, P.(1994). *The family life of schizophrenia: Practical counsel from America's leading experts.* New York: G.P. Putnam's.

Baer, L., Jenike, M. A., Ricciardi, J. N., et al. (1990). Standardized assessment of personality disorders in obsessive-compulsive disorder. *Archives of General Psychiatry, 47*, 826-830.

Barry, P. (1994). *Mental health and mental illness.* Philadelphia: J.B. Lippincott.

Berman, K. F., Torrey, E. F., et al. (1992). Regional cerebral blood flow in monozygotic twins discordant and concordant for schizophrenia. *Archives of General Psychiatry, 49*, 927-934.

Cattell, R. B., & Scheier, I. H. (1963). *IPAT anxiety scale questionnaire manual.* Champaign, IL: Institute for Personality and Ability Testing.

Chalmers, J., Risk, M. T., et al. (1991). Severe amnesia after hypoglycemia, clinical, psychometric and magnetic resonance imaging correlations. *Diabetes Care, 14*, 922-925.

Davis, J. M., et al. (1992). The effects of a support group on grieving and individual's level of perceived support and stress. *Archives of Psychiatric Nursing, 6*(1), 35.

Davis, K. C., Kahn, R. S., Ko, G., et al. (1991). Dopamine in schizophrenia: A review and reconceptualization. *American Journal of Psychiatry, 148*, 1474-1486.

Folstein, M. F. (1975). Mini-mental state: A practical method for grading the cognitive state of patients for the clinician. *Journal of Psychiatric Research, 12*, 189.

Goodman, W., et al. (1989). The Yale-Brown Obsessive Compulsive Scale 1: Development. *Archives of General Psychiatry, 46*(11), 1006-1011.

Goodman, W., et al. (1989). The Yale-Brown Obsessive Compulsive Scale II: Validity. *Archives of General Psychiatry, 46*(11), 1012.

Hales, R. E., Yudofsky, S. C., & Talbott, J. A. (1994). *Textbook of psychiatry.* Washington, DC: American Psychological Association Press.

Houseman, C. (1990). The paranoid person: A biopsychosocial perspective. *Archives of Psychiatric Nursing, 4*(3), 176-181.

Inaba-Roland, K. E., & Maricle, R. A. (1992). Assessing delirium in the acute care setting. *Heart and Lung, 21*(1), 48.

Kaplan, H. I., & Sadock, B. J. (1993). *Pocket handbook of psychiatric drug treatment..* Baltimore: Williams & Wilkins.

Krupnick, S., & Wade, A.(1993). *Psychiatric care planning.* Springhouse, PA: Springhouse.

Lipowski, Z. J.(1990). *Delirium: Acute confusional states.* New York: Oxford University Press.

Mondimore, F. M. (1993). *Depression: The mood disease.* Baltimore: Johns Hopkins University Press.

Paykel, E. S. (Ed.). (1992). *Handbook of affective disorders* (2nd ed.). New York: Guilford Press.

Plante, T. (1990). Social skills training: A program to help schizophrenia clients cope. *Journal of Psychosocial Nursing, 27*(3), 7-10.

Roper, J. M., Shapiro, J., & Change, B. L. (1991). Agitation in the demented patient: A framework for management. *Journal of Gerontological Nursing, 17*(3), 17.

Sherrington, R., et al., (1988). Localization of a susceptibility locus for schizophrenia on chromosomes. *Nature, 336*, 164-166.

Stoudemire, A., & Fogel, B. S. (1993). *Psychiatric care of the medical patient.* New York: Oxford University Press.

Taylor, J. (1953). A personality scale of manifest anxiety. *Journal of Abnormal and Social Psychology, 48*, 235.

Torrey, E. F., Bowen, A., et al. (1994). *Schizophrenia and manic-depressive disorder: The biological roots of mental illness.* New York: Basic Books.

U.S. Department of Health & Human Services. (1993). *Clinical practice guideline. Depression in primary care. Vol. 1: Assessment of major depression. Vol. 2: Treatment of major depression.* Rockville, MD: Agency for Health Care Policy and Research.

Zal, H. M. (1990). *Panic disorders: The great pretender.* New York: Plenum.

Appendices and Index

APPENDIX I ◆

Diagnostic Studies and Their Meaning

Abbreviations

◆ CONVENTIONAL UNITS

kg = kilogram
gm = gram
mg = milligram
μg = microgram
$\mu\mu$g = micromicrogram
ng = nanogram
pg = picogram
dl = 100 milliliters
ml = milliliter
cu mm = cubic millimeter
fL = femtoliter

mM = millimole
nM = nanomole
mOsm = milliosmole
mm = millimeter
μ = micron or micrometer
mm Hg = millimeters of mercury
U = unit
mU = milliunit
μU = microunit
mEq = milliequivalent
IU = International Unit
mIU = milliInternational Unit

◆ SI UNITS

g = gram
L = liter
d = day
h = hour
mol = mole
mmol = millimole
μmol = micromole
nmol = nanomole
pmol = picomole

Reference Ranges—Hematology*

Determination	Reference Range		Clinical Significance
	Conventional Units	SI Units	
A_2 Hemoglobin	1.5%–3.5% of total hemoglobin	Mass fraction: 0.015–0.035 of total hemoglobin	Increased in certain types of thalassemia
Bleeding time	1–9 min	2–8 min	Prolonged in thrombocytopenia, defective platelet function, and aspirin therapy
Factor V assay (proaccelerin factor)	60%–140%		
Factor VIII assay (antihemophiliac factor)	50%–200%		Deficient in classical hemophilia
Factor IX assay (plasma thromboplastin component)	75%–125%		Deficient in Christmas disease (pseudohemophilia)
Factor X (Stuart factor)	60%–140%		Deficient in Stuart clotting defect
Fibrinogen	200–400 mg/dl	2–4 g/dl	Increased in pregnancy, infections accompanied by leukocytosis, nephrosis. Decreased in severe liver disease, abruptio placentae
Fibrin split products	Less than 10 mg/L	Less than 10 mg/L	Increased in disseminated intravascular coagulation

(continued)

Reference Ranges—Hematology* (continued)

Determination	Reference Range		Clinical Significance
	Conventional Units	SI Units	
Fibrinolysins (whole blood clot lysis time)	No lysis in 24 h		Increased activity associated with massive hemorrhage, extensive surgery, transfusion reactions
Partial thromboplastin time (activated)	20–45 sec		Prolonged in deficiency of fibrinogen, factors II, V, VIII, IX, X, XI, and XII, and in heparin therapy
Prothrombin consumption	Over 20 sec		Impaired in deficiency of factors VIII, IX, and X
Prothrombin time INR	9.5–12 sec 1.0		Prolonged by deficiency of factors I, II, V, VII, and X, fat malabsorption, severe liver disease, coumarin-anticoagulant therapy. INR used to standarize the prothrombin time and anticoagulation therapy
Erythrocyte count	Males: 4,600,000–6,200,000/ cu mm	$4.6–6.2 \times 10^{12}$/L	Increased in severe diarrhea and dehydration, polycythemia, acute poisoning, pulmonary fibrosis
	Females: 4,200,000–5,400,000/ cu mm	$4.2–5.4 \times 10^{12}$/L	Decreased in all anemias, in leukemia, and after hemorrhage, when blood volume has been restored
Erythrocyte indices Mean corpuscular volume (MCV)	80–94 (cu μ)	80–94 fL	Increased in macrocytic anemias; decreased in microcytic anemia
Mean corpuscular hemoglobin (MCH)	27–32 $\mu\mu$g/cell	27–32 pg	Increased in macrocytic anemias; decreased in microcytic anemia
Mean corpuscular hemoglobin concentration (MCHC)	33%–38%	Concentration fraction: 0.33–0.38	Decreased in severe hypochromic anemia
Reticulocytes	0.5%–1.5% of red cells	Number fraction: 0.005–0.015	Increased with any condition stimulating increase in bone marrow activity (ie, infection, blood loss [acute and chronic]); following iron therapy in iron-deficiency anemia, polycythemia rubra vera Decreased with any condition depressing bone marrow activity, acute leukemia, late stage of severe anemias
Erythrocyte sedimentation rate (ESR)— Westergren method	Males under 50 yr: <15 mm/h Males over 50 yr: <20 mm/h Females under 50 yr: <20 mm/h Females over 50 yr: <30 mm/h	<15 mm/h <20 mm/h <20 mm/h <30 mm/h	Increased in tissue destruction, whether inflammatory or degenerative; during menstruation and pregnancy; and in acute febrile diseases
Erythrocyte sedimentation ratio—Zeta centrifuge	41%–54% in both sexes	Fraction: 0.41–0.54	Significance similar to ESR
Hematocrit	Males: 42%–50%	Volume fraction: 0.42–0.5	Decreased in severe anemias, anemia of pregnancy, acute massive blood loss
	Females: 40%–48%	Volume fraction: 0.4–0.48	Increased in erythrocytosis of any cause, and in dehydration or hemoconcentration associated with shock

(continued)

Reference Ranges—Hematology* (continued)

| Determination | Reference Range | | Clinical Significance |
	Conventional Units	SI Units	
Hemoglobin	Males: 13–18 g/dl Females: 12–16 gm/dl	2.02–2.79 mmol/L 1.86–2.48 mmol/L	Decreased in various anemias, pregnancy, severe or prolonged hemorrhage, and with excessive fluid intake Increased in polycythemia, chronic obstructive pulmonary disease, failure of oxygenation because of congestive heart failure, and normally in people living at high altitudes
Hemoglobin F	Less than 2% of total hemoglobin	Mass fraction: <0.02	Increased in infants and children, and in thalassemia and many anemias
Leukocyte alkaline phosphatase	Score of 40–100		Increased in polycythemia vera, myelofibrosis, and infections Decreased in chronic granulocytic leukemia, paroxysmal nocturnal hemoglobinuria, hypoplastic marrow, and viral infections, particularly infectious mononucleosis
Leukocyte count Neutrophils Eosinophils Basophils Lymphocytes Monocytes	Total: 5,000–10,000/cu mm 60%–70% 1%–4% 0%–0.5% 20%–30% 2%–6%	$5–10 \times 10^9$/L Number fraction: 0.6–0.7 Number fraction: 0.01–0.04 Number fraction: 0.00–0.05 Number fraction: 0.2–0.3 Number fraction: 0.02–0.06	Elevated in acute infectious diseases, predominantly in the neutrophilic fraction with bacterial diseases, and in the lymphocytic and monocytic fractions in viral diseases Elevated in acute leukemia, following menstruation, and following surgery or trauma Depressed in aplastic anemia, agranulocytosis, and by toxic agents such as chemotherapeutic agents used in treating malignancy Eosinophils elevated in collagen disease, allergy, intestinal parasitosis
Osmotic fragility of red cells	Increased if hemolysis occurs in over 0.5% NaCl Decreased if hemolysis is incomplete in 0.3% NaCl		Increased in congenital spherocytosis, idiopathic acquired hemolytic anemia, isoimmune hemolytic disease, ABO hemolytic disease of newborn Decreased in sickle cell anemia, thalassemia
Platelet count	100,000–400,000/cu mm	$0.1–0.4 \times 10^{12}$/L	Increased in malignancy, myeloproliferative disease, rheumatoid arthritis, and postoperatively; about 50% of patients with unexpected increase of platelet count will be found to have a malignancy Decreased in thrombocytopenic purpura, acute leukemia, aplastic anemia, and during cancer chemotherapy, infections, and drug reactions

* Laboratory values vary according to the techniques used in different laboratories.

Reference Ranges—Serum, Plasma, and Whole Blood Chemistries

Determination	Normal Adult Reference Range		Clinical Significance	
	Conventional Units	SI Units	Increased	Decreased
Acetoacetate	0.2–1.0 mg/dl	19.6–98 μmol/L	Diabetic acidosis Fasting	
Acetone	0.3–2.0 mg/dl	51.6–344.0 μmol/L	Toxemia of pregnancy Carbohydrate-free diet High-fat diet	
Acid, total phosphatase	0–11 UL	0–11 UL	Carcinoma of prostate Advanced Paget's disease Hyperparathyroidism Gaucher's disease	
Acid, phosphatase, prostatic—RIA	0–10 ng/ml Borderline: 2.5–3.3 IU/L	0–10 μg/L	Carcinoma of prostate	
Alkaline phosphatase	Adults: 30–115 mU/ml	30–115 μ/L	Conditions reflecting increased osteoblastic activity of bone Rickets Hyperparathyroidism Liver disease	
Alkaline phosphatase, thermostable fraction	Thermostable fraction >35%: hepatic disease and combined disease with predominant hepatic component Thermostable fraction between 25% and 35%: combined hepatic and skeletal disease Thermostable fraction <25%: skeletal disease with increased osteoblastic activity		Hepatic disease	
Adrenocorticotropic hormone (ACTH) (plasma)—RIA*	Less than 50 pg/ml	Less than 50 mg/L	Pituitary-dependent Cushing's syndrome Ectopic ACTH syndrome Primary adrenal atrophy	Adrenocortical tumor Adrenal insufficiency secondary to hypopituitarism
Aldolase	3–8 Sibley-Lehninger U/dl at 37°C	22–59 mU/L at 37°C	Hepatic necrosis Granulocytic leukemia Myocardial infarction Skeletal muscle disease	
Aldosterone (plasma)—RIA	Supine: 3–10 ng/dl Upright: 5–30 ng/dl Adrenal vein: 200–800 ng/dl	0.08–0.30 nmol/L 0.14–0.90 nmol/L 5.54–22.16 nmol/L	Primary aldosteronism (Conn's syndrome) Secondary aldosteronism	Addison's disease
Alpha-1-antitrypsin	200–400 mg/dl	2–4 g/L		Certain forms of chronic lung and liver disease in young adults
Alpha-1-fetoprotein	None detected		Hepatocarcinoma Metastatic carcinoma of liver Germinal cell carcinoma of the testicle or ovary Fetal neural tube defects—elevation in maternal serum	

(continued)

Reference Ranges—Serum, Plasma, and Whole Blood Chemistries *(continued)*

Determination	Normal Adult Reference Range		Clinical Significance	
	Conventional Units	SI Units	Increased	Decreased
Alpha-hydroxybutyric dehydrogenase	Up to 140 U/ml	Up to 140 U/L	Myocardial infarction Granulocytic leukemia Hemolytic anemias Muscular dystrophy	
Ammonia (plasma)	40–80 μg/dl (enzymatic method); varies considerably with method	22.2–44.3 μmol/L	Severe liver disease Hepatic decompensation	
Amylase	60–160 Somogyi U/dl	111–296 U/L	Acute pancreatitis Mumps Duodenal ulcer Carcinoma of head of pancreas Prolonged elevation with pseudocyst of pancreas Increased by drugs that constrict pancreatic duct sphincters: morphine, codeine, cholinergics	Chronic pancreatitis Pancreatic fibrosis and atrophy Cirrhosis of liver Pregnancy (2nd and 3rd trimesters)
Arsenic	6–20 μg/dl; if 50 μg/dl, suspect toxicity	0.78–2.6 μmol/L	Accidental or intentional poisoning Excessive occupational exposure	
Ascorbic acid (vitamin C)	0.4–1.5 mg/dl	23–85 μmol/L	Large doses of ascorbic acid as a prophylactic against the common cold	
Bilirubin	Total: 0.1–1.2 mg/dl Direct: 0.1–0.2 mg/dl Indirect: 0.1–1 mg/dl	1.7–20.5 μmol/L 1.7–3.4 μmol/L 1.7–17.1 μmol/L	Hemolytic anemia (indirect) Biliary obstruction and disease Hepatocellular damage (hepatitis) Pernicious anemia Hemolytic disease of newborn	

Blood gases
  Oxygen, arterial (whole blood):
    Partial pressure (PaO$_2$)
	95–100 mm Hg	12.64–13.30 kPa	Polycythemia	Anemia

Saturation (SaO$_2$)	94%–100%	Volume fraction: 0.94–1	Anhydremia	Cardiac decompensation Chronic obstructive pulmonary disease
Carbon dioxide, arterial (whole blood): partial pressure (PaCO$_2$)	35–45 mm Hg	4.66–5.99 kPa	Respiratory acidosis Metabolic alkalosis	Respiratory alkalosis Metabolic acidosis
pH (whole blood, arterial)	7.35–7.45	7.35–7.45	Vomiting Hyperpnea Fever Intestinal obstruction	Uremia Diabetic acidosis Hemorrhage Nephritis
Calcitonin	Basal: nondetectable 400 pg/ml	400 ng/L	Medullary carcinoma of the thyroid Some nonthyroid tumors Zollinger-Ellison syndrome	

(continued)

Reference Ranges—Serum, Plasma, and Whole Blood Chemistries *(continued)*

Determination	Normal Adult Reference Range		Clinical Significance	
	Conventional Units	SI Units	Increased	Decreased
Calcium	8.5–10.5 mg/dl	2.125–2.625 mmol/L	Tumor or hyperplasia of parathyroid Hypervitaminosis D Multiple myeloma Nephritis with uremia Malignant tumors Sarcoidosis Hyperthyroidism Skeletal immobilization Excess calcium intake: milk-alkali syndrome	Hypoparathyroidism Diarrhea Celiac disease Vitamin D deficiency Acute pancreatitis Nephrosis After parathyroidectomy
CO_2, venous	Adults 24–32 mEq/L Infants: 18–24 mEq/L	24–32 mmol/L 18–24 mmol/L	Tetany Respiratory disease Intestinal obstruction Vomiting	Acidosis Nephritis Eclampsia Diarrhea Anesthesia
Carcinoembryonic antigen (CEA)—RIA	0–2.5 ng/ml (nonsmoker) 0–5 ng/ml (smoker)	0–2.5 µg/L (nonsmoker) 0–5 µg/L (smoker)	The repeatedly high incidence of this antigen in cancers of the colon, rectum, pancreas, and stomach suggests that CEA levels may be useful in the therapeutic monitoring of these conditions	
Catecholamines (plasma)—RIA	Epinephrine, random: up to 90 pg/ml Norepinephrine, random 100–550 pg/ml Dopamine, random up to 130 pg/ml	Up to 490 pmol/L 590–3240 pmol/L Up to 850 pmol/L	Pheochromocytoma	
Ceruloplasmin	30–80 mg/dl	300–800 mg/L		Wilson's disease (hepatolenticular degeneration)
Chloride	95–105 mEq/L	95–105 mmol/L	Nephrosis Nephritis Urinary obstruction Cardiac decompensation Anemia	Diabetes Diarrhea Vomiting Pneumonia Heavy metal poisoning Cushing's syndrome Burns Intestinal obstruction Febrile conditions
Cholesterol	150–200 mg/dl	3.9–5.2 mmol/L	Lipemia Obstructive jaundice Diabetes Hypothyroidism	Pernicious anemia Hemolytic anemia Hyperthyroidism Severe infection Terminal states of debilitating disease
Cholesterol esters	60%–70% of total	Fraction of total cholesterol 0.6–0.7		The esterified fraction decreases in liver diseases
Cholinesterase	Serum: 0.6–1.6 delta pH Red cells: 0.6–1 delta pH	0.6–1.6 U 0.6–1 U	Nephrosis Exercise	Nerve gas intoxication (greater effect on red cell activity) Insecticides, organic phosphates (greater effect on plasma activity)
Chorionic gonadotropin, beta subunit—RIA	0–5 IU/L	0–5 IU/L	Pregnancy Hydatidiform mole Choriocarcinoma	

(continued)

Reference Ranges—Serum, Plasma, and Whole Blood Chemistries *(continued)*

Determination	Normal Adult Reference Range		Clinical Significance	
	Conventional Units	SI Units	Increased	Decreased
Complement, human C₃	70–150 mg/dl	880–2520 mg/L	Some inflammatory diseases, acute myocardial infarction, cancer	Acute glomerulonephritis Disseminated lupus erythematosus with renal involvement
Complement C₄	16–45 mg/dl	140–510 mg/L	Some inflammatory diseases, acute myocardial infarction, cancer	Often decreased in immunologic disease, especially with active systemic lupus erythematosus Hereditary angioneurotic edema
Complement, total (hemolytic)	90%–94% complement	25–70 U/ml	Some inflammatory diseases	Acute glomerulonephritis Epidemic meningitis Subacute bacterial endocarditis
Copper	70–165 µg/dl	11–25.9 µmol/L	Cirrhosis of liver Pregnancy	Wilson's disease
Cortisol–RIA	8 AM: 7–25 µg/dl 4 PM: 2–9 µg/dl	193–690 nmol/L 55–248 nmol/L	Stress: infectious disease, surgery, burns, *etc.* Pregnancy Cushing's syndrome Pancreatitis Eclampsia	Addison's disease Anterior pituitary hypofunction
C-peptide reactivity	1.5–10 ng/ml	1.5–10 µg/L	Insulinoma	Diabetes
Creatine	0.2–0.8 mg/ml	15.3–61 µmol/L	Pregnancy Skeletal muscle necrosis or atrophy Starvation Hyperthyroidism	
Creatine phosphokinase (CPK)	Males: 50–325 mU/ml Females: 50–250 mU/ml	50–325 U/L 50–250 U/L	Myocardial infarction Skeletal muscle diseases Intramuscular injections Crush syndrome Hypothyroidism Alcohol withdrawal delirium Alcoholic myopathy Cerebrovascular disease	
Creatine phosphokinase isoenzymes	MM band present (skeletal muscle); MB band absent (heart muscle)		MB band increased in myocardial infarction, ischemia	
Creatinine	0.7–1.4 mg/dl	62–124 µmol/L	Nephritis Chronic renal disease	Kidney diseases
Creatinine clearance	100–150 ml of blood cleared of creatinine per min	1.67–2.5 ml/s		
Cryoglobulins, qualitative	Negative		Multiple myeloma Chronic lymphocytic leukemia Lymphosarcoma Systemic lupus erythematosus Rheumatoid arthritis Infective subacute endocarditis Some malignancies Scleroderma	
11-Deoxycortisol	1 µg/dl	<0.029 µmol/L	Hypertensive form of virilizing adrenal hyperplasia due to an 11-β-hydroxylase defect	

(continued)

Reference Ranges—Serum, Plasma, and Whole Blood Chemistries *(continued)*

Determination	Normal Adult Reference Range		Clinical Significance	
	Conventional Units	SI Units	Increased	Decreased
Dibucaine number	Normal: 70%–85% inhibition Heterozygote: 50%–65% inhibition Homozygote: 16%–25% inhibition			Important in detecting carriers of abnormal cholinesterase activity who are susceptible to succinyldicholine anesthetic shock
Dihydrotestosterone	Males: 50–210 ng/dl Females: none detectable	1.72–7.22 nmol/L		Testicular feminization syndrome
Estradiol—RIA	Females: Follicular: 10–90 pg/ml Midcycle: 100–500 pg/ml Luteal: 50–240 pg/ml Follicular phase: 2–20 ng/dl Midcycle: 12–40 ng/dl Luteal phase: 10–30 ng/dl Postmenopausal: 1–5 ng/dl Males: 0.5–5 ng/dl	37–370 pmol/L 367–1835 pmol/L 184–881 pmol/L	Pregnancy	Depressed or failure to peak—ovarian failure
Estriol—RIA	Nonpregnant females: <0.5 ng/ml Pregnant females: 1st trimester: up to 1 ng/ml 2nd trimester: 0.8–7 ng/ml 3rd trimester: 5–25 ng/ml	<1.75 nmol/L Up to 3.5 nmol/L 2.8–24.3 nmol/L 17.4–86.8 nmol/L	Pregnancy	Depressed or failure to peak—ovarian failure
Estrogens, total—RIA	Females: cycle days: Day 1–10: 61–394 pg/ml Day 11–20: 122–437 pg/ml Day 21–30: 156–350 pg/ml Males: 40–115 pg/ml	61–394 ng/L 122–437 ng/L 156–350 ng/L 40–115 ng/L	Pregnancy Measured on a daily basis, can be used to evaluate response of hypogonadotrophic, hypoestrogenic women to human menopausal or pituitary gonadotropin	Fetal distress Ovarian failure
Estrone—RIA	Females: Day 1–10: 4.3–18 ng/dl Day 11–20: 7.5–19.6 ng/dl Day 21–30: 13–20 ng/dl Males: 2.5–7.5 ng/dl	15.9–66.6 pmol/L 27.8–72.5 pmol/L 48.1–74 pmol/L 9.3–27.8 pmol/L		Depressed or failure to peak—ovarian failure
Ferritin—RIA	Males: 29–438 ng/ml Females: 9–219 ng/ml	29–438 µg/L 9–219 µg/L	Nephritis Hemochromatosis Certain neoplastic diseases Acute myelogenous leukemia Multiple myeloma	Iron deficiency

(continued)

Reference Ranges—Serum, Plasma, and Whole Blood Chemistries (continued)

Determination	Normal Adult Reference Range		Clinical Significance	
	Conventional Units	SI Units	Increased	Decreased
Folic acid—RIA	2.5–20 ng/ml	6–46 nmol/L		Megaloblastic anemias of infancy and pregnancy Inadequate diet Liver disease Malabsorption syndrome Severe hemolytic anemia

Follicle stimulating hormone (FSH)—RIA	Males: 2–10 mIU/ml
	Females:
	  Follicular phase: 5–20 mIU/ml
	  Peak of middle cycle: 12–30 mIU/ml
	  Luteinic phase: 5–15 mIU/ml
	  Menopausal females: 40–200 mIU/ml
		5–20 IU/L
		
		12–30 IU/L
		
		5–15 IU/L
		40–200 IU/L
			Menopause and primary ovarian failure	Pituitary failure

Galactose	<5 mg/dl	<0.28 mmol/L		Galactosemia
Gamma glutamyl transpeptidase	Males: <45 IU/L Females: <30 IU/L	45 U/L 30 U/L	Hepatobiliary disease Anicteric alcoholics Drug therapy damage Myocardial infarction Renal infarction	
Gastrin—RIA	Fasting: 50–155 pg/ml Postprandial: 80–170 pg/ml Zollinger-Ellison syndrome: 200–over 2000 pg/ml Pernicious anemia: 130–2260 pg/ml (mean 912)	50–155 ng/L 80–170 ng/L 200–over 2000 ng/L 130–2260 ng/L (mean 912)	Zollinger-Ellison syndrome Peptic ulceration of the duodenum Pernicious anemia	
Glucose	Fasting: 60–110 mg/dl Postprandial (2 h): 65–140 mg/dl	3.3–6.05 mmol/L 3.58–7.7 mmol/L	Diabetes Nephritis Hyperthyroidism Early hyperpituitarism Cerebral lesions Infections Pregnancy Uremia	Hyperinsulinism Hypothyroidism Late hyperpituitarism Pernicious vomiting Addison's disease Extensive hepatic damage

Glucose tolerance (oral)	Features of a normal response:
	1. Normal fasting between 60–110 mg/dl
	2. No sugar in urine
	3. Upper limits of normal:
	  Fasting = 125
	  1 hour = 190
	  2 hours = 140
	  3 hours = 125
		
		3.3–6.05 mmol/L
		
		6.88 mmol/L
		10.45 mmol/L
		7.70 mmol/L
		6.88 mmol/L
			(Flat or inverted curve)
			Hyperinsulinism
			Adrenal cortical insufficiency (Addison's disease)
			Anterior pituitary hypofunction
			Hypothyroidism
			Sprue and celiac diseases
				(High or prolonged curve)
				Diabetes
				Hyperthyroidism
				Primary adrenal cortical tumor or hyperplasia
				Severe anemia
				Certain central nervous system disorders

Glucose-6-phosphate dehydrogenase (red cells)	Screening:
	  Decolorization in 20–100 min
	Quantitative:
	  1.86–2.5 IU/ml RBC
		
		1860–2500 U/L
				Drug-induced hemolytic anemia
				Hemolytic disease of newborn

(continued)

Reference Ranges—Serum, Plasma, and Whole Blood Chemistries *(continued)*

Determination	Normal Adult Reference Range		Clinical Significance	
	Conventional Units	SI Units	Increased	Decreased
Glycoprotein (alpha-1-acid)	40–110 mg/dl	400–1100 mg/L	Neoplasm Tuberculosis Diabetes complicated by degenerative vascular disease Pregnancy Rheumatoid arthritis Rheumatic fever Infectious liver disease Lupus erythematosus	
Growth hormone—RIA	<10 ng/ml	<10 mg/L	Acromegaly	Failure to stimulate with arginine or insulin—hypopituitarism
Haptoglobin	50–250 mg/dl	0.5–2.5 g/L	Pregnancy Estrogen therapy Chronic infections Various inflammatory conditions	Hemolytic anemia Hemolytic blood transfusion reaction
Hemoglobin (plasma)	0.5–5 mg/dl	5–50 mg/L	Transfusion reactions Paroxysmal nocturnal hemoglobinuria Intravascular hemolysis	
Hemoglobin A1 (Glycohemoglobin)	Nondiabetics & diabetics whose control of glucose is: Good: 4.4%–8.2% Fair: 8.3%–9.2% Poor: >9.2%			
Hexosaminidase, total	Controls: 333–375 nM/ml/h	333–375 μmol/L/h	Sandhoff's disease	
Hexosaminidase A	Controls: 49%–68% of total Heterozygotes: 26%–45% of total Tay–Sachs disease: 0%–4% of total Diabetics: 39%–59% of total	Fraction of total: 0.49–0.68 0.26–0.45 0–0.04 0.39–0.59		Tay–Sachs disease and heterozygotes
High-density lipoprotein cholesterol (HDL cholesterol)	Males: 35–70 mg/dL Females: 35-85 mg/dL	0.91-1.81 mmol/L 0.91-220 mmol/L		HDL cholesterol is lower in patients with increased risk for coronary heart disease

Age (yr)	Males (mg/dl)	Females (mg/dl)	Males (mmol/L)	Females (mmol/L)
0–19	30–65	30–70	0.78–1.68	0.78–1.81
20–29	35–70	35–75	0.91–1.81	0.91–1.94
30–39	30–65	35–80	0.78–1.68	0.91–2.07
40–49	30–65	40–85	0.78–1.68	1.04–2.2
50–59	30–65	35–85	0.78–1.68	0.91–2.2
60–69	30–65	35–85	0.78–1.68	0.91–2.2

Determination	Conventional Units	SI Units	Increased	Decreased
17-Hydroxy-progesterone—RIA	Males: 0.4–4 ng/ml Females: 0.1–3.3 ng/ml Children: 0.1–0.5 ng/ml	1.2–12 nmol/L 0.3–10 nmol/L 0.3–1.5 nmol/L	Congenital adrenal hyperplasia Pregnancy Some cases of adrenal or ovarian adenomas	

(continued)

Reference Ranges—Serum, Plasma, and Whole Blood Chemistries (continued)

Determination	Normal Adult Reference Range		Clinical Significance	
	Conventional Units	SI Units	Increased	Decreased
Immunoglobulin A	Adults: 50–300 mg/ dl (in children the normals are lower and vary with age)	0.5–3 g/L	Gamma A myeloma Wiskott-Aldrich syndrome Autoimmune disease Hepatic cirrhosis	Ataxia telangiectasis Agammaglobulinemia Hypogammaglobulinemia, transient Dysgammaglobulinemia Protein-losing enteropathies
Immunoglobulin D	0–30 mg/dl	0–300 mg/L	IgD multiple myeloma Some patients with chronic infectious diseases	
Immunoglublin E	20–740 ng/mL	20–740 µg/L	Allergic patients and those with parasitic infections	
Immonoglublin G	Adults: 565–1765 mg/dl	6.35–14 g/L	IgG myeloma Following hyperimmunization Autoimmune disease states Chronic infections	Congenital and acquired hypogammaglobulinemia IgA myelomas, Waldenström's (IgM) macroglobulinemia Some malabsorption syndromes Extensive protein loss
Immunoglobulin M	Adults: 55–375 mg/dl	0.4–2.8 g/L	Waldenström's macroglobulinemia Parasitic infections Hepatitis	Agammaglobulinemias Some IgG and IgA myelomas Chronic lymphatic leukemia
Insulin—RIA	5–25 µU/ml	0.2–1 µg/L	Insulinoma Acromegaly	Diabetes mellitus
Iron	50–160 µg/dl	9–29 µmol/L	Pernicious anemia Aplastic anemia Hemolytic anemia Hepatitis Hemochromatosis	Iron-deficiency anemia
Iron-binding capacity	IBC: 150–235 µg/dl TIBC: 230–410 µg/dl % Saturation: 20–50	26.9–42.1 µmol/L 41–73 µmol/L Fracton of total iron-binding capacity: 0.2–0.5	Iron deficiency anemia Acute and chronic blood loss Hepatitis	Chronic infectious diseases Cirrhosis
Isocitric dehydrogenase	50–180 U	0.83–3 U/L	Hepatitis: cirrhosis Obstructive jaundice Metastatic carcinoma of the liver Megaloblastic anemia	
Lactic acid (whole blood)	Venous: 5–20 mg/dl Arterial: 3–7 mg/dl	0.6–2.2 mmol/L 0.3–0.8 mmol/L	Increased muscular activity Congestive heart failure Hemorrhage Shock Some varieties of metabolic acidosis Some febrile infections May be increased in severe liver disease	
Lactic dehydrogenase (LDH)	100–225 mU/ml	100–225 U/L	Untreated pernicious anemia Myocardial infarction Pulmonary infarction Liver disease	
Lactic dehydrogenase isoenzymes Total lactic dehydrogenase	100–225 mU/ml	100–225 U/L Fraction of total LDH:	LDH-1 and LDH-2 are increased in myocardial infarction, megaloblastic anemia, and hemoltyic anemia LDH-4 and LDH-5 are increased in pulmonary infarction, congestive heart failure, and liver disease	
LDH-1	20%–35%	0.2–0.35		
LDH-2	25%–40%	0.25–0.4		
LDH-3	20%–30%	0.2–0.3		
LDH-4	0–20%	0–0.2		
LDH-5	0–25%	0–0.25		
Lead (whole blood)	Up to 40 µg/dl	Up to 2 µmol/L	Lead poisoning	

(continued)

Reference Ranges—Serum, Plasma, and Whole Blood Chemistries *(continued)*

Determination	Normal Adult Reference Range		Clinical Significance	
	Conventional Units	SI Units	Increased	Decreased
Leucine aminopeptidase	80–200 U/ml	19.2–48 U/L	Liver or bilary tract diseases Pancreatic disease Metastatic carcinoma of liver and pancreas Biliary obstruction	
Lipase	0.2–1.5 U/ml	55–417 U/L	Acute and chronic pancreatitis Biliary obstruction Cirrhosis Hepatitis Peptic ulcer	
Lipids, total	400–1000 mg/dl	4–10 g/L	Hypothyroidism Diabetes Nephrosis Glomerulonephritis Hyperlipoproteinemias	Hyperthyroidism

Lipoprotein Phenotype: Summary of Findings in the Primary Hyperlipoproteinemias

Type	Frequency	Appearance	Triglyceride	Cholesterol	Lipoprotein Staining				Secondary Causes
					Beta	Pre-Beta	Alpha	Chylomicrons	
Normal		Clear	Normal	Normal	Moderate	Zero to moderate	Moderate	Weak	
I	Very rare	Creamy	Markedly increased	Normal to moderately increased	Weak	Weak	Weak	Markedly increased	Dysglobulinemia
II	Common	Clear	Normal to slightly increased	Slightly to markedly increased	Strong	Zero to strong	Moderate	Weak	Hypothyroidism, myeloma, hepatic syndrome, macroglobulinemia, and high dietary cholesterol
III	Uncommon	Clear, cloudy, or milky	Increased	Increased	Broad intense band	Extends into beta	Moderate	Weak	
IV	Very common	Clear, cloudy, or milky	Slightly to markedly increased	Normal to slightly increased	Weak to moderate	Moderate to strong	Weak to moderate	Weak	Hypothyroidism, diabetes mellitus, pancreatitis, glycogen storage diseases, nephrotic syndrome, myeloma, pregnancy, and oral contraceptives
V	Rare	Cloudy to creamy	Markedly increased	Increased	Weak	Moderate	Weak	Strong	Diabetes mellitus, pancreatitis, and alcoholism

Types I and II are fat induced; types III and IV are carbohydrate induced; type V is fat and carbohydrate induced.

Lithium	Usual maintenance level: 0.5–1 mEq/L	0.5–1 mmol/L		

(continued)

Reference Ranges—Serum, Plasma, and Whole Blood Chemistries (continued)

Determination	Normal Adult Reference Range		Clinical Significance	
	Conventional Units	SI Units	Increased	Decreased
Low-density lipoprotein cholesterol (LDL cholesterol)	mg/dL <130 (desirable) 130–159 (borderline) >160 (high risk)		LDL cholesterol is higher in patients with increased risk for coronary heart disease	

Luteinizing hormone—RIA	Males: 4.9–15 mIU/ml
	Females:
	  Follicular phase: 2–3 mIU/ml
	  Ovulatory peak: 40–200 mIU/ml
	  Luteal phase: 0–20 mIU/ml
	  Postmenopausal: 35–120 mIU/ml
		4.9–15 mg/L
		
		0.5–6.9 mg/L
		
		9.2–46 mg/L
		
		0–5 mg/L
		
		8–27.5 mg/L
			Pituitary tumor
			Ovarian failure
				Depressed or failure to peak—pituitary failure

Lysozyme (muramidase)	2.8–8 µg/ml	2.8–8 mg	Certain types of leukemia (acute monocytic leukemia) Inflammatory states and infections	Acute lymphocytic leukemia
Magnesium	1.3–2.4 mEq/L	0.7–1.2 mmol/L	Excess ingestion of magnesium-containing antacids	Chronic alcoholism Severe renal disease Diarrhea Defective growth
Manganese	0.04–1.4 µg/dl	72.9–255 nmol/L		
Mercury	Up to 10 µg/dl	Up to 0.5 µmol/L	Mercury poisoning	
Myoglobin—RIA	Up to 85 ng/ml	Up to 85 µg/ml	Myocardial infarction Muscle necrosis	
5' Nucleotidase	3.2–11.6 IU/L	3.2–11.6 U/L	Hepatobiliary disease	
Osmolality	280–300 mOsm/kg	280–300 mmol/L	Useful in the study of electrolyte and water balance	Inappropriate secretion of antidiuretic hormone
Parathyroid hormone	160–350 pg/ml	160–350 ng/L	Hyperparathyroidism	
Phenylalanine	1.2–3.5 mg/dl 1st week 0.7–3.5 mg/dl thereafter	0.07–0.21 mmol/L 0.04–0.21 mmol/L	Phenylketonuria	
Phosphohexose isomerase	20–90 IU/L	20–90 U/L	Malignancy Disease of heart, liver, and skeletal muscles	
Phospholipids	125–300 mg/dl	1.25–3 g/L	Diabetes Nephritis	
Phosphorus, inorganic	2.5–4.5 mg/dl	0.8–1.45 mmol/L	Chronic nephritis Hypoparathyroidism	Hyperparathyroidism Vitamin D deficiency
Potassium	3.8–5 mEq/L	3.8–5 mmol/L	Addison's disease Oliguria Anuria Tissue breakdown or hemolysis	Diabetic acidosis Diarrhea Vomiting
Progesterone—RIA	Folliclular phase: up to 0.8 ng/ml Luteal phase: 10–20 ng/ml End of cycle: <1 ng/ml Pregnant: up to 50 ng/ml in 20th week	2.5 nmol/L 31.8–63.6 nmol/L <3 nmol/L Up to 160 nmol/L	Useful in evaluation of menstrual disorders and infertility and in the evaluation of placental function during pregnancies complicated by toxemia, diabetes mellitus, or threatened miscarriage	

(continued)

Reference Ranges—Serum, Plasma, and Whole Blood Chemistries (continued)

Determination	Normal Adult Reference Range		Clinical Significance	
	Conventional Units	SI Units	Increased	Decreased
Prolactin—RIA	6–24 ng/ml	6–24 µg/L	Pregnancy Functional or structural disorders of the hypothalamus Pituitary stalk section Pituitary tumors	
Prostate-specific antigen	<4 ng/ml		Prostatic cancer, benign prostatic hyperplasia, prostatitis	
Protein, total Albumin Globulin	6–8 gm/dl 3.5–5 gm/dl 1.5–3 gm/dl	60–80 g/L 35–50 g/L 15–30 g/L	Hemoconcentration Shock Multiple myeloma (globulin fraction) Chronic infections (globulin fraction) Liver disease (globulin)	Malnutrition Hemorrhage Loss of plasma from burns Proteinuria
Protein Electrophoresis (cellulose acetate) Albumin Alpha-1 globulin Alpha-2 globulin Beta globulin Gamma globulin	 3.5–5 gm/dl 0.2–0.4 gm/dl 0.6–1 gm/dl 0.6–1.2 gm/dl 0.7–1.5 gm/dl	35–50 g/L 2–4 g/L 6–10 g/L 6–12 g/L 7–15 g/L		
Protoporphyrin erythrocyte (whole blood)	15–100 µg/dl	0.27–1.80 µmol/L	Lead toxicity Erythropoietic porphyria	
Pyridoxine	3.6–18 ng/ml			A wide spectrum of clinical conditions, such as mental depression, peripheral neuropathy, anemia, neonatal seizures, and reactions to certain drug therapies
Pyruvic acid (whole blood)	0.3–0.7 mg/dl	34–80 µmol/L	Diabetes Severe thiamine deficiency Acute phase of some infections, possibly secondary to increased glycogenolysis and glycolysis	
Renin (plasma)—RIA	Normal diet: Supine: 0.3–1.9 ng/ml/h Upright: 0.6–3.6 ng/ml/h Low salt diet: Supine: 0.9–4.5 ng/ml/h Upright: 4.1–9.1 ng/ml/h	0.08–0.52 ng/L/S 0.16–1.00 µg/L/S 0.25–1.25 µg/L/S 1.13–2.53 µg/L/S	Renovascular hypertension Malignant hypertension Untreated Addison's disease Primary salt-losing nephropathy Low-salt diet Diuretic therapy Hemorrhage	Frank primary aldosteronism Increased salt intake Salt-retaining steroid therapy Antidiuretic hormone therapy Blood transfusion
Sodium	135–145 mEq/L	135–145 mmol/L	Hemoconcentration Nephritis Pyloric obstruction	Alkali deficit Addison's disease Myxedema
Sulfate (inorganic)	0.5–1.5 mg/dl	0.05–0.15 mmol/L	Nephritis Nitrogen retention	

(continued)

Reference Ranges—Serum, Plasma, and Whole Blood Chemistries *(continued)*

Determination	Normal Adult Reference Range		Clinical Significance	
	Conventional Units	SI Units	Increased	Decreased

Testosterone—RIA	Females: 25–100 ng/dl
	Males: 300–800 ng/dl
		0.9–3.5 nmol/L
		10.5–28 nmol/L
			Females:
			  Polycystic ovary
			  Virilizing tumors
				Males:
				  Orchidectomy for
				    neoplastic disease of
				    the prostate or breast
				  Estrogen therapy
				  Klinefelter's syndrome
				  Hypopituitarism
				  Hypogonadism
				  Hepatic cirrhosis

T_3 (triiodothyronine) uptake	25%–35%	Relative uptake fraction: 0.25–0.35	Hyperthyroidism Thyroxine-binding globulin (TBG) deficiency Androgens and anabolic steroids	Hypothyroidism Pregnancy TBG excess Estrogens and antiovulatory drugs
T_3, total circulating—RIA	75–200 ng/dl	1.15–3.1 nmol/L	Pregnancy Hyperthyroidism	Hypothyroidism
T_4 (thyroxine)—RIA	4.5–11.5 µg/dl	58.5–150 nmol/L	Hyperthyroidism Thyroiditis Elevated thyroxine-binding proteins caused by oral contraceptives Pregnancy	Primary and pituitary hypothyroidism Idiopathic involvement Cases of diminished thyroxine-binding proteins caused by androgenic and anabolic steroids Hypoproteinemia Nephrotic syndrome
T_4, free	1–2.2 ng/dl	13–30 pmol/L	Euthyroid patients with normal free thyroxine levels may have abnormal T_3 and T_4 levels caused by drug preparations	
Thyroid-stimulating hormone (TSH)—RIA		0.3–5 m/IU/L	Hypothyroidism	Hyperthyroidism
Thyroid-binding globulin	10–26 µg/dl	100–260 µg/L	Hypothyroidism Pregnancy Estrogen therapy Oral contraceptives Genetic and idiopathic	Androgens and anabolic steroids Nephrotic syndrome Marked hypoproteinemia Hepatic disease
Transaminase, serum glutamic-oxaloacetate (SGOT, aspartate aminotransferase)	7–40 U/ml	4–20 U/L	Myocardial infarction Skeletal muscle disease Liver disease	
Transaminase, serum glutamic-oxaloacetate (SGPT, alanine aminotransferase)	10–40 U/ml	5–20 U/L	Same conditions as SGOT, but increase is more marked in liver disease than SGOT	
Transferrin	230–320 mg/dl	2.3–3.2 g/L	Pregnancy Iron-deficiency anemia due to hemorrhaging Acute hepatitis Polycythemia Oral contraceptives	Pernicious anemia in relapse Thalassemic and sickle cell anemia Chromatosis Neoplastic and hepatic diseases
Triglycerides	10–150 mg/dl	0.10–1.65 mmol/L	See *Lipoprotein Phenotype*	
Tryptophan	1.4–3 mg/dl	68.6–147 nmol/L		Tryptophan-specific malabsorption syndrome
Tyrosine	0.5–4 mg/dl	27.6–220.8 mmol/L	Tyrosinosis	

(continued)

Reference Ranges—Serum, Plasma, and Whole Blood Chemistries *(continued)*

Determination	Normal Adult Reference Range		Clinical Significance	
	Conventional Units	SI Units	Increased	Decreased
Urea nitrogen (BUN)	10–20 mg/dl	3.6–7.2 mmol/L	Acute glomerulonephritis Obstructive uropathy Mercury poisoning Nephrotic syndrome	Severe hepatic failure Pregnancy
Uric acid	2.5–8 mg/dl	0.15–0.5 mmol/L	Gouty arthritis Acute leukemia Lymphomas treated by chemotherapy Toxemia of pregnancy	Xanthinuria Defective tubular reabsorption
Viscosity	1.4–1.8 relative to water at 37°C (98.6°F)		Patients with marked increases of the gamma globulins	
Vitamin A	50–220 μg/dl	1.75–7.7 μmol/L	Hypervitaminosis A	Vitamin A deficiency Celiac disease Sprue Obstructive jaundice Giardiasis Parenchymal hepatic disease
Vitamin B$_1$ (thiamine)	1.6–4 μg/dl	47.4–135.7 nmol/L		Anorexia Beriberi Polyneuropathy Cardiomyopathies
Vitamin B$_6$ (pyridoxal phosphate)	3.6–18 ng/ml	14.6–72.8 nmol/L		Chronic alcoholism Malnutrition Uremia Neonatal seizures Malabsorption, such as celiac syndrome
Vitamin B$_{12}$—RIA	130–785 pg/ml	100–580 pmol/L	Hepatic cell damage and in association with the myeloproliferative disorders (the highest levels are encountered in myeloid leukemia)	Strict vegetarianism Alcoholism Pernicious anemia Total or partial gastrectomy Ileal resection Sprue and celiac disease Fish tapeworm infestation
Vitamin E	0.5–2 mg/dl	11.6–46.4 μmol/L		Vitamin E deficiency
Xylose absorption test	2 hr, 30–50 mg/dl	2–3.35 mmol/L		Malabsorption syndrome
Zinc	55–150 μg/dl	7.65–22.95 μmol/L	Zinc is essential for the growth and propagation of cell cultures and the functioning of several enzymes	

* By radioimmunoassay.

Reference Ranges—Immunodiagnostic Tests

Determination	Normal Value	Clinical Significance
Acetylcholine receptor binding antibody	Negative or <0.03 nmol/L	Considered to be diagnostic for myasthenia gravis in patients with symptoms.
Anti-ds-DNA antibody	<70 U by enzyme-linked immunosorbent assay (ELISA) <1:20 by indirect fluorescence	Valuable in supporting diagnosis or monitoring disease activity and prognosis of systemic lupus erythematosus (SLE).
Antiglomerular basement membrane antibody	Negative or less than 10 U	Primarily used in the differential diagnosis of glomerular nephritis induced by antiglomerular basement membrane antibodies from other types of glomerular nephritis.
Anti-insulin antibody	<3% binding of labeled beef and pork insulin by patient's serum; or <9 mIU/L	Helpful in determining the best therapeutic agent in diabetics and the cause of allergic manifestations. Also used to identify insulin resistance.
Antimitchondrial antibody and anti–smooth muscle antibody	<1:5 and <1:20, respectively	Increased in cirrhosis, autoimmune disease, thyroiditis, pernicious anemia.
Antinuclear antibody	Negative, <1:20	Increased in SLE, chronic hepatitis, scleroderma, leukemia, and mononucleosis.
Anti–parietal cell antibody	Negative, <1:20	Helpful in diagnosing chronic gastric disease and differentiating autoimmune pernicious anemia from other megaloblastic anemias.
Antiribonucleoprotein antibody	Negative	Helpful in differential diagnosis of systemic rheumatic disease.
Antiscleroderma antibody	Negative	Highly diagnostic for scleroderma.
Anti-Smith antibody	Negative	Highly diagnostic of SLE.
Anti-SS-A anti-SS-B antibody	Negative	SS-A antibodies are found in Sjögren's syndrome alone or associated with lupus. SS-B antibodies are associated with primary Sjögren's syndrome.
Antithyroglobulin and antimicrosomal antibodies	<1:100 titer by gelatin or hemagglutination	Presence and concentration is important in evaluation and treatment of various thyroid disorders, such as Hashimoto's thyroiditis and Graves' disease. May indicate previous autoimmune disorders.
CA 15-3 tumor marker	<22 IU/ml	Increased in metastatic breast cancer.
CA 19-9 tumor marker	<37 IU/ml	Increased in pancreatic, hepatobiliary, gastric, and colorectal cancer; gallstones.
CA 125	0–35 IU/ml	Increased in colon, upper gastrointestinal (GI), ovarian, and other gynecologic cancers; pregnancy, peritonitis.
Cold agglutinins	<1:16	Increased in mycoplasma pneumonia, viral illness, mononucleosis, multiple myeloma, scleroderma.
C-reactive protein	<0.8 mg/dl	Increase indicates active inflammation.
Hepatitis A virus antibodies, IgM (HAV-Ab/IgM)	Negative	Positive in acute-stage hepatitis A; develops early in disease.
Hepatitis A virus antibodies, IgG (HAV-Ab/IgG)	Negative	Positive if previous exposure and immunity to hepatitis A.
Hepatitis B surface antigen (HBsAg)	Negative	Positive in acute-stage hepatitis B.
Hepatitis B surface antibody (HBsAb)	Negative	Positive if previous exposure and immunity to hepatitis B.
Infectious mononucleosis tests (monospot, mono-test, heterophile antigen test, Epstein–Barr virus (EBV), antiviral capsid antigen IgM and IgG)	Negative, <1:80	Positive monospot and monotest are presumptive; positive EBV IgM and IgG indicate acute and recent or past infection, respectively.
Lyme disease titer	Negative, <1:256 by indirect fluorescent antibody method <0.8 by ELISA	Positive results help diagnose Lyme disease. False positive may occur with high rheumatoid factor titers or syphilis. Positive ELISA confirmed by Western blot test.

(continued)

Reference Ranges—Immunodiagnostic Tests *(continued)*

Determination	Normal Value	Clinical Significance
Pyroglobulin test	Negative	These abnormal proteins may be associated with myeloma, lymphoma, polycythemia vera, and SLE.
Rheumatoid factor	Negative or less than 60 IU/ml	Elevated in rheumatoid arthritis, lupus, endocarditis, tuberculosis, syphilis, sarcoidosis, cancer.

T and B cell lymphocyte surface markers T-helper/T-suppressor ratio	T and B surface markers:
	  Percent T cells (CD2) 60–88%
	  Percent helper cells (CD4) 34–67%
	  Percent suppressor cells (CD8) 10–42%
	  Percent B cells (CD19) 3–21%
	Absolute counts:
	  Lymphocytes 0.66–4.60 thou/ml
	  T cells 644–2201 cells/ml
	  Helper cells 493–1191 cells/ml
	  Suppressor T cells 182–785 cells/ml
	  B cells 92–392 cells/ml
	Lymphocyte ratio:
	  T_H/T_S ratio > 1
		Done to evaluate immune system by identifying the specific cells involved in the immune response. Valuable in diagnosis of lymphocytic leukemia, lymphoma, and immunodeficiency diseases including acquired immunodeficiency syndrome, and in the assessment of patient response to chemotherapy and radiation.

Reference Ranges—Urine Chemistry

Determination	Normal Adult Reference Range — Conventional Units	Normal Adult Reference Range — SI Units	Clinical Significance — Increased	Clinical Significance — Decreased
Acetone and acetoacetate	Zero		Uncontrolled diabetes Starvation	
Acid mucopolysaccharides	Negative		Hurler syndrome Marfan syndrome Morquio-Ullrich disease	

Aldosterone	Normal salt:
	  Normal: 4–20 μg/24 h
	  Renovascular: 10–40 μg/24 h
	  Tumor: 20–100 μg/24 h
		11.1–55.5 nmol/24 h
		27.7–111 nmol/24 h
		55.4–277 nmol/24 h
			Primary aldosteronism (adenocortical tumor) Secondary aldosteronism Salt depletion Potassium loading ACTH in large doses Cardiac failure Cirrhosis with ascites formation Nephrosis Pregnancy	

Alpha amino nitrogen	50–200 mg/24 h	3.6–14.3 mmol/24 h	Leukemia Diabetes Phenylketonuria Other metabolic diseases	
Amylase	35–260 units excreted per h	6.5–48.1 U/h	Acute pancreatitis	
Arylsulfatase A	>2.4 U/ml			Metachromatic leukodystrophy
Bence-Jones protein	None detected		Myeloma	
Calcium	<150 mg/24 h	<3.75 mmol/24 h	Hyperparathyroidism Vitamin D intoxication Fanconi's syndrome	Hypoparathyroidism Vitamin D deficiency
Catecholamines	Total: 0–275 μg/24 h Epinephrine: 10%–40% Norepinephrine: 60%–90%	0–275 μg/24 h Fraction total: 0.10–8.4 Fraction total: 0.60–0.90	Pheochromocytoma Neuroblastoma	

(continued)

Reference Ranges—Urine Chemistry (continued)

Determination	Normal Adult Reference Range		Clinical Significance	
	Conventional Units	SI Units	Increased	Decreased
Chorionic gonadotrophin, qualitative (pregnancy test)	Negative		Pregnancy Chorionepithelioma Hydatidiform mole	
Copper	20–70 μg/24 h	0.32–1.12 μmol/24 h	Wilson's disease Cirrhosis Nephrosis	
Coproporphyrin	50–300 μg/24 h	0.075–0.45 μmol/24 h	Poliomyelitis Lead poisoning Porphyria hepatica Porphyria erythropoietica Porphyria cutanea tarda	
Cortisol, free	20–90 μg/24 h	55.2–248.4 nmol/d	Cushing's syndrome	
Creatine	0–200 mg/24 h	0–1.52 mmol/24 h	Muscular dystrophy Fever Carcinoma of liver Pregnancy Hyperthryoidism Myositis	
Creatinine	0.8–2 gm/24 h	7–17.6 mmol/24 h	Typhoid fever Salmonella infections Tetanus	Muscular atrophy Anemia Advanced degeneration of kidneys Leukemia
Creatinine clearance	100–150 ml of blood cleared of creatinine per min	1.67–2.5 ml/s		Measures glomerular filtration rate Renal diseases
Cystine and cysteine	10–100 mg/24 h	0.08–0.83 mmol/24 h	Cystinuria	
Delta aminolevulinic acid	0–0.54 mg/dl	0–40 μmol/L	Lead poisoning Porphyria hepatica Hepatitis Hepatic carcinoma	
11-Desoxycortisol	20–100 μg/24 h	0.6–2.9 μmol/d	Hypertensive form of virilizing adrenal hyperplasia due to an 11-beta hydroxylase defect	
Estriol (placental)	**Weeks of pregnancy** μm/24 h 12 <1 16 2–7 20 4–9 24 6–13 28 8–22 32 12–43 36 14–45 40 19–46	nmol/24 h <3.5 7–24.5 14–32 21–45.5 28–77 42–150 49–158 66.5–160		Decreased values occur with fetal distress of many conditions, including preeclampsia, placental insufficiency, and poorly controlled diabetes mellitus
Estrogens, total (fluorometric)	Females: Onset of menstruation: 4–25 μg/24 h Ovulation peak: 28 μg/24 h Luteal peak: 22–105 μg/24 h Menopausal: 1.4–19.6 μg/24 h Males: 5–18 μg/24 h	4–25 μg/24 h 28 μg/24 h 22–105 μg/24 h 1.4–19.6 μg/24 h 5–18 μg/24 h	Hyperestrogenism due to gonadal or adrenal neoplasm	Primary or secondary amenorrhea

(continued)

Reference Ranges—Urine Chemistry *(continued)*

Determination	Normal Adult Reference Range		Clinical Significance	
	Conventional Units	SI Units	Increased	Decreased
Etiocholanolone	Males: 1.9–6 mg/24 h	6.5–20.6 μmol/24 h	Adrenogenital syndrome	
	Females: 0.5–4 mg/24 h	1.7–13.8 μmol/24 h	Idiopathic hirsutism	
Follicle-stimulating hormone—RIA	Females:		Menopause and primary ovarian failure	Pituitary failure
	Follicular: 5–20 IU/24 h	5–20 IU/d		
	Luteal: 5–15 IU/24 h	5–15 IU/d		
	Midcycle: 15–60 IU/24 h	15–60 IU/d		
	Menopausal: 50–100 IU/24 h	50–100 IU/d		
	Males: 5–25 IU/24 h	5–25 IU/d		
Glucose	Negative		Diabetes mellitus Pituitary disorders Intracranial pressure Lesion in floor of 4th ventricle	
Hemoglobin and myoglobin	Negative		Extensive burns Transfusion of incompatible blood Myoglobin increased in severe crushing injuries to muscles	
Homogentisic acid, qualitative	Negative		Alkaptonuria Ochronosis	
Homovanillic acid	Up to 15 mg/24 h	Up to 82 μmol/d	Neuroblastoma	
17-hydroxycorticosteroids	2–10 mg/24 h	5.5–27.5 μmol/d	Cushing's disease	Addison's disease Anterior pituitary hypofunction
5-Hydroxyindoleacetic acid, qualitative	Negative		Malignant carcinoid tumors	
Hydroxyproline	15–43 mg/24 h	0.11–0.33 μmol/d	Paget disease Fibrous dysplasia Osteomalacia Neoplastic bone disease Hyperparathyroidism	
17-ketosteroids, total	Males: 10–22 mg/24 h	35–76 μmol/d	Interstitial cell tumor of testes	Thyrotoxicosis Female hypogonadism
	Females: 6–16 mg/24 h	21–55 μmol/d	Simple hirsutism, occasionally Adrenal hyperplasia Cushing's syndrome Adrenal cancer, virilism Adrenoblastoma	Diabetes mellitus Hypertension Debilitating disease of mild to moderate severity Eunuchoidism Addison's disease Panhypopituitarism Myxedema Nephrosis
Lead	Up to 150 μg/24 h	Up to 60 μmol/24 h	Lead poisoning	
Luteinizing hormone	Males: 5–18 IU/24 h		Pituitary tumor Ovarian failure	Depressed or failure to peak—pituitary failure
	Females:			
	Follicular phase: 2–25 IU/24 h	2–25 IU/d		
	Ovulatory peak: 30–95 IU/24 h	30–95 IU/d		
	Luteal phase: 2–20 IU/24 h	2–20 IU/d		
	Postmenopausal: 40–110 IU/24 h	40–110 IU/d		

(continued)

Reference Ranges—Urine Chemistry (continued)

Determination	Normal Adult Reference Range		Clinical Significance	
	Conventional Units	SI Units	Increased	Decreased
Metanephrines, total	Less than 1.3 mg/24 h	Less than 6.5 μmol/d	Pheochromocytoma; a few patients with pheochromocytoma may have elevated urinary metanephrines but normal catecholamines and vanillylmandelic acid (VMA)	
Osmolality	Males: 390–1090 mM/kg Females: 300–1090 mM/kg	390–1090 mmol/kg 300–1090 mmol/kg	Useful in the study of electrolyte and water balance	
Oxalate	Up to 40 mg/24 h	Up to 456 μmol/d	Primary hyperoxaluria	
Phenylpyruvic acid qualitative	Negative		Phenylketonuria	
Phosphorus, inorganic	0.8–1.3 gm/24 h	26–42 mmol/24 h	Hyperparathyroidism Vitamin D intoxication Paget disease Metastatic neoplasm to bone	Hypoparathyroidism Vitamin D deficiency
Porphobilinogen, qualitative	Negative		Chronic lead poisoning Acute porphyria Liver disease	
Porphobilinogen, quantitative	0–1 mg/24 h	0–4.4 μmol/24 h	Acute porphyria Liver disease	
Porphyrins, qualitative	Negative		See porphyrins, quantitative	
Porphyrins, quantitative (coproporphyrin and uroporphyrin)	Coproporphyrin: 50–160 μg/24 h Uroporphyrin: up to 50 μg/24 h	0.075–0.24 μmol/24 h Up to 0.06 μmol/24 h	Porphyria hepatica Porphyria erythropoietica Porphyria cutanea tarda Lead poisoning (only coproporphyrin increased)	
Potassium	40–65 mEq/24 h	40–65 mmol/24 h	Hemolysis	
Pregnanediol	Females: Proliferative phase: 0.5–1.5 mg/24 h Luteal phase: 2–7 mg/24 h Menopause: 0.2–1 mg/24 h Pregnancy:	1.6–4.8 μmol/24 h 6–22 μmol/24 h 0.6–3.1 μmol/24 h	Corpus luteum cysts When placental tissue remains in the uterus following parturition Some cases of adrenocortical tumors	Placental dysfunction Threatened abortion Intrauterine death

Pregnanediol Pregnancy table:

Weeks of gestation	mg/24 h	μmol/24 h
10–12	5–15	15.6–47
12–18	5–25	15.6–78.0
18–24	15–33	47.0–103.0
24–28	20–42	62.4–131.0
28–32	27–47	84.2–146.6
Males: 0.1–2 mg/24 h		0.3–6.2 μmol/24 h

Determination	Conventional Units	SI Units	Increased	Decreased
Pregnanetriol	0.4–2.4 mg/24 h	1.2–7.1 μmol/24 h	Congenital adrenal androgenic hyperplasia	

(continued)

Reference Ranges—Urine Chemistry (continued)

Determination	Normal Adult Reference Range		Clinical Significance	
	Conventional Units	SI Units	Increased	Decreased
Protein	Up to 100 mg/24 h	Up to 100 mg/24 h	Nephritis Cardiac failure Mercury poisoning Bence-Jones protein in multiple myeloma Febrile states Hematuria	

Sodium	130–200 mEq/24 h	130–200 mmol/24 h	Useful in detecting gross
			  changes in water and
			  salt balance	

Titratable acidity	20–40 mEq/24 h	20–40 mmol/24 h	Metabolic acidosis	Metabolic alkalosis

Urea nitrogen	9–16 gm/24 h	0.32–0.57 mol/L	Excessive protein
			  catabolism
				Impaired kidney
				  function

Uric acid	250–750 mg/24 h	1.48–4.43 mmol/24 h	Gout	Nephritis

Urobilinogen	Random urine: <0.25
	  mg/dl
	24-hour urine: up to 4
	  mg/24 h
		<0.42 mol/24 h
		
		Up to 6.76 μmol/24 h
			Liver and biliary tract
			  disease
			Hemolytic anemias
				Complete or nearly
				  complete biliary
				  obstruction
				Diarrhea
				Renal insufficiency

Uroporphyrins	Up to 50 μg/24 h	Up to 0.06 μmol/24 h	Porphyria	

Vanillylmandelic acid
  (VMA)
	0.7–6.8 mg/24 h	3.5–34.3 μmol/24 h	Pheochromocytoma
			Neuroblastoma
			Coffee, tea, aspirin,
			  bananas, and several
			  different drugs	

Xylose absorption test
  (5-hour)
	16%–33% of ingested
	  xylose
		Fraction absorbed:
		  0.16–0.33
				Malabsorption
				  syndromes

Zinc	0.15–1.2 mg/24 h	2.3–18.4 μmol/24 h	Zinc is an essential nutritional element	

Reference Ranges—Cerebrospinal Fluid (CSF)

Determination	Normal Adult Reference Range		Clinical Significance	
	Conventional Units	SI Units	Increased	Decreased

Albumin	15–30 mg/dl	150–300 mg/L	Certain neurologic
			  disorders
			Lesion in the choroid
			  plexus or blockage of
			  the flow of CSF
			Damage to the blood–
			  central nervous system
			  (CNS) barrier	

Cell count	0–5 mononuclear cells per cu mm	0–5 × 10^6/L	Bacterial meningitis Neurosyphilis Anterior poliomyelitis Encephalitis lethargica	
Chloride	100–130 mEq/L	100–300 mmol/L	Uremia	Acute generalized meningitis Tuberculous meningitis
Glucose	50–75 mg/dl	2.75–4.13 mmol/L	Diabetes mellitus Diabetic coma Epidemic encephalitis Uremia	Acute meningitides Tuberculous meningitis Insulin shock

(continued)

Reference Ranges—Cerebrospinal Fluid (CSF) *(continued)*

Determination	Normal Adult Reference Range		Clinical Significance	
	Conventional Units	SI Units	Increased	Decreased
Glutamine	6–15 mg/dl	0.41–1 mmol/L	Hepatic encephalopathies, including Reye's syndrome Hepatic coma Cirrhosis	
IgG	0–6.6 mg/dl	0–66 mg/L	Damage to the blood–CNS barrier Multiple sclerosis Neurosyphilis Subacute sclerosing panencephalitis Chronic phases of CNS infections	
Lactic acid	<24 mg/dl	<2.7 mmol/L	Bacterial meningitis Hypocapnia Hydrocephalus Brain abscesses Cerebral ischemia	
Lactic dehydrogenase	$1/10$ that of serum	Activity fraction: 0.1 of serum	CNS disease	

Protein:
  Lumbar
  Cisternal
  Ventricular
	
	15–45 mg/dl
	15–25 mg/dl
	5–15 mg/dl
		
		150–450 mg/L
		150–250 mg/L
		50–150 mg/L
			Acute meningitides
			Tubercular meningitis
			Neurosyphilis
			Poliomyelitis
			Guillain-Barré syndrome	

Protein electrophoresis (cellulose acetate)
  Prealbumin
  Albumin
  Alpha$_1$ globulin
  Alpha$_2$ globulin
  Beta globulin
  Gamma globulin
	% of total:
	3–7
	56–74
	2–6.5
	3–12
	8–18.5
	4–14
		Fraction:
		0.03–0.07
		0.56–0.74
		0.02–0.065
		0.03–0.12
		0.08–0.185
		0.04–0.14
			An increase in the level of albumin alone can be the result of a lesion in the choroid plexus or a blockage of the flow of CSF. An elevated gamma globulin value with a normal albumin level has been reported in multiple sclerosis, neurosyphilis, subacute sclerosing panencephalitis, and the chronic phase of CNS infections. If the blood–CNS barrier has been damaged severely during the course of these diseases, the CSF albumin level may also be elevated.	

Miscellaneous Values

Determinations	Normal Value	Clinical Significance		
		Conventional Units		SI Units
Acetaminophen	Zero	Therapeutic level = 10–20 μg/ml		10–20 mg/L
Aminophylline (theophylline)	Zero	Therapeutic level = 10–20 μg/ml		10–20 mg/L
Bromide	Zero	Therapeutic level = 5–50 mg/dl		50–500 mg/L
Carbamazepine	Zero	Therapeutic level = 8–12 μg/ml		34–51 μmol/L
Carbon monoxide	0%–2%	Symptoms with >20% saturation		
Chlordiazepoxide	Zero	Therapeutic level = 1–3 μg/ml		1–3 mg/L
Diazepam	Zero	Therapeutic level = 0.5–2.5 μg/dl		5–25 μg/L
Digitoxin	Zero	Therapeutic level = 5–30 ng/ml		5–30 μg/L
Digoxin	Zero	Therapeutic level = 0.5–2 ng/ml		0.5–2 μg/L

Ethanol	0%–0.01%	Legal intoxication level = 0.10% or above
		    0.3%–0.4% = marked intoxiciation
		    0.4%–0.5% = alcoholic stupor		

Gentamicin	Zero	Therapeutic level = 4–10 μg/ml		4–10 mg/L
Lithium	Zero	Therapeutic level = 0.6–1.2 mEq/L		0.6–1.2 mmol/L
Methanol	Zero	May be fatal in concentration as low as 10 mg/dl		100 mg/L
Phenobarbital	Zero	Therapeutic level = 15–40 μg/ml		10–20 mg/L
Phenytoin	Zero	Therapeutic level = 10–20 μg/ml		10–20 mg/L
Primidone	Zero	Therapeutic level = 5–12 μg/ml		5–12 mg/L
Quinidine	Zero	Therapeutic level = 0.2–0.5 mg/dl		2–5 mg/L
Salicylate	Zero	Therapeutic level = 2–25 mg/dl Toxic level = >30 mg/dl		20–250 mg/L 300 mg/L

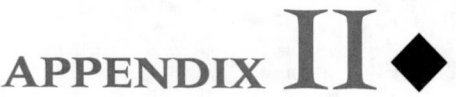

Metric Units and Symbols

Quantity	Unit	Symbol	Equivalent
Length	millimeter	mm	1000 mm = 1 m
	centimeter	cm	100 cm = 1 m
	decimeter	dm	10 dm = 1 m
	meter	m	1000 m = 1 km
Volume	cubic centimeter	cc or cm^3	1000 cc = 1 cm^3 or liter
	milliliter	ml	1000 mL = 1 liter
	cu decimeter	dm^3	1000 dm^3 = 1 m^3
	liter	L	1000 L = 1 m^3
Mass	microgram	μg	1000 μg = 1 mg
	milligram	mg	1000 mg = 1 g
	gram	g	1000 g = 1 kg
	kilogram	kg	1000 kg = 1 metric ton (t)

Table of Metric and Apothecaries' Systems

(Approved *approximate* dose equivalents are enclosed in parentheses. Use exact equivalents in calculations.)

Conversion Factors			
Metric	Apothecaries	Metric	Apothecaries
1 milligram (mg)	$^1/_{64}$ grain	3.888 cubic centimeters or grams	1 dram (4 cc or grams)
64.79 milligrams	1 grain (65 mg)	31.103 cubic centimeters or grams	1 ounce (30 cc or grams)
1 gram	15.43 grains (15 grains)	473.167 cubic centimeters	1 pint (500 cc)
1 cubic centimeter (cc)*	16 minims		

* Note: A cubic centimeter (cc.) is the approximate equivalent of a milliliter (ml.). The terms are used interchangeably in general medicine.

Celsius (Centigrade) and Fahrenheit Temperatures

Celsius (Centigrade) 0°	Fahrenheit 32°
36.0	96.8
36.5	97.7
37.0	98.6
37.5	99.5
38.0	100.4
38.5	101.3
39.0	102.2
39.5	103.1
40.0	104.0
40.5	104.9
41.0	105.8
41.5	106.7
42.0	107.6

CELSIUS

To convert degrees F. to degrees C.
   Subtract 32, then multiply by 5/9
To convert degrees C. to degrees F.
   Multiply by 9/5, then add 32

Nomogram for Estimating Surface Area of Infants and Young Children

HEIGHT		SURFACE AREA	WEIGHT	
feet	centimeters	in square meters	pounds	kilograms

To determine the surface area of the patient, draw a straight line between the point representing the patient's height on the left vertical scale to the point representing the patient's weight on the right vertical scale. The point at which this line intersects the middle vertical scale represents the surface area in square meters. (Courtesy of Abbott Laboratories.)

Nomogram for Estimating Surface Area of Older Children and Adults

HEIGHT		SURFACE AREA	WEIGHT	
feet	centimeters	in square meters	pounds	kilograms

HEIGHT:
7′ — 220, 215, 210
10″ — 205
8″ — 200
6″ — 195
4″ — 190
2″ — 185
6′ — 180
10″ — 175
8″ — 170
6″ — 165
4″ — 160
2″ — 155
5′ — 150
10″ — 145
8″ — 140
6″ — 135
4″ — 130
2″ — 125
4′ — 120
10″ — 115
8″ — 110
6″ — 105
4″ — 100
2″ — 95
3′ — 90
10″ — 85
8″ — 80
6″ — 75

SURFACE AREA:
3.00, 2.90, 2.80, 2.70, 2.60, 2.50, 2.40, 2.30, 2.20, 2.10, 2.00, 1.95, 1.90, 1.85, 1.80, 1.75, 1.70, 1.65, 1.60, 1.55, 1.50, 1.45, 1.40, 1.35, 1.30, 1.25, 1.20, 1.15, 1.10, 1.05, 1.00, .95, .90, .85, .80, .75, .70, .65, .60

WEIGHT pounds:
440, 420, 400, 380, 360, 340, 320, 300, 290, 280, 270, 260, 250, 240, 230, 220, 210, 200, 190, 180, 170, 160, 150, 140, 130, 120, 110, 100, 90, 80, 70, 60, 50

WEIGHT kilograms:
200, 190, 180, 170, 160, 150, 140, 130, 120, 110, 100, 95, 90, 85, 80, 75, 70, 65, 60, 55, 50, 45, 40, 35, 30, 25, 20

See Nomogram for Estimating Surface Area of Infants and Young Children for instructions on use. (Courtesy of Abbott Laboratories.)

Pediatric Laboratory Values

Blood Chemistries

These values are compiled from a review of current published literature, however, normal values vary with the analytic method used. If any doubt exists, consult your laboratory for its analytical method and normal range of values.

Determination	Conventional Units	SI Units	Determination	Conventional Units	SI Units
Acid phosphatase			Bilirubin (total)		
Newborn	7.4–19.4 U/ml	7.4–19.4 U/ml	Cord	<1.8 mg/dl	<30.6 μmol/L
2–13 yr	6.4–15.2 U/ml	6.4–15.2 U/ml	24 h		
Adult	M: 0.5–11 U/ml	0.5–11.0 U/ml	Preterm	≤8 mg/dl	≤103 μmol/L
	F: 0.2–9.5 U/ml	0.2–9.5 U/ml	Term	≤6 mg/dl	≤103 μmol/L
Alanine amino-transferase (ALT)			48 h		
Infants	<54 U/L	<54 U/L	Preterm	<12 mg/dl	<137 μmol/L
Children/adults	1–30 U/L	1–30 U/L	Term	≤ 8 mg/dl	≤120 μmol/L
Aldolase			3–5 days		
Adult	<8 U/L	<8 U/L	Preterm	≤16 mg/dl	≤205 μmol/L
Children	<16 U/L	<16 U/L	Term	≤12 mg/dl	<205 μmol/L
Newborn	<32 U/L	<32 U/L	1 mo-Adult	≤ 2 mg/dl	≤26 μmol/L
Alkaline phosphatase			Conjugated	≤ 1 mg/dl	≤9 μmol/L
Infant	150–420 U/L	150–400 U/L	Calcium (total)		
2–10 yr	100–320 U/L	100–300 U/L	Premature < 1 week	6–10 mg/dl	1.5–2.5 mmol/L
11–18 yr			Full-term < 1 week	7–12 mg/dl	1.75–3 mmol/L
Male	100–390 U/L	50–375 U/L	Child	8–10.5 mg/dl	2–2.6 mmol/L
Female	100–320 U/L	30–300 U/L	Adult	8.5–10.5 mg/dl	2.1–2.6 mmol/L
Adult	30–120 U/L	30–100 U/L	Calcium (ionized)	4.4–5.4 mg/dl	0.1–1.35 mmol/L
Alpha-1-antitrypsin	2.1–5 gm/L		Carbon dioxide (CO_2 content)		
Alpha-fetoprotein	<10 mg/dl	<0.1 g/L	Cord blood	15–20 mmol/L	15–20 mmol/L
Ammonia nitrogen (venous sample: heparinized specimen in ice water and analyzed within 30 min)			Child	18–27 mmol/L	18–27 mmol/L
			Adult	24–35 mmol/L	24–35 mmol/L
			Carbon monoxide (carboxyhemoglobin)		
All ages	13–48 μg/dl	9–34 μmol/L	Nonsmoker	<2% of total hemoglobin	
Amylase					
Newborn	5–65 U/L	5–65 U/L	Smoker	<10% of total hemoglobin	
> 1 yr	0–88 U/L	25–125 U/L	Lethal	>60% of total hemoglobin	
Arsenic	<10 μg/dl	<0.4 mmol/L			
Aspartate aminotransferase (AST)			Carotenoids (carotenes)		
			Infant	20–70 μg/dl	0.37–1.30 μmol/L
			Child	40–130 μg/dl	0.74–2.42 μmol/L
			Adult	60–200 μg/dl	1.12–3.72 μmol/L
Newborn/infant	25–75 U/L	25–75 U/L	Ceruloplasmin	23–58 mg/dl	1.32–3.83 μmol/L
Child/adult	0–40 U/L	0–40 U/L	Chloride	94–106 mEq/L	94–106 mmol/L
Bicarbonate			Cholesterol	See Lipids	
Premature	18–26 mEq/L	18–26 mmol/L	Copper		
Infant	20–26 mEq/L	20–26 mmol/L	0–6 mo	<70 μg/dl	<11 μmol/L
>2 yr	22–26 mEq/L	22–26 mmol/L	6 mo—5 yr	27–153 μg/dl	4.2–24.1 μmol/L
			5–17 yr	94–234 μg/dl	14.2–36.8 μmol/L
			Adult	70–155 μg/dl	11–24.4 μmol/L

(continued)

Blood Chemistries *(continued)*

Creatine Kinase (Creatine Phosphokinase)

	Upper 95th Percentile (U/L)	
Age	Males	Females
1 d	600	500
2–10 d	440	440
<1 yr	170	170
1–7 yr	109	100
7–9 yr	103	85
9–11 yr	109	88
11–13 yr	108	85
13–15 yr	129	85
15–17 yr	247	74
17–19 yr	190	68

Creatinine (serum)

	Upper Limits, mg/dl (μmol/L)	
Age (yr)	Males	Females
1	0.6 (53)	0.5 (44)
2–3	0.7 (62)	0.6 (53)
4–7	0.8 (71)	0.7 (62)
8–10	0.9 (80)	0.8 (71)
11–12	1.0 (88)	0.9 (80)
13–17	1.2 (106)	1.1 (97)
18–20	1.3 (115)	1.1 (97)
Adult	1.2 (106)	1.4 (124)

Ferritin		
Children	7–144 ng/ml	7–144 μg/L
Adult	F: 10–110 ng/ml	10–110 μg/L
	M: 30–265 ng/ml	30–265 μg/L
Fibrin degradation products		
Titer	1:50 = positive	
Fibrinogen	200–400 mg/dl	2–4 g/L
Folic acid (folate)	1.9–14 ng/L	4.3–23.6 nmol/L
Galactose		
Newborn	0–20 mg/dl	0–1.11 mmol/L
Thereafter	<5 mg/dl	<0.28 mmol/L
Gammaglutamyl transferase (GGT)		
Cord	19–270 U/L	19–270 U/L
Premature	56–233 U/L	56–233 U/L
0–3 wk	0–130 U/L	0–130 U/L
3 wk–3 mo	4–120 U/L	4–120 U/L
>3 mo		
M	5–65 U/L	5–65 U/L
F	5–35 U/L	5–35 U/L
1–15 yr	0–23 U/L	0–23 U/L
16 yr—Adult	0–35 U/L	0–35 U/L
Gastrin	<300 pg/ml	<300 ng/L
Glucose (serum)		
Premature	20–65 mg/dl	1.1–3.6 mmol/L
Full term	20–110 mg/dl	1.1–6.4 mmol/L
1 wk–16 yr	60–105 mg/dl	3.3–5.8 mmol/L
>16 yr	70–115 mg/dl	3.9–6.4 nmol/L
Haptoglobin*	400–1800 mg/L	0.4–1.8 g/L

* Detectable in only 10%–20 % of newborns.
† Use of oral contraceptives significantly raises both total serum cholesterol and serum triglyceride levels.

Iron

	Iron		Iron Binding Capacity		% Saturation (μg/dl)
	(μg/dl)	(μmol/L)	(μg/dl)	(μmol/L)	
Newborn	110–270	19.7–48.3	59–175	10.6–31.3	65%
4–10 mo	30–70	5.4–12.5	250–400	45–72	25%
3–10 yr	53–119	9.5–27.0	250–400	45–72	30%
Adult	72–186	12.9–33.3	250–400	45–72	35%

Ketones		
Qualitative	Negative	
Quantitative	up to 3 mg%	
Lactate		
Capillary blood		
Newborn	≤30 mg/dl	<3.0 mmol/L
Child	5–20 mg/dl	0.56–2.25 mmol/L
Venous	5–18 mg/dl	0.5–2.0 mmol/L
Arterial	3–7 mg/dl	0.3–0.8 mmol/L
Lactate dehydrogenase (37°C)		
Newborn	160–1500 U/L	160–1500 U/L
Infant	150–360 U/L	150–360 U/L
Child	150–300 U/L	150–300 U/L
Adult	100–250 U/L	100–250 U/L
Lactate dehydrogenase isoenzymes (% total)		
LD_1 Heart		24–34%
LD_2 Heart, erythrocytes		35–45%
LD_3 Muscle		15–25%
LD_4 Liver, trace muscle		4–10%
LD_5 Liver, muscle		1–9%
Lipase	20–180 U/L	20–180 U/L
Lipids		

Normal Upper Limits

	Total Serum Cholesterol mg/dl (mmol/L)		Serum Triglycerides mg/dl (g/L)	
Age	Males	Females†	Males	Females*
0–4 yr	203 (5.28)	200 (5.2)	99 (0.99)	112 (1.12)
5–9	203 (5.28)	205 (5.33)	101 (1.01)	105 (1.05)
10–14	202 (5.25)	201 (5.22)	125 (1.25)	131 (1.31)
15–19	197 (5.12)	200 (5.2)	148 (1.48)	124 (1.24)

	HDL-Cholesterol mg/dl (mmol/L)		Normal Upper Limits LDL mg/dl (mmol/L)		VLDL mg/dl (mml/L)	
Age	Males	Females	Males	Females	Males	Females
0–4	—	—	—	—	—	—
5–9	74 (1.91)	73 (1.89)	129 (3.34)	140 (3.62)	18 (0.47)	24 (0.62)
10–14	74 (1.91)	70 (1.81)	132 (3.41)	136 (3.52)	22 (0.57)	23 (0.59)
15–19	63 (1.63)	73 (1.89)	130 (3.36)	135 (3.49)	26 (0.67)	24 (0.62)

Magnesium	1.5–2 mEq/L	0.75–1 mmol/L
Manganese (blood)		
Newborn	2.4–9.6 μg/dl	2.44–1.75 μmol/L
2–18 yr	0.8–2.1 μg/dl	0.15–0.38 μmol/L
Methemoglobin	<0.3 g/dl or <3% of total Hb	<46.5 μmol/L
5' Nucleotidase	2.2–15 U/L	2.2–15 U/L
Osmolality	285–295 mOsm/kg	270–285 mOsm/L plasma
Phenylalanine		
Premature	2.0–7.5 mg/dl	
Newborn	<4 mg/dl	<0.24 mmol/L
Child	<3 mg/dl	<0.18 mmol/L

Blood Chemistries (continued)

Phosphorus		
Newborn	4.2–9.0 mg/dl	1.36–2.91 mmol/L
1 yr	3.8–6.2 mg/dl	1.23–2.0 mmol/L
2–5 yr	3.5–6.8 mg/dl	1.13–2.2 mmol/L
Adult	3.0–4.5 mg/dl	0.97–1.45 mmol/L
Porcelain	10–25 mg/dl	No SI conversion factor
Potassium		
<10 days of age	3.5–6 mEq/L	3.5–6 mmol/L
>10 days of age	3.5–5 mEq/L	3.5–5 mmol/L
Prolactin		
Newborn	<200 ng/ml	<200 μg/L
Adult	<20 ng/ml	<20 μg/L

Proteins Average (Range) in gr/dl

Age	Total	Albu-min	Globu-lin	Gamma Globu-lin
Premature	5.5 (4.0–7.0)	3.7 (2.5–4.5)	1.8 (1.2–2.0)	0.7 (0.5–0.9)
FT newborn	6.4 (5.0–7.1)	3.4 (2.5–5.0)	3.1 (1.2–4.0)	0.8 (0.7–0.9)
1-mo	6.6 (4.7–7.4)	3.8 (3.0–4.2)	2.5 (1.0–3.3)	0.3 (0.1–0.5)
3–12 mo	6.8 (5.0–7.5)	3.9 (2.7–5.0)	2.6 (2.0–3.8)	0.6 (0.4–1.2)
1–15 yr	7.4 (6.5–8.6)	4.0 (3.2–5.0)	3.1 (2.0–4.0)	0.9 (0.6–1.2)

Pyruvate	0.3–0.9 mg/dl	50–140 mmol/L
Sodium		
Premature	130–140 mEq/L	130–140 mmol/L
Older	135–145 mEq/L	135–145 mmol/L

Transaminase (SGOT)	*See Aspartate Aminotransferase (AST)*	
Transaminase (SGPT)	*See Alanine Aminotransferase (AT)*	
Triglycerides	*See Lipids*	
Urea nitrogen	5–25 mg/dl	1.8–9 mmol/L
Uric acid		
0–2 yr	2.0–7.0 mg/dl	0.12–0.42 mmol/L
2–12 yr	2.0–6.5 mg/dl	0.12–0.39 mmol/L
12–14 yr	2.0–7.0 mg/dl	0.12–0.42 mmol/L
14–adult		
M	3.0–8.0 mg/dl	0.18–0.48 mmol/L
F	2.0–7.0 mg/dl	0.12–0.42 mmol/L
Vitamin A (retinol)		
0–1 yr	20–90 μg/dl	0.7–3.14 μmol/L
1–5 yr	30–100 μg/dl	1.05–3.50 μmol/L
5–16 yr	60–100 μg/dl	2.09–3.50 μmol/L
Adult	20–80 μg/dl	0.70–2.79 μmol/L
Vitamin B$_1$ (thiamine)	5.3–7.9 μg/dl	0.16–0.23 μmol/L
Vitamin B$_2$ (riboflavin)	3.7–13.7 μg/dl	98–363 mmol/L
Vitamin B$_{12}$ (cobalamin)	130–785 pg/ml	96–579 pmol/L
Vitamin C (ascorbic acid)	0.2–2 mg/dl	11.4–113.6 μmol/L
Vitamin D (1.25 dihydroxy)		
Newborn	21 ± 2 pg/ml	50 ± 4.8 nmol/L
Child	43 ± 3 pg/ml	103 ± 7.2 nmol/L
Adult	29 ± 2 pg/ml	69.6 ± 4.8 nmol/L
Vitamin E	5–20 μg/dl	8.4–23 μmol/L
Zinc	55–150 μg/dl	8.4–23 μmol/L

(From Johns Hopkins Hospital. The Harriet Lane Handbook. 13th ed. Chicago, Year Book Medical Pub, 1993)

Normal Values—Hematology

Age	Hgb (gm %) Mean (−2SD)	HCT (%) Mean (−2SD)	MCV (fl.) Mean (−2SD)	MCHC (gm/% RBC) Mean (−2SD)	Retic (%)	WBC/ mm³ × 100 Mean (−2SD)	Plts (10³/ mm³) Mean (±2SD)
26–30 wk gestation*	13.4 (11)	41.5 (34.9)	118.2 (106.7)	37.9 (30.6)	—	4.4 (2.7)	254 (180–327)
28 wk	14.5	45	120	31	(5–10)	—	275
32 wk	15.0	47	118	32	(3–10)	—	290
Term† (cord)	16.5 (13.5)	51 (42)	108 (98)	33 (30)	(3–7)	18.1 (9–30)‡	290
1–3 days	18.5 (14.5)	56 (45)	108 (95)	33 (29)	(1.8–4.6)	18.9 (9.4–34)	192
2 wk	16.6 (13.4)	53 (41)	105 (88)	31.4 (28.1)		11.4 (5–20)	252
1 mo	13.9 (10.7)	44 (33)	101 (91)	31.8 (28.1)	(0.1–1.7)	10.8 (5–19.5)	
2 mo	11.2 (9.4)	35 (28)	95 (84)	31.8 (28.3)			
6 mo	12.6 (11.1)	36 (31)	76 (68)	35 (32.7)	(0.7–2.3)	11.9 (6–17.5)	
6 mo—2 yr	12 (10.5)	36 (33)	78 (70)	33 (30)		10.6 (6–17)	(150–350)
2–6 yr	12.5 (11.5)	37 (34)	81 (75)	34 (31)	(0.5–1.0)	8.5 (5–15.5)	(150–350)
6–12 yr	13.5 (11.5)	40 (35)	86 (77)	34 (31)	(0.5–1.0)	8.1 (4.5–13.5)	(150–350)
12–18 yr							
Male	14.5 (13)	43 (36)	88 (78)	34 (31)	(0.5–1.0)	7.8 (4.5–13.5)	(150–350)
Female	14 (12)	41 (37)	90 (78)	34 (31)	(0.5–1.0)	7.8 (4.5–13.5)	(150–350)

* Values are from fetal samplings.
† Under 1 month, capillary Hgb exceeds venous: 1 h–3.6 gm difference; 5 days–2.2 gm difference; 3 wks–1.1 gm difference.
‡ Mean (95% confidence limits).
(From Johns Hopkins Hospital. The Harriet Lane Handbook. 13th ed. Chicago, Year Book Medical Pub, 1993)

Normal Serologic Reference Values

Determination	Value
Antinuclear antibody	<1:160
Anti-streptolysin O Titer*	
Preschool	<1:85
School ages and adults	<1:170
Older adults	<1:85
Anti-hyaluronidase	<1:256
Anti-nuclear Antibody	<1:160
C-reactive Protein	Negative
C_1 Esterase inhibitor	17.4–24 mg/dl
C_3	
1–6 mo	53–175 mg/dl
7–12 mo	75–180 mg/dl
1–5 yr	77–166 mg/dl
6–10 yr	88–199 mg/dl
Adult	83–177 mg/dl
C_4	
1–6 mo	7–42 mg/dl
7–12 mo	9.5–39 mg/dl
1–5 yr	9–40 mg/dl
6–10 yr	12–40 mg/dl
Adult	15–45 mg/dl
C_{H50}	75–160 U/ml
Rheumatoid factor	<20 negative
	20–40 suggestive
	≥80 positive
Rheumaton titer (modified Waaler-Rose slide test)	Negative
	≥10 may be significant
Total B cells	5%–20% of lymphocytes
Total T cells	50%–80% of lymphocytes
T helper cells	34%–56% of lymphoyctes
T suppressor cells	18%–32% of lymphocytes
Helper/suppressor ratio	1.1–2.5

* Significant if rising titer can be demonstrated at weekly intervals.
(From Johns Hopkins Hospital. The Harriet Lane Handbook. 13th ed. Chicago, Year Book Medical Pub, 1993)

Cerebrospinal Fluid Values

Determination	Value
Cell Count	
Preterm mean	9.0 (0–25.4 WBC/mm^3) (57% PMNs)
Term mean	8.2 (0–22.4 WBC/mm^3) (61% PMNs)
>1 mo	0–7 (0% PMNs)
Glucose	
Preterm	24–63 mg/dl (mean 50)
Term	34–119 mg/dl (mean 52)
Child	40–80 mg/dl
CSF Glucose/Blood Glucose (%)	
Preterm	55–105
Term	44–128
Child	50%
Lactic acid dehydrogenase	20 U/ml (range 5–30 U/ml)
Myelin basic protein	<4 ng/ml
Pressure (initial lumbar puncture)	
Newborn	80–110 (<110) mm H$_2$O
Infant	<200 (lateral recumbent position) mm H$_2$O
Child	
Respiratory movements	5–10 mm H$_2$O
Protein	
Preterm	65–150 mg/dl (mean 115)
Term	20–170 mg/dl (mean 90)
Children	
Ventricular	5–15 mg/dl
Cisternal	5–25 mg/dl
Lumbar	5–40 mg/dl

(From Johns Hopkins Hospital. The Harriet Lane Handbook. 13th ed. Chicago, Year Book Medical Pub, 1993)

Sample Conversions of Pounds and Ounces to Grams*

Pounds	0	1	2	3	4	5	6	7	8	9	10	11	12	13	14	15
0	—	28	57	85	113	142	170	198	227	255	283	312	340	369	397	425
1	454	482	510	539	567	595	624	652	680	709	737	765	794	822	850	879
2	907	936	964	992	1021	1049	1077	1106	1134	1162	1191	1219	1247	1276	1304	1332
3	1361	1389	1417	1446	1474	1503	1531	1559	1588	1616	1644	1673	1701	1729	1758	1786
4	1814	1843	1871	1899	1928	1956	1984	2013	2041	2070	2098	2126	2155	2183	2211	2240
5	2268	2296	2325	2353	2381	2410	2438	2466	2495	2532	2551	2580	2608	2637	2665	2693
6	2722	2750	2778	2807	2835	2863	2892	2920	2948	2977	3005	3033	3062	3090	3118	3147

(Ounces across top)

* 1 ounce = approximately 30 grams.
(From Avery GB. Neonatology. 4th ed. Philadelphia, JB Lippincott, 1994)

Index

Note: Page numbers in *italics* indicate illustrations; page numbers followed by t indicate tables.

A

ABCs, of cardiopulmonary resuscitation, 942–943
Abdomen
  auscultation of, 481
    in children, 1089
  examination of, 44–46
    in children, *1089*, 1089–1090
    in genitourinary disorders, 588
    in newborn, 1019
    in pregnancy, 981
  incisions in, *73*
  rebound tenderness of, 45
  regions of, *73*
Abdominal aneurysm, 349–351, *350*
Abdominal breathing, 1180
Abdominal distention
  in Hirschsprung's disease, 1266
  in paralytic ileus, 530
Abdominal hernia, surgery for. *See also* Gastrointestinal surgery
Abdominal hernias, 46–47, 506–507, 524–525, 1092
  femoral, 47, 524, 1092
  inguinal, 46–47, 524, 1092
  surgery for, 494, 524–525
Abdominal injuries, emergency care for, 954–956
Abdominal pain. *See also* Pain
  in acute pancreatitis, 557, 558
  in aortic aneurysm, 349, 350–351
  in appendicitis, 520
  assessment of, 480
  in chronic pancreatitis, 558, 559
  in Crohn's disease, 522, 523
  in gallbladder disease, 555, 556
  in liver cancer, 552, 553
  in pancreatic cancer, 560, 561
  in peptic ulcer disease, 515
  in peritonitis, 521, 522
  postoperative, 83
  referred, 954
  traumatic, 954
Abdominal paracentesis, 545, 547–548
Abdominal radiography/imaging, 482–483

Abdominal restraint, 1139
Abdominal striae, in pregnancy, 976, 977, 979
Abdominal thrusts, 944–945
Abducens nerve, assessment of, 52
ABO blood group, 783, 784t
Abortion
  induced, 1027t
    RU-486 for, 650
  spontaneous, 1026t, 1026–1028
Abrasion, corneal, 426, *429*, 438t–439t, 1392–1393
Abruptio placentae, 1030–1032, *1031*, 1032t
Abscess
  anal, 535t
  Bartholin gland, 662–663, *663*
  brain, 385–386
  breast, 694–695
  lung, 229–231
  tubo-ovarian, 679
Absence seizures, 1234. *See also* Seizures
Abuse, child, 1117–1126
Accommodation, visual, 417
ACE inhibitors
  for congestive heart failure, 311
  for hypertension, 354t, 355
Acetaminophen poisoning, 1110
Achalasia, 510–511
Achilles reflex, assessment of, 55
Achilles tendon, injuries of, 866–867
Achondroplasia, 1406t
Acid-fast bacillus precautions, 936
Acidosis
  in children, 1155t
  in renal failure, 612, 612t
Acne vulgaris, 904t
Acoustic impedance evaluation, 451
Acoustic nerve, assessment of, 53
Acoustic neuroma, 405–406
Acoustic stimulation test, 990
Acquired immunodeficiency syndrome (AIDS), 815–821. *See also* Human immunodeficiency virus infection

  in children, 1340–1343
  clinical manifestations of, 815–816
  complications of, 817t, 817–818
  diagnosis of, 816–817
  evaluation in, 821
  management of, 818
  natural history of, 815, *816*
  nursing management in, 818–821
  pathophysiology of, 815
  patient education/health maintenance in, 821
  risk factors for, 815
Acrolentiginous melanoma, 897
ACTH
  assay for, 710
  deficiency of, 729–730
  hypersecretion of, 727–728
ACTH stimulation test, 708
Actinic keratoses, 894–895
Activated charcoal
  for drug overdosage, 967
  for poisoning, 962, 963, 1112
Activities of daily living, assessment of, in elderly, 122, 123t
Activity and exercise. *See also* Exercises
  in asthma, 812
  in burns, 919
  in congenital heart disease, 1207
  in congestive heart failure, 312–313
  in connective tissue disorders, 825
  in elderly, 126, 127
  in hyperthyroidism, 1296
  in juvenile rheumatoid arthritis, 1346
  after myocardial infarction, 296, 297
  in osteoarthritis, 879, 880
  for osteoporosis prevention, 878
  with ostomy, 502
  in pregnancy, 984
  for weight loss, 574
Acute catastrophic reaction, in Alzheimer's disease, 390
Acute (angle-closure) glaucoma, 434–447

Pancreatoduodenectomy, *560, 560–562*
Panic disorder, 1425t
Pantothenic acid deficiency, 581t
Pao₂, in pulse oximetry, 152–153
Pap smear, 647–648
  specimen collection for, *646*
Paracentesis, abdominal, 545, 549
Paraesophageal hernia, 506–507
Paralysis
  in cerebral palsy, 1221t
  facial, 374–375
  in Guillain-Barré syndrome, 393–394
  in muscular dystrophy, 395–397, 396t
  quad cough in, 403
  in spinal cord injury, 399–404, *400*
  in stroke, 379
Paralytic ileus, 530
  in burns, 919, 1375
Parametritis, postpartum, 1049
Paranasal sinuses
  anatomy of, *458*
  examination of, 32–33, 450
    in children, 1085
  inflammation of, 458–459
  surgery of, 451
Paraplegia. *See also* Paralysis
  in spinal cord injury, 399–404, *400*
Parasitic infections, of skin, 900t
Parastomal hernia, 524–525
Parathyroid function, tests of, 707
Parathyroid glands, disorders of, 722–726
Parathyroid hormone
  assay for, 707
  deficiency of, 724–726
  function of, 1296
  hypersecretion of, 722–724
Parenteral nutrition, 570–573
  in burns, 908
Parents. *See also* Mother
  abuse and neglect by, 1117–1126
  of dying child, 1136–1137
  of hospitalized child, 1131, 1132–1133
Parkinsonian effects, of neuroleptics, 1437t
Parkinson's disease, 386–387
Parkland formula, 910–911
Paronychia, 899t
Paroxysmal atrial tachycardia, 321, *321*
Partial rebreathing mask, 177, *177*, 183–184, *184*
Partial seizures, 410, 1234
Partial thromboplastin time, in anticoagulant therapy, 330
Passive immunity, 935

Patau syndrome, 1404t
Patch testing, 887
Patent ductus arteriosus, *1198*, 1200–1201
Pathologic fractures, 951
  bone tumors and, 881
  in osteoporosis, 878
  in steroid therapy, 712
Patient-controlled analgesia, 84–85
Patient rights, 5, 5t
Patient teaching, 10–11. *See also* Health promotion
  for exercise/fitness, 12–13, 16
  for nutrition/diet, 11–12, 16–17
  postoperative, 98
  preoperative, 76–78
    for ambulatory surgery, 73
  for relaxation/stress management, 13, 14–15
  for sexual health, 13–14
  for smoking prevention/cessation, 12, 15
Pavlik harness, 1359, *1359*
PCP. *See also* Substance abuse
  overdosage of, 965–967, 966t
Peak expiratory flow rate (PEFR), 152t
Pediatric primary care, 1098–1126. *See also* Children
Pediculosis, 901t, 1080, 1384t
Pelvic cellulitis, postpartum, 1049
Pelvic examination, 47, 645–647, *646–647*
  in pregnancy, 981–982
  in rape victim, 970
Pelvic exenteration, 674
Pelvic floor exercises, 670–671
  with orthoptic bladder replacement, 609
  postpartum, 1014
Pelvic imaging, 649–650
Pelvic inflammatory disease (PID), 679–680
  nursing care plan for, 681
Pelvic muscle exercises, 134
Pelvic muscle relaxation, 670–672
Pelvic pain, 645
Pelvic thrombophlebitis, postpartum, 1049
Pelvic ultrasonography, 648
Pelvis
  abnormalities of, dystocia and, 1041–1042
  dimension of, 993, *994*
  false, 979, *979*
  fractures of, 873t
  measurement of, 979, *980*
  structure of, *979*, 979–980, *980*
  types of, 979–980, *981*
Pemphigus, *893*, 893–894

Penis
  cancer of, 641–642
  examination of, 46, 588
    in children, 1091
  pain in, 587
  pubertal changes in, *1290*, 1308
    precocious, 1301–1303
Peptic ulcer disease, 515–518
  bleeding in, 514
Percussion, 26–27
  of abdomen, 44–45
    in children, 1089
  of bladder, 587
  of chest, 39, 41, 168, *174*, 174–175
  of flank, for ascites, *546*
  of liver, 41, 45
Percutaneous nephrolithotomy, 623, *623*
Percutaneous stone dissolution, 623
Percutaneous suprapubic bladder aspiration, 1142–1143, *1143*
Percutaneous transhepatic biliary drainage, 541
Percutaneous transhepatic cholangiography, 541
Percutaneous transluminal coronary angioplasty, 278–281, *279*
Percutaneous translumnial coronary angioplasty, 289
Percutaneous umbilical blood sampling, 990
Perez reflex, 1097
Pericardial effusion, 307–308
Pericardiocentesis, 276–278, *277*
Pericarditis, 307–308
Perineal care, 654–655, *655*, *655*
  for body casts, 848
Perineal hematoma, postpartum, 1050
Perineal pain, 587
Perioperative nursing, 72–98. *See also* Surgery
Peripheral circulation
  evaluation of, 43–44, *344*
  postoperative assessment of, 81
Peripheral iridectomy, for glaucoma, 434
Peripheral nerve injury, 404–405
Peripheral neuropathy
  diabetic, 747t
  in megaloblastic anemia, 764
  orthopedic treatment and, 845, 846, 848, 858
Peripheral parenteral nutrition, 570–573
Peripheral stem cell transplantation, 791–797. *See also* Bone marrow transplantation
Peripheral vascular disease
  amputation in, 861–865
  diabetic, 745t

Sources of Further Information

Agency for Health Policy and Research
P.O. Box 8547
Silver Spring, MD 20907
1-800-358-9295

Agoraphobics in Motion
1729 Crooks Road
Royal Oaks, MI 48067
(810) 547-0400

Alexander Graham Bell Association of the Deaf
3417 Volta Place, NW
Washington, DC 20007
(202) 337-5220

The Alzheimer's Association
919 North Michigan Avenue, Suite 1000
Chicago, IL 60611-1676
1-800-272-3900

American Academy of Allergy and Immunology
611 East Wells Street
Milwaukee, WI 53202
1-800-822-2762

American Association of Kidney Patients
100 South Ashley Drive, Suite 280
Tampa, FL 33602
1-800-749-AAKP

The American Brain Tumor Association
2720 River Road
Desplaines, IL 60018
(708) 827-9910

American Cancer Society
1599 Clifton Road, NE
Atlanta, GA 30329-4251
1-800-ACS-2345
(404) 320-3333

American Council for the Blind
1155 15th Street, NW
Washington, DC 20005
1-800-424-8666

American Diabetes Association
1660 Duke Street
Alexandria, VA 22314
(703) 549-1500

American Dietetic Association
216 West Jackson Boulevard
Chicago, IL 60606-6995
1-800-366-1655

American Foundation for Urologic Disease
300 W. Pratt Street, Suite 401
Baltimore, MD 21201-2463
1-800-242-2383

American Foundation for the Prevention of Venereal Disease
799 Broadway, Suite 638
New York, NY 10003
(212) 759-2069

American Heart Association
7272 Greenville Avenue
Dallas, TX 75231-4596
(214) 373-6300

American Juvenile Arthritis Foundation
1314 Spring Street, NW
Atlanta, GA 30309
(404) 872-7100

American Lupus Society
260 Maple Court, Suite 123
Ventura, CA 93003
(805) 339-0443

American Psuedo-Obstruction and Hirschsprung's Disease Society
P.O. Box 772
Medford, MA 02155
(617) 395-4255

American Speech-Language Hearing Association
10801 Rockville Pike
Rockville, MD 20852
(301) 897-5700
1-800-638-TALK

The Amyotrophic Lateral Sclerosis Association
21021 Venture Boulevard, Suite 321
Woodland Hills, CA 91364
1-800-782-4747

Anxiety Disorders Association of America
6000 Executive Boulevard, Suite 513
Rockville, MD 20852
(301) 231-9350

Aplastic Anemia Foundation of America
P.O. Box 22689
Baltimore, MD 21203
(410) 955-2803

ARC (Association for Retarded Citizens)
500 East Border Street, 3rd Floor
Arlington, TX 76010
(817) 261-6003

Association of Birth Defects in Children
827 Irma Avenue
Orlando, FL 32806
(407) 245-7035
800-313-2232

Association of Bladder Extrophy Children
13823 Shavano Downs
San Antonio, TX 78230
(210) 492-6062

Asthma & Allergy Foundation of America
1125 15th Street NW, Suite 502
Washington, DC 20005
(202) 466-7643

Blind Children's Center
4120 Marathon Street
Los Angeles, CA 90029
1-800-222-3566

BMT Newsletter (Bone Marrow Transplant)
c/o Susan Stewart
1985 Spruce Avenue
Highland Park, IL 60035
(708) 831-1913

Celiac Sprue Association
P.O. Box 31700
Omaha, NE 68131-0700
(402) 558-0600

Child Health Foundation
10630 Little Patuxent Parkway, Suite 325
Columbia, MD 21044
(301) 596-4514

Children and Adults With Attention Deficit Disorder
499 NW 70th Avenue, Suite 101
Plantation, FL 33317
(305) 587-3700

Clinical Dietetics Department
Children's Memorial Hospital
2300 Children's Plaza
Chicago, IL 60614
(312) 880-4000

Cooley's Anemia Foundation
129-09 26th Avenue, Suite 203
Flushing, NY 11354
(718) 321-2873
800-522-7222

Coping
Pulse Publications, Inc.
357 Riverside Drive, P.O. Box 682268
Franklin, TN 37086
(615) 790-2400

Corporate Angel Network, Inc.
Westchester County Airport, Building 1
White Plains, NY 10604
(914) 328-1313

Council for Learning Disabilities
P.O. Box 40303
Overland Park, KS 66204
(913) 492-8755

Crohn's and Colitis Foundation of America
444 Park Avenue South
New York, NY 10016
(212) 685-3440

Dissociative Disorder Program
Rush North Shore Medical Center
9600 Grosse Point Road
Skokie, IL 60076
(708) 933-6685

Endometriosis Association
8585 North 76th Place
Milwaukee, WI 53223
1-800-992-3636
(414) 355-2200

The Epilepsy Foundation of America
4351 Garden City Drive
Landover, MD 20785
1-800-332-1000
(301) 459-3700

The Guillain-Barrè Syndrome Foundation International
P.O. Box 262
Wynnewood, PA 19096
(610) 667-0131

International Society for the Study of Multiple Personality and Dissociation
5700 Old Orchard Road, 1st Floor
Skokie, IL 60077
(708) 966-4322

Joseph P. Kennedy Jr. Foundation (Developmental Disabilities)
1325 "G" Street, Suite 500
Washington, DC 20005
(202) 393-1250

Juvenile Diabetes Foundation
120 Wall Street, 19th Floor
New York, NY 10005
1-800-JDF-CURE

Leukemia Society of America
600 Third Avenue
New York, NY 10016
(212) 573-8484

Lupus Foundation of America, Inc.
4 Research Place, Suite 180
Rockville, MD 20850-3226
(301) 670-9292
800-558-0121